THEMATIC REPERTORY

and materia medica of the mind symptoms

From quotations of the Materia Medica

by

Samuel Hahnemann
Timothy Allen
Constantine Hering
Henry Allen
Jeremy Sherr

and

The Complete Repertory

by

Roger van Zandvoort

by

J.A. MIRILLI, MD

ISBN 90-801878-4-4

First edition March 1998

Publishers:
IRHIS b.v.
Annemarie Ekkers
Delftsekade 23, 2266 AJ Leidschendam, The Netherlands
tel. +31703271107, fax. +31703176789
Internet: irhis@pi.net

This publication was made using MS Word™, Nisus Writer™ and Adobe Pagemaker™.
Printed in the Netherlands by Krips, Meppel.

Page layout by Hans Nieuwenhuijs, Baarn.
Bookcover by Ancel Riesener from Studio 4, Amsterdam

Thematic Researches of Materia Medica Pura and Repertories

http://www.geocities.com/HotSprings/Spa/4489
or
http://members.tripod.com/~mirilli/

Dr. José Antonio Mirilli
Rua do Catete, 311 sala 815
Rio de Janeiro, RJ
22220 - 001
Brazil

Tels:
voice: +55212653545
fax: +55212051129

Internet:
mirilli@usa.net

Software version by Miccant Ltd.
14 Mulberry Close, West Bridgford, Nottingham
NG2 7SS, England
Tel / Fax: (+44) 0115 945 5289
internet: dwitko@miccant.co.uk

The Complete Repertory / Roger van Zandvoort
rozand@euronet.nl
info@irhis.nl
http://www.irhis.nl

Aldo Farias Dias
aldo@centroin.com.br
http://www.geocities.com/HotSprings/Spa/5086/index.html

Ariovaldo Ribeiro Filho
tel/fax: +55 11 2735792
email: aribeiro@poboxes.com

Maurizio Castellini
Scuola di Medicina Omeopatica di Verona
castelma@uni.net
http://www.omeoscuolavr.org

Ian Townsend
sheffhom@classic.msn.com

The Homeopathic Recorder / Jasminum
info@jasminum.demon.nl
http://www.jasminum.demon.nl

I would like to thank Roger van Zandvoort for his help since we first met in Brazil. He was the first to offer promoting this work in Europe and the first to offer publishing a European edition. It is a pleasure to have him as a close friend.
I wish also to thank Aldo Farias Dias for his help on conceptual matters in concluding this book.
Thanks to Jeremy Sherr for his encouraging words and the permission for use of his provings for the book.
Thanks to Ariovaldo Ribeiro Filho for his technical support.
Thanks to Ian Townsend for his corrections and support in promoting the book.
Thanks to Frederik Schroyens for his initial support for the book.
Thanks to Maurizio Castellini for his encouraging words and the book's review.
Thanks to Rebecca Preston for her correction of the spelling mistakes.
Thanks to Jorge Biolchini for his review of the first book's version.
Thanks to Luiz Paulo Guanabara for his help in correcting my English translations.
Thanks to Henning Droege for the later technical support and his great ideas on Homeopathy.
Thanks to Hans Nieuwenhuijs for the page layout.
And finally thanks to my publisher, Annemarie Ekkers, for believing in the book's possibilities.

J.A. Mirilli, March 1998

Aldo Farias Dias MD *

Hahnemann used to consider the mental symptoms as the most valuable when choosing a medicine and he says that on paragraphs 210 to 217...and whenever there is a disease that we must heal, the general health must get the same special attention as the totality of the symptoms, so we can get a clear picture of the ailment and treat it successfully by homeophatic mean. (§210) This is so true that the choice of the homeophatic medicine is often determined by the state of mind of the patient which is a very characteristic symptom that should never remain concealed from the physician who is an experienced observer. (§211) The creator of therapeutical agents also observed this main characteristic of all disease, the physical and spiritual altered states, because in the world there is not a single energetic medical substance who changes the physical and mental condition of a sane individual in a way that can not be easily observed. And each medicine does that in a different way. (§212) Thus if we do not see among the other symptoms in each disease, even the grave ones, the symptoms related to changes in mental and moral conditions we will never be able to heal according to nature, that is, homeophatically. Then for the relief of the patient we have to choose a medicine with a pathogenetic potency that besides the similitude with the other symptoms of the disease is capable of producing a similar moral and mental state. Thus the Aconitum will rarely or never produce a fast or permanent healing in a patient who is calm, quiet, and steady. Neither the Nux Vomica in a patient whose temper is gentle and dull; Pulsatilla for persons that are cheerful, live or firm, or Ignatia when he or she is unshakable or with not much sensitivity to feeling frightened or ashamed. (§213)

James Tyler Kent follower of that tradition even suggests in one of his Repertory writings that we should only consider medicines that are in the class of mental symptoms.

Tomas Pablo Paschero, follower of Kent, considers the biopathographic history as a valuable technical to find the Simillimum and follow up the evolution of the patient under treatment. The objective of a dynamic awareness of the Patient and Homeophatical Materia Medica is to discover the sense and intentionality of the symptoms. Since the first writings of Paschero there has been an evolution in the dynamic research of the medicine, the work on the Psora: the only ailment in the discipline of Doctrine and Philosophy, having Professor Masi Elizalde as chairman and the recent improvement in the method of dynamic study of the Homeophatical Materia Medica .

In the center of that research is the concept of THEMES. Masi Elizalde separates ARGUMENT THEMES wherein the experienced describes a whole argument, being a worthless person for example, from WORD THEMES which consists on words the patient or experienced repeats with special delight, words and its synonymous or words and its antonymous. Then the themes are established as constants of vulnerability or constants of reaction. The patient explains that when he feels an aggression, he feels himself offended or hurt regarding this or that. When he reacts, the reaction takes one direction or the other: so we have constants of vulnerability or constants reaction. The themes are classified in Sets and we look for a connection that links the three sets. Then we classify the sensations on the psoric set of vulnerability in the essential parts of loss, guilty, fear of punishment, nostalgia and justification.

To make it possible we need a Materia Medica and a Repertory that classifies the symptoms not in alphabetical order but by themes. Initial works on that direction influenced by those concepts are appearing such as the initial attempts of symptomatic classification on GEHSH (GEHSH Magazine, Aug/86), The Repertory of Modalities by Flora Dabahh, The Repertory of Psoric Centers by Luiz Bernal, The Semiological Guidebook of Ademar Fonseca and the Materia Medica and Thematic Repertory by J.A. Mirilli.

This is the characteristic of Mirilli's work. A compilation and translation of Materia Medica symptoms classified by similar thematic sense making it easier to study the Materia Medica in a dynamic way and allowing the selection of the medicine according to the themes that appear in the Biopathographic History, overcoming in this way the classical repertorial technique. The Repertory can be dealt with in a static form, almost as a dead thing, and in this class are the rubricators who can only manage a Repertory out of a group of rubrics with no meaningful connection. But we will take better advantage of the Repertory as a Guide book to the Materia Medica, its main source. The clinical symptoms may be part of it whenever they are confirmed by clinical healings and to do that we use the resource of medicine punctuation in the rubrics. A rubric is only considered when we understand it within the structure of its pathogenetic or clinical source. Thus the Repertory is a dynamic book and not a sheer catalogue of symptoms. The homeopath that employs it this way is not a mere rubricator and when he uses rubric he is aware of its sense and intentionality, its guidance and indicator for the Materia Medica. So even if he uses the Repertory in a traditional way his repertories will be of superior quality and they will certainly provide the best therapeutical results.

The work of J.A. Mirilli is convenient and necessary and we recommend it to all students of homeopathy who try to meet the requirements of Hahnemann's ideal in search of the Simillimun for a fast, soft, and permanent cure, so the high motive of existence may be fulfilled.

* Aldo Farias, MD, is President of The Samuel Hahnemann Group of Homeophatical Studies.
fax : +55 215561748 internet: Aldo.Dias@bbs.centroin.com.br

Ariovaldo Ribeiro Filho, MD *

About two or three years ago I was walking along the stand of bookstores in a homeophatic congress when my attention was caught by some books that were large and thin. They were home made production which seemed lost in the middle of several "B. Jains" and "Albatros" and I immediately wondered what they were about. What a big surprise when I discovered the titles were in Portuguese. An island of Portuguese in the middle of so much English and Spanish? — A Thematic Medica Materia and a Thematic Repertory of Mental Symptoms— I found that interesting and started to turn over the pages to realize they were thematic studies of the Pure Materia Medica and Barthel's Repertory carefully selected and in English, its original language. At first I disregarded them and thought they were confusing. As I started to go through the pages more attentively, it came to my mind a clinical case I had doubts regarding the symptom "desajuda" or "desvalido" (in Spanish) or "helplessness" (in English). Surprisingly I saw a series of classified medicine such as "acon., agn., alum., am-c., ant-c., bell., bism., etc." that are not in the traditional repertories and even better, they were related to the original terms of the Pure Medica Materia. I found it very interesting, a work like that enlarges the accessibility to the Pure Materia Medica but only to those who are familiar with the language. As I continued to read through the book I was amazed with the quantity of details such as the notation of the bibliographical sources, which is a credit for the book, and the summary of themes and words that really makes it easier to find the terms one is looking for.

I started to consider the practical usefulness of such a work. Back to the "helplessness" issue I began to read what was written in regard to each theme and each medicine. On doing an analysis of its structure and contents I recognized the intuitive work and the struggle attempted by the author on "mining" and studying the relation between the main mental symptoms of the Pure Materia Medica that are so hard to study and, in spite of what the more orthodox homeopaths say, so unattainable in the daily activity of the homeopathist. Now, when we see how the mental symptom is shown on the Pure Materia Medica it has become much easier to relate it to the pattern the patient employed to express it. Thus we can understand through the verbal expression of the experiencer the precise argument of a feeling or sensation, the "feeling of helplessness" of a Lycopodium or Phosphorus patient, with the possibility of making a perceptive distinction of one and the other. This book is a work that introduces into the human world that which was only accessible to the learned. Congratulations, really! But what a shame, it is all written in English.

Recently I got a ride by chance with a doctor from Rio de Janeiro whom I did not know. During our conversation we both realized we were homeopathists. On that same day I had launched the Repertory of Homeopathic Symptoms in the Brazilian Hahnemannian Institute and we talked about Repertory and Materia Medica. Later on I recognized this fellow was Mirilli, MD, the author of theses books I had found earlier. Then I had the opportunity to describe to him the whole work of creating my Repertory which had began with the thematic studying of rubrics from the Kent and Barthel's repertories. I had had not only that experience but also the experience related to the convention of increases taken from the Pure Materia Medica in Barthel

and Kunzli's Repertory, and so I knew how hard it was to realize such a work, which was almost impossible to be done without a computer. Even then it takes a long time to be concluded. I recognized on Mirilli's difficulties our own difficulties and that of all homeopathists who venture

on the detailed research of the Pure Materia Medica. At that point I was informed that the job was being produced in Portuguese. I offered him some technical suggestions and gave him all the support I could so he would conclude the job. Then we would have a real opportunity to introduce it to our publisher. And it happened soon. And just in time because now we have an excellent source of study and Repertory and materia medica research, with publishing quality and national distribution. Much can be done from this work on. We now have the conditions to do some pertinent inclusions in our Repertory, or understand why some medicines are included into it, or research directly the clinical cases through the proposed themes, proceed on word theme analysis, and much more. I congratulate the author for his enthusiasm and idealism on accomplishing the work. It is true that others had already thought about realizing such a project but a canyon separates an idea from its attainment. And a bridge is needed to connect both sides. The energy put on it and the ideal that gives the direction increase the value of the work. It will be useful for all, patients and homeopathists, who will certainly benefit from it.

Ariovaldo Ribeiro Filho, MD, is the author of " Repertório de Sintomas Homeopáticos"
fax: + 55 112735792 internet: aribeiro@link.com.br

Henning Droege

The anatomic order of symptoms from head to foot that Hahnemann and all other authors use is of great help in quickly finding the local symptoms. Even in huge repertories it is a clear thing. For example „Stitching pain in occiput when stooping" has a definite place in all books. It does not matter if the prover called it an awful piercing in the back of head whenever he touches his feet. The symptom is correctly listed as HEAD PAIN; STITCHING; Occiput; stooping, after.

If we assume that the mental sphere in homeopathy and in man is at least as important as the physical sphere, we need a similar helpful order of mental symptoms.

But what do we have? Hahnemann and most other books list mental symptoms indiscriminately as if they were insignificant requiring a small chapter such as „Stool" and did not need a detailed scheme. Only some books, like T.F. Allen's have a rough differentiation between Emotional and Intellectual. But we might even say that mind, soul and body are all aspects of humanity that are of equivalent importance, so that each of these aspects would need a chapter with as many rubrics as the body.

In the repertory the rubric names chosen are listed alphabetically. In the mental sphere there are a lot of words that are not quite synonymous and form a continuum of meanings. It is often highly arbitrary as to where a remedy is listed. Is it more apprehension or anxiety or fear or anguish or nightmare or panic or frightened or sorrow or starting or frightful delusion? Cross-references are certainly helpful, but we have to admit that we have no way of finding mental symptoms and their remedies as assuredly as in the physical sphere. The gift of Kent has not yet worked for the mental symptoms: we still have to know most symptoms or at least rubrics by heart to find what we need. But the purpose of a repertory is to find what we don't know. Kent's mind chapter was still small. But today we have so much information in the Complete Repertory of Mind that it is impossible to survey it all.

A breakthrough was achieved by Mirilli's Thematic Repertory.

He solves the problem in two ways:

First he arranges the symptoms by themes that is according to how we think when we try to understand the patient.

Second he quotes the original provers' words thus differentiating exactly what is really meant by this symptom in this remedy.

Mirilli's book is not only a repertory. It is the first approach to themes of remedies and so to deeper understandig of their cores that is based scientifically, which means in homeopathy: proving without speculation. When reading in Mirilli's book about some symptoms or ideas of a remedy that we knew so far vaguely by a repertory rubric or from a rumour heard in a seminar they suddenly become clear, distinct, coloured. But not by imagining what might be meant behind the shortened words of a rubric or a teacher but by quoting the explicit and vivacious words of the prover. It is amazing to see how much Hahnemann's notes enable us to get a detailed feeling for the suffering of a remedy when arranged by themes. We don't need to speculate!

In this way the so called ideas and themes of remedies that were so far suspicious to be fictive are now based on reliabel and true sources. So Mirilli fulfills what is required in § 144 Organon.

Usually it is tiring work to read the complete literal provers' notes in books such as Hahnemann's, T.F. Allen's or Hughes'. But when reading Mirilli, where the same sentences are arranged by themes comparing the remedies it becomes suddenly exciting and enlightening.

The first editions of the Thematic Repertory were obviously incomplete. Now the fitting rubrics from the Complete Repertory have been added so that the number of remedies listed is nearly complete. The aim must be to give the original prover's words instead of (or in addition to) the rubrics. But unfortunately many items in Kent's Repertory cannot be found in other sources so the two-fold structure of the Thematic Repertory will have to stay.

Henning Droege
Arzt fuer Allgemeinmedizin
Homoeopathie, Naturheilverfahren
Rembrechtser Str. 41 (Haslach)
D-88239 Wangen im Allgaeu
Tel. 07528-9133-3, fax -5
Henning.Droege@t-online.de

Frederik Schroyens MD

Over the past decades, the amount of homeopathic knowledge has been increasing so fast that it has become impossible for any human mind to contain even part of it. There are two attitudes: those who rely on books or computerized databases to check for information or those who believe their memory can hold it all. I regret the latter attitude even more as it often implies that there is no substantial new information coming up. This is no true: so much interesting information is added to the homeopathic library that it takes new initiatives, new technologies to allow anyone to keep in touch with it. The work of my friend Dr. Mirilli is one such interesting initiative in a special way.

With Synthesis I have tried to synthesize all homeopathic knowledge up to date in a repertorial way. This means that symptom stories were split in meaningful bits to allow one to find the symptom back from different angles. The well known and unavoidable disadvantage of the repertorial approach is that the complete symptom is often inperceivable. Therefore several researchers have started to emphasize again the link from the Repertory to the Materia Medica. The present work makes this access even more easy as it sticks to the logic of the Repertory. I recommend this book, and its logic, to improve the knowledge of all those who use it.

Dr. Frederik Schroyens is the author of the Synthesis Repertory
The Radar's Software Homepage
http://www.archibel.com/
Gent, Belgium, July 20, 1996

Ian Townsend M.A., R S Hom, PoCH

The last 10-15 years have seen many improvements in homœopathy. The education and training of future generations of practitioners has changed beyond recognition over that time. The advent of inexpensive electronic international communication has meant it is often easier to get in touch with colleagues a continent away than in the next town. Ideas, resources, co-operative developments are eagerly and willingly being shared, even as you read this book.In a homœopathic world community rapidly changing due to the advantages of modern technology (witness the current plethora of excellently revised repertories offering us even more accurate source documents) such a book as José Mirilli's

Thematic Materia Medica links 20th century homœopathy with that of our illustrious forbears. From the moment I got my copy of Mirilli's original text last year, I knew I had in my hands a work of inestimable value. We will all benefit from the dedication and effort that has gone into making the original proving symptoms even more accessible to us.

The Thematic Materia Medica now occupies a place of high importance on my bookshelf, and I can thoroughly recommend it to my colleagues and students in the knowledge that it is a truly unique and valuable work.

Ian Townsend M.A., R S Hom, PoCH
co-Director, Sheffield School of Homœopathy, England.

Maurizio Castellini MD

When Mirilli asked me to write this preface to the English language edition of his book we had only just met each other and our encounter took place rather oddly and casually in the departure lounge of Naples airport, returning from the LIGA Convention at Capri. I was discussing with my colleague Sforzini the reliability of Pure Materia Medica in the wake of the critical reports presented during the Conference. We were already queuing up at the gate to board the plane when he, Mirilli, arrived and took us to one side. He asked me, breathlessly: "What do you do with Pure Materia Medica? How do you organize yourself? Tell me everything. "Sforzini and I exchanged stunned glances. That was precisely what we were talking about. I'd just asked: "And what should we do with PMM now? What should we do at the School?" and there was Mirilli, appearing from now here like a falcon and asking us exactly the same question.

This amazing coincidence immediately convinced us that something important was taking place! And Mirilli and his work turned out to be exceptional. The theme has essentially remained the one which characterized our first meeting: how important are the symptoms of PMM? How far can we trust them? How can we exploit them?

There are many current and rigorous reports attacking the basic value ofPMM. When, for example, Schroyens and the Versilia Association demonstrate that, in some pathogeny provings, 50% of the modalised symptoms consequently assumed to be valid from an homoeopathic standpoint actually turn out to be symptoms of the placebo, this undermines the credibility of Pure Materia Medica.

The methods used to accumulate the symptoms of PMM have been anything but rigorous and we are therefore authorised to assume that more than half the symptoms in such texts are worthless. Many symptoms of PMM have not even been included in the repertories and therefore have not been verified in clinical terms.

And how many other reports are there which, in more or less rigorous ways ,discuss the same things? If the validity of symptoms is under discussion, then even the immense interpretative work based on these symptoms equally becomes unfounded.

This basic uncertainty also wipes out a large part of the advantages today made available to homoeopaths by computer technology when the symptoms of Pure Materia Medica are made directly available.

The doubt which immediately comes to mind is always the same: "What should we do?"

Abandon these hypertrophic texts and seek refuge in the synthetic materia medica as experienced by these authors? Experiment everything over and again from the beginning? Or, on the other hand, ignore all these reports as if they did not exist? Is there a way out which allows us to exploit the valid aspects of what has already been done?

To all intents and purposes, what we are suggesting are various opportunities which could prove effective in avoiding the loss of the data already available to us. We can more or less summarise such opportunities in two categories:

- a logical review of symptoms in order to coordinate them utilising analysis methods which are not otherwise typical of homoeopathy, such as psychosomatics, psychoanalysis and symbolism
- a thematic re-organisation of PMM symptoms and their possible exegesisand confirmation through other symptoms of the same pathogenesis.

Mirillli's work lies in the field of thematic organisation of symptoms. He has assessed the meaning of symptoms and has grouped them by themes, linking them together and thereby confirming them through other symptoms and their agreements.

This criterion, however, is equally open to criticism: if various similar symptoms are not true then the theme derived from them is equally untrue. But if several symptoms are in agreement, this significantly reduces the margin of error and, therefore, such a criterion undoubtedly diminishes the risk of "untruth".

This is an enormous task and the figures that Mirilli himself supplies in summary demonstrate it clearly: "I have created approximately 300 mental themes..." covering the most important moments in the psychological and relational dynamics of human life "... using the PMM's original words and attempting to classify more than 4000 symptoms selected amongst the 17,000mental symptoms that are in the PMMs."

The first question that immediately comes to mind reading this summary is: "What happened to the other 13,000 symptoms? "The other 13,000 rejected symptoms include common, un-modalised symptoms and those which cannot be referred to themes of particular importance or homoeopathic situations characteristic of various remedies and even, and perhaps above all, to the vast majority of invalid symptoms. This book only deals with symptoms which can be related to themes: this is the task. The selection criteria underlying it are at one and the same timeits advantage and its limitation.

Yet this book offers many important advantages.

First and foremost, thematic re-organisation makes it possible to give greater stability to the pathogenesis of the remedy. The convalidation of the symptoms and their repeated appearance strengthens the pathogenesis itself.

A second advantage of Thematic Materia Medica is its obvious predisposition for clinical application. Thematic organisation in itself is a simplification of research work into the symptoms of the patient in terms of the pathogenesis of the remedy.

For example, we find under ANGER not only "Ailments from anger" but also"... from mortification", "... from rage" and as well as anger all symptoms of a similar nature to anger or, in any case, closely related to it such as "Anguish, anger from", "Cowardice, anger, with sudden ebullition of", "Death; desires, alternating with rage" ... "Despair; rage, cursing and imprecations", "Envy, hate and..." i.e., everything which has anything to do with the various ways, psychological, relational and even physical, of expressing anger as in "Head; pain; anger, from", "Rectum; diarrhea, anger, after", "sleep, sleeplessness, anger after".

This way of presenting symptoms organised by themes satisfies the methodological requirement of escaping from large-scale rubrics to reach smaller and modalised references which are more useful in terms of prescription and more likely to include minor remedies. Thus, when faced by someone who is angry or doubtful, Mirilli makes it possible for us to select from a broad menu the closest and most similar specific rubric to treat each individual patient.

We hope that Mirilli and his work will be publicised as widely and deservedly as possible precisely because of the very special assistance it provides us.

Director, Homoeopathic Medical School of Verona
Piazza S Francesco, 6 - 37123 Verona Italy
tel. 0039.45.8006008 fax 0039.45.8035945
e-mail Castellini = castelma@uni.net

Roger van Zandvoort

When I first saw this book in Curitiba, Brasil, I knew immediately how much work had been involved in the project of making it. This kind of work can only be done by those people that not only invest their time but also give their soul to the project.

If one wants to understand the mental pictures of our most original remedies, of which most are polychrests, this book is the book of choice. In a very careful way José Mirilli has listed keywords/themes, around which a complete network of information has been spun. About 300 themes quoting around 11000 Pure Materia Medica symptoms. First of all there are the Complete Repertory rubrics organized by themes and the complete PMM text remedies around that theme, coming from the original proving MM and indicated as such together with the specific number of the symptom of the original text. This is the basis of the work enriched by lists that indicate relationships between themes, relationships between words belonging to the same and different themes, a analogical-index that can function as a repertory and in doing so reveals a lot of unknown information and last but not least a complete listing of all Repertory's symptoms related to themes.

Since there is not much to add to this work for the sources used we can only ask the author when he is going on, taking this work to it's next step: the same for the other remedies of our MM.

Roger van Zandvoort, author of The Complete Repertory.
homepage: - http://www.irhis.nl/
internet: rozand@euronet.nl
telephone [+31][0]70 327 11 07
telefax [+31][0]70 317 67 89
The Netherlands

J.A. Mirilli , MD *

When I first read a Pure Materia Medica I was amazed by the chaotic organization of the symptoms and so for several years I stayed away from them choosing to study instead the clinical materia medica where the symptoms are organized. During my classes on Kent's and GEHSH's course of studies I could not believe the struggle to study the symptoms, which was something totally unintelligible to me.

By the time I understood the experimental nature of homeopathical symptoms and checked the precise description of the symptoms, a complete change happened on my perception of homeopathy and I became a researcher. Thinking about how hard it was to study the symptoms that are spread along the several volumes of Materia Medica I wondered if there was not an easier way of organizing the symptoms for the homeopathists. When I discovered Bernal's thematic work I foresaw the possibility of organizing the homeopathic symptoms of the pure materia medica by themes.

When I started to use a computer for my homeopathic research I began to classify the mental symptoms by themes into the data bank Micro-Isis. Since in 1989 there were no MMs computer programs, the original idea was to make the PMMs symptoms available to homeopathists. Although today there are many homeopathic programs including several Materia Medica, most homeopathists have no access to computers and for that reason I decided to make a book out of my research.

Initially I attempted on reading the homeopathic symptoms classifying the themes they approached. At the same time I did an analogical research of the key words of the symptoms in English and later on I used those words to create the themes concluding that was the most appropriate method to work with.

I was astonished by the original wealth of the homeopathic symptoms before they are severed and displayed in alphabetical order in the repertories. The living of the homeopathic symptoms expresses itself in the several themes that actually are in the symptom as a whole. We may also see the psychodynamic of each medicine in the successive unfolding of the several themes in each symptom, increasing the conviction that new instruments must be created for us to organize and draw out the essence of the PMMs's symptoms. I have created approximately 300 mental themes using the PMMs's original words attempting to classify more than 4000 symptoms selected amongst the 17000 mental symptoms that are in the PMMs (Hahnemann, Hering, Allen). The repertories were the main attempt to classify the homeopathic symptoms so they could be used by homeopathists for fast medical advice; but they were limited.

The first and probably the most important limitation is related to the symptoms being severed and classified in alphabetical order with no connections in the Repertory, loosing their dynamic expression and their live expression with their succeeding details and following changes that for us, homeopathists, expresses the human suffering.

The second limitation is related to the symptoms being classified in alphabetical order, coming from several repertories of different languages and organizations, and thus similar symptoms are in different places and are not related.

The third limitation is related to the fact that the symptoms described on the Pure Materia Medica are not totally represented on the repertorial rubrics. The symptoms that express helplessness, for example, are represented on the PMMs by a very different medicine than the ones that appear in the helplessness rubric on the Repertory. In my opinion that is due to the fact that the symptoms on the Repertory express the clinical experience of their author or their bibliographical sources with no reference to the experimental PMMs. We can see the same phenomenon in many other symptoms. The work of physician Deniza Futuro confirms that conviction. When she initially tried to realize a bibliographical research over the clinical symptom "Angina pectoris" of Kent's Repertory, comparing its 53 medicines with the symptoms explained on the PMMs and clinical materia medica, she was surprised to see completely contradictory informations. Medicines related to classical angina symptoms and explained in clinical healings described on the PMMs were not represented with enough graduation on the Repertory. And further more, medicines with few or no cardiological symptoms at all are represented on the Repertory with maximum degree. And this may be a shock for you but even among the clinical materia medica and the pure materia medica there were enormous differences regarding the content of the cardiological symptoms for the same medicine. I made a research in the computer of the word "asthma" on the PMMs and I found in Hering dozens of modalities not explained on the repertories. I think new methodologies should be created to provide that such great differences among the several homeopathic sources would not occur. I am not saying the information on the repertories is worthless but we should consider the PMMs sources of experiment and compare them with the clinical symptoms of the repertories to assure that one source may contribute to the other and there may be a coherence between the concepts and contents of the MMs and repertories.

The fourth limit is due to the fact that there is great differences of vocabulary between the Repertory and the classical materia medica. On the materia medica the symptoms are described in a simple language, neither organized nor classified. On the Repertory the symptoms are organized according to an arrangement that I call "conceptual" and not by description, meaning that is the form the author can use to organize the symptoms according to the boundaries of his perception and awareness of reality. Those boundaries are imposed by his conceptual background and are tied up to the values of his time. The idea that the description and understanding of the symptoms should be free of values seems artificial to me. Thus I prefer to think that man can only understand reality from an explanation based on his conceptual values. We can not just accept to be guided by the concepts of understanding the repertorial rubrics without a critical view about the way we consider them as they occur in time and space. That is why I believe the classical classification of the Repertory does not consider the demands of modern man's mentality. It is not enough just to add new medicines in the rubrics but we have to review its concepts and create new rubrics expressing human suffering in modern language. In a modern approach I created the term "supressed", for example, which to me represents the intentional expression of a group of symptoms; the concept did not exist until its creation by psychoanalysis as "repressed", while in the classic texts that behavior is described as "supressed" with no equivalent in the Repertory. It is not necessary to support the concept since it has become a popular fashion on describing and explaining a certain behavior and part of the popular expressions so highly considered by classical homeopathists. I am not saying that psychoanalysis should guide homeopathic classifications but we must be aware of its influence in our understanding of modern man. Classical symptoms such as "anxiety of conscience " are explained nowadays as the "guilt" psychoanalytic concept, even if often unconsciously. Nowadays it is obvious that any classification of the symptoms must be consciously influenced by the conceptual concepts that are part of the expression of modern man's suffering.

We have used several dictionaries. "The American Heritage" gave us the opportunity to know the ethimology of the words while "Webster's" (the old unabridged edition, 1939, 3 volumes - the most complete Webster's) gave us the meaning of obscure words such as "Philoprogenitiveness" (a symptom related to the medicine Ox-ac. - Allen,19), a term not found in modern dictionaries meaning "desire to procreate". We also used the "Aurélio" Portuguese Dictionary, the "Houaiss" English-Portuguese Dictionary, and the CD-ROM "Microsoft Bookshelf" which includes the third edition of "The American Heritage", the "Roget's Thesaurus" Dictionary of synonymous, and the "Columbia Dictionary of Quotations" where you may find samples of words as they appear in classical English textbooks. And finally the "Webster's Collegiate Thesaurus", a Dictionary of synonymous. The thematic research is only beginning and each time I classify the symptoms new themes appear which gives way to classifying them into new themes. That is the reason why I ask for suggestions related to new themes and evaluations of the actual themes, which would make it possible to improve the quality of the book in future editions. I really hope the book may be a new source of research and that your evaluations and suggestions will be useful to the development of homeopathy.

Just in time to explain the nomenclature of the bibliographical references; ever after the abbreviation of the medicine there comes its source (a- "Ha" on the numbering below 200 for the Chronic Diseases' symptoms and above 200 for the Hahnemann's Pure Materia Medica symptoms; b- "Al" for the T.F.Allen's Encyclopedia, "Al-S" for the supplementary symptoms of the tenth volume; c- "Al-N" for the symptoms of the H.C.Allen's Materia Medica of the Nosodes; d- "He" for the symptoms taken from Hering's Guiding Symptoms). Thus when in doubt we may compare the symptom with the original one. And we may also consult the source to know what is the origin of the symptom (experimental, toxic, or clinical cure). After the symptoms there are the themes they motivated so we may observe its possible intentionalities. After the list of the thematic classification there is the list of symptoms for each medicine thus representing their Materia Medica.

Bibliography:

Allen, T.F., Encyclopedia of Pure Materia Medica, New York / Philadelphia , Boericke & Tafel, 1879.

Allen, H.C. The Materia Medica of the Nosodes, Philadelphia, Boericke & Tafel, 1910.

Hahnemann, S. The Chronic Diseases, Translated by Tafel ,Annotations by Hughes Jain Publishing, 1986.

Hahnemann, S. Materia Medica Pura, Translated by Dudgeon, Annotations by Hughes Jain Publishing,1986.

Hering, C. Guiding Symptoms of Our Materia Medica, Philadelphia 1879-1891.

Mirilli, J.A. Repertório Temático English- Portuguese 1993 -1996

Mirilli, J.A. Matéria Médica Temática, English 1994 -1996

Mirilli, J.A. Dicionário Temático English 1994

Mirilli. J.A. Matéria Médica Temática Portuguese - Robe Publisher 1996

Sherr, Jeremy Dynamic Provings, Dynamis school 1997

Zandvoort, Roger van The Complete Repertory, IRHIS 1996

José Antonio Mirilli de Oliveira
Rua do Catete, 311 sala 815
Rio de Janeiro, BRASIL
CEP 22220 -001
Tel / Fax : 055212653545
Internet: jamirilli@ax.apc.org / mirilli@usa.net

Please, feel free to give your opinions
and suggestions on the book.
They will be important to improve the
quality of the next printings.

ABROAD

Confusion of mind; country, as if now in one, now in another: chlol.[36]
Delirium; loquacious, foreign countries, of: cann-i.
Delusions; abroad, being: verat.[30]
- Russia, of being in: lap-mar-c.[194]
- strange, land, as if in a: bry. par. plat. verat.
- voices, hears, strangers, of: bell.[30] ***cham.***[30]

Dreams; country, far off: sil.[1]
➤ country, foreign: ind.[54] ozone[227] plat.[10] sil.[10]
➤ country, native country: ant-c.[1] lach.[36] mur-ac.[36]
➤ fatherland: ant-c.[10] lach.[10] mur-ac.[10]
➤ Indians, being among: jug-c.
➤ journey, China, to: bamb-a.[1184]
➤ journey, countries, in foreign: ind.[54]
➤ journey, cruise around the world: bamb-a.[1184]
➤ journey, distant regions, in: ther.[54]
➤ journey, Peking, to: ozone[227]
➤ mother, flying around the world: hydrog.[222]
Talk; native country, of: aether[36]

ANDROC. Sh, 180 - Desire to be out in the country, intense desire to be on the rocks. Desire to feel the rocks, to stick hand beneath the rocks, to crawl into or behind rocks. (Clinical)
ASTER. He, 2-...hallucinations as if away from home in midst (middle) of strangers; hears voices to which he replies.
CAMPH. Al, 46-...The external world existed for me no longer. (solitude) My thoughts were gone; one single fearful one remained; I imagined myself transferred to another world (estranged, alienated); for me all else was extinguished...
CHLOL. Al, 17-...a feeling as if he were now in one country and now in another, and with an anxious desire to go home.(abroad)
HALI-L. Sh, 948 - I can't identify other bird calls here, as if I'm in the wrong country. All unfamiliar. 20, 30C, 16:XX:XX
IRID. Sh, 114 - Felt I had been given the role of messenger, wasn't always in English. Q3
Sh, 115 - Inner vision, rows upon rows of letters. Thought, "This looks Greek to me." Q8
MAG-C. Al, 932 - Dream of flowers, clothes, and other things; she had to make up the clothes, but had no inclination to do it, and besides did not understand how; she also saw many foreign plants, but during this she became soaked (wet) with rain.
MERC. He, 19 - Homesickness (nostalgia, isolation), or desire to travel; wants to go abroad (absent, nomad); nightly anxiety and perspiration.(wander)
NEON. Sh, 165 - I felt alone and as if everyone perceived me as odd. I felt strange, like an outsider and could not connect on any level. 02, 6C, 22:XX:XX
PLAN. Al, 19 - Feeling great desire to be at home when abroad.
STRAM. He, 130 - Talks in a foreign tongue.

ACCIDENTS

Ailments from; fright or fear, accident, from sight of an: **<u>ACON.</u>**[122] ***calc.*** **<u>OP.</u>**[122]
Ailments from; injuries, accidents: acon.[34] arn.[34] bell.[5] camph.[54] cic.[102] ***glon.***[102] hyos.[5] hyper.[102] mag-c.[102] **NAT-S.**[122] op.[5] rhus-t.[34] ruta[34] stram.[5] sul-ac.[8] verat.[5]
Anxiety; fire were breaking out, as if, morning, on being awakened by noise in the street: tet.[36]
Anxiety; injury, after: ***arn.***[184] chin.[54] op.[28]
Anxiety; motion, from, airplane, of: **BOR.**[122]
Anxiety; motion, from, cable-railway, of: **BOR.**[122]
Anxiety; motion, from, elevator, of: **BOR.**[122]
Anxiety; railroad, when about to journey by, amel. while in train: arg-n.[58] ars.
Anxiety; riding, while: ***arg-n.***[54] ***aur. bor. lach.***[122] psor. sep.
Anxiety; riding, while, closed carriage, in: bor.[172] cimic.[102] nat-m.[172] succ.[137]
Anxiety; riding, while, down hill: **BOR.** ***psor.***
Anxiety; riding, while, hypochondriasis, in: ***arg-n.***[54]
Anxiety; riding, while, rapidly: staph.[172]
Delusions; accidents, fatal, he will have a: alum.[139]
- accidents, of relatives: phos.[1]
- accidents, sees: anac.[5] ars.[5]
- casualties, sees: anac.[10] ars.[10] bell.[10] canth.[10] hep.[10] nat-c.[10] op.[10]
- friend, accident, met with a: ars.
- rainstorm, she is in a terrible, complaining of being so cold, and that carriage has

turned over and hurt her head: naja.[8]
• runs, against something: arg.[139]
• water, disasters by: cann-i.
Dreams; accidents: allox.[119] am-m. androc.[222] ant-c. arg.[36] arn. **ARS.** bamb-a.[1184] bell. calc.[102] cham. chin. cinnb. con. ***dig.***[102] **GRAPH.** ind. iod. iodof. jab. kali-c. kali-m.[192] kali-s.[58] kreos. lyc. mag-m.[1] mand.[144] mez.[1] nat-s. nit-ac.[102] ***nux-v.*** puls. rumx. sars. sil.[102] sul-ac. sulph. thuj. verat.[102] viol-o.[45]
➤ accidents, annoying: ind.[54]
➤ accidents, boat foundering: alum. bamb-a.[1184] lyc. sil.
➤ accidents, car, with: viol-o.[45]
➤ accidents, crash of plane: mand.[144]
➤ accidents, explosion: stann.
➤ accidents, fatal: cham.[54] **GRAPH.**[54] kali-m.[111] **NUX-V.**[54] sars.[54]
➤ accidents, struck by lightning, being: ***arn.***
➤ casualties, of: alum.[10] caust.[10] con.[10] kali-n.[10] mag-c.[10] nat-c.[10] nux-v.[10] plat.[10] rat.[10] rheum[10] sars.[10] sul-ac.[10]
➤ children, about, lying on ice, her little child, and she feared it would fall into water: lipp.[36]
➤ disaster: sars.
➤ disease, injuries: allox.[119] am-m. ant-c. cench.[58] chel.[36] chin. choc.[222] cortico.[119] lob.[54] ***mag-s.***[10] nat-s. nicc.[10] phos. sumb.
➤ driving, up a steep rough track: lap-mar-c.[194]
➤ drowning, mother had been drowned, that her: nicc. rauw.[119]
➤ drowning, people: ***lyc.***[54] mag-s.[10] verat.[36]
➤ falling, elevator is: ozone[227]
➤ injuries, machinery, by: cortico.[119]
➤ misfortune, car, function anymore, does not, brakes: bamb-a.[1184]
➤ misfortune, car, function anymore, does not, while driving: ozone[227]
Fear; accidents, friends, to: ars.[172]
✦ accidents, loved ones, to: phos.[1]
✦ accidents, of: acon. androc.[222] arg-n.[31] carb-an.[1] ***carb-v.*** choc.[222] cupr. gins. graph.[172] hydrog.[222] iod.[8] kali-i.[1] mag-c.[8] mag-s.[54] naja[8] perh.[149] petr.[149] rhus-t.[54] samb-c.[36] tarent.[192]
✦ accidents, of, child, of: ars.[172]
✦ accidents, others, to: osm.[36]
✦ accidents, trifle, from every: iod.[54]
✦ airplanes: ***acon.***[162] arg-n.[162] ars.[162] **CALC.**[162] lup.[162] nat-m.[162]
✦ concussion, of, as if he might run against something: arg.
✦ crossing, streets: acon.[85] ferr-p.[172] gaert.[136] hydr-ac.[137] kali-p.[172] plat.[137]
✦ disable, being: **ARS.**[162] mag-m.[162] psor.[162]
✦ disaster, of: calc.[137] elat. lil-t. psor. ***puls.*** rhus-t.[139] tab. tub.[56] wye.[85] zinc.[139]
✦ disfigured, of being: hep.[30]
✦ friend has met with accident, that a: ars. ***caust.***[184]
✦ going out, alone: ars.[127] ign.[127] pitu-a.[164]
✦ going out, of: pneu.[149] sep.149 tarent.[192]
✦ happen, something will, family, to, or to him: ars.[172] calc.[172] calc-s.[36] caust.[172] phos.[172] psor.[172] sep.[172] tub.[36]
✦ home, away from: ign.[162]
✦ injured, of being: arn.[5] ars.[58] calad. calc-s.[196] cann-i. chin.[137] choc.[222] cupr-acet.[54] gels.[8] hep.[137] hyos. kali-c.[137] lyss.[172] ruta[130] spig.[137] **STRAM.** ***stry.***
✦ motoring: gins.[122]
✦ riding in a carriage, when: acon.[193] androc.[222] arg-n.[185] ***aur.***[193] ***bor.*** bry.[126] carc.[227] cimic.[172] cocc.[172] cupr.[210] gins.[122] ***lach.*** lipp.[36] pitu-a.[164] ***psor.*** sanic.[126] ***sep.***
✦ sea, of the: morbill.[162]
Thoughts; accidents, of, having happened to others: osm.[36]

ACON. Al, 63 - Dread of some accident happening.
ADAM. Sh, 434 - Before a journey, fear of not being able to get home. 8, 6C, 01:09:00
Sh, 436 - Very scared of driving in a car, obsessed with crashing and accidents and death. 20, 1M, XX:XX:XX
Sh, 438 - Nearly backed into another car, which was double-parked, although checking very carefully. Felt as if I was going to have an accident. Didn't feel safe. 6, 30C, 01:16:XX
ANDROC. Sh, 48 - Extremely accident prone, had to avoid driving the car. (10)
Sh, 49 - Accident prone (10, 25) cut fingers frequently. (10)
Sh, 86 - Full of fear when driving, avoided it at all costs. (7)
Sh, 176 - Fear of driving, especially fear of hurting someone else in an accident. (Clinical)

ARG-M. Al, 449 - Anxious dreams; on waking up, he still felt so anxious that he imagined he had suffered the accident he had dreamed about.
He, 19 - Fear of concussion (hurt, injure) as if he might run against something, with pain in testicles.
BRASS. Sh, 8 - Feeling of impending disaster, still cannot settle to anything 3I, 00:08:00
CHOC. Sh, 188 - While walking outside, became anxious in a self-conscious way, anxious and vulnerable as if being watched or observed by something or someone -the attention was on me - anxiety that something would happen. Immediately afterwards I was attacked by four dogs and bitten on the calf. 27, 100C, 01:XX:XX
Sh, 189 - While outside became very weary of cars and people. Felt open and vulnerable. Fear of accidents, cars, or of someone leaping into the road and punching me. This anxiety was worse out of doors. 27, 100C, 01:XX:XX
Sh, 190 - While walking past a block of flats, I worried that it might blow over in the wind and fall on me. 27, 100C, 01:XX:XX
ELAT. He, 3 - Fear of some approaching disaster.
GERM. Sh, 45 - Loss of concentration. Lost my thoughts while driving, nearly causing two accidents. 05, 6C, 08:XX:XX
Sh, 46 - Accident prone at work because of not thinking about what I am doing. Close miss accident driving a fork lift. 16, 30C, 00:04:00
GINS. Al, 3 - Mind generally calm; still there are impatient impulses and fear of accidents, with, at times, disposition to weep, or to be anxious about the future.
GLON. He, 16 - Bad effects of mental excitement, fright, fear, mechanical contusions and their consequences. (ailments from)
HALI-L. Sh, 518 - Feeling obsessed with the question of whether it will rain. I'm planning my son's birthday party outside for tomorrow with 17 children, and am afraid it will rain. 01, 30C, 11:12:30
Sh, 520 - When the rain came down hard, there was a roaring from the creek outside. Awful sleep. I'd wake up with each roar, envisioning the water rising up, fearing the creek was backed up and would overflow its banks. I'd listen till the sound died down, then I could go back to sleep. 08, 30C, 06:XX:XX
Sh, 525 - Big fear on icy road. Scared driving on "Separate Road". Went to see a friend, had a quick hello and good-bye. All wanted to do was go home. 16, 10C, 36:XX:XX
HYDR-AC. He, 3 - Could not remain in middle of road when he saw a vehicle approaching him even at a considerable distance,... (run over)
HYDROG. Sh, 12 - Driving home I felt odd, as if I was hardly in my body. Feel like my body's working on automatic but I'm not really there. Driving along I kept forgetting where I was. Now I feel I'm really more "absent" than normal and feel quite afraid of losing my mind or having an accident. I feel my connection with the physical world is very loose, as though my soul was separated from my body. I have thoughts that this is a bit like dying —not unpleasant. 10, 200C, 13:02:XX
Sh, 194 - Fear I may lose my mind, or even die. Fear about the proving. Feel I could bash the car so I have to make a real effort. 10, 200C, 12:XX:XX
IOD. He, 7 - Apprehends an accident from every trifle.
IRID. Sh, 195 - Panicked about servicing car before a long journey. Felt anxiety that car might break down as it hadn't been running smoothly. However found that car didn't need a service for another two thousand miles. Over-conscientious about getting jobs done on car. A3
Sh, 200 - Waking frequently, every hour, feeling very alert and wide awake, worried that I had forgotten something, not put the guard on the fire, closed down the stove, locked the doors, etc. Feels like I would take ages to get off to sleep. In reality got to sleep quickly. A19
Sh, 203 - Being driven home, I felt the feeling of imminent danger on waking. I kept waking with a start six or seven times during the journey. Nervous because too near the car in front. B7
KALI-BR. Al, 6-...she fancied that the

boarders in the hotel insulted her, and imagined that the weekly bills of the landlord (owner) were evidences of a conspiracy which had been got up against her father; ... while standing on the guards of the boat ...declared she had seen her brother fall overboard;...

KALI-I. Ha, 8 - Whining; apprehensive as from threatened accident.

LIPP. Al, 2 - Feeling of great apprehension, while riding in a carriage; a kind of anxiety in the heart, as of impending misfortune, together with a kind of homesickness.

MAG-C. He, 4 - Trembling, anguish and fear, as if some accident would happen;...

NAJA. He, 5-...imagines she is in a terrible rainstorm, complains of being so cold (coldness), and that the carriage has turned over and hurt her head. (accident)

OP. He, 20-...declares he is not alone in bed; ..desire to escape; says a regiment of horsemen are upon his bed and that he fears to be trodden upon (run over, crushed); when told that horses are very careful, answered that he feared he would be crushed by the wagons that followed them.

OSM. Al, 5 - Thoughts of accidents having happened to others, by a blow, a fall, or being dashed (crushed, hit, knock) to pieces; gradually these thoughts grow upon him, as if he were to do the same injuries to others.

PHOS. Al, 115 - Frightened feeling, as if I was about to be run over by a locomotive. (crushed, smash)

Ha, 5 - Sad and melancholy, as if some accident had happened to his beloved ones.

PSOR. Al, 9 - Unusual anxiety when riding in a carriage.

Al, 32 - Great disinclination to ride in a carriage; then at once she wants to ride all the time, even in bad weather.

PULS. He, 42-...full of anxiety, forebodings of impending (imminent, destined) disaster; ...

SAMB-C. Al, 1-...an indefinable fear as if the horse (a very gentle animal) might run away, or the wagon break at any moment; a dread of some undefined danger.

SEP. Al, 58 - Fearfulness when riding in a carriage.

ACCUSED

Delirium tremens; voices, heard continually on right side of occiput a loud voice, scolding, vituperating and accusing him of ungodliness, and also personifies voices: **STRAM.**[54]

Delirium; accused of theft, after being harshly: ***hyos.***[54]

Delusions; accused, she is: laur. zinc.

- obscene, actions of which she had not been guilty, accuses herself of.: ***phos.***
- thieves, accused of robbing, he has been: kali-br.
- witches, denies having anything to do with them, in delirium after being accused of theft: ***hyos.***[54]

Dreams; accusations: clem.[10] lach.[10] nat-m.[10] thuj.[10]

- ➤ accusations, crime, wrongful of: choc.[222] clem.[10] hydrog.[222] sil.[58]
- ➤ defamatory: mosch.
- ➤ theft, accused of, of being: choc.[222] lach.

GERM. Sh, 153 - Thought nobody understood me and cared for what I felt. Felt it was unfair. I was presented with complaints about something others had done. Felt I was standing between two fighting parts. Felt awkward about it, embarrassed. Difficult to argue about such strong outburst. Thoughts about the day's arguing milling in my head all evening and night. 21, 12C, 32:XX.XX.

HYOS. He, 79 - After being harshly (severe) accused of theft (crime), continual delirium; fancies surrounded by objects of a terrifying nature; not a moment quiet, continual calling out that she saw the devil; denies herself guilty of theft (innocent, injustice), or that she has any concern with witches; ...

KALI-BR. Al, 4 - He imagined that he had been specially singled out (select) for divine vengeance... deploring his sad fate (destiny),...he informed me that he had been accused of robbing a friend, and that the officers were in search of him....

STRAM. He, 107-...heard continually, on r. side of occiput, a loud voice, scolding, vituperating and accusing him of ungodliness (impious, sinful, irreligious, godless, profane); ....prayed expecting, with great anxiety, the flash of lightning which was to kill him;...(redemption, regeneration, salvation)

ALIVE

Delusions; animals abdomen, are in: croc.[162] ***thuj.***
- body, alive, only half alive: crot-h.[36]
- body, mouth, living things were creeping into, at night: merc.
- side, alive on one side and buried on the other, he is: stram.
- talking, inanimate objects with names, t. to but observes no one standing by him: stram.[10]
- vagina, living things creep into (at night): merc.
- voices, hears, abdomen, are in his: thuj.

Discontented; inanimate objects: caps.
Dreams; animals, eating alive: hydrog.[222]
➤ buried alive, being: ***arn.*** chel. ign. pariet.[72]
➤ vivid, images, life like: aster.[54] **NAT-M.**[54]
Fear; buried, alive: atro.[38] tub.[56] ***zinc.***[54]
Thoughts; abdomen, as if from: thuj.[5]
Thoughts; stomach, as if from: acon.[5]

CHOC. Sh, 2 - Feel very excited, very alive, bright and efficient. Had an image of a hedgehog's face.
Sh, 152 - Wanted to eat slugs and grasshoppers. I could feel how they would be in my mouth while they were still alive and wriggling. (Has been vegetarian for twenty years).
CROT-H. He, 13 - Marked indifference, seems only half alive; utter apathy.
NAT-P. Al, 1 - Awakes at night, and imagines pieces of furniture are persons.
PETR. Ha, 27 - The whole day, he is only half conscious, as if only half alive.
STRAM. Al, 122 - For some days the patient was affected with hallucinations and thought that one side of him was alive, while the other side was buried.
THUJ. He, 10 - Fixed ideas: as if a strange person were at his side; as if soul and body were separated (split) ; that body, particularly limbs, are made of glass (frail) and will readily break (weakness); as if a living animal were in abdomen ;talks about being under the influence of a superior power. (possessed)
ZINC. He, 43 - Great fear, as if persecuted by men or the devil, on account of crimes he has never done (injustice); is afraid of becoming imprisoned, or poisoned, or shot, or buried (inter) alive...[0] Delirium tremens.

AMBITION

Achieve; things, desire to: anac.[162] asar.[162] coff.[162] nux-v.[162]
Ailments from; ambition, deceived: bell.[30] merc.[30] ***nux-v.***[54] plat.[30] puls.[30] verat.[30]
Ailments from; ambition, excessive: asar.[187]
Ambition; much, ambitious: acon.[5] alum.[30] anac.[10] ars.[10] asar.[162] aur.[10] bov.[10] calc.[10] camph.[10] carb-an.[10] caust.[5] cina[10] cocain.[102] cocc.[10] coloc.[10] con.[30] cupr.[210] cycl.[10] dros.[10] graph.[30] kali-c.[185] ***lach.***[30] lyc.[10] nat-m.[10] ***nux-v.***[30] pall.[116] phos.[10] plat.[30] puls.[5] ran-b.[10] sars.[10] sil.[10] spig.[10] staph.[30] sulph.[10] tanac.[25] ***verat.***[85]
Ambition; much, fame, for: alum.[30] con.[30] graph.[30] ***lach.***[30] **NUX-V.**[30] staph.[30]
Ambition; much, means, employed every possible: lyc.[30] plat.[30] ***verat.***[30]
Ambition; much, money, for: ars.[30] calc.[30] lyc.[30] nux-v.[30] sulph.[30]
Avarice; wants all for himself: puls.[30]
Bargaining: bry.[122] ***puls.***[122] ***sil.***[122] sulph.[122]
Borrowing of everyone: calc.[30] phos.[30] plat.[30]
Brooding; law suit, over, by which he may gain or loose a million, and takes it in bad part if not allowed to read indictment for said lawsuit, a confused, irrational piece of work, on which he has been working all night, in insanity: ***nux-v.***[54]
Change; desire for, position: pip-m.[102]
Charitable; expectation of recompense, with the: calc.[30] lyc.[30] nat-m.[30] sulph.[30]
Confusion of mind; ambition, from deceived: ***nux-v.***[54]
Delusions; ciphers, sees: ***ph-ac.*** phos. sulph.
- money, counting, he is: alum. bell. cycl. mag-c. zinc.
- money, talks of: calc. carbn-s. kali-br.[25]
- wealth, of: agn. alco. bell. calc. cann-i. kali-br. nit-ac.[5] phos.[102] ***plat.***[102] ***pyrog. sulph.*** verat.

Desires; beautiful things, finery: dat-a.[25] lil-t.[137] sulph.[137]
Desires; everything, for: sant.[36]
Desires; full of: agav-t.[149] bry.[5] cina[10] coff.[5] dulc.[5] ign.[10] ip.[10] nux-m.[10] ***puls.***[5] rheum[10] rhus-t.[5] ***spig.***[30]
Desires; grandeur, for: cur.[36]
Desires; more than she needs: ***ars.***[1] ars-s-f.[58] bar-s.[58] bry.[10] zinc-p.[58]

Desires; numerous, various things: cic.[137] *cina*[36] phos.[36] staph.[137]
Desires; numerous, various things, hard to be had, which are: bry.[160]
Desires; numerous, various things, pleased with nothing: all-s.[137]
Desires; this and that: coff.[36] ***puls.***[36]
Desires; unattainable things: bry.[36] op.[36]
Dictatorial; power, love of: ars.[11] lach.[11] lyc
Dreams; aspiring: zing.[36]
➤ calculating: sel.[8]
➤ lottery, investing in, of: mag-c.[36]
➤ lottery, seeing the numbers he had taken: nat-s.[10]
➤ money: alum. bamb-a.[1184] ***cycl.*** hydrog.[222] mag-c. mag-m. phos. polym.[111] puls. zinc.[5] zinc-o.[10]
➤ money, disputing about money: chin.
➤ money, gold, of: ***cycl.*** puls.
➤ quarrels, money, about: chin.
➤ shooting, someone, who owes him money: ozone[227]
➤ stealing, money: lap-mar-c.[194]
➤ things, desired: sil.[1]
Envy; avidity, and: ***ars.***[30] ***chin.***[30] lyc.[116] nit-ac.[30] nux-v.[30] ph-ac.[30] ***puls.*** rhus-t.[30] sep.[116] stann.[30] staph.[30] sulph.[30]
Gestures; makes, plays, buttons of his clothing, counting money, as if: calc.[30] nux-v.[30] staph.[30]
Greed, cupidity: ***ars.***[30] calc.[122] ***chin.***[122] ***hyos.***[54] iod.[109] ip.[122] ***lyc.***[54] mag-c.[122] merc.[122] nat-c.[122] nit-ac.[30] nux-v.[30] ph-ac.[30] ***puls.***[36] rhus-t.[30] ***sep.***[54] stann.[30] staph.[30] sulph.[30] verat.[122]
Greed; desires are greater than her need, her: ars.[1]
Intuitive; weakness of others, to: sep.[187]
Play; gambling, passion for: ars.[30] bell.[36] calc.[30] caust.[30] chin.[30] lyc.[30] mag-c.[30] mag-m.[30] merc.[30] nux-v.[30] staph.[30] sulph.[30] verat.[30]
Play; passion, making money, for, lotteries: mag-m.[30] merc.[30] staph.[30]
Play; passion, making money, to: bell.[36] calc.[30] lyc.[30] mag-m.[30] ***merc.***[30] ***nat-c.***[30] plat.[30] puls.[30] staph.[30] sulph.[30]
Play; passion, making money, to, staking money: calc.[30] mag-c.[30] merc.[30]
Play; passion, making money, to, stock market: mag-m.[30] merc.[30] staph.[30] ther.[231]
Power, love of: ars.[189] lach.[189] lyc. nux-v.[189] sulph.[189]
Religious affections; spiritual improvement, desires: ***cinnb.***[36]
Selfishness, occupied at first with himself and besides with others for his own profit and loss for others: bell.[30] calc.[30] nux-v.[30]
Talk; money, about: ars.[189] sulph.[189]

ARN. Ha, 627 - Surly, wants to have many things and then refuses them.
ARS. Ha, 1045 - Her desire is greater then her need ; she eats and drinks more than is good for her; she walks further than she need do or can bear. (avidity)
He, 26 - Her desires are greater than her need; she eats and drinks more than is good for her, and walks farther (great distance) than she ought to do.
BRY. Ha, 780 - Too busy; she wishes to undertake and to work at too many things.
He, 15 - Desire for things that cannot be had, which are refused, or not wanted when offered.
CALC-F. Al,S-1-...tendency to look on the dark side of things, with much depression of spirits. Feeling of anxiety about money matters, or thought would come to want (lack), or would soon be "running astern" (reversed, failure) financially...disposition to set a higher value on money than natural to him (avarice?, poverty?).
He, 2 - Depression of spirits and disposition to set a higher value on money than natural to him. (avarice?)
CUR. Al, 5 - Fondness (desire) for luxury (waste) and grandeur.(distinction, fame)
LIL-T. Al, 27 - Symptoms came down on her like a sudden cloud, ...she lost vigor and snap (vitality), ...with all this depression comes a desire for fine (quality) things of all kinds; she is dissatisfied with what she has and is envious of others. (sophistication)
NUX-V. Al, 71 - She wishes to accomplish much, but thinks it will not succeed.
He, 35 - From disappointed ambition, bewildered, (confused) talks incoherently; does everything he attempts (try) to do wrong;..
He, 37-...brooding all night long over a lawsuit by which he may gain or lose a million (megalomania) ; ..replies reluctantly and slowly to physician's questions,

and takes it in bad part (offenses) if not allowed to read indictment (accusation) for said lawsuit, a confused irrational piece of work, on which he has been working all night.

PULS. Al, 9 - Envious, avaricious, unsatisfied, greedy, he would gladly have everything, to himself.

Ha, 1125 - Envious, avaricious, dissatisfied, greedy, wants to have everything for himself.

SEP. Al, 92 - One dose of the medicine takes away my ambition; I simply do not want to do anything, either work or play; it is even an exertion to think.

ANGER

Ailments from; anger, anxiety, with: **ACON.** alum. arg-n.[58] **ARS.** aur. ***bell.*** bry. calc. ***cham.*** cocc. coff. ***cupr.*** **GELS.**[5] hyos. **IGN.** lyc. nat-c. nat-m. **NUX-V.** ***op.*** petr. phos. ***plat. puls.*** rhus-t. samb. sep. stann. stram. sulph. verat.

Ailments from; anger, fright, shock, with: **ACON.** ***aur. bell.*** calc. cocc. coff.[54] cupr. **GELS.**[5] ***glon.***[5] **IGN.** nat-c. ***nux-v. op. petr. phos. plat. puls.*** samb. sep. **STRAM.**[5] sulph. zinc.

Ailments from; anger, grief, with silent: **ACON.**[5] alum. am-m.[116] ars. aur. aur-ar.[58] bell. **BRY.**[5] carc.[210] ***cham.***[5] ***chin.***[116] ***cocc. coloc. gels.***[5] hyos. **IGN. LYC.** nat-c. ***nat-m.*** nux-v. ***ph-ac.*** phos. plat. puls. **STAPH.** verat. ***zinc.***[5]

Ailments from; anger, indignation, with: ars.[5] ***aur.*** **COLOC.**[122] germ.[222] ip. lyc. m-p-a.[5] merc. mur-ac. nat-m. ***nux-v.*** plat. **STAPH.**[122]

Ailments from; anger, suppressed: agar.[198] ***aur.***[54] bamb-a.[1184] ***cand-a.***[239] carc.[207] cham. germ.[222] gink.[149] hep.[5] ***ign.*** ilx-a.[120] **IP.**[54] lachn.[36] **LYC.**[54] lyss.[214] mag-p.[209] ***nat-m.***[54] sep. **STAPH.**[54] 0stram.[185]

Ailments from; anger, vexation: **ACON.** agar. alum. alum-sil.[58] am-c. anac.[30] ***ant-c.***[5] ***ant-t. apis*** arg.[58] arn. ***ars.*** ars-s-f.[58] ***aur.*** aur-ar.[58] ***aur-m.*** aur-m-n.[85] bar-c.[5] ***bell. bry.*** cadm-s. calc. calc-ar. ***calc-p.*** calc-s. calc-sil.[58] camph.[85] ***cand-a.***[239] carc.[210] caust. **CHAM.** chin. cimic. cina[5] cist. **COCC.** ***coch.***[54] ***coff.*** colch.[102] **COLOC.** croc. cupr. ferr. ferr-p.[46] ***gels.*** graph.[58] grat.[102] hecla.[234] hyos. **IGN.** iod.[5] **IP.** kali-br.[85] ***kali-p. lach. lyc.*** m-p-a.[1] mag-c. mag-m. manc. merc.[5] mez. nat-ar.[58] nat-c. ***nat-m.*** nat-p. nat-s. ***nit-ac.***[163] nux-m. **NUX-V.** ol-an.[5] olnd.[5] **OP.** petr. ***ph-ac. phos.*** **PLAT.** ***puls.*** ran-b. rhus-t. sac-alb.[36] samb. scroph-n.[85] sec. sel. sep. sil. stann. **STAPH.**[122] stram. stront-c.[5] sulph. ***tarent.*** verat. vesp.[58] vinc.[85] zinc. zinc-p.[58]

Ailments from; anger; mental ailments: ***acon.***[54] am-m.[85] nux-v.[187] plat.[5] sep.[36]

Ailments from; anger; violence, with: **ACON.**[5] aur.[5] bell.[5] ***bry.***[5] **CHAM.**[5] ***coff.***[5] hyos.[5] lyc.[5] nat-m.[5] **NUX-V.**[5] phos.[5] sep.[5] sulph.[5] verat.[5] zinc.[5]

Ailments from; fright or fear, anger, with: acon.[1]

Ailments from; insults, offenses, from, dignified to fight, too, subdued wrath, went home sick, trembling, exhausted: ***staph.***[54]

Ailments from; love disappointed, jealousy, anger and incoherent talk, with: hyos. nat-m.[122]

Ailments from; love disappointed, rage, with: hyos.[56]

Ailments from; mortification, anger, during: **COLOC.**[122]

Ailments from; rage, fury: ***apis***[54] ***arn.***[54] seq-s.[230]

Anger; absent persons while thinking of them: ***aur.*** kali-c. kali-cy.[36] lyc.

Anger; activity, with great physical: ***plat.***[54]

Anger; alternating with, cares: ran-b.[10]

Anger; alternating with, cheerfulness: ant-t.[10] aur. cann-s.[10] caps. caust.[10] cocc.[10] croc. ign. nat-m.[10] op.[10] seneg.[10] spong.[10] stram. zinc.[10]

Anger; alternating with, indifference: carbn-s.[36] chin.[10]

Anger; alternating with, jesting: caps.[10] cocc.[10] ign.[10]

Anger; alternating with, kindness: cench.[122]

Anger; alternating with, laughing: croc.[10] ***plat.***[54] stram.[10]

Anger; alternating with, repentance, quick: anan.[36] croc. lyss.[54] mez. olnd.[10] ***sulph.***[1] vinc.[10]

Anger; alternating with, sadness: ambr.[10] coff.[10] sumb.[116] zinc.[10]

Anger; alternating with, singing: croc.[10]

Anger; alternating with, timidity: ran-b.[10] zinc.[10]

Anger; answer, when obliged to: ***arn.*** ars.[1] coloc. nat-m. **NUX-V.** ***ph-ac.*** puls.
Anger; approach of a person, on: cham.[109]
Anger; attention, at every little: ant-c.[102]
Anger; bad news: calc-p.[36]
Anger; beating friends: plat.[30]
Anger; business, about: ip.[36]
Anger; caressing, from: chin. ***cina***[179] nit-ac.[193]
Anger; children, in: abrot.[116] ***acon.***[54] anac.[137] ant-t.[137] arn.[8] bac.[62] bell.[10] carb-v.[8] carc.[207] **CHAM.**[54] dros.[70] hep.[54] ip.[116] kali-c.[8] ***lyc.***[8] med.[149] ***phos.***[54] sanic.[85] sil.[53] staph.[70] stram.[101] syph.[149] ***tub.***[70] tub-k.[149]
Anger; coition, after: ***calc.***[10] ***calc-ar.***[36]
Anger; consoled, when: ars. cham. ferr.[162] ***hell.***[54] ign.[137] ***nat-m.*** nux-v.[58] sabal. sep.[137] sil.[137]
Anger; contradiction, from: aesc.[58] aloe am-c. ***anac.*** ars. **AUR.** aur-ar.[58] ***bry.*** cact. calc-p. cocc. ***ferr.*** ***ferr-ar.*** gall-ac.[162] grat. helon. hura **IGN.** **LYC.** med.[212] merc. nat-ar. nat-c. nat-sil.[58] ***nicc.*** nit-ac.[30] ***nux-v.*** olnd. op. petr. pitu-a.[164] prot.[136] **SEP.** ***sil.*** stram. tarent. ***thuj.*** til. ***verat.***[30]
Anger; contradiction, least, from: ***aur.***[54] bry.[54] ferr.[54] nicc.[54] ***nux-v.***[54] petr.[54]
Anger; conversation, from: puls.[36] tarent-c.[36]
Anger; easily: aesc.[54] androc.[222] arg-n.[54] ars.[54] aur.[53] aur-ar.[58] bar-m.[58] bell.[54] calad.[54] calc.[54] calc-hp.[111] calc-s.[58] calc-sil.[58] ***caps.***[54] carbn-s.[144] **CHAM.**[54] chin-ar.[58] ***cocc.***[54] con.[54] ***crot-h.***[54] ***dulc.***[54] ***ferr.***[54] ferr-i.[58] ***gels.***[54] ***graph.***[54] ***hell.***[54] ign.[109] iris[54] kali-m.[192] lap-gr-m.[194] **LYC.**[54] meph.[54] nat-c.[36] **NUX-V.**[54] ***phos.***[54] ***plat.***[54] ***psor.***[54] ran-b.[54] sep.[109] squil.[54] staph.[109] teucr.[122] ***thuj.***[54] valer.[54] ***zinc.***[54]
Anger; easily, consolation agg., does not want to be disturbed: hell.[54]
Anger; easily, contradiction, from least: nicc.[54]
Anger; easily, rheumatism, in cardiac: phos.[54] squil.[54] ***thuj.***[54]
Anger; easily, trifles, at: ***acon.***[54] ***ars.***[54] ***chel.***[54] ***cocc.***[54] ***hep.***[54] mang.[54] ***mez.***[54] ***nat-m.***[54] nat-p.[54] ***nit-ac.***[54] ***plat.***[54]
Anger; eat, when obliged to: ars.[1]
Anger; happen, at what he thinks may: sol-m.[36]
Anger; himself, with: ars.[54] bell.[54] elaps[36] germ.[222] ign.[36] lyc.[1] nux-v.[30] staph.[30] ***sulph.***[54]
Anger; himself, with, spoken to, does not wish to be: elaps[54]
Anger; interruption, from: androc.[222] cench.[58] ***cham.*** cocc. germ.[222] graph.[1] ***hell.***[54] lac-h.[229] lap-mar-c.[194] ***nux-v.***
Anger; introversion, with: lap-gr-m.[194]
Anger; jealousy, with: ***lach.***[54]
Anger; kill, with impulse to: ***prot.***[136]
Anger; laughing, bursts of, with: ***croc.***[54]
Anger; looked at, when: ant-c.[127] ant-t.[47] ***cham.***[102] chin.[91] ***cina***[98] gels.[102] ***iod.***[8] ***nux-v.***[102] sanic.[102] ***sil.***[102]
Anger; mistakes, about his: ars.[54] bell.[54] bry. carc.[193] ***nit-ac.*** nux-v.[30] ***staph.*** ***sulph.***
Anger; noise, at: bamb-a.[1184] hep.[30] ip.[36]
Anger; odors agg.: colch.[137] lac-h.[229]
Anger; paralyzed, felt as: calc-p.[54] ***cist.***[54]
Anger; past events, about: calc. carb-an. sars.[54] sep. sulph.[54]
Anger; past events, about, arise from most indifferent thoughts and from every occurrence in life, unite with new vexations, cannot free herself from them: sulph.[54]
Anger; questioned, on being: coloc.[54]
Anger; recovery, if one spoke of her complete: ***ars.***[36]
Anger; refused, when things he wants are: bry.[56] cham.[56] cina[56] kreos.[56]
Anger; reproaches, from: cadm-s.[144] croc.[36] ***ign.***[10]
Anger; spoken to, when: ***cham.***[54] ***elaps***[54] ***hell.***[54]
Anger; stabbed any one, so that he could have: anac.[10] chin. **HEP.** merc. mosch.[10] nux-v. stront-c.[10] zinc.[10] zinc-acet.[10]
Anger; strangers, at: hep.[109]
Anger; sudden: bar-acet.[36] germ.[222] hep.[109] lyc.[109] merc.[58] phos.[70] prot.[136] puls.[70] tub.[70]
Anger; sudden, cowardice, with: bar-c.[54]
Anger; suffocative attack, with: ***cham.***[54]
Anger; talk, indisposed to: am-m.[10] ***ign.***[10] hydrog.[222] nat-m.[10] petr.[10] puls.[10] stann.[10] stront-c.[144] sul-ac.[10] verat.[144]
Anger; tear himself to pieces, could: sulph.[54]
Anger; temper tantrums: acon.[8] aur.[162] bell.[189] bor.[127] calc.[189] carc.[207] cere-s.[85] cham.[127] chel.[54] cina[148] cocc.[5] cupr.[116] hep.[189] hyos.[8] lach.[189] luna[228] lyss.54 nat-m.[162] ***nux-v.***[5] olnd.[5] phos.[70] prot.[136] puls.[70] sac-alb.[210] sil.[70] ***staph.***[85] stront-c.[137] sulph.[189] tarent.[189] tell.[54] thuj.[8] thyr.[5] tub.[5]
Anger; temper tantrums, falls on the floor kicking and screaming: nat-m.[162]
Anger; temper tantrums, opposed, when at the least: thuj.[8]

Anger; temper tantrums, reprimands, after: nat-m.[162]
Anger; temper tantrums, throw themselves on the floor during, cannot get their breath: thuj.[8]
Anger; thinking of his ailments, when: ***aur-m.***
Anger; touched, when: ***ant-c.*** cham.[162] cina[47] iod. lach.[10] sanic.[137] **TARENT.**
Anger; trembling, with: acon. alum.[122] ambr. arg-n. ***aur.*** cham.[5] chel. cop. daph. ferr-p.[58] gels.[193] lyc. m-aust.[10] merc. ***nit-ac.*** nux-v.[5] pall.[58] petr.[5] phos. ***plat.***[54] ran-b. sep. ***staph.*** yohim.[83] ***zinc.***
Anger; trembling, with, anger, with suppressed: aur.[54]
Anger; understood, when not: ***bufo*** lap-mar-c.[194] laur.[8]
Anger; vex others, inclined to: **CHIN.**[54] ***mez.***[10]
Anger; vexations, thinking about former: ***calc. carb-an.*** lyc.[1] sars.[54] sep. sulph.[54]
Anger; violent: **ACON.** aesc.[102] ambr.[10] **ANAC.** androc.[222] ***apis ars.*** **AUR.** aur-s.[58] bamb-a.[1184] bar-c. bell. bor.[10] ***bry.*** bufo cahin. ***calc.*** camph.[54] cann-s.[10] canth.[54] ***carb-v.*** carbn-s. carc.[207] ***caust.***[10] cere-s.[85] **CHAM.** ***chel.***[54] chin-b.[54] cimx.[85] cocc.[10] coff. ***croc.***[10] cupr.[54] cypr.[54] dros.[54] ferr. ferr-p. germ.[222] ***graph.*** grat. hecla.[234] **HEP.** hydrog.[222] ***hyos.***[122] ictod.[10] ign. iod.[122] ***kali-c.***[10] kali-chl.[10] kali-i. lach.[10] led.[10] ***lyc.*** lyss.[54] ***m-aust.***[10] mag-c.[85] mag-s.[10] med.[212] ***meli.***[54] mez.[10] mosch.[10] ***nat-m.*** nat-s.[10] **NIT-AC. NUX-V.** oena.[116] olnd.[10] ozone[227] pall. ***petr.*** ph-ac.[10] phos. pitu-a.[164] ***plat.***[10] prot.[136] puls.[54] seneg.[10] ***sep.***[122] sil.[10] ***stann.***[10] **STAPH.** stram.[10] stront-c.[10] sulph. **TARENT.** tell.[54] thyr.[5] tub.[5] tub-k.[70] verat. zinc. zinc-p.[58]
Anger; violent, personal, from slight offense: ***anac.***[54]
Anger; violent, takes everything in bad part: ***anac.***[54]
Anger; violent, takes everything in bad part, wishes he might get at some one on whom he might vent it: zinc.[54]
Anger; voices of people, to: con. teucr. zinc.
Anger; will, if things do not go after his: thuj.[1]
Anger; work: nat-m.[36]
Anger; work, aversion: bov.[10] m-aust.[10]
Anger; work, cannot: calc-p.[54]
Anger; worm complaints, in: ***carb-v.***[54] ***cina***[54]
Anguish; anger from: ***plat.***[54]
Answer; violently, as if angry: rhus-t.[60]
Anxiety; alternating with, rage: bell.[10]
Anxiety; anger during: caps.[1] sep. verat.[1]
Anxiety; anger, after: lyc.[10] verat.[10]
Bilious disposition: ars.[36] bol.[36] bufo[36] coca[36] hell.[36] sul-ac.[36]
Bilious disposition, grief, after: tarent.[36]
Contradiction; intolerant of, throw themselves angrily on the floor and cannot get their breath when in the least opposed: thuj.[8]
Cowardice; anger, with sudden fits of: bar-c.[54]
Crawling; floor on, anger, during: prot.[136]
Cursing; rage, after: ***arn.***[54]
Death; desires, alternating with rage: bell.[10]
Death; desires, rage, during intervals from: bell.[54]
Death; presentment of, alternating with, rage: stram.[54]
Delirium tremens; angry rather than anxious, subjects not greatly exhausted: ***graph.***[54]
Delirium; angry: ***cocc.***
Delirium; cheerful, gay, rage, changing to: ***bell.***[54]
Delirium; rabid: bell. canth. lyss. ***stram.***
Delirium; raging, raving: ***acon. act-sp. aeth.*** aether **AGAR.** agar-pa.[36] ail.[48] alco.[36] anac. ant-s. ***ant-t.*** apis[112] ***arg.***[54] arg-n. ars. ars-s-f.[58] atro.[54] **BELL.** bry. calc. ***camph.*** camph-br.[25] cann-i. cann-s.[5] **CANTH.** ***carbn-s.*** cham.[5] chel. chin. chin-s. cic. ***cimic.*** cina clem.[54] colch. coloc. cori-r.[36] ***cupr.*** cupr-acet.[36] dat-f.[36] dig. dulc. glon. graph. ***hell.*** hep. **HYOS.** hyper. jatr. juni-c.[36] ***kali-i.***[54] ***lach.***[5] lob. ***lol.***[5] **LYC.** ***merc.*** merc-cy. morph.[36] mosch. nat-m. **NIT-AC.** nux-m. nux-v.[36] ***oena.*** **OP.** par. phos. ***plb. puls.*** rheum **SEC.** ***sol-n.*** **STRAM.** sul-ac. sulph. ***tab.*** tarent. trach.[36] **VERAT.** verat-v.[54] vip. zinc. zinc-p.[58]
Delirium; raging, raving, alternating with, religious excitement: agar.[36]
Delusions; animals, fierce, with horns and bushy heads: ***bell.***[54]
- doomed, soul cannot be saved, cries and rages: ***ign.***[54].
- grief and anger, from: bell.[10] zinc.[54]
- hated by others, he is: lach.[137] sanic.[144]
- rags, body torn into: phyt.[137]

- toss someone out of the window, he tried to: bry.[36]

Despair; anger, during: tarent.[137]
Despair; rage, bordering on: ***agar.***[54]
Despair; rage, cursing and imprecations: **NIT-AC.**[30]
Discouraged; alternating with, anger: ran-b.[10] zinc.[10]
Discouraged; rage, with: colch.[10] nit-ac.[10]
Dreams; anger: all-c. alum. am-c. ambr.[1] androc.[222] ant-c. apis ***arn.*** asar. aster. aur. bell-p.[149] brom. ***bry.*** calc. calc-sil.[58] canth. carl. cast. caust. cham. convo-d.[36] crot-c.[36] crot-h. dros.[1] kali-n. lach. lipp.[36] ***mag-c.*** mag-m.[10] mag-s. mang.[1] merc-i-r. mosch.[10] myris. nat-ar. nat-m. nicc. **NUX-V.** paeon. peti.[36] ph-ac. ***phos.*** puls. rat. rheum[1] rumx. sabin. salx-am.[36] sars.[1] sel. sep. sil. spong.[1] stann. ***staph.*** sul-ac.[1] tarax. verat. zinc.

➤ anger, pupils, because he has square: ozone[227]
➤ anger, quarreled with his father, that he had, who would not recognize him as a son because he had embraced homeopathy: crot-h.[36]
➤ body, head, runs head against the wall: bamb-a.[1184]
➤ fiends, raging, strong: arg.[36]
➤ heads, picking up half roasted, which opened its eyes and spoke angrily, of: jac-c.[36]
➤ shooting, someone, who owes him money: ozone[227]

Envy; hate and: am-c.[30] am-m.[30] calc.[30] nat-c.[30] nat-m.[30] nit-ac.[30] puls.[30]
Excitement; anger, with inclination to, and to scold: ***petr.***[54]
Fear; alternating with, rage: bell.[10]

✦ death, alternate laughing and weeping, with (after anger): ***plat.***[54]
✦ death, anger, from: ***plat.***[54]
✦ rage, to fly into a: calc.[30] chin.[30] ***nux-v.***[30] staph.[30]

Foolish; behavior, hilarity, with riotous, and subsequent angry savageness, or tearful sorrow: op.[54]
Gestures; makes, angry, somnambulism: meph.[54]
Gestures; makes, fists, doubling as if in furious anger: ***calc.***[54]
Gestures; makes, furious: cann-i. ***hep.*** sep.
Grief; silent, anger, after: ***ign.***[54]
Hatred: acon. ***agar.*** aloe am-c. am-m.[5] **ANAC.** androc.[222] ***aur. calc.*** cand-a.[239] ***cham.***[137] **CIC.**[122] cupr. fl-ac.[5] germ.[222] hep.[5] hydr.[5] kali-c.[122] kali-i. ***lac-c. lach.*** lap-gr-m.[194] ***led.*** mang. merc.[5] mygal.[5] **NAT-M.**[122] ***nit-ac.***[122] **NUX-V.** op.[5] ph-ac.[30] phos. pitu-a.[164] puls.[30] rhus-t. stann. stram.[137] sulph. tarent.[36]
Hatred; bitter feelings for slight offenses, has: ang.
Hatred; children, of: anac.[162] ***lyc.***[162] ***nux-v.***[162] **PLAT.**[162]
Hatred; fellow beings, for: ***led.***[54]
Hatred; men, of: bar-c. ign. led. lyc. phos. stann.
Hatred; morbid ideas, from: sulph.[54]
Hatred; persons, of, absent, amel. on seeing: fl-ac.
Hatred; persons, of, agree with him, who do not: calc-s.
Hatred; persons, of, enjoying life, who are: medus.[168]
Hatred; persons, of, offended him, who had: agar.[60] am-c.[60] anac.[60] ***aur.*** calc.30 cic.[60] lach.[60] led.[60] mang. med.[212] ***merc.***[30] ***nat-m.*** nit-ac. nux-v.[30] ph-ac.[60] sep.[122] stann.[60] staph.[30] sulph.
Hatred; persons, of, offended him, who had, unmoved by apologies: **NIT-AC.**
Hatred; persons, of, owner of dog that bit her, with inclination to utter maledictions which shock her: lyss.[54]
Hatred; persons, of, repels everyone: aloe[54]
Hatred; revenge, and: ***agar.***[5] aloe[5] am-c.[30] am-m.[5] ***anac.***[5] ***aur.***[5] calc.[5] cic.[5] fl-ac.[5] hep.[5] hydr.[5] lach.[58] led.[5] mang.[5] med.[212] mygal.[5] **NAT-M.**[5] **NIT-AC.**[5] op.[5] ***ph-ac.***[30] phos.[5] stann.[5] **SULPH.**[5] vip.[1212]
Hatred; sex, to opposite: sep.[137]
Hatred; women, of: ***puls.*** raph.[36]
Howling; anger, during: arn.[111]
Howling; rage, from, in children: bell.[54]
Hurry; movements, fast enough, cannot do things, angry, making him: sul-ac.[85]
Hysteria; anger, from: ***rhus-t.***[54]
Hysteria; injuring herself, must exert great force to prevent from: ***hydr-ac.***[54]
Hysteria; rage, with: nat-m.[189]
Hysteria; sick, after being insulted and subduing his wrath: ***staph.***[54]
Idiocy; alternating with furor: ***aeth.***[8]
Imbecility; rage, stamps the feet: anac.[122] lyc.[122] nux-v.[122] op.[122] verat.[122]

Indifference; alternating with, anger: carbn-s.[36] foll.[1201] nid.[149]
Indolence; anger, after: ***nux-v.***[54]
Injure; herself, himself, feels could, rage, out of: agar. germ.[222] lyss.[36]
Insanity; anger, from: bell.[10] ***ign. lach.***[30] lyc.[10] op.[10] ***plat.***[122] staph.[30]
Insanity; malicious, malignant: agar.[10] cann-s.[10] ***cupr.*** lyc.[10]
Insanity; rage: ars-s-f.[58] germ.[222] oena.[25] ***tarent.***[54]
Irritability; absent persons, with: aur. fl-ac. kali-cy. lyc.
Irritability; anger, after suppressed: sep.[36]
Irritability; rage, violent, easily producing: bor.[127]
Jealousy; brutal, kind man becoming: calc.[30] lach.[30] nux-v.[30] sulph.[30]
Jealousy; rage, with: **HYOS.**[54]
Jealousy; revenge, desires to take: hyos.[30]
Jesting; alternating with, anger: caps.[10] ign.[10]
Lamenting; alternating with, anger: arn.[5]
Lasciviousness; rage, with: ***hyos.***[54]
Laughing; alternating with, rage, frenzy: acon.[10] stram.[10]
Laughing; anger, after: ***bor.***[8]
Laughing; rage, with: stram.
Loquacity; alternating with, rage: stram.[10]
Malicious; anger, during: anac.[10] bar-c.[10] calc.[54] canth.[10] ***caps.***[10] carb-an.[10] ***chin.***[10] hep.[10] ***lyc.***[10] ***nat-m.***[10] nicc.[10] petr.[30] zinc.[10]
Mania; rage, with: acon.[58] anac.[58] ant-t.[10] arg.[85] ***arn.***[5] ars.[58] ***bell.***[5] **BRY.**[5] camph.[54] cann-i.[116] ***canth.***[10] ***cic.***[5] con.[58] croc.[58] cupr.[58] cur.[8] ***dig.***[8] **HYOS.**[5] kali-c.[58] lach.[58] lyc.[5] merc.[58] ***nat-m.***[8] nux-v.[54] op.[5] phos.[58] plat.[58] plb.[10] puls.[58] sec.[58] sol-n.[10] **STRAM.**[5] tarent.[187] verat.[58]
Mildness; alternating with, anger: kali-c.[30]
Mildness; alternating with, rage: croc.[10]
Pull; desires to, presses her head and pulls her hair: tarent.[36]
Quiet disposition; alternating with, rage: hyos.[1]
Rage; alone, while: bufo.
Rage; alternating with, affectionate disposition: croc.
Rage; alternating with, consciousness: acon. stram.[1]
Rage; alternating with, desire for death: bell.[10]
Rage; alternating with, presentiment of death: stram.[54]
Rage; alternating with, repentance, quick: croc.[60] mez.[60]
Rage; alternating with, tenderness: croc.[10]
Rage; alternating with; religious excitement: agar.
Rage; amorous: **CANTH.**[54]
Rage; amorous, morning when rising: agn.[36]
Rage; beating others: hyos.[1]
Rage; biting, with: bell.[10] ***camph.***[54] canth.[116] croc.[10] cupr.[10] sec.[10] ***stram.***[10] ***verat.***[10]
Rage; chained, had to be: ars.[10] sec.[10]
Rage; consolation, from: ***nat-m.***[54] tarent.[144]
Rage; constant: ***agar. verat.***[54]
Rage; contradiction, from: aur.[127] grat.10 ***ign.***[85] ***lac-c.***[54] lyc.[10] nat-ar.[58] nux-v.[10] olnd.[54] ***thuj.***[36]
Rage; convulsions, fits, after: cocc.[144] op.[102]
Rage; convulsions, fits, after, epileptic: ***arg.*** op.[102]
Rage; convulsions, fits, during: alco.[36] ars.[36] bell.[1] camph.[36] cham.[127] cupr.[54] indg.[171] ***plb.***[8] stram.[36]
Rage; convulsions, fits, during, epileptic: bell. ***canth.***[54] cupr. hyos. nux-v. op. plb. stram.[54]
Rage; convulsive, spasmodic: ars. ***bell. canth.***[54] ***hyos.***[54] ***stram.***
Rage; cursing, with: alco.[36] anac.[116] lac-c.[56] mosch.[58] ***nit-ac.***[10] tub.[189] verat.[10]
Rage; dog that had bitten her, about: lyss.[54]
Rage; eat, when something to, was offered: ars.[54]
Rage; eating, during and after: chlor.[54]
Rage; fury: ***acon.*** acon-c.[36] acon-l.[36] ***aeth.*** **AGAR.** agn.[54] alco.[36] alumn. amyg-am.[54] ***anac.*** androc.[222] ant-t. ***apis***[5] arg.[58] arg-n. ***arn. ars.*** ars-s-f.[58] ***atro.***[54] aur.[54] bar-c. **BELL.** bry. bufo calc. ***camph.*** cann-i. cann-s. **CANTH.** carb-v.[1] ***carbn-s.*** carc.[207] cham. chel. chin. chin-s. cic. cimic. cina cocc.[10] ***colch.*** coloc. cori-r. croc. crot-h. ***cupr.*** cyn-d.[149] dig. dros. dulc. electr.[10] eupi.[36] **FERR.**[5] fl-ac. foll.[1201] glon. graph. ***hell.*** hep. **HYOS.** hyper. ign.[116] jatr. kali-c. ***kali-i.***[54] **LAC-C.** ***lach. led.***[54] lob. ***lol.***[116] **LYC.** m-p-a.[85] meli.[36] ***merc.*** **MOSCH.** ***nat-m. nit-ac.*** nux-m. ***nux-v.***[5] oena. **OP.** ozone[227] par. petr.[10] ph-ac.[116] ***phos.*** plb. psor.[56] ***puls.*** raja-s.[149] raph.[36] ruta sabad. ***sec.*** seneg. sep.[10] ***sol-n.*** staph.[85] **STRAM.** stry.[58] sul-ac. sulo-ac.[36] ***sulph. tab.*** tarent. ter.[144] thyr.[102] **VERAT.** vip. zinc.
Rage; insults, after: sang. stram.

Rage; kill people, tries to: hep. **HYOS.** sec. ***stram.***
Rage; know his relatives, does not: ***bell.***
Rage; laughing, with: ***stram.***[10]
Rage; love, after disappointed: ***hyos.***[54]
Rage; malicious: ***bell.***[10] cann-s.[10] choc.[222] cocc.[10] cupr.[10] lyc.[10] mosch.[10] petr.[10] sec.[10]
Rage; medicine, from forcible administration of: ***bell.***[36]
Rage; menacing: agar.[54]
Rage; mischievous: agar. bell.[10] cann-s.[10] cocc.[10] cupr.[10] lyc.[10] mosch.[10] petr.[10] sec.[10]
Rage; noise, from least: ***zinc.***[54]
Rage; pulls hair of bystanders: ***bell.***
Rage; repentance, followed by: croc.[116] lyss.[54]
Rage; shining objects, from: bell. canth. hyos. ***stram.***
Rage; strength increased: ***agar.*** **BELL.** hyos.[10]
Rage; striking, himself: tarent.[36]
Rage; striking, with: anac.[198] ***arg.***[8] ***bell.***[8] canth.[88] ***carb-v.***[8] cupr.[116] lap-mar-c.[194] lyc.[116] ***stram.***[8]
Rage; suicidal disposition, with: ant-t.[10] sec.[116] stram.[10]
Rage; tears clothing: ***camph.***[54]
Rage; touch, renewed by: ***bell.*** lach.[116] ***op.*** ***stram.***
Rage; uncontrollable, can scarcely be restrained: cere-s.[36] ***hyos.***[54] stram.[54]
Rage; water, at sight of: ***bell.*** ***canth.*** cupr. hyos. lach. merc.[10] ***stram.***
Rage; women, approaching, in a woman: raph.[36]
Remorse; fury, after attacks of, makes earnest apologies: lyss.[54]
Restlessness; anger, from: ***cham.***[116] **COLOC.**[54]
Restlessness; anxious, rage, ending in: ***canth.***[54]
Restlessness; rage, ending in a: canth.
Runs about; madman, like a, from anger: bufo[105]
Sadness; alternating with, anger: kali-fcy.[198] zinc.[10]
Sadness; anger, after: apis ars. bell. foll.[1201] hydrog.[222] nux-v. petr.[1] phos. plat. puls. sep.
Sadness; anger, from: aur.[10] calc-p.[54] ign.[10] lyc.[10] nit-ac.[10] ***puls.***[54] spig.[10]
Shrieking; anger, during: cast.[10] ***cham.***[5] ***iod.***[8] lap-c-b.[194] nux-v.[111] prot.[136] puls.[10] zinc.[111]
Shrieking; looked at, when: ***iod.***[8]
Singing; alternating with, anger and quarrelsomeness: croc.
Singing; alternating with, hatred of work: spong.
Spit, desire to; anger, from: ***calc.***[54]
Striking; anger, from: anan.[36] arg.[214] bufo[36] cina[100] kurch.[192] lap-mar-c.[194] ***nat-c.***[30] tub.[187]
Striking; anger, from, friends his: plat.[30] tarent.[58]
Striking; anger, from, himself: nat-c.[36]
Striking; bystanders, at, grows angry, and: ***lyc.***[54]
Striking; desire to strike: alum.[122] androc.[222] bell. bufo carbn-s. der.[36] elaps hydr. **HYOS.** lil-t. nat-c. **NUX-V.**[122] ***staph.***
Suicidal disposition; anger driving to suicide: carb-v.[10]
Talk; angry: zinc.[54]
Talk; angry, sleep, in: cast.[54]
Talk; indisposed, anger, during: croc.[36]
Talk; sleep, in, angry exclamations, with: cast.[54]
Temperament; choleric: acon.[54] ars.[54] aur.[54] **BRY.**[54] carb-v.[54] ***caust.***[54] **CHAM.**[54] coff.[54] coloc.[85] **FERR.**[54] ***hep.***[54] **HYOS.**[54] kali-p.[54] ***kalm.***[54] ***lach.***[54] ***lyc.***[54] nat-m.[54] ***nit-ac.***[54] **NUX-V.**[54] ***phos.***[54] ***plat.***[54] sec.[54] ***sil.***[54] sulph.[54]
Temperament; choleric, ardent, disposed to anger, spite or deception, always irritable and impatient: **NUX-V.**[54]
Temperament; choleric, bilious, dark hair and complexion, with firm fiber: ***bry.***[54]
Timidity; alternating with, anger: zinc.[10]
Tranquillity; alternating with, anger: aur-ar.[58] ***croc.***[54]
Unconsciousness; alternating with, rage: aloe[54]
Unconsciousness; rage, with: ***stram.***[54]
Violence; crossed, when: prot.[136] ***sil.***[54]
Violence; deeds of, rage leading to: agar.[116] anac. ars.[30] bar-c. ***bell.*** bry.[30] calc.[30] ***camph.***[171] canth.[10] carc.[207] chin. cic.[122] cocc. con. croc.[10] cupr.[10] ***hep.*** hyos. ***ign.*** ***iod.***[122] iodof.[116] kali-ar.[58] lach. lil-t.[116] lyc. mosch. nat-c. nicc.[10] nit-ac.[47] ***nux-v.*** phos.[30] plat. stram. stront-c.[10] tarent. tub.[70] ***verat.***[116] zinc
Weeping; alternating with, rage: acon.[10] cann-s.[10]
Weeping; anger, after: ambr.[10] arn. bell. caust.[10] ***cocc.***[10] ***coff.***[10] luna[228] m-aust.[10] ***mosch.***[54] nat-m.[162] ***nux-v.*** ***plat.*** puls.[10] sabin.[10] spong.[10] staph.[10]

Weeping; anger, with: ant-t.[111] ars.[111] cand-a.[239] ***cham.***[5] lac-c.[5] lil-t.[5] pitu-a.[164] sulph.[111] zinc.[111]
Weeping; anger, with, violent quarreling, even to extreme malice and rage: ***mosch.***[54]
Weeping; children, rage, as from: bell.[54] nat-m.[127]
Weeping; rage, after: ***arn.***[54]
Weeping; rage, maniacal: ***plb.***[54]
Work; aversion to mental, anger after: **NUX-V.**[54]
Work; impossible, anger, after: calc-p.[54]

ADAM. Sh, 130 - I was angry at my house guest and wanted to be left alone, at breakfast.[11], 30C, 12.XX.XX
Sh, 195 - Bad paranoia, that people hate me, anyone just walking down the street hates me. I think they will hit me. 20, 1M, 07:XX:XX
196 - Very nervous and little self-confidence. I think people are laughing at me and hate me. 20, 1M, 07:XX:XX
Sh, 208 - I wanted to sack the receptionist 15 times in the last hour for stupidity. 7, 6C, 03:00:XX
Sh, 213 - Furious cold anger when money stolen from me. 2, 12C, 73:XX:XX
Sh, 214 - I am fidgety and angry and very jealous of people. I feel cold and empty and very angry, almost cruel. 20, 1M, 02:XX:XX
Sh, 215 - I feel very angry and extremely intolerant, cold and hard and I hate myself for feeling these harsh unkind feelings. 20, 1M, 02:XX:XX
Sh, 218 - Red anger with irregularly pounding heart. 2, 12C 73:XX:XX
Sh, 219 - I recognized a familiar uncomfortable feeling as being one of anger. 1, 12C, 00:00:45
Sh, 221 - I felt angry on waking, noise of people upstairs sounds like elephants. I want to kill them. I wanted to complain to them. 7, 6C, 03:06:00
Sh, 223 - Anger with aggressive attitude, short tempered and intolerant. I lashed out verbally when my partner invaded my space. I knew it was out of proportion at the time. 7, 6C, 30:00:XX
Sh, 226 - Angry at my daughter for ignoring that I want my time to do my things. 10, 6C, 17:XX:XX
Sh, 227 - Get very easily angry. Needed to assert myself and pick on someone who I neither know nor respect. My anger was very violent. 20, 1M, 10:XX:XX
Sh, 228 - Resentful towards others. 20, 1M, 10:XX:XX
Sh, 229 - Feeling very angry towards others and hate people. I want to be alone and away from people who upset me. I hate feeling angry and resentful, a lot of it is directed to myself. 20, 1M, XX:XX:XX
Sh, 237 - Quite a lot of anger —a strange kind of energy. I feel like things are changing all around me, like life is speeding along. 20, 1M, 09:XX:XX
Sh, 238 - Quickly felt remorse after anger. 8, 6C, 04:XX:XX
Sh, 240 - Anger from lack of physical or emotional support. 2, 12C, 73:XX:XX
Sh, 241 - I feel angry and want to be comforted. 7, 6C, 03:07:30
Sh, 242 - Feeling very pathetic and scared of people getting angry with me. 20, 1M, 10:XX:XX
Sh, 243 - Anger at people putting lights on instead of opening curtains. 16, 12C, 18:XX:XX
Sh, 244 - Anger with my attraction to P. He's a walker and I wanted to walk with him. I didn't want to be attracted but was, as if enchanted. 16, 12C, 18:XX:XX

AGAR. Al, 2 - He becomes so furious that he can hardly be restrained from ripping up his bowels, as he fancies the mushroom had ordered him to do.
Al, 8-...called for his hatchet; had to be confined alternated with religious excitement.
Al, 56-...grew angry at the servant and felt inclined to fight.

ALOE. Al, 40-...wrap up in himself (introspection), as after a sickness or a fit of anger, which still gnaws (bite) internally, which one cannot express.
Al, 25 - Ill-humor; peevish (angry) about himself, so that he insults and blasphemes; worse afternoons.
He, 11 - Dissatisfied and angry about himself, more so when he is constipated or suffers from pain.
He, 12 - An easily excited, angry, revengeful state of mind, could not brook opposition (contradiction), wanted to destroy object of wrath, relief from tea or milk stimulants;...

ANAN. Al, 7 - Quarrelsome and contrary humor, but after being angry he often regrets (remorse) what he has done.
Al, 6 - Disposition to anger, with desire to strike and destroy.
ANDROC. Sh, 96 - Increased irritability, a "how dare you!" feeling. Felt like tearing offenders to pieces with his bare hands. He felt an enormous surge of violent emotions at trifles, and had to exercise great control to stop outbursts of violence and impulses to hurt someone. Felt that "everyone were creeps", could not be bothered with anyone. (2)
Sh, 97 - Very strong liking and disliking to people —very intense —ranging from immense sexual attraction to extreme hatred. Spoke with hatred and maliciousness about colleagues. (4)
Sh, 99 - Felt angry, did not want to speak to anyone, in the evening with friends he felt very lively, self-confident and forceful, rather biting at times. (4)
Sh, 102 - Assertive, impatient, aggressive. Felt resentful and abused. Had no control over her temper. Bellowed and lashed out at everyone. In the evening, furious for no apparent reason. Wanted to kill her husband and children, banged doors and threw things. By bed-time, she felt fine but the intensity of her evil thoughts was very frightening. (7)
Sh, 104 - By evening, needing to avoid people, anger coming out, no restraint —I look for reasons but there aren't any. (7)
Sh, 108 - Incredibly sensitive to noise, can't bear it, hundreds of thoughts pop in and out of my brain, thoughts of 'why are we here?', deep philosophical issues. Every-day things disappear from my mind. Am free from pressing, nagging responsibilities —just a black thunder sits within me, and I feel afraid of what I might do next. my eyes are staring and full of hate —just looking at the children sends them frantic. I have no control over my emotions. Then after 8:00 p.m., deadness resumes and I feel .k., but the end of myself as I usually am. (7)
Sh, 111 - Short tempered in afternoon, easily excited to anger, worse from being interrupted. (12)
Sh, 112 - Became excited to anger and confrontation. She was not aware of hurting others' feelings and did not seem to care. Could not appreciate anyone else's feeling. Later she reflected on her actions and felt ashamed. (12)
Sh, 115 - When reflecting on her anger and arguments, was filled with remorse, although at the time she believed she was being perfectly reasonable. (12)
Sh, 117 - Angry with her children and family. (7, 12, 17, 28)
Sh, 126 - Great hostility to those around him, which manifested in brooding and stinging observations and comments directed at his friends. (29)
APIS. He, 81 - Ailments from fright, rage, vexation, jealousy, or hearing bad news.
ARN. Ha, 625 - Over-excitability; she could easily laugh when there was no occasion for it, and when one said something annoying to her, she got angry ...
ARS. Al, 91-...she was afraid (fear) of solitude and death; the slightest cause was sufficient to put her into anger and rage, which especially occurred when one spoke of her complete recovery which she considered wholly impossible.
Al, 94 - Very fretful, indignant, capricious; every word offends her, and makes her very angry, when she should answer.
Ha, 1031 - He became furious, must be bound, and seeks to run away.
Ha, 58 - Very peevish and sensitive; the least thing insults him and angers him.
He, 95 - Dissatisfied and angry with himself all day; thinks he has not accomplished enough, and reproaches himself bitterly.
He, 103 - She became furious when something to eat was offered her while complaining of loss of appetite.
He, 101 - The least thing offends him, and moves him to anger.
He, 59 - Very peevish and passionate, capricious, she takes every word ill and is cross when she has to answer.
ATRO. Al, 33 - Mentally either very sad, depressed in constant anxiety and restlessness, fearful of misfortune, or angry and inclined to be alone, seldom lively.
Al, 42 - Morose, quarrelsome the whole day, everything went wrong; trifles usually passed unheeded irritated him to anger.
AUR. Ha, 340 - He sits apart (separated), all by himself in a corner, wrapt up in him-

self, as if in the deepest melancholy, when left undisturbed; but the slightest contradiction excites the greatest heat and anger,...

Ha, 338 - Irascibility; he is very excitable, and the slightest contradiction excites the utmost anger.

He, 80 - Ailments from fright, anger, contradiction, mortification, or vexation with dread, fear, reserved displeasure, or vehemence.

He, 69 - Becomes angry at absent persons while thinking of them.

He, 72 - Contradiction excites wrath; distrust.

BAR-C. He, 36 - Sudden ebullitions of anger, but coupled with cowardice.

BELL. Ha, 1325 - In the momentary intervals, when free from fury, complaints of intolerable anxiety, so that she wished to die.

Ha, 1401 - Peevishness, nothing was right for him; he was angry with himself.

Ha, 1419 - Fury; he injures himself and others and strikes about him. (beat, hit)

Ha, 1422 - Along with burning heat of the body, with open, staring, and fixed eyes, such fury she must constantly be held fast in order to prevent her attacking others,...

He, 115 - Intolerable anguish during time she is free from rage, with desire to die.

BRY. He, 42 - Contradiction easily provoked anger during whole proving.

He, 47 - Bad effects from mortification, violence and anger.

BUFO. Al, 26 - Anger with desire to strike and destroy.

CALC-A. Al, 253 - Dreams vivid, full of strife (quarrel, fight) and anger.

CALC-P. Al, 13 - Grows very violent, if his opinion is differed from, or if contradicted, so that he is vexed not to have been able to control himself.

Al, 16 - Unpleasant news makes him beside himself; sweat breaks out; inclined to indignation and anger.

CALC. Ha, 55 - Thoughts of former vexations irritate him to anger.

CAMPH. Ha, 341 - All external things are repugnant to him, and excite in him a repellent (repulsive) crossness.

CAPS. Al, 1 - He makes reproaches and becomes angry at the faults of others; he becomes offended at trifles and finds fault.

Al, 18 - He is in a contented mood, is jocose, and sings, and still he becomes angry from the slightest causes.

He, 14 - Peevish, irritable angry; easily offended, takes everything in bad part.

He, 7 - He is in a content mood, is jocose, and sings, and still he becomes angry from the slightest cause.

CARB-AN. Al, 28 - Sullen (unsociable, silent) mood and ill-humor about present and past events; this cannot be overcome ; it even amounts to weeping.

CAUST. Ha, 30 - Peevish (angry) all day, at odds (quarrel) with himself, dissatisfied, anxious and yet not indisposed to mental work.

CHAM. Al, 53 - Disposed to anger scorn quarrelsomeness. (after two hours)

He, 68 - All bad effects following anger. (ailments, from) 0Convultions, 0chill, 0fever, 0bilious complaints

CHEL. Al, 55 - Mood very irritable, daily outbreaks of anger without cause (causeless); feels as though she could beat the children, and trembles from rage because she has no reason for doing it.

He, 25 - Is vexed (anger, irritated) about every trifle and has violent attacks of passionate outbursts of temper.

CHIN. Al, 35 - Ill-humor, amounting to the most violent wrath (fury), so that he could have stabbed any one.

Al, 39 - Fretful and irresolute; she is unable to accomplish her aim, and consequently is indignant. (angry)

CHOC. Sh, 7 - In the evening, felt angry with bristling down my back. Irritable with the kids, shouted a lot, slammed doors. Feeling very uncomfortable with my daughter near me. I made a huge issue over something small which I would normally leave. I wanted to leave and walk out of the door on them. Felt very unsympathetic to the children. "You either go, or go to bed". Couldn't cuddle the children and took longer to say "Its all right". I thought that their father should look after them instead of me (very unusual). The feeling I can't be where I want to be because of them. I want to be roaming outside without my possessions. Left kids alone in the house for the first time. I was surprised at how easily I let

them go. My daughter liked it very much.
Sh, 14 - Angry about being in city. When I look, I want to see far distances and sky, not houses. Went to estate agents to look at country houses.
Sh, 302 - Tonight my husband committed a large annoyance. I felt rage rise up in me —he jumped back and cowered! I wanted to beat some sensibility into him, stopping short of actually wanting to kill him, I felt: 'its not fair', 'how inconsiderate and thoughtless to an extreme degree'. However, my will intervened before I made a scene. Its as if I'm more aware of my 'shadow side' and really feeling it, but precisely because I'm more aware of it, I can step in with my will and curb my behaviour if it looks as if I'm likely to hurt someone else.[15], 30C, 03:XX:XX
Sh, 324 - Still snapping and resentful generally.[15], 30C, 36:XX:XX
Sh, 328 - Humourless, intolerant -almost cruel. Scalded a child's hand out of anger, and nothing would make him apologise.[35], 30C, XX:XX:XX:
Sh, 329 - Felt anger at life, I wasn't getting anywhere. The world appeared a cruel place to me, and I felt I had no place in the scheme of things.[35], 30C, XX:XX:XX:
Sh, 331 - I became selfish, impatient and intolerant. Behaved in a strange way -hard and quarrelsome -snapping at people. Could not stand people wasting time or being inefficient, I wanted things done immediately.[35], 30C, XX:XX:XX:
CIMIC. He, 27 - Irritable; the least thing that goes wrong makes her angry.
COCC. Ha, 550 - Everything angers and vexes him; after a few hours he becomes lively and disposed to make jokes.
He, 39 - Angry and indignant form of delirium.
He, 42 - Ill effects of anger and grief. (ailments from)
COFF. He, 33 - Ailments from excessive joy, excessive laughing and playing; from disappointed love; from anger, from vexations with vehemence or fright...
COLOC. He, 10 - Extremely irritable and impatient; nothing seems right; gets angry on being questioned.
He, 12 - Anger with indignation and extreme irritability; throws things out of his hands.
He, 14 - Affections from anger, with indignation, particularly vomiting and diarrhoea ...(ailments from)
CON. Ha, 20 - Peevish mood, he does not know what to do with himself, the time passes too slow for him.
CROC. Al, 24 - A slight cause which would usually have made her laugh, now causes a most violent ill-humor, almost rage, so that she frequently loses her consciousness; afterwards she is astonished at this out break.
Al, 28 - Vacillating (hesitate), peevish mood; the slightest cause excites his anger, for which, next moment, he is sorry (remorse), which however, soon returns, because his calmness frets (disturbs) him and prevents (stop) his exposing his feelings (oppressed); usually he changes a hard word which he has on his tongue to a mild one, but the latter seems too mild, and now chooses a more severe word, ...(sorry, guilty, by anger, mildness, x harsh, rude)
Al, 29 - He takes everything in anger and suddenly repents (apologize) of having injured (offend) others.
Al, 30-...the behavior of relatives and friends excites her to anger,...she is vexed with herself, and her anger becomes greater than ever;..
He, 13 - He takes everything in anger and suddenly repents (sorry) of having injured (offensive) others.
CYCL. Ha, 193 - Peevish, morose disposition; he easily takes every trifle in bad part, and gets angry over it.
ELAPS. Al, 17 - Peevish in the afternoon, did not want to be spoken to, even fretful (irritable) about herself.
He, 6 - Angry about one's self, does not wish to be spoken to.
FERR. Al, 20 - Excited by the slightest opposition; ... even her children's caresses increased her bad temper; she was often rude to those about her, because she hated to see or talk to them, and wanted them to leave her in solitude, which alone was pleasing to her.
He, 14 - Pettish(irritable), quarrelsome, disputative (litigious), easily excited, least contradiction angers.
He, 18 - Ailments from anger.

FL-AC. Al, 15 - During the fourth week very irritable towards people, even to the greatest hatred, which he does not hesitate to give vent to in words, but as soon as he sees them everything is forgotten, and he has an entirely different opinion of them.

Al, 16 - Whilst (while) considering what might happen he gets into a most ungovernable anger, but only in his thoughts;..(lost relation; anger x action)

GERM. Sh, 10 - Reacted very strongly to a very close friend. Something quite small sparked it off and I hung up the phone. Just felt I'd had enough. It's an issuefeeling that's been built up for months, but tonight I flipped inside. Only our third argument in years. I still feel indignant and angry 1 hour later, even after going and working in the garden. Won't answer her calls. 13, 30c, 06:08:30

Sh, 3 - Reacted angrily to husband's demands. 14, 30C, 26:00:00.

Sh, 4 - Desperately angry. So intense that I could barely control it. I made noises like an animal, pushed my arms up and down -instead of hitting my children, which helped. Want to just leave the house and the kids. Felt completely mad, afraid of what the neighbors heard and thought. Very bad conscience afterwards, but no relief - didn't get the anger out. There are a lot of feelings inside that don't come out. 18, 30C, 02:09:00

Sh, 6 - Difficult to accept my own feelings, accusing myself for letting them out, especially anger. Felt a rage, had to use all my power to control it. Lost my patience because of something my son did. I got angry with him, but at the same time despised myself for not having patience with him. I did not want to report this, because I feel unveiled - now everybody can see what awful person I am. I go completely mad of all my thoughts; can't bear it anymore. Inside me everything is chaos. Feel no power. 18, 30C, 18:XX:XX

Sh, 5 - Everything was heavy and felt impossible without meaning. Terrible anger. Bad conscience and crying afterwards. Could not do what I had planned to do, because I felt so terrible and everything was chaos. Was crying, but couldn't get it out - no release in it. 18, 30C, 176:XX:XX

Sh, 112 - Don't see why I am here. I can't bear it. I go mad. I hate myself. I want to beat myself and I do it. Tear my hair. Stop when it hurts too much. It is like hell !!! 18, 30C, 20:XX:XX

Sh, 99 - Came in contact with very much hate and disgust within, and it made a deep impression on me. I have to be reconciled with those parts of me. I think that power can be used in a different way -not so destructive. I am no person. Feel I have no power when I meet people. Sometimes I feel I disappear. I am not in my body. My hands feel gone. My feet are cold; I don't like them. Yet I feel I have great power inside, especially I feel it when I get angry or when I sing. 18, 30C, 46:XX:XX

Sh, 101 - I'm desperate. I want to die. Feel the power to kill. Feel like a wild animal locked in. It's strong, so intense. I hate so strong-feel a terrible disgust and I'm afraid of what I'm able to do. It's completely impossible to be in it and impossible to get out of it. 18, 30C, 190:XX:XX

Sh, 139 - Feel angry hostile and tearful easily. Someone says that I have behaved as if I am from another planet. 08, 12C, 30:00:00

Sh, 151-.... I feel I have no real contact with people, I have no emotion at all except for a feeling of isolation and a concern that people may not like me. I wish someone would cuddle me. By 10 o'clock I have a definite aversion to people, especially certain people- the stubborn or authoritarian kind. I become deeply involved in my own thoughts and can be very irritable and even angry when the thoughts are interrupted by people, but I don't show any signs of anger or irritation. The fate of other people leaves me cold, but I know this is not right. My mind is blank and I feel I could just sit and stare. I have no feelings, no emotions! I think a lot about my state of mind and try to understand it; it puzzles me. What is missing? Eating removes this thoughtful mood. By afternoon and evening I become gradually more involved with what I am doing but still feel isolated even when in the company of other people. I don't mind listening to people, but I contribute little to conversation. This state lasted for three days. 16, 30C, 04:XX:XX

GRAN. Al, 10 - Inclined to get angry at offenses.

GRAPH. He, 22 - Extremely fretful; everything angers and offends him.

GRAT. Al, 8 - Fretful, irritated by every contradiction, angry outbreaks, misanthropic, whith solicitude about his own health.

HALI-L. Sh, 189 - Mad at a friend. Was at his house organizing stuff for him. I had the system organized and then he brought a whole other set of things and dumped them in. I was so furious, I left and got a headache from being angry. 08, 30C, 41:XX:XX

Sh, 205 - Aggravated driving to work. Why don't these people get out of my way? Frustrated with the world, angry with the world. I don't want any red lights. Want everything to be smooth. I used to feel this way years ago when I used to drink. 02, 30C, 10:XX:XX

Sh, 349 - I said I was moody. It wasn't as qualitative as she wanted, and she was asking for more details and I yelled, " A stupid five year old would understand what I was saying." I became sarcastic and very belligerent. I thought I was being simplistic and clear. I gave what I had to give. I was in a depressed state, lost my good feeling and was angry at being asked to explain the depression. She asked me what do you mean and I said, "XXXX off. If you don't understand that, too bad. Do you understand that?! Do you know the English language?" 18, 30C, 04:14:00

Sh, 430 - Get a call from a friend that the utility district is at it again. Don't know what, but expect the worst in negotiations with them. Can't win. So tired of fighting the losing battle. Can't raise the energy to do anything. Rage inside. Hopeless. Daydreams of blowing up the utility district, of shooting them. Only option left to desperate people and I feel desperate. we're a rag-tag group without luck, or leadership, fighting a losing battle. Feels like we're the American Indians. "Here's 24 dollars worth of beads for your island, idiot." In the pit of despair. 09, 6C, 25:XX:XX

Sh, 527 - I was paying attention to the obituaries at this time. Noticed people dying in the newspaper. I would get very angry and frustrated. For a short time, was looking at death notices on a daily basis, during the last week or so of the proving. My anger towards death. How unfair. I don't want it. I shouldn't have to have it. There should never be a day where the morning is taken from me. 18, 30C, 35:XX:XX

Sh, 533 - Boxed in feeling with no way to express anger. Start taking it out on the kids, as if they are trying to break me, to get me. Better getting out, going away from home and family. 09, 6C, 20:XX:XX

Sh, 536 - I have been really pissed off again since the proving ended. Every two months, I get this thing on the 13th to the 16th. Something lightly ruffling happens. It's an unusual amount of anger. An Everest of emotions. 02, 30C, XX:XX:XX

Sh, 565 - Really angry at the swimming club commissioner for planning our morning swim against the tide and not telling me. So angry, I couldn't even look at his face. It was such a hard swim, I knew I couldn't make it and had to be pulled in by a boat. Really furious. 08, 30C, 18:XX:XX

Sh, 569 - About 5:00 p.m. felt an irascibility again about people not paying me, but now it feels like an easily moving type of rage, not suppressed. 13, 30C, 01:11:XX

Sh, 575 - Very angry with the children, who have done no chores. Irritated and yelled at them. I get so angry my nervous system refuses to calm down. I take their behavior personally, plus I'm angry at myself for my own response to them. 09, 6C, 05:04:XX

Sh, 629 - Broke things off with a friend. Felt sad then angry. Felt he degraded me. It was unhealthy to have that energy around me anymore. Very angry. No respect from him. 08, 30C, 36:XX:XX

HELL. Al, 17 - Extremely inclined to be irritable, the most trifling things which goes contrary to his wishes excites anger.

HEP. He, 22 - Temper obstinate and cross, a ferocious spleen (irascible) which would lead to cold blooded murder even among those habitually gay and benevolent.

He, 23 - Wrathful irritability, even to the most extreme violence, threatening to end in murder and arson.(firing pyromania)

HIPP. Al, 6 - Fretful, discontented with himself almost lachrymose, in the morning.

HURA. Al, 28 - Impatience, anger; she bites her hands, and gets into passion because her ideas come too slowly.

HYDR. Al, 16 - Spiteful (cruel), angry disposition, with desire to snub (scorn) any one who differed in anything with me; lasting all day.

Al, 26-...forget, for a few seconds, what was wanted, which makes me very angry and feel like damning (swearing) and cursing (blaspheme) everything and anybody who bothered me the least.

HYDROG. Sh, 107 - Charged around like a bull in a china shop. 22, 12C, 04:XX:XX

Sh, 174 - Emotionally cold and non-communicable with anger felt in stomach. 12, 6C, 17:XX:XX

Sh, 188 - On getting up in the morning, I feel very angry and bad about myself. I feel I can't cope. Whats the use of trying? I feel like giving up. I think for a moment I'd like to die. 10, 200C, 09:XX:XX

Sh, 198 - Growing irritability. Anger below the surface if something is on the floor in my way or if something goes wrong. 12, 6C, 05:00:30

Sh, 202 - The instant I woke I felt angry, felt like throwing the clock at the wall. Didn't feel like talking to anyone and felt a desire to kick the furniture —seemed the only way to let my anger out. 10, 200C, 16:XX:XX

Sh, 253 - I was defensive and angry. I thought my friend didn't understand me. I had to apologise. I felt vulnerable and deeply hurt by her. 16, 30C, 05:XX:XX

HYOS. Ha, 562 - Extreme fury: he rushes at people with knives.

Ha, 545 - Ridiculously solemn acts in improper clothing, mixed with fury. (In a priest's cassock, put on over nothing but a shirt, and in fur boots, he wishes to go to church, in order to preach and perform clerical offices there, and furiously attacks those who try to prevent him.)

Ha, 550 - He displays uncontrollable strength in his fury.

Ha, 559 - Fury; he tries to inflict injury on and hurt others.

He, 62 - Jealousy: with rage and delirium; with attempt (try) to murder.

He, 74 - Disappointed love followed by: epilepsy, melancholy, rage, or inclination to laugh at everything; despair and propensity to drown himself. (ailments from)

IGN. Al, 27 - Slight blame or contradiction excites him to anger, and this makes him angry with himself.

Ha, 765 - From the slight contradiction he is irritated and angry.

He, 30 - Became bilious, nervous, depressed, and would scarce move from the fire, for days together. Morbid grief

He, 53 - Slight blame (censure) or contradiction excites him to anger, and this makes him angry with himself.

He, 55 - Anger, followed by quiet grief or sorrow.

IOD. Al, 28 - Peevish, fretful; nothing is done right.

Al, 27 - Is cross and irascible; feels stupid.(obtuse)

IP. Ha, 227 - He lets (permit) his courage sink (fail), and is greatly given to be vexed and to get angry.

Ha, 229 - He very often gets angry about the merest trifle, and can just as easily and quickly become calm.

IRID. Sh, 300 - I feel snappy, as though I could bite someone's head off. Feel really ratty. I2 At 5.00 a.m., I felt very resentful at having to get up. This mood lasted for at least two hours. At 9.15 a.m., went back to bed, slept for two hours, had frustrating, agitated dreams about the car. Things kept going wrong. Seem to be attracting aggravation. L8

Sh, 320 - Full of anger, like fire burning away inside me. Less tolerant with people. Normally I would say it's okay, but I haven't, and I feel very strong like I could chop any one down who got in the way. Feel very emotional. I would burst into tears if someone said the wrong thing. Similar to the feeling I used to have at school when I was being bullied, a defiant, "I'll show you one day!" type of feeling. I5

Sh, 322 - Had row with partner over work, money, and time off. I was storming about.

I said, "You can't say that to me." I went storming after partner went into another room. I was overwhelmed with fury. I cried with fury. D13

KALI-BR. Al, 4 - He imagined that he had been specially singled out (select) for divine vengeance... deploring his sad fate (destiny),...he informed me that he had been accused of robbing a friend, and that the officers were in search of him....

He, 10 - Imagines he is singled out as an object of divine wrath (fury, rage); extreme drowsiness.

KALI-C. Al, 45 - Disagreeable mood; she longs for things with impetuosity; is contented with nothing, is beside herself, and gets into rage if everything does not go according to her wishes, and frequently does not herself know what she really wishes to have.

Ha, 33 - Contrary mood; she demands (order, command) impetuously; is not satisfied with anything (dissatisfied) ; she is beside herself, and furiously angry; if everything does not go according to her wishes, and often does not herself know what she really wants.

Ha, 49 - Changeful mood, now good and quiet, then passionate and angry about trifles; often hopeful, often despondent.

Ha, 41 - Very peevish, she has no pleasure in anything.

Ha, 44 - Cross and angry thoughts, in the morning, on awaking, so that he gnashes with his teeth.

Ha, 30 - Peevish mood, as if she could not do anything to suit (satisfy) herself.

KALI-CY. Al, 3 - Had occasion to get angry, but could not; felt more like laughing instead.

KALI-I. Al, 16 - Very peevish and excited; everything goes wrong, and she is ready to quarrel with every one.

LACHN. Al, 5 - Became much excited over a trifle; he had suppressed his anger, in the evening.

LED. Ha, 335 - Passionate: he easily gives way to angry expressions.

He, 4 - Discontented; morose; hates his fellow beings.

LYC. Al, 89 - She cannot endure the slightest opposition, and is speedily beside herself from peevishness (cross).

Al, 92 - Easily roused to anger and scorn.

Al, 96 - Quarrelsome rage, partly at herself partly at others.

Al, 94 - Indolent, obstinate (inflexible), rebellious (revolutionary, dissident), passionate, wrathful. (angry)

Al, 2 - Delirious, raging, envious, reproachful, presumptuous, and imperious.

Ha, 59 - Insanity and fury, breaking out in envy, pretensions (inflated) and ordering (dictatorial) others about.

Ha, 60 - As if insane she seeks for quarrels, makes ungrounded reproaches abuses (insulting) most violently and beats the person whom she abuses.

Ha, 56 - Angry fury, partly against himself, and partly against others.

He, 39 - Ailments from fright, anger, mortification, or vexation, with reserved displeasure.

He, 31 - Sensitive, irritable disposition; peevish and cross on getting awake; easily excited to anger; cannot endure slightest opposition, and is speedily beside herself.

LYSS. Al,N-89 - After attacks of fury, evinces (manifest) great regret at his behavior, making earnest (ardent) apologies, warning those about him not to allow him to bite them.

MAG-M. Ha, 18 - He hated to talk; he desired to follow his thought in solitude.

MERC. Ha, 1242 - All day long great seriousness with much indifference; he got angry when others laughed at a trifle, and at the same time was extremely indifferent to all about him.

MEZ. Al, 32 - Is inclined to get angry with others about trifling and perfectly harmless things; everything vexes him, and he wants to say all kinds of annoying and vexatious things.

Al, 33 - Violent outbreak of anger about trifles, which he soon regrets.(remorse)

He, 11 - Inclined to get angry with others about trifles; everything vexes him, he wants to say annoying and vexatious things; is soon sorry for it.

NAT-C. Al, 42 - Very fretful and discontented with whole world; he constantly felt as though he could beat (punish ?) himself, his whole life angered him, and he preferred to have no existence at all; he was solicitous about the future, and inclined to despair, all day.

Al, 48 - He is angry, and inclined to fight and strike, and cannot tolerate contradiction,...

NAT-M. Al, 103 - Hatred of people who had insulted him.

Ha, 68 - Hatred (rancor, resentment) against persons, who had formerly offended him.

He, 11-, ...uttered the most atrocious blasphemes, swore (blaspheme, curse) against God (divine) and the elements (environment), and after raging for awhile became exhausted,...

He, 13 - Taciturnity; offended at every word (easily); avoids company; hates persons because they have offended him; spleen.

He, 48 - Consequences (ailments) of fright, anger, vexation, mortification, or reserved displeasure.

He, 42 - Quarrelsome fretfulness, gets into passion about trifles; passionate vehemence.

He, 43 - Hateful and vindictive nature.

NEON. Sh, 175 - I've been in a rotten mood all day, dwelling on past offenses. I just can't let go, it's making me angry. I feel like I hate that bastard; it's not an emotion I've had before. Now I feel vindictive, really awful; I feel that if I ever found out that he had been lying to me again I would say to him, "I'll kill you," "I'll slit your throat." These violent feelings were much eased when alone. 02, 6C, 04:22:40

Sh, 176 - Got up late in a horrible mood and reproached my partner again. I hurt him but I didn't care. I felt indifferent, malicious and vindictive, full of hate. 02, 6C, 05:22:10

Sh, 182 - Had an explosion for not being the perfect person. I was really pissed off at the situation. I felt out of control, helpless, and lashed out with vehemence and anger at the situation and myself. I'm in the "Valley of Discontent" and want to get out of Sacramento. 31, 12C, 16:XX:XX

NICC. Al, 1 - Very angry and quarrelsome mood; she was inclined to quarrel with and contradict everyone, in the evening.

He, 2 - Vexed and very angry from least contradiction.

NIT-AC. Al, 5 - Long-continued rancor, insensible to apologies and excuses.

Al, 2 - Attacks of rage and despair, with curses and imprecations.(blasphemy)

Ha, 51 - Long-continued rancor; insensible to apology and excuses.

He, 6 - Raving, as if delirious, with coldness of body and inclination to fall.

He, 19-...headstrong (obstinate); trembling while quarreling; fits of rage with curses and maledictions; inveterate ill-will, unmoved by apologies.

NUX-V. Al, 4 - He is hasty; looked angrily at anyone who asked him a question without answering, as though he was obliged to restrain himself to avoid being insulting; he was in such an irritable and unrestrained mood that it seemed as though he would like to strike any one in the face who spoke a word to him.

Ha, 1270 - He is hasty (careless, rapid), looks malignantly (deadly) at any one who asks (asked) him anything, without answering, just as if he must control himself in order to avoid becoming coarse (rude), it seems as if he would like to strike any one in the face who speaks a word to him, so irritable and uncontrollable in his disposition.

He, 8 - Suits very particular, careful,(prudent, meticulous) zealous (conscientious) persons, inclined to get angry or excited, or a spiteful (cruel), malicious disposition.

He, 13 - Irritable, angry disposition, anxious concern about little things. (trifles)

OLND. Ha, 352 - The heat rapidly overcomes him; he breaks out in anger, but repents (sorry) immediately afterwards.

OP. Al, 16-...started up in a fright on account of fancied swordsmen (rival, competitor) who threatened to stab him; became angry if any one argued him or thought him delirious; however, he blamed (reproaches) himself while in delirium for his folly.

OPUN-V. Al, 5 - Fit of swearing (cursing) at evening after coming home; praying in the morning, swearing (cursing) on disappointment in plans; fit of rage, on thwarting (frustrating) of plans.

Al, 6 - In the afternoon, fit of petulance, angry at near relatives, swearing mood, not at all pleased, cannot get over the thought of injuries done by friends.

PETR. He, 6 - Excitable, irritable with

inclination to be angry and to scold; anxious and irresolute.

PH-AC. Ha, 662 - A trifling vexation makes him very angry and hot.

PLAT. Ha, 33 - Very cross and irritated at harmless matters and words; so that she at times would have liked to have beaten herself and friends.

He, 17 - After anger alternate laughing and weeping, with great anguish and fear of death.

PSOR. Al, 22 - She is very irritable, easily angered; thinking always of dying.

Al,N-11 - She is very irritable, easily angered; always thinks of dying.

He, 11 - She is very irritable, easily angered; always thinks of dying.

PULS. Al, 8 - Extremely capricious and peevish at everything, even at himself.

He, 40 - Religious mania; sees the devil coming to take her; the world on fire during night; fear, rage in spells, or weeping... (captured, possessed)

RAN-B. Al, 2 - Vexed and inclined to be angry; quarrels and scolds when the slightest cause is offered (after two hours).

Al, 7 - The objects of his feelings, for instance, chagrin, occupy his mind long after the occurrence took place; one sees that he is thinking of those things; he talks to himself, gesticulates in his anger...

RAPH. Al, 1 - Feeling of aversion towards all women; she is provoked by seeing women going and coming about her; their approach threw her into a fury; the mere contact with a woman's dress caused intolerable distress;...She is attracted to all men without distinction (nymphomania) ; when she gives her hand to a man, she feels great agitation,...When left alone for a hour in the evening, she gave herself a very deep wound in the lips with a penknife, in hopes to put an end to this condition (hurt, punishes). Moral feeling was completely extinct, the physical nature alone ruled and threw her into a frightful state (wild). From morning to noon she would not have been able to resist the advances even of a man for whom she had not the least friendly feeling; from noon to 6 p.m. she could not have held out against any man whatsoever; from 8 to 11 the demands of sense were so importunate as to silence the voice of shame and reason; ... and would have thrown herself into the arms of the first man she met...she was still unable to control her impulses;...

RHUS-T. He, 14 - Fretful; general unhappiness of temper.

SEC. Al, 10 - Raving (talk wildly), whith an attempt to jump into the water.

SEP. Al, 1 - So excited from anger that she fears an apoplectic fit; everything becomes black (evil) before the eyes.

Al, 3 - Attacks of anger over past times come on involuntarily, through which he becomes so excited that he does not know what to do, accompanied by anxiety, palpitation of the heart, and sweat of the whole body.

Al, 76 - Peevish mood, as after suppressed anger.

Ha, 55 - A trifle produces a violent ebullition of anger, with trembling.

STANN. Al, 1 - Excited and inclined to storms of anger.

Ha, 640 - Peevish: nothing was done according to his wish.

Ha, 655 - In the first three days he is rather calm and his vexation quickly passes off, does not fly into a passion, is rather quickly sensitive; the fourth day he is disposed to stormy anger and to fly into a passion...

STAPH. He, 14-...; was insulted (slandered, defamed, calumniated) being too dignified (reserved, lordly,) to fight (contest), subdued (control) his wrath(anger) and went home sick,.. (ailments, from offenses)

STRAM. Al, 23 - Violent delirium; whith was alternately mirthful, furious or dolorous (sad), directed to some imaginary source of pleasure or repugnance, and accompanied which corresponding gesticulations.

Ha, 546 - Furious endeavors to kill people.

Ha, 547 - Furious endeavor to kill himself.

He, 111 - Nymphomania; with diaphragmitis; violent attacks, even to rage; exalted sexual passion.

SULPH. Al, 85 - He could tear himself to pieces from vexation.

Al, 8 - Numerous morbid ideas, extremely disagreeable, causing rancor, though with also joyous thoughts (and melodies)

mostly from the past, take possession of her they throng one upon another so that she cannot free herself from them during the day, with neglect of business,...
Al, 69 - Extremely peevish and ill-humored; nothing seems right to her.
Al, 84 - He is vexed at everything, gets angry and out of humor at every word, thinks he must be defended (protect) and becomes exasperated.
Ha, 38 - He gets vexed about everything, takes every word ill and gets insulted (dishonored, degraded), he imagines he ought (must) to defend himself and gets angry.
Ha, 53 - He is so peevish and obstinate, that he will not give an answer to anybody, he cannot bear to have anyone around him, and cannot get quickly enough what he wants.
He, 8 - Numerous morbid ideas, extremely disagreeable, causing rancor; neglect of business;...
THUJ. Al, 16 - The child is excessively obstinate; on the slightest contradiction it throws itself in the ground in rage and loses its breath.
TIL. Al, 19 - Irritable, critical mood, inclined to quarrel and get angry, even from the slightest difference of opinion.
ZINC. Ha, 26 - He would like to have some one, on whom he might wreak (vent) his (causeless) anger.

ANIMAL

Animal consciousness: choc.[222] germ.[222]
Aversion; animals, to furry: tub.[187]
Barking: ***bell.*** brom.[5] calc. ***canth.*** dros.[5] hyos.[162] nit-ac.[5] ***nux-m.***[30] spong.[5] stann.[5] stram
Cares; full of, nature, for, animals, plants: lap-c-b.[194]
Cruelty, animals to: **ARS.**[162] ***bell.*** calc.[193] med.[162]
Delirium; anxious, dog were attacking her, as if: **STRAM.**[54]
Delirium; bellows like a calf: cupr.
Delirium; wraps up in fur during summer: hyos.
Delusions; animals: absin. aeth. alum.[5] am-c.[5] am-m.[5] arn.[5] ***ars.*** aur. aur-ar.[58] aur-s.[58] ***bell. calc.*** cham. choc.[222] ***cimic.*** cina colch. con. ***crot-h. hyos.*** lac-c. lyc.[5] lyss. mag-m.[5] med. merc.[5] mosch.[5] nux-v.[5] **OP.** phos.[5] puls. sant. sec. sil.[5] ***stram.*** sul-ac.[5] sulph. tarent. thuj. valer. verat.[5] zinc.[5]

- animals abdomen, are in: croc.[162] ***thuj.***
- animals, ants: psil.[164]
- animals, ants, bed seems full of: plb.
- animals, bats, of: bell.[10]
- animals, bear, growling: mag-m.
- animals, bed, on: ars.[10] colch. ***plb.***[122] stram. valer.
- animals, bed, on, dancing: con.
- animals, bed, under the: cham.[54]
- animals, bees sees: puls.
- animals, beetles, worms, etc.: alum.[5] ars. bell. hyos.[58] nep.[149] ***stram.***
- animals, birds, sees: bell. kali-c. lac-c.
- animals, black, on walls and furniture, sees: bell. stram.[162]
- animals, bugs, of: cocain.[102] kres.[144] stram.[54]
- animals, bulls: bell.[10]
- animals, butterflies, of: bell. cann-i.
- animals, cats, see: absin. ***aeth.*** arn. ***bell. calc.*** daph. hyos. hyosin.[102] op.[30] puls. ***stram.***
- animals, cats, see, black: bell. puls.
- animals, centipedes: atro.[54]
- animals, cockroaches: kres.[144] stram.[54]
- animals, corners, coming out of: stram.[116]
- animals, crabs, of: hyos.
- animals, creeping: alum.[5] lac-c.
- animals, creeping, in her (him): ail.[58] cycl.[36] stram.
- animals, creeping, shirt, about in: bell.[54]
- animals, creeping, to her: **OP.**[54]
- animals, cup, moving in a: hyos.
- animals, dark colored: bell.
- animals, devouring him: ***hyos.***
- animals, dogs, attack him: **STRAM.**
- animals, dogs, biting and tearing flesh off his chest: stram.
- animals, dogs, black: ***bell.*** puls.[10]
- animals, dogs, near, that bit her, fought as if to drive it away: lyss.[54]
- animals, dogs, sees: ***aeth.*** arn. aur.[1] **BELL.** ***calc.*** calc-ar.[58] calc-sil.[58] cina[58] lap-c-b.[194] lyc. merc. puls. sil. ***stram.*** sulph. verat. zinc
- animals, dogs, swarm about him: bell. ***calc.***[54] stram.
- animals, dragons, of: op.[36]
- animals, fierce, with horns and bushy heads: ***bell.***[54]
- animals, fire, in the: bell.

- animals, fishes, sees: bell. ***stram.***
- animals, fleas creeping over body, evening: gent-c.[85]
- animals, flies, sees: bell. lyc.[58] ***stram.***
- animals, fowl, sees: hyos.[10] stram.
- animals, fowl, sees: hyos.[10] stram.
- animals, frightful: ***bell.*** cham.[54] ***crot-h.***[54] ***op. stram.*** tarent.
- animals, geese, sees: hyos.
- animals, geese, threw themselves into water, thinking themselves to be: con.
- animals, grasshoppers: choc.[222]
- animals, grotesque: absin.
- animals, he or she is a: choc.[222]
- animals, hedgehogs, sees: choc.[222]
- animals, hens, bound with chains: ***hyos.***[8]
- animals, horses: bell. m-aust.[10] mag-m. zinc
- animals, horses, riding: cann-i.
- animals, ichthyosaurus, seeing an: cann-i.[36]
- animals, insects, creeping on face: croto-t.[36]
- animals, insects, head, on back of, has: hydrog.[222]
- animals, insects, sees: ***abel. aeth.*** **ARS. BELL.** calc. caust. choc.[222] ***cimic.*** cocc.[5] coff.[5] colch.[116] dig. hyos. ***lac-c.*** med. merc. op.[116] phos. plb. puls. ***stram.*** tarent.
- animals, insects, sees, shining: bell.
- animals, jumping at her: ***merc.***[122]
- animals, jumping out of the ground: ***stram.***
- animals, lying near her, which she feels she might hurt: ***valer.***[54]
- animals, mice, bed, on: colch.[10]
- animals, mice, running from under a chair: ***aeth.***[102] calc.[162] ***cimic.***[54] lac-c.[102]
- animals, mice, sees: ***aeth.*** ail.[162] bell. ***calc. cimic.*** colch. cortico.[119] hyos. lac-c. lach.[5] mag-s. ***med.*** op. stram.
- animals, objects are: hyos.[137]
- animals, ox, riding an: bell.
- animals, passing before her: thuj.
- animals, peacocks chasing, he is: hyos.
- animals, persons are: bell.[162] hyos. stram.
- animals, persons are, unclean animals: bell.
- animals, pigeons flying in room which he tries to catch: ***kali-c.***[54]
- animals, rabbits, sees: stram.
- animals, rats, mice, insects etc.: ***aeth. ars.*** bell. calc. choc.[222] ***cimic.*** colch. cortico.[119] hyos. lac-c. lach.[5] mag-s. ***med.*** op.[116] phos. plb. puls. stram. tarent.
- animals, rats, mice, insects etc., colors, of all: absin.
- animals, rats, mice, insects, etc. bed, in: cimic.[54]
- animals, running over her: cycl.[36]
- animals, running, across the room: ***aeth.*** ail. ars. cimic. med.
- animals, running, large, up the legs, feels: ail.[58] ***calc.***[122]
- animals, scorpions, sees: op.
- animals, sheep, bed, in: cimic.[54]
- animals, sheep, driving: acon.
- animals, sheep, sees: ***cimic.***
- animals, snakes, in and around her: abel.[162] ail.[58] anh.[119] bell. calc. gels.[111] ***hyos. lac-c.*** lach. lachn.[111] op. phyt.[30] ***stram.***[8] tub.[56]
- animals, snakes, black: arg-n.[5] cund.[111]
- animals, snakes, crawling up her leg, feels a: ail.[122]
- animals, snakes, crimson, or, fastening around his neck: bell.
- animals, snakes, lying on a large: lac-c. 139
- animals, snakes, white: gels.[5] ign.[111]
- animals, spiders: ***lac-c.***
- animals, suckling: choc.[222]
- animals, surrounded by hideous: ***crot-h.***[54]
- animals, swarmed about the room: bell.
- animals, turtles, sees large, in room: bell.
- animals, unclean: bell.
- animals, vermin, bed is covered with: ars.
- animals, vermin, crawl about, sees: alum. am-c. ***ars.*** bov. calc.[30] kali-c. lac-c.[58] mur-ac. ***nux-v.*** phos. ran-s. sil. sulph.[30]
- animals, wolves, of: bell. stram.
- animals, worms, bed, are in: ars.[36]
- animals, worms, bugs, and: cocain.[102]
- animals, worms, covered with: cocain.
- animals, worms, creeping: alum.[5] am-c.[5] ***ars.***[5] bov.[5] kali-c.[5] mur-ac.[5] **NUX-V.**[5] phos.[5] ran-s.[5] sil.[5]
- animals, worms, vomits is a bunch of: cann-i.
- bird, he is a, runs about, chirping and twittering, until he faints: lyss.[54]
- birds, sees: bell. kali-c. lac-c.
- cat, he is a: lap-mar-c.[194]
- dogs, he is a dog, growls and barks: bell.[54] lyss.[54]
- dogs, others are, barks at them to be understood: stram.[54]

- giraffe, he is a: cann-i.
- goose, he is a: con.
- growling as of a bear, hears: mag-m.
- hedgehog, he or she is: choc.[222]
- hippopotamus, he is a: cann-i.[36]
- nesting, she is: lac-h.[229]
- swine, hogs, people are: hyos.
- tomato is a grasshopper: choc.[222]

Dreams, animals, mule, driving of: chin-b.

Dreams; animals, anxious: ***am-c.***[5] ***am-m.***[5] **ARN.**[5] ***bell.***[5] bov.[5] ***hyos.***[5] ***merc.***[5] **NUX-V.**[5] ran-s.[5] ***sil.***[5] ***sul-ac.***[5]

➤ animals, bat flying in room, causing fear: ham.[36]
➤ animals, bees, driving away: puls.[10]
➤ animals, beetles: coca[36] kres.[149]
➤ animals, birds, of, large, black: choc.[222]
➤ animals, birds, of, singing: com.[36]
➤ animals, biting him: am-m. bov.[10] calc.[10] cench.[58] daph. elaps[136] m-aust.[10] merc. nicc.[10] ***phos.*** puls. sulph.[10] verat.[10] zinc.[10]
➤ animals, black: arn.[10] ***puls.***
➤ animals, boars, wild: merc.[36]
➤ animals, bugs: kres.[119] myric.[36]
➤ animals, bugs, enormous, attacking his head, which he killed one by one: myric.[36]
➤ animals, bulls, chased by: ind. tarent.
➤ animals, bulls, jumped into water and drowned, and: tarent.[36]
➤ animals, bulls, mad: ind.
➤ animals, camels, of: hydrog.[222] ozone[227]
➤ animals, cats: arn. ars. calc-p. ***daph.*** graph. hydrog.[222] hyos. lac-c. mez. nux-v. op.[102] ozone[227] puls. thuj.[111]
➤ animals, cats, army of: calc-p.[36]
➤ animals, cats, black: arn.[36] daph.
➤ animals, cats, frightened: puls.[36]
➤ animals, cats, outside, have to freeze, because of fleas: ozone[227]
➤ animals, cats, pursuing him: ***nux-v.*** sil. verat.
➤ animals, cats, springing at him: hyos.[36]
➤ animals, cats, wild: ozone[227]
➤ animals, cats, without number: graph.[36]
➤ animals, cats, wounded abdomen, with: ozone[227]
➤ animals, copulating: cench.[58]
➤ animals, cows, dying: hydrog.[222]
➤ animals, crocodiles, pursued by, and driving them away by sneezing: sedi.[36]
➤ animals, dead: ptel.[36]
➤ animals, devouring meat in market: hura[36]
➤ animals, dogs: abrot. am-c.[5] ***arn.*** calc. cere-b.[36] cina[58] graph. hyos.[5] lyc. lyss. merc. nux-v. op.[102] paull. pitu-a.[164] puls. rumx. ***sil. sulph.*** verat. zinc.
➤ animals, dogs, bitten, by, of being: calc. lyss. med.[212] merc. ozone[227] ***sulph.*** verat.
➤ animals, dogs, black: ***arn.*** puls.[1] tub.[193]
➤ animals, dogs, frightened by a black dog: puls.
➤ animals, dogs, large dog following him: sil.
➤ animals, dogs, mad dog: abrot. rumx.
➤ animals, dogs, mad dog, killing a: abrot.[85] rumx
➤ animals, dogs, mangy dog approaching her, covered with sores, she takes hold of it and it bites her: paull-p.[36]
➤ animals, dogs, many young dogs, fastening themselves tightly, in constant succession on various parts of his body: lyc.[36]
➤ animals, dogs, pursued by: ***nux-v.*** ozone[227] sil. verat.
➤ animals, dragons: op.
➤ animals, eating alive: hydrog.[222]
➤ animals, elephant, small, very, the size of a dog: ozone[227]
➤ animals, elephants: kali-m.[192]
➤ animals, fights with: staph.[1]
➤ animals, fishes: arg-n.[36] chin-b. kali-c.[5] kali-m.[192] mag-c.[5]
➤ animals, fishes, big as a room: ozone[227]
➤ animals, fishes, gold metal: choc.[222]
➤ animals, fishes, swimming in water: chin-b.
➤ animals, frog in bed: allox.[36]
➤ animals, geese, of being bitten by: zinc.[1]
➤ animals, goats, of: choc.[222]
➤ animals, growing quick, has to destroy them, sticks them into the toilet: ozone[227]
➤ animals, hare, of a white, cannot butcher it: ozone[227]
➤ animals, horses: alum. am-c.[5] am-m. asc-t. atro. bamb-a.[1184] choc.[222] crot-c. hyper.[36] indg. m-aust.[10] mag-m.[10] mag-s. merl. phos. senec.[36] sul-ac.[5] tarent. ther. zinc
➤ animals, horses, bitten by a, in his arm: am-m.
➤ animals, horses, black, with a big white spot on chest: ozone[227]
➤ animals, horses, changing into dogs: zinc.
➤ animals, horses, drowning: crot-c.
➤ animals, horses, eating corn in a garage: ozone[227]
➤ animals, horses, falling from horse: tarent.[36]

- animals, horses, fearing to be bitten by a ferocious black: phos.[36]
- animals, horses, kicking: ***mag-s.***
- animals, horses, pursuing him: allox.[119] alum.
- animals, horses, riding: bamb-a.[1184] nat-c. ther.
- animals, horses, riding, stream, through a: chr-ac.[8]
- animals, horses, running: atro. indg. lipp.[36]
- animals, horses, running, away, waking her: indg.[36]
- animals, horses, running, over her: lipp.[36]
- animals, horses, small, very: ozone[227]
- animals, horses, stealing a horse: aether36
- animals, horses, stealing, his horse: aether[36]
- animals, horses, ugly: merl. phos.
- animals, horses, wild: lap-mar-c.[194]
- animals, insects: arg-n. hist.[149] phos.[36] sphing.[36]
- animals, insects, stung by: lap-mar-c.[194] phos.
- animals, lamas, a zoo full of: bamb-a.[1184]
- animals, lice: am-c. chel. gamb. mur-ac. ***nux-v.*** ped.[36] phos.
- animals, lice, shame, exciting: mur-ac.[36]
- animals, lions: kali-m.[192]
- animals, mice: colch. lap-mar-c.[194] mag-s. sep.
- animals, mice, kill it, had to, and step on it: lap-mar-c.[194]
- animals, mice, yellow: mag-s.
- animals, octopus: ozone[227]
- animals, of: aloe alum.[10] am-c. ***am-m.*** arg-n.[102] **ARN.** bamb-a.[1184] bell. bov. cench.[58] cham. chlorpr.[149] choc.[222] cimic.[56] daph. gran. hura hydr. hydrog.[222] hyos. hyosin.[85] kali-m.[192] lac-c.[102] lyc. mag-m.[10] ***merc.*** merl.[85] nicc.[10] ***nux-v.*** op.[102] ***phos.*** phys. ***puls.*** ran-s. sedi.[36] sil. staph.[1] sul-ac. sulph. tarent. verat.[10] zinc.[10]
- animals, oxen, pursuing him: eupi. hipp.[36] tet.[36]
- animals, oxen, putrid: hura[36]
- animals, playing with: gran.[36]
- animals, poisonous: tarent.[36]
- animals, pursued by: allox.[119] alum. cench.[58] eupi. hipp.[36] hydr.[36] ind. led.[36] nux-v. sil. ***sulph.*** tarent. tet.[36] verat.
- animals, pursued by, wild: allox.[119] alum. cench.[58] eupi. hipp.[36] ind. led.[36] nux-v. sil. ***sulph.*** tet.[36] verat.
- animals, rats: allox.[119] sep.
- animals, rats, creeping under the clothing: menis.[36]
- animals, rhinoceros: ozone[227]
- animals, snakes: alum. ***arg-n.*** bov. carc.[193] cench.[58] colch.[36] daph.[102] grat. indol.[77] iris kali-c. kalm.[54] ***lac-c.*** lach.[122] merl.[36] op.[102] ozone[227] pitu-a.[164] ptel. ran-b.[54] ***ran-s.*** rat. sep. sil. sol-n. sphing.[36] tab. teucr.[111] tub.[56]
- animals, snakes, bed, in: ***lac-c.***[54]
- animals, snakes, bitten by, of being: bov. cench.[58] med.[212] ozone[227]
- animals, snakes, horrifying: ***arg-n.***[36]
- animals, snakes, killing snakes: ptel.[25]
- animals, snakes, splitting in parts that keep moving: ozone[227]
- animals, spiders: cinnb. convo-d.[231] crot-c. sars.[1] ven-m.[149]
- animals, spiders, black, creeping into corner of mouth: ozone[227]
- animals, spiders, hairy, very, which tried to climb on him: crot-c.[36]
- animals, spiders, ox, the size of an: cinnb.
- animals, stags: canth.[10]
- animals, suffering: hydrog.[222]
- animals, terrapin, water turtle: cench.[58]
- animals, toad in bed: allox.[119]
- animals, vampires: psil.[164]
- animals, vermin: alum.[5] am-c. bell.[5] bov.[10] chel. colch. gamb. kali-c.[10] lac-c. mag-s. mur-ac. ***nux-v.*** ped.[85] phos. ran-s.[10] sep. sil.[5]
- animals, wasps: rauw.[119]
- animals, wasps, bitten, by: lap-mar-c.[194]
- animals, wild: hyos.[10] lyc.[36] nux-v. sil. sulph. tarent.[36]
- animals, worms, creeping: alum.[10] am-c. bov.[10] choc.[222] esp-g.[149] kali-c.[10] mur-ac. nux-v. phos. ran-s.[10] sil.[10]
- anxious, pleasant, partly: dros.[54]
- balloon in front of abdomen, has a: ozone[227]
- eating, canine flesh: alum.[10]
- eating, live animals: hydrog.[222]
- journey, horseback, on: nat-c. ther.
- kidnapping, friend is kidnapped by a shepherd dog: ozone[227]
- killing, mad dog, a: rumx.
- leper, of being a: paull.[36]
- lion, that he was a: phys.
- men, transforming into talking animals: sol-t-ae.[85]
- monks, about, singing and dancing: ozone[227]

➤ Noah's ark: bamb-a.[1184]
➤ stealing, someone is stealing his horse: aether.
➤ women, animals, changed into: sol-t-ae.[36]
Fear; alone, of being, starts with a loud cry as if a bird flew towards the window: kali-c.[172]
✦ animals, bats: ham.[36]
✦ animals, bees, of: hep.[162]
✦ animals, birds, of: aesc.[172] apis[162] bufo[36] calc-ar.[162] calc-s.[162] ign.[162] ***nat-m.***[184]
✦ animals, birds, of, mouse, which he thought a: lyss.[54]
✦ animals, bugs: calc.[162]
✦ animals, cats, of: absin.[172] bac.[83] chin.[185] med.[162] plb.[201] sil.[147] syph.[193] ***tub.***[122]
✦ animals, cats, of, rats, and: absin.[172]
✦ animals, chickens, of: chin.[184] ign.[187]
✦ animals, cockroaches, of: alum.[162] manc.[30] ***phos.***[162]
✦ animals, devoured him or her: hyos.[1] stram.
✦ animals, dogs, attacking him, in delirium: **STRAM.**[54]
✦ animals, dogs, black: bac.[149] ***bell.***[54] ***stram.***[54]
✦ animals, dogs, black, malicious: ***stram.***[54]
✦ animals, dogs, hydrocephalic complaints, in: tub.[54]
✦ animals, dogs, of: androc.[222] **BAC.**[62] <u>**BELL.**</u>[122] bufo[179] calc.[30] carc.[193] ***caust.*** **CHIN.** choc.[222] ***hyos.*** lyss.[122] med.[212] nat-m.[162] nat-p.[166] plat.[40] ***puls.***[162] sil.[171] ***stram.*** syc-co.[136] ***tub.*** tub-k.[70] verat.[172]
✦ animals, flies, of: abel.[149]
✦ animals, frogs: carc.[207]
✦ animals, horses, of: hydr-ac.[172] mag-i.[209]
✦ animals, imaginary: **BELL.**
✦ animals, insects, of: abel.[149] bufo[36] **CALC.**[162] calc-ar.[162] cimic.[162] lyc.[162] nat-m.[162] nat-p.[166] phos.[162] puls.[212] sulph.[212]
✦ animals, mice, of: calc.[162] sep.[172]
✦ animals, mice, of, walking, on: colch.[10]
✦ animals, of: abel.[149] aesc.[172] **BELL.**[122] bufo calc.[30] carc.[140] caust. **CHIN.** hyos. lyc.[212] med.[212] nat-m.[172] ***stram.*** syc-co.[136] **TUB.**[122]
✦ animals, rats, of: absin.[172] bell.[172] calc.[172] cimic.[137] op.[172] phos.[172] sep.[172]
✦ animals, reptiles: calc-s.[196]
✦ animals, scorpions: abel.[149] op.[30]
✦ animals, snakes, of: abel.[149] arg-n.[172] bell.[162] calc.[183] calc-s.[196] carc.[207] elaps[152] hep.[162] ign.[187] lac-c.[162] ***lach.***[122] nat-m.[212] puls.[212] ruta[152] sep.[172] spig.[162] sulph.[162] syph.[162]
✦ animals, spiders, of: abel.[149] calc.[162] carc.[210] lac-c.[185] mag-m.[166] nat-m.[162] phos.[155] stram.[172] tarent.[185]
✦ animals, venomous, of, at night: abel.[149]
✦ animals, wasps: hep.[162]
✦ animals, wild, in mania: ***stram.***[54]
✦ animals, wolves, of: bell.[8]
✦ animals, worms, of: aesc.[172] ars.[172] nat-m.[172]
✦ feathers, of: stram.[172] tub.[172]
Foolish; behavior, monkeys, like: **HYOS.**[54]
Growling like a dog: alum. ***bell.*** hell. hyos.[162] lyss. mag-m. phos.[122]
Imitation; voices, motions and gestures of different animals, of: ***stram.***[54]
Insanity; burrows in ground with his mouth, like a pig: stram.[54]
Jealousy; animals and objects, of: caust.[30] hyos.[30] lach.[30] nux-v.[30]
Lasciviousness; animal, as if she were completely, mental power dormant: lach.[54]
Love; animals, for: aeth.[162] calc-p.[184] carc.[193] med.[162] nat-m.[185] phos.[193] psor.[185]
Love; animals, for, cats, for: ***sulph.***[162]
Love; animals, for, pet, his: nat-m.[189]
Love; perversity, animals, with, sodomy: ***plat.***[162]
Rage; dog that had bitten her, about: lyss.[54]
Senses; acute, birds, for: lap-mar-c.[194]
Sensitive; music, bird songs: choc.[222]
Sensitive; noise, birds, of: bamb-a.[1184]
Striking; animals, at: med.[193]
Sympathetic; animals; only for: aeth.[85] carc.[184] med.[187]
Sympathetic; animals; suffering, feels great pain seeing suffering animals: nuph.[36]
Talk; nothing but, murder, fire and rats: ***calc.*** calc-sil.[58]
Thoughts; persistent, thinks of nothing but murder, fire and rats: ***calc.***

ABSIN. Al,S-6 - Terrifying hallucinations, he sees all kinds of animals, cats and rats of all colors, grotesque animals, fancies that he is pursued by soldiers.

ADAM. Sh, 40 - Overwhelmed by beauty of Sumatran tiger on TV, especially his eyes. 16, 12C, 01:XX:XX

Sh, 523 - Delusion animals are changing form, i.e. see a cat and when closer it's actually a dog. 16, 12C, 28:XX:XX

Sh, 554 - Image of reptilian dinosaur skins. Reached up and took his head off. Inside, a human was underneath dinosaur skin. The head was hanging down in shame. 16, 12C, 00:07:30

AETH. Al, 7 - Imagined she saw rats run across the room.

Al, 8 - Delirium; he imagines he sees dogs and cats.

Al,S-1 - Imagined she saw rats run across the room.

ANDROC. Sh, 82 - Absolutely terrified of dog on street, for no apparent reason, with numbness and tingling through every part of his body, followed by a sick feeling in the stomach. He felt shaken for hours later. (2)

ARS. Al, 90 - He sees vermin and bugs crawl about his bed, from which he wants to escape, and constantly throws away whole handfuls of them.

Ha, 34 - He sees nothing but worms and bugs crawling about on his bed, from which he desires to run away (escape) and of which he throws out whole hands full.

He, 17 - He sees all kinds of vermin (insects) on his bed, throws handfuls of them away, and tries to escape from them.

BELL. Al, 81 - He imagines he sees birds flying off through the chimney, and wishes to follow them by the same route. (desire: fly, liberty, freedom)

Al, 87 - Fancied he saw ghosts and animals in the fire.

Al, 82 - Delirious talk of dogs, as if they swarmed (crowd) about him.

Al, 85 - Visions of wolves, dogs, giants, and fire.

Al, 86-...pointing with trembling fingers to swarms (crowd) of unclean (dirty) beasts wich she fancied were scrambling (mix) all over the walls, beds, table, etc. of the wards.

Al, 89 - He imagines he is riding on an ox, or some such thing.

Al,S-2552-...the yellow corpse of a tall man, shrouded (dressed, clothes) in white, tried to share the patient's bed with him, and the unwelcome visitor was promptly ejected. A crimson serpent came from the foot of the bed, with the design of fastening upon the patient's neck...

Al,S-2559 - Seems to see birds flying past and wishes to follow them.

Ha, 1339 - Raves (delirious) about wolves being in the room; at the same time full pulse.

Ha, 1340 - Delirious talk about dogs surrounding him.

Ha, 1433 - Fearful madness; he is afraid (fear) of an imaginary black dog, of the gallows. (hanging)

He, 18 - When closing eyes, though not asleep, patient sees fierce (wild), wicked looking large animals with horns and bushy (scabrous) heads; room seemed to be full of strange men passing in and out, who would snatch (take hold) at her as they passed, which frightened her very much, she thought the men wanted to take her away from home ; she then saw children sitting on low benches (seat) in rows (line) as in a school-room. (purity)

He, 20 - Imagines he sees ghosts, hideous (horrible) faces and various insects.

He, 24 - Fixed ideas, thinks he is riding on an ox, uses a stick for a gun, growling and barking like a dog.

He, 30 - Delirium: with frightful figures and images before eyes; is afraid (fear) of imaginary things; sees monsters; talks of dogs as if they swarmed (crowded) about him; furious.

He, 106 - Anxiety and fear of imaginary objects and hallucinations, ghosts, soldiers which come to take them away (arrest), black animals, rats dogs, wolves, etc.

He, 13 - Timorous anxiety; he is afraid of a an imaginary black dog; of the gallows, etc.

He, 70 - Instead of eating, bit wooden spoon in two, gnawed plate, and growled and barked like a dog.

He, 105 - Anxiety and fear of imaginary objects and hallucinations, ghosts, soldiers which come to take them away, black animals, rats, dogs, wolves, etc.

BERB. Al, 3 - Anxious mood, with great fear and fright...; in the twilight some dogs and children appeared as large again as natural.

BUFO. Al, 14 - Very easily frightened; a bird or insect flying by causes a start.

Al, 15 - Fear of animals.

He, 12 - Fear of disease, of animals, of death.

CALC. Al, 1557 - Anxious dream that he

would be bitten by a dog, which awoke him, after...

He, 22 - Mania; sees many curs (dogs) crowding (compress) around him, fights them off. (surrounded)

He, 28 - She thinks and talks of nothing but murder, fire, rats, etc.

He, 21 - Mania-a-potu, with delirious talk about fire, rats, mice and murder.

CARB-V. Ha, 678-... feeling over the body as if some one stroked him with the hand, and as if ants were running over the skin, at every moment in bed...

CAUST. Ha, 20 - Extreme anxious timidity; she is so much afraid (fear) of a dog near her, which did not harm (hurt, injure) her at all,...every noise in the street made her afraid, and when she saw boys climbing she was very uneasy lest they might get hurt. (care, others)

CHAM. He, 14-..., vows there is some dreadful beast under his bed or in the room, and will not be appeased (calm) until the gas is lit and the room is searched.

CHIN. He, 28 - Dread of dogs and other animals at night.

CHOC. Sh, 2 - Feel very excited, very alive, bright and efficient. Had an image of a hedgehog's face.

Sh, 9 - Had a vivid dream of worms —they were dark and fat, but I wished they were red and thin. I felt very excited by the worms.

Sh, 41 - When hearing talk of babies, breasts aching with a sensation as if filling up with milk —an aching fullness. An image came to me where I found myself suckling young hairy babies, sometimes animals, especially hedgehogs.

Sh, 44 - Dream —coming out of the station a huge black bird the size of a dog with black long soft feathers like those of an ostrich, and a very big beak. It took my left hand in his beak. There were two gypsies there and they stood in front of me and opened their hands and I saw that they held a gold metal flat fish which I saw as a fortune telling object.

Sh, 45 - When I woke from the dream, I had a little panic, an unusual childhood memory came back in which I remembered having read as a child about being covered in clay, baked and eaten. The thought came to me of the spines on my back covered in clay and baked and eaten like a hedgehog.

Sh, 51 - While out walking, saw a dog and became very scared. I felt very uncomfortable and unsympathetic to the dog. All very unusual.

Sh, 57 - Keep getting a picture of the prickles of the start of the hairline of the hedgehog and am aware of this point in me —not discomfort, but keep pushing hair back and pulling my fingers backwards through my hair, thinking its nice that its not in my face. Keep getting pictures of faces of hedgehogs, (rather than the spiny bits) especially the nose, which seems so black and wet.

Sh, 74 - I saw a rat. We stood looking at each other. I felt we both recognised each other. It was very exciting.

Sh, 86 - On seeing a bristly carpet, started laughing excitedly —had a familiar feeling, like meeting a friend. The texture of the carpet was very spiky like a Hedgehog. Told friend that they should come and see it. It's such a wonderful carpet!

Sh, 104 - Rather than hearing the usual music I listen to, I wanted to hear a blackbird sing. The outdoors seems very familiar and my hands get excited at the thought of it.

Sh, 107 - A strange feeling of being an animal, yet having this thinking.

Sh, 114 - When I feel like a hedgehog, my heart is much faster, but when I feel the stillness, I don't feel my heart at all.

Sh, 116-12:30pm -I feel less and less animal at the moment and I desire company. When it comes, its so intense, I almost lose what I am. I've never been there before. I feel very privileged, as if I can be on both sides at the same time.

Sh, 117 - I thought how would an animal be if it had my body. What would they do with thought. I think I'm better off.

Sh, 120 - Felt as if I was hibernating —mouth sealed up perfectly and my tongue seems to fill all the space. I usually sleep with my mouth open as I cannot breathe through my nose, but now my mouth is perfectly sealed and nose free-flowing.

Sh, 121 - I met a dog this morning and felt

that I understood it now and it wasn't a threat, whereas earlier I had been uncertain and wary.

Sh, 127 - Before this, I never felt very comfortable with men. Now I feel much more comfortable. I feel I've lost that extreme feeling of totally female identity. I feel like a female animal, but its not really in my awareness, it just is. Desire to curl up over a man's back. It felt right and comfortable.

Sh, 130 - I feel slightly less like a hedgehog today, but the picture is still in my mind. Human things seem so trivial —so much energy wasted when you are human. Nature is so efficient. It never wastes a seed and we just spend energy everywhere.

Sh, 149 - Hearing and smell still acute — nature seems wonderful. Saw nine magpies and they seemed much bigger than before.

Sh, 151 - Still get images of creatures — thought a tomato was a grasshopper.

Sh, 153 - Since the proving, I know how it feels to be a animal or a plant. I know the feeling of daffodil, of flower, of hedgehog, of dog.

Sh, 191 - I Since the being bitten by the dogs have developed a strong fear of dogs, and have been chased by one dog and growled at by another. This is coupled with a general fear of something happening. These fears are new to me and were better again after the proving. 27, 100C, 05:XX:XX

Sh, 228 - Thoughts about the 'veneer of civilisation' that inhibits how we really feel and keeps us from displaying what we're like beneath the surface. It seems a legitimate layer, but so is the layer beneath it, and I feel amused and happy to meet it. This feeling continued for a few days, a very graphic picture of a veneer -a layer of learned social behaviour lifting and detaching from a basis that is thick, dark, solid, instinctual animal.[15] , 30C, 00:00:30

Sh, 301 - Desire to bite my husband in a playful way. I bit him —I wanted to really sink my teeth in, but willed myself not to. It was an animal need in me.[15], 30C, 00:05:30

Sh, 311 - On stepping out of the shower, a fleeting, momentary imagination of both arms crawling with insects. No physical sensation, purely an imagination.[15], 30C, 00:02:XX

Sh, 312 - While reading small print in materia medica, I had a delusion that tiny insects were crawling down the page. 15, 30C, 03:XX:XX

Sh, 314 - Talking about flying. I would like to be a bird or a bat or in a plane.[01]A, 30C, 00:12:XX

CIMIC. He, 6 - Often startled by illusion of a mouse running from under her chair.

He, 7 - Imagines strange objects about bed, as rats, sheep, etc.

He, 10 - Fear of death; fears those in house will kill him (murdered, by parents); saw wires encasing (lock, imprisoned) him; visions of rats and of strange objects.

CON. Al, 6 - Delirious and stupid; they threw themselves into the water, thinking they were geese; for three years they remained partly paralytic, suffering from much pain.

Al, 10 - The husband, who had been somewhat addicted to liquor, saw all sorts of animals dancing upon the bed, and "picked straws" a little.

CROT-C. Al, 3-... hears a strange voice to her left, and behind her; she follows it, throws herself against closed doors, and scratches them with her nails...She cries out: " He is in the den, but the lions will not eat him"

CROT-H. He, 5-...imagines himself surrounded by enemies or hideous animals;...

GERM. Sh, 101 - I'm desperate. I want to die. Feel the power to kill. Feel like a wild animal locked in. It's strong, so intense. I hate so strong-feel a terrible disgust and I'm afraid of what I'm able to do. It's completely impossible to be in it and impossible to get out of it. 18, 30C, 190:XX:XX

HALI-L. Sh, 7 - My left arm feels like a broken wing. 01, 30C, 21:XX:XX

Sh, 14 - Delusion—Small white animal, sweet and cuddly, has been living in a chair in my living room. 16, 10C, 04:XX:XX

Sh, 592 - Had a peculiar experience during the day. While playing with one of my dogs, I started to wonder what it would be like to crush her. Suddenly I thought how sensual it would be to crush its little head and rip its flesh. There was something very sensual about the idea of crushing flesh and bones of a soft creature that would not be able to fight me off. It was not a strong, powerful impulse, but there was something compelling about the idea. 04, 30C, 02:XX:XX

Sh, 595 - I look at rabbits and birds in a different light. Wondering how a rabbit would taste raw. What would the fur taste like? 20, 30C, XX:XX:XX

Sh, 597 - Reading about the Ring Cycle and how Siegfried tasted the blood of the slain dragon.[16], 10C, 22:XX:XX

Sh, 719 - Not sure whether asleep or not — inner vision. I'm high up and there is water below me and I have an image of a few of my breast feathers floating on the water. Between the breast feathers, the reflection of a very pink dawn. Noticed all birds in pairs. 20, 30C, 00:23:30

Sh, 721 - Inner vision; I was sunning my wings in the dawn sun. I'm not flapping-soaring —not dusk, at dawn — not for dark, of Light. 20, 30C, 00:23:50

Sh, 729 - Delusions —sees eagles. They were rooks and crows really. They looked bigger. 20, 30C, 01:00:58

Sh, 741 - A five year old boy, friend of daughter, said I looked strange, different. He said I was staring at him. I said, "It's all right. I have the eye of an eagle." 20, 30C, 01:12:00

Sh, 862 - Clear and bright, an eagle soared, an amazing bird high up in the sky, when I was lying naked on my back. It wasn't flapping, it just soared. coming from the east towards me then flew into the sun. As I lay there, unbelieving, he soared out again, circled again and then disappeared into the radiance of the sun. I felt like the proving was finished. It felt like a good-bye. My vision had changed. I feel more like me. 20, 30C, 08:08:XX

Sh, 977 - Tears come easily, just on looking at an exhibition of wildlife —sobbing. It was beautiful and lit from the back. It was so beautiful I couldn't contain it. There were pictures of a bald eagle and of a hedgehog right next to each other. 20, 30C, 20:XX:XX

HYDROG. Sh, 169 - Thought there was a large insect, a locust, on the back of my head and put up my hand to check. 16, 30C, 01:XX:XX

Sh, 170 - Sensation as if something is crawling on my head. Checked for lice, but can't find any. 32, 9C, 09:XX:XX

Sh, 189 - As if in a dream, not there, difficult to stay with it all while driving home —very conscious of the blackbirds flying across the motorway. Better taking a nap and fresh air from opening the window. Concomitant to finger abscess. 02, 6C, 54:XX:XX

Sh, 219 - Things seem ridiculous and amusing, ordinary things like birds. Laughing at them. Everything seemed so absurd or futile. 16, 30C, 02:XX:XX

HYOS. Al, 42 - In his delirium he acts as though he were frightening away peacocks whith his hands.

Al, 87 - Remarkable fear that he had been devoured by animals.

Ha, 519 - In the confusion of his fancy he thinks men are swine.(pigs)

Ha, 529 - Comical confusion of mind: they perform all sorts of ridiculous antics (jokes), like monkeys.

Ha, 575 - Peculiar fear of being bitten (hurt) by beasts.

Ha, 535 - In his mania, he acts as if he must drive away peacocks with his hands.(conduct)

He, 59-...constantly pointing to serpents (snakes) which she saw creeping up towards her...

He, 81-...attempts to escape from room; frightful hallucinations of figures coming to seize him, hens (chicken) bound (imprisoned) with chains,...

He, 41 - Comical alienation of mind; ludicrous actions like monkeys; makes ridiculous gestures like a dancing clown;...

He, 90 - Looks at men as hogs.(pigs)

IRID. Sh, 19 - Still didn't feel much like talking. Feel very contained and self contained and my mind feels still. Unintellectual, unthinking, heavy. I wanted to be pre-verbal like the cat. Words too much effort. E1

Sh, 61 - I feel buzzy and vibrating, feels as if my hair is stood on end. I keep talking about being a dog. H1

Sh, 68 - Woke up thinking my alarm clock

was a hedgehog. I wondered what the spiky sound was. I10

Sh, 84 - Morning getting dressed, didn't really want to put clothes on, felt I was taking the first gulp of air that the first breathing animal took as it came out of the water, bursting through the surface, lungs expanding. As with the egg image (day 5), the movement is forceful, BURSTING with great relief. G6

Sh, 99 - Sat at the bus stop. Felt like a really small, frightened rabbit, with a large shadow of this great bird hovering over ready to pounce. G8

Sh, 106 - Mental image: I am inside an egg —a bird, wet feathers, at the point it is smashing through its shell, bursting out; a chick, wet crumpled and hot, shell flying all over. The relief —getting to the air, refreshing, cool. Inside it was humid, stifling. Stretching vast wings, enjoying feeling the air dry them out. G5

Sh, 108 - Realized I had called my ex-partner a chicken for pulling out of an arrangement to go together to a school fundraising event. G5

KALI-C. Al, 25 - She is frightened with a loud cry, by an imaginary apparition (as for example, of a bird flying to the window).

Ha, 26 - She is frightened by an imaginary appearance (e.g. as if a bird was flying toward the window) and she utters a loud scream.

He, 5 - Imagines seeing birds flying in room; he tries to catch them. (seize)

LAC-C. Al,N-18 - After menses, imagines all sorts of things about snakes.

Al,N-19 - Wakes at night with a sensation that she was lying on a large snake.

He, 15 - Sensation or delusion as if surrounded by myriads of snakes, some running like lightning up and down inside the skin ; some that are inside feel long and thin; fears to put her feet on floor, lest she should tread (walk) on them and make them squirm (shake) and wind (round) around her legs; is afraid to look behind her, for fear that she will see snakes there, does not dream of them and is seldom troubled with them after dark; on going to bed she was afraid to shut her eyes for fear that a large snake, the size of her arm, would hit her in the face.

He, 16 - Worries (care) herself lest (fear) pimples (boil) which appear during menses will prove to be little snakes, and twine and twist around each other.

He, 12 - Imagines to see spiders.

LACH. He, 33-...want of self control; lascivious; felt as if she was clear (pure) animal right through, whilst of all mental power was dormant; sensation as if hands of stronger power, as if charmed (enchanted), and as if could not break the spell (charm). (possessed, wildness)

LYSS. Al,N-26 - Thinks he is a dog or a bird, and runs up and down chirping and twittering...(liberty?)

Al,N-46 - After fainting (weak) spell he wrote on paper: I am forsaken by all; even the birds of heaven, they do not look at me (despised), do not fed me if hungry (helplessness) ; I hunger with the young ones and am thirsty with their she ones (starving); my nest (house) is made out of dirt (soiled), not gotten by my own exertions (efforts), but by driving them out of their nests (home) and sitting there with the females and the young.

Al,N-40 - A strong and uncontrollable impulse to do certain acts; to spring at and bite any moving object that came within reach; dog.

He, 26 - Thinks he is a dog or a bird, and runs up and down, chirping and twittering, until he falls down fainting.

MAG-C. Al, 929 - Dream of very small horses, that she exerted herself to reflect upon, after midnight.

Al, 950 - Dream that she burnt her back by some one throwing hot roast (meat) pigeons (bird) at her.

MED. He, 19 - One night saw large (big) people in room; large rats running; felt a delicate hand smoothing her head from front to back. (caressed)

MERC. Ha, 1125 - Anxious dreams; of being bitten by dog, of getting up a revolution (revolutionary, revolting, radical) after midnight.

NEON. Sh, 20 - I had thoughts of albatrosses circumnavigating the earth without having to touch the ground. 20, 6C, 03:02:14

Sh, 109 - Caught sight of a (black and white) cardboard box in the kitchen and momentarily thought it was a black and white dog (day time). 05, 12C, 08:XX:XX

OP. He, 21-...in old, emaciated persons; sees animals coming towards him; people want to hurt him, execute him ; creeping under covers or jumping out of bed; in "old sinners" (criminals) whose long lives of excess have thoroughly destroyed their constitutions; ...; believe themselves to be murderers or criminals to be executed; want to run away (escape) ;...

PLB. Al, 75-..imagined he was going to be poisoned; that his bed was full of ants.

SAMB-C. Al, 1-...an indefinable fear as if the horse (a very gentle animal) might run away, or the wagon break at any moment; a dread of some undefined danger.

SARS. Al, 18 - Extremely ill-humored even vexed " by the fly on the wall".

Ha, 14 - Extremely peevish, the fly on the wall vexes him. (insects)

STRAM. Ha, 562 - His surroundings appear to him quite strange; (unfamiliar) although in the first minutes he knows that he is surrounded by his friends, he forgets this in the second minute, and imagines he is quite alone (solitary, deserted) in a desert (wildness), and is afraid (fearful) ; figures of beasts suddenly spring out of the ground at his side, so that he moves to the other side, where, however, other similar figures pursue him, and he runs forward.

Ha, 551 - She sometimes cries out about cats, dogs and rabbits, which were approaching (pursuing) her from above, from the side and from the middle of the room.

Ha, 565 - Nowhere has he rest, is startled by dream-pictures, even when his eyes are open, which in the form of big dogs, cats and other horrible beasts, grow (expand) out of the ground at his side, and from which he jumps away to the side with signs of terror (fear), and knows not how to save (rescue, free) himself. (cornered, corralled)

Ha, 520 - Loquacious madness; he complains of a dog biting and tearing the flesh off his chest.

He, 40 - Aberration of mind; one carries home all sorts of wood in order to manufacture brandy (cognac) (busy, manufacturing) ; another placed two axes across each other in order to split wood in this way; a third burrowed in ground like a pig with his mouth (animal); a fourth alleged he was a wheelwright and began to bore holes; a fifth ran into forge to catch fish, which he saw swimming there; a lacemaker threw about her bobbins incessantly, and threw everything into confusion; another girl ran about the room and cried out that all evil spirits were pursuing her.(restoration, restitution)

He, 56 - Believes to be in his grave; shrives,(confess) prays, asks to be killed (justified); accuses his wife of infidelity; scolds (cursing), strikes at everybody who wishes to restrain him; thinks they are dogs and barks at them to make himself understood.

He, 65-"There", he replied, "A long train of bedbugs, and after them a procession of beetles and here come crawling over me a host (crowd) of cockroaches"; sank back in alarm, then suddenly said:" I believe I know they are not really bugs, but, except once in a while, they seem real to me. (organization, association, union)

He, 66 - Woke suddenly in night and said there were snakes under and about her; looked wild, screamed and pointed to them.

He, 92 - Mania:... complains that a dog is biting and tearing flesh off his chest; merry exaltation; with pride (haughty) and affectation; runs about, complains of violent headache; ...;steals from his roommates...; disposition to scold persons whom he otherwise loved.

He, 102 - Mania with insomnia ; very talkative; thinks he has every imaginable disease; that he has power (powerful) over all disease; masturbates, fills his pockets with anything he can find (lack?), thinks he has snakes in him.

He, 151 - Making all kinds of faces and imitating motions, gestures and voices of different animals.

He, 14-...thoughts of dying;...fear of wild animals and black dogs.

He, 81-...attempts to stab and bite;...with sexual excitement; fear as if a dog were attacking him;...

He, 94-...fear of malicious animals, black dogs; ...

He, 108-...spoke of lizards and worms being on his clothes,...

He, 114-...seeing rats and cats in room,...wanted a razor;...

He, 119 - His thoughts ran upon obscene things, frequently put his hands to erect penis; sought to bite or to catch flies.

SULPH. Al, 3780 - At night, very vivid anxious dreams, as if was pursued by wild beasts.

Al, 3816 - Frightful dream that he had been bitten by a dog.

TARENT. Al, 11 - Visions of monsters or animals, that frightened him.

THUJ. Al, 8 - At night, while lying awake with closed eyes, she seems to see ghosts, and also now and then all kinds of animals brilliantly illuminated, coming from her...

He, 10 - Fixed ideas: as if a strange person were at his side; as if soul and body were separated (split) ; that body, particularly limbs, are made of glass (frail) and will readily break (weakness); as if a living animal were in abdomen ;talks about being under the influence of a superior power. (possessed)

TUB. Al,N-27 - With every little ailment whines and complains; easily frightened, particularly by dogs; screams in terror when approached by a dog.

He, 2 - Fretful (irritable), ailing (sick), whines (moan) and complains; mind given to be frightened (fearful), particularly by dogs.

VALER. He, 4 - Erroneous ideas; thinks she is some one else,...; imagines animals lying near her which she fears she may hurt.

ANTAGONISM

Anarchist: ***arg-n.*** caust.[30] ***merc.***

Answer; refuses to: ***agar.*** ambr. ***arn.*** ars. ***atro.***[36] bac.[62] bell. calc-sil.[58] ***camph.*** caust. ***chin.*** chin-ar. ***cimic. hell. hyos.*** kali-acet.[58] led. lyss. med.[162] nux-m. nux-v. petr. ph-ac. **PHOS.** sabad. sec. ***stram. sul-ac.*** **SULPH.** tab.[36] tarent. ***verat. verat-v.***[54]

Antagonism; herself, with: acon. **ANAC.** anh.[144] ant-t.[54] aur. bar-c.[137] cann-i.[137] cann-s.[137] caps. irid.[5] ***kali-c.*** lac-c. ***lach.*** lyss. naja op.[5] paro-i.[149] ***sep.***[30] ***sil.***[30] verb.[54]

Aversion; handled, being: abrot.[127] cina[122] nat-m.[127] sep.[127]

Casting off of people against her will: **PLAT.**[36]

Conflict between higher consciousness and worldly existence: hydrog.[222]

Confusion of mind; muscles refuse to obey will, giddy: gels.[8]

Consolation; refuses, for ones own misfortune: nit-ac.[137]

Contemptuous; paroxysms against her will, in: ***plat.***

Contradict, disposition to: alum.[36] **ANAC.**[122] androc.[222] ***apis***[54] arg-n.[162] arn. ***ars.***[30] ***aur.*** aur-m.[36] bar-c.[30] cael.[149] camph. ***canth.*** caps.[5] **CAUST.**[122] ***cupr.***[30] ferr. ferr-ar.[58] grat. **HEP.** hyos. ictod. ign. **LACH.**[122] ***lyc.*** mag-c.[144] mag-s.[119] ***merc.***[122] nat-c. nicc. nit-ac. nux-v. ***olnd.*** ozone[227] ruta sep.[5] staph.[30] sulfonam.[149] sulph.[109] trom.[36] vip-a.[149]

Contradictory; actions are c. to intention: phos.[5] puls.[5] ruta[5] sep.[5] thuj.[5]

Contradictory; intentions are contradictory to speech: acon.[5] alum.[5] am-c.[5] caps.[5] chin.[5] ***lyc.***[5] nux-m.[5] rhus-t.[5] sep.[5]

Contrary: abrot.[116] acon. **ALUM.** alum-p.[58] alum-sil.[58] ambr. **ANAC.** anan. ant-c. ***ant-t.***[5] arag.[102] **ARG-N.** ***arn. ars.***[122] arum-t.[116] aur. aur-ar.[58] bar-c. bell. brom.[10] bry.[5] calad. calc. calc-caust.[10] calc-s. calc-sil.[58] camph. canth.[5] caps. carb-an. caust. **CHAM.**[5] chin.[116] cina[112] ***cocc.*** con. croc. cupr.[5] ferr-acet.[10] guai.[1] **HEP.**[122] hydr-ac.[10] ictod.[10] ign. ip. ***kali-c.*** kali-p. kali-sil.[58] kreos.[116] **LACH.**[30] lact. laur. led. lyc. mag-c. mag-m. ***merc. nit-ac. nux-v.*** olnd.[10] petr. phos. plb. ***puls.*** ruta[5] samb. sars. sep.[30] sil. spong. ***sulph.*** **TARENT.** ***thuj.*** trom. tub.[70] tub-k.[70] ***viol-t.***[5]

Contrary; parents, with: tub.[140]

Contrary; spiteful, just to be: tub.[162]

Delirium; well, declares she is: apis ***arn. ars.*** op.[58]

Delusions; double, he is, another self, there is, and he is not sure which will conquer the other: op.[139]

- opposed by everyone: mosch.[5]
- person; two personalities opposing to each other in himself, who are discussing their disease, there are: paro-i.[149]
- sleeping, while awake, insists that he was: acon. alco.[36] ant-t.[139] rhus-t.[139] ter.[139] visc.[139]
- well, he is: ***apis*** **ARN.** ars. bell.[10] cinnb. hyos. **IOD.** 5 kreos. merc. ***op.***[5] psil.[164] puls.
- wills, possessed of two: anac.[1] lach.[102]

Desires; nothing: ars.[36] cocc.[36] hell.[171] hep.[36]

linu-c.[36] mez.[36] mill.[36] nicc.[36] ***op.***[162] ph-ac.[8] phos.[8]

Desires; numerous, various things, opposed if offered by someone else: caps.[58]

Desires; numerous, various things, refused when offered: ant-t.[56] bry.[56] caps.[137] ***cham.***[10] ***cina***[56] dulc.[137] ferr.[171] hep.[137] ip.[102] kreos.[56] mang.[171] phos.[137] phys.[137] ***staph.***[8]

Desires; present, things not, rejected when offered, which are, playthings, etc.: arn.[5] bry.[160] **CHAM.**[5] ***cina***[54] ***dulc.***[54] hep.[36] kreos.[5] puls.[5] staph.[137]

Disunion with himself: aur.[54]

Dreams; opposite action, contrary to his intention, of: bamb-a.[1184]

➤ students do not obey: ozone[227]

Impulse; contradictory: ***anac.***[137]

Indifference; anosognosia, thinking that he is not ill: thala.[149]

Irritability; sends the, doctor home, says he is not sick: ***apis***[117] **ARN. CHAM.**

Obstinate; declares there is nothing the matter with him: apis **ARN.**

Obstinate; queerest objection, against whatever was proposed, he had the: **ARG-N.**

Obstinate; resists wishes of others: alum.[36] **NUX-V.**[54]

Quarrelsomeness; herself with: merc.[111]

Rage; medicine, from forcible administration of: ***bell.***[36]

Refuses; help: cina.[5]

Refuses; treatment, sick, in spite of being very: ars.[30] caust.[30] nux-v.[30]

Rejects everything offered to him: oena.[36] past.[36]

Seriousness; ludicrous things, when seeing: anac.

Shrieking; obstinate: ***cham.***[116]

Suggestions, will not receive: helon.

Sympathy; compassion, aversion to: ***arn.***[54] carb-ac.[25] cham.[54] sabal.[51] sep.[111]

Talk; himself, to, quarreling with some one, as if, seven p.m.: kali-cy.[36]

Thoughts; two trains of thoughts: acon. **ANAC.** anh.[144] ant-t.[54] aur. bar-c.[137] cann-i.[137] cann-s.[137] caps. irid.[5] ***kali-c.*** lac-c. ***lach.*** lyss. naja op.[5] paro-i.[149] ***sep.***[30] ***sil.***[30] verb.[54]

Undertakes; things opposed to his intentions: phos.[1] sep.

Unmanageable: aether[36] alco.[36] am-c.[1] atro.[36] bell.[36] petr.[36] stram.[36]

Well; fells very: aq-mar.[149] arist-cl.[144] ***ozone***[7]

Well; says he is, when very sick: androc.[222] ***apis*** **ARN.**[122] ars. atro.[36] bac.[62] bell.[10] ***cann-s.***[5] cinnb. ***coff.***[5] hyos. iod.[111] kreos. merc. op.[5] plb.[5] puls.[58] stram.[5] valer.[5]

Will; contradiction of: acon. **ANAC.** anh.[144] ant-t.[54] aq-mar.[231] aur. bar-c.[137] cann-i.[137] cann-s.[137] caps. irid.[5] ***kali-c.*** lac-c. ***lach.*** lyss. naja op.[5] paro-i.[149] sep. ***sil.***[30] verb.[54]

Will; muscles refuse to obey the w. when attention is turned away: ***hell.*** lil-t.[122]

Writing; different alphabets against his will, wrote in, changing from one subject to another: ***nux-m.***[54]

ACON. Al, 27 - Alternate attacks of opposite moral symptoms.

Al, 28 - Variable humour, at one time gay, at another dejected.

ADAM. Sh, 74 - Unbelievable poles, further than I've stretched to before.[16], 12C, 26:XX:XX

Sh, 75 - Feel like a square without corners.[16], 12C, 67:XX:XX

Sh, 106 - Things are very black and white for me. 7, 6C, 04:19:00

Sh, 244 - Anger with my attraction to P. He's a walker and I wanted to walk with him. I didn't want to be attracted but was, as if enchanted. 16, 12C, 18:XX:XX

Sh, 520 - Thoughts of creativity and destruction. One does not exist without the other. 16, 12C, 30:XX:XX

AGAR. Al, 37 - An impulse to laugh overcame him in bed, owing to an indescribably mixed sensation of happiness and misery.(duality)

ALUM. Al, 4 - The boy weeps constantly against his will, for half a hour.

Al, 31 - Is opposed to the wishes of other people.

Ha, 22 - She cannot see blood nor a knife without horrible thoughts pressing in upon her, as if she should, e. g. commit suicide; though she has the greatest horror of it.

He, 10 - Seeing blood on a knife, she has horrid ideas of killing herself, though she abhors the idea.

He, 11 - Crying, against his will.

ANAC. Ha, 25 - He is compelled to laugh, while engaged in very serious matters, ...;in laughable matters he can keep serious. (contrary)

Ha, 24 - He laughs, when he ought to be serious.
Ha, 17 - Passionate and contrary.
He, 67 - Contradiction between reason and will.
He, 68 - Feels as though he had two wills (intentions), one commanding to do what the other forbids.
He, 69 - In one ear a devil, in the other an angel, prompts (incite) him to do murder or acts of benevolence. (homicidal, x helpfulness, kindness)

ANDROC. Sh, 60 - Felt tense and absolutely alone, but sure that the rest of the world was mad, not her. She felt defiant with others and would not be manipulated. (7)
Sh, 167 - Pretended to feel well, although sick. (17)

ANT-T. He, 8 - Contradiction between mind and will.

ARG-N. He, 59 - Against whatever was proposed he had the queerest objections. 0 Melancholia.

ARN. Al, 23 - He is contradictory; nothing can be done to suit him.
Al, 28 - Obstinate and headstrong resistance to other people's opinions.
He, 18 - Says there is nothing the matter with him.

ARS. Al, 91-...she was afraid (fear) of solitude and death; the slightest cause was sufficient to put her into anger and rage, which especially occurred when one spoke of her complete recovery which she considered wholly impossible.
He, 103 - She became furious when something to eat was offered her while complaining of loss of appetite.
He, 22 - In her delirium she thinks she is well; girl, aet.7.

AUR. Ha, 20 - Discouraged (despair) and at odds (quarreling) with himself.(antagonism)
He, 10 - Imagines he cannot succeed (perform, prosper) in anything, (failure) and he does everything wrong; he is in disunion whith himself.

BAR-A. Al, 13 - He wavers for a long time between opposite resolutions.(irresolute, indecision)

BAR-C. Al, 16 - Great irresolution about small things; he wants to drink the cup of coffee, then again not, does not know what he shall do.
Ha, 13 - Long wavering between opposing resolutions.
Ha, 14 - During the day she determines to attend (take care) to some particular matter; but scarcely (just) has the time come, when she is sorry (give up) for it, and she knows not for irresolution what to do to leave undone.
He, 24 - Extremely contrary, irritable humor, passionate about trifles .

BELL. Ha, 1357 - Involuntary, almost loud laughter, without having any laughable thoughts.

CALC-A. Al, 10-...;he performed all his work with aversion and as if compelled (drive) to do so. (compulsive, obsessive)
Ha, 265-...very indifferent to the most important things; he did everything unwillingly (reluctant, averse) as if forced to do them.

CALC-P. He, 11 - Does not want to do what he has to do.

CALC. Ha, 40 - As soon he is idle (unoccupied) and sits still, he becomes peevish and drowsy (tired), and everything goes against him.

CAMPH. Ha, 343 - Quarrelsomeness, insists he is right.

CANN-I. Al, 40 - Had a feeling of duality. One of his minds would be thinking of something, while the other would laugh at it...

CANTH. He, 6 - Strange ideas crowd on him against his will.

CHAM. Ha, 461 - Lachrymose restlessness; the child wants this thing and the other, and when given anything he refuses it or knocks it away from him.
He, 44 - Morose fretfulness; everything that another does is wrong; no one does anything to please him.

CIC. Ha, 232 - When others were gay he was sad.

CINNB. Al, 1 - Illusion of mind; he considers himself well.

CROC. Al, 5 - If any one happens to sing a single musical note, she begins involuntarily to sing, and then is obliged to laugh at herself; she however, soon sings in spite of her determination to stop. (sympathy)
He, 12 - Vexation, contradicted by bursts of laughter.

FL-AC. Al, 15 - During the fourth week very

irritable towards people, even to the greatest hatred, which he does not hesitate to give vent to in words, but as soon as he sees them everything is forgotten, and he has an entirely different opinion of them.

GELS. He, 13 - Confusion; when attempting to move, the muscles refuse to obey the will; head giddy.

GERM. Sh, 153 - Thought nobody understood me and cared for what I felt. Felt it was unfair. I was presented with complaints about something others had done. Felt I was standing between two fighting parts. Felt awkward about it, embarrassed. Difficult to argue about such strong outburst. Thoughts about the day's arguing milling in my head all evening and night. 21, 12C, 32:XX.XX.

Sh, 81 - Wrote red instead of right. Said one word and understood another, husband said physician twice and twice I understood physicist. Talked about a patient who had a need for light and I thought photophobia. Wrote dylexist instead of dyslexic. Said amelioration occupates instead of occupation ameliorates. Quicked instead of quite. V Said nerve underneath sciatica instead of underneath thigh. 05, 6C, 02:XX:XX

GRAPH. Ha, 7 - Very much disposed to grieve and to weep, in the evening; while in the morning, contrary to her wont, she laughs (smile) at every trifle.

HALI-L. Sh, 141 - The drama was clear; the good guy and bad guys. During the proving, I realized it all leads to the same thing. Withdraw. Actingwatching. A Chosen separation. Zen state of watching and witnessing, but I could see how it could become sociopathic. My kids were fighting and I grabbed them and spanked them. Normally, I would be wracked with guilt. It was lovely to be a parent without guilt for awhile. 09, 9C, XX:XX:XX

Sh, 142 - Good guys and bad guys. Drama of evil is set up by the bad guys. They always win, always a struggle to just keep going. That is where I came from. During the proving, I saw that even engaging in that struggle gives it power and meaning. If you stop and watch the game, eventually there won't be anyone playing anymore. Good and bad were still positions, but it was all the same game. 09, 9C, XX:XX:XX

Sh, 144 - Woke feeling fearful, anxious and out of sorts. I thought of what motivates me to be good, and then the ugly feeling. I felt as if the good things were like a mirror to the other side. 08, 30C, 21:XX:XX

Sh, 410 - Feel as low now as I was high. An opposite. More serious. It's a little overbearing. It shouldn't be so serious. I have a place to go. Old issues looked upon detrimentally—maybe. Hard to dispel or find my place with them. Maybe I should lighten up a little. Issues are pressing, weighty. 18, 30C, 03:11:XX

Sh, 434 - Usually I enjoy my exercise; today it's going against what my will wants to do. The exercise practice equals life and health. I feel like going the opposite way. 06, 6C, 10:XX:XX

Sh, 435 - I was feeling very self-destructive. I wanted to do crappy things to myself. The border's breaking loose. I know I have a part of me that does this. It's just rising up. Screw it all, the futility of it all; the futility of working toward the positive, of caring for my health, of doing good things. What for? My big fear is that I'm really crazy, that I'm making all this up, that I'm just crazy (i.e., that the remedy is a placebo). 06, 6C, 11:XX:XX

Sh, 642 - I read prayers for safety before bed because I was afraid of what might happen when I went to sleep. When I came to the phrase "God is One" I realized that was the crux of it—the universe was cracked or split instead of one. Saying that prayer feels healing. Oneness is about caring; the split is about not caring. It's evil in a way. 06, 6C, 01:00:XX

Sh, 649 - Aware of being pulled in two different directions, as if being pulled by two elephants, two strong forces. 02, 30C, 06:XX:XX

Sh, 944 - Big doubts about doing Homeopathy. If you can make people healthy, then the balance must be that someone else gets sicker. 20, 30C, 15:XX:XX

HEP. Al, 19 - Contrary mood, he does not wish to see the members of his own family.

HYOS. Al, 48 - Laughed and said he was exceedingly well.

Al, 139 - He remembers persons and

occurrences which he does not try to recollect.

IGN. Al, 28 - Contrary to his will, thinks of vexatious and peevish things, and dwells upon them.

Ha, 791 - Thinks against his will of annoying, vexatious things, and dwells on them.

KALI-C. Ha, 31 - She is always in antagonism with herself; she knows not what she wants, and feels exceedingly unhappy.

Ha, 32 - Contrary disposition; he is self-willed (obstinate) and often does not know himself what he wishes. (indecision)

Ha, 33 - Contrary mood; she demands (order, command) impetuously; is not satisfied with anything (dissatisfied) ; she is beside herself, and furiously angry; if everything does not go according to her wishes, and often does not herself know what she really wants.

He, 9-...constantly in antagonism which herself; frequently hopeful, frequently despondent; frets (worry) about everything; peevish impatient, contented with nothing.

KALI-CY. Al, 3 - Had occasion to get angry, but could not; felt more like laughing instead.

Al, 5 - At 7 p.m., while walking out of doors, feelings of crossness; carries on a kind of conversation within himself, as if quarreling with someone whith whom he had previously disagreed; thinks what he will reply in case certain things are said to him.

KREOS. He, 4 - Thinks herself well. 0 Metritis

LACH. Al, 34 - So quarrelsome that he disputes with a mother about the age of her daughter, and affirms the younger to be the elder.

LYC. Al, 12 - If one looks at her to say anything serious she is obliged to laugh.

Al, 94 - Indolent, obstinate (inflexible), rebellious (revolutionary, dissident), passionate, wrathful. (angry)

Ha, 50 - He smiles without being merry, capricious.

LYSS. Al,N-12 - The majority of patients have no adequate conception of real origin of their malady, and affirm in decided terms that the scar is of no significance whatever and causes them no pain.

Al,N-64 - Disinclination to change position of head; two distinct trains of thought existing at one time in her mind, the idea that she was unable to move her head (when lying down) with the positive conviction that she has only to make up her mind that she will do it to achieve it.

He, 7 - Thoughts of something terrible going to happen come into his mind against his will; feels impelled to do reckless (impulsive, precipitated) things, such as throwing child, which he carries in his arms, through the window, and the like.

He, 64 - Disinclination to change position of head; two distinct trains of thought existing at one time in her mind, the idea that she is unable to move her head (when lying down) with the positive conviction that she has only to make up her mind that she will do it to achieve it.

MAG-C. Al, 933 - Dream that she has to marry one she did not like, which she violently resisted;...

MED. He, 20 - Is sure that she is worse, knows she is not going to live, cannot see any improvement, even when it is pointed out (antagonism); has no fear of death, speaks calmly about it, and gives directions as to the disposition of her affairs.

MERC. Al, 10 - Great seriousness, with much indifference all day; he was much offended if others laughed over a trifle, and yet was extremely indifferent to everything that took place about him.

NAJA. Al, 13-...I felt that everything that was done was done in a wrong way, and could not be rectified (corrected, revised); if I felt that I had some duty to perform (execute), I had at the same time a strong impulse not to do it, and I am extremely restless in consequence; I seemed to have an increased perception of what I ought to do, but, at the same time, an unaccountable inclination not to do it, to which I was irresistibly compelled to yield "I couldn't help it, didn't know why, but couldn't do it."

NAT-M. Al, 12 - She laughed so immoderately at something not ludicrous, that she could not be quieted, and tears come into her eyes, so that she looked as though she had been weeping.

NICC. Al, 1 - Very angry and quarrelsome mood; she was inclined to quarrel with and contradict everyone, in the evening.

NIT-AC. Al, 43 - She wishes for death and yet dreads it.

Ha, 27 - She wishes to die, and nevertheless she is afraid of death.

NUX-M. Al, 31 - The words he employed to express his sensations remarkable for the merit of being the opposite (contrary) to what he should have used;...

Al, 56-...he went to the theater, which was at some distance; the way seemed to have no end (endless, interminable); ... Although he was, at times, quite unconscious, his limbs did not fail to their service; he went straight on, without recognizing the streets that crossed his way; he was concerned about the time, he feared to come too late..., fancy and reality battle (fight) with each other.

Al, 30 - While writing he omitted letters, wrote in different alphabets against his will and changed from one subject to another.

He, 14 - While writing he omitted letters, wrote in different alphabets against his will, and changed from one subject to another.

He, 24 - Fitful mood, changing from deepest sorrow to most frolicsome (happy) behavior; now grave (serious), now gay.

NUX-V. Ha, 1269 - He obstinately opposes what others wish.

He, 21 - Anxiety with irritability and inclination to commit suicide, but is afraid to die.

He, 16 - Ill-humored, resists obstinately the wishes of others.

OP. Al, 36 - Mind in a state of great confusion; at one moment she was sensible (conscious) to her crime, called for assistance (comfort, aid, help) ; at another she resisted the means used to save her.

Al, 37 - Conscious of being possessed (seized) of two persons (double) of another self besides his real self, the Opium man does things which the real self considers wrong, and it is not always sure which will conquer the other.

PHOS. Ha, 78 - She has to laugh against her will, while she is sad.

PLAT. Al, 11 - Contemptuous, pitiful looking down upon people usually venerated, with a kind of casting (reject, discard) them off in paroxysms, against her will.

Ha, 36 - Contemptuous, pitying looking down on people at other times respected, with a certain disdain (scorn, arrogance), in paroxysms, against her will. (antagonism)

He, 11 - Contemptuous, pitiful, looking down upon people usually venerated, with a kind of casting (forsakes) them off, in paroxysms against her will.

PSOR. Al, 14 - Very melancholy and despairing; he wishes to die in spite of his good luck.

PULS. Al, 10 - Everything disgusts him; he seems averse to everything.

Ha, 1147 - Inattention, acts with precipitancy (hurry), does something different to what he wished to do.

RHUS-T. He, 18 - Disgust of life: thoughts of suicide; wants to drown (immerse) himself; with fear of death: with desire to die, without sadness.

SEP. Al, 96 - He thinks of things which he does not think of, uses expressions which he knows are incorrect, undertakes those things which are opposed to his intentions, and finds such contradictions with himself that it puts him in a very uncomfortable and uneasy mood.

Ha, 68 - He thinks, what he does not wish to think, uses expressions which he himself knows are incorrect; he resolves to do what is against his intention, and is thus in conflict with himself and, therefore in a disagreeable, restless mood. (lost: knowledge, correction)

Ha, 44 - She finds fault with everything, does not wish what others desire; with weeping ...

He, 31 - Contradictory, quarrelsome, complaining about others.

SULPH. Ha, 43 - Ill-humored; she becomes vexed at herself.

TARENT. Al, 65-... Great fear of an imaginary impending calamity (cataclysm, catastrophe) great desire of be alone, fear of being alone...

THUJ. Al, 67 - Sudden unaccountable (strange) anxiety in the head, which against her will, compels her to call some one.

Al, 90 - Excited mood; he is irritable, especially if any one says anything of which he does not exactly approve.

ANTICIPATION

Ailments from; anticipation, foreboding, presentment: ***acon.***[5] aesc.[5] aeth.[122] agn.[5] alum.[116] am-c.[5] ambr.[1189] ***anac.***[122] androc.[222] apis[5] **ARG-N.**[122] arist-cl.[144] **ARS.**[122] aur.[163] bamb-a.[1184] ***bar-c.***[116] bell.[163] bry.[122] **CALC.**[5] ***calc-p.***[163] calc-s.[108] camph.[122] cann-i.[163] canth.[10] carb-v.[5] **CARC.**[122] **CAUST.**[5] cench.[58] chin.[5] chin-s.[137] chlorpr.[149] ***cic.***[122] ***cocc.***[122] coff.[122] crot-h.[36] ***cupr.***[54] dig.[116] dys-co.[136] ***elaps***[117] epip.[85] ferr-p.[163] fl-ac.[122] **GELS.**[54] **GRAPH.**[122] hyos.[122] **IGN.**[122] ***iod.***[163] ***kali-acet.***[163] kali-br.[122] kali-c.[5] kali-i.[163] ***kali-p.***[54] ***lac-c.***[54] lach.[5] lec.[163] levo.[149] **LYC.**[122] lyss.[122] **MED.**[122] merc.[122] **MEZ.**[122] mosch.[10] mur-ac.[163] naja[5] ***nat-c.***[54] nat-m.[5] nat-p.[163] nux-v.[122] ox-ac.[116] ozone[227] petr.[122] ***ph-ac.***[122] phos.[5] plat.[163] plb.[5] **PSOR.**[5] **PULS.**[54] rhus-t.[116] ***sec.***[163] sep.[5] sil.[5] spig.[5] spong.[163] staph.[122] still.[54] ***stram.***[5] stront-c.[122] stroph.[144] sul-ac.[184] sulph.[163] syc-co.[136] thuj.[122] ***tub.***[163] verat.[5] visc.[163]

Ailments from; anticipation, stage-fright: acon.[163] anac.[102] arg-n.[102] ***ars.***[163] bor.[163] calad.[163] calc-p.[163] carb-v.[163] carc.[207] cina[153] coff.[163] crot-c.[163] crot-h.[163] ***cypr.***[163] ***gels.***[102] hyos.[163] ign.[163] ***kali-br.***[163] kali-p.[163] lach.[30] ***lyc.***[163] lyss.[163] ***med.***[163] ***merc.***[163] nat-m.[163] nat-p.[163] nat-s.[163] ox-ac.[163] petr.[163] ***ph-ac.***[163] ***pic-ac.***[163] plb.[163] psor.[163] puls.[163] sep.[163] ***sil.***[163] ***stroph.***[163] sulph.[163] syph.[163] ***thuj.***[163] tub.[163] ***zinc.***[163]

Ailments from; anticipation, stage-fright singers and speakers, in: arg-n.[155] **GELS.**[54]

Anticipation: ***acon.***[10] aeth.[122] ambr.[1189] ***anac.***[122] androc.[222] **ARG-N.**[122] **ARS.**[122] bry.[122] **CALC.**[122] camph.[122] ***carb-v.***[122] **CARC.**[122] ***caust.***[122] ***cic.***[122] ***cocc.***[122] coff.[122] cupr.[210] **GELS.**[122] hydrog.[222] hyos.[122] **IGN.**[122] ***lac-c.***[122] lap-mar-c.[194] **LYC.**[122] lyss.[122] **MED.**[122] merc.[122] nat-c.[122] nat-m.[111] nux-v.[122] petr.[122] ***ph-ac.***[122] **PHOS.**[122] **PLB.**[122] **PSOR.**[122] **PULS.**[122] **SIL.**[122] staph.[122] still.[122] stront-c.[122] thuj.[122] verat.[122]

Anticipation; dentist, physician, before going to: calc.[122] ***gels.***[122] mag-c.[144] ***phos.***[122] ***tub.***[122]

Anticipation; examination, before: ***aeth.***[122] anac.[85] arg-n.[127] carb-v.[137] carc.[207] cupr.[122] ***gels.***[122] hydrog.[222] nux-v.[122] pic-ac.[122] sil.[58] thuj.[137]

Anticipation; impending evil, sensation of: merc.[137]

Anticipation; matters, for, before they occur, and generally correctly: ***med.***[54]

Anxiety; anticipating: aur. canth.[10] carc.[187] choc.[222] dros.[172] dys-co.[136] ***ferr.***[54] levo.[149] mosch.[10]

Anxiety; anticipating, an engagement: <u>**ARG-N.**</u>[122] ***ars.***[162] ***carb-v.***[162] carc.[207] **GELS.**[122] hydrog.[222] ***lyc.*** ***lyss.***[162] <u>**MED.**</u>[122] **NAT-M.**[162] ph-ac.[162] ***sil.***[162] ***thuj.***[162]

Anxiety; anticipating, relatives, for his: carc.[193]

Anxiety; present, about: arn.[144] calc-acet.[36] ***con.***[30] iod.[38]

Anxiety; time is set, if a: alum.[162] ***arg-n.*** gels. med.

Death; presentiment of: **ACON.** aesc.[162] ***agn.*** aloe alum. alum-p.[58] anac. ***anthr.***[54] **APIS** ***arg-n.*** arn. ***ars.***[122] bapt. bar-m. **BELL.**[122] bry. ***cact.***[54] calc. cann-i. canth. carb-v.[58] ***cench.*** ***chel.*** cimic. cupr. dig.[36] ferr-br.[85] gels.[85] ***graph.*** hell.[36] ***hep.*** **HYDR.**[8] kali-ar. kali-br.[25] kali-c. kali-n. lac-d. ***lach.*** lob.[10] ***lyc.*** lyss.[54] ***med.*** **MERC.**[122] mosch. nat-m. ***nit-ac.*** ***nux-v.*** petr. ***phase.***[54] ***phos.*** ***plat.*** podo. ***psor.***[8] puls. ***raph.***[10] rhus-t. sep. staph. stram. sul-ac.[36] sulph.[122] tab.[10] thea.[122] verat. vip. zinc. zinc-p.[58]

Death; presentment of, alternating with, anguish: raph.[54]

Death; presentment of, near, seems, and must settle affairs: petr.[137]

Death; presentment of, soon, believes that she will die, and cannot be helped: ***agn.***

Death; presentment of, sudden death, of a: ***cench.***[122]

Death; thoughts of: **ACON.** agn. aloe[5] am-c. ***apis*** arg-n.[162] arn.[122] ***ars.*** ars-h.[54] aur.[116] aur-m.[162] camph. cann-i. carb-an. caust. ***cham.***[54] chel. clem.[36] ***coff.***[5] ***con.***[122] cortico.[119] cortiso.[119] ***crot-c.*** ***crot-h.*** cupr. ***dig.***[5] ferr. ferr-ar. **GRAPH.** hist.[119] hura hydrog.[222] kali-ar. kali-c. lac-d.[58] ***lach.***[54] lat-m.[119] ***lob.***[5] merc.[5] nux-v.[1] op. ozone[227] phos.[162] plat.[5] ***psor.*** ***puls.***[54] rauw.[119] rhus-t.[10] rob. spong.[10] stram. tarent. thuj.[36] verat. verat-v.[5] vinc.[10] ***zinc.***[122]

Delusions; clock, hears strike of: ph-ac.

Dreams; events, not yet taken place: hydrog.[222] mang. ***sulph.***

Excitement; anticipating events, when: ***arg-n. gels.*** hydrog.[222] kali-br. med.
Forebodings: ***acon.***[5] aesc.[5] agar.[1] agn.[5] alum.[37] am-c.[5] apis[5] ***arg.***[5] ars.[5] **CALC.**[5] carb-v.[5] **CAUST.**[5] cench.[58] chin.[5] ***cimic.***[111] ***dros.***[8] ***elaps***[5] ***ferr.***[8] ***gels.***[5] kali-c.[5] lach.[5] ***lyc.***[5] med.[5] nabal.[36] naja[5] ***nat-m.***[8] nat-p.[36] phos.[5] plb.[5] **PSOR.**[5] sep.[5] sil.[5] spig.[5] ***still.***[36] ***stram.***[5] tab.[85] verat.[5]
Intuitive: acon.[30] cann-i.[36] 0olnd.[30]
Intuitive; weakness of others, to: sep.[187]
Rage; alternating with, presentiment of death: stram.[54]
Sadness; disease, about, sure he, is going to die in twenty four hours: lac-d.[54]

AESC. Al, 9-...he had a feeling as if death was impending (imminent); but this was followed by an exalted condition of brain and nervous system...
AGAR. Ha, 3 - Anxious forebodings (anticipation), as if she were about to experience something disagreeable.
AGN. He, 3 - Low spirited, fears of approaching death.
ALOE. He, 2 - She knew she would die in a week. (predicts, death)
AM-C. Ha, 7 - Sad, dejected, feeling as if a misfortune was imminent,..
He, 5 - Gloomy, depressed, with feeling of impending trouble,...
AML-N. Al, 1 - Anxiety, as if something might happen; must have fresh air.
ANAC. Ha, 3 - Anxiety and apprehension in the evening, after cheerfulness during the day.
He, 57 - Apprehensive (fear) of death being close at hand.
ANG. Al, 14-...internal uneasiness, such as is experienced by those who anticipate some great pleasure, or also owing to all sorts of plans crowding upon his mind.
ANTH. Al, 4 - Feeling as if something was about to happen to him.
ANTHR. He, 5 - Thinks she feels death approaching.
APIS. Al, 15 - She thought she must die, she felt so strangely.(strange)
He, 20 - Anticipation (intuition) of death.
ARG-N. He, 27 - If a time is set, becomes uneasy the day before; is worried and ready long before the time.(anticipation)
ARN. He, 32 - Despondency and conviction of approaching death.
ARS. He, 8 - Gloomy (dark) forebodings (premonition) while lying in bed, in evening, fears something may have happened to his relatives.
BAR-A. Al, 10 - An evil, fearful suspicion suddenly takes possession of her, as if, for example, a loved friend had been taken suddenly deathly ill.
BAR-C. Ha, 7 - An evil fearful foreboding comes suddenly upon his soul, as if, e.g. a beloved friend might suddenly have fallen fatally ill.
BELL. Al, 167 - Events which had been previously anticipated with pleasure appeared to him in an anxious light; he thought them fearful and dreadful.
BRY. He, 29 - Fear of death, which he thinks is near.
CALC-A. Ha, 264 - Very sad humor, as if he had to expect (anticipation) bad news.
CALC. Al, 18 - Despairing mood, with dread of disease and suffering, with foreboding of sad events.
Ha, 23 - Fearful, anxious forebodings, as if evil would befall (happen) him or some one else, and as if he could in no way evade it.
Ha, 29 - Despairing (hopeless) mood with fear of sickness (disease) and misery, with forebodings of sad events. (misfortune)
CANN-I. He, 25 - Great apprehension of approaching (imminent) death.
CANTH. Al, 29 - Anxiety in the morning, as if he expected something very important.
CAST. Al, 2 - Very melancholy and depressed, as if something evil would befall her, in the afternoon.
CAUST. Al, 12 - Anxiety the whole day, as if he had done something bad, or apprehended it, or as if he had been unfortunate (unsuccessful, umprosperous).
Al, 26 - He was busy with thoughts of death, with uneasiness and great solicitude.
Ha, 7 - Anxious, restlessness mood, as if something disagreeable (difficult) was impending (imminent), which keeps him from working.
Ha, 14 - Great apprehensions (forebodings) as to whatever happens.
He, 42 - Great apprehension whenever anything happens; despondent, depressed, most excessive exhaustion and prostration.

CHAM. Al, 15 - Very depressed mood, with anxiety and oppression, as of impending evil.

CHIN-S. Al, 16 - Great anxiety, amounting to an apprehension, as if some evil would happen.

DIRC. Al, 3 - Sense of apprehension, throughout the proving, as of some trouble, which may have depended upon the morbid state of the mind at the same time of the proving.

FERR. He, 8 - Mental depression, gloomy (dark) foreboding thoughts.

GELS. He, 32 - Complaints: (ailments) from exciting or bad news; sudden emotions; the anticipation of any unusual ordeal (difficulty) ; general depression from heat of sun or summer.

GRAPH. Ha, 20 - He often feels as if his end was near (death), or as if the greatest misfortune impended over him.

HELL. Ha, 278 - Restless and anxious, as if anticipating misfortune.

IGN. He, 39 - Anxiety and disquiet as if she had done something wrong, or as if some great misfortune were about to happen, this so overpowers her that she can with difficulty refrain from weeping;...

KALI-C. Al, 15 - At night after lying down, sad forebodings overtake him, on account of which he is unable to sleep.

Al, 13 - He has anxious presentiments, in the evening.

KALI-I. Al, 11 - Very apprehensive and lachrymose, as if some evil were impending, ...

KALI-P. He, 5 - Anxiety, nervous dread without special cause, gloomy moods, fancies, taking dark views of things, dark forebodings.

LACH. Al, 19 - So great apprehensiveness while riding in the open air that it seemed to him some great evil (hurtful, injurious) was impending (imminent), like an evil foreboding; it torments him for more than an hour.

MAG-C. Al, 13 - Tremulous anxiety and fright, as if she apprehended some misfortune, disappearing in the evening in bed.

MANG. Ha, 2 - Constant restlessness, as if he apprehended some sad news.

MED. Al,N-50 - It is always anticipating, fearing evil will happen, loss of reason or suicide.

He, 29 - Is always anticipating; feels most matters sensitively before they occur and generally correctly. (predicts)

He, 30 - Anticipates death. (predicts)

MEZ. Al, 20 - Apprehensiveness in the pit of the stomach, as though expecting something disagreeable.

MOSCH. He, 1 - Great anxiety with palpitation of heart; feeling of anxious expectancy.(anticipation)

MUR-AC. Ha, 269 - Sunk in profound thought, as if something disagreeable were about to happen,...

NAT-C. Ha, 8 - Apprehensive and ennui (tedium, monotony), so that she cannot contain herself; she deems (believe), herself altogether (entirely) lonely (solitary) and forsaken.

He, 13 - Constant fear and forebodings.

NAT-M. He, 32 - Apprehension, feels as if something was going to happen.

He, 33 - Brain fag (weakness), with sleeplessness, gloomy (dark) forebodings, exhaustion after talking, embarrassment (confusion) of brain.

He, 5 - Haunted with thoughts that something unpleasant will happen.

NIT-AC. He, 5 - Fancies she will die soon, yet is not physically ill.

PHOS. Al, 71 - Filled whith gloomy forebodings.

Ha, 21 - Apprehensiveness, like the foreboding (anticipation) of misfortune.

Ha, 59 - When he thinks of anything disagreeable, he is seized with a sort of apprehension, felt most in the scrobiculus cordis.

He, 19 - Weary of life; full of gloomy (dark) forebodings.

PLAT. Ha, 9 - Sensation as if she would have to die soon (immediately), with horror at the thought.

Ha, 11 - Great restlessness of mind, so that she knows not where to stay (indecision), with gloominess (melancholy) which spoils even what should be most enjoyable; she imagines she is not fit (unfit, incapable) for this world, is tired (weary) of life, but has a great horror of the death she believes to be approaching.

PSOR. Al, 8 - Full of forebodings very restless, with trembling of the hands.

Al,N-14 - Anxious, full of fear, melancholic; evil forebodings.

He, 13 - Anxious, full of fear, melancholic; evil forebodings.
PTEL. Al, 2 - Depression of spirits, and a feeling of anxiety about some unknown thing, with the severe headache, in the afternoon.
PULS. He, 42-...full of anxiety, forebodings of impending (imminent, destined) disaster; ...
SEC. Al,N-18 - Anticipated misfortunes, as though about to lose something of great value.(estimate)
SEP. Al, [illegible] - Dark forebodings about his disease in regard to the future.
SPIG. Al, 8 - Anxious forebodings, therewith inclination to a peevish indolent mood.
Ha, 659 - Anxious forebodings (premonition) about the future,...
SPONG. Ha, 382 - Anxious as if misfortune (disaster) threatened (endangered) him and he had a foreboding of it.
He, 25 - He is anxious as if some misfortune would occur of which he has a presentiment.
STRAM. Al, 207 - His whole conduct and countenance was like that of a child severely frightened and apprehending some terrible calamity.
SULPH. Al, 45 - Anxious disposition I could not free myself from the anticipation of some great misfortune, though I had no ground for such fear,...
THUJ. Al, 49 - Sudden rising of dark thoughts (pessimism) causing uneasiness, apprehension (foreboding) of misfortune, with fancied scruples of conscience, ...
Al, 59 - Presentiment of death.
VERAT. Ha, 691 - Anxiety as though he anticipated (expected) misfortune, as if threatened with some calamity.(disaster)

APPROACHED

Ailments from; approach of persons: **ARN.**[5] bry.[162] con.[5] cupr.[210] ign.[5] lyc.[5] op.[56] phos.[162] stry.[5]
Anger; approach of a person, on: cham.[109]
Anxiety; stomach, people, on approach of: lyc.
Anxiety; trifles, about, things coming near him, especially of: ***ign.***[54]
Aversion; approached, of being: arn.[162] aur. bry.[162] caj. canth.[85] cina[83] hell. helon. hipp. ***iod.*** lil-t. ***lyc.***[122] sanic.[85] sulph.
Delirium; anxious, approaching him, of everyone, shrinking from them: ***cupr.***[54]
Delirium; lively active, vivid, alternates in short periods with horrified fright, seeming to dread approach of some monster, appealing for help: stram.[54]
Delusions; death approaching: agn.[85] ***plat.***[54]
• hearing, of, someone approaches his bed: carb-v.[54]
• people, coming out of corners: ***stram.***[54]
Dreams; animals, dogs, mangy dog approaching her, covered with sores, she takes hold of it and it bites her: paull-p.[36]
➤ ghosts, shadow, a, approaching her: ozone[227]
Fear; approaching, of others: acet-ac. ***ambr.*** anac. ant-c.[162] **ARN.**[122] ars.[172] bar-c.[5] ***bell.*** cadm-s. cann-i. caust.[5] cham.[162] con. ***cupr.*** ***cupr-acet.***[54] graph.[146] ***ign.*** iod. ***lyc.*** nux-v.[54] op. petr.[5] phos.[5] plb.[111] rhod.[122] sep.[5] ***stram.*** stry.[5] tarent.[5] ***thuj.*** valer.[172]
✦ approaching, others, of, children cannot bear to have anyone come near them: ambr.[172] ant-c.[162] arn.[172] bell.[172] ***cina cupr.*** ign.[172] kali-c.[172] lach.[172] stram.[172] thuj.[172]
✦ approaching, others, of, delirium, in: cupr. stram. ***thuj.***
✦ approaching, others, of, starting, with: ***bell.***[54]
✦ approaching, others, of, touched, lest he be: **ARN.**[122] ars.[172] chin.[172] coff.[172] colch.[5] kali-c.[172] lach.[172] mag-p.[172] rhod.[122] stram.[172] tell.[172] valer.[172]
✦ approaching, vehicles, of: anth. hydr-ac. lyss.[122] phos.
✦ injured, of being, persons walking towards him, by: arn.[54]
✦ jostling against everyone she meets, during pregnancy: ***acon.***[54]
✦ people, standing near: bell. germ.[222]
✦ struck by those coming toward him, of being, walking behind him, by those: alum.[122]
✦ struck by those coming towards him, of being: **ARN.**[54] bell.[36] ign.[36] kali-c.[36] lach.[36] stram.[36] thuj.[36]
Kill; threatens to k., approach, those who: meli.[85]
Rage; women, approaching, in a woman: raph.[36]
Shrieking; approaches the bed, when anyone: ***ign.***[54]
Starting; fright, from and as from, approach of a person, at: ***bell.***[54]

ARN. He, 34 - Fears being struck (hit, hurt) by those coming towards him; fears even the possibility of being touched.

BELL. Al, 166 - He starts in affright very readily, especially when any one approaches him.

He, 102 - Became fearful when persons approached him in street, and when they had passed, he insisted on it that he had stabbed them.

CARB-V. Ha, 679 - In the evening, during sleep, deception of the hearing; he thought he heard some one approach his bed, this woke him up with anxiety.

CON. Al, 39 - Dread (fear) of men of their approach, yet with dread of being alone.

Ha, 9 - Shyness (timidity) at the approach of people, and yet also dread of being alone.

Ha, 10 - The propinquity (proximity) and the talk of people passing by is very offensive to him, and he feels impelled to assault and maltreat them.

CUPR-A. He, 16 - Afraid of everyone who approaches him, shrinking away from them.

CUPR. He, 5 - Delirium: afraid of every one who approached him, shrinking (retire) away from them; tries to escape; in evening and in the dark.

He, 21 - Afraid of and shrinking away from everyone who approaches him; afraid of falling; clinging tightly to nurse;...

GERM. Sh, 134 - Felt uncomfortable if any one stood close to me. Felt uneasy and paranoid in class. Feel as if done something wrong. 10, 9C, 06:06:00

HYDR-AC. He, 3 - Could not remain in middle of road when he saw a vehicle approaching him even at a considerable distance,... (run over)

IGN. Ha, 762 - Fears every trifle, is specially afraid of objects coming near him.

He, 33 - Dread of every trifle, especially of things coming near him.

KALI-BR. He, 39-...fear and apprehension that she is losing her mind (insanity);...makes her utterly (completely) miserable to be looked at or spoken to; fear to see people; always depressed and lowspirited;...

LYC. Al, 40 - If people come near her, she is immediately attacked with anxiety at the pit of the stomach.

Ha, 8 - When other persons come too near her she feels anguish in the scrobiculus cordis.

LYSS. He, 40 - A strong and uncontrollable impulse to do certain acts; to spring at and to bite any moving object that came within reach; ...

OP. Ha, 638 - He chattered all sorts of unconnected stuff and pointed with his fingers to imaginary masked people approaching him; ...he started at imaginary swordsmen, who might kill him ; ...

He, 12 - Said many disconnected things and pointed to masked people who seemed to approach him.

PH-AC. Ha, 41 - Illusion of the senses, as if he heard the clock strike or as if lofty (tall, elevated) things lying out of his horizon were moving near him.

PLAT. Ha, 18 - Taciturnity and involuntary weeping, even after the most friendly address (communication), so that she gets vexed (anger) about it herself.

RAPH. Al, 1 - Feeling of aversion towards all women; she is provoked by seeing women going and coming about her; their approach threw her into a fury; the mere contact with a woman's dress caused intolerable distress;...She is attracted to all men without distinction (nymphomania) ; when she gives her hand to a man, she feels great agitation,...When left alone for a hour in the evening, she gave herself a very deep wound in the lips with a penknife, in hopes to put an end to this condition (hurt, punishes). Moral feeling was completely extinct, the physical nature alone ruled and threw her into a frightful state (wild). From morning to noon she would not have been able to resist the advances even of a man for whom she had not the least friendly feeling; from noon to 6 p.m. she could not have held out against any man whatsoever; from 8 to 11 the demands of sense were so importunate as to silence the voice of shame and reason; ... and would have thrown herself into the arms of the first man she met...she was still unable to control her impulses;...

STRAM. Al, 136 - Delirium...seeming to

dread the approach of some imaginary monster, and giving utterance in the most piteous appeals for help, protection.
Ha, 551 - She sometimes cries out about cats, dogs and rabbits, which were approaching (pursuing) her from above, from the side and from the middle of the room.
He, 163 - Cries out fearfully, hides face in pillow, is terrified by presence or approach of physician; after attack of typhoid.
He, 51-...converses with spirits who approach his bed, lays hold of a stick and strikes about him,...great sexual excitement.
He, 85-...seemed to dread approach of some imaginary monster, and giving utterance to most piteous appeals for help.
SULPH. Ha, 53 - He is so peevish and obstinate, that he will not give an answer to anybody, he cannot bear to have anyone around him, and cannot get quickly enough what he wants.
THUJ. He, 13 - Nervousness to such a degree that approach of a stranger gave her sudden twitches...
He, 12 - Insane women will not be touched or approached.
TUB. Al,N-27 - With every little ailment whines and complains; easily frightened, particularly by dogs; screams in terror when approached by a dog.

ATTACKED

Ailments from; sexual, abuse, raped, being: acon.[185] caust.[185] foll.[1201] ign.[185] sep.[185] staph.[185]
Anxiety; injury, as from a, received in sleep, morning on waking: plat.[36]
Anxiety; walking, while, people behind him might beat him, as if: alum.[122]
Aversion; approached, of being: arn.[162] aur. bry.[162] caj. canth.[85] cina[83] hell. helon. hipp. ***iod.*** lil-t. ***lyc.***[122] sanic.[85] sulph.
Complaining; injury, of supposed: ***hyos.***
Delirium; anxious, dog were attacking her, as if: **STRAM.**[54]
Delirium; lively active, vivid, alternates in short periods with horrified fright, seeming to dread approach of some monster, appealing for help: stram.[54]
Delusions; animals, dogs, attack him: **STRAM.**
• animals, dogs, near, that bit her, fought as if to drive it away: lyss.[54]
• animals, jumping at her: ***merc.***[122]
• animals, running, large, up the legs, feels: ail.[58] ***calc.***[122]
• animals, snakes, crimson, or, fastening around his neck: bell.
• attacks and insults, defend themselves against imaginary: lyss.[54].
• beaten, he is being: bry.[10] elaps
• bitten, will be: ***hyos.***[10] stram.[5]
• blown at, of being, by persons, some of whom are not present: lyss.[54]
• cut through, he is: ***stram.***
• cut, two, in: ***bell.***[30] plat. stram.[30]
• devoured, of being: cand-a.[239] ***stram.***[10]
• enemy, wait for an, lying in: alco.[36]
• figures, large black, about to jump on him: mosch.
• hand, visions of white, outspread h. coming toward face in the darkness: benz.
• injury, injured, is being: bry. cact. canth. elaps kali-br. lach. lyss. naja[54] phos. rhus-t. stram. sulph.
• injury, injured, sleep, during: plat.[36].
• injury, injured, surroundings, by his: **HYOS.**[122] ***lach. naja***[117]
• injury, receive, will: ars. bell.[58] cann-i. carbn-s. con. hyos.[122] lach. lyc. merc. nux-v. ***op.***[54] sil. stram. sulph.
• injury, receive, will, friends, from: lach.[58]
• jumped upon the ground before her, all sorts of things: brom. ther.[137]
• man, muffled, starts from the wall when walking in the streets: cann-i.
• man, room, in the, intending to perforate his throat with a gimlet: merc-i-f.
• rowdies, brawlers, will break in if she is alone: elaps.[139]
• soldier, sees, cutting him down (amel. on getting cool): bry.
• visions, eyes anxiously fixed sideways on one point where she imagines she sees a terrible hostile figure: ***stram.***[54]
Dreams; abused, being; too weak to defend himself: ambr.[36]
➤ animals, bat flying in room, causing fear: ham.[36]
➤ animals, biting him: am-m. bov.[10] calc.[10] cench.[58] daph. elaps[136] m-aust.[10] merc. nicc.[10] ***phos.*** puls. sulph.[10] verat.[10] zinc.[10]
➤ animals, bugs, enormous, attacking his head, which he killed one by one: myric.[36]
➤ animals, cats, springing at him: hyos.[36]

➤ animals, horses, running, over her: lipp.[36]
➤ animals, spiders, hairy, very, which tried to climb on him: crot-c.[36]
➤ beaten, being: kali-c.[36] kali-n.[58] nat-m.[1]
➤ bitten, arms, into the: am-m.[10] m-aust.[10] nicc.[10]
➤ body, back, burnt, hot roast pigeons thrown at her: mag-c.[36]
➤ body, muscles pierced with arrows: bomb-pr.[36]
➤ bombs: cand-a.[239]
➤ cutting, knife, of being cut with a: frax.[36] guai. nat-s.[36]
➤ dead, bodies, sprang from dissecting table and seized throat: chel.[36]
➤ ill-treatment: ambr.[10] dros.[10]
➤ injuries: allox.[119] am-m. ant-c. cench.[58] chel.[36] chin. choc.[222] cortico.[119] lob.[54] ***mag-s.***[10] nat-s. nicc.[10] phos. sumb.
➤ pursued, man, red skinned, to harm her with his arrows: pitu-a.[164]
➤ radioactivity: ozone[227]
➤ torpedo, of: ozone[227]
➤ wounded, of being: ant-c. chel.[36] lob.[54] ***mag-s.***[10]

Fear; animals, dogs, attacking him, in delirium: **STRAM.**[54]
✦ animals, dogs, of: androc.[222] **BAC.**[62] **BELL.**[122] bufo[179] calc.[30] carc.[193] ***caust.*** **CHIN.** choc.[222] ***hyos.*** lyss.[122] med.[212] nat-m.[162] nat-p.[166] plat.[40] ***puls.***[162] sil.[171] ***stram.*** syc-co.[136] ***tub.*** tub-k.[70] verat.[172]
✦ animals, insects, of: abel.[149] bufo[36] **CALC.**[162] calc-ar.[162] cimic.[162] lyc.[162] nat-m.[162] nat-p.[166] phos.[162] puls.[212] sulph.[212]
✦ animals, rats, of: absin.[172] bell.[172] calc.[172] cimic.[137] op.[172] phos.[172] sep.[172]
✦ animals, snakes, of: abel.[149] arg-n.[172] bell.[162] calc.[183] calc-s.[196] carc.[207] elaps[152] hep.[162] ign.[187] lac-c.[162] ***lach.***[122] nat-m.[212] puls.[212] ruta[152] sep.[172] spig.[162] sulph.[162] syph.[162]
✦ animals, spiders, of: abel.[149] calc.[162] carc.[210] lac-c.[185] mag-m.[166] nat-m.[162] phos.[155] stram.[172] tarent.[185]
✦ attacked, of being: carc.[207] ***stram.***[1]
✦ death, noise of door moving, from, in dark: ozone[227]
✦ door, opening the: cic.[111] con.[111] lyc.[111]
✦ injured, of being, persons walking towards him, by: arn.[54]
✦ people, standing near: bell. germ.[222]
✦ raids, of air: acon.[172] arn.[172] cham.[172] ign.[172] nat-m.[172]
✦ struck by those coming towards him, of being: **ARN.**[54] bell.[36] ign.[36] kali-c.[36] lach.[36] stram.[36] thuj.[36]

Hide; desire to, fear, assaulted, of being: tarent.[58]

ANDROC. Sh, 80 - On occasions experienced fear, especially of being attacked in the street. (1)

ARN. He, 34 - Fears being struck (hit, hurt) by those coming towards him; fears even the possibility of being touched.

ARS. He, 17 - He sees all kinds of vermin (insects) on his bed, throws handfuls of them away, and tries to escape from them.

AUR. Ha, 14 - Anxiousness; even a noise before the door makes him anxious; he is afraid some one might come in; as if afraid of men.

BELL. Al,S-2552-...the yellow corpse of a tall man, shrouded (dressed, clothes) in white, tried to share the patient's bed with him, and the unwelcome visitor was promptly ejected. A crimson serpent came from the foot of the bed, with the design of fastening upon the patient's neck...

He, 18 - When closing eyes, though not asleep, patient sees fierce (wild), wicked looking large animals with horns and bushy (scabrous) heads; room seemed to be full of strange men passing in and out, who would snatch (take hold) at her as they passed, which frightened her very much, she thought the men wanted to take her away from home ; she then saw children sitting on low benches (seat) in rows (line) as in a school-room. (purity)

BROM. He, 3 - Expects to see something jump around floor.

BRY. Al, 5-...a delirious frightful fantasy, as of soldiers cutting him down, that he was on the point of escaping;..

CALC. He, 22 - Mania; sees many curs (dogs) crowding (compress) around him, fights them off. (surrounded)

He, 56 - Feels awe-stricken (terror-injure) at night. 0 Diarrhea

CARB-V. Ha, 678-... feeling over the body as if some one stroked him with the hand, and as if ants were running over the skin, at every moment in bed...

CARBN-S. Al-S, 753 - At one time during the night he seemed to be surrounded by enemies; persons were coming to harm him;...

CHOC. Sh, 189 - While outside became very weary of cars and people. Felt open and vulnerable. Fear of accidents, cars, or of someone leaping into the road and punching me. This anxiety was worse out of doors. 27, 100C, 01:XX:XX

Sh, 191 - I Since the being bitten by the dogs have developed a strong fear of dogs, and have been chased by one dog and growled at by another. This is coupled with a general fear of something happening. These fears are new to me and were better again after the proving. 27, 100C, 05:XX:XX

ELAPS. Al, 2 - Reveries in the daytime; he imagines he is being beaten.

GUAI. Ha, 129 - In the evening in bed (when slumbering?) he felt as if some one threw a towel at his face, so that he started up in a fright at it.

HYDROG. Sh, 243 - Fear that someone was trying to find out if I was home so that they could come and rape and murder me. 16, 30C, XX:XX:XX

HYOS. Ha, 575 - Peculiar fear of being bitten (hurt) by beasts.

He, 59-...constantly pointing to serpents (snakes) which she saw creeping up towards her...

IRID. Sh, 99 - Sat at the bus stop. Felt like a really small, frightened rabbit, with a large shadow of this great bird hovering over ready to pounce. G8

LAC-C. He, 15 - Sensation or delusion as if surrounded by myriads of snakes, some running like lightning up and down inside the skin ; some that are inside feel long and thin; fears to put her feet on floor, lest she should tread (walk) on them and make them squirm (shake) and wind (round) around her legs; is afraid to look behind her, for fear that she will see snakes there, does not dream of them and is seldom troubled with them after dark; on going to bed she was afraid to shut her eyes for fear that a large snake, the size of her arm, would hit her in the face.

He, 17 - On lying down either by day or night begins to think how horrible it would be if a very sharp pain, like a knife, should go through her, and thought of it causes great mental distress.

LACH. He, 9 - Imagines he is followed (pursued) by enemies who are trying to harm (hurt, injure) him; attempts to leave room as if frightened by visions behind him.

He, 21-...imagines he is followed by enemies who are trying to harm him; attempts to leave room as if frightened by visions behind him.

LYSS. Al,N-24 - Fancies he is being blown (hit, hurt) at by several persons, some of whom are not present.

He, 23 - Imagine that they are being abused (hurt, injured), and energetically defend themselves against attacks and insults, which in reality are products of their own fancy.

He, 24 - Fancies he is being blown (strike) at by several persons, some of whom are not present.

MAG-C. Al, 950 - Dream that she burnt her back by some one throwing hot roast (meat) pigeons (bird) at her.

OP. Al, 16-...started up in a fright on account of fancied swordsmen (rival, competitor) who threatened to stab him; became angry if any one argued him or thought him delirious; however, he blamed (reproaches) himself while in delirium for his folly.

Ha, 638 - He chattered all sorts of unconnected stuff and pointed with his fingers to imaginary masked people approaching him; ...he started at imaginary swordsmen, who might kill him ;

He, 20- ...declares he is not alone in bed; ..desire to escape; says a regiment of horsemen are upon his bed and that he fears to be trodden upon (run over, crushed); when told that horses are very careful, answered that he feared he would be crushed by the wagons that followed them.

He, 21-...in old, emaciated persons; sees animals coming towards him; people want to hurt him, execute him ; creeping under covers or jumping out of bed; in "old sinners" (criminals) whose long lives of excess have thoroughly destroyed their constitutions; ...; believe themselves to be murderers or criminals to be executed; want to run away (escape) ;...

PLB. Al, 59-...;he fancied that a cavalry regiment was about to fall upon him (attacked); or that he was in the presence of his employer, who was finding fault with him.

PULS. He, 46 - Dark suspicious and reserved manner; disturbed look on face; sleepless; looks for her bed in the yard (lost?); hides in a corner to escape from a little gray man who wanted to pull out her leg;...

STRAM. Al, 63-...I was assailed (attacked) by imaginary spectres, in the most hideous forms and menacing attitudes; and what was still to my torment my bed was suspended and tantalized (charmed) like a feather (plumage) between two floors.

Al, 136 - Delirium...seeming to dread the approach of some imaginary monster, and giving utterance in the most piteous appeals for help, protection.

Ha, 562 - His surroundings appear to him quite strange; (unfamiliar) although in the first minutes he knows that he is surrounded by his friends, he forgets this in the second minute, and imagines he is quite alone (solitary, deserted) in a desert (wildness), and is afraid (fearful) ; figures of beasts suddenly spring out of the ground at his side, so that he moves to the other side, where, however, other similar figures pursue him, and he runs forward.

Ha, 551 - She sometimes cries out about cats, dogs and rabbits, which were approaching (pursuing) her from above, from the side and from the middle of the room.

Ha, 565 - Nowhere has he rest, is startled by dream-pictures, even when his eyes are open, which in the form of big dogs, cats and other horrible beasts, grow (expand) out of the ground at his side, and from which he jumps away to the side with signs of terror (fear), and knows not how to save (rescue, free) himself. (cornered, corralled)

Ha, 520 - Loquacious madness; he complains of a dog biting and tearing the flesh off his chest.

Ha, 548 - Nonsensical idea, as though he were killed, roasted, and being devoured.

He, 66 - Woke suddenly in night and said there were snakes under and about her; looked wild, screamed and pointed to them.

He, 92 - Mania:... complains that a dog is biting and tearing flesh off his chest; merry exaltation; with pride (haughty) and affectation; runs about, complains of violent headache; ...;steals from his roommates...; disposition to scold persons whom he otherwise loved.

He, 163 - Cries out fearfully, hides face in pillow, is terrified by presence or approach of physician; after attack of typhoid.

He, 81-...attempts to stab and bite;...with sexual excitement; fear as if a dog were attacking him;...

He, 85-...seemed to dread approach of some imaginary monster, and giving utterance to most piteous appeals for help.

SULPH. Al, 3816 - Frightful dream that he had been bitten by a dog.

VALER. Al, 12 - Fearfulness in the evening when sitting in the dark (imagining that some one might hurt him).

AVARICE

Avarice: alum.[30] **ARS.**[122] bar-c.[10] bry. calc. calc-f. carb-an.[30] carb-v.[30] carc.[207] caust.[30] cina coloc. con.[30] ***dulc.***[184] graph.[30] hep.[30] hyos.[30] lach.[30] ***lyc.*** med.[137] meli. merc.[162] nat-c. nat-m.[30] nit-ac.[30] nux-v.[30] petr.[30] ***ph-ac.***[30] phos.[10] plat.[30] **PULS.**[122] rheum ***sep.*** **SIL.**[30] stann.[30] staph.[30] ***sulph.***[111]

Avarice; alternating with squandering: calc.[30] lach.[30] merc.[30] sulph.[30]

Avarice; anxiety about future, from: ***nux-v.***[30] ***ph-ac.***[30] stann.[30]

Avarice; collects carefully the debris of his fortune: stann.[30] staph.[30]

Avarice; generosity towards strangers, as regards his family: carb-v.[30] hyos.[30] nat-m.[30] nux-v.[30]

Avarice; squandering on oneself, but: calc.[30] hyos.[30] lap-mar-c.[194] nux-v.[30] sep.[30]

Avarice; wants all for himself: puls.[30]

Bargaining: bry.[122] ***puls.***[122] ***sil.***[122] sulph.[122]

Desires; everything, for: sant.[36]

Extravagance; sometimes, sometimes miserly: lach.[30] merc.[30]

Extravagance; themselves, for, and miserly as regards others: calc.[30] caust.[30] nux-v.[30] sep.[30]

Gifts to his wife or son, husband making no: **LACH.**[30]
Greed, cupidity: ***ars.***[30] calc.[122] ***chin.***[122] ***hyos.***[54] iod.[109] ip.[122] ***lyc.***[54] mag-c.[122] merc.[122] nat-c.[122] nit-ac.[30] nux-v.[30] ph-ac.[30] ***puls.***[36] rhus-t.[30] ***sep.***[54] stann.[30] staph.[30] sulph.[30] verat.[122]
Greed; constant: merc.[60]
Greed; desires are greater than her need, her: ars.[1]
Greed; grasping greedily with both hands anything offered to him: ***hyos.***[54]
Irresolution; marry, to, avarice, from: lyc.[148]
Selfishness, occupied at first with himself and besides with others for his own profit and loss for others: bell.[30] calc.[30] nux-v.[30]
Ungrateful; avarice, from: bry.[30] puls.[30] sil.[30] sulph.[30]
Usurer: lyc.[30] puls.[30] sulph.[30]

ARS. He, 104 - Obstinacy, avarice, inclined to malice and satire.
CALC-F. Al,S-1-...tendency to look on the dark side of things, with much depression of spirits. Feeling of anxiety about money matters, or thought would come to want (lack), or would soon be "running astern" (reversed, failure) financially...disposition to set a higher value on money than natural to him (avarice?, poverty?).
HALI-L. Sh, 887 - I called Daughter a parasite last night, because of money. 20, 30C, 10:XX:XX
Sh, 900 - It was or is ? As if I'm not really used to domestic duties. I can't really do anything for any other, just hopefully glimpses of illumination. All on own—with everything. Just to give—Does it really help? Doesn't it make others expect, or more needy? They lose freedom—independence. 20, 30C, 10:XX:XX
Sh, 973 - I was told I was an opportunist shopper. I went in at the end of the day and got all the food they were throwing out. 20, 30C, 20:XX:XX
LYC. He, 38 - Parsimonious (economical), greedy (avaricious), malicious (malevolent) and pusillanimous.(cowardice)
PULS. Al, 9 - Envious, avaricious, unsatisfied, greedy, he would gladly have everything, to himself.
Ha, 1125 - Envious, avaricious, dissatisfied, greedy, wants to have everything for himself.
He, 36 - Mistrust; envy; covetousness (avidity); dislike to people.

BETRAYED

Ailments from; jealousy: ***apis***[54] **HYOS.**[5] ***ign.***[5] ***lach.***[5] **NUX-V.**[122] ***ph-ac.***[5] ***phos.***[162] **PULS.**[122] staph.[102]
Children; watchful, they are on the look out for every gesture: phos.[122]
Delirium; jealousy, from: **HYOS.**[54] lach.[162]
Delusions; betrayed, that she is: hydrog.[222]
- conspiracies against her father, the landlord's bills are: kali-br.
- conspiracies, against him, there are: ars. kali-br.[25] lach. plb. puls.[137]
- deceived, is: bamb-a.[1184] dros.[1] ozone[227] ruta[130]
- injury, receive, will, friends, from: lach.[58]
- jealousy, lovers concealed behind stove wife has: ***stram.***[54]
- murder, conspiring to murder him, others are: ars. hydrog.[222] plb. tab.[139]
- murdered, persons are bribed to murder him: cann-i.
- poisoned, about to be, that he is: carc.[207] ***hyos.***[10] kali-br. lach.[102] plb. ***rhus-t.*** verat-v.[102]
- poisoned, has been, he: agar.[139] ang.[139] bufo[139] caj.[85] carb-ac.[139] chin-s.[139] chlor.[139] cic.[139] cimic. cocc.[139] cor-r.[139] croc.[139] culx.[58] cur.[139] euph.[139] ferr.[139] gels.[139] glon.[139] hydr.[139] hydrog.[222] ***hyos.*** iodof.[139] jug-r.[139] kali-br.[139] kali-c.[139] kali-i.[139] ***lach.***[116] lact.[139] lap-mar-c.[194] lil-t.[139] lina.[139] lyc.[139] m-aust.[139] mag-p.[139] med.[139] merl.[139] mez.[139] mill.[139] nicc.[139] nux-m.[139] nux-v.[139] olnd.[139] op.[139] petr.[139] ph-ac.[139] phos.[139] pip-m.[139] plat-m. psor.[139] ptel.[139] puls.[139] ran-b.[139] raph.[139] rat.[139] rheum[139] rhod.[139] rhus-t.[102] sabad.[139] sec.[139] sep.[139] sol-n.[139] spig.[139] squil.[139] staph.[139] stram.[37] sul-ac.[139] sulph.[139] tab.[139] tarax.[139] thuj.[139] valer.[139] verat-v.[102] zinc.[139]
- sold, being: hyos.
- wife is faithless: hyos. stram.

Dreams; betrayed, having been: sil.[1]
➤ conspiracies: mosch.[36] ped.[36]
➤ old gentleman ran away from wife, suspected of having married another: sep.[36]
➤ treason: sil.[1]

Fear; betrayed, of being: hyos. lyss.[172]
✦ death, kill him, that those in the house might: ***cimic.***[54]

✦ knaves, of: alum.[5] ars.[5] chin.[5] hyos.[5] lyss.[5]
✦ sold, of being: ***bell.***[60] bry.[60] ***hyos.*** lyss.[172] rhus-t.[60]

Jealousy; accuses wife of being faithless: ***stram.***[54]

Men; loss of confidence in: cic.[36]

ADAM. Sh, 201 - Sensation of being wronged, of being betrayed, which affects my social relationships. 15, 12C, 08:XX:XX
Sh, 202 - Preoccupied with the past on waking, concerning betrayal of trust in relationships. 15, 12C, 07:XX:XX

APIS. He, 77 - All her ideas turn around jealousy, very talkative (loquacity), sometimes disgusting salacious. (lascivious)

ARS. Al-S, 2879 - Became very nervous, agitated, and delirious, suspecting people were about the house plotting (conspiracy, betrayed) against his life, jumps out of the bed suddenly and reaches after imaginary objects, and stares wildly and suspiciously around him,...

CANN-I. Al, 31 - Imagines men are bribed (suborn) to kill him.

CHAM. Al, 40 - Ill-humor; he suspects that he has been imposed upon.

CIMIC. He, 10 - Fear of death; fears those in house will kill him (murdered, by parents); saw wires encasing (lock, imprisoned) him; visions of rats and of strange objects.
He, 29 - Suspicious of everything, would not take medicine if she knew it.

DROS. Al, 12 - Restless mood and anxiety the whole day; full of distrust, as if he were dealing with none but false men.
Al, 13 - Extremely uneasy, sad mood the whole day; he imagines that he would be deceived by tricky, designing (tricky) men.
Ha, 271 - All day long, uneasiness of disposition and anxiety, full of mistrust (suspicious) as if he had to do with none but false (faithless) people.
Ha, 272 - Extremely uneasy, sad disposition, all day he imagined he was being deceived (deluded, defrauded) by spiteful (hateful), envious people.

GLON. Al, 13-...fear she had been poisoned, and that no one would catch her taking any more.

HALI-L. Sh, 510 - Still having difficulty thinking. Nothing there. In shock about missing court filing deadline. Paralyzed about what to do. Mixes up words when talking. Drifting off. Unable to hold a train of thought. But not getting critical or depressed the way I would have been in the past. It's like fighting an enemy you can't see that keeps hitting you from behind. It's nasty. Observing. Just being, brain completely diffused. Can't keep thoughts on track. 09, 6C, 18:XX:XX

HYDROG. Sh, 249 - I think that no one likes me. I felt betrayed and everything went haywire. 16, 30C,
Sh, 257 - Feeling suspicious all day. Anxious and conscious of vulnerability. (Asked husband to move out if he was thinking of being unfaithful). 12, 6C, 06:XX:XX

HYOS. He, 16 - Fears: being left alone (solitude, deserted); poison, or being bitten (hurt); being poisoned or sold; being betrayed, or injured; wishes to run away. (escape)
He, 64 - Serious illness (ailments) from jealousy and grief about faithless lover;...
He, 65 - Violent and threatening...; mind nearly deranged; disturbed by unfounded jealousy.
He, 66 - A gentle, lovable woman became extremely jealous of her husband, and although fully realizing that she did him injustice, she was so filled with grief that she found no rest day or night... (remorse)
He, 78 - Groundless suspicion of being watched (observed, spied) by members of family with whom he had some slight misunderstanding (dispute); to avoid being recognized by them, clothed himself differently every day,...watching his relations suspiciously and imagining he might be poisoned;... (disguise, camouflage)

KALI-BR. Al, 6-...she fancied that the boarders in the hotel insulted her, and imagined that the weekly bills of the landlord (owner) were evidences of a conspiracy which had been got up against her father; ... while standing on the guards of the boat ...declared she had seen her brother fall overboard;...

LYSS. Al,N-22 - Believe that they are reduced to their present wretched (miserable) condition by the instrumentality

(aid) of those about them.
PLAT. He, 44 - Talks almost continually about fanciful things or such as have really occurred; of faithless love; of her teacher and old school days; ...
PLB. Al, 65 - Often getting out of bed and wishing to go home; sometimes not recognizing his family; thought they were conspiring to kill him.
RUTA. Al, 8 - Peevish and mistrustful (suspicious) all day; he no longer trusted his best friends, he thought that he was constantly deceived.(deluded)
Ha, 286 - All day long cross and suspicious; he would no longer trust (mistrust) his best friend, and imagined he was always being deceived.
STRAM. He, 56 - Believes to be in his grave; shrives,(confess) prays, asks to be killed (justified); accuses his wife of infidelity; scolds (cursing), strikes at everybody who wishes to restrain him; thinks they are dogs and barks at them to make himself understood.
He, 93 - Mania; thinks he is lying on his sepulchre (tomb); confessing, praying, wants to be killed (redemption, salvation, regeneration); laughs as if tickled (excited); wants to be kissed; accuses his wife of being faithless (betrayed); scolding (censure) beating in a rage, will not be taken hold of by attendants (suspicious?) ; takes them for dogs (contemptuous), and barks at them; talking in Jewish jargon; (rank?, stranger?) supposes his house to be surrounded by carts (vehicle), Jews (Judaism) and geese, offending him, ... -(strange, foreign, alien)
He, 103 - Had many strange fancies, such as imagining his wife had lovers concealed (hidden) behind stove; ...afterward had a fit that looked so much like apoplexy that he was bled.(blood)
He, 145 - Wife complains of husband neglecting her; man accuses his wife of being faithless.

BITE

Biting: acon. **AM-BR.**[162] *ant-t.* *anthr.* **ARS.**[162] arum-t.[5] aster. bac.[62] **BAR-C.**[162] **BELL.** bufo *calc.* *camph.* cann-i. *canth.* carb-v. *carbn-s.* carc.[140] choc.[222] cic. cina[152] croc. cub. *cupr.* cupr-acet.[36] cupr-c.[36] cur. gall-ac.[198] hura hydr-ac. *hyos.* ign.[5] *lach.* lil-t.[102] *lyss.* mag-c.[162] **MED.**[162] **NAT-M.**[162] nit-ac.[5] **NUX-V.**[189] op. phos. *phyt.* plb. sanic.[162] sec. senec.[162] squil.[5] **STRAM.** **SULPH.**[162] tarent.[102] tub.[189] *verat.*
Biting; everyone who disturbs him: hyos.[36]
Biting; himself: acon. arum-t.[58] elaps[54] hura lyss. op. plb. stram.[1] tarent.
Delirium; wild, stab and bite, attempts to: **STRAM.**[54]
Delusions; animals, devouring him: *hyos.*
• animals, dogs, biting and tearing flesh off his chest: stram.
• animals, dogs, near, that bit her, fought as if to drive it away: lyss.[54]
• animals, scorpions, sees: op.
• animals, snakes, black: arg-n.[5] cund.[111]
• animals, snakes, crawling up her leg, feels a: ail.[122]
• bitten, will be: *hyos.*[10] stram.[5]
• devoured, of being: cand-a.[239] *stram.*[10]
• murdered, killed, roasted and eaten: stram.
Dreams; animals, biting him: am-m. bov.[10] calc.[10] cench.[58] daph. elaps[136] m-aust.[10] merc. nicc.[10] *phos.* puls. sulph.[10] verat.[10] zinc.[10]
➤ animals, dogs, bitten, by, of being: calc. lyss. med.[212] merc. ozone[227] *sulph.* verat.
➤ animals, dogs, mangy dog approaching her, covered with sores, she takes hold of it and it bites her: paull-p.[36]
➤ animals, geese, of being bitten by: zinc.[1]
➤ animals, horses, bitten by a, in his arm: am-m.
➤ animals, horses, fearing to be bitten by a ferocious black: phos.[36]
➤ animals, insects, stung by: lap-mar-c.[194] phos.
➤ animals, snakes, bitten by, of being: bov. cench.[58] med.[212] ozone[227]
➤ beaten, being, father, by: kali-c.[36]
➤ bitten, arms, into the: am-m.[10] m-aust.[10] nicc.[10]
➤ body, foot, heel, burrowing of insect into, morning: arg-n.[36]
➤ disease, hydrophobia: anan.
➤ water, wading in, serpents, in which are, of which he is afraid: alum.
Fear; animals, dogs, attacking him, in delirium: **STRAM.**[54]
✦ animals, dogs, black, malicious: *stram.*[54]
✦ animals, dogs, of: androc.[222] **BAC.**[62]

BELL.[122] bufo[179] calc.[30] carc.[193] ***caust.*** **CHIN.** choc.[222] ***hyos.*** lyss.[122] med.[212] nat-m.[162] nat-p.[166] plat.[40] ***puls.***[162] sil.[171] ***stram.*** syc-co.[136] ***tub.*** tub-k.[70] verat.[172]
✦ animals, insects, of: abel.[149] bufo[36] **CALC.**[162] calc-ar.[162] cimic.[162] lyc.[162] nat-m.[162] nat-p.[166] phos.[162] puls.[212] sulph.[212]
✦ animals, rats, of: absin.[172] bell.[172] calc.[172] cimic.[137] op.[172] phos.[172] sep.[172]
✦ animals, scorpions: abel.[149] op.[30]
✦ animals, snakes, of: abel.[149] arg-n.[172] bell.[162] calc.[183] calc-s.[196] carc.[207] elaps[152] hep.[162] ign.[187] lac-c.[162] ***lach.***[122] nat-m.[212] puls.[212] ruta[152] sep.[172] spig.[162] sulph.[162] syph.[162]
✦ animals, spiders, of: abel.[149] calc.[162] carc.[210] lac-c.[185] mag-m.[166] nat-m.[162] phos.[155] stram.[172] tarent.[185]
✦ animals, wasps: hep.[162]
✦ animals, wolves, of: bell.[8]
✦ biting, of, lest teeth would fall out: nit-ac.[172]
✦ bitten, of being: choc.[222] ***hyos. lyss.***

Hydrophobia; bitten, after being: lyss.[54]
Idiocy; bite, desire to: **BELL.**[122] **STRAM.**[122]
Liar; deny obstinately that they have been bitten: lyss.[54]
Rage; biting, with: bell.[10] ***camph.***[54] canth.[116] croc.[10] cupr.[10] sec.[10] ***stram.***[10] ***verat.***[10]
Rage; dog that had bitten her, about: lyss.[54]
Shrieking; wild, with disposition to bite and tear: ***verat.***[54]
Tears; things, pillow, with teeth: phos. **STRAM.**

ADAM. Sh, 158 - I feel detached and not sexual. I could bite my partner as a signal I loved her, not in a loving or hungry way. My partner said, "He is looking at me like a piece of steak, he wants to eat me. He looks like a cave man. He wants to nibble me." 7, 6C, 03:22:30

BELL. Ha, 1420 - He tries to bite those about him at night.

He, 70 - Instead of eating, bit wooden spoon in two, gnawed plate, and growled and barked like a dog.

CALC. Al, 1557 - Anxious dream that he would be bitten by a dog, which awoke him, after...

CAUST. Ha, 20 - Extreme anxious timidity; she is so much afraid (fear) of a dog near her, which did not harm (hurt, injure) her at all,...every noise in the street made her afraid, and when she saw boys climbing she was very uneasy lest they might get hurt. (care, others)

CHOC. Sh, 301 - Desire to bite my husband in a playful way. I bit him —I wanted to really sink my teeth in, but willed myself not to. It was an animal need in me.[15], 30C, 00:05:30

CROT-C. Al, 3-... hears a strange voice to her left, and behind her; she follows it, throws herself against closed doors, and scratches them with her nails...She cries out: " He is in the den, but the lions will not eat him"

CUPR. He, 10 - Mania with biting, beating, and tearing things to pieces; insane foolish gestures of imitation and mimicry; full of insane spiteful (cruelty, brutality) tricks (deceitful, false), ..unhappy, despairing...miserable look...

ELAPS. Al, 2 - Reveries in the daytime; he imagines he is being beaten.

HURA. Al, 28 - Impatience, anger; she bites her hands, and gets into passion because her ideas come too slowly.

HYOS. Al, 87 - Remarkable fear that he had been devoured by animals.

Ha, 575 - Peculiar fear of being bitten (hurt) by beasts.

He, 16 - Fears: being left alone (solitude, deserted); poison, or being bitten (hurt); being poisoned or sold; being betrayed, or injured; wishes to run away. (escape)

He, 52 - Bite, scratch (hurt) and nip (pinch) everyone interfering with them.

IRID. Sh, 300 - I feel snappy, as though I could bite someone's head off. Feel really ratty. I[2] At 5.00 a.m., I felt very resentful at having to get up. This mood lasted for at least two hours. At 9.15 a.m., went back to bed, slept for two hours, had frustrating, agitated dreams about the car. Things kept going wrong. Seem to be attracting aggravation. L8

LAC-C. He, 15 - Sensation or delusion as if surrounded by myriads of snakes, some running like lightning up and down inside the skin ; some that are inside feel long and thin; fears to put her feet on floor, lest she should tread (walk) on them and make them squirm (shake) and wind (round) around her legs; is afraid to look behind her, for fear that she will see snakes there, does not dream of them and is seldom troubled with them after dark; on going to bed she was afraid to shut her eyes for fear that a large snake, the size of her arm, would hit her in the face.

LYSS. Al,N-58 - Ordered her husband to go away(forsakes), as she wanted to bite him, and joining (associated) act to threat(menace), she bit herself in arm.

Al,N-40 - A strong and uncontrollable impulse to do certain acts; to spring at and bite any moving object that came within reach; dog.

Al,N-42 - Deny, with great obstinacy, that they have ever been bitten.

Al,N-89 - After attacks of fury, evinces (manifest) great regret at his behavior, making earnest (ardent) apologies, warning those about him not to allow him to bite them.

He, 40 - A strong and uncontrollable impulse to do certain acts; to spring at and to bite any moving object that came within reach; ...

MERC. Ha, 1125 - Anxious dreams; of being bitten by dog, of getting up a revolution (revolutionary, revolting, radical) after midnight.

SEC. He, 4 - Mania; with inclination to bite; with inclination to drown.

STRAM. Ha, 520 - Loquacious madness; he complains of a dog biting and tearing the flesh off his chest.

Ha, 544 - Great desire to bite and tear everything with his teeth that comes near his mouth, even his own limbs.

He, 92 - Mania:... complains that a dog is biting and tearing flesh off his chest; merry exaltation; with pride (haughty) and affectation; runs about, complains of violent headache; ...;steals from his roommates...; disposition to scold persons whom he otherwise loved.

He, 81-...attempts to stab and bite;...with sexual excitement; fear as if a dog were attacking him;...

He, 119 - His thoughts ran upon obscene things, frequently put his hands to erect penis; sought to bite or to catch flies.

SULPH. Al, 3816 - Frightful dream that he had been bitten by a dog.

BLOOD

Anguish; blood, feeling of anguish in the: sep.[1]

Anxiety; wrong, indescribably, of something, in vasomotor affection: ***kali-br.***[54]

Blood or a knife, cannot look at: **ALUM.** nux-m.[137] plat.[137] sac-alb.[210]

Blood; wounds cannot look at: **NUX-V.**[122] staph.[122]

Death; conviction of, epistaxis, in: ***croc.***[54]

Delirium; blood, from profuse loss of: arn.[5] ars.[5] bell.[5] ign.[5] lach.[5] lyc.[5] ph-ac.[5] phos.[5] sep.[5] squil.[5] sulph.[5] verat.[5]

Delusions; blood, ceased to flow, in vertigo: seneg.[139]

- blood, circulate well, does not: ***atro.***[36]
- blood, pouring out of mouth: choc.[222]
- blood, rushed through like roar of many waters: alumn.[58] cann-i.
- body, liver comes out with blood of menses: ozone[227]
- objects, blood covered: stront-c.[137]
- unreal, everything seems, hemorrhage, in post partum: ***cann-s.***[54]

Despair; unwilling to die, in hemoptysis: ***acal.***[54]

Dreams; animals, vampires: psil.[164]

➤ blood: cand-a.[239] kali-m.[192] ***phos.***[111] rad-br.[111] rhus-t.[5] sol-t-ae.[111]

➤ blood, bleeding, that she is, in metrorrhagia: ***sec.***[54]

➤ blood, mangled remains, and: merc.[36]

➤ blood, pools of: cand-a.[239] ***phos.***[5] rhus-t.[102] sol-t-ae.[36]

➤ bloodshed: plat.[10]

➤ body, liver comes out with blood of menses: ozone[227]

➤ disease, haemoptysis: hep. meph. phos.

➤ disease, haemorrhage: phos. sol-t-ae.[122]

➤ hemoptysis, spitting blood: hep. meph. phos.[10] sol-t-ae.[122]

➤ hemorrhage: phos. sol-t-ae.[122]

➤ vomiting, blood and pus: bamb-a.[1184]

Excitement; hemorrhage, after: ***chin.***[54]

Fear; blood, of: **ALUM.**[30] nux-m.[137] phos.[185] plat.[137] sac-alb.[210]

✦ death, abortion, die from hemorrhage, is sure she will: ***acon.***[26]

✦ death, epistaxis. in: ***croc.***[54]

✦ death, hemoptysis, in: **ACON.**[54]

✦ death, hemorrhage, in uterine: acon.[54] coff.[54] nux-m.[54] **PLAT.**[54]

✦ death, metrorrhagia, in: ***coff.***[54]

✦ stoppage of circulation, with sensation of, at night, in angina pectoris: ***lyc.***[54]
Hysteria; hemorrhage, after: ***stict.***[54]
Hysteria; loss of blood, after: ***stict.***[54]
Hysteria; metrorrhagia, during: caul.[102] cimic.[102] mag-m.[102]
Insanity; hemorrhage, after: carb-v. ***chin. cupr.*** kreos. ph-ac. ***sep.*** staph. verat.
Nymphomania; metrorrhagia, during: mosch. murx. plat. sabin.[85] sec.
Restlessness; hemorrhage, during uterine: apis[54] op.[54] pyrog.[54]
Sadness; epistaxis, after: puls.
Suicidal disposition; seeing blood or a knife, she has horrid, thoughts of killing herself, though she abhors the idea: ***alum.***
Suicidal disposition; seeing, blood or a knife, shaving, when: alum.[122]
Thoughts; frightful, seeing blood, or a knife, on: ***alum.***
Time; passes too slowly, post-partum hemorrhage, in: ***cann-s.***[54]
Unconsciousness; blood, sight of: nux-m.

ALUM. Ha, 22 - She cannot see blood nor a knife without horrible thoughts pressing in upon her, as if she should, e. g. commit suicide; though she has the greatest horror of it.
He, 10 - Seeing blood on a knife, she has horrid ideas of killing herself, though she abhors the idea.

ANAC. Al, 16 - Anxiety in all his actions; everything appears to him more terrible; he imagine himself surrounded with enemies; then he feels warm and the blood seems to boil within him.
Ha, 6 - Timorous in all his actions; he views everything more anxiously and timidly, always thinks of being surrounded by enemies, then he becomes hot, his blood seems to boil in his chest.

ATRO. Al, 25 - Insisted repeatedly that her blood did not circulate, and that her feet must put into warm or she should die.

CANN-I. Al, 26 - The idea that he must die returned several times, and seemed to be particularly connected with the sinking and disappearance of the pulse. (blood, circulation)

CROT-H. He, 15 - Oppression as if brain had been intoxicated by carbonic acid, or by degraded or non-oxygenated blood.

HALI-L. Sh, 597 - Reading about the Ring Cycle and how Siegfried tasted the blood of the slain dragon.[16], 10C, 22:XX:XX

HEP. He, 22 - Temper obstinate and cross, a ferocious spleen (irascible) which would lead to cold blooded murder even among those habitually gay and benevolent.

LYSS. Al,N-127 - Thinking of fluids of any kind, even of blood, brings on convulsions.

MERC. Ha, 1234 - Anxiety and apprehension in the blood, he knew not how to compose (control) himself; he felt as if he had committed a crime, without heat, also at the same time as if he was not quite master,(commander). of his senses all day. (lost: mastering, commander)
Ha, 1227 - Much anxiety and ebullition in the blood at night, and shooting in the blood vessels.
Ha, 1263 - Mania; she throws off the clothes at night, tears the straw about, and scolds; by day she leaps (jump) up high like a petulant extravagant person...she talks and scolds much to herself,...spits frequently and spreads the saliva out with her feet, and licks some of it up again; she often licks cowdung (excrements) and the mud of ponds (lake); she often takes little stones in her mouth, without swallowing them, and at the same time complains that they are cutting her bowels; much clotted blood passes with her motion; ...

MUR-AC. Ha, 267-...anxiety and restlessness in the upper extremities (as if in the blood vessels)...

OP. Al, 43 - In walking I was hardly sensible that my feet touched the ground; it seemed as if I slid (floating) along the ground impelled by some invisible agent, and that my blood was composed of some ethereal fluid which rendered my body lighter than air.

RHUS-T. Al, 1382 DREAM-...it seemed to her that the head was hanging out of the bed and the blood was streaming (flow) into it, so that she could hear it flow; together with the appearance of a horrible image which she was obliged to accompany.

SEP. Al, 48 - Great anguish, as if in the blood.

STRAM. He, 103 - Had many strange fancies, such as imagining his wife had lovers concealed (hidden) behind stove; ...afterward had a fit that looked so much like apoplexy that he was bled.(blood)

THUJ. Al, 64 - Frightful anxiety, like death agony; a nameless internal ache, as if the soul were escaping from the body (split), with most terrible uneasiness, frightful orgasm of blood, at night, even to suffocation.

BOTHER

Anger; vex others, inclined to: **CHIN.**[54] ***mez.***[10]

Censorious; nagging: lyc.[137] nux-v.[137] plat.[137]

Fear; burden, of becoming a: raph.

Meddlesome, importunate: alum.[30] atro. con.[30] hyos. hyosin.[36] lyc.[30] plb.[36]

Noise; inclined to make a: acon.[137] **BELL.**[5] cham.[137] cic.[137] merc.[36] op.[36] verat.[36]

Obstinate; children, annoy those about them, with eruption: ***psor.***[54]

Sadness; aversion, children to whom he is devotedly attached become burdensome: **KALI-I.**[54]

Torments; everyone with his complaints: agar.[162] ***psor.***[122] **ZINC.**

Torments; those about him: alumn.[54] **CALC.**[54] lach.[36]

CALC. He, 57 - Anxiety, shuddering and dread (fear) as soon as evening comes on, with fear of death ; torments those around him day and night.

He, 65 - Despairing; hopeless (unhappy, pessimistic) of ever getting well (health); with fear of death, tormenting all around day and night.

CHAM. He, 41 - Peevishness (cross, angry); she seeks a cause for being peevish at everything; can't return a civil (polite) answer.(impolite, rude)

CHIN. Ha, 1110 - Extremely disposed to be vexed, and to take every occasion to get cross; afterwards quarrelsome and disposed to vex others, and to make reproaches and give annoyance(irritation) to others.

He, 31 - Inclined to reproach and vex (annoy, provoke) others.

DROS. Ha, 274 - Anxiety, as if his enemies would not leave him quiet, envied (competition, rivalry, opposition, spite) and persecuted him.

GERM. Sh, 126 - I have a guilty feeling if I get too much attention. I am afraid of bothering others. 18, 30C, 13:XX:XX

Sh, 115 - Very much in doubt whether I should take any more tablets. Whatever I do, I feel that somebody will criticize me, that I do something wrong. Difficult to make a decision. Afraid that other people will laugh at me or say, haven't you understood anything?" Crying. Don't want to get up. Don't want to bother the supervisor so early in the morning. I am a failure. 18, 30C, 01:06:30

HYDR. Al, 26-...forget, for a few seconds, what was wanted, which makes me very angry and feel like damning (swearing) and cursing (blaspheme) everything and anybody who bothered me the least.

LACH. He, 24 - Inclination to be communicative; vivid imagination; extremely impatient at tedious and dry (arid) things.

LYSS. Al, 14 - Feeling as if something annoying was about to happen; goes off when thinking of it.

MYRIC. Al, 12 - Exceedingly irritable; the slightest thing fretted (bother) and irritated him; ungovernable petulance.(rudeness)

NAT-M. Al, 93 - Ill-humored does not want to go into society for fear of vexing others; feels that he could easily give offense.

Ha, 59 - He feels peevish and avoids company, because he foresees that he might easily annoy (bother, molest) others. (intrude)

NUX-V. Al, 4 - He is hasty; looked angrily at anyone who asked him a question without answering, as though he was obliged to restrain himself to avoid being insulting; he was in such an irritable and unrestrained mood that it seemed as though he would like to strike any one in the face who spoke a word to him.

He, 19-...; imagines himself surrounded by persons who carry on all sorts of pranks (joke, jest), or ply (covering) him whith questions which he thinks he is compelled (forced) to answer (proved, questioned, interrogated);..; answers questions rationally and is conscious of his condition; ...appears to be haunted (obsessed) by a great fear.

PSOR. Al,N-10 - Intolerable self-willed

(obstinate), annoys those about him; a boy suffering from an eruption.
Al,N-26 - Greatest despondency (grief), making his own life and that of those about him intolerable;...
He, 26 - Greatest despondency (desperation), making his own life and those about him intolerable;...
RAPH. Al, 2-...she fears she will become a burden (load) to everyone. (flat, tiresome)
SIL. He, 19 - When crossed has to restrain himself to keep from doing violence.

BOTHERED

Anger; attention, at every little: ant-c.[102]
Anger; easily, consolation agg., does not want to be disturbed: hell.[54]
Delusions; enemy, rest, allows him no: dros.[139]
- people, disagreeable, sees: calc-ar.[58] calc-sil.[58]
- people, noise, making: puls.[122]
- people, ply him with questions and he must answers, they: **NUX-V.**[54]

Disturbed, sit or lie in one place, with desire to: chin-ar.[54]
Disturbed; averse to being: adax.[96] agar.[102] ***ant-c.***[102] ant-t.[58] arn.[102] bac.[56] bamb-a.[1184] bell.[102] berb.[30] ***bry.*** cact.[102] carb-an.[102] cench.[58] ***cham.***[102] chin-ar.[54] ***cocc.***[54] ***coloc.***[102] gels. graph.[193] hell.[102] ign.[102] iod.[102] kali-m.[192] lil-t.[58] mur-ac.[102] naja[98] nat-ar.[58] ***nat-m.***[102] nat-s.[102] ***nux-v.***[102] op.[193] oxyt.[102] ***ph-ac.***[102] phos.[102] puls.[193] sars.[102] sil.[102] staph.[193] sulph.[102] tub.[85]
Fear; disturbed, of being: agar.[1]
Morose; questioned: nat-m.[36]
Quarrelsomeness; disturbed, if: **NUX-V.**[54]
Reserved; noise, with sensitivity to: con.[10]
Scratches with hands, everyone interfering with him: ***hyos.***[54] ***stram.***[54]
Temperament; bilious: acon.[54] ***aesc.***[54] ail.[54] ambr.[54] anac.[85] ant-c.[54] ant-t.[54] apis[83] ars.[85] ***bell.***[54] berb.[54] chion.[85] coloc.[85] cub.[85] ***ip.***[54] ***lach.***[54] ***merc.***[54] merc-d.[85] **NUX-V.**[54] petr.[85] plat.[54] plb.[85] **PODO.**[54] ***puls.***[54] sac-alb.[36] sep.[85] ***sulph.***[54]

ACON. He, 53 - Ailments from vexation (worry, care), with fear or vehemence: congestion; palpitation; fever; anxiety, beside himself; threatened miscarriage ; apoplectic congestion.
He, 47 - Vexed at trifles; takes every joke in bad part.
ADAM. Sh, 129 - Irritability about intrusion of space by my house guest. I felt hemmed in. 11, 30C, 07.XX.XX
Sh, 132 - Being told that I'm grumpy really irritates me. Why can't I be let alone and they can just go away. 7, 6C, 05:17:00
AESC. Al, 8 - Feels miserably cross.
AGAR. Al, 57 - She is vexed with herself and pities (compassion) herself.
AM-C. Ha, 5 - Thoughts of previous annoyances torment him.
ANAN. Al, 7 - Quarrelsome and contrary humor, but after being angry he often regrets (remorse) what he has done.
ANDROC. Sh, 63 - Desired company but could not be bothered to see anyone, felt lonely as if he didn't belong. (21)
Sh, 96 - Increased irritability, a "how dare you!" feeling. Felt like tearing offenders to pieces with his bare hands. He felt an enormous surge of violent emotions at trifles, and had to exercise great control to stop outbursts of violence and impulses to hurt someone. Felt that "everyone were creeps", could not be bothered with anyone. (2)
ARN. Ha, 619 - Uncommonly peevish, everything is repugnant to her; everything annoys her.
Ha, 625 - Over-excitability; she could easily laugh when there was no occasion for it, and when one said something annoying to her, she got angry ...
ARS. Ha, 1042 - Irritable state of the disposition, he vexes himself about trifles, and cannot leave off talking about the faults of others.
Ha, 53 - Dissatisfied all day and extremely vexed at himself; he thought he had not worked enough and reproached himself most bitterly.
BELL. He, 119 - Fretfulness; nothing seemed right to him; was vexed with himself.
BOR. Ha, 15 - Passionate, cross, takes offense easily.
CALC. Ha, 41 - Peevish, morose, very cross and most indifferent to the most important things; he also did everything repugnantly and as if by compulsion.
Ha, 46 - Troubled and cross, she looked at the worst side of things, and sought (pursued) out all the evil.

Ha, 55 - Thoughts of former vexations irritate him to anger.

CAMPH. He, 72 - Palpitation; vexed by want of sympathy (compassion, aid), afraid to be alone a moment, fears death.

CAUST. Al, 36 - Extreme irritability of mind; the slightest vexation affects her whole body, so that her knees sink under her.

He, 69 - Injurious (ailments from) effects of fear and vexation. (worry)

CHAM. Ha, 470 - Cannot cease talking about old vexatious things.

Ha, 485 - Quarrelsome crossness; she seeks for everything vexatious.(provoking)

Ha, 476 - He vexes himself inwardly about every trifle.

Ha, 475 - Sulky moroseness; everything others do is displeasing to him; no one does anything to please him.

He, 58 - Insulting, cross and uncivil temper.

CHEL. He, 25 - Is vexed (anger, irritated) about every trifle and has violent attacks of passionate outbursts of temper.

CHIN. Ha, 1113 - Discontented; he thinks himself unfortunate (unsuccessful), and fancies he is opposed (confronted, hostilised), and tormented (molested) by everybody.

Ha, 1110 - Extremely disposed to be vexed, and to take every occasion to get cross; afterwards quarrelsome and disposed to vex others, and to make reproaches and give annoyance(irritation) to others.

He, 11 - She thinks she is very unfortunate and constantly harassed (molested, tormented) by enemies.

CHOC. Sh, 62 - The blackness of the trees is bothering me. They seem dark and leafless.

COCC. Ha, 554 - He is very indignant and annoyed at slight faults and fibs (lie, falsify) of others.

Ha, 550 - Everything angers and vexes him; after a few hours he becomes lively and disposed to make jokes.

Ha, 551 - Easily annoyed; he takes everything in bad part.

Ha, 548 - He cannot bear any interruption in conversation, nor any noise.

COFF. He, 33 - Ailments from excessive joy, excessive laughing and playing; from disappointed love; from anger, from vexations with vehemence or fright...

CON. Ha, 366 - Cross temper; everything about him made a disagreeable impression on him.

CUPR. Ha, 7 - Irresolute (indecisive) and dissatisfied with everything, but only so long as he is peevish. (cross)

DROS. Ha, 281 - He takes insults very resentfully, not without vexation.

GERM. Sh, 3 - Reacted angrily to husband's demands. 14, 30C, 26:00:00.

Sh, 69 - Want to sit alone in front of fire listening to music by myself. Fed up with people everywhere I go irritating me. Want to be looked after. 09, 9C, 01:11:00.

GRAPH. Ha, 35 - Very peevish; everything vexes him and makes him indignant.(anger)

Ha, 36 - He would like to be alone, every disturbance vexes him.

HALI-L. Sh, 347 - In response to a question from the supervisor started yelling, " I'm getting irritated with these conversations . Why can't we just get on with it ?! Why can't you understand what I am saying?!" 02, 30C, 09:XX:XX

Sh, 563 - Patient called and I felt I had no patience for her. Wanted to be more present for her, but felt she was too weepy and needy. Couldn't be bothered. Couldn't be bothered with all the patients the rest of the day. Felt overwhelmed. Trying to be nice at work, hard to do. 02, 30C, 00:06:XX

Sh, 567 - Had to leave my house to study elsewhere, due to an unpleasant visitor at home. Someone I can't stand being around came to visit my partner and see our puppies. He wouldn't ask her to leave. I didn't want to engage with her, because there is no way you can win. If I had said, "It's time to go, now," then I am the ogre. There are no boundaries. 13, 30C, 00:06:00

Sh, 571 - At sacred ceremony, but want to be alone. See a friend there who is rude, disrespectful, and obnoxious at this sacred ceremony, and I feel annoyed. 16, 10C, 15:XX:XX

HELL. Al, 17 - Extremely inclined to be irritable, the most trifling things which goes contrary to his wishes excites anger.

HEP. Ha, 7 - Contrary mood; he does not like to look at his folks. (relatives)

HYDROG. Sh, 145 - Feel that I could get on with everything alright if those around me

would either leave me alone or help constructively. 04, 12C, 19:XX:XX
Sh, 182 - A feeling of boredom and depression at 10:00p.m., whilst in company — very distressful. I didn't talk at all, friends thought something had greatly upset me. 24, 30C, 01:10:XX
IGN. Al, 28 - Contrary to his will, thinks of vexatious and peevish things, and dwells upon them.
Ha, 764 - Slight blame (censuring) or contradiction excites him to quarrel, and he is vexed at himself for doing so.
Ha, 791 - Thinks against his will of annoying, vexatious things, and dwells on them.
IOD. Al, 27 - Is cross and irascible; feels stupid.(obtuse)
Ha, 27 - Peevish, cross, she is not suited by anything...
IP. Ha, 227 - He lets (permit) his courage sink (fail), and is greatly given to be vexed and to get angry.
IRIS. Al, 5 - Vexed, irritable mood, disposed to find fault.
KALI-C. Ha, 44 - Cross and angry thoughts, in the morning, on awaking, so that he gnashes with his teeth.
He, 9-...constantly in antagonism which herself; frequently hopeful, frequently despondent; frets (worry) about everything; peevish impatient, contented with nothing.
KALI-CY. Al, 4 - For two days, desire to find fault; crossness almost uncontrollable on entering the room; while the cold air produces good spirits.
Al, 5 - At 7 p.m., while walking out of doors, feelings of crossness; carries on a kind of conversation within himself, as if quarreling with someone whith whom he had previously disagreed; thinks what he will reply in case certain things are said to him.
KALI-I. Al, 17 - Feelings easily disturbed, as if something was always happening to trouble her.
He, 6 - Very great irritability and unwonted harshness of demeanor (behavior); his children, to whom he is devoted and attached, become burdensome to him; very passionate and spiteful temper;...constant apprehension of impending evil.
LED. Ha, 333 - Cross: he retired into solitude, and almost weeping he longed for death.
LYC. Al, 91 - She is overpowered (defeat) by many unpleasant recollections (memory), about which she becomes vexed; even at night on waking.
Ha, 55 - She cannot bear the least contradiction, and at once gets beside herself for vexation.
Ha, 19 - Great oppression in the scrobiculus cordis from vexation.
He, 39 - Ailments from fright, anger, mortification, or vexation, with reserved displeasure.
He, 31 - Sensitive, irritable disposition; peevish and cross on getting awake; easily excited to anger; cannot endure slightest opposition, and is speedily beside herself.
LYSS. Al, 28 - Very cross, so much that my children expressed great surprise; took offense at the merest trifles; scolded (censorious) my wife and children; ....
Al,N-88 - Very cross, so much... he took offense at veriest trifles, scolding his wife and children, felt wretched, ...
He, 88 - Very cross, so much so that his children expressed great surprise; he took offense at veriest trifles, scolded his wife and children, felt wretched, ...
MANG. Ha, 324 - Cross reflective, silently reserved, wrapped up in himself, with discomfort in the whole body, ...
Ha, 325 - Cross and discontented with himself, and concerned about future..., considers himself very weak (stupid) in mind, and makes mistakes whenever he speaks.
Ha, 330 - Great restlessness of body and disposition, as if something bothered him.
Ha, 7 - Everything she thinks of is annoying (irritating)to her.
MERC. Ha, 1253 - Very cross and intolerant, easily irritated, very suspicious.
Ha, 1257 - During the whole day cross, as if at variance and dissatisfied with himself, and had no inclination for speaking and joking.
MEZ. Al, 32 - Is inclined to get angry with others about trifling and perfectly harmless things; everything vexes him, and he wants to say all kinds of annoying and vexatious things.
He, 11 - Inclined to get angry with others

about trifles; everything vexes him, he wants to say annoying and vexatious things; is soon sorry for it.

NAT-C. Ha, 48 - Peevish and cross, dissatisfied whith all the world; he could have kicked (self sensure) himself; he would rather not live at all ; at the same time solicitous about the future, so that he is ready to despair.

NAT-M. He, 48 - Consequences (ailments) of fright, anger, vexation, mortification, or reserved displeasure.

NIT-AC. Al, 27 - Vexed at the least trifle, even at himself if he makes a mistake.
Ha, 38 - Very ill-humored and vexed at himself.

NUX-V. Ha, 1270 - He is hasty (careless, rapid), looks malignantly (deadly) at any one who asks (asked) him anything, without answering, just as if he must control himself in order to avoid becoming coarse (rude), it seems as if he would like to strike any one in the face who speaks a word to him, so irritable and uncontrollable in his disposition.

PHOS. Al, 100 - She is made anxious by a disagreeable event, mingled with fear and vexation, and inclined to weep.

PLAT. Ha, 18 - Taciturnity and involuntary weeping, even after the most friendly address (communication), so that she gets vexed (anger) about it herself.
Ha, 33 - Very cross and irritated at harmless matters and words; so that she at times would have liked to have beaten herself and friends.

PULS. Ha, 1133 - Cross, takes in bad part what others say.

RAN-B. Al, 2 - Vexed and inclined to be angry; quarrels and scolds when the slightest cause is offered (after two hours).

SAPIN. Al, 5 - Quite ill-natured and inclined to view matters in a disagreeable light; did not seem able to feel settled (decided) enough to know what to do; the crossness became so intense, that I felt myself getting very unreasonable, especially as to food, which seemed all wrong in some way;...

SARS. Al, 18 - Extremely ill-humored even vexed " by the fly on the wall".
Ha, 14 - Extremely peevish, the fly on the wall vexes him. (insects)

SEP. Ha, 51-(Ailments) From vexation, she is so excited that she fears an apoplectic fit, and everything turns black before her eyes.

SPIG. Ha, 665 - Serious humor, he gets cross if the slightest joke is attempted on him.
Ha, 666 - He is very cross and sensitive to everything that he thinks not good, for many hours.

STANN. Ha, 655 - In the first three days he is rather calm and his vexation quickly passes off, does not fly into a passion, is rather quickly sensitive; the fourth day he is disposed to stormy anger and to fly into a passion...

STAPH. Al, 21 - Quiet fretfulness (irritable) ; he is vexed at everything which even does not concern him.
Ha, 700 - All day long peevish and cross; he did not know what to do for ill-humor, and was extremely pensive.
Ha, 701 - Silent peevishness; he gets cross about everything, even what does not concern him.

STRAM. He, 177-...sometimes vexed; neglects her duties, thinks she is not fitted for her position;...

SUL-AC. Ha, 16 - Vexed, peevish, impatient, at once when he does not succeed in his work.

SULPH. Al, 85 - He could tear himself to pieces from vexation.
Al, 84 - He is vexed at everything, gets angry and out of humor at every word, thinks he must be defended (protect) and becomes exasperated.
Ha, 38 - He gets vexed about everything, takes every word ill and gets insulted (dishonored, degraded), he imagines he ought (must) to defend himself and gets angry.
Ha, 60 - Indifferent things and such things as naturally occur in life are attended in her mind with annoying, mortifying ideas from her past, which continually connect themselves with recent annoyances of which she cannot rid herself. This attended (accompanied) with a resoluteness of mind, which is ready for great resolves.(determination)
He, 43 - Vexations and morbid ideas of past arise from most indifferent thoughts, and from every occurrence in life, which

continue to be united with new vexations, so that she cannot free herself from them.
He, 55 - Ill-humored; vexed with herself; everything makes her impatient.
TARENT. Al, 60 - Irritable and cross at the least contradiction.
THUJ. Al, 20 - Uneasiness of mind for many days, everything seems burdensome and distressing.
TUB. Al,N-10 - Does not like to be disturbed by people; trembling of hands.

BRIGHT

Break things, desire to, bright objects: lyss.[85]
Delusions; animals, insects, sees, shining: bell.
• clothes, fly away and become wandering stars, will (on undressing): cann-i
• objects, bright, from: anh.[144] **STRAM.**
• objects, bright, of: canth.[5]
• objects, brilliantly colored: androc.[222] anh.[144] bell. camph.[1] psil.[164]
• objects, glittering: bell.
• stars in his plate, sees: cann-i.
Dreams; fire, burning, brightly: kali-n.[36]
➤ houses, bright, very: ozone[227]
➤ mushrooms, colorful: psil.[164]
➤ star falling: alum.
Excitement; violent, brought on by current of air, bright light, sight of any shining object, slightest touch, even by conversation in vicinity of a patient: lyss.[54]
Fear; brilliant objects, looking-glass, etc., of, or cannot endure: cann-i.[36] canth.[137] lach.[5] lyss.[137] stram.
✦ lightning, of: bell.[5] cycl.[5] dig.[5] lach.[5] phos.[5] phys.[5] sil.[5]
✦ mirrors in room, of: bufo camph. cann-i. ***canth.*** carbn-s.[172] carc.[146] ***lyss.*** puls.[31] ***stram.***
✦ mirrors in room, of, see himself, lest he should: camph.[54]
Light; bright light agg.: colch.[5]
Light; shuns light, brilliant objects: bufo[130]
Rage; shining objects, from: bell. canth. hyos. ***stram.***
Shining objects agg.: anth. **BELL.** bufo camph. cann-i. ***canth.*** cocci-s.[102] glon.[116] ***hyos.*** lach. **LYSS.** mur-ac.[137] phos. ***stram.*** tub.[193]
Shining objects; agg. surface of water: **LYSS.**
Shining objects; amel.: ***stram.***[102] tarent.[102]
Shining objects; aversion to, cannot bear: bufo[22]
Wildness; bright light, strong odors or touch, from: ***colch.***

ADAM. Sh, 31 - The proving experience was very clear. There was a sharpness in both how I felt and what I saw. Mostly this was pleasant: brilliant sunshine through the drops of water in a shower, candlelight bouncing off wine glasses, tiny detail on the chrome-work of cars. 18, 30C, XX:XX:XX
Sh, 33 - Went out to dinner in a restaurant. Was very struck by how everything sparkled. Really dazzling. Asked my friend if it was particularly striking, but she just said it was all of the liquids on the table (water and wine in bottles and glasses.) 18, 30C, 29:XX:XX
Sh, 34 - After taking the remedy again, I was very struck again by sparkling—this time the sun in the shower. Before I took it, I seemed to be surrounded by dark and dirt. 18, 30C, XX:XX:XX
Sh, 36 - White frost this morning. At last some purity in this world. Every ice crystal sparkled like jewels. 16, 12C, 27:XX:XX
Sh, 37 - Great joy at the beauty of the snow, especially at night, reflecting light. Sparkled like jewels, purity. After the snow, joy at seeing greens again, appeared brighter and clearer than before the snow. 16, 12C, 67:XX:XX
Sh, 41 - Desire to see pyrites. 2, 12C, 100:XX:XX
Sh, 42 - Using a lot of words that one might connect with crystals, e.g., clear, cold, shining, crystalline, sparkly, gem, jewel, cut, facet, incisive, penetrating, sharp. 2, 12C, 80:XX:XX
Sh, 43 - Feeling alone and tall and capable, like a beacon beaming out rays of light to all and sundry. 2, 12C, XX:XX:XX
Sh, 44 - Attracted to dark night skies. Stars seem more visible. 16, 12C, 23:XX:XX
Sh, 105 - I went shopping for a red sweater but couldn't find one bright enough. I never wear red. 7, 6C, 12:10:00
Sh, 556 - Feel bright, free and beautiful, more feminine, more fertile and voluptuous. 16, 12C, 24:XX:XX

ANDROC. Sh, 83 - Woke at night to urinate. On going upstairs, all colours seemed incredibly bright and the walls were pulsating — in towards him and out again. This felt similar to an L.S.D. experience years ago. Did not know what to do, was stricken with panic. Terrified, he raced back to bed where he felt hot, so uncovered, then cold so covered, then hot, he uncovered and sat up and immediately felt better — no panic. As soon as he lay down he began to panic. Became afraid in the light and felt better in the dark with the lights off. He wanted to call someone for help, and felt angry about the proving. He then got up and walked around for a few minutes, got back to bed, and fell asleep. (2)

Sh, 118 - Irritability, worse for noise and bright lights. (17)

CAMPH. Al, 40 - Afraid of the mirrors in the room, lest he should see himself in them; so excessive was this fear at times in the night that he would have got up and broken the mirrors, only that he was still more afraid to get up alone in the dark;...

He, 63 - Afraid of mirrors in room, lest he should see himself in them (reflection) ; so excessive was his fear at times in night that he would have got up and broken mirrors, only that he was still (but) more afraid to get up alone in the dark.

CANN-I. Al, 62 - It seemed as though I was transparent; the fire in the grate seemed to shine through me, and to warm the marrow of the bones.

Al, 63 - His body seemed to him become transparent, and he imagined he saw within his breast the hashish he had eaten in the form of an emerald, from which issued millions of little sparks.

CARB-AN. Ha, 32 - The objects on the street seem to him changed, e.g., farther apart and brighter (vivid, brilliant) than usual, as an empty, abandoned city.

CHIN. Ha, 1105 - What formerly appeared to him in a bright genial light, seems now to be lusterless (lifeless), unworthy (inutile), and shallow (superficial, stupid)

CHOC. Sh, 2 - Feel very excited, very alive, bright and efficient. Had an image of a hedgehog's face.

Sh, 309 - A feeling of intoxication with double sensations. Colours are stronger and hearing is sharpened but at the same time feel absent and removed.[29], 200C, 00:XX:XX

Sh, 315 - Been on the move all day — painted a room blue. While lying in the bath looking out the window, the sky is the most glorious, vibrant blue —it seems like the most beautiful colour I've ever seen. Almost wept for the beauty of it. Suddenly, while I'm lying in the bath, the colour blue seems very important — seems very potent. It has the same quality and intensity that I remember colours having on L.S.D. I am very moved by this blue. I wanted to dissolve into it.[15], 30C, 03:05:XX

HALI-L. Sh, 21 - Preoccupied with right eye awareness. Staring at the rainbow colors on the beveling of a stained glass window. Excited to discover what might occur with my right eye. 03, 12C, 03:XX:XX

Sh, 30 - After I looked at the sun, I saw four suns in a ring connected to each other, and another one above with strings of light. One had two lesser ones. 20, 30C, XX:XX:XX

Sh, 847 - The next image (in my head) was of a huge sphere = the sun. Two enormous birds of prey were holding a bright sphere of sun aloft by great talons on either side — beautiful. Then the sphere became a hoop of flames, and they were still holding on. It was very windy outside, and the sky was baby pink. 20, 30C, 06:20:00

Sh, 862 - Clear and bright, an eagle soared, an amazing bird high up in the sky, when I was lying naked on my back. It wasn't flapping, it just soared. coming from the east towards me then flew into the sun. As I lay there, unbelieving, he soared out again, circled again and then disappeared into the radiance of the sun. I felt like the proving was finished. It felt like a good-bye. My vision had changed. I feel more like me. 20, 30C, 08:08:XX

Sh, 975 - As I woke up, the sun had just come up and I felt I had purpose and direction. I really need the sun. 20, 30C, 20:XX:XX

HYDR. Al, 4 - In high spirits; everything looked bright; felt happy, and wanted to sing.

HYDROG. Sh, 165 - I thought I could see energy moving around in the air. Colours looked bright and everything looked beautiful. 16, 30C, 25:XX:XX

IRID. Sh, 118 - Thoughts: Wind is breath of the spirit; love is the greatest of all messages between heaven and earth. Yes, go to heaven, but return to the world transformed by the light of experience, transcend and return; Metals —immortality; need knowledge of their names; Iridescence, oil mother of pearl metal, rainbow, seven plus seven, cosmic joke, messages in other languages —language of angels?; Seven heavens, seven earths. I adore these territories, not so much new as forgotten. Q20

Sh, 125 - Attracted to men with pale skins, appear even more beautiful, luminosity, light shining forth. Q5

Sh, 122 - Sensation as if seven stars in a ring around my head. QXX

Sh, 126 - Euphoric, others look grey, I am many-colored. Q1

Sh, 127 - Bright cold day. My attention was taken by the light reflected off the wet road. The brightness meant I wasn't seeing the tree or road at all. It added to the feeling of detachment. B3

Sh, 128 - People said "You look radiant today." People came and chatted to me. Felt incredibly clear and colourful. Such a big grin on my face, my face hurts. Q1

Sh, 138 - Crossing road, thought wouldn't it be nice to see a rainbow. Saw van belonging to "F. Rainbow and Son" —a removal company. Company I've never seen before. Q17

Sh, 140 - Felt flat, not much energy. Will be glad when it's daylight. When daylight comes you feel lifted. D6

JAMB. He, 4 - Sudden great change in him after micturition, everything seems more beautiful and bright, sky and trees more joyous and clear; but after quarter of an hour everything became gloomy again.

LYSS. Al,N-129 - Hyperesthesia, current of air, bright light, sight of any shining object, slightest touch, even conversation in vicinity of patient, may throw him into a most violent agitation and bring on severe convulsions.

MAG-C. Al, 951 - Frightful dream, that she burnt her cheek by the light.

Al, 942 - Anxious dream of a bright fire, at which she shrieked out violently and cried "fire".

MUR-AC. Al, 15 - The brightness (lively, vivid) of his disposition constantly diminished, until in the evening he became very fretful (irritable).

NEON. Sh, 58 - Image of being inside my iris and looking through. That is, I see a large iris and I was looking through it. From the center of it light was radiating out. 20, 6C, 07:XX:XX

Sh, 97 - Then I had the image like the inside of a body. I was in the dark but it was bright, like an amazing landscape. There were gently undulating folds of membrane. It was shiny and beautiful with bright points (nuclei of each cell) sparkling like tiny jewels. The tiny points of light were like the points of light that sun makes on snow. 'Epithelium' came to mind. 20, 6C, 00:01:30

Sh, 99 - Image of folds of membrane inside a body like a landscape, and it sparkled like tiny jewels, like sun shining in snow. I thought 'epithelium,' and these are the nuclei. 20, 6C, 07:01:30

Sh, 100 - On a cloudy day, I really wanted blue. I looked for the blue sky and remembered the blue flash on the wings of a duck I had seen. I was very excited about anything blue that I could see, especially vibrant blues. I felt I had never seen blues in that way before. Also excited by yellow, limey green fluorescent colors. 20, 6C, 01:03:28

Sh, 102 - My daughter commented that I looked brown and that my eyes looked clear, blue and bright. 20, 6C, 01:09:55

Sh, 108 - I went to the market to buy food and instead I bought lots of material, two pairs of boots and no food. One pair of boots were Canadian arctic boots for 40 degrees below zero. They had a thick felt lining the color of the bright night sky. From a distance I saw the second pair hanging up. It was love at first sight. There they hung under the neon lights. They glowed a fluorescent greenyyellow. They fit perfectly and felt amazing. I thought, "These are my wingless boots." When I unpacked them at home, they were yellow. 20, 6C, 06:04:XX

NUX-V. Ha, 1272 - Over-sensitiveness to impressions of the senses; he cannot bear strong odors and bright light.

PHOS. Al, 86-...; a feeling of dread (fear), as if awaiting something terrible, yet unable to resist or move (terrifying, scaring), overcame me; sometimes it seemed as if I was beginning to bloat (inhalant, inflate, vanity?), and then I could hear a multitude of voices saying in high glee, "Fill him up a little more and he will burst," (blow up) followed by demoniacal laughter, which made the cold chills run over me... I imagined myself an aurora borealis, and could distinctly hear voices shouting, "Beautiful! Oh, was not that splendid?"...

Ha, 76 - Freedom (liberty) of spirit,... everything seems brighter (luminous, vivid) to him.

PSOR. Al, 5 - He pictures the future in the brightest colors.

STRAM. He, 113 - Hydrophobia; water, a mirror, or anything bright, excites convulsion...,afraid to be alone;...

THUJ. Al, 8 - At night, while lying awake with closed eyes, she seems to see ghosts, and also now and then all kinds of animals brilliantly illuminated, coming from her...

BROTHER

Delusions; brother fell overboard in her sight: kali-br.
- dead, corpse, brother and child, c. of: calc-sil.[58] con. plb.

Dreams; death of, brother: plan.[36]
- ➤ stabbed, brother was: chin.[36]
- ➤ visits from brother: nicc.[10]

Sympathetic; felt same pain his brother complained of: ***lyss.***[54]

CHIN. Al, DREAM-1110 - Dreamed that some one had stabbed his brother, and then called for his mother; that his mother was dead, and then he cried; that his mother's arms was hurt;...

CON. Al, 11 - Visions of her brother and child, who had died; at the same time, she saw distinctly persons in the room;...

KALI-BR. Al, 6-...she fancied that the boarders in the hotel insulted her, and imagined that the weekly bills of the landlord (owner) were evidences of a conspiracy which had been got up against her father; ... while standing on the guards of the boat ...declared she had seen her brother fall overboard;...

STRAM. He, 87 - After a dreadful shock, occasioned by death of his brother, who fell dead in his arms,...struck all at around him...spoke at one time in Hungarian, and then in Wallachian language; sang Latin paternosters, declared he was God, and then that he was the devil;...

BURN

Delusions; bed, hot, is: op.[137]
- burnt, everything at home is: bell.[10]
- heat, has a furious, radiating from epigastrium: cann-i.
- roasted, he will be: stram.[5]

Dreams; body, arm, covered with blisters, burning: cast.[10]
- ➤ body, back, burnt, hot roast pigeons thrown at her: mag-c.[36]
- ➤ body, cheek burnt by the light: mag-c.[36]
- ➤ body, hands burning by washing: mag-m.[36]
- ➤ burned, of being: xan.[111]
- ➤ disease, burning blisters: cast.
- ➤ disease, burning hands by washing: mag-m.
- ➤ electrocution, of: hydrog.[222]
- ➤ fire, burning, shrieking out, and: mag-c.[36]
- ➤ heads, picking up half roasted, which opened its eyes and spoke angrily, of: jac-c.[36]
- ➤ thirsty, being, burning: **NAT-M.**[54]
- ➤ vivid, burning thirst, of, unquenchable by beer: nat-m.[36]
- ➤ walking, floor, on hot: apis[36]
- ➤ water, child bathing in boiling: mag-c.
- ➤ water, people, bathing, boiling water, in: mag-c.[58]

Fear; falling, fire, into, when walking by it, and in spite of her willpower she did stagger into the fire: onos.[144] psor.[172]
- ✦ hell, of: manc.[30]
- ✦ roasted, to be: stram.[10]

Fire; throws child into fire, after delivery: merc.[85]

Kill; sudden impulse to, throw child, fire, into: hep.[58] lyss. ***nux-v.*** thea.

BUSY

Activity; work, at: benz-ac.[36]
Ailments from; busy, after being: acon.[30] arn.[30] bry.[30] rhus-t.[30] sulph.[30]
Anxiety; do something, compelled to: ***bry.***[54]
Business; desire for: ars.[36] ***carb-v.***[54] cere-b.[36] con.[36] fel.[36] lach.[36] tarent.[36]
Busy: acon.[116] anac.[116] androc.[222] ***apis*** arn.[10] ars.[36] aur.[10] bar-c.[5] bell.[10] ***bry.*** calad. calc. caps. cere-b.[36] choc.[222] cimic.[36] cina[170] cocc. con.[36] cupr.[210] dig.[10] dulc.[30] fel.[36] ferr-p.[36] ***hyos.***[10] ign. indg.[102] ***iod.***[122] ip.[10] ***kali-br.***[5] kali-i.[116] kalm.[5] lac-h.[229] ***lach.***[5] lil-t.[5] m-arct.[10] mag-c.[10] mag-m.[116] merc.[116] mosch.[5] nat-c.[10] ***nux-m.***[162] nux-v.[30] op.[5] opun-a.[36] phos.[116] rhus-t. ***sep.***[5] sil.[30] stann.[10] staph.[30] stram. stront-c.[116] sul-ac.[10] ***sulph.***[122] ***tarent.***[5] ther.[58] ***valer.***[5] ***verat.*** zinc.[116] zinc-val.[116]
Busy; fruitlessly: absin.[102] adax.[96] ***apis***[5] ***arg-n.***[102] ars.[102] bor.[5] calc.[5] canth.[102] ***kali-bi.***[54] kali-br.[137] lil-t.[122] stann. sulph.[102] tarent.[102] ther.[111] verat.[162]
Busy; himself, with: mag-m.[36] staph.[36]
Busy; illness, after: **ACON.**[30] **ARN.**[30] **BRY.**[30] rhus-t.[30] sulph.[30]
Counting continually: arg-n.[193] cand-a.[239] hyos.[8] phys. sil.[5] verat.[162]
Delirium; busy: arum-t.[58] bapt. bell. ***bry.*** camph. ***hyos.*** kali-cy.[36] rhus-t. ***stram.*** sulph.
Delusions; chairs, he is repairing old: cupr. cupr-acet.[36]
- engaged in some occupation, is: acon. ars. atro. bell. cann-i. cupr. hyos. lyss. plb. rhus-t. stram. verat.
- herbs, gathering: bell. cupr.
- sewing, she is: atro.
- shopping with her sister: atro.
- vegetable, green vegetable, he is selling: cupr.

Dreams; busy, being: ambr. anac. androc.[222] apis bapt.[193] bell. **BRY.** camph. canth. carb-ac. ***carl.*** coca hydr. ***hydrog.***[222] hyos. hyper. ign. kalm. lach. led. lil-t.[36] lyc. mosch. osm. phos. pip-m.[36] polyg.[36] sabad. sabin. sang. sep. spig.[1]
➤ farming: mag-s. merc-i-r.
➤ wedding, busy, at which she was: mag-s.[36]

Hurry; occupation, desires to do several things at once, finish any, but cannot: pin-s.[36] plan.[36]
Hurry; occupation, in: acon. aur. calc-f.[144] camph. carb-v. carc.[227] cimic.[36] hep.[54] ***kali-c.*** kali-p.[58] **LIL-T.** onos.[144] op. ptel.[144] puls. sep. **SUL-AC.** sul-i.[58] ***thuj.*** viol-t.
Impulse; busy, when, amel.: iod.[137]
Insanity; busy: **APIS** bell.[10] hyos.[58] ***iod.***[54] kali-br.
Loquacity; busy: lach.[10] ther.[10]
Mania; action, must be constantly in, in some laborious occupation: ***iod.***[54]
Occupation; diversion amel.: aesc.[58] agar. alum. androc.[222] apis[112] ars.[122] aur. bar-c. calc. calc-p.[102] calc-sil.[58] ***camph.***[5] carc.[207] chin. cic.[5] ***con. croc.***[122] ***cupr. cycl.***[5] ***ferr. hell. helon. ign. iod.*** kali-bi.[5] ***kali-br.*** lac-h.[229] lach.[54] lap-c-b.[194] lap-gr-m.[194] ***lil-t.*** lyc. ***merc-i-f.*** merc-i-r.[137] mez. mur-ac.[5] ***nat-c. nux-v.*** orig.[5] ox-ac.[102] pall.[5] ***pip-m.*** puls.[58] samars.[111] **SEP.** sil. spig.[116] stram. tarent.[102] thuj. verat.
Restlessness; busy: acon.[10] ars.[127] ***aur.***[10] bell.[10] bry.[10] caps.[1] choc.[222] cocc.[1] dig.[10] hyos.[10] ***ign.***[1] ip.[10] ***lach.***[10] m-arct.[10] ***mosch.***[10] nat-c.[10] nux-v.[30] stann.[10] sul-ac.[10] ther.[123] verat.[1]
Restlessness; rest, has none, at any employment: ***chel.***[54]

AGAR. Ha, 28 - Quiet, equable (tranquil), sociable, active, and glad of having done his duty.
ALUM. Ha, 23 - Excited, over-worked (industrious), and yet discontented, because not enough had been done. (duty)
ARN. Ha, 623 - Over-busy, inclination and disposition for great and continuous literary work with no power to do it without injury to the health.
He, 23 - Excessive inclination to hard and long literary labors.(industrious)
ART-V. He, 7 - Gets up every night and does her daily work as a house servant, with closed eyes, lies down again and cannot remember anything next morning.
AUR. Ha, 12 - He is driven to constant activity, and is sorry for his inaction, although he cannot do anything.
BELL. Al, 54 - The delirium was of a busy (engaged, working), restless, vivid character, but generally rather pleasing than otherwise. The patient appeared to think they were pursuing (persevere) their ordinary occupations; one boy appeared eager (animated) in flying a kite (toy),

another pulled tables and chairs about, thinking he was working in a coal-pit, and a woman appeared to be remarkably busy with her household duties...

Al, 109 - A tailor was poisoned with a belladona injection, and for fifteen hours, though speechless and insensible to external objects, went through all the customary operations of his trade with great vivacity and moved his lips as if in conversation.(busy)

Al, 35-...she acts as if she were washing or counting money, or as if she were drinking.

A-S, 2554-..The patients appeared to think that they were pursuing their ordinary occupations;... the woman appeared remarkably busy with her ordinary household duties.

Ha, 1366 - Ridiculous grimaces; ...acts as if she were washing, at another as if counting money, ...

BRY. Al, 37 - Over-busy (industrious); she undertakes and works far too much.

Al, 13 - Anxiety in the whole body, which compelled him to do something constantly, and wherever he went he found no rest.

Ha, 780 - Too busy; she wishes to undertake and to work at too many things.

CALC-A. Ha, 263 - Anxious disposition as if something evil had happened or he had to fear reproaches (censures); at the same time, however, persistent inclination to work. (industrious)

CALC. Al, 22 - Anxious, restless, and busy mood; she is undertaking much things but accomplish nothing...

CAPS. Al, 12 - An excessively busy (occupied) uneasy mood.

CARB-V. Ha, 16 - Excessive excitation, as if she was too much hurried (fast), or over-worked (industrious) in business.

CERE-B. Al, 3 - Felt all day an astonishing (unusual) inclination to be engaged (work, busy) in something useful. (helpful)

Al, 1 - Desire to engage at work.

Al, 2 - Desire to have the time all employed. (work)

CHIN. Ha, 1134 - Liking for work, reading, writing, and thinking; particularly well disposed and industrious.

HALI-L. Sh, 182 - Not doing enough. Feel somewhat critical of myself. Not getting anything done. Want to be in a structured, organized place and can't get there. I'd like to be really busy. I have more ideas in my head than I can do. I need to get active again, structure things, and set goals. 08, 30C, 03:XX:XX

HYOS. Ha, 517 - Over-busy: he thought he was more active and stronger (powerful, Herculean) than he actually was.

IGN. Ha, 755 - Excessively busy: he restlessly sets about doing first one thing then another.

IOD. Ha, 16 - Anxiety and dejection; the patients generally busy themselves with the present.

He, 15 - At night, especially when thinking of real or imaginary wrongs ...dares (try) to go home for fear of doing some dreadful (bad, wicked) deed (action); on one occasion was seized with an almost irresistible impulse to murder a woman who was acting as a guide (direct, conduct) for him, he having lost his way (direction);...must be constantly in action, in some laborious occupation. (lost; direction, correction, control)

KALI-BR. He, 4-...constant worry, fears to see people or to be spoken to;...failure of mental and bodily strength;...constantly busy, tying his shoes, fumbling in his pockets, picking threads, etc.

He, 24 - Hands constantly busy; all sorts of fearful delusions; walks the room groaning, bemoaning his fate (destine, doom); full of fear; unsteady.(inconstant)

LAC-C. Al,N-39 - Wakes distressed, and obliged to rise and occupy herself in some manner; fears she will be crazy.

He, 32 - Wakes distressed, and obliged to rise and occupy herself in some manner; fears she will be crazy.

LACH. Al, 5 - A kind of ecstasy, as after sublime impressions, or excessive joy, throughout the day; he constantly wishes to talk and do much, and even more seems to be at his command.(control, domination)

Al, 41 - Need of being very busy, without the slightest perseverance.

He, 40 - He wishes to do a great deal; begins many things. (undertakes)

STANN. Al, 20 - Fruitlessly busy, as if a rush of ideas prevented him from completing his work at a certain time; all sorts of things occur to him to be done.

Ha, 639 - Busy uselessness (inefficiency): he exerts (use) himself to get a necessary task (duty) done at the appointed hour, and cannot accomplish it, as though prevented (interrupted) by an over-crowding of thoughts, during which one thing and another occur to him which he wishes to do...

Ha, 10 - He is ineffectually (inefficiently) busied, as if he was prevented (obstructed) by super abundance of ideas from finishing his work at a certain time; he thinks of a number of things which he ought yet to attend to.

STRAM. Al, 123-...seemed to herself to be engaged in her usual avocation,...imitate in every respect the routine procedure of one thus engaged.

He, 40 - Aberration of mind; one carries home all sorts of wood in order to manufacture brandy (cognac) (busy, manufacturing) ; another placed two axes across each other in order to split wood in this way; a third burrowed in ground like a pig with his mouth (animal); a fourth alleged he was a wheelwright and began to bore holes; a fifth ran into forge to catch fish, which he saw swimming there; a lacemaker threw about her bobbins incessantly, and threw everything into confusion; another girl ran about the room and cried out that all evil spirits were pursuing her.(restoration, restitution)

VERAT. He, 8 - Attempts (try) a great many things, but accomplishes (achieve) nothing.

CAMOUFLAGE

Fur, wraps up in summer: hep.[111] hyos. ***kali-ar.***[137] ***psor.***[111]

Rover about; wrapped in fur in the Summer: hyos.

HYOS. Ha, 544 - Naked and enveloped in a fur cloak, he senselessly wanders about to a great distance in the summer heat.

He, 78 - Groundless suspicion of being watched (observed, spied) by members of family with whom he had some slight misunderstanding (dispute); to avoid being recognized by them, clothed himself differently every day,...watching his relations suspiciously and imagining he might be poisoned;... (disguise, camouflage)

He, 72 - He lies in bed nude and chatters; walks about insane, naked, wrapped in a skin during summer heat.

PLB. He, 15-...; despair of her salvation...; fixed idea that could only obtain peace and safety though absolution by a priest of the papal church, although she had been a zealous Protestant; ....brooded over any forbidden thing; would steal (leave) from house in servant's cloak (coat, camouflage) and bonnet (hat) to obtain stimulants (drugs), but from the moment their prohibition was withdrawn (retired) ceased to have any desire for them; after being permitted to visit a priest and converse with him ceased to talk and think of the church. (desire; redemption, absolution)

CAPRICIOUS

Absorbed; alternating with frivolity: arg-n.

Anger; refused, when things he wants are: bry.[56] cham.[56] cina[56] kreos.[56]

Anger; temper tantrums, falls on the floor kicking and screaming: nat-m.[162]

Anger; temper tantrums, throw themselves on the floor during, cannot get their breath: thuj.[8]

Aversion; handled, being: abrot.[127] cina[122] nat-m.[127] sep.[127]

Capriciousness: acon. act-sp.[54] agar. alum. alum-sil.[58] am-c. ant-c.[116] ant-t.[102] arn. ***ars.*** ars-s-f.[58] asaf. aur-m. bamb-a.[1184] bar-c. bar-s.[58] ***bell.*** bov.[10] bran.[10] brom. **BRY.** calc. calc-f.[53] calc-s. calc-sil.[58] cand-a.[239] cann-i. cann-s.[10] canth. caps. carb-an. carbn-s. carc.[149] ***caust.***[10] cench.[58] **CHAM.** chap.[149] chin. chin-ar. cimic. **CINA** coca[36] ***cocc.***[10] ***coff.*** coloc.[5] croc. ***cypr.***[54] dig. dros. ***dulc.*** ferr.[116] ferr-acet.[10] fl-ac.[54] goss.[122] grat. hep. ***ign.***[122] ***iod.***[54] **IP.** kali-ar. **KALI-C.** kali-sil.[58] kreos. lach. lap-mar-c.[194] led. lil-t.[58] lyc. m-arct.[10] m-aust.[10] mag-c.[54] mag-m. ***mag-p.***[54] merc. ***merc-i-f.***[36] nat-c.[30] nat-n.[10] nit-ac. nux-m. nux-v. op. ozone[227] par. ***ph-ac.***[30] ***phos.***[122] ***plat.***[10] plb.[54] ***puls.*** raph. ***rheum*** rhod. sac-alb.[85] sanic.[127] sarr. sars.[36] sec. ***sep.***[10] sil. sphing.[36] spong. **STAPH.** stram. ***sul-ac.***[54] ***sulph.*** syph.[149]

thuj. thyr.[149] tub.[149] vac.[149] valer.[10] verat.[30] **VERAT-V.**[162] viol-t. zinc. zinc-p.[58]
Capriciousness; children, in: **CHAM.**[122] **CINA**[122] rheum[1] sac-alb.[85]
Contradiction; intolerant of, throw themselves angrily on the floor and cannot get their breath when in the least opposed: thuj.[8]
Delusions; whimsical: cann-i.[36]
Desires; full of: agav-t.[149] bry.[5] cina[10] coff.[5] dulc.[5] ign.[10] ip.[10] nux-m.[10] ***puls.***[5] rheum[10] rhus-t.[5] ***spig.***[30]
Desires; many things impatiently, dislikes its favorite playthings, child: arn.[5] **CHAM.**[5] cina[56] dulc.[5] kreos.[5] puls.[5] **RHEUM**[54] staph.[56]
Desires; numerous, various things: cic.[137] ***cina***[36] phos.[36] staph.[137]
Desires; numerous, various things, hard to be had, which are: bry.[160]
Desires; numerous, various things, insane: ars.[10] bry.[10] cham.[10] chin.[10] cina[10] coff.[10] dulc.[10] ign.[10] ip.[10] ***puls.***[10] rhus-t.[10]
Desires; numerous, various things, opposed if offered by someone else: caps.[58]
Desires; numerous, various things, pleased with nothing: all-s.[137]
Desires; numerous, various things, refused when offered: ant-t.[56] bry.[56] caps.[137] ***cham.***[10] ***cina***[56] dulc.[137] ferr.[171] hep.[137] ip.[102] kreos.[56] mang.[171] phos.[137] phys.[137] ***staph.***[8]
Desires; numerous, various things, refused when offered, disagree, that: puls.[137]
Desires; numerous, various things, refused when offered, food: rheum[5]
Desires; numerous, various things, refused when offered, throws them away: cham.[103] sec.[137]
Desires; present, things not: bry.[5] calc-sil.[58] puls.[5] rheum[5]
Desires; present, things not, rejected when offered, which are, playthings, etc.: arn.[5] bry.[160] **CHAM.**[5] ***cina***[54] ***dulc.***[54] hep.[36] kreos.[5] puls.[5] staph.[137]
Desires; relish, what cannot: bry.[137] ign.[137] mag-m.[137] puls.[137]
Desires; this and that: coff.[36] ***puls.***[36]
Discontented; always: **HEP.**[30] lach.[30] **MERC.**[30] nit-ac.[30]
Excitement; curses his mother, throws food or medicine across room: ***hydr.***[54]
Fancies; exaltation of, capricious, fitful: acon.[5] viol-o.[5]
Imbecility; rage, stamps the feet: anac.[122] lyc.[122] nux-v.[122] op.[122] verat.[122]
Impatience; cures him at once, the patient insists that the doctor: cham.[85]
Impatience; throws himself about: ***acon.***[54]
Insanity; capricious: raph.[54]
Mania; capricious: raph.[36]
Moaning; children, in, piteous, because he cannot have what he wanted: **CHAM.**[36]
Mood; repulsive, asks for, for what he: arn.[5] bry.[185] cham.[5] dulc.[102] kreos.[102] puls.[5] staph.[144]
Spoiled children: am-c.[30] bar-c.[30] lyc.[30] mosch.[85] op.[30] sulph.[30]
Throws; herself, floor, on: nat-m.[162] nux-v.[189] tub.[70]
Throws; herself, floor, on, opposed, when, and cannot get his breath: thuj.[8]
Throws; herself, forcibly about: ***calc.***[54] naja[36]
Weeping; children, refused, the least thing, when: cham.[8]
Weeping; refused anything, when: bell. cham. ign. tarent.[36] viol-o.[122]

ACT-SP. He, 17 - Irresolution, inconstancy and caprice.
ARN. Ha, 627 - Surly, wants to have many things and then refuses them.
ARS. Al, 94 - Very fretful, indignant, capricious; every word offends her, and makes her very angry, when she should answer.
He, 59 - Very peevish and passionate, capricious, she takes every word ill and is cross when she has to answer.
ASAF. He, 4 - Unsteady (inconstant) and fickle (changeable), cannot persevere in anything; wants now one thing, then another; walks hither and thither.
BRY. He, 15 - Desire for things that cannot be had, which are refused, or not wanted when offered.
CHAM. Al, 13 - Piteous moaning of a child because he cannot have what he wants. (contrariety)
Ha, 460-... The child makes itself stiff and bends backwards, stamps with its feet on the nurse's arm, cries in an uncontrollable way, and throws everything away.
Ha, 461 - Lachrymose restlessness; the child wants this thing and the other, and when given anything he refuses it or knocks it away from him.
He, 17 - Whining (lamenting) restlessness;

the child wants this and that, which, when offered, is refused or pushed away.
He, 15 - Piteous moaning of a child because he cannot have what he wants.
CHIN. Ha, 1103 - She falls time to time into a lachrymose humour, without external cause, from some self-made, trivial whim (caprice), e.q. from some imaginary want (lack, need), such as that she cannot eat enough...
CROC. Al, 3 - An unpleasant sensation, as if he were longing (desire) for something without knowing what, with a kind of apprehension, ...
IGN. Al, 5 - Desires improper (inappropriate) things, and cries aloud when they are refused.
Ha, 775 - When one hesitates in the least to do what she wishes, or remonstrates (censures) much with her, though in a mild friendly manner, or endeavor to persuade her, or wishes differently from what she wishes, she weeps aloud.
Ha, 774 - Desires improper things, and weeps aloud when they are denied him.
IP. Ha, 228 - His disposition is full of wishes and longing he knows not for what.
He, 3 - Full of inexpressible desires.
KALI-C. Al, 45 - Disagreeable mood; she longs for things with impetuosity; is contented with nothing, is beside herself, and gets into rage if everything does not go according to her wishes, and frequently does not herself know what she really wishes to have.
Al, 44 - Disagreeable mood; he is obstinate and frequently does not himself know what he wishes.
LYC. Ha, 50 - He smiles without being merry, capricious.
PHOS. Al, 150 - My wants were numerous and variable.
PLAT. Ha, 37 - During the caprice of contempt, suddenly a voracious hunger...
PULS. Al, 5 - He wishes now for this, now for that employment, but when given to him he will have nothing to do with it.
Al, 8 - Extremely capricious and peevish at everything, even at himself.
He, 13 - Extremely capricious and peevish about everything, himself included.
SEP. Al, 66 - She finds fault and desires nothing which others want, accompanied by weeping and heat of face.
SIL. Al, 37 - Whimsical (capricious) and fault -finding.
Ha, 18 - Capricious and disposed to take things ill.
STANN. Ha, 640 - Peevish: nothing was done according to his wish.
SULPH. Ha, 53 - He is so peevish and obstinate, that he will not give an answer to anybody, he cannot bear to have anyone around him, and cannot get quickly enough what he wants.
THUJ. Al, 16 - The child is excessively obstinate; on the slightest contradiction it throws itself in the ground in rage and loses its breath.

CARES

Ailments from; cares, worries: ***ambr.***[5] arg-n.[85] ars.[85] ***calc.***[122] ***caust.***[122] con.[116] germ.[222] ign.[85] kali-br.[85] kali-p.[5] lyc.[36] mag-c.[102] nat-m.[5] nit-ac.[187] **NUX-V.**[8] ***ph-ac. phos.***[10] pic-ac.[58] sanic.[85] ***staph.***[10]

Ailments from; grief, emotional, mental symptoms from: alum.[36] am-m.[36] ***ars.***[8] ***aur.***[54] bar-s.[58] bell.[10] calc-p.[72] carc.[207] ***caust.***[8] ***cocc.***[54] con.[8] ***gels.***[8] ***ign.***[8] ***kali-br.***[54] lach.[30] lact.[36] lyc.[5] merc.[5] ***nat-m.***[54] ***ph-ac.***[54] phos.[58] phys.[137] ***plat.***[8] zinc.[8]

Ailments from; grief, sorrow, care: alum-p.[58] am-m. ***ambr.***[5] aml-n.[137] anac. ant-c. ***apis arn.***[122] ars. art-v.[85] **AUR.** aur-ar.[58] aur-s.[58] bar-s.[58] bell.[5] **BRY.**[5] cadm-s.[5] cael.[149] ***calc.***[5] ***calc-p.*** caps.[5] carc.[207] **CAUST.** cham.[114] clem. **COCC.** colch. ***coloc. con.***[5] ***crat.***[122] crot-h.[137] cycl. cypr.[54] dig.[58] ***dros.***[122] ***gels. graph. hura***[117] ***hyos.*** **IGN.** ip.[122] ***kali-br.***[54] kali-c.[5] kali-p. **LACH.** laur.[58] lob-c. lob-s.[54] lyc. mag-c.[85] naja nat-c.[5] **NAT-M.** nit-ac. nux-m.[58] ***nux-v.*** op.[5] paull.[8] petr.[5] **PH-AC.** phos.[5] phys.[85] pic-ac.[5] ***plat.*** psor.[185] ***puls.*** pyrus[36] rhus-t.[5] ***samb.***[102] ***sep.***[5] seq-s.[230] ***sol-o.***[122] spig.[162] **STAPH.** stram.[5] sulph.[10] tarent. tub.[193] ***uran-n.***[193] verat. ***zinc.***[5]

Anger; alternating with, cares: ran-b.[10]

Cares, worries, full of: acet-ac.[137] ***ambr.***[5] anac.[10] arn.[10] **ARS.**[5] aur.[1] ***bar-c.***[111] ***calc.***[54] calc-p.[5] calc-sil.[58] cann-i.[36] caust. chel.[10] ***chin.*** cimic.[149] coff. con.[5] cypr.[25] ***dig.***[5] dros.[10] dys-co.[136] fago.[25] graph.[10] hed.[149] ***ign.***[137] ***iod.***[54] ***kali-br.***[54] kali-n.[1] kali-p.[137] lyc.[30] mag-c.[137] mang.[10] med.[54] mur-ac.[1] ***nat-c.***[10] nat-m.[5] nux-v.[116] op.[10] ***ph-ac.***[5]

pic-ac.[116] ***psor.***[5] ***puls.*** ran-b.[172] sal-ac.[54] sep.[1] sil.[30] ***spig.***[10] stann.[10] **STAPH.**[30] ***sulph.***[85] thuj.[10] v-a-b.[149] vac.[54]
Cares; full of, alone, when: hep.[10]
Cares; full of, alternating with, quarrelsomeness: ran-b.[10]
Cares; full of, company, with aversion to: con.[10] nat-m.[10]
Cares; full of, domestic affairs, about: bar-c. ***puls. sep.***
Cares; full of, eat, if he does not: ***cocc.***[54] **IOD.**[54]
Cares; full of, money, about: bamb-a.[1184] ozone[227]
Cares; full of, nature, for, animals, plants: lap-c-b.[194]
Cares; full of, noise, by, or interruption in business: ***lyc.***[54]
Cares; full of, others, about: ars.[5] ***caust.***[30] cocc.[5] ***ign.***[5] lach.[30] lap-c-b.[194] sulph.[10] zinc.[30]
Cares; full of, quietly: ***coff.***[54]
Cares; full of, relatives, about: ars.[10] cand-a.[239] ***caust.***[30] hep.[10] lach.[30] rhus-t.[10] ***spig.***[30] zinc.[30]
Cares; full of, trifles, about: ***ars.*** aur.[58] but-ac.[102] ***chin.***[30] dys-co.[136]
Dementia; business, worry from: lil-t.[137]
Dreams; cares, amel. when seeing the person worrying about: tarent.[36]
➤ cares, full of: alum.[36] am-m.[5] apis[54] ***ars.***[5] caps.[5] carl.[36] cast.[10] caust.[5] croto-t.[10] hydr.[36] ign.[5] laur.[5] lyc.[5] mur-ac.[5] nat-c.[5] nat-m.[5] nux-v.[10] op.[5] phos.[5] ***rheum***[5] rhus-t.[5] sabad.[36] spong.[5] stront-c.[36]
➤ cares, patients, for his: bac.[62]
Dullness; cares for his business, from: ph-ac.[58]
Irritability; alternating with, cares: ran-b.[5]
Prostration; cares, from: ph-ac.[58] pic-ac.[58]
Religious affections; preoccupations: achy.[149]
Restlessness; cares, from: kali-br.[85]
Sadness; preoccupied: ***clem.***[54]
Sighing; worry, from: lyc.[60]

ACET-AC. He, 6 - Anxiety; grieves about his sickness and his children.
ANAC. Al, 1 - Illusions of fancy; he imagines he has his name called by the voice of his far-distant mother and sister, accompanied by an apprehension of misfortune and anxiety.
ARG-M. He, 16 - Anxious about her health; full of care.
BAR-A. Al, 10 - An evil, fearful suspicion suddenly takes possession of her, as if, for example, a loved friend had been taken suddenly deathly ill.
CALC-A. Ha, 262 - Very grave (serious) and full of care (worry); busied with the present and the future; he becomes sad almost to tears.
CALC. Ha, 3 - Mournful (grief), almost to tears, with solicitous occupation with the present and the future.
He, 8 - Mind full of concern about imaginary things that might happen to her. 0 Chlorosis.
CANN-S. Ha, 303 - Dreams of misfortunes happening to others.
CERE-B. Al, 4 - Felt a desire to give something quite necessary to myself to another. (altruism, helpful, sympathetic)
CUPR. Ha, 5 - A kind of timidity; he felt as if he had to step softly, in order not to hurt himself, nor to disturb his room-mates. (friend) (cautious, prudent, gentle, delicate)
HEP. Ha, 5 - Fear about the illness of his family, especially while walking in the open air.
IGN. He, 61 - Melancholia after great grief and domestic trouble; complete sleeplessness; suicidal thoughts and desire to escape.
PH-AC. He, 11 - Ailments from care, grief, sorrow, chagrin, homesickness; or disappointed love;...
STAPH. He, 4 - Sad distressing thoughts about one's illness.

CAUGHT

Delusions; bed, bound to the, by suction: sars.[139]
• bed, drawn from under her: stram.
• body, legs, tied together: syph.[137]
• body, tongue, pulling out his, someone is: bell.
• crowded with arms and legs: ***pyrog.***[122]
• dragged from the lowest abyss of darkness (at night, on waking): thea.
• spectres, sees, clutches at: hyos.
• strangers, snatching at her: ***bell.***[54]
• throat, someone with icy-cold hands took her by the: canth.

Dreams; encircled tightly, being: ruta.
- ➤ finger, of being seized by a: sil.[1]
- ➤ held, tightly by hand, so could not get away: am-m.[36]

ANDROC. Sh, 116 - Impatient, snappy, shouting, felt trapped and despairing. Growled at her children. (12)
BELL. He, 18 - When closing eyes, though not asleep, patient sees fierce (wild), wicked looking large animals with horns and bushy (scabrous) heads; room seemed to be full of strange men passing in and out, who would snatch (take hold) at her as they passed, which frightened her very much, she thought the men wanted to take her away from home ; she then saw children sitting on low benches (seat) in rows (line) as in a school-room. (purity)
CANN-I. Al, 25-...Now demoniac shapes clutched (grasp) at him from the darkness, cloaked (covered) from head to foot in inky (black) palls (mantle), glaring (staring, looking) at him with fiery eyes from beneath their cowls(mantle)....
CANTH. Al, 17 - Visions...something took hold of her hand, and bent it several times up and down, then it seemed as if someone took her by the throat with ice-cold hands.
CHOC. Sh, 50 - Panic feeling of being trapped and enclosed —worse when curtains are closed and the light blocked out. Strong desire to be outside and moving, to be in the bright and warm sunlight. Kept having to move my feet, which I felt I wanted to move.
HYOS. He, 81-...attempts to escape from room; frightful hallucinations of figures coming to seize him, hens (chicken) bound (imprisoned) with chains,...
NIT-AC. Al, 30 - Anxious oppression, like nightmare, as if some one were lying under him and holding him fast with the arms about his abdomen, so that he could not free himself, immediately after falling asleep. (constriction, immobilization)
STRAM. Ha, 559 - She fancies she sees a number of people who are not present, and she grasps at them.
He, 59-...clings to her mother with as much desperation as if she were going to be thrown from a precipice.
He, 79 - Boy seemed to see black objects, spoke of black people and black clouds, and grasped at air.

CENSORIOUS

Censorious, critical: acon. alum. alum-sil.[58] am-c. androc.[222] apis[98] ***arn.*** **ARS.** ars-s-f.[58] aur. aur-ar.[58] aur-s.[58] bac.[62] ***bar-c.*** bar-s.[58] bell. benz. bor. ***brom.***[30] calc. calc-ar.[58] calc-p. calc-sil.[58] caps. carc.[207] carl. ***caust.*** cench. cham. chin. chin-ar. cic. cocc. cupr.[184] cycl. der. dulc. germ.[222] gran. ***graph.***[122] guai. ***helon.***[54] hydrog.[222] hyos. ign. ***ip.*** iris kali-ar.[58] kali-c.[5] kali-cy.[36] kali-s.[184] lac-ac.[58] lac-h.[229] ***lach.*** lap-gr-m.[194] lil-t.[58] ***lyc.*** m-arct.[10] mag-c.[144] med.[212] mez.[58] morph.[102] mosch. myric. naja[5] nat-m. ***nux-v.*** par. petr. ***phos.***[30] ***plat.*** plb. puls.[5] ran-b. rhus-t. sapin.[36] ***sep.*** sil. sol-t-ae. staph. **SULPH.** tarent.[102] til. tus-f.[30] **VERAT.**[122]
Censorious; dearest friends, with: ars-s-f.[58] aur-s.[58] chin-ar. der.
Censorious; find fault or is silent, disposed to: hydrog.[222] ***verat.***
Censorious; nagging: lyc.[137] nux-v.[137] plat.[137]
Censorious; parents, teachers and friends, of: sep.[189]
Censorious; scolding, with: ars.[30] merc.[30]
Censorious; unoccupied, when, close application amel.: sapin.[36]
Complaining; relations and surroundings, of: ***merc.***[54]
Delirium; reproachful: hyos. lyc.
Discontented; wrong, everything another does is: ***cham.***[54]
Insanity; reproaches others: **LYC.**[30]
Jealousy; quarrels, reproaches, scolds, with: gall-ac.[36] ***lach.***[54] ***nux-v.***[54]
Recriminations about trifles: cop.[36]
Reproaches; others: ***acon.*** alum. ambr.[1189] **ARS.** aur. aur-ar.[58] bell.[10] bor.[1] calc.[30] calc-p. caps. ***carc.***[162] caust.[10] cham. **CHIN.** cic. gels.[162] gink.[149] gran. hist.[119] ***hyos.*** ign. ***lach.*** lap-gr-m.[194] lap-mar-c.[194] ***lyc.*** med.[162] merc. mez. mosch.[10] nat-ar. ***nat-m.*** ***nux-v.*** par. petr.[10] rhus-t. sep. ***staph.***[122] sulph.[30] ***verat.***[122]
Reproaches; others, imaginary insult, for: aur-ar.[58]
Sadness; blaming others, with: lil-t.[168]
Slander; disposition to sneak: ars.[30] lach.[30] nat-c.[30]

Slander; disposition to, hypocritical, and: phos.[30] sep.[30]

ACON. Ha, 517 - Piteous (miserable), anxious complaints, with cowardly fears, despair, loud whining weeping, bitter complaints and reproaches.

ADAM. Sh, 205 - Get angry when criticized, yet easily critical of others.[20], 1M, 06:XX:XX

Sh, 207 - I am feeling very critical, casting a critical eye. 7, 6C, 03:00:XX

Sh, 211 - I felt very impatient with my patients. I was making a lot of judgments. 7, 6C, 03:00:XX

ALUM. Ha, 33 - She is extremely peevish, and everything is offensive to her; she only wishes to scold (criticize) and to raise a fuss (trouble) in the afternoon.

AM-C. Al, 33 - She found fault with everything.

ANDROC. Sh, 119 - Critical and irritable. (21)

ARN. Ha, 630 - He contradicts; is opinionative; no one can please him.

ARS. Al, 95 - Very fretful (irritable) and contented with nothing; she finds fault (imperfection, error) with everything; ...

Ha, 1042 - Irritable state of the disposition, he vexes himself about trifles, and cannot leave off talking about the faults of others.

Ha, 1049 - Discontented with everything, finds fault with everything; everything is too strong and too irritating, all conversation, all noise, and all light.

He, 92 - Disposed to discuss the faults of others.

BELL. Ha, 1364 - Unrestrainedly and exuberantly merry, inclined to scold (criticize) without cause, and to insult (affront, offend) in a laughing humor.

Ha, 1401 - Peevishness, nothing was right for him; he was angry with himself.

BOR. Ha, 14-...reproaches people for slight matters, for several days.

CANN-I. Al, 30 - When his friends went out of the room, he thought (delusion) they had left him to his fate (destiny, doom), and wrote "cowards" in his notes.

CAPS. Al, 1 - He makes reproaches and becomes angry at the faults of others; he becomes offended at trifles and finds fault.

Ha, 334 - He makes reproaches, and is indignant (angry) at the faults (errors) of others; he takes trifles ill and finds fault with them.

CARBN-O. Al, 11 - After supper, felt buoyant (happy) and in good humor, an effect never produced by tea; this mental sensation soon passed over into an irritable and sarcastic one, so that I sharply criticized an article in a medical journal, which a few hours ago I hardly thought worth that trouble, and threw away in disgust a book of reference as flat and superficial, which I highly sluggish.(inactive)

CARL. Al, 16 - Very much disposed to take everything in bad part and to be critical.(especially after three weeks and later)

CHAM. He, 55 - In all her sufferings there is a vein of ill humor; she can hardly speak pleasantly; feels like scolding (censorious, offensive) about everything; she often gives vent to her ill humor in spite of all restraint.

CHIN. Ha, 1110 - Extremely disposed to be vexed, and to take every occasion to get cross; afterwards quarrelsome and disposed to vex others, and to make reproaches and give annoyance(irritation) to others.

He, 31 - Inclined to reproach and vex (annoy, provoke) others.

CHOC. Sh, 7 - In the evening, felt angry with bristling down my back. Irritable with the kids, shouted a lot, slammed doors. Feeling very uncomfortable with my daughter near me. I made a huge issue over something small which I would normally leave. I wanted to leave and walk out of the door on them. Felt very unsympathetic to the children. "You either go, or go to bed". Couldn't cuddle the children and took longer to say "Its all right". I thought that their father should look after them instead of me (very unusual). The feeling I can't be where I want to be because of them. I want to be roaming outside without my possessions. Left kids alone in the house for the first time. I was surprised at how easily I let them go. My daughter liked it very much.

Sh, 304 - Feels she has changed her attitude towards herself, less judgmental and pedantic, kinder to herself now. Eating more meat and feeling OK about it, previously had been vegetarian for health and moral reasons.[13], 12C, XX:XX:XX

CIC. Al, 27 - Want of confidence in mankind; with misanthropy; he forsook society, remained alone and reflected upon their errors and about himself.

CON. He, 38 - Very much excited, passionate, domineering (dictatorial), quarrelsome, scolds (censorious) and will not bear contradiction.

GERM. Sh, 171 - Heavy sighing in the morning. Critical and irritable with son. Feel I can't handle him. 21, 12C, 40:XX:XX.

GRAN. Al, 11 - Inclined to criticize and blame.

HALI-L. Sh, 573 - Back into usual blaming and being critical of children and family. Also being very self critical and dissatisfied. 09, 6C, 27—[34]:XX:XX

Sh, 581 - At a meeting for parents and children, I am very critical of my daughter and myself, comparing her to other kids, myself to other moms. Cringe when she sits with her mouth open, pulling on her hair and twisting it into braids. Want to warn her, don't do that! She looks to me like she's bossing someone. Compare myself to other woman who has perfectly put together hair, clothes, nails, boots, bracelets. Very angry and jealous. Make excuses for myself and tear her down inside. 09, 6C, 14:00:XX

HELL. He, 12 - An old woman having been accused of theft by the women around, took it so much to heart that she hanged herself. This suicide produced a profound effect upon the women of the village. One after another accused herself of having caused the death of the old woman by their insinuations; they wept and howled, ran about day and night wringing their hands and despairing of salvation on account of their sin (error); they became quite irrepressible and deranged (disordered) In this way twenty -four or twenty five women were affected, every fresh case being followed by another. Hysterical mania.

HELON. Al, 4-.... could not endure the least contradiction or receive any suggestions in regard to any subject (fixed ideas) ;... what I most desired was to be left alone, reserved to myself the privilege of finding fault (imperfection) with everything around me;....

HYOS. Al, 94 - He reproaches others, and complains of a supposed injury done him.

Ha, 578 - He reproaches others, and complains of injustice that he imagines has been done him.

He, 34 - Scolds (censorious); raves; abuses those about him.

IGN. Al, 30 - Extremely morose, finds fault, and makes reproaches.

Ha, 769 - Is extremely sulky; finds fault and makes reproaches.

IRIS. Al, 5 - Vexed, irritable mood, disposed to find fault.

KALI-AR. He, 1 - Scolding (censorious) morose, retired, quarrelsome and discontented, jealous, indifferent to everything,...

KALI-CY. Al, 4 - For two days, desire to find fault; crossness almost uncontrollable on entering the room; while the cold air produces good spirits.

KALM. Al, 3 - Feels like scolding (censure) everybody...

LAC-AC. He, 2 - Averse to business or what formerly was pleasant to do; lazy (indolent); dislikes to read or think; finds fault, is sarcastic, exacting. (exigent, severe)

LYC. Al, 2 - Delirious, raging, envious, reproachful, presumptuous, and imperious.

Ha, 60 - As if insane she seeks for quarrels, makes ungrounded reproaches abuses (insulting) most violently and beats the person whom she abuses.

He, 37 - Haughty, reproachful and overbearing.(despotic)

LYSS. Al, 28 - Very cross, so much that my children expressed great surprise; took offense at the merest trifles; scolded (censorious) my wife and children; ....

He, 88 - Very cross, so much so that his children expressed great surprise; he took offense at veriest trifles, scolded his wife and children, felt wretched, ...

MERC. He, 35 - Grief, with fear at night; disposition to quarrel; complaining of relations and surroundings.

MEZ. Al, 34 - Inclined to reproach others.

Ha, 14 - Disposed to reproach others.

MYRIC. Al, 9-...a constant desire to find fault (censorious); everything went wrong;

looked upon (contemptuous) this world as a place not fit to live in any longer; considered himself better than the rest (great person, megalomania), in the morning; ...; condemned himself for various imaginary faults; ...

NEON. Sh, 176 - Got up late in a horrible mood and reproached my partner again. I hurt him but I didn't care. I felt indifferent, malicious and vindictive, full of hate. 02, 6C, 05:22:10

Sh, 177 - I feel like writing a letter to Jeremy and reproaching him about the proving. I just realized that I want to reproach people. I reproach my partner as well. 02, 6C, 05:XX:XX

NUX-V. Ha, 1253 - Pains are not borne without loud whining and lamenting, mixed with reproaches and scolding.

Ha, 1266 - Very much given to reproach others severely for their faults.

Ha, 1267 - Scolding, reproaches, abuse, jealous invectives (accusation), mixed with indelicate expressions -then soon howling and loud weeping.

Ha, 1255 - Anxious solicitude and inconsolableness, which breaks out in loud weeping complaints and reproaches...

He, 12 - Inclined to find fault and scold (reprove); morose; stubborn; (obstinate) an insane desire when alone with her husband, whom she adores, to kill him.

He, 37-...betraying (play false, feigning) great moral and physical languor (indifference),..launches into high-flying, fantastic plans, fancies himself rich (rank, position) and wants to make presents of thousands (squanders, waste), and makes large useless purchases; does not consider himself ill; ...,and takes in bad part if not allowed to read indictment (accusation) for said lawsuit, a confused irrational piece of work...

He, 39 - Mania puerperalis...constantly complaining, criticizing or explaining, ... as soon she recognized physician she spoke of imperfection of medical knowledge and declared it an error that one could not live without a heart, inasmuch as she felt very well without one, it having come away with the afterbirth to which it had grown fast, the nurse having separated the two before her eyes; complains of her husband, says he wishes to convince her she is sick, ... nymphomania,... frequently sips at a bowl of warm sugar-water, declaring it will form her a new heart; .(health, healing)...(expert)

He, 17 - He quarrels, reproaches, scolds, insults, from jealousy, mingled with unchaste (obscene) expressions; ...

PH-AC. Ha, 674 - Discontented with himself, self-reproaches.

PLAT. He, 42 - Mania; with great pride; fault-finding; unchaste (sensual) talk; ...(chaste = moral, pure)

PLB. Al, 112 - He is very sad, has no desire to live, and has threatened to destroy himself, and is very fault-finding (severe, critical) with his friends.

RAN-B. Al, 2 - Vexed and inclined to be angry; quarrels and scolds when the slightest cause is offered (after two hours).

SAPIN. Al, 4 - Very irritable; nothing goes right; fault-finding, dissatisfied with everything previously done, no matter how well it was done before; ...

SEP. Al, 66 - She finds fault and desires nothing which others want, accompanied by weeping and heat of face.

Ha, 45 - She finds fault in everything, approves of nothing.

Ha, 44 - She finds fault with everything, does not wish what others desire; with weeping ...

He, 31 - Contradictory, quarrelsome, complaining about others.

SIL. Al, 37 - Whimsical (capricious) and fault -finding.

STRAM. He, 56 - Believes to be in his grave; shrives,(confess) prays, asks to be killed (justified); accuses his wife of infidelity; scolds (cursing), strikes at everybody who wishes to restrain him; thinks they are dogs and barks at them to make himself understood.

He, 92 - Mania:... complains that a dog is biting and tearing flesh off his chest; merry exaltation; with pride (haughty) and affectation; runs about, complains of violent headache; ...;steals from his roommates...; disposition to scold persons whom he otherwise loved.

He, 93 - Mania; thinks he is lying on his sepulchre (tomb); confessing, praying, wants to be killed (redemption, salvation, regeneration); laughs as if tickled (excited); wants to be kissed; accuses his wife of being faithless (betrayed); scolding (censure) beating in a rage, will not be taken hold of by attendants (suspicious?) ; takes them for dogs (contemptuous), and barks at them; talking in Jewish jargon; (rank?, stranger?) supposes his house to be surrounded by carts (vehicle), Jews (Judaism) and geese, offending him, ... -(strange, foreign, alien)

SULPH. Ha, 44 - Ill-humored and in a criticizing mood.

He, 53 - Ill-humored and fault-finding.

TIL. Al, 19 - Irritable, critical mood, inclined to quarrel and get angry, even from the slightest difference of opinion.

VERAT. Al, 62 - He seeks out faults in others and contemplates (examine, inspect) them. (critical)

He, 48 - A crippled girl...; chides (censure) her father for taking part in revolution; thinks she hears drum (timpani) which proclaims his execution; this is followed by silent brooding and occasional starts;...

He, 24 - Disposed to silence, or to talk about faults of others; if irritated scolding and calling names.

CENSURED

Ailments from; admonition: agar.[5] ***bell.*** calc.[10] carc.[193] coloc.[137] germ.[222] ***ign.***[137] kali-c.[5] nit-ac.[5] ***nux-v.***[30] op.[137] ***plat.*** staph.[137] tarent.[137]

Ailments from; admonition, children, in: carc.[85] med.[85]

Ailments from; admonition, kindly: ***bell.***[5] chin.[5] ign.[5] nux-v.[5] ***plat.***[5] ***stann.***[5]

Ailments from; punishment: agar.[137] ambr.[5] con.[5] dam.[85] dig.[5] ign.[5] lach.[5] nat-m.[162] stann.[5] staph.[5] tarent.[85]

Ailments from; reproaches: agar.[5] **AMBR.**[162] bell.[162] cadm-s.[144] calc-sil.[58] carc.[144] cina[58] coloc. croc.[5] dys-co.[136] gels.[5] germ.[222] ***ign.*** med.[144] mosch.[58] **NAT-M.**[193] nit-ac.[10] nux-v.[189] **OP.**[122] ph-ac. ***plat.***[35] sac-alb.[210] ***staph.*** ***stram.***[54] tarent.[85]

Anger; reproaches, from: cadm-s.[144] croc.[36] ***ign.***[10]

Anger; temper tantrums, reprimands, after: nat-m.[162]

Anxiety; reproved, as if he expected to be: dig.[36]

Delusions; criticized, that she is: ***bar-c.*** calc.[185] cocain.[102] germ.[222] hydrog.[222] hyos.[102] ign.[102] lach.[185] lap-mar-c.[194] laur. lyss.[102] pall.[102] plb. rhus-t. staph.[102]

- laughed at, criticized to disadvantage, makes her timid, and she dare not look up while walking in street: bar-c.[54]
- neglected, duty, his, deserves reproach: aur.[54] germ.[222]
- talking, friends talking about her: lach.[58]

Despair; criticism, from the smallest: med.[122]

Fear; get talked about, to: nux-v.[30] pall.[193] puls.[30]

✦ opinion of others, of: **AMBR.**[162] bar-c.[193] germ.[222] nux-v.[30] ozone[227] prot.[136] puls.[30]

✦ reproach, of: caps. carc.[233] dig.[36]

Hysteria; reprimands, after: ign.[189] nat-m.[162]

Indifference; reprimands, to all: ***merc.***[30]

Irritability; criticism, even by mild: dros.[1]

Irritability; reproaches, from: bamb-a.[1184]

Laughing; reprimands, at: bar-c.[184] ***graph.***[54]

Offended; criticism, takes advice as: lil-t.[168]

Quarrelsomeness; recriminations about trifles: cop.[36]

Reproaches; aversion to: carc.[187]

Reproaches; laughing at reproaches: ***graph.***[8]

Sensitive; reprimands, criticism, reproaches, to: ars.[189] bamb-a.[1184] calc.[189] calc-sil.[58] cand-a.[239] caps.[85] ***carc.***[122] cina[130] foll.[1201] ign.[85] lap-mar-c.[194] ***med.***[122] nat-m.[189] nat-s.[146] nux-v.[189] ozone[227] puls.[189] ***sac-alb.***[210] staph.[70]

Striking; reprimanded, when: tub.[193]

Suspiciousness; talking about her, people are: ***bar-c.*** hyos.[137] ign.[137] pall.[137] staph.[137]

Talk; others agg., of, about her: ***bar-c.***[137] hyos.[137] ign.[137] pall.[137] stann.[137] staph.[137]

Violence; reproached, when hearing another: calc-p.[36]

Weeping; admonition, from: bell. ***calc.*** carc.[108] chin. ign. ***kali-c.*** ***lyc.*** nat-m. nit-ac. plat. staph.

Weeping; children, reprimanded, when: nat-m.[70] nit-ac.[10]

Weeping; remonstrated with, when: bell. calc. carc.[193] ign. ***kali-c.*** nit-ac. plat. staph.

Weeping; reproaches, from: calc.[122] cand-a.[239] carc.[184] nat-m.[70] nit-ac.[10] plat.[35]

ADAM. Sh, 181 - I realized I am observing a lot and have a feeling of being observed. The observer bit is female aspect, and the male bit is a critical voice. 7, 6C, 06:06:00

Sh, 205 - Get angry when criticized, yet easily critical of others.[20], 1M, 06:XX:XX

AUR. Ha, 347 - Always very restless and undecided (doubtful) -thought he was neglecting something for which he must incur (obtain) reproach -...he seemed to carry about this restlessness with him in his inmost (deepest) parts ; this condition deprived him of all perseverance, all energy.

Ha, 13 - Restless and undecided, without perceptible ebullition of the blood; he always thinks he is neglecting something for which he will be reproached; he seems to carry with him this internal restlessness, and it took from him all perseverance and energy.

Ha, 33 - He tries his best to quarrel with somebody and to revile (scold) him.

BAR-A. Al, 9 - Dread (fear). When walking in the street, she imagines that people were criticizing her, and judging her wrongfully which makes her anxious, so that she will not look up, will look (aversion) at no one, and sweats all over.

BAR-C. Ha, 4 - She suspected, that when walking in the street, men found fault (defect) with her, and judged her amiss (wrong), which made her anxious, so that she dared not look up, she looked at nobody, and perspired all over.

He, 12 - Walking in street she imagines men are laughing at her, criticizing to disadvantage; this makes her so timid that she dare (venture) not look up or at anybody, and she perspires over whole body.

CALC-A. Ha, 263 - Anxious disposition as if something evil had happened or he had to fear reproaches (censures); at the same time, however, persistent inclination to work. (industrious)

CALC-P. Al, 15 - A communication in which some one is justly reproached concerning his conduct, affects him very disagreeably; he grows violent, and holds up his faults to himself.

CALC. Ha, 13 - Anxious at heart, as if he had done wrong,(immoral) or had to apprehend reproaches (deserves), with constant inclination to work.

CAPS. He, 10 - Fear of censure.

DIG. Al, 24 - Internal anxiety, like pangs of conscience, as though he had committed a crime, or expected to be reproved, continuing nearly three months.

Ha, 9 - Internal anguish, like anguish (anxiety) of conscience, as if he had committed a crime, or had to expect reproaches...

GERM. Sh, 4 - Desperately angry. So intense that I could barely control it. I made noises like an animal, pushed my arms up and down -instead of hitting my children, which helped. Want to just leave the house and the kids. Felt completely mad, afraid of what the neighbors heard and thought. Very bad conscience afterwards, but no relief - didn't get the anger out. There are a lot of feelings inside that don't come out. 18, 30C, 02:09:00

Sh, 115 - Very much in doubt whether I should take any more tablets. Whatever I do, I feel that somebody will criticize me, that I do something wrong. Difficult to make a decision. Afraid that other people will laugh at me or say, haven't you understood anything?" Crying. Don't want to get up. Don't want to bother the supervisor so early in the morning. I am a failure. 18, 30C, 01:06:30

Sh, 118 - Just want to cry. Feeling embarrassed. I do not believe in my own feelings and decisions. So afraid of what others think of me. 18, 30C, 01:09:15

Sh, 146 - Slightest criticism and I am broken hearted. Almost started to cry among all the people, very doubtful about relationships. It kills my confidence. Deep sigh. 21, 12C, 41:XX:XX

HALI-L. Sh, 557 - I feel like everybody's judging me or in my face. 07, 30C, 04:22:30

Sh, 560 - I don't feel cranky, but I have no idea how I'd feel if someone criticized me or tried to lecture me. 07, 30C, 07:06:00

HYDROG. Sh, 242 - Felt vulnerable to criticism —felt people were getting at me. Felt people were not taking notice of poor little me —over-reacting —upset and hurt. 02, 6C, XX:XX:XX

Sh, 256 - Thought someone was telling someone else that I was mad and asking what should be done about it. 16, 30C, 25:XX:XX

IGN. Al, 27 - Slight blame or contradiction excites him to anger, and this makes him angry with himself.

Ha, 764 - Slight blame (censuring) or contradiction excites him to quarrel, and he is vexed at himself for doing so.
Ha, 775 - When one hesitates in the least to do what she wishes, or remonstrates (censures) much with her, though in a mild friendly manner, or endeavor to persuade her, or wishes differently from what she wishes, she weeps aloud.
He, 53 - Slight blame (censure) or contradiction excites him to anger, and this makes him angry with himself.

MED. He, 36 - A word or look of seeming harshness (reproach) put her in despondency for hours. (sensitive)

MERC. Ha, 1261 - He talked nonsense: look! you strike a fly on your hand, and you had previously forbidden me to do so (which was not the case).

NIT-AC. Ha, 9 - At the least admonition (censure), the child begins to weep piteously.

NUX-V. Ha, 1262 - She cannot bear the least contradiction, nor suffer the most reasonable representations (narration) to induce her to alter her conduct; they put her beside herself.

PLAT. Ha, 19 - Tendency to weep and weeping, after a mild reproach.

PLB. Al, 59-...;he fancied that a cavalry regiment was about to fall upon him (attacked); or that he was in the presence of his employer, who was finding fault with him.

RHUS-T. He, 24-...a week later she told her mother to not look at her (observed) ; seemed to be distrustful (suspicious) and did not wish to see any one; she came running in from the street and said people were looking at her; ....; cries without cause, imagines people are finding fault (misconduct, criticized, censured) with her because she is earning (succeed, prosper, reach) nothing, acts in a childish manner;...

SIL. Ha, 5 - The least remark makes her weep.

STRAM. He, 69 - Hallucinations as if near r.mastoid process a voice were scolding (censured, reproved), her < at night, sometimes voice seemed to be under bed.
He, 107-...heard continually, on r. side of occiput, a loud voice, scolding, vituperating and accusing him of ungodliness (impious, sinful, irreligious, godless, profane); ....prayed expecting, with great anxiety, the flash of lightning which was to kill him;...(redemption, regeneration, salvation)

CHILD

Abusive; children insulting parents: am-m.[30] cham.[162] hyos.[30] lach.[176] lyc.[30] nat-m.[30] ***plat.***[30]

Abusive; family and children, to: kali-i.[137]

Abusive; husband insults wife, children, and: lyss.[36]

Ailments from; abuse, childhood, in: carc.[187] stram.[198] thuj.[198]

Ailments from; death, child, of a: calc.[58] caust.[30] ***gels.***[54] **IGN.**[54] ***kali-br.***[54] lach.[30] nat-m.[85] nux-v.[30] ph-ac.[30] plat.[85] staph.[30] sulph.[30]

Ailments from; domination by others, a long history of: carc.[140] foll.[1179] lyc.[193] sep.[193]

Anger; children, in: abrot.[116] ***acon.***[54] anac.[137] ant-t.[137] arn.[8] bac.[62] bell.[10] carb-v.[8] carc.[207] **CHAM.**[54] dros.[70] hep.[54] ip.[116] kali-c.[8] ***lyc.***[8] med.[149] ***phos.***[54] sanic.[85] sil.[53] staph.[70] stram.[101] syph.[149] ***tub.***[70] tub-k.[149]

Anxiety; children, about his: acet-ac. ars.[31] germ.[222] ph-ac.[30] phos.[31] rhus-t.[30] sep.[172] sulph.[31]

Anxiety; children, in, afraid of everything: calc.[137]

Anxiety; children, in, schoolchildren, about their lessons: lyc.[172] sil.[172]

Aversion; husband, and children: ***glon.***[54] verat.[54]

Brooding; constantly over loss of a child: ***gels.***[54] ***kali-br.***[54]

Capriciousness; children, in: **CHAM.**[122] **CINA**[122] rheum[1] sac-alb.[85]

Caressed; caressing husband and child, then pushes away: ***anac.***[54]

Childish behavior, sadness, in: ***kali-br.***[54]

Children; aversion to: **CHOC.**[222] helon.[231] lyc.[137] medus.[231] plat. raph.[36] sep.[162] xan.[231]

Children; aversion, her own: glon. ***lyc.*** nux-v.[162] phos.[137] plat. sep.[162] verat.

Children; aversion, her own, daughter, in a woman: raph

Children; desires to, beat: chel.

Children; desires to, have to beget: ox-ac.

Children; flies from the own: lyc.

Children; watchful, they are on the look out for every gesture: phos.[122]
Company, desire for; children that are rejected, in: carc.[207]
Complaining; childhood, about: ozone[227]
Cruelty; bear, cannot, done to other children: calc.[122]
Delusions; baby, odious looks: puls.[54]
• baby, two in bed: petr.
• bed, strange boy prevents sleep: apis[54]
• born into the world and was overwhelmed with wonder at the novelty of his surroundings, feels as if newly: cori-r.[58]
• child, he is again a, acts like a, and: ***cic.***
• child, is not hers: anac. nit-ac.[88]
• child, sitting on low benches in rows as in a schoolroom: bell.[8]
• childish fantasies, has: lyc.
• children, thinks he must drive, out of the house: fl-ac.
• dead, child was, her: ***kali-bi.***[54] kali-br.
• dead, corpse, brother and child, c. of: calc-sil.[58] con. plb.
• murder, husband and child, she is going to: kali-br.
• nursing her child, she is: atro.
• room, people in, sees, babies, full of white and colored: morph.[85]
Despair; death, separate him from his children, death will: bamb-a.[1184]
Dreams; childbirth, of: choc.[222] ozone[227]
➤ children, about: ***absin.***[102] ***acon.***[102] am-m. ars.[102] bamb-a.[1184] ***bell.***[102] calad.[102] cass.[36] ***cham.***[102] choc.[222] ***cina***[98] ***cypr.***[102] hura hydrog.[222] hyos.[102] kali-br.[102] kali-n. lipp.[36] mag-c. merl. oci.[36] ozone[227] ***passi.***[102] phos.[102] puls.[102] rham-p.[36] sulph.[102]
➤ children, about, babies: choc.[222]
➤ children, about, babies, leukemia, with: ozone[227]
➤ children, about, beaten, had been: kali-c.[36] kali-n. nat-m.[36]
➤ children, about, coma, in: ozone[227]
➤ children, about, danger, in: ozone[227]
➤ children, about, hordes of, disturbing her idyllic fancy: ozone[227]
➤ children, about, lost in crowd: bamb-a.[1184]
➤ children, about, lying on ice, her little child, and she feared it would fall into water: lipp.[36]
➤ children, about, murdered, being: thea.[36]
➤ children, about, neglecting her: bamb-a.[1184]
➤ children, about, protecting them, to save them from falling: ozone[227]
➤ children, about, rescuing them: cass.[36] ***hydrog.***[222]
➤ children, about, something had happened to: hydrog.[222] kali-n.[36]
➤ children, about, younger, were ten years: ozone[227]
➤ children, became a three year old, and rejoiced much: mag-c.[36]
➤ children, wanted to save asphyxiated: cass.[36]
➤ daughter, vexed her, had: nat-s.[36]
➤ dead, bodies, finding a dead child in a churchyard: mag-s.[36]
➤ dead, infants: cench.[58] lap-gr-m.[194]
➤ devils, cooking babies on a vulcano and eating them: ozone[227]
➤ disease, apoplectic fit, daughter has an: nat-s.
➤ evil impending, child, to a: ozone[227]
➤ fit, daughter had a apoplectic: nat-s.
➤ killing, children: thea.[144]
➤ piercing bodies of her children together: dict.[137] phos.[137]
➤ water, child bathing in boiling: mag-c.
➤ water, daughter is in water and crying for help: nat-s.
➤ water, falling into, child, her: eupi.
Escape; attempts to, family, children, from her: am-c.[30] choc.[222] ***lyc.***[122] nux-v.[30] phos.[30] ***sep.***[30] staph.[30]
Escape; attempts to, visit his daughter, wants to: ars.
Estranged; flies her own children: lyc.
Excitement; sexual, children, in: aloe[36] bell.[149] ***orig.***[54] plat.[58] verat.[149]
Fancies; childish: lyc.
Fear; accidents, of, child, of: ars.[172]
✦ broken the arm of her child, that she has, in gastroenteritis during pregnancy: lyc.[172]
✦ disease, child, to: ars.[172]
✦ killing, child, her: ars.[172] coff.[172] manc.[30] ***merc.***[185] ***nux-v.***[185] rhus-t.[172] sep.[185] sil.[172] ***sulph.***[185] **THEA.**[162]
✦ people, of, children, in: **BAR-C.** ***lyc.***
✦ pregnancy, during, child would be deformed, that: acon.[172]
✦ punished, of being, child: camph.[54]
✦ punishment, after, in children, if brought

to bed too soon get convulsions in sleep: ***ign.***[54]
✦ sudden, broken her child's arm by lifting him, that she has: ***lyc.***[54]
Fire; throws child into fire, after delivery: merc.[85]
Forsakes; children, his or her own: lyc.
Gestures; grasping, genitals, children: ***acon.***[54] bell.[122] **BUFO**[171] maland.[171] ***merc.***[54] ***stram.***[54] ***zinc.***[54]
Hatred; children, of: anac.[162] ***lyc.***[162] ***nux-v.***[162] **PLAT.**[162]
Helplessness; feeling of, infant, feels like a: hell.[54]
Hide; desire to, children, run away, and: meli.[137]
Howling; rage, from, in children: bell.[54]
Impatience; children, with: anac.[122] bamb-a.[1184] kali-c.[1]
Impatience; playing of children: anac.
Indifference; children, to her: aur-ar.[58] choc.[222] kali-i. ***lyc.*** nat-c. **PHOS.**[122] **SEP.**[122]
Jealousy; children, between: ars.[30] calc-s.[187] carc.[179] nat-m.[30] nux-v.[30] sep.[30]
Kill; desire to, child, the own: androc.[222] merc.[30] ***plat.***[30]
Kill; desire to, parents, in a child: ***der.***[162]
Kill; sudden impulse to, throw child, fire, into: hep.[58] lyss. ***nux-v.*** thea.
Kill; sudden impulse to, throw child, window, out of: lyss.[54]
Kill; threatens to k, wife and children: ***hep.***[54]
Kisses; caress children, kiss and: ***puls.***[54]
Love; children, for: ***ars.***[10] ***hep.***[10] phos.[10] plat.[10] sep.[10]
Mania; abuses, violent outburst, abuses her child, parturition, after, puerperal: ***camph.***[54]
Moaning; children, in, piteous, because he cannot have what he wanted: **CHAM.**[36]
Moaning; children, in, touched, when: ant-t.[72]
Neglects; children, her: aur-ar.[58]
Obstinate; children, annoy those about them, with eruption: ***psor.***[54]
Religious affections; children, in: ***ars. calc. lach. stram.***[122] ***sulph.***
Rudeness; children, of naughty: ***ant-c.***[5] carc.[207] cham.[5] ***chin.***[54] cina[5] dulc.[5] ***merc.***[5] rheum[5] staph.[5]
Sadness; aversion to see her children from sadness: ***con.***[54]
Sadness; aversion, children to whom he is devotedly attached become burdensome: **KALI-I.**[54]
Sadness; children, want of, from: aur.[91]
Sensitive; crying of children, to: caust. phos.
Spoiled children: am-c.[30] bar-c.[30] lyc.[30] mosch.[85] op.[30] sulph.[30]
Suicidal disposition; mania, in, puerperal, with aversion to husband, baby and coition: agn.[171]
Timidity; bashful, children: bov.[122] bufo[117] tub.[122]
Washing; aversion, children, in: am-c.[58] ant-c.[127] psor.[127] **SULPH.**[54] tub.[106]
Weeping; children, touched, when: ant-t.[102]

ACET-AC. He, 6 - Anxiety; grieves about his sickness and his children.
ADAM. Sh, 277 - Exceptionally strong desire to leave my marriage and children, to live a clear unmuddled life alone. 2, 12C, 74:XX:XX-160:XX:XX
AGAR. Al, 13 - She ran about the yard, romped (playing) with the children, threw them down, even hit them.
ANAC. He, 29 - Has the fixed idea that her husband is not her husband, her child not her child; now she fondles (caress) them and again pushes them away. (reject, repudiate)
He, 13 - After having caressed her husband or child she pushes them away from her, as if they were not what she supposed.
ANDROC. Sh, 102 - Assertive, impatient, aggressive. Felt resentful and abused. Had no control over her temper. Bellowed and lashed out at everyone. In the evening, furious for no apparent reason. Wanted to kill her husband and children, banged doors and threw things. By bed-time, she felt fine but the intensity of her evil thoughts was very frightening. (7)
ANT-T. He, 16 - Child clings (adhere) to those around, calls for help in a hoarse voice, with cough.
APIS. He, 19 - A strange boy lying in bed with him prevents (restrict) sleep.
BELL. He, 18 - When closing eyes, though not asleep, patient sees fierce (wild), wicked looking large animals with horns and bushy (scabrous) heads; room seemed to be full of strange men passing in and out, who would snatch (take hold) at her

as they passed, which frightened her very much, she thought the men wanted to take her away from home ; she then saw children sitting on low benches (seat) in rows (line) as in a school-room. (purity)

BERB. Al, 3 - Anxious mood, with great fear and fright...; in the twilight some dogs and children appeared as large again as natural.

BISM. He, 6 - Desire for company; child holds on to its mother's hand.

BOR. Ha, 5 - The child is timid while being dandled; when it is rocked up and down in the arms it makes a very frightened face...(fear, touch, caresses)

CAMPH. Al, 27 - The child creeps (crawl) into a corner, howls and cries; everything that is said to him is taken as if one were ordering him, and he were considered naughty (disobedient) and should be punished.

CANTH. Al, 22-...; she feels as if newly (recently) born;... (innocent, naive, pure)

CHAM. Al, 13 - Piteous moaning of a child because he cannot have what he wants. (contrariety)

He, 15 - Piteous moaning of a child because he cannot have what he wants.

CHEL. Al, 55 - Mood very irritable, daily outbreaks of anger without cause (causeless); feels as though she could beat the children, and trembles from rage because she has no reason for doing it.

CHOC. Sh, 97 - I feel my kids are ready to go, but I have to get back to the younger ones to feed. Felt I could walk home (300 miles), a feeling that I should never go further than I could walk.

Sh, 145 - My fears around the kids —that they would die, etc. and that they were my total responsibility, like parasites —have gone and I know feel total trust that they will be o.k.

CIC. Ha, 240 - He felt like a child of seven or eight years old, objects were very dear and attractive to him, as toys are to a child. (purity)

He, 7 - He thinks himself a young child. (purity, juvenile, infant)

CON. Al, 11 - Visions of her brother and child, who had died; at the same time, she saw distinctly persons in the room;...

FL-AC. Al, 1 - Great disposition, when alone, to repulsive fantastic imaginations, particularly in regard to persons with whom he stands in near relations, or with whom he is connected (united, joined); it seems, for example, as though he must get rid (discard, repudiate, reject) of all the servants, children must go out of house, a betrothal must be broken off, a marriage should be dissolved. (broke; vows)

GELS. He, 6 - After losing son, inclined to brood over her loss; at times becomes unconscious, or, rather, "rapt"; in imagination thinks herself at the grave; smothered pressure on chest after the spell.

He, 43 - Child dizzy, when carried seizes hold of nurse, fearing that it will fall.

GERM. Sh, 138 - Feeling of revulsion for many people especially young parents with children, while wandering through town. Feel people are stuck in their lives. What a waste. 10, 9C, 00:05:00

GLON. He, 2 - Recognized no one; repulsed her husband and children; raved, screamed, and wished to rush from house; jumped out of bed, but fell because her knees gave way.

HALI-L. Sh, 577 - Children are an obstacle to enlightenment. 09, 6C, 05:XX:XX

HEP. He, 8-...threatened to murder wife and children, attempted to set house on fire, and was with difficulty controlled; ... (pyromaniac) 0Scabies.

HURA. Al, 3 - Every paroxysm of pain excites a nervous laugh, with moanings like those of a sick child.

Al, 700 - Dream about children and the release (liberty) of prisoners.

Al, 709 - Restless night; dream about crimes, dead bodies (corpse), and children lying with their heads half cut off, while others were being decapitated.

HYDROG. Sh, 34 - I felt myself really getting into my yoga and exploring new positions. At one point, I ended up playing with my toes like a baby. 08, 30C, 00:XX:XX

HYOS. He, 68 - Onanism since childhood; has always been greatly attracted by opposite sex and prematurely busied himself with thoughts of marriage;... secretly wrote his love affairs; mania,...one idea rapidly follow another, all in some away concerning love, masturbates at every opportunity...(satyriasis)

IRID. Sh, 58 - Felt child-like, innocent, happy as though seeing things from a child's perspective. Sat watching a milk tanker, it looks just like a child's toy. Felt like I could pick it up and brrrm brrrm it up the lane. I9

KALI-BR. Al, 5 - She had the erroneous idea that she was deserted by all her friends, and as a consequence she passed all her waking moments, which are not many in tears;...delusion that her child was dead, had taken fixed possession of her mind;...she declared that she saw it dead (corpse) before her, and when it was brought to her, she refused to acknowledge that it was hers, or had any resemblance to the one she imagined was dead.

He, 15 - Frightful imaginings at night (in pregnant women during latter months), they are under impression that they have committed, or about to commit, some great crime and cruelty (brutality), such murdering their children or husbands.

He, 17 - Delirium with delusions; thinks he is pursued (hunt); will be poisoned; is selected (designated) for divine vengeance (revenge); that her child is dead, etc.

He, 23-...constantly brooding over loss of a daughter; almost crazy; ... (child)

KALI-I. He, 6 - Very great irritability and unwonted harshness of demeanor (behavior); his children, to whom he is devoted and attached, become burdensome to him; very passionate and spiteful temper;...constant apprehension of impending evil.

LYC. Al, 55 - She flees from her own children.

Ha, 9 - She flees (desert) from her own children.

He, 25 - Anthropophobia (in children); fear of phantoms in evening, with anguish.

He, 35 - Misanthropic; flies even from his own children.

LYSS. Al, 28 - Very cross, so much that my children expressed great surprise; took offense at the merest trifles; scolded (censorious) my wife and children; ....

Al,N-7 - Thoughts of something terrible going to happen come into his mind against his will; feels impelled to do reckless (impulsive) things, such as throwing child, which he carries in his arms, through the window, and the like.

Al,N-45 - Wrote to doctor: I am waiting with impatience that you give me and my young ones something to eat.

Al,N-46 - After fainting (weak) spell he wrote on paper: I am forsaken by all; even the birds of heaven, they do not look at me (despised), do not fed me if hungry (helplessness) ; I hunger with the young ones and am thirsty with their she ones (starving); my nest (house) is made out of dirt (soiled), not gotten by my own exertions (efforts), but by driving them out of their nests (home) and sitting there with the females and the young.

Al,N-88 - Very cross, so much... he took offense at veriest trifles, scolding his wife and children, felt wretched, ...

He, 7 - Thoughts of something terrible going to happen come into his mind against his will; feels impelled to do reckless (impulsive, precipitated) things, such as throwing child, which he carries in his arms, through the window, and the like.

He, 88 - Very cross, so much so that his children expressed great surprise; he took offense at veriest trifles, scolded his wife and children, felt wretched, ...

MAG-C. Al, 923 - Dream that she had become a child three years old, which rejoiced her very much. (youngish)

Al, 945 - Anxious dream, that a child was bathing in boiling water. (purification?)

NAT-M. He, 34 - A pregnant woman saw a man who had a disfiguring nasal cancer; this haunted (obsessed) her, and she was sure her child would be marked; she was melancholy, avoided society, wept continually.

NAT-P. Al, 10 - Awakens; fears his child, who has a trifling ailment (disease), is dead; he goes to her room to relieve the otherwise ineffaceable (perpetual) impression.

NEON. Sh, 63 - I notice a foolish and irresistible desire to spy on my partner through the keyhole in the door to his study. I now remember doing this a couple of times yesterday (on the first day of the proving) as well. I am finding it ridiculous, laughing to myself. I feel like a mischievous child, doing something it

shouldn't do, giggling away to myself. It makes me feel excited in a childish sense. I have never felt compelled to spy on anyone ever -be it through a keyhole or otherwise. Very strange. 02, 6C, 01:06:40
Sh, 69 - Recognized a change in awareness -a vaguely stoned,unreal feeling. Giggly, childish, grinning. Felt light. 05, 12C, 05:05:XX
OX-AC. Al, 19 - Philoprogenitiveness, greater love of his children, in one in whom this feeling was always predominating; a decidedly expressed and clearly distinguishable symptom, it being not traceable to any other cause. (love creation of child)
PETR. He, 5 - Since confinement two weeks ago when in bed, in dark room, at night, delusion that there is another baby (small, tiny) in bed which requires attention also that she has a third leg which would not remain quiet.
PHOS. Ha, 82 - Indifferent to her child, whom at other times she dearly loved.
He, 14 - Apathy; indifferent even to his own children;...
PLAT. He, 36 - While suffering from a slight erysipelas faciei, took leave (quit, abandon) of her children, exhorted her husband to join (unite, combine) church, wanted people to join her in prayer (beg), felt happy to join her Redeemer.
He, 12 - Dislikes her children; calls them too little.
PLB. Al, 66 - Hallucinations of mind, she seemed to see her dead husband and child in a tree out of the window.
PULS. He, 39 - Children are extremely affectionate, which they manifest by kissing and caressing.
SEP. He, 38-...everything seems strange (unusual, unfamiliar) to her;...; it seems as if she could not understand (realize) anything and would have to learn anew everything she wished to do;...(lost: knowledge); greatest indifference to everything, the death of a near relative, or some happy occurrence, leaves her equally unaffected; no trace of her former love for friends or even for her child; aversion for social intercourse amounting to contempt;...
STRAM. Al, 207 - His whole conduct and countenance was like that of a child severely frightened and apprehending some terrible calamity.
THEA. Al, 4 - Sensation as if impelled by some uncontrollable power to commit suicide, to jump out of window, to put her baby in the boiler with the clothes, to cut its throat while cutting bread, to throw it downstairs (in a woman who kept a pot of tea boiling on the stove and drank several bowlfuls every day; cured with tea cm, Finckle)
THUJ. He, 23 - Mental depression, after childbirth (puerperal), in consequence of being told that there had been a slight rupture (division, hurt) of perineum; grows quiet; thinks she must die;...wants to jumps the window; does not care for children or her relatives (careless) ;..(sensitive to disrupt, partition)
VERAT. He, 13 - After severe illness, aversion to husband and children; desire to leave house: hallucinations, room appeared full of people, crowding in, there was no longer room...

CLAIRVOYANCE

Activity; clairvoyant, like that of a: arn.[54]
Activity; prophetical conception, with: **LACH.**[54]
Anticipation; matters, for, before they occur, and generally correctly: ***med.***[54]
Clairvoyance: acon. anac. androc.[222] anh.[102] arn. benz.[85] bry.[10] calc. cann-i. carc.[193] ***crot-c.*** dat-a.[85] hydro-c.[149] hyos. lach. ***lyss.*** m-arct.[10] med. nabal.[102] ***nux-m.*** op. ***phos.*** pyrus sil. stann. stram. tarent. valer.[85] ***verat-v.***[54]
Death; presentiment of, predicts the time: **<u>ACON.</u>**[122] agn.[162] ***aloe***[54] alum.[122] ***arg-n.*** cench.[58] hell.[58] ***lac-d.***[54] thea.[122]
Delusions; bells, hears ringing of, his funeral: aether.
• clairvoyant, she is: pyrus[36]
• experienced before, thought everything had been: kali-br.
Dreams; clairvoyant: **ACON.**[122] asaf. bov. ***cann-i.*** com.[54] cortico.[119] m-arct.[10] mang. ph-ac. phos. rad-br.[111] ***sulph.*** ther.[78]
➤ clairvoyant, solving important questions of the day: ***acon.***[30]
➤ fortune tellers, of: choc.[222]
➤ future events, prophetic: **ACON.**[122] asaf.

bov. ***camph.***[54] ***cann-i.*** cortico.[119] m-arct.[10] mang. ph-ac. phos. rad-br.[111] ***sulph.***
Prophesying: ***acon.*** agar. anh.[119] ant-c.[102] camph. con. **LACH.**[36] med.[36] nux-m.[58] sol-n.[1] stram.
Prophesying; disagreeable events, of: med.[122]
Prophesying; predicts the time of death: **ACON.** ***arg-n.***[122] thea.[122]
Prophesying; rhyming: agar.[102]
Trance; plays on piano with closed eyes, writes letters in an acquired language: ***camph.***[54]

ACON. Ha, 521 - Lucid vision: he says, now my beloved (70 miles away) must have sung the difficult passage (of Beethoven) that I was just singing.
He, 41 - Predicts day of death; bids (offer) her friends good-bye.(farewell)
He, 2 - Clairvoyance; conscious that his beloved, miles away, was singing a certain piece.
AGAR. Ha, 27 - Extravagant fancy, rapture (ecstasy), prophesying, making verses.
ANDROC. Sh, 145 - She found that she was thinking or saying something at the same time or just before someone else was thinking or saying the same thing. (13)
APIS. Al, 13 - Premonition of death arose after a few minutes; "he believes he is going".
ARG-N. He, 13 - Frequently settle (decide, fix) upon time he should die. (death)
ARN. He, 11 - Mind clear like that of a clairvoyant; quiet countenance (expression), pale as chalk, thinks her death unavoidable.(inevitable)
CANN-I. Al, 58 - He imagines that he is possessed of infinite knowledge and power of vision, and then that he is Christ come to restore the world to perfect peace. (redemption, savior, rescuer)
CHOC. Sh, 188 - While walking outside, became anxious in a self-conscious way, anxious and vulnerable as if being watched or observed by something or someone -the attention was on me - anxiety that something would happen. Immediately afterwards I was attacked by four dogs and bitten on the calf. 27, 100C, 01:XX:XX
CROT-C. Al, 9 - While in a clairvoyant state, he speaks to some one who does not answer.
HALI-L. Sh, 16 - Had a superstitious thing happen. A white moth flew up by me in class and I had a strong sense someone close to me had died. 13, 30C, 01:04:XX
Sh, 167 - Clairvoyance about people and what was going on with them. 13, 30C, 12:XX:XX
Sh, 992 - I know things so clearly before they happen. 20, 30C, 31:XX:XX
HYDROG. Sh, 10 - I feel a bit unreal —like taking drugs —a weird spaced-outness. The top of my head feels very clear — seeing and hearing clear and remote, but from the sinus down, I feel muzzy and warm. 08, 30C, 00:01:XX
Sh, 16 - I felt I could see more deeply into people —beyond the roles they were playing. 16, 30C, XX:XX:XX
KALI-BR. Al, 44 - Felt as if everything that I feel, see or think, had been experienced before, as in a dream; this delusion is so strong that I could swear I dreamt it all.
LACH. Al, 7 - It seems to him during the day that he has dreamed everything that has happened, only somewhat different.(dÇj... vu)
He, 5 - Quick comprehension; mental activity, with almost prophetical (oracular, predictive) perception; ecstasy; a kind of trance.
MED. Al,N-47 - It feels the evil coming to it, and the bad news before it arrives (clairvoyance), of course it is selfish, and it is easily hurt by a harsh (rude) word.
He, 29 - Is always anticipating; feels most matters sensitively before they occur and generally correctly. (predicts)
He, 30 - Anticipates death. (predicts)
NEON. Sh, 84 - Repeated prophetic notions of daily events before hearing of them, causing anxiety and discomfort; thoughts of a person not seen for months and found he had phoned a few days before, depression and sadness unexplained until heard of sad family news that had already happened. 10, 6C, 01:XX:XX
PHOS. He, 1 - Excited imagination; zoomagnetic (animal magnetism) condition; ecstasy; clairvoyance.
SPONG. Al, 5 - Anxiety as if a misfortune

would befall him, which he seemed to foresee. (predict, prophesy)

STRAM. He, 49 - After spasms she fell into a trance, says she is under influence(seized) of spirits, and has had conversation with spirits, communications from God; delivers emphatic sermons, prophecies. (missionary)

VIP. Al, 12 - Premonition of death.

CLOTHES

Anguish; clothing too tight when walking in open air, as if: arg.[36]

Anxiety; chest, evening, undressing: chel.

Anxiety; chest, evening, undressing, amel.: ***zinc.***

Anxiety; clothing loosen, must, and open window: nux-v.[122] puls.[122] sulph.[1]

Anxiety; clothing, tight, as if too, walking out doors: arg.[54]

Delusions; abundance, of, destroys clothing: ***sulph.***[54]

- beautiful, old ragged woman is: psil.[164]
- beautiful, rags seem, even: ***sulph.***
- bed, old ragged woman is: psil.[164]
- clothes, beautiful, they are: aeth. sulph.
- clothes, fly away and become wandering stars, will (on undressing): cann-i
- clothes, heavy. too: con.[137] euph.[56] ***lac-c.***[8] merc.[1]
- clothes, rags, clad in: ***cann-i.***
- clothes, tight, too: apis[8] arg.[36] ars-met.[54] benz-ac.[54] chin.[1] glon.[36] paraf.[77] thuj.[36]
- clothes, wet, is: calc.[137] guai.[137] lac-d.[137] lyc.[137] phos.[137] ran-b.[137] sanic.[137] sep.[137] verat-v.[137]
- dresses in strange costumes: iodof.[85]
- hat is a pair of trousers which he tries to put on: stram.
- money, sewed up in clothing, is: kali-br.
- rain; out in the rain, he had been, from having wet cloth on head: atro.
- scratching on linen or similar substance, someone was: asar.
- trees are people in fantastic costume (afternoon, while riding): bell.

Desires; clothing, to wear his best: con.[137]

Desires; rags, clean: alum.[137]

Destructiveness; clothing, cuts them up: ***verat.***

Destructiveness; clothing, of: ***bell. camph.*** hyos.[54] ***ign.*** nux-v.[30] plb.[111] ***stram. sulph.*** **TARENT.** ***verat.***

Dreams; clothes, wearing many layers of: hydrog.[222]

- ➤ clothing, did not wish to make up: mag-c.[36]
- ➤ clothing, hidden her, someone has: bamb-a.[1184]
- ➤ dead, bodies, putting deceased body in shroud: elaps[36]
- ➤ dirt, linen, couple makes love in dirty linen: ozone[227]
- ➤ dirt, linen, dirty: kali-n.[36] ***kreos.***[122] ozone[227]
- ➤ dirt, underwear dirty: lap-mar-c.[194]
- ➤ garment, made the previous day: aeth.[36]
- ➤ ghosts, white, wrapped in scarfs, narcosis, who is under: ozone[227]
- ➤ men, dressed in black: cerv.[36]
- ➤ risen and dressed, having: sumb.[36]
- ➤ theater, but could not get dressed, which woke her, going to: mag-s.[36]
- ➤ unsuccessful efforts to, dress for a ball: mag-c. mag-s.
- ➤ women, naked indecently, she is, and spreads her legs: ozone[227]

Dress; aversion to, in sadness: ***con.***[54]

Dress; unable to: merc.[36]

Eccentricity; dressing: ery-m.[36] hell.[30] sil.[30] sulph.[30]

Elegance; want of: am-c.[30] am-m.[30] caps.[30] nat-c.[30] nat-m.[30] nux-v.[30] sil.[30] sulph.[30]

Finery, luxurious clothing, wants: aeth.[5] cur.[36] lil-t.[111] ***sulph.***[5]

Haughty; clothing, likes to wear his best: ***con.***[54]

Indifference; appearance, about personal: coca[98] **SULPH.**

Insanity; dresses in his bests clothes: con.

Mania; tear clothing: nux-v.[30] ***tarent.***[54] ***verat.***[54]

Monomania; going out, dressing in a grotesque manner: anan.

Rage; tears clothing: ***camph.***[54]

Stupefaction; undressing, while: ***sec.***[54]

Tastelessness in dressing: ***calc.***[30] caust.[30] hell.[1] hyos.[1] lyc.[30] ***nat-m.***[30] nux-v.[30] sec.[1] staph.[30] stram.[1] sulph.[30]

Tears; things, clothing: bell.[36] camph.[171] ***ign.***[54] ***stram.***[54] tarent.[58] verat.[58]

Tears; things, clothing, nightdress and bed clothes: ***bell.***[54]

Tears; things, clothing, nightdress and bed clothes, sadness, in religious: ***kali-p.***[54]

Thoughts; persistent, garment made the previous day, about a: aeth.

Untidy: am-c.[102] androc.[222] aur-ar.[58] caps.[102] carc.[207] lac-h.[229] ***psor.***[102] sil.[102] ***sulph.***[122]
Washing; always, underwear, her: syph.[189]

AETH. Al, 28 - A fixed idea, which she cannot throw off, of a garment (clothes) made the day previous; she also dreamed of it.
Al,S-2 - A fixed idea, from which she could not free herself, of a garment (clothes) made the previous day, of which she also dreamed.
ART-V. He, 11 - Picking (gathering) of bedcovers, making a fold (wrap) of skin on back of her mother's hand, saying that it will not come off (disconnected), wants a knife to cut it off. (stab, wound)
BELL. Al, 55 - The delirium was attended (followed) with phantasms (ghosts), and in this respect resembled that caused by alcohol, but the mind did not run on cats, rats, and mice, ...Sometimes the phantasms appeared to be in the air, and various attempts were made to catch them or chase them with the hands; at other times they were supposed to be on the bed.. One patient (a woman) fancied the sheets (cloths) were covered with cucumbers.
Al,S-2552-...the yellow corpse of a tall man, shrouded (dressed, clothes) in white, tried to share the patient's bed with him, and the unwelcome visitor was promptly ejected. A crimson serpent came from the foot of the bed, with the design of fastening upon the patient's neck...
CON. He, 14 - Likes to wear his best clothes, (vanity) makes useless purchases, (squander) cares very little for things (indifferent), wastes or ruins them; does not want to work, prefers to play. (wanderer)
CUPR-A. He, 17 - Feared bedclothes or house would catch fire.
ERY-A. Al, 1 - Felt very queer (eccentric, inadequate) before completely dressed.
HYOS. Ha, 544 - Naked and enveloped in a fur cloak, he senselessly wanders about to a great distance in the summer heat.
Ha, 545 - Ridiculously solemn acts in improper clothing, mixed with fury. (In a priest's cassock, put on over nothing but a shirt, and in fur boots, he wishes to go to church, in order to preach and perform clerical offices there, and furiously attacks those who try to prevent him.)
He, 78 - Groundless suspicion of being watched (observed, spied) by members of family with whom he had some slight misunderstanding (dispute); to avoid being recognized by them, clothed himself differently every day,...watching his relations suspiciously and imagining he might be poisoned;... (disguise, camouflage)
IRID. Sh, 54 - Getting dressed, didn't want to put clothes on, wanted the freedom of nakedness, chose clothes for their lack of restriction. G 6
KALI-BR. Al, 3 - Decidedly insane; had delusions that lewd women had got into his mother's house; that he was pursued by the police; that his wife was threatened by members of the family; that he had thousands of dollars in gold sewed up in his clothing; (rich, wealth)
LAC-C. He, 24 - When paroxysms of intense nervousness (anxiety) come on, feels like tearing off her clothes; takes off her rings; cannot bear anything to touch her, ...
MAG-C. Al, 930 - Dreams of masks (false) in fools'(idiot) clothes, which they soiled.(dirty)
Al, 931 - Dream that she was at a ball (dance) where they did not dance enough; also at first she could not get ready (fitted) with her dress.
Al, 932 - Dream of flowers, clothes, and other things; she had to make up the clothes, but had no inclination to do it, and besides did not understand how; she also saw many foreign plants, but during this she became soaked (wet) with rain.
MERC. Ha, 1263 - Mania; she throws off the clothes at night, tears the straw about, and scolds; by day she leaps (jump) up high like a petulant extravagant person...she talks and scolds much to herself,...spits frequently and spreads the saliva out with her feet, and licks some of it up again; she often licks cowdung (excrements) and the mud of ponds (lake); she often takes little stones in her mouth, without swallowing them, and at the same time complains that they are cutting her bowels; much clotted blood passes with her motion; ...
PHOS. Ha, 27-....Talks in a vehement, (impetuous) commanding (dictatorial)

tone; spits at nurse, lifts up her clothes (naked) and kisses hotly all who come near her;...

PLB. He, 15-...; despair of her salvation...; fixed idea that could only obtain peace and safety though absolution by a priest of the papal church, although she had been a zealous Protestant; ....brooded over any forbidden thing; would steal (leave) from house in servant's cloak (coat, camouflage) and bonnet (hat) to obtain stimulants (drugs), but from the moment their prohibition was withdrawn (retired) ceased to have any desire for them; after being permitted to visit a priest and converse with him ceased to talk and think of the church. (desire; redemption, absolution)

STRAM. He, 99 - Acute mania; tears his clothing;... threatens to use knife on those about him.

He, 108-...spoke of lizards and worms being on his clothes,...

SULPH. Al, 85 - He could tear himself to pieces from vexation.

Al, 3800-....(DREAM) she walked about like a somnambulist, thought there was a fire, dressed herself, talked out of the window, and was frightened as she heard that it was nothing; for three days afterwards she was very weak, and felt bruised(hurt).

Al, 12 - She fancies that she has beautiful (refined) clothes; old rags look like fine things, a coat like a beautiful jacket, a cap like a beautiful hat.

Ha, 62 - She imagines that she has beautiful clothes, she takes old rags for beautiful clothes, she takes a coat for a jacket, a cap for a hat.

He, 11 - Foolish happiness and pride(haughtiness),thinks himself in possession of beautiful (attractive) things; even rags seem beautiful. (rank, position, distinction)

He, 38 - Destroys clothing; imagines she has everything in abundance. (wealth)

VERAT. He, 21 - Mania; with desire to cut and tear everything, especially clothes; with lewdness and lascivious talk; religious or amorous; de grandeur.

COMPANY

Anxiety; company, in agg.: ***acon.*** ***ambr.*** bell. cadm-s. lac-h.[229] lyc. ***petr.*** plat. stram.

Anxiety; company, shuns, even his doctor: iod.[85]

Aversion; society: anac.[60] bell.[36] caust.[30] cic.[1] clem.[38] coca[38] con.[1] graph.[30] ***kali-c.***[36] lyc.[1] nat-c.[137] stann.[1] syph.[137]

Aversion; visits, to: bell.[36] ferr.[36]

Cares; full of, company, with aversion to: con.[10] nat-m.[10]

Cheerfulness; company, in: bov.

Company desire for; alone, while, agg.: ***act-sp.***[162] aeth.[5] agar.[5] ambr. ant-t.[5] ***apis***[5] **ARS.** asaf.[5] bell.[5] bism.[5] bov. brom. bufo[5] cadm-s. calc. calc-s.[108] calc-sil.[58] ***camph.*** carc.[207] cedr.[5] clem.[5] con. ***dros.*** elaps ***fl-ac.***[5] foll.[1201] gaert.[136] **GALL-AC.**[198] gels.[5] **HEP.**[5] hydrog.[222] ***hyos.***[5] ***kali-c.*** lac-c.[58] lach.[5] lil-t.[5] ***lyc.*** ***merc.***[5] ***mez.*** nat-c.[5] nat-m.[5] ***pall.*** ph-ac.[5] **<u>PHOS.</u>**[122] plb.[5] puls.[160] ran-b.[5] rat. sep.[5] sil. stann.[5] ***stram.*** tab. trif-r.[102] zinc. zinc-p.[58]

Company, aversion to; agg.: absin.[36] achy.[149] acon. agar.[5] allox.[119] ***aloe*** **ALUM.**[122] alum-p.[58] alum-sil.[58] alumn.[36] am-m.[5] ***ambr.*** **ANAC.** anan. androc.[222] ant-c. ant-t. arag.[102] ***arg-n.***[5] arist-cl.[149] arn.[58] ars.[5] ***ars-met.***[54] atro. ***aur.*** aur-i.[58] ***aur-s.*** bamb-a.[1184] **BAR-C.** bar-i.[58] bar-m. bar-s.[58] ***bell.*** bov.[5] ***bry.*** bufo bufo-s. ***cact.*** cadm-s.[144] calc. calc-i.[58] ***calc-p.*** calc-s. camph.[5] cand-a.[239] cann-i. caps.[102] **CARB-AN.** ***carb-v.*** carbn-s. carc.[154] cedr. cench.[58] **CHAM.** ***chin.*** choc.[222] **<u>CIC.</u>**[122] cimic. cinnb. clem. coca ***coloc.*** ***con.*** convo-s.[149] cop. cortico.[119] ***cupr.*** cur. cycl.[58] ***dig.***[122] dios. elaps eug. euphr.[54] ***ferr.*** ferr-i. ferr-p. fl-ac. **GELS.** graph. grat. ham. ***hell.*** helon. ***hep.*** ***hipp.*** hydr. hydrog.[222] ***hyos.*** **IGN.** ***iod.*** jug-c. kali-bi. kali-br. kali-c. kali-i.[5] kali-m.[192] kali-p. kali-s. ***lac-d.*** lac-h.[229] ***lach.*** lap-c-b.[194] lap-gr-m.[194] lap-mar-c.[194] ***led.*** lil-t.[111] luna[228] ***lyc.*** ***m-aust.***[5] mag-c.[5] mag-m. mang. meny. meph.[149] moly.[149] murx.[10] ***nat-c.*** **<u>NAT-M.</u>**[122] nat-p. nat-s.[58] nicc. **NUX-V.** op.[5] ***oxyt.*** ozone[227] ***pall.***[5] pana.[36] petr. ph-ac.[54] phos. pic-ac. ***plat.*** ***plb.***[5] prot.[136] psor. ptel. ***puls.*** ***rhus-t.*** sabal.[144] sanic.[85] sapin.[36] sec. ***sel.*** ***sep.*** sieg.[144] ***stann.*** **STAPH.**[5] stram.[5] sul-ac. sul-i.[58] sulfonam. ***sulph.*** syph.[122] tanac.[25] ***tarent.***[122] tep. thala.[149] thiop.[149] ***thuj.*** til. trinit.[102] ust. ***verat.***[54] wye.[85] x-ray[115]

Company, aversion to; alone, agg. when alone and amel. in company: alum-sil.[58] bism.[10] hep.[10] ph-ac.[10] ran-b.[10]

Company, aversion to; alone, amel. when: allox.[119] alum-sil.[162] ambr. arag.[102] ***bar-c.*** bell.[10] bov. carb-an. choc.[222] coca[15] con. convo-s.[119] cortico.[119] cycl. ferr. ferr-p. germ.[222] halo.[149] hell. hydrog.[222] ign.[102] ipom.[119] iris[152] lac-h.[229] lap-mar-c.[194] ***lyc.*** mag-c.[5] mag-s. meny.[36] ***nat-c. nat-m. oxyt.***[54] ozone[227] petr. ph-ac.[58] phos. plat.[10] ***plb.*** rauw.[119] **SEP.** stann. staph. stram. sulph. trio.[149] visc.[119]

Company, aversion to; alone, dreads being, yet: ars.[5] bufo ***clem. con.*** elaps kali-br. lyc. **NAT-C.**[122] nat-m.[5] ***sep.*** stram.[5] tarent.[5]

Company, aversion to; alternating with bursts of pleasantry and sarcasm: rad-br.[122] rhus-t.

Company, aversion to; avoids the sight of people: acon. ars.[30] calc.[122] **CIC.** ***cupr.*** cur.[122] ferr. ***gels.*** germ.[222] hydrog.[222] ***iod. lac-d.***[122] ***led. nat-c.*** psor.[185] ***sep. thuj.***

Company, aversion to; avoids the sight of people, lies with closed eyes, and: sep.

Company, aversion to; avoids the sight of people, shuts herself up: cur.

Company, aversion to; bear anybody, cannot: merc.[10] nux-v.[10] staph.[10] ***sulph.***[10]

Company, aversion to; country away from people, wants to get into the: androc.[222] calc. calc-p.[58] elaps merc.[137] sep.[137]

Company, aversion to; dizzy, faint in a crowd, or where many gas lights are burning (in agoraphobia): ***nux-v.***[54]

Company, aversion to; friends, meeting of, whom he imagines he has offended, to: ars.

Company, aversion to; friends, meeting them amel.: alum.[162]

Company, aversion to; friends, of intimate: bell. cham.[54] coloc. ***ferr.*** hep.[85] ***iod. nat-c. sel.***

Company, aversion to; loathing at company: bell.[30] ign.[30] lyc.[30] nux-v.[30] sep.[30] staph.[30]

Company, aversion to; presence of, strangers, to: **AMBR.**[122] ***bar-c. bry.*** bufo ***carb-v.*** **CIC.** cina[58] ***con. helon.***[163] ***iod. lach.***[8] lyc. nat-c.[58] petr. ***sep. stram.*** tarent.[193] ***thuj.***

Company, aversion to; solitude, fond of: **ACON.**[5] alum.[10] **AMBR.**[5] ***ant-c.***[8] ***ars.***[8] **AUR.**[5] bamb-a.[1184] bar-c.[1] ***bell.***[5] cact.[25] calc.[10] calc-p.[5] camph.[5] carb-an.[5] ***cham.***[8] chin.[1] cic.[1] coca[25] con.[5] cycl.[5] dig.[5] dios.[25] eug.[10] graph.[10] helon.[25] **IGN.**[5] led.[5] lyc.[5] m-aust.[10] mag-m.[10] meny.[5] nat-c.[5] ***nat-m.***[5] ***nux-v.***[5] op.[10] ozone[227] petr.[5] **PLAT.**[5] ptel.[25] **PULS.**[5] ***rhus-t.***[5] sep.[10] seq-s.[230] stann.[5] staph.[10] sulph.[10] tub.[189] verat.[10]

Company, aversion to; solitude, fond of, desires to practice masturbation: ***bufo*** ust.

Company, aversion to; solitude, fond of; fancy, to indulge her: ***lach.***

Company, aversion to; unpredictable, thinks people are: ozone[227]

Company, desire for; alone, while, yet fear of people: ars.[5] bufo[5] clem.[5] con.[5] tarent.[5]

Company, desire for; angina pectoris, in: ***aur-m.***[54]

Company, desire for; children that are rejected, in: carc.[207]

Company, desire for; dislike to society, with: ***con.***[54]

Company, desire for; friend, of a: lap-gr-m.[194] plb..

Company, desire for; happen, as if something horrible might: ***elaps***[54]

Company, desire for; heart, in organic disease of the: ***apis***[54]

Company, desire for; hold his hand, to: bism.[103] phos.[58] stram.[58]

Company, desire for; treats them outrageously, yet: ***kali-c.***

Company, desire for; wants to be watched constantly: gall-ac.[85]

Company; desire for: acon.[30] act-sp. aeth. all-s. androc.[222] ant-t. ***apis*** **ARG-N. ARS.** ars-h.[54] asaf. aur-m. bell. **BISM.** bov. brom. bry. bufo cadm-s. ***calc.*** calc-ar.[58] calc-p. ***camph.*** cann-s.[5] carb-v. carc.[193] caust. cench. choc.[222] ***clem.*** coca[25] coloc. ***con.*** cot.[36] crot-c.[5] crot-h. cyna.[149] der. dros. dys-co.[136] ***elaps*** fl-ac.[102] foll.[1201] gaert.[136] ***gels.*** hep. hydrog.[222] **HYOS.** ***ign. kali-ar.*** kali-br. **KALI-C.** ***kali-p.*** **LAC-C.** lac-h.[229] lach.[5] lap-c-b.[194] lap-gr-m.[194] ***lil-t.*** lith-c.[25] **LYC.** manc. merc. ***mez.*** mut.[136] naja[98] **NAT-C.**[5] nit-ac.[116] ***nux-v. pall.*** ph-ac.[102] **PHOS.**[122] plb. ***puls.*** rad-br.[102] ran-b. rat. sac-alb.[210] ***sep.*** sil.[102] skat.[102] ***stram. stry.*** sulph.[30] syph.[54] tab. tarent. thymol.[102] verat. verb. zinc. zinc-p.[58]

Confidence, want of self, company, in: lap-gr-m.[194]

Delusions; bed, someone, in with him: anac. apis ***bapt.*** carb-v. graph.[116] nux-v. ***op.***[54] ***petr.***[54] ***puls.*** rhus-t. sec. stram. valer.

- • company, people are averse to her: androc.[222]
- • unreal, felt, in company: psil.[164]

Disgust; society, with the follies, of: cic.[1]
Dreams; body, hair, obliged to dress hair in company: mag-c.
➤ interviews, social, with women: cedr.[36]
➤ people, assembled: apis[54] cere-b.[36] hydrog.[222]
➤ people, companies: canth.[10] phel.[10]
➤ people, occupied, with: bell.[36]
➤ visits, making visits: mag-s.[10]
Dullness; company, in: plat.
Escape; attempts to, society, from: cic.[1]
Excitement; company, in: ambr.[58] ***lec. pall. sep.***
Exhilaration; company, in: pall.[60] sep.[60]
Fancies; exaltation of, company, in: pall.[60] sep.[60]
Fear; alone, of being, company, with aversion to, yet fears to be alone: alum.[35] ars.[5] bufo ***clem. con.*** elaps gels.[111] kali-ar.[58] kali-br. kali-c.[56] lyc. morg.[136] **NAT-C.**[35] ***sep.*** stram.[5] tarent.[111]
✦ alone, of being, disinclined to meet even agreeable company: clem.[172]
✦ alone, of being, light and company, wants: bism.[172] rad-br.[172] stram.[172]
✦ friends, of, meeting: lyc.[172] sep.[85] sil.[172]
✦ going out, alone: ars.[127] ign.[127] pitu-a.[164]
✦ people, of, indisposition to meet: ***kali-br.***[54] kali-p.[102]
✦ satiety of life, with, particularly in company, hysteric: ***lyc.***[54]
Indifference; company, in, agg.: androc.[222] **ARG-N.** bov. kali-c. kali-m.[192] lyc.[54] mez.[85] nat-c. nat-m. **PLAT.** rhus-t.
Insanity; company, with desire for light and: **STRAM.**[54]
Irritability; company, in: allox.[119]
Irritability; sends the, nurse home: ***fl-ac.***
Longing; for, sunshine, light and society, for: grin. stram.
Moral affections; antisocial: aesc.[120] anac.[137] ilx-a.[120] lap-gr-m.[194] sac-alb.[210] syph.[137]
Restlessness; bashful, timid, ill at easy in society: ***coca***[54]
Restlessness; company, in: androc.[222] ***carb-v.*** mez.[162] staph.[162]
Sadness; company, agg. in: agar.[60] euph. ***lyc.***[54]
Sadness; company, aversion to, desire for solitude: alum.[10] aur.[10] bamb-a.[1184] ***con.***[116] cupr.[10] ***helon.***[116] ***led.***[54] murx.[10] nat-c.[10] nat-m.[116] rhus-t.[10] sep.[193]
Sadness; company, desire for: stram.[10]
Shrieking; fainting, with sudden, on going from one room to another full of company: ***plb.***[54]
Suspiciousness; fear of company: ambr.[10] bar-c.[10] ***nat-c.***[10]
Talk; desires to t. to someone: ***arg. arg-n.*** buth-aust.[144] ***cann-i.***[25] caust. eup-pur.[25] lachn.[25] lap-c-b.[194] lil-t. nux-m.[54] petr. phys.[25] ***stict.***[54] tarax.[54]
Talk; indisposed, company, in: arg.[58] hydrog.[222]
Thoughts; vanishing, company, in: ambr.[58]
Weary of life; company, particularly in: ***lyc.***[54]

ADAM. Sh, 115 - Averse company. I wanted to spend time alone, which lasted throughout the entire proving. 1, 12C, 00:00:50
Sh, 121 - Wanting to be alone with own thoughts. Guilt over past event: daughter's back injury that occurred 22 years ago as result of my taking her to a horse riding lesson. 5, 30C, 20:XX:XX
Sh, 124 - I want to be alone with things being done for me. For example, I didn't want to drive so I got a mini-cab. 7, 6C, 06:10:00
Sh, 126 - I feel like I want to hibernate, not to be seen and keep warm. I want to curl up somewhere warm and forget the world. I could easily have stayed in bed. 7, 6C, 06:08:00
Sh, 130 - I was angry at my house guest and wanted to be left alone, at breakfast.[11], 30C, 12.XX.XX
Sh, 132 - Being told that I'm grumpy really irritates me. Why can't I be let alone and they can just go away. 7, 6C, 05:17:00
Sh, 378 - I have lost my enthusiasm, not so much sadness, but a heavy depression. Prefer to be on my own. Everything is an effort, feel I am carrying a heavy weight. 12, 30C, 04:XX:XX.
AETH. He, 22 - After social talking, all symptoms disappear.
AGAR. Ha, 28 - Quiet, equable (tranquil), sociable, active, and glad of having done his duty.
ALOE. Al, 21 - Irritable, he cannot endure the visit of many people, they are repugnant to him.

AMBR. He, 18 - The presence of other people aggravates the symptoms.
He, 16 - Embarrassed (inhibit) manner in company.
ANDROC. Sh, 63 - Desired company but could not be bothered to see anyone, felt lonely as if he didn't belong. (21)
Sh, 150 - Speech slurred, answered with difficulty, was indisposed to talk and averse to company. (16)
ARG-N. He, 23 - Often awakes his wife or child to have some one to talk to.
ASAF. He, 10 - Dislike for solitude.
ATRO. Ha, 17 - Sad and morose, preferring solitude and a dark room to society of friends.
AUR-M. He, 2 - If left alone he thinks about nothing but his ailments,... ; desires company.
BELL. Ha, 1395 - He wishes for solitude and quiet; all noise and visits from others are repugnant to him.
BISM. Ha, 108 - Solitude (isolation) is intolerable to him.
He, 6 - Desire for company; child holds on to its mother's hand.
CALC. Ha, 62 - He is cheerful, and would like to be among men, to walk with them.
CAMPH. He, 45 - Cries for help, takes hold of others, will not be left alone.
He, 72 - Palpitation; vexed by want of sympathy (compassion, aid), afraid to be alone a moment, fears death.
CHOC. Sh, 116-12:30pm -I feel less and less animal at the moment and I desire company. When it comes, its so intense, I almost lose what I am. I've never been there before. I feel very privileged, as if I can be on both sides at the same time.
Sh, 210 - Felt totally isolated and averse to company. Estranged himself from his family and friends and stopped all communication with them for a long period. Did not reply to letters and left no address. He seemed to hide away and literally disappear. The state of Isolation resulted from feeling that "I didn't exist as a human being". This behaviour was in strong contrast to his normal sociable disposition. 35, 30C, XX:XX:XX:
Sh, 213 - Unsociable —averse company and conversation.[15], 30C, 04:XX:XX
CIC. He, 18 - Fondness (desire) for solitude; great disregard and dislike for society of others.
He, 34 - Is afraid (fear) of society, and wants to be alone.
CLEM. He, 5 - Fear of being alone, but disinclined to meet even agreeable company.
CON. He, 17 - Dislike to society and yet a dread to be alone. (solitude)
He, 18 - He is averse to being near people, and to the talk of those passing him (misanthropy); is inclined to seize hold of and abuse them. (insult, offend, curse)
CUPR. Ha, 8 - Peevishness, he himself does not know what he wants, he wishes to be alone;...
CUR. He, 2 - Very much depressed about herself, desire only to shut herself up away from people.
DER. Al, 4 - He dreads pain, and is averse to solitude with great anxiety.
DIOS. Al, 1 - Desire to be alone; do not enjoy society (misanthropy); am usually quite fond of the society of ladies, but they now seem repulsive,...
DROS. Ha, 278 - Anxiety in solitude (alone) he wished to have someone always near him, could not bear to be without companions (friends, company), and was quieter when he had someone to speak to; but when they again left him in solitude, he was all the more anxious, until he fell asleep; on awaking the anxiety returned.
FERR. Al, 4 - Constant desire for solitude; horror of conversation, noise, visits, and even the society of her cherished friends.
GELS. He, 18 - Desires to be quiet, does not wish to speak, nor have any one near her for company, even if the person be silent.
HALI-L. Sh, 327 - I want to sleep. Want to be left alone, like a kid just before he goes to sleep. I don't want to bother with people anymore. 08, 30C, 34:XX:XX
Sh, 401 - Worried feeling. Tearful but can't cry. Want to be with someone. Can't let it go that a friend yelled at me two days ago. I'm more sad than I should be. I don't want to be by myself. Want to cry but can't. Feel better with people and worse being alone. This is happening during my period; usually happens before menses. 08, 30C, 17:XX:XX
Sh, 537 - While asleep in bed, my husband

touched my leg and I started from sleep. Oversensitive to touch and sound. Aversion to being touched. I just wanted to be left alone. Too irritable. 06, 6C, 00:05:00

Sh, 571 - At sacred ceremony, but want to be alone. See a friend there who is rude, disrespectful, and obnoxious at this sacred ceremony, and I feel annoyed. 16, 10C, 15:XX:XX

HEP. Al, 19 - Contrary mood, he does not wish to see the members of his own family.

HYDROG. Sh, 182 - A feeling of boredom and depression at 10:00p.m., whilst in company —very distressful. I didn't talk at all, friends thought something had greatly upset me. 24, 30C, 01:10:XX

HYOS. Al, 14 - Thought he was in his own home, and desire to go out and make visits.

He, 57 - Delirium tremens:...averse to light and company; visions as if persecuted preceded by an epileptic attack;... seeks to escape from men by whom he imagines himself surrounded and who are trying to capture him; does not recognize his wife who is standing by his side, but imagines he sees her under a distant bed.

IGN. He, 35 - Fearfulness; does not like to talk; prefers to be alone.

IRID. Sh, 42 - I wanted to sit with the rest of my family. This is unusual for me; usually sit on my own. I1

Sh, 43 - Overall felt better for animated conversation. O13

Sh, 44 - Better for company. It felt better to be with the family. D2

KALI-C. Al, 7 - Sad, lonely (solitary) ; she seeks society in order to enliven (animate) herself.

Ha, 5 - Sad, she feels lonesome (solitary, lonely); she seeks for company to cheer her up.

Ha, 11 - Anxiety and dislike company.

He, 6 - Great aversion to being alone.

LAC-C. He, 19 - Cannot bear to be left alone for an instant.

LIL-T. He, 10 - Aversion to being alone, and yet no dread felt.

LYSS. Al,N-11-...presentiment of impending death begged them to pray for him and not to leave him alone. (absolution, redemption)

MAG-C. Al, 953 - Dream that she was sadly disturbed in company, where especially her grandmother was taken with spasms, and at last had apoplexy.

Al, 964 - Dream of funeral; she was obliged to dress the hair of the company; also of balls and marriages.

MEZ. Al, 2 - No rest when alone; he desires company.

Ha, 7 - Restless when alone, he wishes to be in company.

He, 5 - No rest when alone; wants to be in company ...unable to repeat what has been learned by heart; looks through window for hours, without being conscious of objects around; knows not what she is about; forgets what she is about to utter (talk); looks ill humored, pale, wretched, fallen away; ......expecting some very unpleasant news.

NAT-M. Al, 93 - Ill-humored does not want to go into society for fear of vexing others; feels that he could easily give offense.

Ha, 59 - He feels peevish and avoids company, because he foresees that he might easily annoy (bother, molest) others. (intrude)

He, 13 - Taciturnity; offended at every word (easily); avoids company; hates persons because they have offended him; spleen.

NIT-AC. He, 8 - Taciturn, disinclined to communicate anything; moody in morning.

PALL. He, 5 - They set great store (deposit) on other people's opinion, and attach great importance to what others think, hence they are very excitable in company and their complaints are worse next day. (sensitive, judgment)

He, 18 - Feels best in company and wants to be flattered.

PETR. Ha, 4 - Anxiety in the bustle (confusion) of many men. crowd

PHOS. He, 18 - Does not like to be alone.

PLAT. Ha, 39 - Indifference, cold (reserved), abstracted (separated) in company of friends,..

SEP. Ha, 19 - He must not be alone for a moment.

STAPH. Al, 1 - He was joyous, enjoyed society, and was good-humored.

STRAM. Al, 48 - She is all the time inconsolable; much affected by trifles; makes much

fuss about trifles; disposed to weep, and sometimes also very easily vexed; now and then neglects her duties; now and then thinks she is not fitted for her position ; after the fall equinox...; she wants light and company.
He, 101 - Mania for light and company, cannot bear to be alone.
ZINC. Ha, 13 - Apprehension and ennui; she seeks company.

COMPASSIONATE

Ailments from; misfortune of others: coloc.[1]
Anguish; others, for: naja[36]
Anxiety; cruelties, after hearing of: ***calc.***
Anxiety; others, losing their protectors or familiar relations, for: bar-c.[162]
Anxiety; others, loved persons, for: aeth.[184] sac-alb.[210]
Benevolence: agar.[10] am-m.[10] anac.[10] aur.[10] bell.[30] calc.[10] cic.[10] coff. coff-t.[36] hydrog.[222] ign.[30] lach.[10] led.[10] mang.[10] nat-m.[10] nit-ac.[10] nux-v.[30] op.[36] phos.[10] sil.[189] stann.[10] sulph.[10]
Benevolence; excited: 0coff-t.[36]
Cares; full of, nature, for, animals, plants: lap-c-b.[194]
Charitable: bell.[30] ign.[30] nux-v.[30]
Charitable; expectation of recompense, with the: calc.[30] lyc.[30] nat-m.[30] sulph.[30]
Cruelty; bear, cannot, done to other children: calc.[122]
Deeds; desire to perform, good: coff-t.[36]
Deeds; desire to perform, useful: ***cere-b.***[36]
Delirium; calls for parents who are present trying to console: **STRAM.**[54]
Delusions; devils, speaking in one ear, angel in the other, prompting to murder, or acts of benevolence, devil: ***anac.***[54]
Desires; nurse all the time, to: calc-p.[102] sanic.[85]
Dreams; animals, hare, of a white, cannot butcher it: ozone[227]
Lamenting; others, about: merc.
Love; animals, for: aeth.[162] calc-p.[184] carc.[193] med.[162] nat-m.[185] phos.[193] psor.[185]
Love; animals, for, cats, for: ***sulph.***[162]
Love; animals, for, pet, his: nat-m.[189]
Love; animals, for, suffering: nuph.[36]
Love; children, for: ***ars.***[10] ***hep.***[10] phos.[10] plat.[10] sep.[10]
Love; overflowing, for humanity: germ.[222] hydrog.[222]
No, cannot say: ***ambr.***[162] murx.[185] ozone[227] staph.[185]
Sadness; family, for his: ars.[10] hep.[10] rhus-t.[10]
Sadness; others, for: cocc.[10] sulph.[10]
Sympathetic, compassionate: aeth.[162] alco.[36] am-c.[5] ambr.[185] androc.[222] arg-n.[162] aur.[146] bac.[62] bell.[30] calc.[146] ***calc-p.***[162] cand-a.[239] ***carc.***[122] carl. ***caust. cic.*** cocc.[5] croc. cupr.[210] ***dulc.***[184] germ.[222] graph.[5] hell.[146] hydrog.[222] ***ign.*** iod. lach.[5] lyc. manc. med.[184] ***nat-c. nat-m. nit-ac.*** nuph. ***nux-v.*** **PHOS.** puls. sep.[146] seq-s.[230] stram.[40] tarent.[5] tarent-c.[116]
Sympathetic; animals; only for: aeth.[85] carc.[184] med.[187]
Sympathetic; animals; suffering, feels great pain seeing suffering animals: nuph.[36]
Sympathetic; felt same pain his brother complained of: ***lyss.***[54]
Sympathetic; misfortune of others, greatly affected by: coloc.[137]
Talk; benevolent: tus-f.[36]
Thoughts; accidents, of, having happened to others: osm.[36]
Weeping; children, misfortune, on hearing of: caust.[109]
Weeping; children, suffering of others, at: caust.[127]
Weeping; hurt, seeing others: carc.[207]
Weeping; sympathy with others, from: carc.[207] carl. caust.

ADAM. Sh, 390 - Sensitive to other people's problems and I feel very sad when people I care about tell me that something bad happened to them. Also people I don't know, I still feel very sorry for their sadness. 20, 1M, XX:XX:XX
AGAR. Al, 57 - She is vexed with herself and pities (compassion) herself.
ANAC. He, 69 - In one ear a devil, in the other an angel, prompts (incite) him to do murder or acts of benevolence. (homicidal, x helpfulness, kindness)
ANDROC. Sh, 43 - Felt she should forgive her parents for any blame of real or imagined slights, at the same time she felt as if knots were untying within her.(25)
Sh, 147 - Sensitive to others' emotions. I feel I know how people are feeling. (25)
Sh, 148 - Sympathetic, took on other people's problems. (29)
BOV. Al, 5 - Very courageous and vigorous; he would like to fight with everybody.

CALC-P. Al, 15 - A communication in which some one is justly reproached concerning his conduct, affects him very disagreeably; he grows violent, and holds up his faults to himself.

CANN-I. Al, 25... The stars seemed to look upon him with pitying (compassion) human aspect, and to bewail (lament) his condition.

Al, 61 - Then he possesses the wealth of the world, and with a benevolence equal to his wealth, showers riches on all the needy around him.

CARL. Al, 4 - His nerves are so much affected that the sorrows of others cause him to weep easily.

CAUST. Al, 11 - Excessively sympathetic; she is beside herself, with weeping and sobbing and cannot be contented when listening to accounts of the hardships (misfortune, difficulty) of others.

Ha, 4 - Excessively compassionate (sympathetic); at the relations of others and of the cruelties inflicted upon them, she is beside herself for weeping and sobbing, and cannot content herself.

Ha, 20 - Extreme anxious timidity; she is so much afraid (fear) of a dog near her, which did not harm (hurt, injure) her at all,...every noise in the street made her afraid, and when she saw boys climbing she was very uneasy lest they might get hurt. (care, others)

He, 54 - Excessive sympathy for others.

CERE-B. Al, 3 - Felt all day an astonishing (unusual) inclination to be engaged (work, busy) in something useful. (helpful)

Al, 4 - Felt a desire to give something quite necessary to myself to another. (altruism, helpful, sympathetic)

CHOC. Sh, 15 - I see plants in the house differently, very aware of them and want to give them more light.

Sh, 103 - On looking at a bird in a cage, felt it should be out.

COFF-T. Al, 5 - Desire to perform good deeds intensified.

COFF. He, 8 - Great loquacity, brain feels clear and is active, he feels strong enough to do anything, feels impelled to push things; veneration for the Supreme Being and love for family; benevolence excited.

GERM. Sh, 21 - Contemplative, like nice things, sees beauty in stones and nature. Good at instinctive understanding, compassionate. 16, 30C, 01:XX:XX

HALI-L. Sh, 25 - While listening to a patient grieve, had a return of increased awareness of right eye, especially the socket. I had a strong image of how my mother's right eye was knocked out when she was hit by a truck and killed 30 years ago. Feel a very strong sense of connection with her. Telling this to my proving supervisor later, I realized I had never said this to anyone. This was an aspect of her death I had suppressed. It had always been so horrifying to me I couldn't deal with it. I cried gently with lots of tears. Feeling very sad and some remorse that I couldn't have been with my mother when she died. Felt very calm with all of this. 03, 12C, 18:XX:XX

Sh, 165 - Tremulous heart center sensation. Feeling for people, puppies and just feel my heart. Emotional pressure over sternum and heart. I was more empathic, feeling other people's pain, almost to the point of weepiness. 13, 30C, 06:XX:XX

Sh, 168 - We are adopting a toddler from China. I want to do it for the girls in China. Three hundred a day are abandoned. 01, 30C, XX:XX:XX

Sh, 208 - Daughter home sick. I'm enjoying just hanging around with her being. "Mom." Realize I still don't feel like her mom. I'm not Mom; I'm just me. But to them, I'm Mom. Does my mom feel the same? 09, 6C, 23:XX:XX

Sh, 212 - Out of the blue, a friend called to see if I want to adopt another child and I said, "Yes I do." It shocked me. 01, 30C, 21:XX:XX

Sh, 937 - I don't know what or who to be. I'm not human. I feel that I'm trapped in a body that's not mine. I related to the birds at the Botanical Gardens more than the people, but felt sad because they are caged. 20, 30C, 15:XX:XX

HYDROG. Sh, 15 - I felt in the presence of a totally pure energy, like meeting God and feeling totally unworthy or like meeting a lover and feeling unworthy — realizing all the mistakes of a lifetime. This pure energy was around for some time protecting me. I feel this unification cleared out lifetimes of symptomatology for me. The joining with this energy was as if a male energy joined with me sexually, but with no desire, pleasure or pain involved. This unification with the male energy lasted quite a few days — I'm not used to seeing myself as a man. The morning after this unifying with the higher presence, I collapsed in emotional overflow. All my grief and pain came out. I was doubled upon the floor and went into a deep state of catharsis. It is not possible to describe where I went as there are no concepts applicable. I felt overflowing love for humanity and wanted to give everything away. My mind turned to the Buddha. It was like seeing the complete picture instead of fragmented bits. (These primary effects lasted about 28 days, then changing to a paranoia state). 16, 30C, 07.XX.XX

Sh, 281 - Felt benevolent —wanted to do something for someone else. Went out and spent a lot of money on food which I then gave to old people. 16, 30C, 03:XX:XX

Sh, 282 - During the proving, developed a true sympathy for the weakness of others. 08, 30C, 100:XX:XX

Sh, 283 - I feel more in touch with people, more sympathetic to the rest of the world. Feel more understanding. 08, 30C, 14:XX:XX

Sh, 284 - While talking to friends, felt less weighed down by their problems. I feel less absorbed into people, more able to let go of things that bother me. (cured symptom). 28, 200C, 00:04:XX

Sh, 285 - More charitable and sympathetic than usual. 08, 30C, 04:XX:XX

Sh, 286 - Generous in my feelings towards my husband. 02, 6C, 04:XX:XX

IRID. Sh, 39 - I am less reserved than normal, more confident; but my boundaries have altered. I get less drawn into other people's emotional problems, less sympathetic. I26

Sh, 101 - Went into pet shop. There was a budgie chirping in a cage. I was so upset. "Oh God, I want to let this bird out." I felt it was crying to be let out. Took me all my control not to let it out or shout at the man to do it. Then thought, "This is silly. It would get hurt, he'll think I'm mad." I slunk out of the shop thinking I'd really let that bird down. Distracted and nearly in tears. Walked round town in a daze, should I go back and ask him to at least open the door, knew that wasn't on. It might get out of the shop and die. Felt a real coward. Set up a train of thought — condor in bird garden —a notice justifying its captivity —it only flies for food —it's quite happy to be there because food comes to it. Weeping as I write this. Birds in cages can't lean on the air currents and be blown away. G6

Sh, 214 - Very strong protective feeling towards daughters. Hen and chicks image. Feel more tender towards them then usual. It feels like they are on the brink of adolescence and very vulnerable. Very strong protective feeling, not felt their vulnerability since they were born and very little. G42

MANC. Al, 5 - feeling of tenderness (friendship) and deep compassion.(sympathy)

NAJA. Al, 14 - Felt melancholy; began to form images of possible wrongs (mistaken) and misfortunes, over which the mind broods; very wretched at times;... a slight cause sets him in a perfect agony of mental suffering on another's behalf (welfare);...makes himself imaginary troubles and wrongs, and frets (bother) over them for two hours...

NEON. Sh, 84 - Repeated prophetic notions of daily events before hearing of them, causing anxiety and discomfort; thoughts of a person not seen for months and found he had phoned a few days before, depression and sadness unexplained until heard of sad family news that had already happened. 10, 6C, 01:XX:XX

Sh, 191 - I suddenly thought about my grandfather and cried over his unfortunate life. Suddenly I was cheerful and joking again. 02, 6C, 16:XX:XX

PHOS. Ha, 71 - Exaltation of the sense of common brotherhood.(fraternity)

PLAT. Al, 11 - Contemptuous, pitiful looking down upon people usually venerated, with a kind of casting (reject, discard) them off in paroxysms, against her will.

Ha, 36 - Contemptuous, pitying looking down on people at other times respected,

with a certain disdain (scorn, arrogance), in paroxysms, against her will. (antagonism)
He, 11 - Contemptuous, pitiful, looking down upon people usually venerated, with a kind of casting (forsakes) them off, in paroxysms against her will.
SUMB. Al, 8-...fond (love) of the society of women; ...sympathy with suffering seems robbed of its pain...nervous excitement and heat, especially in head from listening (hearing) to a disputation, ...humor depressed with despair of future...melancholy despondency, as if ill-treated by everyone purposely... mildness, amiability

CONDUCTED

Delusions; animals, horses, riding: cann-i.
- animals, ox, riding an: bell.
- hand, midnight, at, vision of something taking her: canth.
- nose, takes people by their: merc.

Dreams, animals, mule, driving of: chin-b.
- body, nose, being pulled by the: nat-c.[36]
- driving, car, a: aq-mar.[231] choc.[222] hydrog.[222]
- held, by finger, being: sil.[10]
- held, tightly by hand, so could not get away: am-m.[36]
- journey, horseback, on: nat-c. ther.
- riding: chr-ac.[54] nat-c.[58] ther.[58]
- stream, crossing a stream on horseback: chr-ac.[54]
- water, stream, crossing a, on horseback, and water froze: chr-ac.[36]

Gestures; makes, grasping, bystanders, at, noses: merc.[5]

ACON. Al, 15 - He raves, though awake; jumps out of bed and imagines he is driving sheep.(guide)
BELL. Al, 89 - He imagines he is riding on an ox, or some such thing.
He, 24 - Fixed ideas, thinks he is riding on an ox, uses a stick for a gun, growling and barking like a dog.
CANN-I. Al, 65 - Hallucinations which lead the patient to imagine that he is on horseback, is hunting, that he sees blue water, that he is swimming, or that he is captain of a vessel, that he is traveling, that he has no weight.(lightness)
GELS. He, 42 - When attempting (effort) to move, the muscles refuse to obey the will; giddy, confused, lack of muscular co-ordination.
MERC. Ha, 1264 - When taking a walk he felt a strong inclination to catch (capture) by the nose strangers whom he met.
He, 16 - Great restlessness as if he had committed a great crime; ...considers everybody his enemy;...great inclination when walking to take people by the nose;...(desire: conduct, direct, guide)
SEP. Al, 58 - Fearfulness when riding in a carriage.

CONFIDENCE

Answer; hesitating: sec.[36]
Anxiety; children, in, schoolchildren, about their lessons: lyc.[172] sil.[172]
Anxiety; success, from doubt about: aloe[36] ***lac-c.***[54]
Confidence, want of self, company, in: lap-gr-m.[194]
Confidence, want of self;: agn. alum. am-br.[162] am-c.[30] am-m.[30] **AMBR.** ***aml-n.***[54] **ANAC.** anan. ang. anh.[119] aq-mar.[231] arg-n. arist-cl.[144] ars.[137] ***aur.*** aur-i.[58] aur-s.[58] bamb-a.[1184] bar-acet.[36] ***bar-c.*** bell. ***bry.*** buth-aust.[119] calc. calc-sil.[58] ***cand-a.***[239] canth. carb-an. carb-v. carc.[214] caust. ***chin.*** chlor. choc.[222] cob.[54] cocc.[36] dros. ***dys-co.***[136] foll.[1201] gall-ac.[162] gels. germ.[222] graph.[127] hydrog.[222] hyos. ign. iod. ***kali-c.*** kali-n. kali-s. kali-sil.[58] ***lac-c.*** lac-h.[229] lach. lap-c-b.[194] lap-gr-m.[194] ***lyc.*** manc.[162] ***med.***[162] merc. mur-ac. naja[5] nat-c. ***nat-m.***[54] nat-s.[36] nat-sil.[58] nit-ac. nitro-o.[36] nux-v. olnd. op. ozone[227] pall. ***petr.***[30] ***ph-ac.***[185] phos. pic-ac.[137] plb. prot.[136] ***puls.*** ran-b. rhus-t. ruta ***sac-alb.***[210] sant.[36] **SIL.**[122] spong.[36] staph.[10] stram. sul-ac. sul-i.[58] sulph. sumb.[36] syph.[162] tab. ther. verat.[30] verb. viol-t. zinc.
Confidence, want of self; contradiction, in: anac.[60]
Confidence, want of self; failure, feels himself a: aur-s.[231] bamb-a.[1184] naja[5] sulph.[5]
Confidence, want of self; nobody, feels as if he is: agn.[36]
Confidence; thinks others have none, which makes her unhappy, and: ***aur.***
Confidence; use of voluntary muscles, in, could not finish what he attempted: ang.[54]

Cowardice; opinion, without courage of own: graph.[30] ign.[30] petr.[30]
Delusions; business, unfit for, that he is: ***croc.***
• confidence in him, his friends have lost all: aur. hura.
• disabled, she is: cit-v.
• fail, everything will: act-sp. ***arg-n. aur.*** bamb-a.[1184] cob-n.[144] lac-c.[60] merc. nux-v. sil.
• gave way; ground under him: digin.[139] kali-br.[139] tep.[139]
• insecure, everything is: bamb-a.[1184]
• knees, he walks on: ***bar-c.*** bar-m.
• lose, he will: **CUPR.**[54] ***sulph.***[54]
• position, she is not fitted for her: stram.[54]
• walking, knees, he w. on his: ***bar-c.*** bar-m.
• world, she has her own little, in which things are clear, the outside is uncertain: camph.[54]
Discouraged; irresolution, with: puls.[10]
Doubtful: act-sp.[111] alum.[137] anh.[119] ars.[60] aur.[60] bar-c.[60] ***calc.***[137] **CARB-V.**[30] chin.[60] cic.[5] germ.[222] ***graph.***[30] ***lach.***[30] lap-gr-m.[194] mur-ac.[60] nux-v.[60] ***petr.***[30] psil.[164] sep.[30] sil.[60] staph.[30] sul-i.[137] thuj.[60]
Doubtful, plans, about realizing her: bamb-a.[1184]
Excitement; alternating with indecision: cortiso.[149]
Excitement; stammers when talking to strangers: dig.
Fear; duty, being unable to do her: ***lac-c.***[54]
✦ falling, letting things fall, of, morning, on lifting: coca.
✦ medicine, selecting remedies, when: crot-h.[36]
✦ men, of: 0aloe 0aur. 0bar-c. bar-m. choc.[222] 0con. dios. hypoth.[149] ign. 0lach. lap-mar-c.[194] ***led.*** 0lyc. 0nat-c. 0nat-m. 0phos. ***plat. puls.*** raph. sep. 0stann. 0sulph.
✦ occupation, of: lyc.[172] sel. sil.[172]
✦ operation, of each: aeth.[185] calc.[122]
✦ piano, when playing: ***kali-br.***[54] ***phos.***
✦ say something wrong, lest he should: bamb-a.[1184] germ.[222] ***lil-t.*** med.[85]
✦ undertaking anything: ***arg-n. ars.*** kali-p.[172] ***lyc.*** sil.[58]
✦ undertaking, enterprise, a new: cupr.[210] lyc.[201] plb.[201] ***sil.***[54]
Insecurity, mental: ***aml-n.***[54] anh.[119] ***bry.***[36] cann-s.[5] cham.[5] sumb.[36]
Insecurity; sensation of: ail.[137] aloe[130] bry.[36] sumb.[36]
Irresolution; acts, in: **BAR-C.** chin. hydrog.[222] lyc. nat-c. nat-sil.[58] nux-m. **ONOS.** ozone[227] tarent.
Irresolution; changeable: asaf.[10] bism.[10] cann-s.[10] ign.[10] led.[10] m-aust.[10] nux-v.[10] op.[10] plat.[10] sil.[10] thuj.[10]
Irresolution; evening, obstacles from: ferr-p.[36]
Irresolution; ideas: m-aust.[10] nat-m. sulph. tarent.
Irresolution; marry, to: carb-v.[30] ign.[30] lach.[30] nat-m.[30] nux-v.[30] phos.[30] plat.[30] sil.[30] staph.[30] verat.[30]
Irresolution; projects: ars.[10] asaf.[10] **BAR-C.** bufo-s. cact. cham. cortico.[119] ***nux-m.***[10] rhus-t.
Irresolution; trifles, about: ars.[54] **BAR-C.** ferr-p.[36] graph.[137] lyc. lyss. pic-ac.[144]
Longing; for, good opinion of others: ***pall.***
Postponing everything to next day, business seems so long lasting, or as if it never could be accomplished: med.[54]
Timidity; alternating with, assurance: ***alum.***
Timidity; public, about appearing in: aeth.[122] **AMBR.**[122] anac.[85] arg-n.[36] bamb-a.[1184] ***carb-v.*** chin.[30] cocc.[172] cortico.[119] dys-co.[104] **GELS.**[122] graph.[184] kali-p.[172] ***lyc.***[36] med.[187] ***ph-ac.***[36] **PLB.**[122] **SIL.** staph.[36] thuj.[198]
Timidity; public, talk to: cupr.[122] lach.[30] lyc.[122] med.[187] sil.[122]
Timidity; public, talk to, but capable to: lyc.[1]
Undertakes; nothing lest he fail: ***arg-n.*** nux-v.[36] sil.

ADAM. Sh, 93 - Notice slowness between thought and action. It has been happening for weeks. Have started to hesitate. 16, 12C, 61:XX:XX

Sh, 188 - Lack of confidence. I feel worthless. I haven't got a life. All that I have revolves around boyfriend. If something happened to him I'd be at a loss. No direction. 22, 200C, 01:XX:XX

Sh, 189 - Low self esteem. Felt I am not worthy or not pretty or not interesting enough for people. 20, 1M, XX:XX:XX

196 - Very nervous and little self-confidence. I think people are laughing at me and hate me. 20, 1M, 07:XX:XX

Sh, 198 - I wanted thanks and acknowledgment for a particular act and I didn't get it.

I didn't get resentful but I got hesitant and don't want to repeat the act. 7, 6C, 12:00:XX

AGN. Al, 2 - He sometimes feels as if he were nobody (unimportant, insignificant, worthless), and would rather be dead than have that feeling; when possessed by that feeling he has no courage to undertake anything; and when free from it he feels exalted, would like to read like an orator, etc.

ALOE. Al, 2 - Before taking it, the disposition is apprehensive, speculative, amorous, after taking it, quiet ...reflective, more self sufficient,...

ALUM. Ha, 25 - Varying moods through the day, now confidence, then again faint-heartedness.(timid)

He, 25 - Variable mood, at one time confident, at another timid.

AM-C. Al, 20-...she knows not how to comfort (console) herself, what to do with herself;...

Ha, 9 - Many afternoons she is seized with weakness and timidity, so that she cannot control herself and knew not what to do;...

ANAC. Al, 15 - The future appears dangerous to him, as if nothing but misfortune and danger were reserved for him; want of confidence in his strength (vigor, force) and despondency.

Ha, 8 - The future seems to him very dangerous, as if nothing were imminent but misfortune and danger; distrust in his own power, and despondency.

Ha, 9 - He is at odds (quarreling) with the whole world, and has so little confidence in himself that he despairs of being able to accomplish (succeed) what is demanded of him.

Ha, 20 - Indisposition to work; he is afraid to undertake anything, he has no pleasure in anything.

He, 66 - He is separated (divided, disconnect, estranged) from the whole world and has so little confidence in himself that he despairs of being able to do that which is required of him.

ANG. Al, 16 - Lively mood; he is confident he can achieve everything with vigor.

Ha, 298 - Cheerfulness and self-confidence that he can undertake anything with power.

Ha, 292 - No confidence in himself to undertake and carry through voluntary movements.

ANT-T. Al, 12 - Dreaded (fear) to be left alone even for a few moments, lest he " should be dreadfully nervous and not know what to do with himself."

APIS. Al, 23 - It seems to her as if she did not know what to do, as if she had no volition (desire) of her own, her head feels stupid.

ARG-N. He, 5 - In conversation, forgetting what he wanted to say, he looked around as if expecting some one to help (aid) him out.

AUR. Ha, 356 - Melancholy; he imagines he is unfitted (incompetent, unqualified) for the world ; he is filled (full) with intense delight when he thinks of death, so that he longs to die. (punishment)

He, 61 - Has no confidence in herself, thinks others have none; this makes her unhappy. (merit, value)

BAR-A. Al, 3 - All of self confidence has disappeared.

BAR-C. Al, 2 - Imagine he walks on his knees.

Al, 16 - Great irresolution about small things; he wants to drink the cup of coffee, then again not, does not know what he shall do.

Ha, 4 - She suspected, that when walking in the street, men found fault (defect) with her, and judged her amiss (wrong), which made her anxious, so that she dared not look up, she looked at nobody, and perspired all over.

Ha, 12 - The greatest irresolution; he proposes to himself a brief journey, and as soon as he is to make his preparation, he is sorry for it and prefers to stay at home.

Ha, 15 - All self-confidence has vanished.

He, 11 - Imagines he walks on his knees.

He, 26 - Anxious about most trivial affairs.(duty)

He, 34 - Loss of self confidence; desponding: pusillanimous.(cowardice)

BAR-M. He, 7 - Sense of oppressive anxiety, accompanied by the illusory notion that he is walking on his knees, without legs. (inferiority, dwarf?)

BRY. Al, 25 - Fretful; she imagines that she cannot accomplish (realize) her work;

constantly takes up the wrong piece, and always inclined to change and take another; ...
He, 20 - Great sense of insecurity, with mental depression.
He, 22 - Apprehensive, uneasiness and dread of future.
BUFO-S. Al, 7 - He is unable to act with decision (doubtful) ; he forms projects and does not accomplish (succeed) them.
CALAD. Al, 14 - Fear of cutting himself while shaving.
CAMPH. He, 19 - It was to him as if he moved in his own little world, in which all things were clear (pure, perfect) and defined; outside of which uncertain (doubtful) and undefined. (obscure) (purity x impurity)
CANTH. Al, 26 - Distrust of himself, like a hypochondriac.
CAUST. He, 33 - Anxious uneasy mood, as if something unpleasant impended (threaten, frighten); this unfits (incompetent) him for every kind of work.(lost: competence)
CHAM. Ha, 490 - She has scruples of conscience about everything.
Ha, 465 - Very anxious; nothing she does seems to her to be right; she is irresolute; ...(indecisive)
CHIN. Al, 39 - Fretful and irresolute; she is unable to accomplish her aim, and consequently is indignant. (angry)
COFF. Al, 7 - Great anxiety, so that she does not know what she shall do with herself; she trembles, and cannot hold the pen still.
CON. Ha, 20 - Peevish mood, he does not know what to do with himself, the time passes too slow for him.
CROT-H. Al, 7 - For several days, a certain dread of selecting (choice) remedies, which is usually an agreeable occupation.
CUR. He, 1 - Indecision, no longer (more) wishes to think and act for herself.
DROS. Ha, 287 - Happy steadfast (confiding) disposition; he dreaded no evil, because he was conscious of having acted honorably.
GELS. He, 31 - Nervous dread (fear) of appearing in public; singers and speakers.(talking?, acting?)
He, 32 - Complaints: (ailments) from exciting or bad news; sudden emotions; the anticipation of any unusual ordeal (difficulty) ; general depression from heat of sun or summer.
GERM. Sh, 116 - Blaming myself for having taken too many doses. Was afraid that I would not get the symptoms out strongly enough. Maybe I spoiled the whole proving. Still accusing myself. I felt it does not matter how much I suffer - it's what other think of me that is important. I think that I ought to suffer a good deal. 18, 30C, 01:08:15
Sh, 102 - Everything is my fault -I asked for 'drubbing' (beating) and I have got it. The kids are afraid of me, and I feel insecure about what I'm able to do. I called my sister -the only person I could talk to - but she was not at home. With an enormous effort, with heart palpitations, pain in the stomach, trembling and aggravation of headache I rang another prover. But I didn't get through -it was occupied. 18, 30C, XX:XX:XX
Sh, 118 - Just want to cry. Feeling embarrassed. I do not believe in my own feelings and decisions. So afraid of what others think of me. 18, 30C, 01:09:15
Sh, 111 - If I were me, nobody would like me -so I try to be what I think others expect me to be. I don't think I can be loved with all the parts of me which are ugly and bad. Lonely feelings. Longing for love and understanding. Feel I am so unfriendly to myself. 18, 30C, 04:00:00
Sh, 120 - Easily led of others opinion, and provoked. Sensitive to others attempts at restricting me. Feel like a teenager, but I don't dare to protest. I just feel it inside. 18, 30C, 04:00:00
Sh, 146 - Slightest criticism and I am broken hearted. Almost started to cry among all the people, very doubtful about relationships. It kills my confidence. Deep sigh. 21, 12C, 41:XX:XX
GRAPH. Al, 43 - Extreme hesitation (doubtful); she is unable to make up her mind about anything.
He, 19 - Extreme hesitation; she is unable to make up her mind about anything; timidity.
HALI-L. Sh, 170 - More self confident and self accepting than in the past. Questioning the times I'm not confident, and what

to do about it. Instead of viewing it in a paranoid way, I'm treating it in a more matter of fact way. My feelings changed about certain people at work who have bothered me. Bouncing back quicker. Before, hours and hours would pass thinking about it. 18, 30C, 01:13:30

HELL. Al, 16 - He is doubtful (uncertain) about his own life.

HYDROG. Sh, 131 - Marked tendency to panic at little things that go wrong or small decisions to be made. 08, 30C, 00:XX:XX

Sh, 153 - Insecurity and self doubt. 16, 30C, XX:XX:XX

Sh, 155 - In the afternoon (during the full moon) I felt low and depressed, insecure and vulnerable. Could not cope with work load and didn't want to be alone. 12, 6C, 39:XX:XX

IGN. Al, 20 - Fearfulness timidity; she has no confidence in herself, gives up (desist) everything.

Ha, 759 - Fearfulness, cowardice cannot trust himself to do anything, considers all is lost .

Ha, 757 - He imagines he cannot get on (succeed), cannot walk.

He, 36 - Anxiety as though something terrible had happened cannot speak because of it; hurry, fearfulness, terror, alternating with irresolution and inertness.

He, 31 - A peculiar trembling of hands disturbs her very much in writing, most when she has to write in any one's presence (public), gets worse as soon as she fancies any one might notice it. (observed)

IRID. Sh, 198 - The class I was teaching did not go well and left me feeling upset. I did not perform well and I felt low after it. I identified myself as the problem. I began to doubt the work I'm doing was being valued. Wasn't myself. It was the thirteenth time I'd done similar material and it was as if I had never done it before. I tripped over words, couldn't concentrate on what I was doing. (Added at a later date: "This was like I was pregnant.") No one in class had noticed anything was wrong. It was more my own perception. B2

Sh, 201 - Visited friends and although I was happy, calm, relaxed in their company, I was reticent to put forward my views. Was worried that what I had to say was not relevant or good enough. These women are good friends. I usually feel on a par with them. We chatted easily, up to the point when I felt inadequate in the conversation. (She later added, "I was acting as if this familiar situation was a new one.") B8

KALI-BR. He, 24 - Hands constantly busy; all sorts of fearful delusions; walks the room groaning, bemoaning his fate (destine, doom); full of fear; unsteady.(inconstant)

KALI-C. Ha, 32 - Contrary disposition; he is self-willed (obstinate) and often does not know himself what he wishes. (indecision)

LAC-C. Al,N-15 - Feels very short in morning; while walking; same in evening.

Al,N-33 - Depression of spirits, doubts her ability and success, thinks she will have heart disease and die of it.

He, 26 - Depression of spirits, doubts her ability (competence, aptitude) and success (prospering, progressing, achieving), thinks she will have heart disease and die of it.

LACH. Al, 22 - Sudden doubts (indecision) arise about truths (veracity) of which he had hitherto (before) been convinced (converted), in the afternoon.

LIL-T. Al, 49 - She dreads saying anything to anybody, lest she should say something wrong, and yet she wants to walk.

LYC. Al, 127 - Indecision and loss of confidence.

Al, 128 - He is unable to do anything, cannot think; passes his time with trifles, without being able to make up his mind what to do.

Al, 44 - Loss of confidence in his own vigor.

Ha, 32 - Lack of confidence in his strength.(power, vigor)

He, 29 - Want of self confidence; indecision; timidity; resignation.

He, 30 - Loss (want) of confidence; in his own vigor (vitality, strength); in physician and remedies.

MED. Al,N-43 - Forgetful, cannot remember the least thing any length of time; writes everything down of any importance; cannot trust herself to remember it; great irritability and disgust with life.

He, 13 - Seems to herself to make wrong statements (declaration), because she does not know what to say next, begins all right

but does not know how to finish...
He, 31 - Dread of saying the wrong thing when she has headache.
MERC. He, 29 - Anxiety and apprehension; did not know what to do ; it seemed as though he had committed a crime ; without heat; also with a feeling that he had not control over his senses.
MEZ. Al, 38 - It becomes difficult for him to make a resolution.
NAT-C. Al, 17 - Anxiety and restlessness; he thought he could do nothing properly.(rightly, correctly)
Al, 24 - She does not know what to do, on account of apprehensiveness and ennui and thinks that she is quite lonely (alone, solitary, insulated) and forsaken, all day.
Ha, 13 - Anxious and restless, he thinks he cannot do anything right.
Ha, 23 - Restlessness and unsteadiness (inconstant); he knew not what he wanted, nor what he should do or leave undone.
NAT-M. Al, 132 - Irresolute at work; he could not see his way clearly.
NUX-M. He, 25 - Fickle (capricious); irresolute and wavering in his undertakings.
NUX-V. Al, 68 - Irresolution; constant fickleness in his plans.
Al, 73 - Dread of that kind of literary work at which one must think and employ the ideas, ...
Ha, 1288 - Irresolution, constant hesitation in his intentions.
Ha, 1289 - She wishes to do much, but thinks she will not succeed.
Ha, 1296 - In the morning, dread of those literary occupations in which he must think for himself and unfold ideas from his own mind in order either to commit them to writing or to express them orally; but reading and learning by heart are not distasteful to him.
OLND. Al, 5 - Loss (want) of confidence in himself, and on that account a sad mood.
Ha, 348 - Want of self confidence, and hence serious sad disposition.
He, 6 - Despondency and lack of self-confidence.
PETR. Ha, 9 - Lack of determination.(resolution)
PLAT. Ha, 11 - Great restlessness of mind, so that she knows not where to stay (indecision), with gloominess (melancholy) which spoils even what should be most enjoyable; she imagines she is not fit (unfit, incapable) for this world, is tired (weary) of life, but has a great horror of the death she believes to be approaching.
PSOR. Al,N-24 - Despairing mood; fears he will fail in business.
He, 24 - Despairing mood; fears he will fail in business.
PULS. Al, 44 - Shuns business, is irresolute, with sighing respiration and a feeling as if he were beside himself.
Ha, 1122 - Neglect of his business, hesitancy (indecision), sobbing (cry) respiration and loss of composure.(calm, serenity)
SANT. Al, 6-...irresolution and want of confidence in my own powers as to render me quite unfit for work of any kind;
SAPIN. Al, 5 - Quite ill-natured and inclined to view matters in a disagreeable light; did not seem able to feel settled (decided) enough to know what to do; the crossness became so intense, that I felt myself getting very unreasonable, especially as to food, which seemed all wrong in some way;...
STANN. He, 3 - Uneasy, does not know what to do with himself pains > by walking, yet so weak he soon must die.
STRAM. Al, 48 - She is all the time inconsolable; much affected by trifles; makes much fuss about trifles; disposed to weep, and sometimes also very easily vexed; now and then neglects her duties; now and then thinks she is not fitted for her position ; after the fall equinox...; she wants light and company.
He, 61 - Thinks she is not fitted for her position.
SULPH. Al, 29 - She does not know what to do with herself on account of internal discouragement.
Ha, 24 - She imagines that she might give people something wrong, which might kill them.
Ha, 60 - Indifferent things and such things as naturally occur in life are attended in her mind with annoying, mortifying ideas from her past, which continually connect themselves with recent annoyances of which she cannot rid herself. This attended (accompanied) with a resoluteness of mind, which is ready for great resolves.(determination)

He, 37 - Great dejection,(grief), with thoughts of suicide; feels inferior (mediocre, lower) to everybody; can decide nothing;...
TAB. Al, 41 - From having been one of the most healthy and fearless of men, he had become sick all over, and was timid as a girl; he could not even present a petition in Congress, much less say a word concerning it; ...by any ordinary noise, he was startled or thrown into tremulousness, and afraid to be alone at night.
TARAX. Al, 4 - Without occupation he is quite gloomy; does not know what to do, and cannot make up his mind to do anything.
THEA. Al, 10 - A most uncomfortable state of nervousness and want of confidence, relieved by beer...
THER. Al, 7 - Despair; want of confidence; he gives himself up.
YUC. Al, 6-4 p.m. irresolute, changing mind once in fifteen minutes; don't know what to do; can't keep easy.

CONSCIENCE

Anger; alternating with, repentance, quick: anan.[36] croc. lyss.[54] mez. olnd.[10] ***sulph.***[1] vinc.[10]
Anger; mistakes, about his: ars.[54] bell.[54] bry. carc.[193] ***nit-ac.*** nux-v.[30] ***staph. sulph.***
Anxiety; business, lawsuit, as if engaged in a: ***nit-ac.***[60]
Anxiety; conscience, of: achy.[149] **ALUM.** alum-p.[58] alum-sil.[58] ***am-c.*** anac.[5] androc.[222] arn.[122] **ARS.** ***ars-s-f.***[58] atro.[36] <u>**AUR.**</u>[122] aur-ar.[58] aur-s.[58] bamb-a.[1184] ***bell.***[10] bry.[30] cact. calc.[1] ***cand-a.***[239] canth. carb-an.[54] ***carb-v.*** carbn-s. ***carc.***[187] ***caust.*** cham.[10] **CHEL.** chin.[30] cina cob.[36] ***cocc. coff.***[5] ***con.*** croc.[137] cupr. cycl. **DIG.** ***ferr.*** ferr-ar. ferr-p. ***graph.*** hell.[31] hip-ac.[119] ***hyos. ign. kali-bi.***[54] kali-br.[8] kalm.[111] ***lac-c.***[54] ***lach.***[5] lap-c-b.[194] ***m-arct.***[10] m-aust.[5] mag-c.[144] mag-s. ***med. merc.*** myric.[36] ***nat-m.*** nit-ac. ***nux-v.*** ozone[227] ***ph-ac.***[5] phos. plat.[54] **PSOR.** ***puls.***[5] rheum ***rhus-t.*** rob.[172] ruta sabad. sarr.[36] ***sil.***[5] ***spig.***[30] spirae.[36] staph.[102] ***stram.***[54] stront-c. **SULPH.**[122] ***thuj. verat. zinc.*** zinc-o.[10]
Anxiety; conscience, dreams, in: lach.[10] led.[10]
Anxiety; conscience, masturbation, after: **PH-AC.**[54]
Anxiety; conscience, no rest night or day, prevents lying down: ***phos.***[54]
Anxiety; conscience, unpardonable sin, feels she has done the, and will be eternally lost: ***chel.***[54].
Anxiety; conscience, women and religion, about: puls.[54]
Anxiety; duty, as if had not done his: ars.[36] puls.[172]
Anxiety; duty, as if he had not done his, religious, produced by lascivious impulses: ***orig.***[54]
Anxiety; expected of him, when anything is: ***ars.***
Anxiety; lascivious impulses, from, on account of disinclination of religious duties in a married woman, mother of a family: ***orig.***[54]
Anxiety; murdered someone, as if he had, all night: phos.[36]
Anxiety; murdered someone, as if he had, mania, in: ***ars.***[54]
Anxiety; salvation, about: aq-mar.[149] **ARS.** ars-s-f.[58] ***aur.*** aur-ar.[58] aur-s.[58] ***calc. calc-ar.***[122] calc-s. ***camph.*** cann-i. carbn-s. chel. ***graph.*** hura ign. kali-p. **LACH. LIL-T.** ***lyc. med. mez.*** nat-m. nux-v.[30] ph-ac.[30] plat. plb.[58] podo.[58] ***psor. puls.*** **STAPH.**[30] ***stram. sulph. thuj.*** **VERAT.**
Anxiety; salvation, faith, about loss of his: coloc.[30] merc.[30] nux-v.[30] staph.[30] sulph.[30]
Anxiety; salvation, hell, of: ***plat.***[54]
Anxiety; salvation, scrupulous as to their religious practices, too: ars.[30] ign.[30] lyc.[30] nux-v.[30] ph-ac.[30] puls.[30] **STAPH.**[30] **SULPH.**[30]
Company, aversion to; friends, meeting of, whom he imagines he has offended, to: ars.
Delirium; blames himself for his folly: op.
Delirium; wrongs, of fancied: hyos.
Delusions; accused, she is: laur. zinc.

- arrested, is about to be: arn. ars. ***bell.***[122] cupr. kali-br. meli. plb. ruta[36] tab.[85] ***zinc.***
- blame for her partners bad mood, she is to: bamb-a.[1184]
- called before court, on account of wicked actions during climacteric period: ***zinc.***[54]
- convent, she will have to go to a: lac-d.
- crime, about to commit a: kali-bi.[54] kali-br. thea.[139]
- crime, committed a, he had: alum. alum-sil.[162] am-c.[139] anac. ars.[58] carb-an.[54]

carb-v. chel.[111] chin-s.[139] cina[98] cocc.[139] cycl. dig.[139] hell.[58] ***ign.***[102] kali-bi.[54] kali-br. lach.[58] med.[85] merc.[36] nux-v.[102] plb.[58] puls.[139] rheum[139] rhus-t.[139] ruta[98] sabad. staph.[102] ***verat-v.***[102] zinc.[102] zinc-o.[139]

- criminal, and others know it: cob.
- criminal, executed, to be: **OP.**[54]
- criminal, that he is a: alum.[10] am-c.[10] ars.[10] carb-v.[10] caust.[10] chel.[5] cina[10] cob. coff.[10] cycl. dig. ferr.[10] graph.[10] hyos. ***ign.*** m-arct.[10] ***merc.*** nat-c.[10] nit-ac.[10] nux-v.[10] op. phos. puls.[10] ruta[10] sabad.[139] sarr. sil.[10] stront-c.[10] sulph.[10] thuj. verat.[10]
- criticized, that she is: ***bar-c.*** calc.[185] cocain.[102] germ.[222] hydrog.[222] hyos.[102] ign.[102] lach.[185] lap-mar-c.[194] laur. lyss.[102] pall.[102] plb. rhus-t. staph.[102]
- disgraced, family or his absent friends, he disgraced his: sarr.[36]
- disgraced, family, she disgraced her: ***plat.***[8]
- existence, exist any longer, she cannot: thuj.[139]
- friend, offended: ars.
- gallows, of, with fear: ***bell.***
- hang, wants to hang himself: ***ars.***[116]
- hell, gate of, obliged to confess his sins at: agar.
- honest, he is not: ***stram.***[8]
- murderer, executed to be: **OP.**[54]
- mushroom, he is commanded to fall on his knees and confess his sins and rip up his bowels by a: agar.
- neglected his duty, he has: ars.[36] **AUR.** cur.[137] cycl. hell.[58] hyos. ign. ***lyc.*** naja[36] nat-ar. ptel.[36] puls.
- neglected, duty, his, deserves reproach: aur.[54] germ.[222]
- neglected, duty, his, perfunctory manner, performed in: ptel.[36]
- night, duty, he had been on: conin.[36] ptel.[36]
- obscene, actions of which she had not been guilty, accuses herself of.: ***phos.***
- obstacles, in his way, caused partly by contrary fate, partly by himself: aur.[36]
- offended, people, he has: **ARS.**[122] cere-b.[77] **HYOS.**[30] nit-ac.[30]
- people, sees, connected with the law who will seize him, causing great anxiety, cries like a child: ***cupr-acet.***[54]
- poisoning people, she is: lap-c-b.[194] sulph.[1]
- policeman, calls on him, officers: ***cupr.***[162]
- policeman, come into house, he sees: ars.[58] hyos. kali-br.
- policeman, physician is a: bell.
- pursued, police, by: alco.[36] ars.[58] bell. ***cupr. hyos. kali-br.*** meli. phos. plb. zinc.
- pursued, robbing a friend, for: kali-br.[36]
- read, it seems wrong to: lach.[36]
- reproach, has neglect duty and deserves: ***aur.***
- sinned away his day of grace, unpardonable: ars.[58] aur.[58] kali-p.[58] med.[54] plb.[58] podo.[58] psor.[58] puls.[58] stram.[85] sulph.[58]
- soldier, sees, capture him, that will: bell.[10]
- stolen, somebody thinks it: lach.[58]
- stolen, something, she has: lach.[58]
- thieves, accused of robbing, he has been: kali-br.
- voices, hears, confess things she never did: lach.[58]
- whispering, blasphemic: anac.[85]
- wicked deed, she has committed a: cocc.[139]
- world, rests upon him, the world: tab.[139]
- writing is untidy, her: hydrog.[222]
- wrong, giving wrong things to people, causing their death: sulph.[102]
- wrong, he has done: alum.[36] ***ars. aur.*** aur-ar.[58] cand-a.[239] cina[130] cob.[139] cocc.[85] cycl. dig. digin.[36] germ.[222] ***hell.*** hyos.[122] ***ign. lach. lil-t.***[168] lyc. merc. myric.[144] naja[58] nat-ar. ***nux-m.***[137] puls. ruta[130] sarr.[36] sil.[116] sulph.[1] thuj. verat.[139]
- wrong, he has done, people are therefore against her: lil-t.[168]

Discouraged; reproaches himself: ***m-arct.***[122]

Dreams; accusations: clem.[10] lach.[10] nat-m.[10] thuj.[10]

➤ contraband, of having something, and wanting to snatch and lock it up: mag-c.[36]
➤ crimes, answer, for which he is held to: nat-m.[36]
➤ crimes, committed a crime, having: cocc. nat-s. nit-ac.[36] petr.
➤ crimes, committing: hydrog.[222]
➤ crimes, conscience acquits him of a: thuj.[36]
➤ crimes, discovered by priest: nat-s.[36]
➤ errors, mistakes: am-m.[5] ozone[227]
➤ guilt: androc.[222] asar.[149]
➤ misfortune, woman has legs amputated because of him: ozone[227]
➤ police: bamb-a.[1184] ozone[227]
➤ police, calling for, waking him in last part of night: frax.[36]

➤ pursued, police, by: lap-mar-c.[194]
➤ rape, that he has committed: ***cench.*** kreos.[10] petr. sep.[10]
➤ remorse, God was punishing her for her sins, that: aether[36]
➤ remorse, of: aether[36] arn.[36] ars.[1] elaps[36] fl-ac.[36] hyper.[36] lach.[10] led.[10] nat-c.[10] nat-m.[36] sanic.
➤ remorse, past mistakes, for: nat-m.[36]
➤ remorse, pleading for mercy at bar of judgment: aether[36]
➤ remorse, repudiated by God, of being: hyper.[36]
➤ repentance: ars.[36]
➤ reproaches himself: nat-m.[1]
➤ robbery, of committing: hydrog.[222]
➤ shameful: acon.[36] alum. am-c.[5] arn.[10] ***asar.***[5] con. erech.[36] hydrog.[222] led.[1] mag-m.[1] mosch.[5] mur-ac.[1] ozone[227] staph.[5] tub.[111]
➤ theft, committed, of having: alum. plb.
➤ whipped, getting: ptel.[36]
➤ wrong, doing: cocc.[5] ozone[227]

Escape; attempts to, crime, for a fear of having committed a: ***merc.***[54]

Fear; arrested, of being: ars.[137] bell.[172] meli.[85] plb.[137] ruta[162] tab.[137] zinc.[72]
✦ broken the arm of her child, that she has, in gastroenteritis during pregnancy: lyc.[172]
✦ killing, child, her: ars.[172] coff.[172] manc.[30] ***merc.***[185] ***nux-v.***[185] rhus-t.[172] sep.[185] sil.[172] ***sulph.***[185] **THEA.**[162]
✦ killing, of, delivery, parturition, during: acon.[172] ars.[172] coff.[172] plat.[172]
✦ mischief, he might do (night on waking): canth.[172] ***phys.***
✦ moral obliquity alternating with sexual, excitement: lil-t.
✦ offending his associates, of: tus-f.[36]
✦ punished, of being: plb.[201]
✦ punished, of being, child: camph.[54]
✦ punishment, after, in children, if brought to bed too soon get convulsions in sleep: ***ign.***[54]
✦ sudden, broken her child's arm by lifting him, that she has: ***lyc.***[54]
✦ wrong, commit something, and kill herself: ***merc.***[54]

Grief; consequences, about: **STAPH.**[54]

Grief; neglected duty, over: cycl.[102]

Inconsolable; actions, over all her, which she thinks are evil: sulph.[1]

Inconsolable; heat, with, would rather die on the spot: spong.[54]

Insanity; females, self accusation, from: hell.[137]

Insanity; self-accusation, from: hell.[137]

Irritability; alternating with, remorse: mez.[10]

Irritability; remorse, with easy and quick: ***sulph.***[54] vinc.[54]

Killed, desire to be: ***ars.*** bell. coff-t. ***phyt.***[54] stram.

Killed; desire to be, stabbing heart, by (after midnight): ***ars.***[36]

Mania; destructive efforts, sudden foxlike, requiring utmost vigilance, followed by laughter and apologies: ***tarent.***[54]

Mood; repulsive, food, saying one who does not work should not eat, but driven by hunger he tried to procure it secretly: ***arg-n.***[54]

Morose; repentance, followed by: vinc.[54]

Praying; killed, to be: bell.[30]

Quarrelsomeness; repentance, followed by: vinc.[36]

Rage; alternating with, repentance, quick: croc.[60] mez.[60]

Rage; repentance, followed by: croc.[116] lyss.[54]

Religious affections, sadness, remorse, from: aur.[30] con.[30]

Religious affections; eternal bliss, believes herself unworthy of, because she is unable to perform her duties: stram.[54]

Religious affections; penance, desires to do, wishes to live, in order to mitigate her eternal punishment, in sadness: ***plat.***[54]

Remorse: achy.[149] agn.[58] alum. alum-sil.[58] am-c. anac.[5] androc.[222] ***ars.*** ars-s-f.[58] ***aur.*** aur-ar.[58] ***bell.*** cact.[5] ***calc.***[122] calc-p.[5] cand-a.[239] ***carb-an.***[5] carb-v. carc.[138] caust. cham. chel. chin-b.[54] cina clem.[5] ***cocc.*** **COFF.** con. croc.[88] ***cupr.*** cycl. ***dig.*** ferr. ferr-ar. germ.[222] graph. hell.[187] ***hyos. ign.*** kali-br.[5] lach. ***lil-t.***[187] lyss.[56] ***med.*** merc. mez.[30] nat-c. nat-m. nit-ac. nux-v. olnd.[5] ***ph-ac.***[5] phos.[5] plat. psor.[122] ***puls.*** rheum[5] ruta sabad. sec.[5] sel. ***sep.***[187] ***sil.*** spirae.[36] stram. stront-c. sulph. ***verat.*** vinc.[36] ***zinc.***

Remorse; fury, after attacks of, makes earnest apologies: lyss.[54]

Remorse; indiscretion, over past: spira.[36]

Remorse; masturbation, after: staph.[92]

Remorse; repents quickly: croc. olnd. sulph.[30]

Remorse; repents quickly, apologies, making earnest: lyss.[54]

Remorse; trifles: ***sil.***

Reproaches; himself: ***acon.*** ambr.[162] anac.[116] ***ars. aur.*** aur-ar.[58] calc-p. cand-a.[239] cob. con.[116] cupr.[184] cycl. ***dig.*** germ.[222] gink.[149] hell. hura ***hyos. ign.*** lach.[116] lap-c-b.[194] lyc. ***m-arct.***[10] med.[122] merc. myric.[144] nat-ar. ***nat-m. op.*** ph-ac. plb.[201] ***puls. sarr.*** sil.[116] stram.[111] sulph.[116] ***thuj.*** verat.[116]

Reproaches; accomplished enough, because he had not: ars.[54]

Restlessness; conscience, of: cand-a.[239] ***chel.***[54] merc.[10] ***puls.***[122] zinc-o.[10]

Restlessness; crime, as if he had committed a: ***alum.***[54]

Restlessness; duty, as if he had not done his: ***puls.***[54]

Sadness; brooding over imaginary wrongs and misfortunes, by: naja[130]

Sadness; conscience, of, as if he had committed a bad action, or not done his duty: cycl.[54]

Sadness; criminal as if being the greatest: cycl.[60] sabad.[36]

Sadness; fault, as if in: tarent.[36]

Sadness; wrong way, as if having done everything in, during headache: ***naja***[36]

Self-torture: acon.[111] ***ars.***[111] bell.[111] ***lil-t.***[111] plb.[111] tarent.[111] tub.[111]

Talk; sleep, in, confess themselves loud, they: bell.[30] **HYOS.**[30] stram.[30]

Talk; vexatious things, desire to say, with quick repentance: mez.[36]

Torments; himself: acon.[111] ars.[111] bell.[111] ***lil-t.***[111] nat-m.[36] plb.[111] tarent.[111] tub.[111]

Truth; thinks she does not tell the: macrin.[36]

Violence; suddenly sprang away from attendants and swept everything from mantelpiece, said she was sorry, but could not help it: ***tarent.***[54]

ACON. Al, 53 - Dolorous anxious complaints, with pusillanimous (cowardly) fears, despair, loud wailing (laments) and weeping, and bitter reproaches.

Ha, 516 - Inconsolable anxiety and piteous howling, with complaints and reproaches about (often triflings) evils.

Ha, 517 - Piteous (miserable), anxious complaints, with cowardly fears, despair, loud whining weeping, bitter complaints and reproaches.

He, 28 - Moaning, anxious lamentations; reproaches from trifling causes.

ADAM. Sh, 121 - Wanting to be alone with own thoughts. Guilt over past event: daughter's back injury that occurred 22 years ago as result of my taking her to a horse riding lesson. 5, 30C, 20:XX:XX

Sh, 193 - Felt had spoiled the proving by spraining ankle. Blamed myself. 8, 6C, 02:XX:XX

Sh, 215 - I feel very angry and extremely intolerant, cold and hard and I hate myself for feeling these harsh unkind feelings. 20, 1M, 02:XX:XX

Sh, 238 - Quickly felt remorse after anger. 8, 6C, 04:XX:XX

Sh, 278 - Felt I would create irreparable damage if I said how I feel. Thought I would say the most awful things that the kids would never recover from. Supreme effort to keep silent. Didn't want to be here. The kids were a hassle. I felt old and tired. Desire to get away from the fighting. 16, 12C, 17:XX:XX

Sh, 418 - Anxiety regarding acting irresponsibly about my health. "This might affect the rest of my life." 8, 6C, 01:XX:XX

AGAR. Al, 8-...called for his hatchet; had to be confined alternated with religious excitement.

Al, 14 - He imagines himself at a gate of the hell and that the mushroom commands him to fall on his knees and confess his sins, which he does. (forgiveness, absolution)

ALL-S. He, 3 - Sadness when alone; moral uneasiness; afraid of never getting well; fear of not being able to bear any kind of medicine; fear of being poisoned...

ALUM. Al, 17 - Anxiety with external heat and uneasiness as if she had done something bad.

Al, 19 - Anxiety and fearfulness, as if he had committed a crime.

Ha, 16 - Anxiety with external heat and restlessness, as if she had done something wicked. (immoral, evil)

Ha, 17 - Anxiety and fearfulness, as if he had committed a crime.

Ha, 23 - Excited, over-worked (industrious), and yet discontented, because not enough had been done. (duty)

He, 23 - Anguish, oppressive and vague fearfulness, or uneasiness as if he had committed a crime.

AM-C. Al, 23 - Every afternoon, between

five and six o'clock, she is seized with anguish, as if she had committed the greatest crime; towards evening the anguish passes off.

Ha, 8 - Every afternoon between 5 and 6 o'clock she is seized with anguish, as if she had committed the greatest crime; ...

He, 8 - Anguish as if a crime had been committed.

ANAC. Ha, 4 - Internal anguish, which did not allow him to rest, he troubled himself about every trifle, as if it would cause great injure, with solicitude about the future.

ANAN. Al, 7 - Quarrelsome and contrary humor, but after being angry he often regrets (remorse) what he has done.

ANDROC. Sh, 39 - Cancelled an appointment without any remorse. Thought "maybe I shall feel guilt later". (7)

Sh, 40 - She dreamt that she had murdered her grandfather by poking a knitting needle through his eyes while he slept. Though she felt no remorse, she wanted to be punished but no-one would accept her guilt. Was told by her friends that she had responsibilities and could not go to jail and the police refused to prosecute. Was frightened by the dream. (7)

Sh, 112 - Became excited to anger and confrontation. She was not aware of hurting others' feelings and did not seem to care. Could not appreciate anyone else's feeling. Later she reflected on her actions and felt ashamed. (12)

Sh, 115 - When reflecting on her anger and arguments, was filled with remorse, although at the time she believed she was being perfectly reasonable. (12)

Sh, 121 - When talking to friends felt 'paranoid', suspicious and guilty, when asked questions, he became hot and sweaty. He felt it was a game of who was cleverer, and tried to lie to and outwit his friend, though this gave no satisfaction. His friends reported that he seemed unusually distant and cool. (29)

ARG-N. He, 17 - Refused food, saying one who does not work should not eat (punishment); but driven by hunger he tried to secretly procure it.

ARS-MET. He, 6 - She would very much like to die, or fall asleep (sleep), never to awaken.

ARS. Al, 74 - Continued anxiety, a mental anguish, as if he had not done his duty, without, however, knowing wherein.

Al, 108 - Dissatisfied the whole day, and very fretful at himself for not having done enough.

Ha, 1032 - Mania; first headache, horrible anxiety, noise before the ears, as from a number of large bells, and when he opened the eyes, he always saw a man who had (formerly) hung himself (suicidal, justified) on the ground-floor of the house, who incessantly beckoned (call) him to cut him down (help); he ran thither (there) with a knife, but, as he could not cut him down, (rescue) he became overwhelmed (beaten) with despair (remorse?) and wished (as his friends assured him) to hang himself (punish); but being prevented (stop) from doing so, he became so restless that he could hardly be kept in bed,... and he knelt down and raised his hands in a supplicating manner.

Ha, 1035 - He is cold, shivers and weeps, and thinks, in his despair, (hopelessness, despairing) that nothing can help him, (helplessness) and he must die; followed by general exhaustion.

Ha, 1039 - Persistent anxiety, like a qualm (doubt) of conscience, just as if he had failed (neglected) to do his duty, but without knowing wherein.

Ha, 1064 - All day long discontented with himself and very cross with himself; he imagines he has not done enough, and reproaches himself bitterly.

Ha, 20 - Continual anguish, like remorse of conscience, as if he had acted in violation (transgression, crime) of his duty, without knowing in what particular.

Ha, 53 - Dissatisfied all day and extremely vexed at himself; he thought he had not worked enough and reproached himself most bitterly.

He, 25 - Mania...sees a man who has hanged himself beckoning (call) him to cut him loose (rescue, deliverance, free, saving) on failing to accomplish this he attempts to hang himself (punish, penalize);...finally kneels down and lifts his hands in supplication.(forgiveness, absolution)

He, 48 - Averse to meeting acquaintances,

(friends) because he imagines he has formerly offended them, though knows not how.

He, 76 - Anxiety like that of one who has committed murder; driven from place to place; avoids meeting persons, thinking that he has offended them.

He, 95 - Dissatisfied and angry with himself all day; thinks he has not accomplished enough, and reproaches himself bitterly.

AUR. Ha, 330 - All day long good humor; he was talkative and contented with himself.

Ha, 344 - Discontented with all circumstances; he imagines that he finds everywhere some obstacle (impediment, restriction) in the way; at one time he thinks that this is owing to an unlucky (unfortunate) fate (destiny), at another that he himself is to blame (censured) for it ; when the latter was the case he was particularly mortified and dejected.

Ha, 346 - Remorse about his idleness (indolence), and yet he cannot work at anything; it drives him out of the house, he must always moving.

Ha, 347 - Always very restless and undecided (doubtful) -thought he was neglecting something for which he must incur (obtain) reproach - ...he seemed to carry about this restlessness with him in his inmost (deepest) parts ; this condition deprived him of all perseverance, all energy.

Ha, 11 - Restlessness and hurried impulse to bodily and mental activity; he can not work fast enough; he could not act so as to satisfy himself.

Ha, 12 - He is driven to constant activity, and is sorry for his inaction, although he cannot do anything.

Ha, 13 - Restless and undecided, without perceptible ebullition of the blood; he always thinks he is neglecting something for which he will be reproached; he seems to carry with him this internal restlessness, and it took from him all perseverance and energy.

BAR-C. Al, 9 - Extremely despondent and depressed; she believes that she must die; cries.

BELL. Al, 178 - Fretfulness; nothing seemed right to him; he was vexed with himself.

Ha, 1437 - She tries to strangle herself, and begs those about her to kill her, for this time she must die. (redemption, regeneration, salvation)

He, 85-...patient must do everything violently; she wishes those around her to kill her. (salvation, redemption)

He, 119 - Fretfulness; nothing seemed right to him; was vexed with himself.

BOR. Al, 18-..contented with himself and the world, and looking cheerfully into the future.

CACT. Al, 16 - Feeling of semi remorse at having done something wrong.

CALC-A. Ha, 263 - Anxious disposition as if something evil had happened or he had to fear reproaches (censures); at the same time, however, persistent inclination to work. (industrious)

Ha, 265-...very indifferent to the most important things; he did everything unwillingly (reluctant, averse) as if forced to do them.

CALC-P. Al, 15 - A communication in which some one is justly reproached concerning his conduct, affects him very disagreeably; he grows violent, and holds up his faults to himself.

CALC. Ha, 13 - Anxious at heart, as if he had done wrong,(immoral) or had to apprehend reproaches (deserves), with constant inclination to work.

Ha, 30 - She despairs of her life and believes she has to die (punishment?) ; her heart is sad with weeping, and frequent attacks of sudden, general heat, as if she had hot water poured (flow) over her.

CAMPH. Al, 46-.... As I lay stretched on my couch, as the evil demon, and suffered all the anguish of a condemned and God-forsaken soul, ...I was forever deprived of the Divine protection, and of every consolation and every hope. Nothing remained to me but the conviction of my everlasting damnation...

Al, 46-...And yet I confessed this every morning, and no heavy sin rests upon my conscience. And then came doubts about my doctrinal views, for I had never been of strong faith...

He, 53-...everything that is said is taken as if one was ordering him, and he was considered naughty (disobedient) and would be punished.

CANTH. Al, 36 - He is anxious as if he had committed a murder (homicide); it seems to arise from the stomach.

CARB-V. Ha, 8 - For restlessness and anguish every afternoon, he trembled all over the body; he felt as if he had committed a great crime, this dissolved itself into copious weeping, even before strangers on the street.

He, 18 - Anxiety and uneasiness causing him to tremble all over, as if he had committed a crime, ending in weeping, even before strangers;...

CAUST. Al, 12 - Anxiety the whole day, as if he had done something bad, or apprehended it, or as if he had been unfortunate (unsuccessful, umprosperous).

Ha, 6 - Anxiety the whole day, as if he had done something wrong, or to fear it, or as if a misfortune had happened.

CHAM. Al, 31 - She makes conscientious scruples about everything.

CHEL. Al, 53 - Becomes frightened at the slightest noise, as if he had not a good conscience.

Al, 55 - Mood very irritable, daily outbreaks of anger without cause (causeless); feels as though she could beat the children, and trembles from rage because she has no reason for doing it.

Al, 65 - Fretful depressed, anxious, as if I had committed some evil (crime), which gave me no rest. (remorse)

He, 7 - Thinks she must die.

He, 17 - Restlessness and uneasiness of conscience; feels that she has committed the unpardonable sin (crime, transgression), and that she will be eternally lost.

He, 18 - Anxiety: allowing no rest at any employment (business) ; as if she had committed a crime; fear of getting crazy (insanity), with restlessness and heat.

CHLOL. He, 3 - Fixed despair of recovery; believes he will give his imaginary disease (syphilis) to others.

CHOC. Sh, 193 - Husband wants to go out for a walk. I don't want to go. I feel paranoid that someone will see me and think 'on drugs' and arrest me or cart me off to an institution. 15, 30C, 00:02:00

CLEM. He, 8 - Ailments from homesickness, or contrition (penitence, remorse) of spirit.

COB. Al, 5 - Condemned, mean feeling, as though guilty of some deed (action) of which others knew; as if he could not look one in the face. (shame, dishonored)

COCC. Al, 16 - Anxiety as if she had committed a great crime.

Al, 30 - Great dissatisfaction with himself.

Al, 17 - Great anxiety, as though he had done some evil.

Ha, 536 - Anxiety as if she had committed a great crime.

Ha, 537 - Great anxiety as if he had done something bad.

He, 25 - Melancholy and sadness, with weeping and constant profound absorption in sorrowful thoughts; great apprehensive anxiety of conscience, and feeling at heart as after committing a wicked deed (act), with desire to escape.

CON. Al, 43-...a great guilt weighed upon him, with paralyzed feeling in all the limbs, indifference,..

Ha, 18 - Very morose; ...as if a great guilt weighed him down; at the same time a sensation of paralysis in all the limbs; ...

He, 32 - Discouraged, despondent, and dissatisfied (discontented) with herself and her surrounds.

COP. Al, 9 - Absurd recriminations about trifling and long -past occurrences.

CROC. Al, 28 - Vacillating (hesitate), peevish mood; the slightest cause excites his anger, for which, next moment, he is sorry (remorse), which however, soon returns, because his calmness frets (disturbs) him and prevents (stop) his exposing his feelings (oppressed); usually he changes a hard word which he has on his tongue to a mild one, but the latter seems too mild, and now chooses a more severe word, ...(sorry, guilty, by anger, mildness, x harsh, rude)

Al, 29 - He takes everything in anger and suddenly repents (apologize) of having injured (offend) others.

He, 13 - He takes everything in anger and suddenly repents (sorry) of having injured (offensive) others.

CUPR-A. He, 4 - Fixed idea that he sees persons connected with the law who are about to seize him (imprisoned),...at times sees thieves in the room, spirits, and various other immaterial objects;...

He, 10 - Awoke suddenly from sleep...and wished to escape...thinks she is about to die and desires to see the pastor;...

CUR. Al, 12 - Regrets (remorse) from the past.

CYCL. Al, 10 - Internal grief and anxiety of conscience, as though he had not done his duty, or had committed a crime.

Ha, 196 - Inward grief and anxiety of conscience, as if he had not done his duty or had committed a crime.

Ha, 197 - Excessive sadness, as if he had done something bad and had neglected his duty.

He, 12 - Great sadness, as if he had committed a bad action or not done his duty.

He, 23 - Ailments from inward grief and terrors of conscience.

DIG. Al, 21 - Anxiety, as though he had done wrong.

Al, 24 - Internal anxiety, like pangs of conscience, as though he had committed a crime, or expected to be reproved, continuing nearly three months.

Ha, 425 - An anxious feeling as if he had done something bad.

Ha, 9 - Internal anguish, like anguish (anxiety) of conscience, as if he had committed a crime, or had to expect reproaches...

Ha, 8 - Anxiety as if he had done wrong.

He, 13 - Great anxiety, like from troubled conscience.

FERR. Ha, 272 - Anxiety at night, as she have done something bad; she could not sleep, tossed about the bed.

Ha, 295 - Anxiety as if she had done something bad.

He, 10 - Anxiety as after committing a crime.

GERM. Sh, 4 - Desperately angry. So intense that I could barely control it. I made noises like an animal, pushed my arms up and down - instead of hitting my children, which helped. Want to just leave the house and the kids. Felt completely mad, afraid of what the neighbors heard and thought. Very bad conscience afterwards, but no relief -didn't get the anger out. There are a lot of feelings inside that don't come out. 18, 30C, 02:09:00

Sh, 6 - Difficult to accept my own feelings, accusing myself for letting them out, especially anger. Felt a rage, had to use all my power to control it. Lost my patience because of something my son did. I got angry with him, but at the same time despised myself for not having patience with him. I did not want to report this, because I feel unveiled - now everybody can see what awful person I am. I go completely mad of all my thoughts; can't bear it anymore. Inside me everything is chaos. Feel no power. 18, 30C, 18:XX:XX

Sh, 5 - Everything was heavy and felt impossible without meaning. Terrible anger. Bad conscience and crying afterwards. Could not do what I had planned to do, because I felt so terrible and everything was chaos. Was crying, but couldn't get it out - no release in it. 18, 30C, 176:XX:XX

Sh, 8 - Weeping. Feeling very offended towards father who had objected because I had bought something expensive for myself. Felt anger because of my reaction, but also curiosity to find out why I reacted. Feel anxiety about all my responsibilities. Everything feels like too much. 21, 12C, 26:XX:XX.

Sh, 134 - Felt uncomfortable if any one stood close to me. Felt uneasy and paranoid in class. Feel as if done something wrong. 10, 9C, 06:06:00

Sh, 128 - Afraid of the police of being caught and unveiled. 18, 30C, 02:10:00

Sh, 126 - I have a guilty feeling if I get too much attention. I am afraid of bothering others. 18, 30C, 13:XX:XX

Sh, 117 - I am probably incurable and that's my own fault. The thoughts are repeating themselves again and again in my head. 18, 30C, 46:XX:XX

Sh, 180 - Woke up early 3.30 am. had strong feeling, like a visualization. I picture myself lying on floor in fetal position and being shot in the head like a horse or a dog. Almost welcomed it. Then thought my children still need me. A very strong feeling of failure accompanied this. I felt I did not deserve to live. Better crying next day when talking to husband. This feeling of depression carried on for several nights. As soon as I wake up in the early morning, my mind is active and a feeling of inadequacy comes on strongly. 05 , 6C, 28:XX:XX

Sh, 116 - Blaming myself for having taken too many doses. Was afraid that I would not get the symptoms out strongly enough. Maybe I spoiled the whole proving. Still accusing myself. I felt it does not matter how much I suffer - it's what other think of me that is important. I think that I ought to suffer a good deal. 18, 30C, 01:08:15

Sh, 102 - Everything is my fault -I asked for 'drubbing' (beating) and I have got it. The kids are afraid of me, and I feel insecure about what I'm able to do. I called my sister -the only person I could talk to -but she was not at home. With an enormous effort, with heart palpitations, pain in the stomach, trembling and aggravation of headache I rang another prover. But I didn't get through -it was occupied. 18, 30C, XX:XX:XX

Sh, 123 - Don't understand anything, the meaning of life. Feel also strength somewhere inside. I wish a change could happen, I ought to bring myself together and change. It is silly of me to go on like this. I despise myself. I am hard to myself, but I don't deserve anything else. I think other people are silly too. 18, 30C, 06:XX:XX

Sh, 112 - Don't see why I am here. I can't bear it. I go mad. I hate myself. I want to beat myself and I do it. Tear my hair. Stop when it hurts too much. It is like hell !!! 18, 30C, 20:XX:XX

GLON. Al, 14 - Recalls old grievances...; he was constantly thinking of persons who had offended him, with determination to justify (excuse, defend) his own conduct.

GRAPH. Ha, 22 - Anguish and hurry (quick) chase (pursue, follow) him about, like a criminal.

HALI-L. Sh, 171 - Made a decision to play cards with my friend at work even though a guard who has been hassling me was nearby. She makes me uncomfortable. Decided not to let that person's presence get in the way of my life. Did it very confidently. Very confident! Confidence to accept and to go about my business without making detours. 18, 30C, 03:02:00

Sh, 175 - Date with the local Catholic priest who has a thing for me. I haven't had a date in years and now this—a priest! 16, 10C, 41:XX:XX

Sh, 172 - I have an inner sense of confidence. I feel good about the things I do. I am able to let my friend go and not torment myself about things which haven't working out. 08, 30C, 19:XX:XX

Sh, 598 - Calmness continued, with the exception of seeing ants in my house. They had invaded my house, and I was irritated that I had to kill them and clean them up. I don't like to kill anything. My heart was racing and my face was sweaty while doing this. 03, 12C, 00:XX:XX

Sh, 946 - Inner vision: I was a male Indian. I thought, "I'm not a brave. I don't deserve this feather". 20, 30C, 15:XX:XX

HAM. Al, 9 - Regretful (sorry) in mind for having had emissions at night.

HELL. He, 12 - An old woman having been accused of theft by the women around, took it so much to heart that she hanged herself. This suicide produced a profound effect upon the women of the village. One after another accused herself of having caused the death of the old woman by their insinuations; they wept and howled, ran about day and night wringing their hands and despairing of salvation on account of their sin (error); they became quite irrepressible and deranged (disordered) In this way twenty -four or twenty five women were affected, every fresh case being followed by another. Hysterical mania.

HEP. Al, 4 - Everything of which she only thought was disagreeable and not right.

Al, 16 - Irritable mood; everything that she undertook was wrong; she desired to be alone.

Ha, 4 - Fearful anguish, in the evening, for two hours; he thought he had to perish (die), and was sad even so that he could have committed suicide. (redemption, salvation)

HIPP. Al, 6 - Fretful, discontented with himself almost lachrymose, in the morning.

HURA. Al, 7 - During and after the fainting spell (trance), disposed to love everybody, especially those about him; he often thinks of death, but does not fear it; he feels as though he could die without regret.(fearless)

Al, 8 - He reproaches himself for all his bad actions, even the merest trifles.

Al, 23 - Anxiety about his salvation, during the nervous attack.

HYDROG. Sh, 15 - I felt in the presence of a totally pure energy, like meeting God and feeling totally unworthy or like meeting a lover and feeling unworthy — realizing all the mistakes of a lifetime. This pure energy was around for some time protecting me. I feel this unification cleared out lifetimes of symptomatology for me. The joining with this energy was as if a male energy joined with me sexually, but with no desire, pleasure or pain involved. This unification with the male energy lasted quite a few days — I'm not used to seeing myself as a man. The morning after this unifying with the higher presence, I collapsed in emotional overflow. All my grief and pain came out. I was doubled upon the floor and went into a deep state of catharsis. It is not possible to describe where I went as there are no concepts applicable. I felt overflowing love for humanity and wanted to give everything away. My mind turned to the Buddha. It was like seeing the complete picture instead of fragmented bits. (These primary effects lasted about 28 days, then changing to a paranoia state). 16, 30C, 07.XX.XX

Sh, 75 - Tendency to lose things and blamed myself. Became frantic searching for them. Tore open a friend's bag to find paper and wouldn't have cared if the bag had ripped. 22, 12C, 04:XX:XX

Sh, 114 - I feel quite resentful about having to hurry. 08, 30C, 09:XX:XX

Sh, 248 - While sitting in a restaurant, felt progressively more cut off from friends at the table. I began to feel detached and paranoid. I felt disliked by people. They seemed to look at me menacingly. I became concerned that my lecture this afternoon had created conflict, mayhem and destruction, that my friends in the audience did not like me any more. I became aware of a dull ache in my sacrum making me want to shift backwards and forwards. At the same time, the people round the table seemed further away and smaller, as if I had moved four feet back from the table. I felt very uncomfortable and wanted to get out. I put my head down and rushed out without saying goodbye, feeling a sense of relief at getting away (all very unusual for me). Outside, I felt relief and my mind cleared and I walked home alone. 22, 12C, 04:XX:XX

Sh, 250 - I think I'm dangerous to people and they can't cope with me. 16, 30C, XX:XX:XX

HYOS. Al, 78 - He considers himself a criminal.

Al, 77 - He reproaches himself, and has conscious scruples.

Ha, 577 - He reproaches himself and has scruples of conscience.

Ha, 574 - He considers himself a criminal.

He, 31 - Delirium; talks of business of imaginary wrongs.

He, 66 - A gentle, lovable woman became extremely jealous of her husband, and although fully realizing that she did him injustice, she was so filled with grief that she found no rest day or night... (remorse)

He, 79 - After being harshly (severe) accused of theft (crime), continual delirium; fancies surrounded by objects of a terrifying nature; not a moment quiet, continual calling out that she saw the devil; denies herself guilty of theft (innocent, injustice), or that she has any concern with witches; ...

HYPER. Al,S-3 - For a week past, impure ideas have very seldom presented themselves by day; the mind has been reposing on higher thoughts.

IGN. Al, 27 - Slight blame or contradiction excites him to anger, and this makes him angry with himself.

Al, 15 - Anxiety as if he had committed a crime.

Ha, 749 - Anxiety as if he had done something bad.

Ha, 764 - Slight blame (censuring) or contradiction excites him to quarrel, and he is vexed at himself for doing so.

He, 11-...believes herself married (connected) and pregnant; is tormented by remorse of imagined crimes; seeks constantly to escape to drown (suicide) herself; ...;is only quiet when lying undisturbed and brooding over her troubles, which she rehearses (tell) in a doleful (unhappy) tone ;..." I am neglecting my duty, breaking my vow" (promise, engagement)...;conscientious scruples after eating.

He, 28 - Senseless (illogical) staring at one object, with sighing and moaning; remorse about imaginary crimes, intolerance to noise; great inclination to have fixed ideas.

He, 37 - Tears wept inwardly, the pain and penalty (forfeit) of unrequited (unrecompensed) love; desires solitude so that one may nourish inward grief;...

He, 38 - Anxiety as if he had committed some crime.

He, 39 - Anxiety and disquiet as if she had done something wrong, or as if some great misfortune were about to happen, this so overpowers her that she can with difficulty refrain from weeping;...

IOD. He, 15 - At night, especially when thinking of real or imaginary wrongs ...dares (try) to go home for fear of doing some dreadful (bad, wicked) deed (action); on one occasion was seized with an almost irresistible impulse to murder a woman who was acting as a guide (direct, conduct) for him, he having lost his way (direction);...must be constantly in action, in some laborious occupation. (lost; direction, correction, control)

IRID. Sh, 101 - Went into pet shop. There was a budgie chirping in a cage. I was so upset. "Oh God, I want to let this bird out." I felt it was crying to be let out. Took me all my control not to let it out or shout at the man to do it. Then thought, "This is silly. It would get hurt, he'll think I'm mad." I slunk out of the shop thinking I'd really let that bird down. Distracted and nearly in tears. Walked round town in a daze, should I go back and ask him to at least open the door, knew that wasn't on. It might get out of the shop and die. Felt a real coward. Set up a train of thought — condor in bird garden —a notice justifying its captivity —it only flies for food —it's quite happy to be there because food comes to it. Weeping as I write this. Birds in cages can't lean on the air currents and be blown away. G6

KALI-BR. He, 15 - Frightful imaginings at night (in pregnant women during latter months), they are under impression that they have committed, or about to commit, some great crime and cruelty (brutality), such murdering their children or husbands.

He, 31-...religious delusions and feeling of moral deficiency; ...profound indifference and almost disgust for life.

KALI-C. Al, 4 - Very much depressed; she was obliged to weep much, because it was constantly in her thoughts that she must die.

KALI-P. He, 4 - Says she is eternally and irretrievably damned;...food and medicine must be forcibly administered. 0 Melancholia religious.

LAC-F. Al,N-4 - Morbid conscientiousness; every little fault appeared a crime.

LACH. Al, 23 - It frequently seems to him wrong to read long at a time, although the subject interests him.

He, 12 - Delirium; fears she will be damned.

LAM. Al, 2 - Extraordinary sadness; he thought he had been blamed for reverses (failure) for which he was blameless, and in consequence was obliged to suffer;...

LIL-T. Al, 10 - Profound mental depression; to the prover "the heavens seemed brass and the earth iron;" an apprehension of moral obliquity weighed grievously upon her, for about ten days after the sexual excitement,...

LYSS. Al, 15 - He cannot prevent ideas of something awful (terrible) about to happen, or as if he would do something awful (bad).

Al,N-89 - After attacks of fury, evinces (manifest) great regret at his behavior, making earnest (ardent) apologies, warning those about him not to allow him to bite them.

MACRO. Al, 6 - Suspicious of everybody; thinks she has not told the truth (veracity) in regard to himself. (secretive, pretend)

MAG-C. Al, 937 - Dream she had something contraband, and wanted to snatch (seize) it away from those looking at it, and lock it up.

MANG. Ha, 325 - Cross and discontented with himself, and concerned about future..., considers himself very weak (stupid) in mind, and makes mistakes whenever he speaks.

MED. Al,N-48 - It is also introspective, self-accusative, remorseful. Time moves slowly to it, therefore it is hurried.

He, 35 - Feeling as if he had committed the unpardonable sin and was going to hell.

MENY. Ha, 286 - Cross, ill-humored and discontented with himself and his position (rank); anxiety drives him from one place to another.(restlessness)

MERC. Al, 22 - A feeling as though he had done wrong, with loss of ideas.

Ha, 1222 - Restlessness, he cannot remain quiet in any place; he can neither stand nor lie, and is as if mad, or as if he had committed a great crime.

Ha, 1225 - Imagines he is enduring the tortures (torment) of hell, without being able to account for it (explain). -(lost understanding, judgment)

Ha, 1235 - Anxiety that could drive him far away, as if he had committed a crime or some misfortune were about to happen to him.-(transgression)

Ha, 1237 - With absence of thought, (discernment, knowledge),he feels as if he had done something bad.

Ha, 1229 - Anxiety as if he had committed a crime.

He, 16 - Great restlessness as if he had committed a great crime; ...considers everybody his enemy;...great inclination when walking to take people by the nose;...(desire: conduct, direct, guide)

He, 22 - Great desire to murder (homicidal) or committed suicide ...is fearful that she may commit some wrong and kill herself (punishment); something urges her to kill her husband, of whom she is very fond (loving), and she implores him to hide his razor (knife).

He, 29 - Anxiety and apprehension; did not know what to do ; it seemed as though he had committed a crime ; without heat; also with a feeling that he had not control over his senses.

He, 38 - Great restlessness, must constantly change her place; fear, with desire to escape, as if she had committed some crime.

MEZ. Al, 33 - Violent outbreak of anger about trifles, which he soon regrets.(remorse)

Ha, 16 - Violent boiling over with passion about trifles, for which he is soon sorry.

He, 11 - Inclined to get angry with others about trifles; everything vexes him, he wants to say annoying and vexatious things; is soon sorry for it.

MYRIC. Al, 9-...a constant desire to find fault (censorious); everything went wrong; looked upon (contemptuous) this world as a place not fit to live in any longer; considered himself better than the rest (great person, megalomania), in the morning; ...; condemned himself for various imaginary faults; ...

NAJA. Al, 13-...I felt that everything that was done was done in a wrong way, and could not be rectified (corrected, revised); if I felt that I had some duty to perform (execute), I had at the same time a strong impulse not to do it, and I am extremely restless in consequence; I seemed to have an increased perception of what I ought to do, but, at the same time, an unaccountable inclination not to do it, to which I was irresistibly compelled to yield "I couldn't help it, didn't know why, but couldn't do it."

Al, 14 - Felt melancholy; began to form images of possible wrongs (mistaken) and misfortunes, over which the mind broods; very wretched at times;... a slight cause sets him in a perfect agony of mental suffering on another's behalf (welfare);...makes himself imaginary troubles and wrongs, and frets (bother) over them for two hours...

He, 3 - Melancholy; began to form images of possible wrongs (evils) and misfortunes over which the mind broods; very wretched (miserable) at times.

NAT-C. Al, 42 - Very fretful and discontented with whole world; he constantly felt as though he could beat (punish ?) himself, his whole life angered him, and he preferred to have no existence at all; he was solicitous about the future, and inclined to despair, all day.

Ha, 48 - Peevish and cross, dissatisfied whith all the world; he could have kicked (self sensure) himself; he would rather not live at all ; at the same time solicitous about the future, so that he is ready to despair.

NAT-M. Al, 59 - Anxiety, as if she had done something wrong, with heat and night sweat.

Al, 2761 - In a dream he reproached himself for past mistakes, full of restlessness and anxiety.

Al, 93 - Ill-humored does not want to go into society for fear of vexing others; feels that he could easily give offense.

Ha, 4 - Melancholy mood; he cannot remove from his thoughts injuries (insults) he has inflicted on others, or which have been inflicted on him, which depressed him so much that he had no pleasure in anything. (remorse)

Ha, 8 - He sorrowfully torments (torture) himself, by continually looking for disagreeable ideas, which weakens him.

Ha, 28 - Anxiety, as if she had done something wicked (immoral), with heat and night-sweat.

Ha, 59 - He feels peevish and avoids company, because he foresees that he might easily annoy (bother, molest) others. (intrude)

Ha, 64 - Injuries which he had inflicted on others, or which others had done to him, always dwelled in his thoughts; he could not get rid of them, and this annoyed him, so that he had no pleasure in anything.

NEON. Sh, 85 - Feel out of control, as if time is moving relentlessly and remorselessly forward and I'm stuck behind, unable to keep up. Panic, guilt, constant anxiety that I won't get it all done, including keeping up this journal. 10, 6C, 12:XX:XX

Sh, 198 - Received a long letter from a patient today; haven't even read it, can't be bothered. Very unusual. In terms of indifference, I have felt disgusted with myself; one of these violent and malicious feelings. God, I feel so wretched. 02, 6C, 05:XX:XX

NIT-AC. Al, 20 - Anxiety, like palpitation, with nausea, without efforts to vomit, as if she had committed a crime, at night in bed; ...(conscience)

Al, 27 - Vexed at the least trifle, even at himself if he makes a mistake.

Ha, 44 - Vexed at the least trifle, also at himself, when he does something amiss.(wrong)

NUX-M. Al, 32 - Many ridiculous or extravagant acts or expressions, like idiocy, while she seemed perfectly conscious, and at the next moment would appear chagrined at her conduct, and said she could not control her actions...

NUX-V. Ha, 1236 - Anxiety and anguish as if he had committed some crime.

OLND. Al, 6 - He immediately became overheated; he became passionate, though he immediately repented (sorry) of it.

Ha, 352 - The heat rapidly overcomes him; he breaks out in anger, but repents (sorry) immediately afterwards.

OP. Al, 16-...started up in a fright on account of fancied swordsmen (rival, competitor) who threatened to stab him; became angry if any one argued him or thought him delirious; however, he blamed (reproaches) himself while in delirium for his folly.

Al, 36 - Mind in a state of great confusion; at one moment she was sensible (conscious) to her crime, called for assistance (comfort, aid, help) ; at another she resisted the means used to save her.

Al, 37 - Conscious of being possessed (seized) of two persons (double) of another self besides his real self, the Opium man does things which the real self considers wrong, and it is not always sure which will conquer the other.

Al, 69 - Great strength, courage, contentment with himself.

He, 21-...in old, emaciated persons; sees animals coming towards him; people want to hurt him, execute him ; creeping under covers or jumping out of bed; in "old sinners" (criminals) whose long lives of excess have thoroughly destroyed their constitutions; ...; believe themselves to be murderers or criminals to be executed; want to run away (escape) ;...

OPUN-V. Al, 2 - The mind appears to be much affected, and does not appreciate any of its morbid condition; much tempted to do things one should not do.

PH-AC. Ha, 674 - Discontented with himself, self-reproaches.

Ha, 20 - Discontented with himself, reproaches himself.

PHOS. Al, 101 - Anxiety all night without heat, as if he had murdered some one, with constant tossing about.

He, 29 - Crazy deliria in a young woman who was strictly moral and unhappy in her love; accused herself of the most obscene (immoral, wicked) actions, of which she never was guilty; ....

PLAT. He, 46-...;suffers unspeakable pangs (anxiety) of conscience in consequence of a faux (fault, mistake, embarrassing mistake?) pass when thirty-two years old; says she has brought disgrace upon her family, and that she has incurred the penalty of damnation; (doomed) in order to do penance (penitence) gave away whatever she could lay her hands upon, (redemption) so that she had to be constantly watched; after her confessor asserted that she could not hope for pardon or heaven (condemnable), she seemed in absolute despair ; bemoaned her misery throughout the night, wringing her hands and beseeching (implore) that she might be delivered (free) from the hell of her conscience; twice attempted self-destruction (suicide);...wished to live and do penance (penitence, purgation, purification) in order to mitigate her eternal punishment.

PLB. He, 15-...; despair of her salvation...; fixed idea that could only obtain peace and safety though absolution by a priest of the papal church, although she had been a zealous Protestant; ....brooded over any forbidden thing; would steal (leave) from house in servant's cloak (coat, camouflage) and bonnet (hat) to obtain stimulants (drugs), but from the moment their prohibition was withdrawn (retired) ceased to have any desire for them; after being permitted to visit a priest and converse with him ceased to talk and think of the church. (desire; redemption, absolution)

PULS. Al, 12 - Nightly anxiety on waking as if he had committed a crime.

Ha, 1119 - Cannot think without fretting (anguish) about his affairs (duty, responsibility), in the morning.

Ha, 1120 - Restless state of the disposition, as if did not do his duty properly.

He, 47-...; pangs (pain, anxiety) of conscience about religion and female sex; violent palpitation in the presence of women; abhors (detests, aversion) and hates the sex; must go out of their way for fear of injuring them; looks upon them as evil beings and is afraid (fear; temptation, seduction); considers their presence injurious (insulted, offended) to his soul; ... (sexual loathing)

RAPH. Al, 1 - Feeling of aversion towards all women; she is provoked by seeing women going and coming about her; their approach threw her into a fury; the mere contact with a woman's dress caused intolerable distress;...She is attracted to all men without distinction (nymphomania) ; when she gives her hand to a man, she feels great agitation,...When left alone for a hour in the evening, she gave herself a very deep wound in the lips with a penknife, in hopes to put an end to this condition (hurt, punishes). Moral feeling was completely extinct, the physical nature alone ruled and threw her into a frightful state (wild). From morning to noon she would not have been able to resist the advances even of a man for whom she had not the least friendly feeling; from noon to 6 p.m. she could not have held out against any man whatsoever; from 8 to 11 the demands of sense were so importunate as to silence the voice of shame and reason; ... and would have thrown herself into the arms of the first man she met...she was still unable to control her impulses;...

RHUS-T. He, 22-... great restlessness and anguish as if she had committed a crime or as if she thought some terrible calamity impended; these feelings drove her from one place to another; could not rest quietly at night in bed; was robbed of sleep and all desire to live;...

He, 23 - Restlessness and anxiety about heart as if she had committed a crime or as if some great misfortune was in store (reserved) for her, is driven from one place to another; deprived of sleep and all desire to live; ...

ROB. Al, 3 - Moral agitation, great restlessness; he is always under the impression that he will be disgraced.

Al, 6 - Fear and confusion (anxiety ?) of conscience, as if he had committed a crime,...

RUTA. Al, 3 - Very anxious all day, as

though he had done something wrong; if any one opened the door he feared that some one had come to arrest (imprisonment, jailing) him.

Al, 11 - Much dissatisfied (discontented) by everything that happened to him, and especially with whatever he did himself, and great inclination to weep.

Ha, 276 - Very discontented and very much disposed to weep over everything that happens about him and especially over what he himself has done.

Ha, 280 - All day long very anxious as if he had done something bad; when the door was opened, he feared that someone was coming to take him to prison. (incarcerated, punished)

SABAD. Al, 6 - Gloomy mood, as if he were the greatest criminal,...

SEP. Al, 34 - Feel very much depressed, at 7 A.M.; feel like quarreling with everybody; became very much excited about a mere trifle, and said some very sharp things. (feeling ashamed of it at the same time)

Al, 96 - He thinks of things which he does not think of, uses expressions which he knows are incorrect, undertakes those things which are opposed to his intentions, and finds such contradictions with himself that it puts him in a very uncomfortable and uneasy mood.

SIL. Al, 27 - Most excessive scruples of conscience about trifles frequently, as though he had done a great wrong.

Ha, 8 - He feels the greatest conscientious scruples about trifles; as if he had done a very great wrong.

He, 7 - Compunction (remorse) of conscience about trifles.

SPIRAE. Al, 1 - At 1 A.M. he was attacked with remorse over a long-past slight indiscretion (mistake, wrong), with most fearful qualms (anxiety) of conscience and loathing of himself; ....

STAPH. Ha, 708 - Sad, he apprehends (perceive) the worst consequences from slight (trivial) things and cannot calm himself.

He, 11 - Great indignation about things done by others or by himself; grieves about consequences. (remorse)

STRAM. Al, 48 - She is all the time inconsolable; much affected by trifles; makes much fuss about trifles; disposed to weep, and sometimes also very easily vexed; now and then neglects her duties; now and then thinks she is not fitted for her position ; after the fall equinox...; she wants light and company.

He, 56 - Believes to be in his grave; shrives,(confess) prays, asks to be killed (justified); accuses his wife of infidelity; scolds (cursing), strikes at everybody who wishes to restrain him; thinks they are dogs and barks at them to make himself understood.

He, 93 - Mania; thinks he is lying on his sepulchre (tomb); confessing, praying, wants to be killed (redemption, salvation, regeneration); laughs as if tickled (excited); wants to be kissed; accuses his wife of being faithless (betrayed); scolding (censure) beating in a rage, will not be taken hold of by attendants (suspicious?) ; takes them for dogs (contemptuous), and barks at them; talking in Jewish jargon; (rank?, stranger?) supposes his house to be surrounded by carts (vehicle), Jews (Judaism) and geese, offending him, ... -(strange, foreign, alien)

He, 107-...heard continually, on r. side of occiput, a loud voice, scolding, vituperating and accusing him of ungodliness (impious, sinful, irreligious, godless, profane); ....prayed expecting, with great anxiety, the flash of lightning which was to kill him;...(redemption, regeneration, salvation)

He, 178 - Pangs of conscience; thinks he is not honest. (dishonest)

He, 172 - Downcast and full of anguish, believes herself unworthy of eternal bliss, because she is unable to perform her duties.

He, 177-...sometimes vexed; neglects her duties, thinks she is not fitted for her position;...

STRONT-C. Al, 2 - Apprehensive and anxious, as from a bad conscience.

He, 1 - Apprehensive and anxious as from a bad conscience.

SUL-AC. Al, 35 - Fretful, peevish, impatient, if his work is not done to suit.(unsatisfying)

SULPH. Al, 100 - Thoughts of the business that had been accomplished thronged (crowd) upon her...

Ha, 24 - She imagines that she might give people something wrong, which might kill them.

He, 32 - Melancholy mood; dwelling on religious or philosophic speculations; anxiety about soul's salvation; indifference about lot (destiny) of others.

TARENT. He, 15 - Suddenly sprang (escape) away from her attendants and swept (clean) ornaments from mantelpiece (an ornamental facing around fireplace); said she was sorry, but could not help it; very mischievous and destructive, ...

THUJ. Al, 1 - She herself desires, with anxiety and despair, to be taken to an insane asylum, (imprisonment, confining) and there to be treated very harshly and strictly, (penalized), so that her fixed ideas may be subdued and banished (purified); she knows very well that she does wrong (conscience) and thinks all sorts of bad thoughts (immoral), but she will not take the trouble to banish such thoughts; therewith she indistinctly gives to understand that she is constantly obliged to think of taking her own life, but feels the sinfulness (wicked) of it, in order to avoid it, desires the strict restraint of the asylum;...

Al, 2 - She fancies that she has intentionally represented herself as insane (feigning) in the presence of others in order to palliate a wrong supposed to have been done (penitence, remorse), and that now she is punished, therefore, by real insanity.

Al, 3 - She feels and says that she is deranged (insane, disordered) and unfit (unsuitable) to life, as a punishment for a fault (penitence) which she cannot name, ...

Al, 4 - She fancies that she has committed a sin.(wrong)

Al, 49 - Sudden rising of dark thoughts (pessimism) causing uneasiness, apprehension (foreboding) of misfortune, with fancied scruples of conscience, ...

Al, 72 - Constant anxiety, as if he had committed a great crime, with forgetfulness and general trembling, even to disturbing sleep.

VERAT. Al, 44 - Anxiety as from a bad conscience, as if he had committed a crime.

Ha, 690 - Anxiety as from a bad conscience, as if he had done something bad.

He, 46 - Anxiety as from a bad conscience, as if he had committed a crime.

He, 47 - Anxiety as after committing an evil (immoral) deed (act)...

ZINC. Al, 26 - Very uneasy mood, as though he had committed a crime.

He, 46-...; believed herself to be called before court (judged) on account of her wicked (immoral) actions; ....;believe the devil is after her;...(persecution)

He, 14 - Very uneasy mood as if he had committed a crime.

CONSCIENTIOUS

Activity; thinks of everything: arag.[85]

Anxiety; health, careful about health, therefore very: calad.[54] ***calc.***[54]

Anxiety; salvation, scrupulous as to their religious practices, too: ars.[30] ign.[30] lyc.[30] nux-v.[30] ph-ac.[30] puls.[30] **STAPH.**[30] **SULPH.**[30]

Anxiety; walking, while, slowly, must, otherwise something will happen: cupr.[137]

Avarice; collects carefully the debris of his fortune: stann.[30] staph.[30]

Carefulness: ang.[5] apis[38] ***ars.***[122] ***aur.***[5] ***bar-c.***[122] bry.[5] calc.[30] cham.[5] **CHIN.**[5] cocc.[5] cycl.[5] ***dig.***[5] germ.[222] **GRAPH.**[5] hyos.[5] ***ign.***[5] ***iod.*** ip.[5] ***lach.***[5] ***lyc.***[5] mez.[5] mur-ac.[5] nat-c.[5] nat-m.[155] ***nux-v.*** puls. ran-b. rhus-t.[5] ***sep.***[5] sil.[5] spig.[5] **STRAM.**[5] **SULPH.**[5] thuj.[5] ***verat.***[5]

Cautious: acon.[5] am-c.[10] anac.[10] arn.[10] ars.[5] aur.[10] bar-c.[10] cact.[36] calc.[137] carc.[207] caust. chel.[10] chin.[10] cic.[10] coff.[10] cupr.[5] dros.[10] graph. hyos.[5] ***ign.***[111] ip. kali-n.[10] lach.[10] lact.[10] m-arct. mang.[10] nat-c.[10] nat-m.[10] nit-ac.[10] nux-v.[5] op.[5] ph-ac.[10] puls.[5] spig.[10] stram.[5] thuj.[10] verat.[111]

Cautious, anxiously: am-c.[30] bar-c.[30] carc.[207] caust. lyc.[30] puls.[30] sil.[30] sulph.[30]

Children; watchful, they are on the look out for every gesture: phos.[122]

Conscientious about trifles: ambr.[1189] ang.[5] anh.[144] apis arg.[163] **ARS.**[122] ars-s-f.[58] aur. aur-ar.[58] aur-i.[58] bac.[62] bamb-a.[1184] ***bar-c.*** bry. calc. calc-p.[137] calc-s.[108] carbn-s. carc.[179] caust.[5] cham. chin. chin-ar. cocc.[5] cupr.[210] cycl. ***dig.***[5] dys-co.[136] ferr. ferr-ar. ferr-i. graph. ham.[122] hep. hura[83] hyos. **IGN.** iod. ip.[5] lac-d. lac-f.[85] ***lach.***[5] ***lyc.***

m-p-a.[5] med.[122] mez. ***mur-ac.*** nat-ar. **NAT-C.**[122] nat-sil.[58] ***nux-v.*** ozone[227] ph-ac.[30] plat.[30] plb.[201] ***puls.***[58] rhus-t.[5] samb.[137] sarr. sec. sel.[137] sep. **SIL.** spig. spirae.[102] **STAPH.**[30] ***stram.*** sul-i.[58] ***sulph.*** syc-co.[136] **THUJ.**[122] tub.[5] verat. verat-v.[163] zinc.[137]

Conscientious about trifles; disease, during: pip-m.[184]

Conscientious about trifles; eating, after: ign.

Conscientious about trifles; pedant, too much: plat.[30] puls.[30] sil.[30]

Conscientious about trifles; trifles, occupied with: ars.[5] cocc.[5] ***graph.***[5] lil-t.[5] nit-ac.[5] nux-v.[5] petr.[5] thuj.[5]

Delusions; animals, lying near her, which she feels she might hurt: ***valer.***[54]

• bed, creases, is full of: ***stram.***[54]

• disorder, objects appear in: glon.[122] op.[36]

• forehead, she must look out under: ph-ac.[1]

Dreams; deliberations, with: ***ign.***[54]

Fastidious: alum.[122] ***anac.***[122] androc.[222] arg-n.[193] ***ars.*** asar.[162] aur.[122] cand-a.[239] **CARC.**[122] con.[28] cupr.[210] ***graph.***[122] iod.[162] ***kali-ar.***[184] kali-bi.[184] ***kali-c.***[185] lac-ac.[54] lac-h.[229] ***lob.***[184] med.[164] morg-g.[136] ***nat-m.***[162] nat-s.[58] ***nux-v.*** phos.[164] pip-m.[162] plat.[164] plb.[201] psor. **PULS.**[30] sep.[164] sil.[122] sulph.[162] thuj.[154]

Fear; superstitious: rhus-t.

✦ tread lightly or will injure himself, must: cupr.

Gestures; makes, cautious: pip-m.[36]

Hydrophobia; prophylactic: ***bell.***[137] canth.[137] hyos.[137] lyss.[137] stram.[137]

Rage; alternating with, consciousness: acon. stram.[1]

Responsibility: bamb-a.[1184] carc.[188] cupr.[210] ign.[188] ***lil-t.***[168] nat-ar.[168] nat-m.[189]

Responsibility; strong: aur.[58] ***calc.***[187] carc.[196] cocc.[58] cupr.[210] cycl.[206] ign.[188] kali-c.[162] ***lil-t.***[168] lyc.[206] mag-m.[187] nat-ar.[168] nat-m.[189] nat-s.[162] puls.[206] stront-c.[188]

Responsibility; strong, family, towards his: nat-s.[187]

Responsibility; strong, social: stront-c.[188]

Rest; cannot, when things are not in proper place: anac. ***ars.*** carc.[102] sep.[193] sulph.[58]

Restlessness; careful: **NUX-V.**[54]

Restlessness; zealous: **NUX-V.**[54]

Sensitive; moral impressions, to: all-s. aster.[36] chin.[30] coff.[20] dig. hep.[20] hydrog.[222] ign. nuph.[25] nux-v.[30] plb.[36] psor. ***puls.***[30] staph.[30] upa.[36]

Superstitious: agar.[187] arg-n.[162] bell.[5] carc.[207] ***con.*** kali-ar.[184] ***med.***[162] op.[5] phel.[231] rat.[162] rhus-t.[36] stram.[5] syph.[162] tub.[162] zinc.

Trifles; important, seem: androc.[222] ars.[5] calc.[58] caust.[111] cocc.[5] con.[137] ferr. **GRAPH.**[5] ***hep.***[111] ign.[111] ip. lil-t.[5] nat-m.[111] ***nit-ac.***[5] ***nux-v.***[5] petr.[5] sil.[111] thuj.[5]

Watchfulness: ars.[36] eup-a.[25] stram.[36]

Watchfulness; every movement in the vicinity or every movement of the doctor, of: calc-p.[146] ferr-p.[146] phos.[146]

Watchfulness; everyone eating, of: sulph.[160]

ACON. He, 28 - Moaning, anxious lamentations; reproaches from trifling causes.

ADAM. Sh, 31 - The proving experience was very clear. There was a sharpness in both how I felt and what I saw. Mostly this was pleasant: brilliant sunshine through the drops of water in a shower, candlelight bouncing off wine glasses, tiny detail on the chrome-work of cars. 18, 30C, XX:XX:XX

ANAC. Ha, 4 - Internal anguish, which did not allow him to rest, he troubled himself about every trifle, as if it would cause great injure, with solicitude about the future.

He, 62 - Internal anxiety, which did not leave him any peace; he felt solicitous (careful) on account of every trifle, as if it would lead to some great trouble (misfortune); with apprehension (fear) of future.

ARS. Ha, 45 - Super-sensitiveness and over-tenderness of mind; dejected, sad and lugubrious (unhappy), she is troubled and solicitous about the merest trifles.

BAR-A. Al, 7 - She is very anxious and careful about very insignificant things, which formerly were perfectly indifferent to her.

BAR-C. Ha, 10 - She is very anxious and solicitous about things quite trifling, which are indifferent to her.

He, 24 - Extremely contrary, irritable humor, passionate about trifles .

CACT. Al, 19 - Disposition to do deliberately (resolutely, carefully) whatever was undertaken.

CALAD. He, 12 - Very careful about his health; apprehensive.

CAUST. Ha, 13 - Anxiously careful (cautious, prudent) as to all occurrences.

He, 61 - Very suspicious and distrustful.
CHAM. Al, 31 - She makes conscientious scruples about everything.
Ha, 490 - She has scruples of conscience about everything.
CHIN. Ha, 1095 - Too anxious caution.
Ha, 1096 - An over-anxious concern (care) about trifles.
CHOC. Sh, 73 - Feel I have to be alert, as if my total survival depended on me being alert —exhausting.
Sh, 90 - Concentration very sharp, as if my survival depended on it. I felt very focused. (During a lecture) My understanding was sharper. Normally I have many things going on in my head —too scattered — but in the last few days, narrower attention.
Sh, 331 - I became selfish, impatient and intolerant. Behaved in a strange way -hard and quarrelsome -snapping at people. Could not stand people wasting time or being inefficient, I wanted things done immediately.35, 30C, XX:XX:XX:
CON. He, 31 - Great anxiety; precordial anguish; superstitious (careful, credulous, naive) and full of fear (coward), with frequent thoughts of death...
CUPR. Ha, 5 - A kind of timidity; he felt as if he had to step softly, in order not to hurt himself, nor to disturb his room-mates. (friend) (cautious, prudent, gentle, delicate)
DROS. Al, 1 - Joyful, good courage: he had no fear of evil, because he was conscious of having done right. (moral, virtuous, honest, fearless)
FERR. Al, 3 - My surroundings (material welfare) seem very large (big) and capacious (vast), and I am inclined to attribute great importance to trifles...
GERM. Sh, 39 - Concentration difficult. I lost my pen. I am careful, afraid of doing or saying something silly. 16, 30C, 00:06:00
GRAPH. Ha, 26 - Extreme scrupulousness (careful, prudent); she cannot take anything lightly.(casually)
HALI-L. Sh, 86 - Even now, two years later I have an occasional return of the eagle state. Clarity to my vision. Usually my eyes have a soft focus, but since the proving, every so often they clear up and the focus is sharp. Normally I walk around in a fog, thinking, in my head. In the proving state, there is an outward focus. I'm aware of people, and how they're moving, and what they're doing. Conscious of them and how they might effect me and I might effect them. Normally, I don't care. I like to be in this altered state. The ability to be in that state intensified since taking eagle. An animal awareness, very conscious of other people as animals. 09, 6C, XX:XX:XX
Sh, 187 - I want more from school. Ethics and education are very important. I want things done to a very high standard. To be methodical and well thought out. Want higher quality. 08, 30C, 25:XX:XX
HURA. Al, 8 - He reproaches himself for all his bad actions, even the merest trifles.
HYDROG. Sh, 171 - Feel more patient and accepting during my period. When water poured through the ceiling from an over-full bath, I just sat there and let it flood the floor because I didn't want to disturb the cat sitting on my knee. 12, 6C, 27:XX:XX
HYOS. Al, 60-... Then he wandered into the country and suddenly pulling up a leg, exclaimed, " Take care; give me your hand; that is a very deep step"...
Al, 77 - He reproaches himself, and has conscious scruples.
Ha, 577 - He reproaches himself and has scruples of conscience.
IGN. Ha, 793 - Sensitive disposition, delicate conscientiousness (careful, scrupulous)
Ha, 792 - Delicate disposition (character), with very clear consciousness (justice, judgment, equity)
He, 11-...believes herself married (connected) and pregnant; is tormented by remorse of imagined crimes; seeks constantly to escape to drown (suicide) herself; ...;is only quiet when lying undisturbed and brooding over her troubles, which she rehearses (tell) in a doleful (unhappy) tone ;..." I am neglecting my duty, breaking my vow" (promise, engagement)...;conscientious scruples after eating.
IOD. Al, 8 - Disposition mild, scrupulous (careful) and timid (irresolute), with

blunted (dull) sensibilities.
He, 8 - Fear of evil with over carefulness.
IP. Al, 8 - He is thoughtful, fearful, and thinks trifles are very important.
Ha, 223 - He is scrupulous (careful, conscientious), apprehensive, and thinks trifles of importance.
IRID. Sh, 200 - Waking frequently, every hour, feeling very alert and wide awake, worried that I had forgotten something, not put the guard on the fire, closed down the stove, locked the doors, etc. Feels like I would take ages to get off to sleep. In reality got to sleep quickly. A19
LAC-F. Al,N-4 - Morbid conscientiousness; every little fault appeared a crime.
MUR-AC. Ha, 270 - Anxious scrupulosity (careful) (immediately) all day; he cannot get over the slightest misfortune or become contented; after 72 hours more cheerful, less scrupulous (caution), and more courageous than at ordinary times.
NIT-AC. Al, 27 - Vexed at the least trifle, even at himself if he makes a mistake.
Ha, 44 - Vexed at the least trifle, also at himself, when he does something amiss.(wrong)
NUX-V. He, 8 - Suits very particular, careful,(prudent, meticulous) zealous (conscientious) persons, inclined to get angry or excited, or a spiteful (cruel), malicious disposition.
He, 13 - Irritable, angry disposition, anxious concern about little things. (trifles)
SIL. Al, 27 - Most excessive scruples of conscience about trifles frequently, as though he had done a great wrong.
Ha, 8 - He feels the greatest conscientious scruples about trifles; as if he had done a very great wrong.
He, 7 - Compunction (remorse) of conscience about trifles.
He, 23-...believes she has swallowed pins, and asks those about her whether she has not done so; seeks for hours for lost pins; ...and careful examined her food for fear of pins; very indifferent to friends and former amusements;...
STRAM. He, 175 - Sad; apprehends evil consequences from trifling things.
THUJ. Ha, 628 - Prolonged thoughtfulness about the merest trifle.
He, 27 - Extremely scrupulous (conscientious, careful) about small things.
VALER. He, 4 - Erroneous ideas; thinks she is some one else,...; imagines animals lying near her which she fears she may hurt.
VERAT. He, 28 - Talks much on religious subjects; praying; is overconscientious.

CONSOLATION

Anger; easily, consolation agg., does not want to be disturbed: hell.[54]
Consolation; agg.: ant-c.[127] arg-n.[137] arn. ***ars.*** aur.[5] ***bell.*** cact. calc. ***calc-p.*** calc-sil.[58] ***carc.***[122] cham. chin. con.[58] cupr.[210] graph.[102] hell.[58] hydro-c.[2147] **IGN.** kali-c. ***kali-p.***[5] kali-s.[122] kali-sil.[58] ***lil-t.*** lyc. merc. nat-c.[58] **NAT-M.**[122] ***nit-ac.***[122] nux-v. ***pall.***[193] ***plat.*** sabal.[5] sabin.[5] **SEP.**[122] **SIL.** ***stann.***[5] staph. ***sulph.***[36] **SYPH.**[122] tarent. thuj. visc.[119]
Consolation; agg. friendly advice: calc.[5] calc-p.[5] hell.[5] kali-c.[5] merc.[5]
Consolation; agg. sad and weeping mood, with: **NAT-M.**[54]
Consolation; amel.: ars.[127] asaf.[137] **CAMPH.**[5] carc.[119] cic.[5] gels.[137] hell. lyss.[149] ***phos.***[122] **PULS.** sac-alb.[210]
Consolation; amel. religious: raph.[85]
Consolation; refuses, for ones own misfortune: nit-ac.[137]
Consoled, cannot be, after shock or injury: acon.[54]
Sadness; consoled, cannot be: ars.[54] nat-m.[189] nux-v.[189]
Weeping; consolation, agg.: bell. cact. calc. ***calc-p.*** chin. hell. hydro-c.[2147] ign. kali-c. lil-t. lyc. merc. nat-c.[30] **NAT-M.** nit-ac. nux-v. ***plat.*** **SEP.** **SIL.** stann.[47] staph. sulph. tarent. thuj.

CONSTRICTION

Anguish; clothing too tight when walking in open air, as if: arg.[36]
Anguish; constricted, as if everything become: ***ars.***[36] chel.[25]
Anxiety; constriction of chest: alum.[54] ars.[36] ***cupr.***[54] gins.[36] ozone[227] ***spig.***[54] stann.[1]
Anxiety; contraction in heart region, from: nit-ac.[1]
Anxiety; pressure, chest, on, from: ***acon.***[54] aur.[1] **CARB-V.**[54] coca[54] ***dig.***[54] ign.[162] lach.[162] ph-ac.[54] ***plat.***[54] ***psor.***[54] sabad.[54] **SULPH.** ***tab.***[54]
Delusions; something comes from above which pressing chest: sep.[1]

Dullness; brain, compressed, feels: ***hyper.***[54]
Fear; constipation, with: bell.[54] lach.[10] ***op.***[54]

ADAM. Sh, 112 - Thoughts, on waking, were that I was like a sponge that absorbs in the day and gets squeezed out at night via my dreams. 11, 30C, 06.XX.XX
ARS. He, 75 - Precordial anxiety, feels constricted.
HURA. Al, 19 - Inclination to weep, chest constrict, as from emotion...the least thing disturbs her and makes her sad;...
Al, 26 - Since taking the drug, the least thing irritates her, and then she feels oppressed, with desire to weep;...
IGN. He, 42 - A state of anguish in which she shrieks (scream) for help, with suffocating constriction of throat...
PH-AC. Ha, 654 - Internal heat and anxiety; he feels as if the chest were too narrow.
RHUS-T. Ha, 961 - Very restless disposition, and anxiety and anguish, so that she had always a clutching (grasp) at the heart, with dyspnea.
Ha, 967 - She was inexpressibly anxious; she had pressure at the heart and tearing (cut) in the sacrum.

CONTEMPTUOUS

Abusive; snub one who differed from him, desire to: hydr.[36]
Aversion; men, shuns the foolishness of: cic.
Aversion; society, shuns the foolishness of: cic.
Aversion; women, to, looks upon them as evil beings and is afraid their presence is injurious to his soul: ***puls.***[54]
Company, aversion to; alternating with bursts of pleasantry and sarcasm: rad-br.[122] rhus-t.
Confidence, want of self; nobody, feels as if he is: agn.[36]
Contemptuous: agn.[111] aloe[5] alum. ***androc.*** arn.[5] ***ars.*** bry.[137] calc.[30] canth. caps.[5] cham. ***chin.*** **CIC.** cina[10] com.[36] croc.[10] cycl. germ.[222] gran.[10] guai. hell.[10] hyos. ign. ***ip.*** lac-ac. lac-c.[3087] lach. ***lyc.*** m-arct.[10] merc.[10] mosch.[10] myric.[25] nat-m. nit-ac. ***nux-v.*** **PALL.**[5] par. **PLAT.** puls. sec. sil. spong.[36] stram.[5] verat.[122]
Contemptuous; everything, to: ***chin.*** cina ***ip.***[54] **PLAT.**
Contemptuous; friend, at his: alco.[36]
Contemptuous; hard for subordinates and agreeable or pleasant to superiors or people he has to fear: lach.[30] lyc.[30] plat.[30] verat.[30]
Contemptuous; mankind, for: cic.[36]
Contemptuous; opponents, for: com.[36]
Contemptuous; paroxysms against her will, in: ***plat.***
Contemptuous; ravenous hunger and greed, hasty eating, c. with sudden: ***plat.***[36]
Contemptuous; relations, for: sec.[54]
Contemptuous; self, of: agn. ***aur.***[102] cop. lac-c.[102] thuj.[102]
Contemptuous; self, of, alternating with eccentricity: agn.[10]
Contemptuous; society, mankind, at: cic.[1]
Death; contempt of, in mental derangement: ***op.***[54]
Delusions; animals, persons are: bell.[162] hyos. stram.
• animals, persons are, unclean animals: bell.
• devils, connected to, he is, arrogant towards those who strive to purity, light and love: ozone[227]
• dogs, others are, barks at them to be understood: stram.[54]
• dolls, people are: plb.
• grotesque, people appear: hyos.[36]
• humility and lowers of others, while he is great: germ.[222] plat. staph.
• inferior, on entering house after a walk, people seem mentally and physically: plat.
• insane, everyone but he himself, is: androc.[222]
• nobody, he is: agn.[36]
• shallow, everything is: chin.[36] hell.[36]
• swine, hogs, people are: hyos.
• unworthy to live: nat-s.[137] plat.[137]
• worthless, he is: aur.[137] thuj.[187]
Desires; satire: lach.[36]
Dreams; contempt, of: tarent.[36]
➤ table, tablecloth is too beautiful, for other, special occasions, not for him: ozone[227]
Exclusive, too: calc.[30] nat-m.[30] plat.[30]
Fear; imbecile, that he would become: stram.
✦ men, contempt for: cic.
Gossiping: ars.[30] calc.[30] caust.[30] ***hyos.*** lach.[30] par.[116] stram. verat.
Haughty; races, to other: ars.[10] hep.[10] phos.[10] plat.[10] sep.[10]
Jealousy; images, with frightful, tendency to mock, satire and ridiculous ideas: ***lach.***

Jesting: aeth. aether[36] agav-t.[149] alco.[36] aloe androc.[222] arg. ars. bar-c. bell. bry. calc. cann-i. ***caps.*** carb-v. ***cic. cocc.*** coff.[137] **CROC.**[5] cupr. ferr-p.[58] glon. hyos. ***ign.*** ip. kali-cy.[36] ***kali-i. lach.***[5] lap-c-b.[194] lyc. meny.[5] merc. merl. nat-m. ***nux-m.*** op. peti.[36] phos.[189] plat. psil.[164] psor.[36] rhus-t. sars. sec. spong. ***stann.***[30] staph.[30] ***stram.*** sul-ac. tab. ***tarent.***
Jesting; alternating with, anger: caps.[10] ign.[10]
Jesting; alternating with, taciturnity: plat.[10]
Jesting; facetious, desire to do something: aeth.[36] cact.[36]
Jesting; fun of somebody, making: ***lach.***[30]
Jesting; gravity, after: plat.
Jesting; puns, makes: cann-i. choc.[222]
Jesting; roguish: puls.[10]
Jesting; trifles with everything: alum.[30] con.[30]
Laughing; actions, at his own: iris stram.
Laughing; actions, at his own, stand or walk, at an attempt to: agar.[54]
Laughing; agg., others, of: ambr.[162]
Laughing; contemptuous: alum.
Laughing; ludicrous, everything seems: hydrog.[222] hyos. lyc. ***nux-m.*** sabad.
Laughing; mocking: tarent.[36]
Laughing; reprimands, at: bar-c.[184] ***graph.***[54]
Laughing; sardonic: amyg-am.[36] **BELL.** camph.[5] cann-i.[36] ***caust. colch.*** con. croc.[36] cupr.[210] hydr-ac.[5] hydrog.[222] ***hyos.*** ign. nux-m. ***oena.*** ozone[227] phyt.[5] plb. ran-b.[116] ran-s. ***sec.*** sol-n. ***stram.*** stry. tarent. verat. zinc. zinc-o.[10] zinc-p.[58]
Laughing; scornful: alum.[5]
Laughing; serious matters, over: ***anac.*** apis arg-n. asar.[198] bar-c.[198] bufo[58] cann-i. cast-eq. caust.[198] coff.[198] germ.[222] hydrog.[222] ign. lac-h.[229] lap-gr-m.[194] lil-t. lyc. ***nat-m.*** nux-m. phos.[1] ***plat.*** sil.[198] sulph. viol-o.[45]
Ludicrous, things seem: calc.[10] cann-i. cann-s. hyos.[10] nat-m. ***nux-m.*** plat.[1] stram. sulph.[10] tarent.
Men; contempt for: cic.[36]
Mocking: acon.[5] alum.[5] anh.[119] ars. bac.[62] chin. choc.[222] guai.[5] hyos.[5] ***ign.***[5] ip. ***lach.*** nux-m.[137] ***nux-v.***[5] par. ped.[36] plat. stann.[30] tarent. verat.[5]
Mocking; friends, at his: alco.[36]
Mocking; jealousy, with: ***lach.***[54]
Mocking; relatives, at his: sec.
Mocking; ridicule, passion to: acon. hyos. lach. nux-v. verat.
Mocking; sarcasm: androc.[222] anh.[144] ***ars.***[122] bry.[30] cann-i.[36] **CARB-V.**[30] carbn-o.[36] caust.[30] cham.[193] choc.[222] cinnb.[36] **GRAPH.**[30] hyper.[193] ign.[30] lac-ac.[54] ***lach.***[5] lyc.[155] nit-ac.[137] nux-v.[30] pall.[116] ***par.***[5] petr.[30] rad-br.[122] rhus-t. sac-l.[85] sec.[54] sep.[58] tarent.[137]
Mocking; sarcasm, satire, desire for: ars.[5] lac-ac.[54] ***lach.***[5] sec.[54] stann.[30]
Racism: cocc.[185]
Reproaches; laughing at reproaches: ***graph.***[8]
Ridicule, mania to: acon. hyos. lach. nux-v. verat.
Self-deprecation: ***naja***[5]
Society; shuns the foolishness of society: cic.[1]
Spit, desire to: aeth.[36] ant-t.[111] bar-acet.[36] bar-c.[111] ***bell.***[10] calc.[30] ***cann-s.***[5] carbn-s.[36] ***coc-c.***[36] cupr.[5] dulc.[36] epip.[171] glon.[36] lyc.[30] lyss.[111] merc.[30] ***nux-v.***[30] rhus-t.[36] sec.[36] stram.[111] ***sulph.***[30] ***tab.***[137] ***verat.***[54] ***verat-v.***[54] zinc-chr.[111]
Spit, desire to; anger, from: ***calc.***[54]
Spit, desire to; faces of people, in: ars. **BELL.** bufo[170] ***calc.*** cann-i. cann-s.[10] ***cupr.*** cupr-acet.[36] hyos. merc. phos. plb. ***stram. verat.***
Talk; indisposed, alternating with, jesting: plat.[10]
Teasing; laugh at reprimands: graph.[102]
Unworthy; life, for, feels: ***nat-s.***[137] plat.[137]
Unworthy; objects seem: ***chin.***
Witty: aeth.[36] alco.[36] aran-ix.[144] cann-i.[36] caps. chlol.[36] cocc. ***coff.*** cortiso.[149] croc. ***lach. op.*** spong. sumb. thea.
Witty; indecent, but: ***stram.***[54]
Writing; mean and contemptible things to her friends, all sorts of: ***lac-c.***[54]

AGN. Al, 2 - He sometimes feels as if he were nobody (unimportant, insignificant, worthless), and would rather be dead than have that feeling; when possessed by that feeling he has no courage to undertake anything; and when free from it he feels exalted, would like to read like an orator, etc.
ALOE. Al, 38-...continually mocking the remarks (saying) of others;...
ALUM. Al, 33 - He sneers (mock) at everybody contemptuously.
Ha, 35 - He laughs contemptuously at everything.

ANDROC. Sh, 60 - Felt tense and absolutely alone, but sure that the rest of the world was mad, not her. She felt defiant with others and would not be manipulated. (7)

ARS. Ha, 60 - Inclined to sarcastic mocking.
He, 104 - Obstinacy, avarice, inclined to malice and satire.

CARB-AC. He, 12 - Entire disinclination to study; what he had accomplished seemed very trifling. (unimportant)

CARBN-O. Al, 11 - After supper, felt buoyant (happy) and in good humor, an effect never produced by tea; this mental sensation soon passed over into an irritable and sarcastic one, so that I sharply criticized an article in a medical journal, which a few hours ago I hardly thought worth that trouble, and threw away in disgust a book of reference as flat and superficial, which I highly sluggish.(inactive)

CHAM. Al, 54 - Morose inclined to scorn.
Al, 53 - Disposed to anger scorn quarrelsomeness. (after two hours)

CHIN. Al, 49 - He despises everything.

CHOC. Sh, 327 - My humour has taken a sarcastic turn, mocking people, a bit aggressive in a joking way.[35], 30C, 00:03:XX

CIC. Al, 26 - Contempt and scorn for mankind; he avoided them, abhorred their follies (stupidity) excessively, and his disposition seemed to tend towards misanthropy; he withdrew (retire) himself into solitude.
Ha, 237 - Depreciation and contempt of mankind; he fled (desert) his fellow-creatures, was in the highest degree disgusted with their follies (stupidity), and his disposition seemed to change into misanthropy; he withdrew into solitude.
He, 18 - Fondness (desire) for solitude; great disregard and dislike for society of others.
He, 36 - Mistrust and shunning (avoid) of men; despises others.

COT. Al, 11 - Feels silly (ridiculous) and lost.

CUPR-A. Al, 2 - Attacks of mania; he fancies that he is a military officer; a fancy that he is selling green vegetables; a fancy that he is repairing old chairs...he spits in the faces of the attendants, and laughs heartily at it.

CUPR. Ha, 27 - Fits of insanity, he spits into people's faces, and laughs heartily (soberly) over it.

GERM. Sh, 6 - Difficult to accept my own feelings, accusing myself for letting them out, especially anger. Felt a rage, had to use all my power to control it. Lost my patience because of something my son did. I got angry with him, but at the same time despised myself for not having patience with him. I did not want to report this, because I feel unveiled - now everybody can see what awful person I am. I go completely mad of all my thoughts; can't bear it anymore. Inside me everything is chaos. Feel no power. 18, 30C, 18:XX:XX
Sh, 123 - Don't understand anything, the meaning of life. Feel also strength somewhere inside. I wish a change could happen, I ought to bring myself together and change. It is silly of me to go on like this. I despise myself. I am hard to myself, but I don't deserve anything else. I think other people are silly too. 18, 30C, 06:XX:XX
Sh, 158 - Some persistent feelings coming up. Feel envious of a colleague who I feel manages so well. When I compare with myself I feel worthless and nothing. I feel like talking badly about her to my friends and I do this, even though she is not present. It takes a lot of my attention and energy. 21, 12C, 67:XX:XX.
Sh, 111 - If I were me, nobody would like me -so I try to be what I think others expect me to be. I don't think I can be loved with all the parts of me which are ugly and bad. Lonely feelings. Longing for love and understanding. Feel I am so unfriendly to myself. 18, 30C, 04:00:00
Sh, 113 - Sometimes I don't want to show my strength. I keep it back. I am afraid that others will feel inferior and I don't want them to, because I feel it so much myself. 18, 30C, 26:XX:XX
Sh, 142 - Observe the world as being shabby. I feel separated from people and places. I feel an intense yearning for the feminine. 08, 12C, 08:04:50

HALI-L. Sh, 330 - Bored and superior feeling with an old friend. 16, 10C, 22:XX:XX
Sh, 349 - I said I was moody. It wasn't as

qualitative as she wanted, and she was asking for more details and I yelled, " A stupid five year old would understand what I was saying." I became sarcastic and very belligerent. I thought I was being simplistic and clear. I gave what I had to give. I was in a depressed state, lost my good feeling and was angry at being asked to explain the depression. She asked me what do you mean and I said, "XXXX off. If you don't understand that, too bad. Do you understand that?! Do you know the English language?" 18, 30C, 04:14:00

Sh, 403 - For three weeks I was in a depression, unlike anything I have felt for a long time. Deep sense of low self-worth. Feeling invisible, uncared for and envious. I was lethargic, couldn't do anything. My practice dropped, patients just didn't show up. I felt I sunk as low as I needed to go, unmotivated. Felt unappreciative of all I have. Unappreciative of my life which I usually adore. Anger, dissatisfaction with life, isolating. I wasn't seeing anyone not even my husband, exhaustive. Had no dreams during the depression —unusual. I am emerging from it now. 01, 30C, 30:XX:XX-50:XX:XX

Sh, 580 - Spent most of today thinking about how I am surrounded by idiots, (my family), who are showing no attempts to think for themselves, letting me run the show. They don't care to figure things out. I'm in hyper-drive. I know a lot and I'm right. I've been extremely productive or at least active, balancing several major projects all at the same time, and they can't seem to tidy a table properly. This includes my husband, who continually interrupts me (or so it seems) for some trivial question. I'm coming across with too much force. I find myself shouting at everyone much more than usual. Like a crazy person. Impatient over others' slowness. Almost an arrogance. I want them to THINK! (Obviously, the way I do). or get off the ship and drown yourself. A hard anger, more intense that usual. Feel like leaving them all—they just take and give back little. More trouble than support. This isn't complaining or victimizing talking. This is how it is. I'm healing myself and leaving my family in the dust. I've passed on to them my bad habits, bad parenting. They are content to be idiots. 09, 6C, 13:XX:XX

Sh, 581 - At a meeting for parents and children, I am very critical of my daughter and myself, comparing her to other kids, myself to other moms. Cringe when she sits with her mouth open, pulling on her hair and twisting it into braids. Want to warn her, don't do that! She looks to me like she's bossing someone. Compare myself to other woman who has perfectly put together hair, clothes, nails, boots, bracelets. Very angry and jealous. Make excuses for myself and tear her down inside. 09, 6C, 14:00:XX

Sh, 946 - Inner vision: I was a male Indian. I thought, "I'm not a brave. I don't deserve this feather". 20, 30C, 15:XX:XX

HYDR. Al, 16 - Spiteful (cruel), angry disposition, with desire to snub (scorn) any one who differed in anything with me; lasting all day.

HYDROG. Sh, 210 - I was shouting down the phone, but dead quiet with friends. I thought "Why are they talking? They haven't anything to say". I was very sarcastic. 24, 30C, 01:XX:XX

Sh, 219 - Things seem ridiculous and amusing, ordinary things like birds. Laughing at them. Everything seemed so absurd or futile. 16, 30C, 02:XX:XX

HYOS. Al, 53 - They laughed aloud because all persons seemed ridiculous;...the old woman talked of future,...

Ha, 519 - In the confusion of his fancy he thinks men are swine.(pigs)

He, 90 - Looks at men as hogs.(pigs)

IOD. Al, 27 - Is cross and irascible; feels stupid.(obtuse)

IP. Al, 12 - Ill-humored, quiet, retired in himself, scorning everything.

Ha, 219 - Sullen unsociable moroseness, that makes him disdain (reject) everything.

Ha, 221 - Sulky humor, that despises (scorn, intolerant, antipathy) everything, and he desires that others also should not esteem or care for anything.

He, 12 - Morose mood that scorns everything, and desires also that others shall not appreciate or value anything.

He, 8 - Peevish; irritable; impatient; morose, scornful mood.

He, 9 - Ill humor, despises everything.
IRID. Sh, 108 - Realized I had called my ex-partner a chicken for pulling out of an arrangement to go together to a school fundraising event. G5
LAC-C. Al,N-11 - Thinks that she is looked down upon (despised) by every one, that she is of no importance in life, and feels insulted thereat. (unimportant, worthless)
Al,N-43 - Intense ugliness (repulsiveness, offensiveness) and hatefulness (odiousness, repellently); writes to her best friends all sorts of mean(vulgar) and contemptible things.
He, 9 - Thinks she is looked down (contempted, scorned, despised) upon by everyone, that she is of no importance in life. (self-contemptuous)
He, 37 - Intense ugliness (repulsiveness, hideousness) and hatefulness (offensiveness); writes to her best friends all sorts of mean and contemptible things. (disdainful)
LACH. He, 26 - Jealousy, with frightful images, great tendency to mock, to satire and ridiculous ideas.
LYC. Al, 92 - Easily roused to anger and scorn.
MYRIC. Al, 9-...a constant desire to find fault (censorious); everything went wrong; looked upon (contemptuous) this world as a place not fit to live in any longer; considered himself better than the rest (great person, megalomania), in the morning; ...; condemned himself for various imaginary faults; ...
NAT-M. Al, 11 - Constant laughing; everything in the room looked so ridiculous.
OP. He, 22-... feeling of great strength; contempt of death;...indifference to joy and suffering.
PHOS. Al, 136 - Felt exceedingly petulant (irritable, contemptuous) all day; nothing went right; felt as dissatisfied with myself as with others; seemed as if everybody said or did something to provoke me.
PLAT. Al, 11 - Contemptuous, pitiful looking down upon people usually venerated, with a kind of casting (reject, discard) them off in paroxysms, against her will.
Ha, 35 - Illusion of the imagination; on entering the room after walking for an hour, everything around her seemed very small and all persons physically and bodily inferior to her, but she herself great and lofty (distinguish, elevated) in body;...
Ha, 36 - Contemptuous, pitying looking down on people at other times respected, with a certain disdain (scorn, arrogance), in paroxysms, against her will. (antagonism)
Ha, 21 - She thinks all persons are demons.
Ha, 37 - During the caprice of contempt, suddenly a voracious hunger...
He, 9 - Pride (haughty) and overestimation of one's self, looking down with haughtiness on others.
He, 45-...melancholy with great fear of death, imagines himself superior to his wife;...
He, 11 - Contemptuous, pitiful, looking down upon people usually venerated, with a kind of casting (forsakes) them off, in paroxysms against her will.
PLB. Al, 69 - On first recovering consciousness the people in the ward (hospital) seemed to him as small as dolls (toy, little), and the opposite of the room seemed to be sunk (under, below) forty feet below his own level.
PULS. He, 47-...; pangs (pain, anxiety) of conscience about religion and female sex; violent palpitation in the presence of women; abhors (detests, aversion) and hates the sex; must go out of their way for fear of injuring them; looks upon them as evil beings and is afraid (fear; temptation, seduction); considers their presence injurious (insulted, offended) to his soul; ... (sexual loathing)
SEC. Al,N-13 - Paralytic mental diseases; treats his relations contemptuously and sarcastically.
He, 12 - Paralytic mental diseases; treats his relations contemptuously and sarcastically;...
SEP. He, 38-...everything seems strange (unusual, unfamiliar) to her;...; it seems as if she could not understand (realize) anything and would have to learn anew everything she wished to do;...(lost: knowledge); greatest indifference to everything, the death of a near relative, or some happy occurrence, leaves her equally

unaffected; no trace of her former love for friends or even for her child; aversion for social intercourse amounting to contempt;...

STRAM. Ha, 504 - He appears to himself large and tall, but surrounding objects appear small to him.

He, 56 - Believes to be in his grave; shrives,(confess) prays, asks to be killed (justified); accuses his wife of infidelity; scolds (cursing), strikes at everybody who wishes to restrain him; thinks they are dogs and barks at them to make himself understood.

He, 77 - Patient had a constant vision of an executioner(hangman, lynches) standing before him in spite of which he was lively, talkative, laughed and joked about his hallucination, yet it seemed to him a reality.

He, 93 - Mania; thinks he is lying on his sepulchre (tomb); confessing, praying, wants to be killed (redemption, salvation, regeneration); laughs as if tickled (excited); wants to be kissed; accuses his wife of being faithless (betrayed); scolding (censure) beating in a rage, will not be taken hold of by attendants (suspicious?) ; takes them for dogs (contemptuous), and barks at them; talking in Jewish jargon; (rank?, stranger?) supposes his house to be surrounded by carts (vehicle), Jews (Judaism) and geese, offending him, ... -(strange, foreign, alien)

TARENT. He, 16 - Attacks of hystero-mania... hits and abuses everyone, destroys whatever she can lay hold of,...mocks aged people with their old age, ...

VERAT. Ha, 706 - He searches for faults in others and taunts (ridicule, mockery) them with them.

Ha, 664 - Cursing and making a noise all night, and complains of being stupid, with headache and flow of saliva.

CONTRADICTION

Ailments from; contradiction: anac.[149] **AUR.**[5] aur-ar.[58] bry.[5] cael.[149] cham.[58] elaps[54] ***ferr.***[5] helon.[5] **IGN.**[5] **LYC.**[5] med.[122] ***nux-v.***[5] olnd.[5] ***petr.***[5] sil.[116]

Anger; contradiction, from: aesc.[58] aloe am-c. ***anac.*** ars. **AUR.** aur-ar.[58] ***bry.*** cact. calc-p. cocc. ***ferr. ferr-ar.*** gall-ac.[162] grat. helon. hura **IGN. LYC.** med.[212] merc. nat-ar. nat-c. nat-sil.[58] ***nicc.*** nit-ac.[30] ***nux-v.*** olnd. op. petr. pitu-a.[164] prot.[136] **SEP.** ***sil.*** stram. tarent. ***thuj.*** til. ***verat.***[30]

Anger; contradiction, least, from: ***aur.***[54] bry.[54] ferr.[54] nicc.[54] ***nux-v.***[54] petr.[54]

Anger; easily, contradiction, from least: nicc.[54]

Anger; temper tantrums, opposed, when at the least: thuj.[8]

Anger; will, if things do not go after his: thuj.[1]

Aversion; persons, to, certain, who do not agree with him: calc-s.[137]

Confidence, want of self; contradiction, in: anac.[60]

Contradiction; agg.: ***asar.***[111] **AUR.** bry.[5] cop.[36] ferr.[5] helon.[5] ign.[5] lyc.[5] nux-v.[5] olnd.[5] petr.[5] sep.[111]

Contradiction; intolerant of: acon. aesc.[102] alco.[36] aloe alum. alum-sil.[58] am-c. anac.[162] ***ant-c.***[102] arn.[102] ars. asaf.[102] asar.[102] aster. **AUR.** bell.[102] ***bry.*** cact. calc-p. cann-i. cann-s.[85] canth.[102] ***caps.***[102] carbn-s.[36] carc.[122] cham.[88] chin.[102] ***cina***[98] ***cocc. colch.***[102] coloc.[102] con. echi. ***ferr.*** flav.[149] gall-ac.[162] glon.[102] grat. hecla.[234] hell.[36] ***helon.*** hep.[102] hura hyos.[5] ictod.[10] **IGN.** kali-i.[163] lach.[102] lact.[85] **LYC.** med.[122] merc. mez.[102] morph.[102] mur-ac.[102] ***nat-c.***[122] ***nat-m.***[102] nicc. nit-ac.[5] nuph.[36] nux-v. olnd. ***op.***[54] pall.[102] petr. phos.[102] plan. ***plat.***[102] prot.[136] puls.[102] sars.[102] **SEP.** ***sil. staph.***[102] stram. ***sulph.***[54] syph.[36] tarent. thuj. thyr.[102] til. tub.[212] ***verat.***[30]

Contradiction; intolerant of, restrain himself, has to, to keep from violence: aloe. sil.

Contradiction; intolerant of, shudders, blood boils with prickling: elaps[54]

Contradiction; intolerant of, throw themselves angrily on the floor and cannot get their breath when in the least opposed: thuj.[8]

Delusions; opposed by everyone: mosch.[5]

Excitement; contradiction, from slightest: ***ferr.***[54]

Hatred; persons, of, agree with him, who do not: calc-s.

Impatience; contradiction, during: alco.[36]

Impatience; contradiction, slightest: nuph.[54]

Intolerance; vexation of: ferr-p.[36]

Irritability; contradiction, during: calc-p.[60] ferr.[144] grat.[36] hura[136] *ign.*[36] tarent.[36]

Irritability; contradiction, slightest, at: **IGN.**[54]

Kill; desire to, person that contradicts her: ***merc.***

Moaning; contradicted, when: tarent.

Morose; contradiction, by: ign.[36] tarent.[36] ***verat.***[36]

Rage; contradiction, from: aur.[127] grat.[10] *ign.*[85] ***lac-c.***[54] lyc.[10] nat-ar.[58] nux-v.[10] olnd.[54] ***thuj.***[36]

Weeping; contradiction, from: ign. nux-v.[5] plat.[168] stram. tarent.

ADAM. Sh, 210 - I complained to another therapist who got upset. I thought "I am going nuts." I was upset that he was upset. It was just a little thing. I couldn't see why he couldn't see my point of view. 7, 6C, 03:00:XX

ALOE. Al, 23 - Immediately, strong exhibition of will (disposition); he quarrels with every one who contradicts him; it seems as if he would permit himself to be torn (ruined) in pieces, sooner than give up his will. (lack; will, integration, union)

He, 12 - An easily excited, angry, revengeful state of mind, could not brook opposition (contradiction), wanted to destroy object of wrath, relief from tea or milk stimulants;...

AM-C. Ha, 23 - Can bear no contradiction.

ANAC. He, 67 - Contradiction between reason and will.

ANT-T. He, 8 - Contradiction between mind and will.

ASTER. He, 12 - Paroxysms easily excited by any emotion, especially by contradiction.

AUR-M. Al, 6 - Unreasonable contrariety.

AUR. Ha, 340 - He sits apart (separated), all by himself in a corner, wrapt up in himself, as if in the deepest melancholy, when left undisturbed; but the slightest contradiction excites the greatest heat and anger,...

Ha, 338 - Irascibility; he is very excitable, and the slightest contradiction excites the utmost anger.

He, 80 - Ailments from fright, anger, contradiction, mortification, or vexation with dread, fear, reserved displeasure, or vehemence.

He, 72 - Contradiction excites wrath; distrust.

BRY. He, 42 - Contradiction easily provoked anger during whole proving.

CALC-P. Al, 13 - Grows very violent, if his opinion is differed from, or if contradicted, so that he is vexed not to have been able to control himself.

CALC. Ha, 40 - As soon he is idle (unoccupied) and sits still, he becomes peevish and drowsy (tired), and everything goes against him.

CAUST. Ha, 23 - Extreme excitability of spirit; the least vexation (difficulty) darts through her body, so that her knees give way.

He, 69 - Injurious (ailments from) effects of fear and vexation. (worry)

CIST. He, 3 - Bad effects of vexation; feels as if paralyzed.

COCC. He, 9-...cannot bear least noise or contradiction.

CON. He, 38 - Very much excited, passionate, domineering (dictatorial), quarrelsome, scolds (censorious) and will not bear contradiction.

DROS. Al, 15 - He is very much affected by offenses, with some vexation.

FERR. Al, 20 - Excited by the slightest opposition; ... even her children's caresses increased her bad temper; she was often rude to those about her, because she hated to see or talk to them, and wanted them to leave her in solitude, which alone was pleasing to her.

He, 15 - Excited by slightest opposition; everything irritates or depresses her.

He, 14 - Pettish(irritable), quarrelsome, disputative (litigious), easily excited, least contradiction angers.

GRAT. Al, 8 - Fretful, irritated by every contradiction, angry outbreaks, misanthropic, whith solicitude about his own health.

HELL. Al, 17 - Extremely inclined to be irritable, the most trifling things which goes contrary to his wishes excites anger.

HELON. Al, 4-.... could not endure the least contradiction or receive any suggestions in regard to any subject (fixed ideas) ;... what I most desired was to be left alone, reserved to myself the privilege of finding fault (imperfection) with everything around me;....

He, 5 - Irritable; cannot endure the least contradiction or receive suggestions in relation to any subject.

HURA. Al, 25 - Irritated by the least opposition.

HYOS. He, 52 - Bite, scratch (hurt) and nip (pinch) everyone interfering with them.

IGN. Al, 27 - Slight blame or contradiction excites him to anger, and this makes him angry with himself.

Al, 5 - Desires improper (inappropriate) things, and cries aloud when they are refused.

Ha, 764 - Slight blame (censuring) or contradiction excites him to quarrel, and he is vexed at himself for doing so.

Ha, 775 - When one hesitates in the least to do what she wishes, or remonstrates (censures) much with her, though in a mild friendly manner, or endeavor to persuade her, or wishes differently from what she wishes, she weeps aloud.

Ha, 765 - From the slight contradiction he is irritated and angry.

He, 52 - The slightest contradiction irritates.

He, 53 - Slight blame (censure) or contradiction excites him to anger, and this makes him angry with himself.

IP. He, 13 - Ailments from vexation (worry) and reserved displeasure.

KALI-C. Al, 45 - Disagreeable mood; she longs for things with impetuosity; is contented with nothing, is beside herself, and gets into rage if everything does not go according to her wishes, and frequently does not herself know what she really wishes to have.

Ha, 33 - Contrary mood; she demands (order, command) impetuously; is not satisfied with anything (dissatisfied) ; she is beside herself, and furiously angry; if everything does not go according to her wishes, and often does not herself know what she really wants.

LYC. Al, 89 - She cannot endure the slightest opposition, and is speedily beside herself from peevishness (cross).

Ha, 55 - She cannot bear the least contradiction, and at once gets beside herself for vexation.

He, 31 - Sensitive, irritable disposition; peevish and cross on getting awake; easily excited to anger; cannot endure slightest opposition, and is speedily beside herself.

MERC. He, 21 - Desire to kill the person contradicting her.

NAT-C. Al, 48 - He is angry, and inclined to fight and strike, and cannot tolerate contradiction,...

Ha, 52 - Passionate; disposed to quarrel and fight, and cannot bear any contradiction.

NAT-M. Al, 79 - Easily vexed, pettish; he will not bear opposition for several evenings.

Ha, 58 - Apt to be peevish and abrupt; he does not endure opposition.

NICC. Al, 1 - Very angry and quarrelsome mood; she was inclined to quarrel with and contradict everyone, in the evening.

Al, 2 - Quarrelsome and impatient; she could tolerate no contradiction;...

He, 2 - Vexed and very angry from least contradiction.

NUX-V. Ha, 1262 - She cannot bear the least contradiction, nor suffer the most reasonable representations (narration) to induce her to alter her conduct; they put her beside herself.

He, 26 - Melancholic in consequence of losing his position (rank),...the least contradiction puts him out entirely...(ailments from)

OLND. Al, 7 - He cannot tolerate contradiction.

Ha, 350 - He cannot bear contradiction.

PH-AC. Ha, 662 - A trifling vexation makes him very angry and hot.

RUTA. He, 1 - Inclination to contradict and quarrel.

SEP. Al, 66 - She finds fault and desires nothing which others want, accompanied by weeping and heat of face.

Al, 96 - He thinks of things which he does not think of, uses expressions which he knows are incorrect, undertakes those things which are opposed to his intentions, and finds such contradictions with himself that it puts him in a very uncomfortable and uneasy mood.

STANN. Ha, 640 - Peevish: nothing was done according to his wish.

SULPH. Ha, 39 - He allows himself to be carried away by vexation.

SYPH. Al,N-5-... violent on being opposed,

has tremors, seems on the verge of convulsions,...always washing her hands.

TARENT. Al, 60 - Irritable and cross at the least contradiction.

THUJ. Al, 16 - The child is excessively obstinate; on the slightest contradiction it throws itself in the ground in rage and loses its breath.

Al, 90 - Excited mood; he is irritable, especially if any one says anything of which he does not exactly approve.

THYR. Al,N-1-...at times dangerous and homicidal, would put her arms round the necks of other patients so tightly as almost to strangle them (in this case the insanity was primary and the myxedema secondary; both conditions were removed). Evinced increased vivacity by quarreling with another patient about a trifling difference of opinion.

TIL. Al, 19 - Irritable, critical mood, inclined to quarrel and get angry, even from the slightest difference of opinion.

CONTRARY

ALOE. Al, 23 - Immediately, strong exhibition of will (disposition); he quarrels with every one who contradicts him; it seems as if he would permit himself to be torn (ruined) in pieces, sooner than give up his will. (lack; will, integration, union)

ALUM. Ha, 32 - She does not wish to do what others wish.

ANAC. Ha, 25 - He is compelled to laugh, while engaged in very serious matters, ...;in laughable matters he can keep serious. (contrary)

Ha, 17 - Passionate and contrary.

ANAN. Al, 7 - Quarrelsome and contrary humor, but after being angry he often regrets (remorse) what he has done.

ARN. Ha, 630 - He contradicts; is opinionative; no one can please him.

BAR-C. He, 24 - Extremely contrary, irritable humor, passionate about trifles .

CARB-AN. Ha, 25 - Self-willed; no one can do anything to please him.

HEP. Al, 19 - Contrary mood, he does not wish to see the members of his own family.

Ha, 7 - Contrary mood; he does not like to look at his folks. (relatives)

KALI-C. Ha, 32 - Contrary disposition; he is self-willed (obstinate) and often does not know himself what he wishes. (indecision)

Ha, 33 - Contrary mood; she demands (order, command) impetuously; is not satisfied with anything (dissatisfied) ; she is beside herself, and furiously angry; if everything does not go according to her wishes, and often does not herself know what she really wants.

LYC. He, 32 - Obstinate, defiant (contrary), arbitrary (capricious?); seeks disputes.

NUX-V. He, 10-...every harmless word offends, every little noise frightens, anxious and beside themselves, cannot bear even the least suitable medicine. (contrary)

CORPSE

Delusions; dead, corpse, absent acquaintance on sofa and has dread, of: ars.
- dead, corpse, brother and child, c. of: calc-sil.[58] con. plb.
- dead, corpse, husband: calc-sil.[58] plb.
- dead, corpse, mutilated: ant-c. arn. con. mag-m. merc. nux-v. sep
- dead, corpse, near him: anac.[1]
- dead, corpse, sister, of: agar.
- dead, corpse, tall yellow c. trying to share bed with him and promptly ejected: bell.
- murdered, sees someone: calc.
- mutilated bodies, find, will: lap-mar-c.[194]
- person, coat, shroud, with: psil.[164]
- skeletons, sees: crot-c. op.
- spectres, sees, death appears as a gigantic black skeleton: crot-c.

Dreams; autopsies: rumx.
- ➤ dead, bodies: alum.[10] alumn. am-c. **ANAC.** arn.[10] aur. bar-c.[1] brom.[10] bry.[10] ***calc. calc-sil.*** cand-a.[239] cann-i.[54] cann-s. carb-ac. caust.[10] cedr.[25] ***chel.*** cocc.[10] con.[10] ***crot-c.*** crot-h.[58] dirc. elaps fl-ac.[10] gink.[149] graph.[10] grat.[10] hura hydr-ac.[10] iod.[10] iris jac-c. kali-c.[10] kali-m.[192] lap-gr-m.[194] laur.[10] mag-c.[10] mag-m. mag-s. merc. nat-c. nat-p. nit-ac. ozone[227] peti.[36] ph-ac.[10] phos.[1] plat.[10] ran-s. rumx. sars.[10] sil.[10] sol-t-ae. sul-ac.[10] sulph.[10] tarent. ***thuj.*** verb. zinc
- ➤ dead, bodies, arms cut off, with: hura[36]
- ➤ dead, bodies, bed, in, are put in bed with her: ozone[227]
- ➤ dead, bodies, coming alive after a funeral: allox.[119]
- ➤ dead, bodies, digging knife into wounds of: elaps[36]

➤ dead, bodies, dissecting: cench.[58] chel.[36] iris ped.[36] sang.
➤ dead, bodies, embracing: elaps[36]
➤ dead, bodies, fear, with, wishes to end it by turning on side, but cannot: alumn.[36]
➤ dead, bodies, finding a dead child in a churchyard: mag-s.[36]
➤ dead, bodies, putting deceased body in shroud: elaps[36]
➤ dead, bodies, returning to life: rumx.[36]
➤ dead, bodies, skin taken from: mag-m.[36]
➤ dead, bodies, smell of dead: calc. crot-h.[58]
➤ dead, bodies, sprang from dissecting table and seized throat: chel.[36]
➤ dead, infants: cench.[58] lap-gr-m.[194]
➤ dead, people, of, friends, recently deceased hanging by the legs before him for hours: coca[36]
➤ death, own, his, and orders the rapid removal of the corpse from the house: fl-ac. rauw.[119]
➤ funeral, corpse coming alive after a funeral: allox.[119]
➤ piercing bodies of her children together: dict.[137] phos.[137]
➤ skeletons: op.
Necromania: **AGAR.**[185]
Thoughts; dead bodies, of: hydrog.[222]

ANAC. Al, 8 - Melancholic illusion; he imagines a bier in the side room, upon which either his friend or himself is lying.
Ha, 46 - Melancholy dejection and imagination, as if there was standing in the adjacent room a bier, on which a friend or he himself was lying.
ARS. Al, 78 - Anxiety and fear; he sees a absent acquaintance (friend) lying dead upon the sofa, and has great dread of him.
Ha, 33 - Anguish and fear; he sees an acquaintance who is not present lie dead on sofa, and is much afraid of him.
BELL. Al,S-2552-...the yellow corpse of a tall man, shrouded (dressed, clothes) in white, tried to share the patient's bed with him, and the unwelcome visitor was promptly ejected. A crimson serpent came from the foot of the bed, with the design of fastening upon the patient's neck...
CROT-C. Al, 1 - Magnetic state; she hears nothing, and again sees the spectre of death, as a gigantic black skeleton.
HURA. Al, 709 - Restless night; dream about crimes, dead bodies (corpse), and children lying with their heads half cut off, while others were being decapitated.
HYDROG. Sh, 159 - Thoughts of dead bodies made me feel slightly sick. 10, 200C, 00:XX:XX
Sh, 162 - The remedy "made me think of formaldehyde and dead things". 10, 200C, 00:XX:XX
Sh, 163 - Thoughts of death —thoughts went back to doing dissection as a medical student.[10], 200C, 00:XX:XX
KALI-BR. Al, 5 - She had the erroneous idea that she was deserted by all her friends, and as a consequence she passed all her waking moments, which are not many in tears;...delusion that her child was dead, had taken fixed possession of her mind;...she declared that she saw it dead (corpse) before her, and when it was brought to her, she refused to acknowledge that it was hers, or had any resemblance to the one she imagined was dead.
MAG-M. Al, 715 - Dream that someone cut away one side of her face; that a skin was being taken from a dead body and the like.
NAT-C. Al, 1116 - Dream that she saw a corpse, at which she woke in fright, when it seemed as though a dead acquaintance stood before her, which made her scream aloud, afterwards she fell asleep again .
SABAD. Al, 2 - He imagines all sorts of strange things about his own body, for instance, that it had shrunk (dry, wrinkled) like that of dead persons (corpse), that his stomach was corroded (degeneracy, decomposition), that the scrotum was swollen (enlarged), etc.;...

COWARDICE

Anger; sudden, cowardice, with: bar-c.[54]
Bed; jumps out of, wants to destroy himself but lacks courage: chin.
Courageous; alternating with discouragement: merc.[30] op.[30] staph.[30]
Cowardice: ***acon.*** agar. agn. alco.[36] alum. alum-sil.[58] **AM-C.**[30] ambr.[111] anac. ang. ant-t.[5] ***arg-n.***[5] aur. aur-s.[58] ***bar-c.*** bar-i.[58] bar-m. bar-s.[58] bell. ***bry.*** calc. calc-s. calc-sil.[58] camph. canth. carb-an. carb-v. caust. ***cham.***[5] ***chin.*** chin-b.[54] cocc. coloc. con. cupr. dig. dros. fl-ac.[184] **GELS.** graph. hep.[30] hydr-ac.[5] ign. iod. ip. kali-c. kali-n.

kali-p. kali-sil.[58] kreos.[111] lach.[111] lap-mar-c.[194] laur. led. **LYC.** merc. mur-ac. nat-m. nit-ac. ***nux-m.***[5] ***nux-v.***[5] ol-an.[111] olnd.[5] **OP.**[122] ph-ac. phos. plat. plb. ***puls.*** ran-b.[58] ***rhus-t.***[5] ruta sabin. sec. sep. ***sil.*** spig. stann. staph.[30] **STRAM.** sul-ac. sul-i.[58] sulph. tab. ther.[5] thuj. ***verat.*** verb. viol-t. visc.[119] zinc.[10]

Cowardice; anger, with sudden fits of: bar-c.[54]

Cowardice; opinion, without courage of own: graph.[30] ign.[30] petr.[30]

Cowardice; sadness, with: ***sulph.***[54]

Cowardice; weakness, with, must keep her bed (in pregnancy): ***stann.***[54]

Delusions; coward, he is a: germ.[222]

• cowards, persons leaving him are: cann-i.

Fear; everything, constant of: acet-ac.[54] acon.[172] bell.[36] ***calc.***[54] hydr-ac.[102] ***hyos.***[54] ***lyc.***[54] nat-c.[54] ***puls.***

✦ lifelong: am-c.[30] am-m.[30] calc.[30] lyc.[30] petr.[30] puls.[30] sil.[30] stann.[30] sulph.[30] zinc.[30]

✦ pusillanimous: acon.[36]

✦ shadow, of his own: acon.[137] calad.[72] ***calc.***[54] lyc.[85] staph.[85]

Hide; desire to, fear, assaulted, of being: tarent.[58]

Hide; desire to, fear, on account of: ***ars. bell.*** cupr. ***hyos.***[54]

Irritability; alternating with, cowardice: ran-b.[5] zinc.[10]

Spineless: am-c.[30] bar-c.[30] calc.[30] sil.[155]

Suicidal disposition; courage, but lacks: alum. **CHIN.** nit-ac. **NUX-V.** ozone[227] phos. plat. rhus-t. ***sulph.***[54] tab.

Timidity; bed, about going to: acon. ars. bapt. camph. cann-i. ***caust.*** cench. lach. lyc. nat-c. squil.

ACON. Al, 66 - Great timidity after a severe fright (fear), afraid to go out unattended (abandoned, helplessness) after dark, is unable to control his feelings of apprehensive fear.

Al, 53 - Dolorous anxious complaints, with pusillanimous (cowardly) fears, despair, loud wailing (laments) and weeping, and bitter reproaches.

Ha, 517 - Piteous (miserable), anxious complaints, with cowardly fears, despair, loud whining weeping, bitter complaints and reproaches.

He, 36 - Extreme timidity, especially after a fright; afraid (fear) in dark.

He, 37 - Fears to go where is any excitement (tumult) or many people (crowd); thinks she is jostling (pressing) against everyone she meets (oppressed); countenance (expression) expressive of timidity; constant dread (fear) lest she stagger (vacillated) and fall.

AGN. Al, 2 - He sometimes feels as if he were nobody (unimportant, insignificant, worthless), and would rather be dead than have that feeling; when possessed by that feeling he has no courage to undertake anything; and when free from it he feels exalted, would like to read like an orator, etc.

ALOE. Al, 17 - Great anxiety, timorousness, restlessness, dread (fear) of death, and great anguish, so that she cannot stay anywhere.(restlessness)

AM-C. Ha, 9 - Many afternoons she is seized with weakness and timidity, so that she cannot control herself and knew not what to do;...

ANAC. Ha, 6 - Timorous in all his actions; he views everything more anxiously and timidly, always thinks of being surrounded by enemies, then he becomes hot, his blood seems to boil in his chest.

ASTER. Al, 7-...it seems as if some misfortune was about to happen to him, and that, should it actually (really) come upon him, he would weep, rather than brace (encourage) himself to meet it, or become angry.

BAR-C. Al, 12 - Great fear and cowardice.

Ha, 4 - She suspected, that when walking in the street, men found fault (defect) with her, and judged her amiss (wrong), which made her anxious, so that she dared not look up, she looked at nobody, and perspired all over.

Ha, 17 - Extremely discouraged and pusillanimous ;(cowardice) she thinks she will die, and weeps.

Ha, 16 - Great timidity and cowardice.

He, 29 - A peculiar dread of men.

He, 34 - Loss of self confidence; desponding: pusillanimous.(cowardice)

He, 36 - Sudden ebullitions of anger, but coupled with cowardice.

BELL. Al, 165 - Cowardice, distrust, suspicion, inclination to run away.

CALC. Ha, 22 - Timid and restless, as if evil

(harmful, misfortune) was impending (imminent) over her.

CARB-AN. Ha, 5 - Pusillanimous (cowardice) and sad; everything seems to her so lonely (alone, deserted) and sad, that she would like to weep.

Ha, 15 - Timid and fearful (coward), all day.

CAUST. Al, 27 - Loss of courage.

Ha, 16 - Lack of courage.

Ha, 20 - Extreme anxious timidity; she is so much afraid (fear) of a dog near her, which did not harm (hurt, injure) her at all,...every noise in the street made her afraid, and when she saw boys climbing she was very uneasy lest they might get hurt. (care, others)

CHIN. He, 16-...;wants to destroy himself, but lacks courage.

COFF-T. Al, 9 - Timidity, and fear of sudden death;...

CON. He, 33 - Timid, cannot be persuaded to work ; want of proper will. (lack of: resolution) (vagabond)

CUPR. Al, 8 - Fearful; want of courage.

He, 26 - Loss of spirits (courage); anxiety; fits of anguish and fear of death.

DROS. Al, 4 - He is depressed by the persecutions of others on all sides, and also discouraged and solicitous about the future.

GELS. He, 23 - Fear of death; has no courage. (cowardice)

He, 28 - Great lack of courage.

He, 29 - Every exciting news causes diarrhea ; bad effects from fright and fear. (ailments from)

GERM. Sh, 103 - Felt closed in. My every movement and thought controlled. Didn't know where to go for help. Felt like a coward . Felt afraid of violence. I don't know who I am. 04, 6C, XX:XX:XX

IGN. Al, 20 - Fearfulness timidity; she has no confidence in herself, gives up (desist) everything.

Ha, 759 - Fearfulness, cowardice cannot trust himself to do anything, considers all is lost .

IOD. Al, 8 - Disposition mild, scrupulous (careful) and timid (irresolute), with blunted (dull) sensibilities.

IP. Al, 7 - His courage sinks, and he is extremely inclined to be peevish and ill-humored.

Ha, 227 - He lets (permit) his courage sink (fail), and is greatly given to be vexed and to get angry.

IRID. Sh, 101 - Went into pet shop. There was a budgie chirping in a cage. I was so upset. "Oh God, I want to let this bird out." I felt it was crying to be let out. Took me all my control not to let it out or shout at the man to do it. Then thought, "This is silly. It would get hurt, he'll think I'm mad." I slunk out of the shop thinking I'd really let that bird down. Distracted and nearly in tears. Walked round town in a daze, should I go back and ask him to at least open the door, knew that wasn't on. It might get out of the shop and die. Felt a real coward. Set up a train of thought — condor in bird garden —a notice justifying its captivity —it only flies for food —it's quite happy to be there because food comes to it. Weeping as I write this. Birds in cages can't lean on the air currents and be blown away. G6

Sh, 169 - Did teaching by myself. Bit anxious but nothing like usual. The video didn't work. I would have panicked. I thought, "Let's be systematic about this." Found the problem and it was fine. Much more confident risking it. Very relaxed about how the time was going, not in such a rush. A student called me chicken for taking only one tablet. G4

KALI-BR. Al, 3- ...his character also had undergone a radical change, from having been very frank and brave, he had become excessively timid, and suspicious of every trifling circumstance; ...several times he attempted to throw himself from a window and battered down a door with an axe, in order to escape from some imaginary danger;...

KALI-C. He, 10 - Timid and apprehensive of future and about her disease.

LYC. He, 38 - Parsimonious (economical), greedy (avaricious), malicious (malevolent) and pusillanimous.(cowardice)

MERC. He, 34 - Inexpressive pain of soul and body, anxious restlessness, as if some evil impended ...; disgusted (revolt) with himself, has not courage (cowardice) to live; constant suspicion (distrust), considering everybody his enemy.

NAT-C. Ha, 3 - Dread of men and timidity.

PHOS. Al, 80 - Mental depression, and a most uncommon fearfulness or timidity, with a great sense of fatigue.
Ha, 62 - Very irritable mood, she takes every word ill and becomes pusillanimous (coward) from it.
PSOR. Al,N-48 - Fright caused by the merest trifles; this often causes perspiration and trembling.
RHUS-T. Ha, 972 - From sad thoughts, which she could not get rid of, she became timorous and fainthearted.(coward, fearful)
SOL-T-AE. Al, 1 - She rises in the night, imagining that thieves are hidden behind the curtains; but she not dare (risk) to look for them, and begs some one else to do so.
STANN. He, 6 - A woman, age 39, pregnant in fourth month;...inability to do anything as she cannot muster sufficient courage,...great palpitation of heart and anxiety, especially if she has to give directions in her domestic affairs; thinking makes her feel wretched, ...(unable, incapable)
SULPH. Ha, 5 - Sad pusillanimous, full of weariness (fatigue) of life.
TAB. Al, 34 - Apprehensive, faint-hearted, and despondent, with nausea; she thought she would die, ...
VERAT. He, 51 - Despair; hopeless, loss of courage.

CRAWLING

Crawling; floor on: absin.[137] ***acet-ac.***[36] bell.[5] cann-i.[36] choc.[222] lach.
Crawling; floor on, anger, during: prot.[136]
Delusions; animals, creeping: alum.[5] lac-c.
- animals, creeping, in her (him): ail.[58] cycl.[36] stram.
- animals, creeping, shirt, about in: bell.[54]
- animals, creeping, to her: **OP.**[54]
- animals, fleas creeping over body, evening: gent-c.[85]
- animals, insects, creeping on face: croto-t.[36]
- animals, snakes, crawling up her leg, feels a: ail.[122]
- animals, vermin, crawl about, sees: alum. am-c. ***ars.*** bov. calc.[30] kali-c. lac-c.[58] mur-ac. ***nux-v.*** phos. ran-s. sil. sulph.[30]
- animals, worms, creeping: alum.[5] am-c.[5] ***ars.***[5] bov.[5] kali-c.[5] mur-ac.[5] **NUX-V.**[5] phos.[5] ran-s.[5] sil.[5]
- body, mouth, living things were creeping into, at night: merc.
- creeping things, full of: stram.[54]
- visions, creeping things, of: ***lac-c.***[54]

Dreams; animals, rats, creeping under the clothing: menis.[36]
- ➤ animals, spiders, black, creeping into corner of mouth: ozone[227]
- ➤ animals, worms, creeping: alum.[10] am-c. bov.[10] choc.[222] esp-g.[149] kali-c.[10] mur-ac. nux-v. phos. ran-s.[10] sil.[10]
- ➤ famine, being left in a dungeon to die of; escaping by crawling out: ped.[36]
- ➤ pursued, witch, by a, creeps from under the door like a haze: ozone[227]

Fear; animals, worms, of: aesc.[172] ars.[172] nat-m.[172]
- ✦ creeping out of every corner, of something: med. ***phos.***

ARS. Al, 90 - He sees vermin and bugs crawl about his bed, from which he wants to escape, and constantly throws away whole handfuls of them.
Ha, 34 - He sees nothing but worms and bugs crawling about on his bed, from which he desires to run away (escape) and of which he throws out whole hands full.
BELL. Al, 86-...pointing with trembling fingers to swarms (crowd) of unclean (dirty) beasts wich she fancied were scrambling (mix) all over the walls, beds, table, etc. of the wards.
CARB-V. Ha, 678-... feeling over the body as if some one stroked him with the hand, and as if ants were running over the skin, at every moment in bed...
CHOC. Sh, 311 - On stepping out of the shower, a fleeting, momentary imagination of both arms crawling with insects. No physical sensation, purely an imagination.15, 30C, 00:02:XX
Sh, 312 - While reading small print in materia medica, I had a delusion that tiny insects were crawling down the page. 15, 30C, 03:XX:XX
HYDROG. Sh, 170 - Sensation as if something is crawling on my head. Checked for lice, but can't find any. 32, 9C, 09:XX:XX
HYOS. He, 59-...constantly pointing to serpents (snakes) which she saw creeping up towards her...

LAC-C. He, 15 - Sensation or delusion as if surrounded by myriads of snakes, some running like lightning up and down inside the skin ; some that are inside feel long and thin; fears to put her feet on floor, lest she should tread (walk) on them and make them squirm (shake) and wind (round) around her legs; is afraid to look behind her, for fear that she will see snakes there, does not dream of them and is seldom troubled with them after dark; on going to bed she was afraid to shut her eyes for fear that a large snake, the size of her arm, would hit her in the face.

He, 21 - Sits and looks under chairs, table, sofa and everything in room, expecting yet dreading (fear) to see some terrible monster creep forth and feeling all the time, that if it does, it will drive her raving mad; she is not afraid in dark, it is only in light where she can imagine that she can see them.

PHOS. He, 8 - Fear and dread: in evening; of death; as if something were creeping out of every corner; late in evening as if a horrible face were looking out of every corner.

STRAM. He, 65-"There", he replied, "A long train of bedbugs, and after them a procession of beetles and here come crawling over me a host (crowd) of cockroaches"; sank back in alarm, then suddenly said:" I believe I know they are not really bugs, but, except once in a while, they seem real to me. (organization, association, union)

CRIMINAL

Anxiety; conscience, unpardonable sin, feels she has done the, and will be eternally lost: ***chel.***[54].

Anxiety; murdered someone, as if he had, all night: phos.[36]

Anxiety; murdered someone, as if he had, mania, in: ***ars.***[54]

Delirium; accused of theft, after being harshly: ***hyos.***[54]

Delusions; arrested, is about to be: arn. ars. ***bell.***[122] cupr. kali-br. meli. plb. ruta[36] tab.[85] ***zinc.***

- called before court, on account of wicked actions during climacteric period: ***zinc.***[54]
- crime, about to commit a: kali-bi.[54] kali-br. thea.[139]
- crime, committed a, he had: alum. alum-sil.[162] am-c.[139] anac. ars.[58] carb-an.[54] carb-v. chel.[111] chin-s.[139] cina[98] cocc.[139] cycl. dig.[139] hell.[58] ***ign.***[102] kali-bi.[54] kali-br. lach.[58] med.[85] merc.[36] nux-v.[102] plb.[58] puls.[139] rheum[139] rhus-t.[139] ruta[98] sabad. staph.[102] ***verat-v.***[102] zinc.[102] zinc-o.[139]
- criminal, and others know it: cob.
- criminal, executed, to be: **OP.**[54]
- criminal, that he is a: alum.[10] am-c.[10] ars.[10] carb-v.[10] caust.[10] chel.[5] cina[10] cob. coff.[10] cycl. dig. ferr.[10] graph.[10] hyos. ***ign.*** m-arct.[10] ***merc.*** nat-c.[10] nit-ac.[10] nux-v.[10] op. phos. puls.[10] ruta[10] sabad.[139] sarr. sil.[10] stront-c.[10] sulph.[10] thuj. verat.[10]
- criminals, about: alum. am-c. ***ars.*** bell. carb-v. caust. ***chel.*** cina ***cocc.*** coff. dig. ***ferr.*** graph. ***hyos.*** merc. nat-c. nit-ac. nux-v. puls. ruta sil. stront-c. sulph. verat.
- hell, going to, because he has committed a unpardonable crime: chel.[172] med.[54]
- honest, he is not: ***stram.***[8]
- murderer, executed to be: **OP.**[54]
- people, sees, connected with the law who will seize him, causing great anxiety, cries like a child: ***cupr-acet.***[54]
- policeman, come into house, he sees: ars.[58] hyos. kali-br.
- pursued, police, by: alco.[36] ars.[58] bell. ***cupr. hyos. kali-br.*** meli. phos. plb. zinc.
- pursued, robbing a friend, for: kali-br.[36]
- soldier, sees, capture him, that will: bell.[10]
- stolen, somebody thinks it: lach.[58]
- stolen, something, she has: lach.[58]
- thieves, accused of robbing, he has been: kali-br.
- voices, hears, command him to commit crime: lach.[58]
- witches, denies having anything to do with them, in delirium after being accused of theft: ***hyos.***[54]

Dreams; accusations: clem.[10] lach.[10] nat-m.[10] thuj.[10]

- ➤ accusations, crime, wrongful of: choc.[222] clem.[10] hydrog.[222] sil.[58]
- ➤ contraband, of having something, and wanting to snatch and lock it up: mag-c.[36]
- ➤ crimes: carbn-s.[36] cocc.[10] hura hydrog.[222] nat-m. nat-s. nit-ac. petr.[10] rumx.
- ➤ crimes, answer, for which he is held to: nat-m.[36]
- ➤ crimes, committed a crime, having: cocc. nat-s. nit-ac.[36] petr.

➤ crimes, committing: hydrog.[222]
➤ crimes, conscience acquits him of a: thuj.[36]
➤ crimes, discovered by priest: nat-s.[36]
➤ crimes, witnessed: carbn-s.[36]
➤ drugs, his son is selling: bamb-a.[1184]
➤ guilt: androc.[222] asar.[149]
➤ illegal, is somewhere: ozone[227]
➤ kidnappers: bamb-a.[1184]
➤ money, robbery, he found the money of a: bac.[226]
➤ poisoned, about to be, while innocent of crime: chr-ac.[36]
➤ police: bamb-a.[1184] ozone[227]
➤ pursued, police, by: lap-mar-c.[194]
➤ robbery, of committing: hydrog.[222]
➤ robbing a bank: hydrog.[222]
➤ stealing, fruit: plb.
➤ stealing, money: lap-mar-c.[194]
➤ theft, accused of, of being: choc.[222] lach.
➤ theft, committed, of having: alum. plb.

Escape; attempts to, crime, for a fear of having committed a: ***merc.***[54]

Fear; alone, of being, crime and cruelty would be committed, lest: kali-br.[172]
✦ arrested, of being: ars.[137] bell.[172] meli.[85] plb.[137] ruta[162] tab.[137] zinc.[72]
✦ killing, child, her: ars.[172] coff.[172] manc.[30] ***merc.***[185] ***nux-v.***[185] rhus-t.[172] sep.[185] sil.[172] ***sulph.***[185] **THEA.**[162]
✦ killing, of, mother, her: der.[162]

Inconsolable; actions, over all her, which she thinks are evil: sulph.[1]

Jealousy; crime, to a: hyos.[30] lach.[30]

Jealousy; kill, driving to: **HYOS.**[54] lach.[108]

Kill; desire to, barber wants to k. his customer: ***ars. hep.***

Kill; desire to, sudden impulse to kill: **ALUM.**[162] arg-n.[162] ***ars. ars-i. hep.*** iod. kali-ar. med.[184] merc.[58] ***nux-v. plat.*** rauw.[119] staph.[162] sulfon.[162] sulph.[162] tarent.[137] thea.

Kleptomania: absin. ars. ***art-v.*** **BELL.**[30] bry. calc.[30] carb-v.[30] carc.[207] caust. cic.[102] ***cur.*** hyos.[102] kali-br.[198] kali-c. lach.[189] lyc. mand.[231] nat-m.[30] ***nux-v.*** oxyt.[102] plat.[102] puls. sep. sil.[30] staph. stram. ***sulph.***[122] syph.[5] tarent. thuj.[162]

Kleptomania; boy with epilepsy: ***art-v.***[54]

Kleptomania; goes about house in search of something, not knowing what, but if attracted by any object puts it in his pocket, or hides it in coat: ***staph.***[54]

Kleptomania; steals, dainties: mag-m. nat-c.

Kleptomania; steals, money: calc. puls.

Moral affections; criminal, disposition to become a; without remorse: ars.[30] bell.[30] hep.[30] lach.[30] merc.[30]

Restlessness; crime, as if he had committed a: ***alum.***[54]

Sadness; criminal as if being the greatest: cycl.[60] sabad.[36]

ALUM. Al, 19 - Anxiety and fearfulness, as if he had committed a crime.
Ha, 17 - Anxiety and fearfulness, as if he had committed a crime.
He, 23 - Anguish, oppressive and vague fearfulness, or uneasiness as if he had committed a crime.

AM-C. Al, 23 - Every afternoon, between five and six o'clock, she is seized with anguish, as if she had committed the greatest crime; towards evening the anguish passes off.
Ha, 8 - Every afternoon between 5 and 6 o'clock she is seized with anguish, as if she had committed the greatest crime; ...
He, 8 - Anguish as if a crime had been committed.

ARS. He, 76 - Anxiety like that of one who has committed murder; driven from place to place; avoids meeting persons, thinking that he has offended them.

ART-V. He, 8 - Inclination to steal.(rob, kleptomania)

CALC-P. Al, 15 - A communication in which some one is justly reproached concerning his conduct, affects him very disagreeably; he grows violent, and holds up his faults to himself.

CANTH. Al, 36 - He is anxious as if he had committed a murder (homicide); it seems to arise from the stomach.

CARB-V. Ha, 8 - For restlessness and anguish every afternoon, he trembled all over the body; he felt as if he had committed a great crime, this dissolved itself into copious weeping, even before strangers on the street.
He, 18 - Anxiety and uneasiness causing him to tremble all over, as if he had committed a crime, ending in weeping, even before strangers;...

CHEL. Al, 65 - Fretful depressed, anxious, as if I had committed some evil (crime), which gave me no rest. (remorse)

He, 17 - Restlessness and uneasiness of conscience; feels that she has committed the unpardonable sin (crime, transgression), and that she will be eternally lost.
He, 18 - Anxiety: allowing no rest at any employment (business) ; as if she had committed a crime; fear of getting crazy (insanity), with restlessness and heat.
COCC. Al, 16 - Anxiety as if she had committed a great crime.
Al, 17 - Great anxiety, as though he had done some evil.
Ha, 536 - Anxiety as if she had committed a great crime.
Ha, 537 - Great anxiety as if he had done something bad.
He, 25 - Melancholy and sadness, with weeping and constant profound absorption in sorrowful thoughts; great apprehensive anxiety of conscience, and feeling at heart as after committing a wicked deed (act), with desire to escape.
CUPR-A. He, 4 - Fixed idea that he sees persons connected with the law who are about to seize him (imprisoned),...at times sees thieves in the room, spirits, and various other immaterial objects;...
CYCL. Al, 10 - Internal grief and anxiety of conscience, as though he had not done his duty, or had committed a crime.
Ha, 196 - Inward grief and anxiety of conscience, as if he had not done his duty or had committed a crime.
DIG. Al, 24 - Internal anxiety, like pangs of conscience, as though he had committed a crime, or expected to be reproved, continuing nearly three months.
Ha, 9 - Internal anguish, like anguish (anxiety) of conscience, as if he had committed a crime, or had to expect reproaches...
FERR. He, 10 - Anxiety as after committing a crime.
GERM. Sh, 128 - Afraid of the police of being caught and unveiled. 18, 30C, 02:10:00
GRAPH. Al, 17 - Anxiety and hastiness (hurry) drive him about like an evil-doer.(criminal)
Ha, 22 - Anguish and hurry (quick) chase (pursue, follow) him about, like a criminal.
HURA. Al, 700 - Dream about children and the release (liberty) of prisoners.
Al, 709 - Restless night; dream about crimes, dead bodies (corpse), and children lying with their heads half cut off, while others were being decapitated.
HYOS. Al, 78 - He considers himself a criminal.
Ha, 574 - He considers himself a criminal.
He, 60-... wants to run away for fear of being persecuted by police;...
He, 79 - After being harshly (severe) accused of theft (crime), continual delirium; fancies surrounded by objects of a terrifying nature; not a moment quiet, continual calling out that she saw the devil; denies herself guilty of theft (innocent, injustice), or that she has any concern with witches; ...
IGN. Al, 15 - Anxiety as if he had committed a crime.
He, 11-...believes herself married (connected) and pregnant; is tormented by remorse of imagined crimes; seeks constantly to escape to drown (suicide) herself; ...;is only quiet when lying undisturbed and brooding over her troubles, which she rehearses (tell) in a doleful (unhappy) tone ;..." I am neglecting my duty, breaking my vow" (promise, engagement)...;conscientious scruples after eating.
He, 28 - Senseless (illogical) staring at one object, with sighing and moaning; remorse about imaginary crimes, intolerance to noise; great inclination to have fixed ideas.
He, 38 - Anxiety as if he had committed some crime.
KALI-BR. Al, 4 - He imagined that he had been specially singled out (select) for divine vengeance... deploring his sad fate (destiny),...he informed me that he had been accused of robbing a friend, and that the officers were in search of him....
He, 15 - Frightful imaginings at night (in pregnant women during latter months), they are under impression that they have committed, or about to commit, some great crime and cruelty (brutality), such murdering their children or husbands.
LAC-F. Al,N-4 - Morbid conscientiousness; every little fault appeared a crime.
MAG-C. Al, 937 - Dream she had something contraband, and wanted to snatch (seize) it away from those looking at it, and lock it up.

MERC. Ha, 1222 - Restlessness, he cannot remain quiet in any place; he can neither stand nor lie, and is as if mad, or as if he had committed a great crime.

Ha, 1234 - Anxiety and apprehension in the blood, he knew not how to compose (control) himself; he felt as if he had committed a crime, without heat, also at the same time as if he was not quite master,(commander). of his senses all day. (lost: mastering, commander)

Ha, 1235 - Anxiety that could drive him far away, as if he had committed a crime or some misfortune were about to happen to him.-(transgression)

Ha, 1237 - With absence of thought, (discernment, knowledge),he feels as if he had done something bad.

Ha, 1229 - Anxiety as if he had committed a crime.

He, 16 - Great restlessness as if he had committed a great crime; ...considers everybody his enemy;...great inclination when walking to take people by the nose;...(desire: conduct, direct, guide)

He, 29 - Anxiety and apprehension; did not know what to do ; it seemed as though he had committed a crime ; without heat; also with a feeling that he had not control over his senses.

He, 38 - Great restlessness, must constantly change her place; fear, with desire to escape, as if she had committed some crime.

NIT-AC. Al, 20 - Anxiety, like palpitation, with nausea, without efforts to vomit, as if she had committed a crime, at night in bed; ...(conscience)

NUX-V. Ha, 1236 - Anxiety and anguish as if he had committed some crime.

OP. Al, 36 - Mind in a state of great confusion; at one moment she was sensible (conscious) to her crime, called for assistance (comfort, aid, help) ; at another she resisted the means used to save her.

Al, 68 - Criminals (in India) lose their fear of death and go courageously to their execution.(fearless)

He, 21-...in old, emaciated persons; sees animals coming towards him; people want to hurt him, execute him ; creeping under covers or jumping out of bed; in "old sinners" (criminals) whose long lives of excess have thoroughly destroyed their constitutions; ...; believe themselves to be murderers or criminals to be executed; want to run away (escape) ;...

PHOS. Al, 101 - Anxiety all night without heat, as if he had murdered some one, with constant tossing about.

PLB. He, 15-...; despair of her salvation...; fixed idea that could only obtain peace and safety though absolution by a priest of the papal church, although she had been a zealous Protestant; ....brooded over any forbidden thing; would steal (leave) from house in servant's cloak (coat, camouflage) and bonnet (hat) to obtain stimulants (drugs), but from the moment their prohibition was withdrawn (retired) ceased to have any desire for them; after being permitted to visit a priest and converse with him ceased to talk and think of the church. (desire; redemption, absolution)

PULS. Al, 12 - Nightly anxiety on waking as if he had committed a crime.

RHUS-T. He, 22-... great restlessness and anguish as if she had committed a crime or as if she thought some terrible calamity impended; these feelings drove her from one place to another; could not rest quietly at night in bed; was robbed of sleep and all desire to live;...

He, 23 - Restlessness and anxiety about heart as if she had committed a crime or as if some great misfortune was in store (reserved) for her, is driven from one place to another; deprived of sleep and all desire to live; ...

ROB. Al, 6 - Fear and confusion (anxiety ?) of conscience, as if he had committed a crime,...

RUTA. Ha, 280 - All day long very anxious as if he had done something bad; when the door was opened, he feared that someone was coming to take him to prison. (incarcerated, punished)

SABAD. Al, 6 - Gloomy mood, as if he were the greatest criminal,...

STRAM. He, 92 - Mania:... complains that a dog is biting and tearing flesh off his chest; merry exaltation; with pride (haughty) and affectation; runs about, complains of violent headache; ...;steals from his roommates...; disposition to scold persons whom he otherwise loved.

THUJ. Al, 72 - Constant anxiety, as if he had committed a great crime, with forgetfulness and general trembling, even to disturbing sleep.

VERAT. Al, 44 - Anxiety as from a bad conscience, as if he had committed a crime.

Ha, 690 - Anxiety as from a bad conscience, as if he had done something bad.

He, 46 - Anxiety as from a bad conscience, as if he had committed a crime.

ZINC. Al, 26 - Very uneasy mood, as though he had committed a crime.

He, 43 - Great fear, as if persecuted by men or the devil, on account of crimes he has never done (injustice); is afraid of becoming imprisoned, or poisoned, or shot, or buried (inter) alive...0 Delirium tremens.

He, 46-...; believed herself to be called before court (judged) on account of her wicked (immoral) actions; ....;believe the devil is after her;...(persecution)

He, 14 - Very uneasy mood as if he had committed a crime.

CROWD

Ailments from; crowd, society, in: agar.[5] **AMBR.**[5] **ARG-N.**[5] ars.[5] **BAR-C.**[5] **BELL.**[5] bov.[5] **BRY.**[5] **CALC.**[5] calc-p.[5] ***carb-an.***[5] carb-v.[5] con.[5] ham.[5] ***hell.***[5] ***hydr.***[5] hyos.[10] ***ign.***[5] iod.[5] kali-i.[5] lap-gr-m.[194] **LYC.**[5] ***mag-c.***[5] **NAT-C.**[5] **NAT-M.**[5] pall.[5] ***petr.***[5] ***phos.***[5] ***plat.***[5] **PLB.**[5] **PULS.**[5] ***rhus-t.***[5] **SEP.**[5] ***stann.***[5] ***stram.***[5] sulph.[5] **THUJ.**[5]

Ailments from; crowd, society, in, pleasant: hell.[5]

Company, aversion to; dizzy, faint in a crowd, or where many gas lights are burning (in agoraphobia): ***nux-v.***[54]

Delusions; assembled things, swarms, crowds: acon.[5] ambr.[5] anac.[5] ars.[5] bell.[5] bry.[5] cann-s.[5] con.[5] graph.[5] hell.[5] lyc.[5] merc.[5] nat-acet.[5] op.[5] phos.[5] plb.[5] **STRAM.**[5] sulph.[5] tab.[5]

- • crushed, he is, everybody rushing, by: tub.[139]
- • people in, sees, babies, full of white and colored: morph.[85]

Dreams; animals, cats, without number: graph.[36]

- ➤ animals, lamas, a zoo full of: bamb-a.[1184]
- ➤ assemblies, large: cere-b.[36]
- ➤ children, about, hordes of, disturbing her idyllic fancy: ozone[227]
- ➤ children, about, lost in crowd: bamb-a.[1184]
- ➤ people, assembled: apis[54] cere-b.[36] hydrog.[222]
- ➤ people, crowd: ars-h.[54] choc.[222] coc-c.[36] **EQUIS.**[54] gels.[36] hydrog.[222]
- ➤ piano, playing, in public: lap-mar-c.[194]
- ➤ praying, public meeting with great applause, in: ars-h.[54]
- ➤ row, of getting into a: nat-ar.[36]
- ➤ urinating, desire for, bottle, in a, but could not on account of a crowd: am-br.[36]

Fear; agoraphobia: acon.[5] ***arg-n.***[5] arn.[5] ars.[172] bar-c.[127] calc.[5] carc.[207] 0crot-h.[30] ferr.[30] glon.[5] 0hydr.[30] hydr-ac.[102] hyos.[172] kali-c.[172] ***kali-p.***[5] lac-c.[172] levo.[149] lyc.[172] **LYSS.** merc.[187] morg.[149] nux-v.[5] phos.[172] prot.[136] puls.[30] ***sep.***[137] stram.[187] tab.[38] visc.[5]

- ✦ crowd, in a: **ACON.** aloe am-m. ***ambr.*** ***arg-n.*** arn.[54] ars. ars-s-f.[58] asaf.[5] ***aur.*** aur-ar.[58] aur-i.[58] aur-s.[58] bamb-a.[1184] bar-c. bar-s.[58] bell.[5] bufo calc. carb-an. carc.[187] caust. cic. con. dios. ferr. ferr-ar. ferr-p. graph. hep. hydr-ac. ***kali-ar.*** kali-bi. kali-c. kali-p. led. levo.[149] ***lyc.*** morg.[136] morg-g.[136] nat-ar. nat-c. ***nat-m.*** nat-s.[58] ***nux-v.*** ***petr.*** phos. plat.[102] plb. <u>**PULS.**</u>[122] rhus-t. sel. sil. stann. stram. sulph. tab. til.
- ✦ crowd, public places, of; agoraphobia: acon. ***arg-n.*** ***arn.*** bar-c.[30] ***calc.***[5] crot-h.[30] dys-co.[136] ferr.[30] **GELS.** glon.[5] hydr.[30] hydr-ac.[102] ***kali-ar.***[184] ***kali-p.***[5] levo.[149] morg-g.[136] nux-v.[5] plb.[201] puls.[30] visc.[111]
- ✦ streets, busy: ***acon.***[162] bar-c.[172] carc.[162] caust.[172] **PSOR.**[162]

Impatience; room, in a warm crowded: ***plat.***[54]

Timidity; public, talk to, inapt to talk: ***carb-v.***[30] petr.[30]

Unconsciousness; crowded room, in a: ambr. ars. bar-c. con. ign. ***lyc.*** nat-c. nat-m. ***nux-m.*** ***phos.*** **PULS.** sulph.

ACON. He, 37 - Fears to go where is any excitement (tumult) or many people (crowd); thinks she is jostling (pressing) against everyone she meets (oppressed); countenance (expression) expressive of timidity; constant dread (fear) lest she stagger (vacillated) and fall.

ADAM. Sh, 345 - Lack of irritability in a crowded store and able to focus and be positive, I usually would have left within minutes. Placid and patient although tired and in pain. 12, 30C, 00:07:30

HYDROG. Sh, 164 - Delusion —saw black masses. 24, 30C, 100:XX:XX

PETR. Al, 10 - Anxiety at a noise of a crowd of many people.

Ha, 4 - Anxiety in the bustle (confusion) of many men. crowd

CRUSHED

Delusions; bed, falling on her: stram.[139]
- crushed, he is, bedclothes, by: pic-ac.[139]
- crushed, he is, everybody rushing, by: tub.[139]
- crushed, he is, houses, by: arg-n.[139]
- houses on each side would approach and crush him: ***arg-n.***
- room, falling to pieces, is: cann-i.[139]
- room, walls will crush him: ***arg-n.***
- room, walls, gliding together, seem: cann-i.
- walls, falling: arg-n. cann-i. lyss.[122]
- walls, falling, inward, before epileptic fit: carb-v. lyss.[122]

Dreams; animals, horses, running, over her: lipp.[36]
- ➤ cellar and walls falling in, being in: bov.
- ➤ crushed, he would be: ***sulph.***
- ➤ crushed, people being: choc.[222]
- ➤ earthquake, houses falling: ozone[227]
- ➤ stone lying on him: kali-c.

Fear; falling, high walls and building upon him: ***arg-n.***[54] arn. choc.[222]
- ✦ falling, houses, of: hydr-ac.[137]
- ✦ falling, things falling on her: stram.[54] tarent.[36]

ARG-N. He, 12 - The sight of high houses always made him dizzy (confused) and caused him stagger (hesitation) ; it seemed as if houses on both sides would approach and crush him.

He, 49 - Fears if passing a certain corner or building that he will drop down and create a sensation; is relieved by going in another direction.

GLON. He, 15 - Fear; throat feels swollen; chest as if screwed together; apprehensive of approaching death; fears she has been poisoned.

HALI-L. Sh, 592 - Had a peculiar experience during the day. While playing with one of my dogs, I started to wonder what it would be like to crush her. Suddenly I thought how sensual it would be to crush its little head and rip its flesh. There was something very sensual about the idea of crushing flesh and bones of a soft creature that would not be able to fight me off. It was not a strong, powerful impulse, but there was something compelling about the idea. 04, 30C, 02:XX:XX

MAG-M. Ha, 20-....when she raised her head up she seemed to see great clouds and rocks above her, ...

OP. He, 20-...declares he is not alone in bed; ..desire to escape; says a regiment of horsemen are upon his bed and that he fears to be trodden upon (run over, crushed); when told that horses are very careful, answered that he feared he would be crushed by the wagons that followed them.

OSM. Al, 5 - Thoughts of accidents having happened to others, by a blow, a fall, or being dashed (crushed, hit, knock) to pieces; gradually these thoughts grow upon him, as if he were to do the same injuries to others.

PHOS. Al, 115 - Frightened feeling, as if I was about to be run over by a locomotive. (crushed, smash)

STRAM. He, 71 - Fears; he will lose his senses (insanity); his lips will grow together; to suffocate; of falling; everything is falling on her.

TARENT. Al, 65-...great haste in whatever I undertook, from a constant fear that something would happen to prevent my finishing it;...fear that something would fall on me (doom, disgrace);...fear of striking it against some imaginary object which appeared to be suspended....(hurt)

DAMAGE

Ailments from; punishment: agar.[137] ambr.[5] con.[5] dam.[85] dig.[5] ign.[5] lach.[5] nat-m.[162] stann.[5] staph.[5] tarent.[85]

Ailments from; rudeness of others: anac.[193] bar-m.[40] ***calc.*** carc.[193] cocc. ***colch.*** hyos.[122] lac-c.[122] ***lyc.***[122] mag-m.[162] med.[179] mur-ac.[40] nat-m. nux-v. ph-ac. puls.[162] **STAPH.**

Aversion; women, to, looks upon them as evil beings and is afraid their presence is injurious to his soul: ***puls.***[54]

Delusions; disease, give, to others, that he will: ***chlol.***[54]
- disgraced, family or his absent friends, he disgraced his: sarr.[36]
- disgraced, family, she disgraced her: ***plat.***[8]
- hated by others, he is: lach.[137] sanic.[144]
- women, evil, are, and will injure his soul: puls.
- work, harm, will do him: ***arg-n.***
- wrong, suffered, has: bac.[62] chin.[193] **HYOS.** lach. ***lyss.*** naja

Fear; broken the arm of her child, that she has, in gastroenteritis during pregnancy: lyc.[172]
- ✦ talking, loud talking would kill her, that: meli.
- ✦ work, dread of, persuaded to, cannot be: ***con.***[54]
- ✦ wrong, commit something, and kill herself: ***merc.***[54]

Sadness; blaming others, with: lil-t.[168]

Work; aversion to mental, thinks it will do him harm, he: ***arg-n.***[54]

ADAM. Sh, 201 - Sensation of being wronged, of being betrayed, which affects my social relationships. 15, 12C, 08:XX:XX

Sh, 278 - Felt I would create irreparable damage if I said how I feel. Thought I would say the most awful things that the kids would never recover from. Supreme effort to keep silent. Didn't want to be here. The kids were a hassle. I felt old and tired. Desire to get away from the fighting. 16, 12C, 17:XX:XX

Sh, 426 - Feeling proving is major setback to my long term health. 7, 6C, 43:00:XX

Sh, 429 - Fear something could happen if I had a bath. Want to keep dry. 7, 6C, 20:09:00

ANAC. Ha, 4 - Internal anguish, which did not allow him to rest, he troubled himself about every trifle, as if it would cause great injure, with solicitude about the future.

ARG-N. He, 10-...; does not work because he thinks it will do him harm (hurt), or that he is not able to stand it.

He, 31 - Does not work, thinking it will do him harm or that he is not able to stand it.

ARN. Al, 31 - Excessive inclination to perform many and long literary labors, without possessing the strength which is required to terminate them without injuring health.

Ha, 623 - Over-busy, inclination and disposition for great and continuous literary work with no power to do it without injury to the health.

HALI-L. Sh, 533 - Boxed in feeling with no way to express anger. Start taking it out on the kids, as if they are trying to break me, to get me. Better getting out, going away from home and family. 09, 6C, 20:XX:XX

Sh, 570 - Don't want to do anything but stay underground—"kick a can" around town. Feel angry about people who may be maligning me. 16, 10C, 14:XX:XX

Sh, 612 - Anxious all day. Feel my relationship is on the rocks as if partner is emotionally abusing me. 02, 30C, 05:XX:XX

Sh, 615 - Don't have the guts to tell partner to stick it out a little longer, that it might work out. Feel totally devastated, but have a lot of energy to deal with it, to stick up for my rights. Felt quite centered, as if I can take care of it. Feels like being on a roller coaster, up and down, in and out. Partner wants to be friends, but not sexual. Feeling emotionally abused. 02, 30C, 09:XX:XX

HYDROG. Sh, 194 - Fear I may lose my mind, or even die. Fear about the proving. Feel I could bash the car so I have to make a real effort. 10, 200C, 12:XX:XX

Sh, 247 - I feel people are playing games with me. Everything is out of balance. (prejudiced)[16], 30C, XX:XX:XX

Sh, 248 - While sitting in a restaurant, felt progressively more cut off from friends at the table. I began to feel detached and paranoid. I felt disliked by people. They seemed to look at me menacingly. I became concerned that my lecture this afternoon had created conflict, mayhem and destruction, that my friends in the audience did not like me any more. I became aware of a dull ache in my sacrum making me want to shift backwards and forwards. At the same time, the people round the table seemed further away and smaller, as if I had moved four feet back from the table. I felt very uncomfortable and wanted to get out. I put my head down and rushed out without saying goodbye, feeling a sense of relief at getting away (all very unusual for me). Outside, I felt relief and my mind cleared and I walked home alone. 22, 12C, 04:XX:XX

Sh, 253 - I was defensive and angry. I thought my friend didn't understand me. I had to apologise. I felt vulnerable and deeply hurt by her. 16, 30C, 05:XX:XX

Sh, 278 - Taking very big deep sighs over the last ten to fourteen days. It feels as if the sigh has to go deep down into my lungs so that sometimes it almost hurts. 02, 6C, 109:XX:XX

LACH. Al, 32 - Becomes easily peevish and mistrustful; believes himself intentionally injured (hurt, prejudice) by all his environments, and attaches the most hateful significance to the most innocent occurrences.

LYSS. He, 22 - Believe that they are reduced to their present wretched condition by the instrumentality (aid) of those about them.

He, 62 - He cautioned people around him not to inhale his exhaled air, it was spoiled, stinking like rotten eggs, worse than cholera, and could injure.

NAT-M. Ha, 64 - Injuries which he had inflicted on others, or which others had done to him, always dwelled in his thoughts; he could not get rid of them, and this annoyed him, so that he had no pleasure in anything.

SUMB. Al, 8-...fond (love) of the society of women; ...sympathy with suffering seems robbed of its pain...nervous excitement and heat, especially in head from listening (hearing) to a disputation, ...humor depressed with despair of future...melancholy despondency, as if ill-treated by everyone purposely... mildness, amiability

DANGER

Delirium; crying, help, for: ***canth.*** stram.[54]

Delirium; help, calling for: plat.

Delusions; alarm, of, on waking: agn.[139]

- danger, family, from his: kali-br.
- danger, impression of: camph.[139] fl-ac. kali-br. macrin.[139] ***stram.*** valer.
- danger, life, to his: plb.
- fire, every noise is a cry of fire, she thinks and she trembles: bar-c.
- fire, house, on: bell. hep. stram.
- fire, neighbor's house on (morning, waking in a fright): hep.
- fire, sees, home, on distant: bell.
- happen, something terrible is going to: fl-ac.[36] ***lyss.*** onos.[144] pall.[85]
- help, calling for: plat.
- life, threatened, is: kali-br.
- place, he cannot pass a certain: ***arg-n.*** kali-br.
- runs, away, has to run: ars-met.[139]

Dreams; alarms, that she heard many: hipp.[36]

- ➤ animals, growing quick, has to destroy them, sticks them into the toilet: ozone[227]
- ➤ calling, help, for: kali-c. lil-s.[36] plat.[193]
- ➤ children, about, danger, in: ozone[227]
- ➤ children, about, rescuing them: cass.[36] ***hydrog.***[222]
- ➤ children, wanted to save asphyxiated: cass.[36]
- ➤ danger: aloe am-c. anac. ***ars.*** ars-met.[36] bell. calc-f. calc-p. ***cann-i.*** carbn-s. chin. con. graph. ***hep.*** hydrog.[222] indg.[10] iod. kali-bi. kali-c. kali-i. kali-n. ***lach.*** linu-c.[36] lyc. macrin.[36] mag-c. mag-m.[1] mag-s. mang. nat-c. nat-s.[10] nux-v. ozone[227] phos. psor. puls. ran-b. rumx. sin-a.[36] sul-ac.[1] sulph. tarent. thuj.
- ➤ danger, death, of: bell.[5] mag-m.[10] mang.[36] ran-b.[10] sul-ac.[5] sulph.[5] thuj.[5]
- ➤ danger, drowning, of: bov.[36]
- ➤ danger, escaping from a: hep.
- ➤ danger, escaping, fruitless efforts of: ind.[54]
- ➤ danger, impending: calc-f.[36] nat-c.[36]
- ➤ danger, passing forms, from: kali-c.[36]
- ➤ danger, perils, of encountered: cann-i.[54]
- ➤ danger, want, and: am-c.[54]
- ➤ driving, up a steep rough track: lap-mar-c.[194]
- ➤ drowning, danger of: bov.[36]
- ➤ falling, danger of: alum.[36] am-m.[36] macrin.[36]
- ➤ fire, danger, of: ant-t.[36] bell.[36] clem.[36] merc-acet.[36]
- ➤ hiding from danger, of: lyc.[1]
- ➤ slopes: anac.[10]
- ➤ somersaults, of throwing, at an old man: zing.[36]
- ➤ survival, of: ozone[227]
- ➤ unsuccessful efforts to, escaping from danger, of: ind.

➤ water, danger from: ars. ars-met.[54] ***graph.*** kali-n. ***mag-c.*** mag-m.[1] merc. merc-acet.[10] nat-c.[1] sulph.
➤ water, sailing, dangerous sailing in a small boat: nat-m.[36]
➤ water, swimming in, get out, and cannot: sol-t-ae.[36]
➤ water, wading in, serpents, in which are, of which he is afraid: alum.
➤ wood, being floated down and fearing damage: nat-s.[36]
Fancies; dangerous: raph.[36]
Fear; corners, to walk past certain: ***arg-n. kali-br.***
✦ danger, impending, of: aether camph.[54] caust.[54] choc.[222] ***cic.***[54] cimic. ***cocc.***[54] kali-br.[25] macrin.[36] meli.[85] nat-m.[172] samb.[172] samb-c.[36] sanic.[171]
✦ danger, impending, of, going to sleep, on: coff.
✦ danger, impending, of, night: aether[36] carb-ac.[172]
✦ danger, of impending, urging to stool, with: ***caust.***[54]
✦ fire, catch, things will: cupr. ***cupr-acet.***[54] hep.[187] lyss.[172] onos.[172] psor.[56] stram.[58]
✦ room, entering, on: alum. lyc. plat. til. ***valer.***
Fearlessness; danger menaced him, as if, but without fear: fl-ac.[54]
Runs; about, dangerous place, in most: agar.[36]
Shrieking; calls someone: aloe[130] ***bell.***[5] kali-c.[5] ***plat.***[5]
Shrieking; help, for: camph.[36] ***ign.***[8] kali-c.[1] ***laur.***[54] lepi.[36] levo.[149] plat.

ADAM. Sh, 438 - Nearly backed into another car, which was double-parked, although checking very carefully. Felt as if I was going to have an accident. Didn't feel safe. 6, 30C, 01:16:XX
AGAR. Al, 22 - Some run and walk involuntarily in the most dangerous places.(defiant)
ALUM. Ha, 18 - Restlessness in the evening, as if evil was imminent.
AM-C. He, 5 - Gloomy, depressed, with feeling of impending trouble,...
ANAC. Al, 15 - The future appears dangerous to him, as if nothing but misfortune and danger were reserved for him; want of confidence in his strength (vigor, force) and despondency.
Ha, 8 - The future seems to him very dangerous, as if nothing were imminent but misfortune and danger; distrust in his own power, and despondency.
ANDROC. Sh, 19 - Feeling of separateness, usual sense of urgency gone. (15)
BAR-A. Al, 8 - Solicitous (careful) and fearful. The slightest noise in the street seems to him like a fire alarm, and he is frightened thereat, so that he starts in every limb.
BAR-C. Ha, 11 - Anxious and fearful; a little noise on the street seems to him at once like fire alarm, and he is frightened by it, so that it darts (move quickly) through all his limbs.
CALC. He, 8 - Mind full of concern about imaginary things that might happen to her. 0 Chlorosis.
CAMPH. Al, 46...I started up, ran out, and fell prostrate, with a loud shriek for help, not far from the door of a neighbor....
Al, 46-...I shriek and call for help, because it seems that a murderer stands at my bed side...
He, 45 - Cries for help, takes hold of others, will not be left alone.
He, 61 - Felt a vague sense of impending danger to life,...
CAUST. Al, 24 - Anxious apprehension lest something evil should happen, with urging to stool.
He, 43 - Apprehension of impending danger, with urging to stool.
CHIN. Al, DREAM .[1105]-...;he imagines he is descending a precipice, on which account he awakes, but the dangerous place remains vividly before his fancy...Al, 1109 - At night frightful dreams of falling from a height, whith waking full of uneasiness...
CHOC. Sh, 73 - Feel I have to be alert, as if my total survival depended on me being alert —exhausting.
Sh, 90 - Concentration very sharp, as if my survival depended on it. I felt very focused. (During a lecture) My understanding was sharper. Normally I have many things going on in my head —too scattered — but in the last few days, narrower attention.
CIC. Ha, 231 - Excitement, with concern for the future, he represented to himself as dangerous everything that would happen to him.

He, 35 - Excited, with apprehension concerning the future; everything that could befall him seemed to be dangerous.

COCC. He, 27 - Apprehensive mood; fears death and unknown dangers.

COLCH. He, 5 - Says nothing unless questioned, his condition does not seem to him dangerous. 0Typhus.

CON. He, 31 - Great anxiety; precordial anguish; superstitious (careful, credulous, naive) and full of fear (coward), with frequent thoughts of death...

FL-AC. Al, 13 - Sensation as if dangers did menace (threaten) him, but without being afraid;...

He, 12 - Sensation as if danger menaced (threatened) him, but without fear. (fearless)

GELS. He, 33 - Effects (ailments from) of grief; cannot cry; when thinking of his symptoms (disease), also when spoken to of his loss ; >from diverting talk; oppression and palpitation of heart; feels a sense of peril (danger, harm, risk) ; face flushed; sleeplessness; subdued (subjugate, yielding) manner; ...

HALI-L. Sh, 512 - Feeling slightly hysterical, on and off through the day, as if disconnected and fragile. Not an overpowering sensation, but distinct. It was a sensation as if some danger was near. 04, 30C, 01:XX:XX

Sh, 664 - Feel deflated, calmer and flatter. The feeling of going mad goes back to when I was drinking 15 years ago. That feeling of not being able to decide what to do. Today feeling flat, exhausted; a wonderful day outside, unable to enjoy it. Feeling unenergized, although glad the craziness is gone. I felt I was on speed with emotions. I'm glad I antidoted that thing; feel like an empty balloon. It could have gotten down to a dangerous place. Reminded me of going mad; like the energy it gave me. Felt hooked on the remedy. 02, 30C, 12:XX:XX

HAM. Al, 15 - Was afraid to risk (danger) another dose (medicine); his mind was in a fearful condition.

HYDROG. Sh, 250 - I think I'm dangerous to people and they can't cope with me. 16, 30C, XX:XX:XX

HYOS. Ha, 485 - He is in danger of becoming senseless.

IBER. Al, 2 - Feels frightened; ...as if she had taken a dangerous dose.(medicine)

KALI-BR. Al, 3-...his character also had undergone a radical change, from having been very frank and brave, he had become excessively timid, and suspicious of every trifling circumstance; ...several times he attempted to throw himself from a window and battered down a door with an axe, in order to escape from some imaginary danger;...

MACRO. Al, 4 - Fear of impending danger.

MAG-C. Al, 936 - Dream of the dangerous carrying of glasses.

Al, 943 - Dream of danger by water.

MED. Al,N-41 - Constant state of anguish. Always a feeling of impending danger, but knows not what. There is no cause for such feelings, as she is not obliged to do anything when disinclined; is so situated that nothing need cause her trouble.

MERC. He, 34 - Inexpressive pain of soul and body, anxious restlessness, as if some evil impended ...; disgusted (revolt) with himself, has not courage (cowardice) to live; constant suspicion (distrust), considering everybody his enemy.

NAT-C. Al,DREAM, 1111 - Dream of a flood (current, inundate), and threatening danger.

NUX-M. Al, 60 - State of mind similar to that of the opium-eater, entertaining no apprehension of the result, although aware of the presence of some danger.

He, 26 - Aware of danger, but no apprehension.

NUX-V. Al, 41 - Anxiety; an anxious solicitude, as though something serious (dangerous) were dreaded, in the morning and afternoon..

Al, 54 - She was in great alarm, kept fast hold on her husband and refused to let him go.

Ha, 1235-...anxiety and anxious solicitude (care), as if something important were to be feared (afraid).

OP. He, 20-...declares he is not alone in bed; ..desire to escape; says a regiment of horsemen are upon his bed and that he fears to be trodden upon (run over, crushed); when told that horses are very careful, answered that he feared he would be crushed by the wagons that followed them.

PLB. Al, 23-...His delirium turned chiefly upon the idea that his life was in danger from assassination or poisoning, and that every one about him was a murderer...
He, 13 - Thought his life was in danger from assassination or poison and every one about him was a murderer.

RAPH. Al, 7-...dangerous fancies assail (attacks) her, but she restrains (suppress) herself from putting them into execution.

SAMB-C. Al, 1-...an indefinable fear as if the horse (a very gentle animal) might run away, or the wagon break at any moment; a dread of some undefined danger.

SPONG. Ha, 382 - Anxious as if misfortune (disaster) threatened (endangered) him and he had a foreboding of it.

STRAM. Al, 24 - Much excited and rather delirious, under the impression of some immediate danger, clinging to the person who had him in her lap.
Al, 53-...throw the hands about the head as if attempting to ward off some threatening evil;...escape from the imaginary object ...
He, 85-...seemed to dread approach of some imaginary monster, and giving utterance to most piteous appeals for help.

SULPH. Al, 3802 - Frightful, anxious dreams of danger of death, and of dead people.

VALER. Al, 1 - Extremely delirious, attempting to get out of the window, ... imagined himself away from home, and beset (surrounded) with all sorts of danger, from which he was attempting to escape, although unable to walk without staggering from side to side.

DARK

Anxiety; dark, in: aeth. aur-i.[58] calc.[116] carb-an.[116] carb-v.[58] hypoth.[149] kali-c.[144] nat-m. phos. ***puls.*** rhus-t. **STRAM.**[122] zinc.[116]

Black and somber, everything that is, aversion to: ant-t.[54] rob. stram. ***tarent.***

Concentration, difficult; dark before eyes on attempting: arg-n.

Darkness; agg.: acon. ***aeth.*** am-m.[111] ars. bapt. berb. ***calc.*** camph. ***carb-an. carb-v. caust.*** cupr. graph. hell.[111] ***lyc.*** nat-m. ***phos.*** plat. ***puls.*** rhus-t. sanic. sec.[111] sil.[162] **STRAM.** stront-c.[111] ***valer.*** zinc.[116]

Darkness; amel.: anh.[119] coca[15] con.[137] ***euph.***[137] graph.[137] phos.[137] ***sang.***[137]

Darkness; aversion to: carb-v.[102] sanic.[122]

Darkness; desire for: achy.[149] bry.[58] choc.[222] coca[107]

Darkness; desire for, lie down in the dark and not be talked to, to: aur.[162] aur-m.[162] bry.[162] tarent.

Delirium; dark, in: ***calc-ar. carb-v. cupr. stram.***

Delirium; groping as if in the dark: plb.[36]

Delusions; animals, black, on walls and furniture, sees: bell. stram.[162]
• animals, cats, see, black: bell. puls.
• animals, dark colored: bell.
• animals, dogs, black: ***bell.*** puls.[10]
• animals, snakes, black: arg-n.[5] cund.[111]
• black objects and people, sees: **BELL.**[5] cocc.[5] op.[10] ***plat.***[5] ***puls.***[5] stram. tarent.[185]
• black, thunder sits within her: androc.[222]
• body, black, is: sulph.
• cellar, he is shut in a dark: nat-p.[139]
• clouds, enveloped her, heavy black: arg-n.[102] ***cimic. lac-c.***[102] puls.[102]
• dark: carb-v.[10] cimic.[5] 0form.[5] **STRAM.**[54]
• dark, objects and figures, sees: cimic.[116]
• dragged from the lowest abyss of darkness (at night, on waking): thea.
• faces, dark, in the: chin. **LAC-C.**
• figures, large black, about to jump on him: mosch.
• flying, he is, rock into dark abyss, from a, on going to bed: cann-i.
• images, black: arn. ars. ***bell.*** caust. hydrog.[222] op. plat. puls. **STRAM.**
• images, dark, in the: ***bell. carb-v.*** hell. petr. puls. stram.
• snow, sees black snow blankets: ozone[227]
• spectres, sees, death appears as a gigantic black skeleton: crot-c.
• visions, horrible, dark, in the: ***bell. carb-v.*** hell. petr. puls. stram.
• walk, someone walks behind him, dark, in the: ferr. sanic.

Dreams; actors, turning black, green and yellow: sol-t-ae.[36]
➤ animals, birds, of, large, black: choc.[222]
➤ animals, black: arn.[10] ***puls.***
➤ animals, cats, black: arn.[36] daph.
➤ animals, dogs, black: ***arn.*** puls.[1] tub.[193]
➤ animals, dogs, frightened by a black dog: puls.
➤ animals, horses, black, with a big white spot on chest: ozone[227]
➤ animals, horses, fearing to be bitten by a ferocious black: phos.[36]

➤ black forms: arn. ars. op.[102] puls.
➤ black, forms, darkening the sun: ped.[36]
➤ black, spots in white bathtub: ozone[227]
➤ darkness: ars. aur. choc.[222]
➤ darkness, being in, all night: aur.[36]
➤ fights, generals, with six or seven black, who garroted him and bound him with ropes, causing agony of mind: coca[36]
➤ ghosts, black: ars. cerv.[36]
➤ houses, tarring the floor: ozone[227]
➤ men, dressed in black: cerv.[36]
➤ monstrous, figure, black, that flew up to sky and darkened the sun: ped.[36]
➤ people, black: cimic.[56]
➤ water, black: ***ars.*** lac-c.[193] ozone[227]

Fear; alone, of being, darkness, in: camph.[54] kali-br.[137] kali-p.[172] puls.[212] rad-br.[102] valer.[137]
✦ animals, dogs, black: bac.[149] ***bell.***[54] ***stram.***[54]
✦ animals, venomous, of, at night: abel.[149]
✦ bed, of the, dark, in: carb-v.[127] caust.[47]
✦ black or dark colors, everything: ars.[172] rob. **STRAM.**[122] tarent.[172] verat.[172]
✦ closing eyes, on, lest he should never wake: aeth. ***carb-an. caust.***
✦ danger, impending, of, night: aether[36] carb-ac.[172]
✦ dark: ***acon. aeth.***[122] am-m. arg-n.[137] ars.[58] bapt. bell.[122] brom. calad.[122] ***calc.*** calc-acet.[36] calc-ar.[36] calc-p. calc-s. ***camph.*** **CANN-I.** ***cann-s.***[5] ***carb-an. carb-v.*** carc.[119] caust. chin.[10] chin-s.[162] ***cupr.*** dys-co.[136] gaert.[136] gall-ac.[162] gels.[122] ***grin.***[122] hyos.[102] kali-bi.[122] kali-br.[25] kali-s.[127] lac-c.[56] ***lyc.*** manc.[162] ***med.*** morg.[111] nat-m.[122] nux-m.[122] nux-v.[162] op.[102] ozone[227] ***phos.*** prot.[136] ***puls.*** rad-br.[102] rhus-t. ***sac-alb.***[210] sanic. sep.[127] sil.[122] **STRAM.**[122] ***stront-c.*** sulph.[212] syc-co.[136] tub.[212] tub-k.[70] valer. xan.[111] zinc.[116]
✦ dark, stool and urine, with urging for: ozone[227]
✦ death, noise of door moving, from, in dark: ozone[227]
✦ ghosts, night: ***acon.*** ars. ***carb-v.*** chin. chin-ar.[58] cocc.[1] ***lyc. puls.*** ran-b. ***sulph.***
✦ injured, of being, dark, in: arn.[172] stram.[172] valer.[172]
✦ out of doors, to go, darkness, in, alone: acon.[172]
✦ poisoned, night: ars-met.
✦ robbers, of, midnight, on waking: ars.[172] ***ign.*** nat-m.[1] sulph.
✦ robbers, of, night: cupr.[172] lach.[30]
✦ shadows, of: acon.[137] adax.[96] calad.[137] ***calc.***[5] caust.[47] phos.[30] staph.[137] xan.[111]
✦ suffocation, closing eyes, on: carb-an.
✦ suffocation, dark, in the: aeth.[162]
✦ suffocation, night: agar. ***ant-t.***[122] arn. ars. aur-m.[122] cact. ***chin.***[122] ***dig.***[54] ip.[85] ***lyc.***[54] med.[122] ***puls.***[122] sil.[1] ***spong.***[54] ***sulph.***[122]
✦ tunnels, no light in carriage, with, may cause fainting: stram.[85]
✦ tunnels, of: acon.[162] arg-n.[162] cimic.[172] lyc.[162] nat-m.[172] **STRAM.**[122] succ.[172]

Groping as if in the dark: croc. hyos. op. plb.

Hypochondriasis; weather, in cloudy: aloe[54]

Inconsolable; alone and darkness agg.: stram.

Light; shuns light: achy.[149] ambr. androc.[222] bell.[58] **CON.** hyos. plat.[193] stram.[58] tarent.[5] zinc.

Light; subdued light agg.: nat-s.[137]

Sadness; darkness: am-m.[116] ars.[116] calc. calc-sil.[58] camph. ***phos.*** plat. rhus-t. stram.

Sadness; gloomy: anac.[10] ant-c.[10] ars.[10] aur.[10] bov.[5] calc.[10] cupr.[5] graph.[5] lach.[10] merc.[10] nux-v.[10] sep.[5] sulph.[10]

Sadness; weather, cloudy, in: aloe[140] am-c. bac.[62] plat.[193] sep.[193]

Twilight; agg. mental symptoms: acon.[162] am-m.[116] ambr. androc.[222] ant-c. ars.[8] berb.[5] brom.[127] ***calc.***[5] carb-v. caust.[5] dig. ign. kali-i. lap-c-b.[194] laur. mag-c. nux-v. ***phos.***[5] plat.[116] ***puls.***[5] rhus-t.[5] sep. valer.[116]

ACON. Al, 66 - Great timidity after a severe fright (fear), afraid to go out unattended (abandoned, helplessness) after dark, is unable to control his feelings of apprehensive fear.
He, 36 - Extreme timidity, especially after a fright; afraid (fear) in dark.
He, 51 - Ailments from fright: afraid (fear) in dark; vertigo; faintness; trembling; cardiac weakness; threatened miscarriage (abortion); impending cessation of menstrual flow;..

ACT-SP. He, 14 - Fear of death, especially at night in bed.

ADAM. Sh, 44 - Attracted to dark night skies. Stars seem more visible. 16, 12C, 23:XX:XX

ANAN. Al, 4 - Hypochondria, with dread (fear) of society (people); he seeks solitude and obscurity; does not want to see or hear anything.

ANDROC. Sh, 129 - It seemed as though he was a different person, very similar to the way he had been in adolescence, but in a much more powerful manner. These emotions were so intense he wanted to rip his chest apart to let them out. He lost all control over his emotions, which seemed to come from a deep and distant part of himself, a darker side. He desired to continue the proving for the rest of his life. (29)

ATRO. Ha, 17 - Sad and morose, preferring solitude and a dark room to society of friends.

AUR. He, 41 - All the time a dark, hopeless mood, frequently anxiety and despair; life is a burden (load) to him.

BELL. Ha, 1433 - Fearful madness; he is afraid (fear) of an imaginary black dog, of the gallows. (hanging)

He, 106 - Anxiety and fear of imaginary objects and hallucinations, ghosts, soldiers which come to take them away (arrest), black animals, rats dogs, wolves, etc.

He, 13 - Timorous anxiety; he is afraid of a an imaginary black dog; of the gallows, etc.

He, 105 - Anxiety and fear of imaginary objects and hallucinations, ghosts, soldiers which come to take them away, black animals, rats, dogs, wolves, etc.

BOV. Al, 9 - Anguish; she felt as if enveloped in a black vapor. (cloud, fog)

CALC-A. Al, 5 - Anxious thoughts, which came and went, before going to sleep in the evening; with which the objects seemed like different (strange) objects; he dreaded (fear) the dark, and made an effort to look at the light; all of which was relieved after the passage of flatus.

CAMPH. Al, 37 - Excessively fearful, especially in the dark.

Al, 38 - Dread of being alone in the dark.

Al, 40 - Afraid of the mirrors in the room, lest he should see himself in them; so excessive was this fear at times in the night that he would have got up and broken the mirrors, only that he was still more afraid to get up alone in the dark;...

Al, 46-... The sight increased my despair poor nature extinguished; the sky transparent and lifeless; the earth was still in the dim, dead light. I could not bear it. The sense of touch was gone, and my eyes protruded from their sockets.

He, 62 - Dread of being alone in dark.

He, 63 - Afraid of mirrors in room, lest he should see himself in them (reflection) ; so excessive was his fear at times in night that he would have got up and broken mirrors, only that he was still (but) more afraid to get up alone in the dark.

CANN-I. Al, 25-...Now demoniac shapes clutched (grasp) at him from the darkness, cloaked (covered) from head to foot in inky (black) palls (mantle), glaring (staring, looking) at him with fiery eyes from beneath their cowls(mantle)....

CARB-AN. He, 9 - Fearful in the dark.

CHIN-S. Al, 20-...; felt a gloom (darkness) come over me, as if some evil were impending; relieved by a specific trust in the Almighty;...(divine) (faithful, confiding, devoted)

CHIN. He, 28 - Dread of dogs and other animals at night.

CHOC. Sh, 9 - Had a vivid dream of worms —they were dark and fat, but I wished they were red and thin. I felt very excited by the worms.

Sh, 44 - Dream —coming out of the station a huge black bird the size of a dog with black long soft feathers like those of an ostrich, and a very big beak. It took my left hand in his beak. There were two gypsies there and they stood in front of me and opened their hands and I saw that they held a gold metal flat fish which I saw as a fortune telling object.

Sh, 50 - Panic feeling of being trapped and enclosed —worse when curtains are closed and the light blocked out. Strong desire to be outside and moving, to be in the bright and warm sunlight. Kept having to move my feet, which I felt I wanted to move.

Sh, 62 - The blackness of the trees is bothering me. They seem dark and leafless.

Sh, 110 - I really like my nose. It feels more useful in the dark.

Sh, 146 - I find dark exciting and comfortable, whereas before I was fearful in the dark.

CIMIC. He, 1 - Sensation as if a heavy black cloud (smoke) had settled (descent) all over her, and enveloped (surrounded, wrap) her head, so that all was darkness and confusion, while, at the same time, it weighed (heavy) like lead (metal) on her head.

CROT-C. Al, 1 - Magnetic state; she hears nothing, and again sees the spectre of death, as a gigantic black skeleton.

CUPR. He, 5 - Delirium: afraid of every one who approached him, shrinking (retire) away from them; tries to escape; in evening and in the dark.

FORM. Al, 5-...sudden but momentary spells of unhappiness; everything looks dark.(obscure)

HALI-L. Sh, 648 - Down side, dark side, feels like the gates between the unconscious and conscious are open. Hurricane-like feeling of unconscious energy. Like the gates of hell are open. No barrier. Extreme amount of power. Darkness. Internal pressure. Dogs guard the gates of Hades. A lot of internal pressure-type feeling all day. 13, 30C, 10:XX:XX

HYDROG. Sh, 27 - There is a very fine line at this time between enlightenment and insanity — a split consciousness. The dark side is horrendous, but the positive side of the proving has been well worth it. The positive aspects are beautiful. Its a shame we need to come down. I guess the price of going into the heavens is a trip to hell. 16, 30C, XX:XX:XX

Sh, 164 - Delusion —saw black masses. 24, 30C, 100:XX:XX

IGN. He, 2-...;sees everything as if through a fog (obscurity) ; sits quietly, with a vacant gaze (expression), always thinking of the mortification endured,... prefers to be alone; thinking of the past mortification...0Melancholy after mortification.

LAC-C. He, 15 - Sensation or delusion as if surrounded by myriads of snakes, some running like lightning up and down inside the skin ; some that are inside feel long and thin; fears to put her feet on floor, lest she should tread (walk) on them and make them squirm (shake) and wind (round) around her legs; is afraid to look behind her, for fear that she will see snakes there, does not dream of them and is seldom troubled with them after dark; on going to bed she was afraid to shut her eyes for fear that a large snake, the size of her arm, would hit her in the face.

LYC. Al, 51 - In the evening, in the dark, he is seized with fear when a door that he wishes to open moves with difficulty.

Ha, 26 - In the evening in the dark, he is frightened because a door he wants to open, opens with difficulty. (confined, restricted)

MED. Al,N-44 - The impatience, excitement, wild feelings; the unreal, dazed condition; the gloom (sadness) and fear in the dark;... are marked evidence of functional derangement of the nervous system.

He, 34 - Fear of the dark.

NAT-M. Al, 62 - Woke at 2A.M. in perspiration, and with a distressing anxiety, as though he were shut up (lock) in a dark cellar; this sensation only disappeared on perceiving light through the window.(confined, restricted, incarcerated)

PETR. He, 5 - Since confinement two weeks ago when in bed, in dark room, at night, delusion that there is another baby (small, tiny) in bed which requires attention also that she has a third leg which would not remain quiet.

PH-AC. Ha, 40 - While reading, a thousand other thoughts crowd into his mind (dispersion) ; he could not comprehend anything, what he read was dark to him, and he forgot everything at once, with difficulty in recollecting what he had known a long time already. (lost: memory, concentration, comprehension, knowledge)

PHOS. Al, 40 - As the darkness of night began to enclose (surround) the earth, my peace was disturbed by the most frightful visions and thoughts; constant fear of death, with an almost uncontrollable desire to commit suicide.

POLYG-H. He, 2 - Gloomy (dark) views of life, dislike of change (evolution, transformation) and excessive dread (fear) of death.

ROB. Al, 7 - Dread of everything that is somber and black.

SEP. Al, 1 - So excited from anger that she fears an apoplectic fit; everything becomes black (evil) before the eyes.

Ha, 51-(Ailments) From vexation, she is so

excited that she fears an apoplectic fit, and everything turns black before her eyes.

STAPH. Ha, 703 - Anxious thoughts and things long past come before him as if they were actually present and stood before him, which causes anxiety and the sweat of anguish -Then blackness comes before his eyes; he knows not if what he sees is true (real) or deception (false, unreal), then he regards (suppose) everything as something different to what it is (strange), and he loses all wish to live. (lost; discernment, perception)

STRAM. Al, 206 - Fear of being in the dark and a less extent of being alone, in the evening after sunset.

He, 14-...thoughts of dying;...fear of wild animals and black dogs.

He, 79 - Boy seemed to see black objects, spoke of black people and black clouds, and grasped at air.

He, 94-...fear of malicious animals, black dogs; ...

SYPH. Al,N-12 - Terrible dread (fear) of night, ...death is preferable ; she fears to prepare for night and is positively in abject fear of suffering,...

THUJ. Al, 49 - Sudden rising of dark thoughts (pessimism) causing uneasiness, apprehension (foreboding) of misfortune, with fancied scruples of conscience, ...

VALER. Al, 12 - Fearfulness in the evening when sitting in the dark (imagining that some one might hurt him).

He, 7 - Fear, especially evening in dark,...

DEATH

Ailments from; death, child, of a: calc.[58] caust.[30] ***gels.***[54] **IGN.**[54] ***kali-br.***[54] lach.[30] nat-m.[85] nux-v.[30] ph-ac.[30] plat.[85] staph.[30] sulph.[30]

Ailments from; death, one death after another: ambr.[58]

Ailments from; death, parents or friends, of: ambr.[58] ars.[184] calc.[58] **CAUST.**[30] **IGN.**[122] kali-br.[137] 0nat-m.[184] nit-ac.[54] nux-v.[30] plat.[85] staph.[30]

Anguish; loss of his friend, from: calc.[172] ign.[172] **NIT-AC.**[54]

Anxiety; alone, as if, and all about were dead and still: ***rhus-t.***[54]

Anxiety; sitting, bent over, while, anxiety with fear of death: rhus-t.

Anxiety; sleep, before, fainting would return, as if, and he would die: ***caust.***[54]

Brooding; constantly over loss of a child: ***gels.***[54] ***kali-br.***[54]

Cheerfulness; death, while thinking of: aur.

Death; contempt of, in mental derangement: ***op.***[54]

Death; conviction of: alum-p.[58] ars-h.[54] bapt.[122] bell.[54] ***canth.***[54] ***coff.***[54] ***cupr-acet.***[54] hydr.[137] kali-ar.[58] ***phyt.***[54] ***psor.***[54] ***thuj.***[54]

Death; conviction of, angina pectoris, in: ***ox-ac.***[54]

Death; conviction of, angina pectoris, in: ***ox-ac.***[54]

Death; conviction of, dyspnea, in: lach.[54] ***mosch.***[54]

Death; conviction of, epistaxis, in: ***croc.***[54]

Death; conviction of, erysipelas, facial, in: ***plat.***[54]

Death; conviction of, fever, after, epistaxis amel.: ***psor.***[54]

Death; conviction of, heart, in organic disease of: ***apis***[54]

Death; conviction of, illusions of fancy, with: merc.[54]

Death; desires: agn. alum.[30] alum-sil.[58] ambr.[5] anh.[144] ant-c.[58] apis aran. ars.[58] ars-met. ars-s-f.[58] **AUR.** aur-ar.[58] aur-m.[58] ***aur-s.***[58] bell. berb.[5] calc.[58] caps. carb-v. ***caust.***[122] chel. ***chin.*** clem. cortico.[144] der. euph-c.[116] ***gad.***[36] germ.[222] ***glon.***[54] hep.[5] hura hydr. kali-bi. kali-br. ***kreos.***[122] **LAC-C.** lac-d.[58] ***lach.*** led. lil-t. lyc. ***merc.*** merc-aur.[116] mez. nat-c. ***nat-m.*** nat-s. ***nit-ac.***[122] nux-v. op. orig.[25] ozone[227] phos. phyt. plat. plb. psor. puls.[30] ran-b.[58] rat.[116] ***rhus-t. rob.***[54] sec.[5] sep. ***sil.*** spong. staph. stram.[5] sul-ac. ***sulph.*** thuj. verat-v.[58] vip. xan.[111] zinc.[30]

Death; desires, alternating with laughing: aur.[10]

Death; desires, alternating with rage: bell.[10]

Death; desires, anxiety, anguish, from: acon.[137] bell.[1] caust.[1]

Death; desires, convalescence, during: absin. ***aur.*** lac-c. sep.

Death; desires, convulsions, during: absin.[36]

Death; desires, despair, from: agn.[100] ***kreos.***[116] ozone[227]

Death; desires, fear, with: aur.[122]

Death; desires, hypochondriasis, with: ***aur.***[54]

Death; desires, hysteria, in: ***aur.***[54]

Death; desires, meditates on easiest way of self destruction: lac-d.[8]

Death; desires, morning on waking: hydrog.[222] nat-c. phyt.

Death; desires, rage, during intervals from: bell.[54]

Death; desires, sadness, without, with disgust of life: rhus-t.[54]

Death; dying, fells as if: acon.[54] lyss.[54] ***sep.***[54] ***sil.***[54] ***ther.***[54] vesp.[54]

Death; presentiment of: **ACON.** aesc.[162] ***agn.*** aloe alum. alum-p.[58] anac. ***anthr.***[54] **APIS** ***arg-n.*** arn. ***ars.***[122] bapt. bar-m. **BELL.**[122] bry. ***cact.***[54] calc. cann-i. canth. carb-v.[58] ***cench. chel.*** cimic. cupr. dig.[36] ferr-br.[85] gels.[85] ***graph.*** hell.[36] ***hep.*** **HYDR.**[8] kali-ar. kali-br.[25] kali-c. kali-n. lac-d. ***lach.*** lob.[10] ***lyc.*** lyss.[54] ***med.*** **MERC.**[122] mosch. nat-m. ***nit-ac. nux-v.*** petr. ***phase.***[54] ***phos. plat.*** podo. ***psor.***[8] puls. ***raph.***[10] rhus-t. sep. staph. stram. sul-ac.[36] sulph.[122] tab.[10] thea.[122] verat. vip. zinc. zinc-p.[58]

Death; presentiment of, predicts the time: **ACON.**[122] agn.[162] ***aloe***[54] alum.[122] ***arg-n.*** cench.[58] hell.[58] ***lac-d.***[54] thea.[122]

Death; presentiment of, rejoices and gives directions about funeral: stram.[54]

Death; presentiment of, thinks of death calmly: zinc.

Death; presentment of, alternating with, anguish: raph.[54]

Death; presentment of, alternating with, rage: stram.[54]

Death; presentment of, fear without: lac-d.[85]

Death; presentment of, heart disease, in: ***op.***[54]

Death; presentment of, near, seems, and must settle affairs: petr.[137]

Death; presentment of, soon, believes that she will die, and cannot be helped: ***agn.***

Death; presentment of, sudden death, of a: ***cench.***[122]

Death; sensation of: aesc. aether[36] ***agn.*** anh.[119] apis[5] ***ars.*** camph. cann-i. cench. cic. ***ferr.***[54] gels.[85] ***graph.*** hydrog.[222] kali-br.[36] kali-n. **LAT-M.**[122] morph.[36] nux-v. op. ***phos. plat.*** sil. v-a-b.[149] verat. ***zinc.***[30]

Death; talks about: mosch.[58]

Death; thoughts of: **ACON.** agn. aloe[5] am-c. ***apis*** arg-n.[162] arn.[122] ***ars.*** ars-h.[54] aur.[116] aur-m.[162] camph. cann-i. carb-an. caust. ***cham.***[54] chel. clem.[36] ***coff.***[5] ***con.***[122] cortico.[119] cortiso.[119] ***crot-c. crot-h.*** cupr. ***dig.***[5] ferr. ferr-ar. **GRAPH.** hist.[119] hura hydrog.[222] kali-ar. kali-c. lac-d.[58] ***lach.***[54] lat-m.[119] ***lob.***[5] merc.[5] nux-v.[1] op. ozone[227] phos.[162] plat.[5] ***psor. puls.***[54] rauw.[119] rhus-t.[10] rob. spong.[10] stram. tarent. thuj.[36] verat. verat-v.[5] vinc.[10] ***zinc.***[122]

Death; thoughts of, alone, when: ***crot-c.***

Death; thoughts of, belonging to him, for those, with anxiety: ***ferr.***[54]

Death; thoughts of, calls his friends around and takes leave of them: acon.[172]

Death; thoughts of, calmly: zinc.

Death; thoughts of, fear, without: apis[5] ***coff.***[5] merc.[5] verat-v.[5]

Death; thoughts of, joy, give him: aur.[54]

Death; thoughts of, sadness, with: **GRAPH.**[54] vinc.[54]

Delirium; death, talks about: ***acon.***[54]

Delusions; accidents, fatal, he will have a: alum.[139]

- annihilation, about to sink into: calc.[1] cann-i. carbn-h.
- bells, hears ringing of, his funeral: aether.
- bier, is lying on a: anac. cann-i.
- body, alive, only half alive: crot-h.[36]
- body, shrunken, like the dead, is: ***sabad.***
- danger, life, to his: plb.
- dead, child was, her: ***kali-bi.***[54] kali-br.
- dead, corpse, absent acquaintance on sofa and has dread, of: ars.
- dead, corpse, brother and child, c. of: calc-sil.[58] con. plb.
- dead, corpse, husband: calc-sil.[58] plb.
- dead, corpse, mutilated: ant-c. arn. con. mag-m. merc. nux-v. sep
- dead, corpse, near him: anac.[1]
- dead, corpse, sister, of: agar.
- dead, corpse, tall yellow c. trying to share bed with him and promptly ejected: bell.
- dead, everything is: mez.
- dead, he is: anac. anh.[119] apis camph. cann-i. choc.[222] ***lach.*** mosch.[102] oena.[139] ***op.***[102] phos. raph.[139] sil.[139] stram.
- dead, mother is, his: lach. nat-m.[1]
- dead, persons, morning on waking, frightened by images of: hep.
- dead, persons, sees: agar. alum. am-c. ***anac.*** arg-n. arn. ***ars.*** ars-i. bar-c. bar-i.[58] ***bell.*** brom. bry. calc. calc-ar.[58] calc-i.[58] calc-sil.[58] canth. caust. cocc. con. fl-ac. graph. ***hep.*** hura ***hyos.*** iod. kali-ar. ***kali-br. kali-c.*** kali-p. kali-sil.[58] ***lach.*** laur. ***mag-c.*** mag-m. nat-c. nat-m. nat-p. nit-ac. nux-v. op. paull-p.[36] ***ph-ac. phos. plat.*** plb. ran-s. sars. sil. stram.[5] stry. sul-ac.

sul-i.[58] sulph. thuj. verb. zinc. zinc-p.[58]
• death approaching: agn.[85] ***plat.***[54]
• destruction of all near her, impending: ***kali-br.***[54]
• devoured, of being: cand-a.[239] ***stram.***[10]
• die, about to, will, thinks there is but little time to make his: ***petr.***[54]
• die, about to, exhaustion, from: lach.[139]
• die, about to, exhaustion, from, heart complaints, in: pop.[139]
• die, about to, friend was, his beloved: bar-c.[54]
• die, about to, he is: **ACON.** agn.[85] alum.[36] am-c.[139] ant-t.[139] apis[5] ***arg-n.*** arn.[58] ars.[58] asaf.[139] asar.[139] bac.[62] bar-c. bar-m.[58] bell.[116] cact.[54] calc.[30] cann-i. caps.[139] caust.[139] cench.[58] ***chel.*** chlf.[139] ***croc.*** cupr. gels.[139] glon.[139] graph.[139] hell.[1] iris-t.[85] kali-c. lac-d. ***lach.***[54] lil-t.[139] lyc.[54] lyss.[139] mag-p.[54] magn-gr.[139] med.[85] merc.[10] morph.[139] mur-ac.[139] ***nit-ac.*** nux-v. petr. phos.[36] ***plat.***[54] ***podo.*** psor.[139] pyrus[139] raph.[139] rhus-t. ruta[139] ***sep.***[54] sil.[139] stram. sulph.[139] thea.[139] ther.[54] ***thuj.*** thyr.[139] v-a-b.[149] vesp.[54] ***xan.***[54]
• die, about to, he is, tuberculosis, from: calc.[172] lac-c.[172] paull.[172] sep.[172] tarent.[172]
• die, about to, he is, while walking thinks he will have a fit or die, which makes him walk faster: ***arg-n.***
• die, about to, wishes someone would help her off: ***lach.***[54]
• die, time has come to: ars. bell. lach. med.[85] sabad. thuj.
• die, tuberculosis, from: calc.[172] lac-c.[172] paull.[172] sep.[172] tarent.[172]
• die, will, and soon will be dissected: cann-i.
• disease, throat disease, a horrible, which will end fatally: **SABAD.**[54]
• existence, exist any longer, she cannot: thuj.[139]
• funeral, preparations are made for: ***lach.***[54]
• grave, at a: gels.[8]
• grave, in his: anac.[149] lepi. stram.
• hang, wants to hang himself: ***ars.***[116]
• head, deceased acquaintances without bodies, h. of (at night): nux-v.
• heart, stitches in heart will kill him if they do not cease: psor.[54]
• person, coat, shroud, with: psil.[164]
• sick, a beloved friend is, and dying: bar-c.
• side, alive on one side and buried on the other, he is: stram.
• spectres, sees, death appears as a gigantic black skeleton: crot-c.
• starve, family will: ars. calc-sil.[58] ***sep.*** staph.
• starved, being: naja[36]
• talking, sister, with his dead: bell.[54] ***hyos.***[54]
• talking, sister, with his dead, churchyard, in: bell.[10]
• tetanus must die of, with pain in right leg: ***mag-p.***[54]
• wrong, giving wrong things to people, causing their death: sulph.[102]

Despair; death, separate him from his children, death will: bamb-a.[1184]
Despair; death, with fear of: **CALC.**[54]
Despair; unwilling to die, in hemoptysis: ***acal.***[54]
Dreams; accidents, fatal: cham.[54] **GRAPH.**[54] kali-m.[111] **NUX-V.**[54] sars.[54]
➤ animals, cows, dying: hydrog.[222]
➤ animals, dead: ptel.[36]
➤ body, embalmed: carb-ac.
➤ danger, death, of: bell.[5] mag-m.[10] mang.[36] ran-b.[10] sul-ac.[5] sulph.[5] thuj.[5]
➤ dead, people, of, friends long deceased: arg-n. cedr.[36] coca[36] con.[1] ferr. nat-c.
➤ dead, people, of, friends, talking with deceased: lepi.[36]
➤ dead, people, of, wife: aran-ix.[119]
➤ death of, acquaintance: nicc.[36]
➤ death of, brother: plan.[36]
➤ death of, family, in: plan.[36]
➤ death of, father: alumn.[36] hydrog.[222]
➤ death of, lasting after waking: alum.[36]
➤ death of, mother: chin.[36] mur-ac.[36]
➤ death of, one dear: lach.[36]
➤ death of, parents: cast.[36]
➤ death of, relatives: caust.[1] ferr. fl-ac. hydrog.[222] kali-c.[1] mag-c. mag-s. pitu-a.[164] rheum sars.
➤ death of, sister, of distant: plat.[36]
➤ death, approaching: kali-c. kali-chl. sil. ***sulph.*** tab.
➤ death, dying of: am-c. arn. bov.[10] brom. camph. carc.[227] chel. cocc.[10] cortico.[119] dulc. fl-ac. gels.[85] kali-chl.[10] ozone[227] prot.[136] rauw.[119] sulph. ***thuj.***
➤ death, dying, of, bed surrounded by friends, with his: arn.[36]
➤ death, dying, of, nervous fever, from: kali-chl.[36]

➤ death, far distant: mag-s.[36]
➤ death, friend, of a: allox.[119] bamb-a.[1184] coff. coff-t.[36] con. cortico.[119] fl-ac. kali-n. lach.[36] nicc.
➤ death, friend, of a, dear, which does not abate his mental exhilaration, looking at all with supernatural indifference: coff-t.[36]
➤ death, of: allox.[119] alum. alum-p.[58] alum-sil.[58] alumn. am-c. anac.[85] arn. ars. ars-s-f.[58] aur. aur-ar.[58] aur-s.[58] bell.[5] brom. ***calc.*** calc-f. calc-sil.[58] camph. carb-an.[1] carbn-s.[58] carc.[146] cast. chel. chin. chin-ar. chin-b.[54] chin-s. cocc. coff. con. cortico.[119] crot-c.[102] crot-h.[58] culx.[193] cyt-l.[119] ferr-i. fl-ac. gels.[85] grat. hura ***hydrog.***[222] kali-ar. kali-c. kali-chl. kali-n. kali-s. kali-sil.[58] **LACH.** lyc. mag-m. mag-s. merc-c. nat-m. nat-s.[10] nicc.[10] nit-ac. paeon. plan. plat.[10] raph. rat. rauw.[119] rheum[10] rhus-v. saroth.[119] sil. spong.[1] staph.[1] sul-ac.[5] ***sulph.*** tarent. thuj.[1] ven-m.[149]
➤ death, own, his, and orders the rapid removal of the corpse from the house: fl-ac. rauw.[119]
➤ death, relatives, of: alumn. aran-ix.[149] ***calc-f.*** cast. caust.[1] chin. choc.[222] fl-ac. grat. hydrog.[222] kali-c.[1] levo.[149] mag-s. mur-ac. nicc. paeon. plan. plat.
➤ death, that he is to die: arn.[54] lach.[58] nit-ac. sil.
➤ drowning, danger of: bov.[36]
➤ drowning, drowning man, of a: ***lyc.***[54] ***sil.*** sol-t-ae.
➤ dying: am-c.[54] brom.[54] cortico.[119] rauw.[119]
➤ electrocution, of: hydrog.[222]
➤ falling, high places, men are killed by falling from a height: sabin.[10]
➤ family, own, losing his: choc.[222]
➤ famine, being left in a dungeon to die of; escaping by crawling out: ped.[36]
➤ houses, cold, liveless, nearly threatening: ozone[227]
➤ killing: stram.[54]
➤ nuclear, explosion, about: ozone[227]
➤ piercing bodies of her children together: dict.[137] phos.[137]
➤ quarrels, dead relatives, with: cedr.[25] kali-c.[1]
➤ thrown from carriage, being, grave, into a: mag-c.[36]

Ecstasy; periodical, twice a day, seems to be dying: ***cic.***[54]

Fear; alone, of being, die, lest he: ***arg-n.*** **ARS.**[122] ***ars-h.***[122] bell.[58] ***kali-c. phos.***
✦ buried, alive: atro.[38] tub.[56] ***zinc.***[54]
✦ catalepsy, of: art-v.[172]
✦ cemeteries, of: stram.[187]
✦ death, abortion, abort, is sure she will: nux-m.[26]
✦ death, abortion, die from hemorrhage, is sure she will: ***acon.***[26]
✦ death, alone, evening in bed: act-sp.[162] ***ars. caust.***[54] kali-c.
✦ death, alone, when: ***arg-n. arn.***[122] **ARS.** ars-h. bell. camph.[172] caust.[172] ***kali-ar.***[184] ***kali-c.***[122] menis.[111] ***phos.*** tub.[108]
✦ death, alternate laughing and weeping, with (after anger): ***plat.***[54]
✦ death, anger, from: ***plat.***[54]
✦ death, angina pectoris, in: ***acon.***[54] ***dig.***[54] lat-m.[77] squil.[54]
✦ death, anxiety, with, heart and mind, of: ***psor.***[54]
✦ death, anxiety, with, praecordia, about: **ACON.**[8] ***plat.***[54]
✦ death, bed, fear of going to, with: ***lach.***[54]
✦ death, bed, going to, on: ars.[172] camph.[172] caust.[172]
✦ death, bed, in: nat-m.[1]
✦ death, cholera asiatica, in: ***cupr.***[54] ***cupr-acet.***[54] **VERAT.**[54]
✦ death, convalescence, during: tarent.[54]
✦ death, convulsions, during: acon.[54] kali-br.[54]
✦ death, delirious, from violent beating of carotid and temporal arteries: ***aur-m.***[54]
✦ death, delirium, in: ***acon.***[58] **STRAM.**[54]
✦ death, diarrhea, in: ***ham.***[54]
✦ death, die, fear he will, if he goes to sleep (after night-mare): aeth.[162] ***lach.***[54] led.
✦ death, dream, from: alum.[10] cench.[58]
✦ death, epistaxis. in: ***croc.***[54]
✦ death, excitement, with wild, begs to know if he is to die and before answer drops into heavy sleep: vario.[172]
✦ death, farewell messages, prepares: ***lyc.***[54]
✦ death, fever, during: calc. cocc. ip. mosch. ***nit-ac.*** **RUTA**
✦ death, fright, after: plat.[54]
✦ death, heart symptoms during, death, of instant, with cardiac distress: ***arn.***[54]
✦ death, heart symptoms during, organic: apis[54]
✦ death, heart symptoms, during: **ACON.**[54] ***ang.***[54] ***arn.***[54] asaf. cact.[58] carb-v.[58] cench.[58] **DIG.**[54] ***naja***[54] ***plat.***[54] ***psor.***[54]

✦ death, heat, during: acon.[85] calc. cocc. ip. mosch. ***nit-ac.*** **RUTA**
✦ death, hemoptysis, in: **ACON.**[54]
✦ death, hemorrhage, in uterine: acon.[54] coff.[54] nux-m.[54] **PLAT.**[54]
✦ death, hunger from: calc.[122]
✦ death, impending, of: acon.[30] agn.[48] ***am-c.***[54] ***ars.***[54] asaf.[54] **BELL.**[30] bry.[30] **CANN-I.**[54] caps.[54] carc.[207] ***caust.***[54] cimic.[48] ***croc.***[54] cupr.[30] glon.[54] lach.[30] ***lob.***[54] **MERC.**[30] nit-ac.[48] nux-v.[30] op.[122] **PHOS.**[54] plat.[172] sec.[48] sep.[30] staph.[30] v-a-b.[30]
✦ death, impending, of, reason, and loss of: ***plat.***[54]
✦ death, kill him, that those in the house might: ***cimic.***[54]
✦ death, lying down, on: act-sp.[162] mosch.[58]
✦ death, megrim, in: ***ars.***[54]
✦ death, metrorrhagia, in: ***coff.***[54]
✦ death, night, bed, in, drops into heavy sleep with loud breathing, before sentence is completed: vario.[54]
✦ death, noise of door moving, from, in dark: ozone[227]
✦ death, of: **ACON.**[122] act-sp. ***agn.*** all-s. aloe alum. alum-p.[58] am-br.[162] am-c. anac. anan. anh.[119] ant-c. ant-t. ***apis*** aran.[149] ***arg-n. arn.***[122] **ARS.**[122] ***ars-s-f.***[58] ars-s-r.[54] asaf. aur. aur-ar.[58] aur-s.[58] bapt. bar-c. bar-s.[58] ***bell.*** bol.[54] ***bry.*** bufo ***cact.*** calad. **CALC.** ***calc-ar.***[122] calc-f.[162] calc-s. camph. ***cann-i.*** cann-s.[5] canth. caps. carb-an.[10] carb-v.[58] carbn-s. carc.[207] ***caust.*** chel. chin.[5] **CIMIC.** ***cocc. coff.*** con. cop. croc. ***crot-c.*** culx.[58] ***cupr.*** cur. ***cycl. dig.*** diosm.[72] dros.[36] **ELAPS**[152] fago.[36] ferr. ferr-ar. ***ferr-p. fl-ac.*** **GELS.** glon. ***graph.***[122] ***hell. hep.*** hydr.[102] hydr-ac.[102] hydrog.[222] hyos. ign. iod.[5] iodof.[36] ip. iris kali-ar. ***kali-c.*** kali-fcy.[36] ***kali-i.*** kali-m.[192] ***kali-n.*** kali-p. kali-s. **LAC-C.** ***lach.*** lat-m.[122] led. ***lil-t.***[102] lob. ***lyc.*** mag-s. **MANC.**[184] med. ***merc.***[10] mit.[25] ***mosch.*** mygal. naja[98] nat-c.[10] ***nat-m.***[122] **NIT-AC.** nux-m. ***nux-v. op.*** ox-ac. ozone[227] petr. ***ph-ac.*** phase.[102] **PHOS.** phyt. **PLAT.** pneu.[149] podo. ***psor. puls.*** raph. rheum ***rhus-t.*** rob. ruta[5] sabad.[102] ***sec.*** sep. sium[36] ***spong.*** squil. stann.[102] staph.[102] still.[102] stram. sulph. syph.[102] tab. tarax. tarent. trach.[36] tril. trio.[25] vario.[36] ***verat.*** verat-v. vinc. visc.[119] zinc. zinc-p.[58]
✦ death, pain, from: anan.[36] cact.[58] **COFF.**
✦ death, paralysis, in: ***caust.***[54]
✦ death, predicts the time: **ACON.** apis[162] ***arg-n.***
✦ death, pregnancy, during: **ACON.**
✦ death, pressure in hypochondrium, with: ph-ac.[1]
✦ death, reason, and loss of: ***plat.***[54]
✦ death, sadness with: cupr.[137] ***plat.***[54] vinc.[54]
✦ death, scarlatina, after: ***hell.***[54]
✦ death, sleep, during: aeth.[193] ign.[193]
✦ death, sleep, falling asleep, on: ***nux-v.***[5]
✦ death, sleep, falling asleep, on, nightmare, after: led.[172]
✦ death, sleep, followed by deep: vario.[54]
✦ death, smallpox, in: ***ph-ac.***[54]
✦ death, soon, that she will die: ***agn.*** cench.[58] plat.[168] ***sep.***[30]
✦ death, soul were escaping from body, as if, with utmost terrible uneasiness: thuj.[172]
✦ death, starvation, from: ars.[137]
✦ death, strength, with loss of: ***rhus-t.***[54]
✦ death, sudden, of: ***arn. ars. cench.***[58] lat-m.[77] tab.[144] thea.
✦ death, suffocation, from: ***spong.***[54]
✦ death, suicidal tendency, with: **NUX-V.**[54] ***plat.***[54]
✦ death, talk of death when there is no serious complaint, with trembling and palpitation: mosch.[172]
✦ death, termination, of fatal: ant-t.[54] ***ph-ac.***[54] ***spong.***[54]
✦ death, vexation, after, in cholera Asiatic: **ARS.**[54]
✦ death, vomiting: ***ars.*** mag-c.[1]
✦ death, waking, on: alum. ***ars.***[54] con.[10]
✦ death, walking while: ***dig.***
✦ death, weary of life: ***kali-p.***[54] ***nit-ac.***[54] ***plat.***[54] ***rhus-t.***[54]
✦ death, wires encasing him, saw: ***cimic.***[54]
✦ death, with desire of: ***aur.***[54].
✦ disease, long spell of illness before dying, in old men: ***cic.***[54]
✦ disease, termination, of a fatal: ant-t.[54] calc.[172] kali-c.[172] lil-t.[172] ***ph-ac.***[54] sabad.[172] ***spong.***[54]
✦ heart, disease of, stitches will kill him if they do not cease: psor.[172]
✦ sleep, go to, lest, die, he would: ***lach.***[54] nux-m.[85]
✦ sleep, to go, lest, die he would, nightmare, after: ***led.***[54]
✦ talking, loud talking would kill her, that: meli.

✦ wrong, commit something, and kill herself: ***merc.***[54]
Inconsolable; heat, with, would rather die on the spot: spong.[54]
Indifference; dead, everything seems to him, nothing makes a vivid impression upon his mind: hydrog.[222] **MEZ.**[54]
Insanity; graveyards, visits: bell.[10] stram.[10]
Irritability; anxiety, with, suicide, with inclination to commit, afraid to die: **NUX-V.**[54]
Joy; death, when thinking of: aur.[54]
Laughing; alternating with, anguish, fear of death: ***plat.***[54]
Loathing; general, fear of death, during: cop.[36]
Prophesying; predicts the time of death: **ACON.** ***arg-n.***[122] thea.[122]
Rage; alternating with, desire for death: bell.[10]
Rage; alternating with, presentiment of death: stram.[54]
Sadness; asthma, with, die, thinks he will: ars.[102] phos.[54] psor.[102] spong.[54]
Sadness; disease, about, sure he, is going to die in twenty four hours: lac-d.[54]
Sadness; fear, with, death, of: cupr.[137] ***plat.***[54]
Shrieking; fear, with, death, of, as if in: chlol.[54]
Shrieking; fear, with, death, of, dry convulsive cough, from, in weak nervous children: ***kali-br.***[54]
Suicidal disposition; fear of death, with: alum.[54] **ARS.**[94] aur.[94] ***chin.***[30] hep.[94] kali-ar.[58] **NIT-AC.**[30] nux-v.[94] ***plat.***[54] rhus-t.[58] ***staph.***[30] tab.[36]
Talk; indisposed, die, as if he would: ***mur-ac.***[54]
Testament, refuses to make a: ***calc.***[30] hep.[30] nat-m.[30]
Weary of life; fear of death, but: ***kali-p.***[54] ***nit-ac.***[54] ***plat.***[54] ***rhus-t.***[54]
Weeping; thought of others grief at her own death: lap-c-b.[194]

ACON. Al, 56 - Anxiety he believes he will soon die.
Al, 59 - Feeling as if his last hour had come.
Ha, 538 - Dread of impending death.
Ha, 539 - Mortal anxiety recurring from time to time.
Ha, 540 - Lamentable fears of impending death.
He, 21 - Delirium, with talk about death.
He, 40 - Thrice he became blind and affirmed that death was at hand.
He, 41 - Predicts day of death; bids (offer) her friends good-bye.(farewell)
He, 39 - Fear of death; during pregnancy or confinement; with prolapsus uteri; with great loquacity or anxiety in region of heart.
ACT-SP. He, 14 - Fear of death, especially at night in bed.
ADAM. Sh, 308 - A conversation about death with my children. A feeling that they need some insurance; and I thought I would make a will, to make provisions for them, to clarify the situation. 2, 12C, 05:XX:XX
Sh, 374 - Joyless, desired death. Looked at a pair of scissors and thought of suicide. 16, 12C, 17:XX:XX
Sh, 436 - Very scared of driving in a car, obsessed with crashing and accidents and death. 20, 1M, XX:XX:XX
AESC. Al, 9-...he had a feeling as if death was impending (imminent); but this was followed by an exalted condition of brain and nervous system...
AGN. Al, 2 - He sometimes feels as if he were nobody (unimportant, insignificant, worthless), and would rather be dead than have that feeling; when possessed by that feeling he has no courage to undertake anything; and when free from it he feels exalted, would like to read like an orator, etc.
Al, 3 - She is very sad, and keeps repeating that she will soon die.
He, 3 - Low spirited, fears of approaching death.
He, 4 - Despairing sadness; keeps repeating that she will die, that there is no use doing anything.
ALOE. Al, 17 - Great anxiety, timorousness, restlessness, dread (fear) of death, and great anguish, so that she cannot stay anywhere.(restlessness)
He, 2 - She knew she would die in a week. (predicts, death)
ALUM. He, 21 - Dread (fear) of death, with thoughts of suicide.
AM-C. Al, 22 - At night, attack of great anxiety, as if she had to die, ... she was unable to move her eyes or to speak,...

Al, 7 - Very weeping mood, with thoughts of death.
Ha, 3 - Very lugubrious (sad), with thoughts of death.
AMBR. Al,N-8 - Great sadness; despondent, does not want to live.
ANAC. Al, 8 - Melancholic illusion; he imagines a bier in the side room, upon which either his friend or himself is lying.
Ha, 46 - Melancholy dejection and imagination, as if there was standing in the adjacent room a bier, on which a friend or he himself was lying.
He, 57 - Apprehensive (fear) of death being close at hand.
He, 63 - Despondency (desperation) and fear of approaching death.
ANAN. Al, 2 - Sadness and restlessness, with fear of death and of the future.
Al, 17 - Persistent fear of death during all his sufferings.
ANT-T. He, 6 - Apathy and indifference to everything, even death would have been welcome.
ANTHR. Al,N-6 - Thinks she feels death approaching.
He, 5 - Thinks she feels death approaching.
APIS. Al, 12 - Dread (fear) of death, or sensation as if he should not be able to breathe again.
Al, 13 - Premonition of death arose after a few minutes; "he believes he is going".
Al, 15 - She thought she must die, she felt so strangely.(strange)
Al, 16 - He says, after a few minutes, "I am a dead man".
Al, 5 - Sad thoughts, with longing for death, forenoon.
He, 20 - Anticipation (intuition) of death.
He, 59 - Dread of death or sensation as if he should not be able to breath again.
He, 18 - Thinks he will die. 0 Organic disease of heart.
ARG-N. He, 13 - Frequently settle (decide, fix) upon time he should die. (death)
He, 15 - When walking gets nervous (anxiety), thinks he will have a fit (convulsion?) or die suddenly, which makes him walk faster,(rapid) but soon has to stop, because he gets tired.
He, 42 - Fits of despondency and all kinds of fanciful (unreal) notions for example, that whilst walking along street he could not pass a given point without falling; frequently settled on the time he was to die.
He, 48 - Great nervousness and prostration (lassitude); fears to be alone because he thinks he will die ; is apprehensive of some serious disease, which almost drives him to despair.
ARN. Al, 17 - Horror of instant death.
He, 11 - Mind clear like that of a clairvoyant; quiet countenance (expression), pale as chalk, thinks her death unavoidable.(inevitable)
He, 32 - Despondency and conviction of approaching death.
He, 36 - Horror of instant death. With cardiac distress in night.
ARS-H. Al, 1 - Anxiety he believes his death is near, and despairs of being better...
He, 13 - Afraid (fear) of being alone he thinks he will die.
He, 15 - Anxiety, he believes his death is near, and despairs of being better...
He, 14 - The fear of dying is gone on 3d day, notwithstanding all around him have doubts of his recovery.
ARS-MET. He, 6 - She would very much like to die, or fall asleep (sleep), never to awaken.
ARS. Al, 51 - He despairs and weeps and imagines no one can help him, that he must die;...(unprotected)
Al, 78 - Anxiety and fear; he sees a absent acquaintance (friend) lying dead upon the sofa, and has great dread of him.
Al, 91-...she was afraid (fear) of solitude and death; the slightest cause was sufficient to put her into anger and rage, which especially occurred when one spoke of her complete recovery which she considered wholly impossible.
Al, 83 - Dread of death coming on suddenly when alone, or on going to bed.
Al, 70 - The anxiety and restlessness are indescribable; "Kill me", he cried, "or relieve my pains!".(help)
Ha, 1021 - On account of increasing pains he appeared to lie at the last gasp (breath), with unspeakable anxiety.
Ha, 1035 - He is cold, shivers and weeps, and thinks, in his despair, (hopelessness, despairing) that nothing can help him,

(helplessness) and he must die; followed by general exhaustion.
Ha, 1057 - Uncommonly tranquil disposition; quite unconcerned about their approaching death, they neither hoped nor wished to recover.
Ha, 1065-...extreme anxiety, restlessness; he had a great dread (fear) of the effects of the poison and desired to life.
Ha, 33 - Anguish and fear; he sees an acquaintance who is not present lie dead on sofa, and is much afraid of him.
Ha, 44 - Desponding and weeping, he thinks that nothing can help him, and he would have to die anyhow; (in any way)...
He, 9 - Thoughts of death and the incurability of his complaint. 0Cancerous inoculation
He, 63 - Dread (fear) of death when alone, or on going to bed.
He, 15 - Thinks he must die.
ASAF. He, 5 - Anxious sadness and apprehensions (fear) of dying.
He, 8 - With heart symptoms, fear of death.
ATRO. Al, 25 - Insisted repeatedly that her blood did not circulate, and that her feet must put into warm or she should die.
AUR. Ha, 351 - Great weakness and anxiety, so that he is thought (delusion) to be near death.
Ha, 356 - Melancholy; he imagines he is unfitted (incompetent, unqualified) for the world ; he is filled (full) with intense delight when he thinks of death, so that he longs to die. (punishment)
Ha, 5 - Melancholy; he imagines that he is not fitted for the world, he therefore longs for death, of which he thinks with the most intense delight.
Ha, 7 - Great anxiety and weakness, so that he is thought to be near death.
He, 8 - Looks on dark side, weeps, prays, thinks she is not fit for this world, longs for death, strong inclination to commit suicide; desperate, desires to jump from a height.
He, 12 - Thinking of death, gives him intense joy.
He, 49 - Fearfulness, a longing for death. 0Hyperemia of brain.
BAPT. He, 19 - Hopeless (despair) of recovery, and certain (inevitable) of death.
BAR-A. Al, 10 - An evil, fearful suspicion suddenly takes possession of her, as if, for example, a loved friend had been taken suddenly deathly ill.
BAR-C. Al, 9 - Extremely despondent and depressed; she believes that she must die; cries.
Ha, 7 - An evil fearful foreboding comes suddenly upon his soul, as if, e.g. a beloved friend might suddenly have fallen fatally ill.
Ha, 17 - Extremely discouraged and pusillanimous ;(cowardice) she thinks she will die, and weeps.
He, 27 - She is suddenly overwhelmed with an evil apprehension; she imagines, for instance, that a beloved friend has suddenly fallen sick and is dying.
BAR-M. He, 11 - During an attack of fear, she says in a weak, husky voice, she must die.
BELL. Al, 170 - He feared that death was near.
Al, 153 - She is so anxious and confused that she fears she is about to die.
Al, 160 - In her momentary lucid intervals she complains of intolerable anguish, so that she wishes to die.
Al, 171 - She is so anxious and confused that she fears she is about to die.
Al, 162 - She begs the bystanders to kill her.
Al, 172 - She tries to strangle herself, and begs the bystanders to kill her, because she believes that she will certainly die.
Ha, 1325 - In the momentary intervals, when free from fury, complaints of intolerable anxiety, so that she wished to die.
Ha, 1431 - He fears death in night.
Ha, 1437 - She tries to strangle herself, and begs those about her to kill her, for this time she must die. (redemption, regeneration, salvation)
Ha, 1430 - So anxious and distracted (worried) that she apprehends the approach of death.
He, 49 - She rather (first) desires death than fears it.
He, 115 - Intolerable anguish during time she is free from rage, with desire to die.
He, 109 - Anxious and confused, fears she is about to die.
BRY. He, 29 - Fear of death, which he thinks is near.
He, 46 - Restlessness: wants change; with

fear of future; fear of death, which he thinks is near; with nocturnal heat.

He, 30 - Fear of death.

BUFO. Al, 7 - Desires solitude, and yet is afraid of being left alone and dying forsaken.

Al, 12 - He is anxious about the state of his health; is afraid he will die or that some other misfortune will happen to him.

Al, 22 - He is irritable, anxious about his state of health, with great dread of death.

He, 12 - Fear of disease, of animals, of death.

CACT. Al, 18 - Fear of death extreme and continuous; he believes his disease to be incurable.

He, 4 - Feels she is dying and thinks she will not live till morning, but has no fear of death. (fearless)

He, 14 - Fear of death; he believes his disease, incurable.

He, 16 - During and after attack, great anxiety, fearing some organic lesion of heart which will cause sudden death.

CALC-A. Al, 255 - Dreams of sick people, and dead people, with violent weeping in the sleep.

CALC. Al, 17 - She is very hypochondriac; she thinks that she is deadly sick, nevertheless can complain of nothing.

Al, 19 - She despaired of her life, and believed that she must die, with a most sad mood, and weeping, and frequent sudden attacks of general heat, as if hot water had been dashed over her.

Ha, 28 - Hypochondriac, she conceives herself fatally diseased, and yet cannot complain of anything.

Ha, 30 - She despairs of her life and believes she has to die (punishment?) ; her heart is sad with weeping, and frequent attacks of sudden, general heat, as if she had hot water poured (flow) over her.

He, 53 - Fear: of death; of consumption (decay, waste, tuberculosis); of misfortune (disaster) ; of being alone. (lonely)

He, 57 - Anxiety, shuddering and dread (fear) as soon as evening comes on, with fear of death ; torments those around him day and night.

He, 65 - Despairing; hopeless (unhappy, pessimistic) of ever getting well (health); with fear of death, tormenting all around day and night.

He, 38 - Low-spirited and melancholy, with weeping and despair of life.

CAMPH. Al, 46-..." I am death! No, I am not death! but indeed I must be dead!" And thus I flew round about myself like a top, with no other feeling than for the strong smell of the Camphor. The external world existed for me no longer....

Al, 46-...A fearful terror seized me, and I knew not whither to fly. I cried out aloud, "And so I am indeed dead; that hell I used to think about is no fiction, but a reality which I am doomed to experience forever...

He, 61 - Felt a vague sense of impending danger to life,...

He, 72 - Palpitation; vexed by want of sympathy (compassion, aid), afraid to be alone a moment, fears death.

He, 81 - Thinks he is going to die; < when he thinks about it.

CANN-I. Al, 23 - He seemed to have the one idea that he should die and soon be dissected.

Al, 25 - He became possessed with the idea that he was about to die, from which he cried out, "I am dying; I shall be carried to my death-chamber."

Al, 26 - The idea that he must die returned several times, and seemed to be particularly connected with the sinking and disappearance of the pulse. (blood, circulation)

He, 25 - Great apprehension of approaching (imminent) death.

CANTH. Al, 25 - Extreme despondency and faintheartedness; she says she must die.

Al, 14 - He talked deliriously when lying, sitting and walking, disconnectedly of his business and of people who had long since been dead.

He, 15 - Despondent and low-spirited, says she must die.

CAPS. Al, 6 - Anxiety and apprehensiveness; he imagines that he will die.

He, 13 - Anxiety and fear, as though he was going to die.

CARB-AN. Ha, 17 - Thoughts of death.

CARB-V. Al, 7 - She desired death, she felt so unhappy.

Ha, 11 - She wishes to die, she feels so unhappy.

CAUST. Al, 28 - Fear and anxiety, so that

she does not wish to live. (death)
Al, 26 - He was busy with thoughts of death, with uneasiness and great solicitude.
Ha, 21 - Her fear and anxiety cause her to wish that she might not live.(death)
Ha, 22 - He occupies himself with thoughts of death, with restlessness and great solicitude.(cares)
He, 32 - Hopeless weeping mood, expecting death.
He, 52 - Anxiety before falling asleep, as though attack of fainting would return and he would die.
He, 34 - Becomes anxious, as though he would die.
He, 40 - Fear of death. 0 Paralysis.
CHAM. He, 36 - Thoughts of dying.
CHEL. Al, 43 - Anxiety and fear of death, with desire to eructate, which he cannot do, at night.
Al, 51 - Anxious about death and being a soldier (warrior, disputant), at night.
He, 7 - Thinks she must die.
CHIN. Al, DREAM-1110 - Dreamed that some one had stabbed his brother, and then called for his mother; that his mother was dead, and then he cried; that his mother's arms was hurt;...
Ha, 1119 - Humour gloomy, no wish to live.
CHOC. Sh, 145 - My fears around the kids —that they would die, etc. and that they were my total responsibility, like parasites —have gone and I know feel total trust that they will be o.k.
Sh, 192 - I woke up and could not feel the usual sensation of my heart bulging or beating through my ribs while lying on my left side. I felt shock and thought 'perhaps I'm dead'. Groped for pulse and was reassured to be able to feel it. 15, 30C, 02:02:XX
CIC. Al, 25 - He believes he would die.
He, 33 - Old man fear a long spell (time) of sickness before dying.
CIMIC. He, 10 - Fear of death; fears those in house will kill him (murdered, by parents); saw wires encasing (lock, imprisoned) him; visions of rats and of strange objects.
He, 25 - Fear of death.
CLEM. Al, 19-...dreading to be alone, tired of living, full of thoughts of death, with fear that it would be speedy, longing however, for the repose of death; this mood was soon followed by apprehension, weeping, and homesickness, ...
COCC. Ha, 535 - In the morning, anxiety respecting the incurability of a trifling malady.
He, 27 - Apprehensive mood; fears death and unknown dangers.
He, 28 - Great fear of death.
COFF-T. Al, 9 - Timidity, and fear of sudden death;...
He, 2 - She is greatly excited and sure (inevitable) she will die.
He, 5 - Begs that someone might end her life. (salvation, redemption) (murdered)
COFF. He, 12 - Weeping and complaining, with fear of death; thinks that she will die.
He, 21 - Fear of death.
CON. Al, 11 - Visions of her brother and child, who had died; at the same time, she saw distinctly persons in the room;...
Al, 27 - Frequent thoughts of death.
Al, 36 - Very apprehensive thoughts, almost amounting (whole) to deathly anxiety, after midnight, while half awake.
Al, 45 - Extremely fretful and anxious thoughts about dying, in the morning, with confusion of the head.
Al, 1278 - Many dreams of dead people, and of the death of those living.
Ha, 16 - Frequents thoughts of death.
He, 31 - Great anxiety; precordial anguish; superstitious (careful, credulous, naive) and full of fear (coward), with frequent thoughts of death...
COP. Al, 2 - Disgust (loathing) with life, and at the same time fear of death.
CROC. Al, 10 - Immoderate laughter, as if he would die.
He, 3 - Greatly concerned about his life, believes that he will die, is no longer fit for business.
CROT-C. Al, 1 - Magnetic state; she hears nothing, and again sees the spectre of death, as a gigantic black skeleton.
Al, 19 - Thoughts of death haunt (torment) her everywhere, especially when alone.
Al, 18 - Her thoughts dwell on death; with great sadness.
CROT-H. He, 14 - Sadness, her thoughts dwell on death continually.
CUPR-A. He, 10 - Awoke suddenly from

sleep...and wished to escape...thinks she is about to die and desires to see the pastor;...

CUPR. Al, 5 - Melancholy; she shuns the sight of people (observed), seeks and loves to be alone, and becomes anxious about her death, which she supposes imminent and inevitable.

Ha, 1 - Melancholy; she shuns the sight of men, seeks and loves (desire) solitude, and troubles herself about her imminent death (impending), which she supposes to be unavoidable.

He, 26 - Loss of spirits (courage); anxiety; fits of anguish and fear of death.

CUR. Al, 16 - Excessive fear of death.

CYCL. He, 17-...fear of death, or an illusion of being deserted or persecuted by every one.

DER. Al, 2 - He desires death and will attempt (try) suicide.

DIG. Ha, 424 - Fear of death.

He, 11 - Melancholic, despondent, and constantly tortured by fear of death or loss of reason.

DROS. Ha, 277 - Anxiety; ...,as if he were impelled to jump into the water in order to take his own life by drowning he was not impelled to any other mode of death.

FERR. He, 9 - Mind in highest degree oppressed; despondent (sad); great solicitude (cares) about those belonging to him (relatives, family), with constant thoughts of death.

GELS. He, 6 - After losing son, inclined to brood over her loss; at times becomes unconscious, or, rather, "rapt"; in imagination thinks herself at the grave; smothered pressure on chest after the spell.

He, 23 - Fear of death; has no courage. (cowardice)

GERM. Sh, 109 - Feeling a total failure, I would prefer to die. Very unmotivated. 05, 6C, 360:XX:XX

Sh, 101 - I'm desperate. I want to die. Feel the power to kill. Feel like a wild animal locked in. It's strong, so intense. I hate so strong-feel a terrible disgust and I'm afraid of what I'm able to do. It's completely impossible to be in it and impossible to get out of it. 18, 30C, 190:XX:XX

GLON. Al, 12 - Though naturally cheerful she became apprehensive of her approaching death.

He, 15 - Fear; throat feels swollen; chest as if screwed together; apprehensive of approaching death; fears she has been poisoned.

GRAPH. Al, 3 - Sadness, with thoughts of nothing but death.

Ha, 8 - Mournfulness (sorrowful), with nothing but thoughts of death.

Ha, 20 - He often feels as if his end was near (death), or as if the greatest misfortune impended over him.

He, 6 - Sadness, with thoughts of nothing but death.

He, 13 - It frequently seemed to him as though his end was near, or the greatest misfortunes were impending.

HALI-L. Sh, 16 - Had a superstitious thing happen. A white moth flew up by me in class and I had a strong sense someone close to me had died. 13, 30C, 01:04:XX

Sh, 25 - While listening to a patient grieve, had a return of increased awareness of right eye, especially the socket. I had a strong image of how my mother's right eye was knocked out when she was hit by a truck and killed 30 years ago. Feel a very strong sense of connection with her. Telling this to my proving supervisor later, I realized I had never said this to anyone. This was an aspect of her death I had suppressed. It had always been so horrifying to me I couldn't deal with it. I cried gently with lots of tears. Feeling very sad and some remorse that I couldn't have been with my mother when she died. Felt very calm with all of this. 03, 12C, 18:XX:XX

Sh, 150 - Is this true calm or the calm of the dead? I'm not feeling so much, which is a relief because I was feeling so negative before. 09, 6C, 04:XX:XX

Sh, 350-... "Considered committing suicide. Feeling that life has passed me by. Thinking about my mortality. Terrified of dying. My time has run out." ...18, 30C, 05:XX:XX-16:XX:XX

Sh, 432 - I am deeply in touch with a self—destructive sense inside. The part of me that wants to disintegrate and die. Dis-integrate; the opposite of integral oneness, the opposite direction. I'll have another egg to ground me. 06, 6C, 10:XX:XX

Sh, 507 - Having some trouble speaking. Using the wrong words, or lacking words at times. Just keep it simple. Husband told the kids. We all laughed. I guess that's what you can say for adversity. If it happens enough you learn to get used to it. If it's not too hard. Began thinking about one of my kids dying—that would be too hard. I don't want to do that to find out. 09, 6C, 16:XX:XX

Sh, 521 - Fear of death. 16, 10C, 05:XX:XX

Sh, 522 - Fear for the life of my cat. 16, 10C, 08:XX:XX

Sh, 523 - Sense of fear. Vision: The shadow of death creeping in, like it did in the movie, Ten Commandments". 16, 10C, 09:XX:XX

Sh, 526 - Fear of death came up more than usual during the proving. It wasn't the fear of aging. It was fear of the finality, that one day you won't see the light, or breathe the air, or live to contemplate overcoming your problems. 18, 30C, 35:XX:XX

Sh, 527 - I was paying attention to the obituaries at this time. Noticed people dying in the newspaper. I would get very angry and frustrated. For a short time, was looking at death notices on a daily basis, during the last week or so of the proving. My anger towards death. How unfair. I don't want it. I shouldn't have to have it. There should never be a day where the morning is taken from me. 18, 30C, 35:XX:XX

Sh, 528 - Noticed in the paper all cancer related deaths, particularly prostate, mostly men between 40-60. Seemed to be men who were very loved. Seemed most unfair. Fear that if I drank too much coffee I would get a headache, and the thought was cancer related. 18, 30C, 35:XX:XX

Sh, 604 - Since the remedy, I took over and the physical manifestation of personas splitting off would only come out when I was alone. Did these drawings. The figure in the box was my death — captured, buried and can't get out. The first drawing is a depressed boy, the second is the buried man, the third is an x-ray figure. After that the depression abated. I did another drawing of a negative being laughing at me. It has no arms, no movement. 18, 30C, 35:XX:XX

HELL. Al, 15 - Dread of death (in a sufferer from religious melancholy).

Al, 12 - Such anxiety, nausea, and distress that he thinks he will die.

Al, 19 - Dread of death.(in a sufferer from religious melancholy)

Al, 16 - He is doubtful (uncertain) about his own life.

Ha, 276 - Such anxiety, nausea and suffering, that he thinks he is going to die.

He, 24 - Dread of dying ; feels unhappy in presence of cheerful faces. (spite)

HEP. Al, 1 - Ghostly image of one who was dead, in the morning, in bed, after waking and while conscious, which frightened him; it also seemed as though he saw his neighbor's house burning, which also frightened him.

Ha, 4 - Fearful anguish, in the evening, for two hours; he thought he had to perish (die), and was sad even so that he could have committed suicide. (redemption, salvation)

HURA. Al, 4 - She weeps every little while, and especially for two days past, fancies she sees the dead person before her eyes. (ghost)

Al, 7 - During and after the fainting spell (trance), disposed to love everybody, especially those about him; he often thinks of death, but does not fear it; he feels as though he could die without regret.(fearless)

Al, 12 - Flow of sad thoughts; she fancies she is about to lose a dear friend.

HYDR. He, 5 - Depression of spirits, sure of death and desires it.

HYDROG. Sh, 158 - Thoughts of death and suicide. 16, 30C, 25:XX:XX

Sh, 159 - Thoughts of dead bodies made me feel slightly sick. 10, 200C, 00:XX:XX

Sh, 160 - Wrote a letter to my son, 'to be opened after my death', not morbid, nor do I feel a premonition of death. Its something I've always meant to do —a sort of resolving. Wept with emotion as I wrote it. 12, 6C, 25:XX:XX

Sh, 162 - The remedy "made me think of formaldehyde and dead things". 10, 200C, 00:XX:XX

Sh, 163 - Thoughts of death —thoughts went back to doing dissection as a medical student.10, 200C, 00:XX:XX

Sh, 188 - On getting up in the morning, I feel very angry and bad about myself. I feel I can't cope. Whats the use of trying? I feel like giving up. I think for a moment I'd like to die. 10, 200C, 09:XX:XX

Sh, 194 - Fear I may lose my mind, or even die. Fear about the proving. Feel I could bash the car so I have to make a real effort. 10, 200C, 12:XX:XX

HYOS. Al, 85 - Excessive fear of death, becoming a monomania,...

Al, 87 - Remarkable fear that he had been devoured by animals.

Ha, 582 - Impatient: he thought he should die when he had to wait for something of quite trivial nature.

IGN. He, 26 - Great grief after losing persons or objects very dear.

IRID. Sh-2 - Felt similar to being in water or asleep, as if almost asleep or in a trance, aware, but floating in inner self, uncommunicative; like a near death experience, inner self is primary and separate. E1

KALI-BR. Al, 5 - She had the erroneous idea that she was deserted by all her friends, and as a consequence she passed all her waking moments, which are not many in tears;...delusion that her child was dead, had taken fixed possession of her mind;...she declared that she saw it dead (corpse) before her, and when it was brought to her, she refused to acknowledge that it was hers, or had any resemblance to the one she imagined was dead.

Al, 14 - Great mental depression, a feeling (sensation) of approaching death.

He, 17 - Delirium with delusions; thinks he is pursued (hunt); will be poisoned; is selected (designated) for divine vengeance (revenge); that her child is dead, etc.

He, 23-...constantly brooding over loss of a daughter; almost crazy; ... (child)

KALI-C. Al, 4 - Very much depressed; she was obliged to weep much, because it was constantly in her thoughts that she must die.

Ha, 8 - Very ill-humored; she has to weep much, because it was constantly on her mind that she had to die. (doomed, sentenced)

He, 11 - Fear of being alone; fears she will die.

KALI-FCY. Al, 1 - Feeling of sadness and some disposition to tears, caused by an impression that he was soon to die and leave his friends; disposition to take a sad view of the beauties of autumn; the apprehension of approaching sickness and death can be overcome by reason, but soon returns.

KALI-N. Al, 4 - Depressed; she thinks she must die.

KALI-P. He, 15 - Profound hypochondria and melancholia, weariness of life and fear of death, suspiciousness...

KREOS. Al, 4 - She was depressed; the longing (desire) for death constantly became greater.

He, 5 - Sorrowful mood, inclined to weep or longing (desire) for death;...

LAC-C. Al,N-33 - Depression of spirits, doubts her ability and success, thinks she will have heart disease and die of it.

Al,N-37 - Fear of death, with anxious expression of countenance.

He, 14-..;sometimes imagines heart or breathing are going to stop, or otherwise frightens himself, and this makes heart beat violently; occasionally very depressed, and fancies he is going out of his mind. (insanity)

He, 26 - Depression of spirits, doubts her ability (competence, aptitude) and success (prospering, progressing, achieving), thinks she will have heart disease and die of it.

He, 30 - Fear of death, with anxious expression of countenance.(face)

LAC-D. Al,N-4 - Imagines that all her friends will die and that she must go to a convent. (purification, solitude)

Al,N-9 - Great despondency on account of the disease, is sure he is going to die in 24 hours.

Al,N-10 - Has no fear of death but is sure is going to die.

He, 2 - Depression of spirits; don't care to live, question as to quietest and most certain way of hastening one's death.

He, 5 - Imagines that all her friends will die and that she must go to a convent. (purification, salvation)

He, 9 - Great despondency on account of the disease, is sure he is going to die in twenty-four hours.

He, 10 - Has no fear (fearless) of death but is sure he is going to die.

LACH. He, 8 - Thinks: she is somebody else in the hands (seized) of a stronger power; (supremacy, superiority).or that she is dead, and preparations are made for funeral (cortege) or that she is nearly dead and wishes some one would help her off; herself pursued by enemies, or fears medicine is poison; there are robbers in house and wants to jump out the window; herself under super-human control; visions real, he will die. (helplessness, desire; aid, comfort, salvation)

He, 41 - Dread (fear) of death, fears to go to bed ; fears of being poisoned.

He, 44 - Satiety (loathing?) of life with longing (desiring) for death.

LAUR. Al, 8 - Very lachrymose and despondent (sad) mood; he would rather die than live.

LED. Al, 10 - Fretful; he went by himself, and almost weeping wished to die.

Ha, 333 - Cross: he retired into solitude, and almost weeping he longed for death.

He, 2 - After nightmare, fears to go to sleep lest she die.

LYC. Al, 43 - Anxious thoughts, as if she were about to die, for which she even prepared by thinking of her farewell messages, in the morning...

He, 26 - Anxious thoughts, as if about to die, for which she prepares farewell (departure, adieu) messages.

LYSS. Al,N-11-...presentiment of impending death begged them to pray for him and not to leave him alone. (absolution, redemption)

Al,N-80 - Felt as if she was going to die, as if she was going to sink away.(decline)

He, 10 - They appreciate the formidable (terrible) character of the disease and speak frequently with a remarkable (unusual) quick and sharp articulation of the impending fatal results.

He, 80 - Felt as if she was going to die; as if she was going to sink away.

MAG-C. Al, 955 - Dream that she was weeping about the death of a near relative.

Al, 956 - Dream that her mother had died, at which she woke, and believed that she was still weeping.

Al, 965 - Dream of a grave in a cemetery, into which, after voluntary preparation, she was to be thrown.

Al, 957 - Dream that she saw her dead grandmother.

MAG-M. Al, 715 - Dream that someone cut away one side of her face; that a skin was being taken from a dead body and the like.

MED. Al,N-20 - Fears he is going to die.

He, 20 - Is sure that she is worse, knows she is not going to live, cannot see any improvement, even when it is pointed out (antagonism); has no fear of death, speaks calmly about it, and gives directions as to the disposition of her affairs.

He, 30 - Anticipates death. (predicts)

MERC. Ha, 1236 - He thinks he is losing his reason,(intelligence, capacity) that he is going to die ; with illusions of imagination, e.g. he sees water flowing where there is none (in the morning). (water-1 origin, genesis)

Ha, 1241 - He wished to die, was indifferent to everything, even to what he took most delight in.

He, 30 - Anxiety driving her to suicide ; thoughts of suicide; ...desire for death; great indifference even to those she formerly loved;...

He, 14 - Believes he is losing his reason, thinks he is dying, with illusions of fantasy; sees water running where there is none.

MEZ. Al, 36 - Quiet and contemplative; weary of life, and longing for death.

Ha, 2-...everything seemed to him as if dead, and nothing made a vivid impression on him.

Ha, 8 - Introverted, tired of life and longing for death.

He, 10-...; everything seems to him dead (lifeless, inert) and nothing makes a vivid impression upon his mind.

MOSCH. Al, 11 - He was extremely anxious about the death;...."this is my death" became deathly pale, and in ten minutes fell down in a faint.

Al, 12 - She spoke of nothing but that she must die. (from triturating ten minutes)

He, 4 - Great dread (fear) of death, with paleness of face, fainting; talks only of approaching (nearing) death.

He, 11 - Great tendency to be frightened, trembling, palpitation of heart, and dread of death.

NAT-C. Ha, 48 - Peevish and cross, dissatisfied whith all the world; he could have kicked (self sensure) himself; he would rather not live at all ; at the same time solicitous about the future, so that he is ready to despair.

NAT-M. Al, 72 - Anxious fear of dying.

Ha, 25 - He is afraid he will have to die.

Ha, 97 - Lack of memory, so that he thought his mother (present continually) had died, because he did not remember to have seen her.

NAT-P. Al, 10 - Awakens; fears his child, who has a trifling ailment (disease), is dead; he goes to her room to relieve the otherwise ineffaceable (perpetual) impression.

NIT-AC. Al, 18 - Satiety of life with fear of death.

Al, 43 - She wishes for death and yet dreads it.

Ha, 25 - She imagines she will die soon, but has no bodily indisposition.

Ha, 27 - She wishes to die, and nevertheless she is afraid of death.

He, 10 - Sadness, great fear of death, sensation of extreme weakness, even to trembling.

He, 16 - Anxiety about his disease, with fear of death; morbid fear of cholera.

He, 17 - After continued loss of sleep, long-lasting anxiety, over-exertions of mind and body from nursing the sick, great anguish of mind from loss of his dearest friend.

He, 5 - Fancies she will die soon, yet is not physically ill.

NUX-M. Al, 16 - Great fear of death.

Al, 27 - As soon as she lay down felt a sinking sensation, as though she were going to die, with no fear, however, being perfectly at ease (peace) in mind,...

NUX-V. Al, 53 - She believes that she is near death.

Al, 3 - Rushed into the room, exclaiming that her mother had been murdered.

Al, 39 - Great anxiety; he had to rise from any place and wished rather (first) to die.

Ha, 1237 - Great anxiety; he cannot rest in any place, (restlessness) and would rather die.

Ha, 1246 - He fears death.

Ha, 1247 - She thinks herself near death.

He, 21 - Anxiety with irritability and inclination to commit suicide, but is afraid to die.

OP. Al, 68 - Criminals (in India) lose their fear of death and go courageously to their execution.(fearless)

Al, 78 - Fear of impending death.

Ha, 638 - He chattered all sorts of unconnected stuff and pointed with his fingers to imaginary masked people approaching him; ...he started at imaginary swordsmen, who might kill him ; ...

He, 22-... feeling of great strength; contempt of death;...indifference to joy and suffering.

He, 27 - Anxiety; apprehension; fear of impending death.

OX-AC. Al, 28 - Great distress and fear of death.

PETR. Al, 12 - Fear of death.

PHOS. Al, 40 - As the darkness of night began to enclose (surround) the earth, my peace was disturbed by the most frightful visions and thoughts; constant fear of death, with an almost uncontrollable desire to commit suicide.

Al, 118 - Felt nervous, as if I were going to die.

Al, 1-..this delirium, which preceded death, was erotic, with indications of great, excitement of the sexual system...

Al, 4 - Delirium with fear of death,...

Ha, 20 - Anguish at times in the evening, as if about to die.

He, 7 - Anxious: filled with gloomy (dark) forebodings; as if about to die; about termination (conclude) of her illness (disease); and restless ; at twilight; when alone; about future; during a thunderstorm; ..

He, 8 - Fear and dread: in evening; of death; as if something were creeping out of every corner; late in evening as if a horrible face were looking out of every corner.

He, 21 - Dejection (sadness); thought he would die.

PHYT. He, 4 - Great fear; is sure she will die.

PLAT. Al, 23 - Feeling as if he would die soon, with shuddering (tremor) at the thought.

Ha, 7 - Anguish as if about to die, as if unconsciousness (insensible) would ensue (result),...

Ha, 9 - Sensation as if she would have to

die soon (immediately), with horror at the thought.
Ha, 11 - Great restlessness of mind, so that she knows not where to stay (indecision), with gloominess (melancholy) which spoils even what should be most enjoyable; she imagines she is not fit (unfit, incapable) for this world, is tired (weary) of life, but has a great horror of the death she believes to be approaching.
Ha, 40 - Indifference, he felt unconcerned (careless, insensible) as to whether his absent wife would die or not.
He, 24 - Much anguish; she feels as if she would lose her senses and die soon.
He, 35 - Precordial anguish with palpitation and fear of death and imaginary forms, ghosts.
He, 37-...depressed condition of physical powers; ...fear of approaching death; ... aversion to coition and yet dreams of intense lasciviousness,...
He, 45-...melancholy with great fear of death, imagines himself superior to his wife;...
He, 17 - After anger alternate laughing and weeping, with great anguish and fear of death.
He, 23 - Satiety of life, with taciturnity and fear of death.
He, 29-...thought she had no place in the world; life was wearisome (boring), but had great dread of death, which she believed near at hand.
PLB. Al, 23-...His delirium turned chiefly upon the idea that his life was in danger from assassination or poisoning, and that every one about him was a murderer...
Al, 112 - He is very sad, has no desire to live, and has threatened to destroy himself, and is very fault-finding (severe, critical) with his friends.
Al, 114-...he imagined his disease incurable, and gave way to the gloomy thoughts which the fear of death excited, and to repinings (sadness) caused by the dread of his journey to Valencia.
Al, 118 - Much depressed, fearing to die if left alone.
Al, 66 - Hallucinations of mind, she seemed to see her dead husband and child in a tree out of the window.
He, 13 - Thought his life was in danger from assassination or poison and every one about him was a murderer.
PODO. He, 3 - Depression: imagines he is going to die or be very ill;...
POLYG-H. He, 2 - Gloomy (dark) views of life, dislike of change (evolution, transformation) and excessive dread (fear) of death.
PSOR. Al, 14 - Very melancholy and despairing; he wishes to die in spite of his good luck.
Al, 22 - She is very irritable, easily angered; thinking always of dying.
Al,N-15 - Great fear of death; anxiety about heart ...
Al,N-16 - Believe the stitches in heart will kill him if they do not cease.
Al,N-31 - Despairs of recovery; thinks he will die; hopeless,...
Al,N-11 - She is very irritable, easily angered; always thinks of dying.
He, 11 - She is very irritable, easily angered; always thinks of dying.
He, 15 - Great fear of death; anxiety about heart and dyspnea,...
He, 16 - Believes the stitches in heart will kill him if they do not cease.
He, 31 - Despairs recovery; thinks he will die; hopeless; especially after typhus...
PULS. Al, 19 - Tremulous anxiety, as if death were imminent.(destined)
Al, 16 - Anxiety thinks to die.
Ha, 1116 - Trembling anxiety, as if about to die.
Ha, 1116 - Trembling anxiety, as if about to die.
He, 26 - Anxiety: thinks to die; does not know what to do; as if in a hot atmosphere; in region of heart; even to suicide;...
He, 28 - Tremulous anguish: as if death were near;...
RAPH. Al, 17 - Extreme anxiety, she thought she would die.
Al, 18 - Apprehension and fear of death.
He, 1 - Anguish with dread (fear) of death, which supposed to be near.
RHUS-T. Al, 9 - Satiety (surfeit) of life, with desire to die without sadness.
Al, 27 - Anxiety, with loss of strength (power, energy, force), as if he would die, more after midnight than before.
Al, 41 - Confusion of mind, he thought he would die.

Ha, 953 - Melancholy, sad, and anxious, as if about to hear of a calamity,(misfortune, disaster) or as if she were solitary (lonely, alone) and all around her were dead (lifeless, extinct) and silent (quiet) ; or as if she had bid farewell (separation) to an intimate friend ; worst in the room, diminished by walking in a open air.

Ha, 956 - Along with sinking (descend, submerge) of the strength, (vigor, energy, force) anxiety as if he must die, worse after than before midnight.

Ha, 971 - Confusion of the reason; he thinks he is dying.

Ha, 957 - Without sadness, as if tired of life, with desire to die.

He, 11 - Anxiety: while sitting was obliged to take hold (grasp, keep) of something because she did not think she could keep up (support) on account of the beating and drawing pains in limbs; and apprehension as if he wished to take his own life; with loss of strength (vigor, vitality) as if he would die.

He, 13 - Fear: that he will die; with anxiousness and sighing; of being poisoned.

He, 18 - Disgust of life: thoughts of suicide; wants to drown (immerse) himself; with fear of death: with desire to die, without sadness.

He, 22-... great restlessness and anguish as if she had committed a crime or as if she thought some terrible calamity impended; these feelings drove her from one place to another; could not rest quietly at night in bed; was robbed of sleep and all desire to live;...

He, 23 - Restlessness and anxiety about heart as if she had committed a crime or as if some great misfortune was in store (reserved) for her, is driven from one place to another; deprived of sleep and all desire to live; ...

RHUS-V. Al, 1 - Great sadness, no desire to live, everything seems gloomy.

RUTA. Ha, 270-...anxiety as if he must die,...

SABAD. Al, 2 - He imagines all sorts of strange things about his own body, for instance, that it had shrunk (dry, wrinkled) like that of dead persons (corpse), that his stomach was corroded (degeneracy, decomposition), that the scrotum was swollen (enlarged), etc.;...

Al, 3 - Imagines: himself sick; parts shrunken (small wrinkled) ; that she is pregnant (important?), when she is merely swollen from flatus; that she has some horrible throat disease which will end fatally. (incurable)

SEC. Al, 4 - Muttering delirium, very restless, agitated, and fearful of death.

Al, 28 - Constant moaning and fear of death, with strong desire to live.

Al, 47 - Hypochondria; patient says she must have something to relieve her or she must die.

Al, 45 - Anxiety and fear of death.

Al, 46 - Hypochondria; patient says she must have something to relieve her or she must die.

Al,N-6 - Fear of death.

He, 10 - Constant moaning and fear of death.

SEP. Al, 52 - She is filled with concern about her health; thinks she will have consumption and soon die.

Ha, 9 - She has none but troubled thoughts about her health, thinks she is getting the consumption (tuberculosis, degenerate, decomposition) and will die soon.

He, 38-...everything seems strange (unusual, unfamiliar) to her;...; it seems as if she could not understand (realize) anything and would have to learn anew everything she wished to do;...(lost: knowledge); greatest indifference to everything, the death of a near relative, or some happy occurrence, leaves her equally unaffected; no trace of her former love for friends or even for her child; aversion for social intercourse amounting to contempt;...

SIL. Al, 11 - Gloominess; she felt as if she would die, and for the time lost her memory.

He, 14 - Gloomy, feels as if she would die.

SPONG. Ha, 377 - Every day, several fits of heat, with anxiety, pain in the cardiac region, weeping and inconsolable; she would like to die there and then.

He, 15 - Inconsolability, would rather die on the spot (immediate); with the heat.

He, 19 - She is very fretful and anxious about her condition, fears she will die of suffocation.

He, 24 - Terror and fear: of approaching

death; that she will die of suffocation; with heart disease;...
He, 26 - Apprehension of a fatal termination of his disease.
SQUIL. He, 1 - Great anxiety of mind, with fear of death.
STANN. He, 3 - Uneasy, does not know what to do with himself pains > by walking, yet so weak he soon must die.
STAPH. Ha, 695 - As if dead (decease, lifeless, inert) in mind and sad, but not to weeping.
Ha, 703 - Anxious thoughts and things long past come before him as if they were actually present and stood before him, which causes anxiety and the sweat of anguish -Then blackness comes before his eyes; he knows not if what he sees is true (real) or deception (false, unreal), then he regards (suppose) everything as something different to what it is (strange), and he loses all wish to live. (lost; discernment, perception)
Ha, 707 - Hypochondriacal humor; everything is indifferent to him; he would like to die.
STRAM. Al, 122 - For some days the patient was affected with hallucinations and thought that one side of him was alive, while the other side was buried.
Al-S, 1684-...Constant fear of sudden death. At times believed herself dying...
Ha, 549 - He thinks he is dying, and that he will not live over the evening, he rejoices that he is dying, and gives directions about his funeral, otherwise he is rational and does not feel particularly ill.
Ha, 556 - In the evening after lying in bed very sad, with thoughts of death and violent weeping.
He, 56 - Believes to be in his grave; shrives,(confess) prays, asks to be killed (justified); accuses his wife of infidelity; scolds (cursing), strikes at everybody who wishes to restrain him; thinks they are dogs and barks at them to make himself understood.
He, 93 - Mania; thinks he is lying on his sepulchre (tomb); confessing, praying, wants to be killed (redemption, salvation, regeneration); laughs as if tickled (excited); wants to be kissed; accuses his wife of being faithless (betrayed); scolding (censure) beating in a rage, will not be taken hold of by attendants (suspicious?) ; takes them for dogs (contemptuous), and barks at them; talking in Jewish jargon; (rank?, stranger?) supposes his house to be surrounded by carts (vehicle), Jews (Judaism) and geese, offending him, ... -(strange, foreign, alien)
He, 107-...heard continually, on r. side of occiput, a loud voice, scolding, vituperating and accusing him of ungodliness (impious, sinful, irreligious, godless, profane); ....prayed expecting, with great anxiety, the flash of lightning which was to kill him;...(redemption, regeneration, salvation)
He, 14-...thoughts of dying;...fear of wild animals and black dogs.
He, 55 - He thinks that he is dying and that he will not live over night, rejoices (celebrate) and gives directions about his funeral.
He, 87 - After a dreadful shock, occasioned by death of his brother, who fell dead in his arms,...struck all at around him...spoke at one time in Hungarian, and then in Wallachian language; sang Latin paternosters, declared he was God, and then that he was the devil;...
SUL-AC. Al, 5 - He was roused (waken) with difficulty, and when roused, resisted fiercely, saying in a hoarse muffled (deaden) voice, "Let me alone, let me die".
SULPH. Al, 9 - She imagines that people injure her, and she will die in consequence.
Al, 3772-...it was disturbed by dreams of fire and death.
Al, 3802 - Frightful, anxious dreams of danger of death, and of dead people.
Al, 41 - Frequently during the day she has attacks of melancholy, lasting a few minutes, when she feels extremely unhappy, without cause; she wishes to die.
Al, 44 - Anxiety as if he would cease to live.
Al, 59 - Awoke in a hour in great fright and distress; horror of instant death.
Ha, 4 - Often during the day, attacks lasting for several minutes, when she feels herself utterly (completely) miserable, without any cause, like melancholy; she desires to die.
Ha, 15 - Apprehension, as if he had to lose his life at once.

He, 34-...; profound melancholy; considers herself disgraced (dishonor, degradation) ; speaks of dying, finds life insupportable;...
He, 36-..., feels extremely unhappy without cause, she wishes to die.
He, 21 - Satiety of life, longing for death.
SYPH. Al,N-12 - Terrible dread (fear) of night, ...death is preferable ; she fears to prepare for night and is positively in abject fear of suffering,...
He, 9 - Terrible dread of night, ...it is intolerable, death is preferable. She fears to prepare for night and is positively in abject fear of suffering...
TAB. Al, 20 - Gloom, hypochondria, apprehensions of sudden death.
Al, 34 - Apprehensive, faint-hearted, and despondent, with nausea; she thought she would die, ...
Al, 36 - Apprehension, anxiety, and despondency, as if she dreaded death at 4 p.m. two days in succession.
Al, 38 - Terrible apprehensions (fear) of immediate death.
TARENT. Al, 1-...threatening words of destruction and death; she believes she is insulted; ...
Al, 40 - Excessive grief, accompanied in the afternoon by thoughts of death.
THEA. Al, 19 - Appeared to be actuated by the greatest terror, and said: "I have called upon you to request you would let me in and allow me to die in your house".
THUJ. Al, 58 - Continual thoughts of dying (death), with increasing weakness.
Al, 59 - Presentiment of death.
Al, 64 - Frightful anxiety, like death agony; a nameless internal ache, as if the soul were escaping from the body (split), with most terrible uneasiness, frightful orgasm of blood, at night, even to suffocation.
Al, 34 - While talking, she is unable to go on in spite of every effort; she begins to weep bitterly, and says she can no longer think or live.
He, 23 - Mental depression, after childbirth (puerperal), in consequence of being told that there had been a slight rupture (division, hurt) of perineum; grows quiet; thinks she must die;...wants to jumps the window; does not care for children or her relatives (careless) ;..(sensitive to disrupt, partition)
He, 29 - Feels as if she cannot exist any longer; quiet, shunning everybody.
TUB. Al,N-47 - Despondent, discouraged, feel as if I would rather die than live.
VAC. He, 5 - Fear of death; wild excitement and begging (implore) to know if he was to die,...
VERAT-V. Al, 6 - Great fear of death.
He, 3 - From sudden cerebral congestion: quarrelsome delirium; great mental depression and fear of death;...
VERAT. Ha, 692 - A feeling in his whole being, as if he must gradually come to an end, but with calmness. (death)
He, 26 - Chases (pursue, hunt) his family out of house ; declares the sun travels around the earth (geocentric); fear of death, restlessness, despair...
He, 44 - Cold sweat on forehead, with anguish and fear of death.
VINC. He, 2 - Sadness, with fear of death.
VIP. Al, 12 - Premonition of death.
ZINC. Ha, 15 - Tranquil thoughts of dying, in the afternoon, when weary.

DECEITFUL

Character, lack of: ***caust.*** **LYC.** ***sil.***
Charlatan: calc.[30] plat.[30] sulph.[30]
Deceitful, sly: agar.[5] anac.[5] androc.[222] arg.[111] arg-n. ***ars.***[30] aur-s.[10] bell.[5] bufo calc.[30] chin.[30] chlol. coca ***cupr.***[5] dig.[1] dros. fl-ac.[122] ***hyos.***[5] ***lach.***[5] lap-mar-c.[194] lyc.[30] ***med.***[198] morph.[162] mosch.[58] ***nat-m.***[30] nux-v.[5] ***op.***[5] plat.[30] plb.[58] puls.[30] sep.[30] sil.[30] sulph.[30] ***tarent.***[122] thuj.[58] verat.[5]
Deceitful; corrupt, venal: ars.[30] chin.[30] lyc.[30] puls.[30] sulph.[30]
Deceitful; fraudulent: bell.[30] calc.[30] merc.[30]
Deceitful; perjured: hep.[30] nat-m.[30] nit-ac.[30]
Delusions; honest, he is not: ***stram.***[8]
• juggler, he is a: bell.
• lie, all she said is a: lac-c.
Destructiveness; cunning: ***tarent.***
Dreams; money, counterfeit: zinc-o.
Fear; knaves, of: alum.[5] ars.[5] chin.[5] hyos.[5] lyss.[5]
Liar: alco. androc.[222] arg-n.[122] bell.[30] calc.[30] carb-v.[30] caust.[30] coca[36] con.[30] lyc.[30] med.[212] merc.[30] **MORPH.**[122] nat-m.[30] nux-v.[85] **OP.**[122] phos.[189] puls.[30] sil.[30] staph.[30] sulph.[30] ***syph.***[122] **VERAT.**[122]
Liar; charlatan and: calc.[30] nat-m.[30] puls.[30]
Liar; lie, believes all she says is a: ***lac-c.***

Liar; never speaks the truth, does not know what she is saying: alco.[122] arg-n.[122] ***morph.***[122] **OP.**[122] ***syph.***[122] ***verat.***[122]

Play; dirty trick on others or their teachers, schoolboys p. a: lach.[30] zinc.[30]

Secretive: aur.[5] ***bar-c.***[122] bov.[5] caust.[30] dig. germ.[222] ***ign.*** lap-mar-c.[194] ***lyc.***[122] ***naja***[5] nat-m.[137] nit-ac.[5] phos.[5] plb.[5] ***sep.***[122] syph.[122] thuj.[187] zinc.[36]

Slander; disposition to, hypocritical, and: phos.[30] sep.[30]

Temperament; choleric, ardent, disposed to anger, spite or deception, always irritable and impatient: **NUX-V.**[54]

Truth; thinks she does not tell the: macrin.[36]

Truth; want of: ferr.[30] iod.[30] mag-c.[30] nux-v.[30] sep.[30] sulph.[30]

Unreliable: act-sp.[162] anh.[119]

Unsympathetic, unscrupulous: am-c.[1] ***anac.***[5] androc.[222] ars.[30] calc.[1] carb-an.[1] carb-v.[1] ***cham.*** chin.[5] con.[1] **DIG.**[91] lac-h.[229] lap-gr-m.[194] lap-mar-c.[194] mag-m.[5] nat-m.[5] nit-ac.[5] op.[5] ozone[227] 0pall.[185] ***plat.*** puls.[30] ***sep.*** staph.[1] sumb.[36]

ANDROC. Sh, 121 - When talking to friends felt 'paranoid', suspicious and guilty, when asked questions, he became hot and sweaty. He felt it was a game of who was cleverer, and tried to lie to and outwit his friend, though this gave no satisfaction. His friends reported that he seemed unusually distant and cool. (29)

CUPR. He, 10 - Mania with biting, beating, and tearing things to pieces; insane foolish gestures of imitation and mimicry; full of insane spiteful (cruelty, brutality) tricks (deceitful, false), ..unhappy, despairing...miserable look...

GERM. Sh, 158 - Some persistent feelings coming up. Feel envious of a colleague who I feel manages so well. When I compare with myself I feel worthless and nothing. I feel like talking badly about her to my friends and I do this, even though she is not present. It takes a lot of my attention and energy. 21, 12C, 67:XX:XX.

LAC-C. Al,N -8 - Is impressed with the idea that all she says is a lie; it seems to be very difficult to speak the truth (liar, dissimulator), but continually distrusts things (suspicious); when reading anything she rapidly changes the meaning, omitting or adding things. (mischievous)

MAG-C. Al, 930 - Dreams of masks (false) in fools'(idiot) clothes, which they soiled.(dirty)

VERAT. He, 5 - Never speaks the truth; does not know herself what she is saying.

DEFIANT

Defiant: acon. alum.[116] am-c.[116] anac. androc.[222] ***arn.*** **BAR-C.**[30] bell.[116] bufo canth. **CAUST.**[122] ***cina***[5] guai. ***ign.***[5] kreos.[116] ***lyc.*** merc.[193] nux-v. ph-ac.[116] puls.[30] ruta[152] ***sac-alb.***[210] sec.[116] sep.[122] sil.[116] spong. sulph.[116] tub.[193]

Inciting others: hyos.

Insolence; servants to chiefs, of: lyc.[30] nat-m.[30]

Rudeness; children, of naughty: ***ant-c.***[5] carc.[207] cham.[5] ***chin.***[54] cina[5] dulc.[5] ***merc.***[5] rheum[5] staph.[5]

Rudeness; employees to the chiefs, of: lyc.[30] nat-m.[30]

AGAR. Al, 22 - Some run and walk involuntarily in the most dangerous places.(defiant)

ANDROC. Sh, 60 - Felt tense and absolutely alone, but sure that the rest of the world was mad, not her. She felt defiant with others and would not be manipulated. (7)
Sh, 112 - Became excited to anger and confrontation. She was not aware of hurting others' feelings and did not seem to care. Could not appreciate anyone else's feeling. Later she reflected on her actions and felt ashamed. (12)

BUFO. Al, 25 - Defiance (disobedience, challenger), duplicity (hypocrisy), spitefulness.(cruelty)

CHAM. He, 59 - Great tendency to quarrel, to speak in an obstreperous (rude, vulgar) manner.

LYC. He, 32 - Obstinate, defiant (contrary), arbitrary (capricious?); seeks disputes.

MERC. Ha, 1263 - Mania; she throws off the clothes at night, tears the straw about, and scolds; by day she leaps (jump) up high like a petulant extravagant person...she talks and scolds much to herself,...spits frequently and spreads the saliva out with her feet, and licks some of it up again; she often licks cowdung (excrements) and the mud of ponds (lake); she often takes little stones in her mouth, without swallowing them, and at the same time complains that they are cutting her bowels; much clotted blood passes with her motion; ...

DESPAIR

Anxiety; health, despair of getting well: ***ars.***[54]
Cheerfulness; alternating with, despair: acon.[1]
Consoled, cannot be, after shock or injury: acon.[54]
Death; desires, despair, from: agn.[100] ***kreos.***[116] ozone[227]
Delusions; lost, salvation, world, to the, beyond hope: ***arg-n.***[54]
Despair: ***acon.*** act-sp.[54] aesc.[5] agar. agn. all-c. aloe alum. alum-sil.[58] am-c. am-m.[5] ***ambr.*** ***anac.***[5] androc.[222] ant-c.[102] ant-t. apis[5] ***arg-n.*** arn. **ARS.** ars-h.[36] ***ars-i.*** ars-s-f.[58] aster. **AUR.** aur-ar.[58] bac.[62] bad. bamb-a.[1184] ***bar-c.***[5] bell. benz. bov. brom. bry. bufo[58] **CALC.** calc-i.[58] calc-s. ***calc-sil.***[58] camph.[1] cand-a.[239] ***cann-i.*** canth. carb-an. ***carb-v.***[122] carbn-s. ***caust.*** cham. chel. chin. chin-ar. chin-s.[10] choc.[222] clem. ***cocc.*** coch.[8] **COFF.** colch. ***con.*** crat.[116] crot-c.[2016] crot-h.[54] ***croto-t.*** cupr. ***cupr-acet.***[54] cur. der. dig. eup-per. fago.[25] ***gad.***[122] gamb. gels.[102] germ.[222] ***graph.*** **HELL.** helon. hep. hura hydr-ac. hydrog.[222] hyos. **IGN.** iod. kali-ar. kali-br. kali-i.[5] kali-n. ***kali-p.*** kreos.[10] ***lach.*** laur.[5] ***lept.***[5] ***lil-t.*** lith-c. **LYC.**[122] med.[58] ***merc.*** ***mez.*** morph. naja ***nat-ar. nat-c. nat-m.*** nat-s. nat-sil.[58] ***nit-ac.*** nitro-o.[36] nux-v. op.[5] orig. ozone[227] petr. ph-ac.[5] phos.[5] pic-ac.[102] plat. plb. podo. **PSOR.** ***puls.*** ***rhus-t.*** rhus-v.[25] ruta[5] sec. sel.[85] sep. sil. spig.[5] ***spong.***[5] stann. ***staph.***[30] ***stram.*** ***sul-ac.***[5] sul-i.[58] **SULPH.**[122] sumb. syph.[5] tab.[5] ther. thuj. thymol.[102] tub. valer. **VERAT.**[122] verb. vip.[5]
Despair; alternating with hope: acon.[10] bov.[10]
Despair; anger, during: tarent.[137]
Despair; comforted, wants to be: ozone[227]
Despair; concussion, after: **ARN.**[54]
Despair; criticism, from the smallest: med.[122]
Despair; death, separate him from his children, death will: bamb-a.[1184]
Despair; death, with fear of: **CALC.**[54]
Despair; destiny, everything is controlled by: bamb-a.[1184]
Despair; existence, about miserable: ***sep.***[122]
Despair; future, about: carb-v.[30] ***nat-m.***[54] sumb.[36]
Despair; health, of: calc. staph.
Despair; heart disease or liver disease, in: aur.[58]
Despair; heaven or hell, did not care whether he went to: med.[54]
Despair; hypochondriasis, in: agn.[54]
Despair; injury, from: verat.[54]
Despair; insanity, as of incipient: ***med.***[54]
Despair; itching of the skin, from: **PSOR.**
Despair; life, of: ***ars.***[1] calc.[36] cimic.[149]
Despair; lost, thinks everything is: aur.[10] ign.[10]
Despair; love, from disappointed: caust.[30] ***hyos.***[54]
Despair; masturbation, in: ***op.***[54]
Despair; others and oneself: ***arg-n.***[54] aur.[54]
Despair; others, about: ***aur.***
Despair; pains, with the: acon. aloe[58] arn.[102] ***ars.*** **AUR.** aur-ar.[58] ***bell-p.***[102] calc.[122] carb-v. ***cham.*** chin.[58] chin-ar. coch.[102] ***coff.*** colch. coloc.[58] hyper. **IGN.** lach. lil-t. mag-c. med.[102] morph.[102] naja[36] **NAT-M.**[185] **NAT-S.**[185] nux-v. psil.[164] stram.[122] ***verat.*** vip.[5] zinc-val.[102]
Despair; rage, bordering on: ***agar.***[54]
Despair; rage, cursing and imprecations: **NIT-AC.**[30]
Despair; recovery, ague, in: ***tarent.***[54]
Despair; recovery, convalescence, during: **ALUM.**[122] **ARS.**[122] **CALC.**[122] ***psor.*** **SYPH.**[122]
Despair; recovery, convulsions, after: calc.[193]
Despair; recovery, mania, in: ***verat.***[54]
Despair; recovery, of: ***acon.*** all-s.[36] alum.[5] am-c.[10] anac.[137] ant-t.[36] **ARS.** aur-ar.[58] aur-i.[58] ***aur-s.***[58] bac.[62] bapt. bar-c. bor.[10] ***bry.*** cact.[58] calad.[10] **CALC.** calc-ar.[58] calc-s. cann-i. carc.[207] caust.[30] cham. chlol. cimic.[149] **COLOC.**[162] dig.[172] germ.[222] ***hell.*** hep.[30] hura ***ign.***[122] kali-ar. kali-br. kali-c. kreos. lac-c.[116] lach.[10] lil-t.[172] lyc.[1] m-arct.[10] mag-c.[144] ***med.***[72] ***merc.***[30] nat-c.[10] nat-m.[10] nat-s. nit-ac.[58] nux-v. ph-ac.[10] phos.[10] plat.[172] ***psor.*** puls.[10] ***sep.*** sil. sulph.[10] **SYPH.**[122] ther. ***thyr.***[162] verat.[58] zinc.
Despair; recovery, thinks it is useless to take medicine: ars.[102]
Despair; religious: ***arg-n.*** **ARS. AUR.** aur-ar.[58] aur-i.[58] aur-s.[58] ***calc.*** calc-ar.[58] calc-i.[58] ***camph. chel.*** cycl.[116] hell. hura ign. ***kali-p.*** **LACH. LIL-T.** ***lyc.*** med. ***mez.***

nat-m. ozone[227] plat. plb. podo. ***psor.*** **PULS.**[122] ***stram. sulph. thuj.*** **VERAT.**
Despair; religious, alternating with sexual excitement: ***lil-t.***
Despair; religious, constant prayer: ***puls.***[54]
Despair; religious, suicidal tendency, with: verat.[54]
Despair; sad thoughts, on account of: rhus-t.[54]
Despair; salvation of soul, of eternal, after fright: stram.[54]
Despair; sexual craving, from: aster.[54]
Despair; social position, of: calc.[30] ign.[30] puls.[30] rhus-t.[30] sep.[30] staph.[30] sulph.[30] **VERAT.**
Despair; support, wants: bamb-a.[1184]
Despair; trifles, over: ***graph.***
Despair; unwilling to die, in hemoptysis: ***acal.***[54]
Despair; work, over his: anac.[58]
Discouraged; alternating with, confidence: alum.[10]
Discouraged; alternating with, hope: alum.[10] kali-c.[10] ***merc.***[30] ***op.***[30] ***staph.***[30]
Doubtful; recovery, medicine is useless: alumn.[54] ars.[10]
Dreams; loss, disheartening: ***meph.***[36]
Euphoria; alternating with, despair: ozone[227]
Hopefulness; alternating with despair: acon.[10] kali-c.[122] kali-p.[29]
Impatience; suicidal desperation, with: carb-v.[1]
Insanity; black insanity with despair and weariness of life from fear of mortification or of loss of position: calc.[30] ign.[30] puls.[30] rhus-t.[30] staph.[30] sulph.[30] verat.[30]
Jumping; impulse to, window, from, pain makes her so despaired that she would like to: ***aur.***[54]
Mania; business, discouragement, from: ***lil-t.***[54]
Sadness; despairing: ***agn.***[54] **HELL.**[54] ***plat.***[54] ***sars.***[54]
Shrieking; despair, from, before during and after paroxysm: lyss.[54]
Suicidal disposition; despair, about his miserable existence: ***sep.***[54]
Suicidal disposition; despair, from: ambr.[116] ant-c.[54] carb-v.[116] hyos.[116]
Suicidal disposition; despair, from, religious: verat.[54]
Suicidal disposition; despair, from, spells of asthma, during: ***rumx.***[54]
Weeping; despair, from: arg-n.[137] chel.[5] ***cupr-acet.***[54] hell.[5] sil.[5]

ACON. Al, 53 - Dolorous anxious complaints, with pusillanimous (cowardly) fears, despair, loud wailing (laments) and weeping, and bitter reproaches.
Ha, 510 - Sometimes he despairs of his recovery, sometimes he is full of hope.
Ha, 517 - Piteous (miserable), anxious complaints, with cowardly fears, despair, loud whining weeping, bitter complaints and reproaches.
ACT-SP. He, 16 - Desperation of success of every, even most trifling undertaking.
ADAM. Sh, 246 - Cried with despair. Nothing I do is right. Rocking from side to side, sobbing. Desire to stab with a knife or scissors. Felt very different from other humans. Long, late phone call ameliorates. 16, 12C, 43:XX:XX
Sh, 376 - Cried with despair. Nothing I do is right. Rocking from side to side sobbing. Desire to stab with a knife or scissors. Felt very different from other humans. Long, late phone call ameliorates. 16, 12C, 43:XX:XX
AGN. He, 4 - Despairing sadness; keeps repeating that she will die, that there is no use doing anything.
ALUM. Ha, 5 - He thinks that he cannot get well again.
ANAC. Ha, 8 - The future seems to him very dangerous, as if nothing were imminent but misfortune and danger; distrust in his own power, and despondency.
Ha, 9 - He is at odds (quarreling) with the whole world, and has so little confidence in himself that he despairs of being able to accomplish (succeed) what is demanded of him.
He, 63 - Despondency (desperation) and fear of approaching death.
He, 66 - He is separated (divided, disconnect, estranged) from the whole world and has so little confidence in himself that he despairs of being able to do that which is required of him.
He, 64 - Anxiousness; despairs of getting well.
ANDROC. Sh, 116 - Impatient, snappy, shouting, felt trapped and despairing. Growled at her children. (12)

ANT-C. He, 20 - Is driven to despair, resolved to drown himself.
ANT-T. Al, 5 - Despondent and apprehensive about his recovery. (despair)
He, 22 - Despondent and apprehensive (fear) that he would not recover.
He, 25 - Hopeless and despairing when awake.
He, 29 - Despair of his recovery.
He, 38 - Despair and hopelessness, with lethargy, with cold sweat.
APIS. He, 53 - Eccentric cheerfulness, despondency, or hopelessness.
ARG-N. He, 14 - Thinks he has softening of brain, or some other incurable affection (disease), which almost drives him to despair.
He, 19 - He wept and assured every one that he has lost beyond hope for this world; that no one could delude him in that respect, and no one could reason him out of it.
He, 41 - Despaired of help from himself or others.
He, 42 - Fits of despondency and all kinds of fanciful (unreal) notions for example, that whilst walking along street he could not pass a given point without falling; frequently settled on the time he was to die.
He, 48 - Great nervousness and prostration (lassitude); fears to be alone because he thinks he will die ; is apprehensive of some serious disease, which almost drives him to despair.
ARS-H. Al, 1 - Anxiety he believes his death is near, and despairs of being better...
ARS. Al, 50 - He despairs of his life.(recovery?)
Al, 51 - He despairs and weeps and imagines no one can help him, that he must die;...(unprotected)
Al, 56 - Anguish and despair driving from one place to another for relief.
Ha, 1035 - He is cold, shivers and weeps, and thinks, in his despair, (hopelessness, despairing) that nothing can help him, (helplessness) and he must die; followed by general exhaustion.
Ha, 44 - Desponding and weeping, he thinks that nothing can help him, and he would have to die anyhow; (in any way)...
He, 1033 - He despairs of his life.
He, 9 - Thoughts of death and the incurability of his complaint. 0Cancerous inoculation
He, 61 - Religious melancholy; hopelessness, despair.
AUR. Ha, 18 - Dispirited ill-humor; he thinks he cannot succeed in anything.
Ha, 19 - Dispirited and despondent; he thinks that everything goes awkwardly (incapacity, unfit) with him, and nothing will succeed with him.
He, 41 - All the time a dark, hopeless mood, frequently anxiety and despair; life is a burden (load) to him.
He, 8 - Looks on dark side, weeps, prays, thinks she is not fit for this world, longs for death, strong inclination to commit suicide; desperate, desires to jump from a height.
He, 57 - Despair of self and others.
BAR-C. Ha, 17 - Extremely discouraged and pusillanimous ;(cowardice) she thinks she will die, and weeps.
He, 34 - Loss of self confidence; desponding: pusillanimous.(cowardice)
BELL. He, 67-...suffered greatest anxiety and despaired of recovery.
BRY. He, 33 - Despair of recovery.
CACT. He, 3 - Thinks she will not recover; weeps much; despondent.
CALC. Al, 19 - She despaired of her life, and believed that she must die, with a most sad mood, and weeping, and frequent sudden attacks of general heat, as if hot water had been dashed over her.
Al, 18 - Despairing mood, with dread of disease and suffering, with foreboding of sad events.
Ha, 29 - Despairing (hopeless) mood with fear of sickness (disease) and misery, with forebodings of sad events. (misfortune)
Ha, 30 - She despairs of her life and believes she has to die (punishment?) ; her heart is sad with weeping, and frequent attacks of sudden, general heat, as if she had hot water poured (flow) over her.
He, 18 - Mental aberration with horrid visions before eyes and cardiac anxiety; he despairs of his salvation (pardon, rescue) and wants to stab himself.
He, 43 - Hopelessness; despair.
He, 38 - Low-spirited and melancholy, with weeping and despair of life.

CAMPH. Al, 46-... The sight increased my despair poor nature extinguished; the sky transparent and lifeless; the earth was still in the dim, dead light. I could not bear it. The sense of touch was gone, and my eyes protruded from their sockets.

CANN-I. Al, 35 - Despair, and fear of being eternally lost.

CANTH. He, 15 - Despondent and low-spirited, says she must die.

CARB-AN. Al, 10 - Discouraged and sad (unhappy); everything seems so sad and lonely that she desires to weep.

CARB-V. Ha, 714 - Peevish, impatient and desperate, so much so that he would like to shoot himself.

Ha, 9 - He felt like weeping, everything seemed to him dreadful (fearful), and he felt in despair.

Ha, 21 - Peevish, impatient, desperate, so that he would like to shoot himself.

CARL. Al, 10 - Discouraged and anxious in the discharge (execution) of his domestic duties.

CAUST. He, 32 - Hopeless weeping mood, expecting death.

CHEL. Al, 25 - Sadness, even to weeping, and despondency (desperation) about the present and future.

CHLOL. He, 3 - Fixed despair of recovery; believes he will give his imaginary disease (syphilis) to others.

COCC. Ha, 535 - In the morning, anxiety respecting the incurability of a trifling malady.

DER. Al, 3 - He is discouraged and despairs of a cure (recovery), declaring himself a hypochondriac.

DIG. Ha, 14-..he is much affected by everything, but especially by sad things, and the least trifle can throw him into disconsolate despair.(sensitive)

He, 11 - Melancholic, despondent, and constantly tortured by fear of death or loss of reason.

DROS. Ha, 275 - He is sad and dejected about the ills (evil) of life, which people cause one another and himself, respecting which he is anxious and concerned;...(ethical)

FERR. He, 9 - Mind in highest degree oppressed; despondent (sad); great solicitude (cares) about those belonging to him (relatives, family), with constant thoughts of death.

GERM. Sh, 7 - Recurrent rows triggered by my detachment. Felt despair and utter confusion about what was related to the proving and what was reality. 04, 6C, 14.00.00.

Sh, 101 - I'm desperate. I want to die. Feel the power to kill. Feel like a wild animal locked in. It's strong, so intense. I hate so strong-feel a terrible disgust and I'm afraid of what I'm able to do. It's completely impossible to be in it and impossible to get out of it. 18, 30C, 190:XX:XX

GRAPH. Al, 12 - Grief about the slightest occurrences (trifle), even to despair.

Ha, 6 - Grief even to despair, about the most trifling matters.

HALI-L. Sh, 430 - Get a call from a friend that the utility district is at it again. Don't know what, but expect the worst in negotiations with them. Can't win. So tired of fighting the losing battle. Can't raise the energy to do anything. Rage inside. Hopeless. Daydreams of blowing up the utility district, of shooting them. Only option left to desperate people and I feel desperate. we're a rag-tag group without luck, or leadership, fighting a losing battle. Feels like we're the American Indians. "Here's 24 dollars worth of beads for your island, idiot." In the pit of despair. 09, 6C, 25:XX:XX

HELL. Ha, 281 - He despairs of his life.

He, 12 - An old woman having been accused of theft by the women around, took it so much to heart that she hanged herself. This suicide produced a profound effect upon the women of the village. One after another accused herself of having caused the death of the old woman by their insinuations; they wept and howled, ran about day and night wringing their hands and despairing of salvation on account of their sin (error); they became quite irrepressible and deranged (disordered) In this way twenty -four or twenty five women were affected, every fresh case being followed by another. Hysterical mania.

HELON. Al, 2 - Reaction (from feeling of general wellness) began, and for a fortnight I was in a mental hell; it was the most profound mental depression I have ever known; I was plunged into the most abject despair.

HEP. Al, 15 - Extremely discontented and fretful about his pains, and discouraged (unhappy).

HURA. Al, 10 - Sadness, melancholy; she thinks despondingly of the future.

HYDROG. Sh, 180 - Indifference, despair and hopelessness—no way out. 32, 9C, 03:XX:XX

Sh, 259 - Fear and desperation about being pregnant —period 16 days late —felt terrible all day. So despairing. 08, 30C, 50:XX:XX

HYOS. Al, 82 - In despair, he wishes to drown himself.

Ha, 579 - In despair he wishes to take his life, and throw himself into the water.(suicidal)

He, 74 - Disappointed love followed by: epilepsy, melancholy, rage, or inclination to laugh at everything; despair and propensity to drown himself. (ailments from)

IGN. He, 40 - Anxiety, sleeplessness, despair; severe palpitation; loss of appetite; constipation.

KALI-BR. Al, 24 - The patient, who has been violently excited, glorying (adoration) in his imaginary power of body and mind, becomes desponding sullen, melancholic, and frequently lachrymose, often even despairing.

He, 30 - Great despondency; "feel as if they should go out of their minds."

KALI-C. Al, 22 - Faint-hearted and despondent to an excessive degree.

He, 9-...constantly in antagonism which herself; frequently hopeful, frequently despondent; frets (worry) about everything; peevish impatient, contented with nothing.

MED. Al,N-23 - Wild desperate feeling, as of incipient insanity.

Al,N-52 - Feeling of desperation; did not care if he went to heaven or hell.

He, 22 - Wild and desperate feeling, as of incipient insanity.

He, 36 - A word or look of seeming harshness (reproach) put her in despondency for hours. (sensitive)

He, 37 - Feeling of desperation, did not care if he went to heaven or hell.

MEZ. He, 8 - Despairs of eternal salvation.

NAT-C. Al, 42 - Very fretful and discontented with whole world; he constantly felt as though he could beat (punish ?) himself, his whole life angered him, and he preferred to have no existence at all; he was solicitous about the future, and inclined to despair, all day.

NAT-M. Al, 51 - Attacks of complete hopelessness and internal despair, that deprived him of all power.

Ha, 21 - Attacks of entire hopelessness (despairing) and internal despondency (despair) which take away all her strength.

Ha, 5 - Melancholy dejection and sorrowful anxious despondency all day, without any known cause, with unceasing palpitation,...

He, 36 - Despairing, hopeless feeling about the future.

NAT-S. Al, 5 - Very much disheartened; tired (weary) of life; despairs of getting well. (recovery)

NICC. Al, 6 - Apprehensive and despondent, as if some misfortune were impending.

NIT-AC. Al, 33 - Depressed, as if despondent and as if in deep thought.

Al, 2 - Attacks of rage and despair, with curses and imprecations.(blasphemy)

Ha, 2 - Dejected, as if desponding and as if lost in thoughts.

He, 13 - Hopeless despair.

PHOS. Al, 108 - Anxiously solicitous concerning the unfortunate termination of her illness.

Al, 109 - Discouraged about his health.

Al, 38 - Told those about him repeatedly that he could not possibly recover, and gave some disjointed directions about his business affairs.

He, 22- ...uneasy about one's health; paroxysms of anguish, when alone or in a stormy weather, with timorous disposition; told those about him repeatedly that he could not possibly recover, and gave some disjointed (incoherent) directions about his business affairs.

PHYS. He, 3-...feels as if she must lose her mind and become insane or despondent;...;thinks she is a castaway (repudiated, discarded, rejected, forsaken);....fears she is crazy or will certainly lose her mind;...

PLB. He, 15-...; despair of her salvation...; fixed idea that could only obtain peace and safety though absolution by a priest of the papal church, although she had been a zealous Protestant; ....brooded over any forbidden thing; would steal (leave) from house in servant's cloak (coat, camouflage) and bonnet (hat) to obtain stimulants (drugs), but from the moment their prohibition was withdrawn (retired) ceased to have any desire for them; after being permitted to visit a priest and converse with him ceased to talk and think of the church. (desire; redemption, absolution)

He, 16 - Mental disturbance of eight or ten years' duration in a man addicted to masturbation; has several times attempted suicide; has been in seclusion (solitude); greatest dejection and despair;...; believes himself lost (condemned) ; has the sounds of hell constantly in his ears; hears voices and sees shadows of demons, great disposition to make away (suicide) with himself or do himself some bodily injury;

PSOR. Al, 14 - Very melancholy and despairing; he wishes to die in spite of his good luck.

Al, 19 - Despairing mood; he fears to fail in business.

Al,N-24 - Despairing mood; fears he will fail in business.

Al,N-32 - Melancholy after suppressed itch;...seeks solitude, despairs of recovery; ...

Al,N-35 - Driving to despair with excessive itching.

He, 24 - Despairing mood; fears he will fail in business.

He, 26 - Greatest despondency (desperation), making his own life and those about him intolerable;...

He, 32 - Melancholy after suppressed itch;...seeks solitude, despair of recovery;...

PULS. Al, 28 - He sinks into a condition of sadness and despondency from disagreeable news.

Ha, 1131 - On hearing some disagreeable news he became affected with sadness and despondency.

He, 48-...despaired of her soul's salvation; did not believe she would be restored to health ; ...

He, 53-...afraid of everybody; considers every one her enemy, despairs of everything; ...;trusts no one;.. (suspicious)

RHUS-T. Al, 31 - Fear and despair on account of sad thoughts, which she could not get rid of.

Ha, 963 - Ill-humored, dejected, and as if in despair.

He, 12 - Fear and despair on account of sad thoughts, which she could not get rid of. (fixed ideas)

SCROPH-N. Al, 1 - Desponding (sad), much troubled (worried) about the past, and very apprehensive of the future, which passed off after a few days, and left the intellect clear.

SEP. Ha, 10 - All her troubles present themselves in a very sad light to her mind, so that she is despondent.(sad, depressed)

He, 28 - Propensity to suicide from despair about his miserable (wretched, unfortunate) existence.

SPONG. He, 29 - Nervous; despondent about loss of sexual power.

STRAM. Ha, 363 - He feels his hands and feet as if separated in the joints, and he is inconsolable on account of this sensation.

He, 59-...clings to her mother with as much desperation as if she were going to be thrown from a precipice.

He, 112 - Religious mania; pious (divine) looks, praying; restless nights; inspired talking, singing; despairs of her salvation.

SULPH. He, 29-...is filled with anxious, despondent (sad) thoughts, from which she cannot free herself, they make her suspicious, peevish and lachrymose.

SUMB. Al, 8-...fond (love) of the society of women; ...sympathy with suffering seems robbed of its pain...nervous excitement and heat, especially in head from listening (hearing) to a disputation, ...humor depressed with despair of future...melancholy despondency, as if ill-treated by everyone purposely... mildness, amiability

TAB. Al, 35 - Great apprehension with oppression of the chest, and a very despondent, sad mood, as if apprehended some misfortune,...

THER. Al, 7 - Despair; want of confidence; he gives himself up.

THUJ. Al, 1 - She herself desires, with

anxiety and despair, to be taken to an insane asylum, (imprisonment, confining) and there to be treated very harshly and strictly, (penalized), so that her fixed ideas may be subdued and banished (purified); she knows very well that she does wrong (conscience) and thinks all sorts of bad thoughts (immoral), but she will not take the trouble to banish such thoughts; therewith she indistinctly gives to understand that she is constantly obliged to think of taking her own life, but feels the sinfulness (wicked) of it, in order to avoid it, desires the strict restraint of the asylum;...

Al, 74 - Constant great despair changes at last to complete indifference.

TUB. Al,N-47 - Despondent, discouraged, feel as if I would rather die than live.

VERAT. He, 10 - Suicidal tendency from religious despair.

He, 26 - Chases (pursue, hunt) his family out of house ; declares the sun travels around the earth (geocentric); fear of death, restlessness, despair...

He, 52 - Despair about his position in society, feels very unlucky.

He, 53 - Despair of her salvation;...

He, 54 - Despair of his recovery; attempts suicide.

He, 19 - A woman, ...hopeless despair, ...brought on by sexual excitement.

He, 51 - Despair; hopeless, loss of courage.

ZINC. He, 29-...;sad, weeps frequently; despairs of her recovery;...

DESPISED

Ailments from; mortification, humiliation, chagrin, emotional or mental ailments from: anac.[8] ***apoc.***[8] ***aur.***[8] bell.[5] ***coloc.***[8] con.[103] cur.[11] ***ign.***[8] lach.[30] lyc.[58] lyss.[56] nat-m.[10] ***nux-v.***[10] pall.[116] plat.[30] ***puls.***[8] ran-b.[36] ***staph.***[54] verat.[30] zinc.[10]

Ailments from; pride of others: grat.[85]

Ailments from; scorn, being scorned: acon. alum.[58] ***aur.*** bell. **BRY. CHAM.** coff. ***coloc.*** ferr. hyos. ip. lyc. ***nat-m.*** **NUX-V.** olnd. ***par. phos. plat.*** sep. ***staph.*** stront-c. sulph. verat.

Ailments from; scorn, looked down upon by everyone, feels he is: ***lac-c.***[54]

Confidence; thinks others have none, which makes her unhappy, and: ***aur.***

Delusions; alone, castaway, being a: germ.[222] ***phys.***[54]

- appreciated, she is not: arg-n.[185] aur.[185] lap-c-b.[194] ***pall.*** plat. puls.[162] seq-s.[230]
- despised, is: **ARG-N.** cob.[144] hura hydrog.[222] lac-c. lach.[137] ***orig.***[54]
- faces, doctor is making faces at her, she looked black: puls.[54]
- insane, people think her: **CALC.** germ.[222] hydrog.[222]
- laughed at, criticized to disadvantage, makes her timid, and she dare not look up while walking in street: bar-c.[54]
- laughed at, hides behind furniture, therefore: ***bar-c.***[122]
- laughed at, mocked, she is: aq-mar.[231] ***bar-c.*** germ.[222] ***ign.***[30] lach.[162] nux-v.[30] ***ph-ac.***[30] psor.[185] ***sep.***[30]
- looked down upon, she is: ***lac-c.***
- lost, salvation, despised, and, in erotomania: ***orig.***[54].
- neglected, he is: ***arg-n.*** lap-mar-c.[194] naja nat-m.[189] **PALL.** puls.[58] sac-alb.[210] sep.[189]
- neglected, he is, despised by his family, and: ***arg-n.***[54]
- neglected, husband, by her: ***stram.***[8]
- people, prank with him, carry on all sorts of: hydrog.[222] **NUX-V.**[54]
- repudiated by relatives, he is: arg-n. hura.
- repudiated, society, he is repudiated by: hydrog.[222]
- talking, friends talking about her: lach.[58]

Dreams; humiliation: alum. am-c. arn. ***asar.*** con. ign. led. mag-m. mosch. mur-ac. ***sil.*** staph.

➤ table, tablecloth is too beautiful, for other, special occasions, not for him: ozone[227]
➤ throw away, being to: rhus-t.[10]
➤ wedding, everyone is going to a, except her: hydrog.[222]

Fear; humiliated, of being: puls.[30] ***sep.***[30]

✦ looked at: aq-mar.[231] ars.[193] bar-c.[193] calc.[172] meli.[193] rhus-t.[193]
✦ neglected, of being: cand-a.[239] puls.[58]
✦ ridiculed, of being: calc.[127]

Forsaken; feeling, isolation, sensation of, talking, on, people do not hear him: cortico.[119]

Hide; desire to, children, thinks all visitors laugh at it and hides behind furniture: ***bar-c.***

Humiliation, painful sense of: chin-b.[54]

Jealousy; neglect, accuses husband of: ***stram.***[54]

Jesting; aversion to: ***acon.*** am-c. ang. apis ars. bor. bov. caps. carb-an. ***cina*** cocc. cycl. ***merc.***[122] nat-m. nux-v. puls. sabin. sil. spig. staph.[30] sulph. thuj.
Lamenting; appreciated, because he is not: calc-s.
Misunderstood, feels: ign.[155] lap-c-b.[194]
Mocking; others at him, thinks: ign.[30] nux-v.[30] ph-ac.[30] sep.[30]
Offended; jokes, by: nat-m.[36]
Sadness; slight or treat, from an undeserved: arg-n.
Sensitive; laughed at, to being: calc.[127]
Suspiciousness; talking about her, people are: ***bar-c.*** hyos.[137] ign.[137] pall.[137] staph.[137]
Violence; observed, when he thinks he is not: tarent.[146]
Weeping; neglect, from the slightest: coff.[58]
Weeping; ungratefulness, at: ***lyc.***[30]

ADAM. 196 - Very nervous and little self-confidence. I think people are laughing at me and hate me. 20, 1M, 07:XX:XX
197 - Suspiciousconfusion that people are making a fool of me, laughing at me. 2, 12C, XX:XX:XX
Sh, 200 - I felt like I had been treated badly, a mixture of insult and humiliation. 15, 12C, 01:09:45
ARG-N. He, 40 - Melancholy since an undeserved slight (scorn); fixed idea that he was neglected and despised by his family; his callings (job, work) became indifferent to him.
AUR. Ha, 3 - He believes that he has lost the love of others, and this mortifies him even to tears.
Ha, 353 - He imagines he has forfeited (penalty, lost,) the affections of others, and this grieves him to tears.
BAR-C. He, 12 - Walking in street she imagines men are laughing at her, criticizing to disadvantage; this makes her so timid that she dare (venture) not look up or at anybody, and she perspires over whole body.
BRASS. Sh, 12 - Called on a friend who was busy with funeral arrangements. Felt rejected when she had not time to talk to me; my head was saying "don't be silly" but my eyes filled with tears, and my wee heart felt very unloved 3I, 00:06:30
CAMPH. Al, 46-...I sat up in bed, but all about me had indeed disappeared. I was alone in the great universe, the last of all things. My ideas of the world, God and religion, now seemed to me to have existed only in my imagination; the earth upon which yesterday I lived and moved, had run its appointed course, and I was the final and solitary fragment of the whole creation...(meaningless, unimportant, neglected, forsaken, loneliness, deserted) (godless)
CANN-I. Al, 25... The stars seemed to look upon him with pitying (compassion) human aspect, and to bewail (lament) his condition.
CHIN-B. He, 5 - Feels abandoned and deserted.
COCC. He, 24 - Melancholy and sad; indulges in sad reveries (daydream); is sensitive to insults, slights (despises) and disappointment.
GERM. Sh, 115 - Very much in doubt whether I should take any more tablets. Whatever I do, I feel that somebody will criticize me, that I do something wrong. Difficult to make a decision. Afraid that other people will laugh at me or say, haven't you understood anything?" Crying. Don't want to get up. Don't want to bother the supervisor so early in the morning. I am a failure. 18, 30C, 01:06:30
Sh, 111 - If I were me, nobody would like me - so I try to be what I think others expect me to be. I don't think I can be loved with all the parts of me which are ugly and bad. Lonely feelings. Longing for love and understanding. Feel I am so unfriendly to myself. 18, 30C, 04:00:00
Sh, 141 - Painfully aware of the feelings of being an outcast. 08, 12C, 02:00:10
Sh, 151-.... I feel I have no real contact with people, I have no emotion at all except for a feeling of isolation and a concern that people may not like me. I wish someone would cuddle me. By 10 o'clock I have a definite aversion to people, especially certain people- the stubborn or authoritarian kind. I become deeply involved in my own thoughts and can be very irritable and even angry when the thoughts are interrupted by people, but I don't show any signs of anger or irritation. The fate of other people leaves

me cold, but I know this is not right. My mind is blank and I feel I could just sit and stare. I have no feelings, no emotions! I think a lot about my state of mind and try to understand it; it puzzles me. What is missing? Eating removes this thoughtful mood. By afternoon and evening I become gradually more involved with what I am doing but still feel isolated even when in the company of other people. I don't mind listening to people, but I contribute little to conversation. This state lasted for three days. 16, 30C, 04:XX:XX

Sh, 153 - Thought nobody understood me and cared for what I felt. Felt it was unfair. I was presented with complaints about something others had done. Felt I was standing between two fighting parts. Felt awkward about it, embarrassed. Difficult to argue about such strong outburst. Thoughts about the day's arguing milling in my head all evening and night. 21, 12C, 32:XX.XX.

HALI-L. Sh, 55 - I usually relate to people who make a lot less money than me. I had an argument with a friend who is in a high class about money. Am thinking about taking a job that would put me in a high class, but don't know if I would want to work with those kind of people—downtown people into their careers who make hundreds of thousands. They make me nervous. Afraid they will snub me. So much to do with worth. What am I worth? 08, 30C, 42:XX:XX

Sh, 337 - Talked to a friend who didn't understand me and didn't understand my goals. I felt degraded and wanted to really yell at him. In the end, he understood me, and I expressed my frustration with him. Frustrated that I couldn't make him get what I was saying. So furious. They didn't give me any respect. I deserve more. Frustrated. I do so much more than he thought, and he didn't understand. 08, 30C, 37:XX:XX

Sh, 427 - Luckily, this legal dispute is not happening to me personally. But I feel it is. I imagine them laughing at us and doing their worst to squash us. Never felt so helpless in my life. 09, 6C, 26:XX:XX

Sh, 431 - The first thing that happened was I became very depressed and fearful. I was weak and couldn't resolve my issues. I became a laughable matter. The next thing I knew, I became embittered at all those I thought were laughing at me. During the last week of the proving, the vindictive side of reacting to that depression came out. 18, 30C, 7:XX:XX

Sh, 604 - Since the remedy, I took over and the physical manifestation of personas splitting off would only come out when I was alone. Did these drawings. The figure in the box was my death — captured, buried and can't get out. The first drawing is a depressed boy, the second is the buried man, the third is an x-ray figure. After that the depression abated. I did another drawing of a negative being laughing at me. It has no arms, no movement. 18, 30C, 35:XX:XX

Sh, 629 - Broke things off with a friend. Felt sad then angry. Felt he degraded me. It was unhealthy to have that energy around me anymore. Very angry. No respect from him. 08, 30C, 36:XX:XX

HURA. Al, 15 - Hypochondria, sadness, despair; he fancies he is repudiated and deserted by his relations. (rejected, refused)

HYDROG. Sh, 235 - Feel a bit depressed and frustrated by present circumstances. Feel like the unappreciated victim. 04, 12C, 14:XX:XX

Sh, 254 - When shopping, felt people did not accept me as belonging to the community. Felt isolated in the shop. Feeling unacceptable, 'as if I was a marked person' —but later felt better on my own. 12, 6C, 19:XX:XX

Sh, 255 - Very worried that people don't like me and can't cope with me —that they will think I am insane. I think maybe I am insane. This is frightening me. 16, 30C, 25:XX:XX

LAC-C. Al,N-11 - Thinks that she is looked down upon (despised) by every one, that she is of no importance in life, and feels insulted thereat. (unimportant, worthless)

He, 9 - Thinks she is looked down (contempted, scorned, despised) upon by everyone, that she is of no importance in life. (self-contemptuous)

He, 36 - Feels insulted because she thinks she is looked down (scorn, despised) upon by everyone.

LYSS. Al,N-46 - After fainting (weak) spell he wrote on paper: I am forsaken by all; even the birds of heaven, they do not look at me (despised), do not fed me if hungry (helplessness) ; I hunger with the young ones and am thirsty with their she ones (starving); my nest (house) is made out of dirt (soiled), not gotten by my own exertions (efforts), but by driving them out of their nests (home) and sitting there with the females and the young.

NAT-M. Al, 109 - Offended by a joke.

NEON. Sh, 44 - Dreamed that I was knocking on many different doors. Nobody opened them. 20, 6C, 19:XX:XX

NUX-V. He, 19-...; imagines himself surrounded by persons who carry on all sorts of pranks (joke, jest), or ply (covering) him with questions which he thinks he is compelled (forced) to answer (proved, questioned, interrogated);..; answers questions rationally and is conscious of his condition; ...appears to be haunted (obsessed) by a great fear.

PALL. He, 8 - Imagines herself neglected (scorned, despised); wounded pride.

PHYS. He, 3-...feels as if she must lose her mind and become insane or despondent;...;thinks she is a castaway (repudiated, discarded, rejected, forsaken);....fears she is crazy or will certainly lose her mind;...

RHUS-T. He, 24-...a week later she told her mother to not look at her (observed) ; seemed to be distrustful (suspicious) and did not wish to see any one; she came running in from the street and said people were looking at her; ....; cries without cause, imagines people are finding fault (misconduct, criticized, censured) with her because she is earning (succeed, prosper, reach) nothing, acts in a childish manner;...

SPIG. Ha, 665 - Serious humor, he gets cross if the slightest joke is attempted on him.

STRAM. He, 145 - Wife complains of husband neglecting her; man accuses his wife of being faithless.
He, 176 - Melancholia,...complains her husband has neglecting her.

SULPH. He, 37 - Great dejection,(grief), with thoughts of suicide; feels inferior (mediocre, lower) to everybody; can decide nothing;...

SUMB. Al, 8-...fond (love) of the society of women; ...sympathy with suffering seems robbed of its pain...nervous excitement and heat, especially in head from listening (hearing) to a disputation, ...humor depressed with despair of future...melancholy despondency, as if ill-treated by everyone purposely... mildness, amiability

DEVIL

Delusions; bed, surrounded by devils, is: op.[10]

- demoniacal, he is: ***anac.***[54] **HYOS.**[30]
- devils, after her: ***hyos. manc. zinc.***[54]
- devils, after her, climacteric period, during: zinc.[54]
- devils, blasphemous words, devil whispers: ***anac.***[54]
- devils, connected to, he is, arrogant towards those who strive to purity, light and love: ozone[227]
- devils, erotic mania, in: orig.[54]
- devils, he is a devil: anac. camph. cann-i. *hyos.* kali-br. stram.
- devils, persons are, all: **PLAT.** plb.[54]
- devils, possessed of a devil, is: bor.[58] cann-i.[36] hyos. plat.[30] stram.[85]
- devils, possessed, everyone is: meli.
- devils, present, are: anac. cann-i. op. phos. **PLAT.**
- devils, sees: absin.[172] ambr. ***anac.*** ars. ***bell.*** cann-i. cupr. dulc. ***hell.*** hyos. kali-c. lach. ***manc.*** nat-c. ***op.***[122] ***plat. puls.*** stram. sulph. ***zinc.***
- devils, sits in his neck, and tells him offensive things: ***anac.***[54]
- devils, speaking in one ear, angel in the other, prompting to murder, or acts of benevolence, devil: ***anac.***[54]
- devils, taken by the devil, he will be: bell.[30] manc. ***puls.***[54]
- devils, taken by, that he will be, mania, in religious: ***puls.***[54]
- faces, diabolical, crowd upon him: ***ambr.*** carb-an. caust. tarent.[58]
- faces, diabolical, get rid of them, cannot: ambr.
- God, he is, then he is devil: **STRAM.**[54]
- incubus, being weighted down by: cere-b.[36]
- possessed, God and the devil, alternately by: psil.[164]

- pursued, satan, by: vip.[1212]
- pursued, spirits, evil, are pursuing him, runs around room, cries out: stram.[54]
- religious, redemption and devil, about: ***anac.***[54]
- spectres, sees, night, evil ones: ***hell.***[54]

Dreams; devils: apis arg. cand-a.[239] carc.[227] kali-c. lac-c. nat-c. nicc. op.[30] ozone[227] sin-n.

➤ devils, cooking babies on a vulcano and eating them: ozone[227]
➤ devils, seeing an acquaintance coming and mistaking him for the devil: nicc.[36]
➤ fiends: apis[36]
➤ fiends, raging, strong: arg.[36]

Fear; devil, of being taken by the: anac.[116] manc. puls.[172]

Mania; demoniacal: ***anac.***[116] arge.[149] bell.[116] ***hell.***[54] hyos.[116] op.[116] plat.[116] sil.[116] sulph.[116] verat.[116]

AMBR. Al, N-6 - Distorted images, grimaces; diabolical faces crowd upon his fancy.

Ha, 478 - Distorted fancies, grimaces, satanic faces take possession of the mind, and he cannot get rid of them.

ANAC. He, 25 - Has a devil in his ear whispering blasphemous words.

He, 28 - Fixed ideas: that mind and body are separated ; about redemption (salvation) of soul and about the devil; that a stranger is constantly by his side (pursued); that strange forms accompany him, one to his right and one to his left.

He, 30 - Hallucination; delirium a demon sits on his neck and tells him most offensive things.

He, 40 - Uses profane language, swears, thinks himself a demon.

He, 69 - In one ear a devil, in the other an angel, prompts (incite) him to do murder or acts of benevolence. (homicidal, x helpfulness, kindness)

CAMPH. Al, 46-... My misery was boundless; time itself was no more; in short, I suffered such fearful anguish as no fancy can comprehend. What soul could paint to itself my everlasting (eternal) dwelling as the Evil One (devil), alone in a vast universe, without faith or hope, and my heart forever broken by unimaginable tortures? (miserable, timeless, endless, solitude, forsaken, faithless, hopeless)

Al, 46-...For a moment I resolved to throw myself from the window and sweep through the domain of my infernal kingdom, but a weak glimmer of reason held me back...

Al, 46-.... As I lay stretched on my couch, as the evil demon, and suffered all the anguish of a condemned and God-forsaken soul, ...I was forever deprived of the Divine protection, and of every consolation and every hope. Nothing remained to me but the conviction of my everlasting damnation...

CANN-I. Al, 25-...Now demoniac shapes clutched (grasp) at him from the darkness, cloaked (covered) from head to foot in inky (black) palls (mantle), glaring (staring, looking) at him with fiery eyes from beneath their cowls(mantle)....

HALI-L. Sh, 589 - I wanted to really hurt somebody or something, no respect for the person, anyway that I could. There was another part of me that couldn't believe I was doing that. It was like a horror movie. I got to that place of no boundaries or responsibility to life. It didn't matter what I did. Indifferent. Like ice, no feeling. Just like if I killed someone there would be no regrets. Just the thought: This is what I have to do now. Desire to kill. It did not matter. Just do it. You've got to. I had no fear. I could do anything, whatever I was asked to do, I could do it then. I was a strong person. The me was the only thing that kept me from doing it. That's where I got scared. The last five days of the proving were in a black hole. I refused to write anything down. A god-like place or a devil-like place. Why do I have these things? Human things. 02, 30C, XX:XX:XX

Sh, 650 - It was like a horror movie. That's where I got scared. The last five days of the proving were in a black hole. A god-like place or a devil-like place. Why do I have these things? Human things. 02, 30C, XX:XX:XX

HELL. He, 9 - Mania demoniac; sees evil (harmful) spirits at night.

HYOS. Al, 9 - Madness as if possessed by a devil.

Ha, 541 - Mania, as if possessed by the devil.

He, 79 - After being harshly (severe) accused of theft (crime), continual delirium; fancies surrounded by objects of a terrifying nature; not a moment quiet, continual calling out that she saw the devil; denies herself guilty of theft (innocent, injustice), or that she has any concern with witches; ...

KALI-BR. He, 11 - Imagines she is a devil; cannot sleep; fears to be alone.

LIL-T. Al, 351 - The sexual desire, dormant hitherto, was so strongly aroused that the prover said, "I am afraid of myself, I seem possessed of a demon."

MANC. He, 3 - Fear of getting crazy; of evil spirits; of being taken (possessed) by the devil.

He, 5-...about midnight attacks of fear and trembling; afraid of evil spirits, of being taken (possessed) hold of by the devil;...

OP. Ha, 637 - She was troubled when awake with the supposed sight of ghosts, devils and spectres, which she believed to be surrounding her bed...

PHOS. Al, 86-...; a feeling of dread (fear), as if awaiting something terrible, yet unable to resist or move (terrifying, scaring), overcame me; sometimes it seemed as if I was beginning to bloat (inhalant, inflate, vanity?), and then I could hear a multitude of voices saying in high glee, "Fill him up a little more and he will burst," (blow up) followed by demoniacal laughter, which made the cold chills run over me... I imagined myself an aurora borealis, and could distinctly hear voices shouting, "Beautiful! Oh, was not that splendid?"...

PLAT. Ha, 21 - She thinks all persons are demons.

PLB. Al, 63 - The patient imagined that he was constantly followed (persecuted), and that he heard voices coming from the chimney... ; this man after a few days wished to leave the hospital and go home, because he was convinced that there were fiends in the building that pursued him and sought (want) his life.

He, 16 - Mental disturbance of eight or ten years' duration in a man addicted to masturbation; has several times attempted suicide; has been in seclusion (solitude); greatest dejection and despair;...; believes himself lost (condemned) ; has the sounds of hell constantly in his ears; hears voices and sees shadows of demons, great disposition to make away (suicide) with himself or do himself some bodily injury;

PULS. He, 40 - Religious mania; sees the devil coming to take her; the world on fire during night; fear, rage in spells, or weeping... (captured, possessed)

He, 47-...; pangs (pain, anxiety) of conscience about religion and female sex; violent palpitation in the presence of women; abhors (detests, aversion) and hates the sex; must go out of their way for fear of injuring them; looks upon them as evil beings and is afraid (fear; temptation, seduction); considers their presence injurious (insulted, offended) to his soul; ... (sexual loathing)

STRAM. He, 40 - Aberration of mind; one carries home all sorts of wood in order to manufacture brandy (cognac) (busy, manufacturing) ; another placed two axes across each other in order to split wood in this way; a third burrowed in ground like a pig with his mouth (animal); a fourth alleged he was a wheelwright and began to bore holes; a fifth ran into forge to catch fish, which he saw swimming there; a lacemaker threw about her bobbins incessantly, and threw everything into confusion; another girl ran about the room and cried out that all evil spirits were pursuing her.(restoration, restitution)

He, 87 - After a dreadful shock, occasioned by death of his brother, who fell dead in his arms,...struck all at around him...spoke at one time in Hungarian, and then in Wallachian language; sang Latin paternosters, declared he was God, and then that he was the devil;...

ZINC. He, 43 - Great fear, as if persecuted by men or the devil, on account of crimes he has never done (injustice); is afraid of becoming imprisoned, or poisoned, or shot, or buried (inter) alive...0 Delirium tremens.

He, 46-...; believed herself to be called before court (judged) on account of her wicked (immoral) actions; ....;believe the devil is after her;...(persecution)

DICTATORIAL

Answer; dictatorial: lach.[162] ***lyc.***[54] plat.[162] sulph.[162]
Change; aversion to: caps.[188] cupr.[210] ***kali-c.***[187] medus.[168] polyg.[8]
Delirium; imperious: lyc.[36]
Delusions; council, holding a: arn.[5] cham.[5]
• general, he is a: cupr.
Desires; captivating others: lap-mar-c.[194]
Desires; order: lap-mar-c.[194]
Desires; servants: lap-mar-c.[194]
Dictatorial: allox.[119] ***androc.*** apis[117] arn.[10] ars.[189] bamb-a.[1184] ***camph.*** caust. cham. chel.[193] chin.[30] con. cupr.[5] ***dulc.***[187] ferr. gall-ac.[198] lach. lil-t.[137] ***lyc.*** med.[212] ***merc.*** nux-v.[189] ozone[227] pall.[137] phos.[54] plat.[111] sulph.[137] thymol.[102] thyr.[77] verat.[5]
Dictatorial; abortion, in threatening: lyc.[26]
Dictatorial; command, talking with air of: arn.[10] cupr.[10] ***lyc.***[10] ***phos.***[54]
Dictatorial; control others, wants to: lach.[162] merc.[162]
Dictatorial; power, love of: ars.[11] lach.[11] lyc
Dogmatic: camph.[5] caust.[5] ferr.[5] kali-c.[162] lach.[5] lyc.[60] merc.[5]
Dreams; preaching: allox.[119] anac. ant-t.
Insanity; dictatorial: **LYC.**[10]
Loquacity; domineering: ozone[227]
Power, love of: ars.[189] lach.[189] lyc. nux-v.[189] sulph.[189]
Talk; dictatorial: ***lyc.***[54] ***phos.***[54]

AGAR. Al, 2 - He becomes so furious that he can hardly be restrained from ripping up his bowels, as he fancies the mushroom had ordered him to do.
Al, 9 - Delirium; he imagines himself a military (martial) officer, commanding (dominant) at a drill (training) and directing the various maneuvers.
Al, 14 - He imagines himself at a gate of the hell and that the mushroom commands him to fall on his knees and confess his sins, which he does. (forgiveness, absolution)

ANDROC. Sh, 41 - Feels much more self centred —have given up all the permanent favours I do for people —I don't want to do any more. Feel I need more time for me. I must feel guilt but I don't think I do. I feel the nasty side of my character is emerging much more aggressive and domineering. I don't want peoples' good opinion of me as someone who is nice — very unusual. (7)

ARN. Al, 27 - Sullen (morose) insolence and imperiousness. (dictatorial)
Ha, 634 - Surly insolence and imperiousness. (domineering)

CAMPH. Ha, 343 - Quarrelsomeness, insists he is right.
He, 73 - Dogmatical, easily offended.

CON. He, 38 - Very much excited, passionate, domineering (dictatorial), quarrelsome, scolds (censorious) and will not bear contradiction.

CUPR. Ha, 23 - Fits of insanity, imagines he is a military commander.

FERR. He, 16 - Vehement; quarrelsome; anxious.

HALI-L. Sh, 582 - Enforcing deadlines and rules with kids. Son wants to sing me a song but his work's not done so I "don't have time" to listen. Feel I am neglecting my family. 09, 6C, 15:00:XX
Sh, 610 - Want to stay in integrity with myself and not run after my lover. We talked about commitment and she got scared. I got angry. This is it. I told her I'm not going all over the place with you. Want you XX per cent here. Feel angry at her indecision and confusion. Feel I want to hit and shake her. Ran on the beach instead. 02, 30C, 02:09:XX
Sh, 619 - Explosive fight. Communication not good. I felt trapped. We didn't have a common language and we usually do. It was like two needy babies. I had my plan and he wasn't playing his part, and he had his plan and I wasn't playing my part. 01, 30C, 03:XX:XX

HYDROG. Sh, 240 - I feel life is a serious thing. When putting children to bed, I felt serious and uncompromising. I wanted them to do exactly as I said and, if not, threatened to hit them. 32, 9C, 03:XX:XX

KALI-C. Ha, 33 - Contrary mood; she demands (order, command) impetuously; is not satisfied with anything (dissatisfied) ; she is beside herself, and furiously angry; if everything does not go according to her wishes, and often does not herself know what she really wants.

LYC. Al, 2 - Delirious, raging, envious, reproachful, presumptuous, and imperious.
Ha, 59 - Insanity and fury, breaking out in envy, pretensions (inflated) and ordering (dictatorial) others about.
He, 17-...imperiousness(domineering, despotic) ; speaks with an air of command (ordering, domination) ; manner stiff (severe, obstinate) and pretentious;...
He, 37 - Haughty, reproachful and overbearing.(despotic)
He, 32 - Obstinate, defiant (contrary), arbitrary (capricious?); seeks disputes.
LYSS. Al,N-33-...Thinks he is a man of great authority.(power, command, expert)
He, 33 - Makes speeches in delirium; thinks he is a man of great authority.
MERC. Ha, 1254 - Quarreling with everyone, opinionative, (doctrinal) quarrelsome.
PHOS. Ha, 27-....Talks in a vehement, (impetuous) commanding (dictatorial) tone; spits at nurse, lifts up her clothes (naked) and kisses hotly all who come near her;...
SEP. He, 23 - Is easily offended and inclined to be vehement.(intense)

DIRTY

Anxiety; bathing the feet, after: nat-c. sep.[172]
Delirium; feces, swallows his own: verat.[60]
Delirium; spits and licks it up or rubs it over the floor: merc.[36]
Delusions; animals, persons are, unclean animals: bell.
• animals, unclean: bell.
• black objects and people, sees: **BELL.**[5] cocc.[5] op.[10] ***plat.***[5] ***puls.***[5] stram. tarent.[185]
• body, black, is: sulph.
• body, head, transparent and speckled brown: bell.
• body, mouth, stinking odor from: ***hyos.***[54]
• body, spotted brown, is: bell.
• contaminates everything she touches: ars.
• dirt, eating dirt, he is: verat.
• dirty, everything is: cur.
• dirty, he is: hydrog.[222] ***lac-c.*** lap-c-b.[194] lycps. rhus-t. ***syph.***[111]
• faces, doctor is making faces at her, she looked black: puls.[54]
• feces, swallows: verat.[5]
• flatus, everyone notices his: zinc-p.[162]
• foul, everything appears: cur.
• resin, exuding from every pore: cann-s.[36]
• snow, polluted by industry, poisonous: ozone[227]
• soot, shower of, fell on him: cann-i.
• washing, of: bell. syph.[5]
Desires; rags, clean: alum.[137]
Dirtiness: ***am-c.***[102] calc-s.[108] ***caps.***[102] chel.[137] coca[161] crot-h.[30] ***graph.***[137] ***lac-c.***[137] lac-h.[229] lach.[137] lycps.[137] merc.[102] nux-v.[30] petr.[30] phos.[137] ***plat.***[162] ***psor.***[102] rhus-t.[137] sep.[137] sil.[102] staph.[30] ***sulph.***[102] verat.[102]
Dirtiness; aversion to, especially of the hands: syph.[212]
Dirtiness; dirtying everything: am-c.[30] bry.[30] ***nat-m.***[30]
Dirtiness; urinating and defecating everywhere, children: ***sep.***[30] sil.[30] sulph.[30]
Discomfort; bath, after: phys.[36]
Disgust; odor of his own, body: lac-c.[137] pyrog.[137] ***sulph.***[54]
Disgust; odor of his own, stool: ambr.[1189]
Dreams; ashamed, dirty and sloppy house, because of her: ozone[227]
➤ body, hands burning by washing: mag-m.[36]
➤ cleaning: hydrog.[222]
➤ closet, being on: psor.[36]
➤ dirt: kreos.[10] prun.[10]
➤ dirt, bathtub dirty, with black border: ozone[227]
➤ dirt, linen, couple makes love in dirty linen: ozone[227]
➤ dirt, linen, dirty: kali-n.[36] ***kreos.***[122] ozone[227]
➤ dirt, roads: apis.[36]
➤ dirt, table, dirty: prun.
➤ dirt, toilets dirty: ozone[227]
➤ dirt, underwear dirty: lap-mar-c.[194]
➤ disease, burning hands by washing: mag-m.
➤ excrements: aloe[58] cast-v.[58] iod.[58] psor.[58] sars.[58] zinc.[58]
➤ excrements, large amounts: hydrog.[222]
➤ excrements, smeared with excrements, being: iod.[10] zinc.[36].
➤ excrements, soiling himself with excrements: aloe cast-v. iod. sars.[58] zinc.
➤ excrements, wading in excrements: iod.[10]
➤ excrements, youths defecating enormous amounts of: hydrog.[222]
➤ houses, dirty: ozone[227]
➤ houses, tarring the floor: ozone[227]

➤ mud, walking in: iod.
➤ room full of water closets: ozone[227]
➤ rubbish is falling on her, lying in a strange house: mag-m.
➤ smelling sulphur, tinder: anac.
➤ snow, polluted by industry, poisonous: ozone[227]
➤ stool: aloe androc.[222] cast-v. psor. sars. zinc.
➤ stool, diarrheal: allox.[119] apis[36] psil.[164]
➤ walking, roads, over dirty wet: apis[36]
➤ water, black: ***ars.*** lac-c.[193] ozone[227]
➤ water, black, tar, like: ozone[227]
➤ water, child bathing in boiling: mag-c.
➤ water, dirty, bathing impossible: ozone[227]
➤ water, people, bathing: chin-b.
➤ water, people, bathing, boiling water, in: mag-c.[58]
➤ water, people, bathing, lake, in a: ozone[227]
➤ water, people, bathing, swimming pool of hotel, in, naked: ozone[227]
➤ water, poisoned: ozone[227]
➤ water, poured upon him, is: ox-ac.
➤ water, putrid: arg-n.
➤ water, yellow: hura.
➤ writing, dirty table and paper becoming smeared, on: prun.

Excitement; bath, during: gast.[36]
Fear; bath, of: ant-c.[172] rhus-t.[172] sep.[172] spig.[172] sulph.[172]
✦ stool, escape, should, with flatus or urination: aloe[162] carb-v.[172] nat-m.[172] nat-p.[172] nat-s.[172] olnd.[172] ph-ac.[172] podo.[172] sulph.[172] verat.[172]
✦ stool, involuntary, of: ***phos.***[54] sep.[1]
✦ washed, being: ant-c.[172] sulph.[58]

Feces; licks up cow-dung, mud, saliva: hyos.[162] merc.
Feces; passed on the floor: cupr. hyos.[162] sulph.[122]
Feces; swallows his own: ***camph.***[54] merc.[5] verat. visc.[5]
Feces; urinating and going to stool everywhere, children: ***sep.***[30] sil.[30] sulph.[30]
Insanity; burrows in ground with his mouth, like a pig: stram.[54]
Insanity; eats, dung or lapping up of saliva: merc.[5]
Insanity; eats, filth: ***camph.***[54] sulph.[10]
Insanity; passes her feces on the floor: cupr.
Rolling; filth, in his own: camph.[137]
Sensitive; odors, to, dirty clothing: ***carb-an.***[137]
Washing; always, face, her: puls.[102]
Washing; always, hands, her: ars.[111] coca[122] cur.[162] ***lac-c.***[122] ***med.***[122] merc.[184] ***nat-m.***[162] plat.[126] psor.[111] sep.[162] sil.[185] ***sulph.***[162] syph. thuj.[162]
Washing; always, underwear, her: syph.[189]
Washing; as if: bell.[58]
Washing; aversion to: lap-mar-c.[194] phys.[60]
Washing; aversion, children, in: am-c.[58] ant-c.[127] psor.[127] **SULPH.**[54] tub.[106]
Washing; bathing, mania for: zea-i.[122]
Washing; cleanness, mania for: ars.[58] sep.[193] sil.[30] sulph.[30]
Washing; desire for: tarent.[60]
Washing; desire for, cold water, in: meph.[60] phyt.[60]

ADAM. Sh, 34 - After taking the remedy again, I was very struck again by sparkling—this time the sun in the shower. Before I took it, I seemed to be surrounded by dark and dirt. 18, 30C, XX:XX:XX

Sh, 36 - White frost this morning. At last some purity in this world. Every ice crystal sparkled like jewels. 16, 12C, 27:XX:XX

Sh, 47 - Need air—fresh, cold, clean. I feel stuffy inside. This feeling is related to the feeling of food being dirty. 20, 1M, 06:XX:XX

Sh, 51 - Wanted to clean windows and wash clothes, enjoyed the cleaning. Most unusual. 12, 30C, 01.XX:XX

Sh, 156 - The weekend started with me locking myself and the boys and one dog out of the house, and the keys and one dog still inside. I got very upset then and the weekend just got worse and worse. I had blazing rows with everybody. Thought I was getting the flu. Thought I was surrounded by dirt. Wanted to just go to bed and take my boys and the dogs with me. Couldn't or wouldn't go to work on Monday. 18, 30C, 31:XX:XX

Sh, 277 - Exceptionally strong desire to leave my marriage and children, to live a clear unmuddled life alone. 2, 12C, 74:XX:XX-160:XX:XX

BELL. Al, 90 - It seems to her that her nose is transparent, and a spot on the left side of the head transparent and colored brown.

Al, 86-...pointing with trembling fingers to swarms (crowd) of unclean (dirty) beasts wich she fancied were scrambling (mix) all over the walls, beds, table, etc. of the wards.

Al, 35-...she acts as if she were washing or counting money, or as if she were drinking.

Ha, 1366 - Ridiculous grimaces; ...acts as if she were washing, at another as if counting money, ...

CANN-I. Al, 65 - Hallucinations which lead the patient to imagine that he is on horseback, is hunting, that he sees blue water, that he is swimming, or that he is captain of a vessel, that he is traveling, that he has no weight.(lightness)

Al, 67 - Illusion that he was an inkstand, and that, as he lay on the bed, the ink might spill over the white counterpane.

CUR. Al, 4 - Everything he sees appears foul and nasty. (dirty, dishonest, offensive, injurious, indecent)

HALI-L. Sh, 15 - My pillow smelled like mouse excrement. 16, 10C, XX:XX:XX

Sh, 186 - I've never been this clean for this long. I want to use up everything, all the leftovers. Everything has to be done and clean. Very methodically using up old things, like old jars of beans. I want everything to be in order and neat. 08, 30C, 22:XX:XX

Sh, 402 - I felt pathetic, defeated and vulnerable. I was reaching on a high shelf for pots for plants. All the pots and soil came tumbling down. Was knocked on the head, on the vertex. Dirt all over me, and I thought, "This is perfect. This is exactly how I feel." I felt like I had to just give up — give up the bravado. I'm exhausted, I'm just going to rest. I just wanted to go into a little ball and lick my wounds. Felt very much like childhood symptoms. I felt very young. 01, 30C, 18:XX:XX

Sh, 414 - Every thing back to yucky normal. 09, 6C, 00:15:XX

Sh, 433 - Feel self-destructive, like eating greasy fatty junk food, not exercising, slowly kill myself that way. Why care? 06, 6C, 10:XX:XX

HYDROG. Sh, 45 - Feel grubby even after a shower. 16, 30C, 02:XX:XX

HYOS. He, 84-...constant talking, particularly on religious subjects; believes himself poisoned, or that there is a stinking odor from his mouth;...

HYPER. Al,S-3 - For a week past, impure ideas have very seldom presented themselves by day; the mind has been reposing on higher thoughts.

LAC-C. He, 11 - Imagines to be dirty. (obscene, vulgar, dishonorable)

LYSS. Al,N-46 - After fainting (weak) spell he wrote on paper: I am forsaken by all; even the birds of heaven, they do not look at me (despised), do not fed me if hungry (helplessness) ; I hunger with the young ones and am thirsty with their she ones (starving); my nest (house) is made out of dirt (soiled), not gotten by my own exertions (efforts), but by driving them out of their nests (home) and sitting there with the females and the young.

Al,N-62 - He cautioned people around him not to inhale his exhaled air, it was spoiled (dirty), stinking (smelling) like rotten (putrefying) eggs, worse than cholera, and could injure. (contaminates, infects)

MAG-C. Al, 930 - Dreams of masks (false) in fools'(idiot) clothes, which they soiled.(dirty)

Al, 945 - Anxious dream, that a child was bathing in boiling water. (purification?)

MAG-M. Al, 711 - An anxious dream; she was lying in a strange house, where rubbish (garbage) was constantly falling upon her; she tried to cry out and could not, because there was too great heaviness on the chest.

Al, 714 - Frightful dreams; that she was pursued by robbers; that she burned her hand by washing ...

MERC. Ha, 1263 - Mania; she throws off the clothes at night, tears the straw about, and scolds; by day she leaps (jump) up high like a petulant extravagant person...she talks and scolds much to herself,...spits frequently and spreads the saliva out with her feet, and licks some of it up again; she often licks cowdung (excrements) and the mud of ponds (lake); she often takes little stones in her mouth, without swallowing them, and at the same time complains that they are cutting her bowels; much clotted blood passes with her motion; ...

NEON. Sh, 1 - I was overwhelmingly agitated, amazed, confused, and upset about a neon tube discarded across the road. I couldn't believe that people could use these things. Where would the dustmen throw it? I thought, "It's the worst kind of light possible." I could not believe people would want it. 20, 6C, 00:03:05
Sh, 2 - I took a deep breath of relief as I saw the dustmen come for the neon strip light. 20, 6C, 00:04:30
Sh, 33 - I had intense pleasure at hearing the wind and I thought, "It will clear the skies." 20, 6C, 05:00:XX
Sh, 197 - This morning I felt indifference about the dirty house. I left the dishes, and dirty hair in the bath. 02, 6C, 05:XX:XX
SULPH. He, 51 - Dread of being washed.
SYPH. Al,N-[5]-... violent on being opposed, has tremors, seems on the verge of convulsions,...always washing her hands.

DISAPPOINTMENT

Ailments from; ambition, deceived: bell.[30] merc.[30] ***nux-v.***[54] plat.[30] puls.[30] verat.[30]
Ailments from; disappointment, deception: acon.[102] alum.[85] apis[98] ars.[102] **AUR.**[8] ***bry.***[102] caps.[83] carb-v.[58] carc.[214] caust.[102] cham.[28] ***cocc.***[8] colch.[102] ***coloc.***[102] dig.[36] ***gels.***[102] grat.[102] hyos.[102] **IGN.**[122] ***lach.***[122] **LYC.**[122] ***merc.***[122] **NAT-M.**[122] ***nux-v.***[122] op.[122] **PH-AC.**[122] phos.[28] plat.[58] **PULS.**[122] sep.[102] **STAPH.**[122] verat.[122]
Ailments from; disappointment, deception, new: **IGN.**[122]
Ailments from; disappointment, deception, old: **NAT-M.**[122]
Ailments from; friendship, deceived: aur.[8] ign.[30] mag-c.[30] mag-m.[30] nux-v.[30] ph-ac.[30] sil.[30] sulph.[30]
Ailments from; love disappointed, drowsiness, with: **PH-AC.**[54]
Ailments from; love disappointed, emotional and mental symptoms from: ant-c.[8] ***aur.***[8] bell.[30] calc-p.[31] caust.[30] ***cimic.***[8] dig.[91] ***hyos.***[8] **IGN.**[8] ***lach.***[8] ***nat-m.***[54] ***ph-ac.***[8] ***phos.***[8] staph.[137] ***verat.***[8]
Ailments from; love disappointed, grief, with silent: **IGN. NAT-M. PH-AC.** phos.
Ailments from; love disappointed, jealousy, anger and incoherent talk, with: hyos. nat-m.[122]
Ailments from; love disappointed, laugh, with inclination to: hyos.[54]
Ailments from; love disappointed, rage, with: hyos.[56]
Ailments from; love disappointed, sadness, with: ***aur.***[54] bell.[30] ***hyos.***[54] **IGN.**[54] ***nat-m.***[54]
Ailments from; love, disappointed, unhappy: ***acon.***[5] am-c.[5] androc.[222] ant-c. **AUR.**[5] ***bell.***[30] ***bufo***[117] cact.[5] ***calc-p.*** ***caust.***[5] ***cimic.*** ***coff.*** com.[5] ***con.***[116] dig.[85] ***hell.*** **HYOS.** **IGN.**[122] iod.[85] kali-c. ***kali-p.***[5] ***lach.*** **NAT-M.** nux-m. nux-v. orig.[187] ozone[227] **PH-AC.** phos.[5] pitu-a.[164] psor.[185] ***sac-alb.***[210] sep. seq-s.[230] **STAPH.**[122] stram.[37] sulph.[122] tarent. til.[36] verat.[54]
Ambition; loss of, disappointment, from: nux-v.[137]
Ambition; loss of, fame, for: am-m.[30] ars.[30] sep.[30]
Ambition; loss of, money, to make: chin-ar.[30] kali-c.[30] merc.[30] nat-c.[30] sep.[30]
Brooding; disappointment, cardiac weakness, with: ***ph-ac.***[54]
Brooding; disappointment, love: ***ph-ac.***[54]
Brooding; disappointment, over: **BELL.**[122] ***ph-ac.***[54]
Confusion of mind; ambition, from deceived: ***nux-v.***[54]
Cursing; disappointment in plans, on: opun-a.[36]
Delirium; maniacal, love, from disappointed: ***phos.***[54]
Despair; love, from disappointed: caust.[30] ***hyos.***[54]
Dreams; disappointments: cann-s. echi.[111] ign. rumx. ust.
➤ hope, of disappointed: ***ign.***[5]
Dwells; disappointments, on: ***ph-ac.***[54]
Grief; deception, from: **AUR.**[162] **IGN.**[122] lach.[30] **LYC.**[162] merc.[30] **NAT-M.**[122] ***nux-v.***[162] op.[162] ph-ac.[30] puls.[30] sep.[162] verat.[162]
Grief; silent, love, with disappointed: **IGN.**[54]
Indolence; disappointment, from: nux-v.[137]
Insanity; love, on account of unfortunate: tarent.[36]
Irritability; disappointment, from: carc.[207] nit-ac.[58]
Jealousy; love disappointment, in: ***hyos.***[54]
Laughing; love, from disappointed: ***hyos.***[54]
Rage; love, after disappointed: ***hyos.***[54]
Sadness; disappointment, from: dig.[36] ign.[109]
Sadness; love, from disappointed: ***aur.***[54] bell.[30] dig.[137] ***hyos.***[54] **IGN.**[54] ***nat-m.***[54]

Suicidal disposition; drowning, by, love, from disappointed: ***hyos.***[54]
Suicidal disposition; love, from disappointed: ant-c.[188] ***aur.***[54] bell.[137] caust.[137] ***hyos.***[54] staph.[137]
Suicidal disposition; love, from disappointed, weeping, with: ***aur.***[54]
Weeping; disappointments, about: dig.[36]
Weeping; love, from unrequited: ***ign.***[54]

ANDROC. Sh, 59 - Felt disappointed with people. (7)
ANT-C. Ha, 28 - Consequences of (ailments from) disappointed love.
AUR. He, 59 - Disappointed love, with weeping and inclination to commit suicide.
He, 79 - Ailments from grief, disappointed love.
CALC-P. He, 19 - Ailments from grief, disappointed love.
CHIN. Ha, 1105 - What formerly appeared to him in a bright genial light, seems now to be lusterless (lifeless), unworthy (inutile), and shallow (superficial, stupid)
CIMIC. He, 34 - Mind disturbed by disappointed love, business failures.
COCC. He, 24 - Melancholy and sad; indulges in sad reveries (daydream); is sensitive to insults, slights (despises) and disappointment.
COFF. He, 33 - Ailments from excessive joy, excessive laughing and playing; from disappointed love; from anger, from vexations with vehemence or fright...
DIG. Al, 19 - Weeping sadness about many things which have disappointed him.
GERM. Sh, 121 - Very strong longing for excitement and some love adventure. I planned to go out, but though I probably would be disappointed, so I stayed at home and was depressed instead. Feel like drinking - to get away from myself and everything. 18, 30C, 04:00:00
HYOS. He, 74 - Disappointed love followed by: epilepsy, melancholy, rage, or inclination to laugh at everything; despair and propensity to drown himself. (ailments from)
IGN. He, 37 - Tears wept inwardly, the pain and penalty (forfeit) of unrequited (unrecompensed) love; desires solitude so that one may nourish inward grief;...
He, 62 - Ill effects (ailments) from hearing bad news; from vexation with reserved displeasure ; from grief, or suppressed mental sufferings; of shame and disappointed love.
He, 24 - Melancholy after disappointed love, always combined with spinal symptoms.
He, 27 - Unhappy love with silent grief.
He, 50 - Jealousy, disappointed love.
KALI-BR. He, 39-...fear and apprehension that she is losing her mind (insanity);...makes her utterly (completely) miserable to be looked at or spoken to; fear to see people; always depressed and lowspirited;...
LACH. He, 59 - Ailments from fright (fear), disappointed love or jealousy.
OPUN-V. Al, 5 - Fit of swearing (cursing) at evening after coming home; praying in the morning, swearing (cursing) on disappointment in plans; fit of rage, on thwarting (frustrating) of plans.
PH-AC. He, 11 - Ailments from care, grief, sorrow, chagrin, homesickness; or disappointed love;...
PHOS. He, 29 - Crazy deliria in a young woman who was strictly moral and unhappy in her love; accused herself of the most obscene (immoral, wicked) actions, of which she never was guilty; ....
PLAT. He, 44 - Talks almost continually about fanciful things or such as have really occurred; of faithless love; of her teacher and old school days; ...
TARENT. Al, 2 - Insanity on account of an unfortunate love.
VERAT. He, 22 - Nymphomania, with violence and destructiveness; had been disappointed in love; melancholia; ...great desire for sexual intercourse; void (empty) of shame; obscenity; ....

DISCONTENTED

Discontented; always: **HEP.**[30] lach.[30] **MERC.**[30] nit-ac.[30]
Discontented; coition, after: ***calc.*** sel.[116]
Discontented; eating, after: bov. fl-ac.
Discontented; health, about: phos.[1]
Discontented; himself, with: act-sp.[111] ***agn.*** aloe ***ars.***[122] asaf.[137] aur. bamb-a.[1184] bell. bry. calc-p. cand-a.[239] caust. cham. cinnam.[36] cinnb. cob. cocc. con.[137] germ.[222]

hep. kali-c. lac-h.[229] lyc. m-aust.[10] mang. meny. merc. mez. mur-ac. ***nit-ac.*** nux-v.[30] ozone[227] pana.[36] ph-ac. ***puls.***[122] ruta ***sac-alb.***[210] staph.[58] ***sulph.*** tarent. ther. viol-t. ziz.[54]

Discontented; life, cut off from: bamb-a.[1184]

Discontented; others, with: cham.[127] hep.[137] ruta[130]

Discontented; revolutionary: **MERC.**[30]

Discontented; surroundings, with: ang.[36] bac.[149] ***cham.***[36] chel.[36] meny.[36] merc.[36] mez.[36] par.[36] plat.[36]

Discontented; weather, in rainy: aloe.

Discontented; wrong, everything another does is: ***cham.***[54]

Quarrelsomeness; alternating with, care and discontentment: ran-b.

Weeping; discontent with himself: ***nit-ac.***[54] ziz.[54]

AGN. Al, 1-,...he feels as if nothing existed around him; he is dissatisfied with himself all the time; he is incapable of attending to any business; the things around him are entirely indifferent to him;...

APIS. Al, 17-... would have liked to kill a dog that barked at him, etc. ; everything went wrong; nothing could be done to please him.

Al, 19-...nothing appeared to satisfy him; everything out of place.

ARN. Ha, 630 - He contradicts; is opinionative; no one can please him.

ARS. Ha, 1049 - Discontented with everything, finds fault with everything; everything is too strong and too irritating, all conversation, all noise, and all light.

Ha, 53 - Dissatisfied all day and extremely vexed at himself; he thought he had not worked enough and reproached himself most bitterly.

AUR. Ha, 344 - Discontented with all circumstances; he imagines that he finds everywhere some obstacle (impediment, restriction) in the way; at one time he thinks that this is owing to an unlucky (unfortunate) fate (destiny), at another that he himself is to blame (censured) for it ; when the latter was the case he was particularly mortified and dejected.

Ha, 355 - He is discontented with himself and depressed in spirits.

Ha, 4 - Discontented with all conditions; he thinks that he everywhere finds an impediment, caused now by an opposing fate,(destiny) then again by himself, which latter mortifies him and renders him dejected.(sad)

Ha, 11 - Restlessness and hurried impulse to bodily and mental activity; he can not work fast enough; he could not act so as to satisfy himself.

BISM. Al, 3 - He is morose and discontented with his condition (health, position) and complains about it.

He, 11 - Ill humor; he is morose and discontented with his condition (position), and complains about it.

CAUST. Ha, 24 - Discontented with himself, of gloomy (melancholic) countenance.

Ha, 30 - Peevish (angry) all day, at odds (quarrel) with himself, dissatisfied, anxious and yet not indisposed to mental work.

CHIN. Al, 47 - Discontent; he considers himself unhappy and thinks he is hindered (obstructed) and tormented by everyone. (after five hours)

COCC. Al, 30 - Great dissatisfaction with himself.

Ha, 529 - Great discontent with himself.

CUPR. Al, 13 - Irresolute; satisfied with nothing; this only lasts as long as he is fretful.

Ha, 7 - Irresolute (indecisive) and dissatisfied with everything, but only so long as he is peevish. (cross)

FL-AC. Al, 18 - In the evening he is very discontented; he looks at everything in the worst light; ...

HEP. Ha, 13 - Whatever she thought about was unsatisfactory (disappointed) and did not suit (satisfy) her.

Ha, 9 - Irritable mood; whatever she started to do, was not satisfactory, she wished to be alone.

Ha, 11 - Dissatisfied with oneself.

IGN. Al, 32 - He is discontented, morose, and obstinate towards evening; no one can do anything right or please him.

Ha, 768 - Towards evening he is discontented, sulky, stubborn (obstinate), no one can do anything right, anything to please him.

IP. Ha, 215 - He has no pleasure in nothing, nothing is agreeable to him.

KALI-AR. He, 1 - Scolding (censorious) morose, retired, quarrelsome and discontented, jealous, indifferent to everything,...

KALI-C. Al, 45 - Disagreeable mood; she longs for things with impetuosity; is contented with nothing, is beside herself, and gets into rage if everything does not go according to her wishes, and frequently does not herself know what she really wishes to have.

Ha, 30 - Peevish mood, as if she could not do anything to suit (satisfy) herself.

He, 9-...constantly in antagonism which herself; frequently hopeful, frequently despondent; frets (worry) about everything; peevish impatient, contented with nothing.

KALI-N. Al, 19 - Perverse hypochondriac mood; discontented with himself and the world, peevish irritable, ...

LED. Al, 12 - Discontented all day with his companions, which at last amounts to misanthropy.

Ha, 329 - All day long; discontented with his fellow-creatures (friend, relations), which at last amounted to misanthropy.

He, 4 - Discontented; morose; hates his fellow beings.

MENY. Ha, 286 - Cross, ill-humored and discontented with himself and his position (rank); anxiety drives him from one place to another.(restlessness)

MERC. Al, 31 - Fretful all day; very much out of sorts and discontented with himself; he had no desire to talk or joke.

Ha, 1248 - Without cause he is very discontented with himself and his position.

Ha, 1257 - During the whole day cross, as if at variance and dissatisfied with himself, and had no inclination for speaking and joking.

He, 35 - Grief, with fear at night: disposition to quarrel; complaining of relations and surroundings. (living conditions)

He, 35 - Grief, with fear at night; disposition to quarrel; complaining of relations and surroundings.

MEZ. Al, 10 - Great discontent with himself and his surroundings (living, conditions, position) for several weeks...

MUR-AC. Ha, 1 - Sad taciturn and discontented with his fate. (destiny, doom)

NAT-C. Al, 42 - Very fretful and discontented with whole world; he constantly felt as though he could beat (punish ?) himself, his whole life angered him, and he preferred to have no existence at all; he was solicitous about the future, and inclined to despair, all day.

NIT-AC. Al, 62 - Discontented, despising (scorn) life.

Ha, 28 - Discontented despising life.

Ha, 33 - Discontented with oneself, dissolving in tears, which gives relief.

He, 22 - Discontent with himself induces violent weeping.

PH-AC. Ha, 674 - Discontented with himself, self-reproaches.

Ha, 20 - Discontented with himself, reproaches himself.

PHOS. Al, 136 - Felt exceedingly petulant (irritable, contemptuous) all day; nothing went right; felt as dissatisfied with myself as with others; seemed as if everybody said or did something to provoke me.

PULS. Ha, 1142 - Everything disgusts him; everything is repugnant to him.

RAN-B. Al, 3 - Ill humored, and disposed to quarrel and scold the first forenoon; in the evening is desponding, apprehensive, sensitive, discontented; on the second day he again inclines to be provoked by innocent jests of his friends, etc.;...

RUTA. Ha, 276 - Very discontented and very much disposed to weep over everything that happens about him and especially over what he himself has done.

He, 2 - Dissatisfied with himself and others.

SAPIN. Al, 4 - Very irritable; nothing goes right; fault-finding, dissatisfied with everything previously done, no matter how well it was done before; ...

SEP. He, 11 - Sad about her health and domestic affairs, discontented with everything.

SULPH. Al, 42-...discontented with himself and all about him, which made him unfit for any serious occupations...whole evening he was absorbed in himself and unable to command his thoughts to read...

Ha, 55-...cannot do anything to please herself, is obstinate and unyielding (rigorous), without herself knowing why.

DISCUSSION

Ailments from; discords between chief and subordinates: graph.[30] ***lyc.*** mag-m.[162] merc.[30] nat-m.[30] nit-ac.[30] nux-v.[30] sulph.[30]
Ailments from; discords between, relatives, friends: ars.[30] graph.[8] hep.[30] lach.[30] mag-m.[162] merc.[30] ***nat-m.***[162] nit-ac.[30] nux-v.[162] sulph.[30]
Anxiety; business, lawsuit, as if engaged in a: ***nit-ac.***[60]
Anxiety; conversation, from: alum. ***ambr.*** androc.[222] plat. stram.
Anxiety; lawsuit or dispute, as if he was engaged in: ***nit-ac.***[54]
Brooding; law suit, over, by which he may gain or loose a million, and takes it in bad part if not allowed to read indictment for said lawsuit, a confused, irrational piece of work, on which he has been working all night, in insanity: ***nux-v.***[54]
Delusions; contests, sees: bell.[10]
- debate, of being in: hyos.
- lawsuit, being engaged in a: ***nit-ac.***[36]
- person; two personalities opposing to each other in himself, who are discussing their disease, there are: paro-i.[149]

Discuss, desire to: trio.[149]
Discuss, her symptoms with everyone: arg-n.[193] pop-c.[122]
Dreams; contests: ferr.[10] hyos.[10] plat.[10] ran-s.[10] thuj.[10] verb.[10]
➤ court, stands before: bamb-a.[1184]
➤ political: asc-t.[36]
➤ quarrels, strife: alum. alum-sil.[58] am-c. am-m.[5] anan. ant-c. apis aran-ix.[149] ***arn.*** ars.[5] astra-me.[36] aur. aza.[36] ***bapt.*** bar-c. ***bell.*** brom. ***bry.*** calc. calc-acet.[36] canth. carl. cast. ***caust.*** cedr.[36] ceph.[36] cere-b.[36] cham. chin.[5] con. convo-d.[36] crot-c.[36] ***crot-h.*** culx.[58] echi.[111] ferr-p.[5] guai. guare. hep. hydr.[5] indg.[10] kali-c.[10] ***kali-n.*** lach.[85] lyc.[5] m-aust.[1] ***mag-c.*** mag-s. maland.[56] ***merc.***[10] mosch. nat-ar.[36] nat-c. nat-m. nat-s. nicc. ***nit-ac.***[5] **NUX-V.** op. oxyt.[51] ozone[227] paeon. peti.[36] ph-ac. ***phos.*** plat. ***puls.*** raph.[111] rat.[10] rheum[5] sabin. ***sel.*** sep. sil. sol-a.[36] spig. ***stann.*** staph. **STRAM.**[5] tarax. verat. x-ray[56] zinc.

Excitement; debate, during: ***caust. nit-ac.***
Insanity; dispute, to: camph.[60]
Restlessness; conversation, from: ***ambr.***
Sadness; quarrel with husband, after: ***anac.***[54]

AGAR. He, 25 - Protracted (postponed) mental application or exciting debates brought on vertigo.

ANDROC. Sh, 113 - Argumentative. Pursued conflict almost with relish. (12)
Sh, 121 - When talking to friends felt 'paranoid', suspicious and guilty, when asked questions, he became hot and sweaty. He felt it was a game of who was cleverer, and tried to lie to and outwit his friend, though this gave no satisfaction. His friends reported that he seemed unusually distant and cool. (29)
Sh, 125 - Desire to pick an argument or fight. (29)

ARS. He, 92 - Disposed to discuss the faults of others.

ATRO. Al, 15 - The patient is busied with subjects which at other times occupy his mind, politics and struggles consequent on his relations in life.
Al, 22 - Expostulates with those who try to lead him to bed; says he will lose the train, that all things are packed up, and that he must start immediately.

GERM. Sh, 11 - Feeling detached when involved in a row with husband. No guilt that I'm not pleasing him . 04, 6C, 09:XX:XX

HALI-L. Sh, 152 - I used to always be ready to tangle. Loved to argue even if it was a topic I didn't care about. Since the proving that is gone. I now actually enjoy listening to people express opinions I don't necessarily agree with. I continue to feel calm, able to listen, and not get caught up in the fray. 03, 12C, 62:XX:XX
Sh, 517 - Dread of upcoming legal battle. 09, 6C, 15:XX:XX

HYOS. Al, 90-...called on various absent persons by name, with whom imagined himself to be in debate.
He, 78 - Groundless suspicion of being watched (observed, spied) by members of family with whom he had some slight misunderstanding (dispute); to avoid being recognized by them, clothed himself differently every day,...watching his relations suspiciously and imagining he might be poisoned;... (disguise, camouflage)

KALI-CY. Al, 5 - At 7 p.m., while walking out of doors, feelings of crossness; carries on a kind of conversation within himself, as if quarreling with someone whith whom he had previously disagreed; thinks what he will reply in case certain things are said to him.

LACH. Al, 33 - Unusually contentious (hostile) and obstinate, so that he quarrels with everything about him.

Al, 34 - So quarrelsome that he disputes with a mother about the age of her daughter, and affirms the younger to be the elder.

MERC. He, 35 - Grief, with fear at night: disposition to quarrel; complaining of relations and surroundings. (living conditions)

NIT-AC. Ha, 16 - Anxiety, as if he was engaged in a disquieting lawsuit or contest. (conflict, debate, competition)

Ha, 47 - He is inclined to be passionate and contentious.(quarrelsome)

Ha, 46 - When disputing (debate), there is trembling in all the limbs.

Ha, 6 - Inclined to be violent and to quarrel.

He, 15 - Anxiety as if he was engaged in a lawsuit or dispute, causing uneasiness.

NUX-V. He, 37-...brooding all night long over a lawsuit by which he may gain or lose a million (megalomania) ; ..replies reluctantly and slowly to physician's questions, and takes it in bad part (offenses) if not allowed to read indictment (accusation) for said lawsuit, a confused irrational piece of work, on which he has been working all night.

SUMB. Al, 8-...fond (love) of the society of women; ...sympathy with suffering seems robbed of its pain...nervous excitement and heat, especially in head from listening (hearing) to a disputation, ...humor depressed with despair of future...melancholy despondency, as if ill-treated by everyone purposely... mildness, amiability

TAX. Al, 5 - Impatient disposition, which scarcely allows of the least intellectual contest.(discussion)

THUJ. Al, 91 - Morose, quarrels about a harmless joke.

THYR. Al,N-1-...at times dangerous and homicidal, would put her arms round the necks of other patients so tightly as almost to strangle them (in this case the insanity was primary and the myxedema secondary; both conditions were removed). Evinced increased vivacity by quarreling with another patient about a trifling difference of opinion.

DISEASE

Anger; easily, rheumatism, in cardiac: phos.[54] squil.[54] ***thuj.***[54]

Anger; recovery, if one spoke of her complete: ***ars.***[36]

Anger; thinking of his ailments, when: ***aur-m.***

Anguish; cardiac: ***acon.***[54] **ARN.**[54] ***ars.***[54] aur.[1] ***bell.***[54] ***carb-v.***[54] ***dig.***[54] **SPONG.**[54]

Anticipation; dentist, physician, before going to: calc.[122] ***gels.***[122] mag-c.[144] ***phos.***[122] ***tub.***[122]

Anxiety; chest, heart, region of, insupportable, almost, in heart disease: ***ferr-m.***[54]

Anxiety; chest, heart, region of, pain in heart, with: ***aur.***[54] ***kalm.***[54] mill.[54] ***op.***[54]

Anxiety; chest, stitching in: ruta.[1]

Anxiety; congestion, heart in: nit-ac.[1]

Anxiety; future, disease, and of her: kali-c.[54]

Anxiety; health, about: acet-ac. acon. aeth.[162] agar.[54] agn.[162] aloe[37] alum. alum-p.[58] alum-sil.[58] am-c.[36] androc.[222] ant-t.[36] ***arg.*** arg-n. arn. ars. ars-h.[54] aur-m.[162] bar-c.[187] bell.[10] blatta[152] bor.[10] bov.[162] brom.[116] bry. bufo[36] ***calad.***[122] ***calc.*** calc-ar.[58] calc-f.[103] ***calc-p.***[162] calc-s. calc-sil.[58] cand-a.[239] cann-i.[162] canth.[10] carc.[187] ***chin-ar.***[54] choc.[222] cocc. cop.[36] cub.[36] cupr.[10] euph.[60] germ.[222] glon.[116] grat. hyos.[10] ign. **KALI-AR.** kali-br.[137] kali-c. kali-m.[192] kali-p. kali-sil.[58] kreos.[5] lac-c. lach. lob.[10] ***lyc.*** m-arct.[10] mag-m. med.[162] merc.[10] morg.[136] nat-c. nat-m.[10] nat-p. **NIT-AC.** nux-m. nux-v. ozone[227] ***ph-ac.***[122] **PHEL.**[162] ***phos.*** podo.[116] psor. ***puls.***[122] ruta[152] sel.[116] ***sep.*** sil. spong.[54] staph. sulph.

Anxiety; health, despair of getting well: ***ars.***[54]

Anxiety; health, loved persons, of: carc.[193] hep.[30] merc.[30]

Anxiety; health, recovery, concerning: ***ph-ac.***[54]

Anxiety; health, relatives: ***ars.***[162] bar-c.[162] cand-a.[239] carb-v.[172] caust.[172] cocc.[36] **HEP.**[30] merc.[30] nat-c.[172] ***phos.***[162] puls.[172]

Anxiety; heart, complains of in: **ACON.**[137] arn.[137] ars.[137] ***aur.***[137] calc.[137] carb-v.[137]

dig.[137] ign.[137] ip.[137] nux-v.[10] ***phos.***[137] plat.[137] ***puls.***[137] spig.[137] spong.[10] stroph.[137] sulph.[137] ther.[137] verat.[137]
Anxiety; hypochondriacal: ***acon.***[10] **AGAR.** agn.[162] aloe[54] alum.[10] am-c. anac. arg-n.[54] ***arn. ars.*** asaf. asar.[5] bar-c.[162] ***bell.***[10] bry.[10] calad. calc.[1] calc-sil.[185] cann-i.[162] canth. caust.[10] cham. ***con.***[10] cupr.[10] dros. ferr-p. graph.[10] ***grat.*** hyos.[10] ign.[10] ***iod.***[10] kali-ar.[162] ***kali-c.***[10] kali-chl. kali-p. lach.[10] lob.[162] lyc.[10] m-arct.[10] med.[193] mosch. nat-c.[5] **NAT-M.** ***nit-ac. nux-v.***[10] ol-an.[31] ox-ac.[116] ph-ac. **PHOS.** plat.[10] psor.[122] ***puls.***[10] ***raph.***[10] ***rhus-t.***[10] ***sep.***[10] squil.[10] staph.[10] sulph.[10] **SYPH.**[162] valer.
Anxiety; hypochondriacal, mania to read medical books: **CALC.**[30] ***nux-v.***[30] ***puls.***[30] staph.[30] sulph.[30]
Anxiety; ill, as if he would be: ph-ac.[36] ***podo.***[54] tarent.[36]
Anxiety; motion, from, heart disease, in: **DIG.**[54]
Anxiety; pneumonia, in: ***ant-t.***[54] ***chel.***[54] squil.[54]
Anxiety; tuberculosis, in: agar.[54] ***chin-ar.***[54]
Anxiety; typhus, in: **ARS.**[54] **CALC.**[54] ***chin-s.***[54] **SPONG.**[54]
Anxiety; vertigo, during, apoplexy, as if he would have: ***zinc.***[54]
Anxiety; wrong, indescribably, of something, in vasomotor affection: ***kali-br.***[54]
Anxiety; wrong, with him, as if it went: mang.[36]
Begging; relief, for: plb.[36]
Brooding; condition, illness, over one's: aur.[114] kali-p.[58] ***ph-ac.***[1]
Brooding; imaginary troubles, disease: cycl.[137] lil-t.[137] ***naja***[117]
Brooding; imaginary troubles, over, disease: cycl.[137] **IGN.**[54] lil-t.[137] ***naja***[117]
Busy; illness, after: **ACON.**[30] **ARN.**[30] **BRY.**[30] rhus-t.[30] sulph.[30]
Cheerfulness; heart disease, laughs, sings and dances: ***nat-m.***[54]
Cheerfulness; heart disease, with: ***cact.***[54]
Company, desire for; heart, in organic disease of the: ***apis***[54]
Complaining; condition, of his: bism.[54]
Complaining; disease, of: ***ant-t.***[54] cham.[1] **LACH.**[10] ***nux-v.***[10] ph-ac.[36]
Complaining; symptoms, about his numerous, in pneumonia: ***ant-t.***[54]
Confusion of mind; identity, sick, as if someone else were: gels.[5]
Confusion of mind; stitching in chest, from: sep.[1]
Conscientious about trifles; disease, during: pip-m.[184]
Deafness; pretended: verat.
Death; conviction of, angina pectoris, in: ***ox-ac.***[54]
Death; conviction of, angina pectoris, in: ***ox-ac.***[54]
Death; conviction of, epistaxis, in: ***croc.***[54]
Death; conviction of, erysipelas, facial, in: ***plat.***[54]
Death; conviction of, fever, after, epistaxis amel.: ***psor.***[54]
Death; conviction of, heart, in organic disease of: ***apis***[54]
Death; presentment of, heart disease, in: ***op.***[54]
Delirium; well, declares she is: apis ***arn. ars.*** op.[58]
Delusions; apoplexy, he has: arg. carb-v.[36]
- blind, that he is: bell.[1] hyos.[10] mosch. stram.[10] verat.
- blood, circulate well, does not: ***atro.***[36]
- blood, pouring out of mouth: choc.[222]
- body, brain, cracking, is: nux-m.[122]
- body, brain, decaying, is: crot-h.[72]
- body, brain, dissolving: calc.[139]
- body, brain, softening: abrot. ***arg-n.***[8] cann-i.[58]
- body, brittle, bones are: ther.[102]
- body, goiter, he has a: indg.
- body, goiter, that he cannot see over when sitting down: zinc.
- body, limbs, crooked: sabad.[58]
- body, lip lower, is swollen, lower: glon.
- body, putrefy, will: ***ars.*** bell.
- body, shrunken, like the dead, is: ***sabad.***
- body, spotted brown, is: bell.
- body, stomach, has corrosion of: acet-ac.[54] ign. sabad.
- breath is spoiled, his exhaled, cautions people not to inhale: lyss.[54]
- cancer, he has a: verat.
- contaminates everything she touches: ars.
- crippled old man, that he is: hydrog.[222]
- deaf and dumb: verat.
- die, about to, he is, tuberculosis, from: calc.[172] lac-c.[172] paull.[172] sep.[172] tarent.[172]

- die, about to, he is, while walking thinks he will have a fit or die, which makes him walk faster: ***arg-n.***
- die, tuberculosis, from: calc.[172] lac-c.[172] paull.[172] sep.[172] tarent.[172]
- disease, deaf, dumb and has cancer, is: verat.
- disease, every, that he has: ***aur-m.*** stram.
- disease, give, to others, that he will: ***chlol.***[54]
- disease, heart disease, has: calc.[1] graph.[5] ***nat-c.***[54] podo.[58]
- disease, incurable, has: acon.[116] alum.[1] ***arg-n.*** arn.[116] cact. calc.[116] calc-sil.[58] chel. ***ign.***[116] lac-c.[102] ***lach.***[116] ***lil-t.***[116] macrin.[36] mag-c.[144] nit-ac.[116] ***phos.***[8] plb. podo.[58] ***sabad.*** stann.[116] ***syph.***[171]
- disease, incurable, heart: ***phos.***[54]
- disease, she has some organic disease nobody understands: ***lil-t.***[8]
- disease, throat disease, a horrible, which will end fatally: **SABAD.**[54]
- disease, unrecognized, has an: raph.
- disease, yellow fever, that he will have: camph.[54]
- dumb, he is: verat.
- emaciation, of: ***anh.***[144] nat-m.[5] sabad.[5] sulph.
- epilepsy, he has: atro.
- epilepsy, he will have a fit: alum.[139] cina[139] lyss.[139]
- fit, she will have a fit and walks faster: ***arg-n.***
- head, disease will break out of h.: stram.
- headache, has: bamb-a.[1184]
- health, he has ruined his: bamb-a.[1184] chel.
- hear, he cannot: hyos.[10] mosch. verat.
- heart disease, will have and die: arn.[58] germ.[222] ***kali-ar.***[162] ***lac-c.***[54] lach.[122] podo.[58]
- heart, stitches in heart will kill him if they do not cease: psor.[54]
- hollow, whole body is: aur. ***kali-c.*** nux-v. pall.
- hydrothorax, he has a: alco.[36] phos.[36]
- insane, become, that she will: ***acon.*** act-sp.[162] agar.[139] ail.[139] alum.[5] ambr.[5] ars.[5] brom.[139] ***calc.***[5] cann-i. cann-s.[5] ***chel.*** chlor.[5] **CIMIC.** colch.[5] con.[58] cupr.[139] cycl.[139] ***eup-per.***[54] gels.[139] glon.[139] ham.[5] hydrog.[222] hyos.[139] ***ign.***[54] iod.[54] iris-t.[139] kali-bi.[123] ***kali-br.***[5] kali-p.[123] ***lac-c.***[5] lam.[36] lil-t. ***manc.*** med. merc. nat-m. nat-s.[139] nitro-o.[36] nux-v.[5] pall.[8] phys.[5] plat.[5] psor.[85] sil.[139] sulph.[139] ***syph.***[102] tanac. tarent.[36] vario.[123]
- insane, become, that she will, delivery, parturition, during: cimic.[54] coff.[54]
- liver disease, he will have: podo.[58]
- paralyzed, being: agar.[139] cist.[139] con.[139] cycl.[139] sac-alb.[139] ***sang.***[171] syph.[85]
- person; two personalities opposing to each other in himself, who are discussing their disease, there are: paro-i.[149]
- power over all disease, has: ***stram.***[54]
- seasick, he is: der. magn-gr.[139] nitro-o.[36] tab.[139]
- sick, a beloved friend is, and dying: bar-c.
- sick, going to be, that he was: bell.[5] hell.[5] nat-p. nicc.[139] podo.
- sick, he is: ambr.[5] arg-n. ***ars. asar.***[5] bar-c. bell. ***calc.*** caust.[30] cham.[5] ***chel.***[5] ***cic.***[5] **COLCH.**[5] graph. hell.[58] ***iod. kali-c.*** lac-c.[58] laur.[5] led.[5] ***lyc.*** merc.[60] mosch.[58] murx. nat-c. nat-m. nit-ac. nux-m.[5] **NUX-V.**[5] petr. phos. podo. psor. **PULS.**[5] ***sabad.*** sel.[5] ***sep.*** spig.[5] spong.[5] **STAPH.**[5] stram. tarax.[139] ***tarent.***[122] valer.[5] verat.[5]
- sick, he is, mind and body, in: merc.[60]
- sick, he is, work, and for this reason will not: calc.[30] caust.[30] nux-v.[30] sep.[30]
- sick, members of the family are: hep.
- sick, someone else is: gels.[111]
- sick, two sick people were in bed, one of whom got well and the other did not: sec.
- strange, symptoms, his, are: bamb-a.[1184]
- swollen, is: acon.[102] ***aran.***[102] ***arg-n.***[102] asaf.[102] bapt.[102] ***bov.***[102] ***cann-i.*** carbn-s. glon.[102] op.[102] plat.[102]
- tetanus must die of, with pain in right leg: ***mag-p.***[54]
- thin, is getting: lap-c-b.[194] sulph.
- typhoid fever, he will have: nat-p.
- warts, he has: mez.
- wasting away, he is: naja[36]
- well, he is: ***apis*** **ARN.** ars. bell.[10] cinnb. hyos. **IOD.** 5 kreos. merc. ***op.***[5] psil.[164] puls.

Desires; recover, to: sec.[36]

Despair; heart disease or liver disease, in: aur.[58]

Despair; hypochondriasis, in: agn.[54]

Despair; pains, stomach, in the: ant-c. ***coch.***[8] ***coff.***

Despair; pains, with the: acon. aloe[58] arn.[102] ***ars.*** **AUR.** aur-ar.[58] ***bell-p.***[102] calc.[122] carb-v. ***cham.*** chin.[58] chin-ar. coch.[102] ***coff.*** colch. coloc.[58] hyper. **IGN.** lach. lil-t.

mag-c. med.[102] morph.[102] naja[36] **NAT-M.**[185] **NAT-S.**[185] nux-v. psil.[164] stram.[122] ***verat.*** vip.[5] zinc-val.[102]
Despair; recovery, ague, in: ***tarent.***[54]
Despair; recovery, convalescence, during: **ALUM.**[122] **ARS.**[122] **CALC.**[122] ***psor.*** **SYPH.**[122]
Despair; recovery, of: ***acon.*** all-s.[36] alum.[5] am-c.[10] anac.[137] ant-t.[36] **ARS.** aur-ar.[58] aur-i.[58] ***aur-s.***[58] bac.[62] bapt. bar-c. bor.[10] ***bry.*** cact.[58] calad.[10] **CALC.** calc-ar.[58] calc-s. cann-i. carc.[207] caust.[30] cham. chlol. cimic.[149] **COLOC.**[162] dig.[172] germ.[222] ***hell.*** hep.[30] hura ***ign.***[122] kali-ar. kali-br. kali-c. kreos. lac-c.[116] lach.[10] lil-t.[172] lyc.[1] m-arct.[10] mag-c.[144] ***med.***[72] ***merc.***[30] nat-c.[10] nat-m.[10] nat-s. nit-ac.[58] nux-v. ph-ac.[10] phos.[10] plat.[172] ***psor.*** puls.[10] ***sep.*** sil. sulph.[10] **SYPH.**[122] ther. ***thyr.***[162] verat.[58] zinc.
Despair; recovery, thinks it is useless to take medicine: ars.[102]
Discontented; health, about: phos.[1]
Discuss, her symptoms with everyone: arg-n.[193] pop-c.[122]
Disgust; consciousness of his unnatural state mind: tarent.[54]
Doubtful; recovery, climacteric period, during: sars.[54]
Doubtful; recovery, medicine is useless: alumn.[54] ars.[10]
Doubtful; recovery, of: ***acon.*** agn. alum.[1] arn.[116] ***ars.***[10] ars-h.[54] aur.[122] bry. calc. calc-sil.[58] cecr.[149] ***ign.***[122] kali-c. kreos.[10] lac-c.[116] lach. ***lept.***[116] lil-t.[116] ***lyc.***[116] mag-c.[193] ***merc.***[30] nat-s.[10] nit-ac.[116] nux-v. ph-ac. phos. psor. puls. sep. ***stann.***[116] sulph. syph.[122]
Dreams; blind, that he was: phys.
➤ body, abdomen, covered with warts and ulcers: choc.[222] junc.[36]
➤ body, abdomen, cut, a big cut in, blood and pus, under which amounts of: ozone[227]
➤ body, abdomen, cut, a big cut in, tumor, under which grows a: ozone[227]
➤ body, abdomen, painful: apis[36] choc.[222]
➤ body, arm, covered with blisters: cast.[10]
➤ body, arm, covered with blisters, burning: cast.[10]
➤ body, arm, hurt, mother's arm: chin.[36]
➤ body, arm, painful: nicc.[36]
➤ body, arm, paralyzed: nicc.[36]
➤ body, back, covered with warts: mez.[36]
➤ body, cheek, swollen: kali-n.[1]
➤ body, emaciated, becoming: kali-n.[36] kreos.[58]
➤ body, eyelids itching: upa.[36]
➤ body, eyes, violent stitches in: calc.[54]
➤ body, face covered with pustules: anac.[36]
➤ body, face, swollen: kali-n.[10]
➤ body, fingers stiff: calc-s.[10]
➤ body, foot, stitching in the: asar.[36]
➤ body, knee, painful: zinc.[36]
➤ body, knee, swollen: cocc.
➤ body, penis, prepuce sloughed off: linu-c.
➤ body, rash, covered with: am-m.
➤ body, teeth breaking off: kali-n. rauw.[119] sul-ac.[10] ther. thuj.
➤ body, teeth falling, filling is falling out: nux-v.[36]
➤ body, teeth, falling out: bamb-a.[1184] coca[36] cocc. convo-d.[36] nicc. nux-v. sul-ac.[10] tab.
➤ body, throat, having a lump in the: cinnb.[36]
➤ body, throat, sore throat: bar-c.[36] bor.[1] pip-m.[36]
➤ boils: prun.
➤ cancer, of: halo.[149]
➤ children, about, babies, leukemia, with: ozone[227]
➤ children, about, coma, in: ozone[227]
➤ cholera, of: linu-c.[36]
➤ cough, dry, chronic and consumptive: eupi.[36]
➤ daughter, struck by paralysis, had been: nat-s.[36]
➤ diphtheria, of: bac.[62]
➤ disease: am-c.[122] am-m. anac. anan. apis asar. bar-c. bor. both-a.[3070] ***calc.*** calc-acet.[36] calc-sil.[58] cast-eq.[36] caust. cocc.[5] con. dros. eupi. fago. graph. hep. kali-c. kali-n. kali-s. ***kreos.*** lac-c. ***lyc.*** mag-c. meph. nat-m.[5] nat-s. **NUX-V.** peti.[36] phos. prun. rat. sil. squil.[5] sulph. sumb. syph. upa. ven-m.[149] zinc.[5]
➤ disease, acquaintance, of a: nat-s.[36]
➤ disease, aids: bamb-a.[1184]
➤ disease, apoplectic fit, daughter has an: nat-s.
➤ disease, blind, being: phys.
➤ disease, boils: phys.
➤ disease, burning blisters: cast.
➤ disease, cancer: halo.
➤ disease, cholera: linu-c.
➤ disease, convulsions: calc-s.
➤ disease, cough: eupi.

➤ disease, diarrhea: allox. apis.
➤ disease, discharge, watery, nose: ped.
➤ disease, emaciation: kreos.
➤ disease, epilepsy: iris-foe, mag-c, sil.
➤ disease, eruption: am-c. am-m. anac. cast.
➤ disease, excrescencies: mez.
➤ disease, expectoration, purulent: hep.
➤ disease, fainting: bamb-a.[1184] graph.
➤ disease, family, of: peti.[36]
➤ disease, fever: kali-chl. sulph.
➤ disease, fracture of jaw: rauw.
➤ disease, fracture, limbs, of: cimic.
➤ disease, haemoptysis: hep. meph. phos.
➤ disease, haemorrhage: phos. sol-t-ae.[122]
➤ disease, hair falling out: mag-c.
➤ disease, headache: pip-m. polyg-h.
➤ disease, hydrophobia: anan.
➤ disease, injuries: allox.[119] am-m. ant-c. cench.[58] chel.[36] chin. choc.[222] cortico.[119] lob.[54] ***mag-s.***[10] nat-s. nicc.[10] phos. sumb.
➤ disease, injuries, self-inflicted: nicc.
➤ disease, insane, becoming: aloe ferr-p.
➤ disease, leper, being: paull.[36]
➤ disease, lethargy: graph.[1] op.[10]
➤ disease, loathsome: anac.
➤ disease, lump in throat and ear: cinnb.
➤ disease, miscarriage: m-arct.
➤ disease, nausea: ***arg.***
➤ disease, own disease, his: ***syph.***[54]
➤ disease, pain, abdomen: apis.
➤ disease, pain, about: asar.[5] bry.[36] cahin.[54] carbn-h.[36] cocc.[5] lyc.[1] ***med.***[54] ozone[227]
➤ disease, pain, maxillary joint: agar.
➤ disease, pain, temples: lyc.
➤ disease, plague: ozone[227]
➤ disease, pustules, face: anac.
➤ disease, rash: am-c
➤ disease, sick people: both-a.[3070] calc. calc-sil.[58] cast-eq.[36] ign. mosch. nat-s.[36] peti.[36] rat. rheum staph.
➤ disease, sick people, help them, cannot: ozone[227]
➤ disease, sick people, mother, his: cast-eq.[36]
➤ disease, sore throat: bar-c. bor. pip-m.
➤ disease, stitches, eyes: ***calc.***
➤ disease, stitches, foot: asar.
➤ disease, stoppage, throat: kreos.
➤ disease, strangury: chr-ac.
➤ disease, suffocation: arn. chel.[193] ign.[162] iris kali-bi. kali-c.[1] sang.[193] xan.[85]
➤ disease, ulcers, abdomen: junc-e.
➤ disease, variola: anac.
➤ disease, vertigo: ***sil.***
➤ disease, vomiting worms: ***chin-b.***
➤ disease, warts: mez.
➤ disease, wind-colic: fago.
➤ disease, wounded by shot: lob.[54]
➤ emaciated, becoming: kali-n.[36] kreos.
➤ epilepsy, of: iris-foe. mag-c. sil.
➤ eruptions: am-c.[10] am-m.[5] anac.[10] bamb-a.[1184] cast.[10]
➤ excrescencies: hydrog.[222] mez.[10]
➤ expectoration, purulent: hep.[1]
➤ fever, of: kali-chl.[10] sulph.
➤ feverish: euphr.[36] lachn.[36]
➤ fit, daughter had a apoplectic: nat-s.
➤ fit, he had a: iris mag-c. sil.
➤ frightful, heart disease, in: ***dig.***[54]
➤ funeral, people who had died of scarlatina, in trying to avoid wind blowing from procession toward him he awoke: form.[102]
➤ hemoptysis, spitting blood: hep. meph. phos.[10] sol-t-ae.[122]
➤ pains, about: asar.[5] bry.[36] cahin.[54] carbn-h.[36] cocc.[5] lyc.[1] ***med.***[54] ozone[227]
➤ physician: canna[36] mang.[36]
➤ poisoned, of being: chr-ac.[36] kali-n.[36] ***kreos.*** nat-m. oci.
➤ pus spitting: hep.[1]
➤ smallpox: anac.[10]
➤ stool, diarrheal: allox.[119] apis[36] psil.[164]
➤ suffering: cimic.[36]
➤ vomiting, blood and pus: bamb-a.[1184]
➤ warts: mez.
➤ women, leprous: paull-p.[36]

Dwells; health, his broken: aur-m.[58]

Excitement; frantic, hypochondriasis, in: ***arg-n.***[54]

Excitement; heart, organic disease of, in: ***apis***[54]

Fear; apoplexy, night with feeling as if head would burst, at: ***aster.***
✦ apoplexy, of: abel.[149] acon.[162] ***alum.***[36] apis ***arg.*** arg-n. arn. ***aster.*** bell. brom.[5] calc.[184] carb-v. cench. ***coff.*** elaps ***ferr.*** ferr-p. ferr-t.[36] fl-ac. glon.[5] kali-br.[5] lach. nat-c. nux-v.[185] phos. plat.[162] psor.[56] ***puls.***[30] sel.[116] sep.[1] staph.[30] ter. thuj. verat. ***zinc.***[122]
✦ apoplexy, palpitation, with: arg.
✦ apoplexy, stool, during: verat.
✦ apoplexy, waking, on: arn.[10] carb-v.[1] glon.
✦ blind, of becoming: arge.[149] atro.[172] ***nux-v.***[54] ***sulph.***[54]
✦ brain, disease, in: acon.[8]
✦ brain, disease, of, incurable: arg-n.[47]

- ✦ brain, inflammation of, from dullness in head, amel. by epistaxis: psor.[54]
- ✦ brain, of softening of: abrot. ***arg-n.***[8] asaf. calc-sil.[58]
- ✦ cancer, brain tumor: bamb-a.[1184]
- ✦ cancer, of: agar.[162] **ARS.**[162] bac.[62] bamb-a.[1184] bar-c.[162] **CALC.**[162] calc-f.[162] calc-p.[162] carc.[187] chin-ar.[162] fl-ac.[122] ign.[162] ***kali-ar.***[162] lac-c.[172] ***lob.***[184] **MANC.**[184] med.[122] nat-m.[172] ***nit-ac.***[162] phos.[162] **PLAT.**[8] **PSOR.**[122] ruta[152] sep.[172] verat.[172]
- ✦ cancer, rectum, of, although examination shows nothing abnormal: ***plat.***[8]
- ✦ catalepsy, of: art-v.[172]
- ✦ chlorosis, in: ***calc.***[122]
- ✦ choking, of, inflammation of throat, in: ***hep.***[54]
- ✦ cholera, of: arg-n.[172] ars.[30] jatr.[54] **LACH.**[122] **NIT-AC.** ph-ac.[54] verat.[30]
- ✦ cholera, of the, cramps in calves would set in, as if: ***jatr.***[54]
- ✦ cold, of taking: nat-c. sulph. syph.[193]
- ✦ consumption, of: ***calc.*** kali-c.[149] lac-c. paull. puls.[172] sep. tarent. ***tub.***[54]
- ✦ cough, of, burst, something will burst: apis[162]
- ✦ death, cholera asiatica, in: ***cupr.***[54] ***cupr-acet.***[54] **VERAT.**[54]
- ✦ death, fever, during: calc. cocc. ip. mosch. ***nit-ac.*** **RUTA**
- ✦ death, heart symptoms, during: **ACON.**[54] ***ang.***[54] ***arn.***[54] asaf. cact.[58] carb-v.[58] cench.[58] **DIG.**[54] ***naja***[54] ***plat.***[54] ***psor.***[54]
- ✦ death, heat, during: acon.[85] calc. cocc. ip. mosch. ***nit-ac.*** **RUTA**
- ✦ death, pain, from: anan.[36] cact.[58] **COFF.**
- ✦ death, scarlatina, after: ***hell.***[54]
- ✦ death, smallpox, in: ***ph-ac.***[54]
- ✦ death, termination, of fatal: ant-t.[54] ***ph-ac.***[54] ***spong.***[54]
- ✦ death, vexation, after, in cholera Asiatic: **ARS.**[54]
- ✦ diarrhea from: arg-n.[54] **GELS.**[54] ign.[54] ***kali-p.***[54] **OP.**[54] ***verat.***[54]
- ✦ diarrhea, with f.: acon.[58] aeth.[116] ant-t.[172] arg-n.[54] coff.[172] ***croto-t.***[54] **GELS.**[54] ign.[54] ***kali-p.***[54] **OP.**[54] phos.[172] ***puls.***[54] verat.[172]
- ✦ diphtheria, of: bac.[62]
- ✦ disable, being: **ARS.**[162] mag-m.[162] psor.[162]
- ✦ disease, child, to: ars.[172]
- ✦ disease, contagious, epidemic diseases, of: bar-c.[10] ***bor.*** bov.[36] bufo calad. **CALC.**[30] cur.[193] lach. nat-m.[185] sil.[193] **SULPH.**[193] syph.[193]
- ✦ disease, diarrhea, in: ***croto-t.***[54]
- ✦ disease, ill, that he would be very, when waking in morning, with dull pulsating headache in bilious remittent fever: ***podo.***[54]
- ✦ disease, incurable, of being: acon.[5] agn.[102] all-s.[36] alum.[5] anac.[102] ant-t.[36] apis[102] ***arg-n.***[8] arn.[5] ars.[36] aur.[102] bac.[62] cact.[58] calc.[5] calc-sil.[58] cann-i.[102] carc.[207] cecr.[149] cimic.[149] cocc.[1] dig.[102] graph.[102] hep.[30] hydr.[102] ign.[5] kali-c.[102] lac-c.[5] lach.[5] lil-t.[5] med.[102] naja[102] nat-m.[102] nit-ac.[102] nux-v.[102] phase.[102] phos.[172] plat.[102] podo.[102] psor.[102] puls.[102] raph.[172] rhus-t.[102] sabad.[102] sec.[102] sep.[47] stann.[5] still.[102] syph.[56] verat.[102]
- ✦ disease, long spell of illness before dying, in old men: ***cic.***[54]
- ✦ disease, of impending: acet-ac.[54] acon. aether agar. ***alum.***[122] alum-p.[58] am-c. ambr.[172] anac.[172] ant-t.[5] ***arg-n. arn.***[5] ars. bac.[62] bamb-a.[1184] ***bor.*** bov.[122] bry. bufo calad. ***calc. calc-ar.***[122] calc-f.[162] calc-s.[108] calc-sil.[58] cand-a.[239] carb-ac. carb-an. carc.[214] ***chin-ar.***[54] chlor.[116] cic. cimic.[149] dros.[172] elaps elat.[111] eup-pur.[58] hep. hydr. ign. iod.[172] iris kali-br.[25] **KALI-C.** ***kali-p.***[58] kali-tel.[36] kreos. ***lac-c.*** lach. ***lec. lil-t.*** lyc.[1] m-arct.[10] med.[102] merc. morg.[136] nat-ar. nat-c. nat-m. nat-p. ***nit-ac. nux-v.*** ozone[227] paull. ***ph-ac.*** **PHOS.** ***plat.***[5] pneu.[149] podo. psor.[111] ***puls.***[5] sabad.[5] ***sep.***[122] ***spong.***[8] stann.[5] staph.[30] sulph. tab.[111] tarent. thuj. tril.
- ✦ disease, symptoms indicate internal organic, that: ***lil-t.***[54]
- ✦ disease, termination, of a fatal: ant-t.[54] calc.[172] kali-c.[172] lil-t.[172] ***ph-ac.***[54] sabad.[172] ***spong.***[54]
- ✦ disease, unrecognized: lil-t.[172] raph.[172]
- ✦ disease; viral: nux-v.[172]
- ✦ epilepsy, of: alum. arg-n. bamb-a.[1184] merc.[10]
- ✦ examination, medical: ant-t.[103] phos.[146] puls.[70] sanic.[141] tub.[70]
- ✦ examination, medical, will not let you feel the pulse: ant-t.[103] sanic.[141]
- ✦ exposure night in bed, of: mag-c.
- ✦ fever, going to bed, on: hura
- ✦ fever, of (while chilly): calc.[122] sulph.
- ✦ fever, typhus: cham.[54] nat-p.[172] tarent.
- ✦ fever, yellow: ***merc.***[54] ***sulph.***[54]

✦ head, something wrong in her: bamb-a.[1184]
✦ health, ruined her, that she has: calc.[122] chel. staph.[122]
✦ heart, cease to beating, unless constantly on the move, h. will: ***gels.***
✦ heart, disease of: acon.[52] arg-n.[162] ***arn.***[91] ***aur.*** bapt. cact. ***calc.***[54] calc-p.[162] calc-s.[58] caust.[172] cupr.[210] daph.[36] germ.[222] hed.[119] hydrog.[222] ***kali-ar.***[162] lac-c. lach. ***lil-t.*** lob.[162] meny.[85] mez.[179] nat-m.[162] nux-m.[54] ***phos.***[162] podo.[58] psor.[172] rhus-t.[172] sars.[162] sin-n.[54] ***spong.*** tarent.[172]
✦ heart, disease of, organic: ***apis***[117] ***aur.***[54] calc.[36]
✦ heart, disease of, stitches will kill him if they do not cease: psor.[172]
✦ heart, pain about h., from: daph.
✦ heat, during: acon. ***ars.*** cham.[54] nux-m. spong.
✦ imbecile, that he would become: stram.
✦ invaded, of being: lap-gr-m.[194]
✦ joints are weak, that: sep.
✦ liver, complaints of, in: ***mag-m.***[54] podo.[58]
✦ lumps in mamma, of: bamb-a.[1184]
✦ lung disease, of: anh.[122] aral.[36] arg-n.[172]
✦ memory will fail, that his: nat-m.[172]
✦ operation, before: phos.[146]
✦ osteoporosis: calc.[185]
✦ pain, of: aur.[127] bry.[172] calc.[122] clem.[122] coff.[172] cor-r.[172] cori-r.[36] der.[36] eup-per.[172] lil-t.[172] lyc.[5] phos.[172] pip-m.[36] pip-n.[172]
✦ pancreas problems, with: ***atro.***[54]
✦ paralysis, of: ***anac.*** arn. asaf. bapt.[85] bell. kali-p.[172] syph.
✦ pneumonia, of: chel.
✦ pregnancy, during: ***acon.***[54] ***ant-t.***[54] bar-c.[54] ***caul.***[122] ***cimic.*** con.[5] ign.[54] lyc.[54] ***lyss.***[54] ***nux-m.***[54] psor.[54] stann.
✦ pregnancy, during, child would be deformed, that: acon.[172]
✦ prolapse, of, anus: ign.[172] nit-ac.[172]
✦ prolapse, uterus, everything dropping through: ***lil-t.***[54]
✦ pulsation in, head, from: aml-n.[54]
✦ smallpox, of: ***vac.***[54] ***vario.***[72]
✦ stomach, ulcer in, of: ign. nat-m.[172] sabad.[10]
✦ stoppage of circulation, with sensation of, at night, in angina pectoris: ***lyc.***[54]
✦ suffering, of: achy.[149] acon.[172] aur.[127] bry. calc. cham.[184] clem.[122] coff.[172] cor-r. cori-r.[36] der. eup-per. fl-ac.[162] hep.[162] lil-t. merc-br.[36] phos.[172] pip-m. pip-n.[172] spig.[58] stram.[172]
✦ suffocation, asthma, with: ***phos.***[54]
✦ suffocation, goiter, in: ***merc-i-f.***[122]
✦ suffocation, heart disease, in: ***dig.***[122] lach.[162] ***spong.***[122]
✦ syphilis, of: ***hyos.*** merc.[30] syph.[162]
✦ throat, sensation of swelling of, from: ***glon.*** nat-m.[1]
✦ tuberculosis, incipient, in: ***tub.***[54]
✦ tuberculosis, of: calc.[137]
✦ urination, retention of, from: ***op.***[54]
✦ vision, of losing his: euphr.[36] ***nux-v.***[54]
✦ worm diseases, with: stann.[8]

Feigning; paroxysms, faintness: ***tarent.***
Feigning; sick: arg-n. bell. ign.[5] mosch.[162] plb.[58] sabad.[137] sil.[30] ***tarent.*** verat.
Grief; condition, about his: staph.
Groping as if in the dark: croc. hyos. op. plb.
Haughty; sick, when: lyc.[102]
Helplessness; feeling of, heart complaints, with: am-c.[1]
Hopefulness; recovery, of: sang.[54]
Hydrophobia; bitten, after being: lyss.[54]
Hydrophobia; frequently speaks with a remarkably quick and sharp articulation of the impending result: lyss.[54]
Hypochondriasis: abies-n.[85] ***acon.***[5] agn.[5] alf.[102] aloe[5] alum.[5] ***ambr.***[5] anac.[5] anag.[54] anan.[54] ***ant-t.***[54] arg.[149] arg-n.[5] ***arn.***[5] ***ars.***[5] arum-m.[54] ***asaf.***[5] **AUR.**[5] ***aur-m.***[54] aur-s.[10] aven.[102] aza.[149] bamb-a.[1184] ***bell.***[5] **BENZ-AC.**[54] bism.[5] both-l.[3070] bran.[10] brom.[5] bry.[5] **CACT.**[54] **CALC.**[5] ***cann-s.***[5] canth.[5] ***caps.***[122] carc.[207] card-m.[25] caust.[5] ***cham.***[5] chin.[5] ***cimic.***[102] coca[25] cocc.[5] coff.[5] ***colch.***[54] **CON.**[5] croc.[5] cupr.[5] ***cycl.***[5] dig.[5] esp-g.[149] euphr.[5] ferr.[5] ferr-p.[58] gels.[5] gran.[10] **GRAPH.**[5] ***grat.***[54] ***hell.***[5] helon.[102] hep.[5] hydr-ac.[102] ***hyos.***[54] **IGN.**[5] iod.[5] ***ip.***[54] kali-br.[102] kali-c.[5] kali-chl.[10] kali-hp.[25] kali-p.[5] **LACH.**[5] lath.[102] ***lil-t.***[54] ***lyc.***[5] lycps.[85] mag-c.[144] **MAG-M.**[5] merc.[5] merc-d.[5] ***mez.***[5] ***mill.***[54] ***mosch.***[5] murx.[54] ***nat-c.***[5] **NAT-M.**[5] nep.[144] nit-ac.[5] nux-m.[5] **NUX-V.**[5] ***ol-an.***[5] op.[5] ***petr.***[5] ***ph-ac.***[5] ***phos.***[5] ***plat.***[5] plb.[5] podo.[5] ***puls.***[5] ***rhus-t.***[5] sabad.[5] sabin.[5] sac-alb.[85] ***sel.***[5] seneg.[5] ***sep.***[5] sin-n.[54] ***spong.***[5] ***stann.***[5] ***staph.***[5] stram.[5] sul-ac.[5] ***sulph.***[5] sumb.[102] tab.[5] tarent.[102] ***ter.***[54] thuj.[102] v-a-b.[149] **VALER.**[5] ***verat.***[5] vib-t.[85] ***viol-o.***[5] **ZINC.**[5] zinc-o.[102] zinc-val.[85] ***zing.***[54] ziz.[102]

Hypochondriasis; abdominal complaints, with: aur.[10] calc.[10] ***graph.***[54] lach.[10] nat-c.[10] nux-v.[10] sil.[10] sulph.[10]

Hypochondriasis; alone: ars.[10]

Hypochondriasis; continence in unmarried men, from: con.[1]

Hypochondriasis; eating, after: anac.[54] chin.[54] ***nat-c.***[54] ***nux-v.***[10] zinc.[10]

Hypochondriasis; grief, inclined to: **IGN.**[54] **PULS.**[54]

Hypochondriasis; insults, from: ***staph.***[54]

Hypochondriasis; masturbation, after: ***tarent.***[54]

Hypochondriasis; sexual: ***mosch.***[54]

Hypochondriasis; sexual, abstinence, from: **CON.**[54] mosch.[54]

Hypochondriasis; sexual, abuse, after: ***ph-ac.***[54]

Hypochondriasis; sexual, dwelling on sexual subjects: ***staph.***[54]

Hypochondriasis; sexual, excesses, from: anac.[10] calc.[10] chin.[10] **CON.**[54] nat-m.[10] nux-v.[10] ***ph-ac.***[54] sep.[10] **STAPH.**[54] sulph.[10]

Hypochondriasis; suicide, leading to: alum.[30] aur.[30] calc.[30] caust.[30] chin.[30] con.[30] graph.[30] hep.[10] ***nat-m.***[30] sep.[30] **STAPH.**[30] sulph.[30]

Hypochondriasis; weather, in cloudy: aloe[54]

Hysteria; sick, after being insulted and subduing his wrath: ***staph.***[54]

Impatience; cures him at once, the patient insists that the doctor: cham.[85]

Indifference; condition does not seem dangerous to him, in typhus: colch.[54]

Indifference; illness, to his: gels.[72]

Indifference; recovery, about his: ars.[1] aur-m-n.[162] ***calc.***

Indifference; typhoid, in: ail.[58] ***apis***[54] ***arn.*** chin. ***chin-s.***[54] ***colch.***[54] ***nit-s-d.***[54] ***ph-ac.*** ***verat.***[54]

Indolence; sad, making him, with feeling of deep-seated inward trouble: sabin.[54]

Irritability; disease, before: caps.[193]

Irritability; sends the, doctor home, says he is not sick: ***apis***[117] **ARN. CHAM.**

Irritability; sick, when: bell.[137] ***lyc.***[122]

Lamenting; disease, about his: arg-n. **LACH.**[30] nux-v.[30] ph-ac.

Loquacity; excited, heart disease, in: ***op.***[54]

Loquacity; health, about his: **NUX-V.**[122]

Mood; repulsive, treatment, every, sick, in spite of being very: ars.[30] caust.[30] nux-v.[30]

Morose; thinking of his ailments when alone, on: **AUR-M.**[54]

Narrating her symptoms agg.: **CALC.** cic. ign. ***kali-c.***[163] ***med.***[163] ***puls.*** ***sep.***[163] teucr.

Pities herself; sick, desire to show being: tarent.[36]

Quiet disposition; hypochondriasis, in: puls.[10] valer.[54]

Rage; convulsions, fits, after, epileptic: ***arg.*** op.[102]

Rage; convulsions, fits, during, epileptic: bell. ***canth.***[54] cupr. hyos. nux-v. op. plb. stram.[54]

Reading; desire for, medical books: ***calc.***[30] ***nux-v.***[30] ***puls.***[30] staph.[30] sulph.[30]

Refuses; treatment, sick, in spite of being very: ars.[30] caust.[30] nux-v.[30]

Religious affections; happy to join her Redeemer, felt, in facial erysipelas: ***plat.***[54]

Restlessness; angina pectoris, in: ***aur-m.***[54]

Restlessness; hypochondriacal: ars.[10] ***asaf.***[54] graph.[36] valer.[10]

Sadness; asthma, with, die, thinks he will: ars.[102] phos.[54] psor.[102] spong.[54]

Sadness; disease, about: alum.[36] cecr.[149] sin-n.[54] ***sulph.***[54] syph.[54]

Sadness; disease, about, incurable, of heart, which makes him reckless: ***phos.***[54]

Sadness; disease, about, sure he would not recover, in bronchial asthma: ***sin-n.***[54]

Sadness; disease, about, sure he, is going to die in twenty four hours: lac-d.[54]

Sadness; disease, as from, approaching: ph-ac.[36]

Sadness; disease, sure he, would not recover, in bronchial asthma: ***sin-n.***[54]

Sadness; dwell constantly over her condition, inclination to: ***sulph.***[54]

Sadness; epilepsy, with: ***atro.***[54] ***indg.***[54] ***sulph.***[54] tarent.[54]

Sadness; gonorrhea, in: ***hydr.***[54] ***merc.***[54] ***thuj.***[54]

Sadness; health, about the: acon.[54] ***sep.***[36] staph.[54]

Sadness; hypochondriacal: ***arg-n.***[54] caust.[1] con.[36b]

Shrieking; cardiac rheumatism, in: ***cact.***[54]

Suicidal disposition; cancer patients, in: carc.[85] scirr.[85]

Talk; indisposed, illness or injuries, about: **BAPT.**[54]

Talk; indisposed, sufferings, over his: ign.[5]

Thinking; ailments, complaints, of, constantly to his: ***ham.***[122]

Thinking; ailments, of, alone, when left: ars.[54]
Thinking; ailments, of, angina pectoris, in: ***aur-m.***[54]
Thoughts; disease, incurable, of some: ***ars.***[8] merc.[36]
Thoughts; disease, of: alum. ***ars.***[122] chel. lepi.[36] murx. nat-m. nat-p. ph-ac. phos. sep. sulph.
Thoughts; morbid, evening, in bed: ***sulph.***[36]
Tranquillity; fears she would not recover, yet, during climacteric period: sars.[54]
Violence; sick, when: bell.[85]
Vivacious; heart disease, in: ***cact.***[54]
Washing; always, hands, her: ars.[111] coca[122] cur.[162] ***lac-c.***[122] ***med.***[122] merc.[184] ***nat-m.***[162] plat.[126] psor.[111] sep.[162] sil.[185] ***sulph.***[162] syph. thuj.[162]
Weeping; disease, with progression of the: aeth.[31]
Weeping; heart disease, in: ***aur.***[54] ***op.***[54]
Weeping; hypochondriasis, in: ***arg-n.***[54] mez.[54]
Weeping; telling of her illness, when: aster.[231] bry.[122] carc.[122] ign.[162] ***kali-c. med. nat-m.***[189] prot.[136] **PULS. SEP.**
Well; feels very, ill, before falling: bry.[111] helon.[85] nux-v.[111] phos.[111] ***psor.***[111] sep.[111]
Well; says he is, when very sick: androc.[222] ***apis*** **<u>ARN.</u>**[122] ars. atro.[36] bac.[62] bell.[10] ***cann-s.***[5] cinnb. ***coff.***[5] hyos. iod.[111] kreos. merc. op.[5] plb.[5] puls.[58] stram.[5] valer.[5]

ABROT. He, 3 - Thinks her brain is softening. (dissolving)
ACET-AC. He, 6 - Anxiety; grieves about his sickness and his children.
He, 3 - Fancies he has an ulcer in his stomach.
ACON-F. Al, 3 - In the intervals of relief from distressing symptoms, he laughed and joked about his very comical condition;...(proper disease)
ACON. Al, 30 - Now he doubts his recovery, now he is full of hope. (despair x hopeful)
Ha, 510 - Sometimes he despairs of his recovery, sometimes he is full of hope.
Ha, 516 - Inconsolable anxiety and piteous howling, with complaints and reproaches about (often triflings) evils.
He, 23 - Pains are so intolerable, they drive him crazy; he becomes very restless.
He, 35 - Sadness with solicitude; concerned about future; about her recovery or fears loss of reason. (insanity)
He, 40 - Thrice he became blind and affirmed that death was at hand.
He, 51 - Ailments from fright: afraid (fear) in dark; vertigo; faintness; trembling; cardiac weakness; threatened miscarriage (abortion); impending cessation of menstrual flow;..
He, 53 - Ailments from vexation (worry, care), with fear or vehemence: congestion; palpitation; fever; anxiety, beside himself; threatened miscarriage ; apoplectic congestion.
He, 39 - Fear of death; during pregnancy or confinement; with prolapsus uteri; with great loquacity or anxiety in region of heart.
ADAM. Sh, 419 - Fear of breast cancer because of aching in the breast and arm. Feel a certainty of breast cancer. 2, 12C, 08:XX:XX
Sh, 420 - Informed that my father has cancer of cardiac sphincter. Feel sure I have cancer of the lymph nodes of interior axilla. Don't feel any emotion for my father, but weep with anger. 2, 12C, 26:XX:XX
Sh, 422 - I am concerned about my health. Think I have TB or pneumonia. I am sure I will die. 7, 6C, 28:00:XX
Sh, 423 - Extreme weakness, painful cough, weak chest. Feels like TB or wasting disease. 22, 200C, 01:XX:XX
Sh, 429 - Fear something could happen if I had a bath. Want to keep dry. 7, 6C, 20:09:00
AETH. He, 22 - After social talking, all symptoms disappear.
ALL-S. Al, 5 - Fears he will never get well.
He, 3 - Sadness when alone; moral uneasiness; afraid of never getting well; fear of not being able to bear any kind of medicine; fear of being poisoned...
ALOE. Al, 40-...wrap up in himself (introspection), as after a sickness or a fit of anger, which still gnaws (bite) internally, which one cannot express.
ALUM. Al, 9 - He believes he will not be able to recover his health.
Al, 10 - He feels low-spirited on account of his disease.

Ha, 4 - Dejected (depressed, unhappy) as to his disease._
Ha, 20 - In the morning, anxiety as if he were to have an attack of epilepsy in a few hours.(convulsion)
Ha, 5 - He thinks that he cannot get well again.
He, 20 - Fears he is not to recover.
ALUMN. Al, 3 - Great anxiety, and disbelief (doubt, suspicious) in the power of medicine to relieve him.
Al, 13 - When thinking about his disease, he feels the heart beating.
He, 5 - Thinking about her disease causes palpitation.
AM-C. Al, 19 - She is anxious on account of her illness.
Ha, 6 - Anxious and distressed about her diseased condition.
He, 6 - Anxious concern about one's sickness.
AML-N. He, 13 - Haunted (obsessed) many times a day with an indescribable dread and sensation as of an oncoming fit, although it came on only once or twice a week.
ANAC. He, 64 - Anxiousness; despairs of getting well.
ANDROC. Sh, 167 - Pretended to feel well, although sick. (17)
ANT-T. Al, 5 - Despondent and apprehensive about his recovery. (despair)
Al, 19-...anxious thoughts about the future; she thinks she will remain in her present condition.
He, 22 - Despondent and apprehensive (fear) that he would not recover.
He, 30 - Depression of mind and fear that he will never get well.
He, 29 - Despair of his recovery.
APIS. He, 60 - Dread (fear) of apoplexy.
He, 66 - When asked if sick, he says: "Nothing is the matter".
He, 18 - Thinks he will die. 0 Organic disease of heart.
ARG-M. He, 2-...as if he might have an apoplectic stroke, and could not finish this proving; with spasmodic contraction of heart.
He, 16 - Anxious about her health; full of care.
ARG-N. He, 14 - Thinks he has softening of brain, or some other incurable affection (disease), which almost drives him to despair.
He, 46 - Easily frightened; fears disease may result seriously; weeping mood.
He, 48 - Great nervousness and prostration (lassitude); fears to be alone because he thinks he will die ; is apprehensive of some serious disease, which almost drives him to despair.
He, 24 - Constantly talking about his sufferings. 0Hypochondriasis
He, 31 - Does not work, thinking it will do him harm or that he is not able to stand it.
He, 35 - Sad; fear of apoplexy.
He, 44 - Apprehension of some serious disease.
He, 29 - Frequently remains in bed on slightest pretext of being "indisposed". 0 Hypochondriasis.
ARN. Al, 31 - Excessive inclination to perform many and long literary labors, without possessing the strength which is required to terminate them without injuring health.
He, 47 - All occupation had to be relinquished (quit) for the time, so intense were the sufferings. (impediment)
He, 18 - Says there is nothing the matter with him.
ARS-H. Al, 1 - Anxiety he believes his death is near, and despairs of being better...
He, 12 - Full of care and fear about his complaint (disease) when he gets awake at night.
He, 15 - Anxiety, he believes his death is near, and despairs of being better...
He, 23 - Thinking of water irritates him, as if he would have to vomit; it nauseates him.
He, 14 - The fear of dying is gone on 3d day, notwithstanding all around him have doubts of his recovery.
ARS. Al, 50 - He despairs of his life.(recovery?)
Al, 91-...she was afraid (fear) of solitude and death; the slightest cause was sufficient to put her into anger and rage, which especially occurred when one spoke of her complete recovery which she considered wholly impossible.
Al, 70 - The anxiety and restlessness are indescribable; "Kill me", he cried, "or relieve my pains!".(help)

Ha, 1034 - Hypochondriac anxiety, ...as if it came from the upper part of the chest; without palpitation of the heart.

Ha, 1038 - When he is alone he is beset by thoughts about disease and other thoughts of an indifferent character, of which he cannot get rid.

Ha, 1057 - Uncommonly tranquil disposition; quite unconcerned about their approaching death, they neither hoped nor wished to recover.

Ha, 42 - When he is alone he falls into thoughts about disease and other things, from which he can not easily tear himself away.

He, 7 - When alone, he falls to thinking about disease and other things, which he can scarcely keep out of his mind.

He, 9 - Thoughts of death and the incurability of his complaint. 0Cancerous inoculation

He, 22 - In her delirium she thinks she is well; girl, aet.7.

ART-V. He, 18 - Fright (fear) and other emotions are followed by epilepsy.

ASAF. He, 9 - Fear paralysis or softening of brain.

ASTER. He, 7 - Fear of apoplexy, followed by fever.

ATRO. Al, 3-...the mind would become filled with strange and fanciful ideas ...fits of wild, uncontrollable laughter...I fancied myself afflicted with epilepsy, and was constantly fearful lest others should discover my unfortunate condition; ...

AUR-M. He, 1-...he imagines he has all possible diseases.

He, 2 - If left alone he thinks about nothing but his ailments,... ; desires company.

He, 15 - Thinking about his disease brings on palpitation.

BAPT. He, 16 - Aversion... to hear conversation about sickness or injuries; feeble mind. (impressionable) 0Spasmodic stricture of esophagus.

He, 19 - Hopeless (despair) of recovery, and certain (inevitable) of death.

BAR-A. Al, 10 - An evil, fearful suspicion suddenly takes possession of her, as if, for example, a loved friend had been taken suddenly deathly ill.

BAR-C. Ha, 7 - An evil fearful foreboding comes suddenly upon his soul, as if, e.g. a beloved friend might suddenly have fallen fatally ill.

He, 27 - She is suddenly overwhelmed with an evil apprehension; she imagines, for instance, that a beloved friend has suddenly fallen sick and is dying.

He, 39 - Thinking of one's complaints makes them worse.

BELL. Ha, 1434 - Madness; he thinks that his living body is putrefying. (decay, degeneracy)

He, 67-...suffered greatest anxiety and despaired of recovery.

BISM. Al, 3 - He is morose and discontented with his condition (health, position) and complains about it.

He, 11 - Ill humor; he is morose and discontented with his condition (position), and complains about it.

BOR. Al, 14 - Dread and fear of contagion.

Ha, 6 - Apprehension and fear of infection.

BRY. He, 33 - Despair of recovery.

BUFO. Al, 12 - He is anxious about the state of his health; is afraid he will die or that some other misfortune will happen to him.

Al, 16 - Fear of catching diseases.

Al, 22 - He is irritable, anxious about his state of health, with great dread of death.

He, 12 - Fear of disease, of animals, of death.

CACT. Al, 18 - Fear of death extreme and continuous; he believes his disease to be incurable.

Al, 6 - Decided repugnance to take any more medicine.

He, 3 - Thinks she will not recover; weeps much; despondent.

He, 14 - Fear of death; he believes his disease, incurable.

He, 16 - During and after attack, great anxiety, fearing some organic lesion of heart which will cause sudden death.

CALAD. Al, 3 - He is very apprehensive about his health, and about everything...

He, 12 - Very careful about his health; apprehensive.

He, 13 - Fear of catching scarlet fever when attending a case; a fear he never had before.

CALC-A. Al, 255 - Dreams of sick people, and dead people, with violent weeping in the sleep.

CALC-P. He, 17 - Feel complaints more when thinking about them.

CALC. Al, 17 - She is very hypochondriac; she thinks that she is deadly sick, nevertheless can complain of nothing.

Al, 30 - Dread and anxiety of the future, with fear of consumption.

Al, 18 - Despairing mood, with dread of disease and suffering, with foreboding of sad events.

Ha, 25 - His heart is agitated with fear and anxiety for the future, with fear of consumption.(tuberculosis, ruin)

Ha, 28 - Hypochondriac, she conceives herself fatally diseased, and yet cannot complain of anything.

Ha, 29 - Despairing (hopeless) mood with fear of sickness (disease) and misery, with forebodings of sad events. (misfortune)

He, 48 - Anxious about getting well, during the intervals. (Epilepsy)

He, 50 - Apprehensive (fearful, worried) mood ; as if some misfortune was about to happen; about his health (vigour) ; that he might have an organic disease of the heart.

He, 53 - Fear: of death; of consumption (decay, waste, tuberculosis); of misfortune (disaster) ; of being alone. (lonely)

He, 65 - Despairing; hopeless (unhappy, pessimistic) of ever getting well (health); with fear of death, tormenting all around day and night.

He, 34 - Does not care to get well, or to do anything to assist (aid) recovery.

CAMPH. He, 21 - Very nervous; imagined various things; that he would get yellow fever.

CANTH. Al, 26 - Distrust of himself, like a hypochondriac.

CARB-AC. He, 17 - Fear of impending sickness...

CARB-V. Ha, 677 - At night he wakes up several times on account of pulsation in the head and anxiety as if about to have a fit of apoplexy; ...and he felt that if he put off awaking longer he would have fainted.

CAUST. Al, 18 - Anxiety with the physical troubles.

Ha, 9 - Anxiety about bodily ailments.(disease)

He, 39 - Ill effects of sudden emotions, fright, fear, etc. (ailments from)

He, 62 - Thinking of complains aggravates them.

CHEL. Al, 24 - Sad mood; she fears that she has ruined her health by the proving.

Al, 54 - Fear that pneumonia is coming on.

CHLOL. Al, 24-...knew that she was very ill, and herself insisted upon my being sent for...(ordered, dictatorial)

He, 3 - Fixed despair of recovery; believes he will give his imaginary disease (syphilis) to others.

CIC. Ha, 235-...; everything appeared to him strange and almost frightful; it was as if he woke up out of an acute fever and saw all sorts of figures, and yet he did not feel corporeally ill.

He, 33 - Old man fear a long spell (time) of sickness before dying.

CIMIC. He, 21 - Mental depression, with suicidal mood; also after checked neuralgia.

CINNB. Al, 1 - Illusion of mind; he considers himself well.

COCC. Al, 15 - Anxiety concerning the curability of a slight complaint, in the morning.

Ha, 531 - Serious, and though caring little about his own health, he is very anxious about the illnesses of others.

Ha, 535 - In the morning, anxiety respecting the incurability of a trifling malady.

COLCH. He, 5 - Says nothing unless questioned, his condition does not seem to him dangerous. 0Typhus.

CON. Al, 1277 - Dreams of wretched (miserable) diseases.

He, 29 - Hypochondriasis and hysteria from suppression of, or too free indulgence in, sexual instinct,...(ailments from)

COP. Al, 7 - Anxiety about his health.

CROT-C. Al, 6 - She fancies her eyes are falling out (tenth day).

CROT-H. He, 15 - Oppression as if brain had been intoxicated by carbonic acid, or by degraded or non-oxygenated blood.

He, 10 - Mania in zymotic (infectious) disease and when connected with puerperal or ovary-uterine disease.

DER. Al, 1 - He fancies he is seasick. (nauseated)

Al, 3 - He is discouraged and despairs of a cure (recovery), declaring himself a hypochondriac.

Al, 4 - He dreads pain, and is averse to solitude with great anxiety.

DIG. Ha, 421 - He is sad and has a feeling of being very ill; all objects appear to him as in fever, just as if he had a perversion of the visual faculty as in fever.

DIRC. Al, 3 - Sense of apprehension, throughout the proving, as of some trouble, which may have depended upon the morbid state of the mind at the same time of the proving.

ELAPS. He, 4 - Fearful and apprehensive of some fatal disease.

EUP-PUR. He, 9 - Has a great fear of sickness.

FERR. He, 12 - Nervous, hysterical feeling; fear of apoplexy.

FL-AC. He, 14 - Fear of apoplexy.

GELS. He, 33 - Effects (ailments from) of grief; cannot cry; when thinking of his symptoms (disease), also when spoken to of his loss ; >from diverting talk; oppression and palpitation of heart; feels a sense of peril (danger, harm, risk) ; face flushed; sleeplessness; subdued (subjugate, yielding) manner; ...

GERM. Sh, 15 - Wake feeling anxious, increasingly. Legs tremble and shake. I have to get out of bed. I am scared that a heart attack is imminent and cannot be prevented. It's to late to do anything. I walk from room to room, thirsty, chilly and in turmoil. Accompanied by a desire for stool and flatulence. 08, 12C, 80:00:00

Sh, 117 - I am probably incurable and that's my own fault. The thoughts are repeating themselves again and again in my head. 18, 30C, 46:XX:XX

Sh, 174 - Hopeless. There no hope for me. My fate is not to get well. 18, 30C, 36:XX:XX

GRAT. Al, 8 - Fretful, irritated by every contradiction, angry outbreaks, misanthropic, whith solicitude about his own health.

HALI-L. Sh, 528 - Noticed in the paper all cancer related deaths, particularly prostate, mostly men between 40-60. Seemed to be men who were very loved. Seemed most unfair. Fear that if I drank too much coffee I would get a headache, and the thought was cancer related. 18, 30C, 35:XX:XX

HELL. Al, 16 - He is doubtful (uncertain) about his own life.

HEP. Al, 15 - Extremely discontented and fretful about his pains, and discouraged (unhappy).

Al, 10 - Fearful concerning sickness in the family, especially when walking alone in the open air.

Ha, 5 - Fear about the illness of his family, especially while walking in the open air.

HURA. Al, 3 - Every paroxysm of pain excites a nervous laugh, with moanings like those of a sick child.

HYDROG. Sh, 103 - Feel like a crippled old man. 38, 200C, 18:XX:XX

Sh, 192 - During palpitations, extreme fear —thought I was having a heart attack. Frightened the living daylights out of me. 24, 30C, 100:XX:XX

Sh, 264 - Talking to God about the state of my heart and asking for it to be healed. 16, 30C, XX:XX:XX

HYOS. Al, 48 - Laughed and said he was exceedingly well.

He, 64 - Serious illness (ailments) from jealousy and grief about faithless lover;...

IGN. Al, 22 - She fears that she will have an ulcer in the stomach.

Ha, 758 - She fears she will get an ulceration of the stomach.

INDG. Al, 1 - Illusion of sensation; it constantly seems to her as though she had a large goitre, which was very prominent; she was constantly obliged to look down and feel whether it was so.

IRIS. Al, 3 - Despondency; thinks he is going to be very sick, then a disposition to laugh at his fears, which, however, soon return.

He, 2 - Fears approaching illness.

KALI-BR. He, 38 - Much concerned (anxiety) about health; complains without cause;...uncontrollable sensation of fear and anxiety, thinks she is becoming deranged (insanity) ; change of life.

KALI-C. Al, 19 - Fears that she cannot recover.

Al, 17 - Fearful and anxious about her disease.

Ha, 14 - He is afraid that he might not get well.

Ha, 15 - Apprehensive and anxious about her disease.

He, 10 - Timid and apprehensive of future and about her disease.

KALI-FCY. Al, 1 - Feeling of sadness and some disposition to tears, caused by an impression that he was soon to die and leave his friends; disposition to take a sad view of the beauties of autumn; the apprehension of approaching sickness and death can be overcome by reason, but soon returns.

KREOS. Al, 5 - Towards evening her spirits were much depressed, and she was doubtful whether she would ever be well again.

He, 4 - Thinks herself well. 0 Metritis

LAC-C. Al,N-28 - Fear of disease; of consumption; of heart disease. (tuberculosis)

Al,N-33 - Depression of spirits, doubts her ability and success, thinks she will have heart disease and die of it.

He, 7 - Every time a symptom appears she feels very confident that it is not attributable to medicine, but that it is some settled disease.

He, 13 - Woke at daylight feeling that she is a loathsome (repulsive), horrible mass of disease (while the breasts were affected); could not bear to look at any portion of her body (loathing, himself), not even hands, as it intensified feeling of disgust and horror; could not bear to have any part of her body touch another, had to keep even fingers apart; felt that if she could not in some way get out of her body, she should soon become crazy .

He, 16 - Worries (care) herself lest (fear) pimples (boil) which appear during menses will prove to be little snakes, and twine and twist around each other.

He, 26 - Depression of spirits, doubts her ability (competence, aptitude) and success (prospering, progressing, achieving), thinks she will have heart disease and die of it.

LAC-D. Al,N-9 - Great despondency on account of the disease, is sure he is going to die in 24 hours.

He, 9 - Great despondency on account of the disease, is sure he is going to die in twenty-four hours.

LACH. He, 55 - Nightly attacks of anxiety; afraid of chorea, gets cramps in calves from fear; nausea, heavy feeling in abdomen...

He, 60 - After a jealous quarrel, she put both hands to her chest and cried out "Oh! my heart!" then fell down and was in an asphyctic state for nearly twenty-four hours;...

He, 25 - Is morbidly talkative and gives a rambling (discursive) account of her ailments.

LEPI. Al, 6 - Deep melancholy; with thoughts of sickness.

LIL-T. Al, 15 - Apprehensive as from impending disease or calamity (misfortune); fears insanity; fears heart disease; fears she is incurable; often with moderate or sub acute uterine or ovarian inflammation.

Al, 9 - Depression of spirits; constant inclination to weep, with fearfulness, and apprehension of suffering from some terrible internal disease, already seated.

Al, 24-..a feeling of irritation and of something wrong in abdomen and pelvic organs (disease); feels hurried (fast) and yet incapable (incompetent), as if she had a great deal (busy) to do and cannot do it.

Al, 19 - Apprehension of some calamity or serious disease very much increased.

He, 4 - Believes her disease to be incurable; that she has some organic disease that nobody understands. (misunderstanding, misjudged)

He, 14 - Anxiety; fearful that the symptoms indicate an internal organic disease; very marked in both male and female.

LOB-S. He, 2 - Bad effects from grief.(ailments from)

LYC. He, 30 - Loss (want) of confidence; in his own vigor (vitality, strength); in physician and remedies.

He, 40 - Nervous action weakened; threatened softening of brain from overwork, or metastasis of ulcers suddenly healed.

LYSS. Al,N-62 - He cautioned people around him not to inhale his exhaled air, it was spoiled (dirty), stinking (smelling) like rotten (putrefying) eggs, worse than cholera, and could injure. (contaminates, infects)

Al,N-127 - Thinking of fluids of any kind, even of blood, brings on convulsions.

Al,N-129 - Hyperesthesia, current of air, bright light, sight of any shining object,

slightest touch, even conversation in vicinity of patient, may throw him into a most violent agitation and bring on severe convulsions.
Al,N-10 - They appreciate the formidable character of the disease and speak frequently with a remarkable quick and sharp articulation of the impending fatal results.
Al,N-12 - The majority of patients have no adequate conception of real origin of their malady, and affirm in decided terms that the scar is of no significance whatever and causes them no pain.
Al,N-31-...Fancies doctors were two young girls who had come in to see her.
Al,N-42 - Deny, with great obstinacy, that they have ever been bitten.
He, 10 - They appreciate the formidable (terrible) character of the disease and speak frequently with a remarkable (unusual) quick and sharp articulation of the impending fatal results.
He, 62 - He cautioned people around him not to inhale his exhaled air, it was spoiled, stinking like rotten eggs, worse than cholera, and could injure.
MACRO. Al, 5 - More or less fear; apprehensive; thinks she has some incurable disease.
MAG-C. Al, 952 - Dream that he had an epileptic fit.
Al, 953 - Dream that she was sadly disturbed in company, where especially her grandmother was taken with spasms, and at last had apoplexy.
MED. He, 20 - Is sure that she is worse, knows she is not going to live, cannot see any improvement, even when it is pointed out (antagonism); has no fear of death, speaks calmly about it, and gives directions as to the disposition of her affairs.
MERC. Ha, 1224. Indescribable sensation of an internal, intolerable ill, during which he remains silent and will not get up from bed.
Ha, 1263 - Mania; she throws off the clothes at night, tears the straw about, and scolds; by day she leaps (jump) up high like a petulant extravagant person...she talks and scolds much to herself,...spits frequently and spreads the saliva out with her feet, and licks some of it up again; she often licks cowdung (excrements) and the mud of ponds (lake); she often takes little stones in her mouth, without swallowing them, and at the same time complains that they are cutting her bowels; much clotted blood passes with her motion; ...
MOSCH. He, 5 - Hypochondriacal complaints having their origin in sexual system.
MUR-AC. Al, 637 - Dream that she had lice, which made her very much ashamed.(shame)
MURX. Al, 2 - Great depression of spirits; it seemed to her that she was hopelessly ill.
He, 2 - Deep sadness at approach of menses, all her symptoms gave her great concern (care); seemed to her she was hopelessly ill; she gave up everything.
NAT-M. Al, 35 - Sad as if sick (suffering), in the afternoon.
Al, 119 - The patient's mind was much weakened by disease and poison; her moral perceptions, her once keen (sharp) sense of honor, and of right and wrong, seemed blunted (dull); she was in turns vehement (angry) and passionate, and moody and silent.
NAT-P. Al, 6 - Very despondent; imagined he was going to be sick, to have typhoid fever.
Al, 8 - Worries (cares) about the health, about the future.
Al, 10 - Awakens; fears his child, who has a trifling ailment (disease), is dead; he goes to her room to relieve the otherwise ineffaceable (perpetual) impression.
NAT-S. Al, 5 - Very much disheartened; tired (weary) of life; despairs of getting well. (recovery)
NIT-AC. Al, 17 - At once she is taken which peculiar anguish, runs to her physician, but he is not at home, hires a carriage to drive to the house where she expects to find him; during her ride all the anguish is gone; arrived at home she feels as bad as ever, and feels herself thus forced to drive about the whole day, till all the effects of the Nitric acid have passed off.
Ha, 25 - She imagines she will die soon, but has no bodily indisposition.
He, 14 - Often anxious about his illness; constantly thinks about his past troubles; mind weak and wandering.

He, 16 - Anxiety about his disease, with fear of death; morbid fear of cholera.
He, 5 - Fancies she will die soon, yet is not physically ill.
NUX-V. Al, 6 - The usual pain seems intolerable; she would rather take her life.
Ha, 1239 - She deems (believe) the pain she suffers intolerable and will rather take her own life.
He, 39 - Mania puerperalis...constantly complaining, criticizing or explaining, ... as soon she recognized physician she spoke of imperfection of medical knowledge and declared it an error that one could not live without a heart, inasmuch as she felt very well without one, it having come away with the afterbirth to which it had grown fast, the nurse having separated the two before her eyes; complains of her husband, says he wishes to convince her she is sick, ... nymphomania,... frequently sips at a bowl of warm sugar-water, declaring it will form her a new heart; .(health, healing)...(expert)
He, 20 - Desire to talk about one's condition, with anxious reflections about it.
PETR. Ha, 1 - Sad and dispirited, with a sick (suffering) feeling owing (due) to weakness of the heart.
Ha, 14 - Ill-humor; strong tendency to be hypochondriac with a feverish condition for fourteen days.
PH-AC. Al, 17 - He was constantly complaining about his illness.
Al, 10 - Sadness and feeling of solitude, as if she would be sick.
Ha, 3 - Sad and full of solicitude (anxiety), afraid she might fall ill.
Ha, 5 - Continually brooding over his disease.
Ha, 22 - He looks very ill-humored and peevish, so that everyone asks him what is the matter with him; but he was not sick. (appearance)
Ha, 4 - Restless and full of anxiety, that she might get ill.
He, 12 - Anxiety and doubt concerning his recovery...
He, 18 - Dread (fear) of the future; brooding over one's condition.
PHOS. Al, 46 - Imagines he has hydrothorax.
Al, 108 - Anxiously solicitous concerning the unfortunate termination of her illness.
Al, 109 - Discouraged about his health.
Al, 38 - Told those about him repeatedly that he could not possibly recover, and gave some disjointed directions about his business affairs.
Ha, 23 - Anxiously solicitous, about the unfortunate (unlucky) issue (subject) of her disease.
Ha, 43 - Depressed on account of his health.
He, 7 - Anxious: filled with gloomy (dark) forebodings; as if about to die; about termination (conclude) of her illness (disease); and restless ; at twilight; when alone; about future; during a thunderstorm; ..
He, 22-...uneasy about one's health; paroxysms of anguish, when alone or in a stormy weather, with timorous disposition; told those about him repeatedly that he could not possibly recover, and gave some disjointed (incoherent) directions about his business affairs.
PLAT. He, 36 - While suffering from a slight erysipelas faciei, took leave (quit, abandon) of her children, exhorted her husband to join (unite, combine) church, wanted people to join her in prayer (beg), felt happy to join her Redeemer.
PLB. Al, 114-...he imagined his disease incurable, and gave way to the gloomy thoughts which the fear of death excited, and to repinings (sadness) caused by the dread of his journey to Valencia.
PODO. He, 3 - Depression: imagines he is going to die or be very ill;...
PSOR. Al,N-16 - Believe the stitches in heart will kill him if they do not cease.
Al,N-31 - Despairs of recovery; thinks he will die; hopeless,...
Al,N-46 - Attacks of fear; fear of fire, of being alone, of apoplexy, of becoming insane.
Al,N-32 - Melancholy after suppressed itch;...seeks solitude, despairs of recovery; ...
Al,N-34-....thinks he will not recover; has lost all hope;...formication and crawling, with pricking and smarting on scalp, and some on extremities; tongue white.
Al,N-25 - Much depression on account of an eruption on dorsum of hand which appears over night.

Al,N-28 - Great depression of mind during climaxes, with chronic abdominal disorders.

He, 16 - Believes the stitches in heart will kill him if they do not cease.

He, 31 - Despairs recovery; thinks he will die; hopeless; especially after typhus...

He, 34-...;thinks he will not recover; has lost all hope; cannot apply his mind to business;...

He, 32 - Melancholy after suppressed itch;...seeks solitude, despair of recovery;...

PTEL. Al, 43 - Goes about his professional duties in a perfunctory (indifference) manner, very unlike (contradictory) his fiery (passionate) zeal with which he usually combats disease and his allopathic step-brethren (brotherhood).

PULS. Al, 18 - Anxiety as if would have apoplexy, in the evening, after lying down, ...

Al, 22 - Anxious solicitude about his health.

Ha, 1115 - Anxiety, as if threatened with apoplexy, in the evening after lying down, ...

Ha, 1117 - Anxious solicitude about his health.

He, 48-...despaired of her soul's salvation; did not believe she would be restored to health ; ...

PYROG. Al,N-9 - Increased buoyancy (happy) of spirits, although he felt ill.

RAPH. Al, 16 - Her condition troubles her, and for a moment cannot believe it to be owing to the medicine; she forgets it entirely, and believes she has a disease which is not recognized. (unknown, undiscovered)

SABAD. Al, 2 - He imagines all sorts of strange things about his own body, for instance, that it had shrunk (dry, wrinkled) like that of dead persons (corpse), that his stomach was corroded (degeneracy, decomposition), that the scrotum was swollen (enlarged), etc.;...

Al, 3 - Imagines: himself sick; parts shrunken (small wrinkled) ; that she is pregnant (important?), when she is merely swollen from flatus; that she has some horrible throat disease which will end fatally. (incurable)

He, 2 - Erroneous impressions as to the state of his body.

SABIN. Al, 7 - Ill-humor, with sensation as if he had taken cold.

He, 4 - Great tiredness and laziness, with a feeling of deep-seated inward trouble, which makes him melancholy and sad.

SANG. He, 9-..."what will become of my condition, shall I have typhoid fever, inflammation of the brain, or shall I remain paralyzed?".

SARS. He, 6 - Thinking about the food he has been eating makes him sick. (indigestion)

He, 8 - She thinks she cannot bear (support, endure) the headache.

SEC. Al, 19-...There were two sick persons in the bed, one of whom recovered and the other did not.

Al, 47 - Hypochondria; patient says she must have something to relieve her or she must die.

Al, 27 - Strong desire to recover.

Al, 36 - The greatest depression of mind and loss of strength, a very sick feeling.

Al, 46 - Hypochondria; patient says she must have something to relieve her or she must die.

SEP. Al, 1 - So excited from anger that she fears an apoplectic fit; everything becomes black (evil) before the eyes.

Al, 22 - Sadness about her health.

Al, 29 - Dark forebodings about his disease in regard to the future.

Al, 33 - Received news of the slight illness of a friend, which caused great mental depression (at another time it would not have made slightest impression); this condition grew on me until I became so nervous that I felt that unless I held on something, I should scream.

Al, 52 - She is filled with concern about her health; thinks she will have consumption and soon die.

Al, 53 - Concerned about her health, anxious, irritated, and very weak.

Ha, 5 - Sad (despair) about her health.(vitality)

Ha, 6 - Troubled (worries) thoughts about his disease and about the future.(destine)

Ha, 8 - Troubled (worried) about her health (vigor) anxious, irritated and very weak.

Ha, 9 - She has none but troubled thoughts about her health, thinks she is getting the consumption (tuberculosis, degenerate,

decomposition) and will die soon.
Ha, 51-(Ailments) From vexation, she is so excited that she fears an apoplectic fit, and everything turns black before her eyes.
He, 11 - Sad about her health and domestic affairs, discontented with everything.
He, 13 - Dark forebodings about his disease in regard to the future.
SPONG. He, 19 - She is very fretful and anxious about her condition, fears she will die of suffocation.
He, 24 - Terror and fear: of approaching death; that she will die of suffocation; with heart disease;...
He, 26 - Apprehension of a fatal termination of his disease.
STAPH. He, 4 - Sad distressing thoughts about one's illness.
He, 14-...; was insulted (slandered, defamed, calumniated) being too dignified (reserved, lordly,) to fight (contest), subdued (control) his wrath(anger) and went home sick,.. (ailments, from offenses)
STRAM. Al, 126 - The boy repeatedly said there were" big sores" on him.
Ha, 550 - At night he jumps out of the bed and cries out that the disease is breaking out of his head.
He, 102 - Mania with insomnia ; very talkative; thinks he has every imaginable disease; that he has power (powerful) over all disease; masturbates, fills his pockets with anything he can find (lack?), thinks he has snakes in him.
He, 103 - Had many strange fancies, such as imagining his wife had lovers concealed (hidden) behind stove; ...afterward had a fit that looked so much like apoplexy that he was bled.(blood)
STRY. Al, 5 - A peculiar nervous erethism, almost resembling what I had seen in a case of hydrophobia ...wandering when left to himself, and begged most piteously (miserable) that I would not hurt him...fear of being injured...
SULPH. Al, 57 - During the proving I was much concerned (anxiety) about my state of health, and feared lest I might really get ill.
Al, 60 - Fear that he would take cold in the open air; he did not know whether it was illusive or physical.
Al, 28 - Depressed about his illness and out of humor.
Al, 11 - She fancies that she is becoming emaciated.(skeletal)
Ha, 35 - He imagines he is getting thin (weak).
He, 31 - Depressed about her illness, and out of humor.
SYPH. Al,N-7 - Very despondent, does not think he will ever get better.
Al,N-12 - Terrible dread (fear) of night, ...death is preferable ; she fears to prepare for night and is positively in abject fear of suffering,...
He, 8 - Very despondent, does not think will ever get better. (hopeless)
He, 9 - Terrible dread of night, ...it is intolerable, death is preferable. She fears to prepare for night and is positively in abject fear of suffering...
TAB. Al, 42 - Evenness and mildness of temper, notwithstanding he felt very uneasy about his health.
Al, 51 - Exalted action of the brain; copious flow of ideas; ...leaving me in the morning worn-out and sick, I would conceive and elaborate about twenty undertakings, of which probably not one would ever come to light.
TARENT. Al, 14 - Feigned (simulate) paroxysms; a girl simulating fainting and insensibility, looks sideways to watch the effect produced on those around her. (manipulation)
Al, 57 - Fear of getting "typhus fever".
TER. He, 14 - Fears apoplexy; fullness and pressure in head.
THUJ. Al, 57 - Apprehension of becoming sick.
Al, 76 - Dread that she would be attacked with apoplexy, ...
He, 9 - Sensation as if whole body were thin and delicate, (weak, fragile, frail) and could not resist least attack (illness); as if continuity of body would be dissolved.
He, 23 - Mental depression, after childbirth (puerperal), in consequence of being told that there had been a slight rupture (division, hurt) of perineum; grows quiet; thinks she must die;...wants to jumps the window; does not care for children or her relatives (careless) ;..(sensitive to disrupt, partition)

TUB. Al,N-45 - Insanity; acute or chronic, with a family history of tubercular affections.
Al,N-46 - When the best selected remedy fails to relieve or permanently cure in a marked tubercular diathesis, with a tubercular family history.
VERAT. Al, 49 - Anxiety with fear of apoplexy during an evacuation of the bowels.
Al, 12 - He thinks that he is dumb and blind, and has a cancer.
Ha, 673 - He asserts (declare) that he is deaf and blind (obstructed) and that he has got cancer.
He, 54 - Despair of his recovery; attempts suicide.
ZINC. Ha, 47 - Illusion of fancy, when holding down her head, as if she had a large goitre, which prevented her looking beyond it.
He, 29-...;sad, weeps frequently; despairs of her recovery;...

DISINTEGRATION

Delusions; body, abdomen, fallen in, his stomach devoured, his scrotum swollen: **SABAD.**
- body, back, loosened, is: bamb-a.[1184]
- body, brain, balanced on a slight point and is likely to be turned over at any moment: camph.[139]
- body, brain, cracking, is: nux-m.[122]
- body, brain, dissolving: calc.[139]
- body, brain, softening: abrot. ***arg-n.***[8] cann-i.[58]
- body, brain, turns around: bry.[139] sabad.[139]
- body, continuity of, will be dissolved: thuj.[139]
- body, dashed to pieces, being: calc.[36].
- body, diffused, has: lap-c-b.[194]
- body, disintegrating: ***lach.***[36] lap-mar-c.[194]
- body, disintegrating, internally: lap-mar-c.[194]
- body, divided, is: cann-i. choc.[222] lil-t.[36] ***petr.*** sil. ***stram.***[10]
- body, fiber in her right side, feels every: sep.[122]
- body, head, divided, is: psor.[116] ther.[116] xan.[102]
- body, head, lift it off, can: ther.
- body, limbs, separated from body: bapt.[122] stram.[1]
- body, liver comes out with blood of menses: ozone[227]
- body, parts, separated, are: daph.[72]
- body, pieces, in danger of coming in: thuj.[36]
- body, scattered about bed, limbs talking with each other: bapt.[85]
- body, scattered about bed, tossed about to get the pieces together: ***bapt.*** caj.[102] daph.[102] petr. ***phos.*** pyrog.[58] stram.[102]
- body, separated, body and thoughts are: anac. sabad.[5] thuj.
- body, stomach, has corrosion of: acet-ac.[54] ign. sabad.
- body, threads, inside is made of (afternoon on lying): nux-v.[36]
- bones in fragments and cannot fit pieces together: phos.[54]
- die, will, and soon will be dissected: cann-i.
- dissected, he will be: cann-i.
- divided, four parts, into: choc.[222]
- falling, pieces, to: lac-c.[5] xan.[139]
- flesh was off bones and edges were separated and sticking out: lac-d.[85]
- head, disease will break out of h.: stram.
- ideas floating outside of brain: dat-a.[36]
- melting away, he or she is, agg. from change, amel. in recumbent position: sumb.
- rags, body torn into: phyt.[137]
- room, falling to pieces, is: cann-i.[139]
- separated, thoughts are: sabad.[122]
- space, decomposition of space and shape: anh.[119]

Dreams; animals, snakes, splitting in parts that keep moving: ozone[227]
- ➤ blood, mangled remains, and: merc.[36]
- ➤ body, hands cut to pieces, being: sol-t-ae.[36]
- ➤ body, liver comes out with blood of menses: ozone[227]
- ➤ body, pieces, in: dict.[111]
- ➤ body, prepuce sloughed off: linu-c.
- ➤ body, teeth breaking off: kali-n. rauw.[119] sul-ac.[10] ther. thuj.
- ➤ body, teeth falling, filling is falling out: nux-v.[36]
- ➤ body, teeth, falling out: bamb-a.[1184] coca[36] cocc. convo-d.[36] nicc. nux-v. sul-ac.[10] tab.
- ➤ buildings, demolished: hura[36]
- ➤ cars, automobiles, of, wheels detaching from body: choc.[222]

- ➤ cutting, knife, of being cut with a, to pieces: lil-s.[36]
- ➤ excrements, soiling himself with excrements: aloe cast-v. iod. sars.[58] zinc.
- ➤ listeners explode like balloons: ozone[227]
- ➤ nightmare, left side from neck to knee were jerking up and down like a mass of jelly, as if, this motion extending into chest and centering at heart: gels.[36]
- ➤ nuclear, explosion, about: ozone[227]
- ➤ storms, destroying palaces: jac-c.[36]
- ➤ window, smashing the window: bry.[10]

Fear; apoplexy, night with feeling as if head would burst, at: ***aster.***

- ✦ biting, of, lest teeth would fall out: nit-ac.[172]
- ✦ brain, of softening of: abrot. ***arg-n.***[8] asaf. calc-sil.[58]
- ✦ cough, of, burst, something will burst: apis[162]
- ✦ death, soul were escaping from body, as if, with utmost terrible uneasiness: thuj.[172]
- ✦ falling, high walls and building upon him: ***arg-n.***[54] arn. choc.[222]
- ✦ osteoporosis: calc.[185]

Forgetfulness; connection of consecutive thoughts, of, after apoplexy: ***op.***[54]

Thoughts; intrude and crowd around each other, closing eyes, on, a mass of subjects, some scientific, cross each other: spong.[54]

Thoughts; one thought excludes all other: androc.[222]

Thoughts; persistent, separated, will, thoughts separated from: anh.[119]

ABROT. He, 3 - Thinks her brain is softening. (dissolving)

ADAM. 54 - Holding together, connecting, bonding. Interconnection in body, had body bonding points. Feel full, connected again.[16], 12C, 03:07:45

Sh, 60 - After waking, pattern on walls became fluid in movement, in air. The wall lost solidity, could easily move through it. 16, 12C, 26:XX:XX

Sh, 61 - Material objects appear to lack substance. I see molecules.[16], 12C, 34:XX:XX

Sh, 62 - Wondered, if I dematerialized would I be able to regain the same form? 16, 12C, 26:XX:XX

Sh, 110 - Intense feeling of wanting to break through. Felt it around the solar plexus. Just felt like I wanted to burst out. 6, 30C, 10:XX:XX

Sh, 111 - Sense of waiting for things to explode, more in others than in me. 7, 6C, 59:00:XX

Sh, 113 - Waking, my hands were together, but I did not know which one was holding which; which fingers were next to each other. I did not know where everything was. I lay for several seconds wondering where my hands were, or what they were doing. Could hardly get together. 5, 30C, 00:12:50

Sh, 165 - I feel like I'm looking at the world through half-closed eyes, like slits. 7, 6C, 09:00:XX

Sh, 519 - mages of nuclear mushroom clouds. 16, 12C, 00:04:25

Sh, 521 - After waking, pattern on walls became fluid in movement, in air. The wall lost solidity; could easily move through it. 16, 12C, 26:XX:XX

Sh, 522 - Wondered if I dematerialized, would I be able to regain the same form? 16, 12C, 26:XX:XX

ALUM. Al, 41 - Incapacity for connected thought.

He, 4 - Inability to recollect things or follow up a train of thought.

ANDROC. Sh, 76 - Mind blank when concentrating. Unable to think of more than one thing at a time. The current thought excludes all others, I often forget what I am doing and am easily side tracked. (25)

BAPT. He, 7 - Feels scattered about, and tosses about to get the pieces together. (dispersed, separated, reparation.)

CALC. Al, 21 - Anxious at night as she would become insane, followed by shuddering chilliness for a few minutes, and a sensation as if the body were dashed (hit) to pieces.

CANN-I. Al, 23 - He seemed to have the one idea that he should die and soon be dissected.

CERE-B. Al, 5 - Desire to be dissolved, (evaporate, disintegrate) especially the trunk.

CHOC. Sh, 179 - Apprehensive about the shift in consciousness and nervous someone would notice. It is reminiscent of L.S.D., the 'shifting edges', before the full blown trip arrives — an uneasiness and unsureness about which way things will go. A desire to hide in case things go to pieces. 15, 30C, 00:00:50

Sh, 209 - A desire to hide in case things go to pieces. 15, 30C, 00:00:50

COT. Al, 14 - After taking the medicine, she feels lost; cannot collect herself; forgets what she is doing and saying; difficulty in expressing herself.

Al, 1-...a feeling as if there was no foot. The head felt exceeding light, as if there were no solid head, and she could not articulate for some time, although she endeavored to do so....

GELS. Al, 22-...I could not pursue one train of thought for any time, the ideas would vanish (disappear) and leave a vacancy (empty) of mind...(lost, ideas, thoughts)

He, 10 - Unconnected (disconnection, separation) ideas, cannot follow any idea for any length of time; if he attempts to think consecutively (step by step), he is attacked by a painful, vacant feeling of the mind.

He, 42 - When attempting (effort) to move, the muscles refuse to obey the will; giddy, confused, lack of muscular co-ordination.

GERM. Sh, 179 - Sensation of being very slightly aware of having a brain. A kind of fuzzy sensation around the periphery of where I imagined my brain to be in my head i.e. just below the surface. 02, 6C, 01:XX:XX

Sh, 177 - Twice while driving I had an illusion -part of a stationery car on the right moved through my field of vision. 02, 6C, 01:XX:XX

Sh, 7 - Recurrent rows triggered by my detachment. Felt despair and utter confusion about what was related to the proving and what was reality. 04, 6C, 14.00.00.

Sh, 99 - Came in contact with very much hate and disgust within, and it made a deep impression on me. I have to be reconciled with those parts of me. I think that power can be used in a different way - not so destructive. I am no person. Feel I have no power when I meet people. Sometimes I feel I disappear. I am not in my body. My hands feel gone. My feet are cold; I don't like them. Yet I feel I have great power inside, especially I feel it when I get angry or when I sing. 18, 30C, 46:XX:XX

Sh, 178 - Generally a sense of unreality. A kind of fuzzy sensation around the periphery of where I imagined my brain to be in my head i.e. just below the surface. 02, 6C, 01:XX:XX

HALI-L. Sh, 432 - I am deeply in touch with a self—destructive sense inside. The part of me that wants to disintegrate and die. Dis-integrate; the opposite of integral oneness, the opposite direction. I'll have another egg to ground me. 06, 6C, 10:XX:XX

Sh, 601 - Back feels split as if two planes are pulled apart, like after an earthquake; the planes are off with a sharp delineation between the two. 09, 6C, 03:XX:XX

Sh, 602 - Have had experience of split personas before, but during the proving all the bits and pieces that seemingly had unique personalities of their own were simply more broken up. I call it a movement. It happened only when I was alone. 18, 30C, 35:XX:XX

Sh, 603 - The remedy brought up episodes from the past. After each episode I'd create and act out. I'd step to the side and say, "This is not you. You can't do this. You know you can't do this." And as it went on, I pulled things together and got integrated. 18, 30C, 35:XX:XX

Sh, 605 - The remedy accelerated the personas out of me, and along with them, all these other problems. It forced me to look at all of it. Then my "I" came out! Has happened before but this was much more magnified. With the remedy, none of the fragmented personalities were willing to get behind the wheel and drive. It was like being driven, without going anywhere. Then, I slowly started seeing that these personas were just rationalizations that just didn't suffice. It helped me to come out to face them. With the remedy, I quickly pulled them together. 18, 30C, 35:XX:XX

Sh, 604 - Since the remedy, I took over and the physical manifestation of personas splitting off would only come out when I was alone. Did these drawings. The figure in the box was my death — captured, buried and can't get out. The first drawing is a depressed boy, the second is the buried man, the third is an x-ray figure. After that the depression abated. I did another drawing of a negative being laughing at me. It has no arms, no movement. 18, 30C, 35:XX:XX

Sh, 632 - In the body a lot of splits. Lower lumbar, felt a definite line. Same split with my vision, a break. We were having a lot of earthquakes, the huge earthquake in Kobe the day the proving started. I am very connected to Japan, having lived there. Felt a shift, along a fault line, along the spine. Split was at the waist lower back. Vision was split on horizon. 09, 9C, XX:XX:XX

Sh, 634 - Like being in the edge of an abyss, a crevice that's cracking deeper all the time. A crack that gets deeper and longer. 06, 6C, 00:12:30

Sh, 640 - A lot of agitation and irritability on the surface. Underneath there was a crevice, a crack... in my soul or the universe. Dread or anticipation of what else could happen if this process went on. If the process went on, it could lead to complete insanity, completely being out of touch with reality. 06, 6C, 01:00:XX

Sh, 642 - I read prayers for safety before bed because I was afraid of what might happen when I went to sleep. When I came to the phrase "God is One" I realized that was the crux of it— the universe was cracked or split instead of one. Saying that prayer feels healing. Oneness is about caring; the split is about not caring. It's evil in a way. 06, 6C, 01:00:XX

Sh, 645 - Caring equals oneness. A scary point about that acute phase yesterday— there was no caring. It didn't matter. Nothing mattered. I was alone and wanted to be that way. To have caring, there must be an attunement with the oneness of the universe. Is that where Hitler came from? The crack in the universe? 06, 6C, 01:09:00

Sh, 670 - When I was alone in my apartment with the lights on, I manifested many fragmented personalities, probably around five or six. Never did before like this. What was different was nobody was in the room to make a chain reaction. I was alone. Needed no provocation to make a change, or experience a change. I talk outloud, and talk to the person in a number of different ways. Fearful Joe, Vindictive Joe, One That's Just Like Someone Else Joe —each will act out in a number of different ways. 18, 30C, 35:XX:XX

Sh, 676 - The remedy worked very directly on my will. Fragmentation is the denial of will. Integration is the use of will. All separate states under a unified country. 18, 30C, 35:XX:XX

HYDROG. Sh, 11 - I felt I had gone mad, possessed, hysterical laughter, singing and a feeling of non-reality, as if in a dream, out of the body — like my mind went out of the window. High one minute and then low. People asked if I was on speed. After seven hours, in the evening (7:30p.m.), the feeling changed to an angry mood and very irritable with a dry furry mouth,...l. 24, 30C, 00:00:45

Sh, 12 - Driving home I felt odd, as if I was hardly in my body. Feel like my body's working on automatic but I'm not really there. Driving along I kept forgetting where I was. Now I feel I'm really more "absent" than normal and feel quite afraid of losing my mind or having an accident. I feel my connection with the physical world is very loose, as though my soul was separated from my body. I have thoughts that this is a bit like dying —not unpleasant. 10, 200C, 13:02:XX

Sh, 23 - Feel as if I've been somewhere else and coming back into my body is a shock. 16, 30C, 10:XX:XX

Sh, 25 - A hovering numbness hit with a sensation that my mind was being pulled from the top of the head downwards, like internal pressure being pulled down inside of me —as after a fright. Incredible sensation. 24, 30C, 00:XX:45

Sh, 27 - There is a very fine line at this time between enlightenment and insanity — a split consciousness. The dark side is horrendous, but the positive side of the proving has been well worth it. The positive aspects are beautiful. Its a shame we need to come down. I guess the price of going into the heavens is a trip to hell. 16, 30C, XX:XX:XX

Sh, 63-"Oh God, what shall I do? Where do

things go from here? What way shall I go? Feel I'm cracking up". Emotional confusion. Try to find a path to be happy, but unsure of what I'm doing. 24, 30C, 100:XX:XX

IRID. Sh, 195 - Panicked about servicing car before a long journey. Felt anxiety that car might break down as it hadn't been running smoothly. However found that car didn't need a service for another two thousand miles. Over-conscientious about getting jobs done on car. A3

MAG-C. Ha, 16 - Lack of tone (character, personality) in spirit, mind and body.

NAT-C. Al, 18 - Anxiety and hasty (fast) restlessness all day; he could not keep the limbs still, especially the arms; obliged to stretch them; it seemed as though they would be torn (cut) asunder. (in two divided).

NEON. Sh, 31 - On closing eyes to relieve a bad headache, sensation that top of head and headache seemed to rise as I and the rest of my body sank, like a horizontal separation. Felt sick and exhausted 7:30 PM. 06, 12C, 18:XX:XX

Sh, 46 - Had the strong thought, "my connection with the past is dissolving" at 2.15 pm. 05, 12C, 05:05:35

Sh, 47 - Lay in bed and body felt insubstantial starting with hands and forearms -as if I was dematerializing "beaming down." 05, 12C, 00:14:20

Sh, 48 - A phrase from a Lewis Carroll poem repeated itself over and over in my mind: "Come tell me aged man he cried, come tell me how you live. And his answer trickled through my brain like water through a sieve." I felt this was about dissolving, which related to my feeling in the proving. 05, 12C, 05:05:XX

Sh, 55 - Looking out of the window at the night sky, it suddenly cracked open and a great darkness revealed itself. Infinity was blackness. It was deeply disturbing. 02, 6C, 67:XX:XX

Sh, 91 - I'm finding it hard to judge how long ago recent events were. Can't seem to judge time in the past. Can't think back through the days. It's as if I've lost the thread with the past that connects all past days together. It has dissolved. I seem to be more in the moment and less hurried. I usually look at my watch often, but today I forgot I had put it on, and kept asking a friend the time. Was surprised when I discovered I'd been wearing it all day. Very unusual. 05, 12C, 05:XX:XX

NUX-V. He, 4 - Cannot read or calculate, for she loses the connection of ideas; thinks she will lose her reason.

He, 30 - Ailments after continued mental exertion; indisposition to it, particularly to that form which involves elaboration and connection of subjective ideas independently of external objects.

PH-AC. Ha, 34 - He cannot get his ideas into their proper connection.

PHOS. Al, 86-...; a feeling of dread (fear), as if awaiting something terrible, yet unable to resist or move (terrifying, scaring), overcame me; sometimes it seemed as if I was beginning to bloat (inhalant, inflate, vanity?), and then I could hear a multitude of voices saying in high glee, "Fill him up a little more and he will burst," (blow up) followed by demoniacal laughter, which made the cold chills run over me... I imagined myself an aurora borealis, and could distinctly hear voices shouting, "Beautiful! Oh, was not that splendid?"...

He, 28-...;erotic with indications of great excitement of sexual system; ... fancied he was in several pieces and could not get the fragments properly adjusted.(disconnection, fragmentation, split, disconnected, divided)

PYROG. Al,N-5 - Sensation as if she covered the whole bed; knew her head was on pillow, but did not know where the rest of her body was.

SPONG. He, 11 - Crazy feeling, head feels blown up.

STRAM. Ha, 550 - At night he jumps out of the bed and cries out that the disease is breaking out of his head.

Ha, 360 - Sensation in the arms and legs as if the limbs were completely severed (separated, detached, cut of) from the body.

Ha, 361 - Sensation as if every portion of the limbs were completely severed in the joints from the other parts and could not be joined together again.

Ha, 363 - He feels his hands and feet as if

separated in the joints, and he is inconsolable on account of this sensation.
He, 57 - Strange absurd ideas; thinks herself tall, double or lying crosswise; one half of body cut off (divided); bed is full of creases (wrinkle) (disorganization); that he was killed roasted and being eaten.

THUJ. Al, 64 - Frightful anxiety, like death agony; a nameless internal ache, as if the soul were escaping from the body (split), with most terrible uneasiness, frightful orgasm of blood, at night, even to suffocation.
He, 9 - Sensation as if whole body were thin and delicate, (weak, fragile, frail) and could not resist least attack (illness); as if continuity of body would be dissolved.
He, 10 - Fixed ideas: as if a strange person were at his side; as if soul and body were separated (split) ; that body, particularly limbs, are made of glass (frail) and will readily break (weakness); as if a living animal were in abdomen ;talks about being under the influence of a superior power. (possessed)
He, 23 - Mental depression, after childbirth (puerperal), in consequence of being told that there had been a slight rupture (division, hurt) of perineum; grows quiet; thinks she must die;...wants to jumps the window; does not care for children or her relatives (careless) ;..(sensitive to disrupt, partition)

VIOL-O. Al, 10 - He seems able to recognize only half an idea; he puts it in the proper place but cannot hold to it; he makes great effort to grasp (understand) the other half, but at the same moment half of another incomplete idea presses upon him, and so on; thoughts chase one another, but he always has only half a thought ...
He, 7 - Disconnected (separated) thoughts thronged (crowd) one upon the other, he was able to grasp none of them;...

DISPERSION

Hurry; occupation, desires to do several things at once, finish any, but cannot: pin-s.[36] plan.[36]

Inconstancy: acon.[1] acon-l.[36] act-sp. agar. alum.[10] am-c.[10] ***ambr.***[30] anh.[144] apis[58] arn.[30] ars. asaf. bell.[1] bism. bor.[58] cand-a.[239] cann-s.[1] canth. cimic. coff. dros. ***graph.***[10] **IGN. KALI-BR.**[54] lac-c. lach. led. lil-t.[5] lyc.[30] m-arct.[85] m-aust.[10] nat-c. ***nux-m.***[54] olnd.[1] op. opun-a.[36] petr.[30] plan. plat.[30] sil. sphing. stann.[30] stram.[36] syph.[122] thuj. v-a-b.[85] valer.[58] verat.[30] voes.[36] zinc.

Obstinate; purpose, but difficulty in way of carrying out its: ***phys.***[54]

Persists in nothing: alum.[111] asaf.[137] aur.[1] bar-c.[10] calc.[189] grat.[54] lac-c. lach. lyc.[36] nux-v.[155] plan. ***sil.***[111] stann.[1] sulph.[111]

Undertakes; many things, perseveres in nothing: ***acon.*** alum.[30] androc.[222] ant-c.[102] apis[83] bism.[1] bor.[1] canth.[85] cortico.[119] graph.[30] grat.[137] ign.[58] ***lac-c. lach.*** **LIL-T.**[36] lyc.[36] med.[179] ***nux-m.***[54] petr.[30] phos.[189] pin-s.[36] plan. sanic.[108] stann.[30] sulph.[81] verat.[1]

Writing; different alphabets against his will, wrote in, changing from one subject to another: ***nux-m.***[54]

ACON. Al, 21 - Unsteadiness (inconstant) of ideas; on attempting to think of one thing, another forces it out of the mind and this is supplanted by another, and so on, until he becomes quite confused.

ACT-SP. He, 17 - Irresolution, inconstancy and caprice.

ALUM. He, 4 - Inability to recollect things or follow up a train of thought.

ANDROC. Sh, 50 - Did the shopping in a very disorganised way, started one thing, forgot it, then started something else. (25)

ARG-N. He, 8 - To fix thoughts in anything, or to give his business any consideration, was impossible for him; on attempting it, it immediately got dark before his eyes and headache increased.

ASAF. He, 4 - Unsteady (inconstant) and fickle (changeable), cannot persevere in anything; wants now one thing, then another; walks hither and thither.

BISM. Al, 5 - He commences one thing and then another, but keeps to one thing only a short time.
He, 10 - Unstable-minded; begin now this, again that, holds but short time to any one thing.

BOR. Ha, 21 - He fritters away the afternoon, without getting to any real work, goes from one work to another, from one room to another, without remaining in one thing.

BRY. Ha, 777 - Cross; imagined she could not finish her work (obstruction) ; she always took hold (continued) of the wrong thing and constantly wished to take something else ; then a pressing aching headache in the forehead.

Al, 25 - Fretful; she imagines that she cannot accomplish (realize) her work; constantly takes up the wrong piece, and always inclined to change and take another; ...

Ha, 780 - Too busy; she wishes to undertake and to work at too many things.

CALC. Al, 22 - Anxious, restless, and busy mood; she is undertaking much things but accomplish nothing...

CANTH. He, 14 - Constantly attempting (try) to do something, but accomplishing nothing.

CERE-B. Al, 16 - Difficult to keep employed.

CYCL. Ha, 188 - He is always in a reverie (meditation, air castles), and not inclined to speak. (talk, aversion)

GRAT. He, 1 - Irresolute (wavering); want of perseverance. (determination)

HALI-L. Sh, 316 - I start something and get bored with it. I need three things going on at the same time and rotate from one to the other. Can't stick to anything. 08, 30C, 34:XX:XX

IGN. Ha, 755 - Excessively busy: he restlessly sets about doing first one thing then another.

Ha, 770 - Fickle, impatient, irresolute, quarrelsome.

KALI-C. Ha, 51 - Lack of presence of mind; he cannot proceed right along in his business.

LACH. Al, 45 - No sooner does one idea occur to him then a number of others follow in succession while he is writing down, so that he is unable to finish the record.

Al, 41 - Need of being very busy, without the slightest perseverance.

He, 30 - Undertakes many things, perseveres in nothing.

LYC. Al, 113 - Excited, busy mood in the evening, without perseverance, changing from one subject to another, with difficulty of fixing the thoughts, and greater difficulty in accomplishing anything; while reading fell asleep...

Ha, 78 - He cannot do nor think anything; he spends his time in trifling, and is not able to resolve to do what he has to do.

MEZ. Al, 14 - Indifferent to everything; he could scarcely compel himself to note the symptoms beyond brief annotations (as a sea-sickness)

NAT-C. Al, 56 - He has no desire to do anything, and can keep at nothing long.

NIT-AC. He, 14 - Often anxious about his illness; constantly thinks about his past troubles; mind weak and wandering.

NUX-M. Al, 48 - He never accomplishes what she undertakes, but remains standing in one place, absent minded; he appears quite changed to his companions.

He, 6 - Never accomplishes what he undertakes, but remains standing in one place, absent-minded...

PH-AC. Ha, 40 - While reading, a thousand other thoughts crowd into his mind (dispersion) ; he could not comprehend anything, what he read was dark to him, and he forgot everything at once, with difficulty in recollecting what he had known a long time already. (lost: memory, concentration, comprehension, knowledge)

PULS. Al, 5 - He wishes now for this, now for that employment, but when given to him he will have nothing to do with it.

Ha, 1123 - Sometimes he wants to do one thing, sometimes another, and when he is given something to do, he will not do it.

STANN. Al, 20 - Fruitlessly busy, as if a rush of ideas prevented him from completing his work at a certain time; all sorts of things occur to him to be done.

Ha, 639 - Busy uselessness (inefficiency): he exerts (use) himself to get a necessary task (duty) done at the appointed hour, and cannot accomplish it, as though prevented (interrupted) by an over-crowding of thoughts, during which one thing and another occur to him which he wishes to do...

Ha, 7 - Dawdling (indolent) and irritated, with heat in the face; she wanted to do a number of things, but accomplished (complete) nothing.

Ha, 10 - He is ineffectually (inefficiently)

busied, as if he was prevented (obstructed) by super abundance of ideas from finishing his work at a certain time; he thinks of a number of things which he ought yet to attend to.

Ha, 8 - Restless and distracted, no perseverance in her work (at once).

SULPH. Ha, 26 - Anxiety with heat in the head and cold feet, so that he does not know what to do; he forgets every moment what he desired to do.

TAB. Al, 51 - Exalted action of the brain; copious flow of ideas; ...leaving me in the morning worn-out and sick, I would conceive and elaborate about twenty undertakings, of which probably not one would ever come to light.

VERAT. Ha, 713 - Busy restlessness; he undertakes many things, but becomes always tired of them, nothing succeeds with him.

DISTANCES

Delusions; distances, of: ***cann-i.*** cann-s. nux-m.
- enlarged, distances are: acon.[102] agar.[102] ***arg-n.***[102] atro.[102] bov.[102] camph. **CANN-I.** cann-s. cob-n.[144] ***gels.***[102] glon. hydrog.[222] ***hyos.***[102] nux-m. op.[102] par.[102] stann.
- hearing, of, sounds, distant, are: coca[25] lac-c.[137] sabal.[137]
- hearing, of, sounds, remained longer: ptel.[122]
- hearing, talk seems distant: aran.[149]
- living, locality three hours distant from his house, in a: ***op.***[54]
- road is long: ozone[227]
- runs, long way, he can run a: coca[139]
- runs, never before, she can run like: agar.[139]
- space, carried into, that he is, orbit, and compelled to describe a vast: cann-i.[36]
- space, expansion of.: cann-i. nux-m.[122]
- space, few rods are an immense distance: **CANN-I.**[54]
- space, he is in: germ.[222]

Distance; desire to see great distances: choc.[222]

Distance; exaggerated, is: anac.[58] ***cann-i.*** cann-s.[122] glon. nux-m.[122] ox-ac.[116] stram.[54] sulph.[116] ther.[116]

Distance; exaggerated, is, runs against things which appear to him distant: stram.[54]

Distance; exaggerated, is, time during sleepiness, and: nux-v.[10]

Distance; inaccurate judge of: agar.[5] anac.[5] ***arg-n.***[5] atro.[25] ***cann-i.*** cann-s.[5] carb-an.[85] coca[25] dat-m.[85] glon.[5] hyos.[1] lac-h.[229] magn-gr.[139] ***nux-m.***[122] onos.[137] op.[5] ozone[227] stann.[5] ***stram.***

Distance; inaccurate judge of, walking, while, cannot judge distance to ground: ozone[227]

Dreams; distant, things: fl-ac.[36]
- ➤ distant, things, strange, on closing eyes: plat.[1]
- ➤ journey, distant regions, in: ther.[54]
- ➤ jumping, leaps, great: apis[36] hydrog.[222]
- ➤ unsuccessful efforts to, reach a distant place: croc. plat.

Size; incorrect judge of: agar. calc.[137] cann-i.[137] cann-s.[137] chin-s.[36] onos.[137] plat.[137] stram.

Talk; village, of a far distant, in dream: merc.[36]

CHOC. Sh, 14 - Angry about being in city. When I look, I want to see far distances and sky, not houses. Went to estate agents to look at country houses.

Sh, 313 - Desire to see far —to a distant horizon. Desire to be outside more.[01]A, 30C, 00:XX:XX

HALI-L. Sh, 637 - If I had known this was going to happen, I wonder if I would have taken the remedy. I thought I must be crazy (after taking remedy last night). I would like to fling that vial of remedy to the ends of the universe. 06, 6C, 00:12:30

HYDROG. Sh, 20 - Distortion of reality — that other places seemed a million times more real than the real world. Everything seemed a long way away. 16, 30C, 04:XX:XX

IRID. Sh, 15 - Don't feel like reading paper or working on the train. Very unusual; just want to look out of window at the snow. E2

Sh, 85 - Have noticed a difference in my spatial awareness. Am misjudging distances when driving not to a dangerous degree. Keep bumping into things and people in the house and street. B ?

NEON. Sh, 20 - I had thoughts of albatrosses circumnavigating the earth without having to touch the ground. 20, 6C, 03:02:14

DIVIDED

Conflict between higher consciousness and worldly existence: hydrog.[222]

Confusion of mind; identity, head separated from body, as if: allox.[119] cocc.[58] ***daph.***[122] **PSOR.**[122] ther.[58]

Delusions; body, alive, only half alive: crot-h.[36]

- body, brain, far from skull, as if too: staph.
- body, divided, is: cann-i. choc.[222] lil-t.[36] ***petr.*** sil. ***stram.***[10]
- body, feet, belong to her, do not: carc.[227]
- body, feet, separated from body, are: stram.[1]
- body, fiber in her right side, feels every: sep.[122]
- body, hand, belong to her, do not: carc.[227]
- body, hand, separated from body: daph.[171] germ.[222] stram.[1]
- body, head, belongs to another: alum.[5] cann-i.[122] cann-s.[5] nat-m.[111] ther. thuj.[5]
- body, head, divided, is: psor.[116] ther.[116] xan.[102]
- body, head, lift it off, can: ther.
- body, head, separated from body, is: allox.[119] alum.[122] anac.[162] ant-t.[122] cann-i.[139] daph.[36] nat-c.[122] psor.[8]
- body, legs, belong to her, don't: ***agar.***[122] ***bapt.***[122] coll.[137] hydrobr-ac.[102] op.[122] sumb.[122]
- body, legs, separated on standing: phos.[137]
- body, limbs, separated from body: bapt.[122] stram.[1]
- body, parts, separated, are: daph.[72]
- body, parts, take away: ***bapt.***[122] daph.[122]
- body, scattered about bed, tossed about to get the pieces together: ***bapt.*** caj.[102] daph.[102] petr. ***phos.*** pyrog.[58] stram.[102]
- body, separated, body and thoughts are: anac. sabad.[5] thuj.
- body, smaller, left side of body is: cinnam.
- companions are half men, half plants: cann-i.
- cut, two, in, could not tell of which part he had possession on waking: thuj.
- divided, four parts, into: choc.[222]
- divided, two parts, into: anac.[162] ***bapt.*** bell.[30] cann-i. lil-t.[36] ozone[227] petr. plat. puls. sil. stram. thuj.
- flesh was off bones and edges were separated and sticking out: lac-d.[85]
- flying, out of his skin: thuj.[5]
- head, rising up, tearing neck: bamb-a.[1184]
- headless: asar. calc-i. cocc.[8] cot.[139] nit-ac. nux-v.[10]
- hearing, of, ear, not his own, with: psor.[137]
- mind, going out of his, he is: ambr.[85] calc.[31] cot.[36] eup-per.[8] ham.[8] ***kali-br.***[8] ***lac-c.***[56] nit-ac.[85] ol-j.[139] paraf.[38] petr.[85] visc.[77]
- outside his body: anh.[119] sabad.[5]
- sees anything, as if another person had seen it, or as if he could transfer himself into another and only then could see: alum.
- separated, mind and body are: anac. cann-i.[58] hyos.[102] lap-c-b.[194] nit-ac.[102] ozone[227] sabad.[5] thuj.
- side, alive on one side and buried on the other, he is: stram.
- side, left and right side are not the same: bamb-a.[1184]
- side, own her left, she did not: sil.
- soul, body is too small for, or that it is separated from: anac. cann-i. hydrog.[222] nit-ac.[102] sabad.[5] thuj.
- space, empty space between brain and skull, that there is: caust.
- talking, to another part of body, one part is: bapt. 58

Detached; ego, from: lac-h.[229]

Detached; headache and nausea, with: androc.[222]

Dreams; wedding, repeated, has to be, since only one half of the body has been married: bamb-a.[1184]

Fear; death, soul were escaping from body, as if, with utmost terrible uneasiness: thuj.[172]

Mirror, all thoughts appear in a moment as if seen in an inner: carbn-h.[102]

Thoughts; mirror, all thoughts appear in a moment as if seen in an inner: carbn-h.[102]

Thoughts; persistent, separated, mind and body are: anac. sabad.[5] thuj.

Thoughts; persistent, separated, will, thoughts separated from: anh.[119]

ALUM. Ha, 55 - A numb (insensibility) feeling in the head as if his consciousness was outside of his body; when he says anything, he feels as if another person had said it; and when he sees anything, as if another person had seen it, or as if he could transfer himself into another, and only then could see. (transmigration)

ANAC. He, 2 - Feeling as if spirit was separated from the body.

He, 28 - Fixed ideas: that mind and body are separated ; about redemption (salvation) of soul and about the devil; that a stranger is constantly by his side (pursued); that strange forms accompany him, one to his right and one to his left.

He, 68 - Feels as though he had two wills (intentions), one commanding to do what the other forbids.

ANDROC. Sh, 20 - Felt detached from her stomach cramps. (6)

Sh, 129 - It seemed as though he was a different person, very similar to the way he had been in adolescence, but in a much more powerful manner. These emotions were so intense he wanted to rip his chest apart to let them out. He lost all control over his emotions, which seemed to come from a deep and distant part of himself, a darker side. He desired to continue the proving for the rest of his life. (29)

Sh, 179 - Extreme anguish and restlessness, but at the same time felt like an observer of my condition, watching it all transpire without being able to change anything. Mind fixed on the physical anguish. It dominates my senses. (21)

BAPT. He, 7 - Feels scattered about, and tosses about to get the pieces together. (dispersed, separated, reparation.)

CALC. Al, 21 - Anxious at night as she would become insane, followed by shuddering chilliness for a few minutes, and a sensation as if the body were dashed (hit) to pieces.

CAMPH. Al, 46-...I feel a tendency to self contemplation; outer things vanish, and I behold myself in spirit freed from matter.

CHOC. Sh, 228 - Thoughts about the 'veneer of civilisation' that inhibits how we really feel and keeps us from displaying what we're like beneath the surface. It seems a legitimate layer, but so is the layer beneath it, and I feel amused and happy to meet it. This feeling continued for a few days, a very graphic picture of a veneer - a layer of learned social behaviour lifting and detaching from a basis that is thick, dark, solid, instinctual animal.[15] , 30C, 00:00:30

Sh, 306 - Her usual sensation of left right body split has been much more defined. Later on during the proving this "split" became more balanced than usual and felt much more integrated, (curative).[13], 12C, 02:XX:XX

GERM. Sh, 130 - While standing felt my spirit step backwards. The kitchen seems smaller and lower down. 04, 6C, 00.[10].[00].

HALI-L. Sh, 632 - In the body a lot of splits. Lower lumbar, felt a definite line. Same split with my vision, a break. We were having a lot of earthquakes, the huge earthquake in Kobe the day the proving started. I am very connected to Japan, having lived there. Felt a shift, along a fault line, along the spine. Split was at the waist lower back. Vision was split on horizon. 09, 9C, XX:XX:XX

Sh, 733 - Upper body feels strong, chest and shoulders. Lower back feels weak and tired. 20, 30C, 01:02:00

HYDROG. Sh, 23 - Feel as if I've been somewhere else and coming back into my body is a shock. 16, 30C, 10:XX:XX

Sh, 25 - A hovering numbness hit with a sensation that my mind was being pulled from the top of the head downwards, like internal pressure being pulled down inside of me —as after a fright. Incredible sensation. 24, 30C, 00:XX:45

Sh, 27 - There is a very fine line at this time between enlightenment and insanity — a split consciousness. The dark side is horrendous, but the positive side of the proving has been well worth it. The positive aspects are beautiful. Its a shame we need to come down. I guess the price of going into the heavens is a trip to hell. 16, 30C, XX:XX:XX

Sh, 259 - Fear and desperation about being pregnant —period 16 days late —felt terrible all day. So despairing. 08, 30C, 50:XX:XX

Sh, 261 - Almost the impression that I am pregnant —many old sensations and emotions from previous pregnancies recurred. Like having another person inside of me. All physical symptoms of pregnancy. Went for a test. 08, 30C, 01:XX:XX

NAT-C. Al, 18 - Anxiety and hasty (fast) restlessness all day; he could not keep the limbs still, especially the arms; obliged to stretch them; it seemed as though they would be torn (cut) asunder. (in two divided).

NEON. Sh, 30 - I had a fleeting image of being split down the middle (left and right sides split). 06, 12C, 01:22:XX

PETR. Ha, 27 - The whole day, he is only half conscious, as if only half alive.

PHOS. He, 28-...;erotic with indications of great excitement of sexual system; ... fancied he was in several pieces and could not get the fragments properly adjusted.(disconnection, fragmentation, split, disconnected, divided)

PYROG. Al,N-5 - Sensation as if she covered the whole bed; knew her head was on pillow, but did not know where the rest of her body was.

STRAM. He, 57 - Strange absurd ideas; thinks herself tall, double or lying cross-wise; one half of body cut off (divided); bed is full of creases (wrinkle) (disorganization); that he was killed roasted and being eaten.

TAB. Al, 2 - He went to sleep in the cabin, which was full of large packages of tobacco, ...His inability to move was not accompanied by any pain or uneasiness but he felt as if the principle of life had entirely departed from his frame.(body)

THUJ. Al, 5 - She has a decided sensation that her soul is separated from her body (split), and in such a condition hears and feels everything as from distance.

Al, 64 - Frightful anxiety, like death agony; a nameless internal ache, as if the soul were escaping from the body (split), with most terrible uneasiness, frightful orgasm of blood, at night, even to suffocation.

He, 10 - Fixed ideas: as if a strange person were at his side; as if soul and body were separated (split) ; that body, particularly limbs, are made of glass (frail) and will readily break (weakness); as if a living animal were in abdomen ;talks about being under the influence of a superior power. (possessed)

He, 23 - Mental depression, after childbirth (puerperal), in consequence of being told that there had been a slight rupture (division, hurt) of perineum; grows quiet; thinks she must die;...wants to jumps the window; does not care for children or her relatives (careless) ;..(sensitive to disrupt, partition)

DOOMED

Anxiety; conscience, unpardonable sin, feels she has done the, and will be eternally lost: ***chel.***[54].

Anxiety; salvation, hell, of: ***plat.***[54]

Begging, pray for him, to, and not to leave him alone: lyss.[54]

Death; conviction of: alum-p.[58] ars-h.[54] bapt.[122] bell.[54] ***canth.***[54] ***coff.***[54] ***cupr-acet.***[54] hydr.[137] kali-ar.[58] ***phyt.***[54] ***psor.***[54] ***thuj.***[54]

Death; presentment of, soon, believes that she will die, and cannot be helped: ***agn.***

Delusions; criminal, executed, to be: **OP.**[54]

- die, time has come to: ars. bell. lach. med.[85] sabad. thuj.
- doomed, being: acon.[102] ars.[58] aur.[58] bell.[30] cycl.[102] hell.[58] hyos.[58] ***ign.***[54] ***kali-br.***[54] ***kali-p.***[54] ***lach.***[102] ***lil-t.***[54] lyc.[102] med.[54] meli.[102] nat-m.[30] op.[102] plat.[54] psor.[102] puls.[102] stram.[102] sulph.[10] ***verat.***[102]
- doomed, expiated her sins and those of her family, to: ***lil-t.***[54].
- doomed, soul cannot be saved, cries and rages: ***ign.***[54].
- happy is his own house, he will never be: ars.
- hell, chains, in erotomania: ***orig.***[54]
- hell, gate of, obliged to confess his sins at: agar.
- hell, going to, because he has committed a unpardonable crime: chel.[172] med.[54]
- hell, is in: camph. cann-i. germ.[222] hydrog.[222] lyss.[54] merc. ***orig.***[54]
- hell, suffers the torments of, without being able to explain: lyss.[54] ***merc.***[122]
- helped, cannot be: nat-p.[168]
- lost, salvation for: ars.[58] ***aur.*** hell.[58] hura plb.
- lost, salvation, despised, and, in erotomania: ***orig.***[54].
- lost, salvation, predestination, from: ***lach.***[30]
- lost, salvation, world, to the, beyond hope: ***arg-n.***[54]
- obstacles, in his way, caused partly by contrary fate, partly by himself: aur.[36]
- sinned away his day of grace, unpardonable: ars.[58] aur.[58] kali-p.[58] med.[54] plb.[58] podo.[58] psor.[58] puls.[58] stram.[85] sulph.[58]

• troubles, great troubles have come over him: cycl.[139]
• vengeance, thinks he is singled out for Divine: **KALI-BR.**

Despair; destiny, everything is controlled by: bamb-a.[1184]
Despair; religious, constant prayer: ***puls.***[54]
Despair; religious, suicidal tendency, with: verat.[54]
Despair; salvation of soul, of eternal, after fright: stram.[54]
Dreams; fire, house on, neighbors, which could not be saved: mag-s.[36]
➤ remorse, God was punishing her for her sins, that: aether[36]
➤ remorse, pleading for mercy at bar of judgment: aether[36]
➤ remorse, repudiated by God, of being: hyper.[36]
Fear; damned, of being: arg-n.[172] ***lach.***[54] med.[172] psor.[172] verat.[58]
✦ death, night, bed, in, drops into heavy sleep with loud breathing, before sentence is completed: vario.[54]
Moaning; fate, about the: ***kali-br.***[54]
Reconciled to fate: cham.[36]
Religious affections; penance, desires to do, wishes to live, in order to mitigate her eternal punishment, in sadness: ***plat.***[54]
Religious affections; sadness, doubt about salvation, with: ***lyc.***[54]
Sadness; fate, bemoaning: ***kali-br.***[54]
Tranquillity; reconciled to fate: aloe[36] cham.[36]

AGN. He, 4 - Despairing sadness; keeps repeating that she will die, that there is no use doing anything.

AM-C. Al, 22 - At night, attack of great anxiety, as if she had to die, ... she was unable to move her eyes or to speak,...

ANAC. Al, 15 - The future appears dangerous to him, as if nothing but misfortune and danger were reserved for him; want of confidence in his strength (vigor, force) and despondency.

APIS. Al, 16 - He says, after a few minutes, "I am a dead man".

ARG-N. He, 16 - Possessed of distressing idea that all his undertakings will and must fail.

ARN. He, 11 - Mind clear like that of a clairvoyant; quiet countenance (expression), pale as chalk, thinks her death unavoidable.(inevitable)

ARS. Al, 51 - He despairs and weeps and imagines no one can help him, that he must die;...(unprotected)

Ha, 1032 - Mania; first headache, horrible anxiety, noise before the ears, as from a number of large bells, and when he opened the eyes, he always saw a man who had (formerly) hung himself (suicidal, justified) on the ground-floor of the house, who incessantly beckoned (call) him to cut him down (help); he ran thither (there) with a knife, but, as he could not cut him down, (rescue) he became overwhelmed (beaten) with despair (remorse?) and wished (as his friends assured him) to hang himself (punish); but being prevented (stop) from doing so, he became so restless that he could hardly be kept in bed,... and he knelt down and raised his hands in a supplicating manner.

Ha, 1035 - He is cold, shivers and weeps, and thinks, in his despair, (hopelessness, despairing) that nothing can help him, (helplessness) and he must die; followed by general exhaustion.

He, 25 - Mania...sees a man who has hanged himself beckoning (call) him to cut him loose (rescue, deliverance, free, saving) on failing to accomplish this he attempts to hang himself (punish, penalize);...finally kneels down and lifts his hands in supplication.(forgiveness, absolution)

He, 58 - Melancholy; after financial losses; cannot be consoled; thinks he will have to die (sentenced), with his family, from starvation (hunger); sleepless nights; walks about wringing his hands, with moaning and groaning.

AUR. Ha, 344 - Discontented with all circumstances; he imagines that he finds everywhere some obstacle (impediment, restriction) in the way; at one time he thinks that this is owing to an unlucky (unfortunate) fate (destiny), at another that he himself is to blame (censured) for it ; when the latter was the case he was particularly mortified and dejected.

Ha, 347 - Always very restless and undecided (doubtful) -thought he was neglecting something for which he must incur (obtain) reproach -...he seemed to carry about this restlessness with him in his inmost (deepest) parts ; this condition deprived him of all perseverance, all energy.

Ha, 352 - Amid (in the middle) howling and crying she imagines herself to be irretrievably lost.

Ha, 353 - He imagines he has forfeited (penalty, lost,) the affections of others, and this grieves him to tears.

Ha, 4 - Discontented with all conditions; he thinks that he everywhere finds an impediment, caused now by an opposing fate,(destiny) then again by himself, which latter mortifies him and renders him dejected.(sad)

Ha, 21 - Crying and wailing (lamenting); she thinks that she is irretrievably lost.

BAR-C. Ha, 4 - She suspected, that when walking in the street, men found fault (defect) with her, and judged her amiss (wrong), which made her anxious, so that she dared not look up, she looked at nobody, and perspired all over.

BELL. Al, 172 - She tries to strangle herself, and begs the bystanders to kill her, because she believes that she will certainly die.

Ha, 1437 - She tries to strangle herself, and begs those about her to kill her, for this time she must die. (redemption, regeneration, salvation)

CALC. Al, 25 - Frightened apprehensive mood, as if some misfortune were about to happen to him, or some one else, which he could in no way overcome.

Ha, 23 - Fearful, anxious forebodings, as if evil would befall (happen) him or some one else, and as if he could in no way evade it.

Ha, 30 - She despairs of her life and believes she has to die (punishment?) ; her heart is sad with weeping, and frequent attacks of sudden, general heat, as if she had hot water poured (flow) over her.

He, 18 - Mental aberration with horrid visions before eyes and cardiac anxiety; he despairs of his salvation (pardon, rescue) and wants to stab himself.

CAMPH. Al, 46-... There was no other feeling in my soul than that of my hopeless endless damnation (condemnation). I sank back upon the bed, believing that I was the spirit of evil in a world forsaken of God.

Al, 46-.... As I lay stretched on my couch, as the evil demon, and suffered all the anguish of a condemned and God-forsaken soul, ...I was forever deprived of the Divine protection, and of every consolation and every hope. Nothing remained to me but the conviction of my everlasting damnation...

Al, 27 - The child creeps (crawl) into a corner, howls and cries; everything that is said to him is taken as if one were ordering him, and he were considered naughty (disobedient) and should be punished.

Al, 46-...A fearful terror seized me, and I knew not whither to fly. I cried out aloud, "And so I am indeed dead; that hell I used to think about is no fiction, but a reality which I am doomed to experience forever...

CANN-I. Al, 35 - Despair, and fear of being eternally lost.

CHAM. Al, 6 - Earnest (serious) and taciturn mood; reconciled to his fate (destiny), about which he is deeply affected (later action).

Ha, 491 - Serious reservedness; calm submission to his profoundly felt fate (destiny).

CHEL. He, 17 - Restlessness and uneasiness of conscience; feels that she has committed the unpardonable sin (crime, transgression), and that she will be eternally lost.

COB. Al, 5 - Condemned, mean feeling, as though guilty of some deed (action) of which others knew; as if he could not look one in the face. (shame, dishonored)

CUPR. Al, 5 - Melancholy; she shuns the sight of people (observed), seeks and loves to be alone, and becomes anxious about her death, which she supposes imminent and inevitable.

Ha, 1 - Melancholy; she shuns the sight of men, seeks and loves (desire) solitude, and troubles herself about her imminent death (impending), which she supposes to be unavoidable.

FL-AC. He, 13 - Felt certain (inevitable) that something dreadful would happen,...

GERM. Sh, 180 - Woke up early 3.30 am. had strong feeling, like a visualization. I picture myself lying on floor in fetal position and being shot in the head like a horse or a dog. Almost welcomed it. Then thought my children still need me. A very strong feeling of failure accompanied this. I felt I did not deserve to live. Better crying next day when talking to husband. This feeling of depression carried on for several nights. As soon as I wake up in the early morning, my mind is active and a feeling of inadequacy comes on strongly. 05 , 6C, 28:XX:XX

Sh, 108 - Hopeless, helpless, gloom and doom. Weeping and self pity. 14, 30C, 23:00:00.

Sh, 174 - Hopeless. There no hope for me. My fate is not to get well. 18, 30C, 36:XX:XX

HELL. He, 12 - An old woman having been accused of theft by the women around, took it so much to heart that she hanged herself. This suicide produced a profound effect upon the women of the village. One after another accused herself of having caused the death of the old woman by their insinuations; they wept and howled, ran about day and night wringing their hands and despairing of salvation on account of their sin (error); they became quite irrepressible and deranged (disordered) In this way twenty - four or twenty five women were affected, every fresh case being followed by another. Hysterical mania.

HEP. Ha, 4 - Fearful anguish, in the evening, for two hours; he thought he had to perish (die), and was sad even so that he could have committed suicide. (redemption, salvation)

HYDROG. Sh, 275 - Sexually totally closed when my girlfriend kissed me. I felt as if it was a sin. 24, 30C, 00:08:XX

IGN. He, 10 - Spasms and insanity after fright; imagines her soul cannot be saved (rescued), and cries very much; ...(lost, sentenced)

KALI-BR. Al, 4 - He imagined that he had been specially singled out (select) for divine vengeance... deploring his sad fate (destiny),...he informed me that he had been accused of robbing a friend, and that the officers were in search of him....

He, 10 - Imagines he is singled out as an object of divine wrath (fury, rage); extreme drowsiness.

He, 17 - Delirium with delusions; thinks he is pursued (hunt); will be poisoned; is selected (designated) for divine vengeance (revenge); that her child is dead, etc.

He, 24 - Hands constantly busy; all sorts of fearful delusions; walks the room groaning, bemoaning his fate (destine, doom); full of fear; unsteady.(inconstant)

KALI-C. Ha, 8 - Very ill-humored; she has to weep much, because it was constantly on her mind that she had to die. (doomed, sentenced)

KALI-P. He, 4 - Says she is eternally and irretrievably damned;...food and medicine must be forcibly administered. 0 Melancholia religious.

LAC-D. He, 9 - Great despondency on account of the disease, is sure he is going to die in twenty-four hours.

LACH. He, 17 - Religious monomania, fear of being damned (condemned to eternal punishment).

He, 12 - Delirium; fears she will be damned.

LIL-T. He, 16 - Doubts her salvation; thinks she is doomed to expiate her sins and those of her family; ... (redemption, salvation) (sacrifice)

LYSS. Al,N-50 - Declares amid violent sobs that she is suffering the torments of hell.

MED. He, 35 - Feeling as if he had committed the unpardonable sin and was going to hell.

MERC. Ha, 1225 - Imagines he is enduring the tortures (torment) of hell, without being able to account for it (explain). -(lost understanding, judgment)

MUR-AC. Ha, 1 - Sad taciturn and discontented with his fate. (destiny, doom)

NAT-M. He, 34 - A pregnant woman saw a man who had a disfiguring nasal cancer; this haunted (obsessed) her, and she was sure her child would be marked; she was melancholic, avoided society, wept continually.

PHOS. Al, 108 - Anxiously solicitous concerning the unfortunate termination of her illness.

PLAT. Ha, 9 - Sensation as if she would have to die soon (immediately), with horror at the thought.

He, 46-...;suffers unspeakable pangs (anxiety) of conscience in consequence of a faux (fault, mistake, embarrassing mistake?) pass when thirty-two years old; says she has brought disgrace upon her family, and that she has incurred the penalty of damnation; (doomed) in order to do penance (penitence) gave away whatever she could lay her hands upon, (redemption) so that she had to be constantly watched; after her confessor asserted that she could not hope for pardon or heaven (condemnable), she seemed in absolute despair ; bemoaned her misery throughout the night, wringing her hands and beseeching (implore) that she might be delivered (free) from the hell of her conscience; twice attempted self-destruction (suicide);...wished to live and do penance (penitence, purgation, purification) in order to mitigate her eternal punishment.

PLB. He, 15-...; despair of her salvation...; fixed idea that could only obtain peace and safety though absolution by a priest of the papal church, although she had been a zealous Protestant; ....brooded over any forbidden thing; would steal (leave) from house in servant's cloak (coat, camouflage) and bonnet (hat) to obtain stimulants (drugs), but from the moment their prohibition was withdrawn (retired) ceased to have any desire for them; after being permitted to visit a priest and converse with him ceased to talk and think of the church. (desire; redemption, absolution)

He, 16 - Mental disturbance of eight or ten years' duration in a man addicted to masturbation; has several times attempted suicide; has been in seclusion (solitude); greatest dejection and despair;...; believes himself lost (condemned) ; has the sounds of hell constantly in his ears; hears voices and sees shadows of demons, great disposition to make away (suicide) with himself or do himself some bodily injury;

PULS. Al, 19 - Tremulous anxiety, as if death were imminent.(destined)

Ha, 1113 - Anxiety, thinks he will be ruined.(decay, perdition)

He, 48-...despaired of her soul's salvation; did not believe she would be restored to health ; ...

STANN. Ha, 659 - Calm, collected disposition: he was reconciled to his fate (destiny) and was perfectly contented with his lot. (destiny, doom)

THUJ. Al, 1 - She herself desires, with anxiety and despair, to be taken to an insane asylum, (imprisonment, confining) and there to be treated very harshly and strictly, (penalized), so that her fixed ideas may be subdued and banished (purified); she knows very well that she does wrong (conscience) and thinks all sorts of bad thoughts (immoral), but she will not take the trouble to banish such thoughts; therewith she indistinctly gives to understand that she is constantly obliged to think of taking her own life, but feels the sinfulness (wicked) of it, in order to avoid it, desires the strict restraint of the asylum;...

Al, 2 - She fancies that she has intentionally represented herself as insane (feigning) in the presence of others in order to palliate a wrong supposed to have been done (penitence, remorse), and that now she is punished, therefore, by real insanity.

Al, 3 - She feels and says that she is deranged (insane, disordered) and unfit (unsuitable) to life, as a punishment for a fault (penitence) which she cannot name, ...

He, 29 - Feels as if she cannot exist any longer; quiet, shunning everybody.

VERAT. Al, 45 - Anxiety as if he dread a misfortune, as if some evil were impending.

He, 48 - A crippled girl...; chides (censure) her father for taking part in revolution; thinks she hears drum (timpani) which proclaims his execution; this is followed by silent brooding and occasional starts;...

DOUBLE

Conflict between higher consciousness and worldly existence: hydrog.[222]

Confusion of mind; identity, duality, sense of: ***alum.***[5] **ANAC.**[5] anh.[149] arg-n.[137] **BAPT.**[5] calc-p.[137] cann-i.[36] cann-s.[5] cycl.[5] des-ac.[149] **GELS.**[5] lach.[5] lil-t.[5] lyc.[5] mosch.[5] naja[117] nat-m.[5] ***nux-m.***[5] op.[5] paro-i.[149] petr.[5] ***phos.***[5] plb.[5] psor.[5] puls.[5] pyrog.[111] sec.[5] sil.[5] ***stram.***[5] ther.[5] thuj.[5] tril.[137] xan.[137]

Confusion of mind; identity, head separated from body, as if: allox.[119] cocc.[58] ***daph.***[122] **PSOR.**[122] ther.[58]

Delusions; baby, two in bed: petr.
- body, able to go out of b. and walk around, looking down upon: agar.[162] anh.[144] cann-i.[162] pyrus[36]
- body, arms, belong to her, do not: agar. bapt.[122] carc.[140] ign.[137] op.[137]
- body, arms, four, she has: sulfon.[30]
- body, arms, many, has: pyrog.[137]
- body, arms, separated, from body: bapt.[137] daph.[137] psor.[137]
- body, arms, three, that she has: petr.
- body, divided, is: cann-i. choc.[222] lil-t.[36] ***petr.*** sil. ***stram.***[10]
- body, feet, belong to her, do not: carc.[227]
- body, feet, separated from body, are: stram.[1]
- body, halves, left half does not belong to her: sil.
- body, hand, belong to her, do not: carc.[227]
- body, hand, separated from body: daph.[171] germ.[222] stram.[1]
- body, head, belongs to another: alum.[5] cann-i.[122] cann-s.[5] nat-m.[111] ther. thuj.[5]
- body, head, divided, is: psor.[116] ther.[116] xan.[102]
- body, head, double: sulfon.[30]
- body, head, separated from body, is: allox.[119] alum.[122] anac.[162] ant-t.[122] cann-i.[139] daph.[36] nat-c.[122] psor.[8]
- body, head, two, he has: mosch.[48] nux-m. sulfon.[30]
- body, legs, belong to her, don't: ***agar.***[122] ***bapt.***[122] coll.[137] hydrobr-ac.[102] op.[122] sumb.[122]
- body, legs, four, has: sulfon.[30]
- body, legs, talking, one is talking with the other: bapt.
- body, legs, three, has: petr. stram.
- body, legs, toe, first, is in controversy with first finger, thumb: bapt.[58]
- body, limbs, double, one is: petr.
- body, limbs, four or eight, has: ***sulfon.***[162]
- body, mouth, double, is: choc.[222]
- body, nose, double, is: merl.
- body, scattered about bed, limbs talking with each other: bapt.[85]
- body, separated, body and thoughts are: anac. sabad.[5] thuj.
- body, threefold, has a: ars. petr.
- companions are half men, half plants: cann-i.
- consciousness belongs to another: alum.
- cut, two, in, could not tell of which part he had possession on waking: thuj.
- divided, two parts, into: anac.[162] ***bapt.*** bell.[30] cann-i. lil-t.[36] ozone[227] petr. plat. puls. sil. stram. thuj.
- double, he is: alum. ***anac.*** anh.[119] ***bapt.*** calc-p.[137] cann-i. cann-s.[5] corn-f.[102] cycl.[5] ***gels.***[5] glon. lach. lil-t. lyc.[5] mosch. nat-m.[5] ***nux-m.*** op.[5] ***petr.*** phos.[1] plb.[5] psil.[164] psor.[5] puls.[5] pyrog.[5] rhus-t.[47] sec. sil.[1] ***stram.*** ther.[5] thuj. valer.[102]
- double, he is, another self, there is, and he is not sure which will conquer the other: op.[139]
- double, lying on one side, she is one, and lying on the other side she is another person: pyrog.[139]
- double, objects are: ***anh.***[144] zinc.[116]
- double, of being: alum. ***anac.*** anh.[119] ***bapt.*** calc-p.[137] cann-i. cann-s.[5] corn-f.[102] cycl.[5] ***gels.***[5] glon. lach. lil-t. lyc.[5] mosch. nat-m.[5] ***nux-m.*** op.[5] ***petr.*** phos.[1] plb.[5] psil.[164] psor.[5] puls.[5] pyrog.[5] rhus-t.[47] sec. sil.[1] ***stram.*** ther.[5] thuj. valer.[102]
- double, sensations present themselves in a double form: cann-i.
- dreams have been stolen or belong to another: choc.[222]
- existence, two existences, to have: cann-i.[58]
- flying, out of his skin: thuj.[5]
- hearing, of, ear, not his own, with: psor.[137]
- hearing, of, sounds, double, whistling, are: med.[8]
- hearing, tone, split, is: anh.[119]
- mind, going out of his, he is: ambr.[85] calc.[31] cot.[36] eup-per.[8] ham.[8] ***kali-br.***[8] ***lac-c.***[56] nit-ac.[85] ol-j.[139] paraf.[38] petr.[85] visc.[77]
- outside his body: anh.[119] sabad.[5]
- person, existed in another person, she: pyrog.[139]
- person, three persons that he is: anac.[116] bapt.[122] cann-i.[36] nux-m. ***petr.***[116] psil.[164]

- person; two personalities opposing to each other in himself, who are discussing their disease, there are: paro-i.[149]
- places, being in different, at a time: anac.[5] brom.[5] cann-i. ***cench. lyc.*** plb. raph. ***sil.***
- places, two at the same time, of being in: anac.[5] brom.[5] cann-i. ***cench. lyc.*** plb. raph. ***sil***
- pregnant, is, birth to a blue eyed baby, that she is about to give: ***verat.***[54]
- pregnant, is, distension of flatus, if there is: ign.[85] ozone[227] **SABAD.**[54]
- pregnant, is, menses, after: ***ign.***[54]
- says something, it seems to him as though somebody else has said it, when he: alum.
- sees anything, as if another person had seen it, or as if he could transfer himself into another and only then could see: alum.
- separated, mind and body are: anac. cann-i.[58] hyos.[102] lap-c-b.[194] nit-ac.[102] ozone[227] sabad.[5] thuj.
- sick, two sick people were in bed, one of whom got well and the other did not: sec.
- side, left and right side are not the same: bamb-a.[1184]
- side, own her left, she did not: sil.
- standing by oneself: anh.[119]
- talking, someone else is, when he speaks: alum.[36] cann-s.[58]
- talking, to another part of body, one part is: bapt. 58
- voices, hears, abdomen, are in his: thuj.
- voices, hears, abusive and filthy language, voices from within him speaking in: ***zinc.***[54]
- walk, he sees the same one walking after him that he sees walking before him: euph.
- wills, possessed of two: anac.[1] lach.[102]

Dreams; another person lying in bed with him: petr.

- ➤ lying, bed, in, with another person: petr.[58]
- ➤ wedding, repeated, has to be, since only one half of the body has been married: bamb-a.[1184]
- ➤ wedding, women, with two: nat-c.[10]

Mirror, all thoughts appear in a moment as if seen in an inner: carbn-h.[102]

Thoughts; abdomen, as if from: thuj.[5]

Thoughts; mirror, all thoughts appear in a moment as if seen in an inner: carbn-h.[102]

Thoughts; persistent, separated, mind and body are: anac. sabad.[5] thuj.

Thoughts; stomach, as if from: acon.[5]

Thoughts; two trains of thoughts: acon. **ANAC.** anh.[144] ant-t.[54] aur. bar-c.[137] cann-i.[137] cann-s.[137] caps. irid.[5] ***kali-c.*** lac-c. ***lach.*** lyss. naja op.[5] paro-i.[149] ***sep.***[30] ***sil.***[30] verb.[54]

ADAM. Sh, 63 - Thought of female twins producing male twins. 16, 12C, 00:00:20

Sh, 64 - In Tai Chi asked to get into a pair, but formed a foursome which felt comfortable. We laughed. We all wanted to be together. I couldn't pair, needed to be four —very unusual. 16, 12C, 07:14:00

Sh, 66 - Delusion that I can see four sides, as if four faces. 16, 12C, 38:03:14

Sh, 67 - Delusion of galaxies spiraling. One, then two, then four. 16, 12C, 39:XX:XX

Sh, 68 - Delusion; I have two pairs of hands. 16, 12C, 45:XX:XX

Sh, 71 - Extremely irritable and it seems as if I have a lot of work to do —the work of two.[16], 12C, 35:XX:XX

Sh, 73 - Feels like doing two things at once all the time.[16], 12C, 67:XX:XX

ALUM. Ha, 55 - A numb (insensibility) feeling in the head as if his consciousness was outside of his body; when he says anything, he feels as if another person had said it; and when he sees anything, as if another person had seen it, or as if he could transfer himself into another, and only then could see. (transmigration)

ANAC. He, 2 - Feeling as if spirit was separated from the body.

He, 27 - Thinks he is double.

He, 28 - Fixed ideas: that mind and body are separated ; about redemption (salvation) of soul and about the devil; that a stranger is constantly by his side (pursued); that strange forms accompany him, one to his right and one to his left.

He, 68 - Feels as though he had two wills (intentions), one commanding to do what the other forbids.

ARS. He, 16 - Tormenting hallucination, as if there was one by his side who did that he was doing, eating, washing etc.

BAPT. He, 6 - Sensation as if there was a second self outside of patient. 0Typhus.

He, 8 - He thinks his legs are holding a

conversation with each other. 0Gout.
He, 9 - He thinks his gouty toe is holding a confab (conversation, talk) with his gouty thumb.
CANN-I. Al, 40 - Had a feeling of duality. One of his minds would be thinking of something, while the other would laugh at it...
Al, 41 - Felt as if he was a third person looking at himself and his friend.
Al, 42 - The soul seemed to be separated from the body, and to look down upon it, and view all the motions of the vital processes, and to be able to pass and repass though the solid walls of the room, and to view the landscape (view) beyond.
He, 18 - A sense of having two existences; double consciousness.
CHOC. Sh, 116-12:30pm -I feel less and less animal at the moment and I desire company. When it comes, its so intense, I almost lose what I am. I've never been there before. I feel very privileged, as if I can be on both sides at the same time.
Sh, 307 - Talking to a friend, noticed her mouth felt strange, almost as if she had two mouths, one on top of the other. No other part appeared double.27, 100C, 00:22:15
Sh, 309 - A feeling of intoxication with double sensations. Colours are stronger and hearing is sharpened but at the same time feel absent and removed.29, 200C, 00:XX:XX
EUPH. He, 4 - Imagines he sees the same man walking after him that he sees walking before him.
GERM. Sh, 130 - While standing felt my spirit step backwards. The kitchen seems smaller and lower down. 04, 6C, 00.10.00.
GUAI. Ha, 131 - Whilst he lay asleep on his back, he dreamt that some one was lying on him; from anxiety he could not fetch his breath nor cry out; ...
HALI-L. Sh, 140 - Went to co-counseling feeling happy and suddenly started crying. I was focused while I was crying. A part of me was above myself crying, watching me crying. 08, 30C, 21:XX:XX
Sh, 216 - Had an extreme emotional shift about my Dad and what he did to me in the past. Cried and cried and cried. Went into a deep place of far past stuff that I've rarely talked about. Surprised, because I didn't think I had anything to say. Went to co-counseling feeling happy and suddenly started crying. I was focused while I was crying. I had to tell everything and not stop until I was done, even though it went overtime. A part of me was above myself crying, watching me crying. 08, 30C, 21:XX:XX
Sh, 670 - When I was alone in my apartment with the lights on, I manifested many fragmented personalities, probably around five or six. Never did before like this. What was different was nobody was in the room to make a chain reaction. I was alone. Needed no provocation to make a change, or experience a change. I talk outloud, and talk to the person in a number of different ways. Fearful Joe, Vindictive Joe, One That's Just Like Someone Else Joe —each will act out in a number of different ways. 18, 30C, 35:XX:XX
Sh, 679 - Sun rose over house, felt there should be two suns. Desire for symmetry in the sky. 20, 30C, 00:00:20
Sh, 683 - I am parallel to myself, with myself; dual, but not divided. 20, 30C, 00:00:50
HYDROG. Sh, 11 - I felt I had gone mad, possessed, hysterical laughter, singing and a feeling of non-reality, as if in a dream, out of the body —like my mind went out of the window. High one minute and then low. People asked if I was on speed. After seven hours, in the evening (7:30p.m.), the feeling changed to an angry mood and very irritable with a dry furry mouth,...l. 24, 30C, 00:00:45
Sh, 12 - Driving home I felt odd, as if I was hardly in my body. Feel like my body's working on automatic but I'm not really there. Driving along I kept forgetting where I was. Now I feel I'm really more "absent" than normal and feel quite afraid of losing my mind or having an accident. I feel my connection with the physical world is very loose, as though my soul was separated from my body. I have thoughts that this is a bit like dying —not unpleasant. 10, 200C, 13:02:XX
Sh, 259 - Fear and desperation about being pregnant —period 16 days late —felt

terrible all day. So despairing. 08, 30C, 50:XX:XX
Sh, 261 - Almost the impression that I am pregnant —many old sensations and emotions from previous pregnancies recurred. Like having another person inside of me. All physical symptoms of pregnancy. Went for a test. 08, 30C, 01:XX:XX

LAC-C. He, 10 - Imagine he wears some one's nose.

LIL-T. Al, 2 - Excitement, weeping, feeling as if she were two persons, at night.
Al, 32 - Perceptive and reflexive faculties seem benumbed (confused), whereas at first she was overactive and seemed to be two individuals.

LYC. Al, 4 - A kind of living (presence) outside of herself, as in the commencement of fever.
He, 9 - Absent minded; supposes to be in two places at a time.

LYSS. Al, 34 - There seems to be two distinct trains of thought operating at one and the same time.
Al,N-15 - It seems to her as if two entirely different trains of thought influenced her at the same time.
Al,N-64 - Disinclination to change position of head; two distinct trains of thought existing at one time in her mind, the idea that she was unable to move her head (when lying down) with the positive conviction that she has only to make up her mind that she will do it to achieve it.
He, 15 - It seems to her as if two entirely different trains of thought influenced her at the same time.
He, 64 - Disinclination to change position of head; two distinct trains of thought existing at one time in her mind, the idea that she is unable to move her head (when lying down) with the positive conviction that she has only to make up her mind that she will do it to achieve it.

MAG-M. He, 6 - While reading, felt as if some one was reading after her and she must read faster and faster. (imitated)

NEON. Sh, 13 - Thoughts of twos and water. Saw images of Noah's ark. 20, 6C, 08:01:30
Sh, 30 - I had a fleeting image of being split down the middle (left and right sides split). 06, 12C, 01:22:XX

OP. Al, 37 - Conscious of being possessed (seized) of two persons (double) of another self besides his real self, the Opium man does things which the real self considers wrong, and it is not always sure which will conquer the other.

PETR. Ha, 27 - The whole day, he is only half conscious, as if only half alive.
He, 5 - Since confinement two weeks ago when in bed, in dark room, at night, delusion that there is another baby (small, tiny) in bed which requires attention also that she has a third leg which would not remain quiet.
He, 4 - Delirium; thinks another person lies alongside (close) of him, or that one limb is double.

PYROG. Al,N-6 - Feels when lying on one side that she is one person, and another person when turning on the other side.
Al,N-7 - Sensation as though crowded with arms and legs.

SEC. Al, 19-...There were two sick persons in the bed, one of whom recovered and the other did not.

SIL. Al, 58 - Distraction of mind; he is almost always trying to think of two things at the same time.
Ha, 34 - Distracted, he is almost always, as to his mind, in two places at time.

STRAM. Al, 122 - For some days the patient was affected with hallucinations and thought that one side of him was alive, while the other side was buried.
Ha, 499 - In this slumber he hears two persons talking but knows not who they are.
He, 57 - Strange absurd ideas; thinks herself tall, double or lying crosswise; one half of body cut off (divided); bed is full of creases (wrinkle) (disorganization); that he was killed roasted and being eaten.

THUJ. Al, 5 - She has a decided sensation that her soul is separated from her body (split), and in such a condition hears and feels everything as from distance.
Al, 6 - She often fancies that someone is sitting near her, with whom she talks aloud while she is lying quite wide awake with open eyes, and wonders when she is asked with whom she is talking, then she does not know what to think of it. (double)
Al, 64 - Frightful anxiety, like death agony;

a nameless internal ache, as if the soul were escaping from the body (split), with most terrible uneasiness, frightful orgasm of blood, at night, even to suffocation.
He, 10 - Fixed ideas: as if a strange person were at his side; as if soul and body were separated (split) ; that body, particularly limbs, are made of glass (frail) and will readily break (weakness); as if a living animal were in abdomen ;talks about being under the influence of a superior power. (possessed)

DOUBTFUL

Anxiety; success, from doubt about: aloe[36] *lac-c.*[54]
Delusions; existence, doubt if anything had: agn.
Discouraged; irresolution, with: puls.[10]
Doubtful: act-sp.[111] alum.[137] anh.[119] ars.[60] aur.[60] bar-c.[60] *calc.*[137] **CARB-V.**[30] chin.[60] cic.[5] germ.[222] *graph.*[30] *lach.*[30] lap-gr-m.[194] mur-ac.[60] nux-v.[60] *petr.*[30] psil.[164] sep.[30] sil.[60] staph.[30] sul-i.[137] thuj.[60]
Doubtful; recovery, climacteric period, during: sars.[54]
Doubtful; recovery, of: *acon.* agn. alum.[1] arn.[116] *ars.*[10] ars-h.[54] aur.[122] bry. calc. calc-sil.[58] cecr.[149] *ign.*[122] kali-c. kreos.[10] lac-c.[116] lach. *lept.*[116] lil-t.[116] *lyc.*[116] mag-c.[193] *merc.*[30] nat-s.[10] nit-ac.[116] nux-v. ph-ac. phos. psor. puls. sep. *stann.*[116] sulph. syph.[122]
Doubtful; soul's welfare, of: **ARS. AUR.** bell. calc. chel. croc. cycl.[5] dig. hyos. **LACH.** *lil-t.* lyc. nux-v. **PULS.** sel. stram. *sulph.*[5] *verat.*
Excitement; alternating with indecision: cortiso.[149]
Irresolution, indecision: act-sp. *agar. alum.* alum-p.[58] alum-sil.[58] alumn. am-c. *anac.* androc.[222] ang. anh.[119] apis *aran-ix.*[144] *arg-n.* arn. *ars.* ars-i. asaf. aur. aur-ar.[58] aur-i.[58] aur-s.[58] bar-acet.[36] **BAR-C.**[122] bar-i.[58] *bar-m.* bism. bry. bufo[30] bufo-s. buth-aust.[119] cact. *calc.* calc-ar.[58] calc-f. calc-i.[58] calc-p. calc-s. *calc-sil.*[122] camph. cand-a.[239] cann-i. cann-s. canth. *carbn-s.* carc.[207] caust. cench.[58] cham. chel. chin. chin-s. *chlol.* cimic.[149] cina clem. coca *cocc.* coch.[8] coff. coll. coloc.[10] *con.* cortico.[119] croc.[5] crot-h.[54] cub.[36] cupr. *cur.* daph. dig. dros. dulc. ferr. ferr-ar. ferr-i. ferr-m.[10] ferr-ma. foll.[1201] germ.[222] *graph.* grat. guare. guat.[119] **HELL.** hydrog.[222] hyos. hypoth.[149] **IGN.** iod. *ip.* kali-ar. kali-br. kali-c. kali-chl.[58] kali-p. kali-s. *kali-sil.*[58] kiss.[36] lac-c.[58] lac-d. lac-h.[229] **LACH.** laur. led. *lyc.* lyss. *m-arct.*[10] m-aust.[10] m-p-a.[1] mag-m. mand.[144] mang. med.[137] *merc. mez.* mur-ac. *naja* nat-c. *nat-m.* nat-sil.[58] nit-ac. *nux-m. nux-v.* **ONOS. OP.** ozone[227] pall. **PETR.**[122] *phos.* pic-ac. plat. plb. *psor. puls.* rad-br.[119] rauw.[119] rheum rhus-t. ruta *sac-alb.*[210] sanic. sant.[36] seneg. *sep. sil.* spig. *stann.*[30] staph.[30] sul-ac.[58] *sulph.* tab. tarax. tarent. ther.[25] thuj. zinc. zinc-p.[58]
Irresolution; accomplish or finish anything, cannot, pupils contracted: *cocc.*[54]
Irresolution; acts, in: **BAR-C.** chin. hydrog.[222] lyc. nat-c. nat-sil.[58] nux-m. **ONOS.** ozone[227] tarent.
Irresolution; changeable: asaf.[10] bism.[10] cann-s.[10] ign.[10] led.[10] m-aust.[10] nux-v.[10] op.[10] plat.[10] sil.[10] thuj.[10]
Irresolution; ideas: m-aust.[10] nat-m. sulph. tarent.
Irresolution; marry, to: carb-v.[30] ign.[30] lach.[30] nat-m.[30] nux-v.[30] phos.[30] plat.[30] sil.[30] staph.[30] verat.[30]
Irresolution; projects: ars.[10] asaf.[10] **BAR-C.** bufo-s. cact. cham. cortico.[119] *nux-m.*[10] rhus-t.
Irresolution; trifles, about: ars.[54] **BAR-C.** ferr-p.[36] graph.[137] lyc. lyss. pic-ac.[144]
Unsettled: carb-an.[36] guare.[36] sapin.[36]

ACON. Al, 30 - Now he doubts his recovery, now he is full of hope. (despair x hopeful)
ACT-SP. He, 17 - Irresolution, inconstancy and caprice.
ALUM. Al, 44 - Great absence of mind and irresolution.(undecided)
AM-C. Al, 20-...she knows not how to comfort (console) herself, what to do with herself;...
ARS. Ha, 1044 - Recurring fits of irresolution; he wishes something and when one attempts (try) to gratify his wish the merest trifle will alter his resolution, and he wishes it no longer.
Ha, 40 - Lack determination (indetermination); he desires something, and when the endeavor (try) is made to fulfill his desire; the merest trifle will change his determi-

nation and he is not willing to have it so.

AUR. Ha, 347 - Always very restless and undecided (doubtful) -thought he was neglecting something for which he must incur (obtain) reproach - ...he seemed to carry about this restlessness with him in his inmost (deepest) parts ; this condition deprived him of all perseverance, all energy.

Ha, 13 - Restless and undecided, without perceptible ebullition of the blood; he always thinks he is neglecting something for which he will be reproached; he seems to carry with him this internal restlessness, and it took from him all perseverance and energy.

BAR-A. Al, 13 - He wavers for a long time between opposite resolutions.(irresolute, indecision)

Al, 14 - During the day she resolves to undertake a certain matter in the evening, but scarcely is the time come when she repents it, and is undecided whether she shall do it or not.

Al, 15 - Extreme irresolution ; he proposes a short journey, but as soon as he makes preparation he changes his mind, and is inclined to remain at home.

BAR-C. Al, 16 - Great irresolution about small things; he wants to drink the cup of coffee, then again not, does not know what he shall do.

Ha, 12 - The greatest irresolution; he proposes to himself a brief journey, and as soon as he is to make his preparation, he is sorry for it and prefers to stay at home.

Ha, 13 - Long wavering between opposing resolutions.

Ha, 14 - During the day she determines to attend (take care) to some particular matter; but scarcely (just) has the time come, when she is sorry (give up) for it, and she knows not for irresolution what to do to leave undone.

BRY. Al, 25 - Fretful; she imagines that she cannot accomplish (realize) her work; constantly takes up the wrong piece, and always inclined to change and take another; ...

CALC. He, NERVES, Sensation of power with lack (loss, want) of will (command, resolution, intention), force.

CHAM. Ha, 490 - She has scruples of conscience about everything.

Ha, 465 - Very anxious; nothing she does seems to her to be right; she is irresolute; ...(indecisive)

He, 32 - Very anxious; everything she undertakes is very unsatisfactory (disappointed) ; she is irresolute,...(indecision)

CIC. Ha, 226 - He became indifferent to everything, and began to doubt whether this was really the condition in which he was.

CON. Al, 46 - Fretful mood; he does not knows how he shall busy himself; the times passes too slowly. (tedium)

CUPR. Ha, 7 - Irresolute (indecisive) and dissatisfied with everything, but only so long as he is peevish. (cross)

CUR. He, 1 - Indecision, no longer (more) wishes to think and act for herself.

FERR-MA. Al-S, 4 - Irresolute; he considers for a long time before commencing anything .

GERM. Sh, 115 - Very much in doubt whether I should take any more tablets. Whatever I do, I feel that somebody will criticize me, that I do something wrong. Difficult to make a decision. Afraid that other people will laugh at me or say, haven't you understood anything?" Crying. Don't want to get up. Don't want to bother the supervisor so early in the morning. I am a failure. 18, 30C, 01:06:30

Sh, 42 - Can't decide what to buy. Don't know where to put things. Head in the clouds. 09, 9C, 01:09:00.

GRAPH. He, 19 - Extreme hesitation; she is unable to make up her mind about anything; timidity.

GRAT. He, 1 - Irresolute (wavering); want of perseverance. (determination)

HALI-L. Sh, 317 - Feel overwhelmed when deciding what art supplies to order. Hard to make limited choices among many good things. Usually very decisive. 03, 12C, 08:XX:XX

Sh, 319 - Very difficult to decide what to eat. 03, 12C, 15:XX:XX

HYDROG. Sh, 63-"Oh God, what shall I do? Where do things go from here? What way shall I go? Feel I'm cracking up". Emotional confusion. Try to find a path to be happy, but unsure of what I'm doing. 24, 30C, 100:XX:XX

Sh, 153 - Insecurity and self doubt. 16, 30C, XX:XX:XX

IGN. Ha, 770 - Fickle, impatient, irresolute, quarrelsome.

IRID. 199 - Feelings of self-doubt crept in during the morning. Helped out at school and found myself checking with others over little things. Unable to make small decisions, spellings, etc., things I wouldn't be concerned about normally, usually feel sure of my own judgment. B4

KALI-C. Ha, 31 - She is always in antagonism with herself; she knows not what she wants, and feels exceedingly unhappy.

Ha, 32 - Contrary disposition; he is self-willed (obstinate) and often does not know himself what he wishes. (indecision)

Ha, 33 - Contrary mood; she demands (order, command) impetuously; is not satisfied with anything (dissatisfied) ; she is beside herself, and furiously angry; if everything does not go according to her wishes, and often does not herself know what she really wants.

KREOS. Al, 5 - Towards evening her spirits were much depressed, and she was doubtful whether she would ever be well again.

LACH. Al, 22 - Sudden doubts (indecision) arise about truths (veracity) of which he had hitherto (before) been convinced (converted), in the afternoon.

He, 34-...repugnance to society and dislike to talk; solicitude about future, whith disgust of life; inclination to doubt everything; mistrusts (suspicious) and misconstrues (misjudge) ...[0] Melancholia.

LYC. Al, 127 - Indecision and loss of confidence.

Al, 128 - He is unable to do anything, cannot think; passes his time with trifles, without being able to make up his mind what to do.

He, 29 - Want of self confidence; indecision; timidity; resignation.

LYSS. Al, 36 - Undecided about little things.

MED. He, 13 - Seems to herself to make wrong statements (declaration), because she does not know what to say next, begins all right but does not know how to finish...

NAT-C. Al, 24 - She does not know what to do, on account of apprehensiveness and ennui and thinks that she is quite lonely (alone, solitary, insulated) and forsaken, all day.

Ha, 23 - Restlessness and unsteadiness (inconstant); he knew not what he wanted, nor what he should do or leave undone.

NAT-M. He, 2 - Absent minded or distracted while talking; does not know what he ought (have to) say; awkward in talking; easily makes mistakes.

NUX-M. He, 25 - Fickle (capricious); irresolute and wavering in his undertakings.

NUX-V. Al, 69 - Dawdles (delay) and is irresolute.

Ha, 1288 - Irresolution, constant hesitation in his intentions.

PETR. Ha, 10 - He does not know how to stop talking about a thing.

He, 6 - Excitable, irritable with inclination to be angry and to scold; anxious and irresolute.

PH-AC. He, 12 - Anxiety and doubt concerning his recovery...

PULS. Ha, 1122 - Neglect of his business, hesitancy (indecision), sobbing (cry) respiration and loss of composure.(calm, serenity)

He, 26 - Anxiety: thinks to die; does not know what to do; as if in a hot atmosphere; in region of heart; even to suicide;...

SAPIN. Al, 5 - Quite ill-natured and inclined to view matters in a disagreeable light; did not seem able to feel settled (decided) enough to know what to do; the crossness became so intense, that I felt myself getting very unreasonable, especially as to food, which seemed all wrong in some way;...

STANN. He, 3 - Uneasy, does not know what to do with himself pains > by walking, yet so weak he soon must die.

SULPH. He, 37 - Great dejection,(grief), with thoughts of suicide; feels inferior (mediocre, lower) to everybody; can decide nothing;...

TAB. Al, 45 - He was incapacitated for business of any kind, weak irresolute, and despondent.

TARAX. Al, 4 - Without occupation he is quite gloomy; does not know what to do, and cannot make up his mind to do anything.

Al, 6 - Irresolution and dread of work, though it progresses well as soon as he undertakes it.
VERAT. Al, 23 - He groans, is beside himself; does not know what to do with himself.

DROWNING

Delirium; water, jumping into: bell. sec.
Delusions; brother fell overboard in her sight: kali-br.
• water, under water, he is: lap-c-b.[194]
Dreams; animals, bulls, jumped into water and drowned, and: tarent.[36]
➤ animals, horses, drowning: crot-c.
➤ children, about, lying on ice, her little child, and she feared it would fall into water: lipp.[36]
➤ danger, drowning, of: bov.[36]
➤ drowned, being: ign.[10] rumx.[36] verat-v.[25]
➤ drowning: aether[36] alum. bov. ign. kali-c. lyc. mag-s.[10] merc. merc-acet.[10] merc-i-f. nicc. ran-b. rauw.[119] rumx. samb. sil. verat. verat-v.[54] zinc.
➤ drowning, danger of: bov.[36]
➤ drowning, drowning man, of a: ***lyc.***[54] ***sil.*** sol-t-ae.
➤ drowning, foundering boat, on a: alum. lyc.
➤ drowning, mother had been drowned, that her: nicc. rauw.[119]
➤ drowning, people: ***lyc.***[54] mag-s.[10] verat.[36]
➤ drowning, someone trying to open her mouth, and: aether[36]
➤ falling, flood, into a: am-m.
➤ murdering, drowning two people in pool: ozone[227]
➤ water, daughter is in water and crying for help: nat-s.
➤ water, falling into: ***am-m. dig.*** eupi. ***ferr.*** ign. iod. mag-m. mag-s. merc. mez.[10] nicc. ph-ac.[1] plb.[10] puls.[10] sars.[10] sep.[10] sulph.[10] zinc.[10]
➤ water, falling into, child, her: eupi.
➤ water, falling into, daughter: iod.
➤ water, falling into, mother: nicc.
Fear; drowned, of being: cann-i.
✦ falling, water, into: perh.[149]
✦ sea, of the: morbill.[162]
✦ walking, of, canal by a: ang.[137]
✦ water, fossets, of: lyss.[122]
Jumping; impulse to, river, into: ***arg-n.*** sec. sil.
Suicidal disposition; drowning, by: ant-c. ***arg-n.***[122] ***aur.***[5] ***bell. dros. hell.*** hep.[116] ***hyos.*** ign. ***lach.*** nux-v.[30] ped.[122] ***puls. rhus-t.*** sec. ***sil.*** staph.[30] sulph. ***ust.***[184] verat.
Suicidal disposition; drowning, by, love, from disappointed: ***hyos.***[54]
Suicidal disposition; drowning, by, mania, in: sec.[54]
Suicidal disposition; drowning, by, seeks to escape, after menses: ***ign.***[54]
Suicidal disposition; drowning, by, thinks with pleasure of: ***puls.***[54]

DUTY

Ailments from; responsibility, early, too: carc.[210]
Ailments from; responsibility, unusual: aur.[58]
Anxiety; anticipating, an engagement: **ARG-N.**[122] ***ars.***[162] ***carb-v.***[162] carc.[207] **GELS.**[122] hydrog.[222] ***lyc. lyss.***[162] **MED.**[122] **NAT-M.**[162] ph-ac.[162] ***sil.***[162] ***thuj.***[162]
Anxiety; duty, as if had not done his: ars.[36] puls.[172]
Anxiety; duty, as if he had not done his, religious, produced by lascivious impulses: ***orig.***[54]
Anxiety; expected of him, when anything is: ***ars.***
Anxiety; household matters, about: ars.[172] bar-c.[60] carl.[102] hyos.[172] nux-v.[172] ph-ac.[172] puls.[60] rhus-t.[60] sep.[60] sulph.[5]
Anxiety; lascivious impulses, from, on account of disinclination of religious duties in a married woman, mother of a family: ***orig.***[54]
Anxiety; time is set, if a: alum.[162] ***arg-n.*** gels. med.
Business; neglects his: opun-a.[36] ptel.[144] ***sulph.***[36]
Carefree: ham.[5] laur.[5] op.[5] phos.[5] tarax.[5] zinc.[5]
Cares; full of, domestic affairs, about: bar-c. ***puls. sep.***
Confusion of mind; daily affairs, about: lyc.[137]
Death; presentment of, near, seems, and must settle affairs: petr.[137]
Delusions; business, doing, is: bell. ***bry.*** canth. cupr. op.[102] ***phos.*** rhus-t. verat.
• murdered, someone, he has: ars.[58] phos.[1]
• neglected his duty, he has: ars.[36] **AUR.** cur.[137] cycl. hell.[58] hyos. ign. ***lyc.*** naja[36] nat-ar. ptel.[36] puls.

• neglected, duty, his, deserves reproach: aur.[54] germ.[222]
• neglected, duty, his, headache, during: naja[36]
• neglected, duty, his, perfunctory manner, performed in: ptel.[36]
• night, duty, he had been on: conin.[36] ptel.[36]
• people, ply him with questions and he must answers, they: **NUX-V.**[54]
• reproach, has neglect duty and deserves: ***aur.***
• vow, breaking her: ign.
• vow, keep it, must: verat.[10]
• work, advance fast enough, does not: gamb.[36]
• work, works too much, all work comes to him: ozone[227]
• world, rests upon him, the world: tab.[139]

Dereliction, sensation of: bar-c.[10] carb-an.[10] nat-c.[10] plat.[10] stram.[10]

Dreams; business, forgot during day, he: sel.[102]
➤ responsibility, of: carc.[227]
➤ unsuccessful efforts to, do various things, get cooking ready for brother and father: am-m.[36]

Duty; aversion to domestic: cench.[58] cit-l.[54] sul-i.[58]

Duty; want of sense of: alum.[30] ambr.[30] anac.[30] ars.[30] **CALC.**[36] cench.[58] coloc.[30] hep.[30] lach.[30] merc.[30] nat-m.[30] ptel.[36] sil.[30] sulph.[30]

Fear; duty, being unable to do her: ***lac-c.***[54]
✦ duty, neglect her, to: aur.[30]
✦ responsibility, of: arg-n.[172] ars.[172] aur.[137] kali-p.[172] lyc.[109] sil.[172]

Freedom remarkable, in doing what he had to do: op.[36] ozone[227]

Grief; neglected duty, over: cycl.[102]

Handle things anymore, cannot, housewives: bamb-a.[1184] sep.[187]

Handle things anymore, cannot, responsible for everything, does not want to be: bamb-a.[1184]

Handle things anymore, cannot, support, looks for: bamb-a.[1184]

Handle things anymore, cannot, weight, wants to throw off the: bamb-a.[1184]

Hurry; duties, as by imperative: **LIL-T.**[36]

Hurry; occupation, desires to do several things at once: aur. **LIL-T.** petr.[102] plan.

Hurry; time, for the appointed, to arrive: **ARG-N.** carc.[138] cupr.[210]

Indifference; conscience, to the dictates of: cann-i. caust.[30] con.[30] graph.[30] petr.[30]

Indifference; duties, domestic, to: androc.[222] aur-ar.[58] brom.[58] ***cimic.***[54] cit-l.[54] sep.[81] sul-i.[58]

Indifference; duties, to: ars.[30] **CALC.**[54] carb-v.[122] cench.[58] lach.[30] merc.[30] nat-m.[30] ***ptel.***[54] sil.[30] sul-i.[58] sulph.[30]

Indolence; housework, aversion to her usual: bamb-a.[1184] cench.[58] ***cit-ac.*** cit-l.[54] sep.[137] sul-i.[58]

Kill; desire to, somebody, thought he ought to k.: camph. ***hyos.***[54]

Neglects; household, the: aur-ar.[58] sul-i.[58]

Neglects; important things: alum.[30] con.[30] kali-m.[192]

Obstinate; pertinacity, duties, in performing irksome: lim.[36]

Punctuality, always on time: arg-n.[214] aur-ar.[214] kali-n.[222]

Religious affections; eternal bliss, believes herself unworthy of, because she is unable to perform her duties: stram.[54]

Reproaches; accomplished enough, because he had not: ars.[54]

Responsibility: bamb-a.[1184] carc.[188] cupr.[210] ign.[188] ***lil-t.***[168] nat-ar.[168] nat-m.[189]

Responsibility; strong: aur.[58] ***calc.***[187] carc.[196] cocc.[58] cupr.[210] cycl.[206] ign.[188] kali-c.[162] ***lil-t.***[168] lyc.[206] mag-m.[187] nat-ar.[168] nat-m.[189] nat-s.[162] puls.[206] stront-c.[188]

Responsibility; strong, family, towards his: nat-s.[187]

Responsibility; strong, social: stront-c.[188]

Responsibility; wants to give up her: sep.[187]

Restlessness; duty, as if he had not done his: ***puls.***[54]

Sadness; conscience, of, as if he had committed a bad action, or not done his duty: cycl.[54]

Sadness; domestic affairs, over: bar-c.[10] puls.[10] rhus-t.[10] ***sep.***[54] viol-t.[8]

Talk; domestic affairs, of: hyos.[54]

Unreliable; promises, in his: bell.[30] calc.[30] con.[30] lyc.[30] merc.[30] op.[30] sil.[30] sulph.[30]

ADAM. Sh, 76 - Felt rushed; so much to do. Overwhelmed. 8, 6C, 04:XX:XX

AGAR. Ha, 28 - Quiet, equable (tranquil), sociable, active, and glad of having done his duty.

ALUM. Ha, 23 - Excited, over-worked (industrious), and yet discontented, because not enough had been done. (duty)

ARN. Al, 39-...;one feels as if one were prevented (suspend) from doing something which is extremely necessary, accompanied by a total want of disposition for any kind of work.

Ha, 620 - Restlessness of body and mind, as if he was prevented (obstructed) doing something necessary, whith complete indisposition for occupation.

ARS. Al, 74 - Continued anxiety, a mental anguish, as if he had not done his duty, without, however, knowing wherein.

Al, 108 - Dissatisfied the whole day, and very fretful at himself for not having done enough.

Ha, 1039 - Persistent anxiety, like a qualm (doubt) of conscience, just as if he had failed (neglected) to do his duty, but without knowing wherein.

Ha, 1064 - All day long discontented with himself and very cross with himself; he imagines he has not done enough, and reproaches himself bitterly.

Ha, 20 - Continual anguish, like remorse of conscience, as if he had acted in violation (transgression, crime) of his duty, without knowing in what particular.

Ha, 53 - Dissatisfied all day and extremely vexed at himself; he thought he had not worked enough and reproached himself most bitterly.

He, 95 - Dissatisfied and angry with himself all day; thinks he has not accomplished enough, and reproaches himself bitterly.

ART-V. He, 7 - Gets up every night and does her daily work as a house servant, with closed eyes, lies down again and cannot remember anything next morning.

AUR. Ha, 345 - An urging to activity, bodily as well as mental; when he did anything, he thought he did not do it quick enough, and that he had a great deal (much) more to do; he could not live to his liking. (desire, aspiration)

Ha, 347 - Always very restless and undecided (doubtful) -thought he was neglecting something for which he must incur (obtain) reproach -...he seemed to carry about this restlessness with him in his inmost (deepest) parts ; this condition deprived him of all perseverance, all energy.

Ha, 13 - Restless and undecided, without perceptible ebullition of the blood; he always thinks he is neglecting something for which he will be reproached; he seems to carry with him this internal restlessness, and it took from him all perseverance and energy.

BAR-C. He, 28 - Solicitude, about his future; about domestic affairs.

He, 26 - Anxious about most trivial affairs.(duty)

BELL. Al, 54 - The delirium was of a busy (engaged, working), restless, vivid character, but generally rather pleasing than otherwise. The patient appeared to think they were pursuing (persevere) their ordinary occupations; one boy appeared eager (animated) in flying a kite (toy), another pulled tables and chairs about, thinking he was working in a coal-pit, and a woman appeared to be remarkably busy with her household duties...

Al, 109 - A tailor was poisoned with a belladona injection, and for fifteen hours, though speechless and insensible to external objects, went through all the customary operations of his trade with great vivacity and moved his lips as if in conversation.(busy)

A-S, 2554-..The patients appeared to think that they were pursuing their ordinary occupations;... the woman appeared remarkably busy with her ordinary household duties.

BOR. Ha, 20 - Disinclination to work, he only does what he has to do, as if compulsorily.

BROM. He, 6 - Aversion to any kind of work, even reading; takes no interest in household duties.

CACT. Al, 19 - Disposition to do deliberately (resolutely, carefully) whatever was undertaken.

CALAD. He, 4 - Very forgetful; he cannot remember if what he ought to have done and written during the day is really accomplished until he convinces himself of it.

CALC-A. Al, 10-...;he performed all his work with aversion and as if compelled (drive) to do so. (compulsive, obsessive)

Ha, 265-...very indifferent to the most important things; he did everything unwillingly (reluctant, averse) as if forced to do them.

CALC-P. He, 11 - Does not want to do what he has to do.

CARB-V. Ha, 711 - Excessive irritation, as if she were too much hurried, or had too much to do.

CARL. Al, 10 - Discouraged and anxious in the discharge (execution) of his domestic duties.

CAUST. Ha, 61 - A sort of absent-mindedness; while doing one thing, he always felt as if he had to do something else, more importance, (duty) and yet he knew not what ; he reflected about it, and yet thought nothing. (lost: signification, value, purpose)

CHOC. Sh, 145 - My fears around the kids —that they would die, etc. and that they were my total responsibility, like parasites —have gone and I know feel total trust that they will be o.k.

CIMIC. He, 26 - Indifferent, taciturn, takes no interest in household matters.

CYCL. Al, 10 - Internal grief and anxiety of conscience, as though he had not done his duty, or had committed a crime.

Ha, 196 - Inward grief and anxiety of conscience, as if he had not done his duty or had committed a crime.

Ha, 197 - Excessive sadness, as if he had done something bad and had neglected his duty.

He, 12 - Great sadness, as if he had committed a bad action or not done his duty.

CYPR. He, 2 - Profound indifference to everything, even to his studies, duties and common courtesies (kindness, compassion) of life.

DROS. Ha, 287 - Happy steadfast (confiding) disposition; he dreaded no evil, because he was conscious of having acted honorably.

GERM. Sh, 8 - Weeping. Feeling very offended towards father who had objected because I had bought something expensive for myself. Felt anger because of my reaction, but also curiosity to find out why I reacted. Feel anxiety about all my responsibilities. Everything feels like too much. 21, 12C, 26:XX:XX.

Sh, 180 - Woke up early 3.30 am. had strong feeling, like a visualization. I picture myself lying on floor in fetal position and being shot in the head like a horse or a dog. Almost welcomed it. Then thought my children still need me. A very strong feeling of failure accompanied this. I felt I did not deserve to live. Better crying next day when talking to husband. This feeling of depression carried on for several nights. As soon as I wake up in the early morning, my mind is active and a feeling of inadequacy comes on strongly. 05 , 6C, 28:XX:XX

HALI-L. Sh, 157 - Called into work a half an hour early, for an emergency. Went into automatic overwhelm. Felt a lot of responsibilities. I didn't have the time to do all the things I wanted to do. 01, 30C, 01:23:XX

Sh, 182 - Not doing enough. Feel somewhat critical of myself. Not getting anything done. Want to be in a structured, organized place and can't get there. I'd like to be really busy. I have more ideas in my head than I can do. I need to get active again, structure things, and set goals. 08, 30C, 03:XX:XX

Sh, 390 - While making the schedule, instead of working hard to fill every spot, I left some blanks to be filled in at the staff meeting. It felt good to let go of the responsibility. 02, 30C, 01:04:XX

Sh, 391 - Staff meeting was awful. Everyone feeling frustrated due to extra work, but I did not feel any blame. Normally I would have felt responsible, but this time I felt it was not my fault. 02, 30C, 01:10:XX -01:12:XX

Sh, 575 - Very angry with the children, who have done no chores. Irritated and yelled at them. I get so angry my nervous system refuses to calm down. I take their behavior personally, plus I'm angry at myself for my own response to them. 09, 6C, 05:04:XX

HAM. Al, 14 - I became impatient, and resolved not to take anymore of the medicine; felt as if I did not care whether I attended (guard) to my practice or not; did not want any one to call at the office for medicine.

IGN. He, 11-...believes herself married (connected) and pregnant; is tormented by remorse of imagined crimes; seeks constantly to escape to drown (suicide) herself; ...;is only quiet when lying undisturbed and brooding over her troubles, which she rehearses (tell) in a doleful (unhappy) tone ;..." I am neglecting my duty, breaking my vow" (promise, engagement)...;conscientious scruples after eating.

He, 61 - Melancholia after great grief and domestic trouble; complete sleeplessness; suicidal thoughts and desire to escape.

IOD. Al, 31 - Mind feels tired, and does not care to work.

IP. Ha, 224 - He is morose and vexed that his business is not performed quick enough. (time)

LAC-C. Al,N-36 - Fears she will become unable to perform her duties.

Al,N-39 - Wakes distressed, and obliged to rise and occupy herself in some manner; fears she will be crazy.

He, 29 - Fears she will become unable to perform (achieve, accomplish) her duties.(responsibility)

LACH. He, 14 - Delirium from overwatching, overfatigue; loss of fluids; excessive study.

LIL-T. Al, 24-..a feeling of irritation and of something wrong in abdomen and pelvic organs (disease); feels hurried (fast) and yet incapable (incompetent), as if she had a great deal (busy) to do and cannot do it.

Al, 30 - Constant hurried (precipitation) feeling as of imperative duties and utter inability to perform them; during the sexual excitement.

Al, 40-...I can see around me any number of things I must do, but cannot force myself to do anything.

He, 12 - Listless, inert, yet does not want to sit still (quiet); restless, yet does not want to walk; hurried manner, desire to do something, yet feels no ambition; feeling as of imperative duties and utter (complete) inability (incapacity, incompetence) to perform them; sexual excitement.

LIM. Al, 3 - The great disinclination to work, and inability to accomplish much, which he had experienced since the sea-bath, disappeared completely during the day, and gave place to mental quiet and steadiness, with constancy and perseverance in performing very irksome duties.

LYC. Ha, 78 - He cannot do nor think anything; he spends his time in trifling, and is not able to resolve to do what he has to do.

MAG-C. Al, 932 - Dream of flowers, clothes, and other things; she had to make up the clothes, but had no inclination to do it, and besides did not understand how; she also saw many foreign plants, but during this she became soaked (wet) with rain.

MAG-M. Al, 709 - She becomes anxious in a dream about the work that she could not accomplish.

MED. Al,N-40 - Always wakens tired in the morning; hates to do anything that must be done (duty), even nice things; gets nervous and excited about riding and driving as soon the time is fixed.

He, 2 - Dullness of memory and desire to procrastinate (delay), because business seemed so long lasting (permanent), or as if it never could be accomplished. (postponing)

NAJA. Al, 13-...I felt that everything that was done was done in a wrong way, and could not be rectified (corrected, revised); if I felt that I had some duty to perform (execute), I had at the same time a strong impulse not to do it, and I am extremely restless in consequence; I seemed to have an increased perception of what I ought to do, but, at the same time, an unaccountable inclination not to do it, to which I was irresistibly compelled to yield "I couldn't help it, didn't know why, but couldn't do it."

NAT-AR. Al, 15 - Requires an effort to attend to accustomed duties; feels dull; tries to write, but it requires an effort to form each word.

NAT-C. Ha, 23 - Restlessness and unsteadiness (inconstant); he knew not what he wanted, nor what he should do or leave undone.

NEON. Sh, 85 - Feel out of control, as if time is moving relentlessly and remorselessly forward and I'm stuck behind, unable to keep up. Panic, guilt, constant anxiety that I won't get it all done, including keeping up this journal. 10, 6C, 12:XX:XX

NUX-M. He, 17 - The outer world had no

existence for her; automatically she attended to her household duties, and on awaking from this condition she had not the slightest recollection of what she had done; ...

OP. Al, 70 - Sensation of courage with activity, as if he could forcibly accomplish whatever was required without dread or fear, with a peculiar sensation of lustiness. (strong)

Ha, 601 - Tranquil indifference to earthly things; she cared for nothing in comparison with ecstasies of the fantasy.

OPUN-V. Al, 2 - The mind appears to be much affected, and does not appreciate any of its morbid condition; much tempted to do things one should not do.

PHOS. Al, 38 - Told those about him repeatedly that he could not possibly recover, and gave some disjointed directions about his business affairs.

PLB. Al, 20 - He was at time delirious, very restless, and manifested great concern (care) for his affairs.

PTEL. Al, 43 - Goes about his professional duties in a perfunctory (indifference) manner, very unlike (contradictory) his fiery (passionate) zeal with which he usually combats disease and his allopathic step-brethren (brotherhood).

PULS. Ha, 1118 - Solicitude about his domestic concerns, in the morning.

Ha, 1119 - Cannot think without fretting (anguish) about his affairs (duty, responsibility), in the morning.

Ha, 1120 - Restless state of the disposition, as if did not do his duty properly.

Ha, 1122 - Neglect of his business, hesitancy (indecision), sobbing (cry) respiration and loss of composure.(calm, serenity)

RHUS-T. Al, 40 - Impatient desire to accomplish several kinds of business, chiefly intellectual,...

SEP. He, 11 - Sad about her health and domestic affairs, discontented with everything.

STANN. Al, 20 - Fruitlessly busy, as if a rush of ideas prevented him from completing his work at a certain time; all sorts of things occur to him to be done.

Al, 21 - Indolent and irritable, with heat in the face; would do everything, but really does nothing.

Ha, 639 - Busy uselessness (inefficiency): he exerts (use) himself to get a necessary task (duty) done at the appointed hour, and cannot accomplish it, as though prevented (interrupted) by an over-crowding of thoughts, during which one thing and another occur to him which he wishes to do...

He, 6 - A woman, age 39, pregnant in fourth month;...inability to do anything as she cannot muster sufficient courage,...great palpitation of heart and anxiety, especially if she has to give directions in her domestic affairs; thinking makes her feel wretched, ...(unable, incapable)

STRAM. Al, 48 - She is all the time inconsolable; much affected by trifles; makes much fuss about trifles; disposed to weep, and sometimes also very easily vexed; now and then neglects her duties; now and then thinks she is not fitted for her position ; after the fall equinox...; she wants light and company.

He, 172 - Downcast and full of anguish, believes herself unworthy of eternal bliss, because she is unable to perform her duties.

He, 177-...sometimes vexed; neglects her duties, thinks she is not fitted for her position;...

SUL-AC. Al, 9 - Hasty (hurried, fast) mood; nothing that she does can be finished quickly enough, though she makes unusual effort.

Al, 35 - Fretful, peevish, impatient, if his work is not done to suit.(unsatisfying)

He, 2 - Must do everything in a great hurry; nothing can be finished quickly enough.

SULPH. Al, 8 - Numerous morbid ideas, extremely disagreeable, causing rancor, though with also joyous thoughts (and melodies) mostly from the past, take possession of her they throng one upon another so that she cannot free herself from them during the day, with neglect of business,...

Al, 94 - He sits for hours immovable and indolent, without definite thought, though he has much to accomplish.

Al, 100 - Thoughts of the business that had been accomplished thronged (crowd) upon her...

Ha, 51 - For hours he sits motionless and indolent, without any definite thoughts, though he has many things to attend to.
He, 3-...feels as if crazy; does not know whether she has done what she intended (planned) or whether objects seen are really there, or whether she only imagines them to be, until she has touched them;...
SUMB. Al, 2 - More cheerful in humor and more disposed for intellectual occupation; he felt in the happy enthusiastic state of mind that accompanies the consciousness of having performed a noble (generous, virtuous) deed; this sort of medicinal intoxication went away in a few hours.
TELL. Al, 3 - He forgets and neglects (ignores, indifference) much; also the writing down, and even the observing of symptoms ...when thinking of the one, or of any business, he forgets everything else, and on account of this he neglects much that is necessary.
VERAT. Al, 2 - Slight delirium; ...he prattles about religious subjects and about vows to be performed, prays, believes that he is not in his own house.
He, 16-... prattles about religious subjects and about vows (promise) to be performed, prays, believes that he is not in his own house.
VIOL-T. He, 2 - Low spirited about domestic affairs.

DWELLS

Absorbed; become of him, as to what would: nat-m.
Brooding: acon.[1] agar.[162] alum. androc.[222] anh.[119] arn. aur. aur-s.[58] bamb-a.[1184] bar-i.[58] bell. calc.[58] calc-s. cann-s.[5] canth. caps. carb-an.[1] carc.[207] caust. cham. chel.[58] chin.[5] clem.[116] cocc. con.[8] cycl. euphr. ***gels.*** goss.[122] hell. **IGN.** ip. kali-p. lach.[10] lil-t.[58] lyc.[58] mez. mosch.[5] mur-ac. ***naja*** nit-ac.[36] ***nux-m.***[137] nux-v. olnd. op. ozone[227] ***ph-ac.*** plat.[58] ran-b.[5] ***rheum***[10] rhus-t.[5] sep.[1] spig.[1] stram.[36] sulph. ***verat.*** viol-o.[5]
Brooding; constantly over loss of a child: ***gels.***[54] ***kali-br.***[54]
Brooding; corner, brooding or moping in a: aur.[5] aur-s.[58] bar-c.[5] bar-i.[58] bell.[5] camph.[5] cocc.[54] con.[58] cupr.[5] hyos.[5] ph-ac.[5] **VERAT.**[5]
Brooding; disappointment, cardiac weakness, with: ***ph-ac.***[54]
Brooding; forbidden things, over: ***plb.***[54]
Brooding; imaginary troubles, disease: cycl.[137] lil-t.[137] ***naja***[117]
Brooding; imaginary troubles, over, disease: cycl.[137] **IGN.**[54] lil-t.[137] ***naja***[117]
Brooding; imaginary troubles, over, sadness, with: naja[54]
Brooding; law suit, over, by which he may gain or loose a million, and takes it in bad part if not allowed to read indictment for said lawsuit, a confused, irrational piece of work, on which he has been working all night, in insanity: ***nux-v.***[54]
Brooding; silence, in: bell.[54] ***verat.***[54]
Brooding; unpleasant things: kiss.[36]
Delusions; images, dwells upon: arn. nux-m. sil.
• troubles, broods over imaginary: ***ign.***[54] ***naja***[117]
Dreams; fixed upon one subject: acon. ign. puls. stann.
➤ fixed upon one subject, leave him on waking, does not: ign.[54]
Dwells on past disagreeable occurrences: am-c. arg-n. asar.[149] calc.[10] ***cham. chin.*** cob-n.[119] ***cocc. con.*** cop. form. glon. goss.[122] hep. hydrog.[222] hyos.[111] ***ign.***[54] kali-c.[108] ***kali-p.***[54] kiss.[36] lil-t.[58] luna[228] lyc. meny. mez. **NAT-M.** nit-ac. op.[30] opun-a.[36] phos.[111] ***plat.*** psor.[111] rhus-t. sars.[54] ***sep.*** spong.[1] staph.[30] ***sulph.*** syph.[122] thuj.[5] verat.[116] visc.[119]
Dwells; disappointments, on: ***ph-ac.***[54]
Dwells; grief from past offenses: calc.[30] staph.[30]
Dwells; grieve therefore, to: nat-m.[30]
Dwells; health, his broken: aur-m.[58]
Dwells; on past disagreeable occurrences, night, on: ambr.[58] benz-n.[36] caust. chin. graph. kali-c. kali-p.[122] lyc. nat-m.[116] ***plat. rhus-t. sulph.***
Dwells; on past disagreeable occurrences, recalls old grievances: glon. sars.[54] sulph.[54]
Dwells; on past disagreeable occurrences, sexual matters, on: staph.[102]
Dwells; on past disagreeable occurrences, thinking of everything which others have done to displease him, lies awake all night to lay plans to talk to them about it, but forgets it in the morning: am-c.[58]
Dwells; unpleasant, disagreeable things: ***ambr. benz-ac.*** kreos.

Fear; thinking of, when, disagreeable things: phos.
Hypochondriasis; sexual, dwelling on sexual subjects: ***staph.***[54]
Irritability; recollection of unpleasant circumstances, during: sep.[36]
Meditation; deep, profound: acon.[5] cocc.[10] **SEP.**[5] staph.[5]
Religious affections; speculations, dwells on: **SULPH.**[54]
Sadness; brooding over imaginary wrongs and misfortunes, by: naja[130]
Sadness; dwell constantly over her condition, inclination to: ***sulph.***[54]
Sit; wrapped in deep, sad thoughts and notices nothing, as if: alum-sil.[58] ***ambr.***[122] aur. cench.[58] cham.[1] cimic.[58] ***cocc.*** con.[58] elaps ***hipp. ign.***[54] ozone[227] plat.[137] psor.[137] ***puls. stram.***[54] ***verat.***
Theorizing; philosophic, mind dwells on: hydrog.[222] **SULPH.**[54]
Thoughts; persistent, alone: ars. kali-c. zinc.
Thoughts; repetition, of: mag-m.[58] stram.

ACON. He, 8 - Ideas haunt (obsess) him, cannot get rid of them.
AETH. Al, 28 - A fixed idea, which she cannot throw off, of a garment (clothes) made the day previous; she also dreamed of it.
Al,S-2 - A fixed idea, from which she could not free herself, of a garment (clothes) made the previous day, of which she also dreamed.
AMBR. Al,N-9 - Forced to dwell upon most disagreeable things; ...
Ha, 478 - Distorted fancies, grimaces, satanic faces take possession of the mind, and he cannot get rid of them.
ANDROC. Sh, 126 - Great hostility to those around him, which manifested in brooding and stinging observations and comments directed at his friends. (29)
ANG. Al, 15-,...prevented by the intrusion upon his mind of a rather agreeable project which he almost believes to be real and feasible, and which exclusively absorbs all his attention; it is a sort of waking dream.
He, 8 - Thinks about one project and nothing else, with great activity of mind.
ANT-C. He, 6 - Inclined to suicide by shooting; at night he is obliged to get out of bed, because he cannot free himself of the idea.
ARS. Ha, 1038 - When he is alone he is beset by thoughts about disease and other thoughts of an indifferent character, of which he cannot get rid.
He, 7 - When alone, he falls to thinking about disease and other things, which he can scarcely keep out of his mind.
CALC-A. Ha, 261 - Not without inclination to work, but indifferent to all external things; sunk in thought about the present and future.
CALC. He, 5 - Buried in deep thought; anxiety about present and future.(destine)
CAMPH. He, 16 - Monomania, with horrible visions and torturing ideas about religion, which he cannot shake off, although he is conscious that they are morbid.; is< at night.
COCC. Al, 10 - She is absorbed in the saddest thoughts, and affronts (indignity) sink deep into her heart.
Al, 11 - Thoughts directed to an unpleasant object; she is absorbed in herself, and notices nothing about her.
Ha, 520 - The thoughts are fixed on a single disagreeable subject; she is absorbed in thought and notices nothing about her.
CON. Al, 38 - Sunk in deep thought; he apprehensively considered the present and the future, and sought (wanted) to be alone.
CROT-C. Al, 18 - Her thoughts dwell on death; with great sadness.
CROT-H. He, 14 - Sadness, her thoughts dwell on death continually.
GELS. He, 6 - After losing son, inclined to brood over her loss; at times becomes unconscious, or, rather, "rapt"; in imagination thinks herself at the grave; smothered pressure on chest after the spell.
HELL. He, 20 - After typhoid, ...sits quietly in bed and seems lost in brooding;...constantly seeks (try) to escape, ...;without a word quietly climbs out of the window, and if she succeeds in escaping goes in direction of river; finally threw herself into privy (toilet), from which she was rescued.
HYDROG. Sh, 236 - Dwells on past disagreeable occurrences. 16, 30C, XX:XX:XX
Sh, 261 - Almost the impression that I am

pregnant —many old sensations and emotions from previous pregnancies recurred. Like having another person inside of me. All physical symptoms of pregnancy. Went for a test. 08, 30C, 01:XX:XX

IGN. Al, 28 - Contrary to his will, thinks of vexatious and peevish things, and dwells upon them.

Ha, 791 - Thinks against his will of annoying, vexatious things, and dwells on them.

He, 6 - Brooding over imaginary or real troubles; is wrappd in thought.

KALI-BR. Al, 5 - She had the erroneous idea that she was deserted by all her friends, and as a consequence she passed all her waking moments, which are not many in tears;...delusion that her child was dead, had taken fixed possession of her mind;...she declared that she saw it dead (corpse) before her, and when it was brought to her, she refused to acknowledge that it was hers, or had any resemblance to the one she imagined was dead.

He, 23-...constantly brooding over loss of a daughter; almost crazy; ... (child)

KREOS. He, 11 - Seeks for unpleasant things and broods over them.

MANG. Ha, 324 - Cross reflective, silently reserved, wrapped up in himself, with discomfort in the whole body, ...

MENY. Ha, 290 - Melancholy humor; his thoughts are disposed to dwell on past sad disagreeable things.

NAJA. Al, 14 - Felt melancholy; began to form images of possible wrongs (mistaken) and misfortunes, over which the mind broods; very wretched at times;... a slight cause sets him in a perfect agony of mental suffering on another's behalf (welfare);...makes himself imaginary troubles and wrongs, and frets (bother) over them for two hours...

He, 3 - Melancholy; began to form images of possible wrongs (evils) and misfortunes over which the mind broods; very wretched (miserable) at times.

NAT-M. Ha, 9 - For hours, immersed in thoughts, as to what would become of him.

Ha, 64 - Injuries which he had inflicted on others, or which others had done to him, always dwelled in his thoughts; he could not get rid of them, and this annoyed him, so that he had no pleasure in anything.

He, 21 - Gloomy thoughts, recalls (remember),insults long since suffered; likes to dwell upon past unpleasant occurrences.

NAT-P. Al, 10 - Awakens; fears his child, who has a trifling ailment (disease), is dead; he goes to her room to relieve the otherwise ineffaceable (perpetual) impression.

NIT-AC. Ha, 12 - She falls to thinking over an anxious occurrence long past, and cannot rid herself of it, almost like as if in a waking dream; from time to time she, as it were, awakes from it startled, but is always absorbed in these ideas, without being able, in spite of strenuous efforts of thinking of anything else.

NUX-V. He, 37-...brooding all night long over a lawsuit by which he may gain or lose a million (megalomania) ; ..replies reluctantly and slowly to physician's questions, and takes it in bad part (offenses) if not allowed to read indictment (accusation) for said lawsuit, a confused irrational piece of work, on which he has been working all night.

PH-AC. Ha, 5 - Continually brooding over his disease.

Ha, 35 - He cannot get rid of one thought, and the other thoughts to be connected therewith do not come in.

He, 18 - Dread (fear) of the future; brooding over one's condition.

PLB. He, 15-...; despair of her salvation...; fixed idea that could only obtain peace and safety though absolution by a priest of the papal church, although she had been a zealous Protestant; ....brooded over any forbidden thing; would steal (leave) from house in servant's cloak (coat, camouflage) and bonnet (hat) to obtain stimulants (drugs), but from the moment their prohibition was withdrawn (retired) ceased to have any desire for them; after being permitted to visit a priest and converse with him ceased to talk and think of the church. (desire; redemption, absolution)

PULS. Al, 47 - He cannot at all get rid of a thought that he once grasped.

RAN-B. Al, 7 - The objects of his feelings,

for instance, chagrin, occupy his mind long after the occurrence took place; one sees that he is thinking of those things; he talks to himself, gesticulates in his anger...

STAPH. He, 6 - Hypochondriasis (depression);...;caused by unmerited insults (offenses, affronts, abuses) sexual excesses, or by persistently dwelling on sexual subjects.

SULPH. Al, 10 - Vexatious and morbid ideas of the past arise from the most indifferent thoughts, and from every occurrence in life, which continue to be united with new vexations, so that she cannot free herself from them, together with a courageous mood which is ready for great resolution.

He, 32 - Melancholy mood; dwelling on religious or philosophic speculations; anxiety about soul's salvation; indifference about lot (destiny) of others.

EATING

Anger; eat, when obliged to: ars.[1]
Anxiety; chest, breakfast, after: con.[172] kali-c.[172] valer.
Anxiety; food, about: lac-h.[229]
Conscientious about trifles; eating, after: ign.
Conscientious about trifles; eating, during: plat.[30] puls.[30] sil.[30]
Delusions; animals, devouring him: ***hyos.***
• dirt, eating dirt, he is: verat.
• eating, he is: lap-c-b.[194]
Discomfort; eating, after: bar-acet.[36] bry.[36] clem.[36] olnd.[36] ph-ac.[36] zinc.[36]
Discontented; eating, after: bov. fl-ac.
Dreams; animals, devouring meat in market: hura[36]
➤ animals, eating alive: hydrog.[222]
➤ animals, horses, eating corn in a garage: ozone[227]
➤ banquet, of being at a: mag-c.[10] mag-s. nit-ac.[10] ph-ac.
➤ coffin, eating moldy sausage, after: form.[36]
➤ devils, cooking babies on a vulcano and eating them: ozone[227]
➤ eating: ***iod.***
➤ eating, canine flesh: alum.[10]
➤ eating, human flesh: sol-t-ae.
➤ eating, live animals: hydrog.[222]
➤ feasting: anan. ant-c. asaf. hura m-p-a.[1] mag-s. nit-ac. ph-ac. tril. zinc.
➤ food: choc.[222] ptel.[36]
➤ fruit: cast-eq. choc.[222] jac-c.[36] mag-c.[5]
➤ meat, roasted, gets, to feed vegetarians: ozone[227]
➤ table is being set for him: ozone[227]
Fear; eating, agg., while: bran.[36] caust. grat. op. puls. tarent.
✦ eating, agg., while, offered, what is: hyos.[172]
Hurry; eating, while: anac.[102] androc.[222] arg-n.[122] aur.[1] bell.[54] berb.[54] calad. **CAUST.** clem.[5] ***coff.*** cupr.[1] graph.[5] **HEP.** kali-c.[122] ***lach.*** lyc.[1] nux-m.[5] ***olnd.***[5] pip-m. **PLAT.**[5] plect.[36] ***rhus-t.***[162] sabad.[5] **SUL-AC.** sulph.[1] zinc.[1]
Hurry; eating, while, eat fast enough, cannot: zinc.[137]
Indifference; eating, after: aloe lach.[137] lyc.[137] ***ph-ac.***[137] sel.[137]
Lasciviousness; eating, after, with feeling of weakness in parts: lyss.[54]
Rage; eating, during and after: chlor.[54]
Revelry, feasting: agar.[5] ambr.[5] ang.[5] ant-c.[5] ip.[30] kali-c.[30] ***lach.***[5] ***nat-c.***[30] **NUX-V.**[5] sel.[5] sulph.[5]
Sadness; eating, after: alum. ***anac.*** ant-c.[85] arg-n. ***ars.*** asaf. bar-c. canth. caust. cham. ***chin. cinnb.*** con. graph.[111] hyos. iod. mosch. ***nat-c.*** **NUX-V.** ol-an. podo. ptel.[36] ***puls.*** til. zinc.
Sadness; eating, amel.: am-c. am-m. clem. kali-bi. mag-m. tarent.
Sadness; eating, desire for, with: ign.[193]
Sadness; errors of diet, from: **NAT-C.**
Sadness; food, with aversion of: ***plat.***[54]
Secretive; eating, while: lac-h.[229]
Talk; indisposed, eating after: aloe arg-n. ferr-ma. mez. plb.
Thoughts; eating, of, unpleasant: tanac.[25]
Unconsciousness; appetite, before want of: ***calad.***[54]
Watchfulness; everyone eating, of: sulph.[160]

CHOC. Sh, 41 - When hearing talk of babies, breasts aching with a sensation as if filling up with milk — an aching fullness. An image came to me where I found myself suckling young hairy babies, sometimes animals, especially hedgehogs.

Sh, 96 - Everything seems right and in order now. I feel much better. Only survival matters, simpler. All the trivial affairs and worries of humans are irrelevant. The only things that matter are food and warmth. I need just enough to eat — red berries. On a walk I saw red berries and thought everything is there, no problem. I have no worries like humans have —no decision making —there isn't any choice.

Sh, 97 - I feel my kids are ready to go, but I have to get back to the younger ones to feed. Felt I could walk home (300 miles), a feeling that I should never go further than I could walk.

Sh, 106 - I feel excited —a purpose in me — as if geared up and something is about to happen. Is nice. There is no choice involved. It just is. A feeling that you know that every part of you is right and must be right to go forward. All the senses must be there, not like my old blithering-around in distraction. Just one objective —find food!

Sh, 152 - Wanted to eat slugs and grasshoppers. I could feel how they would be in my mouth while they were still alive and wriggling. (Has been vegetarian for twenty years).

HALI-L. Sh, 595 - I look at rabbits and birds in a different light. Wondering how a rabbit would taste raw. What would the fur taste like? 20, 30C, XX:XX:XX

Sh, 867 - Memories of being fed as a child and having no choice of what to eat. 20, 30C, 08:23:50

Sh, 869 - Realized that the wind is more nourishing than food. 20, 30C, 09:XX:XX

EGOTISM

Ailments from; egotism: ***calc. lach. lyc.*** med.[162] merc. ***pall. plat.*** sil. ***sulph.***

Ambition; much, fame, for: alum.[30] con.[30] graph.[30] ***lach.***[30] **NUX-V.**[30] staph.[30]

Avarice; wants all for himself: puls.[30]

Busy; himself, with: mag-m.[36] staph.[36]

Delusions; sun, travels around earth: ***verat.***[54]

Egotism, self-esteem: act-sp.[54] agar.[162] alco.[36] anac.[116] anan.[54] androc.[222] arn.[30] aur.[116] bufo[171] ***calc.*** cimic.[54] croto-t.[102] cur.[36] hydrog.[222] ***lach.*** lap-gr-m.[194] lap-mar-c.[194] ***lyc.***[30] med. merc. nux-v.[5] ***pall.*** par.[10] phos.[62] **PLAT.** ***sil.*** staph.[30] stram.[116] ***sulph. verat.***[30]

Egotism; self-esteem, nymphomania, in: ***agar.***[54]

Egotism; self-esteem, over-estimation of him self: cic.[137]

Egotism; self-esteem, reciting their exploits: agar.[36]

Egotism; self-esteem, speaking always about themselves in company: lach.[30] par.[10] staph.[30]

Haughty; look self-contented: ferr.[54] ferr-ma.[10]

Hysteria; attention, from: tarent.[47]

Love; herself, towards: germ.[222]

Love; self, of, excessive: plat.[10]

Selfishness, egotism: agar. androc.[222] anh.[119] ars.[102] asaf. bell.[30] ***calc.***[30] calc-f.[53] caust.[30] cench.[58] chin.[185] choc.[222] cic.[137] croto-t. hydrog.[222] ign. lach.[58] lap-mar-c.[194] lyc.[30] med. merc.[30] mosch. nat-m.[189] nux-v.[30] ozone[227] pall.[5] phos.[189] plat.[5] ***puls.*** pyrus senec.[111] sep.[102] sil.[30] ***sulph.*** tarent.[137] tub.[162] valer.

Selfishness, express oneself, desire to: anh.[119]

Selfishness, occupied at first with himself and besides with others for his own profit and loss for others: bell.[30] calc.[30] nux-v.[30]

Smiling; self-satisfied: anan.[36]

Talk; pleasure in his own talking: nat-m. par. stram. sulph.[189]

Thoughts; himself, about, think of anyone besides, cannot: croto-t.[54]

Thoughts; himself, desires to be diverted from thoughts of himself: camph.[54]

Thoughts; suffering, of his own: sabal.[137]

Thoughts; thoughtful, himself, about: cic.[36] viol-o.[36]

Unsympathetic; unscrupulous, friends and family, even towards closest: lap-gr-m.[194]

Unsympathetic; unscrupulous, idleness, from: con.[54]

ADAM. 154 - Very selfish to other peoples needs and cares —unseeing in that way. I do not want to listen to my mother's problems, or my friends'. 20, 1M, 11:XX:XX

AGAR. He, 23 - Great selfishness. 0 Nymphomania.

ANDROC. Sh, 41 - Feels much more self centred —have given up all the permanent favours I do for people —I don't want to do any more. Feel I need more time for me. I must feel guilt but I don't think I do. I feel the nasty side of my character is emerging much more aggressive and domineering. I don't want peoples' good opinion of me as someone who is nice — very unusual. (7)

Sh, 112 - Became excited to anger and confrontation. She was not aware of hurting others' feelings and did not seem to care. Could not appreciate anyone else's feeling. Later she reflected on her actions and felt ashamed. (12)

CHOC. Sh, 331 - I became selfish, impatient and intolerant. Behaved in a strange way -hard and quarrelsome -snapping at people. Could not stand people wasting time or being inefficient, I wanted things done immediately.[35], 30C, XX:XX:XX:

CUR. Al, 9 - Melancholy, egotistical, envious, obstinate...

HYDROG. Sh, 29 - I've experienced a lot more egotism in the last few weeks. I feel frustrated by the limitations of the ego. 16, 30C, XX:XX:XX

LYC. He, 38 - Parsimonious (economical), greedy (avaricious), malicious (malevolent) and pusillanimous.(cowardice)

MERC. He, 44 - Ailments from mortification; from insults; from egotism.

He, 49 - Ailments from mortification; from insults; from egotism.

SIL. He, 6 - Affections from egotism. (ailments from)

SULPH. He, 59 - Egotism.

THUJ. Al, 11 - He often dreamed in a clear day, with open eyes...; in this he especially reveled in a overpowering selfishness, himself the central point about which everything must turn, with an intoxicated feeling of the most joyous self-satisfaction, ... (egotism)

VERAT. He, 26 - Chases (pursue, hunt) his family out of house ; declares the sun travels around the earth (geocentric); fear of death, restlessness, despair...

EMPTY

Confusion of mind; identity, own, as if it were not his: alum.[5] lach.[5] nat-m.[5] thuj.[5]

Delusions; body, brain, far from skull, as if too: staph.
- body, hollow, body, whole: aur.[5] ***kali-c.***[8] nux-v.[162] pall.[36]
- body, hollow, organs, in: ***cocc.***[102] oxyt.[102]
- emptiness: ***calad.***[122] **COCC.**[122] ign.[122] ***kali-c.***[122] ***mur-ac.***[122] ***olnd.***[122] **PULS.**[122] sars.[122] **SEP.**[122] stann.[122] ***sulph.***[122] ***zing.***[122]
- emptiness, around him and under him, on standing: kali-br.[139]
- emptiness, behind him on turning around: kali-c.[139]
- emptiness, fainting sensation, with: **SEP.**[122]
- emptiness, internal: aur.[122]
- hollow, whole body is: aur. ***kali-c.*** nux-v. pall.
- space, empty space between brain and skull, that there is: caust.
- stepping, empty space, on: dubin.[72]

Ego, feels devoid of: lap-c-b.[194]

Emptiness of the mind, sensation of: am-c.[137] asar. calad.[122] cand-a.[239] cann-i.[36] **COCC.**[122] ***gels.***[54] germ.[222] **IGN.**[122] ***kali-c.***[122] mur-ac.[122] oena.[36] ***olnd.***[122] ozone[227] ***plat.***[54] **PULS.**[122] sars.[122] **SEP.**[122] **STANN.**[122] stry.[36] ***sulph.***[122] ***zing.***[122]

Staring; thoughtless: androc.[222] brom.[54] carbn-s.[54] carc.[227] cench.[58] choc.[222] cic.[5] **HELL.**[54] ***hydr-ac.***[54] hyos.[58] ign.[8] lap-mar-c.[194] ***merc-c.***[54] ***puls.***[54] ran-b.[54] stram.[58]

Thoughts; vacancy of: chlol.[36] ***gels.***[36] hydrog.[222] lyc.[10] oena.[36] phos.[1]

ENEMY

Affability; enemy, to an: alco.[36]

Anxiety; pursued, as if, enemies, by: dros.[36]

Contemptuous; opponents, for: com.[36]

Delusions; enemy, everyone is an: ***merc.*** plat. ***puls.***[54]
- enemy, rest, allows him no: dros.[139]
- enemy, surrounded by enemies: ***anac.*** cand-a.[239] carbn-s. ***crot-h.*** dros.[1] lap-mar-c.[194] ***merc.***
- enemy, under the bed, is: am-m.
- pursued by enemies: absin. ***anac.***[102] ars. aur. ***bell. chin.*** cic. ***cocain.***[102] con. crot-h. cupr. cycl.[162] dros. hell. ***hyos.*** kali-br. ***lach.*** lepi. lyc. med.[108] meli. merc. nat-c. nux-v.[102] plb. ***puls.*** rhus-t. sil. stram. stry. zinc.

Dreams; enemies: arg. con. hydrog.[222] ptel.
- ➤ pursued, enemies, by: con.
- ➤ stab, antagonist, his: nat-c.[36] ozone[227]
- ➤ stabbed, antagonist in chest, with large knife, his: nat-c.[36]

Fear; enemies, of: anac.[149] dros.[172] hyos.[102]
- ✦ enemies, pursuing: bell.[172] sil.[172]

ABSIN. Al,S-7 - Hallucination of vision and of hearing, that is pursued by imaginary enemies; hallucinations of various kinds, of naked women, etc.

ANAC. Al, 16 - Anxiety in all his actions; everything appears to him more terrible; he imagine himself surrounded with enemies; then he feels warm and the blood seems to boil within him.

Ha, 6 - Timorous in all his actions; he views everything more anxiously and timidly, always thinks of being surrounded by enemies, then he becomes hot, his blood seems to boil in his chest.

CARBN-S. Al-S, 753 - At one time during the night he seemed to be surrounded by enemies; persons were coming to harm him;...

CHIN. He, 10 - Fixed idea that he is unhappy, persecuted by enemies.

He, 11 - She thinks she is very unfortunate and constantly harassed (molested, tormented) by enemies.

CROT-H. He, 5-...imagines himself surrounded by enemies or hideous animals;...

DROS. Al, 11 - Anxiety as if his enemies allowed him no rest, but persecuted and pursued him.

Ha, 274 - Anxiety, as if his enemies would not leave him quiet, envied (competition, rivalry, opposition, spite) and persecuted him.

LACH. He, 8 - Thinks: she is somebody else in the hands (seized) of a stronger power; (supremacy, superiority).or that she is dead, and preparations are made for funeral (cortege) or that she is nearly dead and wishes some one would help her off; herself pursued by enemies, or fears medicine is poison; there are robbers in house and wants to jump out the window; herself under super-human control; visions real, he will die. (helplessness, desire; aid, comfort, salvation)

He, 9 - Imagines he is followed (pursued) by enemies who are trying to harm (hurt, injure) him; attempts to leave room as if frightened by visions behind him.

He, 21-...imagines he is followed by enemies who are trying to harm him; attempts to leave room as if frightened by visions behind him.

MERC. Ha, 1256 - All day long sulky and distrustful (suspicious); he almost insulted those about him, and regarded them all as his greatest enemies.(opponent, rival)

He, 16 - Great restlessness as if he had committed a great crime; ...considers everybody his enemy;...great inclination when walking to take people by the nose;...(desire: conduct, direct, guide)

He, 34 - Inexpressive pain of soul and body, anxious restlessness, as if some evil impended ...; disgusted (revolt) with himself, has not courage (cowardice) to live; constant suspicion (distrust), considering everybody his enemy.

He, 37 - Morose and mistrustful; treated his associates almost insultingly, looked upon every one as his worst enemy.

NAT-C. Al, 1114 - Dream of a quarrel, in which he stabbed his antagonist (enemy) in the chest with a large knife.

PULS. He, 53-...afraid of everybody; considers every one her enemy, despairs of everything; ...;trusts no one;.. (suspicious)

RHUS-T. Al, 32 - He thought an enemy want to poison him.

Ha, 965 - He imagines an enemy seeks to poison him.

ENERGY

Anxiety; weakness, with: acon.[10] aeth.[54] agn.[10] alum.[10] am-c.[1] ang.[54] ars.[60] aur.[1] bor.[10] calc.[1] carb-an.[10] carb-v.[10] caust.[1] cic.[10] ign.[10] kali-n.[10] mag-c.[10] nit-s-d.[60] phos.[10] rhus-t.[1] sil.[10] verat.[10]

Brooding; disappointment, cardiac weakness, with: ***ph-ac.***[54]

Buoyancy: arum-d.[25] cimic.[25] eucal.[54] ***fl-ac.***[54] phys.[25] sarr.[54] scut.[25]

Cowardice; weakness, with, must keep her bed (in pregnancy): ***stann.***[54]

Delirium; exaltation of strength, with: ***agar.*** ***aur.*** hyos. sec.[162] stram. tarent.[162]

Delusions; blood, rushed through like roar of many waters: alumn.[58] cann-i.

- energy is moving around in the air: hydrog.[222]
- prostration, cannot endure such utter: ***chin-ar.***[54] eup-per.[139]
- runs, never before, she can run like: agar.[139]
- strong, he is: androc.[222] germ.[222] hydrog.[222]
- vitality, vivid conscious of usually unnoticed operations of: cann-i.[36]

Desires; strength, feats of: coca[36]

Dreams; amorous, weakness, with, in both sexes: plat.[54]

➤ steam: com.[58]

➤ weakness: ambr.[10]
Exhilaration; strength, with increased: ziz.[85]
Fancies; power, increased, of: **LACH.**[5] op.[5] viol-o.[5]
Fancies; power, wanting of, decreased: cann-s.[5] sel.[5]
Fear; death, strength, with loss of: ***rhus-t.***[54]
✦ joints are weak, that: sep.
✦ stress, of breaking down under: lyc.[102]
Handle things anymore, cannot, overwhelmed by stress: anh.[204] ***bamb-a.***[1184] bar-n.[209] calc.[198] calc-p.[198] caust.[198] cocc.[187] lac-eq.[204] med.[198] nat-n.[209] ph-ac.[188] sulph.[198]
Helplessness; feeling of, weakness, from, in mental exertion: ***gels.***[54]
Indifference; emaciation and weakness, especially with: **PH-AC.**[54]
Insanity; strength increased, with: agar. ***bell.*** canth. cori-r. hyos. ***plb.***[162] ***stram.*** **TARENT.**
Irritability; coition, after, agg., weakness, with: calc.[102]
Irritability; sexual, weakness, with: ***pic-ac.***
Lasciviousness; eating, after, with feeling of weakness in parts: lyss.[54]
Magnetic state, feeling of personal power increased: androc.[222] crot-c.[36] phos.[8]
Memory; weakness, business, for: agn. androc.[222] chel. fl-ac. hyos. kali-c. kreos. mag-c.[10] phos. sabin. sel. sulph. tell. tep
Memory; weakness, coition, after exhausting: ***sec.***[54]
Memory; weakness, fear, from: ***anac.***[54] ***cupr.***[54]
Memory; weakness, sexual excesses, from: agn.[102] anac.[102] arg-n.[102] aur.[102] calad. **CALC.**[54] chin.[102] **DIG.**[54] kali-br.[72] ***nat-ar.*** nat-m.[102] nux-v.[102] ***ph-ac.***[102] **PHOS.**[54] **STAPH.**[54]
Memory; weakness, time, for: bamb-a.[1184] ***lach.***[10] merc.
Prostration; cares, from: ph-ac.[58] pic-ac.[58]
Prostration; coition, after: ***calc.***[122] coca[54] sep.[5]
Prostration; grief, from: ign.[137] **NUX-M.**[137] phys.[137]
Prostration; grief, from long: **IGN.**[54] kali-br.[137]
Prostration; sexual excesses, after: sel.[58]
Prostration; shock, from, feels so tired, wants to lie down and sleep: ***pic-ac.***[54]
Rage; strength increased: ***agar.*** **BELL.** hyos.[10]
Sadness; alternating with, energy, physical: ***aur.*** hir.[149]
Strength increased, mental: anag.[36] anh.[119] ars.[36] camph.[36] cann-i.[36] clem.[36] cod.[36] dig.[36] eaux[36] ferr.[36] hyper.[122] lach.[116] nep.[144] op.[36] pip-m.[36] thea.[36] thuj.[36] verat.[36] visc.[119]
Strength increased, mental; sensation: calc.[5] ozone[227]
Strength increased, mental; sensation, alternating with sadness and weeping: ozone[227]

ABROT. He, 2 - No capacity for thinking, as if all bodily and mental power were gone.
ACON. Ha, 505 - Morose, as though she had no life in her. (animation)
Ha, 514 - Palpitation of the heart with great anxiety, oppression of the breathing and great weariness (lassitude) in all limbs...
Ha, 511 - After vomiting, immediate revival of hope.
Ha, 535 - Lively power of imagination.
ADAM. Sh, 122 - I do not want to go out at all, just need to be on my own. Unusual for me and I feel drained. 12, 30C, 22:XX:XX.
Sh, 313, I feel very tall and large. I am a giant, 12:30 a.m. -powerful feeling. 20, 1M, 09:XX:XX
Sh, 317 - Enjoy the powerful night force. I can fly in the dark. 16, 12C, 35:XX:XX
Sh, 423 - Extreme weakness, painful cough, weak chest. Feels like TB or wasting disease. 22, 200C, 01:XX:XX
AGAR. Al, 3 - Fearless, menacing, mischievous (rude) frenzy; also, frenzy which causes the patient to assail and injure himself, with great exertion of power.
Al, 16-.... reciting (enumerate) before the beauties of the tribe their exploits (adventures) in war or the chase.(hunting) Their physical strength is increased...(boasting)
Al, 19 - During the intoxication they lift and carry the heaviest loads, take long steps and jump over small objects, as if trunks of trees lay in their way.
Al, 29 - Taken in moderation it excites the intellect and inspires cheerfulness and courage.
Ha, 23 - Fearless, threatening, destructive frenzy, also such as turns against itself and injures itself, combined with great exertion of strength.
ALUM. Ha, 52 - Everything is easy to him, the powers of his understanding and of his body seem excited.

AM-C. Ha, 9 - Many afternoons she is seized with weakness and timidity, so that she cannot control herself and knew not what to do;...

AMBR. Ha, 483 - Sad thoughts take possession of him, with sinking feeling about the heart; he is for a long time depressed in spirits.

ANAC. Al, 15 - The future appears dangerous to him, as if nothing but misfortune and danger were reserved for him; want of confidence in his strength (vigor, force) and despondency.

ANDROC. Sh, 45 - Incredible upsurge of energy —laughing, felt very high, then low, then high again. (4, 29)

Sh, 99 - Felt angry, did not want to speak to anyone, in the evening with friends he felt very lively, self-confident and forceful, rather biting at times. (4)

Sh, 124 - In the street, he felt aggressive and very strong, that his umbrella was a knife, and desired to smash people up. (29)

Sh, 129 - It seemed as though he was a different person, very similar to the way he had been in adolescence, but in a much more powerful manner. These emotions were so intense he wanted to rip his chest apart to let them out. He lost all control over his emotions, which seemed to come from a deep and distant part of himself, a darker side. He desired to continue the proving for the rest of his life. (29)

ANG. Al, 16 - Lively mood; he is confident he can achieve everything with vigor.

Ha, 298 - Cheerfulness and self-confidence that he can undertake anything with power.

ARG-N. He, 52 - Frequent attacks of anxiety with weakness in legs, ... (walking?)

He, 56 - Was utterly (complete) bereft(deprived) of all power of will.

He, 18 - Feels as if everything at home had changed and that his mind is weak.

He, 43 - Alarmed by vertigo and weakness of left side.

ARN. Al, 31 - Excessive inclination to perform many and long literary labors, without possessing the strength which is required to terminate them without injuring health.

ARS. Al, 57 - Anguish from the heart, interrupted by attacks of weakness.

Al-S, 2893 - The whole head sick, the heart faint, she awoke in the morning wretched, her life a burden (load) weariness the day's portion, and each succeeding day like its predecessor, unless (except) physic (laxative) helped her with its little aid.

Ha, 1035 - He is cold, shivers and weeps, and thinks, in his despair, (hopelessness, despairing) that nothing can help him, (helplessness) and he must die; followed by general exhaustion.

ASTER. Al, 5 - Melancholy, alternating with almost intolerable cerebral excitement; she is inclined to give herself up to mental or bodily work, to walk, or engage in a violent exercise;...

AUR-M. He, 11 - Loss of energy; diminished virility; unrefreshing sleep.

AUR. Ha, 347 - Always very restless and undecided (doubtful) -thought he was neglecting something for which he must incur (obtain) reproach -...he seemed to carry about this restlessness with him in his inmost (deepest) parts ; this condition deprived him of all perseverance, all energy.

Ha, 351 - Great weakness and anxiety, so that he is thought (delusion) to be near death.

Ha, 7 - Great anxiety and weakness, so that he is thought to be near death.

Ha, 13 - Restless and undecided, without perceptible ebullition of the blood; he always thinks he is neglecting something for which he will be reproached; he seems to carry with him this internal restlessness, and it took from him all perseverance and energy.

BAPT. He, 16 - Aversion... to hear conversation about sickness or injuries; feeble mind. (impressionable) 0Spasmodic stricture of esophagus.

BELL. Al, 109 - A tailor was poisoned with a belladona injection, and for fifteen hours, though speechless and insensible to external objects, went through all the customary operations of his trade with great vivacity and moved his lips as if in conversation.(busy)

Al, 134 - Great mirthfulness (happy) after supper; the vital powers were increased to an extraordinary degree for a quarter of an hour, after which came drowsiness.

Ha, 1422 - Along with burning heat of the body, with open, staring, and fixed eyes, such fury she must constantly be held fast in order to prevent her attacking others,...
Ha, 1365 - Excessive gaiety (happiness) after supper, the vital powers extraordinarily increased for a quarter of a hour, followed by drowsiness.
BOV. Al, 5 - Very courageous and vigorous; he would like to fight with everybody.
BRY. He, 4 - So weak in mind that his ideas vanish (empty) as if he would faint, ...
CALC. Ha, 65 - Great weakness of the imaginative (creative) faculty; with a very slight exertion in speaking, he felt as if his brain was paralyzed, ...;he could not think, nor recollect what was spoken of, with muddled (confused) feeling in the head.(lost: imagination, thoughts)
CANN-I. Al, 42 - The soul seemed to be separated from the body, and to look down upon it, and view all the motions of the vital processes, and to be able to pass and repass though the solid walls of the room, and to view the landscape (view) beyond.
Al, 62 - It seemed as though I was transparent; the fire in the grate seemed to shine through me, and to warm the marrow of the bones.
Al, 63 - His body seemed to him become transparent, and he imagined he saw within his breast the hashish he had eaten in the form of an emerald, from which issued millions of little sparks.
CARB-AN. He, 1 - Unclouded consciousness and great anguish with sinking of vital forces.
CAUST. He, 42 - Great apprehension whenever anything happens; despondent, depressed, most excessive exhaustion and prostration.
CHOC. Sh, 2 - Feel very excited, very alive, bright and efficient. Had an image of a hedgehog's face.
Sh, 52 - My right hand feels bigger and wider and I feel more powerful. But my wrists feel weaker and flatter. Sensation of opening of hands and tightness in the forearm.
COFF-T. Al, 15 - It gives rise to a need of creative activity, a vivacity of thought, a versatility and ardor of desire, more favorable to the exaggerated expression of ideas previously formed, than to the quiet examination of new conceptions.
COFF. He, 8 - Great loquacity, brain feels clear and is active, he feels strong enough to do anything, feels impelled to push things; veneration for the Supreme Being and love for family; benevolence excited.
CON. Al, 15 - Tendency to laugh, with loss of vital energy.
CROC. Al, 18 - Irresistible inclination to joke and laugh, with great prostration, and great dilatation of the pupils.
DROS. Ha, 269 - Anxiety with feeling of heat quickly running all over the body, but especially all over the face, as though he were about to receive bad news ...rigor all over the body, without heat and without thirst.
EUCAL. He, 2 - Irresistible desire to move about, with a feeling of buoyancy (happiness) and increased strength.
GELS. Al, 2 - General vivacity after rising.
He, 27 - Mental exertions cause a sense of helplessness (disability) from brain-weakness; inability to attend to anything requiring thought.
GERM. Sh, 99 - Came in contact with very much hate and disgust within, and it made a deep impression on me. I have to be reconciled with those parts of me. I think that power can be used in a different way - not so destructive. I am no person. Feel I have no power when I meet people. Sometimes I feel I disappear. I am not in my body. My hands feel gone. My feet are cold; I don't like them. Yet I feel I have great power inside, especially I feel it when I get angry or when I sing. 18, 30C, 46:XX:XX
Sh, 113 - Sometimes I don't want to show my strength. I keep it back. I am afraid that others will feel inferior and I don't want them to, because I feel it so much myself. 18, 30C, 26:XX:XX
Sh, 100 - Cannot feel pleasure or sorrow. Everything is Chaos. Cannot restore my energy. Totally meaningless. Feels like an empty battery. Cannot take care of the kids as I should. 18, 30C, 183:XX:XX
GLON. Al, 18 - Immediate effect, confusion of ideas, and loss of strength; with diminished power of tongue.
HALI-L. Sh, 84 - Sensitive to energy. A lot of

synchronicity going on. At a seminar, the teacher talked about the same topic I wrote a paper on. I met people from the same town I grew up in. When I wanted to get on to another subject, someone else would bring it up. I'd just answer the teacher's questions and it would be right. 08, 30C, 12:XX:XX

Sh, 185 - I have a higher energy and things happen. I think of something and immediately someone hands it to me. The power is greater so I have to make sure the goals are right. Have to be in perfect order because goals will happen. 08, 30C, 12:XX:XX

Sh, 614 - Full of energy in the morning. Run and walk in the sea, amazed at my high energy. Feel like I have to let out lack of sex. Want partner badly but mad at her and at myself for being so open. Feel speedy. 02, 30C, 08:03:XX

Sh, 648 - Down side, dark side, feels like the gates between the unconscious and conscious are open. Hurricane-like feeling of unconscious energy. Like the gates of hell are open. No barrier. Extreme amount of power. Darkness. Internal pressure. Dogs guard the gates of Hades. A lot of internal pressure-type feeling all day. 13, 30C, 10:XX:XX

Sh, 659 - Less maniacal type feeling but still high amount of energy. Excessive energy but not uncontrollable. Strong sense of well being. Meditation very strong. 13, 30C, 08:XX:XX

Sh, 664 - Feel deflated, calmer and flatter. The feeling of going mad goes back to when I was drinking 15 years ago. That feeling of not being able to decide what to do. Today feeling flat, exhausted; a wonderful day outside, unable to enjoy it. Feeling unenergized, although glad the craziness is gone. I felt I was on speed with emotions. I'm glad I antidoted that thing; feel like an empty balloon. It could have gotten down to a dangerous place. Reminded me of going mad; like the energy it gave me. Felt hooked on the remedy. 02, 30C, 12:XX:XX

Sh, 728 - Felt a tremendous power. Me in bed with my arms stretched out in the shape of a cross. The horizontal line across was powerful. 20, 30C, 01:00:58

HELL. He, 11 - Psychical conditions occupying a place between melancholia and mania, and in conditions where true depression and weakness is present, in which the patient is governed by a fixed idea.

HYDROG. Sh, 15 - I felt in the presence of a totally pure energy, like meeting God and feeling totally unworthy or like meeting a lover and feeling unworthy — realizing all the mistakes of a lifetime. This pure energy was around for some time protecting me. I feel this unification cleared out lifetimes of symptomatology for me. The joining with this energy was as if a male energy joined with me sexually, but with no desire, pleasure or pain involved. This unification with the male energy lasted quite a few days — I'm not used to seeing myself as a man. The morning after this unifying with the higher presence, I collapsed in emotional overflow. All my grief and pain came out. I was doubled upon the floor and went into a deep state of catharsis. It is not possible to describe where I went as there are no concepts applicable. I felt overflowing love for humanity and wanted to give everything away. My mind turned to the Buddha. It was like seeing the complete picture instead of fragmented bits. (These primary effects lasted about 28 days, then changing to a paranoia state). 16, 30C, 07.XX.XX

Sh, 165 - I thought I could see energy moving around in the air. Colours looked bright and everything looked beautiful. 16, 30C, 25:XX:XX

Sh, 167 - Thought or vision that I was taller or stronger than I was. 28, 200C, 02:01:XX

Sh, 294 - Spirits uplifted by wonderful weather. Felt strong, positive and adventurous. 04, 12C, 32:XX:XX

HYOS. Ha, 517 - Over-busy: he thought he was more active and stronger (powerful, Herculean) than he actually was.

Ha, 550 - He displays uncontrollable strength in his fury.

IOD. Al, 6 - Remarkably lively and talkative, no one else is able to get in a word.

Ha, 26 - Her phlegmatic disposition has disappeared; she has become blooming (growing), stronger and more lively.

IRID. Sh, 140 - Felt flat, not much energy. Will be glad when it's daylight. When daylight comes you feel lifted. D6

KALI-BR. Al, 16 - A consciousness that the currents or sources of psychical force are hampered...(obstructed) sometimes makes an intellectual patient who is moderately bromized, reason himself into depression....

He, 4-...constant worry, fears to see people or to be spoken to;...failure of mental and bodily strength;...constantly busy, tying his shoes, fumbling in his pockets, picking threads, etc.

LAC-C. He, 40 - Feels weak, and nerves so thoroughly out of order, that she cannot bear one finger touch another.

LACH. Al, 43 - He is impelled to productive work in the evening, although he had been much fatigued during the day ... writes with the greatest freedom and increased vigor about everything he knows;...

He, 33-...want of self control; lascivious; felt as if she was clear (pure) animal right through, whilst of all mental power was dormant; sensation as if hands of stronger power, as if charmed (enchanted), and as if could not break the spell (charm). (possessed, wildness)

He, 14 - Delirium from overwatching, overfatigue; loss of fluids; excessive study.

LIL-T. Al, 27 - Symptoms came down on her like a sudden cloud, ...she lost vigor and snap (vitality), ...with all this depression comes a desire for fine (quality) things of all kinds; she is dissatisfied with what she has and is envious of others. (sophistication)

LYC. Al, 44 - Loss of confidence in his own vigor.

Ha, 32 - Lack of confidence in his strength.(power, vigor)

He, 30 - Loss (want) of confidence; in his own vigor (vitality, strength); in physician and remedies.

LYSS. Al,N-46 - After fainting (weak) spell he wrote on paper: I am forsaken by all; even the birds of heaven, they do not look at me (despised), do not fed me if hungry (helplessness) ; I hunger with the young ones and am thirsty with their she ones (starving); my nest (house) is made out of dirt (soiled), not gotten by my own exertions (efforts), but by driving them out of their nests (home) and sitting there with the females and the young.

Al,N-72 - An attack of mental depression and indifference quite (very) strange to him; feels as if he could do nothing; if he forces himself he lacks mental power.

He, 72 - An attack of mental depression and indifference quite strange to him; feels as if he could do nothing; if he forces himself he lacks mental power.

MANG. Ha, 325 - Cross and discontented with himself, and concerned about future..., considers himself very weak (stupid) in mind, and makes mistakes whenever he speaks.

MERC. He, 3 - Loss of will (command, intentions, resolutions,) power.(vigor)

MUR-AC. Al, 15 - The brightness (lively, vivid) of his disposition constantly diminished, until in the evening he became very fretful (irritable).

MURX. Al, 4 - It made me miserable; I was so low-spirited that I gave up everything; I had no strength left.

NAT-C. Al, 53 - Sensation of loss of will power, in the morning on waking.

NAT-M. Al, 51 - Attacks of complete hopelessness and internal despair, that deprived him of all power.

Ha, 8 - He sorrowfully torments (torture) himself, by continually looking for disagreeable ideas, which weakens him.

Ha, 21 - Attacks of entire hopelessness (despairing) and internal despondency (despair) which take away all her strength.

NEON. Sh, 37 - On walking in the fresh air I suddenly felt as if I was cruising along on an energy which was not of my own muscular power. It seemed as if it was coming from somewhere else. It seemed effortless and unreal. I felt as if I was passing everyone else. 02, 6C, 13:XX:XX

Sh, 193 - Feel sad and depressed while walking outside in the cold, clear, open air. I don't want to be outside, and walk with head down. On returning inside, I feel in suspended animation. Listless, low energy. Want to close my eyes, which are dry, with heavy, slightly numb lids. I don't feel like working and would just like to go to sleep or read a good book in bed under covers. I still feel chilly from 5 minute walk outside though I've been inside and dressed warmly for 5 minutes. 06, 12C, 00:01:00

NIT-AC. He, 10 - Sadness, great fear of death, sensation of extreme weakness, even to trembling.

He, 14 - Often anxious about his illness; constantly thinks about his past troubles; mind weak and wandering.

He, 7 - Feels as though he had partly lost his will-power.

OP. Al, 69 - Great strength, courage, contentment with himself.

Al, 70 - Sensation of courage with activity, as if he could forcibly accomplish whatever was required without dread or fear, with a peculiar sensation of lustiness. (strong)

Al, 187 - The memory and mental powers generally became greatly impaired, attended by a miserable depression of spirits.

Ha, 621 - Feeling of courage and merriment (joy), so that he is as if he would carry out what was required with energy, without repugnance or fear, with a peculiar feeling of voluptuousness...(sensuality)

He, 22-... feeling of great strength; contempt of death;...indifference to joy and suffering.

PALL. He, 1 - Extremely fatigued in evening; feels mentally gone; is averse to speaking a foreign language which at other times he speaks fluently; it is too much of an exertion, he is tired of it. (lack of communication)

PETR. Ha, 1 - Sad and dispirited, with a sick (suffering) feeling owing (due) to weakness of the heart.

PHOS. Al, 80 - Mental depression, and a most uncommon fearfulness or timidity, with a great sense of fatigue.

He, 9 - Mental depression and a most uncommon fearfulness or timidity with great sense of fatigue.

He, 1 - Excited imagination; zoomagnetic (animal magnetism) condition; ecstasy; clairvoyance.

PLAT. He, 3 - Attacks of cheerfulness; increased feeling of strength.

He, 37-...depressed condition of physical powers; ...fear of approaching death; ... aversion to coition and yet dreams of intense lasciviousness,...

RHUS-T. Al, 27 - Anxiety, with loss of strength (power, energy, force), as if he would die, more after midnight than before.

Al, 4 - Full of sad thoughts, anxious and fearful, wherewith she gradually lost strength, and was obliged to lie down for hours in order to regain vigor.

Ha, 956 - Along with sinking (descend, submerge) of the strength, (vigor, energy, force) anxiety as if he must die, worse after than before midnight.

Ha, 964 - Full of sad thoughts, anxious and timorous (timid), during which she always lost her strength, (power) and must lie down for hours; in order to recover her strength. (inert, motionless)

He, 11 - Anxiety: while sitting was obliged to take hold (grasp, keep) of something because she did not think she could keep up (support) on account of the beating and drawing pains in limbs; and apprehension as if he wished to take his own life; with loss of strength (vigor, vitality) as if he would die.

SABIN. Al, 5-...music was intolerable, it penetrated marrow and bone,...feeling of weakness, debility.

SANT. Al, 6-...irresolution and want of confidence in my own powers as to render me quite unfit for work of any kind;

SEC. Al, 36 - The greatest depression of mind and loss of strength, a very sick feeling.

SEP. Al, 53 - Concerned about her health, anxious, irritated, and very weak.

Ha, 8 - Troubled (worried) about her health (vigor) anxious, irritated and very weak.

Ha, 59 - Great indifference to everything, no real vital feeling.

SIL. Ha, 36 - Even from little conversation, his head at once becomes muddled (confusion) and there is general exhaustion,...

He, 4 - Reading and writing fatigue, cannot bear to think.

SPIG. Al, 3 - Lively contented, and trustful mood, alternating with palpitation and anxious oppression of the chest.

STANN. He, 3 - Uneasy, does not know what to do with himself pains > by walking, yet so weak he soon must die.

STAPH. Ha, 693 - Phlegmatic (indifferent), prostrate mind and sad disposition, unsympathetic, indifferent to all externals, yet not cross or exhausted.

STRAM. Ha, 542 - Exertion of strength: a strong man could scarcely hold him down in bed.

He, 11 - Stupor: weakened intellect; torpor and fits; extreme excitement of sexual parts,...

SULPH. Al, 3800-....(DREAM) she walked about like a somnambulist, thought there was a fire, dressed herself, talked out of the window, and was frightened as she heard that it was nothing; for three days afterwards she was very weak, and felt bruised(hurt).

TAB. Al, 45 - He was incapacitated for business of any kind, weak irresolute, and despondent.

Al, 51 - Exalted action of the brain; copious flow of ideas; ...leaving me in the morning worn-out and sick, I would conceive and elaborate about twenty undertakings, of which probably not one would ever come to light.

TARAX. Al, 4 - Without occupation he is quite gloomy; does not know what to do, and cannot make up his mind to do anything.

THUJ. Al, 58 - Continual thoughts of dying (death), with increasing weakness.

Ha, 630 - Walking is performed with extreme ease; she feels as though her body were borne up by wings; she ran many miles in an uncommonly short time, and with unusual high spirits.

THYR. Al,N-[1]-...at times dangerous and homicidal, would put her arms round the necks of other patients so tightly as almost to strangle them (in this case the insanity was primary and the myxedema secondary; both conditions were removed). Evinced increased vivacity by quarreling with another patient about a trifling difference of opinion.

TUB. Al,N-36 - Somnolence; loss of vital power; great physical weakness. (vigor)

UST. He, 2 - Very sad, cries frequently; excessively prostrated from sexual abuse and loss of semen; sleep restless.

VERAT-V. He, 6 - Loquacity, with exaltation of ideas, or an exalted opinion of her own ideas and powers; everything seems clear to her; now clearly understands former mysterious things; wants no medicine, as that will restore her to former condition;...

VERAT. Ha, 709 - He is too lively (energetic), eccentric, extravagant.(wasteful)

He, 29-...prays says it is a secret (secretive, mysterious) and a misfortune; ...saying she must strengthen (encourage) herself, ...imagines herself in heaven (elevated, sublime, noble) talking with God.

ENVY

Aversion; faces, to laughing: m-aust.[85]

Break things, desire to, possession, parents most prized: tub.[189]

Delirium; envy, with: lyc.[36]

Disgust; exhilaration, of others, at: m-aust.[10]

Disgust; laughing of others, at: ambr.[10]

Envy: ***am-c.***[30] ars. bry. calc. cench.[58] cub. cur. germ.[222] hell. lach. lap-mar-c.[194] lil-t. lyc. nat-c. nux-v.[30] ***plat.***[30] ***puls.*** sac-alb.[210] sarr. sep. spig.[30] ***staph.*** sulph.[30] zinc.[36]

Envy; avidity, and: ***ars.***[30] ***chin.***[30] lyc.[116] nit-ac.[30] nux-v.[30] ph-ac.[30] ***puls.*** rhus-t.[30] sep.[116] stann.[30] staph.[30] sulph.[30]

Envy; hate and: am-c.[30] am-m.[30] calc.[30] nat-c.[30] nat-m.[30] nit-ac.[30] puls.[30]

Envy; qualities of others, at: ars.[122] calc.[122] lach.[122] lyc.[122] puls.[122] sulph.[122]

Evil to others, wishes: nat-c.[1]

Happy; seeing others, agg.: hell.[137] helon.[137]

Hatred; persons, of, enjoying life, who are: medus.[168]

Insanity; envy, with: **LYC.**[30]

Jealousy; children, in, when a new baby takes the attention of the family away: ***hyos.***[8] ign.[8]

Jealousy; happy, seeing others: hell.[137]

Jealousy; others getting all attention: ozone[227]

Jealousy; value or appreciate anything, desires that others shall not: ***ip.***[54]

Sadness; happy, on seeing others: cic.[36] hell.[1] helon.

Slander; disposition to, denounce, and: ars.[30] lach.[30] nat-c.[30] nat-m.[30]

CIC. Ha, 232 - When others were gay he was sad.

CUR. Al, 9 - Melancholy, egotistical, envious, obstinate...

DROS. Ha, 272 - Extremely uneasy, sad disposition, all day he imagined he was being deceived (deluded, defrauded) by spiteful (hateful), envious people.

Ha, 274 - Anxiety, as if his enemies would not leave him quiet, envied (competition, rivalry, opposition, spite) and persecuted him.

GERM. Sh, 158 - Some persistent feelings coming up. Feel envious of a colleague who I feel manages so well. When I compare with myself I feel worthless and nothing. I feel like talking badly about her to my friends and I do this, even though she is not present. It takes a lot of my attention and energy. 21, 12C, 67:XX:XX.

HALI-L. Sh, 213 - I wanted to do more mothering while I was being mothered and at the same time not mothering the son I do have. Feeling envy of all families who had more children. Constant state of desire for something other than what I had. If busy, I wanted to be not busy. If no one calls, I felt nobody cares about me. Could find no comfort anywhere and felt isolatedalone. 01, 30C,, 21:XX:XX

Sh, 403 - For three weeks I was in a depression, unlike anything I have felt for a long time. Deep sense of low self-worth. Feeling invisible, uncared for and envious. I was lethargic, couldn't do anything. My practice dropped, patients just didn't show up. I felt I sunk as low as I needed to go, unmotivated. Felt unappreciative of all I have. Unappreciative of my life which I usually adore. Anger, dissatisfaction with life, isolating. I wasn't seeing anyone not even my husband, exhaustive. Had no dreams during the depression — unusual. I am emerging from it now. 01, 30C, 30:XX:XX-50:XX:XX

HELL. Al, 10 - He becomes melancholy on beholding (observe) a cheerful person, and then, for the first time, feels very unhappy.

Ha, 284 - On seeing a happy person he becomes melancholy and then only he feels very unhappy.

He, 24 - Dread of dying ; feels unhappy in presence of cheerful faces. (spite)

IP. Ha, 221 - Sulky humor, that despises (scorn, intolerant, antipathy) everything, and he desires that others also should not esteem or care for anything.

He, 12 - Morose mood that scorns everything, and desires also that others shall not appreciate or value anything.

IRID. Sh, 60 - Patient said she was going to get married, I thought "big mistake." Q17

LIL-T. Al, 27 - Symptoms came down on her like a sudden cloud, ...she lost vigor and snap (vitality), ...with all this depression comes a desire for fine (quality) things of all kinds; she is dissatisfied with what she has and is envious of others. (sophistication)

LYC. Al, 2 - Delirious, raging, envious, reproachful, presumptuous, and imperious.

Ha, 59 - Insanity and fury, breaking out in envy, pretensions (inflated) and ordering (dictatorial) others about.

PULS. Al, 9 - Envious, avaricious, unsatisfied, greedy, he would gladly have everything, to himself.

Ha, 1125 - Envious, avaricious, dissatisfied, greedy, wants to have everything for himself.

He, 36 - Mistrust; envy; covetousness (avidity); dislike to people.

STAPH. He, 7 - Suffering from pride, envy (spite) or chagrin (shame, dishonor) .

ESCAPE

Anxiety; fly away, as if she must, no peace anywhere: ***bell.***[54]

Anxiety; night, escape, with desire to: merc.[54]

Delirium tremens; escape, attempts to: ***bell.***[116] stram.[116]

Delirium; anxious, approaching him, of everyone, shrinking from them: ***cupr.***[54]

Delirium; quiet, alternating with restlessness and desire to run away: ***chlor.***[54]

Delusions; creep into himself, has to, he could not sufficiently crouch together: ***cimx.***[54]

- fly, run away, must: ars-s-f.[139] bell.[139] verat.[139]
- pursued, spirits, evil, are pursuing him, runs around room, cries out: stram.[54]
- runs, away, has to run: ars-met.[139]
- runs, backward, is chased and runs: sep.[139]
- thieves, jump out of window, therefore wants to: ***lach.***[54]
- visions, hide, wishes to: bell.[54]
- visions, leave the room, attempts to, as if frightened by visions behind him: ***lach.***[54]
- wife, will run away from him: staph.

Desires; skip, to: pip-m.[36]

Dreams; animals, crocodiles, pursued by, and driving them away by sneezing: sedi.[36]
➤ animals, horses, running, away, waking her: indg.[36]
➤ danger, escaping from a: hep.
➤ danger, escaping, fruitless efforts of: ind.[54]
➤ escape, Buddhist monastery, from: lap-mar-c.[194]
➤ escape, of: hydrog.[222] ozone[227]
➤ famine, being left in a dungeon to die of; escaping by crawling out: ped.[36]
➤ fleeing, of: zinc.
➤ nightmare, inability to see, as if he could not escape from: cot.[36]
➤ pursued, run backwards, must: sep.[58]
➤ pursued, witch, by a, creeps from under the door like a haze: ozone[227]
➤ running: bell.[36]
➤ unsuccessful efforts to, escaping from danger, of: ind.
➤ window, jumping from: mag-m.
➤ window, trying to get out of, from a dream: calc-f.

Escape, attempts to: acon. ***aesc. agar.*** agar-st.[36] alco.[36] all-s. androc.[222] ***ars.*** ars-met. arum-t. bapt. bar-c. **BELL.**[122] ***bry.*** camph. caust. cham. chel.[5] chin. chlor. choc.[222] cic. ***cocc.*** coloc. ***crot-h. cupr. dig.*** germ.[222] ***glon.*** hell. **HYOS.** ign. iod.[5] kali-br.[5] lach. lap-c-b.[194] lil-t. lyc.[5] meli. merc. merc-c. mez.[5] ***nux-v. oena. op.*** oper.[102] ozone[227] phos. plb. puls. ran-b. rhus-t. rib-ac.[149] samb. sol-n. ***stram.*** sul-ac. sulph. tub. valer.[5] ***verat.*** zinc. zinc-p.[58]

Escape; attempts to, crime, for a fear of having committed a: ***merc.***[54]

Escape; attempts to, delirium, during: alco.[36] bell.[36] ***cupr.***[54] dig.[36] merc.[36] oena.[36] phos.[36] sol-m.[85] ***stram.***[36] sul-ac.[36] verat.[36]

Escape; attempts to, delusions, during: ars.[54] ***hyos.***[8] merc.[36] op.[5] puls.[5]

Escape; attempts to, dreams, in a world of: anh.[149]

Escape; attempts to, family, children, from her: am-c.[30] choc.[222] ***lyc.***[122] nux-v.[30] phos.[30] ***sep.***[30] staph.[30]

Escape; attempts to, house, wants to get out of: germ.[222] ***verat.***[54]

Escape; attempts to, house, wants to get out of, fright, after: merc.[54]

Escape; attempts to, night, anxiety at night, with: bell.[54] hyos.[54] ***merc.***[54]

Escape; attempts to, restrained with difficulty, is: ***stram.***[54] zinc.

Escape; attempts to, run away, to: alum.[58] bar-c.[54] ***bell.*** bry. chel.[111] ***cupr.*** dig. glon. hydrog.[222] hyos. ***merc.***[54] mez.[122] nux-v. op. ozone[227] rhus-t. ***verat.***

Escape; attempts to, run away, to, wants, and hide as she insists that everyone is looking at her: meli.[85]

Escape; attempts to, society, from: cic.[1]

Escape; attempts to, surrounded and captured from men, as if: ***hyos.***[54]

Escape; attempts to, throw himself into the river, tries to: ***hell.***[54]

Escape; attempts to, visit his daughter, wants to: ars.

Fear; escape, with desire to: ***bell.***[10] ***bry.***[10] coloc.[10] cupr.[10] dig.[10] merc.[54] puls.[10] stram.[10] verat.[10]
✦ jumps, out of the window: ars.
✦ shrinks back, seeing anyone: ***stram.***[54]

Hide; desire to, children, run away, and: meli.[137]

Hide; desire to, corner, in: camph.[8] elaps[36] puls.[8]

Impulse; run, to, away, hide and: meli.[102]

Impulse; run, to, followed, thinks he is: anac.[109]

Insanity; escape, desire to: ars.[10] ***bell.***[10] cupr.[10] dig.[10] nux-v.[10] ***op.***[30] stram.[30] verat.[10]

Loquacity; escape, with desire to: crot-h.[102]

Play; desire to, hide and seek, at: bell.[54]

Runs about; away from home: stram.[109] tub.[189]

Stupor; alternating with, escape, desire to: ***coloc.***[54]

Suicidal disposition; drowning, by, seeks to escape, after menses: ***ign.***[54]

Unconsciousness; alternating with, escape, desire to: ***coloc.***[54]

ADAM. Sh, 128 - I really need to escape, booked trip to France. 7, 6C 14:00:xx
Sh, 190 - Very unhappy with my body, I want to escape from it, to run away from myself. I want to go from me. 20, 1M, 08:XX:XX

ANDROC. Sh, 128 - Desired alcohol and drugs, a feeling of wanting to escape. (29)

ARS-MET. He, 5 - Feels as if she had to run away (escape), far away, and as if she would hardly touch ground.

He, 5 - Feels as if she had to run away, far away, and as if she would hardly touch ground.

ARS. Al, 88 - He has so much fear that he jumps out of his bed and hides himself in the wardrobe, which he can hardly be induced to leave.

Al, 89 - He sees thieves in his room, and therefore hides himself under the bed.

Al, 90 - He sees vermin and bugs crawl about his bed, from which he wants to escape, and constantly throws away whole handfuls of them.

Ha, 34 - He sees nothing but worms and bugs crawling about on his bed, from which he desires to run away (escape) and of which he throws out whole hands full.

Ha, 1031 - He became furious, must be bound, and seeks to run away.

He, 17 - He sees all kinds of vermin (insects) on his bed, throws handfuls of them away, and tries to escape from them.

He, 42 - Fear drives him out of bed; he hides in a closet.

BELL. Al, 81 - He imagines he sees birds flying off through the chimney, and wishes to follow them by the same route. (desire: fly, liberty, freedom)

Al, 165 - Cowardice, distrust, suspicion, inclination to run away.

Al, 174 - He escaped, under some pretext, into the open field.(run away)

Al, 156 - By day great anxiety; she has no peace anywhere; it seems to her as if she must flee away.(escape)

Ha, 1312 - By day great anxiety; she cannot rest (restlessness) anywhere; she feels as if she should run away.

Ha, 1436 - He makes an excuse (pretext) and runs out into the open fields.

He, 104 - Fear of imaginary things, wants to run away from them.

BRY. Al, 5-...a delirious frightful fantasy, as of soldiers cutting him down, that he was on the point of escaping;..

CALC. Ha, 69 - Unconsciousness and delusion about her abode (home) as if her room were a hall (passage) in a garden.

CAMPH. Al, 46-...A fearful terror seized me, and I knew not whither to fly. I cried out aloud, "And so I am indeed dead; that hell I used to think about is no fiction, but a reality which I am doomed to experience forever...

CAUST. He, 17 - Great restlessness, which prompts him to run away.

CHLOL. He, 7-...inclined to wander and hide herself, avoiding shrewdly (astute) the vigilance of her friends...

CHOC. Sh, 7 - In the evening, felt angry with bristling down my back. Irritable with the kids, shouted a lot, slammed doors. Feeling very uncomfortable with my daughter near me. I made a huge issue over something small which I would normally leave. I wanted to leave and walk out of the door on them. Felt very unsympathetic to the children. "You either go, or go to bed". Couldn't cuddle the children and took longer to say "Its all right". I thought that their father should look after them instead of me (very unusual). The feeling I can't be where I want to be because of them. I want to be roaming outside without my possessions. Left kids alone in the house for the first time. I was surprised at how easily I let them go. My daughter liked it very much.

Sh, 209 - A desire to hide in case things go to pieces. 15, 30C, 00:00:50

CIC. Ha, 238 - Want of trust (mistrust, skepticism) in people and anthrophoby,(misanthropy) he fled (escape) from them remained solitary, and thought seriously about their errors and about himself.

COCC. He, 25 - Melancholy and sadness, with weeping and constant profound absorption in sorrowful thoughts; great apprehensive anxiety of conscience, and feeling at heart as after committing a wicked deed (act), with desire to escape.

CUPR-A. He, 10 - Awoke suddenly from sleep...and wished to escape...thinks she is about to die and desires to see the pastor;...

CUPR. He, 5 - Delirium: afraid of every one who approached him, shrinking (retire) away from them; tries to escape; in evening and in the dark.

He, 21 - Afraid of and shrinking away from everyone who approaches him; afraid of falling; clinging tightly to nurse;...

He, 8 - Mania characterized by a wild look and fear; tries to escape.

DIG. He, 10 - Profound melancholy,...great fear of future; insane obstinacy and disobedience, with desire to escape.

ELAPS. Al, 9 - She wishes to leave the house just when she is going to bed.

GLON. He, 2 - Recognized no one; repulsed her husband and children; raved, screamed, and wished to rush from house; jumped out of bed, but fell because her knees gave way.

He, 12 - Great mental agitation; attempts to run away; attempted to spring from window.

HALI-L. Sh, 192 - Ran up an down a beach yelling and screaming to get it out of me. 02, 30C, XX:XX:XX

Sh, 529 - There was definitely someone else inside of me. The essence of that person was trying to get out, escaping, trying to get away. It felt like I was in prison or the thing in me was in prison. I was saying, "go," and it wouldn't get out of there. My supervisor got worried about me. On purpose, I made sure I was unavailable. If anyone asked me details, I would get angry. I won't explain it to you. I'm feeling that now a little, talking about it. 02, 30C, XX:XX:XX

Sh, 530 - Trying to do the work schedule; it won't click in like normal. Get stuck, then go away from it, get stuck again. Want to run away. Left the schedule until the next morning. 02, 30C, 00:04:XX

Sh, 532 - I started to speed up emotionally, got really pissed off at supervisor for getting in touch with me, beeping me. Wanted to escape and fly away. Phoned the airlines, trying to fly away. Hiding. Difficult to be with patients, with their stupid emotions. 02, 30C, XX:XX:XX

Sh, 663 - In a total frenzy, like steaming horses that had escaped, running down the road. Very hard to keep any control, to be patient in traffic, or the grocery store. Couldn't handle it any longer. Put lip balm with camphor on, every ten minutes, and would feel calm momentarily. Finally got some tiger balm at a friend's house and used it two times. I was instantly calmer. Came back to being me. 02, 30C, 11:XX:XX

HELL. He, 20 - After typhoid, ...sits quietly in bed and seems lost in brooding;...constantly seeks (try) to escape, ...;without a word quietly climbs out of the window, and if she succeeds in escaping goes in direction of river; finally threw herself into privy (toilet), from which she was rescued.

He, 19 - Tries to escape, to throw herself into the river.

HYOS. He, 16 - Fears: being left alone (solitude, deserted); poison, or being bitten (hurt); being poisoned or sold; being betrayed, or injured; wishes to run away. (escape)

He, 60-... wants to run away for fear of being persecuted by police;...

He, 81-...attempts to escape from room; frightful hallucinations of figures coming to seize him, hens (chicken) bound (imprisoned) with chains,...

He, 87-...; refused medicine, and cunningly (skill) evaded all stratagems to give it; escaped from room, ...

He, 57 - Delirium tremens:...averse to light and company; visions as if persecuted preceded by an epileptic attack;... seeks to escape from men by whom he imagines himself surrounded and who are trying to capture him; does not recognize his wife who is standing by his side, but imagines he sees her under a distant bed.

IGN. He, 11-...believes herself married (connected) and pregnant; is tormented by remorse of imagined crimes; seeks constantly to escape to drown (suicide) herself; ...;is only quiet when lying undisturbed and brooding over her troubles, which she rehearses (tell) in a doleful (unhappy) tone ;..." I am neglecting my duty, breaking my vow" (promise, engagement)...;conscientious scruples after eating.

He, 61 - Melancholia after great grief and domestic trouble; complete sleeplessness; suicidal thoughts and desire to escape.

KALI-BR. Al, 3-...his character also had undergone a radical change, from having been very frank and brave, he had become excessively timid, and suspicious of every trifling circumstance; ...several times he attempted to throw himself from a window and battered down a door with an axe, in order to escape from some imaginary danger;...

LACH. He, 9 - Imagines he is followed (pursued) by enemies who are trying to harm (hurt, injure) him; attempts to leave room as if frightened by visions behind him.

He, 21-...imagines he is followed by enemies who are trying to harm him; attempts to leave room as if frightened by visions behind him.

MAG-C. Al, 816 - Dream that some one came to murder her; that she jumped from a window,...

MERC. He, 38 - Great restlessness, must constantly change her place; fear, with desire to escape, as if she had committed some crime.

MEZ. Al, 23 - Very irritable mood; very averse to everything; desire to run away.

OP. He, 21-...in old, emaciated persons; sees animals coming towards him; people want to hurt him, execute him ; creeping under covers or jumping out of bed; in "old sinners" (criminals) whose long lives of excess have thoroughly destroyed their constitutions; ...; believe themselves to be murderers or criminals to be executed; want to run away (escape) ;...

PULS. He, 46 - Dark suspicious and reserved manner; disturbed look on face; sleepless; looks for her bed in the yard (lost?); hides in a corner to escape from a little gray man who wanted to pull out her leg;...

STRAM. Al, 53-...throw the hands about the head as if attempting to ward off some threatening evil;...escape from the imaginary object ...

Ha, 565 - Nowhere has he rest, is startled by dream-pictures, even when his eyes are open, which in the form of big dogs, cats and other horrible beasts, grow (expand) out of the ground at his side, and from which he jumps away to the side with signs of terror (fear), and knows not how to save (rescue, free) himself. (cornered, corralled)

He, 63 - An old lady had a vision every night since six weeks, in which many persons, all strangers, came into her room and to her bedside, causing her such fear that she had to leave bed.

He, 156 - Endeavors to escape, imagines he is alone all the time, and is afraid. (loneliness, isolation)

SULPH. He, 46 - Great anxiety, fear lest she should come to ruin (destruction); ..tried to run away...

TARENT. Al, 56 - Fear and shaking; the patient cannot find a suitable place where to hide himself; thinks he is going to be assaulted.

He, 15 - Suddenly sprang (escape) away from her attendants and swept (clean) ornaments from mantelpiece (an ornamental facing around fireplace); said she was sorry, but could not help it; very mischievous and destructive, ...

VALER. Al, 1 - Extremely delirious, attempting to get out of the window, ... imagined himself away from home, and beset (surrounded) with all sorts of danger, from which he was attempting to escape, although unable to walk without staggering from side to side.

EXECUTED

Delusions; criminal, executed, to be: **OP.**[54]
- execute him, people want to: ***op.***[54]
- executioner, visions of an: stram.
- hearing, of, drums which proclaim his execution, chides father for taking part in revolutions: verat.[54]
- murderer, executed to be: **OP.**[54]

Dreams; decapitation of people: ozone[227]
➤ hung, seeing persons: merc-s.[36]

ARS. Al, 70 - The anxiety and restlessness are indescribable; "Kill me", he cried, "or relieve my pains!".(help)

BELL. Al, 162 - She begs the bystanders to kill her.

Al, 172 - She tries to strangle herself, and begs the bystanders to kill her, because she believes that she will certainly die.

Ha, 1433 - Fearful madness; he is afraid (fear) of an imaginary black dog, of the gallows. (hanging)

Ha, 1437 - She tries to strangle herself, and begs those about her to kill her, for this time she must die. (redemption, regeneration, salvation)

He, 85-...patient must do everything violently; she wishes those around her to kill her. (salvation, redemption)

He, 13 - Timorous anxiety; he is afraid of a an imaginary black dog; of the gallows, etc.

COFF-T. He, 5 - Begs that someone might end her life. (salvation, redemption) (murdered)

HURA. Al, 709 - Restless night; dream about crimes, dead bodies (corpse), and children lying with their heads half cut off, while others were being decapitated.

OP. Al, 68 - Criminals (in India) lose their fear of death and go courageously to their execution.(fearless)

He, 21-...in old, emaciated persons; sees animals coming towards him; people want to hurt him, execute him ; creeping under covers or jumping out of bed; in "old sinners" (criminals) whose long lives of excess have thoroughly destroyed their constitutions; ...; believe themselves to be murderers or criminals to be executed; want to run away (escape) ;...

STRAM. He, 56 - Believes to be in his grave; shrives,(confess) prays, asks to be killed (justified); accuses his wife of infidelity; scolds (cursing), strikes at everybody who wishes to restrain him; thinks they are dogs and barks at them to make himself understood.

He, 77 - Patient had a constant vision of an executioner(hangman, lynches) standing before him in spite of which he was lively, talkative, laughed and joked about his hallucination, yet it seemed to him a reality.

He, 93 - Mania; thinks he is lying on his sepulchre (tomb); confessing, praying, wants to be killed (redemption, salvation, regeneration); laughs as if tickled (excited); wants to be kissed; accuses his wife of being faithless (betrayed); scolding (censure) beating in a rage, will not be taken hold of by attendants (suspicious?) ; takes them for dogs (contemptuous), and barks at them; talking in Jewish jargon; (rank?, stranger?) supposes his house to be surrounded by carts (vehicle), Jews (Judaism) and geese, offending him, ... -(strange, foreign, alien)

He, 107-...heard continually, on r. side of occiput, a loud voice, scolding, vituperating and accusing him of ungodliness (impious, sinful, irreligious, godless, profane); ....prayed expecting, with great anxiety, the flash of lightning which was to kill him;...(redemption, regeneration, salvation)

VERAT. He, 48 - A crippled girl...; chides (censure) her father for taking part in revolution; thinks she hears drum (timpani) which proclaims his execution; this is followed by silent brooding and occasional starts;...

FAILURE

Ailments from; ambition, deceived: bell.[30] merc.[30] ***nux-v.***[54] plat.[30] puls.[30] verat.[30]

Ailments from; business, cares: ambr.[137] calc.[58] caust.[137] kali-br.[85] nux-v.[36] ph-ac.[58] puls.[8] rhus-t.[1] sep.[8] sulph.[36]

Ailments from; business, failure: ***ambr.***[30] aur.[187] calc.[58] ***cimic.***[8] coloc.[30] ***hyos.***[8] ign.[8] kali-br.[56] nat-m.[30] nux-v.[30] ph-ac.[30] puls.[30] rhus-t.[30] sep.[30] sulph.[30] verat.[30]

Ailments from; disappointment, deception: acon.[102] alum.[85] apis[98] ars.[102] **AUR.**[8] ***bry.***[102] caps.[83] carb-v.[58] carc.[214] caust.[102] cham.[28] ***cocc.***[8] colch.[102] ***coloc.***[102] dig.[36] ***gels.***[102] grat.[102] hyos.[102] **IGN.**[122] ***lach.***[122] **LYC.**[122] ***merc.***[122] **NAT-M.**[122] ***nux-v.***[122] op.[122] **PH-AC.**[122] phos.[28] plat.[58] **PULS.**[122] sep.[102] **STAPH.**[122] verat.[122]

Ailments from; disappointment, deception, new: **IGN.**[122]

Ailments from; disappointment, deception, old: **NAT-M.**[122]

Ailments from; financial loss: ***arn.***[122] ars.[8] aur.[58] calc.[30] ign.[30] mez.[58] nat-m.[30] nux-v.[30] puls.[193] ***rhus-t.***[30] ***sars.***[8] stann.[30] verat.[30]

Ailments from; friendship, deceived: aur.[8] ign.[30] mag-c.[30] mag-m.[30] nux-v.[30] ph-ac.[30] sil.[30] sulph.[30]

Ailments from; literary, scientific failure: calc.[30] ign.[30] lyc.[30] nux-v.[30] puls.[30] sulph.[30]

Ailments from; position, job, loss of: ***ign.***[30] ***nux-v.***[8] pers.[149] ***plat.***[30] staph.[30]

Ailments from; reversal of fortune: ambr.[116] con.[116] dig.[116] lach.[116] stann.[116] staph.[116]

Avarice; collects carefully the debris of his fortune: stann.[30] staph.[30]

Business; man, in worn out: ***coca***[54] kali-p.[85] **NUX-V.**[54] zinc-p.[137]

Confidence, want of self; failure, feels himself a: aur-s.[231] bamb-a.[1184] naja[5] sulph.[5]

Confidence; use of voluntary muscles, in, could not finish what he attempted: ang.[54]

Confusion of mind; ambition, from deceived: ***nux-v.***[54]

Cursing; disappointment in plans, on: opun-a.[36]

Delusions; business, accomplished, can not be: med.[139]

- fail, everything will: act-sp. ***arg-n. aur.*** bamb-a.[1184] cob-n.[144] lac-c.[60] merc. nux-v. sil.
- failure, he is a: germ.[222] naja[130] sulph.[137]
- fortune, he was going to lose his: psor. staph.
- lose, he will: **CUPR.**[54] ***sulph.***[54]
- lost, everything is: ign.[144]
- succeed, he cannot; does everything wrong: anac. ***arg-n.*** arn.[114] ***aur.***[122] bamb-a.[1184] bapt.[58] bar-c.[162] gels.[114] naja[130] nat-c. nat-m.[114] ozone[227] phos.[114] sulph.[137]
- succeed, that he cannot, unfit for this world: ***aur.***[54]
- unfit for, world, the: ***aur.***[54]

Despair; lost, thinks everything is: aur.[10] ign.[10]

Despair; work, over his: anac.[58]

Dreams; business, accomplish, cannot: mag-m. ***phos.*** sabad.

➤ coition, unsuccessful: ind.[36]

➤ coition, unsuccessful, men, with, in men: ind.[36]

➤ danger, escaping, fruitless efforts of: ind.[54]

➤ destination, not reaching her: cadm.[144]

➤ failures: fago.[36] ign.[10] mosch.[10] op.[10]

➤ flying, apparatus, whose wings will not work: apis[36]

➤ money, left behind without, he is: ozone[227]

➤ unsuccessful efforts to, coition, in: ind.[36]

➤ unsuccessful efforts to, do various things: am-m. androc.[222] cadm.[149] calc. calc-f. cann-s.[10] carl. cham.[10] choc.[222] croc. dig. ign. mag-c. mag-s. mosch. mur-ac.[1] nat-c.[10] op. ozone[227] ph-ac. plat. polym.[111] stann.[10] tab. vanad.[209]

➤ unsuccessful efforts to, do various things, get cooking ready for brother and father: am-m.[36]

➤ unsuccessful efforts to, do various things, jumping long distance contest: ozone[227]

➤ unsuccessful efforts to, escaping from danger, of: ind.

➤ unsuccessful efforts to, finding way in his own house: mag-c.

➤ unsuccessful efforts to, open the mouth, to: agar.

➤ unsuccessful efforts to, running, of: croc. ind.

➤ unsuccessful, efforts to, reach a distant place, to: croc. plat.

➤ visits, making visits, friend, to a, who is not at home: ozone[227]

➤ wrong, everything goes: fago.[36]

Fancies; misfortune, all his efforts would miscarry: merc.[36]

Fear; destination, of being unable to reach his: lyc.

✦ failure, business or work, in: acon.[172] arg-n.[58] arn.[162] ***aur.***[184] bry.[172] calc.[172] carb-an.[162] cimic.[172] gels.[162] iod.[162] ***kali-c.***[184] kali-p.[172] lac-c.[162] lyc.[58] nat-m.[162] nux-v.[172] phos.[162] ***psor.*** sil.[162] sulph.[162]

✦ failure, of: act-sp.[162] aloe[36] arg-n.[5] arn.[5] carc.[193] cob-n.[144] cupr.[210] gels.[5] iod.[116] ***lac-c.***[54] lyc.[172] naja[141] nat-m.[5] phos.[5] plb.[201] ***sac-alb.***[210] sil.[58] sulph.[5]

✦ failure, of, examinations, in: anac.[185]

✦ memory will fail, that his: nat-m.[172]

✦ position, to lose his lucrative: calc.[30] ign.[30] puls.[30] rhus-t.[30] sep.[30] staph.[30] sulph.[30] verat.[30]

✦ social position, about his: chel.[172] cub.[36] sep.[30] staph.[30] verat.

✦ undertaking anything: ***arg-n. ars.*** kali-p.[172] ***lyc.*** sil.[58]

✦ undertaking, enterprise, a new: cupr.[210] lyc.[201] plb.[201] ***sil.***[54]

Grief; financial loss: arn.[137] aur.[137]

Insanity; black insanity with despair and weariness of life from fear of mortification or of loss of position: calc.[30] ign.[30] puls.[30] rhus-t.[30] staph.[30] sulph.[30] verat.[30]

Insanity; business, from failure in: ***cimic.***[54] ***lil-t.***[54]

Insanity; fortune, losing, after: calc.[30] ign.[30] rhus-t.[30] verat.[30]

Insanity; position, from fear to lose the: calc.[30] ign.[30] puls.[30] rhus-t.[30] staph.[30] sulph.[30] verat.[30]

Mania; business, failure, from: ***cimic.***[54]

Sadness; loss, after financial: arn.[137] ars.[54] aur.[137] mez.[137] psor.[137]

Succeeds, never: am-c. asar. aur. canth. merc.[1] mur-ac. nat-c. nat-s. nux-v. spong.[1]

Undertakes; nothing lest he fail: ***arg-n.*** nux-v.[36] sil.

ACT-SP. He, 16 - Desperation of success of every, even most trifling undertaking.

ADAM. Sh, 189 - Low self esteem. Felt I am not worthy or not pretty or not interesting enough for people. 20, 1M, XX:XX:XX

ALOE. Al, 20 - Little inclination to labor; discouraged, apprehensive about his success.

ANAC. Ha, 9 - He is at odds (quarreling) with the whole world, and has so little confidence in himself that he despairs of being able to accomplish (succeed) what is demanded of him.
Ha, 20 - Indisposition to work; he is afraid to undertake anything, he has no pleasure in anything.
APIS. Al, 17-... would have liked to kill a dog that barked at him, etc. ; everything went wrong; nothing could be done to please him.
ARG-N. Al, 6 - He fells very much affected bodily and mentally; he does not undertake anything lest he should not succeed.
He, 16 - Possessed of distressing idea that all his undertakings will and must fail.
ARS. Ha, 1039 - Persistent anxiety, like a qualm (doubt) of conscience, just as if he had failed (neglected) to do his duty, but without knowing wherein.
Ha, 1064 - All day long discontented with himself and very cross with himself; he imagines he has not done enough, and reproaches himself bitterly.
He, 25 - Mania...sees a man who has hanged himself beckoning (call) him to cut him loose (rescue, deliverance, free, saving) on failing to accomplish this he attempts to hang himself (punish, penalize);...finally kneels down and lifts his hands in supplication.(forgiveness, absolution)
He, 58 - Melancholy; after financial losses; cannot be consoled; thinks he will have to die (sentenced), with his family, from starvation (hunger); sleepless nights; walks about wringing his hands, with moaning and groaning.
He, 95 - Dissatisfied and angry with himself all day; thinks he has not accomplished enough, and reproaches himself bitterly.
AUR. Ha, 342 - Peevish (irritable) dejection; (sadness) he thinks nothing will succeed (prosper) with him.
Ha, 18 - Dispirited ill-humor; he thinks he cannot succeed in anything.
Ha, 19 - Dispirited and despondent; he thinks that everything goes awkwardly (incapacity, unfit) with him, and nothing will succeed with him.
He, 10 - Imagines he cannot succeed (perform, prosper) in anything, (failure) and he does everything wrong; he is in disunion whith himself.
BOV. Al, 2 - Very open-hearted; she spoke of her own failings, contrary to her custom.
CALC-F. Al,S-1-...tendency to look on the dark side of things, with much depression of spirits. Feeling of anxiety about money matters, or thought would come to want (lack), or would soon be "running astern" (reversed, failure) financially...disposition to set a higher value on money than natural to him (avarice?, poverty?).
He, 3 - Feeling of anxiety about money matters; thought he would come to want (poverty) or would soon be "running astern" financially (entirely without occasion)
CANN-S. Ha, 304 - Dreams of disagreeable and frightful character, in which he is unsuccessful (unproductive, frustrated) in everything, which causes him great anxiety.
CARB-AC. He, 12 - Entire disinclination to study; what he had accomplished seemed very trifling. (unimportant)
CHAM. He, 32 - Very anxious; everything she undertakes is very unsatisfactory (disappointed) ; she is irresolute,...(indecision)
CHLOR. He, 3 - A horrible state of mind, fears he will go crazy, fears he cannot make a living.(subsistence)
CIMIC. He, 34 - Mind disturbed by disappointed love, business failures.
DIG. Ha, 4 - Tearful sorrow (grief) over many things which have failed (disappointment, frustration) with him.
Ha, 420 - Lachrymose sadness about many things in which he has been unsuccessful.
GERM. Sh, 180 - Woke up early 3.30 am. had strong feeling, like a visualization. I picture myself lying on floor in fetal position and being shot in the head like a horse or a dog. Almost welcomed it. Then thought my children still need me. A very strong feeling of failure accompanied this. I felt I did not deserve to live. Better crying next day when talking to husband. This feeling of depression carried on for several nights. As soon as I wake up in the early morning, my mind is active and a feeling of inadequacy comes on strongly. 05 , 6C, 28:XX:XX

Sh, 109 - Feeling a total failure, I would prefer to die. Very unmotivated. 05, 6C, 360:XX:XX

HALI-L. Sh, 402 - I felt pathetic, defeated and vulnerable. I was reaching on a high shelf for pots for plants. All the pots and soil came tumbling down. Was knocked on the head, on the vertex. Dirt all over me, and I thought, "This is perfect. This is exactly how I feel." I felt like I had to just give up — give up the bravado. I'm exhausted, I'm just going to rest. I just wanted to go into a little ball and lick my wounds. Felt very much like childhood symptoms. I felt very young. 01, 30C, 18:XX:XX

Sh, 417 - Frustrated and depressed. Feeling lonely, friendless and unaccomplished. 18, 30C, 15:XX:XX

Sh, 430 - Get a call from a friend that the utility district is at it again. Don't know what, but expect the worst in negotiations with them. Can't win. So tired of fighting the losing battle. Can't raise the energy to do anything. Rage inside. Hopeless. Daydreams of blowing up the utility district, of shooting them. Only option left to desperate people and I feel desperate. we're a rag-tag group without luck, or leadership, fighting a losing battle. Feels like we're the American Indians. "Here's 24 dollars worth of beads for your island, idiot." In the pit of despair. 09, 6C, 25:XX:XX

Sh, 624 - Companionship. The idea that you had your chance and it didn't work out, and you're just going to be alone, and there's nothing you can do about it. 18, 30C, 17:XX:XX

HEP. Al, 16 - Irritable mood; everything that she undertook was wrong; she desired to be alone.

HYDROG. Sh, 188 - On getting up in the morning, I feel very angry and bad about myself. I feel I can't cope. Whats the use of trying? I feel like giving up. I think for a moment I'd like to die. 10, 200C, 09:XX:XX

IGN. Ha, 754-,... he cannot express himself in talking, write, or do anything as quickly as he wishes; ...he makes mistakes in speaking and writing, and does everything awkwardly...

Ha, 759 - Fearfulness, cowardice cannot trust himself to do anything, considers all is lost .

IRID. Sh, 197 - There's a slight element of confusion and a faint glimmer of not being able to cope. The feeling of not coping came on this afternoon. I've got lots to do and I've done nothing. I don't feel like doing anything but the concern is will I ever be able to focus my mind long enough to get anything done! M4

LIL-T. He, 7 - Dementia produced by business discouragements and sexual excesses.

MERC. Al, 30 - Fretful and peevish all day; he imagined that all his efforts would at last miscarry. (fail)

Ha, 1251 - All day long cross and peevish; he believed that all his efforts (endeavor) would finally fail.

NAJA. Al, 9 - Considerable depression of spirits, and a feeling of inability to exertion of any kind, and a conviction that all is going wrong;...

Al, 10 - Great depression of spirits this morning; everything for two or three hours appeared to go wrong with me, and to be without remedy;...

NAT-C. Al, 22 - His fancy is mostly busy with apprehensions of the future; he often makes plans for half an hour at a time as if it would go wrong with him, wherewith he seeks to be alone for several days together.

NAT-S. Al, 12 - Nothing that she undertakes succeeds well, and she does not know why.

NUX-V. Al, 60 - Everything miscarriages (failure) with him; it seems to go contrary.

Al, 71 - She wishes to accomplish much, but thinks it will not succeed.

Ha, 1289 - She wishes to do much, but thinks she will not succeed.

Ha, 1290 - He thinks that everything will go wrong.(failure)

Ha, 1291 - Everything goes wrong with him. (everything goes contrary)

Ha, 1289 - She wishes to do much, but thinks she will not succeed.

He, 23 - Great anxiety of mind without particular cause; thinks she will not be able to get along (prosper) in life; caducity; (senility)...

He, 26 - Melancholic in consequence of losing his position (rank),...the least contradiction puts him out entirely...(ailments from)

He, 35 - From disappointed ambition, bewildered, (confused) talks incoherently; does everything he attempts (try) to do wrong;..

OPUN-V. Al, 5 - Fit of swearing (cursing) at evening after coming home; praying in the morning, swearing (cursing) on disappointment in plans; fit of rage, on thwarting (frustrating) of plans.

PSOR. Al, 19 - Despairing mood; he fears to fail in business.

Al,N-24 - Despairing mood; fears he will fail in business.

He, 24 - Despairing mood; fears he will fail in business.

SPONG. Al, 11 - She is dissatisfied with what she accomplishes; she cannot rightly help herself at work (helpless) (incompetent) ; she does not succeed.

Ha, 384 - She is not satisfied with her work; she cannot do her work properly, she is not successful with it.

STANN. Ha, 639 - Busy uselessness (inefficiency): he exerts (use) himself to get a necessary task (duty) done at the appointed hour, and cannot accomplish it, as though prevented (interrupted) by an over-crowding of thoughts, during which one thing and another occur to him which he wishes to do...

STAPH. He, 15-...; firmly believed he would lose his fortune, constantly told his wife to be careful that they did not starve; thinks his wife will run away from him (deserted) (lost: position, rank), ... amuses himself by throwing into the fire any article near at hand, regardless of value; at times more violent, strikes at any one coming near him, ...tells his wife he will try not kill any one;...

SUL-AC. Al, 35 - Fretful, peevish, impatient, if his work is not done to suit.(unsatisfying)

Ha, 16 - Vexed, peevish, impatient, at once when he does not succeed in his work.

TARENT. Al, 52 - Worried (troubled) and greatly vexed (disturbing), with much weeping, as if one could not realize (accomplish, complete) something earnestly (ardently) desired.

Al, 65-...great haste in whatever I undertook, from a constant fear that something would happen to prevent my finishing it;...fear that something would fall on me (doom, disgrace);...fear of striking it against some imaginary object which appeared to be suspended....(hurt)

FALL

Anxiety; ascending stairs, on: ***nit-ac.*** onos.[144] ox-ac.[36]

Anxiety; fall, as if he would, during walking: nat-m.[36]

Anxiety; motion, from, downward: **BOR.** coff-t.[54] ***gels.*** sanic.

Bed; fall out, as if he would: ars-s-f.[54]

Clinging; children of, grasp the nurse when carried: bor.[58] cupr.[8] cupr-acet.[8] ***gels.***[122]

Clinging; children of, take the hand of mother, will always: ***bism.***[85] gels.[116] kali-c.[56] lil-t.[56] lyc.[56] phos.[162]

Clinging; convulsions, before: ***cic.***[54]

Clinging; grasps at others: agar.[185] ars.[5] ***camph.***[54] op.[30] phos.[5]

Clinging; persons or furniture, to: bar-c.[162] bism.[122] bor.[1] coff. gels. phos.[1] stram.

Delusions; abyss: ozone[227]

- abyss behind him: kali-c.[122]
- abyss, fear of falling down an: alco.[36] carbn-s.[85]
- bed, small, too, to hold him: germ.[222] sulph.[137]
- body, brain, balanced on a slight point and is likely to be turned over at any moment: camph.[139]
- body, eyes, falling out: crot-c.
- body, head, falls off: nux-m.[85]
- brother fell overboard in her sight: kali-br.
- elevated in air, fall, and will: mosch.[139]
- falling, bed, out of: arg-n.[5] ars.[5] ars-s-f.[54] crot-c.[5]
- falling, bed, through the: bell.[139] chin-s.[139] dulc.[139] lach.[139] rhus-t.[139] sac-alb.[139] sec.[139]
- falling, forward, she is: alum-sil.[58] elaps mosch.[10] stram.[58]
- falling, he is: alum-sil.[58] ambro.[139] apis[139] aran.[139] bell.[139] bism.[139] calc.[139] caust.[139] chen-a.[139] clem.[139] coloc.[139] cupr.[139] equis.[139] gels.[139] lappa[139] lyss.[139] mag-m.[139] mag-p.[139] med.[139] mosch.[10] puls.[139] rhus-t.[139] sabin.[139] sep.[139] spig.[139] stram. tub.[139] upa.[139] visc.[139] wies.[139] zinc.[139]

• falling, he is, clings and asks to be held: stram.[54]
• falling, he will be, if he stands: alum-sil.[58]
• falling, height, from a: calen.[139] mosch.[85]
• falling, hole, in a: carbn-s.[85]
• falling, things will be: hyos. stram.
• flying, he is, rock into dark abyss, from a, on going to bed: cann-i.
• gave way, everything under him: sanic.[139]
• gave way; ground under him: digin.[139] kali-br.[139] tep.[139]
• heavy, is, fall, and he will: eup-pur.[54]
• hole, small, is a frightful chasm: agar.
• knees, he walks on: ***bar-c.*** bar-m.
• lifted up, falling, with fear of: hyper.[172] mosch.[172]
• rising, then falling, of: bar-c.[162] lach.[162]
• sitting on a sofa, she is falling off, keeps holding on to everything: ***stram.***[54]
• walking, knees, he w. on his: ***bar-c.*** bar-m.
• walls, falling, inward, before epileptic fit: carb-v. lyss.[122]

Dreams; animals, horses, falling from horse: tarent.[36]
➤ body, hair, falling out: mag-c.
➤ body, teeth falling, filling is falling out: nux-v.[36]
➤ body, teeth, falling out: bamb-a.[1184] coca[36] cocc. convo-d.[36] nicc. nux-v. sul-ac.[10] tab.
➤ cellar and walls falling in, being in: bov.
➤ children, about, lying on ice, her little child, and she feared it would fall into water: lipp.[36]
➤ children, about, protecting them, to save them from falling: ozone[227]
➤ disease, hair falling out: mag-c.
➤ earthquake, houses falling: ozone[227]
➤ falling: acon. all-c.[163] allox.[119] alum. alum-p.[58] ***am-m.*** ange-s.[149] ars.[163] aur. **BELL.** bism. ***cact.*** cahin. calc. canth. caps. cham.[163] chel. chin. choc.[222] cimic.[5] cob-n.[149] coff.[163] ***dig.*** dulc. elaps eupi. ferr. ferr-p. ***guai.*** hell.[111] ***hep.***[122] ign. kali-c. kali-i. kali-n.[5] kali-p. ***kreos.*** lyc.[102] m-arct.[10] mag-m. ***merc.*** mez. nat-s. nicc. nit-ac.[102] nux-m. nux-v. op. ph-ac. phos.[5] plb. ***puls.*** rumx. sabad. sabin. sang. ***sars.*** sep. sil.[102] sol-t-ae. ***sulph.*** sumb. tab.[5] **THUJ.** verat.[102] zinc. zinc-o.[10] zinc-p.[58]
➤ falling, abyss, into an: ***cham.*** elaps eupi. ozone[227]
➤ falling, danger of: alum.[36] am-m.[36] macrin.[36]
➤ falling, elevator is: ozone[227]
➤ falling, flood, into a: am-m.
➤ falling, hammock, from a: phos.[36]
➤ falling, high places, from: acon. alum. am-m. anan. aur. chin. cimic.[111] ***dig.*** guai. hep. kali-c. kali-m.[192] kali-n.[36] ***kreos.*** merc. merc-c.[36] ***mez.*** nat-s. nicc. nux-m. op. ph-ac.[1] phos. sep. sin-a.[36] sol-n.[25] ***sulph.*** sumb. **THUJ.** zinc.
➤ falling, high places, men are killed by falling from a height: sabin.[10]
➤ falling, loft, from: nicc.[36]
➤ falling, pit, into a: elaps.[36]
➤ falling, window, from, friends: choc.[222]
➤ friends, falling from window: choc.[222]
➤ frightful, falling downstairs, after: ***rhus-t.***[54]
➤ graves, falling into a grave, waking her: iris.
➤ graves, thrown into a grave, being: mag-c.[36]
➤ hung, hanged man falling down an interminable lift shaft: choc.[222]
➤ precipices: ***all-c.***[54] ***lac-ac.***[54]
➤ precipices, abysses, in cramp: ***lac-ac.***[54]
➤ slipping: ox-ac.[36] sars.[36]
➤ slopes: anac.[10]
➤ star falling: alum.
➤ thrown from a carriage, being: nat-s.[36]
➤ waking, falling into a pit with grotesque figures: narcot.[36]
➤ water, falling into: ***am-m. dig.*** eupi. ***ferr.*** ign. iod. mag-m. mag-s. merc. mez.[10] nicc. ph-ac.[1] plb.[10] puls.[10] sars.[10] sep.[10] sulph.[10] zinc.[10]
➤ water, falling into, child, her: eupi.
➤ water, falling into, daughter: iod.
➤ water, falling into, ice, through: ozone[227]
➤ water, falling into, mother: nicc.
➤ wells, let down into, of being: ***all-s.*** merc-c.

Fear; airplanes: ***acon.***[162] arg-n.[162] ars.[162] **CALC.**[162] lup.[162] nat-m.[162]
✦ ascending, of: ***nit-ac.***[122]
✦ carried, being, or raised: ***bor.***[102] bry.[102] sanic.[102]
✦ crossing a bridge or place, of: ang.[137] arg-n.[58] bar-c.[30] ***bor.***[162] ferr.[30] puls.[30] sulph.[137] ter.[162]
✦ drawn upward, of being: calc-p.[184] camph.
✦ falling, child holds on to mother, nurse: bor.[56] ***cupr-acet.***[54] **GELS.**[54] sanic.[56]
✦ falling, downstairs: lac-f.[56] ovi-g-p.[85]

- ✦ falling, fire, into, when walking by it, and in spite of her willpower she did stagger into the fire: onos.[144] psor.[172]
- ✦ falling, height, from: aur.[172] hyos.[137] thuj.[172]
- ✦ falling, high walls and building upon him: ***arg-n.***[54] arn. choc.[222]
- ✦ falling, houses, of: hydr-ac.[137]
- ✦ falling, letting things fall, of, morning, on lifting: coca.
- ✦ falling, looking down, on: bor.[172] gels.[172] lac-c.[172] onos.[172]
- ✦ falling, of: acon. alum. alumn. arg-n. ars.[1] ***bor.*** calc.[30] caust.[172] chin.[5] coca[98] coff.[5] ***cupr.*** cur. ***gels.*** graph.[172] hyper.[5] kali-c.[5] kali-s. ***lac-c.*** ***lil-t.*** lyc.[172] lyss.[5] med.[58] nux-v. onos.[5] ovi-g-p.[85] phos.[172] prim-v.[72] prot.[136] sanic.[111] sil.[5] ***stram.***[122] tab.[5] tub.[162] zinc.[5]
- ✦ falling, sleep, on going to: coff.
- ✦ falling, things falling on her: stram.[54] tarent.[36]
- ✦ falling, turning the head, on: der.
- ✦ falling, walking, when: coca cocc.[172] gels.[172] hura[36] lyss.[36] nat-m.
- ✦ falling, water, into: perh.[149]
- ✦ high places, of: ***arg-n.*** ***aur.***[137] calc.[162] calc-f.[179] carc.[193] cob-n.[119] coca[130] gels.[137] manc.[162] morg-g.[102] nat-m.[189] phos.[162] psor.[54] puls. staph. stram.[182] sulph. zinc.[162]
- ✦ motion, downward: **BOR.**[122] calc.[58] coca[117] cupr.[122] gels. hyper.[102] lac-c.[122] lil-t.[122] ***sanic.***[102] sil.[137] zinc.[137]
- ✦ prolapse, of, anus: ign.[172] nit-ac.[172]
- ✦ prolapse, uterus, everything dropping through: ***lil-t.***[54]
- ✦ walking, of, canal by a: ang.[137]
- ✦ water, fossets, of: lyss.[122]

Frightened; easily, night, starting up as if falling from a height into water: ph-ac.[36]

High places agg.: ***arg-n.*** ***aur.*** gels. puls. staph. ***sulph***

ACON. Al, 65 - Fear that he might stagger and fall.
Ha, 518 - Fear lest he should fall.
He, 37 - Fears to go where is any excitement (tumult) or many people (crowd); thinks she is jostling (pressing) against everyone she meets (oppressed); countenance (expression) expressive of timidity; constant dread (fear) lest she stagger (vacillated) and fall.

APIS. He, 11 - Lets everything fall out of her hand, or breaks things and laughs over it.

ARG-N. He, 42 - Fits of despondency and all kinds of fanciful (unreal) notions for example, that whilst walking along street he could not pass a given point without falling; frequently settled on the time he was to die.
He, 49 - Fears if passing a certain corner or building that he will drop down and create a sensation; is relieved by going in another direction.

BAR-C. Al, 2 - Imagine he walks on his knees.
He, 11 - Imagines he walks on his knees.

BAR-M. He, 7 - Sense of oppressive anxiety, accompanied by the illusory notion that he is walking on his knees, without legs. (inferiority, dwarf?)

BOR. Ha, 4 - Very timid, in driving down a mountain (elevation); quite at variance with his customary bearing; he felt as if it would take his breath away.
Ha, 8 - Timid, an anxious scream causes terror to fall on all his limbs.

CAMPH. Al, 39 - Indescribable dread of being drawn upwards.

CANN-S. Ha, 289 - He fears he will fall to the ground...

CAUST. Al, 36 - Extreme irritability of mind; the slightest vexation affects her whole body, so that her knees sink under her.
Ha, 23 - Extreme excitability of spirit; the least vexation (difficulty) darts through her body, so that her knees give way.

CHIN. Al, DREAM .[1105]-...;he imagines he is descending a precipice, on which account he awakes, but the dangerous place remains vividly before his fancy...Al, 1109 - At night frightful dreams of falling from a height, whith waking full of uneasiness...

COCA. Al, 17 - When lifting anything, fear lest I should let it fall, in the morning (dropping)

CROT-C. Al, 6 - She fancies her eyes are falling out (tenth day).

CUPR-A. He, 15 - Afraid of falling; holds on to his nurse's hair, hugs up to her, afraid of being injured,...

CUPR. He, 21 - Afraid of and shrinking away from everyone who approaches him; afraid of falling; clinging tightly to nurse;...

ELAPS. Al, 4 - She fancies she is falling forward, thought really quite still.
FERR. Al, 766 - Dreams he is in battle, that he has fallen into the water, etc.
Ha, 270 - Dreams that he is in battle, that he has fallen into the water...
GELS. He, 43 - Child dizzy, when carried seizes hold of nurse, fearing that it will fall.
GERM. Sh, 187 - Head jumped inside when there was a sudden noise. 07, 30C, 00.09.30
GLON. He, 2 - Recognized no one; repulsed her husband and children; raved, screamed, and wished to rush from house; jumped out of bed, but fell because her knees gave way.
GUAI. Ha, 130 - Frequent waking from sleep, as from a fright; he felt as if he were falling.
HALI-L. Sh, 10 - Sensation as if floor suddenly dropped down another few inches, after left foot landed on the floor. 09, 6C, 16:XX:XX
Sh, 306 - When I'm focused I bring it all in, in the present, There. like meditating, or seeing God. When I'm unfocussed it's like I'll go into the abyss, and won't come back, go crazy. 08, 30C, 31:XX:XX
Sh, 634 - Like being in the edge of an abyss, a crevice that's cracking deeper all the time. A crack that gets deeper and longer. 06, 6C, 00:12:30
Sh, 651 - When I'm focused, I bring it all in, in the present. There, like meditating, or seeing God. When I'm unfocussed, it's like I'll go into the abyss, and won't come back; go crazy. 08, 30C, 31:XX:XX
HYOS. Ha, 539 - They cried out that near objects were going to fall, and seized hold of them.
KALI-BR. Al, 6-...she fancied that the boarders in the hotel insulted her, and imagined that the weekly bills of the landlord (owner) were evidences of a conspiracy which had been got up against her father; ... while standing on the guards of the boat ...declared she had seen her brother fall overboard;...
LAC-C. Al,N-40 - Has a great fear of falling down stairs at times.
He, 33 - Has a great fear of falling down stairs at times.
LAC-F. Al,N-3 - Fear falling down stairs, but without vertigo.
MAG-C. Al, 935 - Dream of her hair falling out, which made her very sad.
NAT-M. Al, 61 - Very anxious, as if he would fall, while walking.
NIT-AC. Ha, 15 - Apprehensiveness, with stitches above the heart, and a fancy as if he was talking deliriously, with coldness of the body and a tendency to fall down.
He, 6 - Raving, as if delirious, with coldness of body and inclination to fall.
OSM. Al, 5 - Thoughts of accidents having happened to others, by a blow, a fall, or being dashed (crushed, hit, knock) to pieces; gradually these thoughts grow upon him, as if he were to do the same injuries to others.
STRAM. Ha, 561 - In the moments of consciousness he begged to be held as he was falling.
He, 71 - Fears; he will lose his senses (insanity); his lips will grow together; to suffocate; of falling; everything is falling on her.
He, 59-...clings to her mother with as much desperation as if she were going to be thrown from a precipice.
He, 161 - While sitting on a sofa, fancied she was falling off, kept holding on to everything; while in bed said that bed was being drawn from under her.
He, 162 - In his conscious moments, he asked to be held because he was falling.

FAMILY

Abusive; family and children, to: kali-i.[137]
Abusive; husband insults wife, in front of children or vice versa: anac.[30] ars.[30] lach.[30] nux-v.[30] verat.[30]
Ailments from; death, parents or friends, of: ambr.[58] ars.[184] calc.[58] **CAUST.**[30] **IGN.**[122] kali-br.[137] 0nat-m.[184] nit-ac.[54] nux-v.[30] plat.[85] staph.[30]
Ailments from; discords between, relatives, friends: ars.[30] graph.[8] hep.[30] lach.[30] mag-m.[162] merc.[30] ***nat-m.***[162] nit-ac.[30] nux-v.[162] sulph.[30]
Anxiety; anticipating, relatives, for his: carc.[193]
Anxiety; evening, family, about his, which he left behind while on a journey: ***petr.***[54]
Anxiety; family, about his: acet-ac.[54] aeth.[193] ***ars.***[10] calc-sil.[58] carb-an.[184] carc.[140] ***caust.***[30] cupr.[210] germ.[222] hep.[1] lach.[30] petr.[54] phos.[10] **RHUS-T.**[10] ***spig.***[30] sulph.[10] zinc.[30]

Anxiety; health, loved persons, of: carc.[193] hep.[30] merc.[30]
Anxiety; health, relatives: *ars.*[162] bar-c.[162] cand-a.[239] carb-v.[172] caust.[172] cocc.[36] **HEP.**[30] merc.[30] nat-c.[172] *phos.*[162] puls.[172]
Anxiety; health, relatives, little concerned about his own: cocc.[54]
Avarice; generosity towards strangers, as regards his family: carb-v.[30] hyos.[30] nat-m.[30] nux-v.[30]
Aversion; family members, to: am-c.[5] am-m.[5] aran.[192] aur.[5] *calc.* calc-s.[108] cit-ac.[65] con.[5] *crot-h. fl-ac.* hep.[5] iod.[137] kali-c.[122] kali-p.[5] lyc.[5] *merc.*[5] *nat-c.* nat-m.[30] *phos.*[5] plat.[5] plb.[162] senec.[137] *sep.*
Aversion; family, talks pleasantly to others: fl-ac.[137]
Aversion; parents, to: fl-ac.[30]
Cares; full of, relatives, about: ars.[10] cand-a.[239] *caust.*[30] hep.[10] lach.[30] rhus-t.[10] *spig.*[30] zinc.[30]
Censorious; parents, teachers and friends, of: sep.[189]
Complaining; relations and surroundings, of: *merc.*[54]
Contemptuous; relations, for: sec.[54]
Contrary; parents, with: tub.[140]
Cruelty; family, to her: kali-p.[58]
Death; thoughts of, belonging to him, for those, with anxiety: *ferr.*[54]
Delirium; abandons her relatives: sec.
Delirium; calls for parents who are present trying to console: **STRAM.**[54]
Delusions; accidents, of relatives: phos.[1]
- danger, family, from his: kali-br.
- disgraced, family or his absent friends, he disgraced his: sarr.[36]
- disgraced, family, she disgraced her: *plat.*[8]
- doomed, expiated her sins and those of her family, to: *lil-t.*[54].
- family, does not belong to her own: plat.
- family, get along without her, cannot: lil-t.[168]
- injury, receive, will, friends, from: lach.[58]
- loved by parents, is not: sac-alb.[210]
- murder, family with a hatchet, that she will: jab.
- neglected, he is, despised by his family, and: *arg-n.*[54]
- repudiated by relatives, he is: arg-n. hura.
- sick, members of the family are: hep.
- starve, family will: ars. calc-sil.[58] *sep.* staph.

Dreams; dead, people, of, relatives: caust.[1] ferr. fl-ac. hydrog.[222] kali-c.[1] mag-c. mag-s. pitu-a.[164] rheum sars.
- ➤ dead, people, of, relatives, long ago deceased: ferr.[36] sars.[36]
- ➤ death of, family, in: plan.[36]
- ➤ death of, one dear: lach.[36]
- ➤ death of, parents: cast.[36]
- ➤ death of, relatives: caust.[1] ferr. fl-ac. hydrog.[222] kali-c.[1] mag-c. mag-s. pitu-a.[164] rheum sars.
- ➤ death, relatives, of: alumn. aran-ix.[149] *calc-f.* cast. caust.[1] chin. choc.[222] fl-ac. grat. hydrog.[222] kali-c.[1] levo.[149] mag-s. mur-ac. nicc. paeon. plan. plat.
- ➤ disease, family, of: peti.[36]
- ➤ family, own: androc.[222] ant-c.[10] choc.[222] lap-gr-m.[194]
- ➤ family, own, losing his: choc.[222]
- ➤ house, family, for a big: ozone[227]
- ➤ household affairs: bell. *bry.*
- ➤ quarrels, dead relatives, with: cedr.[25] kali-c.[1]
- ➤ relatives: merc-i-r.[36] oci.[36]

Escape; attempts to, family, children, from her: am-c.[30] choc.[222] *lyc.*[122] nux-v.[30] phos.[30] *sep.*[30] staph.[30]
Estranged; family, from her: am-c.[30] anac. arn.[85] ars. choc.[222] con. hep. hydrog.[222] lap-c-b.[194] *nat-c. nat-m.* nat-s. *nit-ac.* nux-v.[30] phos. plat. psor.[58] *sep.* staph.[30]
Estranged; forgetful of relatives and friends: lap-c-b.[194] lyss.[54]
Estranged; ignores his relatives: bell.[5] hyos.[5] merc.[5] verat.[5]
Estranged; strangers, being kind with, but not with his family and entourage: lyc.[30] nux-v.[30] puls.[30] verat.[30]
Fear; accidents, loved ones, to: phos.[1]
- ✦ death, kill him, that those in the house might: *cimic.*[54]
- ✦ family matters, about: calc-sil.[58]
- ✦ happen, something will, family, to, or to him: ars.[172] calc.[172] calc-s.[36] caust.[172] phos.[172] psor.[172] sep.[172] tub.[36]

Forgetfulness; friends and relatives, of: lyss.[54]
Forsaken; feeling, beloved by his parents, wife, friends, feels of not being: *ars.*[30] calc.[30] lyc.[30] *mag-c.*[122] sep.[30] sil.[30] sulph.[30]
Forsakes; relations: sec.

Inconsolable; anxiety about his family, from, which he left behind while going on a short journey: ***petr.***[54]
Indifference; family, to his: carb-v.[58] hell.[36] lap-gr-m.[194] nat-p.[58] nit-ac.[116] **<u>PHOS.</u>**[122] **<u>SEP.</u>**[122]
Indifference; loved ones, to: ***acon.*** allox.[119] ars. ars-i.[58] bell.[193] carb-v.[58] carc.[193] ***fl-ac.*** **HELL.** kali-p.[58] kali-sil.[58] lil-t.[168] merc. myric.[25] nat-p. nat-sil.[58] **PHOS.** plat. **SEP.** ***syph.***[122]
Indifference; parents, to: phos.[10] sep.[146]
Indifference; relations, to: acon.[58] bac.[62] ***fl-ac.*** **HELL.** hep. hydrog.[222] kali-p.[58] lap-gr-m.[194] nat-c. nat-p.[58] **<u>PHOS.</u>**[122] plat. **<u>SEP.</u>**[122] ***syph.***[122]
Insanity; domestic calamity, after: ***lach.***[54]
Irritability; family, to her: kali-fcy.[198] lac-h.[229] opun-a.[36] thuj.[58]
Kill; desire to, loved ones: ars.[102] chin.[102] hep.[58] jab.[137] kali-br.[137] merc.[102] ***nux-v.***[102] ***plat.***[102]
Kill; desire to, parents, in a child: ***der.***[162]
Love; family, for: coff.[8] coff-t.[36]
Malicious; loved ones, to: germ.[222] sep.[58]
Mania; domestic calamity, after: ***lach.***[54]
Mocking; relatives, at his: sec.
Quarrelsomeness; family, with her: kali-c.[58] kali-m.[192] kali-p.[58] thyr.[149]
Relatives; ignore his: bell.[5] hyos.[5] merc.[5] verat.[5]
Responsibility; strong, family, towards his: nat-s.[187]
Sadness; family, for his: ars.[10] hep.[10] rhus-t.[10]
Suspiciousness; family, towards: ars-s-f.[58]
Unfeeling; family, with his: kali-i.[58]
Unsympathetic; unscrupulous, friends and family, even towards closest: lap-gr-m.[194]
Violence; chases family out of house: ***verat.***[54]

ADAM. Sh, 183 - I couldn't get involved in the conversation at family supper. I didn't feel the need to. I spent most of the evening being there, but observing. It was a strange experience but I felt very calm and present. 7, 6C, 12:22:00
Sh, 234 - Swearing and cursing. A lot to do, finding it hard to set priorities in my work and the needs of my family. 10, 6C, 19:XX:XX
ANDROC. Sh, 117 - Angry with her children and family. (7, 12, 17, 28)
ARG-N. He, 40 - Melancholy since an undeserved slight (scorn); fixed idea that he was neglected and despised by his family; his callings (job, work) became indifferent to him.
ARS. Ha, 1036 - In the evening, in bed, anxious sad fancies, e.g. that something bad (misfortune) must have happened to his relatives.
Ha, 3 - Sad, sorrowful ideas, in the evenings in bed, as if some misfortune (disaster, accident) might have happened to one's relatives.
He, 8 - Gloomy (dark) forebodings (premonition) while lying in bed, in evening, fears something may have happened to his relatives. He, 10 - Fixed idea that he and his family will die of starvation. (hunger, privation, want)
He, 58 - Melancholy; after financial losses; cannot be consoled; thinks he will have to die (sentenced), with his family, from starvation (hunger); sleepless nights; walks about wringing his hands, with moaning and groaning.
CHOC. Sh, 210 - Felt totally isolated and averse to company. Estranged himself from his family and friends and stopped all communication with them for a long period. Did not reply to letters and left no address. He seemed to hide away and literally disappear. The state of Isolation resulted from feeling that "I didn't exist as a human being". This behaviour was in strong contrast to his normal sociable disposition. 35, 30C, XX:XX:XX:
CIMIC. He, 10 - Fear of death; fears those in house will kill him (murdered, by parents); saw wires encasing (lock, imprisoned) him; visions of rats and of strange objects.
CROC. Al, 30-...the behavior of relatives and friends excites her to anger,...she is vexed with herself, and her anger becomes greater than ever;..
EUP-PUR. He, 7-... feeling like homesickness, though occupying her own home and surrounded by her own family,...
FERR. He, 9 - Mind in highest degree oppressed; despondent (sad); great solicitude (cares) about those belonging to him (relatives, family), with constant thoughts of death.
FL-AC. Al, 1 - Great disposition, when

alone, to repulsive fantastic imaginations, particularly in regard to persons with whom he stands in near relations, or with whom he is connected (united, joined); it seems, for example, as though he must get rid (discard, repudiate, reject) of all the servants, children must go out of house, a betrothal must be broken off, a marriage should be dissolved. (broke; vows)

He, 7 - Aversion to his own family, bordering on insanity.

FORM. Al, 7 - Sudden and unexpected return of sense of mortification and grief, with vivid recollection of circumstances long since passed, which had caused great mortification and pain, and which had rendered several years of his life unhappy; this was caused by the transactions (doing) of a near relative; this grief continues...

GERM. Sh, 138 - Feeling of revulsion for many people especially young parents with children, while wandering through town. Feel people are stuck in their lives. What a waste. 10, 9C, 00:05:00

HALI-L. Sh, 213 - I wanted to do more mothering while I was being mothered and at the same time not mothering the son I do have. Feeling envy of all families who had more children. Constant state of desire for something other than what I had. If busy, I wanted to be not busy. If no one calls, I felt nobody cares about me. Could find no comfort anywhere and felt isolatedalone. 01, 30C,, 21:XX:XX

Sh, 215 - Made up a meditation before going to bed. Felt both parents at the bedside. I am being totally held and loved by my father, wrapped up in blankets like I'm a baby. He is adoring me, cooing over me with my mother looking on. This calms my nerves and the sad feeling moves outward. This feels the same as swimming to me. The water on my skin calms my nerves. 08, 30C, 23:XX:XX

Sh, 507 - Having some trouble speaking. Using the wrong words, or lacking words at times. Just keep it simple. Husband told the kids. We all laughed. I guess that's what you can say for adversity. If it happens enough you learn to get used to it. If it's not too hard. Began thinking about one of my kids dying—that would be too hard. I don't want to do that to find out. 09, 6C, 16:XX:XX

HELL. Al,S-1 Happy carelessness about everything; feel indifferent to family.

HEP. Al, 19 - Contrary mood, he does not wish to see the members of his own family.

Al, 10 - Fearful concerning sickness in the family, especially when walking alone in the open air.

Ha, 5 - Fear about the illness of his family, especially while walking in the open air.

Ha, 7 - Contrary mood; he does not like to look at his folks. (relatives)

HURA. Al, 15 - Hypochondria, sadness, despair; he fancies he is repudiated and deserted by his relations. (rejected, refused)

HYDROG. Sh, 175 - At the family celebration, I could not feel that I belonged. 12, 6C, 34:XX:XX

HYOS. He, 78 - Groundless suspicion of being watched (observed, spied) by members of family with whom he had some slight misunderstanding (dispute); to avoid being recognized by them, clothed himself differently every day,...watching his relations suspiciously and imagining he might be poisoned;... (disguise, camouflage)

IRID. Sh, 42 - I wanted to sit with the rest of my family. This is unusual for me; usually sit on my own. I1

Sh, 44 - Better for company. It felt better to be with the family. D2

KALI-BR. Al, 3 - Decidedly insane; had delusions that lewd women had got into his mother's house; that he was pursued by the police; that his wife was threatened by members of the family; that he had thousands of dollars in gold sewed up in his clothing; (rich, wealth)

LIL-T. He, 16 - Doubts her salvation; thinks she is doomed to expiate her sins and those of her family; ... (redemption, salvation) (sacrifice)

MERC. He, 35 - Grief, with fear at night: disposition to quarrel; complaining of relations and surroundings. (living conditions)

MAG-C. Al, 948 - Anxious dreams of the misfortune of relatives.

Al, 955 - Dream that she was weeping about the death of a near relative.

NAT-C. He, 4 - Aversion to mankind and society; estrangement (separation, alienation) from individuals and society; even from her husband and family.

OPUN-V. Al, 6 - In the afternoon, fit of petulance, angry at near relatives, swearing mood, not at all pleased, cannot get over the thought of injuries done by friends.

PETR. He, 13 - Towards evening anxiety and apprehension about his family which he left behind while going on a short journey; the anxiety increases until he becomes inconsolable.

PLAT. Ha, 41 - She feels as if she did not at all belong to her family (stranger); after a short absence everything appears to be quite changed. (unfamiliar)

He, 39 - It seems to her as if she does not belong to her own family; ...

PLB. Al, 65 - Often getting out of bed and wishing to go home; sometimes not recognizing his family; thought they were conspiring to kill him.

SEC. Al, 1 - Delirium; she abandons (reject, forsakes) her relatives and does absurd things.

SEP. He, 38-...everything seems strange (unusual, unfamiliar) to her;...; it seems as if she could not understand (realize) anything and would have to learn anew everything she wished to do;...(lost: knowledge); greatest indifference to everything, the death of a near relative, or some happy occurrence, leaves her equally unaffected; no trace of her former love for friends or even for her child; aversion for social intercourse amounting to contempt;...

SEP. He, 19 - Aversion to one's occupation (work) and family.

He, 22 - Great indifference to one's family, to those they love best.

SIL. He, 9 - Longing for his relations and home.

THUJ. He, 23 - Mental depression, after childbirth (puerperal), in consequence of being told that there had been a slight rupture (division, hurt) of perineum; grows quiet; thinks she must die;...wants to jumps the window; does not care for children or her relatives (careless) ;..(sensitive to disrupt, partition)

FATHER

Delusions; hearing, of, drums which proclaim his execution, chides father for taking part in revolutions: verat.[54]

Dreams; anger, quarreled with his father, that he had, who would not recognize him as a son because he had embraced homeopathy: crot-h.[36]

➤ death of, father: alumn.[36] hydrog.[222]

➤ father is an Arab: ozone[227]

➤ murdering, father, her: cast.[36]

Fear; father, to become like his: ozone[227]

ADAM. Sh, 203 - Insulted. The worst insult is being told I've become like my father. 7, 6C, 05:17:00

FEARFUL

Absorbed; horrid: psor.[137]

Ailments from; alone, being, fear of people, yet: ars.[5] bufo[5] ***clem.***[5] ***con.***[5] tarent.[5]

Ailments from; anger, fright, shock, with: **ACON.** ***aur.*** ***bell.*** calc. cocc. coff.[54] cupr. **GELS.**[5] ***glon.***[5] **IGN.** nat-c. ***nux-v.*** ***op.*** ***petr.*** ***phos.*** ***plat.*** ***puls.*** samb. sep. **STRAM.**[5] sulph. zinc.

Ailments from; fright or fear: **ACON.**[122] act-sp.[54] agar.[5] anac. androc.[222] ***apis*** arg.[58] ***arg-n.*** arn. ars. ***art-v.*** ***aur.*** aur-m. ***bell.*** bry. ***bufo***[117] calc.[5] calc-sil.[58] camph.[30] canth.[30] carb-v.[5] carbn-s. carc.[119] **CAUST.**[5] cham. cic.[5] cimic.[85] cina[5] cocc.[5] ***coff.*** coloc.[5] crot-h.[85] ***cupr.*** ***gels.***[5] ***glon.*** ***graph.*** hep.[5] ***hyos.*** ***hyper.*** **IGN.** iod. ***kali-br.***[5] kali-c.[5] ***kali-p.***[116] ***lach.*** laur.[5] **LYC.** lyss.[54] mag-c. merc. morph.[102] nat-c. **NAT-M.** nicc.[163] nit-ac. nux-m.[58] ***nux-v.*** **OP.**[122] ***petr.***[54] **PH-AC.** **PHOS.** ***plat.*** psor.[58] **PULS.** ran-b.[58] ***rhus-t.*** sabad. samb. sec. ***sep.*** **SIL.** spong.[5] stann.[5] ***stram.***[5] sulph.[5] tarent.[54] **VERAT.**[5] verb.[5] vib.[137] visc.[85] zinc. zinc-p.[58]

Ailments from; fright or fear, anger, with: acon.[1]

Ailments from; fright or fear, fear of the fright still remaining: ***acon.***[58] bell.[54] merc.[54] nat-m.[54] **OP.**[8] ***verat.***[54]

Ailments from; fright or fear, grief, with: ign.[1]

Ailments from; fright or fear, long lasting: carc.[207]

Ailments from; fright or fear, menses,

during: ***acon.***[22] bell.[162] ***coff.***[54] ign.[51] ***lach.***[162] ***nux-v.***[8] ***op.***[8] ph-ac.[162] phos.[162] staph.[162] verat.[5]
Ailments from; fright or fear, ordeal, of an: **ARG-N.**[5] **GELS.**[5]
Ailments from; unusual, anything: ambr.[102]
Anxiety; chest, heart, region of, fear, with: rhus-t.[10]
Anxiety; children, in, afraid of everything: calc.[137]
Anxiety; fright, after: acon. both-a.[139] ***cupr.***[54] gels. ***ign.***[54] ***kali-br.***[116] lyc. merc. nat-m. op. rob. samb.[1] ***sil. verat.***[54]
Anxiety; waking, on, screams and remains full of fear: caps.[172]
Bed; get out of, wants to, fear, from: ars.[172] **BELL.**[54]
Cheerfulness; fearful, but: ***nat-c.***[137]
Clinging; children of, awakes terrified, knows no one, screams, clings to those near: **BOR.**[122] cina[36] ***stram.***[122]
Confusion of mind; images, from terrifying: stram.[36]
Courageous; alternating with, fear: ***alum.***[10]
Delirium; frightful: ***acon.*** anac. ***atro.*** bar-c.[54] **BELL.** calc. canth. carb-v.[10] caust.[10] chin.[10] cic. colch. coloc. dig. hep.[30] ***hyos.*** lyc.[10] merc.[10] nat-m. nit-ac.[10] nux-v. ***op.*** phos.[58] ***plb.***[122] ***puls.*** rhod.[36] samb.[10] sec. sil. **STRAM.** sulph.[10] ***verat.*** zinc. zinc-p.[58]
Delirium; lively active, vivid, alternates in short periods with horrified fright, seeming to dread approach of some monster, appealing for help: stram.[54]
Delirium; terror, expression of: bell.[36]
Delusions; animals, frightful: ***bell.*** cham.[54] ***crot-h.***[54] ***op. stram.*** tarent.
- dead, persons, morning on waking, frightened by images of: hep.
- figures, old repulsive persons, which fill her with fear, in hysteria: ***kali-c.***[54]
- heart or respiration is going to stop, or otherwise frightens herself causing heart to beat violently: ***lac-c.***[54]
- images, frightful: absin.[54] ***ambr.*** anac. arg-n. arn. ars. atro. bar-c. ***bell.*** bry.[1] **CALC.** calc-s. camph. ***carb-an. carb-v. caust.*** chin. chin-ar. cina[58] coca con. croc. gels. graph. ***hep.*** hyos. ign. kali-ar. ***kali-br.*** kali-c. ***kali-p.*** kali-sil.[58] ***lac-c. lach.*** lap-mar-c.[194] laur. lyc. mang. ***merc.*** mur-ac. nat-c. nat-p. nit-ac. nux-v. ***op.*** petr. ph-ac. ***phos.*** puls. rhod. rhus-t. samb. sars. sec. sil. spong. ***stram.*** sulph. tab. tarent.
- images, frightful, night, while trying to sleep: calc-s. sil.[1]
- mystery, everything around seems a terrifying: aether[36] androc.[222] cann-i.
- night, terrifying: berb.[85]
- people threatening her, screams horrible: ars-met.[54]
- people, threatening her, screams horrible: ars-met.[54]
- persecuted, that he is, tormented by some frightful scene of some mournful event of the past, and: spong.[54]
- scream, obliging to: ars.[54] kali-c.[10] plat.[10] puls.[10] stram.[10]
- scream, with: canth.[10] hyos.[10] ***stram.***[10] verat.[10]
- strangers, sees, every night since six weeks, causing fear, had to leave bed, a old woman: ***stram.***[54]
- thieves, dreams of robbers is frightened on waking, and thinks dream is true: verat.
- visions, eyes anxiously fixed sideways on one point where she imagines she sees a terrible hostile figure: ***stram.***[54]
- visions, horrible, fright, from: bell.[54] nat-m.[54] samb.[54]
- visions, leave the room, attempts to, as if frightened by visions behind him: ***lach.***[54]

Despair; salvation of soul, of eternal, after fright: stram.[54]
Dreams; animals, cats, frightened: puls.[36]
➤ animals, dogs, frightened by a black dog: puls.
➤ bullying: peti.[36]
➤ dead, bodies, fear, with, wishes to end it by turning on side, but cannot: alumn.[36]
➤ frightful: abrot. acon. adon.[102] aeth. aether[36] agar. agn. alco.[36] alet.[102] all-c. all-s. ***alum.***[5] alumn. am-c. **AM-M.** ambr.[5] ammc. ***anac.***[5] androc.[222] ang. ***ant-c. ant-t.***[5] apis ***aran.*** aran-ix.[119] ***arg. arg-n. arn.*** **ARS.** ars-i.[58] ars-s-f.[58] asar.[5] asc-t.[25] atro. **AUR.** aur-ar.[58] aur-i.[58] aur-m. ***aur-s.***[58] bad. ***bapt.*** bar-c. bar-m. bar-s.[58] ***bell. bism.*** bol.[36] **BOR.** bov. bruc.[10] ***bry.*** bufo cact. **CALC.** calc-acet.[36] **CALC-AR.** ***calc-f. calc-p. calc-s. calc-sil.***[58] ***camph.*** cann-i. ***cann-s.*** canth.[5] caps.[5] carb-an. **CARB-V.** carbn-s. ***carl.***[122] casc. cast. caust. ***cench.***[122] ***cham. chel. chin.*** chin-ar. chin-s. ***chlol.*** cimic.

CINA clem. coca[25] **COCC.** cod. coff. *colch.* coloc. **CON.** cop. corn. *croc.* **CROT-C.** crot-h.[58] *cycl.* dig. digin.[36] digox.[36] dios. dor. dros. dulc. echi.[111] elaps *erig.*[144] *eup-pur.* euph.[5] euphr. eupi.[102] ferr.[5] fl-ac. **GRAPH.** grat. guai. ham.[36] hell.[5] hep. hipp.[36] hydr. hydrog.[222] *hyos.* hyper. iber. ign. indg. *iod.*[5] ip. iris jac-c. jug-c. jug-r. **KALI-AR.** kali-bi. **KALI-BR.** **KALI-C.** kali-chl.[58] kali-cy.[36] *kali-i.* kali-n. kali-p. *kali-s.* *kali-sil.*[58] kalm. kiss.[36] kreos. lach. *laur.* *led.*[5] lil-s.[36] lil-t. **LYC.** lyss. *mag-c.* *mag-m.* mag-s.[10] manc. mand.[149] mang. *med.* *merc.* merc-c. merc-i-f. merc-i-r. merc-s. mez. mit.[36] morph.[36] mosch. mur-ac. myric. naja *nat-ar.* *nat-c.* **NAT-M.** *nat-p.*[58] *nat-s.* nat-sil.[58] **NICC.** *nit-ac.* nux-m. *nux-v.* op. ox-ac. paeon. par.[5] ped.[85] petr. ph-ac. phel. *phos.* phys. pitu-a.[164] plan. plat. *plb.*[5] psil.[164] *psor.*[122] ptel. **PULS.** *pyrog.*[5] *ran-b.*[5] *ran-s.* rat. *rheum*[5] rhod.[5] rhus-t. sabad. sabin.[5] sang. sarr. sars. scroph-n.[36] scut.[36] sec. sel.[54] sep. serp.[36] **SIL.** sin-n. sol-n.[36] spig. **SPONG.**[5] squil.[5] stann. staph. stram. stront-c. **SUL-AC.**[5] *sulph.* tab. *tarax.*[5] teucr.[5] thea. thuj. til. tub.[111] ust. valer.[5] verat. verat-v. verb. viol-o.[45] *zinc.* zinc-p.[58] zing.

➤ frightful, alone, when: kali-c.[58]
➤ frightful, blow on head, after: *nat-m.*[54]
➤ frightful, falling downstairs, after: *rhus-t.*[54]
➤ frightful, fear, followed by: alum.[10] *am-m.*[10] *chin.*[10] *cocc.*[10] *con.*[10] hep.[10] lyc.[10] mag-s.[10] mur-ac.[10] nat-c.[10] ph-ac.[10] sil.[10] sulph.[10] zinc.[10]
➤ frightful, figure, presenting a bottle to her: merc-c.[36]
➤ frightful, heart disease, in: *dig.*[54]
➤ frightful, hypochondriasis, in: *arg-n.*[54]
➤ frightful, impression, making a painful: *tarax.*[54]
➤ frightful, laborious: lil-t.[54]
➤ frightful, sadness, in: *naja*[54]
➤ ghosts, white, frightening him: sars.
➤ hydrophobia, of: anan.
➤ robbers, anxious, wakes frequently, with violent palpitation and screaming: *zinc.*[54]
➤ robbers, waking, with frightened, and a fixed idea that dream is true: verat.[54]
➤ storms, frightful: sil.[36]
➤ weeping, frightful or sad: *puls.*[54]

Dullness; fright, after: hyos.[172] op.[172]

Escape; attempts to, house, wants to get out of, fright, after: merc.[54]

Excitement; frightened, as if, on waking: *merc.*[54]

Fancies; exaltation of, frightful: **CALC.** *caust.* hydr. hydr-ac. *lac-c.* merc. *op.* *sil.* **STRAM.**

Fear; abortion, in threatening: bell.[26] *cimic.*[54] kali-c.[26] *op.*[54] *sabin.*[54]

✦ bed, of the, sit up and wander about the house as for them the nights are too long and restlessness comes with approaching day: syph.[172]
✦ called by his name, being: sulph.[172]
✦ death, fright, after: plat.[54]
✦ driving him from place to place, dyspnea, in: *acet-ac.*[54] acon-f.[36] ars.[60] astac.[54] bism.[54] *carb-an.*[54] hydr-ac.[60] *kalm.*[54] kreos.[60] *lyc.*[54] *phos.*[54] plat.[60] seneg.[60] **SPONG.**[54] viol-o.[54]
✦ endure, cannot: lyss.[137]
✦ events, of sudden: cocc.[1]
✦ everything, constant of: acet-ac.[54] acon.[172] bell.[36] *calc.*[54] hydr-ac.[102] *hyos.*[54] *lyc.*[54] nat-c.[54] *puls.*
✦ everything, constant of, ringing of a door bell, even at: *lyc.*[54]
✦ gnawing of fist, with: acon.[137]
✦ imaginary things: *acon.*[5] ars. bad.[5] **BELL.** brom.[5] calc-sil.[122] cham.[5] chin.[5] dros.[5] **HELL.**[5] hydr-ac.[102] hyos.[5] iod. laur. lyc. **MED.**[122] merc. nat-c.[172] *phos.* rhus-t.[5] sep.[172] **STRAM.**[5] verat.[5] zinc.[5]
✦ jumps, out of the window: ars.
✦ lifelong: am-c.[30] am-m.[30] calc.[30] lyc.[30] petr.[30] puls.[30] sil.[30] stann.[30] sulph.[30] zinc.[30]
✦ long lasting: *acon.*[111] carc.[184] hyos.[111] op.[111] petr.[137]
✦ mania, fright, after: *ign.*[54] *plat.*[54] *stram.*[54]
✦ panic attacks, dreams of fights, from: coca[36]
✦ panic attacks, overpowering: acon.[5] androc.[222] arg-n.[5] ars.[5] ars-i.[162] aur.[5] bamb-a.[1184] bell.[5] calc.[162] *cann-i.*[187] carb-v.[5] carc.[207] caust.[5] cham.[5] chin.[5] cocc.[5] coff.[5] cycl.[206] dig.[5] foll.[1201] germ.[222] hydrog.[222] hyos.[20] kali-ar.[188] kali-br.[162] kali-c.[162] lap-gr-m.[194] levo.[149] meli.[56] merc.[187] nux-v.[5] phos.[5] plat.[5] plb.[201] puls.[5] rhus-t.[5] stry.[188] sulph.[5] verat.[5]
✦ physician, surgeon: *coff.*[54]
✦ physician, will not see her; he seems to terrify her: arg-n.[172] arn.[162] dys-co.[136]

ign.[162] iod. nat-m.[162] ***nux-v.***[54] ***phos.***[162] ***sep.***[162] ***stram.***[54] thuj. tub.[172] verat.[172] verat-v.

✦ pulsation in, body, with: carb-v.[10]

✦ shadows, of, candle light, from: calc.[172]

✦ shrinks back, seeing anyone: ***stram.***[54]

✦ sleep, to go, lest, nightmare, he would have a: nux-v.[8]

✦ trembling of joints, as from electricity, from: paraf.[77]

✦ unknown, of the: ars.[127] aur.[172] med.[214] morg.[136] sac-alb.[210]

✦ urination, involuntary, of, at night: alum. ***phos.***[54] pitu-p.[149]

Frightened; easily, hideous objects, cries as if being frightened by seeing: stram.[8]

Frightened; easily, pollutions, after: aloe[1]

Frightened; easily, surprise, from every little: merc.[54]

Frightened; easily, touch, from: ***kali-c.*** ruta[36]

Frightened; easily, waking, in a fright from least noise: nux-v.

Hide; desire to, fear, on account of: ***ars. bell.*** cupr. ***hyos.***[54]

Hydrophobia; water, could not hear mentioned without shudder of fear: ***lyss.***[54] phys.[137]

Hypochondriasis; timid, fearful: cocc.[54]

Hysteria; fright, after: sabad.[54] ***stram.***[54] ***tarent.***[54] valer.[54]

Ideas; frightful, in evening: **CAUST.**[54]

Insanity; fright, from: **ARS.**[30] **BELL.**[30] ***ign.*** lach.[54] merc.[54] plat. sabad.[137] stram.[54]

Restlessness; thunderstorm, thunderbolt, after heavy, with terrific screams: ***gels.***[54]

Sadness; fear, from: cimic.[58] nux-m.[54] sec.[137] ***stram.***[54]

Shrieking; approaches the bed, when anyone: ***ign.***[54]

Shrieking; cardiac rheumatism, in: ***cact.***[54]

Shrieking; fear with, happened, of what suddenly: lap-c-b.[194]

Shrieking; fear, with: ***acon.***[137] rhus-t.[54] ***verat.***[54]

Shrieking; fear, with, death, of, as if in: chlol.[54]

Shrieking; fear, with, death, of, dry convulsive cough, from, in weak nervous children: ***kali-br.***[54]

Somnambulism; fright, after, in plethoric subjects: acon.[172]

Starting; fright, from and as from, approach of a person, at: ***bell.***[54]

Suicidal disposition; fear of death, with: alum.[54] **ARS.**[94] aur.[94] ***chin.***[30] hep.[94] kali-ar.[58] **NIT-AC.**[30] nux-v.[94] ***plat.***[54] rhus-t.[58] ***staph.***[30] tab.[36]

Thoughts; arrested by thrills caused by imagining something unpleasant: asar.[54]

Thoughts; frightful: androc.[222] calc. ***caust.*** hydr-ac. ***iod.***[54] lac-c. lap-c-b.[194] lyss. phos. phys. ***plat.***[54] psor.[137] ***rhus-t.*** stram. thea. ***visc.***

Thoughts; frightful, seeing blood, or a knife, on: ***alum.***

ACON. Al, 66 - Great timidity after a severe fright (fear), afraid to go out unattended (abandoned, helplessness) after dark, is unable to control his feelings of apprehensive fear.

Ha, 540 - Lamentable fears of impending death.

He, 36 - Extreme timidity, especially after a fright; afraid (fear) in dark.

He, 51 - Ailments from fright: afraid (fear) in dark; vertigo; faintness; trembling; cardiac weakness; threatened miscarriage (abortion); impending cessation of menstrual flow;..

ADAM. Sh, 242 - Feeling very pathetic and scared of people getting angry with me. 20, 1M, 10:XX:XX

ALOE. Al, 17 - Great anxiety, timorousness, restlessness, dread (fear) of death, and great anguish, so that she cannot stay anywhere.(restlessness)

ALUM. Al, 19 - Anxiety and fearfulness, as if he had committed a crime.

Ha, 17 - Anxiety and fearfulness, as if he had committed a crime.

Ha, 25 - Varying moods through the day, now confidence, then again faint-heartedness.(timid)

He, 23 - Anguish, oppressive and vague fearfulness, or uneasiness as if he had committed a crime.

ALUMN. Al, 4 - Feared to leave her sit in church, after feeling faint.

AML-N. He, 13 - Haunted (obsessed) many times a day with an indescribable dread and sensation as of an oncoming fit, although it came on only once or twice a week.

ANAC. Ha, 6 - Timorous in all his actions; he views everything more anxiously and timidly, always thinks of being surrounded by enemies, then he becomes hot, his blood seems to boil in his chest.

ANAN. Al, 2 - Sadness and restlessness, with fear of death and of the future.

ANDROC. Sh, 81 - Felt out of control, his emotions took over. Felt terror, panic, fear and that he could not cope. (2)

Sh, 82 - Absolutely terrified of dog on street, for no apparent reason, with numbness and tingling through every part of his body, followed by a sick feeling in the stomach. He felt shaken for hours later. (2)

Sh, 83 - Woke at night to urinate. On going upstairs, all colours seemed incredibly bright and the walls were pulsating —in towards him and out again. This felt similar to an L.S.D. experience years ago. Did not know what to do, was stricken with panic. Terrified, he raced back to bed where he felt hot, so uncovered, then cold so covered, then hot, he uncovered and sat up and immediately felt better — no panic. As soon as he lay down he began to panic. Became afraid in the light and felt better in the dark with the lights off. He wanted to call someone for help, and felt angry about the proving. He then got up and walked around for a few minutes, got back to bed, and fell asleep. (2)

Sh, 84 - Overwhelmed by terror, panic and fear, like a psychic attack. Then specifically became fear of being psychically tested as if confronted by something absolutely horrible, as in a "cult initiation ordeal". He felt so scared he had to shut the door, with a feeling that something would appear from behind it if he left it open. (4)

Sh, 87 - Panic stricken with her customers. (7)

Sh, 88 - Intense but very rapid fear, immensely powerful and very upsetting. Avery deep fear and panic felt in abdomen. (10)

Sh, 122 - When his friends were talking, he became very suspicious and fearful, but had no fear of strangers or the police. (29)

ANT-T. Al, 12 - Dreaded (fear) to be left alone even for a few moments, lest he " should be dreadfully nervous and not know what to do with himself."

He, 30 - Depression of mind and fear that he will never get well.

ANTH. Al, 6 - On going out of doors, in evening, felt nervous, and exceedingly afraid of being run over.

APIS. He, 81 - Ailments from fright, rage, vexation, jealousy, or hearing bad news.

ARG-N. He, 46 - Easily frightened; fears disease may result seriously; weeping mood.

He, 47 - Fear or thinking brings on diarrhea.(ailments from)

ARN. Ha, 611 - Fright and starting at unexpected (accidental) trifles.

ARS-MET. He, 4 - Fearful visions of spectres (ghosts) in bright daylight; she sees threatening people after her,...

ARS. Al, 78 - Anxiety and fear; he sees a absent acquaintance (friend) lying dead upon the sofa, and has great dread of him.

Al, 84 - The greatest fear and anguish; sees ghosts day and night.

Al, 87 - He imagines that the whole house, and the space under the bed, are full of thieves, which causes, from fright, anxious cold sweat to break out over his body.

Ha, 33 - Anguish and fear; he sees an acquaintance who is not present lie dead on sofa, and is much afraid of him.

He, 42 - Fear drives him out of bed; he hides in a closet.

He, 63 - Dread (fear) of death when alone, or on going to bed.

AUR. He, 80 - Ailments from fright, anger, contradiction, mortification, or vexation with dread, fear, reserved displeasure, or vehemence.

He, 49 - Fearfulness, a longing for death. 0Hyperemia of brain.

BAR-A. Al, 8 - Solicitous (careful) and fearful. The slightest noise in the street seems to him like a fire alarm, and he is frightened thereat, so that he starts in every limb.

Al, 10 - An evil, fearful suspicion suddenly takes possession of her, as if, for example, a loved friend had been taken suddenly deathly ill.

BAR-C. Al, 12 - Great fear and cowardice.

Ha, 11 - Anxious and fearful; a little noise on the street seems to him at once like fire alarm, and he is frightened by it, so that it darts (move quickly) through all his limbs.

BAR-M. He, 11 - During an attack of fear, she says in a weak, husky voice, she must die.

BELL. Ha, 1432 - Fearful mistrust.

Al, 127 - Aversion to all fluids (liquid, water) so that she demeaned (conduct) herself frightfully (fear) at the sight of them.

Al, 165 - Cowardice, distrust, suspicion, inclination to run away.

Al, 167 - Events which had been previously anticipated with pleasure appeared to him in an anxious light; he thought them fearful and dreadful.

Al, 166 - He starts in affright very readily, especially when any one approaches him.

Ha, 1433 - Fearful madness; he is afraid (fear) of an imaginary black dog, of the gallows. (hanging)

He, 22 - Frightful visions; she wishes (desires) to hide herself.(veil, cover)

He, 30 - Delirium: with frightful figures and images before eyes; is afraid (fear) of imaginary things; sees monsters; talks of dogs as if they swarmed (crowded) about him; furious.

He, 102 - Became fearful when persons approached him in street, and when they had passed, he insisted on it that he had stabbed them.

He, 104 - Fear of imaginary things, wants to run away from them.

He, 13 - Timorous anxiety; he is afraid of a an imaginary black dog; of the gallows, etc.

BERB. Al, 3 - Anxious mood, with great fear and fright...; in the twilight some dogs and children appeared as large again as natural.

BOR. Ha, 4 - Very timid, in driving down a mountain (elevation); quite at variance with his customary bearing; he felt as if it would take his breath away.

Ha, 5 - The child is timid while being dandled; when it is rocked up and down in the arms it makes a very frightened face...(fear, touch, caresses)

Ha, 8 - Timid, an anxious scream causes terror to fall on all his limbs.

BRY. He, 22 - Apprehensive, uneasiness and dread of future.

BUFO. Al, 15 - Fear of animals.

Al, 16 - Fear of catching diseases.

Al, 22 - He is irritable, anxious about his state of health, with great dread of death.

CACT. Al, 18 - Fear of death extreme and continuous; he believes his disease to be incurable.

CALAD. Al, 3 - He is very apprehensive about his health, and about everything...

CALC-P. He, 12 - Feels as if he had been frightened.(terrorized)

CALC. Al, 25 - Frightened apprehensive mood, as if some misfortune were about to happen to him, or some one else, which he could in no way overcome.

Ha, 23 - Fearful, anxious forebodings, as if evil would befall (happen) him or some one else, and as if he could in no way evade it.

Ha, 25 - His heart is agitated with fear and anxiety for the future, with fear of consumption.(tuberculosis, ruin)

He, 56 - Feels awe-stricken (terror-injure) at night. 0 Diarrhea

CAMPH. Al, 46-... My misery was boundless; time itself was no more; in short, I suffered such fearful anguish as no fancy can comprehend. What soul could paint to itself my everlasting (eternal) dwelling as the Evil One (devil), alone in a vast universe, without faith or hope, and my heart forever broken by unimaginable tortures? (miserable, timeless, endless, solitude, forsaken, faithless, hopeless)

Al, 37 - Excessively fearful, especially in the dark.

Al, 38 - Dread of being alone in the dark.

Al, 39 - Indescribable dread of being drawn upwards.

Al, 46-...A fearful terror seized me, and I knew not whither to fly. I cried out aloud, "And so I am indeed dead; that hell I used to think about is no fiction, but a reality which I am doomed to experience forever...

CANN-I. Al, 34 - All around and within seems to be a great mystery, and is terrifying.

CANTH. Al, 25 - Extreme despondency and faintheartedness; she says she must die.

CAPS. He, 12 - Awakens with fright, screams, and remains full of fear.

CARB-AN. Ha, 16 - He feels horror in the evening, even to shivering and weeping.
Ha, 15 - Timid and fearful (coward), all day.
He, 9 - Fearful in the dark.

CARB-V. Ha, 9 - He felt like weeping, everything seemed to him dreadful (fearful), and he felt in despair.

CARBN-O. Al, 7 - Frightful anxiety, and instinctive impulse to seek change of air, while he felt powerless to overcome the paralysis of his muscles and move from where he sat.

CAUST. Ha, 20 - Extreme anxious timidity; she is so much afraid (fear) of a dog near her, which did not harm (hurt, injure) her at all,...every noise in the street made her afraid, and when she saw boys climbing she was very uneasy lest they might get hurt. (care, others)
Ha, 21 - Her fear and anxiety cause her to wish that she might not live.(death)
He, 36 - Fearfulness and distressed (anguish) feeling about heart.
He, 37 - Full of timorous fancies, evenings; child fears to go to bed alone.
He, 42 - Great apprehension whenever anything happens; despondent, depressed, most excessive exhaustion and prostration.
He, 69 - Injurious (ailments from) effects of fear and vexation. (worry)
He, 39 - Ill effects of sudden emotions, fright, fear, etc. (ailments from)

CEDR. Al, 5 - Dread of friends.(in females, particularly)

CHEL. Al, 53 - Becomes frightened at the slightest noise, as if he had not a good conscience.

CHOC. Sh, 51 - While out walking, saw a dog and became very scared. I felt very uncomfortable and unsympathetic to the dog. All very unusual.

COFF. He, 20-...anxiety of mind and conscience filled with many fears.

CON. Al, 39 - Dread (fear) of men of their approach, yet with dread of being alone.
Ha, 365 - Sunk in deep thought, he cogitated timorously about the present and the future and sought (wants) solitude.
He, 31 - Great anxiety; precordial anguish; superstitious (careful, credulous, naive) and full of fear (coward), with frequent thoughts of death...

COP. Al, 2 - Disgust (loathing) with life, and at the same time fear of death.

CUPR. Al, 8 - Fearful; want of courage.
He, 21 - Afraid of and shrinking away from everyone who approaches him; afraid of falling; clinging tightly to nurse;...
He, 8 - Mania characterized by a wild look and fear; tries to escape.

ELAPS. Al, 13 - Fearfulness, dread (fear) of being alone, as though something would happen, or as though rowdies (revolution, rebellious) would break in.
Al, 14 - Excessive horror of rain.
He, 4 - Fearful and apprehensive of some fatal disease.
He, 5 - Fear of being left alone, as if something horrible might happen; horror of rain.

EUP-PUR. He, 9 - Has a great fear of sickness.

GELS. He, 29 - Every exciting news causes diarrhea ; bad effects from fright and fear. (ailments from)
He, 30 - Bad effects (ailments) from suddenly hearing bad news; from fright(fear); diarrhea, abortion etc.

GERM. Sh, 15 - Wake feeling anxious, increasingly. Legs tremble and shake. I have to get out of bed. I am scared that a heart attack is imminent and cannot be prevented. It's to late to do anything. I walk from room to room, thirsty, chilly and in turmoil. Accompanied by a desire for stool and flatulence. 08, 12C, 80:00:00
Sh, 103 - Felt closed in. My every movement and thought controlled. Didn't know where to go for help. Felt like a coward . Felt afraid of violence. I don't know who I am. 04, 6C, XX:XX:XX

GLON. Al, 12 - Though naturally cheerful she became apprehensive of her approaching death.
He, 16 - Bad effects of mental excitement, fright, fear, mechanical contusions and their consequences.(ailments from)

GRAPH. Al, 27 - Extreme apprehensiveness, so that she did not know how to overcome (succeed) it, disappearing after weeping.
Ha, 14 - Extraordinary apprehensiveness, so that she cannot compose (calm) herself; it goes off on weeping.

GUAI. Ha, 129 - In the evening in bed (when slumbering?) he felt as if some one threw a towel at his face, so that he started up in affright at it.

HALI-L. Sh, 350-... "Considered committing suicide. Feeling that life has passed me by. Thinking about my mortality. Terrified of dying. My time has run out." ...[18], 30C, 05:XX:XX-[16]:XX:XX

Sh, 670 - When I was alone in my apartment with the lights on, I manifested many fragmented personalities, probably around five or six. Never did before like this. What was different was nobody was in the room to make a chain reaction. I was alone. Needed no provocation to make a change, or experience a change. I talk outloud, and talk to the person in a number of different ways. Fearful Joe, Vindictive Joe, One That's Just Like Someone Else Joe —each will act out in a number of different ways. 18, 30C, 35:XX:XX

HAM. Al, 15 - Was afraid to risk (danger) another dose (medicine); his mind was in a fearful condition.

HELL. Al, 19 - Dread of death.(in a sufferer from religious melancholy)

HEP. Al, 1 - Ghostly image of one who was dead, in the morning, in bed, after waking and while conscious, which frightened him; it also seemed as though he saw his neighbor's house burning, which also frightened him.

Al, 10 - Fearful concerning sickness in the family, especially when walking alone in the open air.

Ha, 298 - In the morning in bed after waking, when conscious, he had the visionary appearance of a deceased (dead, defunct) person, which frightened him, and he also imagined he saw a neighboring house in flames, which terrified him.

He, 5 - Frightful visions of fire and of dead persons.

HYDROG. Sh, 192 - During palpitations, extreme fear —thought I was having a heart attack. Frightened the living daylights out of me. 24, 30C, 100:XX:XX

Sh, 195 - Apprehensive, panicky, with cold sweat on palms. Feel extremely vulnerable emotionally —like an egg that has just broken. Frightened, anything can happen. 16, 30C, 05:XX:XX

Sh, 255 - Very worried that people don't like me and can't cope with me —that they will think I am insane. I think maybe I am insane. This is frightening me. 16, 30C, 25:XX:XX

HYOS. Al, 85 - Excessive fear of death, becoming a monomania,...

Al, 87 - Remarkable fear that he had been devoured by animals.

Ha, 575 - Peculiar fear of being bitten (hurt) by beasts.

IBER. Al, 1 - Frightened mood; fears she has taken too much of the drug; in the evening.(medicine)

Al, 2 - Feels frightened; ...as if she had taken a dangerous dose.(medicine)

IGN. Al, 20 - Fearfulness timidity; she has no confidence in herself, gives up (desist) everything.

Ha, 759 - Fearfulness, cowardice cannot trust himself to do anything, considers all is lost .

Ha, 762 - Fears every trifle, is specially afraid of objects coming near him.

He, 35 - Fearfulness; does not like to talk; prefers to be alone.

He, 36 - Anxiety as though something terrible had happened cannot speak because of it; hurry, fearfulness, terror, alternating with irresolution and inertness.

He, 33 - Dread of every trifle, especially of things coming near him.

IP. Al, 8 - He is thoughtful, fearful, and thinks trifles are very important.

IRID. Sh, 99 - Sat at the bus stop. Felt like a really small, frightened rabbit, with a large shadow of this great bird hovering over ready to pounce. G8

Sh, 204 - All day, woke with sense of foreboding as if something bad was going to happen. Feeling quite shaky, butterflies in tummy, a bit nauseous. I14

IRIS. Al, 3 - Despondency; thinks he is going to be very sick, then a disposition to laugh at his fears, which, however, soon return.

KALI-BR. He, 37 - Timid, suspicious, full of fear.

He, 38 - Much concerned (anxiety) about health; complains without cause;...uncontrollable sensation of fear and anxiety, thinks she is becoming deranged (insanity) ; change of life.

He, 39-...fear and apprehension that she is losing her mind (insanity);...makes her utterly (completely) miserable to be looked at or spoken to; fear to see people; always depressed and lowspirited;...

He, 24 - Hands constantly busy; all sorts of fearful delusions; walks the room groaning, bemoaning his fate (destine, doom); full of fear; unsteady.(inconstant)

KALI-C. Al, 17 - Fearful and anxious about her disease.

Al, 25 - She is frightened with a loud cry, by an imaginary apparition (as for example, of a bird flying to the window).

Ha, 26 - She is frightened by an imaginary appearance (e.g. as if a bird was flying toward the window) and she utters a loud scream.

Ha, 25 - Readily frightened, especially by a slight touch of the body.

He, 16 - Very easily frightened; shrieks about imaginary appearances; starts when touched.

He, 17 - Is frightened and cries out whenever he is touched lightly on his feet.

LAC-C. He, 8 - Sensation as if she was going deranged, when sitting still and thinking; sometimes she has most horrible sights presented to her mental vision (not always snakes), feels horribly afraid that they will take objective form and show themselves to her natural eye.

He, 21 - Sits and looks under chairs, table, sofa and everything in room, expecting yet dreading (fear) to see some terrible monster creep forth and feeling all the time, that if it does, it will drive her raving mad; she is not afraid in dark, it is only in light where she can imagine that she can see them.

LACH. He, 41 - Dread (fear) of death, fears to go to bed ; fears of being poisoned.

He, 59 - Ailments from fright (fear), disappointed love or jealousy.

LED. He, 2 - After nightmare, fears to go to sleep lest she die.

LIL-T. Al, 9 - Depression of spirits; constant inclination to weep, with fearfulness, and apprehension of suffering from some terrible internal disease, already seated.

LYC. Al, 49 - Fear of going to bed in the evening. (sleep?)

Al, 50 - In the evening on entering a room he is attacked with fear, as though he saw some one; even during the day he believes that he hears some one in the room.

Al, 52 - Great fear of frightful images which her fancy conjures(charm) up, in the evening, and lachrymose during the day.

Ha, 26 - In the evening in the dark, he is frightened because a door he wants to open, opens with difficulty. (confined, restricted)

Ha, 27 - He is afraid (fear) in the evening, on entering a room, as if he saw somebody; by day also he sometimes imagines he hears somebody in the room.

He, 14 - Dread (fear) of men ; of solitude, irritability and melancholy.

He, 24 - Easily frightened (afraid) and starts up; feels frightened at everything, even ringing of door bell.

He, 39 - Ailments from fright, anger, mortification, or vexation, with reserved displeasure.

He, 36 - Distrustful, suspicious and fault (mistake) finding. (judgment)

LYSS. Al,N-78 - Feels as if he cannot physically endure his fears much longer, and shall be compelled to go into an insane asylum.

He, 78 - Feels he cannot physically endure his fears much longer, and shall be compelled to go into an insane asylum.

MAG-C. Al, 951 - Frightful dream, that she burnt her cheek by the light.

MAG-M. Al, 714 - Frightful dreams; that she was pursued by robbers; that she burned her hand by washing ...

MED. He, 33 - Woke at an early hour with a frightened sensation, as if something dreadful had happened;... as if she must do something to rid her mind of this torture.

MERC. He, 28 - Anxiety and restless change of place; ebullitions, sweat; apprehensive, imaginary fears; fears he will lose his mind;...(sanity).

MOSCH. He, 4 - Great dread (fear) of death, with paleness of face, fainting; talks only of approaching (nearing) death.

He, 11 - Great tendency to be frightened, trembling, palpitation of heart, and dread of death.

NAT-C. Al,DREAM, 1113 - Anxious, vivid, frightful dreams of thieves, from which he

started up with loud cry, and when awake could scarcely realize that his fears were groundless.
Al, 28 - He is very timid, and starts at the slightest noise.
Al, 29 - Anthropophobia and fearfulness.
He, 13 - Constant fear and forebodings.

NAT-M. Al, 70 - In the evening it seemed as though he became paralyzed from a fright (terrify) ; afterwards he seemed horrified, and apprehended some misfortune.
Al, 71 - Fear of insanity.
Ha, 54 - In the evening, he was, as it were, paralyzed by a fright, then he became horrified and apprehensive.
He, 48 - Consequences (ailments) of fright, anger, vexation, mortification, or reserved displeasure.

NICC. Al, 9 - Tremulous, fearful, with inclination to be alone all day.

NUX-V. Al, 41 - Anxiety; an anxious solicitude, as though something serious (dangerous) were dreaded, in the morning and afternoon..
Al, 54 - She was in great alarm, kept fast hold on her husband and refused to let him go.
Ha, 1235-...anxiety and anxious solicitude (care), as if something important were to be feared (afraid).
Ha, 1246 - He fears death.
Ha, 1257 - Anxiety from suspicious and timorous (timidity) solicitude, especially in the hours after midnight.
He, 19-...; imagines himself surrounded by persons who carry on all sorts of pranks (joke, jest), or ply (covering) him whith questions which he thinks he is compelled (forced) to answer (proved, questioned, interrogated);..; answers questions rationally and is conscious of his condition; ...appears to be haunted (obsessed) by a great fear.

OP. He, 13 - Sees frightful ghosts; easily frightened.

PHOS. Al, 80 - Mental depression, and a most uncommon fearfulness or timidity, with a great sense of fatigue.
Al, 111 - Horrible fearfulness, late in the evening, as if a horrible face were looking out from every corner.
Al, 116 - The world was frightful (fearful, offensive) to him, only weeping could relieve him;...
Ha, 31 - Dreadful fearfulness, late in the evening, as if a horrid face was looking out of every corner.
Ha, 62 - Very irritable mood, she takes every word ill and becomes pusillanimous (coward) from it.
Ha, 79 - In the evening, usually of so vivid an imagination that the mere representation of disagreeable things causes horror with her.
Ha, 12 - The world seemed dreadful to him; only weeping could relieve him, soon afterward apathy and indifference.
He, 22-...uneasy about one's health; paroxysms of anguish, when alone or in a stormy weather, with timorous disposition; told those about him repeatedly that he could not possibly recover, and gave some disjointed (incoherent) directions about his business affairs.
He, 9 - Mental depression and a most uncommon fearfulness or timidity with great sense of fatigue.
He, 34-...full of fear, especially at piano; constantly on lookout (look carefully) for something to happen; ...sexual dreams and violent sexual excitement.

PSOR. Al,N-46 - Attacks of fear; fear of fire, of being alone, of apoplexy, of becoming insane.
Al,N-14 - Anxious, full of fear, melancholic; evil forebodings.
Al,N-48 - Fright caused by the merest trifles; this often causes perspiration and trembling.
He, 13 - Anxious, full of fear, melancholic; evil forebodings.

PULS. He, 29 - When evening comes begins to dread ghosts.
He, 53-...afraid of everybody; considers every one her enemy, despairs of everything; ...;trusts no one;.. (suspicious)
He, 43 - Sleepless nights on account of great fear and anxious restlessness; despairs of her salvation and seeks aid in constant prayer;...
He, 50 - After slight emotions, difficult breathing; bad effects from fright, mortification or excessive joy.(ailments from)

RHUS-T. Al, 33 - He is frightened (afraid, fear) by a trifle (insignificance) (on falling asleep) as if he had dreaded (worry) the greatest misfortune.

Al, 1385 - Fearful dreams, for example, that the world was on fire, with palpitation on waking.

Al, 4 - Full of sad thoughts, anxious and fearful, wherewith she gradually lost strength, and was obliged to lie down for hours in order to regain vigor.

Ha, 962 - She did not sleep half the night, was timorous (timid, fearful) full of anguish and cardiac anxiety.

Ha, 964 - Full of sad thoughts, anxious and timorous (timid), during which she always lost her strength, (power) and must lie down for hours; in order to recover her strength. (inert, motionless)

Ha, 972 - From sad thoughts, which she could not get rid of, she became timorous and fainthearted.(coward, fearful)

RUTA. Ha, 275 - Very frequent anxiety with desponding (sad) thoughts and fears.

SEL. Al, 4 - Dread of people and of his occupation, but overcoming this he is able to continue his work.

SEP. Al, 30 - All her troubles appear to her mind in a very gloomy light, so that she is fearful.

Al, 58 - Fearfulness when riding in a carriage.

SIL. He, 16 - Yielding, faint-hearted, anxious mood.

SPONG. Al, 6 - She is very fearful, and tormented by a frightful image of a past sad event.

Ha, 381 - She is timorous (fearful) and particularly pursued and incessantly plagued (disturbed, bothered) by a frightful picture out of a melancholic past.

He, 21 - She is very timid, and is especially pursued and incessantly tormented by a frightful scene of some mournful (unhappy) event of the past.

He, 22 - She is very timorous (fearful), and starts at every trifle, which affects her feet, so as to make them feel heavy.

STRAM. Al, 207 - His whole conduct and countenance was like that of a child severely frightened and apprehending some terrible calamity.

Ha, 564 - He always imagines he is alone (solitary, lonely) and is afraid.

Ha, 565 - Nowhere has he rest, is startled by dream-pictures, even when his eyes are open, which in the form of big dogs, cats and other horrible beasts, grow (expand) out of the ground at his side, and from which he jumps away to the side with signs of terror (fear), and knows not how to save (rescue, free) himself. (cornered, corralled)

Ha, 553 - Frightful pictures of the imagination; he fancies he sees ghosts.

Ha, 563 - As a rule he has more imaginary figures at his side than in front of him, they all inspire him with horror.

He, 65-"There", he replied, "A long train of bedbugs, and after them a procession of beetles and here come crawling over me a host (crowd) of cockroaches"; sank back in alarm, then suddenly said:" I believe I know they are not really bugs, but, except once in a while, they seem real to me. (organization, association, union)

He, 156 - Endeavors to escape, imagines he is alone all the time, and is afraid. (loneliness, isolation)

He, 163 - Cries out fearfully, hides face in pillow, is terrified by presence or approach of physician; after attack of typhoid.

He, 58 - Imagines he is alone, and is frightened.

He, 94-...fear of malicious animals, black dogs; ...

SUL-AC. Al, 28 - Very fearful; extremely mistrustful.

Ha, 10 - So irritable and affected that she gets frightened at everything.

SULPH. Al, 3800-....(DREAM) she walked about like a somnambulist, thought there was a fire, dressed herself, talked out of the window, and was frightened as she heard that it was nothing; for three days afterwards she was very weak, and felt bruised(hurt).

Al, 3816 - Frightful dream that he had been bitten by a dog.

Al, 59 - Awoke in a hour in great fright and distress; horror of instant death.

He, 33 - Sleepless, disgusted with life, fears the future, where she sees nothing but misery (wretchedness, poverty) and suffering (misfortune). 0 Melancholia.

SYPH. Al,N-12 - Terrible dread (fear) of night, ...death is preferable ; she fears to prepare for night and is positively in abject fear of suffering,...

He, 9 - Terrible dread of night, ...it is

intolerable, death is preferable. She fears to prepare for night and is positively in abject fear of suffering...

TAB. Al, 38 - Terrible apprehensions (fear) of immediate death.

Al, 41 - From having been one of the most healthy and fearless of men, he had become sick all over, and was timid as a girl; he could not even present a petition in Congress, much less say a word concerning it; ...by any ordinary noise, he was startled or thrown into tremulousness, and afraid to be alone at night.

TARENT. Al, 11 - Visions of monsters or animals, that frightened him.

Al, 55 - Fear, which could not be stopped, in a young lady; questioned about it, she tried to find a cause, and leaves others to think there is one; but really there was none.

THEA. Al, 19 - Appeared to be actuated by the greatest terror, and said: "I have called upon you to request you would let me in and allow me to die in your house".

TUB. Al,N-27 - With every little ailment whines and complains; easily frightened, particularly by dogs; screams in terror when approached by a dog.

He, 2 - Fretful (irritable), ailing (sick), whines (moan) and complains; mind given to be frightened (fearful), particularly by dogs.

VALER. Al, 12 - Fearfulness in the evening when sitting in the dark (imagining that some one might hurt him).

VERAT. He, 45-... he is tormented by fearful anxiety, wherewith forehead becomes covered with cold sweat and he becomes sick to vomiting.

ZINC. He, 7 - Stares (look) as if frightened on waking, head rolls (turn) from side to side.

FEARLESS

Audacity: acon. agar. alum.[5] ant-t.[5] ***arn.***[122] aur.[137] bamb-a.[1184] bell.[102] bov.[5] calad.[5] carc.[187] cic.[137] cocain.[102] guai.[5] hep.[30] **IGN.**[5] lach.[5] m-arct.[10] merc. mez.[5] nat-c.[5] nitro-o.[36] op. ozone[227] plat.[30] ***puls.***[5] sil.[102] squil.[5] staph.[30] sulph.[5] tarax.[5] tub.[137] verat.[5]

Confidence; future, in: androc.[222] ferr-ma.[36]

Courageous: acon. agar. alco.[36] alum. ant-t. berb. ***bov.***[122] ***calad.***[122] calc-s.[108] dros. ferr-p.[36] gins. ***ign.*** m-arct.[10] merc. mez. nat-c. ***op.*** phos. ***puls.***[122] squil. sulph. tab. tarax. ter.[122] ***tub.***[137] valer. verat.

Courageous; alternating with discouragement: merc.[30] op.[30] staph.[30]

Courageous; alternating with, fear: ***alum.***[10]

Courageous; alternating with, timidity: ***alum.***[30]

Courageous; foolish: calad.[137]

Death; presentiment of, thinks of death calmly: zinc.

Death; presentment of, fear without: lac-d.[85]

Death; thoughts of, calmly: zinc.

Death; thoughts of, fear, without: apis[5] ***coff.***[5] merc.[5] verat-v.[5]

Delusions; jump from a height and land safely, she can: lap-mar-c.[194]

• tall, he is, fright, from: plat.[54]

Dreams; acrobats, swinging from trapezes: hydrog.[222]

➤ adventurous: bar-c.[10] ozone[227] senec.[36] sulph.[10]

➤ somersaults, of throwing, at an old man: zing.[36]

Fearlessness: agar.[36] bell.[72] calad.[172] cocain.[102] coff-t.[102] gels.[102] hell.[36] **IGN.**[8] mosch.[36] op.[1] ozone[227] sil.[102]

Fearlessness; danger menaced him, as if, but without fear: fl-ac.[54]

High-spirited: hydr. hyos. op. spig. spong. verat. verb

Impetuous: acon. ***anac.*** arg-n.[187] arn.[37] aur.[117] ***bry.*** calc.[117] calc-s.[108] ***carb-v.*** caust. ***cham.*** cocain.[38] croc. ferr-p. glon.[137] **HEP.** ***hyos.***[8] ictod.[8] ***iod.***[184] ***kali-c.*** kali-i. kali-p. kali-s.[58] lach.[58] laur. led. mag-c.[85] med.[102] nat-c. ***nat-m.*** **NIT-AC. NUX-V.** olnd. phos. rheum **SEP.** ***staph.*** stront-c. sul-ac.[117] ***sulph.*** tab.[137] ***zinc.*** zinc-p.[58]

Improvident: alum.[30] caust.[30] nat-m.[30]

Indifference; traffic, in: pull-g.[181]

Plans; bold: agar.[36]

Rashness: ***aur.*** caps. cic.[137] meny. op.[137] puls. tub.[137]

Runs; about, dangerous place, in most: agar.[36]

AGAR. Al, 4 - He is intoxicated with fearless frenzy; forming bold (courageous, brave) and revengeful projects.

Al, 22 - Some run and walk involuntarily in the most dangerous places.(defiant)

Al, 3 - Fearless, menacing, mischievous (rude) frenzy; also, frenzy which causes the patient to assail and injure himself, with great exertion of power.

Ha, 23 - Fearless, threatening, destructive frenzy, also such as turns against itself and injures itself, combined with great exertion of strength.

Ha, 20 - Drunken fearless frenzy with bold (courageous), vengeful determinations.

ARS-H. He, 14 - The fear of dying is gone on 3d day, notwithstanding all around him have doubts of his recovery.

BOV. Al, 5 - Very courageous and vigorous; he would like to fight with everybody.

CACT. He, 4 - Feels she is dying and thinks she will not live till morning, but has no fear of death. (fearless)

DROS. Al, 1 - Joyful, good courage: he had no fear of evil, because he was conscious of having done right. (moral, virtuous, honest, fearless)

FL-AC. Al, 12 - During the tottering (tremble) sensation he has a decided though not anxious expectation, as if there was to happen something awful (horrible), but he feels no anxiety.

Al, 13 - Sensation as if dangers did menace (threaten) him, but without being afraid;...

He, 12 - Sensation as if danger menaced (threatened) him, but without fear. (fearless)

HURA. Al, 7 - During and after the fainting spell (trance), disposed to love everybody, especially those about him; he often thinks of death, but does not fear it; he feels as though he could die without regret.(fearless)

HYDROG. Sh, 294 - Spirits uplifted by wonderful weather. Felt strong, positive and adventurous. 04, 12C, 32:XX:XX

LAC-D. Al,N-10 - Has no fear of death but is sure is going to die.

He, 10 - Has no fear (fearless) of death but is sure he is going to die.

NUX-M. Al, 27 - As soon as she lay down felt a sinking sensation, as though she were going to die, with no fear, however, being perfectly at ease (peace) in mind,...

Al, 60 - State of mind similar to that of the opium-eater, entertaining no apprehension of the result, although aware of the presence of some danger.

He, 26 - Aware of danger, but no apprehension.

OP. Al, 68 - Criminals (in India) lose their fear of death and go courageously to their execution.(fearless)

Al, 70 - Sensation of courage with activity, as if he could forcibly accomplish whatever was required without dread or fear, with a peculiar sensation of lustiness. (strong)

ZINC. Ha, 15 - Tranquil thoughts of dying, in the afternoon, when weary.

FEIGNING

Affectation: alum.[30] carb-v.[30] caust.[30] con.[30] graph.[30] hyos.[30] lyc.[30] mez.[1] nat-m.[30] 0pall.[185] petr.[30] plat.[30] ***stram.*** verat.[30]

Affectation; gestures and acts, in: hyos.[30] mez.[1] stram.[108] verat.[30]

Affectation; mania, in: ***stram.***[54]

Affectation; words and expressions, in: lyc.[30] plat.[30] verat.[30]

Blindness pretended: verat.

Charlatan: calc.[30] plat.[30] sulph.[30]

Cheerfulness; appears, but looks down when on street: ***dios.***[54]

Cheerfulness; simulates hilarity, while feels wretched: apis.[58]

Contemptuous; hard for subordinates and agreeable or pleasant to superiors or people he has to fear: lach.[30] lyc.[30] plat.[30] verat.[30]

Deafness; pretended: verat.

Delirium; groping as if in the dark: plb.[36]

Delirium; wraps up in fur during summer: hyos.

Delusions; faces, mask-like: anh.[119] op.[10]

- faces, scheming: anh.[119]
- harlequin, he is a: hyos.
- juggler, he is a: bell.
- labor, pretends to be in, or thinks she has pains: verat.
- magician, is a: bell.
- pregnant; she is: apis[36] berb.[85] carc.[146] ***caul.***[54] ***croc.***[54] cycl.[102] hydrog.[222] ign. nux-v.[85] ***op.***[102] ozone[227] ***puls.***[54] ***sabad.*** sulph.[102] thuj. ***verat.***
- sensations, misrepresents his: bell.
- shoot with a stick, tries to: bell.[5] merc.

Destructiveness; cunning: ***tarent.***

Dreams; masks: kali-c.[1] mag-c.[36] ran-r.

Fear; pregnancy, during, conception, in false: ***caul.***[54]

Feigning; looking to others in distress: tarent.[137]
Feigning; paroxysms, faintness: ***tarent.***
Feigning; pregnancy: croc.[171] verat.
Feigning; sick: arg-n. bell. ign.[5] mosch.[162] plb.[58] sabad.[137] sil.[30] ***tarent.*** verat.
Fur, wraps up in summer: hep.[111] hyos. ***kali-ar.***[137] ***psor.***[111]
Gestures; makes, actor, like an: hyos.[36]
Groping as if in the dark: croc. hyos. op. plb.
Hypocrisy: bar-c.[30] caust.[30] lap-mar-c.[194] lyc.[148] merc.[30] nux-v.[30] phos. ***puls.*** sep.[30] ***sil.***[30] ***sulph.***[30]
Liar; describes some symptoms truly, misrepresents others: ***cupr-acet.***[54]
Mildness; violence, masking the: carc.[207]
Mirth; simulates hilarity while he feels wretched: apis[58]
Pities herself; sick, desire to show being: tarent.[36]
Sadness; smiling, with: coffin.[1] lyc.[1]
Secretive: aur.[5] ***bar-c.***[122] bov.[5] caust.[30] dig. germ.[222] ***ign.*** lap-mar-c.[194] ***lyc.***[122] ***naja***[5] nat-m.[137] nit-ac.[5] phos.[5] plb.[5] ***sep.***[122] syph.[122] thuj.[187] zinc.[36]

ANDROC. Sh, 167 - Pretended to feel well, although sick. (17)

ARG-N. He, 29 - Frequently remains in bed on slightest pretext of being "indisposed". 0 Hypochondriasis.

BELL. Al, 54 - The delirium was of a busy (engaged, working), restless, vivid character, but generally rather pleasing than otherwise. The patient appeared to think they were pursuing (persevere) their ordinary occupations; one boy appeared eager (animated) in flying a kite (toy), another pulled tables and chairs about, thinking he was working in a coal-pit, and a woman appeared to be remarkably busy with her household duties...

Ha, 1366 - Ridiculous grimaces; ...acts as if she were washing, at another as if counting money, ...

CHOC. Sh, 228 - Thoughts about the 'veneer of civilisation' that inhibits how we really feel and keeps us from displaying what we're like beneath the surface. It seems a legitimate layer, but so is the layer beneath it, and I feel amused and happy to meet it. This feeling continued for a few days, a very graphic picture of a veneer -a layer of learned social behaviour lifting and detaching from a basis that is thick, dark, solid, instinctual animal.15 , 30C, 00:00:30

HYDROG. Sh, 222 - Feel that the things we do are on different levels. Some of them are on higher and more meaningful levels —the real me —and others are just a trivial game. Laughing at the absurdity of notions — everything seems ridiculous. 16, 30C, 09:XX:XX

HYOS. Ha, 529 - Comical confusion of mind: they perform all sorts of ridiculous antics (jokes), like monkeys.

Ha, 533 - He gesticulates like a harlequin. (buffoon) (foot-note: "like an actor" -Hughes). (feigning)

Ha, 545 - Ridiculously solemn acts in improper clothing, mixed with fury. (In a priest's cassock, put on over nothing but a shirt, and in fur boots, he wishes to go to church, in order to preach and perform clerical offices there, and furiously attacks those who try to prevent him.)

He, 78 - Groundless suspicion of being watched (observed, spied) by members of family with whom he had some slight misunderstanding (dispute); to avoid being recognized by them, clothed himself differently every day,...watching his relations suspiciously and imagining he might be poisoned;... (disguise, camouflage)

He, 87-...; refused medicine, and cunningly (skill) evaded all stratagems to give it; escaped from room, ...

He, 41 - Comical alienation of mind; ludicrous actions like monkeys; makes ridiculous gestures like a dancing clown;...

LAC-C. Al,N -8 - Is impressed with the idea that all she says is a lie; it seems to be very difficult to speak the truth (liar, dissimulator), but continually distrusts things (suspicious); when reading anything she rapidly changes the meaning, omitting or adding things. (mischievous)

LACH. He, 60 - After a jealous quarrel, she put both hands to her chest and cried out "Oh! my heart!" then fell down and was in an asphyctic state for nearly twenty-four hours;...

LYC. Ha, 50 - He smiles without being merry, capricious.

MERC. Ha, 1262 - He is silly, acts like a

buffoon, ...he lit (burning) his fire, laid swords across one another, and put candles in one corner of the room, in the other boots (shoe),all this quite gravely...(serious)

NUX-V. He, 37-...betraying (play false, feigning) great moral and physical languor (indifference),..launches into high-flying, fantastic plans, fancies himself rich (rank, position) and wants to make presents of thousands (squanders, waste), and makes large useless purchases; does not consider himself ill; ...,and takes in bad part if not allowed to read indictment (accusation) for said lawsuit, a confused irrational piece of work...

PALL. He, 14 - She tries to appear as amiable as possible, but is obstinate.

PLB. He, 15-...; despair of her salvation...; fixed idea that could only obtain peace and safety though absolution by a priest of the papal church, although she had been a zealous Protestant; ....brooded over any forbidden thing; would steal (leave) from house in servant's cloak (coat, camouflage) and bonnet (hat) to obtain stimulants (drugs), but from the moment their prohibition was withdrawn (retired) ceased to have any desire for them; after being permitted to visit a priest and converse with him ceased to talk and think of the church. (desire; redemption, absolution)

STRAM. Al, 123-...seemed to herself to be engaged in her usual avocation,...imitate in every respect the routine procedure of one thus engaged.

He, 40 - Aberration of mind; one carries home all sorts of wood in order to manufacture brandy (cognac) (busy, manufacturing) ; another placed two axes across each other in order to split wood in this way; a third burrowed in ground like a pig with his mouth (animal); a fourth alleged he was a wheelwright and began to bore holes; a fifth ran into forge to catch fish, which he saw swimming there; a lacemaker threw about her bobbins incessantly, and threw everything into confusion; another girl ran about the room and cried out that all evil spirits were pursuing her.(restoration, restitution)

He, 98 - Mania; affects (pretend) being a distinguished (label) person, of high rank (position, nobility) ; is full of fear.

He, 151 - Making all kinds of faces and imitating motions, gestures and voices of different animals.

He, 29 - Talking in Jewish jargon.(clichÇ)

He, 112 - Religious mania; pious (divine) looks, praying; restless nights; inspired talking, singing; despairs of her salvation.

SULPH. Ha, 62 - She imagines that she has beautiful clothes, she takes old rags for beautiful clothes, she takes a coat for a jacket, a cap for a hat.

TARENT. Al, 14 - Feigned (simulate) paroxysms; a girl simulating fainting and insensibility, looks sideways to watch the effect produced on those around her. (manipulation)

Al, 55 - Fear, which could not be stopped, in a young lady; questioned about it, she tried to find a cause, and leaves others to think there is one; but really there was none.

THUJ. Al, 2 - She fancies that she has intentionally represented herself as insane (feigning) in the presence of others in order to palliate a wrong supposed to have been done (penitence, remorse), and that now she is punished, therefore, by real insanity.

VERAT. Ha, 672 - He pretends (simulate, feigning) he is a prince, and gives himself airs (affectation, pretentious) accordingly.

Ha, 673 - He asserts (declare) that he is deaf and blind (obstructed) and that he has got cancer.

Ha, 674 - She asserts that she has labour pains (pregnant).(important?)

Ha, 676 - She announces her imminent confinement.

Ha, 675 - She boasts (exult, triumph) that she is pregnant.

He, 3 - Fancies herself pregnant, or that she will be delivered (liberation) soon; that she is in throes (spasms) of childbirth.(labor)

FIGHT

Ailments from; quarrels: berb.[5] chion.[5] cic.[5] germ.[222] glon.[5] hydrog.[222] kali-chl.[5] spig.[5] thuj.[5]

Beside oneself; fight, from: coff.[54]

Cares; full of, alternating with, quarrelsomeness: ran-b.[10]

Cheerfulness; alternating with, quarrel: croc.[10] spong.[10] staph.[10]
Cheerfulness; quarrelsome, and: ***bell.***[54] ***staph.***[116]
Confusion of mind; arouse himself, compelled to: **CARB-V.** choc.[222] hydrog.[222] ***sulph.***[122]
Delusions; animals, dogs, near, that bit her, fought as if to drive it away: lyss.[54]
• contests, sees: bell.[10]
• double, he is, another self, there is, and he is not sure which will conquer the other: op.[139]
• fighting, that people are: op. stram.
• war, being at: bell.[10] ***ferr.***[5] hyos.[5] plat.[5] ran-b.[5] thuj.[5] verb.[5]
Discouraged; alternating with, quarrelsomeness: ran-b.[10]
Disputatious: camph.[54] ferr.[54] hyos.[36] lach.[60] ***lyc.***[54] merc.[60]
Dreams; air attacks: visc.[119]
➤ anger, quarreled with his father, that he had, who would not recognize him as a son because he had embraced homeopathy: crot-h.[36]
➤ animals, cats, army of: calc-p.[36]
➤ animals, fights with: staph.[1]
➤ battles: ***all-c.*** bamb-a.[1184] bell. bry. crot-c.[36] ferr. guai. hyos.[10] ***meny.***[162] nat-m.[36] nat-s.[171] plat. ran-s. rat.[36] sil. sol-t-ae.[36] stann. thuj. verb.
➤ bloodshed: plat.[10]
➤ bombs: cand-a.[239]
➤ cannonading: menis.[36]
➤ dead, people, of, quarreling with: cedr.[36]
➤ duels: asc-t.
➤ fights: aesc. ***all-c.*** allox.[119] aza.[149] bapt. bell. brom. bry. calad. ceph.[36] coca con. crot-c. culx.[58] echi.[111] elaps ***ferr.*** ferr-i. guai. guare. hyper. indg. iris jab. jac-c. kali-bi. kali-c.[10] kali-m.[192] kali-n.[10] lyc. lyss.[54] m-aust.[10] mag-c. mag-s.[10] mosch. nat-ar. nat-c.[10] ***nat-m.*** nat-s. nicc.[10] phel.[10] phos. pip-m. plat. ptel. puls.[10] ***ran-s.*** rat. sars.[10] senec. sil. sol-t-ae. stann. ***staph.*** ***stram.***[54] verb.
➤ fights, conquers, and: bapt.
➤ fights, fitful slumbers, in: phos.[36]
➤ fights, galley slave, with: elaps[36]
➤ fights, generals, with six or seven black, who garroted him and bound him with ropes, causing agony of mind: coca[36]
➤ fights, joining in: mag-c.[36]
➤ fights, karate with his teacher: ozone[227]
➤ fights, suggested by reading: coca[36]
➤ ghosts, fighting with: sars. sep. sil.[10]
➤ gun, shots: hura[36]
➤ guns: choc.[222] hep.[85]
➤ money, disputing about money: chin.
➤ quarrels, changing suddenly to happy conversation with another person: ferr-p.[85]
➤ quarrels, dead relatives, with: cedr.[25] kali-c.[1]
➤ quarrels, money, about: chin.
➤ quarrels, strife: alum. alum-sil.[58] am-c. am-m.[5] anan. ant-c. apis aran-ix.[149] ***arn.*** ars.[5] astra-me.[36] aur. aza.[36] ***bapt.*** bar-c. ***bell.*** brom. ***bry.*** calc. calc-acet.[36] canth. carl. cast. ***caust.*** cedr.[36] ceph.[36] cere-b.[36] cham. chin.[5] con. convo-d.[36] crot-c.[36] ***crot-h.*** culx.[58] echi.[111] ferr-p.[5] guai. guare. hep. hydr.[5] indg.[10] kali-c.[10] ***kali-n.*** lach.[85] lyc.[5] m-aust.[1] ***mag-c.*** mag-s. maland.[56] ***merc.***[10] mosch. nat-ar.[36] nat-c. nat-m. nat-s. nicc. ***nit-ac.***[5] **NUX-V.** op. oxyt.[51] ozone[227] paeon. peti.[36] ph-ac. ***phos.*** plat. ***puls.*** raph.[111] rat.[10] rheum[5] sabin. ***sel.*** sep. sil. sol-a.[36] spig. ***stann.*** staph. **STRAM.**[5] tarax. verat. x-ray[56] zinc.
➤ revolution: hura[36] merc.[36]
➤ riots: bry. con. guai. indg. kali-c. kali-n.[10] lyc. m-aust.[10] merc.[10] nat-c. nat-m. ped.[36] phos. puls. sars.[10] stann.
➤ robbers, fighting, with: ferr-i. jac-c.[36] mag-c. nat-c. psil.[164] sil.
➤ ships, wartime, in: hydrog.[222]
➤ shooting: ***am-m.*** hep. mag-s.[10] ***merc.*** merc-i-r.[36] spong.[10]
➤ shooting, hears: hep.
➤ shooting, shot, soldier is shot, a: am-m.[58]
➤ shooting, someone, who owes him money: ozone[227]
➤ shots: cerv.[36] hura[36] ozone[227]
➤ soldiers, seeing a soldier shot: am-m.
➤ tanks, battle tanks: bamb-a.[1184]
➤ torpedo, of: ozone[227]
➤ war: ferr.[5] ***meny.***[162] ozone[227] pitu-a.[164] plat.[5] stann.[149] **THUJ.** ***verb.***[5] visc.[149]
➤ war, civil war: op.[30]
Euphoria; alternating with, quarrel: thyr.[149]
Fear; panic attacks, dreams of fights, from: coca[36]
✦ raids, of air: acon.[172] arn.[172] cham.[172] ign.[172] nat-m.[172]
Fight, wants to: ***androc.*** atro.[36] bell. bov.

cocc.[36] hipp. hyos. lap-gr-m.[194] med.[212] merc. sec. sulo-ac.[102] tub.[36]
Insanity; quarrelsome: hyos.[137] ***verat.***[8]
Irritability; querulous: ***zinc.***[54]
Jealousy; quarrels, reproaches, scolds, with: gall-ac.[36] ***lach.***[54] ***nux-v.***[54]
Laughing; alternating with, quarrelsomeness: croc.[10]
Quarrelsomeness, scolding: acon. agar. alco.[36] aloe[5] alum. am-c. ambr. ***anac.*** anan. androc.[222] ang.[5] anh.[116] ant-t. ***arn. ars.*** ars-s-f.[58] **ASAF.**[5] asar.[149] aster. atro.[36] **AUR.** aur-ar.[58] aur-s.[58] bamb-a.[1184] bar-c. ***bell.*** bor. ***bov. brom. bry.*** bufo cael.[149] calc. calc-s. ***camph.*** cand-a.[239] cann-s.[10] canth. caps. carb-an.[10] carb-v.[10] ***caust.*** cench. ***cham.*** chap.[149] chel. chin. choc.[222] cocc.[10] coff.[5] colch.[5] ***con.*** cor-r. ***croc.*** crot-h. culx.[58] ***cupr.*** cycl.[10] cyn-d.[149] dig. ***dulc.*** elaps ferr. ferr-acet.[10] ferr-ar. fl-ac. germ.[222] gran.[10] graph.[10] hell.[10] ***hep.***[58] hipp. hir.[144] ***hist.***[119] hydrog.[222] **HYOS.**[122] ictod.[10] **IGN.** iod.[10] ip. kali-ar. kali-bi.[5] ***kali-c.*** kali-chl.[5] kali-i. kali-p.[58] ***lach.*** lap-gr-m.[194] lap-mar-c.[194] led.[10] lepi. ***lyc.*** lyss. m-aust.[10] mag-c.[144] mag-s.[119] mang.[10] med.[189] meph.[149] ***merc.*** merl. mez. ***mosch.*** mur-ac.[10] nat-ar. ***nat-c. nat-m.*** nat-s. nicc. ***nit-ac. nit-s-d.***[10] **NUX-V.** olnd. op.[5] ozone[227] pall. **PETR.** ***ph-ac. phos. plat.*** plb. prot.[136] ***psor.*** puls.[30] ***ran-b.*** rat. reser.[149] rheum **RHUS-T.**[5] rib-ac.[149] ruta sabad.[10] sac-alb.[36] seneg. ***sep. sil.***[5] spong. stann. ***staph. stram.*** stront-c. sul-ac. sulfonam.[149] **SULPH.** **TARENT.**[122] thea. ***thuj.*** til. tub.[36] tub-k.[70] upa.[85] ***verat. verat-v.*** viol-t. wye.[85] zinc.
Quarrelsomeness; alternating with, care and discontentment: ran-b.
Quarrelsomeness; alternating with, sadness, silent: ***con.***
Quarrelsomeness; alternating with, singing: croc.
Quarrelsomeness; causeless: stram.[10]
Quarrelsomeness; disputes with absent persons: lyc.
Quarrelsomeness; disturbed, if: **NUX-V.**[54]
Quarrelsomeness; family, with her: kali-c.[58] kali-m.[192] kali-p.[58] thyr.[149]
Quarrelsomeness; herself with: merc.[111]
Quarrelsomeness; jealousy, from: ***cench. hyos.***[10] ***lach.*** nux-v.
Quarrelsomeness; jealousy, from, unchaste expressions, with: ***nux-v.***[54]
Quarrelsomeness; litigious: ars.[30] caust.[30] lach.[30] nux-v.[30] plat.[30] staph.[30]
Quarrelsomeness; pugnacious: bell.[10] nat-c.[10] nicc.[10]
Quarrelsomeness; recriminations about trifles: cop.[36]
Quarrelsomeness; repentance, followed by: vinc.[36]
Quarrelsomeness; sadness, in: ***kali-ar.***[54]
Quarrelsomeness; staring of eyes, heat of face, bluish lips, dry mouth, with: mosch.[10]
Quarrelsomeness; vexation, with tearful: ***mosch.***[54]
Sadness; alternating with, quarrelsomeness: ***con.***[54] sulfonam.[149]
Sadness; quarrel with husband, after: ***anac.***[54]
Sensitive; disharmony and quarrel, home, in: nat-m.[162]
Singing; alternating with, anger and quarrelsomeness: croc.
Talk; battles, about: bell. hyos.
Talk; himself, to, quarreling with some one, as if, seven p.m.: kali-cy.[36]
Talk; indisposed, alternating with, quarrelsomeness: ***con.***
Talk; sleep, in war, of: hyos.[1]
Talk; war, of: agar. bell. hyos.
Timidity; alternating with, quarrelsomeness: ran-b.[10]
Weeping; aloud, quarrelsome attack, after: ***nux-v.***[36]
Weeping; anger, with, violent quarreling, even to extreme malice and rage: ***mosch.***[54]

ADAM. Sh, 156 - The weekend started with me locking myself and the boys and one dog out of the house, and the keys and one dog still inside. I got very upset then and the weekend just got worse and worse. I had blazing rows with everybody. Thought I was getting the flu. Thought I was surrounded by dirt. Wanted to just go to bed and take my boys and the dogs with me. Couldn't or wouldn't go to work on Monday. 18, 30C, 31:XX:XX
AGAR. Al, 16-.... reciting (enumerate) before the beauties of the tribe their exploits (adventures) in war or the chase.(hunting) Their physical strength is increased...(boasting)
Al, 56-...grew angry at the servant and felt inclined to fight.

ALOE. Al, 23 - Immediately, strong exhibition of will (disposition); he quarrels with every one who contradicts him; it seems as if he would permit himself to be torn (ruined) in pieces, sooner than give up his will. (lack; will, integration, union)
Al, 11 - In the afternoon, he is disposed to become reconciled (pacify) where he would not otherwise have been so.
ALUM. Al, 32 - She is excessively peevish, and everything is offensive to her; she desires nothing but to quarrel and make a fuss,...
Ha, 33 - She is extremely peevish, and everything is offensive to her; she only wishes to scold (criticize) and to raise a fuss (trouble) in the afternoon.
ANAC. Ha, 9 - He is at odds (quarreling) with the whole world, and has so little confidence in himself that he despairs of being able to accomplish (succeed) what is demanded of him.
ANAN. Al, 7 - Quarrelsome and contrary humor, but after being angry he often regrets (remorse) what he has done.
ANDROC. Sh, 112 - Became excited to anger and confrontation. She was not aware of hurting others' feelings and did not seem to care. Could not appreciate anyone else's feeling. Later she reflected on her actions and felt ashamed. (12)
Sh, 113 - Argumentative. Pursued conflict almost with relish. (12)
Sh, 125 - Desire to pick an argument or fight. (29)
ATRO. Al, 15 - The patient is busied with subjects which at other times occupy his mind, politics and struggles consequent on his relations in life.
Al, 42 - Morose, quarrelsome the whole day, everything went wrong; trifles usually passed unheeded irritated him to anger.
AUR. Ha, 33 - He tries his best to quarrel with somebody and to revile (scold) him.
BOV. Al, 5 - Very courageous and vigorous; he would like to fight with everybody.
CALC-A. Al, 253 - Dreams vivid, full of strife (quarrel, fight) and anger.
CALC. He, 22 - Mania; sees many curs (dogs) crowding (compress) around him, fights them off. (surrounded)
CAMPH. Ha, 343 - Quarrelsomeness, insists he is right.
CAUST. Ha, 30 - Peevish (angry) all day, at odds (quarrel) with himself, dissatisfied, anxious and yet not indisposed to mental work.
CHAM. Al, 53 - Disposed to anger scorn quarrelsomeness. (after two hours)
Ha, 485 - Quarrelsome crossness; she seeks for everything vexatious.(provoking)
He, 59 - Great tendency to quarrel, to speak in an obstreperous (rude, vulgar) manner.
CHIN. Ha, 1110 - Extremely disposed to be vexed, and to take every occasion to get cross; afterwards quarrelsome and disposed to vex others, and to make reproaches and give annoyance(irritation) to others.
CHOC. Sh, 331 - I became selfish, impatient and intolerant. Behaved in a strange way -hard and quarrelsome -snapping at people. Could not stand people wasting time or being inefficient, I wanted things done immediately.[35], 30C, XX:XX:XX:
CON. He, 38 - Very much excited, passionate, domineering (dictatorial), quarrelsome, scolds (censorious) and will not bear contradiction.
ELAPS. Al, 13 - Fearfulness, dread (fear) of being alone, as though something would happen, or as though rowdies (revolution, rebellious) would break in.
Al, 16 - Inclination to strike and pick a quarrel.
FERR. Al, 21 - Violence, quarrelsomeness; insists that he is right.
Al, 766 - Dreams he is in battle, that he has fallen into the water, etc.
Ha, 270 - Dreams that he is in battle, that he has fallen into the water...
Ha, 291 - Violence, quarrelsomeness (litigious, combative), positiveness (obstinate, emphatic, resolute)
He, 14 - Pettish(irritable), quarrelsome, disputative (litigious), easily excited, least contradiction angers.
He, 16 - Vehement; quarrelsome; anxious.
GERM. Sh, 153 - Thought nobody understood me and cared for what I felt. Felt it was unfair. I was presented with complaints about something others had done. Felt I was standing between two fighting parts. Felt awkward about it, embarrassed. Difficult to argue about such strong outburst. Thoughts about the day's

arguing milling in my head all evening and night. 21, 12C, 32:XX.XX.
GUAI. Ha, 126 - Dreams of fighting.
HALI-L. Sh, 349 - I said I was moody. It wasn't as qualitative as she wanted, and she was asking for more details and I yelled, " A stupid five year old would understand what I was saying." I became sarcastic and very belligerent. I thought I was being simplistic and clear. I gave what I had to give. I was in a depressed state, lost my good feeling and was angry at being asked to explain the depression. She asked me what do you mean and I said, "XXXX off. If you don't understand that, too bad. Do you understand that?! Do you know the English language?" 18, 30C, 04:14:00
Sh, 430 - Get a call from a friend that the utility district is at it again. Don't know what, but expect the worst in negotiations with them. Can't win. So tired of fighting the losing battle. Can't raise the energy to do anything. Rage inside. Hopeless. Daydreams of blowing up the utility district, of shooting them. Only option left to desperate people and I feel desperate. we're a rag-tag group without luck, or leadership, fighting a losing battle. Feels like we're the American Indians. "Here's 24 dollars worth of beads for your island, idiot." In the pit of despair. 09, 6C, 25:XX:XX
HIPP. Al, 15 - He feels as though he would fight with any one.
HYDROG. Sh, 207 - Stormy and acrimonious (hash) row (fight) with girlfriend. Quarrelling continued throughout the day. Cried a lot —generally feeling rough with loss of appetite — heart pounding and sunk feeling in abdomen though I can't eat. 04, 12C, 01:00:30
Sh, 234 - Developed a self pitying, very tearful depression through the morning. I was unable to communicate any of these feelings and this led to a fierce row with girlfriend. 04, 12C, 30:XX:XX
IGN. Ha, 764 - Slight blame (censuring) or contradiction excites him to quarrel, and he is vexed at himself for doing so.
Ha, 770 - Fickle, impatient, irresolute, quarrelsome.
IRID. Sh, 322 - Had row with partner over work, money, and time off. I was storming about. I said, "You can't say that to me." I went storming after partner went into another room. I was overwhelmed with fury. I cried with fury. D13
Sh, 327 - Had a massive argument with friend. For first time in my life really stood my ground. Went hot. Said, "This is my point and I am sticking to it." Burst into floods of tears. It was as though a volcano had erupted. Anger and grief were coming out. My friend had done this on purpose. I got on high horse. We parted friends and sorted it all out. I4
KALI-AR. He, 1 - Scolding (censorious) morose, retired, quarrelsome and discontented, jealous, indifferent to everything,...
KALI-CY. Al, 5 - At 7 p.m., while walking out of doors, feelings of crossness; carries on a kind of conversation within himself, as if quarreling with someone whith whom he had previously disagreed; thinks what he will reply in case certain things are said to him.
KALI-I. Al, 16 - Very peevish and excited; everything goes wrong, and she is ready to quarrel with every one.
LACH. Al, 33 - Unusually contentious (hostile) and obstinate, so that he quarrels with everything about him.
Al, 34 - So quarrelsome that he disputes with a mother about the age of her daughter, and affirms the younger to be the elder.
He, 60 - After a jealous quarrel, she put both hands to her chest and cried out "Oh! my heart!" then fell down and was in an asphyctic state for nearly twenty-four hours;...
LYC. Al, 96 - Quarrelsome rage, partly at herself partly at others.
Al, 97 - As if out of her mind, she seeks quarrels, makes unfounded reproaches, is most exceedingly violent, and strikes those whom she thus insults.
Ha, 60 - As if insane she seeks for quarrels, makes ungrounded reproaches abuses (insulting) most violently and beats the person whom she abuses.
Ha, 58 - He quarrels in mind with absent persons.
He, 32 - Obstinate, defiant (contrary), arbitrary (capricious?); seeks disputes.

MAG-C. Al, 958 - Anxious dream of a fight with robbers.
Al, 969 - Dream...he quarreled with a beggar.
MERC. Al, 36 - Quarrels with everything; would above all have everything right; quarrelsome.
Ha, 1254 - Quarreling with everyone, opinionative, (doctrinal) quarrelsome.
He, 35 - Grief, with fear at night; disposition to quarrel; complaining of relations and surroundings.
NAT-C. Al, 1114 - Dream of a quarrel, in which he stabbed his antagonist (enemy) in the chest with a large knife.
Al, 48 - He is angry, and inclined to fight and strike, and cannot tolerate contradiction,...
Ha, 52 - Passionate; disposed to quarrel and fight, and cannot bear any contradiction.
NAT-M. He, 42 - Quarrelsome fretfulness, gets into passion about trifles; passionate vehemence.
NICC. Al, 1 - Very angry and quarrelsome mood; she was inclined to quarrel with and contradict everyone, in the evening.
Al, 2 - Quarrelsome and impatient; she could tolerate no contradiction;...
NIT-AC. Ha, 16 - Anxiety, as if he was engaged in a disquieting lawsuit or contest. (conflict, debate, competition)
Ha, 47 - He is inclined to be passionate and contentious.(quarrelsome)
Ha, 6 - Inclined to be violent and to quarrel.
He, 19-...headstrong (obstinate); trembling while quarreling; fits of rage with curses and maledictions; inveterate ill-will, unmoved by apologies.
NUX-V. He, 17 - He quarrels, reproaches, scolds, insults, from jealousy, mingled with unchaste (obscene) expressions; ...
PLAT. Ha, 15 - At odds (quarreling) with all the world, everything is too close (near, intimate) for her, with inclination to weep. (persecution)
RAN-B. Al, 2 - Vexed and inclined to be angry; quarrels and scolds when the slightest cause is offered (after two hours).
Al, 3 - Ill humored, and disposed to quarrel and scold the first forenoon; in the evening is desponding, apprehensive, sensitive, discontented; on the second day he again inclines to be provoked by innocent jests of his friends, etc.;...
RUTA. He, 1 - Inclination to contradict and quarrel.
SENEG. Al, 13 - Phlegmatic; inclines to quarrel and give offense.
SEP. Al, 34 - Feel very much depressed, at 7 A.M.; feel like quarreling with everybody; became very much excited about a mere trifle, and said some very sharp things. (feeling ashamed of it at the same time)
He, 31 - Contradictory, quarrelsome, complaining about others.
STAPH. He, 14-...; was insulted (slandered, defamed, calumniated) being too dignified (reserved, lordly,) to fight (contest), subdued (control) his wrath(anger) and went home sick,.. (ailments, from offenses)
STRAM. He, 110-...frightful dreams about fighting and killing; takes offensive in imaginary quarrels, and attacks aggressor; runs against supposed object to attack it;...
SULPH. Ha, 57 - His mood is quarrelsome and contentious (hostile) about everything.
THUJ. Al, 91 - Morose, quarrels about a harmless joke.
THYR. Al,N-1-...at times dangerous and homicidal, would put her arms round the necks of other patients so tightly as almost to strangle them (in this case the insanity was primary and the myxedema secondary; both conditions were removed). Evinced increased vivacity by quarreling with another patient about a trifling difference of opinion.
TIL. Al, 19 - Irritable, critical mood, inclined to quarrel and get angry, even from the slightest difference of opinion.
TUB. Al,N-13 - Very irritable, want to fight; no hesitancy in throwing anything at anyone, even without cause.
VERAT-V. He, 3 - From sudden cerebral congestion: quarrelsome delirium; great mental depression and fear of death;...

FINE

Delusions; beautiful, old ragged woman is: psil.[164]
• beautiful, rags seem, even: ***sulph.***
Desires; beautiful things, finery: dat-a.[25] lil-t.[137] sulph.[137]
Desires; clothing, to wear his best: con.[137]
Dreams; Latin, he admires his own skill in speaking: lyss.[36]

Dress; best, at his: con.[137]
Finery, luxurious clothing, wants: aeth.[5] cur.[36] lil-t.[111] ***sulph.***[5]
Gourmand: calc.[30] chin.[30] ip.[30] mag-c.[30] merc.[30] nat-c.[30] **VERAT.**[30]
Imbecility; old rags are as fine as silk: **SULPH.**
Insanity; dresses in his bests clothes: con.
Loquacity; selected expressions, in: lach.[10]
Restlessness; mild, amiable, refined, sensitive, intellectual: chim-m.[54]
Talk; fine: hyos.

IRID. Sh, 56 - Delight at seeing my own female form in mirror, desire to shave legs so they would be smooth. Highly sexual, more refined, dressed in best clothes today. Desire to dance naked in moonlight. Q6

FIRE

Anxiety; fire were breaking out, as if, morning, on being awakened by noise in the street: tet.[36]
Delirium; loquacious, fire, of: ***calc.*** cupr.[162]
Delusions; animals, fire, in the: bell.
- burnt, everything at home is: bell.[10]
- fire, balls of fire rolling over bedclothes: stram.[36]
- fire, every noise is a cry of fire, she thinks and she trembles: bar-c.
- fire, flame of fire is passing through him: phos.
- fire, head is surrounded by: am-m.
- fire, house, on: bell. hep. stram.
- fire, neighbor's house on (morning, waking in a fright): hep.
- fire, room is on: stram.
- fire, sees: alum. am-m. anac. ant-t. ars. ***bell. calc.*** calc-ar.[58] calc-p. clem. croc. daph. ***hep.*** kali-n. kreos. lach.[72] laur. lyss. mag-m. mez.[5] nat-m. op.[58] phos. plat. ***puls.*** rhod. rhus-t. spig. spong. stann. stram. sulph. tet.[36] zinc. zinc-p.[58]
- fire, sees, home, on distant: bell.
- fire, warms hands before, sees: hyosin.[102]
- fire, world is on: ***hep. puls.***[54] verat.[58]
- spectres, sees, fire, in: bell.
- stove, heats the, in heat of summer: merc.

Dreams; cities, destroyed by fire: sol-t-ae.[36]
- ➤ fire: alum. am-c.[5] **ANAC.** ant-t. ***ars.*** aur.[137] bar-c. ***bell.*** calc. ***calc-p.*** calc-sil.[58] cann-i.[116] cann-s.[5] ***carb-ac.*** carb-v. cass.[36] cench.[58] chin. choc.[222] clem. ***croc. cur.*** daph. euph.[54] euphr. fl-ac. graph. **HEP.** hyos.[137] iris kali-ar. kali-c. kali-n. kali-sil.[58] kiss.[36] ***kreos.*** lach.[102] **LAUR.** lyc.[137] ***m-aust.***[10] **MAG-C. MAG-M.** ***mag-s.*** meny.[137] ***meph.*** merc. merc-acet.[36] merc-c. naja nat-c. ***nat-m.*** nat-p. nat-s. nit-s-d.[36] osm. ***phos.*** pip-m.[36] plat. rad-br.[111] rham-p.[36] rhod. ***rhus-t.*** sel.[149] sil. sol-t-ae.[36] spig. spong. stann. stront-c. sul-ac. ***sulph.*** tub.[137] zinc. zinc-o.[10] zing.
- ➤ fire, blow on head, after: ***nat-m.***[54]
- ➤ fire, boiling lard into fire, pouring: nat-s.[36]
- ➤ fire, burning, brightly: kali-n.[36]
- ➤ fire, burning, shrieking out, and: mag-c.[36]
- ➤ fire, cathedral on: kali-c.[36]
- ➤ fire, coming down from heaven: ***sulph.***
- ➤ fire, danger, of: ant-t.[36] bell.[36] clem.[36] merc-acet.[36]
- ➤ fire, destroying a city: sol-t-ae.[36]
- ➤ fire, house on, her: kali-c.[36]
- ➤ fire, house on, neighbors, which could not be saved: mag-s.[36]
- ➤ fire, lightning, from: euphr.[36]
- ➤ fire, nervous weakness, in: ***cur.***[54]
- ➤ fire, small flames, with: cass.[36]
- ➤ fire, vivid, exerting himself to extinguish them: merc-s.[54]
- ➤ fire, wants to go to, but cannot get there: plat.[54]
- ➤ fire, world on fire: ***rhus-t.***
- ➤ stove, hot: apis.[36]
- ➤ torches in the sea: ozone[227]
- ➤ world on fire: ***rhus-t.***

Fear; falling, fire, into, when walking by it, and in spite of her willpower she did stagger into the fire: onos.[144] psor.[172]
- ✦ fire, catch, things will: cupr. ***cupr-acet.***[54] hep.[187] lyss.[172] onos.[172] psor.[56] stram.[58]
- ✦ fire, loss by, of: bell.[10]

Fire; desire to be near to: naja[36]
Fire; thinks and talks of: ***calc.***[54]
Fire; throws child into fire, after delivery: merc.[85]
Fire; throws things into: hep.[172] staph
Fire; wants to set things on, or house on: alco.[36] ant-t.[1] **BELL.**[122] **HEP.**[122] hyos.[30] phos.[122] staph.[122] stram.[30]
Kill; sudden impulse to, throw child, fire, into: hep.[58] lyss. ***nux-v.*** thea.
Suicidal disposition; fire, to set oneself on: ***ars.***[122] hep.[58]
Talk; nothing but, murder, fire and rats: ***calc.*** calc-sil.[58]

Thoughts; persistent, thinks of nothing but murder, fire and rats: ***calc.***

ADAM. Sh, 108 - I feel like burying myself in grass and earth. I love touching and covering my hands with earth. I want to be enclosed and hidden in the earth. 20, 1M, 08:XX:XX
BAR-A. Al, 8 - Solicitous (careful) and fearful. The slightest noise in the street seems to him like a fire alarm, and he is frightened thereat, so that he starts in every limb.
BAR-C. Ha, 11 - Anxious and fearful; a little noise on the street seems to him at once like fire alarm, and he is frightened by it, so that it darts (move quickly) through all his limbs.
BELL. Al, 87 - Fancied he saw ghosts and animals in the fire.
Al, 91 - He raves as in a dream, and cries he must go home, because everything is burning up there. (rescue, saving)
Al, 85 - Visions of wolves, dogs, giants, and fire.
Ha, 1338 - He is delirious, and cries out in his dreams that he must go home, because everything is on fire there.
CALC. He, 28 - She thinks and talks of nothing but murder, fire, rats, etc.
He, 21 - Mania-a-potu, with delirious talk about fire, rats, mice and murder.
CANN-I. Al, 25-...Now demoniac shapes clutched (grasp) at him from the darkness, cloaked (covered) from head to foot in inky (black) palls (mantle), glaring (staring, looking) at him with fiery eyes from beneath their cowls(mantle)....
Al, 62 - It seemed as though I was transparent; the fire in the grate seemed to shine through me, and to warm the marrow of the bones.
CHOC. Sh, 172 - Dreams of fire.
CUPR-A. He, 17 - Feared bedclothes or house would catch fire.
HALI-L. Sh, 18 - Woke up and thought I smelled burnt wood. 08, 30C, 16:XX:XX
Sh, 513 - On my way home, while it was dark, I saw a glow in the sky and immediately I thought my house was burning. I was very scared and I should have realized that the glow came from the town behind the ridge, but it took me a while to get that. 04, 30C, 03:XX:XX
HEP. Al, 1 - Ghostly image of one who was dead, in the morning, in bed, after waking and while conscious, which frightened him; it also seemed as though he saw his neighbor's house burning, which also frightened him.
Ha, 298 - In the morning in bed after waking, when conscious, he had the visionary appearance of a deceased (dead, defunct) person, which frightened him, and he also imagined he saw a neighboring house in flames, which terrified him.
He, 5 - Frightful visions of fire and of dead persons.
He, 8-...threatened to murder wife and children, attempted to set house on fire, and was with difficulty controlled; ... (pyromaniac) 0Scabies.
He, 23 - Wrathful irritability, even to the most extreme violence, threatening to end in murder and arson.(firing pyromania)
IGN. He, 30 - Became bilious, nervous, depressed, and would scarce move from the fire, for days together. Morbid grief
IRID. Sh, 200 - Waking frequently, every hour, feeling very alert and wide awake, worried that I had forgotten something, not put the guard on the fire, closed down the stove, locked the doors, etc. Feels like I would take ages to get off to sleep. In reality got to sleep quickly. A19
LIL-T. Al, 25 - While attending a lecture (speech), desire to hit the lecturer, and in the evening desirous of swearing and damning the fire and things generally, and to think and speak obscene things; disposed to strike and hit persons; as these feelings came, the uterine pains passed away.
LYSS. Al,N-28 - Complains bitterly that a fire has been lighted and that the stove is smoking, although there is no fire; another continually directed a window to be closed, which was not opened. (fear suffocation?)
He, 28 - Complains bitterly that a fire has been lighted and that the stove is smoking, although there is no fire; another continually directed a window to be closed, which was not opened.
MAG-C. Al, 940 - Dream of a fire, at which she was present.

Al, 941 - Anxious dream of a fire, being arrested etc.
Al, 945 - Anxious dream, that a child was bathing in boiling water. (purification?)
Al, 950 - Dream that she burnt her back by some one throwing hot roast (meat) pigeons (bird) at her.
Al, 951 - Frightful dream, that she burnt her cheek by the light.
Al, 942 - Anxious dream of a bright fire, at which she shrieked out violently and cried "fire".
MAG-M. Al, 714 - Frightful dreams; that she was pursued by robbers; that she burned her hand by washing ...
MERC. Ha, 1262 - He is silly, acts like a buffoon, ...he lit (burning) his fire, laid swords across one another, and put candles in one corner of the room, in the other boots (shoe),all this quite gravely...(serious)
PSOR. Al,N-46 - Attacks of fear; fear of fire, of being alone, of apoplexy, of becoming insane.
PULS. He, 40 - Religious mania; sees the devil coming to take her; the world on fire during night; fear, rage in spells, or weeping... (captured, possessed)
RHUS-T. Al, 1385 - Fearful dreams, for example, that the world was on fire, with palpitation on waking.
STAPH. He, 15-...; firmly believed he would lose his fortune, constantly told his wife to be careful that they did not starve; thinks his wife will run away from him (deserted) (lost: position, rank), ... amuses himself by throwing into the fire any article near at hand, regardless of value; at times more violent, strikes at any one coming near him, ...tells his wife he will try not kill any one;...
STRAM. Al, 130 - The apartment seemed all on fire.
SULPH. Al, 3772-...it was disturbed by dreams of fire and death.
Al, 3799 - An anxious dream, that fire came down from heaven.
Al, 3800-....(DREAM) she walked about like a somnambulist, thought there was a fire, dressed herself, talked out of the window, and was frightened as she heard that it was nothing; for three days afterwards she was very weak, and felt bruised(hurt).
THEA. Al, 4 - Sensation as if impelled by some uncontrollable power to commit suicide, to jump out of window, to put her baby in the boiler with the clothes, to cut its throat while cutting bread, to throw it downstairs (in a woman who kept a pot of tea boiling on the stove and drank several bowlfuls every day; cured with tea cm, Finckle)

FIT

Abusive; scolds until the lips are blue and eyes stared and she falls down fainting: ***mosch.***
Affectionate; love for everyone about him, during and after fainting: hura[60]
Anguish; convulsions of extremities, with: cocc.[54]
Anguish; convulsive, spasmodic: nux-v.[36]
Anguish; fainting, followed by: nux-v.[54] verat.[54]
Anxiety; alternating with, fainting: vip.[36]
Anxiety; faintness, with: ***arg-n.***[54] ars.[10] cic.[10] ***crot-h.***[122] ***dig.***[54] ign.[10] mag-m.[60] nit-ac.[60] nux-v.[10] op.[60] ***plb.***[122] ran-b.[60] **SPONG.**[54]
Anxiety; fits, with: alum. ars.[54] bell. calc.[54] caust. cocc. crot-h.[54] cupr. ferr. ***hyos.*** ign. stram.[54]
Anxiety; inexpressible, with fainting: ***dig.***[54]
Anxiety; sleep, before, fainting would return, as if, and he would die: ***caust.***[54]
Anxiety; vertigo, during: acon. aloe alum. arn. asar. bamb-a.[1184] bar-m.[60] bell. ***cact.*** caps.[5] ***caust.*** coff. ***dig.*** graph.[10] ign. ***lach.***[5] lyc.[5] merc. nux-m. nux-v. ***op.*** rhod. rhus-t. sel.[5] seneg.[60] ***sep.***[36] sil.[60] ***sulph.*** verat.[60] vip.[85] ***zinc.***[5]
Anxiety; vertigo, during, apoplexy, as if he would have: ***zinc.***[54]
Clinging; convulsions, before: ***cic.***[54]
Company, aversion to; dizzy, faint in a crowd, or where many gas lights are burning (in agoraphobia): ***nux-v.***[54]
Cursing; laughing, with, convulsive, spasmodic: oena.[36]
Death; desires, convulsions, during: absin.[36]
Delusions; apoplexy, he has: arg. carb-v.[36]
- bird, he is a, runs about, chirping and twittering, until he faints: lyss.[54]
- body, expanded, is, convulsions, before: arg-n.[91]
- body, head, forehead is swelling suddenly, during headache, before convulsions: bac.[55]

• die, about to, he is, while walking thinks he will have a fit or die, which makes him walk faster: ***arg-n.***
• emptiness, fainting sensation, with: **SEP.**[122]
• epilepsy, he has: atro.
• epilepsy, he will have a fit: alum.[139] cina[139] lyss.[139]
• faintness, of: ang.[139] bry.[139] calc.[139] calen.[139] cocc.[139] **CUPR.**[54] dig.[139] kali-c.[139] lappa[139] levo.[149] mag-c.[139] med.[139] mosch.[36] nat-m.[139] sabad.[139] sep.[139] sil.[139] spong.[139] stann.[139] sulph.[54] thea.[139] upa.[139] zing.[139]
• fit, she will have a fit and walks faster: ***arg-n.***
• man, huge drunk man coming toward her, who lies down beside her, she begs him to retire, falls into convulsions and turns over on her abdomen: cic.[54]
• smaller, he is, epileptic fit, before: carb-v.
• vanish, senses: cann-s.[58] plat.[85]
• vanish, she will: lap-c-b.[194]
• walls, falling, inward, before epileptic fit: carb-v. lyss.[122]

Despair; recovery, convulsions, after: calc.[193]

Dreams; amorous, pollutions, with, waking him, headache, with, dim sight, prostration and vertigo: ***sars.***[54]
➤ convulsions, of: calc-s.[54]
➤ disease, apoplectic fit, daughter has an: nat-s.
➤ disease, convulsions: calc-s.
➤ disease, fainting: bamb-a.[1184] graph.
➤ disease, vertigo: ***sil.***
➤ epilepsy, of: iris-foe. mag-c. sil.
➤ fainting: bamb-a.[1184] graph.
➤ fit, daughter had a apoplectic: nat-s.
➤ fit, he had a: iris mag-c. sil.
➤ water, waves, head, in, causing vertigo: bamb-a.[1184]

Fear; apoplexy, night with feeling as if head would burst, at: ***aster.***
✦ apoplexy, of: abel.[149] acon.[162] ***alum.***[36] apis ***arg.*** arg-n. arn. ***aster.*** bell. brom.[5] calc.[184] carb-v. cench. ***coff.*** elaps ***ferr.*** ferr-p. ferr-t.[36] fl-ac. glon.[5] kali-br.[5] lach. nat-c. nux-v.[185] phos. plat.[162] psor.[56] ***puls.***[30] sel.[116] sep.[1] staph.[30] ter. thuj. verat. ***zinc.***[122]
✦ apoplexy, palpitation, with: arg.
✦ apoplexy, stool, during: verat.
✦ apoplexy, waking, on: arn.[10] carb-v.[1] glon.
✦ breakdown, of: kali-p.[172] nat-m.[172] sil.[172]
✦ catalepsy, of: art-v.[172]
✦ convulsions, before: aml-n.[54] arg-n.[54] cic.[58] **CUPR.**[162] nat-m.[54]
✦ convulsions, during: cocc.[54] stram.[54]
✦ convulsions, of: bamb-a.[1184] cann-i.[54] op.[172]
✦ death, convulsions, during: acon.[54] kali-br.[54]
✦ death, excitement, with wild, begs to know if he is to die and before answer drops into heavy sleep: vario.[172]
✦ epilepsy, of: alum. arg-n. bamb-a.[1184] merc.[10]
✦ fainting, of: ***acon.***[162] ***arg-n.*** ars-s-f.[54] aster. carb-an. cimic.[198] **LAC-C.** ***plat.***[36] sac-alb.[210]
✦ fit, of having a: agar. alum. aml-n.[54] ***arg-n.*** cann-i. carb-an. carb-v.[139] grat.[54] helon.[172] lach.[10] lyss.[54] med.[184] merc.[10] nux-m. phos. puls.
✦ punishment, after, in children, if brought to bed too soon get convulsions in sleep: ***ign.***[54]
✦ tunnels, no light in carriage, with, may cause fainting: stram.[85]
✦ unconsciousness, of: alumn.[36] til.[36]
✦ vertigo, of: acon.[172] bamb-a.[1184] op.[172] sumb.

Feigning; paroxysms, faintness: ***tarent.***

Forgetfulness; connection of consecutive thoughts, of, after apoplexy: ***op.***[54]

Hydrophobia; convulsions, during: canth.[54] lyss.[54]

Hydrophobia; idea of fluids may cause a paroxysm, the mere: lyss.[54]

Hydrophobia; spasms renewed by contact: ***bell.***[54]

Hysteria; fainting hysterical: ***acon.***[102] am-c.[58] apisin.[102] arn.[54] ars. asaf.[102] cench.[58] ***cham.*** cimic. **COCC.** cupr.[102] ***dig.***[54] **IGN.** kali-ar.[58] lac-d. lach.[102] ***mosch. nat-m. nux-m. nux-v.*** puls. ***sep.***[54] ***stict.***[54] sumb. ter.

Impatience; convulsions before attack, in: ***mosch.***[54]

Impulse; run, to, convulsive paroxysms came on, when: agar-st.[36]

Insanity; alternating with, depressive narcosis: apis[130] ***hyos.***[137]

Kleptomania; boy with epilepsy: ***art-v.***[54]

Lasciviousness; convulsions, before: ***lach.***[54]

Love; everybody around him, for, during and after fainting: hura[36]

Malicious; convulsions, after: ***cupr.***[54]

Malicious; convulsions, during: cham.[54]

Rage; convulsions, fits, after: cocc.[144] op.[102]

Rage; convulsions, fits, after, epileptic: ***arg.*** op.[102]

Rage; convulsions, fits, during: alco.[36] ars.[36] bell.[1] camph.[36] cham.[127] cupr.[54] indg.[171] ***plb.***[8] stram.[36]
Rage; convulsions, fits, during, epileptic: bell. ***canth.***[54] cupr. hyos. nux-v. op. plb. stram.[54]
Rage; convulsive, spasmodic: ars. ***bell.*** ***canth.***[54] ***hyos.***[54] ***stram.***
Restlessness; alternating with, fainting: vip.[36]
Restlessness; fainting, followed by: calc.
Sadness; epilepsy, with: ***atro.***[54] ***indg.***[54] ***sulph.***[54] tarent.[54]
Sadness; fainting, with: ars.[10] ***lach.***[54] mosch.[10]
Shrieking; fainting, with sudden, on going from one room to another full of company: ***plb.***[54]
Shrieking; fear, with, death, of, dry convulsive cough, from, in weak nervous children: ***kali-br.***[54]
Smiling; convulsions, during: ***bell.***[10]
Talk; indisposed, convulsions, during: plb.[36] sul-ac.[36]
Thoughts; vanishing, blackness before eyes, with, in paroxysms: ***lach.***[54]
Unconsciousness; alone, when: ***ph-ac.***
Unconsciousness; alternating with, dangerous violence: absin.
Unconsciousness; alternating with, escape, desire to: ***coloc.***[54]
Unconsciousness; alternating with, rage: aloe[54]
Unconsciousness; alternating with, sadness: thyr.[102]
Unconsciousness; angina pectoris, in: ***arn.***[54] ***chim-m.***[54] ***cimic.***[54]
Unconsciousness; appetite, before want of: ***calad.***[54]
Unconsciousness; blood, sight of: nux-m.
Unconsciousness; coition, after: ***agar.*** asaf. ***dig.***
Unconsciousness; crowded room, in a: ambr. ars. bar-c. con. ign. ***lyc.*** nat-c. nat-m. ***nux-m. phos.*** **PULS.** sulph.
Unconsciousness; dream; as in a: ambr. anac. cann-i. carb-an. con. **NUX-M.** phos. rheum stram. valer. ***verat.***
Unconsciousness; emotion, after: ***acon.*** am-c. camph. ***caust. cham.*** **COFF. IGN. LACH.** mosch.[116] nux-m. ***op. ph-ac.*** phos.[189] verat.
Unconsciousness; erotomania, in: apis[98] ***orig.***[54]
Unconsciousness; music, from: cann-i. sumb.
Unconsciousness; rage, with: ***stram.***[54]
Unconsciousness; sadness, from: aur.[184] visc.[184]
Unconsciousness; sexual excitement, with: ***orig.***[54] ***stram.***[54]
Unconsciousness; trance, as in a: **LACH.** ***laur.*** tab.

ACON. He, 51 - Ailments from fright: afraid (fear) in dark; vertigo; faintness; trembling; cardiac weakness; threatened miscarriage (abortion); impending cessation of menstrual flow;..
AGAR. He, 25 - Protracted (postponed) mental application or exciting debates brought on vertigo.
ALUM. Ha, 20 - In the morning, anxiety as if he were to have an attack of epilepsy in a few hours.(convulsion)
Ha, 54 - Numb (paralyzed) feeling in the head, with a fear that he would become unconscious.
ALUMN. Al, 4 - Feared to leave her sit in church, after feeling faint.
AML-N. He, 13 - Haunted (obsessed) many times a day with an indescribable dread and sensation as of an oncoming fit, although it came on only once or twice a week.
ARG-M. He, 2-...as if he might have an apoplectic stroke, and could not finish this proving; with spasmodic contraction of heart.
ARG-N. He, 12 - The sight of high houses always made him dizzy (confused) and caused him stagger (hesitation) ; it seemed as if houses on both sides would approach and crush him.
He, 15 - When walking gets nervous (anxiety), thinks he will have a fit (convulsion?) or die suddenly, which makes him walk faster,(rapid) but soon has to stop, because he gets tired.
He, 53 - When walking, becomes faint (weak, fall?) with anxiety, which makes him walk faster.
He, 43 - Alarmed by vertigo and weakness of left side.
ARS. Ha, 1013 - Anxiety so that he frequently fainted, besides a violent pain in the place, and black pocks on the spot .

Ha, 1017 - Precordial anxiety, interrupted by the occurrence of faintings.
ART-V. He, 18 - Fright (fear) and other emotions are followed by epilepsy.
ASAF. He, 17 - If he thinks of having taken drug, it brings on faintness. (medicine)
ASTER. He, 15 - Fear of fainting, with sensation of fullness in chest.(fit)
BRY. He, 4 - So weak in mind that his ideas vanish (empty) as if he would faint, ...
CACT. He, 16 - During and after attack, great anxiety, fearing some organic lesion of heart which will cause sudden death.
CALC. Ha, 70 - In the evening, two fits of loss of consciousness in walking; she would have fallen down, if she had not been held up.
He, 16 - Feels as if she would lose her senses.0Megrim
CAMPH. Al, 17 - He beats himself on the chest, and falls into a faint.
He, 42 - Was found much excited, screaming loudly, " I shall not faint! I can't faint, for if I do, I will have fits and never come out of them.
He, 52 - He beats himself on chest, and falls into a faint.
CARB-V. Ha, 677 - At night he wakes up several times on account of pulsation in the head and anxiety as if about to have a fit of apoplexy; ...and he felt that if he put off awaking longer he would have fainted.
CAUST. He, 52 - Anxiety before falling asleep, as though attack of fainting would return and he would die.
CHAM. Ha, 460-... The child makes itself stiff and bends backwards, stamps with its feet on the nurse's arm, cries in an uncontrollable way, and throws everything away.
CROC. Al, 24 - A slight cause which would usually have made her laugh, now causes a most violent ill-humor, almost rage, so that she frequently loses her consciousness; afterwards she is astonished at this out break.
CUPR. He, 26 - Loss of spirits (courage); anxiety; fits of anguish and fear of death.
FL-AC. He, 14 - Fear of apoplexy.
GERM. Sh, 15 - Wake feeling anxious, increasingly. Legs tremble and shake. I have to get out of bed. I am scared that a heart attack is imminent and cannot be prevented. It's to late to do anything. I walk from room to room, thirsty, chilly and in turmoil. Accompanied by a desire for stool and flatulence. 08, 12C, 80:00:00
HYOS. Ha, 485 - He is in danger of becoming senseless.
He, 74 - Disappointed love followed by: epilepsy, melancholy, rage, or inclination to laugh at everything; despair and propensity to drown himself. (ailments from)
He, 54 - Tries to injure those around him; convulsions after trying to swallow.
He, 57 - Delirium tremens:...averse to light and company; visions as if persecuted preceded by an epileptic attack;... seeks to escape from men by whom he imagines himself surrounded and who are trying to capture him; does not recognize his wife who is standing by his side, but imagines he sees her under a distant bed.
LAC-C. He, 31 - Very nervous; constant dread; a feeling as if she was going to become unconscious (faint, fit)
LYC. Al, 45 - While walking in open air, apprehensiveness and attacks of vertigo.
LYSS. Al,N-76 - Felt as if she was going to get a fit.
Al,N-127 - Thinking of fluids of any kind, even of blood, brings on convulsions.
Al,N-129 - Hyperesthesia, current of air, bright light, sight of any shining object, slightest touch, even conversation in vicinity of patient, may throw him into a most violent agitation and bring on severe convulsions.
He, 26 - Thinks he is a dog or a bird, and runs up and down, chirping and twittering, until he falls down fainting.
He, 76 - Felt as if she was going to get a fit; at 11 p.m.
MAG-C. Al, 952 - Dream that he had an epileptic fit.
Al, 953 - Dream that she was sadly disturbed in company, where especially her grandmother was taken with spasms, and at last had apoplexy.
MOSCH. Al, 11 - He was extremely anxious about the death;...."this is my death" became deathly pale, and in ten minutes fell down in a faint.
He, 4 - Great dread (fear) of death, with

paleness of face, fainting; talks only of approaching (nearing) death.
He, 3 - Scolding; keeps it up till her lips turn blue, eyes stare, and she falls down fainting.
NAT-C. Al, 3 - Every event makes a strong impression upon her; a wavy trembling in the nerves, with a sensation of faintness.
NAT-M. He, 51 - After violent fits of passion, paralysis.
OP. He, 30 - Grief over insults is followed by convulsions.
PLAT. Ha, 7 - Anguish as if about to die, as if unconsciousness (insensible) would ensue (result),...
He, 24 - Much anguish; she feels as if she would lose her senses and die soon.
He, 15 - Deadly anxiety, as if her senses would vanish, ...(disappear)
PULS. Al, 18 - Anxiety as if would have apoplexy, in the evening, after lying down, ...
Ha, 1115 - Anxiety, as if threatened with apoplexy, in the evening after lying down, ...
SEP. Al, 1 - So excited from anger that she fears an apoplectic fit; everything becomes black (evil) before the eyes.
Ha, 51-(Ailments) From vexation, she is so excited that she fears an apoplectic fit, and everything turns black before her eyes.
SPONG. Ha, 377 - Every day, several fits of heat, with anxiety, pain in the cardiac region, weeping and inconsolable; she would like to die there and then.
STRAM. He, 103 - Had many strange fancies, such as imagining his wife had lovers concealed (hidden) behind stove; ...afterward had a fit that looked so much like apoplexy that he was bled.(blood)
He, 113 - Hydrophobia; water, a mirror, or anything bright, excites convulsion...,afraid to be alone;...
He, 11 - Stupor: weakened intellect; torpor and fits; extreme excitement of sexual parts,...
SYPH. Al,N-5-... violent on being opposed, has tremors, seems on the verge of convulsions,...always washing her hands.
TARENT. Al, 14 - Feigned (simulate) paroxysms; a girl simulating fainting and insensibility, looks sideways to watch the effect produced on those around her. (manipulation)
THUJ. Al, 76 - Dread that she would be attacked with apoplexy, ...

FLATTERY

Contemptuous; hard for subordinates and agreeable or pleasant to superiors or people he has to fear: lach.[30] lyc.[30] plat.[30] verat.[30]
Desires; flowers: ars.[189] nat-m.[189]
Desires; respect, due to him shown: ham.[137]
Flatterer: arn.[30] carb-v.[30] **LYC.**[30] petr.[30] puls.[30] staph.[30]
Flattery; desires: carb-v.[193] lap-mar-c.[194] ***pall.***
Flattery; gives everything, when flattered.: lyc.[30] puls.[30] sulph.[30]
Haughty; wounded, wishes to be flattered: **PALL.**[54]
Hypocrisy: bar-c.[30] caust.[30] lap-mar-c.[194] lyc.[148] merc.[30] nux-v.[30] phos. ***puls.*** sep.[30] ***sil.***[30] ***sulph.***[30]
Longing; for, good opinion of others: ***pall.***
Opinions, expects others to pay respect to her: ham.
Reverence; those around him, for: cocc.[30] ham. ***hyos.***[54] nat-m.[30] nux-v.[30] plat.[30] puls.[30] sil.[30] sulph.[30]

HAM. Al, 1 - Feeling that she ought (have) to be reverenced (honored, venerated) by all around her and have great respect (regard) paid to her opinions; lasting about an hour.
PALL. He, 18 - Feels best in company and wants to be flattered.
ROB. Al, 12 - Anxiety to seek honors (distinction) ; excessive pride (haughtiness, arrogance) ; he considers himself better than an emperor.

FLOATING

Delusions; air, he is hovering in, like a spirit: asar. lac-c.[58] lach.[58] psil.[164]
- bed, raised, is: canth.
- bed, swimming: bell.[1]
- body, brain, swimming, is: sol-n.[139]
- body, feet, touching scarcely the ground: dat-a.[36]
- body, legs, floating: acon.[137] ph-ac.[137] spig.[137] zinc-i.[137]
- body, lighter than air, is, embrace, after: agn.[36]

- body, lighter than air, is, masturbation, from, or hysterical subjects, in: gels.[137]
- chair is rising up: phos.
- clouds, rocks, and, in the air: mag-m.
- elevated in air: nitro-o.[36] phos.[139] rhus-t.[139] sil.[139]
- elevated in air, fall, and will: mosch.[139]
- elevated, bed is raised: canth.
- figures, marching in the air (evening while half asleep): nat-c.
- floating in air: ***acon.*** agar.[162] ***ambr.***[162] anh.[119] ***arg.***[162] arn.[193] asar. bell.[116] bry.[139] calc.[85] calc-ar.[58] camph. cand-a.[239] cann-i. canth. chlf.[36] cocain.[139] cocc.[137] coff.[137] dat-a.[36] euon.[122] euon-a.[85] germ.[222] hura hyos.[85] hyper.[102] jug-r.[85] kali-br. ***lac-c.***[72] ***lach.*** lact.[85] lat-k.[102] m-aust.[85] manc.[139] mosch.[139] nat-ar.[102] nat-m.[137] ***nux-m. op.***[137] ozone[227] passi.[85] pen.[85] ph-ac.[85] phos. phys.[85] pip-m.[139] rhus-g.[102] sep.[48] spig.[162] ***stach.***[116] ***stict.***[72] stram.[137] stroph.[85] ***tarent.***[85] tell.[85] tep.[139] ter.[5] thuj.[137] ***valer.*** visc.[149] xan.[85] zinc-i.[137]
- floating, bed, resting in is not: ***lach.*** stict.
- floating, bed, swimming in: bell. stram.
- floating, maze, in a wavy: keroso.[36]
- hanging, or standing high, seems as if: phos.
- hanging, three feet from the ground (on falling asleep): hura.
- head, captive balloon, is a: bamb-a.[1184]
- ideas floating outside of brain: dat-a.[36]
- skull is raised and lowered: stict.[85]
- space, carried into, that he is, while lying: cann-i.[58] coca germ.[222] ***lach.***
- space, he is in: germ.[222]
- spectres, sees, hovering in the air: aur. lach.[58]
- stepping, empty space, on: dubin.[72]
- swimming, air, in the: calc-ar.[139] lac-c.[58] lact.[139] manc.[139] valer.[139]

Dreams; air, sleeping in, with nothing under him: acon.[36]

- ➤ air, that she was in: kreos.[36]
- ➤ ascending a height: brom.[54] hydrog.[222] rhus-t.[54]
- ➤ floating: hell.
- ➤ flying: aether[36] ***apis*** asc-t.[36] atro. bell.[111] cann-i.[36] choc.[222] convo-d.[36] indg. ***lat-m.***[36] lyc. nat-s. ***rhus-g.***[122] stict.[8] xan.
- ➤ sleeping in air: acon.[36]
- ➤ swimming, air, in: lact.[85]
- ➤ walking, ground, above the: lact.[85]

Fear; upward, of being drawn: camph.

ADAM. Sh, 3 - Feeling like a cloud is lifting, world becoming clearer again and not feeling so irritable and grumpy. 7, 6C, 48:00:XX

Sh, 45 - Sensation as if I am bubbling under the surface 7, 6C, 59:00:XX

ARS-MET. He, 5 - Feels as if she had to run away (escape), far away, and as if she would hardly touch ground.

ASAR. Al, 1 - He imagines he is hovering (floating) in the air, when walking, like a spirit.

BELL. Al, 92 - Lying in bed in the evening, it appears to him as if he were floating away with his couch; ten evenings in succession, he imagined, immediately after lying down, that he was floating in his bed.

He, 86 - Sensation of floating or gliding along, as if in a boat; as if the body, or part of it was greatly enlarged.

CANTH. Al, 16 - Visions at night, when half awake; she heard soft steps in the room, then knocking under the bed, and the bed was raised up.

CHOC. Sh, 139 - Meditation is much smoother —an effortless zooming in. I feel much more comfortable in the world. Before I always wanted to get out. During meditation, felt a floating feeling, felt an opening and upwards movement in my back, as if wings were forming and I was just light.

GERM. Sh, 132 - Feeling of being pushed backwards, floating backwards in space, as if weightless. 10, 9C, 00:00:10

HALI-L. Sh, 12 - Returning home after dropping kids off at school, I feel light, my legs feel springy, the weight on my feet more forward, feel like I am floating around the house. Still calm. 09, 6C, 03:XX:XX

Sh, 197 - I was flowing in the car. Driving to a destination and not being driven. More a sense like floating without the tension of driving. 09, 9C, XX:XX:XX

HYDROG. Sh, 25 - A hovering numbness hit with a sensation that my mind was being pulled from the top of the head downwards, like internal pressure being pulled down inside of me —as after a fright. Incredible sensation. 24, 30C, 00:XX:45

IRID. Sh, 102 - Just before sleep, image came into head from nowhere. Sitting on an air current as if it was a soft comfy settee foam cushion. Started to move over a landscape, took me high up, trees, towns, like the flying sequence from The Snowman. The air was so supportive, like floating on water. It had real substance but unlike water it was bouncy. There was no way I was going to fall. I was sitting back, not floating, tummy down. Felt like a child bouncing on the air. Fun —at the same time sense of awe, experiencing something for the first time. No sense of danger — trust. Floatiness experienced before with cannabis but then I was anxious, "Would I get back into body?" With this I was still in my body — no separation. G44

Sh, 103 - Felt light and young, found things fun and amusing. Walking effortlessly, easy, as if not touching the ground. Q1

KEROSE. Al, 1 - As you breathe the vapor you seem to float into a wavy maze (labyrinth, puzzle), with a sense of complete loneliness; there appears to be but one object in the universe, and that object is yourself; on recovery the first thing seen is deemed (judge, conclude) the next only existence in the universe; ...

NEON. Sh, 50 - I have superbly fluid and graceful motions, as if I were moving in water instead of air. I have much pleasure in the right shoulder being free. 20, 6C, 05:XX:XX

Sh, 49 - I have lost the delusion, which I have always had, that I could walk on water. 20, 6C, 04:XX:XX

OP. Al, 43 - In walking I was hardly sensible that my feet touched the ground; it seemed as if I slid (floating) along the ground impelled by some invisible agent, and that my blood was composed of some ethereal fluid which rendered my body lighter than air.

Al, 44 - He seems to be flying or floating in the air, and to whirl (rotate) with everything about him.

STRAM. Al, 63-...I was assailed (attacked) by imaginary spectres, in the most hideous forms and menacing attitudes; and what was still to my torment my bed was suspended and tantalized (charmed) like a feather (plumage) between two floors.

THUJ. Ha, 630 - Walking is performed with extreme ease; she feels as though her body were borne up by wings; she ran many miles in an uncommonly short time, and with unusual high spirits.

VALER. He, 11 - Feels light as if flying in air.

FLY

Anxiety; motion, from, airplane, of: **BOR.**[122]

Delusions; animals, butterflies, of: bell. cann-i.

- animals, pigeons flying in room which he tries to catch: ***kali-c.***[54]
- body, back, opens and wings are forming: choc.[222]
- body, head, lift it off, can: ther.
- clothes, fly away and become wandering stars, will (on undressing): cann-i
- clouds, rocks, and, in the air: mag-m.
- flight from objects: ***stram.***[36]
- fly, he can: camph.[139] lil-t.[139] tub.[139]
- flying, away, what he holds in his hands: coloc.[5] dulc.[5] **STAPH.**[5]
- flying, he is, rock into dark abyss, from a, on going to bed: cann-i.
- flying, he or she is: anh.[119] asar. bell.[116] calc-ar.[54] camph. ***cann-i.*** euon.[116] jug-r.[139] lach. lact.[139] lat-k.[102] manc.[139] nitro-o.[36] oena. op. valer.[171]
- flying, out of his skin: thuj.[5]
- head, captive balloon, is a: bamb-a.[1184]
- objects, flight from: **STRAM.**[36]
- space, carried into, that he is, orbit, and compelled to describe a vast: cann-i.[36]
- space, carried into, that he is, while lying: cann-i.[58] coca germ.[222] ***lach.***
- wings, her body is borne upon wings, after laughing: thuj.[54]

Dreams; animals, bat flying in room, causing fear: ham.[36]

- ➤ animals, birds, of, large, black: choc.[222]
- ➤ animals, birds, of, singing: com.[36]
- ➤ box, flying: ozone[227]
- ➤ cask races from the sky, a big white, with a green lid: ozone[227]
- ➤ flying: aether[36] ***apis*** asc-t.[36] atro. bell.[111] cann-i.[36] choc.[222] convo-d.[36] indg. ***lat-m.***[36] lyc. nat-s. ***rhus-g.***[122] stict.[8] xan.
- ➤ flying, airplane, in: allox.[119] hydrog.[222]
- ➤ flying, apparatus, whose wings will not work: apis[36]
- ➤ flying, lighted street, along: convo-d.[36]

➤ flying, people: hydrog.[222]
➤ flying, tops of houses, over: xan.[54]
➤ journey, airplane, by: ozone[227]
➤ mother, flying around the world: hydrog.[222]

Fear; airplanes: ***acon.***[162] arg-n.[162] ars.[162] **CALC.**[162] lup.[162] nat-m.[162]
✦ alone, of being, starts with a loud cry as if a bird flew towards the window: kali-c.[172]
✦ animals, bats: ham.[36]
✦ animals, bees, of: hep.[162]
✦ animals, cockroaches, of: alum.[162] manc.[30] ***phos.***[162]
✦ night, fly, with desire to: ***merc.***[54]

Fly, desire to: choc.[222]

ADAM. Sh, 317 - Enjoy the powerful night force. I can fly in the dark. 16, 12C, 35:XX:XX

BELL. Al, 81 - He imagines he sees birds flying off through the chimney, and wishes to follow them by the same route. (desire: fly, liberty, freedom)

Al,S-2559 - Seems to see birds flying past and wishes to follow them.

BUFO. Al, 14 - Very easily frightened; a bird or insect flying by causes a start.

CANN-I. Al, 32 - He thinks he can fly through the air like the birds.

CHOC. Sh, 139 - Meditation is much smoother —an effortless zooming in. I feel much more comfortable in the world. Before I always wanted to get out. During meditation, felt a floating feeling, felt an opening and upwards movement in my back, as if wings were forming and I was just light.

Sh, 314 - Talking about flying. I would like to be a bird or a bat or in a plane.[01]A, 30C, 00:12:XX

HALI-L. Sh, 637 - If I had known this was going to happen, I wonder if I would have taken the remedy. I thought I must be crazy (after taking remedy last night). I would like to fling that vial of remedy to the ends of the universe. 06, 6C, 00:12:30

Sh, 720 - Thoughts of flying —Icarus! 20, 30C, 00:23:30

Sh, 721 - Inner vision; I was sunning my wings in the dawn sun. I'm not flapping-soaring —not dusk, at dawn — not for dark, of Light. 20, 30C, 00:23:50

Sh, 862 - Clear and bright, an eagle soared, an amazing bird high up in the sky, when I was lying naked on my back. It wasn't flapping, it just soared. coming from the east towards me then flew into the sun. As I lay there, unbelieving, he soared out again, circled again and then disappeared into the radiance of the sun. I felt like the proving was finished. It felt like a good-bye. My vision had changed. I feel more like me. 20, 30C, 08:08:XX

Sh, 901 - Sensation of such harmonious balance when on the wing, Such power in these almost weightless wings. Sensation of deep warmth echoing the sun. 20, 30C, 10:XX:XX

HYDROG. Sh, 189 - As if in a dream, not there, difficult to stay with it all while driving home —very conscious of the blackbirds flying across the motorway. Better taking a nap and fresh air from opening the window. Concomitant to finger abscess. 02, 6C, 54:XX:XX

IRID. Sh, 102 - Just before sleep, image came into head from nowhere. Sitting on an air current as if it was a soft comfy settee foam cushion. Started to move over a landscape, took me high up, trees, towns, like the flying sequence from The Snowman. The air was so supportive, like floating on water. It had real substance but unlike water it was bouncy. There was no way I was going to fall. I was sitting back, not floating, tummy down. Felt like a child bouncing on the air. Fun —at the same time sense of awe, experiencing something for the first time. No sense of danger — trust. Floatiness experienced before with cannabis but then I was anxious, "Would I get back into body?" With this I was still in my body —no separation. G44

Sh, 106 - Mental image: I am inside an egg —a bird, wet feathers, at the point it is smashing through its shell, bursting out; a chick, wet crumpled and hot, shell flying all over. The relief —getting to the air, refreshing, cool. Inside it was humid, stifling. Stretching vast wings, enjoying feeling the air dry them out. G5

Sh, 109 - Sensation as if wings 3 —4 p.m. Q5

Sh, 112 - Sensation as if winged ankles, while wind blowing through house. Thought, "back to earth." Q17

KALI-C. Al, 25 - She is frightened with a loud cry, by an imaginary apparition (as for example, of a bird flying to the window).
Ha, 26 - She is frightened by an imaginary appearance (e.g. as if a bird was flying toward the window) and she utters a loud scream.
He, 5 - Imagines seeing birds flying in room; he tries to catch them. (seize)

NEON. Sh, 20 - I had thoughts of albatrosses circumnavigating the earth without having to touch the ground. 20, 6C, 03:02:14

OENA. Al, 14 - It seemed to her as if she were flying.

OP. Al, 44 - He seems to be flying or floating in the air, and to whirl (rotate) with everything about him.

STICT. Al, 1 - She got very lively (active), told her father she felt as if she would like to strike out, only for fun; she would like it just for fun of it. After awhile she lay down on the lounge, and began, to use a common expression, to kick up her heels; her mother reproaching, said, " Bella, do behave, that is not ladylike"; when child responded: " Ma, I cannot help it; I feel exactly as if I want to fly away"...

THUJ. Ha, 630 - Walking is performed with extreme ease; she feels as though her body were borne up by wings; she ran many miles in an uncommonly short time, and with unusual high spirits.

VALER. He, 11 - Feels light as if flying in air.

FORSAKEN

Anxiety; forsaken her, as if a friend had: ***rhus-t.***[54]

Blackmail, emotional, says "you don't love me" when refused: puls.[189] tub.[189]

Company, desire for; children that are rejected, in: carc.[207]

Confidence; thinks others have none, which makes her unhappy, and: ***aur.***

Delusions; alone, always: puls. stram.
- alone, castaway, being a: germ.[222] ***phys.***[54]
- alone, world, she is a. in the: ***androc.*** bamb-a.[1184] camph. choc.[222] ***cycl.***[122] germ.[222] hura ***plat. puls.***
- appreciated, she is not: arg-n.[185] aur.[185] lap-c-b.[194] ***pall.*** plat. puls.[162] seq-s.[230]
- asylum, insane, sent to: lach.[58]
- asylum, she will be sent to: cench.
- company, people are averse to her: androc.[222]
- confidence in him, his friends have lost all: aur. hura.
- cowards, persons leaving him are: cann-i.
- deserted, forsaken, is: **ARG-N.** ***aur.***[116] bamb-a.[1184] bar-c. camph. cann-i. carb-an. carb-v. chin. ***cycl.*** hura hyos. ***kali-br.*** lach.[139] lap-c-b.[194] lap-gr-m.[194] lap-mar-c.[194] lil-t. lyss. **MAG-C.**[185] nat-c. ozone[227] pall. ***plat.*** puls. rhus-t.[139] sac-alb.[210] sanic.[85] ***stram.***
- friend, affection of, has lost the: ***aur.*** hura hydrog.[222] hyos.[58]
- friend, she is about to lose a: hura.
- lost, salvation, despised, and, in erotomania: ***orig.***[54].
- lost, salvation, world, to the, beyond hope: ***arg-n.***[54]
- loved by parents, is not: sac-alb.[210]
- neglected, he is: ***arg-n.*** lap-mar-c.[194] naja nat-m.[189] **PALL.** puls.[58] sac-alb.[210] sep.[189]
- neglected, he is, despised by his family, and: ***arg-n.***[54]
- neglected, husband, by her: ***stram.***[8]
- places, none in the world, she has: germ.[222] ***plat.***[54]
- repudiated by relatives, he is: arg-n. hura.
- repudiated, society, he is repudiated by: hydrog.[222]
- room, desolated, is: valer.[36]
- town, he is in desert: carb-an.[10]
- wife, will run away from him: staph.

Despair; others and oneself: ***arg-n.***[54] aur.[54]

Despair; others, about: ***aur.***

Dreams; anger, quarreled with his father, that he had, who would not recognize him as a son because he had embraced homeopathy: crot-h.[36]
➤ remorse, repudiated by God, of being: hyper.[36]
➤ throw away, being to: rhus-t.[10]
➤ wedding, everyone is going to a, except her: hydrog.[222]

Fear; neglected, of being: cand-a.[239] puls.[58]

Forsaken feeling: allox.[119] alum. anac.[185] androc.[222] ***arg-n.*** asar.[162] **AUR.** bamb-a.[1184] bar-c. calc. calc-s.[36] camph. cand-a.[239] cann-i. carb-an. carb-v. carc.[207] chin. chin-b.[54] 0coff.[5] cortico.[119] ***cycl.*** dros.[5] germ.[222] hell.[5] hura hydrog.[222] hyosin.[123]

ip.[5] kali-br. kali-c. keroso.[36] lac-d. ***lach.*** lact. lam. lap-c-b.[194] lap-gr-m.[194] laur.[5] lil-t. lith-c. lyss. m-aust. ***mag-c.***[122] mag-m. **MENY.**[5] ***merc.***[122] ***nat-c.***[122] ***nat-m.***[193] ozone[227] pall. ***plat.*** plb.[201] **PSOR. PULS.** rhus-t. sabin.[5] ***sac-alb.***[210] sanic.[85] sars.[5] sec.[5] sep.[5] spig.[5] ***stram.*** sulph.[176] valer. verat. wye.[77]

Forsaken; feeling, air, amel. in open: rhus-t.

Forsaken; feeling, beloved by his parents, wife, friends, feels of not being: ***ars.***[30] calc.[30] lyc.[30] ***mag-c.***[122] sep.[30] sil.[30] sulph.[30]

Forsaken; feeling, evening: androc.[222] bar-c. ***puls.***

Forsaken; feeling, friendless, feels: arg-n.[58] ***lach.***[8] pip-n.[2103]

Forsaken; feeling, heat of sun, or in Summer, from: gels.[8]

Forsaken; feeling, isolation, sensation of: allox.[119] ***anac. androc. anh.***[119] ***arg-n.*** arist-cl.[149] camph. cann-i. cann-s.[36] choc.[222] coca cortico.[144] germ.[222] hura ***hydrog.*** lac-h.[229] lap-mar-c.[194] merc.[187] op.[231] ozone[227] pip-m.[231] plat. psil.[231] puls.[193] sac-alb.[210] stram. tab.[231]

Forsaken; feeling, isolation, sensation of, talking, on, people do not hear him: cortico.[119]

Forsaken; feeling, morning: carb-an. carb-v. ***lach.***

Forsaken; feeling, night, with weeping: bamb-a.[1184]

Forsaken; feeling, old people, in: aur.[193] psor.[193]

Forsaken; feeling, sighing, with: lith-c.[60]

Forsaken; feeling, thinks she is left alone in the world: plat.[60]

Forsaken; feeling, waking, on: ***arg-n. lach.***

Forsaken; headache, with: meny.[122]

Helplessness, feeling of: aether[36] anac.[1] ant-t.[36] arg-n.[162] ars.[1] bamb-a.[1184] ***calad.***[122] cand-a.[239] ***gels.***[8] germ.[222] hecla.[234] hell. hydrog.[222] jasm.[36] kali-br. lith-c.[25] **LYC.**[122] ozone[227] petr. phos. puls.[189] rhus-t.[137] stram. tax.

Irritability; carelessness of others, about: lap-gr-m.[194]

Jealousy; neglect, accuses husband of: ***stram.***[54]

Lamenting; appreciated, because he is not: calc-s.

Misunderstood, feels: ign.[155] lap-c-b.[194]

Weeping; goes off alone and weeps as if she had no friends: bar-c.

Weeping; love, from unrequited: ***ign.***[54]

Weeping; neglect, from the slightest: coff.[58]

ANDROC. Sh, 61 - Felt constrained and had a gloomy approach to everything, averse company, desire to be alone. I feel people will not want to talk or be with me. (28)

Sh, 63 - Desired company but could not be bothered to see anyone, felt lonely as if he didn't belong. (21)

ARG-N. He, 40 - Melancholy since an undeserved slight (scorn); fixed idea that he was neglected and despised by his family; his callings (job, work) became indifferent to him.

AUR-M. He, 6 - Everything is disagreeable, dreary (lugubrious, desolate, deserted), even nature around.

AUR. Ha, 3 - He believes that he has lost the love of others, and this mortifies him even to tears.

Ha, 353 - He imagines he has forfeited (penalty, lost,) the affections of others, and this grieves him to tears.

BAR-C. Ha, 6 - Sad and anxious; all manner of gloomy (sad) ideas as to his future fate (destiny) rise in his mind, and believes himself totally forsaken (deserted); in the evening.

BRASS. Sh, 12 - Called on a friend who was busy with funeral arrangements. Felt rejected when she had not time to talk to me; my head was saying "don't be silly" but my eyes filled with tears, and my wee heart felt very unloved 3I, 00:06:30

BUFO. Al, 7 - Desires solitude, and yet is afraid of being left alone and dying forsaken.

CAMPH. Al, 46-...I sat up in bed, but all about me had indeed disappeared. I was alone in the great universe, the last of all things. My ideas of the world, God and religion, now seemed to me to have existed only in my imagination; the earth upon which yesterday I lived and moved, had run its appointed course, and I was the final and solitary fragment of the whole creation...(meaningless, unimportant, neglected, forsaken, loneliness, deserted) (godless)

Al, 46-... There was no other feeling in my soul than that of my hopeless endless damnation (condemnation). I sank back upon the bed, believing that I was the spirit of evil in a world forsaken of God.

Al, 46-... My misery was boundless; time itself was no more; in short, I suffered such fearful anguish as no fancy can comprehend. What soul could paint to itself my everlasting (eternal) dwelling as the Evil One (devil), alone in a vast universe, without faith or hope, and my heart forever broken by unimaginable tortures? (miserable, timeless, endless, solitude, forsaken, faithless, hopeless)

Al, 46-.... As I lay stretched on my couch, as the evil demon, and suffered all the anguish of a condemned and God-forsaken soul, ...I was forever deprived of the Divine protection, and of every consolation and every hope. Nothing remained to me but the conviction of my everlasting damnation...

CANN-I. Al, 30 - When his friends went out of the room, he thought (delusion) they had left him to his fate (destiny, doom), and wrote "cowards" in his notes.

Al, 57 - Strange feeling of isolation (solitude) from all around him, with great sense of loneliness (isolation), though surrounded by his friends.

CARB-AN. Al, 11 - In the morning, he felt abandoned and homesick.

Ha, 1 - Extremely melancholy (depression, grief) mood, with a sensation of being deserted.

Ha, 2 - He feels in the morning, as if he was deserted, and full of homesickness.(nostalgia, loneliness, isolation)

Ha, 5 - Pusillanimous (cowardice) and sad; everything seems to her so lonely (alone, deserted) and sad, that she would like to weep.

Ha, 32 - The objects on the street seem to him changed, e.g., farther apart and brighter (vivid, brilliant) than usual, as an empty, abandoned city.

CHIN-B. He, 5 - Feels abandoned and deserted.

CHOC. Sh, 208 - Felt rejected and oversensitive. Hid away from the world, felt my life would fall apart. 35, 30C, XX:XX:XX:

CYCL. He, 17-...fear of death, or an illusion of being deserted or persecuted by every one.

GERM. Sh, 111 - If I were me, nobody would like me -so I try to be what I think others expect me to be. I don't think I can be loved with all the parts of me which are ugly and bad. Lonely feelings. Longing for love and understanding. Feel I am so unfriendly to myself. 18, 30C, 04:00:00

Sh, 140 - Feel I am in an impossible situation. Nobody to talk to who understands me. I can't say things as they are because I have to take others feelings into consideration. I need comfort and encouragement, but no one can give me. Weeping. 18, 30C, 36:XX:XX

Sh, 141 - Painfully aware of the feelings of being an outcast. 08, 12C, 02:00:10

Sh, 138 - Feeling of revulsion for many people especially young parents with children, while wandering through town. Feel people are stuck in their lives. What a waste. 10, 9C, 00:05:00

Sh, 153 - Thought nobody understood me and cared for what I felt. Felt it was unfair. I was presented with complaints about something others had done. Felt I was standing between two fighting parts. Felt awkward about it, embarrassed. Difficult to argue about such strong outburst. Thoughts about the day's arguing milling in my head all evening and night. 21, 12C, 32:XX.XX.

HALI-L. Sh, 213 - I wanted to do more mothering while I was being mothered and at the same time not mothering the son I do have. Feeling envy of all families who had more children. Constant state of desire for something other than what I had. If busy, I wanted to be not busy. If no one calls, I felt nobody cares about me. Could find no comfort anywhere and felt isolatedalone. 01, 30C,, 21:XX:XX

HURA. Al, 15 - Hypochondria, sadness, despair; he fancies he is repudiated and deserted by his relations. (rejected, refused)

Al, 16 - She fancies she is left alone (lonely, solitary, forsaken) in the world and is lost.

HYDROG. Sh, 248 - While sitting in a restaurant, felt progressively more cut off from friends at the table. I began to feel detached and paranoid. I felt disliked by people. They seemed to look at me menacingly. I became concerned that my lecture this afternoon had created conflict, mayhem and destruction, that my friends in the audience did not like me any more. I became aware of a dull ache in my sacrum making me want to shift backwards and forwards. At the same time, the people round the table seemed further away and smaller, as if I had moved four feet back from the table. I felt very uncomfortable and wanted to get out. I put my head down and rushed out without saying goodbye, feeling a sense of relief at getting away (all very unusual for me). Outside, I felt relief and my mind cleared and I walked home alone. 22, 12C, 04:XX:XX

Sh, 249 - I think that no one likes me. I felt betrayed and everything went haywire. 16, 30C,

Sh, 254 - When shopping, felt people did not accept me as belonging to the community. Felt isolated in the shop. Feeling unacceptable, 'as if I was a marked person' —but later felt better on my own. 12, 6C, 19:XX:XX

Sh, 255 - Very worried that people don't like me and can't cope with me —that they will think I am insane. I think maybe I am insane. This is frightening me. 16, 30C, 25:XX:XX

Sh, 258 - Felt cut off from people and suspicious. 22, 12C, 06:XX:XX

HYOS. He, 16 - Fears: being left alone (solitude, deserted); poison, or being bitten (hurt); being poisoned or sold; being betrayed, or injured; wishes to run away. (escape)

IRID. Sh, 318 - Still feeling down, irritable, restless, frustrated and bored. I Feel heavy, everything is an effort. Feel totally unloved, dejected, unwanted, "nobody likes me" feeling. I34

KALI-BR. Al, 5 - She had the erroneous idea that she was deserted by all her friends, and as a consequence she passed all her waking moments, which are not many in tears;...delusion that her child was dead, had taken fixed possession of her mind;...she declared that she saw it dead (corpse) before her, and when it was brought to her, she refused to acknowledge that it was hers, or had any resemblance to the one she imagined was dead.

LAC-D. He, 5 - Imagines that all her friends will die and that she must go to a convent. (purification, salvation)

LACH. He, 39 - Weak and unhappy, particularly in morning, when she feels, on awaking, friendless and forsaken; ...(deserted) has had domestic troubles. 0 Melancholia

LAM. Al, 1 - Weeping mood; she wept as if she had been abandoned. (forsaken)

LIL-T. Al, 16 - Worse on going to bed; can't go to sleep; wild (tumultuous, uncontrollable) feeling in the head as though I should go crazy (insane) and no one would take care of me (forsaken, helpless); thoughts of suicide; how much opium would put me to sleep forever, and who would find my body, and who would care; ... (friendless, abandoned, deserted)

LYSS. Al,N-46 - After fainting (weak) spell he wrote on paper: I am forsaken by all; even the birds of heaven, they do not look at me (despised), do not fed me if hungry (helplessness) ; I hunger with the young ones and am thirsty with their she ones (starving); my nest (house) is made out of dirt (soiled), not gotten by my own exertions (efforts), but by driving them out of their nests (home) and sitting there with the females and the young.

NAT-C. Al, 24 - She does not know what to do, on account of apprehensiveness and ennui and thinks that she is quite lonely (alone, solitary, insulated) and forsaken, all day.

Ha, 8 - Apprehensive and ennui (tedium, monotony), so that she cannot contain herself; she deems (believe), herself altogether (entirely) lonely (solitary) and forsaken.

NEON. Sh, 200 - I feel that nobody is there for me when I need them; I'm there for everyone when they need me but no one is ever there for me. 13, 30C, 07:00:00

PALL. He, 8 - Imagines herself neglected (scorned, despised); wounded pride.

PHOS. Ha, 89 - Delirious fantasies, while slumbering (sleep) and when awake, as if she was on a distant island (isolation, segregation), as if she had a large business, was a distinguished (important, rank) lady, etc.

PHYS. He, 3-...feels as if she must lose her mind and become insane or despondent;...;thinks she is a castaway (repudiated, discarded, rejected, forsaken);....fears she is crazy or will certainly lose her mind;...

PLAT. Ha, 2 - She imagines herself deserted (abandoned) and standing alone in the world.

He, 28 - Thinks she is left entirely to herself and stands alone in the world. (loneliness)

He, 29-...thought she had no place in the world; life was wearisome (boring), but had great dread of death, which she believed near at hand.

PULS. Ha, 1143 - Her head is so quiet and all about her is so empty as if she were alone (solitude, loneliness) in the house and in the world; she does not wish to talk to any one, just as if all around her were no concern (relation) of hers and she belonged to nobody. (lonely, missed)

RHUS-T. Al, 5 - Melancholy, ill-humor, and anxiety, as if a misfortune (disgrace) would happen, or as if she were alone (solitary), and all about her were dead (lifeless, inert) and still (silent, quiet), or as if she had been forsaken by a near friend; worse in the house, relieved by walking in the open air.

Ha, 953 - Melancholy, sad, and anxious, as if about to hear of a calamity,(misfortune, disaster) or as if she were solitary (lonely, alone) and all around her were dead (lifeless, extinct) and silent (quiet) ; or as if she had bid farewell (separation) to an intimate friend ; worst in the room, diminished by walking in a open air.

STAPH. He, 15-...; firmly believed he would lose his fortune, constantly told his wife to be careful that they did not starve; thinks his wife will run away from him (deserted) (lost: position, rank), ... amuses himself by throwing into the fire any article near at hand, regardless of value; at times more violent, strikes at any one coming near him, ...tells his wife he will try not kill any one;...

STRAM. Ha, 562 - His surroundings appear to him quite strange; (unfamiliar) although in the first minutes he knows that he is surrounded by his friends, he forgets this in the second minute, and imagines he is quite alone (solitary, deserted) in a desert (wildness), and is afraid (fearful) ; figures of beasts suddenly spring out of the ground at his side, so that he moves to the other side, where, however, other similar figures pursue him, and he runs forward.

Ha, 564 - He always imagines he is alone (solitary, lonely) and is afraid.

He, 145 - Wife complains of husband neglecting her; man accuses his wife of being faithless.

He, 176 - Melancholia,...complains her husband has neglecting her.

VALER. Al, 11 - Anxious, hypochondriac feeling, as if the objects around him had been estranged from him; the room appears to him desolate (isolated), he does not feel at home in the room, he is impelled to leave it.

FORSAKES

Affection; rejects: sep.[189]

Aversion; family members, to: am-c.[5] am-m.[5] aran.[192] aur.[5] ***calc.*** calc-s.[108] cit-ac.[65] con.[5] ***crot-h.*** ***fl-ac.*** hep.[5] iod.[137] kali-c.[122] kali-p.[5] lyc.[5] ***merc.***[5] ***nat-c.*** nat-m.[30] ***phos.***[5] plat.[5] plb.[162] senec.[137] ***sep.***

Aversion; family, talks pleasantly to others: fl-ac.[137]

Aversion; husband, and children: ***glon.***[54] verat.[54]

Aversion; husband, to: agn.[171] bamb-a.[1184] choc.[222] ***glon.*** kali-c.[122] kali-p. ***nat-c.*** nat-m. pitu-a.[164] **SEP.** thuj.[137] verat.

Aversion; parents, to: fl-ac.[30]

Aversion; wife, to his: ars.[137] ***fl-ac.***[122] nat-s.[137] plat.[137] staph.[137]

Caressed; caressing husband and child, then pushes away: ***anac.***[54]

Casting off of people against her will: **PLAT.**[36]

Children; aversion, her own: glon. ***lyc.*** nux-v.[162] phos.[137] plat. sep.[162] verat.

Children; aversion, her own, daughter, in a woman: raph

Children; flies from the own: lyc.

Delirium; abandons her relatives: sec.

Delusions; baby, odious looks: puls.[54]

- betrothal, engagement, must be broken: fl-ac.
- child, is not hers: anac. nit-ac.[88]
- children, thinks he must drive, out of the house: fl-ac.
- husband, he is not her: ***anac.***
- marriage, must dissolve: fl-ac.

- neglected, friends, his: ***aur.***[58]
- servants, he must get rid of: fl-ac.

Dreams; abortion, efforts and plans: ign.[36]
➤ children, about, neglecting her: bamb-a.[1184]
➤ old gentleman ran away from wife, suspected of having married another: sep.[36]
Escape; attempts to, family, children, from her: am-c.[30] choc.[222] ***lyc.***[122] nux-v.[30] phos.[30] ***sep.***[30] staph.[30]
Estranged; flies her own children: lyc.
Estranged; forgetful of relatives and friends: lap-c-b.[194] lyss.[54]
Estranged; friends, from: hydrog.[222] nat-c.[58]
Estranged; ignores his relatives: bell.[5] hyos.[5] merc.[5] verat.[5]
Estranged; strangers, being kind with, but not with his family and entourage: lyc.[30] nux-v.[30] puls.[30] verat.[30]
Estranged; wife, from his: ars. nat-c.[58] plat. staph.
Forsakes; children, his or her own: lyc.
Forsakes; relations: sec.
Hatred; persons, of, repels everyone: aloe[54]
Indifference; children, to her: aur-ar.[58] choc.[222] kali-i. ***lyc.*** nat-c. **PHOS.**[122] **SEP.**[122]
Indifference; family, to his: carb-v.[58] hell.[36] lap-gr-m.[194] nat-p.[58] nit-ac.[116] **PHOS.**[122] **SEP.**[122]
Indifference; loved ones, to: ***acon.*** allox.[119] ars. ars-i.[58] bell.[193] carb-v.[58] carc.[193] ***fl-ac.*** **HELL.** kali-p.[58] kali-sil.[58] lil-t.[168] merc. myric.[25] nat-p. nat-sil.[58] **PHOS.** plat. **SEP.** ***syph.***[122]
Indifference; loved ones; to, strangers, but animated to: ***fl-ac.***[54]
Indifference; others, about lot of: lap-mar-c.[194] plat.[185] sabad.[185] sulph.
Indifference; relations, to: acon.[58] bac.[62] ***fl-ac.*** **HELL.** hep. hydrog.[222] kali-p.[58] lap-gr-m.[194] nat-c. nat-p.[58] **PHOS.**[122] plat. **SEP.**[122] ***syph.***[122]
Indifference; welfare of others, to: androc.[222] ars.[30] cand-a.[239] caust.[30] lach.[30] lap-mar-c.[194] nat-m.[30] ***nux-v.***[30] ozone[227] plat.[30] sep.[30] **SULPH.**
Irritability; sends the, nurse home: ***fl-ac.***
Neglects; children, her: aur-ar.[58]
Relatives; ignore his: bell.[5] hyos.[5] merc.[5] verat.[5]
Sadness; aversion to see her children from sadness: ***con.***[54]
Sadness; aversion, children to whom he is devotedly attached become burdensome: **KALI-I.**[54]
Unfeeling; family, with his: kali-i.[58]

ADAM. Sh, 277 - Exceptionally strong desire to leave my marriage and children, to live a clear unmuddled life alone. 2, 12C, 74:XX:XX-160:XX:XX
ANAC. He, 29 - Has the fixed idea that her husband is not her husband, her child not her child; now she fondles (caress) them and again pushes them away. (reject, repudiate)
He, 13 - After having caressed her husband or child she pushes them away from her, as if they were not what she supposed.
BRASS. Sh, 15 - Feeling of "leave me alone" if John or the children came near. 3I, 00:06:30
CHOC. Sh, 7 - In the evening, felt angry with bristling down my back. Irritable with the kids, shouted a lot, slammed doors. Feeling very uncomfortable with my daughter near me. I made a huge issue over something small which I would normally leave. I wanted to leave and walk out of the door on them. Felt very unsympathetic to the children. "You either go, or go to bed". Couldn't cuddle the children and took longer to say "Its all right". I thought that their father should look after them instead of me (very unusual). The feeling I can't be where I want to be because of them. I want to be roaming outside without my possessions. Left kids alone in the house for the first time. I was surprised at how easily I let them go. My daughter liked it very much.
Sh, 210 - Felt totally isolated and averse to company. Estranged himself from his family and friends and stopped all communication with them for a long period. Did not reply to letters and left no address. He seemed to hide away and literally disappear. The state of Isolation resulted from feeling that "I didn't exist as a human being". This behaviour was in strong contrast to his normal sociable disposition. 35, 30C, XX:XX:XX:
CIC. Al, 27 - Want of confidence in mankind; with misanthropy; he forsook

society, remained alone and reflected upon their errors and about himself.

Ha, 237 - Depreciation and contempt of mankind; he fled (desert) his fellow-creatures, was in the highest degree disgusted with their follies (stupidity), and his disposition seemed to change into misanthropy; he withdrew into solitude.

Ha, 238 - Want of trust (mistrust, skepticism) in people and anthrophoby,(misanthropy) he fled (escape) from them remained solitary, and thought seriously about their errors and about himself.

FERR. Al, 20 - Excited by the slightest opposition; ... even her children's caresses increased her bad temper; she was often rude to those about her, because she hated to see or talk to them, and wanted them to leave her in solitude, which alone was pleasing to her.

FL-AC. Al, 1 - Great disposition, when alone, to repulsive fantastic imaginations, particularly in regard to persons with whom he stands in near relations, or with whom he is connected (united, joined); it seems, for example, as though he must get rid (discard, repudiate, reject) of all the servants, children must go out of house, a betrothal must be broken off, a marriage should be dissolved. (broke; vows)

He, 6 - Feeling of indifference towards those he loves best; has no objection to their presence but does not care to converse with them, yet if strangers or mere acquaintances come in will enter into animated conversation....

GERM. Sh, 4 - Desperately angry. So intense that I could barely control it. I made noises like an animal, pushed my arms up and down -instead of hitting my children, which helped. Want to just leave the house and the kids. Felt completely mad, afraid of what the neighbors heard and thought. Very bad conscience afterwards, but no relief - didn't get the anger out. There are a lot of feelings inside that don't come out. 18, 30C, 02:09:00

GLON. He, 2 - Recognized no one; repulsed her husband and children; raved, screamed, and wished to rush from house; jumped out of bed, but fell because her knees gave way.

HALI-L. Sh, 580 - Spent most of today thinking about how I am surrounded by idiots, (my family), who are showing no attempts to think for themselves, letting me run the show. They don't care to figure things out. I'm in hyper-drive. I know a lot and I'm right. I've been extremely productive or at least active, balancing several major projects all at the same time, and they can't seem to tidy a table properly. This includes my husband, who continually interrupts me (or so it seems) for some trivial question. I'm coming across with too much force. I find myself shouting at everyone much more than usual. Like a crazy person. Impatient over others' slowness. Almost an arrogance. I want them to THINK! (Obviously, the way I do). or get off the ship and drown yourself. A hard anger, more intense that usual. Feel like leaving them all—they just take and give back little. More trouble than support. This isn't complaining or victimizing talking. This is how it is. I'm healing myself and leaving my family in the dust. I've passed on to them my bad habits, bad parenting. They are content to be idiots. 09, 6C, 13:XX:XX

Sh, 582 - Enforcing deadlines and rules with kids. Son wants to sing me a song but his work's not done so I "don't have time" to listen. Feel I am neglecting my family. 09, 6C, 15:00:XX

HYOS. He, 85-...repelled with rage and seeming disgust his mother, of whom, in natural state, he was dotingly (loving) fond, did not know her, said she was not his mama;...0Maniacal fury.

IGN. He, 44-...;indifference to things she loved best ; sits alone and weeps, imagines things, a especially that she might go crazy; ..

IP. Ha, 219 - Sullen unsociable moroseness, that makes him disdain (reject) everything.

KALI-I. He, 6 - Very great irritability and unwonted harshness of demeanor (behavior); his children, to whom he is devoted and attached, become burdensome to him; very passionate and spiteful temper;...constant apprehension of impending evil.

LYC. Al, 55 - She flees from her own children.

Ha, 9 - She flees (desert) from her own children.
He, 35 - Misanthropic; flies even from his own children.
LYSS. Al,N-58 - Ordered her husband to go away(forsakes), as she wanted to bite him, and joining (associated) act to threat(menace), she bit herself in arm.
MERC. He, 30 - Anxiety driving her to suicide ; thoughts of suicide; ...desire for death; great indifference even to those she formerly loved;...
NAT-C. He, 4 - Aversion to mankind and society; estrangement (separation, alienation) from individuals and society; even from her husband and family.
PHOS. Ha, 82 - Indifferent to her child, whom at other times she dearly loved.
He, 14 - Apathy; indifferent even to his own children;...
PLAT. Al, 11 - Contemptuous, pitiful looking down upon people usually venerated, with a kind of casting (reject, discard) them off in paroxysms, against her will.
Ha, 39 - Indifference, cold (reserved), abstracted (separated) in company of friends,..
He, 36 - While suffering from a slight erysipelas faciei, took leave (quit, abandon) of her children, exhorted her husband to join (unite, combine) church, wanted people to join her in prayer (beg), felt happy to join her Redeemer.
He, 11 - Contemptuous, pitiful, looking down upon people usually venerated, with a kind of casting (forsakes) them off, in paroxysms against her will.
He, 12 - Dislikes her children; calls them too little.
SEC. Al, 1 - Delirium; she abandons (reject, forsakes) her relatives and does absurd things.
SEP. He, 38-...everything seems strange (unusual, unfamiliar) to her;...; it seems as if she could not understand (realize) anything and would have to learn anew everything she wished to do;...(lost: knowledge); greatest indifference to everything, the death of a near relative, or some happy occurrence, leaves her equally unaffected; no trace of her former love for friends or even for her child; aversion for social intercourse amounting to contempt;...
He, 22 - Great indifference to one's family, to those they love best.
THUJ. He, 23 - Mental depression, after childbirth (puerperal), in consequence of being told that there had been a slight rupture (division, hurt) of perineum; grows quiet; thinks she must die;...wants to jumps the window; does not care for children or her relatives (careless) ;..(sensitive to disrupt, partition)
UPA. Al, 4 - Melancholic; has to force the tears back; cold towards his friends, repelling everyone.
VERAT. He, 13 - After severe illness, aversion to husband and children; desire to leave house: hallucinations, room appeared full of people, crowding in, there was no longer room...

FRAGILE

Delicacy, feeling of: ign.[5] nux-v.[5]
Delusions; body, brain, glass, made of: ***dig.***[8]
- body, brittle, bones are: ther.[102]
- body, brittle, is: sars.[5] seq-s.[230] ***thuj.***
- body, dashed to pieces, being: calc.[36].
- body, delicate, is: ***thuj.***
- body, disintegrating: ***lach.***[36] lap-mar-c.[194]
- body, head, transparent and speckled brown: bell.
- body, immaterial, is: anh.[119]
- body, jelly, as made out of: ***eupi.***[102]
- body, nose, transparent, is: bell.
- body, skin is very thin: bamb-a.[1184]
- body, thin, body is: lap-c-b.[194] thuj.
- emaciation, of: ***anh.***[144] nat-m.[5] sabad.[5] sulph.
- faces, every ones face in a glass except his own: anac.[85]
- glass, she is made of: eupi.[102] rhus-t.[102] thuj.
- hollow, whole body is: aur. ***kali-c.*** nux-v. pall.
- protection, defense, has no: carc.[227]
- thin, is getting: lap-c-b.[194] sulph.
- transparent, he is: anh.[149] bell.[10] cann-i.
- womb is soft and feeble and would cause abortion: abies-c.[85]

Dreams; abused, being; too weak to defend himself: ambr.[36]
➤ body, emaciated, becoming: kali-n.[36] kreos.[58]

➤ disease, emaciation: kreos.
➤ emaciated, becoming: kali-n.[36] kreos.
➤ houses, walls of glass, with: ozone[227]
Fancies; power, wanting of, decreased: cann-s.[5] sel.[5]
Fear; biting, of, lest teeth would fall out: nit-ac.[172]
✦ joints are weak, that: sep.
Injure; herself, himself, feels could: germ.[222] sep.
Vulnerable, emotionally: am-m.[209] am-s.[209] anac.[187] ars.[187] bamb-a.[1184] calc.[198] calc-f.[214] calc-p.[198] carc.[227] ***caust.***[198] choc.[222] hep.[187] hydrog.[222] hyos.[198] lap-gr-m.[194] mag-p.[209] med.[198] merc.[187] ***nat-c.***[98] nat-m.[187] nat-p.[209] nat-s.[187] nat-sil.[198] ph-ac.[209] puls.[187]

ADAM. Sh, 365 - I am obsessed about the future and what's going to happen to me. A feeling, nothing specific, of vulnerability. 7, 6C, 05:07:00
Sh, 379 - Tearful and vulnerable. A situation I would normally cope with seemed threatening. 8, 6C, 01:20:00
ARS. Ha, 45 - Super-sensitiveness and over-tenderness of mind; dejected, sad and lugubrious (unhappy), she is troubled and solicitous about the merest trifles.
BELL. Al, 90 - It seems to her that her nose is transparent, and a spot on the left side of the head transparent and colored brown.
CHOC. Sh, 19 - I feel very vulnerable in the base of the spine.
Sh, 188 - While walking outside, became anxious in a self-conscious way, anxious and vulnerable as if being watched or observed by something or someone -the attention was on me - anxiety that something would happen. Immediately afterwards I was attacked by four dogs and bitten on the calf. 27, 100C, 01:XX:XX
Sh, 189 - While outside became very weary of cars and people. Felt open and vulnerable. Fear of accidents, cars, or of someone leaping into the road and punching me. This anxiety was worse out of doors. 27, 100C, 01:XX:XX
GERM. Sh, 120 - Easily led of others opinion, and provoked. Sensitive to others attempts at restricting me. Feel like a teenager, but I don't dare to protest. I just feel it inside. 18, 30C, 04:00:00
HALI-L. Sh, 334 - Sad. Can't break from therapist. Don't want to go out because I feel like I would be over exposed. 16, 10C, 10:XX:XX
Sh, 402 - I felt pathetic, defeated and vulnerable. I was reaching on a high shelf for pots for plants. All the pots and soil came tumbling down. Was knocked on the head, on the vertex. Dirt all over me, and I thought, "This is perfect. This is exactly how I feel." I felt like I had to just give up — give up the bravado. I'm exhausted, I'm just going to rest. I just wanted to go into a little ball and lick my wounds. Felt very much like childhood symptoms. I felt very young. 01, 30C, 18:XX:XX
Sh, 512 - Feeling slightly hysterical, on and off through the day, as if disconnected and fragile. Not an overpowering sensation, but distinct. It was a sensation as if some danger was near. 04, 30C, 01:XX:XX
HYDROG. Sh, 150 - Feeling weepy and vulnerable —want someone to "manage" things for me. Feel so fed up of having to do it all myself. 18, 200C, 26:XX:XX
Sh, 155 - In the afternoon (during the full moon) I felt low and depressed, insecure and vulnerable. Could not cope with work load and didn't want to be alone. 12, 6C, 39:XX:XX
Sh, 195 - Apprehensive, panicky, with cold sweat on palms. Feel extremely vulnerable emotionally —like an egg that has just broken. Frightened, anything can happen. 16, 30C, 05:XX:XX
Sh, 242 - Felt vulnerable to criticism —felt people were getting at me. Felt people were not taking notice of poor little me — over-reacting —upset and hurt. 02, 6C, XX:XX:XX
Sh, 253 - I was defensive and angry. I thought my friend didn't understand me. I had to apologise. I felt vulnerable and deeply hurt by her. 16, 30C, 05:XX:XX
Sh, 257 - Feeling suspicious all day. Anxious and conscious of vulnerability. (Asked husband to move out if he was thinking of being unfaithful). 12, 6C, 06:XX:XX
Sh, 276 - Feelings of vulnerability and anxiety about being masculine, both in looks and in behaviourroles. Hope it doesn't get more. To counteract this, I

have been stressing the feminine. I spent lots of money on silk clothing and spent a lot of time making myself up, curling hair, etc. People comment that I look softer, but I feel harder inside. I feel confused about my sexual identity. This is in contrast to my previous proving of the remedy, when people commented that my moustache disappeared and breasts grew. 12, 6C, 30:XX:XX (homosexuality)

Sh, 287 - Feel relaxed, like a jellyfish —no bones in my body. 16, 30C, 00:XX:XX

IRID. Sh, 214 - Very strong protective feeling towards daughters. Hen and chicks image. Feel more tender towards them then usual. It feels like they are on the brink of adolescence and very vulnerable. Very strong protective feeling, not felt their vulnerability since they were born and very little. G42

NEON. Sh, 29 - While drifting in and out of sleep between 6:30 and 7:30 am, I had a fleeting sensation that part of me was parchment-like, i.e., thin, somewhat stiff, somewhat brittle in appearance but actually not brittle. Appearing weak but not weak. 06, 12C, 01:22:XX

SULPH. Al, 2 - Delirium; she destroys her things, throws them away, thinking that she has a superfluity (excess) of everything, wherewith she wastes(thin) to a skeleton.(wealth?)

Al, 11 - She fancies that she is becoming emaciated.(skeletal)

Ha, 35 - He imagines he is getting thin (weak).

THUJ. He, 9 - Sensation as if whole body were thin and delicate, (weak, fragile, frail) and could not resist least attack (illness); as if continuity of body would be dissolved.

He, 10 - Fixed ideas: as if a strange person were at his side; as if soul and body were separated (split) ; that body, particularly limbs, are made of glass (frail) and will readily break (weakness); as if a living animal were in abdomen ;talks about being under the influence of a superior power. (possessed)

FRIEND

Abusive; friends, even to his best: gall-ac.[36]

Ailments from; death, parents or friends, of: ambr.[58] ars.[184] calc.[58] **CAUST.**[30] **IGN.**[122] kali-br.[137] 0nat-m.[184] nit-ac.[54] nux-v.[30] plat.[85] staph.[30]

Ailments from; discords between, relatives, friends: ars.[30] graph.[8] hep.[30] lach.[30] mag-m.[162] merc.[30] ***nat-m.***[162] nit-ac.[30] nux-v.[162] sulph.[30]

Ailments from; friendship, deceived: aur.[8] ign.[30] mag-c.[30] mag-m.[30] nux-v.[30] ph-ac.[30] sil.[30] sulph.[30]

Anger; beating friends: plat.[30]

Anguish; loss of his friend, from: calc.[172] ign.[172] **NIT-AC.**[54]

Anxiety; forsaken her, as if a friend had: ***rhus-t.***[54]

Anxiety; friends at home, about: bar-c. ***phos.*** phys. puls.[172] ***sulph.***

Aversion; friends, to: anac.[60] aur-m.[162] cedr. coloc.[137] ferr. fl-ac.[58] kali-m.[192] ***led.*** pitu-a.[164]

Censorious; dearest friends, with: ars-s-f.[58] aur-s.[58] chin-ar. der.

Censorious; parents, teachers and friends, of: sep.[189]

Company, aversion to; friends, meeting of, whom he imagines he has offended, to: ars.

Company, aversion to; friends, meeting them amel.: alum.[162]

Company, aversion to; friends, of intimate: bell. cham.[54] coloc. ***ferr.*** hep.[85] ***iod. nat-c. sel.***

Company, desire for; friend, of a: lap-gr-m.[194] plb..

Contemptuous; friend, at his: alco.[36]

Death; thoughts of, calls his friends around and takes leave of them: acon.[172]

Delusions; companions are half men, half plants: cann-i.
- companions, companions of his youth, is with the: aether.
- confidence in him, his friends have lost all: aur. hura.
- dead, corpse, absent acquaintance on sofa and has dread, of: ars.
- die, about to, friend was, his beloved: bar-c.[54]
- disgraced, family or his absent friends, he disgraced his: sarr.[36]
- friend, accident, met with a: ars.

- friend, affection of, has lost the: ***aur.*** hura hydrog.[222] hyos.[58]
- friend, fantasy world of imaginary friends, lives in a: calc.[189]
- friend, he had never seen them (after waking): stram.[54]
- friend, offended: ars.
- friend, she is about to lose a: hura.
- friend, surrounded by friends, shaking hands and calling them by name: ***hydr-ac.***[54]
- head, friend's head stick out of a bottle, sees: bell.
- injury, receive, will, friends, from: lach.[58]
- murder, struck friends who came to help him: ***stram.***[54]
- neglected, friends, his: ***aur.***[58]
- pursued, by fiends (Allen, 63): plb.
- pursued, robbing a friend, for: kali-br.[36]
- sick, a beloved friend is, and dying: bar-c.
- strangers, friends appears as: bry. stram.
- surrounded by friends, is: bell. cann-i.

Dreams; acquaintances, distant: choc.[222] fl-ac. plat.[36] plb. sel.

➤ acquaintances, strange things: plat.[1]
➤ companies: canth.[10] phel.[10]
➤ dead, people, of, friends long deceased: arg-n. cedr.[36] coca[36] con.[1] ferr. nat-c.
➤ dead, people, of, friends, talking with deceased: lepi.[36]
➤ death of, acquaintance: nicc.[36]
➤ death, dying, of, bed surrounded by friends, with his: arn.[36]
➤ death, friend, of a: allox.[119] bamb-a.[1184] coff. coff-t.[36] con. cortico.[119] fl-ac. kali-n. lach.[36] nicc.
➤ death, friend, of a, dear, which does not abate his mental exhilaration, looking at all with supernatural indifference: coff-t.[36]
➤ devils, seeing an acquaintance coming and mistaking him for the devil: nicc.[36]
➤ disease, acquaintance, of a: nat-s.[36]
➤ distant, acquaintances, midnight, after: fl-ac.[36]
➤ falling, window, from, friends: choc.[222]
➤ friends: ferr.[58] oci.[36] ozone[227] rumx.[58]
➤ friends, apartment, in wrong: ozone[227]
➤ friends, falling from window: choc.[222]
➤ friends, loses friend in the city, cannot find her: ozone[227]
➤ friends, meeting of: calc-p.[36]
➤ friends, old: ant-c.[1] bamb-a.[1184] ferr. lap-gr-m.[194] ozone[227] rumx.
➤ friends, seeing friends: rumx.[36]
➤ kidnapping, friend is kidnapped by a shepherd dog: ozone[227]
➤ killing, friend, a: allox.[119]
➤ parties, giving surprise to friend: pip-m.[36]
➤ schoolmate, meeting of old: ant-c.[10] ferr.[36]
➤ stab, friend, his: allox.[119]
➤ visits, making visits, friend, to a, who is not at home: ozone[227]
➤ water, walking on, acquaintances: ped.[11]

Embraces; companions, his: agar. ***phos.***[8] plat.

Estranged; forgetful of relatives and friends: lap-c-b.[194] lyss.[54]

Estranged; friends, from: hydrog.[222] nat-c.[58]

Fear; accidents, friends, to: ars.[172]

✦ friend has met with accident, that a: ars. ***caust.***[184]
✦ friends, of: androc.[222] ars.[172] cedr. phos.[172] phys.[172] sulph.[172]
✦ friends, of, female: cedr.[25]
✦ friends, of, meeting: lyc.[172] sep.[85] sil.[172]

Forgetfulness; friends and relatives, of: lyss.[54]

Forsaken; feeling, beloved by his parents, wife, friends, feels of not being: ***ars.***[30] calc.[30] lyc.[30] ***mag-c.***[122] sep.[30] sil.[30] sulph.[30]

Forsaken; feeling, friendless, feels: arg-n.[58] ***lach.***[8] pip-n.[2103]

Indifference; friends, to: ars-i.[58]

Mocking; friends, at his: alco.[36]

Striking; anger, from, friends his: plat.[30] tarent.[58]

Suspiciousness; friends, to: ars-s-f.[58] kali-ar.[58]

Unsympathetic; unscrupulous, friends and family, even towards closest: lap-gr-m.[194]

Violence; friends, to his: kali-ar.[58]

Writing; mean and contemptible things to her friends, all sorts of: ***lac-c.***[54]

ACON. He, 41 - Predicts day of death; bids (offer) her friends good-bye.(farewell)

ADAM. Sh, 150 - Felt separate from friends today, which was unusual. I felt outside them. I was quiet. Definitely unusual. 5, 30C, 00:06:50

ANAC. Al, 8 - Melancholic illusion; he imagines a bier in the side room, upon which either his friend or himself is lying.
Ha, 46 - Melancholy dejection and imagination, as if there was standing in the adjacent room a bier, on which a friend or he himself was lying.

ANDROC. Sh, 58-. Felt more love for her

mother, friends and husband. (7)
Sh, 123 - In the evening he became manic, stalked the streets and visited many friends for a short time only, but could not relax or relate to them. Was pleased when he found his friends were not at home. Spoke nonsense and tried to squeeze a laugh out of anything. (29)
Sh, 126 - Great hostility to those around him, which manifested in brooding and stinging observations and comments directed at his friends. (29)
ARS. Al, 78 - Anxiety and fear; he sees a absent acquaintance (friend) lying dead upon the sofa, and has great dread of him.
Ha, 33 - Anguish and fear; he sees an acquaintance who is not present lie dead on sofa, and is much afraid of him.
He, 48 - Averse to meeting acquaintances, (friends) because he imagines he has formerly offended them, though knows not how.
ATRO. Ha, 17 - Sad and morose, preferring solitude and a dark room to society of friends.
BAR-A. Al, 10 - An evil, fearful suspicion suddenly takes possession of her, as if, for example, a loved friend had been taken suddenly deathly ill.
BAR-C. Ha, 7 - An evil fearful foreboding comes suddenly upon his soul, as if, e.g. a beloved friend might suddenly have fallen fatally ill.
He, 27 - She is suddenly overwhelmed with an evil apprehension; she imagines, for instance, that a beloved friend has suddenly fallen sick and is dying.
CANN-I. Al, 30 - When his friends went out of the room, he thought (delusion) they had left him to his fate (destiny, doom), and wrote "cowards" in his notes.
Al, 41 - Felt as if he was a third person looking at himself and his friend.
Al, 57 - Strange feeling of isolation (solitude) from all around him, with great sense of loneliness (isolation), though surrounded by his friends.
Al, 66 - Illusion that he was a pump-log, through which a stream of hot water was playing, and threatening his friend with a wetting.
CEDR. Al, 5 - Dread of friends.(in females, particularly)
CHLOL. He, 7-...inclined to wander and hide herself, avoiding shrewdly (astute) the vigilance of her friends...
CHOC. Sh, 86 - On seeing a bristly carpet, started laughing excitedly —had a familiar feeling, like meeting a friend. The texture of the carpet was very spiky like a Hedgehog. Told friend that they should come and see it. It's such a wonderful carpet!
Sh, 210 - Felt totally isolated and averse to company. Estranged himself from his family and friends and stopped all communication with them for a long period. Did not reply to letters and left no address. He seemed to hide away and literally disappear. The state of Isolation resulted from feeling that "I didn't exist as a human being". This behaviour was in strong contrast to his normal sociable disposition. 35, 30C, XX:XX:XX:
CROC. Al, 30-...the behavior of relatives and friends excites her to anger,...she is vexed with herself, and her anger becomes greater than ever;..
CUPR. Ha, 5 - A kind of timidity; he felt as if he had to step softly, in order not to hurt himself, nor to disturb his room-mates. (friend) (cautious, prudent, gentle, delicate)
DER. Al, 6 - He is disposed to strike, and inveighs against his dearest friends.
FERR. Al, 764 - Did not sleep well, as sleep was much disturbed by dreams of old friends.
Al, 769 - Rested well, but dreamed a great deal of meeting with old schoolmates, of student life, etc.
Al, 4 - Constant desire for solitude; horror of conversation, noise, visits, and even the society of her cherished friends.
HALI-L. Sh, 56 - Lately thinking over my worth and friendships. Who are my friends and where am I wasting my time. What is my position in society in relationship to career, how friends view me and relationships with men? I find myself going back to having older friends and finding them to be true to me. 08, 30C, 42:XX:XX
Sh, 330 - Bored and superior feeling with an old friend. 16, 10C, 22:XX:XX
HURA. Al, 12 - Flow of sad thoughts; she fancies she is about to lose a dear friend.

IRID. Sh, 36 - Went to a 40th birthday celebration. One very good friend said I didn't seem to be there. They seemed like strangers to me. I was looking at the situation, which needed jollying up, but was unable to do anything about it because I felt distanced from them. It felt strange as if I'd gone out with people I didn't want to be with. H3

KALI-BR. Al, 4 - He imagined that he had been specially singled out (select) for divine vengeance... deploring his sad fate (destiny),...he informed me that he had been accused of robbing a friend, and that the officers were in search of him....

Al, 5 - She had the erroneous idea that she was deserted by all her friends, and as a consequence she passed all her waking moments, which are not many in tears;...delusion that her child was dead, had taken fixed possession of her mind;...she declared that she saw it dead (corpse) before her, and when it was brought to her, she refused to acknowledge that it was hers, or had any resemblance to the one she imagined was dead.

KALI-FCY. Al, 1 - Feeling of sadness and some disposition to tears, caused by an impression that he was soon to die and leave his friends; disposition to take a sad view of the beauties of autumn; the apprehension of approaching sickness and death can be overcome by reason, but soon returns.

LAC-C. Al,N-43 - Intense ugliness (repulsiveness, offensiveness) and hatefulness (odiousness, repellently); writes to her best friends all sorts of mean(vulgar) and contemptible things.

He, 37 - Intense ugliness (repulsiveness, hideousness) and hatefulness (offensiveness); writes to her best friends all sorts of mean and contemptible things. (disdainful)

LAC-D. Al,N-4 - Imagines that all her friends will die and that she must go to a convent. (purification, solitude)

He, 5 - Imagines that all her friends will die and that she must go to a convent. (purification, salvation)

LED. Al, 12 - Discontented all day with his companions, which at last amounts to misanthropy.

LYSS. Al-N, 37 - Inclined to use insulting language, scold his friends, beat and abuse those near him.

MYRIC. Al, 8-...;did not care about anything or for any friends; was perfectly wretched, beyond description.

NAT-C. Al, 1116 - Dream that she saw a corpse, at which she woke in fright, when it seemed as though a dead acquaintance stood before her, which made her scream aloud, afterwards she fell asleep again .

NIT-AC. He, 17 - After continued loss of sleep, long-lasting anxiety, over-exertions of mind and body from nursing the sick, great anguish of mind from loss of his dearest friend.

OP. He, 11 - Thinks he is not in his own house; imagines himself living in a locality three hours distant from his house; detains all passers-by and wishes to take them into his house; ...he does not recognize friends;... (estranged, alien)

OPUN-V. Al, 6 - In the afternoon, fit of petulance, angry at near relatives, swearing mood, not at all pleased, cannot get over the thought of injuries done by friends.

PHOS. He, 31-...; indifference even towards dearest friends;... ; monomania de grandeur et de la richesse;...

PHYS. Al, 3 - Felt great anxiety about friends at home; could not get them out of mind.

PLAT. Ha, 39 - Indifference, cold (reserved), abstracted (separated) in company of friends,..

Ha, 33 - Very cross and irritated at harmless matters and words; so that she at times would have liked to have beaten herself and friends.

PLB. Al, 112 - He is very sad, has no desire to live, and has threatened to destroy himself, and is very fault-finding (severe, critical) with his friends.

Al, 127 - Longing (deprived, wanting) for a distant friend, in the evening...

RAN-B. Al, 3 - Ill humored, and disposed to quarrel and scold the first forenoon; in the evening is desponding, apprehensive, sensitive, discontented; on the second day he again inclines to be provoked by innocent jests of his friends, etc.;...

RHUS-T. Al, 5 - Melancholy, ill-humor, and

anxiety, as if a misfortune (disgrace) would happen, or as if she were alone (solitary), and all about her were dead (lifeless, inert) and still (silent, quiet), or as if she had been forsaken by a near friend; worse in the house, relieved by walking in the open air.

Ha, 953 - Melancholy, sad, and anxious, as if about to hear of a calamity,(misfortune, disaster) or as if she were solitary (lonely, alone) and all around her were dead (lifeless, extinct) and silent (quiet) ; or as if she had bid farewell (separation) to an intimate friend ; worst in the room, diminished by walking in a open air.

RUTA. Al, 8 - Peevish and mistrustful (suspicious) all day; he no longer trusted his best friends, he thought that he was constantly deceived.(deluded)

Ha, 286 - All day long cross and suspicious; he would no longer trust (mistrust) his best friend, and imagined he was always being deceived.

SEP. Al, 33 - Received news of the slight illness of a friend, which caused great mental depression (at another time it would not have made slightest impression); this condition grew on me until I became so nervous that I felt that unless I held on something, I should scream.

He, 38-...everything seems strange (unusual, unfamiliar) to her;...; it seems as if she could not understand (realize) anything and would have to learn anew everything she wished to do;...(lost: knowledge); greatest indifference to everything, the death of a near relative, or some happy occurrence, leaves her equally unaffected; no trace of her former love for friends or even for her child; aversion for social intercourse amounting to contempt;...

SIL. He, 23-...believes she has swallowed pins, and asks those about her whether she has not done so; seeks for hours for lost pins; ...and careful examined her food for fear of pins; very indifferent to friends and former amusements;...

STRAM. Ha, 562 - His surroundings appear to him quite strange; (unfamiliar) although in the first minutes he knows that he is surrounded by his friends, he forgets this in the second minute, and imagines he is quite alone (solitary, deserted) in a desert (wildness), and is afraid (fearful) ; figures of beasts suddenly spring out of the ground at his side, so that he moves to the other side, where, however, other similar figures pursue him, and he runs forward.

Ha, 503 - After waking all objects seem to him new (strange, unusual) even his friends as though he had never in his life seen them before.

UPA. Al, 4 - Melancholic; has to force the tears back; cold towards his friends, repelling everyone.

FRIENDLESS

Delusions; confidence in him, his friends have lost all: aur. hura.

- friend, affection of, has lost the: ***aur.*** hura hydrog.[222] hyos.[58]
- friend, she is about to lose a: hura.

Despair; others and oneself: ***arg-n.***[54] aur.[54]

Despair; others, about: ***aur.***

Forsaken; feeling, friendless, feels: arg-n.[58] ***lach.***[8] pip-n.[2103]

Helplessness, feeling of: aether[36] anac.[1] ant-t.[36] arg-n.[162] ars.[1] bamb-a.[1184] ***calad.***[122] cand-a.[239] ***gels.***[8] germ.[222] hecla.[234] hell. hydrog.[222] jasm.[36] kali-br. lith-c.[25] **LYC.**[122] ozone[227] petr. phos. puls.[189] rhus-t.[137] stram. tax.

Weeping; goes off alone and weeps as if she had no friends: bar-c.

ALUM. Al, 6 - Depressed and friendless; he wishes only to be left alone, in the forenoon.

ARS. Al, 51 - He despairs and weeps and imagines no one can help him, that he must die;...(unprotected)

GERM. Sh, 150 - I only want to cry. Don't know what to do. Feel terrible and lonely. Cannot describe how I feel. Want attention, but don't dare to ask for it. Soon there is no more energy left. 18, 30C, 182:XX:XX

HALI-L. Sh, 417 - Frustrated and depressed. Feeling lonely, friendless and unaccomplished. 18, 30C, 15:XX:XX

Sh, 625 - I find that I don't have a real friend. I have acquaintances, but not a friend. That has been bothering me. A new realization. The friends I have cultivated are caught up in their own lives, and they don't have time for me. This is different—now I have time to think about it. I'm seeing for myself. At times I'm extremely lonely. I like my own place but sometimes it's nice to have a friend. 18, 30C, 17:XX:XX

LACH. He, 39 - Weak and unhappy, particularly in morning, when she feels, on awaking, friendless and forsaken; ...(deserted) has had domestic troubles. 0 Melancholia

LIL-T. Al, 16 - Worse on going to bed; can't go to sleep; wild (tumultuous, uncontrollable) feeling in the head as though I should go crazy (insane) and no one would take care of me (forsaken, helpless); thoughts of suicide; how much opium would put me to sleep forever, and who would find my body, and who would care; ... (friendless, abandoned, deserted)

FRIENDLY

Abrupt; affectionate, yet: aur-m.[162] lyc.[30] nux-v.[30] **PULS.**[30]
Affability: apis[36] hypoth.[149]
Affability; enemy, to an: alco.[36]
Affection; children craving for: carc.[207]
Affection; responds to, returns: phos.[155]
Affectionate: acon. alum.[30] anac. ant-c. ***ars.***[10] bar-c.[30] bor. bry.[30] calc-p.[146] carb-an. carb-v. carc.[146] caust.[30] choc.[222] coff. ***croc.*** graph.[30] hura hydr.[36] ***ign.*** lach.[30] lyc.[30] murx.[102] ***nat-m.*** nit-ac.[30] ***nux-v.***[122] op.[36] ox-ac. par. ph-ac.[30] ***phos.***[122] plat. ***puls.*** seneg. sil.[122] staph.[30] stram.[36] thea.[36] verat.
Affectionate; children kiss and caress: ***puls.***[54]
Affectionate; love for everyone about him, during and after fainting: hura[60]
Affectionate; returns affection: ***phos.***[122]
Anger; alternating with, kindness: cench.[122]
Caressed; propensity for being: cann-i.[36] carc.[140] germ.[222] lap-mar-c.[194] puls.[102] ***sac-alb.***[210]
Carried; desires to be, caressed and: acon.[122] kreos.[5] puls.[5]
Communicative, expansive: acon.[30] alum.[30] bar-c.[30] choc.[222] germ.[222] hydrc.[36] ***lach.***[5] lap-c-b.[194] lap-mar-c.[194]
Company; desire for: acon.[30] act-sp. aeth. all-s. androc.[222] ant-t. ***apis*** **ARG-N. ARS.** ars-h.[54] asaf. aur-m. bell. **BISM.** bov. brom. bry. bufo cadm-s. ***calc.*** calc-ar.[58] calc-p. ***camph.*** cann-s.[5] carb-v. carc.[193] caust. cench. choc.[222] ***clem.*** coca[25] coloc. ***con.*** cot.[36] crot-c.[5] crot-h. cyna.[149] der. dros. dys-co.[136] ***elaps*** fl-ac.[102] foll.[1201] gaert.[136] ***gels.*** hep. hydrog.[222] **HYOS.** ***ign. kali-ar.*** kali-br. **KALI-C.** ***kali-p.*** **LAC-C.** lac-h.[229] lach.[5] lap-c-b.[194] lap-gr-m.[194] ***lil-t.*** lith-c.[25] **LYC.** manc. merc. ***mez.*** mut.[136] naja[98] **NAT-C.**[5] nit-ac.[116] ***nux-v. pall.*** ph-ac.[102] **PHOS.**[122] plb. ***puls.*** rad-br.[102] ran-b. rat. sac-alb.[210] ***sep.*** sil.[102] skat.[102] ***stram. stry.*** sulph.[30] syph.[54] tab. tarent. thymol.[102] verat. verb. zinc. zinc-p.[58]
Consolation; agg. friendly advice: calc.[5] calc-p.[5] hell.[5] kali-c.[5] merc.[5]
Delusions; delightful, she is, or wants to be: stram.[122]
- friend, surrounded by friends, shaking hands and calling them by name: ***hydr-ac.***[54]
- smooth, being: alum.[137]

Desires; cheerful, to be: chin.[36]
Dreams; conciliation: bamb-a.[1184]
- dead, bodies, embracing: elaps[36]
- embrace: cand-a.[239]
- friendly, being: ped.[36]
- parties, giving surprise to friend: pip-m.[36]
- quarrels, changing suddenly to happy conversation with another person: ferr-p.[85]
- reconciliation: mang.[1]
- visits, making visits: mag-s.[10]

Embraces anything, in morning, agg. in open air: plat.[36]
Embraces; companions, his: agar. ***phos.***[8] plat.
Embraces; inanimate objects, even: ***verat.***[54]
Embraces; trees, wants to embrace: ozone[227]
Fraternized with the whole world: aloe.[36]
Harshness; affectionate, yet: lyc.[30] nux-v.[30] **PULS.**[30]
Kissed, wants to be: ***stram.***[54]
Kisses; caress children, kiss and: ***puls.***[54]
Kisses; everyone: caps. ***croc.*** hyos.[5] kres.[144] mand.[144] phos. plat.[54] stram. ***verat.***
Kisses; hands, his companions: agar. anac.
Love; everybody around him, for, during and after fainting: hura[36]
Morose; alternating with, tenderness: plat.[10]
Political: choc.[222] sulph.[5]
Rage; alternating with, affectionate disposition: croc.
Rage; alternating with, tenderness: croc.[10]
Sadness; alternating with, tenderness: plat.[10]
Sociability: agar.[5] alco.[36] carc.[214] lach.[5] nat-c.[5] nat-p.[162] stann.[5]

Social; inhibition, lack of: choc.[222] germ.[222] med.[162] merc.[162] staph.[162]

ADAM. Sh, 307 - Still an enormous desire to nurture and feed people. In the last month I have fed sixty people weekly during a political campaign. Made many friends. 2, 12C, 57:XX:XX

ANDROC. Sh, 58-. Felt more love for her mother, friends and husband. (7)

Sh, 65 - Desired comfort and sympathy. (29)

CHOC. Sh, 150 - People keep stopping me and saying they don't recognise me. I still have a silly grin on my face. Laugh more —so much joy inside and a sense of freedom very different to before the proving. Dogs seem to like me more and babies seem to like me more, and this was noticed by others too.

Sh, 218 - Had a deep conversation with a friend and felt more mature, as if being detached, is helping me to understand her more.[35], 30C, 04:XX:XX

Sh, 418 - Feel affectionate and quiet in evening, less restless than usual.[11], 6C, 00:XX:XX

GERM. Sh, 154 - When outside and looking at people thought to myself I know them. People were friendlier to me. Thought I could start a conversation with strangers . 07, 30C, 00.06.00.

Sh, 135 - I see a stranger who looks so familiar . 08, 12C, 11:04:20

Sh, 159 - People seem friendlier in the streets in London. Felt like I'd made some sort of contact -people smile at me and were chatty. 13, 30C, 02:XX:XX

Sh, 148 - The last days I have had moments when I have felt I have been united to the world and people -to humanity. Have felt more love and reconciliation towards myself and other people. Started to be more conscious about the environment and what I can do to our mutual benefit. Something is happening within me. I wish to get more contact with my feelings. 18, 30C, 64:XX:XX

Sh, 163 - Felt lack of romance in my life. Desired romantic love, to be loved. 05, 6C, 41:XX:XX

HYDROG. Sh, 283 - I feel more in touch with people, more sympathetic to the rest of the world. Feel more understanding. 08, 30C, 14:XX:XX

Sh, 286 - Generous in my feelings towards my husband. 02, 6C, 04:XX:XX

FUNERAL

Dancing; desire for, night, in churchyard: cic.[36] stram.[36]

Death; presentiment of, rejoices and gives directions about funeral: stram.[54]

Delusions; alone, graveyard, she is: lepi sep.
- bells, hears ringing of, his funeral: aether.
- bier, is lying on a: anac. cann-i.
- churchyard, dancing in, he is: cic.[36] stram.
- churchyard, visits a: anac. arn. ***bell.*** stram.
- funeral, preparations are made for: ***lach.***[54]
- grave, at a: gels.[8]
- grave, in his: anac.[149] lepi. stram.
- person, coat, shroud, with: psil.[164]
- pursued, phantom in a churchyard, by: lepi.[85]
- talking, sister, with his dead, churchyard, in: bell.[10]

Dreams; armies, rising from their graves: ptel.[36]
- ➤ buried alive, being: ***arn.*** chel. ign. pariet.[72]
- ➤ churchyard: crot-h.[58] hura[36]
- ➤ coffin, eating moldy sausage, after: form.[36]
- ➤ coffins: brom. form.[36] lipp.[36] merc-i-f.
- ➤ dead, bodies, coming alive after a funeral: allox.[119]
- ➤ dead, bodies, finding a dead child in a churchyard: mag-s.[36]
- ➤ dead, bodies, putting deceased body in shroud: elaps[36]
- ➤ funeral, corpse coming alive after a funeral: allox.[119]
- ➤ funeral, funeral knell, his own: aether[36]
- ➤ funeral, people who had died of scarlatina, in trying to avoid wind blowing from procession toward him he awoke: form.[102]
- ➤ funeral, procession, after eating moldy sausage: form.[102]
- ➤ funerals: allox.[119] alum. ange-s.[149] bart. brom. ***chel.*** form. hura mag-c. nat-c.[1] nicc. rat.
- ➤ grave, armies rising from their graves: ptel.[36]
- ➤ graves: anac. ***arn.*** guare.[54] hura iris mag-c. ptel.
- ➤ graves, falling into a grave, waking her: iris.

➤ graves, living in tombs: nicc.
➤ graves, putting tapers on tombs: hura.
➤ graves, thrown into a grave, being: mag-c.[36]
➤ thrown from carriage, being, grave, into a: mag-c.[36]
Fear; buried, alive: atro.[38] tub.[56] ***zinc.***[54]
✦ cemeteries, of: stram.[187]
Insanity; graveyards, visits: bell.[10] stram.[10]

ANAC. Al, 8 - Melancholic illusion; he imagines a bier in the side room, upon which either his friend or himself is lying.
Ha, 46 - Melancholy dejection and imagination, as if there was standing in the adjacent room a bier, on which a friend or he himself was lying.
CANN-I. Al, 25 - He became possessed with the idea that he was about to die, from which he cried out, "I am dying; I shall be carried to my death-chamber."
GELS. He, 6 - After losing son, inclined to brood over her loss; at times becomes unconscious, or, rather, "rapt"; in imagination thinks herself at the grave; smothered pressure on chest after the spell.
LACH. He, 8 - Thinks: she is somebody else in the hands (seized) of a stronger power; (supremacy, superiority).or that she is dead, and preparations are made for funeral (cortege) or that she is nearly dead and wishes some one would help her off; herself pursued by enemies, or fears medicine is poison; there are robbers in house and wants to jump out the window; herself under super-human control; visions real, he will die. (helplessness, desire; aid, comfort, salvation)
LEPI. Al, 1 - She fancies herself alone in a graveyard, pursued by a ghost, and screams so that her voice is lost next day; yet nobody hears her. (helpless)
MAG-C. Al, 964 - Dream of funeral; she was obliged to dress the hair of the company; also of balls and marriages.
Al, 965 - Dream of a grave in a cemetery, into which, after voluntary preparation, she was to be thrown.
STRAM. Ha, 549 - He thinks he is dying, and that he will not live over the evening, he rejoices that he is dying, and gives directions about his funeral, otherwise he is rational and does not feel particularly ill.
Ha, 524 - He dances at night in the churchyard.
He, 56 - Believes to be in his grave; shrives,(confess) prays, asks to be killed (justified); accuses his wife of infidelity; scolds (cursing), strikes at everybody who wishes to restrain him; thinks they are dogs and barks at them to make himself understood.
He, 93 - Mania; thinks he is lying on his sepulchre (tomb); confessing, praying, wants to be killed (redemption, salvation, regeneration); laughs as if tickled (excited); wants to be kissed; accuses his wife of being faithless (betrayed); scolding (censure) beating in a rage, will not be taken hold of by attendants (suspicious?) ; takes them for dogs (contemptuous), and barks at them; talking in Jewish jargon; (rank?, stranger?) supposes his house to be surrounded by carts (vehicle), Jews (Judaism) and geese, offending him, ... -(strange, foreign, alien)
He, 55 - He thinks that he is dying and that he will not live over night, rejoices (celebrate) and gives directions about his funeral.
ZINC. He, 43 - Great fear, as if persecuted by men or the devil, on account of crimes he has never done (injustice); is afraid of becoming imprisoned, or poisoned, or shot, or buried (inter) alive...[0] Delirium tremens.

FUTURE

Absorbed; become of him, as to what would: nat-m.
Absorbed; future, about: spig.[1]
Anxiety; future, about: acon. aeth.[10] agar. allox.[119] alum. alum-p.[58] aml-n.[25] ***anac.*** anan.[36] ant-c. ant-t. arg-n.[58] arist-cl.[149] arn. ***ars.***[54] aster.[137] aur.[10] bamb-a.[1184] ***bar-c.*** ***bar-m.*** bar-s.[58] **BRY.** bufo[58] buth-aust.[119] calad. **CALC.** calc-acet.[36] ***calc-ar.*** calc-f.[149] calc-s. carb-an.[10] carb-v.[10] carbn-s. ***caust.*** cham. chel. ***chin.*** **CHIN-S.** choc.[222] **CIC.** cimic.[137] clem.[172] cocc. coff.[10] ***con.***[122] cupr.[5] cycl. ***dig.*** dirc. ***dros.*** ***dulc.*** euph. euphr.[5] ferr. ferr-acet. ferr-c. ***ferr-p.*** fl-ac. ***gels.*** gins. ***graph.*** grat. hep.[30] hipp. hura[36] ***iod.*** kali-br.[25] kali-c. kali-m.[192] kali-p. kalm. ***lach.*** laur.[137] lil-t. lyc.[172] m-arct.[10] mag-c.[10] mang. meny.[10] merc.[10] ***mur-ac.*** nat-acet.[36]

nat-ar. ***nat-c.*** ***nat-m.*** nat-p. nat-s.[58] ***nit-ac.***[10] ***nux-v.*** ***op.***[10] ozone[227] petr. ***ph-ac.*** **PHOS.** plat.[137] psor. ***puls.*** ran-b. ***rhus-t.*** ***sabin.*** scroph-n.[36] ***sep.***[10] ***sil.***[30] sol-t-ae.[36] ***spig.***[122] **SPONG.**[122] ***stann.***[122] ***staph.*** stram. sul-ac.[10] ***sulph.***[122] tab.[10] tarent. thuj. tub.[5] verat. vichy-h.[36] viol-t.[36] wies.[36] xan. viol-t.[36] wies.[36] xan.

Anxiety; future, disease, and of her: kali-c.[54]

Anxiety; future, disgust of life, with: ***lach.***[54]

Anxiety; future, sadness, with: ***sulph.***[54]

Anxiety; health, future, in regard to the: ***sep.***[54]

Avarice; anxiety about future, from: ***nux-v.***[30] ***ph-ac.***[30] stann.[30]

Day-dreaming; poetical, about the future: olnd.[60]

Despair; future, about: carb-v.[30] ***nat-m.***[54] sumb.[36]

Discouraged; future about: ***dros.***[54] merc.[10]

Dream, as if in a; future, poetical: olnd.

Dreams; as if in a; future, about the: ***staph.***[54]

➤ future events, prophetic: **ACON.**[122] asaf. bov. ***camph.***[54] ***cann-i.*** cortico.[119] m-arct.[10] mang. ph-ac. phos. rad-br.[111] ***sulph.***

Far away; as if, with apathy and indifference to the future: med.[137] syph.[54]

Grief; future, for the: mang.[1] nat-c. ***nat-m.*** stann.[1]

Howling; future trouble, about: lyc.[36]

Indifference; future, to, far away feeling: syph.[54]

Lamenting; future, about: lyc.

Plans; future, for the: ***coff.***[54]

Talk; future, about: hyos.

Thoughts; future, of the: chin-b.[54] cycl. iod. senec. sep. spig.

Thoughts; himself, become of him, what would: nat-m.[137]

Thoughts; profound, future, about his: cycl. spig.

Weary of life; future, from solicitude about: ***lach.***[54]

Weeping; future, about the: lyc.

ACON. He, 35 - Sadness with solicitude; concerned about future; about her recovery or fears loss of reason. (insanity)

ADAM. Sh, 365 - I am obsessed about the future and what's going to happen to me. A feeling, nothing specific, of vulnerability. 7, 6C, 05:07:00

AGAR. Al, 46 - His mind is uneasy and anxious; he was constantly concerned only about himself, his present and future condition.

Ha, 5 - The mind is restless and troubled; he was always solely occupied with his present and his future condition.

AIL. Al, 4 - Recklessness (careless) in regard (respect) to present and future.

ANAC. Al, 15 - The future appears dangerous to him, as if nothing but misfortune and danger were reserved for him; want of confidence in his strength (vigor, force) and despondency.

Ha, 4 - Internal anguish, which did not allow him to rest, he troubled himself about every trifle, as if it would cause great injure, with solicitude about the future.

Ha, 7 - Anxious apprehension and deep thoughts, on meditating over his present and his future fate. (destiny)

Ha, 8 - The future seems to him very dangerous, as if nothing were imminent but misfortune and danger; distrust in his own power, and despondency.

Ha, 47 - He mixes up the present with the future.

He, 46 - Estrangement (separation) from individuals and society, with fear of future.

He, 62 - Internal anxiety, which did not leave him any peace; he felt solicitous (careful) on account of every trifle, as if it would lead to some great trouble (misfortune); with apprehension (fear) of future.

ANAN. Al, 2 - Sadness and restlessness, with fear of death and of the future.

ANT-C. Ha, 7 - Anxious meditation, during the day, about himself, his present and future fate. (doom, destine).

Ha, 23 - Ecstasy and exalted love, with great anxiety about his fate (destiny, doom), and inclination to shoot himself;...

He, 18 - Anxiety in relation to his present and future condition.

ANT-T. Al, 19-...anxious thoughts about the future; she thinks she will remain in her present condition.

He, 32 - Great concern (care) about future with beating in stomach.

He, 41 - Gaiety, wild mirthfulness, with subsequent ill humor and anxiety for future.

ARN. Al, 16 - Apprehension of future evils.
Al, 13 - Anxiety about the present and the future.
Ha, 609 - Anxious concern (care) about the present and the future.
BAR-C. Al, 5 - Sad and fearful; he has all kinds of sad thoughts about his future state, and thinks that he is lost entirely; in the evening.
Ha, 6 - Sad and anxious; all manner of gloomy (sad) ideas as to his future fate (destiny) rise in his mind, and believes himself totally forsaken (deserted); in the evening.
He, 28 - Solicitude, about his future; about domestic affairs.
BOR. Al, 18-..contented with himself and the world, and looking cheerfully into the future.
BRY. Al, 39 - Imagination very sluggish (slow); it is impossible to make any plan for the future, even for the next day; the judgment (discernment), however, is unimpaired .
Ha, 770 - Anxiety; he is apprehensive about the future.
He, 26 - Anxiety about future, particularly in childbed (puerperal) or after.
He, 46 - Restlessness: wants change; with fear of future; fear of death, which he thinks is near; with nocturnal heat.
He, 22 - Apprehensive, uneasiness and dread of future.
CALC-A. Al, 3 - Sadness, almost to weeping, with solicitous cares for the present and future.
Ha, 261 - Not without inclination to work, but indifferent to all external things; sunk in thought about the present and future.
Ha, 262 - Very grave (serious) and full of care (worry); busied with the present and the future; he becomes sad almost to tears.
CALC. Al, 30 - Dread and anxiety of the future, with fear of consumption.
Ha, 3 - Mournful (grief), almost to tears, with solicitous occupation with the present and the future.
Ha, 12 - Anxious about the present and the future, with deep reflection, at the same time indifferent to things outside...
Ha, 25 - His heart is agitated with fear and anxiety for the future, with fear of consumption.(tuberculosis, ruin)
He, 5 - Buried in deep thought; anxiety about present and future.(destine)
CAUST. He, 24 - Chilly, with sad mood and apprehension of the future < in evening.
He, 25 - Sorrowful thoughts during night, during day weeping, anxiety and misgiving (doubt) about the future.
CHEL. Al, 25 - Sadness, even to weeping, and despondency (desperation) about the present and future.
Al, 27 - Extremely depressed; full of sad thoughts about the present and future, even to weeping; he had no rest of any kind.
Ha, 154 - Extraordinarily depressed, full of gloomy (dark) thoughts about the present and future, causing him to weep;...
Ha, 155 - Sad to weeping and depressed about the present and future.
CHIN. Ha, 1135 - He makes a number of grand (great) plans for the future.
CIC. Ha, 228 - He thought with anxiety of the future and was always sad.
Ha, 231 - Excitement, with concern for the future, he represented to himself as dangerous everything that would happen to him.
He, 35 - Excited, with apprehension concerning the future; everything that could befall him seemed to be dangerous.
He, 16 - Thinks of the future with anxiety, and is constantly sad.
COFF. He, 5 - Lively fancies; full of plans for the future.
CON. Al, 38 - Sunk in deep thought; he apprehensively considered the present and the future, and sought (wanted) to be alone.
Ha, 365 - Sunk in deep thought, he cogitated timorously about the present and the future and sought (wants) solitude.
Ha, 8 - Lost in deep meditation, he anxiously thought over the present and the future, and sought solitude.
He, 10 - Buried in thought; apprehensive (anxiety) respecting the present or future.
He, 28 - Solicitude (anxiety) concerning the future; great concern (cares) about any little thing that may happen.
CYCL. Ha, 194 - Sunk in deep thought (meditation), he sought (desire) solitude and thought about his future fate (destine, doom).

Ha, 195 - Deep thought about the present and future, so that he almost wept.
He, 4 - Absorbed in deep thought, seeks solitude, thinks about his future.
DIG. Al, 22 - Anxiety with great dread of the future, worse about 6 p.m. with sadness and weeping, which bring relief.
Ha, 7 - Anxiousness, with great apprehension of the future...
He, 10 - Profound melancholy,...great fear of future; insane obstinacy and disobedience, with desire to escape.
DROS. Al, 4 - He is depressed by the persecutions of others on all sides, and also discouraged and solicitous about the future.
Ha, 276 - He is dejected (unhappy) about the malice (rancor, hostility) of others on all hands, and at the same time disheartened (discouraged) and concerned about the future.(disgusted, revolted)
He, 2 - Depressed by persecutions of others on all sides, and also discouraged and solicitous about future.
DULC. Al, 8 - Anxiety and fear of the future after midnight.
GELS. He, 22 - Solicitude (anxiety) about the present and the future.
GINS. Al, 3 - Mind generally calm; still there are impatient impulses and fear of accidents, with, at times, disposition to weep, or to be anxious about the future.
GRAT. He, 6 - Ill humor, tired (weary) of life, apprehensive of the future.
HIPP. Al, 3 - Apprehensiveness, anxiety about the future, in the evening.
HURA. Al, 10 - Sadness, melancholy; she thinks despondingly of the future.
HYOS. Al, 53 - They laughed aloud because all persons seemed ridiculous;...the old woman talked of future,...
IOD. Al, 16 - Anxiety and prostration; the patients busy themselves for the most part about the future.
KALI-BR. Al, 11-...gloomy ideas relative to his present and future condition, if an opinion could be formed from the signs of distress, such as weeping, moaning, and wringing his hands,...
KALI-C. Al, 14 - Sad presentiments of the future.
Ha, 17 - Troubled ideas about the future.
He, 10 - Timid and apprehensive of future and about her disease.
LACH. He, 34-...repugnance to society and dislike to talk; solicitude about future, whith disgust of life; inclination to doubt everything; mistrusts (suspicious) and misconstrues (misjudge) ...0 Melancholia.
LYC. Al, 10 - He cries and howls, at first about past and then about future troubles.
MANG. Ha, 325 - Cross and discontented with himself, and concerned about future..., considers himself very weak (stupid) in mind, and makes mistakes whenever he speaks.
MUR-AC. Ha, 266 - Silent reserve, with anxious concern about the present and future.
He, 2 - Taciturn, introverted and quiet; anxious care about future.
NAT-C. Al, 22 - His fancy is mostly busy with apprehensions of the future; he often makes plans for half an hour at a time as if it would go wrong with him, wherewith he seeks to be alone for several days together.
Al, 42 - Very fretful and discontented with whole world; he constantly felt as though he could beat (punish ?) himself, his whole life angered him, and he preferred to have no existence at all; he was solicitous about the future, and inclined to despair, all day.
Ha, 10 - His fancy is mostly anxiously occupied with the future; he paints to himself what misfortunes might happen to him; and he seeks solitude for several days.
Ha, 48 - Peevish and cross, dissatisfied whith all the world; he could have kicked (self sensure) himself; he would rather not live at all ; at the same time solicitous about the future, so that he is ready to despair.
NAT-M. Al, 65 - Extremely solicitous about the future.
Al, 66 - Lost for hours in thought as to what would become of him.
Ha, 9 - For hours, immersed in thoughts, as to what would become of him.
Ha, 23 - Anxiously solicitous about the future.
He, 36 - Despairing, hopeless feeling about the future.
NAT-P. Al, 8 - Worries (cares) about the health, about the future.
OLND. Al, 15 - While studying he had

constantly other thoughts; he found himself dreaming of the future, and busying himself with beautiful images concerning it.

PH-AC. Al, 9 - Sad and solicitous concerning the future.

Ha, 670 - Sad humor, on account of concern for the future.

Ha, 6 - Sad and solicitous about the future.

He, 18 - Dread (fear) of the future; brooding over one's condition.

PHOS. He, 7 - Anxious: filled with gloomy (dark) forebodings; as if about to die; about termination (conclude) of her illness (disease); and restless ; at twilight; when alone; about future; during a thunderstorm; ..

PLAT. He, 10 - Cold, haughty, too well satisfied with one's self, and not at all anxious about the future. (presumptuous, egotistic, inexpugnable, safe)

PSOR. Al, 5 - He pictures the future in the brightest colors.

PULS. Ha, 1113 - Anxiety, thinks he will be ruined.(decay, perdition)

SCROPH-N. Al, 1 - Desponding (sad), much troubled (worried) about the past, and very apprehensive of the future, which passed off after a few days, and left the intellect clear.

SEP. Al, 29 - Dark forebodings about his disease in regard to the future.

Al, 94 - Inclination of the mind to wonder over future events.

Al, 101 - Dullness of comprehension; inability to collect or express his thoughts; constantly building air-castles or running on future events.

Ha, 6 - Troubled (worries) thoughts about his disease and about the future.(destine)

He, 13 - Dark forebodings about his disease in regard to the future.

SOL-T-AE. Al, 5 - She is much concerned (care, anxiety) about her future, destiny, which she fancies will be wretched.(miserable)

SPIG. Al, 9 - Anxiety and apprehensive solicitude for the future.

Al, 10 - Deep thought about his future.

Ha, 657 - Anxiety and anxious concern about the future.

Ha, 658 - Profound reflection about his future fate. (destiny)

Ha, 659 - Anxious forebodings (premonition) about the future,...

He, 3 - Restless and anxious; solicitude about the future.

SPONG. He, 6 - Fear of future, tired of life.(ennui)

STANN. Al, 7 - Quite absorbed in himself, solicitous for the future.

Ha, 648 - Silent reserved disposition; he thought about the present and the future and was much concerned (care) about the latter.

Ha, 16 - The mind is quiet, introverted, solicitous (anxiety) about the future.

STAPH. Ha, 706 - Great anxiety; he dreads the future.

He, 13 - Continual concern about the future.

SULPH. Al, 58 - The condition seems very distressing, and she is apprehensive of the future.

Ha, 11 - She finds her state very agonizing and she is apprehensive about the future.

He, 33 - Sleepless, disgusted with life, fears the future, where she sees nothing but misery (wretchedness, poverty) and suffering (misfortune). 0 Melancholia.

SUMB. Al, 8-...fond (love) of the society of women; ...sympathy with suffering seems robbed of its pain...nervous excitement and heat, especially in head from listening (hearing) to a disputation, ...humor depressed with despair of future...melancholy despondency, as if ill-treated by everyone purposely... mildness, amiability

SYPH. He, 11 - A far-away feeling, with apathy and indifference to future.

THUJ. Al, 62 - Averse to everything; anxious and solicitous about the future.

Ha, 629 - Everything is distasteful (unpleasant) to him; he is anxious and concerned about the future.

TUB. Al,N-16 - Great anxiety for future, otherwise marked indifference.

GHOSTS

Anxiety; apparition, from horrible, while awake: ***camph.***[54] zinc.

Delusions; dead, persons, morning on waking, frightened by images of: hep.

- dead, persons, sees: agar. alum. am-c. ***anac.*** arg-n. arn. ***ars.*** ars-i. bar-c. bar-i.[58]

bell. brom. bry. calc. calc-ar.[58] calc-i.[58] calc-sil.[58] canth. caust. cocc. con. fl-ac. graph. ***hep.*** hura ***hyos.*** iod. kali-ar. ***kali-br. kali-c.*** kali-p. kali-sil.[58] ***lach.*** laur. ***mag-c.*** mag-m. nat-c. nat-m. nat-p. nit-ac. nux-v. op. paull-p.[36] ***ph-ac. phos. plat.*** plb. ran-s. sars. sil. stram.[5] stry. sul-ac. sul-i.[58] sulph. thuj. verb. zinc. zinc-p.[58]
- head, deceased acquaintances without bodies, h. of (at night): nux-v.
- images, phantoms, sees: acon. alum.[10] ***ambr. apis arg-n. ars.*** bar-c. **BELL.** berb. brom. calc. calc-ar.[58] calc-s. calc-sil.[58] camph. ***cann-s.***[5] canth. carb-an. ***carb-v.*** caust. cham. chin. chin-ar. cic. cimic.[5] coca ***crot-h.*** cupr. dros. dulc. graph. hell. ***hep. hyos.*** ign. kali-ar. kali-br. kali-c. kali-p. kali-sil.[58] lac-c.[58] **LACH.** lachn.[54] led. ***lyc.*** mag-m.[5] ***merc.*** nat-c. ***nat-m.*** nat-p. nit-ac. nux-m.[10] nux-v. ***op.*** ph-ac. ***phos.*** plat. puls. pyrog.[137] rhod.[10] rhus-t. ruta[5] ***samb.*** sep. sil. spong. ***stram.*** sulph. tab. ***tarent. thuj.*** valer.[58] verat. ***zinc.***
- people, talks with, dead: bell. **CALC-SIL.** canth. chol.[54] hell. ***hyos.*** nat-m. stram.
- pursued, ghosts, by: lepi plat. stram.
- pursued, phantom in a churchyard, by: lepi.[85]
- skeletons, sees: crot-c. op.
- spectres, ghosts, spirits, sees: acon.[102] agar. alum. am-c. ambr. ant-t. ***ars.***[58] ars-met.[54] ***atro.***[54] aur. **BELL.** bov. brom.[102] calc.[162] ***camph.*** cann-i.[25] **CANN-S.**[5] carb-an.[5] carb-v. caust.[5] cimic.[5] coca[25] cocc. crot-c.[103] ***cupr. cupr-acet.***[54] dig.[85] dros.[5] dulc. hell. hep. hura ***hyos.*** hyper. ign. ***kali-br.***[5] kali-c. kali-i.[5] kali-sil.[58] lach. lepi. lyc. mag-m.[5] merc. ***nat-c. nat-m.*** nit-ac. **NUX-V.**[5] ***op.***[122] orig.[25] ph-ac.[5] phos.[5] phys. plat. psor.[54] puls. ran-b.[5] rhus-t.[5] ruta[5] sars. sep. sil. spig. ***stram. sulph.*** tarent. thuj. verat.[5] verb.[54] visc.[36] zinc.
- spectres, sees, behind him: lach.[85]
- spectres, sees, bright daylight, in: ars.[54]
- spectres, sees, closing eyes, on: apis arg-n. bell. ***bry. calc.*** chin. ign. ***lach.*** led. nat-m. samb. sep. spong. stram. ***sulph. thuj.***
- spectres, sees, clutches at: hyos.
- spectres, sees, death appears as a gigantic black skeleton: crot-c.
- spectres, sees, fire, in: bell.
- spectres, sees, hovering in the air: aur. lach.[58]
- spectres, sees, morning on waking, a spectre continues to enlarge until it disappears: dulc.
- spectres, sees, night, evil ones: ***hell.***[54]
- spectres, sees, poltergeist: anh.[119]
- spectres, sees, talking with, he is: nat-m.[30] nit-ac.[137] plat.[30]
- spectres, sees, throng upon him: ***psor.***[54] verb.[54]
- spectres, sees, twilight, in: berb. phos.[172]
- spectres, sees, waking, on: dulc. zinc.
- talking, dead people, with: bell. **CALC-SIL.** canth. hell. ***hyos.*** med.[58] nat-m. stram.
- talking, sister, with his dead: bell.[54] ***hyos.***[54]
- talking, sister, with his dead, churchyard, in: bell.[10]
- talking, spirits, with: bell.[10] **NAT-M.**[122] nit-ac.[137] ***plat.***[122] stram.
- voices, hears, dead people, of: anac.[102] ***bell.*** calc-sil.[58] hyper.[122] nat-m. stram.

Dreams; dead, people, of: alum.[5] am-c.[54] ***anac.*** ange-s.[149] ant-c.[5] ***arg-n. arn.*** **ARS.** ars-i. ars-s-f.[58] aur. aur-ar.[58] aur-s.[58] bar-c. bry. calad. ***calc.*** calc-ar. calc-f. calc-i.[58] ***calc-sil.*** cann-i. cann-s.[5] carbn-s. caust. cench. ***chel.*** chin-s. coca[36] cocc.[5] cod.[36] con. convo-d.[36] ***crot-h.*** culx.[58] cyt-l.[119] elaps ferr. ferr-i.[58] goss.[122] ***graph.*** hydrog.[222] iod. iris kali-ar. ***kali-c.*** kali-n.[10] kali-sil.[58] laur. lepi.[36] lipp.[36] lyc. **MAG-C.** mag-m. mag-s. ***med.*** mur-ac.[5] nat-c.[10] nat-p.[36] nat-s.[10] nicc.[10] nit-ac.[5] nux-v.[10] ol-an. ozone[227] paull.[36] ph-ac. ***phos.*** plat. plumbg.[36] prot.[136] ran-b.[5] ran-s.[5] rat. rauw.[119] rheum[5] saroth.[119] ***sars.***[5] sil. sin-n. spong.[5] sul-ac. sul-i.[58] ***sulph.*** syc-co.[136] **THUJ.** ***verb.***[5] viol-o.[45] vip-a.[149] zinc.[5]
- ➤ dead, people, of, grandmother: mag-c.[36]
- ➤ dead, people, of, mother: mag-s.[36]
- ➤ dead, people, of, quarreling with: cedr.[36]
- ➤ dead, people, of, relatives: caust.[1] ferr. fl-ac. hydrog.[222] kali-c.[1] mag-c. mag-s. pitu-a.[164] rheum sars.
- ➤ dead, people, of, relatives, long ago deceased: ferr.[36] sars.[36]
- ➤ dead, people, of, talking with: lepi.[36]
- ➤ dead, people, of, woman coming back to life: hydrog.[222]
- ➤ fiends: apis[36]
- ➤ fiends, raging, strong: arg.[36]
- ➤ ghosts, black: ars. cerv.[36]

➤ ghosts, distorted images: ***graph.***[54]
➤ ghosts, fighting with: sars. sep. sil.[10]
➤ ghosts, horrid: cham.[54]
➤ ghosts, moving about room: mag-s.[36]
➤ ghosts, outside of window: sep.[36]
➤ ghosts, pursued, by: sil.
➤ ghosts, retreating when approached: arg-n.[36]
➤ ghosts, shadow, a, approaching her: ozone[227]
➤ ghosts, spectres: aesc. alum. am-c. ant-t.[10] ***arg-n.*** asc-t. atro. bell. bov. ***camph. carb-v.*** carbn-s. cham. chlol.[54] cina[58] convo-d.[36] ***crot-c.*** eupi. ***graph.*** ign. ***kali-c. kali-s.***[58] kali-sil.[58] lach.[10] lact.[10] mag-c. mag-s. manc. ***med.*** nat-c. nat-m. nat-sil.[58] nit-ac.[10] ***ol-j.***[54] op. paeon. puls. sars. sep. ***sil.*** spig. ***sulph.***
➤ ghosts, white, frightening him: sars.
➤ ghosts, white, wrapped in scarfs, narcosis, who is under: ozone[227]
➤ ghosts, woman, of old: eupi.[36]
➤ pursued, ghosts, by: sil.

Fear; ghosts, night: ***acon.*** ars. ***carb-v.*** chin. chin-ar.[58] cocc.[1] ***lyc. puls.*** ran-b. ***sulph.***
✦ ghosts, of: absin.[172] ***acon.*** agar.[162] ***ars.*** ars-s-f.[58] bell. berb.[172] brom. calc.[30] cann-i. ***carb-v.*** carc.[207] ***caust.*** chin. chin-ar. clem.[30] cocc.[1] crot-c.[103] dros. gall-ac.[198] ***hyos.***[102] ***kali-br.***[116] kali-c. ***lyc. manc.*** med.[102] nat-m.[172] op.[102] ***phos. plat. puls.*** rad-br.[102] ran-b. rhus-t. sep. spong. ***stram. sulph. valer.***[5] zinc. zinc-p.[58]
✦ ghosts, praecordial anguish, with: ***plat.***[54]
✦ ghosts, waking, on: cocc.[5] phos.[162] sulph.[10]
✦ shadows, of: acon.[137] adax.[96] calad.[137] ***calc.***[5] caust.[47] phos.[30] staph.[137] xan.[111]

ACON. Al, 67 - Fear of ghosts.
He, 38 - fear of ghosts.

ARS-MET. He, 4 - Fearful visions of spectres (ghosts) in bright daylight; she sees threatening people after her,...

ARS. Al, 84 - The greatest fear and anguish; sees ghosts day and night.
Ha, 38 - The greatest fear and anguish; night and day he sees ghosts.

BELL. Al, 55 - The delirium was attended (followed) with phantasms (ghosts), and in this respect resembled that caused by alcohol, but the mind did not run on cats, rats, and mice, ...Sometimes the phantasms appeared to be in the air, and various attempts were made to catch them or chase them with the hands; at other times they were supposed to be on the bed.. One patient (a woman) fancied the sheets (cloths) were covered with cucumbers.
Al, 87 - Fancied he saw ghosts and animals in the fire.
Al, 124 - Dread (fear) of solitude, of ghosts and thieves.
Al, 58-... Passed a restless night, her sleep, she says, being disturbed by "miserable phantoms"...
He, 20 - Imagines he sees ghosts, hideous (horrible) faces and various insects.
He, 106 - Anxiety and fear of imaginary objects and hallucinations, ghosts, soldiers which come to take them away (arrest), black animals, rats dogs, wolves, etc.
He, 105 - Anxiety and fear of imaginary objects and hallucinations, ghosts, soldiers which come to take them away, black animals, rats, dogs, wolves, etc.

CALC-A. Al, 255 - Dreams of sick people, and dead people, with violent weeping in the sleep.

CARB-V. He, 14 - Nightly fear of ghosts.

CON. Al, 11 - Visions of her brother and child, who had died; at the same time, she saw distinctly persons in the room;...
Al, 1278 - Many dreams of dead people, and of the death of those living.

CUPR-A. He, 4 - Fixed idea that he sees persons connected with the law who are about to seize him (imprisoned),...at times sees thieves in the room, spirits, and various other immaterial objects;...

DROS. He, 4 - Dread (fear) of ghosts and of being alone.

DULC. Al, 3 - She wakes early, as if called and sees the form of a ghost, which keeps enlarging until it disappears.

HELL. He, 9 - Mania demoniac; sees evil (harmful) spirits at night.

HEP. Al, 1 - Ghostly image of one who was dead, in the morning, in bed, after waking and while conscious, which frightened him; it also seemed as though he saw his neighbor's house burning, which also frightened him.
Ha, 298 - In the morning in bed after waking, when conscious, he had the visionary appearance of a deceased (dead, defunct) person, which frightened him,

and he also imagined he saw a neighboring house in flames, which terrified him.

He, 5 - Frightful visions of fire and of dead persons.

HURA. Al, 4 - She weeps every little while, and especially for two days past, fancies she sees the dead person before her eyes. (ghost)

HYOS. He, 83-...imagining that her deceased sister was sitting by her bedside, and talking with this imaginary person...

KALI-C. He, 16 - Very easily frightened; shrieks about imaginary appearances; starts when touched.

LEPI. Al, 1 - She fancies herself alone in a graveyard, pursued by a ghost, and screams so that her voice is lost next day; yet nobody hears her. (helpless)

LYC. Ha, 25 - Great fear of phantoms, (ghosts) which crowd upon her fancy in the evening; during the day she is disposed to weep.

He, 25 - Anthropophobia (in children); fear of phantoms in evening, with anguish.

MANC. He, 3 - Fear of getting crazy; of evil spirits; of being taken (possessed) by the devil.

He, 5-...about midnight attacks of fear and trembling; afraid of evil spirits, of being taken (possessed) hold of by the devil;...

NAT-C. Al, 1116 - Dream that she saw a corpse, at which she woke in fright, when it seemed as though a dead acquaintance stood before her, which made her scream aloud, afterwards she fell asleep again .

OP. Ha, 637 - She was troubled when awake with the supposed sight of ghosts, devils and spectres, which she believed to be surrounding her bed...

He, 13 - Sees frightful ghosts; easily frightened.

PLAT. He, 35 - Precordial anguish with palpitation and fear of death and imaginary forms, ghosts.

PLB. Al, 63 - The patient imagined that he was constantly followed (persecuted), and that he heard voices coming from the chimney... ; this man after a few days wished to leave the hospital and go home, because he was convinced that there were fiends in the building that pursued him and sought (want) his life.

PSOR. Al, 13 - She is so downhearted (unhappy) that she could commit suicide, then is full of phantasms.

He, 27 - Is so downhearted she could committed suicide, then is full of phantasms.

PULS. Ha, 1110 - When it becomes evening ... he began to be afraid of ghosts; ...

He, 29 - When evening comes begins to dread ghosts.

RAN-B. Al, 1 - Fearfulness in the evening, she does not want to remain alone, she is afraid she may be haunted (seized) by ghosts.

He, 4 - Afraid of ghosts; does not like to remain alone.

RHUS-T. Al, 1382 DREAM-...it seemed to her that the head was hanging out of the bed and the blood was streaming (flow) into it, so that she could hear it flow; together with the appearance of a horrible image which she was obliged to accompany.

STRAM. Al, 63-...I was assailed (attacked) by imaginary spectres, in the most hideous forms and menacing attitudes; and what was still to my torment my bed was suspended and tantalized (charmed) like a feather (plumage) between two floors.

Ha, 553 - Frightful pictures of the imagination; he fancies he sees ghosts.

Ha, 563 - As a rule he has more imaginary figures at his side than in front of him, they all inspire him with horror.

He, 53 - Hallucinations which terrify patient; sees ghosts, hears voices back his ear; sees strangers.

He, 51-...converses with spirits who approach his bed, lays hold of a stick and strikes about him,...great sexual excitement.

SULPH. Al, 3802 - Frightful, anxious dreams of danger of death, and of dead people.

THUJ. Al, 8 - At night, while lying awake with closed eyes, she seems to see ghosts, and also now and then all kinds of animals brilliantly illuminated, coming from her...

ZINC. Ha, 11 - Fear of thieves or of horrible phantoms, seen while waking as if in a feverish fancy.

GO OUT

Dreams; theater, but could not get dressed, which woke her, going to: mag-s.[36]
➤ unsuccessful efforts to, theater, for going to: mag-s.[54]
Escape; attempts to, house, wants to get out of: germ.[222] ***verat.***[54]
Fear; away from home: ign.[162]
✦ bed, go out of, to: acon.[172]
✦ bed, of the, raised himself in, when he: ox-ac.[36]
✦ church or opera, when ready to go: **ARG-N.** dys-co.[136] ***gels.*** plb.[201]
✦ going out, alone: ars.[127] ign.[127] pitu-a.[164]
✦ going out, of: pneu.[149] sep.[149] tarent.[192]
✦ home, away from: ign.[162]
✦ out of doors, to go: acon.[172] anth. bar-c.[127] dys-co.[136] kali-p.[172] ***lyss.***[184]
✦ out of doors, to go, darkness, in, alone: acon.[172]
✦ run over, of being (on going out): anth.[172] hydr-ac. lyss. op.[8] phos.
Going out, aversion to: agar.[137] am-c. anth. clem. ***cycl.*** hydr. ign.[137] sep.[127]
Going out, aversion, happy when she does, but: sep.[127]
Home; desires to go, go out, and when there: ***bry.***[54] ***calc.***[54] **CALC-P.**[54] ***cupr-acet.***[54]
Home; desires to, leave: arag.[102] ***bry.***[102] elat. fl-ac.[58] lach.[102] merc.[102] verat.[102]
Home; desires to, leave, retiring, when: elaps[36]
House; aversion to being kept in: lyc.[36]
Wander, desires to, home, from, and ranges in woods: ***elat.***[54]

ACON. Al, 66 - Great timidity after a severe fright (fear), afraid to go out unattended (abandoned, helplessness) after dark, is unable to control his feelings of apprehensive fear.
ADAM. Sh, 46 - Feel need to be outdoors, in air surrounded by trees even when raining, need air and space and beauty all around. 20, 1M, 04:XX:XX
Sh, 122 - I do not want to go out at all, just need to be on my own. Unusual for me and I feel drained. 12, 30C, 22:XX:XX.
Sh, 127 - I don't want to go out of the flat 7, 6C, 08:00:XX
Sh, 297 - I didn't want to go away to teach. Wanted to be at home. Feel happy at home with children. 2, 12C, 05:XX:XX
AM-C. Al, 13 - Kind of sadness not usual with me; no inclination to go out.
ANTH. Al, 5 - Dislike to go out of doors.
Al, 6 - On going out of doors, in evening, felt nervous, and exceedingly afraid of being run over.
ARG-N. He, 45 - Apprehension when ready to go to church or to opera; diarrhea sets in.
BAR-C. Ha, 12 - The greatest irresolution; he proposes to himself a brief journey, and as soon as he is to make his preparation, he is sorry for it and prefers to stay at home.
He, 15 - Mania; talks much and confusedly; wants to go out of house. 0during pregnancy.
BELL. Ha, 1436 - He makes an excuse (pretext) and runs out into the open fields.
CHOC. Sh, 189 - While outside became very weary of cars and people. Felt open and vulnerable. Fear of accidents, cars, or of someone leaping into the road and punching me. This anxiety was worse out of doors. 27, 100C, 01:XX:XX
Sh, 313 - Desire to see far —to a distant horizon. Desire to be outside more.01A, 30C, 00:XX:XX
CLEM. He, 6 - Irritable, taciturn, does not want to go out.
CYCL. He, 6-...love of (desire) solitude;....;sensation as if room was too small, with reluctance to go into open air;...
ELAPS. Al, 9 - She wishes to leave the house just when she is going to bed.
HALI-L. Sh, 229 - Walk at night in the moonlight; hard to come back into the house. I have no fear, it's so beautiful. 16, 10C, 30:XX:XX
Sh, 300 - Like being outside at night. 16, 10C, 33:XX:XX
Sh, 312 - Eyes feel nearsighted. Don't want to look far away. Don't want to go far out of my house either, not even to the market. Don't want to go far outside my territory. 08, 30C, 15:XX:XX
Sh, 333 - Aversion to going out of the house. 16, 10C, 07:XX:XX
Sh, 567 - Had to leave my house to study elsewhere, due to an unpleasant visitor at home. Someone I can't stand being around came to visit my partner and see our

puppies. He wouldn't ask her to leave. I didn't want to engage with her, because there is no way you can win. If I had said, "It's time to go, now," then I am the ogre. There are no boundaries. 13, 30C, 00:06:00

HYDROG. Sh, 241 - I'm afraid to go out because I think I frighten people. 16, 30C, XX:XX:XX

HYOS. Al, 14 - Thought he was in his own home, and desire to go out and make visits.

IRID. Sh, 5 - I want to be a home-bird this week. I don't want to go out at all. D9

NEON. Sh, 193 - Feel sad and depressed while walking outside in the cold, clear, open air. I don't want to be outside, and walk with head down. On returning inside, I feel in suspended animation. Listless, low energy. Want to close my eyes, which are dry, with heavy, slightly numb lids. I don't feel like working and would just like to go to sleep or read a good book in bed under covers. I still feel chilly from 5 minute walk outside though I've been inside and dressed warmly for 5 minutes. 06, 12C, 00:01:00

NIT-AC. Al, 17 - At once she is taken which peculiar anguish, runs to her physician, but he is not at home, hires a carriage to drive to the house where she expects to find him; during her ride all the anguish is gone; arrived at home she feels as bad as ever, and feels herself thus forced to drive about the whole day, till all the effects of the Nitric acid have passed off.

OPUN-V. Al, 4 - In a few minutes, desire to be at prayer; go there, and in a minute or two desire to go out and "tidy" up; soon went out on an errand downstairs, then come up and go again to prayer.

VALER. Al, 11 - Anxious, hypochondriac feeling, as if the objects around him had been estranged from him; the room appears to him desolate (isolated), he does not feel at home in the room, he is impelled to leave it.

VERAT. He, 13 - After severe illness, aversion to husband and children; desire to leave house: hallucinations, room appeared full of people, crowding in, there was no longer room...

GOD

HALI-L. Sh, 306 - When I'm focused I bring it all in, in the present, There. like meditating, or seeing God. When I'm unfocussed it's like I'll go into the abyss, and won't come back, go crazy. 08, 30C, 31:XX:XX

Sh, 645 - Caring equals oneness. A scary point about that acute phase yesterday—there was no caring. It didn't matter. Nothing mattered. I was alone and wanted to be that way. To have caring, there must be an attunement with the oneness of the universe. Is that where Hitler came from? The crack in the universe? 06, 6C, 01:09:00

Sh, 650 - It was like a horror movie. That's where I got scared. The last five days of the proving were in a black hole. A god-like place or a devil-like place. Why do I have these things? Human things. 02, 30C, XX:XX:XX

Sh, 651 - When I'm focused, I bring it all in, in the present. There, like meditating, or seeing God. When I'm unfocussed, it's like I'll go into the abyss, and won't come back; go crazy. 08, 30C, 31:XX:XX

HYDROG. Sh, 15 - I felt in the presence of a totally pure energy, like meeting God and feeling totally unworthy or like meeting a lover and feeling unworthy — realizing all the mistakes of a lifetime. This pure energy was around for some time protecting me. I feel this unification cleared out lifetimes of symptomatology for me. The joining with this energy was as if a male energy joined with me sexually, but with no desire, pleasure or pain involved. This unification with the male energy lasted quite a few days — I'm not used to seeing myself as a man. The morning after this unifying with the higher presence, I collapsed in emotional overflow. All my grief and pain came out. I was doubled upon the floor and went into a deep state of catharsis. It is not possible to describe where I went as there are no concepts applicable. I felt overflowing love for humanity and wanted to give everything away. My mind turned to the Buddha. It was like seeing the complete picture instead of fragmented bits. (These primary effects lasted about 28 days, then changing to a paranoia state). 16, 30C, 07.XX.XX

Sh, 264 - Talking to God about the state of my heart and asking for it to be healed. 16, 30C, XX:XX:XX

GODLESS

Anxiety; salvation, faith, about loss of his: coloc.[30] merc.[30] nux-v.[30] staph.[30] sulph.[30]
Delirium tremens; voices, heard continually on right side of occiput a loud voice, scolding, vituperating and accusing him of ungodliness, and also personifies voices: **STRAM.**[54]
Fear; faith, to lose his religious: coloc.[162] merc.[162] nux-v.[162] staph.[162] ***sulph.***[162]
Godless, want of religious feeling: ***anac.***[122] calc.[30] coloc. croc. kali-br.[137] **LACH.**[30] laur.[137] ***lyc.***[30] merc.[30] plat.[30] sil.[30] ***sulph.***[30]
Indifference; religion, to his: anac. coloc. med.[179] sil.[137]
Religious affections; feeling, want of: anac. coloc. croc.[122] kali-br.[137] laur.[137]

CAMPH. Al, 46-...I sat up in bed, but all about me had indeed disappeared. I was alone in the great universe, the last of all things. My ideas of the world, God and religion, now seemed to me to have existed only in my imagination; the earth upon which yesterday I lived and moved, had run its appointed course, and I was the final and solitary fragment of the whole creation...(meaningless, unimportant, neglected, forsaken, loneliness, deserted) (godless)
Al, 46-... Faith and hope were gone. There was here no longer any God, or rather the Infinite himself, like all his works, had ceased to be... (hopeless, faithless, godless, privation, want, destitution)
Al, 46-... My misery was boundless; time itself was no more; in short, I suffered such fearful anguish as no fancy can comprehend. What soul could paint to itself my everlasting (eternal) dwelling as the Evil One (devil), alone in a vast universe, without faith or hope, and my heart forever broken by unimaginable tortures? (miserable, timeless, endless, solitude, forsaken, faithless, hopeless)
Al, 46-.... As I lay stretched on my couch, as the evil demon, and suffered all the anguish of a condemned and God-forsaken soul, ...I was forever deprived of the Divine protection, and of every consolation and every hope. Nothing remained to me but the conviction of my everlasting damnation...
NAT-M. He, 11-, ...uttered the most atrocious blasphemes, swore (blaspheme, curse) against God (divine) and the elements (environment), and after raging for awhile became exhausted,...
STRAM. He, 107-...heard continually, on r. side of occiput, a loud voice, scolding, vituperating and accusing him of ungodliness (impious, sinful, irreligious, godless, profane); ....prayed expecting, with great anxiety, the flash of lightning which was to kill him;...(redemption, regeneration, salvation)

GREAT

Delusions; animals, turtles, sees large, in room: bell.
- body, arms, enlarged: lap-c-b.[194]
- body, chin is too long: glon. sabad.[58]
- body, enlarged: arg-n.[139] bell.[139] bov.[123] caj.[123] cench.[58] cic.[139] hydrog.[222] lap-c-b.[194] mim-p.[149] op.[1] par.[139]
- body, fingers, longer: kali-n.[1] tab.[5]
- body, greatness of, as to: ***cann-i. coca hell. plat.*** staph.
- body, head, large, heads make grimaces evening on closing eyes: euphr.
- body, head, large, is too: acon. sil.[1]
- body, heart, large, too: bov.[116] lach. sulph.[137]
- body, legs, long, too: alum.[111] aster.[36] cann-i. coloc.[137] kreos. lac-c.[111] phos.[111] rhus-t.[137] stram. tab.[111] tep.[36] thuj.
- body, lip lower, is swollen, lower: glon.
- body, mammae are too big or too small: bar-c.[162]
- body, tongue, long, too: aeth.
- body, tongue, seems to reach the clouds (when going to sleep): pic-ac.
- dead, corpse, tall yellow c. trying to share bed with him and promptly ejected: bell.
- diminished, everything in room is, while she is tall and elevated: plat.
- enlarged: acon. agar.[102] alum. apis[36] aran.[102] ***arg-n.***[102] asaf.[102] atro.[102] bapt.[102] bell. berb. bov.[102] caj.[85] **CANN-I.** coc-c. euph. ferr.[36] ***gels.***[102] glon. hoit.[72] hydrog.[222] ***hyos.***[102] kali-br.[85] laur. nat-c. nux-v. ***op.*** par.[102] pic-ac. ***plat.*** sabad. stram. zinc.

- enlarged, objects are: acon.[102] agar.[102] ***anh.***[144] ***arg-n.***[102] atro.[102] bov.[102] **CANN-I.** ***gels.***[102] glon.[102] ***hyos.***[102] nux-m. op.[102] par.[102]
- enlarged, persons are: cann-i. caust. tub.
- eyes, big, of: ***lac-c.***[54] op.[1] ***puls.***[54]
- faces, reaching the clouds, when falling asleep: pic-ac.[36]
- figures, gigantic: atro.
- figures, large black, about to jump on him: mosch.
- flowers, of gigantic: cann-i.[36]
- giants, sees: bell.
- giraffe, he is a: cann-i.
- hall, of a gigantic: cann-i.
- humility and lowers of others, while he is great: germ.[222] plat. staph.
- large, he or she is too: pyrog. staph.[1] stram.
- large, he or she is too, entering the house after walking, on: plat.
- large, surroundings are too: ferr.
- large, to grow too: kali-br.[56]
- lower, surrounding objects are, he is much taller: staph.[85]
- man, huge drunk man coming toward her, who lies down beside her, she begs him to retire, falls into convulsions and turns over on her abdomen: cic.[54]
- objects, large: nux-m.[85]
- people, large, in room at night, saw: ***med.***[54]
- road is long: ozone[227]
- room, large, is too: tub.[139]
- saw, he was a huge, darting up and down: cann-i.
- spectres, sees, death appears as a gigantic black skeleton: crot-c.
- square, of a colossal, surrounded by houses a hundred stories high: cann-i.
- surroundings are capacious: ferr.
- tall, he is: cop. eos.[122] hydrog.[222] iodof.[36] lap-c-b.[194] op. pall. plat. staph.[1] stram.
- tall, things, objects grow taller: berb.[10] camph. dros. kreos. nit-ac. sulph.
- water, lake, a spoonful of water is a: agar.

Distance; exaggerated, is, runs against things which appear to him distant: stram.[54]

Distance; exaggerated, is, time during sleepiness, and: nux-v.[10]

Dreams; animals, bugs, enormous, attacking his head, which he killed one by one: myric.[36]

➤ animals, dogs, large dog following him: sil.
➤ animals, spiders, ox, the size of an: cinnb.
➤ body, tongue too large: tab.[10]
➤ buildings: androc.[222] choc.[222] hura[36] myris.[36] pall.[36]
➤ giants: bamb-a.[1184] bell. lyc.
➤ giants, pursued by: bell.
➤ house, family, for a big: ozone[227]
➤ monstrous, figure, black, that flew up to sky and darkened the sun: ped.[36]
➤ monuments, huge: bamb-a.[1184]
➤ pursued, giants, by: bell.
➤ tall, of being very: ferr-i.
➤ things, bigger and overpowering: bamb-a.[1184]
➤ unsuccessful efforts to, talk, large tongue which extended out of her mouth and up her nose, on account of: tab.[36]

ACON. Al,S-2 - Some few hallucinations, such as imagining his head was three times its original size.

ADAM. Sh, 313, I feel very tall and large. I am a giant, 12:30 a.m. -powerful feeling. 20, 1M, 09:XX:XX

BELL. Al, 85 - Visions of wolves, dogs, giants, and fire.

Al,S-2552-...the yellow corpse of a tall man, shrouded (dressed, clothes) in white, tried to share the patient's bed with him, and the unwelcome visitor was promptly ejected. A crimson serpent came from the foot of the bed, with the design of fastening upon the patient's neck...

He, 18 - When closing eyes, though not asleep, patient sees fierce (wild), wicked looking large animals with horns and bushy (scabrous) heads; room seemed to be full of strange men passing in and out, who would snatch (take hold) at her as they passed, which frightened her very much, she thought the men wanted to take her away from home ; she then saw children sitting on low benches (seat) in rows (line) as in a school-room. (purity)

He, 86 - Sensation of floating or gliding along, as if in a boat; as if the body, or part of it was greatly enlarged.

BERB. Al, 3 - Anxious mood, with great fear and fright...; in the twilight some dogs and children appeared as large again as natural.

CANN-I. Al, 44 - Extreme exaggerations of the duration of time and extent of space-a few seconds seem ages-the utterance (declaration) of a word seems as long as a whole drama, and a few rods are a distance which can never be passed it is so great.(distances)

Al, 64 - Imagines he is gradually swelling, his body becoming larger and larger.

He, 15-...he is gradually swelling, his body becomes larger and larger; that someone calls him; that he hears numberless bells ringing most sweetly; imagines he hears music; shuts his eyes, and is lost for some time in the most delicious thoughts and dreams.

CHOC. Sh, 44 - Dream —coming out of the station a huge black bird the size of a dog with black long soft feathers like those of an ostrich, and a very big beak. It took my left hand in his beak. There were two gypsies there and they stood in front of me and opened their hands and I saw that they held a gold metal flat fish which I saw as a fortune telling object.

Sh, 52 - My right hand feels bigger and wider and I feel more powerful. But my wrists feel weaker and flatter. Sensation of opening of hands and tightness in the forearm.

Sh, 149 - Hearing and smell still acute — nature seems wonderful. Saw nine magpies and they seemed much bigger than before.

Sh, 310 - On bending my head back, a sensation, or imagination, that the back of my head is horribly elongated. I can't get it out of my mind.15, 30C, 03:13:30

CROT-C. Al, 1 - Magnetic state; she hears nothing, and again sees the spectre of death, as a gigantic black skeleton.

FERR. Al, 3 - My surroundings (material welfare) seem very large (big) and capacious (vast), and I am inclined to attribute great importance to trifles...

GERM. Sh, 186 - While walking felt round-shoulder like a bodybuilder, worse after rising. 15, 30C,

GLON. He, 6 - The chin (jaw) feels too long.

HALI-L. Sh, 3 - Feel like abdomen is much bigger, but husband says it's not. 09, 6C, 00:XX:XX

Sh, 729 - Delusions —sees eagles. They were rooks and crows really. They looked bigger. 20, 30C, 01:00:58

HYDROG. Sh, 166 - Sensation of being larger. 10, 200C, 11:XX:XX

Sh, 167 - Thought or vision that I was taller or stronger than I was. 28, 200C, 02:01:XX

Sh, 169 - Thought there was a large insect, a locust, on the back of my head and put up my hand to check. 16, 30C, 01:XX:XX

IRID. Sh, 88 - Forgot to race downhill again. Voice sounded deeper. My immediate reaction, "Oh God, I'm turning into a man." Felt I was overwhelming colleague so didn't ask if I really was. I seemed to take up a lot of space in the room so I drew back and left. G5

Sh, 89 - Sensation as if tall. Q3

Sh, 90 - Feeling extremely tall. Feeling as if kitchen table too low. Q6

KALI-AR. He, 2 - Thought her head felt larger.

LAC-C. Al,N-19 - Wakes at night with a sensation that she was lying on a large snake.

MED. He, 19 - One night saw large (big) people in room; large rats running; felt a delicate hand smoothing her head from front to back. (caressed)

NEON. Sh, 10 - Walking up a long gradual incline, I felt every stride was covering great distances. I felt I was doing the usual 20 minute walk in seconds. I felt like a titan in 7 - league boots, but then I couldn't decide which league boots they were and I wanted an even number. My thoughts went titan-titanium-uranium-Uranus-clouds-clouds-where is the sky? 20, 6C, 01:12:20

Sh, 14 - After a shower, I felt enormous, massive, yet in proportion. I was amazed at how huge I was. 20, 6C, 03:00:00

Sh, 15 - I've been feeling huge the last few days, due to eating biscuits. Feel like my legs have gone all fleshy. 02, 6C, 07:XX:XX

OP. He, 16 - Imagines parts of body very large.

PALL. He, 3 - When walking in street in evening, it seems to him as if he had grown taller. (enlarged, grow)

PHOS. Al, 86-...; a feeling of dread (fear), as if awaiting something terrible, yet unable to resist or move (terrifying, scaring), overcame me; sometimes it seemed as if I was beginning to bloat (inhalant, inflate, vanity?), and then I could hear a multitude of voices saying in high glee, "Fill him up a little more and he will burst," (blow up) followed by demoniacal laughter, which made the cold chills run over me... I imagined myself an aurora borealis, and could distinctly hear voices shouting, "Beautiful! Oh, was not that splendid?"...

PLAT. Ha, 35 - Illusion of the imagination; on entering the room after walking for an hour, everything around her seemed very small and all persons physically and bodily inferior to her, but she herself great and lofty (distinguish, elevated) in body;...

STRAM. Ha, 504 - He appears to himself large and tall, but surrounding objects appear small to him.

He, 57 - Strange absurd ideas; thinks herself tall, double or lying crosswise; one half of body cut off (divided); bed is full of creases (wrinkle) (disorganization); that he was killed roasted and being eaten.

GREATNESS

Boaster, braggart: agn.[162] alco.[36] arn.[30] ars.[30] bell.[30] hydrog.[222] lach.[30] lil-t.[184] lyc.[162] med.[162] merc.[30] nat-m.[30] nux-v.[30] plat.[30] stram.[30] sulph.[189]

Boaster; belongings, toys, about his: sulph.[127]

Boaster; rich, wishes to be considered as: lach.[30] lyc.[30] verat.[30]

Boaster; squander through ostentation: calc.[30] nux-v.[30] plat.[30] puls.[30]

Confidence; self, in: ang.[36] choc.[222] hell.[36] nitro-o.[36] nux-v.[58]

Contemptuous; mankind, for: cic.[36]

Contemptuous; society, mankind, at: cic.[1]

Deeds; desire to perform, great: cocain.[102]

Deeds; he could do great, as if: cocain.[162] hell.

Delirium; presumptuous: lyc.[36]

Delirium; speeches, makes: lyss.[54]

Delusions; argument, making an eloquent: cann-i.

- beautiful, she is b. and wants to be: stram.[122]
- better than others, that he is: germ.[222] lap-gr-m.[194] myric.
- body, greatness of, as to: ***cann-i. coca hell. plat.*** staph.
- castles and palaces, sees: plb.
- Christ, himself to be: cann-i. verat.[58]
- creative power, has: cann-i. psil.[164]
- diminished, everything in room is, while she is tall and elevated: plat.
- distinguish, squanders money, proud of his position: ***verat.***[54]
- distinguished, is: lap-mar-c.[194] phos.[1] stram. verat.
- divine, he is: cann-i. glon.[116] stram.
- emperor, thought himself an: cann-i.
- emperor, talked of: carbn-s.
- faces, distinguished people, of: cann-i.
- general, he is a: cupr.
- God, communication with, he is in: psil.[164] stram. verat.
- God, he is, then he is devil: **STRAM.**[54]
- God, sees: aether.[36]
- great person, is a: aeth. ***agar.*** alum.[122] bell. ***cann-i.*** coca[162] cupr. cur.[36] glon.[5] ***graph.***[54] ***hyos.***[5] ***lach.***[5] lap-mar-c.[194] lyc.[5] ***lycpr.***[30] lyss. phos. ***plat.*** stram.[5] sulph. ***syph.***[122] verat. ***verat-v.***[54]
- humility and lowers of others, while he is great: germ.[222] plat. staph.
- knowledge, he possesses infinite: cann-i. psil.[164] verat-v.[171]
- large, he or she is too, entering the house after walking, on: plat.
- lower, surrounding objects are, he is much taller: staph.[85]
- mandarin, his friend is a: cann-i.
- noble person, he is a: lap-mar-c.[194] phos. plat.[58]
- power over all disease, has: ***stram.***[54]
- presumptuous: lyc.[10]
- prince, is a: verat.
- proud: lach.[10] plat. stram. verat.
- queen, she is a: cann-i.
- rank, he is a person of: cupr. phos. ***stram.***[54] verat.
- runs, long way, he can run a: coca[139]
- runs, never before, she can run like: agar.[139]
- squanders money: ***verat.***[54]
- statue, poses as: ***stram.***
- strong, he is: androc.[222] germ.[222] hydrog.[222]
- superhuman, is: cann-i. psil.[164]
- superiority, of: germ.[222] lap-gr-m.[194] ***plat.***
- tall, has grown, while walking: pall.
- tall, he is: cop. eos.[122] hydrog.[222] iodof.[36] lap-c-b.[194] op. pall. plat. staph.[1] stram.
- understands everything: verat-v.[171]
- Virgin Mary, she is: cann-i.
- visions, grandeur, of magnificent: cann-i.[54] carbn-s. coff.

• visions, imaginary power of: cann-i. psil.[164]
• wealth, makes useless purchases, and: ***nux-v.***[54]
• wealth, of: agn. alco. bell. calc. cann-i. kali-br. nit-ac.[5] phos.[102] ***plat.***[102] ***pyrog. sulph.*** verat.

Desires; grandeur, for: cur.[36]
Desires; great things, to do: cocain.[137]
Desires; respect, due to him shown: ham.[137]
Dignity: caj.[25] calc.[36] guare.[25] nat-c.[188] nat-m.[187] staph.[188]
Dreams; banquet, of being at a: mag-c.[10] mag-s. nit-ac.[10] ph-ac.
➤ boasting: asc-t.[36] m-p-a.[1]
➤ buildings, admirable: graph.[30]
➤ coronation: upa.[36]
➤ feasting: anan. ant-c. asaf. hura m-p-a.[1] mag-s. nit-ac. ph-ac. tril. zinc.
➤ glorification of oneself: saroth.[144]
➤ greatness: bufo[5] stann.[1]
➤ important events, of: osm.[36]
➤ lion, that he was a: phys.
➤ money, gold, of: ***cycl.*** puls.
➤ nuclear, power plant, about: ozone[227]
➤ people, influential persons, to whom he occupies position of servant or subordinate: lyss.[54]
➤ praying, public meeting with great applause, in: ars-h.[54]
➤ queen Victoria: rumx.[36]
➤ solemnities: ant-c.[36]
➤ splendor: stann.[10]
➤ triumph: bapt.[36]
➤ visionary: acon.[5] aloe am-c. ambr.[5] ***anh.***[119] ant-t.[5] arn. ars.[5] ***bar-c.***[5] bell. **BRY.**[5] bufo[5] ***calc.*** calc-sil.[58] camph. carb-an. ***carb-v.***[5] cham. chin. coloc. **CON.**[5] graph. hell.[5] ***kali-c. kali-n.*** kali-sil.[58] ***lach.*** lachn. ***lyc.*** meny.[5] merc.[5] mur-ac. nat-c. ***nat-m.*** nicc. nit-ac.[5] ***nux-v. op. petr.*** plan. prun.[10] ***puls.*** rheum[5] sep. ***sil. spong. stram.***[5] sulph. zinc.[5] zinc-o.[10]
➤ women, arrogant, of a, with exaggerated confidence: ozone[227]

Egotism; self-esteem, over-estimation of him self: cic.[137]
Egotism; self-esteem, reciting their exploits: agar.[36]
Elated; alternating with sadness: caust.[198] senec.[36] ***sul-ac.***[209] visc.[119]
Exaggerates her symptoms: asaf.[137] cham.[137] plb.[137]
Exclusive, too: calc.[30] nat-m.[30] plat.[30]
Fancies; power, increased, of: **LACH.**[5] op.[5] viol-o.[5]
Gestures; makes, sublime: hyos.[36] nitro-o.[36]
Gourmand: calc.[30] chin.[30] ip.[30] mag-c.[30] merc.[30] nat-c.[30] **VERAT.**[30]
Haughty; stiff and pretentious: ***lyc.***[54]
Ideas; exaggerated: glon.[5] pall.[5] petr.[36] plat.[5]
Importance; feels his, pompous: alco.[36] arn.[5] bell.[5] calc.[137] cann-i.[36] cupr.[5] ferr.[60] ferr-ma.[36] glon.[5] hyos.[60] ***lyc.***[5] phos.[5] **PLAT.**[5] stram.[5] sulph.[5] ***verat.***[5]
Indifference; superiority, with feeling of: ozone[227]
Loquacity; exalted opinion of her own ideas and powers, with, in insanity: ***verat-v.***[54]
Loquacity; speeches, makes: arn. cham. ign.[5] ***lach.*** lachn.[102]
Magnetic state, feeling of personal power increased: androc.[222] crot-c.[36] phos.[8]
Plans; fantastic, in insanity: ***nux-v.***[54]
Plans; gigantic: op.
Power, love of: ars.[189] lach.[189] lyc. nux-v.[189] sulph.[189]
Presumptuous: arn.[30] calc.[30] ***lyc.***[122] plat.[30] staph.[30]
Reading; desire for, orator, like a: agn.[36]
Respect, thinks he earns: ham.[36]
Self-sufficient; overly confident: ferr-ma.[10]
Talk; bombast, worthless: crot-h.[30] ***lach.***[30] nux-v.[30] staph.[30]
Talk; extravagant: aether ***cann-i.*** lach.[36] ***nux-m.*** plb. stram.
Theorizing; gigantic: ***cann-i.***[36] op.[36]
Thoughts; sublime: lach.[60]
Walk; self-sufficient impression of importance, walks along with a: ferr-ma.[36]
Walk; slowly and dignified, walks: caj.

ADAM. Sh, 35 - Delusion of being an Indian prince, with a turban and jewel on his Third Eye. 16, 12C, 31:XX:XX
Sh, 43 - Feeling alone and tall and capable, like a beacon beaming out rays of light to all and sundry. 2, 12C, XX:XX:XX
Sh, 313, I feel very tall and large. I am a giant, 12:30 a.m. -powerful feeling. 20, 1M, 09:XX:XX
Sh, 314 - Feeling of absolute power, invincible. 16, 12C, 14:14:00
Sh, 536 - With my eyes closed after meditating, to my right appeared a huge Tibetan deity. He appeared to know who I was.

Felt it would be rude to ask his name. He said, "Do you want to know how powerful I am?" He was not friendly but powerful.... 16, 12C, 00:07:30

AGAR. Al, 9 - Delirium; he imagines himself a military (martial) officer, commanding (dominant) at a drill (training) and directing the various maneuvers.

AGN. Al, 2 - He sometimes feels as if he were nobody (unimportant, insignificant, worthless), and would rather be dead than have that feeling; when possessed by that feeling he has no courage to undertake anything; and when free from it he feels exalted, would like to read like an orator, etc.

ALOE. Al, 9 - Contented with his station (position, rank) in life; it involuntarily occurs to him, that he is really much better off than many other people.

BELL. Al, 203-..;he imagined himself rich, owner of a large house, etc. (great person)

CANN-I. Al, 58 - He imagines that he is possessed of infinite knowledge and power of vision, and then that he is Christ come to restore the world to perfect peace. (redemption, savior, rescuer)

Al, 59 - He believes there is creative power in his own word, and that he has only to speak, and it will be done.

Al, 61 - Then he possesses the wealth of the world, and with a benevolence equal to his wealth, showers riches on all the needy around him.

CARBN-S. Al-S, 754 - Hallucinations (delirium) of vision and hearing, he seemed to see splendid spectacles of carriages, with magnificent objects, talked of the emperor, of money, and of grandeur, often incoherently.

CHIN. Ha, 1135 - He makes a number of grand (great) plans for the future.

Ha, 1137 - He has many ideas, undertakes (begin, try) to carry out (achieve, perform, execute) all sorts of things, builds castles in air.(fanciful)

COFF-T. Al, 15 - It gives rise to a need of creative activity, a vivacity of thought, a versatility and ardor of desire, more favorable to the exaggerated expression of ideas previously formed, than to the quiet examination of new conceptions.

COFF. He, 8 - Great loquacity, brain feels clear and is active, he feels strong enough to do anything, feels impelled to push things; veneration for the Supreme Being and love for family; benevolence excited.

CUPR-A. Al, 2 - Attacks of mania; he fancies that he is a military officer; a fancy that he is selling green vegetables; a fancy that he is repairing old chairs...he spits in the faces of the attendants, and laughs heartily at it.

CUPR. Ha, 23 - Fits of insanity, imagines he is a military commander.

CUR. Al, 5 - Fondness (desire) for luxury (waste) and grandeur.(distinction, fame)

Al, 6 - He would like to go travel in a great style.(luxury)

FERR-MA. Al-S, 1 - Walking along with a self-sufficient impression of importance.

GERM. Sh, 186 - While walking felt round-shoulder like a bodybuilder, worse after rising. 15, 30C,

Sh, 113 - Sometimes I don't want to show my strength. I keep it back. I am afraid that others will feel inferior and I don't want them to, because I feel it so much myself. 18, 30C, 26:XX:XX

Sh, 149 - Feel lonely. I nearly always feel special -always on the sideoutside of others. Either better or smaller than others. 18, 30C, 46:XX:XX

HALI-L. Sh, 301 - Want to move to mountains, but I can't do it in one day. 08, 30C, 30:XX:XX

Sh, 330 - Bored and superior feeling with an old friend. 16, 10C, 22:XX:XX

Sh, 580 - Spent most of today thinking about how I am surrounded by idiots, (my family), who are showing no attempts to think for themselves, letting me run the show. They don't care to figure things out. I'm in hyper-drive. I know a lot and I'm right. I've been extremely productive or at least active, balancing several major projects all at the same time, and they can't seem to tidy a table properly. This includes my husband, who continually interrupts me (or so it seems) for some trivial question. I'm coming across with too much force. I find myself shouting at everyone much more than usual. Like a crazy person. Impatient over others' slowness. Almost an arrogance. I want them to THINK! (Obviously, the way I do).

or get off the ship and drown yourself. A hard anger, more intense that usual. Feel like leaving them all—they just take and give back little. More trouble than support. This isn't complaining or victimizing talking. This is how it is. I'm healing myself and leaving my family in the dust. I've passed on to them my bad habits, bad parenting. They are content to be idiots. 09, 6C, 13:XX:XX

Sh, 581 - At a meeting for parents and children, I am very critical of my daughter and myself, comparing her to other kids, myself to other moms. Cringe when she sits with her mouth open, pulling on her hair and twisting it into braids. Want to warn her, don't do that! She looks to me like she's bossing someone. Compare myself to other woman who has perfectly put together hair, clothes, nails, boots, bracelets. Very angry and jealous. Make excuses for myself and tear her down inside. 09, 6C, 14:00:XX

Sh, 817 - I feel regal and generous. 20, 30C, 05:01:XX

Sh, 913-6:30 a.m. Sitting up in bed to meditate. The dawn came and I felt majestic. 20, 30C, 12:00:30

HAM. Al, 1 - Feeling that she ought (have) to be reverenced (honored, venerated) by all around her and have great respect (regard) paid to her opinions; lasting about an hour.

HYDROG. Sh, 167 - Thought or vision that I was taller or stronger than I was. 28, 200C, 02:01:XX

HYOS. Al, 73 - In speaking, used very fine language, so that the usually quiet and indolent peasant (farmer) was scarcely recognized.

Ha, 517 - Over-busy: he thought he was more active and stronger (powerful, Herculean) than he actually was.

Ha, 545 - Ridiculously solemn acts in improper clothing, mixed with fury. (In a priest's cassock, put on over nothing but a shirt, and in fur boots, he wishes to go to church, in order to preach and perform clerical offices there, and furiously attacks those who try to prevent him.)

IRID. Sh, 30 - Feel as if I am the only person. E3

KALI-BR. Al, 3 - Decidedly insane; had delusions that lewd women had got into his mother's house; that he was pursued by the police; that his wife was threatened by members of the family; that he had thousands of dollars in gold sewed up in his clothing; (rich, wealth)

Al, 24 - The patient, who has been violently excited, glorying (adoration) in his imaginary power of body and mind, becomes desponding sullen, melancholic, and frequently lachrymose, often even despairing.

LACH. Al, 5 - A kind of ecstasy, as after sublime impressions, or excessive joy, throughout the day; he constantly wishes to talk and do much, and even more seems to be at his command.(control, domination)

He, 8 - Thinks: she is somebody else in the hands (seized) of a stronger power; (supremacy, superiority).or that she is dead, and preparations are made for funeral (cortege) or that she is nearly dead and wishes some one would help her off; herself pursued by enemies, or fears medicine is poison; there are robbers in house and wants to jump out the window; herself under super-human control; visions real, he will die. (helplessness, desire; aid, comfort, salvation)

He, 16 - Most extraordinary loquacity, making speeches in very select (finest, excellent) phrases (pretentious), but jumping off to most heterogeneous subjects; at the same time proud (haughty), full of mistrust. 0Mania.

He, 33-...want of self control; lascivious; felt as if she was clear (pure) animal right through, whilst of all mental power was dormant; sensation as if hands of stronger power, as if charmed (enchanted), and as if could not break the spell (charm). (possessed, wildness)

He, 54 - A girl, after excessive study, uses exalted language; exceedingly particular about language she uses, often correcting after using a word, and substituting another of very similar meaning, talking about being under influence of a superior power. (possessed) 0 Mania.

LYC. Al, 2 - Delirious, raging, envious, reproachful, presumptuous, and imperious.

Ha, 59 - Insanity and fury, breaking out in envy, pretensions (inflated) and ordering (dictatorial) others about.
He, 17-...imperiousness(domineering, despotic) ; speaks with an air of command (ordering, domination) ; manner stiff (severe, obstinate) and pretentious;...
LYSS. Al, 2 - Exaltation; thinks he has something of importance.
Al,N-33-...Thinks he is a man of great authority.(power, command, expert)
He, 33 - Makes speeches in delirium; thinks he is a man of great authority.
MYRIC. Al, 9-...a constant desire to find fault (censorious); everything went wrong; looked upon (contemptuous) this world as a place not fit to live in any longer; considered himself better than the rest (great person, megalomania), in the morning; ...; condemned himself for various imaginary faults; ...
NEON. Sh, 10 - Walking up a long gradual incline, I felt every stride was covering great distances. I felt I was doing the usual 20 minute walk in seconds. I felt like a titan in 7 - league boots, but then I couldn't decide which league boots they were and I wanted an even number. My thoughts went titan-titanium-uranium-Uranus-clouds-clouds-where is the sky? 20, 6C, 01:12:20
Sh, 12 - I had many thoughts of the second day of creation. 20, 6C, 03:XX:XX
Sh, 39 - During the night, in a semi-sleep state, I had many thoughts of the second day of creation. I was aware that my form and weight were appropriate. 20, 6C, 03:XX:XX
Sh, 49 - I have lost the delusion, which I have always had, that I could walk on water. 20, 6C, 04:XX:XX
NUX-V. He, 37-...betraying (play false, feigning) great moral and physical languor (indifference),..launches into high-flying, fantastic plans, fancies himself rich (rank, position) and wants to make presents of thousands (squanders, waste), and makes large useless purchases; does not consider himself ill; ...,and takes in bad part if not allowed to read indictment (accusation) for said lawsuit, a confused irrational piece of work...
OP. Al, 19-...; all the actors are happy, and each retires home in a total state of irrationality, but likewise in the entire and full enjoyment of happiness not to be procured by reason. Disregarding the ridicule of those they meet, who divert themselves by making them talk absurdly, each imagines looks and feels himself possessed of whatever he wishes...
Al, 148-...his mind to be not only clear and active, but filled with gigantic schemes and theories, the realization of which seems to him quite natural and easy; his faculties are remarkably keen (sharp)...
He, 22-... feeling of great strength; contempt of death;...indifference to joy and suffering.
PHOS. Al, 86-...; a feeling of dread (fear), as if awaiting something terrible, yet unable to resist or move (terrifying, scaring), overcame me; sometimes it seemed as if I was beginning to bloat (inhalant, inflate, vanity?), and then I could hear a multitude of voices saying in high glee, "Fill him up a little more and he will burst," (blow up) followed by demoniacal laughter, which made the cold chills run over me... I imagined myself an aurora borealis, and could distinctly hear voices shouting, "Beautiful! Oh, was not that splendid?"...
Ha, 89 - Delirious fantasies, while slumbering (sleep) and when awake, as if she was on a distant island (isolation, segregation), as if she had a large business, was a distinguished (important, rank) lady, etc.
He, 31-...; indifference even towards dearest friends;... ; monomania de grandeur et de la richesse;...
PLAT. Ha, 35 - Illusion of the imagination; on entering the room after walking for an hour, everything around her seemed very small and all persons physically and bodily inferior to her, but she herself great and lofty (distinguish, elevated) in body;...
Ha, 38 - Haughty, proud feelings.
He, 8 - Arrogant, reserved, absent-minded.
He, 9 - Pride (haughty) and overestimation of one's self, looking down with haughtiness on others.
He, 41 - Delirium, with fear of men (people); often changing, with overestimation (haughty) of oneself.
He, 45-...melancholy with great fear of death, imagines himself superior to his wife;...

He, 42 - Mania; with great pride; fault-finding; unchaste (sensual) talk; ...(chaste = moral, pure)

He, 50 - Puerperal mania...assumed or seemed to feel herself a person of great superiority;...

PLB. Al, 61 - He had, some time back, illusions of vision; saw castles, palaces, but these have ceased since he entered the hospital.

PYROG. Al,N-8 - Hallucination that he is very wealthy (rich); remaining after fever.

ROB. Al, 12 - Anxiety to seek honors (distinction) ; excessive pride (haughtiness, arrogance) ; he considers himself better than an emperor.

STRAM. Ha, 504 - He appears to himself large and tall, but surrounding objects appear small to him.

He, 49 - After spasms she fell into a trance, says she is under influence(seized) of spirits, and has had conversation with spirits, communications from God; delivers emphatic sermons, prophecies. (missionary)

He, 92 - Mania:... complains that a dog is biting and tearing flesh off his chest; merry exaltation; with pride (haughty) and affectation; runs about, complains of violent headache; ...;steals from his roommates...; disposition to scold persons whom he otherwise loved.

He, 98 - Mania; affects (pretend) being a distinguished (label) person, of high rank (position, nobility) ; is full of fear.

He, 87 - After a dreadful shock, occasioned by death of his brother, who fell dead in his arms,...struck all at around him...spoke at one time in Hungarian, and then in Wallachian language; sang Latin paternosters, declared he was God, and then that he was the devil;...

SULPH. Al, 2 - Delirium; she destroys her things, throws them away, thinking that she has a superfluity (excess) of everything, wherewith she wastes(thin) to a skeleton.(wealth?)

Al, 12 - She fancies that she has beautiful (refined) clothes; old rags look like fine things, a coat like a beautiful jacket, a cap like a beautiful hat.

Ha, 62 - She imagines that she has beautiful clothes, she takes old rags for beautiful clothes, she takes a coat for a jacket, a cap for a hat.

Ha, 63 - Insanity; she spoils (ruin) her things and throws them away, imagining she has an abundance of everything; at the same time she becomes emaciated, like a skeleton.-(wealthy, rich X miserable, poor, destitute)

He, 11 - Foolish happiness and pride(haughtiness),thinks himself in possession of beautiful (attractive) things; even rags seem beautiful. (rank, position, distinction)

He, 38 - Destroys clothing; imagines she has everything in abundance. (wealth)

TAB. Al, 51 - Exalted action of the brain; copious flow of ideas; ...leaving me in the morning worn-out and sick, I would conceive and elaborate about twenty undertakings, of which probably not one would ever come to light.

THUJ. He, 10 - Fixed ideas: as if a strange person were at his side; as if soul and body were separated (split) ; that body, particularly limbs, are made of glass (frail) and will readily break (weakness); as if a living animal were in abdomen ;talks about being under the influence of a superior power. (possessed)

VERAT-V. He, 6 - Loquacity, with exaltation of ideas, or an exalted opinion of her own ideas and powers; everything seems clear to her; now clearly understands former mysterious things; wants no medicine, as that will restore her to former condition;...

VERAT. Al, 4 - He imagines that he is a prince (noble) and behaves in a very haughty manner. (proud, arrogant)

Ha, 672 - He pretends (simulate, feigning) he is a prince, and gives himself airs (affectation, pretentious) accordingly.

Ha, 675 - She boasts (exult, triumph) that she is pregnant.

He, 11 - Thinks himself distinguished (classify) ; squanders (futile) his money; proud (haughty) of his position.

He, 29-...prays says it is a secret (secretive, mysterious) and a misfortune; ...saying she must strengthen (encourage) herself, ...imagines herself in heaven (elevated, sublime, noble) talking with God.

He, 4 - Erroneous and haughty notions.

He, 21 - Mania; with desire to cut and tear

everything, especially clothes; with lewdness and lascivious talk; religious or amorous; de grandeur.

GRIEF

Ailments from; anger, grief, with silent: **ACON.**[5] alum. am-m.[116] ars. aur. aur-ar.[58] bell. **BRY.**[5] carc.[210] ***cham.***[5] ***chin.***[116] ***cocc. coloc. gels.***[5] hyos. **IGN. LYC.** nat-c. ***nat-m.*** nux-v. ***ph-ac.*** phos. plat. puls. **STAPH.** verat. ***zinc.***[5]

Ailments from; fright or fear, grief, with: ign.[1]

Ailments from; grief, cry, cannot: aeth.[162] am-m.[85] apis[36] carc.[146] crot-c.[36] ***gels.*** ign.[36] kali-fcy.[198] **NAT-M.** nux-v.[5] op.[36] puls.[36]

Ailments from; grief, drowsiness, particularly with: ***op.***[54] **PH-AC.**[54]

Ailments from; grief, emotional, mental symptoms from: alum.[36] am-m.[36] ***ars.***[8] ***aur.***[54] bar-s.[58] bell.[10] calc-p.[72] carc.[207] ***caust.***[8] ***cocc.***[54] con.[8] ***gels.***[8] ***ign.***[8] ***kali-br.***[54] lach.[30] lact.[36] lyc.[5] merc.[5] ***nat-m.***[54] ***ph-ac.***[54] phos.[58] phys.[137] ***plat.***[8] zinc.[8]

Ailments from; grief, prolonged and unresolved: carc.[207]

Ailments from; grief, sorrow, care: alum-p.[58] am-m. ***ambr.***[5] aml-n.[137] anac. ant-c. ***apis arn.***[122] ars. art-v.[85] **AUR.** aur-ar.[58] aur-s.[58] bar-s.[58] bell.[5] **BRY.**[5] cadm-s.[5] cael.[149] ***calc.***[5] ***calc-p.*** caps.[5] carc.[207] **CAUST.** cham.[114] clem. **COCC.** colch. ***coloc. con.***[5] ***crat.***[122] crot-h.[137] cycl. cypr.[54] dig.[58] ***dros.***[122] ***gels. graph. hura***[117] ***hyos.*** **IGN.** ip.[122] ***kali-br.***[54] kali-c.[5] kali-p. **LACH.** laur.[58] lob-c. lob-s.[54] lyc. mag-c.[85] naja nat-c.[5] **NAT-M.** nit-ac. nux-m.[58] ***nux-v.*** op.[5] paull.[8] petr.[5] **PH-AC.** phos.[5] phys.[85] pic-ac.[5] ***plat.*** psor.[185] ***puls.*** pyrus[36] rhus-t.[5] ***samb.***[102] ***sep.***[5] seq-s.[230] ***sol-o.***[122] spig.[162] **STAPH.** stram.[5] sulph.[10] tarent. tub.[193] ***uran-n.***[193] verat. ***zinc.***[5]

Ailments from; love disappointed, grief, with silent: **IGN. NAT-M. PH-AC.** phos.

Ailments from; mortification, humiliation, chagrin, emotional or mental ailments from: anac.[8] ***apoc.***[8] ***aur.***[8] bell.[5] ***coloc.***[8] con.[103] cur.[11] ***ign.***[8] lach.[30] lyc.[58] lyss.[56] nat-m.[10] ***nux-v.***[10] pall.[116] plat.[30] ***puls.***[8] ran-b.[36] ***staph.***[54] verat.[30] zinc.[10]

Anxiety; chagrin, after: lyc.

Anxiety; chest, heart, region of, grief, from: ***naja***[54]

Anxiety; future, disgust of life, with: ***lach.***[54]

Anxiety; grief, as from internal: am-m.[54]

Bilious disposition, grief, after: tarent.[36]

Cheerfulness; alternating with, grief: calc-s.[54] graph.[10] ***op.***[30]

Cheerfulness; evening, grief, changes to: calc-s.[36]

Delirium; sorrowful: acon. bell. dulc. lyc. puls.

Delusions; grief and anger, from: bell.[10] zinc.[54]

- grief, weighed upon him: am-m.[139] con.[139]
- pitied on account of his misfortune and he weeps, he is: nat-m.[1]
- sorrow, everyone he meets has a secret: cann-i.

Discouraged; disgust, with: caust.[10]

Dreams; grief: all-c.[36] carl.[36] stront-c.[36]

➤ mortification: asar.[54] ign.[54] mosch.[54] rheum[54] staph.[54]

Dullness; chagrin, vexation; from: ign. lach.

Dullness; grief, from: ign.[58] lach.[58]

Dwells; on past disagreeable occurrences, recalls old grievances: glon. sars.[54] sulph.[54]

Fear; death, megrim, in: ***ars.***[54]

✦ grief, as from: am-m.[54] phos.

✦ grief, followed by: ***ign.***[54]

✦ night, grief, with: ***merc.***[54]

Foolish; behavior, hilarity, with riotous, and subsequent angry savageness, or tearful sorrow: op.[54]

Grief: acet-ac. acon. agar. ail.[102] alum. am-c. am-m. **AMBR.**[5] ***anac.***[10] ant-c. ***arn.***[10] ***ars.***[122] **AUR.** aur-ar.[58] bar-c. benz-ac.[5] bov.[5] cael.[149] calc. calc-f.[103] calc-p.[102] caps.[5] carb-an. carc.[214] card-m.[5] **CAUST.** chel.[10] chin.[30] choc.[222] ***cic.***[10] cimic.[102] ***cocc.***[5] coff.[10] ***coloc.*** con.[30] croc.[5] cycl. dig.[102] ***dros.***[10] foll.[1201] ***graph.*** **HELL.**[5] hyos. ***iber.***[102] **IGN.** kali-bi.[5] kali-br.[5] kali-n.[10] kali-p.[58] ***lach.*** lact. lap-c-b.[194] ***laur.***[5] ***lyc.*** mag-m.[5] mang.[10] meny.[5] ***merc.*** mez.[5] mur-ac.[5] naja[130] nat-c.[5] **NAT-M.** nit-ac.[30] ***nux-v. op.***[122] paull.[54] petr.[137] ***ph-ac.*** phos.[30] **PULS.** ran-s.[5] rhus-t.[162] ***sep.***[122] sil.[30] ***spig.***[54] stann.[91] **STAPH.**[122] stram.[5] stront-c.[5] sul-ac. ***sulph.***[30] ***tarent.*** thuj.[10] verat. zinc.[137]

Grief; boisterous: nat-m.[137]

Grief; business, when thinking of his, in morning: ***puls.***[54]

Grief; complaining, with: caust.[30]

Grief; condition, about his: staph.

Grief; consequences, about: **STAPH.**[54]

Grief; constant and chronic: ***graph.***[30]
Grief; deception, from: **AUR.**[162] **<u>IGN.</u>**[122] lach.[30] **LYC.**[162] merc.[30] **<u>NAT-M.</u>**[122] ***nux-v.***[162] op.[162] ph-ac.[30] puls.[30] sep.[162] verat.[162]
Grief; fear at night, with: ***merc.***[54]
Grief; feelings, from wounded: ***cham.***[54] ***ign.***[54]
Grief; financial loss: arn.[137] aur.[137]
Grief; future, for the: mang.[1] nat-c. ***nat-m.*** stann.[1]
Grief; hunting for something to grieve oneself: lil-t.
Grief; jealousy, with: ***hyos.***[54]
Grief; long past offenses: calc.[1]
Grief; losing persons or objects, after: **IGN.**[54]
Grief; neglected duty, over: cycl.[102]
Grief; offenses, from long past: calc.[1] ***cham.***[54] ***ign.***[54] ***op.***[54] ***staph.***[30]
Grief; paralytic state of body and mind, from: phys.[137]
Grief; past events, about: ***plat.***[54]
Grief; prolonged: carc.[207] nat-m.[111] phos.[111]
Grief; punishment, after: ***ign.***[54]
Grief; sensitiveness to: ***cocc.***[54]
Grief; silent: am-m.[54] anthr.[162] apis[117] aq-mar.[231] aur-ar.[58] carc.[146] ***coff.***[54] coloc.[5] crot-c.[36] cycl.[58] ***gels.*** **IGN.** ***indg.***[8] ip.[122] kali-fcy.[198] lach.[5] lap-gr-m.[194] lyc.[5] **<u>NAT-M.</u>**[122] nux-v.[1] peti.[36] ph-ac.[137] ***puls.*** sal-ac.[54]
Grief; silent, anger, after: ***ign.***[54]
Grief; silent, indignation, with: ***coloc.***[54]
Grief; silent, love, with disappointed: **IGN.**[54]
Grief; silent, submissiveness, with: **PULS.**[54]
Grief; undemonstrative: cycl. ***ign.***
Hydrophobia; grief agg.: lyss.[54]
Hypochondriasis; grief, inclined to: **IGN.**[54] **PULS.**[54]
Hysteria; grief, from: bar-s.[58] ***gels.***[54] ***ign.***[54]
Injure; satiety of life, must use self-control to prevent shooting himself: ***nat-s.***
Insanity; black insanity with despair and weariness of life from fear of mortification or of loss of position: calc.[30] ign.[30] puls.[30] rhus-t.[30] staph.[30] sulph.[30] verat.[30]
Insanity; grief, from: **ARS.**[30] **BELL.**[30] ***cocc.***[54] ***plat.***[54]
Irritability; grief, as if a great, weighted on him, five p.m. -six p.m.: ***con.***[54]
Irritability; grief, from: ***kali-br.***[54] mag-c.[116]
Irritability; grief, from, long: carc.[207]
Memory; weakness, grief, after: con.[58] ign.[10]
Prostration; grief, from: ign.[137] **NUX-M.**[137] phys.[137]
Prostration; grief, from long: **IGN.**[54] kali-br.[137]
Quiet disposition; grief, in: ***gels.***[54]
Roaring; grief, after, involuntary: ***ars.***[54]
Sadness; grief, after: am-m.[54] ***aur.***[54] ***ign.***[8] ***nat-m.***[54] ***ph-ac.***[54]
Sadness; grief, with: alum.[54] ***ign.***[54] ***lyc.***[54]
Sighing; grief, with: acet-ac.[85] ail.[162] **CIMIC.**[54] ***iber.***[102] ign.[5] nat-m.[102] orni.[120] ***puls.***[102]
Talk; indisposed, grief, during: peti.[36]
Talk; sleep, in, grief, after: ***anac.***[54]
Tranquillity; alternating with, sorrowfulness: cann-s.[60] casc.[60] graph.[60] nit-ac.[60] petr.[60] plat.[60] sep.[60] zinc.[60]
Vivaciousness; alternating with, sorrow: tarent.
Vivaciousness; evening, grief, changes to: calc-s.[36]
Weeping; thought of others grief at her own death: lap-c-b.[194]
ACET-AC. He, 6 - Anxiety; grieves about his sickness and his children.

ADAM. Sh, 387 - Got terribly distressed. Sharp and keen sense of grief (over past issues) with a lot of words. 18, 30C, 05:XX:XX
AM-M. Ha, 2 - Anxious and melancholy, as if internal grief or sorrow were gnawing in her heart.
ARS. Ha, 3 - Sad, sorrowful ideas, in the evenings in bed, as if some misfortune (disaster, accident) might have happened to one's relatives.
AUR-M. He, 17 - Ailments from violent chagrin.
AUR. Ha, 353 - He imagines he has forfeited (penalty, lost,) the affections of others, and this grieves him to tears.
He, 79 - Ailments from grief, disappointed love.
BAR-A. Al, 5 - Grief at every trifle.
CALC-P. He, 19 - Ailments from grief, disappointed love.
CALC. Al, 16 - Sorrowful and peevish; she looked upon everything from the worst side, and imagined everything evil.
Ha, 3 - Mournful (grief), almost to tears, with solicitous occupation with the present and the future.
Ha, 9 - Grief and complains over insults long past.

Ha, 56 - Aversion, dislike and repugnance to most men.

CARB-V. Ha, 9 - He felt like weeping, everything seemed to him dreadful (fearful), and he felt in despair.

CARBN-O. Al, 11 - After supper, felt buoyant (happy) and in good humor, an effect never produced by tea; this mental sensation soon passed over into an irritable and sarcastic one, so that I sharply criticized an article in a medical journal, which a few hours ago I hardly thought worth that trouble, and threw away in disgust a book of reference as flat and superficial, which I highly sluggish.(inactive)

CIC. Ha, 237 - Depreciation and contempt of mankind; he fled (desert) his fellow-creatures, was in the highest degree disgusted with their follies (stupidity), and his disposition seemed to change into misanthropy; he withdrew into solitude.

CLEM. Al, 14 - He seemed oppressed by some grief or sorrow, or the shadow of impending misfortune.

COCC. He, 22 - Great sorrowfulness, with constant inclination to sit in a corner buried in thought.

He, 25 - Melancholy and sadness, with weeping and constant profound absorption in sorrowful thoughts; great apprehensive anxiety of conscience, and feeling at heart as after committing a wicked deed (act), with desire to escape.

He, 33 - Tearful chagrin about least trifle.

He, 42 - Ill effects of anger and grief. (ailments from)

COLCH. He, 15 - Ailments from grief of misbehavior of others.

COLOC. He, 13 - Indignation, with silent internal grief.

CON. He, 35-...a great grief weighed upon him, with paralyzed feeling in all the limbs, indifference and taking no interest in anything.

COP. Al, 2 - Disgust (loathing) with life, and at the same time fear of death.

CYCL. Al, 10 - Internal grief and anxiety of conscience, as though he had not done his duty, or had committed a crime.

Ha, 196 - Inward grief and anxiety of conscience, as if he had not done his duty or had committed a crime.

He, 23 - Ailments from inward grief and terrors of conscience.

DIG. Ha, 4 - Tearful sorrow (grief) over many things which have failed (disappointment, frustration) with him.

FORM. Al, 7 - Sudden and unexpected return of sense of mortification and grief, with vivid recollection of circumstances long since passed, which had caused great mortification and pain, and which had rendered several years of his life unhappy; this was caused by the transactions (doing) of a near relative; this grief continues...

GELS. He, 33 - Effects (ailments from) of grief; cannot cry; when thinking of his symptoms (disease), also when spoken to of his loss ; >from diverting talk; oppression and palpitation of heart; feels a sense of peril (danger, harm, risk) ; face flushed; sleeplessness; subdued (subjugate, yielding) manner; ...

GRAPH. Al, 12 - Grief about the slightest occurrences (trifle), even to despair.

Ha, 7 - Very much disposed to grieve and to weep, in the evening; while in the morning, contrary to her wont, she laughs (smile) at every trifle.

Ha, 8 - Mournfulness (sorrowful), with nothing but thoughts of death.

Ha, 6 - Grief even to despair, about the most trifling matters.

He, 27 - Ailments from grief.

HALI-L. Sh, 216 - Had an extreme emotional shift about my Dad and what he did to me in the past. Cried and cried and cried. Went into a deep place of far past stuff that I've rarely talked about. Surprised, because I didn't think I had anything to say. Went to co-counseling feeling happy and suddenly started crying. I was focused while I was crying. I had to tell everything and not stop until I was done, even though it went overtime. A part of me was above myself crying, watching me crying. 08, 30C, 21:XX:XX

HYDROG. Sh, 15 - I felt in the presence of a totally pure energy, like meeting God and feeling totally unworthy or like meeting a lover and feeling unworthy — realizing all the mistakes of a lifetime. This pure energy was around for some time protecting me. I feel this unification cleared out lifetimes of symptomatology for me. The joining with this energy was as if a male energy joined with me sexually, but with no desire, pleasure or pain involved. This unification with the male energy lasted quite a few days — I'm not used to seeing myself as a man. The morning after this unifying with the higher presence, I collapsed in emotional overflow. All my grief and pain came out. I was doubled upon the floor and went into a deep state of catharsis. It is not possible to describe where I went as there are no concepts applicable. I felt overflowing love for humanity and wanted to give everything away. My mind turned to the Buddha. It was like seeing the complete picture instead of fragmented bits. (These primary effects lasted about 28 days, then changing to a paranoia state). 16, 30C, 07.XX.XX

HYOS. He, 64 - Serious illness (ailments) from jealousy and grief about faithless lover;...

He, 66 - A gentle, lovable woman became extremely jealous of her husband, and although fully realizing that she did him injustice, she was so filled with grief that she found no rest day or night... (remorse)

IGN. He, 22 - Melancholia from suppressed mental sufferings, with much sighing; desire to be alone (solitude) so as to give way to her real or imaginary grief; weeps bitterly.

He, 37 - Tears wept inwardly, the pain and penalty (forfeit) of unrequited (unrecompensed) love; desires solitude so that one may nourish inward grief;...

He, 61 - Melancholia after great grief and domestic trouble; complete sleeplessness; suicidal thoughts and desire to escape.

He, 62 - Ill effects (ailments) from hearing bad news; from vexation with reserved displeasure ; from grief, or suppressed mental sufferings; of shame and disappointed love.

He, 27 - Unhappy love with silent grief.

He, 30 - Became bilious, nervous, depressed, and would scarce move from the fire, for days together. Morbid grief

He, 55 - Anger, followed by quiet grief or sorrow.

IP. He, 13 - Ailments from vexation (worry) and reserved displeasure.

IRID. Sh, 344 - Feels like I have lost something, feels like I am grieving. It is a bit of a swine really. I11

KALI-BR. Al, 19 - Painful sadness, profound indifference, and almost disgust for life.

He, 31-...religious delusions and feeling of moral deficiency; ...profound indifference and almost disgust for life.

LACH. He, 34-...repugnance to society and dislike to talk; solicitude about future, whith disgust of life; inclination to doubt everything; mistrusts (suspicious) and misconstrues (misjudge) ...[0] Melancholia.

LOB-S. He, 2 - Bad effects from grief.(ailments from)

LYC. He, 39 - Ailments from fright, anger, mortification, or vexation, with reserved displeasure.

MED. Al,N-43 - Forgetful, cannot remember the least thing any length of time; writes everything down of any importance; cannot trust herself to remember it; great irritability and disgust with life.

MERC. He, 35 - Grief, with fear at night: disposition to quarrel; complaining of relations and surroundings. (living conditions)

He, 35 - Grief, with fear at night; disposition to quarrel; complaining of relations and surroundings.

NAT-M. Al, 47 - Full of grief; he tormented himself; he seemed to prefer disagreeable thoughts, which prostrated him very much.

Ha, 8 - He sorrowfully torments (torture) himself, by continually looking for disagreeable ideas, which weakens him.

Ha, 5 - Melancholy dejection and sorrowful anxious despondency all day, without any known cause, with unceasing palpitation,...

He, 48 - Consequences (ailments) of fright, anger, vexation, mortification, or reserved displeasure.

He, 6 - Tries to recollect past disagreeable occurrences for the purpose of thinking on them and indulging (suffer) the grief which it causes.

NUX-M. Al, 32 - Many ridiculous or extravagant acts or expressions, like idiocy, while she seemed perfectly conscious, and at the next moment would appear chagrined at her conduct, and said she could not control her actions...

He, 24 - Fitful mood, changing from deepest sorrow to most frolicsome (happy) behavior; now grave (serious), now gay.

NUX-V. Ha, 1248 - Wrapped up in sorrow and care.

OP. He, 30 - Grief over insults is followed by convulsions.

PH-AC. He, 11 - Ailments from care, grief, sorrow, chagrin, homesickness; or disappointed love;...

PHOS. Al, 90 - Apprehensive, as if were grieving about something, frequently recurring.

Ha, 17 - Apprehension, as if she was grieved about something, frequently recurring.

PSOR. Al,N-26 - Greatest despondency (grief), making his own life and that of those about him intolerable;...

PULS-N. Al, 3 - Great depression of spirits, in the afternoon; a kind of homesickness, with despondency. (grief)

PULS. He, 19 - Silent mood; inclined to silent grief with submissiveness.

He, 51 - Sinks into a condition of sadness and despondency (grief) from disagreeable news.(ailments from)

RAN-B. Al, 7 - The objects of his feelings, for instance, chagrin, occupy his mind long after the occurrence took place; one sees that he is thinking of those things; he talks to himself, gesticulates in his anger...

RHUS-T. He, 18 - Disgust of life: thoughts of suicide; wants to drown (immerse) himself; with fear of death: with desire to die, without sadness.

ROB. Al, 13 - Hypochondriac grief; he seeks pleasures and tries to divert his mind, without succeeding.

SEP. Al, 36 - The greatest loathing of life; it seemed to him as if he could not endure so miserable an existence any longer, and as if he would pine away (longing, wanting) if he did not kill himself. (pine = intense longing or grief)

Ha, 37 - Sorrowful mood, as after secret vexation.

SIL. Ha, 16 - Internal surfeit (satiety) of life.

STAPH. He, 7 - Suffering from pride, envy (spite) or chagrin (shame, dishonor) .

He, 12 - Ailments from indignation and vexation, or reserved displeasure ;sleeplessness.

SULPH. He, 33 - Sleepless, disgusted with life, fears the future, where she sees nothing but misery (wretchedness, poverty) and suffering (misfortune). 0 Melancholia.

He, 37 - Great dejection,(grief), with thoughts of suicide; feels inferior (mediocre, lower) to everybody; can decide nothing;...

TARENT. Al, 40 - Excessive grief, accompanied in the afternoon by thoughts of death.

GROW

Confusion of mind; inflated, as if: merl.[36]

Delusions; body, abdomen, fallen in, his stomach devoured, his scrotum swollen: **SABAD.**

- body, arms, enlarged: lap-c-b.[194]
- body, arms, forearm is enlarged: aran.[36]
- body, arms, reach the clouds when falling asleep: pic-ac.
- body, back, opens and wings are forming: choc.[222]
- body, covered whole, bed: pyrog
- body, covered whole, earth: cann-i.
- body, enlarged: arg-n.[139] bell.[139] bov.[123] caj.[123] cench.[58] cic.[139] hydrog.[222] lap-c-b.[194] mim-p.[149] op.[1] par.[139]
- body, enlarged, right side: cann-i.[36]
- body, expanded, is: xan.[85]
- body, expanded, is, convulsions, before: arg-n.[91]
- body, eyelashes are enlarged: cann-i.
- body, eyes, enlarged, are: bell. levo.[149] op.
- body, fingernails seem as large as plates during drowsiness: cann-i.
- body, fingers, longer: kali-n.[1] tab.[5]
- body, hand, enlarged: choc.[222] lap-c-b.[194]
- body, head, enlarged, is: acon. ***bapt.***[116] berb.[116] ***bov.***[116] caj.[123] cann-i. ***gels.***[116] glon.[116] kali-ar. lap-c-b.[194] mang.[116] meph.[116] nux-m.[116] ***par.***[116] pip-m.[116] ***plat.***[162] sil.[1] zinc.
- body, head, forehead is swelling suddenly, during headache, before convulsions: bac.[55]
- body, head, longer, back of: choc.[222]
- body, legs, growing larger and longer: ***plat.***[54]
- body, neck is too large: kali-c
- body, nose, longer, is: choc.[222] ***glon.***[54] ***verat.***[54]

- body, parts, enlarged: acon.[116] alum. anh.[149] aran.[116] bad.[137] bapt.[47] bell.[8] bov.[116] cann-i.[58] carb-v.[58] ***hyos.*** mang.[116] nux-m.[116] op. pic-ac. stram.
- body, parts, enlarged, growing too long, as if: kali-br.[85]
- body, parts, thick, are: acon.[102]
- body, scrotum is swollen: sabad.
- body, toes, longer: thuj.[111]
- diminished, everything in room is, while she is tall and elevated: plat.
- enlarged: acon. agar.[102] alum. apis[36] aran.[102] ***arg-n.***[102] asaf.[102] atro.[102] bapt.[102] bell. berb. bov.[102] caj.[85] **CANN-I.** coc-c. euph. ferr.[36] ***gels.***[102] glon. hoit.[72] hydrog.[222] ***hyos.***[102] kali-br.[85] laur. nat-c. nux-v. ***op.*** par.[102] pic-ac. ***plat.*** sabad. stram. zinc.
- enlarged, everything is: euph.[102]
- enlarged, he is: aur.[139] op. pall. plat. pyrog. staph.[1] stram.
- enlarged, he is, entering the house after walking, on: plat.
- enlarged, objects are: acon.[102] agar.[102] ***anh.***[144] ***arg-n.***[102] atro.[102] bov.[102] **CANN-I.** ***gels.***[102] glon.[102] ***hyos.***[102] nux-m. op.[102] par.[102]
- enlarged, objects are, diminished and, letters are: ***anh.***[122]
- enlarged, objects are, diminished, and: ***anh.***[122]
- enlarged, persons are: cann-i. caust. tub.
- enlarged, surroundings seemed: ferr.
- expanding, passers-by are: cann-i.
- faces, elongated: stram.
- faces, grow larger: acon. aur.
- faces, reaching the clouds, when falling asleep: pic-ac.[36]
- figures, rising out of earth: stram.[5]
- images, increasing and decreasing, sees: nit-ac.[1]
- images, rising out of the earth: stram.
- large, he or she is too: pyrog. staph.[1] stram.
- large, he or she is too, entering the house after walking, on: plat.
- large, surroundings are too: ferr.
- large, to grow too: kali-br.[56]
- longer, things are: berb. camph. dros. kreos. nit-ac. sulph. zinc.[116]
- space, expansion of.: cann-i. nux-m.[122]
- spectres, sees, morning on waking, a spectre continues to enlarge until it disappears: dulc.
- swollen, is: acon.[102] ***aran.***[102] ***arg-n.***[102] asaf.[102] bapt.[102] ***bov.***[102] ***cann-i.*** carbn-s. glon.[102] op.[102] plat.[102]
- tall, has grown, while walking: pall.
- tall, things, objects grow taller: berb.[10] camph. dros. kreos. nit-ac. sulph.
- tall, things, objects grow taller, pulse is throbbing, as the: camph.[10]
- tall, things, objects grow taller, pulse is throbbing, as the, diminish, and: berb.[10]
- water, lake, a spoonful of water is a: agar.

Dreams; animals, growing quick, has to destroy them, sticks them into the toilet: ozone[227]

- ➤ body, face, swollen: kali-n.[10]
- ➤ body, swollen: squil.
- ➤ excrescencies: hydrog.[222] mez.[10]
- ➤ growing things: choc.[222] kreos.[10]
- ➤ large, of growing: ferr.[36]
- ➤ things, growing: kreos.[10]
- ➤ throat grows up: xan.[85]
- ➤ unsuccessful efforts to, talk, large tongue which extended out of her mouth and up her nose, on account of: tab.[36]

ACON. Al,S-2 - Some few hallucinations, such as imagining his head was three times its original size.

ADAM. Sh, 528 - Feeling as if right side bigger than the left. 16, 12C, 05:03:55

Sh, 527 - Walking lopsided, sensation as if right side is elongated. 16, 12C, 00:13:20

BELL. He, 86 - Sensation of floating or gliding along, as if in a boat; as if the body, or part of it was greatly enlarged.

BERB. Al, 3 - Anxious mood, with great fear and fright...; in the twilight some dogs and children appeared as large again as natural.

CANN-I. Al, 64 - Imagines he is gradually swelling, his body becoming larger and larger.

He, 15-...he is gradually swelling, his body becomes larger and larger; that someone calls him; that he hears numberless bells ringing most sweetly; imagines he hears music; shuts his eyes, and is lost for some time in the most delicious thoughts and dreams.

CHOC. Sh, 23 - A sensation of my back being larger and wider than what I know it to be. The sensation developed so that it seemed that my back moved higher up

and outwards towards the scapula —as if opening out.
Sh, 310 - On bending my head back, a sensation, or imagination, that the back of my head is horribly elongated. I can't get it out of my mind.15, 30C, 03:13:30
DULC. Al, 3 - She wakes early, as if called and sees the form of a ghost, which keeps enlarging until it disappears.
GERM. Sh, 129 - Felt not enough space in bed. It's a big bed. I felt spacy, out of focus, odd, slightly, not there. Maybe in a dream. 05 , 6C, 06.00.00
Sh, 186 - While walking felt round-shoulder like a bodybuilder, worse after rising. 15, 30C,
GLON. He, 6 - The chin (jaw) feels too long.
HALI-L. Sh, 11 - Sensation that my right leg was lengthening. 16, 10C, 00:XX:XX
Sh, 722 - Looking out the window, on waking, and a huge bird outside the window. Birds look bigger than they really are. 20, 30C, 00:23:50
Sh, 889 - I'm ripping all my clothes. I'm so much fatter that I'm not aware of my width, and I'm catching on things. 20, 30C, 10:XX:XX
HYDROG. Sh, 166 - Sensation of being larger. 10, 200C, 11:XX:XX
IRID. Sh, 88 - Forgot to race downhill again. Voice sounded deeper. My immediate reaction, "Oh God, I'm turning into a man." Felt I was overwhelming colleague so didn't ask if I really was. I seemed to take up a lot of space in the room so I drew back and left. G5
Sh, 89 - Sensation as if tall. Q3
Sh, 90 - Feeling extremely tall. Feeling as if kitchen table too low. Q6
Sh, 98 - Feeling as if my right and left were equal, previously feeling as if my right side bigger. Q1
KALI-AR. He, 2 - Thought her head felt larger.
NEON. Sh, 10 - Walking up a long gradual incline, I felt every stride was covering great distances. I felt I was doing the usual 20 minute walk in seconds. I felt like a titan in 7 - league boots, but then I couldn't decide which league boots they were and I wanted an even number. My thoughts went titan-titanium-uranium-Uranus-clouds-clouds-where is the sky? 20, 6C, 01:12:20
Sh, 14 - After a shower, I felt enormous, massive, yet in proportion. I was amazed at how huge I was. 20, 6C, 03:00:00
Sh, 15 - I've been feeling huge the last few days, due to eating biscuits. Feel like my legs have gone all fleshy. 02, 6C, 07:XX:XX
NUX-V. He, 39 - Mania puerperalis...constantly complaining, criticizing or explaining, ... as soon she recognized physician she spoke of imperfection of medical knowledge and declared it an error that one could not live without a heart, inasmuch as she felt very well without one, it having come away with the afterbirth to which it had grown fast, the nurse having separated the two before her eyes; complains of her husband, says he wishes to convince her she is sick, ... nymphomania,... frequently sips at a bowl of warm sugar- water, declaring it will form her a new heart; .(health, healing)...(expert)
PALL. He, 3 - When walking in street in evening, it seems to him as if he had grown taller. (enlarged, grow)
PHOS. Al, 86-...; a feeling of dread (fear), as if awaiting something terrible, yet unable to resist or move (terrifying, scaring), overcame me; sometimes it seemed as if I was beginning to bloat (inhalant, inflate, vanity?), and then I could hear a multitude of voices saying in high glee, "Fill him up a little more and he will burst," (blow up) followed by demoniacal laughter, which made the cold chills run over me... I imagined myself an aurora borealis, and could distinctly hear voices shouting, "Beautiful! Oh, was not that splendid?"...
SABAD. Al, 2 - He imagines all sorts of strange things about his own body, for instance, that it had shrunk (dry, wrinkled) like that of dead persons (corpse), that his stomach was corroded (degeneracy, decomposition), that the scrotum was swollen (enlarged), etc.;...
STRAM. Ha, 565 - Nowhere has he rest, is startled by dream-pictures, even when his eyes are open, which in the form of big dogs, cats and other horrible beasts, grow (expand) out of the ground at his side, and from which he jumps away to the side with signs of terror (fear), and knows not how to save (rescue, free) himself. (cornered, corralled)

HALF

Delusions; body, alive, only half alive: crot-h.[36]
- body, halves, left half does not belong to her: sil.
- body, one half cut off: ***stram.***[54]
- body, smaller, left side of body is: cinnam.
- companions are half men, half plants: cann-i.
- cut through, he is: ***stram.***
- cut, two, in: ***bell.***[30] plat. stram.[30]
- cut, two, in, could not tell of which part he had possession on waking: thuj.
- divided, two parts, into: anac.[162] ***bapt.*** bell.[30] cann-i. lil-t.[36] ozone[227] petr. plat. puls. sil. stram. thuj.
- insane, he is, half: sanic.[139]
- side, alive on one side and buried on the other, he is: stram.
- side, own her left, she did not: sil.

Dreams; cars, automobiles, of, split in half, passing houses: hydrog.[222]
- ➤ wedding, repeated, has to be, since only one half of the body has been married: bamb-a.[1184]

CHOC. Sh, 306 - Her usual sensation of left right body split has been much more defined. Later on during the proving this "split" became more balanced than usual and felt much more integrated, (curative).[13], 12C, 02:XX:XX

CROT-H. He, 13 - Marked indifference, seems only half alive; utter apathy.

CYCL. Al, 28-...he constantly feels as though he had just suffered from an overwhelming (remarkable) affliction; only when he becomes excited is his mind somewhat clearer, and then he acts like one who has just awakened from slumber (sleep), and only half understands what is going on about him.

HALI-L. Sh, 928 - I'm only half aware. When I was doing things wrong, I was half aware I was doing them. 20, 30C, 14:XX:XX

NEON. Sh, 4 - I have been living without a partner for 10 years, which I really enjoyed. Now I have an uncomfortable feeling of needing a partner. Usually I only want a partner because I have so much that I want to share it. This is a feeling of only being half and needing another. 20, 6C, 01:03:40

Sh, 6 - Occasional thoughts about numbers: I had always felt comfortable with odd numbers. Now, being both gave a whole other dimension. To have had half missing for so long! What is different? From 3 to 1, slight tension. From 2 to 1, effortless natural progression. I had many thoughts on potency. It was important to chose the potency precisely, not to be so random in choosing a 9, 12, 15 etc. 20, 6C, 02:01:02

Sh, 11 - Doing research on Uranus, I found that the planet has a tilt. For 42 years one side is in the dark and then comes into the light for 42 years. Interesting that I am now 43. Uranus feels very near, like a friend. The quasars are much further out and it was a real stretch for me to go so far. 20, 6C, XX:XX:XX

PETR. Ha, 27 - The whole day, he is only half conscious, as if only half alive.

STRAM. Al, 122 - For some days the patient was affected with hallucinations and thought that one side of him was alive, while the other side was buried.

He, 57 - Strange absurd ideas; thinks herself tall, double or lying crosswise; one half of body cut off (divided); bed is full of creases (wrinkle) (disorganization); that he was killed roasted and being eaten.

VIOL-O. Al, 10 - He seems able to recognize only half an idea; he puts it in the proper place but cannot hold to it; he makes great effort to grasp (understand) the other half, but at the same moment half of another incomplete idea presses upon him, and so on; thoughts chase one another, but he always has only half a thought ...

HANGED

Delusions; gallows, of, with fear: ***bell.***
- hang, wants to hang himself: ***ars.***[116]
- hanging, sees persons, beckoning him to cut them loose: ars.[54]
- man, hung himself, saw, who: ars.

Dreams; dead, people, of, friends, recently deceased hanging by the legs before him for hours: coca[36]
- ➤ hung, being: am-m.
- ➤ hung, hanged man falling down an interminable lift shaft: choc.[222]
- ➤ hung, seeing persons: merc-s.[36]

Fear; gallows, of the: ***bell.***
- ✦ hanged, to be: **PLAT.**[122]

Suicidal disposition; hanging, by: **ARS.**[122] aur.[58] ***bell.***[122] carb-v.[30] hell.[58] nat-s. ter.

HARD

Delusions; body, brain, hard, is: mez.[1]
- body, tongue, made of wood: apis.
- building stones, appearance of: thuj.
- comfortable, that he is, while sitting on something hard: psil.[164]
- hard, everything is, while lying or sitting: lyc.[36] petr.[36]
- wood, is made of: eupi.[102] kali-n. petr.[137] rhus-t.[102] ***thuj.***[102]

Dreams; metal, about: bamb-a.[1184]

BELL. Al, 34 - He took a piece of bread for a stone, and threw it far away, laughing violently and running about the room.
He, 80 - The boy ran around room laughing immoderately, desired neither food nor drink; a piece of bread, which he took to be a stone, he threw far from him;...

HALI-L. Sh, 217 - Skin feels softer, a hardness is gone from it. Feels squishier, more pliable. It reminds me of my mother's skin, which gives me the creeps. Not wanting to be like my mother. 09, 6C, 02:XX:XX

MAG-C. Al, 8 - She was very anxious several nights in succession, and the bed felt as hard as though she were lying upon stones,...

PETR. He, 12 - Sensation as if there were a cold stone in heart.(indifferent, careless)

HAUGHTY

Abusive; snub one who differed from him, desire to: hydr.[36]

Boaster, braggart: agn.[162] alco.[36] arn.[30] ars.[30] bell.[30] hydrog.[222] lach.[30] lil-t.[184] lyc.[162] med.[162] merc.[30] nat-m.[30] nux-v.[30] plat.[30] stram.[30] sulph.[189]

Boaster; belongings, toys, about his: sulph.[127]

Boaster; rich, wishes to be considered as: lach.[30] lyc.[30] verat.[30]

Business; talk of, exploits, their: agar.[36]

Deeds; he could do great, as if: cocain.[162] hell.

Delusions; beautiful, rags seem, even: ***sulph.***
- better than others, that he is: germ.[222] lap-gr-m.[194] myric.
- clothes, beautiful, they are: aeth. ***su***lph.
- devils, connected to, he is, arrogant towards those who strive to purity, light and love: ozone[227]
- diminished, everything in room is, while she is tall and elevated: plat.
- distinguish, squanders money, proud of his position: ***verat.***[54]
- distinguished, is: lap-mar-c.[194] phos.[1] stram. verat.
- humility and lowers of others, while he is great: germ.[222] plat. staph.
- inferior, on entering house after a walk, people seem mentally and physically: plat.
- knowledge, he possesses infinite: cann-i. psil.[164] verat-v.[171]
- noble person, he is a: lap-mar-c.[194] phos. plat.[58]
- proud: lach.[10] plat. stram. verat.
- queen, she is a: cann-i.
- rank, he is a person of: cupr. phos. ***stram.***[54] verat.
- superiority, of: germ.[222] lap-gr-m.[194] ***plat.***

Dignity: caj.[25] calc.[36] guare.[25] nat-c.[188] nat-m.[187] staph.[188]

Discouraged; alternating with, haughtiness: agn.
- ➤ glorification of oneself: saroth.[144]
- ➤ women, arrogant, of a, with exaggerated confidence: ozone[227]

Egotism; self-esteem, over-estimation of him self: cic.[137]

Egotism; self-esteem, reciting their exploits: agar.[36]

Exclusive, too: calc.[30] nat-m.[30] plat.[30]

Foolish; behavior, happiness and pride: **SULPH.**

Haughty: acon.[5] agar. alum. anac. arn. ars.[189] asar.[162] aur. bac.[56] bell.[102] calc.[30] cann-i. cann-s.[5] carc.[207] ***caust.*** chin. cic. cina[10] coloc.[58] con. cupr. dulc. ferr. ferr-ma. gran.[122] grat.[5] guai. ham. hell.[5] ***hyos.*** ign. ***ip.*** kali-i.[5] ***lach.*** lap-gr-m.[194] lap-mar-c.[194] lil-t.[122] <u>**LYC.**</u>[122] merc. myric.[25] nat-m.[122] nitro-o.[36] nux-v. ***pall.*** par. phos. <u>**PLAT.**</u>[122] puls.[5] rob. sabad. sec. sil.[30] squil. ***staph. stram.*** stront-c. **SULPH.** thuj. **VERAT.**

Haughty; clothing, likes to wear his best: ***con.***[54]

Haughty; fright, after: plat.[54]

Haughty; intelligent, but very: lach.[30] nux-v.[30] ***plat.***[30] verat.[30]

Haughty; introverted, and: lap-gr-m.[194]

Haughty; look self-contented: ferr.[54] ferr-ma.[10]

Haughty; mania, in: ***graph.***[54] ***lach.***[54] **PLAT.**[54] ***verat.***[54] ***verat-v.***[54]
Haughty; pregnancy, during: ***verat.***[54]
Haughty; races, to other: ars.[10] hep.[10] phos.[10] plat.[10] sep.[10]
Haughty; religiousness, with: ***plat.***[54]
Haughty; sick, when: lyc.[102]
Haughty; stiff and pretentious: ***lyc.***[54]
Haughty; stupid and haughty: bell.[30] calc.[30] lyc.[30] plat.[30] stram.[30] verat.[30]
Haughty; weaning, over: grat.[137]
Imbecility; old rags are as fine as silk: **SULPH.**
Importance; feels his, pompous: alco.[36] arn.[5] bell.[5] calc.[137] cann-i.[36] cupr.[5] ferr.[60] ferr-ma.[36] glon.[5] hyos.[60] ***lyc.***[5] phos.[5] **PLAT.**[5] stram.[5] sulph.[5] ***verat.***[5]
Indifference; superiority, with feeling of: ozone[227]
Insanity; haughty: **HYOS.**[5] lach.[10] **LYC.**[5] ***stram.***[5] **VERAT.**[5]
Loquacity; self-satisfied: par.[10]
Presumptuous: arn.[30] calc.[30] ***lyc.***[122] plat.[30] staph.[30]
Religious affections; taciturnity, haughtiness, voluptuousness, cruelty, r. a with: ***plat.***[54]
Vanity: ***bell.***[30] lap-mar-c.[194] lil-t.[137] lyc.[30] ***merc.***[30] nux-v.[30] plat.[30] ***puls.***[30] sulph.[30] ***verat.***[137]
Walk; self-sufficient impression of importance, walks along with a: ferr-ma.[36]
Walk; slowly and dignified, walks: caj.

ACT-SP. He, 4 - Self-deception; self-satisfaction.

ALOE. Al, 9 - Contented with his station (position, rank) in life; it involuntarily occurs to him, that he is really much better off than many other people.

CAJ. Al,S-60 - Want to walk in a low and a very dignified (nobility, honored, proud, refined) manner, and prefer to walk alone.

CIC. Al, 26 - Contempt and scorn for mankind; he avoided them, abhorred their follies (stupidity) excessively, and his disposition seemed to tend towards misanthropy; he withdrew (retire) himself into solitude.

CUPR. He, 6 - Craziness (insanity); attacks with savage malice (evil), with proud (arrogant) bearing (posture),...

FERR-MA. Al-S, 1 - Walking along with a self-sufficient impression of importance.

FERR. He, 17 - Haughtiness; proud, self-contented look.

GRAT. He, 9 - Mental troubles from overweening (presumptuous, arrogant, haughty) pride. (ailments)

HALI-L. Sh, 580 - Spent most of today thinking about how I am surrounded by idiots, (my family), who are showing no attempts to think for themselves, letting me run the show. They don't care to figure things out. I'm in hyper-drive. I know a lot and I'm right. I've been extremely productive or at least active, balancing several major projects all at the same time, and they can't seem to tidy a table properly. This includes my husband, who continually interrupts me (or so it seems) for some trivial question. I'm coming across with too much force. I find myself shouting at everyone much more than usual. Like a crazy person. Impatient over others' slowness. Almost an arrogance. I want them to THINK! (Obviously, the way I do). or get off the ship and drown yourself. A hard anger, more intense that usual. Feel like leaving them all—they just take and give back little. More trouble than support. This isn't complaining or victimizing talking. This is how it is. I'm healing myself and leaving my family in the dust. I've passed on to them my bad habits, bad parenting. They are content to be idiots. 09, 6C, 13:XX:XX

Sh, 610 - Want to stay in integrity with myself and not run after my lover. We talked about commitment and she got scared. I got angry. This is it. I told her I'm not going all over the place with you. Want you XX per cent here. Feel angry at her indecision and confusion. Feel I want to hit and shake her. Ran on the beach instead. 02, 30C, 02:09:XX

HAM. Al, 1 - Feeling that she ought (have) to be reverenced (honored, venerated) by all around her and have great respect (regard) paid to her opinions; lasting about an hour.

LACH. He, 16 - Most extraordinary loquacity, making speeches in very select (finest, excellent) phrases (pretentious), but jumping off to most heterogeneous subjects; at the same time proud (haughty), full of mistrust. 0Mania.

He, 51 - Proud; jealous, suspicious; developing into mania.

LYC. Al, 2 - Delirious, raging, envious, reproachful, presumptuous, and imperious.

Ha, 59 - Insanity and fury, breaking out in envy, pretensions (inflated) and ordering (dictatorial) others about.

He, 37 - Haughty, reproachful and overbearing.(despotic)

LYSS. Al, 2 - Exaltation; thinks he has something of importance.

Al,N-33-...Thinks he is a man of great authority.(power, command, expert)

He, 33 - Makes speeches in delirium; thinks he is a man of great authority.

PLAT. Ha, 35 - Illusion of the imagination; on entering the room after walking for an hour, everything around her seemed very small and all persons physically and bodily inferior to her, but she herself great and lofty (distinguish, elevated) in body;...

Ha, 36 - Contemptuous, pitying looking down on people at other times respected, with a certain disdain (scorn, arrogance), in paroxysms, against her will. (antagonism)

Ha, 38 - Haughty, proud feelings.

He, 8 - Arrogant, reserved, absent-minded.

He, 9 - Pride (haughty) and overestimation of one's self, looking down with haughtiness on others.

He, 10 - Cold, haughty, too well satisfied with one's self, and not at all anxious about the future. (presumptuous, egotistic, inexpugnable, safe)

He, 41 - Delirium, with fear of men (people); often changing, with overestimation (haughty) of oneself.

He, 40 - Disturbed state of mind; religious, with taciturnity, haughtiness, voluptuousness (sensual) and cruelty.

He, 42 - Mania; with great pride; fault-finding; unchaste (sensual) talk; ...(chaste = moral, pure)

He, 49 - Affections from pride. (ailments from)

He, 50 - Puerperal mania...assumed or seemed to feel herself a person of great superiority;...

ROB. Al, 12 - Anxiety to seek honors (distinction) ; excessive pride (haughtiness, arrogance) ; he considers himself better than an emperor.

STAPH. He, 7 - Suffering from pride, envy (spite) or chagrin (shame, dishonor) .

He, 14-...; was insulted (slandered, defamed, calumniated) being too dignified (reserved, lordly,) to fight (contest), subdued (control) his wrath(anger) and went home sick,.. (ailments, from offenses)

STRAM. He, 92 - Mania:... complains that a dog is biting and tearing flesh off his chest; merry exaltation; with pride (haughty) and affectation; runs about, complains of violent headache; ...;steals from his roommates...; disposition to scold persons whom he otherwise loved.

SULPH. He, 11 - Foolish happiness and pride(haughtiness),thinks himself in possession of beautiful (attractive) things; even rags seem beautiful. (rank, position, distinction)

VERAT. Al, 4 - He imagines that he is a prince (noble) and behaves in a very haughty manner. (proud, arrogant)

Ha, 672 - He pretends (simulate, feigning) he is a prince, and gives himself airs (affectation, pretentious) accordingly.

He, 11 - Thinks himself distinguished (classify) ; squanders (futile) his money; proud (haughty) of his position.

He, 4 - Erroneous and haughty notions.

HEALING

Anxiety; future, disease, and of her: kali-c.[54]

Anxiety; health, despair of getting well: ***ars.***[54]

Anxiety; health, recovery, concerning: ***ph-ac.***[54]

Death; desires, convalescence, during: absin. ***aur.*** lac-c. sep.

Desires; recover, to: sec.[36]

Despair; recovery, ague, in: ***tarent.***[54]

Despair; recovery, convalescence, during: **ALUM.**[122] **ARS.**[122] **CALC.**[122] ***psor.*** **SYPH.**[122]

Despair; recovery, of: ***acon.*** all-s.[36] alum.[5] am-c.[10] anac.[137] ant-t.[36] **ARS.** aur-ar.[58] aur-i.[58] ***aur-s.***[58] bac.[62] bapt. bar-c. bor.[10] ***bry.*** cact.[58] calad.[10] **CALC.** calc-ar.[58] calc-s. cann-i. carc.[207] caust.[30] cham. chlol. cimic.[149] **COLOC.**[162] dig.[172] germ.[222] ***hell.*** hep.[30] hura ***ign.***[122] kali-ar. kali-br. kali-c. kreos. lac-c.[116] lach.[10] lil-t.[172] lyc.[1] m-arct.[10] mag-c.[144] ***med.***[72] ***merc.***[30] nat-c.[10] nat-m.[10] nat-s. nit-ac.[58] nux-v. ph-ac.[10] phos.[10]

plat.[172] ***psor.*** puls.[10] ***sep.*** sil. sulph.[10] **SYPH.**[122] ther. ***thyr.***[162] verat.[58] zinc.
Despair; recovery, thinks it is useless to take medicine: ars.[102]
Doubtful; recovery, climacteric period, during: sars.[54]
Dreams; body, arm, cauterizing: bomb-pr.[36]
Fear; death, convalescence, during: tarent.[54]
Impatience; cures him at once, the patient insists that the doctor: cham.[85]
Indifference; recovery, about his: ars.[1] aur-m-n.[162] ***calc.***
Indifference; well, to getting: ***calc.***[54]
Mood; repulsive, medicine, to take the: ***arn.***[122] calad.[137] cimic.[58] hyos. ***kali-p.***[54] **LACH.**[122] ***stram.***[54] tub.[160] ***verat-v.***[54] visc.[119]
Mood; repulsive, medicine, to take the, religious insanity, in: ***kali-p.***[54]
Mood; repulsive, treatment, every: bell.[30] caust.[30] lach.[30] plat.[30]
Mood; repulsive, treatment, every, sick, in spite of being very: ars.[30] caust.[30] nux-v.[30]
Sadness; disease, about, sure he would not recover, in bronchial asthma: ***sin-n.***[54]
Tranquillity; fears she would not recover, yet, during climacteric period: sars.[54]

HEALTH

Anger; recovery, if one spoke of her complete: ***ars.***[36]
Anxiety; health, about: acet-ac. acon. aeth.[162] agar.[54] agn.[162] aloe[37] alum. alum-p.[58] alum-sil.[58] am-c.[36] androc.[222] ant-t.[36] ***arg.*** arg-n. arn. ars. ars-h.[54] aur-m.[162] bar-c.[187] bell.[10] blatta[152] bor.[10] bov.[162] brom.[116] bry. bufo[36] ***calad.***[122] ***calc.*** calc-ar.[58] calc-f.[103] ***calc-p.***[162] calc-s. calc-sil.[58] cand-a.[239] cann-i.[162] canth.[10] carc.[187] ***chin-ar.***[54] choc.[222] cocc. cop.[36] cub.[36] cupr.[10] euph.[60] germ.[222] glon.[116] grat. hyos.[10] ign. **KALI-AR.** kali-br.[137] kali-c. kali-m.[192] kali-p. kali-sil.[58] kreos.[5] lac-c. lach. lob.[10] ***lyc.*** m-arct.[10] mag-m. med.[162] merc.[10] morg.[136] nat-c. nat-m.[10] nat-p. **NIT-AC.** nux-m. nux-v. ozone[227] ***ph-ac.***[122] **PHEL.**[162] ***phos.*** podo.[116] psor. ***puls.***[122] ruta[152] sel.[116] ***sep.*** sil. spong.[54] staph. sulph.
Anxiety; health, careful about health, therefore very: calad.[54] ***calc.***[54]
Anxiety; health, despair of getting well: ***ars.***[54]
Anxiety; health, future, in regard to the: ***sep.***[54]
Anxiety; health, loved persons, of: carc.[193] hep.[30] merc.[30]
Anxiety; health, recovery, concerning: ***ph-ac.***[54]
Anxiety; health, relatives, little concerned about his own: cocc.[54]
Anxiety; ill, as if he would be: ph-ac.[36] ***podo.***[54] tarent.[36]
Brooding; condition, illness, over one's: aur.[114] kali-p.[58] ***ph-ac.***[1]
Delusions; abundance, of, destroys clothing: ***sulph.***[54]
• health, he has ruined his: bamb-a.[1184] chel.
Desires; recover, to: sec.[36]
Despair; health, of: calc. staph.
Despair; recovery, convulsions, after: calc.[193]
Despair; recovery, mania, in: ***verat.***[54]
Discontented; health, about: phos.[1]
Dreams; physician: canna[36] mang.[36]
Dwells; health, his broken: aur-m.[58]
Fear; health, ruined her, that she has: calc.[122] chel. staph.[122]
Hopefulness; recovery, of: sang.[54]
Indifference; health, as to his: cocc.[60]
Loquacity; health, about his: **NUX-V.**[122]
Medicine; drugs, desire to swallow large doses of: cact.[36]
Sadness; health, about the: acon.[54] ***sep.***[36] staph.[54]
Talk; health, about his: nux-v.[60]
Talk; indisposed, condition, about her: chel.[36]
Theorizing; health, about: kali-c.[215]
Well; feels very, ill, before falling: bry.[111] helon.[85] nux-v.[111] phos.[111] ***psor.***[111] sep.[111]

ADAM. Sh, 418 - Anxiety regarding acting irresponsibly about my health. "This might affect the rest of my life." 8, 6C, 01:XX:XX
Sh, 425 - Despair about my health. 7, 6C, 31:22:00
Sh, 426 - Feeling proving is major setback to my long term health. 7, 6C, 43:00:XX
Sh, 428 - Despair about health as I feel I am taking a long time to recover and I'm still coughing. 7, 6C, 75:00:XX
HALI-L. Sh, 944 - Big doubts about doing Homeopathy. If you can make people healthy, then the balance must be that someone else gets sicker. 20, 30C, 15:XX:XX

Sh, 953 - Memories triggered off by the sensation in my head back and feet. Twenty three years ago in the States, I fell off a wall and smashed lots of vertebrae together. I was told I would never walk again. At the time, I got an internal explosion in my head opposite to what happened yesterday with the lightning in my vertex. 20, 30C, 18:XX:XX

HYDROG. Sh, 264 - Talking to God about the state of my heart and asking for it to be healed. 16, 30C, XX:XX:XX

HEART

Anger; easily, rheumatism, in cardiac: phos.[54] squil.[54] ***thuj.***[54]

Anguish; angina pectoris, in: aml-n.[25]

Anguish; cardiac: ***acon.***[54] **ARN.**[54] ***ars.***[54] aur.[1] ***bell.***[54] ***carb-v.***[54] ***dig.***[54] **SPONG.**[54]

Anguish; heart complaints, in: aesc.[25]

Anguish; palpitation, with: **ARS.**[36] aur.[54] ***calc.***[54] ***mosch.***[54] plat.[1] ***puls.***[54] ***verat.***[54]

Anxiety; chest, heart, region of: **ACON.** ***aeth.*** agar. alum. alum-p.[58] am-c. ***ambr.*** ***aml-n.*** anac. anh.[119] **ANT-T.** apis ***arg-n.*** arn. **ARS.** ***ars-i.*** aster. **AUR.** aur-ar.[58] aur-i.[58] ***aur-m.*** **BELL.** bov. ***brom.*** bry.[54] ***cact.*** ***calc.*** calc-i.[58] calc-s.[58] **CAMPH.** cann-i.[25] cann-s. ***canth.*** **CARB-V.** ***carbn-o.*** ***carbn-s.*** carl. ***caust.*** **CENCH.** ***cham.*** chel. chin. chin-ar. chin-s. cic. cimic.[25] cina ***cocc.*** ***coff.*** colch. ***con.*** croc. ***crot-c.***[122] ***cupr.*** cycl. ***dig.*** echi. elaps electr.[10] ***euon.*** ***ferr.*** ***ferr-i.*** ferr-p. ***gels.*** ***glon.*** gran. graph. hed.[119] hell. ***helo.***[5] hep.[30] hydr. hydr-ac. hyos. **IGN.** ***iod.*** ***IP.*** ***kali-c.***[5] kali-chl.[58] **KALM.** ***kreos.*** ***lach.*** lachn.[85] ***lact.*** ***lat-m.***[111] ***led.***[5] lob. ***lyc.*** lyss.[172] m-aust.[5] med.[172] **MENY.** ***merc.*** ***merc-c.*** mez. mosch. ***naja*** ***nat-m.***[5] nat-s. nit-ac. ***nux-v.*** olnd. op. ox-ac. petr. **PHOS.** ***plat.*** ***plb.*** ***prun.*** psil.[164] ***psor.*** ***puls.*** pyrog.[58] ran-b. ***rhus-t.*** rob.[172] sabad. salx-n. scol.[36] sec. sep. sil. sol-n.[25] ***spig.*** ***spong.*** stann. staph.[137] stict. stram. sulph. ***tab.*** ***tarent.*** **THER.** thuj. ***verat.*** viol-t. vip.

Anxiety; chest, heart, region of, driving him from place to place: ars.[172] aur.[172]

Anxiety; chest, heart, region of, evil was going to happen, as if something: meny.[137]

Anxiety; chest, heart, region of, fear, with: rhus-t.[10]

Anxiety; chest, heart, region of, grief, from: ***naja***[54]

Anxiety; chest, heart, region of, hurry, with: **NAT-M.**[54]

Anxiety; chest, heart, region of, insupportable, almost, in heart disease: ***ferr-m.***[54]

Anxiety; chest, heart, region of, pain in heart, with: ***aur.***[54] ***kalm.***[54] mill.[54] ***op.***[54]

Anxiety; chest, heart, region of, vexation, after: lyc.

Anxiety; congestion, heart in: nit-ac.[1]

Anxiety; contraction in heart region, from: nit-ac.[1]

Anxiety; heart, about his: hed.[119] xan.[111]

Anxiety; heart, complains of in: **ACON.**[137] arn.[137] ars.[137] ***aur.***[137] calc.[137] carb-v.[137] dig.[137] ign.[137] ip.[137] nux-v.[10] ***phos.***[137] plat.[137] ***puls.***[137] spig.[137] spong.[10] stroph.[137] sulph.[137] ther.[137] verat.[137]

Anxiety; heart, evil was going to happen, as if something: meny.[137]

Anxiety; motion, from, heart disease, in: **DIG.**[54]

Anxiety; sudden, angina pectoris, in: ***tab.***[54]

Brooding; disappointment, cardiac weakness, with: ***ph-ac.***[54]

Cheerfulness; heart disease, laughs, sings and dances: ***nat-m.***[54]

Cheerfulness; heart disease, with: ***cact.***[54]

Company, desire for; angina pectoris, in: ***aur-m.***[54]

Company, desire for; heart, in organic disease of the: ***apis***[54]

Death; conviction of, angina pectoris, in: ***ox-ac.***[54]

Death; conviction of, angina pectoris, in: ***ox-ac.***[54]

Death; conviction of, heart, in organic disease of: ***apis***[54]

Death; presentment of, heart disease, in: ***op.***[54]

Delusions; body, heart, has no: ozone[227]

- body, heart, has no, muscle, only feels a thin: ozone[227]
- body, heart, large, too: bov.[116] lach. sulph.[137]
- body, heart, stops beating, when sitting: ***arg-n.***[54] gels.[162]
- body, heart, turning around, is: aur.
- die, about to, exhaustion, from, heart complaints, in: pop.[139]
- disease, heart disease, has: calc.[1] graph.[5] ***nat-c.***[54] podo.[58]
- disease, incurable, heart: ***phos.***[54]
- heart disease, will have and die: arn.[58] germ.[222] ***kali-ar.***[162] ***lac-c.***[54] lach.[122] podo.[58]

- heart or respiration is going to stop, or otherwise frightens herself causing heart to beat violently: ***lac-c.***[54]
- heart, live without, he can: ***nux-v.***[54]
- heart, stitches in heart will kill him if they do not cease: psor.[54]

Despair; heart disease or liver disease, in: aur.[58]

Dreams; frightful, heart disease, in: ***dig.***[54]

➤ nightmare, left side from neck to knee were jerking up and down like a mass of jelly, as if, this motion extending into chest and centering at heart: gels.[36]

Excitement; heart, organic disease of, in: ***apis***[54]

Excitement; heart, vexation, trembling and fluttering, with, painful to shoulders, in valvular insufficiency: ***lith-c.***[54]

Fear; death, angina pectoris, in: ***acon.***[54] ***dig.***[54] lat-m.[77] squil.[54]

✦ death, anxiety, with, heart and mind, of: ***psor.***[54]

✦ death, anxiety, with, praecordia, about: **ACON.**[8] ***plat.***[54]

✦ death, heart symptoms during, death, of instant, with cardiac distress: ***arn.***[54]

✦ death, heart symptoms during, organic: apis[54]

✦ death, heart symptoms, during: **ACON.**[54] ***ang.***[54] ***arn.***[54] asaf. cact.[58] carb-v.[58] cench.[58] **DIG.**[54] ***naja***[54] ***plat.***[54] ***psor.***[54]

✦ ghosts, praecordial anguish, with: ***plat.***[54]

✦ heart, cease beating, unless, not moving: coca[162] dig.[102]

✦ heart, cease beating, will: both-a.[3070]

✦ heart, cease beating, will, lying down, on: lach.[137]

✦ heart, cease to beating, unless constantly on the move, h. will: ***gels.***

✦ heart, disease of: acon.[52] arg-n.[162] ***arn.***[91] ***aur.*** bapt. cact. ***calc.***[54] calc-p.[162] calc-s.[58] caust.[172] cupr.[210] daph.[36] germ.[222] hed.[119] hydrog.[222] ***kali-ar.***[162] lac-c. lach. ***lil-t.*** lob.[162] meny.[85] mez.[179] nat-m.[162] nux-m.[54] ***phos.***[162] podo.[58] psor.[172] rhus-t.[172] sars.[162] sin-n.[54] ***spong.*** tarent.[172]

✦ heart, disease of, organic: ***apis***[117] ***aur.***[54] calc.[36]

✦ heart, disease of, stitches will kill him if they do not cease: psor.[172]

✦ heart, pain about h., from: daph.

✦ pregnancy, during, praecordia, with anxiety in: **ACON.**[54]

✦ stoppage of circulation, with sensation of, at night, in angina pectoris: ***lyc.***[54]

✦ suffocation, heart disease, in: ***dig.***[122] lach.[162] ***spong.***[122]

Helplessness; feeling of, heart complaints, with: am-c.[1]

Killed; desire to be, stabbing heart, by (after midnight): ***ars.***[36]

Loquacity; excited, heart disease, in: ***op.***[54]

Mania; heart, affected, with: cupr.[54]

Restlessness; angina pectoris, in: ***aur-m.***[54]

Restlessness; sensitive, hysterical people, anomalous functional disorders of the heart: sumb.[54]

Sadness; cardiac rheumatism, in: ***cact.***[54]

Sadness; cardialgia, in: ***kali-c.***[54]

Sadness; disease, about, incurable, of heart, which makes him reckless: ***phos.***[54]

Sadness; heart sensations, from: asaf.[54] lyc.[1]

Sadness; heart sensations, from, oppression: ***caust.***[54]

Sadness; pain, from, heart, in region of: both-a.[139] crot-h.[36]

Shrieking; cardiac rheumatism, in: ***cact.***[54]

Sighing; heart, anxiety in, with: ***plb.***[54]

Sighing; heart, pain in, with: **LYSS.**[54]

Singing; monotonous, in heart disease: ***op.***[54]

Starting; alternating with sadness and faintness of heart: zinc.[10]

Starting; sleep, falling asleep, on, heart failure, as from: op.[1]

Thinking; ailments, of, angina pectoris, in: ***aur-m.***[54]

Unconsciousness; angina pectoris, in: ***arn.***[54] ***chim-m.***[54] ***cimic.***[54]

Vivacious; heart disease, in: ***cact.***[54]

Weeping; anxiety, after, praecordial: **PULS.**[54]

Weeping; heart disease, in: ***aur.***[54] ***op.***[54]

ACON. Ha, 514 - Palpitation of the heart with great anxiety, oppression of the breathing and great weariness (lassitude) in all limbs...

He, 51 - Ailments from fright: afraid (fear) in dark; vertigo; faintness; trembling; cardiac weakness; threatened miscarriage (abortion); impending cessation of menstrual flow;..

He, 53 - Ailments from vexation (worry, care), with fear or vehemence: congestion; palpitation; fever; anxiety, beside himself; threatened miscarriage ; apoplectic congestion.

He, 39 - Fear of death; during pregnancy or confinement; with prolapsus uteri; with great loquacity or anxiety in region of heart.

ACT-SP. He, 13 - Anxiety with urging in heart.

ADAM. Sh, 218 - Red anger with irregularly pounding heart. 2, 12C 73:XX:XX

AETH. He, 15 - Anxiousness sensation as if a heavy load was lying on chest.

ALUMN. Al, 13 - When thinking about his disease, he feels the heart beating.

He, 5 - Thinking about her disease causes palpitation.

AM-C. Ha, 10 - Severe compression of the heart, he knows not how to help himself.

AM-M. Ha, 2 - Anxious and melancholy, as if internal grief or sorrow were gnawing in her heart.

AMBR. Ha, 483 - Sad thoughts take possession of him, with sinking feeling about the heart; he is for a long time depressed in spirits.

APIS. He, 18 - Thinks he will die. 0 Organic disease of heart.

ARG-M. He, 2-...as if he might have an apoplectic stroke, and could not finish this proving; with spasmodic contraction of heart.

ARN. He, 36 - Horror of instant death. With cardiac distress in night.

ARS. Al, 6 - After midnight, a frequent desire to kill himself, by stabbing his heart through and through.

Al, 57 - Anguish from the heart, interrupted by attacks of weakness.

Al-S, 2893 - The whole head sick, the heart faint, she awoke in the morning wretched, her life a burden (load) weariness the day's portion, and each succeeding day like its predecessor, unless (except) physic (laxative) helped her with its little aid.

Ha, 1017 - Precordial anxiety, interrupted by the occurrence of faintings.

Ha, 1034 - Hypochondriac anxiety, ...as if it came from the upper part of the chest; without palpitation of the heart.

He, 89 - Irritable, despondent (despairing) and anxious ; cardiac anxiety, with insupportable pain.

ASAF. He, 8 - With heart symptoms, fear of death.

AUR-M. He, 13 - Insurmountable mental or bodily restlessness; he has to spend hours in street and in open air. 0 Angina pectoris.

AUR. Ha, 350 - Great anxiety that has its origin in the praecordial region; ...

Ha, 6 - Great anxiety springing from the region of the heart, and which drives him from one place to another, so that he cannot long remain in a place. (restlessness)

He, 55 - Great anguish coming from precordial region, and driving him from place to place, so that he can remain nowhere.

CACT. He, 16 - During and after attack, great anxiety, fearing some organic lesion of heart which will cause sudden death.

CALC. Al, 15 - Melancholy, not exactly a sad feeling, about the heart, without cause, with a kind of voluptuous trembling of the body.

Ha, 2 - Melancholy, not really mournful (unhappy) feeling, about the heart, without cause, with a sort of voluptuous tremor all over the body.

Ha, 13 - Anxious at heart, as if he had done wrong,(immoral) or had to apprehend reproaches (deserves), with constant inclination to work.

Ha, 25 - His heart is agitated with fear and anxiety for the future, with fear of consumption.(tuberculosis, ruin)

Ha, 30 - She despairs of her life and believes she has to die (punishment?) ; her heart is sad with weeping, and frequent attacks of sudden, general heat, as if she had hot water poured (flow) over her.

He, 18 - Mental aberration with horrid visions before eyes and cardiac anxiety; he despairs of his salvation (pardon, rescue) and wants to stab himself.

He, 50 - Apprehensive (fearful, worried) mood ; as if some misfortune was about to happen; about his health (vigour) ; that he might have an organic disease of the heart.

He, 61 - Anguish, with palpitation of heart.

CAMPH. Al, 46-... My misery was boundless; time itself was no more; in short, I suffered such fearful anguish as no fancy can comprehend. What soul could paint to itself my everlasting (eternal) dwelling as the Evil One (devil), alone in a vast universe, without faith or hope, and my heart forever broken by unimaginable tortures? (miserable, timeless, endless, solitude, forsaken, faithless, hopeless)

CARB-V. Al, 12 - Anxiety in the evening after lying down, as from oppression of the chest, ...,a sensation as if the heart would be pressed downward; objects about her seem to become constantly narrower and smaller,...

CAUST. He, 36 - Fearfulness and distressed (anguish) feeling about heart.

CHAM. Ha, 458 - He feels a sinking in the precordium; he is beside himself with anxiety,...

CHOC. Sh, 109 - In the night, heart stops beating. All very still inside.

Sh, 114 - When I feel like a hedgehog, my heart is much faster, but when I feel the stillness, I don't feel my heart at all.

Sh, 192 - I woke up and could not feel the usual sensation of my heart bulging or beating through my ribs while lying on my left side. I felt shock and thought 'perhaps I'm dead'. Groped for pulse and was reassured to be able to feel it. 15, 30C, 02:02:XX

COCC. Al, 10 - She is absorbed in the saddest thoughts, and affronts (indignity) sink deep into her heart.

He, 25 - Melancholy and sadness, with weeping and constant profound absorption in sorrowful thoughts; great apprehensive anxiety of conscience, and feeling at heart as after committing a wicked deed (act), with desire to escape.

CON. He, 31 - Great anxiety; precordial anguish; superstitious (careful, credulous, naive) and full of fear (coward), with frequent thoughts of death...

GELS. He, 33 - Effects (ailments from) of grief; cannot cry; when thinking of his symptoms (disease), also when spoken to of his loss ; >from diverting talk; oppression and palpitation of heart; feels a sense of peril (danger, harm, risk) ; face flushed; sleeplessness; subdued (subjugate, yielding) manner; ...

GERM. Sh, 15 - Wake feeling anxious, increasingly. Legs tremble and shake. I have to get out of bed. I am scared that a heart attack is imminent and cannot be prevented. It's to late to do anything. I walk from room to room, thirsty, chilly and in turmoil. Accompanied by a desire for stool and flatulence. 08, 12C, 80:00:00

HALI-L. Sh, 676 - The remedy worked very directly on my will. Fragmentation is the denial of will. Integration is the use of will. All separate states under a unified country. 18, 30C, 35:XX:XX

Sh, 951 - Phoned a friend to hear what I already knew. As I heard the words, I felt a sensation as if hit by a thunderbolt through the vertex, down to hit my heart then spread up and across my shoulders out to my hands. (Drawing shows hands like wing tips). 20, 30C, 17:XX:XX

HELL. Ha, 277 - He could neither sit, stand nor lie, and always pointed to his heart.

HYDROG. Sh, 192 - During palpitations, extreme fear —thought I was having a heart attack. Frightened the living daylights out of me. 24, 30C, 100:XX:XX

Sh, 264 - Talking to God about the state of my heart and asking for it to be healed. 16, 30C, XX:XX:XX

LAC-C. Al,N-28 - Fear of disease; of consumption; of heart disease. (tuberculosis)

Al,N-33 - Depression of spirits, doubts her ability and success, thinks she will have heart disease and die of it.

He, 14-..;sometimes imagines heart or breathing are going to stop, or otherwise frightens himself, and this makes heart beat violently; occasionally very depressed, and fancies he is going out of his mind. (insanity)

He, 26 - Depression of spirits, doubts her ability (competence, aptitude) and success (prospering, progressing, achieving), thinks she will have heart disease and die of it.

LACH. He, 60 - After a jealous quarrel, she put both hands to her chest and cried out "Oh! my heart!" then fell down and was in an asphyctic state for nearly twenty-four hours;...

LIL-T. Al, 15 - Apprehensive as from impending disease or calamity (misfortune); fears insanity; fears heart disease; fears she is incurable; often with moderate or sub acute uterine or ovarian inflammation.

LIPP. Al, 2 - Feeling of great apprehension, while riding in a carriage; a kind of anxiety in the heart, as of impending misfortune, together with a kind of homesickness.

MENY. Al, 8 - Apprehensive sensation about the heart, as of impending evil, and as if

he had to endure some hardship. (adversity, privation, suffering)
Ha, 285 - Anxious feeling about the heart, as if something bad were about to happen, and he had to undergo (experience) a calamity. (cataclysm, disaster)
He, 2 - Anxiety about heart, as if some evil was going to happen.
MOSCH. He, 1 - Great anxiety with palpitation of heart; feeling of anxious expectancy.(anticipation)
He, 11 - Great tendency to be frightened, trembling, palpitation of heart, and dread of death.
NIT-AC. Ha, 15 - Apprehensiveness, with stitches above the heart, and a fancy as if he was talking deliriously, with coldness of the body and a tendency to fall down.
NUX-V. Ha, 1238 - After midnight very violent palpitation of the heart with extreme anxiety, which urges (impulse) him to commit suicide.
He, 39 - Mania puerperalis...constantly complaining, criticizing or explaining, ... as soon she recognized physician she spoke of imperfection of medical knowledge and declared it an error that one could not live without a heart, inasmuch as she felt very well without one, it having come away with the afterbirth to which it had grown fast, the nurse having separated the two before her eyes; complains of her husband, says he wishes to convince her she is sick, ... nymphomania,... frequently sips at a bowl of warm sugar-water, declaring it will form her a new heart; .(health, healing)...(expert)
PETR. Ha, 1 - Sad and dispirited, with a sick (suffering) feeling owing (due) to weakness of the heart.
He, 12 - Sensation as if there were a cold stone in heart.(indifferent, careless)
PLAT. He, 35 - Precordial anguish with palpitation and fear of death and imaginary forms, ghosts.
PSOR. Al,N-15 - Great fear of death; anxiety about heart ...
Al,N-16 - Believe the stitches in heart will kill him if they do not cease.
He, 15 - Great fear of death; anxiety about heart and dyspnea,...
He, 16 - Believes the stitches in heart will kill him if they do not cease.
PULS. Ha, 1114 - Anxiety in the region of the heart, with suicidal impulse, and feeling or inclination to vomit in the scrobiculus cordis.
He, 26 - Anxiety: thinks to die; does not know what to do; as if in a hot atmosphere; in region of heart; even to suicide;...
He, 27 - Anguish in region of heart, sometimes increasing to a desire for suicide.
RHUS-T. Ha, 959-...;true cardiac anxiety; she could not to sleep half the night on account of great anguish, and was always so anxious that she perspired.
Ha, 961 - Very restless disposition, and anxiety and anguish, so that she had always a clutching (grasp) at the heart, with dyspnea.
Ha, 962 - She did not sleep half the night, was timorous (timid, fearful) full of anguish and cardiac anxiety.
Ha, 967 - She was inexpressibly anxious; she had pressure at the heart and tearing (cut) in the sacrum.
SEP. Al, 3 - Attacks of anger over past times come on involuntarily, through which he becomes so excited that he does not know what to do, accompanied by anxiety, palpitation of the heart, and sweat of the whole body.
SPONG. Ha, 377 - Every day, several fits of heat, with anxiety, pain in the cardiac region, weeping and inconsolable; she would like to die there and then.
He, 24 - Terror and fear: of approaching death; that she will die of suffocation; with heart disease;...
STANN. He, 6 - A woman, age 39, pregnant in fourth month;...inability to do anything as she cannot muster sufficient courage,...great palpitation of heart and anxiety, especially if she has to give directions in her domestic affairs; thinking makes her feel wretched, ...(unable, incapable)
SULPH. Al, 3815 - At night, horrible dreams, with great palpitation or heart, and on awaking, sometimes rigor, sometimes heat and fear of robbers.
TARENT. Al, 34 - Lamentation, with oppressive pain in the heart, as if a misfortune had befallen her.
Al, 35 - Weeping, with oppression and pain in the heart, as from misfortune;...

HEAVY

Anxiety; body would become thick and heavy, as if, at night: nat-c.[36]
Delusions; body, head, heavy, his own is too: bry.
- body, heavy and thick, has become (at night): nat-c.[1]
- body, thick, is: nat-c.[1]
- building stones, appearance of: thuj.
- clothes, heavy. too: con.[137] euph.[56] ***lac-c.***[8] merc.[1]
- clouds, enveloped her, heavy black: arg-n.[102] ***cimic. lac-c.***[102] puls.[102]
- fat internally, she gets: conv.[38]
- grief, weighed upon him: am-m.[139] con.[139]
- heavy, is: aran.[102] atro.[54] chr-ac.[54] nat-c. ***nit-ac.***[54] sarr.[54] thuj.
- heavy, is, fall, and he will: eup-pur.[54]
- wood, is made of: eupi.[102] kali-n. petr.[137] rhus-t.[102] ***thuj.***[102]
- world, rests upon him, the world: tab.[139]

Dreams; stone lying on him: kali-c.
Handle things anymore, cannot, weight, wants to throw off the: bamb-a.[1184]
Irritability; grief, as if a great, weighted on him, five p.m. -six p.m.: ***con.***[54]
Irritability; heaviness, during: aeth.[36] ***phos.***[36]
Obstinate; children, fat, inclined to grow: **CALC.**
Sadness; heaviness of, body, with: ***cedr.***[54] graph.[10]
Sadness; heaviness of, feet, with: graph.[10]
Sadness; heaviness of, legs, with: calc.[1]
Sensitive; want of sensitiveness, stone, feels like a dead, insensitive: ozone[227]

ADAM. Sh, 1 - I felt as if a heavy, grey cloud with red specks descended down to my chest entering into me. 7, 6C, 02:00:XX
Sh, 192 - Feel fat!!! 25SA, 5MMb, 09:XX:XX
Sh, 378 - I have lost my enthusiasm, not so much sadness, but a heavy depression. Prefer to be on my own. Everything is an effort, feel I am carrying a heavy weight. 12, 30C, 04:XX:XX.
AETH. He, 15 - Anxiousness sensation as if a heavy load was lying on chest.
AGAR. Al, 19 - During the intoxication they lift and carry the heaviest loads, take long steps and jump over small objects, as if trunks of trees lay in their way.
ALOE. He, 3 - life is a burden. (load)
ALUMN. Al, 2-...felt very much oppressed, anxious, and heavy, like a stone on the chest, with inclination to take a long breath.
AMBR. Al, 3 - She is excited, loquacious; talking fatigues her; she was enable to sleep at night; got a headache, as if she carried a large load upon her head...
BELL. Al, 34 - He took a piece of bread for a stone, and threw it far away, laughing violently and running about the room.
CHOC. Sh, 9 - Had a vivid dream of worms —they were dark and fat, but I wished they were red and thin. I felt very excited by the worms.
CIMIC. He, 1 - Sensation as if a heavy black cloud (smoke) had settled (descent) all over her, and enveloped (surrounded, wrap) her head, so that all was darkness and confusion, while, at the same time, it weighed (heavy) like lead (metal) on her head.
CON. He, 35-...a great grief weighed upon him, with paralyzed feeling in all the limbs, indifference and taking no interest in anything.
GERM. Sh, 191 - Feeling in a rather poetical mood. I feel I can almost capture the essence of the feeling I have been going through: it's an eructation! As if a marble lands somewhere, chest, stomach, brain and sucks to it all the matter around it in a radius of 3-4 cm and packs it tighter and tighter. It gets hard and brittle, then suddenly it grows with a zoomy feeling, steadily becoming less dense and suddenly it bursts and spreads a cloud of relief. I think the remedy is Champagne. 16, 30C, 03:14:00
HALI-L. Sh, 4 - Feel fat. 16, 10C, 18:XX:XX
Sh, 5 - Feel like I'm gaining weight, but am actually losing weight. 08, 30C, 05:XX:XX
Sh, 221 - I feel heavy and earthbound — why don't I fit? 20, 30C, XX:XX:XX
Sh, 812 - My bones feel lighter than the outside of me. I don't like this fat anymore. 20, 30C, 04:XX:XX
Sh, 889 - I'm ripping all my clothes. I'm so much fatter that I'm not aware of my width, and I'm catching on things. 20, 30C, 10:XX:XX
Sh, 938 - I feel so heavy and earthbound, stuck with human desires that are not my own. Why don't I fit? Where is the truth

and justice they talk about? Why do humans lie and deceive? I feel a big thing about truth and justice. "Why don't these people just tell me the truth?" It feels like a game, not telling me what they really want and need. 20, 30C, 15:XX:XX

Sh, 966 - I'm so slow and heavy on earth and so light and swift in the air. 20, 30C, 19:XX:XX

IRID. Sh, 3 - The heavy feeling is more earthed than spaced. I don't feel spacey, more interior, like in a dream or under water. E1

Sh, 91 - Felt very low again, like being covered by a heavy blanket. I felt weighed down by it. B3

Sh, 93 - Felt the blanket descending on me again (happened exactly one week ago), and I suddenly felt exhausted. Lay down and slept for half an hour. Woke and felt heavy feelings in arms and legs. Felt panicky as I recognized same feelings of despair that characterized events of last week. B9

MAG-M. Al, 711 - An anxious dream; she was lying in a strange house, where rubbish (garbage) was constantly falling upon her; she tried to cry out and could not, because there was too great heaviness on the chest.

MED. He, 28 - Spirits in the depths, weighed down with heavy, solid gloom (sadness),> by torrents of tears.

RAPH. Al, 2-...she fears she will become a burden (load) to everyone. (flat, tiresome)

SPONG. Al, 7 - She was very easily frightened, and started at every trifle; it always seemed to shoot (discharge) into her feet, and afterwards they seemed to remain heavy.

He, 22 - She is very timorous (fearful), and starts at every trifle, which affects her feet, so as to make them feel heavy.

THUJ. Al, 9 - While half awake...cannot move a limb (paralyzed), with a sensation as though the whole body were as heavy as lead (heaviness), then she tries to call for help; can utter no sound, and lies with open eyes ...

HEIGHT

Delirium; throwing from windows: ***aeth.***[54] calc.[58] sil.[58]

Delusions; abyss: ozone[227]
- clouds, rocks, and, in the air: mag-m.
- falling, height, from a: calen.[139] mosch.[85]
- hole, small, is a frightful chasm: agar.
- lifted up, falling, with fear of: hyper.[172] mosch.[172]
- lifted up, he or she is: hyper.[72] ozone[227] phos.[137] stront-c.[137]
- mountain, descending a: cycl.[139]
- mountain, he stands on the ridge of a: cann-i.
- saw, he was a huge, darting up and down: cann-i.

Dreams; falling, high places, from: acon. alum. am-m. anan. aur. chin. cimic.[111] ***dig.*** guai. hep. kali-c. kali-m.[192] kali-n.[36] ***kreos.*** merc. merc-c.[36] ***mez.*** nat-s. nicc. nux-m. op. ph-ac.[1] phos. sep. sin-a.[36] sol-n.[25] ***sulph.*** sumb. **THUJ.** zinc.
- ➤ falling, high places, men are killed by falling from a height: sabin.[10]
- ➤ high places: all-c. anac. brom. calc.[185] chin. cortico.[119] hydrog.[222] laur. lyss. macrin.[36]
- ➤ jumping, height, from a, and landing easily: lap-mar-c.[194]
- ➤ precipices: ***all-c.***[54] ***lac-ac.***[54]
- ➤ stairs, has to climb countless: ozone[227]
- ➤ tossing someone out of window: bry.[36]

Fear; ascending, of: ***nit-ac.***[122]
- ✦ falling, height, from: aur.[172] hyos.[137] thuj.[172]
- ✦ high places, of: ***arg-n. aur.***[137] calc.[162] calc-f.[179] carc.[193] cob-n.[119] coca[130] gels.[137] manc.[162] morg-g.[102] nat-m.[189] phos.[162] psor.[54] puls. staph. stram.[182] sulph. zinc.[162]
- ✦ high places, throw himself down, lest he: arg-n.[172]
- ✦ places, buildings: arg-n.[111] calc.[137] carc.[207] iod.[172] kali-p.[111] phos.[172] visc.[111]

Frightened; easily, night, starting up as if falling from a height into water: ph-ac.[36]

High places agg.: ***arg-n. aur.*** gels. puls. staph. ***sulph***

Jumping; impulse to, height, from a: anac. ***arg-n.*** **AUR.** gels. lap-mar-c.[194] staph.

Jumping; impulse to, window, from, dash herself down, or, during parturition: aur.[54]

Kill; sudden impulse to, throw child, window, out of: lyss.[54]

Suicidal disposition; seeing, an open window or knives: arg-n. camph. chin. ***merc.***
Suicidal disposition; seeing, open windows or knife: arg-n. camph. chin. ***merc.***
Suicidal disposition; throwing himself from, height, a: anac. ***arg-n.*** ars. **AUR. BELL.**[122] camph. crot-h. gels. glon.[5] hydrog.[222] hyos.[30] ign.[122] iod.[5] iodof.[116] lach.[5] ***lyss.***[162] ***nux-v.*** orig. sec.[30] ***sel.***[162] sil.[30] staph.[58] stram. ***sulph.***[54] x-ray[152]
Suicidal disposition; throwing, windows, from: ***aeth.*** arg-n.[122] ***ars.***[122] **AUR.** aur-ar.[58] bell. camph. ***carbn-s.*** chin. crot-c. gels. ***glon. iod.***[116] ***iodof.***[116] nux-v.[116] ***sulph.***[54] thea. thuj. verat.

AETH. Al, 9 - Delirium; he jumps out of window.

ARG-N. He, 12 - The sight of high houses always made him dizzy (confused) and caused him stagger (hesitation) ; it seemed as if houses on both sides would approach and crush him.
He, 22 - On crossing a bridge, almost irresistible desire to jump into river; meeting some one prevented it.

AUR. He, 8 - Looks on dark side, weeps, prays, thinks she is not fit for this world, longs for death, strong inclination to commit suicide; desperate, desires to jump from a height.

BELL. Al, 96 - In his delirium he threw himself down from a height.
Ha, 1439 - Throws herself down from a height.(in delirium)

CAMPH. Al, 46-...For a moment I resolved to throw myself from the window and sweep through the domain of my infernal kingdom, but a weak glimmer of reason held me back...
Al, 39 - Indescribable dread of being drawn upwards.
Al, 19 - Stripped naked, he danced wildly about, and attempted to jump out of the window.
He, 36 - Impulse to jump out the window.
He, 51 - Strips (undress) himself (naked), and tries to jump out of window.

CHIN. Al, DREAM .1105-...;he imagines he is descending a precipice, on which account he awakes, but the dangerous place remains vividly before his fancy...Al, 1109 - At night frightful dreams of falling from a height, whith waking full of uneasiness...
Ha, 1093-...;he jumps out of the bed and wants to make away whith himself (suicide), and yet he fears to go near and open window or to approach a knife.

CROT-C. Al, 5 - She stands for ten minutes on the window-sill, and is arrested when on the point of throwing herself off.

GLON. He, 9 - Frantic; attempted to jump from the window.

HALI-L. Sh, 651 - When I'm focused, I bring it all in, in the present. There, like meditating, or seeing God. When I'm unfocussed, it's like I'll go into the abyss, and won't come back; go crazy. 08, 30C, 31:XX:XX

HYDROG. Sh, 33 - About two months after beginning the proving, developed an extreme range of mental symptoms that he had never had before. These included severe depression with strong alternations of moods, & high then low &, with suicidal tendency, desire to jump from a high building or cut wrist, confusion of identity (especially concerning sex and homosexuality) and became more religious. He moved away from his parents home (which he had never before been able t o do) and shut himself away in a small flat. This condition lasted for another six or seven months and was finally antidoted by Phosphorus 200. Before that, he had tried to anti-dote it with acupuncture, to no avail. 24, 30C, 60:XX:XX

IRID. Sh, 77 - A sudden, very deep desire for wilderness, space and air and height. E15

KALI-BR. Al, 3-...his character also had undergone a radical change, from having been very frank and brave, he had become excessively timid, and suspicious of every trifling circumstance; ...several times he attempted to throw himself from a window and battered down a door with an axe, in order to escape from some imaginary danger;...

LAC-C. He, 33 - Has a great fear of falling down stairs at times.

LYSS. Al,N-7 - Thoughts of something terrible going to happen come into his mind against his will; feels impelled to do reckless (impulsive) things, such as throwing child, which he carries in his arms, through the window, and the like.

He, 7 - Thoughts of something terrible going to happen come into his mind against his will; feels impelled to do reckless (impulsive, precipitated) things, such as throwing child, which he carries in his arms, through the window, and the like.

MERC. He, 20 - After suppression of foot sweat, whenever he sees an open window or cutting instruments breaks into a sweat, with great heat of head, and is seized with an almost uncontrollable desire to commit suicide.

NUX-V. Al, 5-(Suicide; she throws herself down from a height)

Ha, 1241-(Suicide; she throws herself from a height.)

OENA. Al, 21 - She thought that she was transported to a very great elevation.(elevated)

PH-AC. Ha, 41 - Illusion of the senses, as if he heard the clock strike or as if lofty (tall, elevated) things lying out of his horizon were moving near him.

STRAM. He, 59-...clings to her mother with as much desperation as if she were going to be thrown from a precipice.

He, 100-...threatens to knock everybody down, to break furniture, to throw himself out of window.

SULPH. He, 35-...,strong impulsive tendency to suicide, by drowning or by precipitating herself from window;...(high, water)

THEA. Al, 4 - Sensation as if impelled by some uncontrollable power to commit suicide, to jump out of window, to put her baby in the boiler with the clothes, to cut its throat while cutting bread, to throw it downstairs (in a woman who kept a pot of tea boiling on the stove and drank several bowlfuls every day; cured with tea cm, Finckle)

THUJ. He, 23 - Mental depression, after childbirth (puerperal), in consequence of being told that there had been a slight rupture (division, hurt) of perineum; grows quiet; thinks she must die;...wants to jumps the window; does not care for children or her relatives (careless) ;..(sensitive to disrupt, partition)

HELL

Anxiety; salvation, hell, of: ***plat.***[54]

Delusions; hell, chains, in erotomania: ***orig.***[54]

- hell, gate of, obliged to confess his sins at: agar.
- hell, going to, because he has committed a unpardonable crime: chel.[172] med.[54]
- hell, is in: camph. cann-i. germ.[222] hydrog.[222] lyss.[54] merc. *orig.*[54]
- hell, shadows of, in, midnight on waking: cann-i.
- hell, suffers the torments of, without being able to explain: lyss.[54] ***merc.***[122]

Despair; heaven or hell, did not care whether he went to: med.[54]

Dreams; hell: cand-a.[239]

Fear; hell, of: manc.[30]

AGAR. Al, 14 - He imagines himself at a gate of the hell and that the mushroom commands him to fall on his knees and confess his sins, which he does. (forgiveness, absolution)

BELL. Ha, 1422 - Along with burning heat of the body, with open, staring, and fixed eyes, such fury she must constantly be held fast in order to prevent her attacking others,...

CAMPH. Al, 46-...For a moment I resolved to throw myself from the window and sweep through the domain of my infernal kingdom, but a weak glimmer of reason held me back...

Al, 46-...A fearful terror seized me, and I knew not whither to fly. I cried out aloud, "And so I am indeed dead; that hell I used to think about is no fiction, but a reality which I am doomed to experience forever...

GERM. Sh, 112 - Don't see why I am here. I can't bear it. I go mad. I hate myself. I want to beat myself and I do it. Tear my hair. Stop when it hurts too much. It is like hell !!! 18, 30C, 20:XX:XX

HALI-L. Sh, 647 - Life seems like hell. The beauty and order are gone. I feel awful, tense, overwhelmed, anxious with nausea. My sense of well being is gone.[06], 6C, 16:XX:XX

Sh, 648 - Down side, dark side, feels like the gates between the unconscious and conscious are open. Hurricane-like feeling of unconscious energy. Like the gates of hell are open. No barrier. Extreme amount of power. Darkness. Internal pressure. Dogs guard the gates of Hades. A lot of internal pressure-type feeling all day. 13, 30C, 10:XX:XX

HELON. Al, 2 - Reaction (from feeling of general wellness) began, and for a fortnight I was in a mental hell; it was the most profound mental depression I have ever known; I was plunged into the most abject despair.

HYDROG. Sh, 27 - There is a very fine line at this time between enlightenment and insanity —a split consciousness. The dark side is horrendous, but the positive side of the proving has been well worth it. The positive aspects are beautiful. Its a shame we need to come down. I guess the price of going into the heavens is a trip to hell. 16, 30C, XX:XX:XX

LYSS. Al,N-50 - Declares amid violent sobs that she is suffering the torments of hell.
He, 50 - Declares amid violent sobs that she is suffering the torments of hell.

MED. Al,N-52 - Feeling of desperation; did not care if he went to heaven or hell.
He, 35 - Feeling as if he had committed the unpardonable sin and was going to hell.
He, 37 - Feeling of desperation, did not care if he went to heaven or hell.

MERC. Ha, 1225 - Imagines he is enduring the tortures (torment) of hell, without being able to account for it (explain). -(lost understanding, judgment)

PLAT. He, 46-...;suffers unspeakable pangs (anxiety) of conscience in consequence of a faux (fault, mistake, embarrassing mistake?) pass when thirty-two years old; says she has brought disgrace upon her family, and that she has incurred the penalty of damnation; (doomed) in order to do penance (penitence) gave away whatever she could lay her hands upon, (redemption) so that she had to be constantly watched; after her confessor asserted that she could not hope for pardon or heaven (condemnable), she seemed in absolute despair ; bemoaned her misery throughout the night, wringing her hands and beseeching (implore) that she might be delivered (free) from the hell of her conscience; twice attempted self-destruction (suicide);...wished to live and do penance (penitence, purgation, purification) in order to mitigate her eternal punishment.

PLB. He, 16 - Mental disturbance of eight or ten years' duration in a man addicted to masturbation; has several times attempted suicide; has been in seclusion (solitude); greatest dejection and despair;...; believes himself lost (condemned) ; has the sounds of hell constantly in his ears; hears voices and sees shadows of demons, great disposition to make away (suicide) with himself or do himself some bodily injury;

HELPFUL

Avarice; generosity towards strangers, as regards his family: carb-v.[30] hyos.[30] nat-m.[30] nux-v.[30]

Benevolence: agar.[10] am-m.[10] anac.[10] aur.[10] bell.[30] calc.[10] cic.[10] coff. coff-t.[36] hydrog.[222] ign.[30] lach.[10] led.[10] mang.[10] nat-m.[10] nit-ac.[10] nux-v.[30] op.[36] phos.[10] sil.[189] stann.[10] sulph.[10]

Benevolence; excited: 0coff-t.[36]

Charitable: bell.[30] ign.[30] nux-v.[30]

Charitable; expectation of recompense, with the: calc.[30] lyc.[30] nat-m.[30] sulph.[30]

Constructive: cupr.[10]

Deeds; desire to perform, good: coff-t.[36]

Deeds; desire to perform, useful: ***cere-b.***[36]

Dreams; children, about, protecting them, to save them from falling: ozone[227]
- ➤ children, about, rescuing them: cass.[36] ***hydrog.***[222]
- ➤ children, wanted to save asphyxiated: cass.[36]
- ➤ disease, sick people, help them, cannot: ozone[227]
- ➤ fire, house on, neighbors, which could not be saved: mag-s.[36]
- ➤ fire, vivid, exerting himself to extinguish them: merc-s.[54]
- ➤ help: sabad.[10]

Generous; too much: cere-b.[36] nux-v.[30] op.[36] staph.[30] sulph.[189]

Responsibility; strong, family, towards his: nat-s.[187]

Responsibility; strong, social: stront-c.[188]

Selflessness: anh.[119] iod.[30] nat-c.[62] puls.[30] rhus-t.[30]

Talk; benevolent: tus-f.[36]

Useful, desire to be: ***cere-b.***[36]

ADAM. Sh, 269 - The beginning of many "help me" phone calls from people in difficult relationships which they need to leave and can't. 2, 12C, 00:00:10

Sh, 307 - Still an enormous desire to nurture and feed people. In the last month I have fed sixty people weekly during a political campaign. Made many friends. 2, 12C, 57:XX:XX

Sh, 308 - A conversation about death with my children. A feeling that they need some insurance; and I thought I would make a will, to make provisions for them, to clarify the situation. 2, 12C, 05:XX:XX

Sh, 357 - I have a great desire to feed huge nourishing meals to my family; to spend money in the achievement of their dreams. 2, 12C, 26:XX:XX

Sh, 359 - Feeling a sense of wealth of prosperity of a beneficent universe. 32SA, 200C, XX:XX:XX

ANAC. He, 69 - In one ear a devil, in the other an angel, prompts (incite) him to do murder or acts of benevolence. (homicidal, x helpfulness, kindness)

CERE-B. Al, 3 - Felt all day an astonishing (unusual) inclination to be engaged (work, busy) in something useful. (helpful)

Al, 4 - Felt a desire to give something quite necessary to myself to another. (altruism, helpful, sympathetic)

COFF-T. Al, 5 - Desire to perform good deeds intensified.

COFF. He, 8 - Great loquacity, brain feels clear and is active, he feels strong enough to do anything, feels impelled to push things; veneration for the Supreme Being and love for family; benevolence excited.

HALI-L. Sh, 519 - I was anxious about so much rain. There was severe flooding in our valley, washing the bridge out that connected us to the rest of the world. I felt isolated; lives were decimated. I felt frantic because I couldn't be helpful. 01, 30C, 30:XX:XX—53:XX:XX

Sh, 817 - I feel regal and generous. 20, 30C, 05:01:XX

HYDROG. Sh, 281 - Felt benevolent — wanted to do something for someone else. Went out and spent a lot of money on food which I then gave to old people. 16, 30C, 03:XX:XX

Sh, 285 - More charitable and sympathetic than usual. 08, 30C, 04:XX:XX

HYOS. Al, 60-... Then he wandered into the country and suddenly pulling up a leg, exclaimed, " Take care; give me your hand; that is a very deep step"...

IRID. Sh, 101 - Went into pet shop. There was a budgie chirping in a cage. I was so upset. "Oh God, I want to let this bird out." I felt it was crying to be let out. Took me all my control not to let it out or shout at the man to do it. Then thought, "This is silly. It would get hurt, he'll think I'm mad." I slunk out of the shop thinking I'd really let that bird down. Distracted and nearly in tears. Walked round town in a daze, should I go back and ask him to at least open the door, knew that wasn't on. It might get out of the shop and die. Felt a real coward. Set up a train of thought — condor in bird garden —a notice justifying its captivity —it only flies for food —it's quite happy to be there because food comes to it. Weeping as I write this. Birds in cages can't lean on the air currents and be blown away. G6

NUX-V. He, 37-...betraying (play false, feigning) great moral and physical languor (indifference),..launches into high-flying, fantastic plans, fancies himself rich (rank, position) and wants to make presents of thousands (squanders, waste), and makes large useless purchases; does not consider himself ill; ...,and takes in bad part if not allowed to read indictment (accusation) for said lawsuit, a confused irrational piece of work...

PLB. Al, 53-...; he fancied one of the patients called to him, ran headlong (hurry) to help him, ...

SUMB. Al, 2 - More cheerful in humor and more disposed for intellectual occupation; he felt in the happy enthusiastic state of mind that accompanies the consciousness of having performed a noble (generous, virtuous) deed; this sort of medicinal intoxication went away in a few hours.

HELPLESSNESS

Anguish; evening, paralyzing, impossible to call and move, with heat in head: cob-n.[144]

Anguish; night, paralyzing, impossible to call and move, with heat in head: cob-n.[144]

Anxiety; alone, watched, desires to be: gall-ac.[36]

Anxiety; night, helplessness, with feeling of: lith-c.[54]

Anxiety; others, losing their protectors or familiar relations, for: bar-c.[162]

Carried; desires to be: acet-ac. acon. ant-c.[5] ant-t. ***ars.*** aspar.[122] bell.[5] benz-ac. bor.[111] brom. **BRY.**[36] calc.[193] carb-v. **CHAM.**[122] chel.[5] ***cina*** coff.[122] coloc.[116] cupr.[210] ign. ip.[36] jal.[163] ***kali-c.*** kreos.[5] ***lyc.*** merc.[5] oci.[109] podo.[5] puls. rheum[153] ***rhus-t.*** sac-alb.[210] sanic. staph. sulph. vac.[54] ***verat.***

Carried; desires to be, fast: acon.[111] **ARS.** bell. brom. cham.[127] rhus-t. verat.

Clinging; children of, awakes terrified, knows no one, screams, clings to those near: **BOR.**[122] cina[36] ***stram.***[122]

Clinging; children of, grasp the nurse when carried: bor.[58] cupr.[8] cupr-acet.[8] ***gels.***[122]

Clinging; children of, mother: bar-c.[162] puls.[189] sil.[53]

Clinging; children of, take the hand of mother, will always: ***bism.***[85] gels.[116] kali-c.[56] lil-t.[56] lyc.[56] phos.[162]

Clinging; convulsions, before: ***cic.***[54]

Clinging; grasps at others: agar.[185] ars.[5] ***camph.***[54] op.[30] phos.[5]

Clinging; persons or furniture, to: bar-c.[162] bism.[122] bor.[1] coff. gels. phos.[1] stram.

Company, desire for; happen, as if something horrible might: ***elaps***[54]

Company, desire for; hold his hand, to: bism.[103] phos.[58] stram.[58]

Company, desire for; wants to be watched constantly: gall-ac.[85]

Death; presentment of, soon, believes that she will die, and cannot be helped: ***agn.***

Delirium; crying, help, for: ***canth.*** stram.[54]

Delirium; help, calling for: plat.

Delirium; lively active, vivid, alternates in short periods with horrified fright, seeming to dread approach of some monster, appealing for help: stram.[54]

Delusions; calls, absent peoples, for: hyos.

• calls, him with name, the absent mother or sister: anac.[10]

• calls, him, someone: ***cann-i.***[54] rhod.[54] ***sep.***[54] sulph.[30]

• calls, someone: anac. ant-c. bell.[111] cann-i. dros. hyos.[185] kali-c. med.[185] plat.[10] ***plb.*** ruta[10] stram.[185] thuj. verat.[185]

• calls, waking, someone calls on: ant-c. ars. bell.[111] dulc.[1] rhod.[137] rhus-t. sep.

• die, about to, wishes someone would help her off: ***lach.***[54]

• falling, he is, clings and asks to be held: stram.[54]

• hanging, sees persons, beckoning him to cut them loose: ars.[54]

• help, calling for: plat.

• helped, cannot be: nat-p.[168]

• people, say, "come": med.[54]

• people, seized them, sees a number of strangers and tries to: stram.[54]

• railway train, she is in a car, begs others to hold her: ***sang.***[54]

• rowdies, brawlers, will break in if she is alone: elaps.[139]

• voices, hears, absent people, of: anac.[1] cham.[1]

• voices, hears, bed, in, ceases when listening intently: abrot.

• voices, hears, distant: bell. ***cann-s.***[54] cham. nat-m. sabal.[137] stram.

Desires; attended, to be: lap-mar-c.[194]

Desires; understood, to be: lap-c-b.[194]

Despair; comforted, wants to be: ozone[227]

Despair; support, wants: bamb-a.[1184]

Dreams; called, that some one: ant-c. merc. sep.

➤ calling out: kali-c. thuj.

➤ calling, help, for: kali-c. lil-s.[36] plat.[193]

➤ children, about, lost in crowd: bamb-a.[1184]

➤ help: sabad.[10]

➤ helpless feeling, as if the end of the world: hydrog.[222]

➤ water, daughter is in water and crying for help: nat-s.

Fear; alone, of being, child wants mother to hold her hand: bism.[172] kali-c.[172] lil-t.[172] lyc.[172] sac-alb.[210] stram.[172]

✦ falling, child holds on to mother, nurse: bor.[56] ***cupr-acet.***[54] **GELS.**[54] sanic.[56]

✦ going out, alone: ars.[127] ign.[127] pitu-a.[164]

✦ physician, will not see her; he seems to terrify her: arg-n.[172] arn.[162] dys-co.[136] ign.[162] iod. nat-m.[162] ***nux-v.***[54] ***phos.***[162] ***sep.***[162] ***stram.***[54] thuj. tub.[172] verat.[172] verat-v.

Forsaken; feeling, thinks she is left alone in the world: plat.[60]

Gestures; makes, grasping, bystanders, at: **ANT-T.**[36] ars.[5] bell.[1] ***camph.***[54] cocc.[36] merc.[10] phos. stram.[10]

Help, shrieking for: androc.[222] ant-t.[8] bov.[36] ***camph. canth.*** cham.[31] cic.[38] hep.[1] ***ign.***[8] kali-c.[1] ***laur.***[54] lev.[149] plat. plb.[36] pyrog.[85] pyrus[85] rhus-t.[10] sabad.[36] sil.[1] stram.[54]

Helplessness, feeling of: aether[36] anac.[1] ant-t.[36] arg-n.[162] ars.[1] bamb-a.[1184] ***calad.***[122] cand-a.[239] ***gels.***[8] germ.[222] hecla.[234] hell. hydrog.[222] jasm.[36] kali-br. lith-c.[25] **LYC.**[122] ozone[227] petr. phos. puls.[189] rhus-t.[137] stram. tax.
Helplessness; feeling of, afternoon: kali-br.
Helplessness; feeling of, heart complaints, with: am-c.[1]
Helplessness; feeling of, infant, feels like a: hell.[54]
Helplessness; feeling of, mental exertion, from: gels.[8]
Helplessness; feeling of, night: ***lith-c.***[54]
Helplessness; feeling of, weakness, from, in mental exertion: ***gels.***[54]
Helplessness; feeling, of paralyzed, from sensation of being: ***sang.***[171]
Holding or being held; amel.: ars.[137] ***bry.***[137] calc-p.[5] carb-an.[137] diph.[137] dros.[137] eup-per.[137] ***gels.***[137] glon.[137] **LACH.**[5] lil-t.[137] murx.[137] nat-s.[137] nux-m.[137] nux-v.[137] rhus-t.[137] sang.[137] sep.[5] ***sil.***[5] stram.[5] sul-ac.[137] sulph.[137]
Holding or being held; desire for: ***ars.***[5] coff.[5] diph.[111] ***gels.***[5] iod.[5] iodof.[36] kali-p.[5] **LACH.**[5] ***nux-m.***[5] ***nux-v.***[5] phos.[5] plb.[5] rhus-t.[5] sac-alb.[210] ***sang.***[5] ***sep.***[5] **STRAM.**[5] sul-ac.[111] ***sulph.***[5]
Injure; fears to be left alone, lest he should, himself: alum. arg-n. ars. ***cimic.***[54] ***merc. nat-s.*** sep.
Mania; held, wants to be: **ARS.**
Praying; begged others to pray for him: lyss.[54]
Protection, constantly wants mothers: sil.[53]
Sadness; awkward and helpless manner, with: anac.[1]
Shrieking; calls someone: aloe[130] ***bell.***[5] kali-c.[5] ***plat.***[5]
Shrieking; help, for: camph.[36] ***ign.***[8] kali-c.[1] ***laur.***[54] lepi.[36] levo.[149] plat.
Shrieking; help, for, hysteria, in: ***ign.***[54]
Shrieking; help, for, sleep, in: hep.[10] kali-c.[10] rhus-t.[10]
Shrieking; help, for, Springing up from bed: hep.[10] rhus-t.[10]
Shrieking; holds on to something, unless she: **SEP.**
Shrieking; sleep, during, jumping out of sleep and shrieks for help: hep.[10] rhus-t.[10]
Sympathy; compassion, desire, for: alco.[36] anac.[54] androc.[222] asaf.[111] **BELL.**[5] **CAMPH.**[5] carc.[146] caust.[36] cic.[5] germ.[222] **HELL.**[5] nat-c.[36] nat-m.[91] ***olnd.***[54] ozone[227] **PHOS.**[122] puls.[5] rhod.[36] sac-alb.[210] ***sep.***[36] thuj.[36] ***tub.***[189]
Weeping; constant, wants: ail.[58]

ACON. Al, 66 - Great timidity after a severe fright (fear), afraid to go out unattended (abandoned, helplessness) after dark, is unable to control his feelings of apprehensive fear.

ADAM. Sh, 239 - Would like some support. Cannot tolerate the emotional demands made on me. I ask for help or remedy. 2, 12C, 72:XX:XX
Sh, 240 - Anger from lack of physical or emotional support. 2, 12C, 73:XX:XX
Sh, 241 - I feel angry and want to be comforted. 7, 6C, 03:07:30
Sh, 310 - Feel orphaned after an angry phone call from my parents. Feel unparented. Oh well, what the hell. 2, 12C, 26:XX:XX

ALUM. Al, 6 - Depressed and friendless; he wishes only to be left alone, in the forenoon.

AM-C. Ha, 10 - Severe compression of the heart, he knows not how to help himself.

ANAC. Ha, 10 - In the forenoon, extremely hypochondriac, discouraged and despondent, with awkward (unskillful), helpless manner; ...
Ha, 45 - Delusions of fancy, he thought his name was called by the voice of his (far distant) mother and sister; at the same time an apprehension and anguish foreboding misfortune.
He, 39 - Every five minutes he screams loudly, as if he would call someone.

ANDROC. Sh, 83 - Woke at night to urinate. On going upstairs, all colours seemed incredibly bright and the walls were pulsating —in towards him and out again. This felt similar to an L.S.D. experience years ago. Did not know what to do, was stricken with panic. Terrified, he raced back to bed where he felt hot, so uncovered, then cold so covered, then hot, he uncovered and sat up and immediately felt better — no panic. As soon as he lay down he began to panic. Became afraid in the light and felt better in the dark with the lights off. He wanted to call someone for help, and felt angry about the proving. He then got up and walked around for a few minutes, got back to bed, and fell asleep. (2)

ANT-T. Al, 12 - Dreaded (fear) to be left alone even for a few moments, lest he " should be dreadfully nervous and not know what to do with himself."

He, 16 - Child clings (adhere) to those around, calls for help in a hoarse voice, with cough.

ARG-N. He, 5 - In conversation, forgetting what he wanted to say, he looked around as if expecting some one to help (aid) him out.

He, 41 - Despaired of help from himself or others.

ARS. Al, 51 - He despairs and weeps and imagines no one can help him, that he must die;...(unprotected)

Al, 70 - The anxiety and restlessness are indescribable; "Kill me", he cried, "or relieve my pains!".(help)

Ha, 1032 - Mania; first headache, horrible anxiety, noise before the ears, as from a number of large bells, and when he opened the eyes, he always saw a man who had (formerly) hung himself (suicidal, justified) on the ground-floor of the house, who incessantly beckoned (call) him to cut him down (help); he ran thither (there) with a knife, but, as he could not cut him down, (rescue) he became overwhelmed (beaten) with despair (remorse?) and wished (as his friends assured him) to hang himself (punish); but being prevented (stop) from doing so, he became so restless that he could hardly be kept in bed,... and he knelt down and raised his hands in a supplicating manner.

Ha, 1035 - He is cold, shivers and weeps, and thinks, in his despair, (hopelessness, despairing) that nothing can help him, (helplessness) and he must die; followed by general exhaustion.

Ha, 44 - Desponding and weeping, he thinks that nothing can help him, and he would have to die anyhow; (in any way)...

He, 24 - Delirium during heat, unconsciousness, mania, wants to be held; with a tearing headache.

He, 25 - Mania...sees a man who has hanged himself beckoning (call) him to cut him loose (rescue, deliverance, free, saving) on failing to accomplish this he attempts to hang himself (punish, penalize);...finally kneels down and lifts his hands in supplication.(forgiveness, absolution)

BISM. He, 6 - Desire for company; child holds on to its mother's hand.

CAMPH. Al, 46-...I sat up in bed, but all about me had indeed disappeared. I was alone in the great universe, the last of all things. My ideas of the world, God and religion, now seemed to me to have existed only in my imagination; the earth upon which yesterday I lived and moved, had run its appointed course, and I was the final and solitary fragment of the whole creation...(meaningless, unimportant, neglected, forsaken, loneliness, deserted) (godless)

Al, 46-.... As I lay stretched on my couch, as the evil demon, and suffered all the anguish of a condemned and God-forsaken soul, ...I was forever deprived of the Divine protection, and of every consolation and every hope. Nothing remained to me but the conviction of my everlasting damnation...

Al, 46...I started up, ran out, and fell prostrate, with a loud shriek for help, not far from the door of a neighbor....

Al, 46-...I shriek and call for help, because it seems that a murderer stands at my bed side...

He, 45 - Cries for help, takes hold of others, will not be left alone.

He, 72 - Palpitation; vexed by want of sympathy (compassion, aid), afraid to be alone a moment, fears death.

CANN-I. Al, 30 - When his friends went out of the room, he thought (delusion) they had left him to his fate (destiny, doom), and wrote "cowards" in his notes.

CHAM. Al, 3 - At night, it seems as though he hears the voices of absent persons.

CROT-C. Al, 7 - He fancies he hears groans. (laments)

CUPR-A. He, 15 - Afraid of falling; holds on to his nurse's hair, hugs up to her, afraid of being injured,...

GELS. He, 27 - Mental exertions cause a sense of helplessness (disability) from brain-weakness; inability to attend to anything requiring thought.

GERM. Sh, 103 - Felt closed in. My every movement and thought controlled. Didn't know where to go for help. Felt like a coward . Felt afraid of violence. I don't know who I am. 04, 6C, XX:XX:XX

Sh, 111 - If I were me, nobody would like me -so I try to be what I think others expect me to be. I don't think I can be loved with all the parts of me which are ugly and bad. Lonely feelings. Longing for love and understanding. Feel I am so unfriendly to myself. 18, 30C, 04:00:00

Sh, 140 - Feel I am in an impossible situation. Nobody to talk to who understands me. I can't say things as they are because I have to take others feelings into consideration. I need comfort and encouragement, but no one can give me. Weeping. 18, 30C, 36:XX:XX

Sh, 153 - Thought nobody understood me and cared for what I felt. Felt it was unfair. I was presented with complaints about something others had done. Felt I was standing between two fighting parts. Felt awkward about it, embarrassed. Difficult to argue about such strong outburst. Thoughts about the day's arguing milling in my head all evening and night. 21, 12C, 32:XX.XX.

Sh, 69 - Want to sit alone in front of fire listening to music by myself. Fed up with people everywhere I go irritating me. Want to be looked after. 09, 9C, 01:11:00.

Sh, 108 - Hopeless, helpless, gloom and doom. Weeping and self pity. 14, 30C, 23:00:00.

HALI-L. Sh, 403 - For three weeks I was in a depression, unlike anything I have felt for a long time. Deep sense of low self-worth. Feeling invisible, uncared for and envious. I was lethargic, couldn't do anything. My practice dropped, patients just didn't show up. I felt I sunk as low as I needed to go, unmotivated. Felt unappreciative of all I have. Unappreciative of my life which I usually adore. Anger, dissatisfaction with life, isolating. I wasn't seeing anyone not even my husband, exhaustive. Had no dreams during the depression —unusual. I am emerging from it now. 01, 30C, 30:XX:XX-50:XX:XX

Sh, 417 - Frustrated and depressed. Feeling lonely, friendless and unaccomplished. 18, 30C, 15:XX:XX

Sh, 427 - Luckily, this legal dispute is not happening to me personally. But I feel it is. I imagine them laughing at us and doing their worst to squash us. Never felt so helpless in my life. 09, 6C, 26:XX:XX

Sh, 437 - Remedy brought up tendency to look at my lack of self-benefaction, and I became depressed looking at that picture. "What you need to do is do it. Get on with your life. Concentrate on the moves for your future." 18, 30C, 35:XX:XX

HYDROG. Sh, 150 - Feeling weepy and vulnerable —want someone to "manage" things for me. Feel so fed up of having to do it all myself. 18, 200C, 26:XX:XX

Sh, 152 - Feel helpless, as if I may need to be looked after because I don't feel I can do anything. 16, 30C, 00:00:30

Sh, 242 - Felt vulnerable to criticism —felt people were getting at me. Felt people were not taking notice of poor little me — over-reacting —upset and hurt. 02, 6C, XX:XX:XX

IGN. He, 42 - A state of anguish in which she shrieks (scream) for help, with suffocating constriction of throat...

IRID. Sh, 45-"I want you to hold my hand." B3

Sh, 46 - Went to bed and clung to husband, needed him to hold me (due to depression). We made love out of need rather than passion. B9

KALI-FCY. Al, 1 - Feeling of sadness and some disposition to tears, caused by an impression that he was soon to die and leave his friends; disposition to take a sad view of the beauties of autumn; the apprehension of approaching sickness and death can be overcome by reason, but soon returns.

LACH. He, 8 - Thinks: she is somebody else in the hands (seized) of a stronger power; (supremacy, superiority).or that she is dead, and preparations are made for funeral (cortege) or that she is nearly dead and wishes some one would help her off; herself pursued by enemies, or fears medicine is poison; there are robbers in house and wants to jump out the window; herself under super-human control; visions real, he will die. (helplessness, desire; aid, comfort, salvation)

LED. Al, 10 - Fretful; he went by himself, and almost weeping wished to die.

LEPI. Al, 1 - She fancies herself alone in a graveyard, pursued by a ghost, and screams so that her voice is lost next day; yet nobody hears her. (helpless)

LIL-T. Al, 16 - Worse on going to bed; can't go to sleep; wild (tumultuous, uncontrollable) feeling in the head as though I should go crazy (insane) and no one would take care of me (forsaken, helpless); thoughts of suicide; how much opium would put me to sleep forever, and who would find my body, and who would care; ... (friendless, abandoned, deserted)

Al, 3 - A sense as if she were going to be crazy, if she did not hang on to herself, and hold tight.

LYSS. Al,N-45 - Wrote to doctor: I am waiting with impatience that you give me and my young ones something to eat.

Al,N-46 - After fainting (weak) spell he wrote on paper: I am forsaken by all; even the birds of heaven, they do not look at me (despised), do not fed me if hungry (helplessness) ; I hunger with the young ones and am thirsty with their she ones (starving); my nest (house) is made out of dirt (soiled), not gotten by my own exertions (efforts), but by driving them out of their nests (home) and sitting there with the females and the young.

NAJA. Al, 13-...I felt that everything that was done was done in a wrong way, and could not be rectified (corrected, revised); if I felt that I had some duty to perform (execute), I had at the same time a strong impulse not to do it, and I am extremely restless in consequence; I seemed to have an increased perception of what I ought to do, but, at the same time, an unaccountable inclination not to do it, to which I was irresistibly compelled to yield "I couldn't help it, didn't know why, but couldn't do it."

NEON. Sh, 182 - Had an explosion for not being the perfect person. I was really pissed off at the situation. I felt out of control, helpless, and lashed out with vehemence and anger at the situation and myself. I'm in the "Valley of Discontent" and want to get out of Sacramento. 31, 12C, 16:XX:XX

Sh, 200 - I feel that nobody is there for me when I need them; I'm there for everyone when they need me but no one is ever there for me. 13, 30C, 07:00:00

NIT-AC. Al, 17 - At once she is taken which peculiar anguish, runs to her physician, but he is not at home, hires a carriage to drive to the house where she expects to find him; during her ride all the anguish is gone; arrived at home she feels as bad as ever, and feels herself thus forced to drive about the whole day, till all the effects of the Nitric acid have passed off.

NUX-V. Al, 54 - She was in great alarm, kept fast hold on her husband and refused to let him go.

OP. Al, 36 - Mind in a state of great confusion; at one moment she was sensible (conscious) to her crime, called for assistance (comfort, aid, help) ; at another she resisted the means used to save her.

He, 11 - Thinks he is not in his own house; imagines himself living in a locality three hours distant from his house; detains all passers-by and wishes to take them into his house; ...he does not recognize friends;... (estranged, alien)

PETR. He, 5 - Since confinement two weeks ago when in bed, in dark room, at night, delusion that there is another baby (small, tiny) in bed which requires attention also that she has a third leg which would not remain quiet.

PLAT. He, 28 - Thinks she is left entirely to herself and stands alone in the world. (loneliness)

PLB. Al, 53-...; he fancied one of the patients called to him, ran headlong (hurry) to help him, ...

PULS. He, 43 - Sleepless nights on account of great fear and anxious restlessness; despairs of her salvation and seeks aid in constant prayer;...

RHUS-T. Al, 26 - Anxiety at night; he would flee (leave) from bed and seek help (aid), on account of an indescribable distressing sensation.

He, 11 - Anxiety: while sitting was obliged to take hold (grasp, keep) of something because she did not think she could keep up (support) on account of the beating and drawing pains in limbs; and apprehension as if he wished to take his own life; with loss of strength (vigor, vitality) as if he would die.

SANG. He, 11 - It seems to her ...she is in a railroad car and begs others to hold her.

SEP. Al, 33 - Received news of the slight illness of a friend, which caused great mental depression (at another time it would not have made slightest impression); this condition grew on me until I became so nervous that I felt that unless I held on something, I should scream.

He, 14 - Felt that unless he held on to something he should scream.

SOL-T-AE. Al, 1 - She rises in the night, imagining that thieves are hidden behind the curtains; but she not dare (risk) to look for them, and begs some one else to do so.

SPONG. Al, 11 - She is dissatisfied with what she accomplishes; she cannot rightly help herself at work (helpless) (incompetent) ; she does not succeed.

STRAM. Al, 24 - Much excited and rather delirious, under the impression of some immediate danger, clinging to the person who had him in her lap.

Al, 136 - Delirium...seeming to dread the approach of some imaginary monster, and giving utterance in the most piteous appeals for help, protection.

Ha, 559 - She fancies she sees a number of people who are not present, and she grasps at them.

Ha, 561 - In the moments of consciousness he begged to be held as he was falling.

He, 59-...clings to her mother with as much desperation as if she were going to be thrown from a precipice.

He, 79 - Boy seemed to see black objects, spoke of black people and black clouds, and grasped at air.

He, 85-...seemed to dread approach of some imaginary monster, and giving utterance to most piteous appeals for help.

He, 161 - While sitting on a sofa, fancied she was falling off, kept holding on to everything; while in bed said that bed was being drawn from under her.

He, 162 - In his conscious moments, he asked to be held because he was falling.

STRY. Al, 30 - He had a feeling of dread, and begged he might not be left alone.

TAX. Al, 10 - State of profound stupor and helplessness.

THEA. Al, 19 - Appeared to be actuated by the greatest terror, and said: "I have called upon you to request you would let me in and allow me to die in your house".

THUJ. Al, 1 - She herself desires, with anxiety and despair, to be taken to an insane asylum, (imprisonment, confining) and there to be treated very harshly and strictly, (penalized), so that her fixed ideas may be subdued and banished (purified); she knows very well that she does wrong (conscience) and thinks all sorts of bad thoughts (immoral), but she will not take the trouble to banish such thoughts; therewith she indistinctly gives to understand that she is constantly obliged to think of taking her own life, but feels the sinfulness (wicked) of it, in order to avoid it, desires the strict restraint of the asylum;...

Al, 9 - While half awake...cannot move a limb (paralyzed), with a sensation as though the whole body were as heavy as lead (heaviness), then she tries to call for help; can utter no sound, and lies with open eyes ...

Al, 67 - Sudden unaccountable (strange) anxiety in the head, which against her will, compels her to call some one.

HIDE

Delirium; shy, hides himself: **STRAM.**[54]

Delusions; bed, someone, under it: am-m. ars. bell. calc. canth. colch.

- bed, someone, under it, knocking: bell.[5] calc. canth. colch.[5]
- creep into himself, has to, he could not sufficiently crouch together: ***cimx.***[54]
- enemy, under the bed, is: am-m.
- laughed at, hides behind furniture, therefore: ***bar-c.***[122]
- noise, hears, bed, under: bell.[1]
- noise, hears, clattering above the bed when going to sleep: calc.
- thieves, house, and space under bed are full of that: ***ars.***
- visions, hide, wishes to: bell.[54]
- voices, hears, mastoid process, as if near right, a voice were scolding her, night agg., voice seems sometimes to be under bed: ***stram.***[54]

Dreams; clothing, hidden her, someone has: bamb-a.[1184]

➤ contraband, of having something, and wanting to snatch and lock it up: mag-c.[36]
➤ hiding from danger, of: lyc.[1]
➤ lying, someone is lying under him: nit-ac.[1]
Escape; attempts to, run away, to, wants, and hide as she insists that everyone is looking at her: meli.[85]
Hide, desire to: ars. aur.[58] **BELL.** camph. chlol. choc.[222] coca[25] cupr. eug.[10] ***hell.*** hyos. ***ign.***[54] lach. lap-c-b.[194] lap-mar-c.[194] meli.[72] ***puls.*** staph.[10] ***stram.*** tarent.
Hide; desire to, children, strangers, from: bar-c.[85]
Hide; desire to, children, thinks all visitors laugh at it and hides behind furniture: ***bar-c.***
Hide; desire to, corner, in: camph.[8] elaps[36] puls.[8]
Hide; desire to, fear, assaulted, of being: tarent.[58]
Hide; desire to, fear, on account of: ***ars. bell.*** cupr. ***hyos.***[54]
Hides things: bell. ***staph.***[8] tarent.[58]
Impulse; run, to, away, hide and: meli.[102]
Play; desire to, hide and seek, at: bell.[54]

ARS. Al, 88 - He has so much fear that he jumps out of his bed and hides himself in the wardrobe, which he can hardly be induced to leave.
Al, 89 - He sees thieves in his room, and therefore hides himself under the bed.
Ha, 39 - He jumps out of bed for fear, and hides away in a wardrobe.(closed)
Ha, 35 - He sees nothing but rogues in his room, and therefore always creeps under the bed.
He, 42 - Fear drives him out of bed; he hides in a closet.
BELL. He, 22 - Frightful visions; she wishes (desires) to hide herself.(veil, cover)
CHLOL. He, 7-...inclined to wander and hide herself, avoiding shrewdly (astute) the vigilance of her friends...
CHOC. Sh, 39 - Felt a need to be covered up.
Sh, 179 - Apprehensive about the shift in consciousness and nervous someone would notice. It is reminiscent of L.S.D., the 'shifting edges', before the full blown trip arrives —an uneasiness and unsureness about which way things will go. A desire to hide in case things go to pieces. 15, 30C, 00:00:50
Sh, 208 - Felt rejected and oversensitive. Hid away from the world, felt my life would fall apart. 35, 30C, XX:XX:XX:
Sh, 209 - A desire to hide in case things go to pieces. 15, 30C, 00:00:50
Sh, 210 - Felt totally isolated and averse to company. Estranged himself from his family and friends and stopped all communication with them for a long period. Did not reply to letters and left no address. He seemed to hide away and literally disappear. The state of Isolation resulted from feeling that "I didn't exist as a human being". This behaviour was in strong contrast to his normal sociable disposition. 35, 30C, XX:XX:XX:
ELAPS. Al, 6 - Desire to be alone; she takes refuge for days together in a corner of the antechamber.
HALI-L. Sh, 375 - Just wants to crawl away, hide in a hole, do something else. Hard to get motivated. This feeling about one job she has to do spills over into everything else and she doesn't want to do anything. 09, 6C, 03:XX:XX
Sh, 532 - I started to speed up emotionally, got really pissed off at supervisor for getting in touch with me, beeping me. Wanted to escape and fly away. Phoned the airlines, trying to fly away. Hiding. Difficult to be with patients, with their stupid emotions. 02, 30C, XX:XX:XX
Sh, 570 - Don't want to do anything but stay underground—"kick a can" around town. Feel angry about people who may be maligning me. 16, 10C, 14:XX:XX
HYOS. He, 78 - Groundless suspicion of being watched (observed, spied) by members of family with whom he had some slight misunderstanding (dispute); to avoid being recognized by them, clothed himself differently every day,...watching his relations suspiciously and imagining he might be poisoned;... (disguise, camouflage)
OP. He, 21-...in old, emaciated persons; sees animals coming towards him; people want to hurt him, execute him ; creeping under covers or jumping out of bed; in "old sinners" (criminals) whose long lives of excess have thoroughly destroyed their constitutions; ...; believe themselves to be murderers or criminals to be executed; want to run away (escape) ;...

PULS. He, 46 - Dark suspicious and reserved manner; disturbed look on face; sleepless; looks for her bed in the yard (lost?); hides in a corner to escape from a little gray man who wanted to pull out her leg;...
SOL-T-AE. Al, 1 - She rises in the night, imagining that thieves are hidden behind the curtains; but she not dare (risk) to look for them, and begs some one else to do so.
STRAM. He, 163 - Cries out fearfully, hides face in pillow, is terrified by presence or approach of physician; after attack of typhoid.
TARENT. Al, 56 - Fear and shaking; the patient cannot find a suitable place where to hide himself; thinks he is going to be assaulted.

HIMSELF

Anger; himself, with: ars.[54] bell.[54] elaps[36] germ.[222] ign.[36] lyc.[1] nux-v.[30] staph.[30] ***sulph.***[54]
Anger; himself, with, spoken to, does not wish to be: elaps[54]
Anger; mistakes, about his: ars.[54] bell.[54] bry. carc.[193] ***nit-ac.*** nux-v.[30] ***staph. sulph.***
Anger; tear himself to pieces, could: sulph.[54]
Antagonism; herself, with: acon. **ANAC.** anh.[144] ant-t.[54] aur. bar-c.[137] cann-i.[137] cann-s.[137] caps. irid.[5] ***kali-c.*** lac-c. ***lach.*** lyss. naja op.[5] paro-i.[149] ***sep.***[30] ***sil.***[30] verb.[54]
Anxiety; himself, about: nat-c.[36] ***sil.***[54]
Avarice; squandering on oneself, but: calc.[30] hyos.[30] lap-mar-c.[194] nux-v.[30] sep.[30]
Aversion; herself, to: crot-h.[111] fl-ac.[111] iod.[111] kali-p.[111] lac-c.[122] lyc.[111] phos.[111] pitu-a.[164] plat.[111] senec.[111] sep.[111] spirae.[36]
Aversion; sex, her own, to: raph.
Biting; himself: acon. arum-t.[58] elaps[54] hura lyss. op. plb. stram.[1] tarent.
Busy; himself, with: mag-m.[36] staph.[36]
Confusion of mind; arouse himself, compelled to: **CARB-V.** choc.[222] hydrog.[222] ***sulph.***[122]
Contemptuous; self, of: agn. ***aur.***[102] cop. lac-c.[102] thuj.[102]
Contemptuous; self, of, alternating with eccentricity: agn.[10]
Cursing; herself, to: merc.[122]
Delusions; dead, he is: anac. anh.[119] apis camph. cann-i. choc.[222] ***lach.*** mosch.[102] oena.[139] ***op.***[102] phos. raph.[139] sil.[139] stram.
• nobody, he is: agn.[36]
• obscene, actions of which she had not been guilty, accuses herself of.: ***phos.***
• obstacles, in his way, caused partly by contrary fate, partly by himself: aur.[36]
• unworthy to live: nat-s.[137] plat.[137]
Despair; others and oneself: ***arg-n.***[54] aur.[54]
Discontented; himself, with: act-sp.[111] ***agn.*** aloe ***ars.***[122] asaf.[137] aur. bamb-a.[1184] bell. bry. calc-p. cand-a.[239] caust. cham. cinnam.[36] cinnb. cob. cocc. con.[137] germ.[222] ***hep.*** kali-c. lac-h.[229] lyc. m-aust.[10] mang. meny. merc. mez. mur-ac. ***nit-ac.*** nux-v.[30] ozone[227] pana.[36] ph-ac. ***puls.***[122] ruta ***sac-alb.***[210] staph.[58] ***sulph.*** tarent. ther. viol-t. ziz.[54]
Discouraged; reproaches himself: ***m-arct.***[122]
Disgust; himself, with: germ.[222] lap-gr-m.[194]
Disgust; himself, with; courage to live, has none: ***merc.***[54]
Dreams; body, head, runs head against the wall: bamb-a.[1184]
➤ disease, injuries, self-inflicted: nicc.
➤ glorification of oneself: saroth.[144]
➤ injures, self-inflicted: nicc.
➤ reproaches himself: nat-m.[1]
Fear; alone, of being, injure himself, and: ars. merc.[137] nat-s.[137]
✦ cutting himself when shaving: **CALAD.**[122]
✦ mirrors in room, of, see himself, lest he should: camph.[54]
✦ thoughts, of his own: androc.[222] camph.
✦ tread lightly or will injure himself, must: cupr.
Haughty; look self-contented: ferr.[54] ferr-ma.[10]
Hysteria; injuring herself, must exert great force to prevent from: ***hydr-ac.***[54]
Impulse; stab his flesh with the knife he holds, to: ***lyss.***.
Indifference; himself, to: phos.[111] sep.[111] thuj-l.[149]
Irritability; himself, with: ars.[36] aur.[36] bell.[60]
Morose; oneself, with: ars.[36] aur.[36]
Mutilating his body, inclination to: agar.[102] ars. bell.[102] hyos.[102] med.[212] stram.[102]
Pull; desires to, presses her head and pulls her hair: tarent.[36]
Quarrelsomeness; herself with: merc.[111]
Rage; striking, himself: tarent.[36]
Reproaches; himself: ***acon.*** ambr.[162] anac.[116] ***ars. aur.*** aur-ar.[58] calc-p. cand-a.[239] cob. con.[116] cupr.[184] cycl. ***dig.*** germ.[222] gink.[149]

hell. hura ***hyos. ign.*** lach.[116] lap-c-b.[194] lyc. ***m-arct.***[10] med.[122] merc. myric.[144] nat-ar. ***nat-m. op.*** ph-ac. plb.[201] ***puls. sarr.*** sil.[116] stram.[111] sulph.[116] ***thuj.*** verat.[116]
Restlessness; internal, beat about herself with hands and feet, as if he would: lyc.
Sadness; diverted from thoughts of himself, desires to be: ***aur.***[54] camph.[54]
Scratches with hands, himself, raw: arum-t.[137] psor.[137]
Self-deception: act-sp.[54]
Self-torture: acon.[111] ***ars.***[111] bell.[111] ***lil-t.***[111] plb.[111] tarent.[111] tub.[111]
Striking; abdomen, his: bell.
Striking; anger, from, himself: nat-c.[36]
Striking; chest, his: camph. verat-v.
Striking; himself: ars. bac.[55] bell. camph. cur. germ.[222] plat.[1] **TARENT.** ***verat-v.***
Striking; himself, head, his: ars. bac.[55] hyos.[5] stram. **TARENT.**
Talk; himself, to, quarreling with some one, as if, seven p.m.: kali-cy.[36]
Talk; indisposed, condition, about her: chel.[36]
Tears; himself: ars. bell. cur. lach.[189] plb. sec. **STRAM.**
Tears; himself, hair, his: ***ars.***[137] bac.[55] ***bell. cupr.***[137] dig.[137] ***lil-t.*** med.[137] tarent. tub.[8] xan.[137]
Thoughts; himself, become of him, what would: nat-m.[137]
Thoughts; himself, desires to be diverted from thoughts of himself: camph.[54]
Thoughts; thoughtful, himself, about: cic.[36] viol-o.[36]
Torments; himself: acon.[111] ars.[111] bell.[111] ***lil-t.***[111] nat-m.[36] plb.[111] tarent.[111] tub.[111]
Weeping; discontent with himself: ***nit-ac.***[54] ziz.[54]

ACT-SP. He, 4 - Self-deception; self-satisfaction.
ADAM. Sh, 190 - Very unhappy with my body, I want to escape from it, to run away from myself. I want to go from me. 20, 1M, 08:XX:XX
Sh, 191 - I feel like vomiting out all my insides. I want to get rid of everything inside me I physically feel like vomiting all my stomach and even all my breath. I want everything to get out of me. 20, 1M, 07:XX:XX
Sh, 194 - Felt ugly, miserable and generally fed up with myself during menses, more intensely than I usually would at this time. 8, 6C, 17:XX:XX
Sh, 229 - Feeling very angry towards others and hate people. I want to be alone and away from people who upset me. I hate feeling angry and resentful, a lot of it is directed to myself. 20, 1M, XX:XX:XX
AGAR. Al, 46 - His mind is uneasy and anxious; he was constantly concerned only about himself, his present and future condition.
Al, 57 - She is vexed with herself and pities (compassion) herself.
AGN. Al, 1-,...he feels as if nothing existed around him; he is dissatisfied with himself all the time; he is incapable of attending to any business; the things around him are entirely indifferent to him;...
ALOE. Al, 25 - Ill-humor; peevish (angry) about himself, so that he insults and blasphemes; worse afternoons.
He, 11 - Dissatisfied and angry about himself, more so when he is constipated or suffers from pain.
ANT-C. Ha, 7 - Anxious meditation, during the day, about himself, his present and future fate. (doom, destine).
ARS. Ha, 1064 - All day long discontented with himself and very cross with himself; he imagines he has not done enough, and reproaches himself bitterly.
Ha, 53 - Dissatisfied all day and extremely vexed at himself; he thought he had not worked enough and reproached himself most bitterly.
He, 95 - Dissatisfied and angry with himself all day; thinks he has not accomplished enough, and reproaches himself bitterly.
AUR. Ha, 330 - All day long good humor; he was talkative and contented with himself.
Ha, 20 - Discouraged (despair) and at odds (quarreling) with himself.(antagonism)
Ha, 355 - He is discontented with himself and depressed in spirits.
He, 57 - Despair of self and others.
BELL. Al, 178 - Fretfulness; nothing seemed right to him; he was vexed with himself.
Ha, 1401 - Peevishness, nothing was right for him; he was angry with himself.
Ha, 1419 - Fury; he injures himself and others and strikes about him. (beat, hit)

He, 119 - Fretfulness; nothing seemed right to him; was vexed with himself.

BISM. He, 11 - Ill humor; he is morose and discontented with his condition (position), and complains about it.

BOR. Al, 18-..contented with himself and the world, and looking cheerfully into the future.

CACT. Al, 17 - Feeling of doing violence (injury) to myself.

CAMPH. Al, 40 - Afraid of the mirrors in the room, lest he should see himself in them; so excessive was this fear at times in the night that he would have got up and broken the mirrors, only that he was still more afraid to get up alone in the dark;...

Al, 17 - He beats himself on the chest, and falls into a faint.

He, 63 - Afraid of mirrors in room, lest he should see himself in them (reflection) ; so excessive was his fear at times in night that he would have got up and broken mirrors, only that he was still (but) more afraid to get up alone in the dark.

CHOC. Sh, 304 - Feels she has changed her attitude towards herself, less judgmental and pedantic, kinder to herself now. Eating more meat and feeling OK about it, previously had been vegetarian for health and moral reasons.[13], 12C, XX:XX:XX

CIC. Ha, 238 - Want of trust (mistrust, skepticism) in people and anthrophoby,(misanthropy) he fled (escape) from them remained solitary, and thought seriously about their errors and about himself.

Ha, 241 - Tranquillity of mind; he was extremely satisfied with his position, and with himself, and very cheerful.

COB. Al, 4 - Low-spirited; thinks too little of himself.

COCC. Al, 30 - Great dissatisfaction with himself.

Ha, 529 - Great discontent with himself.

CON. He, 32 - Discouraged, despondent, and dissatisfied (discontented) with herself and her surrounds.

He, 36 - Morose mood; everything about him impresses him unpleasantly.

COT. Al, 11 - Feels silly (ridiculous) and lost.

CROC. Al, 30-...the behavior of relatives and friends excites her to anger,...she is vexed with herself, and her anger becomes greater than ever;..

CUR. Al, 1 - Paroxysm of insanity impelling him to attack himself; he strikes, scratches, and tears himself with a sort of relish, (enjoy) and without feeling any pain.

He, 2 - Very much depressed about herself, desire only to shut herself up away from people.

ELAPS. He, 6 - Angry about one's self, does not wish to be spoken to.

GERM. Sh, 123 - Don't understand anything, the meaning of life. Feel also strength somewhere inside. I wish a change could happen, I ought to bring myself together and change. It is silly of me to go on like this. I despise myself. I am hard to myself, but I don't deserve anything else. I think other people are silly too. 18, 30C, 06:XX:XX

Sh, 112 - Don't see why I am here. I can't bear it. I go mad. I hate myself. I want to beat myself and I do it. Tear my hair. Stop when it hurts too much. It is like hell !!! 18, 30C, 20:XX:XX

Sh, 99 - Came in contact with very much hate and disgust within, and it made a deep impression on me. I have to be reconciled with those parts of me. I think that power can be used in a different way -not so destructive. I am no person. Feel I have no power when I meet people. Sometimes I feel I disappear. I am not in my body. My hands feel gone. My feet are cold; I don't like them. Yet I feel I have great power inside, especially I feel it when I get angry or when I sing. 18, 30C, 46:XX:XX

Sh, 158 - Some persistent feelings coming up. Feel envious of a colleague who I feel manages so well. When I compare with myself I feel worthless and nothing. I feel like talking badly about her to my friends and I do this, even though she is not present. It takes a lot of my attention and energy. 21, 12C, 67:XX:XX.

Sh, 111 - If I were me, nobody would like me -so I try to be what I think others expect me to be. I don't think I can be loved with all the parts of me which are ugly and bad. Lonely feelings. Longing for love and understanding. Feel I am so unfriendly to myself. 18, 30C, 04:00:00

HEP. Ha, 11 - Dissatisfied with oneself.
HIPP. Al, 6 - Fretful, discontented with himself almost lachrymose, in the morning.
HYDROG. Sh, 188 - On getting up in the morning, I feel very angry and bad about myself. I feel I can't cope. Whats the use of trying? I feel like giving up. I think for a moment I'd like to die. 10, 200C, 09:XX:XX
IGN. Al, 27 - Slight blame or contradiction excites him to anger, and this makes him angry with himself.
He, 53 - Slight blame (censure) or contradiction excites him to anger, and this makes him angry with himself.
IOD. Al, 27 - Is cross and irascible; feels stupid.(obtuse)
KALI-C. Ha, 31 - She is always in antagonism with herself; she knows not what she wants, and feels exceedingly unhappy.
Ha, 30 - Peevish mood, as if she could not do anything to suit (satisfy) herself.
He, 9-...constantly in antagonism which herself; frequently hopeful, frequently despondent; frets (worry) about everything; peevish impatient, contented with nothing.
KALI-CY. Al, 5 - At 7 p.m., while walking out of doors, feelings of crossness; carries on a kind of conversation within himself, as if quarreling with someone whith whom he had previously disagreed; thinks what he will reply in case certain things are said to him.
KALI-N. Al, 19 - Perverse hypochondriac mood; discontented with himself and the world, peevish irritable, ...
LAC-C. Al,N-11 - Thinks that she is looked down upon (despised) by every one, that she is of no importance in life, and feels insulted thereat. (unimportant, worthless)
He, 9 - Thinks she is looked down (contempted, scorned, despised) upon by everyone, that she is of no importance in life. (self-contemptuous)
LYC. Al, 96 - Quarrelsome rage, partly at herself partly at others.
Ha, 56 - Angry fury, partly against himself, and partly against others.
MANG. He, 6 - Everything she even thinks of makes her fretful.
MENY. Ha, 286 - Cross, ill-humored and discontented with himself and his position (rank); anxiety drives him from one place to another.(restlessness)
MERC. Al, 31 - Fretful all day; very much out of sorts and discontented with himself; he had no desire to talk or joke.
Ha, 1248 - Without cause he is very discontented with himself and his position.
Ha, 1257 - During the whole day cross, as if at variance and dissatisfied with himself, and had no inclination for speaking and joking.
He, 34 - Inexpressive pain of soul and body, anxious restlessness, as if some evil impended ...; disgusted (revolt) with himself, has not courage (cowardice) to live; constant suspicion (distrust), considering everybody his enemy.
MEZ. Al, 10 - Great discontent with himself and his surroundings (living, conditions, position) for several weeks...
NAT-C. Al, 42 - Very fretful and discontented with whole world; he constantly felt as though he could beat (punish ?) himself, his whole life angered him, and he preferred to have no existence at all; he was solicitous about the future, and inclined to despair, all day.
Al, 14 - Anxious, solicitous about himself.(cares)
Ha, 48 - Peevish and cross, dissatisfied whith all the world; he could have kicked (self sensure) himself; he would rather not live at all ; at the same time solicitous about the future, so that he is ready to despair.
Ha, 14 - Anxiously solicitous about himself.
NAT-M. Al, 63 - When alone, she becomes uneasy (discontent) about herself, and must weep.
Al, 2761 - In a dream he reproached himself for past mistakes, full of restlessness and anxiety.
NIT-AC. Al, 27 - Vexed at the least trifle, even at himself if he makes a mistake.
Ha, 44 - Vexed at the least trifle, also at himself, when he does something amiss.(wrong)
Ha, 33 - Discontented with oneself, dissolving in tears, which gives relief.
Ha, 38 - Very ill-humored and vexed at himself.
Ha, 49 - He gets violently excited about

trifles, all the day, and has then to laugh at himself.
He, 22 - Discontent with himself induces violent weeping.
NUX-V. He, 20 - Desire to talk about one's condition, with anxious reflections about it.
OP. Al, 69 - Great strength, courage, contentment with himself.
PH-AC. Ha, 674 - Discontented with himself, self-reproaches.
PLAT. Ha, 18 - Taciturnity and involuntary weeping, even after the most friendly address (communication), so that she gets vexed (anger) about it herself.
Ha, 33 - Very cross and irritated at harmless matters and words; so that she at times would have liked to have beaten herself and friends.
He, 10 - Cold, haughty, too well satisfied with one's self, and not at all anxious about the future. (presumptuous, egotistic, inexpugnable, safe)
PSOR. Al,N-44 - Mania of self-destruction.
PULS. Al, 8 - Extremely capricious and peevish at everything, even at himself.
He, 13 - Extremely capricious and peevish about everything, himself included.
RUTA. Al, 11 - Much dissatisfied (discontented) by everything that happened to him, and especially with whatever he did himself, and great inclination to weep.
He, 2 - Dissatisfied with himself and others.
SEP. Ha, 68 - He thinks, what he does not wish to think, uses expressions which he himself knows are incorrect; he resolves to do what is against his intention, and is thus in conflict with himself and, therefore in a disagreeable, restless mood. (lost: knowledge, correction)
SIL. He, 8 - Overanxious about himself; low-spirited...
SPIRAE. Al, 1 - At 1 A.M. he was attacked with remorse over a long-past slight indiscretion (mistake, wrong), with most fearful qualms (anxiety) of conscience and loathing of himself; ....
STRAM. Ha, 544 - Great desire to bite and tear everything with his teeth that comes near his mouth, even his own limbs.
SULPH. Al, 42-...discontented with himself and all about him, which made him unfit for any serious occupations...whole evening he was absorbed in himself and unable to command his thoughts to read...
Ha, 43 - Ill-humored; she becomes vexed at herself.
He, 50 - Irritable mood; easily excited and always absorbed in himself.
He, 55 - Ill-humored; vexed with herself; everything makes her impatient.
He, 56 - He could tear himself to pieces with vexation.
TARENT. He, 2 - Great taciturnity and irritability; desire to strike himself and others.
THER. Al, 7 - Despair; want of confidence; he gives himself up.
TUB. Al,N-11 - Felt positively ugly (repulsive, spiteful); personal aversions became almost a mania.
VERAT. Ha, 664 - Cursing and making a noise all night, and complains of being stupid, with headache and flow of saliva.

HOME

Anxiety; friends at home, about: bar-c. ***phos.*** phys. puls.[172] ***sulph.***
Anxiety; home, about: nat-p.[36]
Anxiety; house, in agg.: alum. ars. aster. ***bry.*** carl. chel. kali-c. **LYC.** ***mag-m.*** plat. **PULS. RHUS-T.** spong. ***til.*** valer.
Anxiety; household matters, about: ars.[172] bar-c.[60] carl.[102] hyos.[172] nux-v.[172] ph-ac.[172] puls.[60] rhus-t.[60] sep.[60] sulph.[5]
Cares; full of, domestic affairs, about: bar-c. ***puls. sep.***
Delirium; home, wants to go: bell.[36] bry.[72] ***cupr-acet.***[54]
Delusions; burnt, everything at home is: bell.[10]
- door, someone was coming in at the (at night): con.
- fire, house, on: bell. hep. stram.
- fire, neighbor's house on (morning, waking in a fright): hep.
- fire, room is on: stram.
- fire, sees, home, on distant: bell.
- happy is his own house, he will never be: ars.
- home, at, when not: cann-i. hyos.
- home, away from, is: acon. aster.[8] bell. **BRY.** calc. calc-p.[102] cic. cimic.[102] ***coff.*** germ.[222] ***hyos.*** lach. lap-c-b.[194] meli. merc.[15] ***nux-v.***[30] ***op.*** par.[10] plb.[5] puls.[122] ***rhus-t.*** valer. verat. vip.

- • home, away from, is, abortion, in threatening: op.[26]
- • home, away from, must go there: ***bry.***[102] calc-p.[102] cimic.[102] hyos.[102] ***op.***[102]
- • home, changed, everything at h., has: arg-n.
- • house, his own, is not in: ***op.***[54] verat.[54]
- • house, movable, is: cann-i.
- • house, people, full of: ars. cann-i. con. lach. lyc. merc. nat-m. nux-v. sil. stram.
- • house, place, not in right (while walking in the street after headache): glon.
- • house, surrounded, is: stram.
- • living, locality three hours distant from his house, in a: ***op.***[54]
- • nesting, she is: lac-h.[229]
- • people, entering the house at night: con.
- • places, wrong, in, but does not want to go home: hyos.
- • policeman, come into house, he sees: ars.[58] hyos. kali-br.
- • room, foam of a troubled sea, is the: sec.
- • room, hall in a garden, a bower, is a: calc.[1]
- • room, sees people bedside in: atro. con.
- • thieves, house, and space under bed are full of that: ***ars.***
- • thieves, house, in: ars. cann-i. con.[30] ***cupr-acet.***[54] ***lach.*** merc. ***nat-m.*** sil. sol-t-ae.

Desires; removal: form.[36]

Dreams; ashamed, dirty and sloppy house, because of her: ozone[227]

- ➤ fire, house on, her: kali-c.[36]
- ➤ friends, apartment, in wrong: ozone[227]
- ➤ home: lach.[36] mur-ac.[36]
- ➤ house, family, for a big: ozone[227]
- ➤ house, looses his way in his: mag-c.[1]
- ➤ house, mothers, her: ozone[227]
- ➤ houses: ozone[227] pall.[54]
- ➤ houses, bright, very: ozone[227]
- ➤ houses, buildings or, beside which he stands, or in which he stands before a window, or walks over wide stairs through many rooms: pall.[8]
- ➤ houses, cold, liveless, nearly threatening: ozone[227]
- ➤ houses, crystal and marble, built of: ozone[227]
- ➤ houses, dirty: ozone[227]
- ➤ houses, find house where he wants to go, cannot: ozone[227]
- ➤ houses, like the house of her youth: ozone[227]
- ➤ houses, tarring the floor: ozone[227]
- ➤ houses, walls of glass, with: ozone[227]
- ➤ lost, home, at: choc.[222] mag-c.[1]
- ➤ men, rough men put out of house: frax.[36]
- ➤ robbers, house, want to go into: ozone[227]
- ➤ unsuccessful efforts to, finding way in his own house: mag-c.

Duty; aversion to domestic: cench.[58] cit-l.[54] sul-i.[58]

Escape; attempts to, house, wants to get out of: germ.[222] ***verat.***[54]

Escape; attempts to, house, wants to get out of, fright, after: merc.[54]

Fear; away from home: ign.[162]

- ✦ door, closed, lest the d. should be: lac-d.[122]
- ✦ happen, something will, home, before he got: ***zing.***[54]
- ✦ home, away from: ign.[162]
- ✦ out of doors, to go: acon.[172] anth. bar-c.[127] dys-co.[136] kali-p.[172] ***lyss.***[184]

Going out, aversion to: agar.[137] am-c. anth. clem. ***cycl.*** hydr. ign.[137] sep.[127]

Handle things anymore, cannot, housewives: bamb-a.[1184] sep.[187]

Home, desires to go: acon.[111] bell. **BRY.** ***calc.*** calc-p. ***carb-an.***[36] chlol. cic. cimic.[111] clem.[36] coff.[111] cupr. ***cupr-acet.***[54] eup-per.[36] germ.[222] hell.[36] hyos. ***lach.*** lap-c-b.[194] lipp.[36] mag-c.[36] meli.[111] merc.[36] nit-ac.[36] ***op.*** plan. psor.[58] puls.[36] rhus-t. sac-alb.[36] senec.[36] sil.[36] valer.[111] verat. vip.

Home; desires to go, go out, and when there: ***bry.***[54] ***calc.***[54] **CALC-P.**[54] ***cupr-acet.***[54]

Home; desires to, leave: arag.[102] ***bry.***[102] elat. fl-ac.[58] lach.[102] merc.[102] verat.[102]

Home; desires to, leave, retiring, when: elaps[36]

Home; talks of h.: bell. ***bry.***

House-keeping, women inapt to: cit-l.[54] lyc.[30] nux-v.[30] pitu-a.[164] sil.[30] sulph.[30]

House; aversion to being kept in: lyc.[36]

Indifference; duties, domestic, to: androc.[222] aur-ar.[58] brom.[58] ***cimic.***[54] cit-l.[54] sep.[81] sul-i.[58]

Irritability; house, in, agg.: anac.[10] ign.[60] **RHUS-T.**[36]

Neglects; household, the: aur-ar.[58] sul-i.[58]

Recognize; does not, house, his own: cic.[58] meli. merc. psor.

Runs about; away from home: stram.[109] tub.[189]

Sadness; domestic affairs, over: bar-c.[10] puls.[10] rhus-t.[10] ***sep.***[54] viol-t.[8]

Sadness; house, driving out of: laur.[10]
Sadness; house, entering, on: plat.[36] tarent.[36]
Sadness; house, in, agg.: ***plat.***[36] **RHUS-T.**[36]
Talk; domestic affairs, of: hyos.[54]
Time; passes too slowly, way home too long: **GLON.**[54]
Violence; chases family out of house: ***verat.***[54]

ADAM. Sh, 296 - Thinking a lot about a cottage in Hampshire that I'd wanted to buy and feeling sad that I hadn't. Feeling that it would have been so blissful to be alone there, and be creative in the garden. No sound except birds, just to relax and be alone. 1, 12C, 01:XX:XX
Sh, 297 - I didn't want to go away to teach. Wanted to be at home. Feel happy at home with children. 2, 12C, 05:XX:XX
ARS. Al, 87 - He imagines that the whole house, and the space under the bed, are full of thieves, which causes, from fright, anxious cold sweat to break out over his body.
Al, 86 - He runs through the whole house at night in search of thieves.
Ha, 36 - His whole house, also under his bed, is full of rogues, which causes a cold sweat to break out, which runs down cold over his body.
Ha, 37 - In the night he runs all about the house, looking for thieves.
ASTER. He, 2-...hallucinations as if away from home in midst (middle) of strangers; hears voices to which he replies.
BAR-A. Al, 15 - Extreme irresolution ; he proposes a short journey, but as soon as he makes preparation he changes his mind, and is inclined to remain at home.
BAR-C. He, 28 - Solicitude, about his future; about domestic affairs.
BELL. Al, 54 - The delirium was of a busy (engaged, working), restless, vivid character, but generally rather pleasing than otherwise. The patient appeared to think they were pursuing (persevere) their ordinary occupations; one boy appeared eager (animated) in flying a kite (toy), another pulled tables and chairs about, thinking he was working in a coal-pit, and a woman appeared to be remarkably busy with her household duties...
Al, 91 - He raves as in a dream, and cries he must go home, because everything is burning up there. (rescue, saving)
Al, 203-..;he imagined himself rich, owner of a large house, etc. (great person)
A-S, 2554-..The patients appeared to think that they were pursuing their ordinary occupations;... the woman appeared remarkably busy with her ordinary household duties.
Ha, 1338 - He is delirious, and cries out in his dreams that he must go home, because everything is on fire there.
Ha, 1337 - He makes preparation to go home.
He, 18 - When closing eyes, though not asleep, patient sees fierce (wild), wicked looking large animals with horns and bushy (scabrous) heads; room seemed to be full of strange men passing in and out, who would snatch (take hold) at her as they passed, which frightened her very much, she thought the men wanted to take her away from home ; she then saw children sitting on low benches (seat) in rows (line) as in a school-room. (purity)
BROM. He, 6 - Aversion to any kind of work, even reading; takes no interest in household duties.
BRY. He, 13 - The patient desires to go home.
CALC. Ha, 69 - Unconsciousness and delusion about her abode (home) as if her room were a hall (passage) in a garden.
He, 23 - Desire to go home.
CANN-I. Al, 29 - Looks under beds and tables, unlocks and relocks doors, for the fancies he hears strange noises, and that thieves are in the house.
CARL. Al, 10 - Discouraged and anxious in the discharge (execution) of his domestic duties.
CHLOL. Al, 17-...a feeling as if he were now in one country and now in another, and with an anxious desire to go home.(abroad)
CIMIC. He, 26 - Indifferent, taciturn, takes no interest in household matters.
COFF. He, 7 - Delirium tremens: unsteady running about; imagines he is not at home,...
CUPR-A. He, 17 - Feared bedclothes or house would catch fire.
FL-AC. Al, 1 - Great disposition, when alone, to repulsive fantastic imaginations,

particularly in regard to persons with whom he stands in near relations, or with whom he is connected (united, joined); it seems, for example, as though he must get rid (discard, repudiate, reject) of all the servants, children must go out of house, a betrothal must be broken off, a marriage should be dissolved. (broke; vows)

GLON. He, 2 - Recognized no one; repulsed her husband and children; raved, screamed, and wished to rush from house; jumped out of bed, but fell because her knees gave way.

He, 3 - She could not remember which side of the street her house was on.

HALI-L. Sh, 184 - Totally in gear. Cleaned and organized my whole house. Wanted everything in order. If everything is in order then life will be great. It will go well. 08, 30C, 08:XX:XX

Sh, 513 - On my way home, while it was dark, I saw a glow in the sky and immediately I thought my house was burning. I was very scared and I should have realized that the glow came from the town behind the ridge, but it took me a while to get that. 04, 30C, 03:XX:XX

Sh, 993 - I was traveling around inside my head last night — Israel, the States, New Zealand and Scotland. All places I've never been, but all the same sort of terrain, like barren, down South, New Zealand. I was looking for a new home. 20, 30C, 31:XX:XX

HEP. Al, 1 - Ghostly image of one who was dead, in the morning, in bed, after waking and while conscious, which frightened him; it also seemed as though he saw his neighbor's house burning, which also frightened him.

Ha, 298 - In the morning in bed after waking, when conscious, he had the visionary appearance of a deceased (dead, defunct) person, which frightened him, and he also imagined he saw a neighboring house in flames, which terrified him.

He, 8-...threatened to murder wife and children, attempted to set house on fire, and was with difficulty controlled; ... (pyromaniac) 0Scabies.

HYOS. Al, 14 - Thought he was in his own home, and desire to go out and make visits.

IGN. He, 61 - Melancholia after great grief and domestic trouble; complete sleeplessness; suicidal thoughts and desire to escape.

IOD. He, 15 - At night, especially when thinking of real or imaginary wrongs ...dares (try) to go home for fear of doing some dreadful (bad, wicked) deed (action); on one occasion was seized with an almost irresistible impulse to murder a woman who was acting as a guide (direct, conduct) for him, he having lost his way (direction);...must be constantly in action, in some laborious occupation. (lost; direction, correction, control)

KALI-BR. Al, 3 - Decidedly insane; had delusions that lewd women had got into his mother's house; that he was pursued by the police; that his wife was threatened by members of the family; that he had thousands of dollars in gold sewed up in his clothing; (rich, wealth)

LACH. He, 8 - Thinks: she is somebody else in the hands (seized) of a stronger power; (supremacy, superiority).or that she is dead, and preparations are made for funeral (cortege) or that she is nearly dead and wishes some one would help her off; herself pursued by enemies, or fears medicine is poison; there are robbers in house and wants to jump out the window; herself under super-human control; visions real, he will die. (helplessness, desire; aid, comfort, salvation)

He, 39 - Weak and unhappy, particularly in morning, when she feels, on awaking, friendless and forsaken; ...(deserted) has had domestic troubles. 0 Melancholia

LYSS. Al,N-46 - After fainting (weak) spell he wrote on paper: I am forsaken by all; even the birds of heaven, they do not look at me (despised), do not fed me if hungry (helplessness) ; I hunger with the young ones and am thirsty with their she ones (starving); my nest (house) is made out of dirt (soiled), not gotten by my own exertions (efforts), but by driving them out of their nests (home) and sitting there with the females and the young.

MAG-C. Al, 947 - Anxious dream as if he was unable to find his way in his own house.

MAG-M. Al, 711 - An anxious dream; she

was lying in a strange house, where rubbish (garbage) was constantly falling upon her; she tried to cry out and could not, because there was too great heaviness on the chest.

Ha, 3 - Apprehensive and melancholic, lonely (isolated, abandoned) ; she is homesick and weeps.

MERC. Ha, 1130 - Frightful dreams, in which he started up; he imagined he was not in his own house, sat up in bed and spoke about a distant village.

NAT-P. Al, 7 - Felt anxious about home (homesickness?); had misgivings (worry) ; feared bad news.

NIT-AC. Al, 17 - At once she is taken which peculiar anguish, runs to her physician, but he is not at home, hires a carriage to drive to the house where she expects to find him; during her ride all the anguish is gone; arrived at home she feels as bad as ever, and feels herself thus forced to drive about the whole day, till all the effects of the Nitric acid have passed off.

NUX-M. He, 17 - The outer world had no existence for her; automatically she attended to her household duties, and on awaking from this condition she had not the slightest recollection of what she had done; ...

OP. He, 11 - Thinks he is not in his own house; imagines himself living in a locality three hours distant from his house; detains all passers-by and wishes to take them into his house; ...he does not recognize friends;... (estranged, alien)

He, 17 - Thinks she is not at home.

PH-AC. Ha, 8 - Sad serious, disheartened (depressed), only while walking in the open air, increasing the longer he walks; at home it gradually passed of and he became more serene.

PLB. Al, 60-...; he hears everywhere threatening voices, officers come to arrest him, to seize his furniture (movables), (confiscated, expropriated) and to expel (eject) him from his lodgings (home) (expulsion, exiled) ; the voices come from the pillow, the mattress (bed); they enter by the window, where he sees people, and they consult about him with closed doors (secretive) ; ...

PULS. Al, 25 - It seems so quiet (silent) in her head and everything feels so empty that she seems alone in the house and in the world; she will speak to no one, just as if her surroundings did not exist (estrange), and she paid attention to no one. (left, solitary)

Ha, 1118 - Solicitude about his domestic concerns, in the morning.

Ha, 1143 - Her head is so quiet and all about her is so empty as if she were alone (solitude, loneliness) in the house and in the world; she does not wish to talk to any one, just as if all around her were no concern (relation) of hers and she belonged to nobody. (lonely, missed)

He, 46 - Dark suspicious and reserved manner; disturbed look on face; sleepless; looks for her bed in the yard (lost?); hides in a corner to escape from a little gray man who wanted to pull out her leg;...

SEP. He, 11 - Sad about her health and domestic affairs, discontented with everything.

SIL. Ha, 3 - Longing for home.

He, 9 - Longing for his relations and home.

STANN. He, 6 - A woman, age 39, pregnant in fourth month;...inability to do anything as she cannot muster sufficient courage,...great palpitation of heart and anxiety, especially if she has to give directions in her domestic affairs; thinking makes her feel wretched, ...(unable, incapable)

THEA. Al, 19 - Appeared to be actuated by the greatest terror, and said: “I have called upon you to request you would let me in and allow me to die in your house”.

VALER. Al, 1 - Extremely delirious, attempting to get out of the window, ... imagined himself away from home, and beset (surrounded) with all sorts of danger, from which he was attempting to escape, although unable to walk without staggering from side to side.

Al, 11 - Anxious, hypochondriac feeling, as if the objects around him had been estranged from him; the room appears to him desolate (isolated), he does not feel at home in the room, he is impelled to leave it.

VERAT. Al, 2 - Slight delirium; ...he prattles about religious subjects and about vows to be performed, prays, believes that he is not in his own house.

He, 16-... prattles about religious subjects and about vows (promise) to be performed, prays, believes that he is not in his own house.
He, 26 - Chases (pursue, hunt) his family out of house ; declares the sun travels around the earth (geocentric); fear of death, restlessness, despair...
He, 13 - After severe illness, aversion to husband and children; desire to leave house: hallucinations, room appeared full of people, crowding in, there was no longer room...
VIOL-T. He, 2 - Low spirited about domestic affairs.

HOMESICKNESS

Ailments from; homesickness: ***caps.*** carc.[233] ***clem.*** eup-pur.[102] hell.[102] ***ign.***[102] mag-m.[102] **PH-AC.**[54] senec.[102]
Ailments from; homesickness, drowsiness, particularly with: **PH-AC.**[54]
Anxiety; evening, family, about his, which he left behind while on a journey: ***petr.***[54]
Anxiety; home, about: nat-p.[36]
Delirium; home, wants to go: bell.[36] bry.[72] ***cupr-acet.***[54]
Delusions; calls, him with name, the absent mother or sister: anac.[10]
• home, away from, is: acon. aster.[8] bell. **BRY.** calc. calc-p.[102] cic. cimic.[102] ***coff.*** germ.[222] ***hyos.*** lach. lap-c-b.[194] meli. merc.[15] ***nux-v.***[30] ***op.*** par.[10] plb.[5] puls.[122] ***rhus-t.*** valer. verat. vip.
• home, away from, is, abortion, in threatening: op.[26]
• home, away from, must go there: ***bry.***[102] calc-p.[102] cimic.[102] hyos.[102] ***op.***[102]
• house, his own, is not in: ***op.***[54] verat.[54]
Dreams; country, native country: ant-c.[1] lach.[36] mur-ac.[36]
➤ dead, people, of, friends long deceased: arg-n. cedr.[36] coca[36] con.[1] ferr. nat-c.
➤ dead, people, of, friends, talking with deceased: lepi.[36]
➤ death of, relatives: caust.[1] ferr. fl-ac. hydrog.[222] kali-c.[1] mag-c. mag-s. pitu-a.[164] rheum sars.
➤ distant, beloved one: plb.[36]
➤ distant, people: sel.[36]
➤ homesickness: ***glon.***[36]
➤ houses: ozone[227] pall.[54]
➤ parting people: ozone[227]
➤ people, seen for years, not: hydrog.[222]
➤ people, seen for years, not, twenty years: calad.[54] calc-ar.[54]
➤ schoolmate, meeting of old: ant-c.[10] ferr.[36]
Ennui; homesickness, with: alum.[162] ***caps.***[122] ***clem.***[122]
Escape; attempts to, visit his daughter, wants to: ars.
Hatred; persons, of, absent, amel. on seeing: fl-ac.
Home, desires to go: acon.[111] bell. **BRY.** ***calc.*** calc-p. ***carb-an.***[36] chlol. cic. cimic.[111] clem.[36] coff.[111] cupr. ***cupr-acet.***[54] eup-per.[36] germ.[222] hell.[36] hyos. ***lach.*** lap-c-b.[194] lipp.[36] mag-c.[36] meli.[111] merc.[36] nit-ac.[36] ***op.*** plan. psor.[58] puls.[36] rhus-t. sac-alb.[36] senec.[36] sil.[36] valer.[111] verat. vip.
Home; desires to go, old, deteriorated people: cic.[193]
Home; talks of h.: bell. ***bry.***
Homesickness: acon.[5] ant-c.[5] ***aur.*** bar-c.[1] ***bell.***[122] **BRY.**[5] ***calc.***[163] calc-p. **CAPS.**[122] **CARB-AN.** carc.[233] carl. ***caust.*** cent. cimic.[5] ***clem. cocc.***[122] ***coff.***[122] dros. elaps elat.[122] eup-pur. germ.[222] ***hell.***[5] hyos. **IGN.**[122] iris-t.[85] kali-m.[192] ***kali-p.*** kreos.[5] lach. lap-c-b.[194] lipp.[36] mag-c. **MAG-M.**[122] manc.[8] ***meny.***[5] **MERC.**[122] ***nat-m.*** nit-ac. op.[5] petr. **PH-AC.** ***phos.***[122] plan. plb.[5] puls. puls-n.[83] ***ran-s.***[5] sac-alb.[56] sac-l. senec. sep. ***sil. staph.*** valer.[5] verat. ***zinc.***[163]
Homesickness; anguish, with: merc.[10]
Homesickness; evening: hipp.
Homesickness; hot feeling in fauces, with: **CAPS.**[54]
Homesickness; house, even when in her own: eup-pur.[85]
Homesickness; mental derangement, in: manc.[54]
Homesickness; morning: carb-an.
Homesickness; red cheeks, with: *caps.*
Homesickness; silent ill humor, with: nit-ac. *ph-ac.*
Homesickness; sleeplessness, with: caps.[122]
Homesickness; weep, with inclination to: ph-ac.[8]
Hysteria; homesickness: eup-pur.[25]
Inconsolable; anxiety about his family, from, which he left behind while going on a short journey: ***petr.***[54]
Suicidal disposition; homesickness, from: caps.[5]

Talk; native country, of: aether[36]
Weeping; homesickness, as from: ph-ac.[36]

ADAM. Sh, 100 - Sensitive to music that I know and like —very nostalgic. 20, 1M, 11:XX:XX
Sh, 299 - Want desperately to be at home. 8, 6C, 01:10:00
AETH. Al, 15 - The disposition becomes retiring (reserved) and tearful, as in nostalgia.
ANAC. Al, 1 - Illusions of fancy; he imagines he has his name called by the voice of his far-distant mother and sister, accompanied by an apprehension of misfortune and anxiety.
He, 24 - Imagines he hears voice of mother or sister, who are far away.
AUR-M. He, 7 - Sadness as when homesick; sad as though a great misfortune impended.
BELL. Ha, 1337 - He makes preparation to go home.
BRY. He, 13 - The patient desires to go home.
He, 14 - Desire to get out of bed and go home.
CALC. He, 23 - Desire to go home.
CAPS. He, 8 - Homesickness; with red cheeks and sleeplessness; ...
CARB-AN. Al, 11 - In the morning, he felt abandoned and homesick.
Ha, 2 - He feels in the morning, as if he was deserted, and full of homesickness.(nostalgia, loneliness, isolation)
Ha, 3 - Homesickness.
He, 13 - Homesick.
CARL. Al, 5 - Mood very much depressed, like an excessive homesickness; at last violent weeping.(second day) (after four glasses)
CHLOL. Al, 17-...a feeling as if he were now in one country and now in another, and with an anxious desire to go home.(abroad)
CLEM. Al, 19-...dreading to be alone, tired of living, full of thoughts of death, with fear that it would be speedy, longing however, for the repose of death; this mood was soon followed by apprehension, weeping, and homesickness, ...
He, 8 - Ailments from homesickness, or contrition (penitence, remorse) of spirit.
EUP-PUR. He, 7-... feeling like homesickness, though occupying her own home and surrounded by her own family,...
GERM. Sh, 143 - I Don't belong. I don't feel at home any place. Strong desire for finding a place to stay, to make a home for me and my kids. 18, 30C, 30:XX:XX
HALI-L. Sh, 227 - Pictures of the mountains make me homesick. Deeper than homesick. Feeling low, remembering the freedom of going to them. Missing mountains and the outdoors. 02, 30C, 07:01:XX
Sh, 228 - Homesick for home before I go away to NY—I don't want to go. 16, 10C, 27:XX:XX
HELL. Al, 5 - Homesickness.
HIPP. Al, 2 - Homesickness in the evening.
IRID. Sh, 42 - I wanted to sit with the rest of my family. This is unusual for me; usually sit on my own. I1
KALI-P. He, 17 - Homesickness, morbid activity of memory, haunted (obsessed) by visions of past, and longing after them.
LIPP. Al, 2 - Feeling of great apprehension, while riding in a carriage; a kind of anxiety in the heart, as of impending misfortune, together with a kind of homesickness.
MAG-M. Ha, 3 - Apprehensive and melancholic, lonely (isolated, abandoned) ; she is homesick and weeps.
He, 2 - Tearful, inclined to weep; sad and homesick.
MERC. He, 19 - Homesickness (nostalgia, isolation), or desire to travel; wants to go abroad (absent, nomad); nightly anxiety and perspiration.(wander)
NIT-AC. Ha, 5 - homesickness.
OP. He, 11 - Thinks he is not in his own house; imagines himself living in a locality three hours distant from his house; detains all passers-by and wishes to take them into his house; ...he does not recognize friends;... (estranged, alien)
PH-AC. Al, 8 - Lachrymose, as from homesickness.
Ha, 673 - Disposition lachrymose, as from homesickness.
Ha, 7 - Tendency to weep, as from homesickness.
He, 11 - Ailments from care, grief, sorrow, chagrin, homesickness; or disappointed love;...

He, 8 - Homesickness, with inclination to weep.
PLAN. Al, 19 - Feeling great desire to be at home when abroad.
PLB. Al, 127 - Longing (deprived, wanting) for a distant friend, in the evening...
PULS-N. Al, 3 - Great depression of spirits, in the afternoon; a kind of homesickness, with despondency.(grief)
SIL. Ha, 3 - Longing for home.
He, 9 - Longing for his relations and home.
VERAT. He, 16-... prattles about religious subjects and about vows (promise) to be performed, prays, believes that he is not in his own house.

HOMICIDAL

Anger; kill, with impulse to: ***prot.***[136]
Anger; stabbed any one, so that he could have: anac.[10] chin. **HEP.** merc. mosch.[10] nux-v. stront-c.[10] zinc.[10] zinc-acet.[10]
Anxiety; murdered someone, as if he had, all night: phos.[36]
Anxiety; murdered someone, as if he had, mania, in: ***ars.***[54]
Cursing; threatening destruction and death: tarent.[54]
Cut, mutilate, slit others, desire to: lyss. verat.[58]
Delirium; attacks people with knife: hyos.
Delusions; devils, speaking in one ear, angel in the other, prompting to murder, or acts of benevolence, devil: ***anac.***[54]
• murder, family with a hatchet, that she will: jab.
• murder, husband and child, she is going to: kali-br.
• murder, someone, that he has to: ars. hyos.[58] lach.[58]
• murder, struck friends who came to help him: ***stram.***[54]
• murdered, someone, he has: ars.[58] phos.[1]
• murderer, executed to be: **OP.**[54]
• poisoning people, she is: lap-c-b.[194] sulph.[1]
• stabbed a person who passed on the street, he had: ***bell.***
• toss someone out of the window, he tried to: bry.[36]
• voices, hears, steal and kill, that she must: lach.[58]
• wrong, giving wrong things to people, causing their death: sulph.[102]

Dreams; cutting, woman, of cutting a woman up for salting: calc-f.
➤ killing: stram.[54]
➤ killing, children: thea.[144]
➤ killing, friend, a: allox.[119]
➤ murdering, Arab, an, with four stabs in chest: ozone[227]
➤ murdering, drowning two people in pool: ozone[227]
➤ murdering, father, her: cast.[36]
➤ murdering, some one, at noon nap: petr.[36]
➤ murdering, young boys and girls in cold blood: thea.[36]
➤ shooting, someone, who owes him money: ozone[227]
➤ stab others, will: lach.[10]
➤ stab, antagonist, his: nat-c.[36] ozone[227]
➤ stab, friend, his: allox.[119]
➤ stabbed, antagonist in chest, with large knife, his: nat-c.[36]
➤ tossing someone out of window: bry.[36]
Fear; impulses, of his own: alum.[111] androc.[222] germ.[222] osm.[36]
✦ killing, child, her: ars.[172] coff.[172] manc.[30] ***merc.***[185] ***nux-v.***[185] rhus-t.[172] sep.[185] sil.[172] ***sulph.***[185] **THEA.**[162]
✦ killing, of: absin. alumn. am-m. arg-n.[184] ***ars. chin.***[30] der. kali-br.[8] merc.[58] ***nux-v.***[122] ***rhus-t.*** sulph. thea.
✦ killing, of, delivery, parturition, during: acon.[172] ars.[172] coff.[172] plat.[172]
✦ killing, of, knife, with a: ars. der. ***nux-v.***
✦ killing, of, mother, her: der.[162]
Fire; throws child into fire, after delivery: merc.[85]
Heedless; impelled to do reckless things, such as throwing child which he carries in his arms, out of window: lyss.[54]
Insanity; threatens destruction and death: ***tarent.***
Jealousy; crime, to a: hyos.[30] lach.[30]
Jealousy; kill, driving to: **HYOS.**[54] lach.[108]
Jealousy; murder, with attempt to: **HYOS.**[54]
Kill, desire to: agar. alco.[36] alum.[116] anac. androc.[222] ***ars. ars-i.*** bell. calc. camph. chin. cupr. cur. **HEP.**[122] **HYOS.** ***iod.*** kali-ar.[58] lach. ***lyc.***[30] lyss. ***med.***[184] merc. ***nux-v.*** op. ***petr. phos. plat.*** prot.[136] sec. sil.[122] ***staph.***[54] ***stram.*** syph.[122] thea. thyr.[85] x-ray[115]
Kill; desire to, barber wants to k. his customer: ***ars. hep.***

Kill; desire to, child, the own: androc.[222] merc.[30] ***plat.***[30]
Kill; desire to, everyone he sees: hyos.[30]
Kill; desire to, hysterical sadness, with: ***merc.***[54]
Kill; desire to, knife, at sight of a: ***alum.*** ars.[172] ***merc.***[30] nux-v.[30] plat.
Kill; desire to, knife, at sight of a knife or a gun: ***alum.***
Kill; desire to, knife, with a: ***alum.*** ars.[1] chin.[54] ***hep.***[54] ***hyos.***[30] **LYC.**[30] lyss.[5] ***merc.***[54] ***nux-v.***[54] plat. ***stram.***[54]
Kill; desire to, loved ones: ars.[102] chin.[102] hep.[58] jab.[137] kali-br.[137] merc.[102] ***nux-v.***[102] ***plat.***[102]
Kill; desire to, parents, in a child: ***der.***[162]
Kill; desire to, person that contradicts her: ***merc.***
Kill; desire to, poison, impulse to: ars.[30] lach.[30] nux-v.[30]
Kill; desire to, somebody, thought he ought to k.: camph. ***hyos.***[54]
Kill; desire to, sudden impulse to kill: **ALUM.**[162] arg-n.[162] ***ars. ars-i. hep.*** iod. kali-ar. med.[184] merc.[58] ***nux-v. plat.*** rauw.[119] staph.[162] sulfon.[162] sulph.[162] tarent.[137] thea.
Kill; desire to, walking in open air and street, while: camph. hyos.[30]
Kill; sudden impulse to, husband, her beloved: ***merc. nux-v. plat.***
Kill; sudden impulse to, husband, her beloved, menses, particularly during, implores him to hide his razor: ***merc.***[54]
Kill; sudden impulse to, offense, for a slight: ***hep. merc. nux-v.***
Kill; sudden impulse to, throw child, fire, into: hep.[58] lyss. ***nux-v.*** thea.
Kill; sudden impulse to, throw child, window, out of: lyss.[54]
Kill; sudden impulse to, woman, a, almost irresistible: ***iod.***[54]
Kill; threatens to k, wife and children: ***hep.***[54]
Kill; threatens to k.: ***hep.*** meli.[85] ***tarent.***
Kill; threatens to k., approach, those who: meli.[85]
Malicious; murder someone, as if she could: ***hep.***[54]
Mania; abuses, violent outburst, abuses her child, parturition, after, puerperal: ***camph.***[54]
Rage; kill people, tries to: hep. **HYOS.** sec. ***stram.***
Sadness; hysteria, in, inclination to murder, with: ***merc.***[54]
Striking; tells his wife he will try not to kill anyone: ***staph.***[54]
Thoughts; frightful, seeing blood, or a knife, on: ***alum.***
Thoughts; murder, of: ***calc.***[54]
Thoughts; persistent, homicide: calc. iod. op. phos. stram.
Thoughts; persistent, thinks of nothing but murder, fire and rats: ***calc.***
Threatening; kill, threatens to: ***hep.***[122] ***tarent.***[54]

ADAM. Sh, 221 - I felt angry on waking, noise of people upstairs sounds like elephants. I want to kill them. I wanted to complain to them. 7, 6C, 03:06:00

ANAC. He, 69 - In one ear a devil, in the other an angel, prompts (incite) him to do murder or acts of benevolence. (homicidal, x helpfulness, kindness)

ANDROC. Sh, 40 - She dreamt that she had murdered her grandfather by poking a knitting needle through his eyes while he slept. Though she felt no remorse, she wanted to be punished but no-one would accept her guilt. Was told by her friends that she had responsibilities and could not go to jail and the police refused to prosecute. Was frightened by the dream. (7)

Sh, 102 - Assertive, impatient, aggressive. Felt resentful and abused. Had no control over her temper. Bellowed and lashed out at everyone. In the evening, furious for no apparent reason. Wanted to kill her husband and children, banged doors and threw things. By bed-time, she felt fine but the intensity of her evil thoughts was very frightening. (7)

Sh, 124 - In the street, he felt aggressive and very strong, that his umbrella was a knife, and desired to smash people up. (29)

APIS. Al, 17-... would have liked to kill a dog that barked at him, etc. ; everything went wrong; nothing could be done to please him.

ARS. Al, 85 - He is anxious and trembling, and is afraid he shall not be able to prevent himself from killing a person with a knife.

Ha, 1027 - Trembling, anxious, he is afraid (fear) that he cannot refrain (restrain) from killing some one with a sharp knife.

He, 28 - A barber felt inclination to cut his customer's throats.

He, 76 - Anxiety like that of one who has committed murder; driven from place to place; avoids meeting persons, thinking that he has offended them.

BELL. He, 102 - Became fearful when persons approached him in street, and when they had passed, he insisted on it that he had stabbed them.

CAMPH. Al, 6 - Often felt as if he ought (must) to kill people, when in the street, never felt the disposition to kill any of his own family, but thought he ought to kill somebody.

He, 35 - Often felt as if he ought (must) to kill people, when in the street; never felt a disposition to kill any of his own family, but thought he ought to kill somebody.

CANTH. Al, 36 - He is anxious as if he had committed a murder (homicide); it seems to arise from the stomach.

CHIN. Al, 35 - Ill-humor, amounting to the most violent wrath (fury), so that he could have stabbed any one.

CHOC. Sh, 302 - Tonight my husband committed a large annoyance. I felt rage rise up in me — he jumped back and cowered! I wanted to beat some sensibility into him, stopping short of actually wanting to kill him, I felt: 'its not fair', 'how inconsiderate and thoughtless to an extreme degree'. However, my will intervened before I made a scene. Its as if I'm more aware of my 'shadow side' and really feeling it, but precisely because I'm more aware of it, I can step in with my will and curb my behaviour if it looks as if I'm likely to hurt someone else.[15], 30C, 03:XX:XX

CUR. Al, 17 - Irascibility, wicked disposition; desires to lie in wait in order to assault others, and even to kill and rob them.

DER. Al, 5 - He is afraid of killing some one with a knife.

GERM. Sh, 101 - I'm desperate. I want to die. Feel the power to kill. Feel like a wild animal locked in. It's strong, so intense. I hate so strong-feel a terrible disgust and I'm afraid of what I'm able to do. It's completely impossible to be in it and impossible to get out of it. 18, 30C, 190:XX:XX

HALI-L. Sh.589 - I wanted to really hurt somebody or something, no respect for the person, anyway that I could. There was another part of me that couldn't believe I was doing that. It was like a horror movie. I got to that place of no boundaries or responsibility to life. It didn't matter what I did. Indifferent. Like ice, no feeling. Just like if I killed someone there would be no regrets. Just the thought: This is what I have to do now. Desire to kill. It did not matter. Just do it. You've got to. I had no fear. I could do anything, whatever I was asked to do, I could do it then. I was a strong person. The me was the only thing that kept me from doing it. That's where I got scared. The last five days of the proving were in a black hole. I refused to write anything down. A god-like place or a devil-like place. Why do I have these things? Human things. 02, 30C, XX:XX:XX

Sh, 590 - While I was in the shower, I just wanted to kill. 02, 30C, 11:XX:XX

Sh, 591 - I have to kill the children. They are not obeying me. 09, 6C, 06:XX:XX

Sh, 662 - I can't stand it any longer. Spiraled and spiraled and spiraled. Feel like I'm going mad, like there's no escaping out of this. Pull, pull, like a hypoglycemic who hasn't eaten, and just wants to scream and yell. While I was in the shower I just wanted to kill. Feel like I'm going to lose it. Going stir crazy;...[02], 30C, 11:XX:XX

HEP. Ha, 289 - The slightest thing put him into a violent passion, he could have murdered any one without hesitation.

He, 8-...threatened to murder wife and children, attempted to set house on fire, and was with difficulty controlled; ... (pyromaniac) 0Scabies.

He, 9 - Malicious (vindictive, malevolent) mood; feels as if he could murder someone whith pleasure.

He, 22 - Temper obstinate and cross, a ferocious spleen (irascible) which would lead to cold blooded murder even among those habitually gay and benevolent.

He, 23 - Wrathful irritability, even to the most extreme violence, threatening to end

in murder and arson.(firing pyromania)
HYDROG. Sh, 161 - I am aware of some ridiculous thoughts coming into my mind, odd unconnected sentences such as about killing a 13 year old girl. 12, 6C, 22:XX:XX
HYOS. Ha, 562 - Extreme fury: he rushes at people with knives.
Ha, 563 - He strikes and tries to murder those he meets.
He, 50 - Tendency to action: wants to kill somebody or himself.
He, 62 - Jealousy: with rage and delirium; with attempt (try) to murder.
IOD. He, 15 - At night, especially when thinking of real or imaginary wrongs ...dares (try) to go home for fear of doing some dreadful (bad, wicked) deed (action); on one occasion was seized with an almost irresistible impulse to murder a woman who was acting as a guide (direct, conduct) for him, he having lost his way (direction);...must be constantly in action, in some laborious occupation. (lost; direction, correction, control)
KALI-BR. He, 15 - Frightful imaginings at night (in pregnant women during latter months), they are under impression that they have committed, or about to commit, some great crime and cruelty (brutality), such murdering their children or husbands.
LYSS. Al, 32 - Thought came into his mind to attack others in a mean way; to cut others with a knife he holds; to throw water he has in a tumbler into another's face.
Al,N-7 - Thoughts of something terrible going to happen come into his mind against his will; feels impelled to do reckless (impulsive) things, such as throwing child, which he carries in his arms, through the window, and the like.
He, 7 - Thoughts of something terrible going to happen come into his mind against his will; feels impelled to do reckless (impulsive, precipitated) things, such as throwing child, which he carries in his arms, through the window, and the like.
MERC. He, 22 - Great desire to murder (homicidal) or committed suicide ...is fearful that she may commit some wrong and kill herself (punishment); something urges her to kill her husband, of whom she is very fond (loving), and she implores him to hide his razor (knife).
He, 21 - Desire to kill the person contradicting her.
He, 33 - Hysterical melancholia, with inclination to murder.
NAT-C. Al, 1114 - Dream of a quarrel, in which he stabbed his antagonist (enemy) in the chest with a large knife.
NEON. Sh, 175 - I've been in a rotten mood all day, dwelling on past offenses. I just can't let go, it's making me angry. I feel like I hate that bastard; it's not an emotion I've had before. Now I feel vindictive, really awful; I feel that if I ever found out that he had been lying to me again I would say to him, "I'll kill you," "I'll slit your throat." These violent feelings were much eased when alone. 02, 6C, 04:22:40
NUX-V. He, 12 - Inclined to find fault and scold (reprove); morose; stubborn; (obstinate) an insane desire when alone with her husband, whom she adores, to kill him.
He, 38 - Three months ago mental shock, since then fears to be alone,...fears as if she would choke (suffocation)...fears to be alone, fear of knives and the like, (similar) lest she should kill herself or others...
PHOS. Al, 101 - Anxiety all night without heat, as if he had murdered some one, with constant tossing about.
ROB. Al, 10 - Love and excited passions, leading him to the grossest (obscene, rude) excesses, even to homicide.
STAPH. He, 15-...; firmly believed he would lose his fortune, constantly told his wife to be careful that they did not starve; thinks his wife will run away from him (deserted) (lost: position, rank), ... amuses himself by throwing into the fire any article near at hand, regardless of value; at times more violent, strikes at any one coming near him, ...tells his wife he will try not kill any one;...
STRAM. Ha, 546 - Furious endeavors to kill people.
He, 81-...attempts to stab and bite;...with sexual excitement; fear as if a dog were attacking him;...
He, 99 - Acute mania; tears his clothing;... threatens to use knife on those about him.

He, 110-...frightful dreams about fighting and killing; takes offensive in imaginary quarrels, and attacks aggressor; runs against supposed object to attack it;...

SULPH. Ha, 24 - She imagines that she might give people something wrong, which might kill them.

TARENT. Al, 1-...threatening words of destruction and death; she believes she is insulted; ...

He, 14 - Paroxysms of insanity; restlessness of legs; threatening words of destruction and death.

THEA. Al, 4 - Sensation as if impelled by some uncontrollable power to commit suicide, to jump out of window, to put her baby in the boiler with the clothes, to cut its throat while cutting bread, to throw it downstairs (in a woman who kept a pot of tea boiling on the stove and drank several bowlfuls every day; cured with tea cm, Finckle)

THYR. Al,N-1-...at times dangerous and homicidal, would put her arms round the necks of other patients so tightly as almost to strangle them (in this case the insanity was primary and the myxedema secondary; both conditions were removed). Evinced increased vivacity by quarreling with another patient about a trifling difference of opinion.

HOPELESS

Anxiety; inconsolable: ***acon.***[54] cham.[10] chin.[10] cic.[172] graph.[10] m-arct.[10] nux-v.[10] spong.[10] verat.[172]

Discouraged; alternating with, anger: ran-b.[10] zinc.[10]

Discouraged; alternating with, courage: merc.[30] op.[30] staph.[30]

Discouraged; alternating with, quarrelsomeness: ran-b.[10]

Discouraged; ambition, from loss of: nux-v.[137]

Discouraged; cursing, with: nit-ac.[10]

Discouraged; disgust, with: caust.[10]

Discouraged; impatience, with: ***calc.***[10]

Discouraged; quiet, and: lyc.[10]

Discouraged; rage, with: colch.[10] nit-ac.[10]

Inconsolable; dreams, in his: tab.[10]

ACON. Ha, 510 - Sometimes he despairs of his recovery, sometimes he is full of hope.

ACT-SP. He, 12 - Hopeless; constant apprehension; anxious solicitude when quiet.

ALUMN. Al, 3 - Great anxiety, and disbelief (doubt, suspicious) in the power of medicine to relieve him.

AMBR. Al,N-8 - Great sadness; despondent, does not want to live.

ANT-T. He, 23 - Hopelessness. despondency.

He, 38 - Despair and hopelessness, with lethargy, with cold sweat.

APIS. He, 53 - Eccentric cheerfulness, despondency, or hopelessness.

ARG-N. He, 19 - He wept and assured every one that he has lost beyond hope for this world; that no one could delude him in that respect, and no one could reason him out of it.

ARN. He, 32 - Despondency and conviction of approaching death.

ARS-H. He, 15 - Anxiety, he believes his death is near, and despairs of being better...

ARS. He, 61 - Religious melancholy; hopelessness, despair.

AUR. He, 41 - All the time a dark, hopeless mood, frequently anxiety and despair; life is a burden (load) to him.

BAPT. He, 19 - Hopeless (despair) of recovery, and certain (inevitable) of death.

CALC. He, 65 - Despairing; hopeless (unhappy, pessimistic) of ever getting well (health); with fear of death, tormenting all around day and night.

He, 43 - Hopelessness; despair.

CAMPH. Al, 46-... There was no other feeling in my soul than that of my hopeless endless damnation (condemnation). I sank back upon the bed, believing that I was the spirit of evil in a world forsaken of God.

Al, 46-... Faith and hope were gone. There was here no longer any God, or rather the Infinite himself, like all his works, had ceased to be... (hopeless, faithless, godless, privation, want, destitution)

Al, 46-... My misery was boundless; time itself was no more; in short, I suffered such fearful anguish as no fancy can comprehend. What soul could paint to itself my everlasting (eternal) dwelling as the Evil One (devil), alone in a vast universe, without faith or hope, and my heart forever broken by unimaginable tortures? (miserable, timeless, endless, solitude, forsaken, faithless, hopeless)

Al, 46-.... As I lay stretched on my couch, as the evil demon, and suffered all the anguish of a condemned and God-forsaken soul, ...I was forever deprived of the Divine protection, and of every consolation and every hope. Nothing remained to me but the conviction of my everlasting damnation...

CAUST. He, 27 - Melancholy mood; sadness; hopelessness.

CON. He, 32 - Discouraged, despondent, and dissatisfied (discontented) with herself and her surrounds.

DIG. Al, 31 - Great irritability; everything especially sad things affected him very much, and the merest trifle can make him hopelessly despondent; lasting more than three months.

Ha, 11 - Anxious apprehension (fear) of a sad kind, with great dejection, extremely aggravated by music.

He, 12 - Desponding (sad) and irresolute.(indecisive)

GERM. Sh, 108 - Hopeless, helpless, gloom and doom. Weeping and self pity. 14, 30C, 23:00:00.

Sh, 172 - Sad, indifferent and hopeless feeling. Want to cry but it won't come. 18, 30C, 00:14:00

Sh, 174 - Hopeless. There no hope for me. My fate is not to get well. 18, 30C, 36:XX:XX

HALI-L. Sh, 430 - Get a call from a friend that the utility district is at it again. Don't know what, but expect the worst in negotiations with them. Can't win. So tired of fighting the losing battle. Can't raise the energy to do anything. Rage inside. Hopeless. Daydreams of blowing up the utility district, of shooting them. Only option left to desperate people and I feel desperate. we're a rag-tag group without luck, or leadership, fighting a losing battle. Feels like we're the American Indians. "Here's 24 dollars worth of beads for your island, idiot." In the pit of despair. 09, 6C, 25:XX:XX

HYDROG. Sh, 180 - Indifference, despair and hopelessness—no way out. 32, 9C, 03:XX:XX

KALI-C. Ha, 49 - Changeful mood, now good and quiet, then passionate and angry about trifles; often hopeful, often despondent.

LAC-D. Al,N-9 - Great despondency on account of the disease, is sure he is going to die in 24 hours.

LAUR. Al, 8 - Very lachrymose and despondent (sad) mood; he would rather die than live.

LIL-T. He, 7 - Dementia produced by business discouragements and sexual excesses.

MURX. Al, 2 - Great depression of spirits; it seemed to her that she was hopelessly ill.

He, 2 - Deep sadness at approach of menses, all her symptoms gave her great concern (care); seemed to her she was hopelessly ill; she gave up everything.

NAT-M. Al, 51 - Attacks of complete hopelessness and internal despair, that deprived him of all power.

Ha, 21 - Attacks of entire hopelessness (despairing) and internal despondency (despair) which take away all her strength.

He, 36 - Despairing, hopeless feeling about the future.

NIT-AC. He, 13 - Hopeless despair.

OLND. He, 6 - Despondency and lack of self-confidence.

PSOR. Al,N-22 - Depressed in spirits and hopeless.

Al,N-31 - Despairs of recovery; thinks he will die; hopeless,...

Al,N-34-....thinks he will not recover; has lost all hope;...formication and crawling, with pricking and smarting on scalp, and some on extremities; tongue white.

He, 31 - Despairs recovery; thinks he will die; hopeless; especially after typhus...

He, 34-...;thinks he will not recover; has lost all hope; cannot apply his mind to business;...

He, 22 - Depressed in spirits and hopeless.

PULS. He, 48-...despaired of her soul's salvation; did not believe she would be restored to health ; ...

SIL. He, 13 - Desponding, melancholy, tired of life.

SYPH. Al,N-7 - Very despondent, does not think he will ever get better.

He, 8 - Very despondent, does not think will ever get better. (hopeless)

TAB. Al, 36 - Apprehension, anxiety, and despondency, as if she dreaded death at 4 p.m. two days in succession.
THEA. Al, 20 - Nocturnal fright; sinister thoughts; invincible propensity to analyze his life, to look at it on the dark side, and to resolve it into its most hopeless realities.
VERAT. He, 19 - A woman, ...hopeless despair, ...brought on by sexual excitement.
He, 51 - Despair; hopeless, loss of courage.

HORRIBLE

Anguish; horrible things, after hearing: calc.[30]
Anxiety; apparition, from horrible, while awake: ***camph.***[54] zinc.
Company, desire for; happen, as if something horrible might: ***elaps***[54]
Cruelty; children cannot bear to see cruelty in cinema: calc.[122]
Delusions; animals, grotesque: absin.
• animals, surrounded by hideous: ***crot-h.***[54]
• faces, doctor is making faces at her, she looked black: puls.[54]
• faces, hideous: ***ambr. bell.*** **CALC.**[122] calc-sil. cann-i. carb-an. caust. cocc.[116] ***kali-c.***[54] lac-c. lyc.[10] merc. nux-v. **OP.** phos.[111] stram.[116] stry. sulph.[10] ***tarent.***
• grotesque: cann-i.[36] plb.[36] sulph.[5]
• head, monstrous h. on distant wall of room: aur.[1] cann-i.
• horrible, everything is: **CALC.**[54] lac-c.[137] ***plat.***
• images, frightful: absin.[54] ***ambr.*** anac. arg-n. arn. ars. atro. bar-c. ***bell.*** bry.[1] **CALC.** calc-s. camph. ***carb-an. carb-v. caust.*** chin. chin-ar. cina[58] coca con. croc. gels. graph. ***hep.*** hyos. ign. kali-ar. ***kali-br.*** kali-c. ***kali-p.*** kali-sil.[58] ***lac-c. lach.*** lap-mar-c.[194] laur. lyc. mang. ***merc.*** mur-ac. nat-c. nat-p. nit-ac. nux-v. ***op.*** petr. ph-ac. ***phos.*** puls. rhod. rhus-t. samb. sars. sec. sil. spong. ***stram.*** sulph. tab. tarent.
• people, threatening her, screams horrible: ars-met.[54]
• pursued, horrid thing, by some: anac.
• room, walls, horrible things on the, sees: bell. cann-i. hyos. samb.
• strange, everything is, terrible, and: cic.[137] ***plat.***[54]
• strange, familiar things seem horrible: plat.
• visions, eyes anxiously fixed sideways on one point where she imagines she sees a terrible hostile figure: ***stram.***[54]
• visions, horrible: absin. ambr.[58] atro.[36] **BELL. CALC.**[122] calc-sil.[58] camph. carb-an. carb-v. ***caust.*** hep.[116] ign.[54] ***kali-br.*** lac-c. lyc. merc. nicot.[36] ***nux-v.***[54] op. phos. ***puls.*** rhod.[36] samb. sil. ***stram.*** sulph. tarent.
• visions, horrible, afraid they will take objective form: ***lac-c.***[54]
• visions, horrible, behind him: ***lach.***[54]
• visions, horrible, beside him: ***stram.***[10]
• visions, horrible, dark, in the: ***bell. carb-v.*** hell. petr. puls. stram.
• visions, horrible, events, of past: spong.[36]
• visions, horrible, eyes, when opening: calc.[102]
• visions, horrible, fright, from: bell.[54] nat-m.[54] samb.[54]
• visions, monsters, delirium, in: ***bell.***[54]
• visions, monsters, of: ***bell.*** camph. cann-i. cic. lac-c. op.[10] samb. ***stram.*** tarent.
• visions, monsters, sleep, on falling asleep, and on waking: ign.
Dreams; animals, snakes, horrifying: ***arg-n.***[36]
➤ figures, grotesque, dancing before her: narcot.[36]
➤ figures, horrid, presenting a bottle: merc-c.[36]
➤ ghosts, horrid: cham.[54]
➤ grimaces, horrible: op.[10]
➤ grotesque: cina[1] coca[38] lil-t. squil.[1] sulph.[38]
➤ hideous: alum.[5] ***am-m.***[5] arn.[5] ars.[5] bar-c.[5] bell.[5] carb-an.[5] **CHAM.**[5] **CHIN.**[5] croc.[5] **GRAPH.**[5] guai.[5] laur.[5] led.[5] lyc.[5] mang.[5] merc.[5] mur-ac.[5] ***nux-v.***[5] op.[5] phos.[36] **PULS.**[5] rhus-t.[5] sars.[5] stann.[5] sul-ac.[5] sulph.[5] verat.[5]
➤ monsters: aloe cann-i.[36] hydr. ped.[85] sedi.[36]
➤ monstrous: arg-n.[85]
➤ monstrous, figure, black, that flew up to sky and darkened the sun: ped.[36]
➤ shocking: bell.[102] hyos.[102] ph-ac.[36]
➤ waking, falling into a pit with grotesque figures: narcot.[36]
Excitement; horrible things, after hearing: ***calc. chin.***[122] cic.[58] cocc. gels. ign. ***lach.*** nat-c. nux-v. ***teucr. zinc.***
Fear; cruelties, from report of, excite: calc.
✦ dreams, of terrible: **NUX-V.**[54] spong.[193] ***sulph.***[54]

✦ happen, something will, terrible, horrible: aml-n.[139] ***calc.***[54] ***calen.***[162] carc.[207] elaps[139] fl-ac.[54] ***ign.***[54] lap-c-b.[194] lappa[139] **LYSS.**[162] mang.[172] med.[139] onos.[139] pall.[54] psor.[36] pyrus[139] ***scut.***[102] ***sep.***[36] thea.[139]

Frightened; easily, hideous objects, cries as if being frightened by seeing: stram.[8]

Horrible things sad stories, affected her profoundly: ars.[122] ***aur.***[122] ***aur-m.***[122] benz-ac.[58] **CALC.**[122] calc-s.[108] cand-a.[239] carb-v.[193] carc.[146] ***caust.***[122] cench.[58] chin.[162] **CIC.** coca[153] cocc. con.[122] ferr.[122] gels. ***hep.***[122] ign. **IOD.**[122] ***kali-c.***[184] ***lach.*** lap-c-b.[194] lap-mar-c.[194] ***lyc.***[122] manc.[162] nat-c. nat-m.[162] ***nit-ac.***[122] ***nux-v.*** op.[163] ozone[227] ***phos.***[122] plat.[137] prot.[193] ***puls.***[122] ***sep.***[122] ***sil.***[122] staph.[1] ***sulph.***[122] ***teucr. zinc.***

Horrible things sad stories, affected her profoundly, thoughts, her own, during labor: plat.[54]

Jealousy; images, with frightful, tendency to mock, satire and ridiculous ideas: ***lach.***

Sensitive; cruelties, when hearing of: **CALC.** hep.[162]

Sensitive; sad stories, to: cic.

Thoughts; terrible, taking possession of him, in mania: ***iod.***[54]

ABSIN. Al,S-6 - Terrifying hallucinations, he sees all kinds of animals, cats and rats of all colors, grotesque animals, fancies that he is pursued by soldiers.

ALUM. Ha, 22 - She cannot see blood nor a knife without horrible thoughts pressing in upon her, as if she should, e. g. commit suicide; though she has the greatest horror of it.

AMBR. Al,N-6 - Distorted images, grimaces; diabolical faces crowd upon his fancy.

ANDROC. Sh, 84 - Overwhelmed by terror, panic and fear, like a psychic attack. Then specifically became fear of being psychically tested as if confronted by something absolutely horrible, as in a "cult initiation ordeal". He felt so scared he had to shut the door, with a feeling that something would appear from behind it if he left it open. (4)

ARG-N. Al, 1-... visions and distorted (deform) faces hover before his imagination...

BELL. Al, 48 - Very delirious; she would persist that there were very horrid monsters all over the room, staring at her.

Ha, 1324 - Events which hitherto he had hoped for with pleasure, now appear to him in an anxious light; they appear to him frightful and horrible. (attractive x horrible, terrible)

He, 18 - When closing eyes, though not asleep, patient sees fierce (wild), wicked looking large animals with horns and bushy (scabrous) heads; room seemed to be full of strange men passing in and out, who would snatch (take hold) at her as they passed, which frightened her very much, she thought the men wanted to take her away from home ; she then saw children sitting on low benches (seat) in rows (line) as in a school-room. (purity)

He, 20 - Imagines he sees ghosts, hideous (horrible) faces and various insects.

BENZ-AC. Al, 2-...If he saw any one who was deformed (disfigured) it made him shudder. (tremor)

CALC. He, 18 - Mental aberration with horrid visions before eyes and cardiac anxiety; he despairs of his salvation (pardon, rescue) and wants to stab himself.

He, 62 - Fear excited by reports (news) of cruelties.(brutality, barbarity).

CAUST. Ha, 19 - When she closes her eyes, she always sees frightful visages and distorted human faces before her.

CHAM. He, 14-..., vows there is some dreadful beast under his bed or in the room, and will not be appeased (calm) until the gas is lit and the room is searched.

CIC. Al, 9 - He did not believe that he was living under ordinary relations; everything seemed strange and almost fearful to him; it seemed as though he has awakened from an acute fever...

CROT-H. He, 5-...imagines himself surrounded by enemies or hideous animals;...

ELAPS. He, 5 - Fear of being left alone, as if something horrible might happen; horror of rain.

GLON. He, 10-...looked as if he were contemplating some afflicting (torment) sight,...

HALI-L. Sh, 25 - While listening to a patient grieve, had a return of increased awareness of right eye, especially the socket. I had a strong image of how my mother's right eye was knocked out when she was hit by a truck and killed 30 years ago. Feel a very strong sense of connection with her. Telling this to my proving supervisor later, I realized I had never said this to anyone. This was an aspect of her death I had suppressed. It had always been so horrifying to me I couldn't deal with it. I cried gently with lots of tears. Feeling very sad and some remorse that I couldn't have been with my mother when she died. Felt very calm with all of this. 03, 12C, 18:XX:XX

Sh, 650 - It was like a horror movie. That's where I got scared. The last five days of the proving were in a black hole. A god-like place or a devil-like place. Why do I have these things? Human things. 02, 30C, XX:XX:XX

HYOS. Al, 28 - The people in the room seemed to assume grotesque appearances; ...

LAC-C. He, 8 - Sensation as if she was going deranged, when sitting still and thinking; sometimes she has most horrible sights presented to her mental vision (not always snakes), feels horribly afraid that they will take objective form and show themselves to her natural eye.

He, 13 - Woke at daylight feeling that she is a loathsome (repulsive), horrible mass of disease (while the breasts were affected); could not bear to look at any portiòn of her body (loathing, himself), not even hands, as it intensified feeling of disgust and horror; could not bear to have any part of her body touch another, had to keep even fingers apart; felt that if she could not in some way get out of her body, she should soon become crazy .

He, 17 - On lying down either by day or night begins to think how horrible it would be if a very sharp pain, like a knife, should go through her, and thought of it causes great mental distress.

He, 21 - Sits and looks under chairs, table, sofa and everything in room, expecting yet dreading (fear) to see some terrible monster creep forth and feeling all the time, that if it does, it will drive her raving mad; she is not afraid in dark, it is only in light where she can imagine that she can see them.

LYC. Al, 52 - Great fear of frightful images which her fancy conjures(charm) up, in the evening, and lachrymose during the day.

NAT-M. He, 34 - A pregnant woman saw a man who had a disfiguring nasal cancer; this haunted (obsessed) her, and she was sure her child would be marked; she was melancholy, avoided society, wept continually.

PALL. He, 6 - Apprehension (fear) as if something horrible would happen.

PHOS. Al, 111 - Horrible fearfulness, late in the evening, as if a horrible face were looking out from every corner.

Ha, 31 - Dreadful fearfulness, late in the evening, as if a horrid face was looking out of every corner.

Ha, 79 - In the evening, usually of so vivid an imagination that the mere representation of disagreeable things causes horror with her.

He, 8 - Fear and dread: in evening; of death; as if something were creeping out of every corner; late in evening as if a horrible face were looking out of every corner.

PLAT. He, 20 - Everything seems strange and horrible to her.

RHUS-T. Al, 1382 DREAM-...it seemed to her that the head was hanging out of the bed and the blood was streaming (flow) into it, so that she could hear it flow; together with the appearance of a horrible image which she was obliged to accompany.

SPONG. Al, 6 - She is very fearful, and tormented by a frightful image of a past sad event.

STRAM. Al, 63-...I was assailed (attacked) by imaginary spectres, in the most hideous forms and menacing attitudes; and what was still to my torment my bed was suspended and tantalized (charmed) like a feather (plumage) between two floors.

Ha, 565 - Nowhere has he rest, is startled by dream-pictures, even when his eyes are open, which in the form of big dogs, cats and other horrible beasts, grow (expand) out of the ground at his side, and from which he jumps away to the side with signs of terror (fear), and knows not how

to save (rescue, free) himself. (cornered, corralled)
SULPH. Al, 3815 - At night, horrible dreams, with great palpitation or heart, and on awaking, sometimes rigor, sometimes heat and fear of robbers.
TARENT. Al, 11 - Visions of monsters or animals, that frightened him.
ZINC. Ha, 11 - Fear of thieves or of horrible phantoms, seen while waking as if in a feverish fancy.
He, 10 - Anxiety on account of thieves or horrible apparitions, while awake, like a feverish fancy.

HUNTER

Delusions; animals, peacocks chasing, he is: hyos.
• animals, pigeons flying in room which he tries to catch: ***kali-c.***[54]
• hunter, he is a: cann-i. verat.
Desires; forage for food, to: choc.[222]
Dreams; fishing: arg-n. chin-b. mag-c. verat-v.
➤ hunting: hura hyper. junc.[36] merc-i-r. verat.
Play; desire to, hide and seek, at: bell.[54]

AGAR. Al, 16-.... reciting (enumerate) before the beauties of the tribe their exploits (adventures) in war or the chase.(hunting) Their physical strength is increased...(boasting)
CANN-I. Al, 65 - Hallucinations which lead the patient to imagine that he is on horseback, is hunting, that he sees blue water, that he is swimming, or that he is captain of a vessel, that he is traveling, that he has no weight.(lightness)
STRAM. He, 40 - Aberration of mind; one carries home all sorts of wood in order to manufacture brandy (cognac) (busy, manufacturing) ; another placed two axes across each other in order to split wood in this way; a third burrowed in ground like a pig with his mouth (animal); a fourth alleged he was a wheelwright and began to bore holes; a fifth ran into forge to catch fish, which he saw swimming there; a lacemaker threw about her bobbins incessantly, and threw everything into confusion; another girl ran about the room and cried out that all evil spirits were pursuing her.(restoration, restitution)
He, 119 - His thoughts ran upon obscene things, frequently put his hands to erect penis; sought to bite or to catch flies.
VERAT. Ha, 671 - Mania: he alleges that he is a hunter.(pursue)

HURRY

Activity; bodily, and, cannot do things fast enough: ***aur.***[60]
Ailments from; hurry: ***acon.***[30] ***alum.*** am-c.[30] ***arn.***[30] benz-ac.[5] ***bry.***[30] ***nit-ac.***[30] nux-v.[30] ***puls.***[30] rhus-t.[30] sulph.[30]
Anxiety; chest, heart, region of, hurry, with: **NAT-M.**[54]
Anxiety; hurry, with: alum.[162] **NAT-M.**[54]
Anxiety; walking, while, faster, which makes him walk: arg.[1] **ARG-N.** ars.[60] fl-ac.[5] lil-t.[60] sep.[5] sul-ac.[60] tarent-c.[77]
Awkwardness; hurry, because he is in a: alum.[30] ambr.[30] nat-m.[127] nat-s.[30] sulph.[30]
Contemptuous; ravenous hunger and greed, hasty eating, c. with sudden: ***plat.***[36]
Delusions; car stands still, although driving fast: ozone[227]
• die, about to, he is, while walking thinks he will have a fit or die, which makes him walk faster: ***arg-n.***
• fit, she will have a fit and walks faster: ***arg-n.***
• reading after her, someone is, which makes her read the faster: mag-m.
• slow, bus goes: cortiso.[119]
• talking, rapidly, all around her are t.: ***sang.***[54]
• time, working against: nat-ar.[168]
• walk, cannot walk, must run or hop: apis. hell.
• work, advance fast enough, does not: gamb.[36]
Dreams; hurried: choc.[222] coca hydrog.[222] merc-c. ***nux-v.***[54] zinc.[85]
➤ moped, driving one hundred kilometers an hour: ozone[227]
Excitement; hurried, as if: carb-v. coff.
Fear; hurry, after: benz-ac.
✦ hurry, with: **NAT-M.**[54]
Handle things anymore, cannot, fast, when happening fast: arg.[209]
Hurry; aimless: lil-t.[162] **SUL-AC.**[162]
Hurry; always in: ars-s-f.[58] dulc.[30] kali-ar.[58] nux-v.[30] sil.[30] staph.[30] sul-i.[58]
Hurry; breath, with short: caust.[54]

Hurry; drinking, unconsciousness, during: hell.[137]

Hurry; duties, as by imperative: **LIL-T.**[36]

Hurry; eating, while: anac.[102] androc.[222] arg-n.[122] aur.[1] bell.[54] berb.[54] calad. **CAUST.** clem.[5] *coff.* cupr.[1] graph.[5] **HEP.** kali-c.[122] *lach.* lyc.[1] nux-m.[5] *olnd.*[5] pip-m. **PLAT.**[5] plect.[36] *rhus-t.*[162] sabad.[5] **SUL-AC.** sulph.[1] zinc.[1]

Hurry; eating, while, eat fast enough, cannot: zinc.[137]

Hurry; everybody moves too slowly: med.[58]

Hurry; everybody must hurry: arg-n.[102] cann-i.[102] *lach.* nat-p.[58] *nux-m.*[102] **TARENT.**

Hurry; mental work, in: ambr. aur. ign. *kali-c.* laur. op. *sul-ac.* *thuj.*

Hurry; movements, fast enough, cannot do things: aur. **SUL-AC.**

Hurry; movements, fast enough, cannot do things, angry, making him: sul-ac.[85]

Hurry; movements, is: acon. arg-n.[137] ars. ars-s-f.[58] atro.[36] *bell.* camph. cann-i. coca coff. con. gins. *hyos.* kali-c. meny. merc. merl. **STRAM.** **SUL-AC.** *sulph.* **TARENT.** *thuj.* viol-t.

Hurry; occupation, desires to do several things at once: aur. **LIL-T.** petr.[102] plan.

Hurry; occupation, desires to do several things at once, finish any, but cannot: pin-s.[36] plan.[36]

Hurry; occupation, in: acon. aur. calc-f.[144] camph. carb-v. carc.[227] cimic.[36] hep.[54] *kali-c.* kali-p.[58] **LIL-T.** onos.[144] op. ptel.[144] puls. sep. **SUL-AC.** sul-i.[58] *thuj.* viol-t.

Hurry; tendency: *acon.* aloe alum. alum-p.[58] am-c.[30] ambr. anac.[5] anan. androc.[222] apis *aran-ix.*[149] arg.[102] *arg-n.* *ars.* *ars-i.* ars-s-f.[58] aur. aur-ar.[58] aur-i.[58] aur-s.[58] *bar-c.* bar-i.[58] bar-s.[58] *bell.* benz-ac. bov. *bry.* cact. calad. calc. *calc-f.*[149] calc-s. calc-sil.[58] *camph.* cand-a.[239] cann-i. cann-s.[1] canth. caps. carb-an. carb-v. *carbn-s.* carc.[227] caust.[30] chlol.[54] cimic.[122] coca[5] cocc. *coff.* con. *crot-c.* cur.[5] dig. **DULC.**[122] esp-g.[1158] fl-ac.[5] graph. grat. *hep.* hydrog.[222] hyos. *ign.* *iod.* ip.[137] kali-ar. *kali-c.* kali-p. kali-s. *lach.* laur. **LIL-T.** lob-p.[85] lyc. lycps.[137] *m-arct.*[10] m-aust.[10] m-p-a.[1] mag-m.[58] **MED.** meny. **MERC.** merl. mez.[36] morph. mosch. nat-ar. nat-c. **NAT-M.** nat-p. *nit-ac.*[30] *nux-v.* op. ox-ac. *ph-ac.* phos. *plat.*[5] plb.[5] prot.[136] psor.[185] ptel. *puls.* ran-b.[85] rheum[130] rhus-t.[10] sep. **SIL.**[30] staph.[30] *stram.* **SUL-AC.** sul-i.[58] **SULPH.** sumb. **TARENT.** *thuj.* verat. viol-t. zinc-val.[102]

Hurry; time, for the appointed, to arrive: **ARG-N.** carc.[138] cupr.[210]

Hurry; walking, while: acon. **ARG-N.** canth. carb-an.[1] fl-ac.[5] iod. mosch. prun. sep.[5] stram. **SUL-AC.** sul-i.[58] *sulph.* **TARENT.** *thuj.*

Hurry; writing, in: alum.[10] anac.[54] coca[36] ign.[30] lyc.[10] ped.[36] ptel. **SUL-AC.**

Impatience; slowly, everything goes too: androc.[222] *cham.*[54]

Impulse; run, to, violence, and to: iod.[102]

Irritability; business; proceed fast, when does not: ip.[36]

Irritability; hurriedness, with: alum.[193] merc.[187] thuj.[54]

Irritability; travel goes too slow, when: cortiso.[119]

Morose; business does not proceed fast, when: ip.[36]

Quick to act: androc.[222] choc.[222] *coff.* eup-a.[102] hydrog.[222] ign.[137] lac-h.[229] *lach.* lyss.[54] op.[36]

Restlessness; anxious, has to, walk rapidly: androc.[222] *arg-n.* **ARS.** cimic.[144] lil-t. sul-ac. **TARENT.**

Walk; rapidly from anxiety: arg-n. fl-ac.[111] *sep.*[5]

ACON. Al, 23 - Excessive restlessness, all movements and actions are performed with great haste and hurry.

Al, 14 - Excessive disagreeable restlessness; without occasion for hurrying, he is in the greatest haste, every obstacle that delays his rapid pace is excessively annoying; he knocks against some people who do not get out of his way fast enough, and runs in breathless haste up the steps;...

Ha, 502 - He does everything in a hurry (quick), and runs about the house.

He, 31 - Restlessness, agony, internal anxiety; does everything in great haste (rapidity); must move about or change position often.

ADAM. Sh, 76 - Felt rushed; so much to do. Overwhelmed. 8, 6C, 04:XX:XX

Sh, 78 - Hurried. Family tells me to stop rushing. On a high, but I don't feel hurried inside.[10], 6C, 05:XX:XX

Sh, 79 - Hurriedwild. Husband says I look

wild, like a jungle child moving rapidly, jerky movements in different directions. Very excitable as if about to lose control. 10, 6C, 19:XX:XX

Sh, 81 - I'm feeling impatient with patients. I'm using intuition more as I have a sense of not wanting to waste time. 7, 6C, 17:18:00

Sh, 82 - Finding it difficult to treat, finding I'm there for my patients too much. Sensation as if there's no time to wait to let them finish their story. 7, 6C, 18:00:XX

Sh, 83 - Impatience for plans to come to fruition, but can't hurry the process. 2, 12C, 60:XX:XX

Sh, 86 - Feels like cycle of life has speeded up, with no way of stopping. 16, 12C, 51:XX:XX

Sh, 97 - At times, my awareness is not at the same speed as my head, it's faster.[16], 12C, 29:XX:XX

Sh, 533 - Feels like cycle of life has speeded up with no way of stopping. 16, 12C, 51:XX:XX

AMBR

He, 15 - Hurries too much while engaged in mental labor.

ANDROC. Sh, 90 - Impatient, expected to be able to do everything immediately. (1)

Sh, 91 - Impatient watching others, wanted to speed them up. (7)

ARG-N. Ha, 16 - Anxiety that compels him to walk quickly.

He, 15 - When walking gets nervous (anxiety), thinks he will have a fit (convulsion?) or die suddenly, which makes him walk faster,(rapid) but soon has to stop, because he gets tired.

He, 25 - Impulsive, must walk very fast; frequent turns of anxiety.

He, 53 - When walking, becomes faint (weak, fall?) with anxiety, which makes him walk faster.

AUR. Ha, 345 - An urging to activity, bodily as well as mental; when he did anything, he thought he did not do it quick enough, and that he had a great deal (much) more to do; he could not live to his liking. (desire, aspiration)

Ha, 11 - Restlessness and hurried impulse to bodily and mental activity; he can not work fast enough; he could not act so as to satisfy himself.

CARB-V. Al, 25 - Exceedingly irritable; she seems to be overhurried (quick, fast) in her business.

Ha, 16 - Excessive excitation, as if she was too much hurried (fast), or over-worked (industrious) in business.

Ha, 711 - Excessive irritation, as if she were too much hurried, or had too much to do.

CHAM. He, 49 - Great impatience, everything seems to go too slowly.

CHOC. Sh, 82 - Dream that my daughter was there drying her hair. She was late for school and I was very distressed with her slowness. I felt she should be brushing her hair and not drying it. I went to switch off the drier, but the wall socket was open and exposed, with electrical bits everywhere, so I couldn't switch it off.

Sh, 331 - I became selfish, impatient and intolerant. Behaved in a strange way -hard and quarrelsome -snapping at people. Could not stand people wasting time or being inefficient, I wanted things done immediately.[35], 30C, XX:XX:XX:

Sh, 420 - Urgency and strong desire to travel decreased since proving, (curative).[11], 6C, XX:XX:XX

GRAPH. Al, 17 - Anxiety and hastiness (hurry) drive him about like an evil-doer.(criminal)

Ha, 22 - Anguish and hurry (quick) chase (pursue, follow) him about, like a criminal.

HALI-L. Sh, 191 - Frustration. Slight feeling of being hurried. 11, 30C, 15:XX:XX

Sh, 201 - Very speedy feeling, anxious inside regarding relationship. Trying to get car fixed so I can go see her. 02, 30C, 07:XX:XX

203 - Feel like a rushing train. Like diving from a high dive and there is no water in the pool. 02, 30C, 16:XX:XX

Sh, 205 - Aggravated driving to work. Why don't these people get out of my way? Frustrated with the world, angry with the world. I don't want any red lights. Want everything to be smooth. I used to feel this way years ago when I used to drink. 02, 30C, 10:XX:XX

Sh, 206 - Feeling on an emotional roller coaster. 02, 30C, 05:XX:XX

Sh, 532 - I started to speed up emotionally, got really pissed off at supervisor for getting in touch with me, beeping me.

Wanted to escape and fly away. Phoned the airlines, trying to fly away. Hiding. Difficult to be with patients, with their stupid emotions. 02, 30C, XX:XX:XX

Sh, 580 - Spent most of today thinking about how I am surrounded by idiots, (my family), who are showing no attempts to think for themselves, letting me run the show. They don't care to figure things out. I'm in hyper-drive. I know a lot and I'm right. I've been extremely productive or at least active, balancing several major projects all at the same time, and they can't seem to tidy a table properly. This includes my husband, who continually interrupts me (or so it seems) for some trivial question. I'm coming across with too much force. I find myself shouting at everyone much more than usual. Like a crazy person. Impatient over others' slowness. Almost an arrogance. I want them to THINK! (Obviously, the way I do). or get off the ship and drown yourself. A hard anger, more intense that usual. Feel like leaving them all—they just take and give back little. More trouble than support. This isn't complaining or victimizing talking. This is how it is. I'm healing myself and leaving my family in the dust. I've passed on to them my bad habits, bad parenting. They are content to be idiots. 09, 6C, 13:XX:XX

Sh, 614 - Full of energy in the morning. Run and walk in the sea, amazed at my high energy. Feel like I have to let out lack of sex. Want partner badly but mad at her and at myself for being so open. Feel speedy. 02, 30C, 08:03:XX

HYDROG. Sh, 17 - Feeling of great release —catharsis —my whole time scale has changed since taking the remedy. Even my work on Homoeopathy has opened up — boundaries have disappeared. Lost a lot of boundaries on time. All sorts of things have clicked into place since yesterday. Feel wonderful. Now I don't actually feel slowed down. Didn't hurry, just did things in my own time. Normally would have pulled out all the stops and rushed around. It doesn't matter if I'm late. 08, 30C, 06:XX:XX

Sh, 97 - My whole time scale has changed since taking the remedy, I've lost a lot of boundaries on time. Don't hurry, just do things in my own time. 08, 30C, 06:XX:XX

Sh, 105 - I felt better when driving the car fast with company and loud music. 24, 30C, 03:XX:XX

Sh, 108 - Doing everything faster —driving faster than usual. 24, 30C, 100:XX:XX

Sh, 114 - I feel quite resentful about having to hurry. 08, 30C, 09:XX:XX

IGN. Ha, 754-,... he cannot express himself in talking, write, or do anything as quickly as he wishes; ...he makes mistakes in speaking and writing, and does everything awkwardly...

He, 36 - Anxiety as though something terrible had happened cannot speak because of it; hurry, fearfulness, terror, alternating with irresolution and inertness.

IP. Al, 11 - Ill-humored and vexed that his business does not proceed fast enough.

Ha, 224 - He is morose and vexed that his business is not performed quick enough. (time)

IRID. Sh, 76 - Twice now I have overtaken cars going up the hill out of town which were going only marginally slower than me. Had to get past them, urgency to get to the top out of the valley. G7

Sh, 154 - Felt quick and was frustrated at the slowness of others. Q4

LIL-T. Al, 24-..a feeling of irritation and of something wrong in abdomen and pelvic organs (disease); feels hurried (fast) and yet incapable (incompetent), as if she had a great deal (busy) to do and cannot do it.

Al, 30 - Constant hurried (precipitation) feeling as of imperative duties and utter inability to perform them; during the sexual excitement.

Al, 45 - She can't think; acts without thought; keeps walking fast as though by instinct; feels hurried, but doesn't know why; is forgetful, can't decide for herself; must depend on others.

He, 12 - Listless, inert, yet does not want to sit still (quiet); restless, yet does not want to walk; hurried manner, desire to do something, yet feels no ambition; feeling as of imperative duties and utter (complete) inability (incapacity, incompetence) to perform them; sexual excitement.

MAG-M. Ha, 20 - Fanciful (fantastic) delusions: As if while she was reading in a book, another person was reading after her, and compelled her to read more quickly, with humming and buzzing (murmur) around her...(faster)

He, 6 - While reading, felt as if some one was reading after her and she must read faster and faster. (imitated)

MED. Al,N-48 - It is also introspective, self-accusative, remorseful. Time moves slowly to it, therefore it is hurried.

He, 25 - Is in a great hurry; when doing anything is in such a hurry that she gets fatigued.

NAT-C. Al, 18 - Anxiety and hasty (fast) restlessness all day; he could not keep the limbs still, especially the arms; obliged to stretch them; it seemed as though they would be torn (cut) asunder. (in two divided).

NEON. Sh, 86 - A friend observed that my eyes were wider open, not so soft. She said they looked very forward and excited. She also observed that I seemed excited in company. I felt very speedy, and could not get words out fast enough, tripping over my words. I was speaking faster than I could articulate the words. 20, 6C, 01:08:45

NUX-V. Al, 4 - He is hasty; looked angrily at anyone who asked him a question without answering, as though he was obliged to restrain himself to avoid being insulting; he was in such an irritable and unrestrained mood that it seemed as though he would like to strike any one in the face who spoke a word to him.

Ha, 1270 - He is hasty (careless, rapid), looks malignantly (deadly) at any one who asks (asked) him anything, without answering, just as if he must control himself in order to avoid becoming coarse (rude), it seems as if he would like to strike any one in the face who speaks a word to him, so irritable and uncontrollable in his disposition.

PH-AC. Ha, 13 - Hurried in talking; he cannot get anything fast enough.

PLB. Al, 53-...; he fancied one of the patients called to him, ran headlong (hurry) to help him, ...

PTEL. Al, 20 - In writing a letter, felt a curious and unusual disposition to hurry (run, hasten, speed) through with it as quickly as possible, hardly taking time to write the words.

Al, 21 - Able to examine the papers, but inclined to hurry with it, and in selecting the remedy, inclined to follow Fred Humphrey's rule, "First impressions are the best". (hastily, rapidly, quickly) (heedless)

PULS. Ha, 1147 - Inattention, acts with precipitancy (hurry), does something different to what he wished to do.

RHUS-T. Al, 40 - Impatient desire to accomplish several kinds of business, chiefly intellectual,...

SEP. Ha, 27 - Great internal restlessness, for many days, with hastiness (hurried); he wants to be done with his work even as he begins it.

STAPH. Ha, 697 - When he walks quickly he feels as if some one were following him; this caused anxiety and fear, and he must always look about him.

SUL-AC. Al, 9 - Hasty (hurried, fast) mood; nothing that she does can be finished quickly enough, though she makes unusual effort.

Ha, 12 - Hastiness (fast) ; everything she does, she cannot accomplish fast enough; but it fatigues her exceedingly.

He, 2 - Must do everything in a great hurry; nothing can be finished quickly enough.

SULPH. Ha, 53 - He is so peevish and obstinate, that he will not give an answer to anybody, he cannot bear to have anyone around him, and cannot get quickly enough what he wants.

TARENT. Al, 65-...great haste in whatever I undertook, from a constant fear that something would happen to prevent my finishing it;...fear that something would fall on me (doom, disgrace);...fear of striking it against some imaginary object which appeared to be suspended....(hurt)

HURT

Ailments from; abuse, childhood, in: carc.[187] stram.[198] thuj.[198]

Ailments from; injuries, accidents: acon.[34] arn.[34] bell.[5] camph.[54] cic.[102] ***glon.***[102] hyos.[5] hyper.[102] mag-c.[102] **NAT-S.**[122] op.[5] rhus-t.[34] ruta[34] stram.[5] sul-ac.[8] verat.[5]

Ailments from; sexual, abuse, raped, being: acon.[185] caust.[185] foll.[1201] ign.[185] sep.[185] staph.[185]

Anger; tear himself to pieces, could: sulph.[54]
Anguish; shock from injury, in: ***op.***[54]
Anxiety; injury, after: ***arn.***[184] chin.[54] op.[28]
Anxiety; injury, as from a, received in sleep, morning on waking: plat.[36]
Anxiety; walking, while, people behind him might beat him, as if: alum.[122]
Biting; himself: acon. arum-t.[58] elaps[54] hura lyss. op. plb. stram.[1] tarent.
Complaining; injury, of supposed: ***hyos.***
Consoled, cannot be, after shock or injury: acon.[54]
Delusions; animals, devouring him: ***hyos.***
- animals, dogs, biting and tearing flesh off his chest: stram.
- attacks and insults, defend themselves against imaginary: lyss.[54].
- beaten, he is being: bry.[10] elaps
- bitten, will be: ***hyos.***[10] stram.[5]
- blown at, of being, by persons, some of whom are not present: lyss.[54]
- body, abdomen, fallen in, his stomach devoured, his scrotum swollen: **SABAD.**
- body, parts, take away: ***bapt.***[122] daph.[122]
- body, tongue, pulling out his, someone is: bell.
- corners of houses project so that he fears he will run against then while walking in the street: ***arg-n.***
- cut through, he is: ***stram.***
- cut, two, in: ***bell.***[30] plat. stram.[30]
- devoured, of being: cand-a.[239] ***stram.***[10]
- injury, injured, head: naja[54]
- injury, injured, is being: bry. cact. canth. elaps kali-br. lach. lyss. naja[54] phos. rhus-t. stram. sulph.
- injury, injured, sleep, during: plat.[36].
- injury, injured, surroundings, by his: **HYOS.**[122] ***lach. naja***[117]
- injury, receive, will: ars. bell.[58] cann-i. carbn-s. con. hyos.[122] lach. lyc. merc. nux-v. ***op.***[54] sil. stram. sulph.
- injury, receive, will, friends, from: lach.[58]
- man, room, in the, intending to perforate his throat with a gimlet: merc-i-f.
- murder, struck friends who came to help him: ***stram.***[54]
- rainstorm, she is in a terrible, complaining of being so cold, and that carriage has turned over and hurt her head: naja.[8]
- runs, against something: arg.[139]
- soldier, sees, cutting him down (amel. on getting cool): bry.

Despair; concussion, after: **ARN.**[54]
Dreams; abused, being; too weak to defend himself: ambr.[36]
- ➤ animals, biting him: am-m. bov.[10] calc.[10] cench.[58] daph. elaps[136] m-aust.[10] merc. nicc.[10] ***phos.*** puls. sulph.[10] verat.[10] zinc.[10]
- ➤ animals, cats, wounded abdomen, with: ozone[227]
- ➤ animals, dogs, mangy dog approaching her, covered with sores, she takes hold of it and it bites her: paull-p.[36]
- ➤ animals, geese, of being bitten by: zinc.[1]
- ➤ beaten, being: kali-c.[36] kali-n.[58] nat-m.[1]
- ➤ bitten, arms, into the: am-m.[10] m-aust.[10] nicc.[10]
- ➤ blood, mangled remains, and: merc.[36]
- ➤ blow on the mouth: menth-pu.[85] meny.[36]
- ➤ body, abdomen, cut, a big cut in: ozone[227]
- ➤ body, abdomen, cut, a big cut in, blood and pus, under which amounts of: ozone[227]
- ➤ body, abdomen, cut, a big cut in, tumor, under which grows a: ozone[227]
- ➤ body, arm, hurt, mother's arm: chin.[36]
- ➤ body, back, pinched, back and breast are: phos.[36]
- ➤ body, head, runs head against the wall: bamb-a.[1184]
- ➤ body, jaw broken: rauw.[119]
- ➤ body, limbs broken: cimic.
- ➤ body, muscles pierced with arrows: bomb-pr.[36]
- ➤ bruising himself: nicc.[36]
- ➤ children, about, abused: ozone[227]
- ➤ children, about, beaten, had been: kali-c.[36] kali-n. nat-m.[36]
- ➤ crushed, he would be: ***sulph.***
- ➤ cutting: androc.[222] calc-f. chin. hura mag-m. nat-c. nicc. op.
- ➤ cutting, knife, of being cut with a: frax.[36] guai. nat-s.[36]
- ➤ cutting, trying to cut off finger of acquaintance: nicc.[36]
- ➤ disease, fracture of jaw: rauw.
- ➤ disease, fracture, limbs, of: cimic.
- ➤ disease, injuries: allox.[119] am-m. ant-c. cench.[58] chel.[36] chin. choc.[222] cortico.[119] lob.[54] ***mag-s.***[10] nat-s. nicc.[10] phos. sumb.
- ➤ disease, injuries, self-inflicted: nicc.
- ➤ disease, wounded by shot: lob.[54]
- ➤ falling, window, from, friends: choc.[222]
- ➤ fire, blow on head, after: ***nat-m.***[54]
- ➤ flayed persons, about, frightening: arn.[1]

➤ frightful, blow on head, after: ***nat-m.***[54]
➤ frightful, falling downstairs, after: ***rhus-t.***[54]
➤ harassing: thuj.[36]
➤ ill-treatment: ambr.[10] dros.[10]
➤ injures, self-inflicted: nicc.
➤ injuries: allox.[119] am-m. ant-c. cench.[58] chel.[36] chin. choc.[222] cortico.[119] lob.[54] ***mag-s.***[10] nat-s. nicc.[10] phos. sumb.
➤ injuries, machinery, by: cortico.[119]
➤ lightning, struck by lightning, being: ***arn.***
➤ maltreated, of being: dros.[36]
➤ murder, blow on the head, after: ***nat-m.***[54]
➤ rape: cand-a.[239] ***cench.***[58] kreos.[10] lap-gr-m.[194] petr. sep.[10]
➤ rape, pursued for the purpose of: ***cench.***[122] kreos.
➤ rape, seeing, of: ***cench.***
➤ rape, threats of rape: cench.[58] sep.
➤ robbers, blow on the head, after: ***nat-m.***[54]
➤ shooting, shot, being: bell. lact.[10] lob. mag-s. mang.[1]
➤ shooting, shot, soldier is shot, a: am-m.[58]
➤ soldiers, seeing a soldier shot: am-m.
➤ stabbed, acquaintance was: lil-s.[36]
➤ stabbed, being: chin. guai. lil-s.[36] nat-c. op.
➤ stabbed, fear of being stabbed: lach.
➤ threats of rape: sep.[36]
➤ whipped, getting: ptel.[36]
➤ wood, being floated down and fearing damage: nat-s.[36]
➤ wounded, of being: ant-c. chel.[36] lob.[54] ***mag-s.***[10]
➤ wounded, of being, shot, by: lob.[54]

Fear; accidents, of: acon. androc.[222] arg-n.[31] carb-an.[1] ***carb-v.*** choc.[222] cupr. gins. graph.[172] hydrog.[222] iod.[8] kali-i.[1] mag-c.[8] mag-s.[54] naja[8] perh.[149] petr.[149] rhus-t.[54] samb-c.[36] tarent.[192]
✦ alone, of being, injure himself, and: ars. merc.[137] nat-s.[137]
✦ animals, birds, of: aesc.[172] apis[162] bufo[36] calc-ar.[162] calc-s.[162] ign.[162] ***nat-m.***[184]
✦ animals, cats, of: absin.[172] bac.[83] chin.[185] med.[162] plb.[201] sil.[147] syph.[193] ***tub.***[122]
✦ animals, devoured him or her: hyos.[1] stram.
✦ animals, dogs, attacking him, in delirium: **STRAM.**[54]
✦ animals, dogs, of: androc.[222] **BAC.**[62] **BELL.**[122] bufo[179] calc.[30] carc.[193] ***caust.*** **CHIN.** choc.[222] ***hyos.*** lyss.[122] med.[212] nat-m.[162] nat-p.[166] plat.[40] ***puls.***[162] sil.[171] ***stram.*** syc-co.[136] ***tub.*** tub-k.[70] verat.[172]
✦ animals, wolves, of: bell.[8]
✦ approaching, vehicles, of: anth. hydr-ac. lyss.[122] phos.
✦ bitten, of being: choc.[222] ***hyos. lyss.***
✦ broken the arm of her child, that she has, in gastroenteritis during pregnancy: lyc.[172]
✦ coition, thought of, in a woman, rape: arn.[162] ***kreos.*** ozone[227]
✦ concussion, of, as if he might run against something: arg.[8]
✦ cutting himself when shaving: **CALAD.**[122]
✦ disfigured, of being: hep.[30]
✦ electricity, of: ran-b.[172]
✦ injured, of being: arn.[5] ars.[58] calad. calc-s.[196] cann-i. chin.[137] choc.[222] cupr-acet.[54] gels.[8] hep.[137] hyos. kali-c.[137] lyss.[172] ruta[130] spig.[137] **STRAM.** ***stry.***
✦ injured, of being, dark, in: arn.[172] stram.[172] valer.[172]
✦ injured, of being, persons walking towards him, by: arn.[54]
✦ injured, of being, sewing, when: sep.[172]
✦ injured, of being, stay in bed, would not: ***cupr-acet.***[54]
✦ injured, of being, traumatic shock, in: ***gels.***[54]
✦ jostling against everyone she meets, during pregnancy: ***acon.***[54]
✦ knives, of, thinks how horrible it would be if a sharp pain like a knife should go through her, on lying down: lac-c.[54]
✦ people, standing near: bell. germ.[222]
✦ sports, doing: calc-s.[196]
✦ struck by those coming toward him, of being, walking behind him, by those: alum.[122]
✦ struck by those coming towards him, of being: **ARN.**[54] bell.[36] ign.[36] kali-c.[36] lach.[36] stram.[36] thuj.[36]
✦ sudden, broken her child's arm by lifting him, that she has: ***lyc.***[54]
✦ torturing, of: ars-s-f.[54]
✦ tread lightly or will injure himself, must: cupr.
✦ wounds, to see: calc.[30]

Frightened; easily, shock, at a distant: ***bor.***[36]

Hysteria; injuring herself, must exert great force to prevent from: ***hydr-ac.***[54]

Injure; fears to be left alone, lest he should, himself: alum. arg-n. ars. ***cimic.***[54] ***merc. nat-s.*** sep.

Injure; herself, himself, feels could: germ.[222] sep.

Injure; herself, himself, feels could, rage, out of: agar. germ.[222] lyss.[36]
Jealousy; tearing the hair: lach.[30]
Malicious; injure someone, desire to: androc.[222] levo.[149] osm.[36]
Mania; abuses, violent outburst, abuses her child, parturition, after, puerperal: ***camph.***[54]
Mutilating his body, inclination to: agar.[102] ars. bell.[102] hyos.[102] med.[212] stram.[102]
Pull; desires to, hair, ones: ars. **BELL.** ***cupr.*** dig.[137] lach. ***lil-t.*** med.[5] mez.[5] tarent. tub.[5] xan.[137]
Pull; desires to, noses of strangers, in the street: merc.
Pull; desires to, presses her head and pulls her hair: tarent.[36]
Rage; striking, himself: tarent.[36]
Restlessness; cutting himself while shaving: calad.[54]
Restlessness; internal, beat about herself with hands and feet, as if he would: lyc.
Restlessness; sensitive, remains long impressed by even slight mechanical injuries: ***arn.***[54]
Sadness; injuries, from: ***hyper.***[54]
Sadness; injuries, from, head, of the: arn. ***cic.*** con. ***nat-s.*** puls. rhus-t. sul-ac.[8] sulph.
Scratches with hands, everyone interfering with him: ***hyos.***[54] ***stram.***[54]
Scratches with hands, himself, raw: arum-t.[137] psor.[137]
Sighing; injure, after: cupr.[54] ***lach.***[54]
Somnambulism; strike sleepers, from vengeance, to: **NAT-M.**[30] nit-ac.[30]
Striking; abdomen, his: bell.
Striking; anger, from, himself: nat-c.[36]
Striking; chest, his: camph. verat-v.
Striking; himself: ars. bac.[55] bell. camph. cur. germ.[222] plat.[1] **TARENT.** ***verat-v.***
Striking; himself, head, his: ars. bac.[55] hyos.[5] stram. **TARENT.**
Stupefaction; shock of injury, from: camph.[54]
Talk; indisposed, sexual abuse, after: **STAPH.**[54]
Tears; himself: ars. bell. cur. lach.[189] plb. sec. **STRAM.**
Tears; himself, genitals, his: sec. tab.[5]
Tears; himself, hair his, headache, during: bac.[55]
Tears; himself, hair, his: ***ars.***[137] bac.[55] ***bell.*** ***cupr.***[137] dig.[137] ***lil-t.*** med.[137] tarent. tub.[8] xan.[137]
Tears; himself, skin around nails: carc.[149]
Thoughts; persistent, injury to others, of doing: osm.[54]

ADAM. Sh, 193 - Felt had spoiled the proving by spraining ankle. Blamed myself. 8, 6C, 02:XX:XX
Sh, 195 - Bad paranoia, that people hate me, anyone just walking down the street hates me. I think they will hit me. 20, 1M, 07:XX:XX
AGAR. Al, 3 - Fearless, menacing, mischievous (rude) frenzy; also, frenzy which causes the patient to assail and injure himself, with great exertion of power.
Al, 13 - She ran about the yard, romped (playing) with the children, threw them down, even hit them.
Ha, 23 - Fearless, threatening, destructive frenzy, also such as turns against itself and injures itself, combined with great exertion of strength.
ANDROC. Sh, 49 - Accident prone (10, 25) cut fingers frequently. (10)
Sh, 176 - Fear of driving, especially fear of hurting someone else in an accident. (Clinical)
ARG-M. He, 19 - Fear of concussion (hurt, injure) as if he might run against something, with pain in testicles.
ARG-N. He, 10-...; does not work because he thinks it will do him harm (hurt), or that he is not able to stand it.
ARN. Ha, 623 - Over-busy, inclination and disposition for great and continuous literary work with no power to do it without injury to the health.
He, 34 - Fears being struck (hit, hurt) by those coming towards him; fears even the possibility of being touched.
BELL. Ha, 1419 - Fury; he injures himself and others and strikes about him. (beat, hit)
BRY. Al, 5-...a delirious frightful fantasy, as of soldiers cutting him down, that he was on the point of escaping;..
CACT. Al, 17 - Feeling of doing violence (injury) to myself.
CALAD. Al, 5 - Fear of cutting himself while shaving.
Al, 14 - Fear of cutting himself while shaving.
CALC. He, 56 - Feels awe-stricken

(terror-injure) at night. 0 Diarrhea

CAMPH. Al, 17 - He beats himself on the chest, and falls into a faint.

CARB-V. Ha, 678-... feeling over the body as if some one stroked him with the hand, and as if ants were running over the skin, at every moment in bed...

CARBN-S. Al-S, 753 - At one time during the night he seemed to be surrounded by enemies; persons were coming to harm him;...

CAUST. Ha, 20 - Extreme anxious timidity; she is so much afraid (fear) of a dog near her, which did not harm (hurt, injure) her at all,...every noise in the street made her afraid, and when she saw boys climbing she was very uneasy lest they might get hurt. (care, others)

CHIN. Al, DREAM-1110 - Dreamed that some one had stabbed his brother, and then called for his mother; that his mother was dead, and then he cried; that his mother's arms was hurt;...

CHOC. Sh, 189 - While outside became very weary of cars and people. Felt open and vulnerable. Fear of accidents, cars, or of someone leaping into the road and punching me. This anxiety was worse out of doors. 27, 100C, 01:XX:XX

Sh, 190 - While walking past a block of flats, I worried that it might blow over in the wind and fall on me. 27, 100C, 01:XX:XX

Sh, 191 - I Since the being bitten by the dogs have developed a strong fear of dogs, and have been chased by one dog and growled at by another. This is coupled with a general fear of something happening. These fears are new to me and were better again after the proving. 27, 100C, 05:XX:XX

CUPR-A. He, 15 - Afraid of falling; holds on to his nurse's hair, hugs up to her, afraid of being injured,...

CUPR. Ha, 5 - A kind of timidity; he felt as if he had to step softly, in order not to hurt himself, nor to disturb his room-mates. (friend) (cautious, prudent, gentle, delicate)

CUR. Al, 1 - Paroxysm of insanity impelling him to attack himself; he strikes, scratches, and tears himself with a sort of relish, (enjoy) and without feeling any pain.

DROS. Al, 266 - Vivid frightful dreams about being maltreated (insulted, injured).

ELAPS. Al, 2 - Reveries in the daytime; he imagines he is being beaten.

Al, 16 - Inclination to strike and pick a quarrel.

GERM. Sh, 180 - Woke up early 3.30 am. had strong feeling, like a visualization. I picture myself lying on floor in fetal position and being shot in the head like a horse or a dog. Almost welcomed it. Then thought my children still need me. A very strong feeling of failure accompanied this. I felt I did not deserve to live. Better crying next day when talking to husband. This feeling of depression carried on for several nights. As soon as I wake up in the early morning, my mind is active and a feeling of inadequacy comes on strongly. 05 , 6C, 28:XX:XX

Sh, 112 - Don't see why I am here. I can't bear it. I go mad. I hate myself. I want to beat myself and I do it. Tear my hair. Stop when it hurts too much. It is like hell !!! 18, 30C, 20:XX:XX

GLON. He, 16 - Bad effects of mental excitement, fright, fear, mechanical contusions and their consequences.(ailments from)

HALI-L. Sh, 7 - My left arm feels like a broken wing. 01, 30C, 21:XX:XX

Sh, 139 - During a massage on her abdomen, felt as if she were going into shock. Had this feeling before at age 19 when she had a bad fall with broken ribs, and punctures to the liver, with internal bleeding, which resulted in surgery and the unnecessary removal of her spleen. Never had this kind of experience during massage before... 09, 6C, 04:XX:XX

Sh, 954 - My feet hurt —sharp —down the inside, all along the big toe joint when I started walking again 23 years ago. I had the same pain again last night. 20, 30C, 18:XX:XX

HURA. Al, 28 - Impatience, anger; she bites her hands, and gets into passion because her ideas come too slowly.

HYDROG. Sh, 243 - Fear that someone was trying to find out if I was home so that they could come and rape and murder me. 16, 30C, XX:XX:XX

HYOS. Ha, 575 - Peculiar fear of being

bitten (hurt) by beasts.
Ha, 559 - Fury; he tries to inflict injury on and hurt others.
Ha, 563 - He strikes and tries to murder those he meets.
He, 16 - Fears: being left alone (solitude, deserted); poison, or being bitten (hurt); being poisoned or sold; being betrayed, or injured; wishes to run away. (escape)
He, 54 - Tries to injure those around him; convulsions after trying to swallow.

LAC-C. He, 17 - On lying down either by day or night begins to think how horrible it would be if a very sharp pain, like a knife, should go through her, and thought of it causes great mental distress.

LAC-F. Al,N-5 - Mental illusion that the corners of furniture, or any pointed object near her, were about to run into eyes;...

LACH. He, 9 - Imagines he is followed (pursued) by enemies who are trying to harm (hurt, injure) him; attempts to leave room as if frightened by visions behind him.
He, 21-...imagines he is followed by enemies who are trying to harm him; attempts to leave room as if frightened by visions behind him.

LIL-T. Al, 25 - While attending a lecture (speech), desire to hit the lecturer, and in the evening desirous of swearing and damning the fire and things generally, and to think and speak obscene things; disposed to strike and hit persons; as these feelings came, the uterine pains passed away.
He, 9 - Disposed to curse, to strike, to think of obscene things; as these mental states came, uterine irritation abated.(reduced)

LYC. Al, 97 - As if out of her mind, she seeks quarrels, makes unfounded reproaches, is most exceedingly violent, and strikes those whom she thus insults.

LYSS. Al,N-24 - Fancies he is being blown (hit, hurt) at by several persons, some of whom are not present.
Al,N-34-....to stab his flesh with the knife he is holding, and the like.
Al,N-58 - Ordered her husband to go away(forsakes), as she wanted to bite him, and joining (associated) act to threat(menace), she bit herself in arm.
Al-N, 37 - Inclined to use insulting language, scold his friends, beat and abuse those near him.
He, 23 - Imagine that they are being abused (hurt, injured), and energetically defend themselves against attacks and insults, which in reality are products of their own fancy.
He, 24 - Fancies he is being blown (strike) at by several persons, some of whom are not present.

MERC. Al, 37 - While taking a walk, he has a strong inclination to pinch the noses of the strangers he meets.
Al, 1......she puts small stones into her mouth without swallowing them, and complains that they cut her intestines; ...
Ha, 1263 - Mania; she throws off the clothes at night, tears the straw about, and scolds; by day she leaps (jump) up high like a petulant extravagant person...she talks and scolds much to herself,...spits frequently and spreads the saliva out with her feet, and licks some of it up again; she often licks cowdung (excrements) and the mud of ponds (lake); she often takes little stones in her mouth, without swallowing them, and at the same time complains that they are cutting her bowels; much clotted blood passes with her motion; ...

NAJA. He, 5-...imagines she is in a terrible rainstorm, complains of being so cold (coldness), and that the carriage has turned over and hurt her head. (accident)

NAT-C. Al, 42 - Very fretful and discontented with whole world; he constantly felt as though he could beat (punish ?) himself, his whole life angered him, and he preferred to have no existence at all; he was solicitous about the future, and inclined to despair, all day.

OP. Al, 16-...started up in a fright on account of fancied swordsmen (rival, competitor) who threatened to stab him; became angry if any one argued him or thought him delirious; however, he blamed (reproaches) himself while in delirium for his folly.
Al, 39-...threatened alternately self-destruction and injury to others.
He, 21-...in old, emaciated persons; sees animals coming towards him; people want to hurt him, execute him ; creeping under covers or jumping out of bed; in "old

sinners" (criminals) whose long lives of excess have thoroughly destroyed their constitutions; ...; believe themselves to be murderers or criminals to be executed; want to run away (escape) ;...

OSM. Al, 5 - Thoughts of accidents having happened to others, by a blow, a fall, or being dashed (crushed, hit, knock) to pieces; gradually these thoughts grow upon him, as if he were to do the same injuries to others.

PLAT. Ha, 33 - Very cross and irritated at harmless matters and words; so that she at times would have liked to have beaten herself and friends.

He, 16 - Very peevish and easily excited; he could have beaten any one without provocation.

PLB. He, 16 - Mental disturbance of eight or ten years' duration in a man addicted to masturbation; has several times attempted suicide; has been in seclusion (solitude); greatest dejection and despair;...; believes himself lost (condemned) ; has the sounds of hell constantly in his ears; hears voices and sees shadows of demons, great disposition to make away (suicide) with himself or do himself some bodily injury;

PSOR. Al,N-44 - Mania of self-destruction.

RAPH. Al, 1 - Feeling of aversion towards all women; she is provoked by seeing women going and coming about her; their approach threw her into a fury; the mere contact with a woman's dress caused intolerable distress;...She is attracted to all men without distinction (nymphomania) ; when she gives her hand to a man, she feels great agitation,...When left alone for a hour in the evening, she gave herself a very deep wound in the lips with a penknife, in hopes to put an end to this condition (hurt, punishes). Moral feeling was completely extinct, the physical nature alone ruled and threw her into a frightful state (wild). From morning to noon she would not have been able to resist the advances even of a man for whom she had not the least friendly feeling; from noon to 6 p.m. she could not have held out against any man whatsoever; from 8 to 11 the demands of sense were so importunate as to silence the voice of shame and reason; ... and would have thrown herself into the arms of the first man she met...she was still unable to control her impulses;...

SPIG. He, 5 - Afraid (fear) of pointed things, pins, etc.

STRAM. Ha, 544 - Great desire to bite and tear everything with his teeth that comes near his mouth, even his own limbs.

He, 87 - After a dreadful shock, occasioned by death of his brother, who fell dead in his arms,...struck all at around him...spoke at one time in Hungarian, and then in Wallachian language; sang Latin paternosters, declared he was God, and then that he was the devil;...

He, 100-...threatens to knock everybody down, to break furniture, to throw himself out of window.

He, 110-...frightful dreams about fighting and killing; takes offensive in imaginary quarrels, and attacks aggressor; runs against supposed object to attack it;...

STRY. Al, 5 - A peculiar nervous erethism, almost resembling what I had seen in a case of hydrophobia ...wandering when left to himself, and begged most piteously (miserable) that I would not hurt him...fear of being injured...

SULPH. Al, 9 - She imagines that people injure her, and she will die in consequence.

Al, 3800-....(DREAM) she walked about like a somnambulist, thought there was a fire, dressed herself, talked out of the window, and was frightened as she heard that it was nothing; for three days afterwards she was very weak, and felt bruised(hurt).

TARENT. Al, 65-...great haste in whatever I undertook, from a constant fear that something would happen to prevent my finishing it;...fear that something would fall on me (doom, disgrace);...fear of striking it against some imaginary object which appeared to be suspended....(hurt)

Al, 16 - Great taciturnity and irritability; desire to strike himself and others.

He, 2 - Great taciturnity and irritability; desire to strike himself and others.

TUB. Al,N-13 - Very irritable, want to fight; no hesitancy in throwing anything at anyone, even without cause.

VALER. Al, 12 - Fearfulness in the evening when sitting in the dark (imagining that some one might hurt him).

He, 4 - Erroneous ideas; thinks she is some one else,...; imagines animals lying near her which she fears she may hurt.

HUSBAND

Abusive; husband, to: thuj.[137]
Aversion; husband, and children: ***glon.***[54] verat.[54]
Aversion; husband, to: agn.[171] bamb-a.[1184] choc.[222] ***glon.*** kali-c.[122] kali-p. ***nat-c.*** nat-m. pitu-a.[164] **SEP.** thuj.[137] verat.
Caressed; caressing husband and child, then pushes away: ***anac.***[54]
Delusions; dead, corpse, husband: calc-sil.[58] plb.
- husband, he is not her: ***anac.***
- murder, husband and child, she is going to: kali-br.
- neglected, husband, by her: ***stram.***[8]

Fear; happen, something will, husband will not return home: ars.[172] bar-c.[172] caust.[172] ***plat.*** sep.[172]
Indifference; husband, towards: luna[228]
Irritability; husband, towards: bamb-a.[1184] luna[228]
Jealousy; brutal, kind man becoming: calc.[30] lach.[30] nux-v.[30] sulph.[30]
Kill; sudden impulse to, husband, her beloved: ***merc. nux-v. plat.***
Kill; sudden impulse to, husband, her beloved, menses, particularly during, implores him to hide his razor: ***merc.***[54]
Sadness; quarrel with husband, after: ***anac.***[54]
Suicidal disposition; mania, in, puerperal, with aversion to husband, baby and coition: agn.[171]

ANAC. He, 29 - Has the fixed idea that her husband is not her husband, her child not her child; now she fondles (caress) them and again pushes them away. (reject, repudiate)
He, 13 - After having caressed her husband or child she pushes them away from her, as if they were not what she supposed.

ANDROC. Sh, 58-. Felt more love for her mother, friends and husband. (7)
Sh, 102 - Assertive, impatient, aggressive. Felt resentful and abused. Had no control over her temper. Bellowed and lashed out at everyone. In the evening, furious for no apparent reason. Wanted to kill her husband and children, banged doors and threw things. By bed-time, she felt fine but the intensity of her evil thoughts was very frightening. (7)

GLON. He, 2 - Recognized no one; repulsed her husband and children; raved, screamed, and wished to rush from house; jumped out of bed, but fell because her knees gave way.

HYDROG. Sh, 177 - Upset husband by telling him what I thought of the way he'd been behaving. I felt curiously uninvolved. Indifference to husband. Felt a little 'dead', uninvolved, wasn't really responding in any way — not in a good way or a bad way. Didn't feel cross, affectionate or anything. Very peculiar, like I was watching and its nothing to do with me. Like looking at somebody else, almost as if I wasn't there. Felt emotionally numb and unable to respond —as if I wasn't there. Like a living dead being alive and not being able to make the appropriate responses. Real total detachment. 08, 30C, 10:XX:XX

HYOS. He, 66 - A gentle, lovable woman became extremely jealous of her husband, and although fully realizing that she did him injustice, she was so filled with grief that she found no rest day or night... (remorse)

KALI-BR. He, 15 - Frightful imaginings at night (in pregnant women during latter months), they are under impression that they have committed, or about to commit, some great crime and cruelty (brutality), such murdering their children or husbands.

LYSS. Al,N-58 - Ordered her husband to go away(forsakes), as she wanted to bite him, and joining (associated) act to threat(menace), she bit herself in arm.

MERC. He, 22 - Great desire to murder (homicidal) or committed suicide ...is fearful that she may commit some wrong and kill herself (punishment); something urges her to kill her husband, of whom she is very fond (loving), and she implores him to hide his razor (knife).

NAT-C. He, 4 - Aversion to mankind and society; estrangement (separation, alienation) from individuals and society; even from her husband and family.

NUX-V. He, 12 - Inclined to find fault and

scold (reprove); morose; stubborn; (obstinate) an insane desire when alone with her husband, whom she adores, to kill him.
He, 39 - Mania puerperalis...constantly complaining, criticizing or explaining, ... as soon she recognized physician she spoke of imperfection of medical knowledge and declared it an error that one could not live without a heart, inasmuch as she felt very well without one, it having come away with the afterbirth to which it had grown fast, the nurse having separated the two before her eyes; complains of her husband, says he wishes to convince her she is sick, ... nymphomania,... frequently sips at a bowl of warm sugar-water, declaring it will form her a new heart; .(health, healing)...(expert)
PLB. Al, 66 - Hallucinations of mind, she seemed to see her dead husband and child in a tree out of the window.
STRAM. He, 145 - Wife complains of husband neglecting her; man accuses his wife of being faithless.
He, 176 - Melancholia,...complains her husband has neglecting her.
VERAT. He, 13 - After severe illness, aversion to husband and children; desire to leave house: hallucinations, room appeared full of people, crowding in, there was no longer room...

IDENTITY

Confounding; objects and ideas: calc. cann-s. colch.[54] hyos. nux-v. phos.[189] plat. ***sulph.***
Confusion of mind; identity, as to his: **ALUM.** ***anh.***[119] ant-c. aur.[54] bapt. camph.[30] cand-a.[239] cann-s. cic.[58] foll.[1201] germ.[222] kali-br. lach. med. nat-m.[5] petr. phos. plb. pyrus stram. sulph. thuj. valer.
Confusion of mind; identity, depersonalization: anh.[119] halo.[149] thuj.[198]
Confusion of mind; identity, duality, sense of: ***alum.***[5] **ANAC.**[5] anh.[149] arg-n.[137] **BAPT.**[5] calc-p.[137] cann-i.[36] cann-s.[5] cycl.[5] des-ac.[149] **GELS.**[5] lach.[5] lil-t.[5] lyc.[5] mosch.[5] naja[117] nat-m.[5] ***nux-m.***[5] op.[5] paro-i.[149] petr.[5] ***phos.***[5] plb.[5] psor.[5] puls.[5] pyrog.[111] sec.[5] sil.[5] ***stram.***[5] ther.[5] thuj.[5] tril.[137] xan.[137]
Confusion of mind; identity, head separated from body, as if: allox.[119] cocc.[58] ***daph.***[122] **PSOR.**[122] ther.[58]
Confusion of mind; identity, own, as if it were not his: alum.[5] lach.[5] nat-m.[5] thuj.[5]
Confusion of mind; identity, paralysis, in: alum.[54]
Confusion of mind; identity, sexual: hydrog.[222]
Confusion of mind; identity, sick, as if someone else were: gels.[5]
Delirium; bellows like a calf: cupr.
Delusions; animals, geese, threw themselves into water, thinking themselves to be: con.
- animals, he or she is a: choc.[222]
- bird, he is a, runs about, chirping and twittering, until he faints: lyss.[54]
- blind, that he is: bell.[1] hyos.[10] mosch. stram.[10] verat.
- body, arms, belong to her, do not: agar. bapt.[122] carc.[140] ign.[137] op.[137]
- body, black, is: sulph.
- body, erroneous ideas as to the state of his: cot.[102] germ.[222] pyrog.[58] **SABAD.** stram.[58]
- body, legs, belong to her, don't: ***agar.***[122] ***bapt.***[122] coll.[137] hydrobr-ac.[102] op.[122] sumb.[122]
- body, legs, talking, one is talking with the other: bapt.
- body, legs, toe, first, is in controversy with first finger, thumb: bapt.[58]
- body, nose, someone else's, has: lac-c.
- body, sweets, is made of: merc.
- body, threefold, has a: ars. petr.
- cat, he is a: lap-mar-c.[194]
- child, he is again a, acts like a, and: ***cic.***
- Christ, himself to be: cann-i. verat.[58]
- consciousness belongs to another: alum.
- criminal, and others know it: cob.
- criminal, that he is a: alum.[10] am-c.[10] ars.[10] carb-v.[10] caust.[10] chel.[5] cina[10] cob. coff.[10] cycl. dig. ferr.[10] graph.[10] hyos. ***ign.*** m-arct.[10] ***merc.*** nat-c.[10] nit-ac.[10] nux-v.[10] op. phos. puls.[10] ruta[10] sabad.[139] sarr. sil.[10] stront-c.[10] sulph.[10] thuj. verat.[10]
- demoniacal, he is: ***anac.***[54] **HYOS.**[30]
- devils, he is a devil: anac. camph. cann-i. ***hyos.*** kali-br. stram.
- distinguished, is: lap-mar-c.[194] phos.[1] stram. verat.
- divine, he is: cann-i. glon.[116] stram.
- dogs, he is a dog, growls and barks: bell.[54] lyss.[54]
- dogs, others are, barks at them to be understood: stram.[54]

- dolls, people are: plb.
- double, he is: alum. ***anac.*** anh.[119] ***bapt.*** calc-p.[137] cann-i. cann-s.[5] corn-f.[102] cycl.[5] ***gels.***[5] glon. lach. lil-t. lyc.[5] mosch. nat-m.[5] ***nux-m.*** op.[5] ***petr.*** phos.[1] plb.[5] psil.[164] psor.[5] puls.[5] pyrog.[5] rhus-t.[47] sec. sil.[1] ***stram.*** ther.[5] thuj. valer.[102]
- double, lying on one side, she is one, and lying on the other side she is another person: pyrog.[139]
- double, of being: alum. ***anac.*** anh.[119] ***bapt.*** calc-p.[137] cann-i. cann-s.[5] corn-f.[102] cycl.[5] ***gels.***[5] glon. lach. lil-t. lyc.[5] mosch. nat-m.[5] ***nux-m.*** op.[5] ***petr.*** phos.[1] plb.[5] psil.[164] psor.[5] puls.[5] pyrog.[5] rhus-t.[47] sec. sil.[1] ***stram.*** ther.[5] thuj. valer.[102]
- dreams have been stolen or belong to another: choc.[222]
- emperor, thought himself an: cann-i.
- general, he is a: cupr.
- giraffe, he is a: cann-i.
- gnome, he is a: cann-i.[36]
- God, he is, then he is devil: **STRAM.**[54]
- goose, he is a: con.
- harlequin, he is a: hyos.
- hat is a pair of trousers which he tries to put on: stram.
- hearing, of, ear, not his own, with: psor.[137]
- hearing, of, his own voice seems changed: alum.[1]
- hedgehog, he or she is: choc.[222]
- hippopotamus, he is a: cann-i.[36]
- hunter, he is a: cann-i. verat.
- identity, errors of personal: alum. androc.[222] anh.[149] ant-c. bapt. cann-i.[72] cann-s. cic.[58] gels. kali-br.[25] lac-c. ***lach.*** lil-t.[25] mosch.[122] myric.[25] naja[25] nat-m.[5] ol-j.[25] orig.[25] petr. phos. plb. pyrog.[58] pyrus raja-s.[149] stram. syph.[137] thuj. ***valer.*** ***verat.***[187]
- juggler, he is a: bell.
- locomotive, he is a: cann-i.
- magician, is a: bell.
- marble statue, he is a: cann-i.
- noble person, he is a: lap-mar-c.[194] phos. plat.[58]
- officer, he is an: agar. bell. cann-i. ***cupr.*** cupr-acet.[36]
- old, he looks: mag-m.[187]
- person, existed in another person, she: pyrog.[139]
- person, three persons that he is: anac.[116] bapt.[122] cann-i.[36] nux-m. ***petr.***[116] psil.[164]
- poor, he is: bamb-a.[1184] bell. bry.[185] calc-f. hep. mez. nux-v. psor.[58] ***sep.*** stram. valer.
- pregnant, is, birth to a blue eyed baby, that she is about to give: ***verat.***[54]
- prince, is a: verat.
- pure, that she is: stram.[122]
- saw, he was a huge, darting up and down: cann-i.
- says something, it seems to him as though somebody else has said it, when he: alum.
- sees anything, as if another person had seen it, or as if he could transfer himself into another and only then could see: alum.
- side, own her left, she did not: sil.
- soda water, being a bottle of: arg-n.[91] cann-i.[36]
- soldier, he is a, (at night): chel.[36]
- stranger, he is a: germ.[222] nat-m.[111] valer.
- talking, someone else is, when he speaks: alum.[36] cann-s.[58]
- tomato is a grasshopper: choc.[222]
- wild, he will go: lob.[139]
- wood, is made of: eupi.[102] kali-n. petr.[137] rhus-t.[102] ***thuj.***[102]

Dreams; body, chest, wished to open the chest and look in: paull.[36]

- ➤ devils, seeing an acquaintance coming and mistaking him for the devil: nicc.[36]
- ➤ fairytale, as in a: ozone[227]
- ➤ girl, that he is a: apis.
- ➤ leper, of being a: paull.[36]
- ➤ lion, that he was a: phys.
- ➤ physician: canna[36] mang.[36]
- ➤ soldier, being a: chel.[36]
- ➤ women, animals, changed into: sol-t-ae.[36]

Ego, feels devoid of: lap-c-b.[194]

Fear; imbecile, that he would become: stram.

Memory; active, past events, remembered as belonging to someone else, or as matter read: ail.[54]

ACON. Al, 92-...feels that all the mental operations transpire (develop) in the region of the stomach; after two hours,...the thinking power returns again to the head.

ADAM. Sh, 166 - I felt confused and not myself. 7, 6C, 02:00:XX

AIL. He, 1 - Past events are forgotten, remembered as belonging to someone else, or as matters read.

ALUM. Ha, 55 - A numb (insensibility)

feeling in the head as if his consciousness was outside of his body; when he says anything, he feels as if another person had said it; and when he sees anything, as if another person had seen it, or as if he could transfer himself into another, and only then could see. (transmigration)

He, 2 - Consciousness (knowledge) of his personal identity (personality) confused.

ANAC. He, 29 - Has the fixed idea that her husband is not her husband, her child not her child; now she fondles (caress) them and again pushes them away. (reject, repudiate)

He, 40 - Uses profane language, swears, thinks himself a demon.

ANDROC. Sh, 62 - A friend commented that she "looked strange and not at all like herself". (7)

Sh, 129 - It seemed as though he was a different person, very similar to the way he had been in adolescence, but in a much more powerful manner. These emotions were so intense he wanted to rip his chest apart to let them out. He lost all control over his emotions, which seemed to come from a deep and distant part of himself, a darker side. He desired to continue the proving for the rest of his life. (29)

BAPT. He, 8 - He thinks his legs are holding a conversation with each other. 0Gout.

He, 9 - He thinks his gouty toe is holding a confab (conversation, talk) with his gouty thumb.

BELL. He, 24 - Fixed ideas, thinks he is riding on an ox, uses a stick for a gun, growling and barking like a dog.

CAMPH. Al, 46-... There was no other feeling in my soul than that of my hopeless endless damnation (condemnation). I sank back upon the bed, believing that I was the spirit of evil in a world forsaken of God.

CANN-I. Al, 66 - Illusion that he was a pump-log, through which a stream of hot water was playing, and threatening his friend with a wetting.

Al, 67 - Illusion that he was an inkstand, and that, as he lay on the bed, the ink might spill over the white counterpane.

Al, 69 - He seems to himself to be transformed into a vegetable existence, as a huge fern, and to be surrounded by clouds of music and perfume.

CANN-S. He, 1 - Seems to be in a dream, as if things were not real; feels as if she did not know where she was; objects seem strange; feels at times as if she was somebody else;...

He, 5 - Voices including her own, seem to come from a distance; her own voice seems strange, as if it was somebody else speaking.

CANTH. Al, 22-...; she feels as if newly (recently) born;... (innocent, naive, pure)

CHOC. Sh, 32 - When I look in the mirror, I don't recognise myself. I look different, especially around and over the eyes —my face doesn't seem familiar. The area around my forehead feels more congested and bigger.

Sh, 45 - When I woke from the dream, I had a little panic, an unusual childhood memory came back in which I remembered having read as a child about being covered in clay, baked and eaten. The thought came to me of the spines on my back covered in clay and baked and eaten like a hedgehog.

Sh, 57 - Keep getting a picture of the prickles of the start of the hairline of the hedgehog and am aware of this point in me —not discomfort, but keep pushing hair back and pulling my fingers backwards through my hair, thinking its nice that its not in my face. Keep getting pictures of faces of hedgehogs, (rather than the spiny bits) especially the nose, which seems so black and wet.

Sh, 74 - I saw a rat. We stood looking at each other. I felt we both recognised each other. It was very exciting.

Sh, 86 - On seeing a bristly carpet, started laughing excitedly —had a familiar feeling, like meeting a friend. The texture of the carpet was very spiky like a Hedgehog. Told friend that they should come and see it. It's such a wonderful carpet!

Sh, 107 - A strange feeling of being an animal, yet having this thinking.

Sh, 114 - When I feel like a hedgehog, my heart is much faster, but when I feel the stillness, I don't feel my heart at all.

Sh, 116-12:30pm -I feel less and less animal at the moment and I desire company. When it comes, its so intense, I almost lose what I am. I've never been there before. I feel very privileged, as if I can be on both sides at the same time.

Sh, 117 - I thought how would an animal be if it had my body. What would they do with thought. I think I'm better off.

Sh, 127 - Before this, I never felt very comfortable with men. Now I feel much more comfortable. I feel I've lost that extreme feeling of totally female identity. I feel like a female animal, but its not really in my awareness, it just is. Desire to curl up over a man's back. It felt right and comfortable.

Sh, 130 - I feel slightly less like a hedgehog today, but the picture is still in my mind. Human things seem so trivial —so much energy wasted when you are human. Nature is so efficient. It never wastes a seed and we just spend energy everywhere.

Sh, 134 - I felt small enough to get into a drawer in a desk full of rubbish and rout around under things, a kind of curiosity.

Sh, 151 - Still get images of creatures — thought a tomato was a grasshopper.

Sh, 153 - Since the proving, I know how it feels to be a animal or a plant. I know the feeling of daffodil, of flower, of hedgehog, of dog.

Sh, 210 - Felt totally isolated and averse to company. Estranged himself from his family and friends and stopped all communication with them for a long period. Did not reply to letters and left no address. He seemed to hide away and literally disappear. The state of Isolation resulted from feeling that "I didn't exist as a human being". This behaviour was in strong contrast to his normal sociable disposition. 35, 30C, XX:XX:XX:

CIC. Ha, 240 - He felt like a child of seven or eight years old, objects were very dear and attractive to him, as toys are to a child. (purity)

He, 7 - He thinks himself a young child. (purity, juvenile, infant)

CON. Al, 6 - Delirious and stupid; they threw themselves into the water, thinking they were geese; for three years they remained partly paralytic, suffering from much pain.

GERM. Sh, 110 - I don't like to be me. Want to be different. Have a distant feeling to myself yet long for physical contact, a boyfriend. Not able to do something about it. 18, 30c, 02:10:00

Sh, 101 - I'm desperate. I want to die. Feel the power to kill. Feel like a wild animal locked in. It's strong, so intense. I hate so strong-feel a terrible disgust and I'm afraid of what I'm able to do. It's completely impossible to be in it and impossible to get out of it. 18, 30C, 190:XX:XX

HALI-L. Sh, 7 - My left arm feels like a broken wing. 01, 30C, 21:XX:XX

Sh, 208 - Daughter home sick. I'm enjoying just hanging around with her being. "Mom." Realize I still don't feel like her mom. I'm not Mom; I'm just me. But to them, I'm Mom. Does my mom feel the same? 09, 6C, 23:XX:XX

Sh, 326 - Unconsciously, I have taken on the characteristics of the speech of a guy I work with; an actual copying of a certain vernacular. When he talks, he stretches a word. I don't do it consciously, but when it happens, I'm aware I've adopted a small part of that personality. The way he gestures, the way he uses his teeth—enunciates—the gestures of his language. I feel I'm malleable. I don't like it. It feels like I don't have my own personality, no true identity. In fact I might even believe that. I'm more outward with actual copying. It's something I like in him, so when I do it, it makes me feel good about myself. I realize it then try to combat it. I don't want to be like a piece of clay that can be pressed this way and that way. 18, 30C, 17:XX:XX

Sh, 719 - Not sure whether asleep or not — inner vision. I'm high up and there is water below me and I have an image of a few of my breast feathers floating on the water. Between the breast feathers, the reflection of a very pink dawn. Noticed all birds in pairs. 20, 30C, 00:23:30

Sh, 721 - Inner vision; I was sunning my wings in the dawn sun. I'm not flapping-soaring —not dusk, at dawn — not for dark, of Light. 20, 30C, 00:23:50

Sh, 741 - A five year old boy, friend of daughter, said I looked strange, different. He said I was staring at him. I said, "It's all right. I have the eye of an eagle." 20, 30C, 01:12:00

Sh, 783 - On waking, my arms felt like wings. I was spread-eagled across the bed, front and back. Normally I would sleep on my side, but I can't get the right position on my arms. 20, 30C, 03:23:00

Sh, 933 - I don't recognize myself as human. I don't know who I am. 20, 30C, 15:XX:XX

Sh, 937 - I don't know what or who to be. I'm not human. I feel that I'm trapped in a body that's not mine. I related to the birds at the Botanical Gardens more than the people, but felt sad because they are caged. 20, 30C, 15:XX:XX

Sh, 942 - Don't feel part of the human race. Overwhelming gratitude that I could walk and not be in a wheelchair. 20, 30C, 15:XX:XX

Sh, 950 - This morning a friend brought me three condor feathers. I was standing wrapped in a towel, wet from the bath and the friend said I looked like a wet fledgling. 20, 30C, 17:XX:XX

HYDROG. Sh, 1 - It dawned on me that it was as if there was a shift in the universe. 12, 6C, 07:XX:XX

Sh, 2 - I can honestly say I'll never be the same again —a bit like having a baby. Amazing how my whole perception seems to have altered one degree, which makes everything different. 08, 30C, 100:XX:XX

Sh, 28 - I felt an incredible clarity before and now I feel it may all have been a illusion. I am uncertain, don't know how I am anymore. I don't recognize what is happening. It's as if I have made a step into the unknown. I feel I'm in an unknown area without protection. Fear is the biggest limitation. 16, 30C, 05:XX:X

Sh, 33 - About two months after beginning the proving, developed an extreme range of mental symptoms that he had never had before. These included severe depression with strong alternations of moods, & high then low &, with suicidal tendency, desire to jump from a high building or cut wrist, confusion of identity (especially concerning sex and homosexuality) and became more religious. He moved away from his parents home (which he had never before been able t o do) and shut himself away in a small flat. This condition lasted for another six or seven months and was finally antidoted by Phosphorus 200. Before that, he had tried to anti-dote it with acupuncture, to no avail. 24, 30C, 60:XX:XX

Sh, 274 - Developed an aversion to the idea of sex —confused about sexual issues and identity. Became aware of being bi-sexual or homosexual (in a man). "I want to find out who I am. I should know at 23. I used to know. What am I sexually?" Very confused. This led to suicidal depression. 24, 30C, 100:XX:XX

Sh, 276 - Feelings of vulnerability and anxiety about being masculine, both in looks and in behaviourroles. Hope it doesn't get more. To counteract this, I have been stressing the feminine. I spent lots of money on silk clothing and spent a lot of time making myself up, curling hair, etc. People comment that I look softer, but I feel harder inside. I feel confused about my sexual identity. This is in contrast to my previous proving of the remedy, when people commented that my moustache disappeared and breasts grew. 12, 6C, 30:XX:XX (homosexuality)

HYOS. Ha, 519 - In the confusion of his fancy he thinks men are swine.(pigs)

IRID. Sh, 25 - Feeling of being on the outside. F9

Sh, 57 - On the bus a woman turned to me and said, "Your eyes are the same as my daughter's." Baby like me. I knew we had met before, knew that I knew her. She knew me as well. A wonderful moment. Q7

Sh, 58 - Felt child-like, innocent, happy as though seeing things from a child's perspective. Sat watching a milk tanker, it looks just like a child's toy. Felt like I could pick it up and brrrm brrrm it up the lane. I9

Sh, 61 - I feel buzzy and vibrating, feels as if my hair is stood on end. I keep talking about being a dog. H1

Sh, 83 - It feels like my personality has been invaded, taken over. I7

Sh, 99 - Sat at the bus stop. Felt like a really small, frightened rabbit, with a large shadow of this great bird hovering over ready to pounce. G8

Sh, 106 - Mental image: I am inside an egg —a bird, wet feathers, at the point it is smashing through its shell, bursting out; a chick, wet crumpled and hot, shell flying all over. The relief —getting to the air, refreshing, cool. Inside it was humid, stifling. Stretching vast wings, enjoying feeling the air dry them out. G5

Sh, 116 - On going to sleep, asked the question, "Who am I." Message on waking, that my name was Iris. QXX

KALI-BR. He, 11 - Imagines she is a devil; cannot sleep; fears to be alone.

LAC-C. He, 10 - Imagine he wears some one's nose.

LACH. He, 8 - Thinks: she is somebody else in the hands (seized) of a stronger power; (supremacy, superiority).or that she is dead, and preparations are made for funeral (cortege) or that she is nearly dead and wishes some one would help her off; herself pursued by enemies, or fears medicine is poison; there are robbers in house and wants to jump out the window; herself under super-human control; visions real, he will die. (helplessness, desire; aid, comfort, salvation)

He, 33-...want of self control; lascivious; felt as if she was clear (pure) animal right through, whilst of all mental power was dormant; sensation as if hands of stronger power, as if charmed (enchanted), and as if could not break the spell (charm). (possessed, wildness)

LIL-T. Al, 2 - Excitement, weeping, feeling as if she were two persons, at night.

LYSS. Al, 34 - There seems to be two distinct trains of thought operating at one and the same time.

Al,N-26 - Thinks he is a dog or a bird, and runs up and down chirping and twittering...(liberty?)

He, 26 - Thinks he is a dog or a bird, and runs up and down, chirping and twittering, until he falls down fainting.

PHOS. Al, 12-...; wherever he turned his eyes he saw faces; they swarmed (crowded, surrounded) by him in long panoramic succession; they leered (look lecherous) at him over the footboard of the bed; they squinted (look) at him though the windows, or came trooping (crowd) in when the doors were left ajar (open) (invade);..he fancied he was some one else, ...

Al, 86-...; a feeling of dread (fear), as if awaiting something terrible, yet unable to resist or move (terrifying, scaring), overcame me; sometimes it seemed as if I was beginning to bloat (inhalant, inflate, vanity?), and then I could hear a multitude of voices saying in high glee, "Fill him up a little more and he will burst," (blow up) followed by demoniacal laughter, which made the cold chills run over me... I imagined myself an aurora borealis, and could distinctly hear voices shouting, "Beautiful! Oh, was not that splendid?"...

PYROG. Al,N-6 - Feels when lying on one side that she is one person, and another person when turning on the other side.

Al,N-7 - Sensation as though crowded with arms and legs.

SABAD. He, 2 - Erroneous impressions as to the state of his body.

VALER. He, 4 - Erroneous ideas; thinks she is some one else,...; imagines animals lying near her which she fears she may hurt.

VERAT. Ha, 671 - Mania: he alleges that he is a hunter.(pursue)

Ha, 672 - He pretends (simulate, feigning) he is a prince, and gives himself airs (affectation, pretentious) accordingly.

IMITATED

Delusions; man, does all the things he does: ars.

- people, beside him, doing as he does: ***ars.***
- reading after her, someone is, which makes her read the faster: mag-m.

Imitation, mimicry: bell.[5] calc.[109] caust.[148] cupr.[5] hyos.[5] lach.[137] nux-m.[137] sars.[5] stram.[5] verat.[5]

Imitation; voices, motions and gestures of different animals, of: ***stram.***[54]

Imitation; writing, in, without knowing signification: ***lyc.***[54]

ARS. He, 16 - Tormenting hallucination, as if there was one by his side who did that he was doing, eating, washing etc.

CROC. Al, 5 - If any one happens to sing a single musical note, she begins involuntarily to sing, and then is obliged to laugh at herself; she however, soon sings in spite of her determination to stop. (sympathy)

CUPR. He, 10 - Mania with biting, beating, and tearing things to pieces; insane foolish gestures of imitation and mimicry; full of insane spiteful (cruelty, brutality) tricks (deceitful, false), ..unhappy, despairing...miserable look...

MAG-M. Ha, 20 - Fanciful (fantastic) delusions: As if while she was reading in a book, another person was reading after her, and compelled her to read more quickly, with humming and buzzing (murmur) around her...(faster)

He, 6 - While reading, felt as if some one was reading after her and she must read faster and faster. (imitated)

STRAM. Al, 120...all his ideas seemed to consist of mere reproductions (duplication); there was nothing original (creative) and there were no new combinations.

Al, 123-...seemed to herself to be engaged in her usual avocation,...imitate in every respect the routine procedure of one thus engaged.

He, 151 - Making all kinds of faces and imitating motions, gestures and voices of different animals.

IMPATIENCE

Cheerfulness; alternating with, impatience: tell.[149]

Delusions; wait, he had to: anh.[119]

Desires; many things impatiently, dislikes its favorite playthings, child: arn.[5] **CHAM.**[5] cina[56] dulc.[5] kreos.[5] puls.[5] **RHEUM**[54] staph.[56]

Discouraged; impatience, with: ***calc.***[10]

Impatience: ***acon.*** act-sp. aeth.[10] agar-ph.[36] alco.[36] all-s. allox.[119] ambr. amph.[85] anac. androc.[222] ant-c.[102] ***apis*** aral.[5] ***ars. ars-h. ars-i.*** ars-s-f.[58] aster. aur. aur-ar.[58] aur-i.[58] aur-m-n. bad.[1] bamb-a.[1184] bar-c. bar-i.[58] bar-s.[58] bell. bor.[161] ***bry.*** bufo ***calc.*** calc-f.[119] calc-i.[58] calc-s. calc-sil.[58] ***carb-ac.***[54] carb-v. carc.[227] **CHAM.** chin. chin-ar. choc.[222] cimic. ***cina***[5] colch. ***coloc.*** cub. culx.[58] digin.[36] dros. ***dulc.*** ferul.[36] gels. germ.[222] gins.[10] goss.[122] graph.[58] hell. ***hep.*** hist.[119] hura hydrog.[222] ***hyos.*** **IGN.** ***iod. ip.*** kali-ar. ***kali-bi. kali-c.*** kali-p. kali-s. kali-sil.[58] ***kreos.***[5] ***lach.*** lil-t. luna[228] ***lyc.*** lyss. manc. ***med.*** menis.[25] merc. ***morg-g.***[136] mosch.[54] murx.[54] nat-ar. nat-c. ***nat-m.*** nat-p. nep.[149] nicc. nid.[149] nit-ac. nuph.[54] nux-m.[5] **NUX-V.** onos. op. osm. pall. ph-ac. pitu-a.[164] ***plan. plat. psor. puls.*** pulx.[102] rheum ***rhus-t.*** sang. sars. **SEP. SIL.**[122] spig. spong. stann. staph. ***sul-ac.*** sul-i.[58] **SULPH.** tarax.[119] tarent. tax. thal.[85] thiop.[149] thuj. uran-n.[25] vac. viol-t. vip-a.[149] wies.[36] wye.[85] zinc. zinc-p.[58]

Impatience; always: merc.[30] sil.[30]

Impatience; children, with: anac.[122] bamb-a.[1184] kali-c.[1]

Impatience; contradiction, during: alco.[36]

Impatience; contradiction, slightest: nuph.[54]

Impatience; convulsions before attack, in: ***mosch.***[54]

Impatience; cures him at once, the patient insists that the doctor: cham.[85]

Impatience; pain, from, herself and others, at: ***murx.***[54]

Impatience; playing of children: anac.

Impatience; room, in a warm crowded: ***plat.***[54]

Impatience; runs about, never sits or sleeps at night: ***iod.***[54]

Impatience; sadness, in: ***kali-c.***[54]

Impatience; slowly, everything goes too: androc.[222] ***cham.***[54]

Impatience; suicidal desperation, with: carb-v.[1]

Impatience; throws himself about: ***acon.***[54]

Impatience; trifles, about: kali-p. ***med.*** merc. nat-m. sang.[36] sol-a.[36] ***sul-ac. sulph.***

Impatience; work, for: ***ip.***[54]

Impatience; work, in: ***nux-v.***[116] sep.[30]

Temperament; choleric, ardent, disposed to anger, spite or deception, always irritable and impatient: **NUX-V.**[54]

Weeping; impatience, from: dulc.[5]

ACON. Al, 14 - Excessive disagreeable restlessness; without occasion for hurrying, he is in the greatest haste, every obstacle that delays his rapid pace is excessively annoying; he knocks against some people who do not get out of his way fast enough, and runs in breathless haste up the steps;...

ADAM. Sh, 83 - Impatience for plans to come to fruition, but can't hurry the process. 2, 12C, 60:XX:XX

Sh, 211 - I felt very impatient with my patients. I was making a lot of judgments. 7, 6C, 03:00:XX

Sh, 217 - Impatient and intolerant with others. 20, 1M, 00:XX:XX

ALUM. He, 7 - Time passes too slowly; intolerable ennui; an hour seems half a day.

ANDROC. Sh, 90 - Impatient, expected to be able to do everything immediately. (1)

Sh, 91 - Impatient watching others, wanted to speed them up. (7)

Sh, 101 - Can't avoid shouting at people she was intolerant of, could not hide her feelings. More impatient with others and herself. (7)

Sh, 102 - Assertive, impatient, aggressive. Felt resentful and abused. Had no control over her temper. Bellowed and lashed out at everyone. In the evening, furious for no apparent reason. Wanted to kill her husband and children, banged doors and threw things. By bed-time, she felt fine but the intensity of her evil thoughts was very frightening. (7)

Sh, 116 - Impatient, snappy, shouting, felt trapped and despairing. Growled at her children. (12)

CHAM. He, 49 - Great impatience, everything seems to go too slowly.

CHOC. Sh, 331 - I became selfish, impatient and intolerant. Behaved in a strange way -hard and quarrelsome -snapping at people. Could not stand people wasting time or being inefficient, I wanted things done immediately.[35], 30C, XX:XX:XX:

COLOC. He, 10 - Extremely irritable and impatient; nothing seems right; gets angry on being questioned.

GINS. Al, 3 - Mind generally calm; still there are impatient impulses and fear of accidents, with, at times, disposition to weep, or to be anxious about the future.

HALI-L. Sh, 205 - Aggravated driving to work. Why don't these people get out of my way? Frustrated with the world, angry with the world. I don't want any red lights. Want everything to be smooth. I used to feel this way years ago when I used to drink. 02, 30C, 10:XX:XX

HAM. Al, 14 - I became impatient, and resolved not to take anymore of the medicine; felt as if I did not care whether I attended (guard) to my practice or not; did not want any one to call at the office for medicine.

HURA. Al, 28 - Impatience, anger; she bites her hands, and gets into passion because her ideas come too slowly.

HYDROG. Sh, 171 - Feel more patient and accepting during my period. When water poured through the ceiling from an over-full bath, I just sat there and let it flood the floor because I didn't want to disturb the cat sitting on my knee. 12, 6C, 27:XX:XX

Sh, 266 - While talking, restless, impatient and ill at ease, as if wanting to leave. 22, 12C, 06:XX:XX

HYOS. Ha, 582 - Impatient: he thought he should die when he had to wait for something of quite trivial nature.

IGN. Ha, 770 - Fickle, impatient, irresolute, quarrelsome.

IOD. He, 13 - Excessive kind of impatience, she is running about all the time and never sits down or sleeps at night.

IP. He, 8 - Peevish; irritable; impatient; morose, scornful mood.

KALI-C. Al, 45 - Disagreeable mood; she longs for things with impetuosity; is contented with nothing, is beside herself, and gets into rage if everything does not go according to her wishes, and frequently does not herself know what she really wishes to have.

He, 9-...constantly in antagonism which herself; frequently hopeful, frequently despondent; frets (worry) about everything; peevish impatient, contented with nothing.

LACH. Al, 30 - Impatient; desires positive answers when this is not practicable.

He, 24 - Inclination to be communicative; vivid imagination; extremely impatient at tedious and dry (arid) things.

LYSS. Al,N-45 - Wrote to doctor: I am waiting with impatience that you give me and my young ones something to eat.

MED. Al,N-44 - The impatience, excitement, wild feelings; the unreal, dazed condition; the gloom (sadness) and fear in the dark;... are marked evidence of functional derangement of the nervous system.

NICC. Al, 2 - Quarrelsome and impatient; she could tolerate no contradiction;...

RHUS-T. Al, 40 - Impatient desire to accomplish several kinds of business, chiefly intellectual,...

SEP. Ha, 27 - Great internal restlessness, for many days, with hastiness (hurried); he wants to be done with his work even as he begins it.

Ha, 28 - Restless and lacking serenity, for many days; occupied with sad memories, and anxious, she has not the patience to stay long in place.
SUL-AC. Al, 35 - Fretful, peevish, impatient, if his work is not done to suit.(unsatisfying)
SULPH. He, 55 - Ill-humored; vexed with herself; everything makes her impatient.
TAX. Al, 5 - Impatient disposition, which scarcely allows of the least intellectual contest.(discussion)

IMPRISONED

Delusions; animals, hens, bound with chains: ***hyos.***[8]
- arrested, is: cand-a.[239]
- arrested, is about to be: arn. ars. ***bell.***[122] cupr. kali-br. meli. plb. ruta[36] tab.[85] ***zinc.***
- body, adherent to woolen sack (night while half awake): coc-c.
- body, arms, bound to her body: caj.[85] cimic.
- body, hand, bound with chains: hyos.[54]
- cellar, he is shut in a dark: nat-p.[139]
- enclosed, she is: germ.[222]
- enslaved, is: lap-c-b.[194]
- hell, chains, in erotomania: ***orig.***[54]
- net, he is in a: nat-m.[139]
- people, sees, connected with the law who will seize him, causing great anxiety, cries like a child: ***cupr-acet.***[54]
- room, close and hot, is, oppressing: plan.
- soldier, sees, capture him, that will: bell.[10]
- trapped, he is: lap-c-b.[194]
- walls, surrounded by high: cann-i.
- wires, is caught in: **CACT.** ***cimic.*** 0ust.[102]

Dreams; arrested, imprisonment: bov.[10] cerv.[36]
- ➤ arrested, of being: clem. mag-c.
- ➤ bound, with chain across mouth, being: bapt.[36]
- ➤ famine, being left in a dungeon to die of; escaping by crawling out: ped.[36]
- ➤ fights, galley slave, with: elaps[36]
- ➤ fights, generals, with six or seven black, who garroted him and bound him with ropes, causing agony of mind: coca[36]
- ➤ finger, of being seized by a: sil.[1]
- ➤ kidnappers: bamb-a.[1184]
- ➤ kidnapping, friend is kidnapped by a shepherd dog: ozone[227]
- ➤ prisoner, being taken a: allox.[119] nat-m.
- ➤ prisoner, release of prisoners: hura.[36]
- ➤ robbers, laying snares for him: jac-c.[36]

Escape; attempts to, surrounded and captured from men, as if: ***hyos.***[54]

Fear; arrested, of being: ars.[137] bell.[172] meli.[85] plb.[137] ruta[162] tab.[137] zinc.[72]
- ✦ death, wires encasing him, saw: ***cimic.***[54]

Rage; chained, had to be: ars.[10] sec.[10]

HALI-L. Sh, 604 - Since the remedy, I took over and the physical manifestation of personas splitting off would only come out when I was alone. Did these drawings. The figure in the box was my death — captured, buried and can't get out. The first drawing is a depressed boy, the second is the buried man, the third is an x-ray figure. After that the depression abated. I did another drawing of a negative being laughing at me. It has no arms, no movement. 18, 30C, 35:XX:XX
AGAR. Al, 8-...called for his hatchet; had to be confined alternated with religious excitement.
ANDROC. Sh, 40 - She dreamt that she had murdered her grandfather by poking a knitting needle through his eyes while he slept. Though she felt no remorse, she wanted to be punished but no-one would accept her guilt. Was told by her friends that she had responsibilities and could not go to jail and the police refused to prosecute. Was frightened by the dream. (7)
BELL. He, 106 - Anxiety and fear of imaginary objects and hallucinations, ghosts, soldiers which come to take them away (arrest), black animals, rats dogs, wolves, etc.
He, 105 - Anxiety and fear of imaginary objects and hallucinations, ghosts, soldiers which come to take them away, black animals, rats, dogs, wolves, etc.
CANN-I. Al, 25-...He seemed to be walking in a vast arena, encircled by tremendous walls... (confined, limited)
CHOC. Sh, 50 - Panic feeling of being trapped and enclosed —worse when curtains are closed and the light blocked out. Strong desire to be outside and moving, to be in the bright and warm sunlight. Kept having to move my feet, which I felt I wanted to move.

Sh, 103 - On looking at a bird in a cage, felt it should be out.

Sh, 193 - Husband wants to go out for a walk. I don't want to go. I feel paranoid that someone will see me and think 'on drugs' and arrest me or cart me off to an institution. 15, 30C, 00:02:00

CIMIC. He, 10 - Fear of death; fears those in house will kill him (murdered, by parents); saw wires encasing (lock, imprisoned) him; visions of rats and of strange objects.

CROT-T. He, 5 - Feeling as though one cannot think outside of himself, "feels all pent up" (restricted, limited, confined, circumscribed) inside, and no chance for thoughts to flow out; as if hide-bound.(obstinate)

CUPR-A. He, 4 - Fixed idea that he sees persons connected with the law who are about to seize him (imprisoned),...at times sees thieves in the room, spirits, and various other immaterial objects;...

GERM. Sh, 128 - Afraid of the police of being caught and unveiled. 18, 30C, 02:10:00

Sh, 127 - Feel like a prisoner. 18, 30C, 15:XX:XX

Sh, 101 - I'm desperate. I want to die. Feel the power to kill. Feel like a wild animal locked in. It's strong, so intense. I hate so strong-feel a terrible disgust and I'm afraid of what I'm able to do. It's completely impossible to be in it and impossible to get out of it. 18, 30C, 190:XX:XX

HALI-L. Sh, 386 - I feel removed and everything is in slow motion and I couldn't really contact reality. I felt like I was compensating for the lack of motion. (On this page of her journal she has doodled a picture of a slanted cube with vertical bars on it. It looks like an animal cage leaning to the right.) 01, 30C, 15:XX:XX

Sh, 428 - Realizing we haven't had any fun as a family in forever. Haven't had any fun myself either. Like a caged animal, snarling. I'm in a pressure cooker. Can't even imagine what would get me out of this mood, what actually would be fun. Don't want to do anything, or talk to anyone. Like a porcupine or sea urchin. "Don't tread on me." 09, 6C, 30:XX:XX

Sh, 529 - There was definitely someone else inside of me. The essence of that person was trying to get out, escaping, trying to get away. It felt like I was in prison or the thing in me was in prison. I was saying, "go," and it wouldn't get out of there. My supervisor got worried about me. On purpose, I made sure I was unavailable. If anyone asked me details, I would get angry. I won't explain it to you. I'm feeling that now a little, talking about it. 02, 30C, XX:XX:XX

Sh, 534 - The thing about the proving, I see now, was the intense trapped feeling. I felt trapped by people and situations. People who are being weird. Before, I would just let things slide, or roll off of me, like water off a duck's back. During the proving, I needed to break out, a screeching feeling. I had to speak out to change the situation. I had to stop letting things slide. 13, 30C, 7 months

HURA. Al, 700 - Dream about children and the release (liberty) of prisoners.

HYOS. He, 81-...attempts to escape from room; frightful hallucinations of figures coming to seize him, hens (chicken) bound (imprisoned) with chains,...

He, 57 - Delirium tremens:...averse to light and company; visions as if persecuted preceded by an epileptic attack;... seeks to escape from men by whom he imagines himself surrounded and who are trying to capture him; does not recognize his wife who is standing by his side, but imagines he sees her under a distant bed.

IRID. Sh, 65 - Motivation difficult, Sensation as if trapped in magnetic fields. Curled up stroking body, especially legs, feet together, Feeling as if they were magnetic. Desire for a young man. Thought that the feminine form is rounded and curved due to magnetism; arcs due to magnetic forces. Q2

Sh, 78 - Today I noticed how narrow my life feels, and what I feel like doing is making my life even narrower. E2

Sh, 79 - Had this longing to find real wilderness. Britain is too full, nothing is really alive anymore except people. The world really feels too oppressed with people and roofs. I kept saying to partner, "Why do we live in this dreary, ugly place, where people know nothing about freedom, and certainly nothing about discovery or mystery, just tarmac and roofs." It struck me that the world was too small for me, and thought "That's got to be something about the remedy, something around pressure." E5

Sh, 80 - I felt all closed in like I couldn't move, I couldn't breathe. I felt oppressed by being in this room, there's no space. It's funny but I felt like that tonight when I was sitting outside. There were lots of clouds in the sky and it felt like they were coming down on me. Like the sky had been really close and the clouds in the sky were nearer to me; I noticed it because I was watching the moon waxing. It was like I hadn't really noticed the clouds at night before. J5

Sh, 81 - Feel hemmed in by ex-partner's needs, feel I'm being fitted into the little spaces in his life. Can no longer shrug and say, "Well this is how it is." G5

Sh, 106 - Mental image: I am inside an egg —a bird, wet feathers, at the point it is smashing through its shell, bursting out; a chick, wet crumpled and hot, shell flying all over. The relief —getting to the air, refreshing, cool. Inside it was humid, stifling. Stretching vast wings, enjoying feeling the air dry them out. G5

LYC. Al, 51 - In the evening, in the dark, he is seized with fear when a door that he wishes to open moves with difficulty.

Ha, 26 - In the evening in the dark, he is frightened because a door he wants to open, opens with difficulty. (confined, restricted)

MAG-C. Al, 941 - Anxious dream of a fire, being arrested etc.

NAT-M. Al, 62 - Woke at 2A.M. in perspiration, and with a distressing anxiety, as though he were shut up (lock) in a dark cellar; this sensation only disappeared on perceiving light through the window.(confined, restricted, incarcerated)

NIT-AC. Al, 30 - Anxious oppression, like nightmare, as if some one were lying under him and holding him fast with the arms about his abdomen, so that he could not free himself, immediately after falling asleep. (constriction, immobilization)

PLB. Al, 60-...; he hears everywhere threatening voices, officers come to arrest him, to seize his furniture (movables), (confiscated, expropriated) and to expel (eject) him from his lodgings (home) (expulsion, exiled) ; the voices come from the pillow, the mattress (bed); they enter by the window, where he sees people, and they consult about him with closed doors (secretive) ; ...

Al, 38 - Begged and prayed to be released from the strait-waistcoat, "for", he said, "I am not mad; but the idea of being forcibly restrained is enough to drive me crazy".

RUTA. Al, 3 - Very anxious all day, as though he had done something wrong; if any one opened the door he feared that some one had come to arrest (imprisonment, jailing) him.

Ha, 280 - All day long very anxious as if he had done something bad; when the door was opened, he feared that someone was coming to take him to prison. (incarcerated, punished)

SEP. Al, 100-...seems as if my mind were hedged (enclose) in, as if it were circumscribed,...(encircle, confined)

THUJ. Al, 1 - She herself desires, with anxiety and despair, to be taken to an insane asylum, (imprisonment, confining) and there to be treated very harshly and strictly, (penalized), so that her fixed ideas may be subdued and banished (purified); she knows very well that she does wrong (conscience) and thinks all sorts of bad thoughts (immoral), but she will not take the trouble to banish such thoughts; therewith she indistinctly gives to understand that she is constantly obliged to think of taking her own life, but feels the sinfulness (wicked) of it, in order to avoid it, desires the strict restraint of the asylum;...

ZINC. He, 43 - Great fear, as if persecuted by men or the devil, on account of crimes he has never done (injustice); is afraid of becoming imprisoned, or poisoned, or shot, or buried (inter) alive...[0] Delirium tremens.

INDIFFERENCE

Activity; alternating with, indifference: sarr.[36]
Affection; none, has, during pregnancy: acon.[54]
Amusement; nothing gives him: sep.[109]
Anger; alternating with, indifference: carbn-s.[36] chin.[10]
Answer; questioned, when, says nothing, indifferent, does not answer: alum.[36] apom.[36] chlol.[36] cocc.[36] ***colch.***[162] hyos.[36] juni-c.[36] mosch.[36] op.[36] ozone[227] tarent.[58] thuj.[8] zinc.[171]
Anxiety; alternating with, indifference: nat-m.
Ascetic: diosm.[72]
Autism, mutinism: agra.[137] kali-br.[187] lyc.[137] tub.[187]
Cheerfulness; alternating with, indifference: tarent.[36]
Delusions; detached: hydrog.[222] lap-gr-m.[194]
• neglected, duty, his, perfunctory manner, performed in: ptel.[36]
Dreams; death, friend, of a, dear, which does not abate his mental exhilaration, looking at all with supernatural indifference: coff-t.[36]
Dullness; world, the outer, has no existence for her: ***nux-m.***[54]
Estranged; climacteric period, in: ***aster.***[122] cycl.[122] hipp.[122] ***lach.***[122] ***lil-t.***[122] ***puls.***[122] ***sep.***[122] ***sulph.***[122] ther.[122] ***verat.***[122]
Estranged; convulsions, during: cimic.[54]
Euphoria; alternating with, indifference: ozone[227]
Far away; as if, with apathy and indifference to the future: med.[137] syph.[54]
Fear; insensible, of becoming: lyc.[5] nux-v.[5] sulph.[5]
Feeling, loss of: anh.[119]
Hypochondriasis; inert, takes no interest in his surroundings: euphr.[54]
Indifference, apathy: absin. acet-ac.[36] ***acon. agar. agn.*** ail. allox.[119] aloe[5] **ALUM.**[122] alum-p.[58] alum-sil.[58] alumn.[36] am-c.[10] am-m. ambr. amor-r.[149] **ANAC.**[122] ***anac-oc.***[54] anan.[36] androc.[222] ***anh.***[119] ant-t. **APIS** aq-mar.[149] arag.[162] ***arg-n. arn. ars.*** ars-h.[54] ars-i. ars-s-f.[58] arum-t.[54] asaf. asar. aster. atro.[36] ***bac.***[62] ***bamb-a.***[1184] bapt. ***bar-c.*** bar-i.[58] bar-m. bar-s.[58] ***bell.*** berb. bism. bor.[1] ***bov.*** brom. bry.[102] bufo but-ac.[119] buth-aust.[119] cadm.[119] calad.[54] ***calc.*** calc-ar.[58] calc-f.[149] calc-i.[58] ***calc-p.*** calc-s. camph. cand-a.[239] cann-i. cann-s. caps. ***carb-an.*** **CARB-V.** carbn-o.[36] ***carbn-s.*** carc.[122] caust. ***cham. chel.*** **CHIN.** ***chin-ar. chin-s.*** chlf.[54] chloram.[149] chlorpr.[149] choc.[222] cic. ***cimic.*** cina clem. coca[36] ***cocc.*** cod.[36] coloc.[10] colos.[39] **CON.**[122] conin-br.[85] corn. croc. **CROT-C.** ***crot-h.*** cupr. cupr-s.[36] ***cycl.*** cypr. cyt-l.[102] dig. dros.[1] ***dulc.***[54] elaps esp-g.[1158] euphr. fago.[25] ferr. ferr-ar. ferr-i. ferr-p. fl-ac. ***gels.*** germ.[222] glon. glyc.[102] ***graph.*** guai. guare.[54] gymn. ham.[5] harp.[149] **HELL.** helo. hep. hura hydr-ac.[10] hydrc.[36] hydrog.[222] ***hyos. ign.*** ind.[149] indol.[102] iod. ip. jatr. jug-r.[122] ***kali-ar.*** kali-bi. kali-br. ***kali-c.*** kali-chl.[5] kali-n.[10] ***kali-p.*** kali-s. kali-sil.[58] kres.[149] lac-c. lac-d.[58] ***lach.*** lap-c-b.[194] laur. lepi. levo.[149] lil-s.[36] **LIL-T.** linu-c.[36] luf-op.[144] luna[228] ***lyc.*** lyss.[36] mag-c.[36] mag-m. manc. mand.[58] ***meli.*** meny. meph.[94] ***merc.*** merc-i-f.[36] merc-i-r.[54] **MEZ.** moly.[149] morph.[36] mur-ac. myric.[25] naja narz.[36] nat-ar.[54] **NAT-C. NAT-M. NAT-P.** nat-s.[58] nep.[149] nid.[149] ***nit-ac.*** nit-s-d.[116] ***nux-m.*** nux-v. olnd. onop.[149] **ONOS. OP.** ozone[227] ped.[85] petr. **PH-AC. PHOS.** ***phyt. pic-ac.*** pitu-a.[164] **PLAT.** plb. prun. psil.[149] ***psor.*** ptel.[5] **PULS.** ran-b.[10] raph. rauw.[119] rheum rhod. rhus-g.[36] rhus-t. rhus-v.[25] ric.[36] rumx. ruta sabad. sabin. sac-alb.[36] ***sang.***[5] sapo.[102] saroth.[119] sarr.[85] sars. ***sec.*** sel. seneg. **SEP.** seq-s.[230] sieg.[144] ***sil.*** spong. squil. stann. **STAPH.** stram. sul-ac.[54] sul-i.[58] sulfa.[149] ***sulph. syph.***[122] **TAB.**[5] tarax.[149] tarent. tax.[36] tell.[5] thal.[149] ther. thiop.[149] ***thuj. thuj-l.***[149] **THYR.**[162] trinit.[102] tub.[5] ven-m.[149] ***verat.*** verb. ***viol-t.*** vip.[5] visc.[119] xan. zinc. zinc-p.[58] ziz.
Indifference; act for herself, no longer wishes to, in nervous weakness: ***cur.***[54]
Indifference; agreeable things, to: ambr. anac. apis[58] cina corn. merc.[30] op. rhod. staph. stram.
Indifference; alternating with, anger: carbn-s.[36] foll.[1201] nid.[149]
Indifference; alternating with, anxiety and restlessness: ant-t.[54] nat-m.
Indifference; alternating with, timidity: stram.[10]
Indifference; alternating with, vexation: cham. chin.

Indifference; anosognosia, thinking that he is not ill: thala.[149]
Indifference; appearance, about personal: coca[98] **SULPH.**
Indifference; business affairs, to: aesc.[162] agar. ***arg-n.*** ***arn.***[10] bamb-a.[1184] ***fl-ac.*** ham.[122] ***kali-bi.*** kali-p.[58] myris. nat-ar. ***ph-ac.*** phys. phyt.[58] psil.[164] ***ptel.*** ***puls.*** rhus-t.[162] ***sep.*** ***stram.*** ***sulph.***
Indifference; children, to her: aur-ar.[58] choc.[222] kali-i. ***lyc.*** nat-c. **PHOS.**[122] **SEP.**[122]
Indifference; coition, after: ***calc.***[137]
Indifference; coition, after, menses, before: sep.[26]
Indifference; coition, during: lyss.[36]
Indifference; company, in, agg.: androc.[222] **ARG-N.** bov. kali-c. kali-m.[192] lyc.[54] mez.[85] nat-c. nat-m. **PLAT.** rhus-t.
Indifference; condition does not seem dangerous to him, in typhus: colch.[54]
Indifference; conscience, to the dictates of: cann-i. caust.[30] con.[30] graph.[30] petr.[30]
Indifference; dead, everything seems to him, nothing makes a vivid impression upon his mind: hydrog.[222] **MEZ.**[54]
Indifference; desires, has no, no action of the will: hell. ***verat.***[54]
Indifference; done for her, about anything being: **LIL-T.**[54]
Indifference; duties, domestic, to: androc.[222] aur-ar.[58] brom.[58] ***cimic.***[54] cit-l.[54] sep.[81] sul-i.[58]
Indifference; duties, to: ars.[30] **CALC.**[54] carb-v.[122] cench.[58] lach.[30] merc.[30] nat-m.[30] ***ptel.***[54] sil.[30] sul-i.[58] sulph.[30]
Indifference; eating, after: aloe lach.[137] lyc.[137] ***ph-ac.***[137] sel.[137]
Indifference; eating, to: bac.[62] chin.[1] lac-h.[229] merc.[30] nat-c.[30] nat-m.[30] ***rhus-t.***[5] ***staph.***[30] valer.[5]
Indifference; emaciation and weakness, especially with: **PH-AC.**[54]
Indifference; ennui, with: alum.[10] choc.[222] con.[10] ***kali-n.***[10] lach.[10] lyc.[10] ***nat-c.***[10] ***nux-v.***[10] petr.[10] ***plb.***[10] zinc.[10]
Indifference; everything, of: acet-ac. ***acon.*** agar. agn.[102] ail. ambr.[58] anac. androc.[222] ***apis***[98] arg-n.[102] arn. ***ars.***[54] asaf.[10] bac.[62] bamb-a.[1184] bapt.[122] bell. bism.[10] bov. bry.[102] buth-aust.[144] cadm.[119] calc.[8] cann-s. canth. caps. **CARB-V.** carc.[149] cham.[10] chin.[10] choc.[222] cic.[10] cimic.[102] ***cina*** con.[58] croc. crot-h.[36] cub.[36] cur.[36] cypr. dig. ferr.[36] fl-ac.[102] ***gels.***[102] glyc.[102] ***hell.*** hydr. hydr-ac.[102] hyos.[10] ign. indol.[102] iod.[137] kali-ar. kali-c.[36] kali-chl.[10] kali-m.[192] lac-h.[229] lach.[102] lap-gr-m.[194] lepi. lil-t.[102] ***lyc.***[10] meny.[85] ***merc.*** merl. mez. nat-c.[10] ***nat-m.***[10] nat-p.[58] nit-ac.[58] ***nit-s-d.***[54] nux-m. ***nux-v.***[54] ***op.***[10] ozone[227] **PH-AC.** ***phos.*** ***pic-ac.***[102] ***pitu-p.***[162] ***plat.***[54] psil.[149] ***puls.***[10] ***rheum***[10] rib-ac.[149] sec. ***sep.*** sima.[102] stann.[10] **STAPH.**[122] sulph. syph.[58] **THYR.**[162] verat.[10] ziz.
Indifference; external things, to: agn. am-c.[30] am-m.[30] bac.[62] berb.[10] bov.[10] buth-aust.[119] cann-i. cham. choc.[222] cic. con.[36] euphr.[10] ***hell.***[122] lyc. merl. op. ozone[227] plat.[10] rumx. stann. staph. **SULPH.** tarent. thuj.[10] verat. vip.[10]
Indifference; fine feeling, to: op.[10]
Indifference; friends, to: ars-i.[58]
Indifference; future, to, far away feeling: syph.[54]
Indifference; happiness, to: ars-i.[58]
Indifference; health, as to his: cocc.[60]
Indifference; himself, to: phos.[111] sep.[111] thuj-l.[149]
Indifference; husband, towards: luna[228]
Indifference; illness, to his: gels.[72]
Indifference; important, news, to: ars-h.[54]
Indifference; important, things, to: calc. fl-ac.
Indifference; life, to: absin.[36] ***ars.***[36] bov.[36] cham.[116] fago.[25] lap-gr-m.[194] lyc.[54] ***merc.***[30] phos.[116] ***phyt.***[36] rhus-v.[25] ***sep.***[54] sulph.[116] ***tab.***[116] ***xan.***[54]
Indifference; loved ones, to: ***acon.*** allox.[119] ars. ars-i.[58] bell.[193] carb-v.[58] carc.[193] ***fl-ac.*** **HELL.** kali-p.[58] kali-sil.[58] lil-t.[168] merc. myric.[25] nat-p. nat-sil.[58] **PHOS.** plat. **SEP.** ***syph.***[122]
Indifference; loved ones; to, strangers, but animated to: ***fl-ac.***[54]
Indifference; masturbation, after: **STAPH.**
Indifference; money-making, to: chin.[30] kali-c.[30] merc.[30] nat-c.[30] sep.[30]
Indifference; music, to, loves, which she: ***carb-v.*** caust.[10]
Indifference; neighbors, towards: phos.[10] ***sep.***[10]
Indifference; opinion of others, to: androc.[222]
Indifference; opposite sex, to: ***puls.***[162] **SEP.**[162] thuj.
Indifference; others, about lot of: lap-mar-c.[194] plat.[185] sabad.[185] sulph.

Indifference; parents, to: phos.[10] sep.[146]
Indifference; persons, to all: kali-m.[192] mez.[36]
Indifference; pleasure: alum. anac. androc.[222] ***apis***[170] ***arg-n.*** ***ars.*** ars-i.[58] calc-ar.[58] cench.[58] ***cham.*** chin-ar.[58] ***chin-s.*** cocc. croc. ferr-p. germ.[222] graph. **HELL.** hep. hura ip. kali-ar. kali-c. kali-chl.[58] kali-sil.[58] mag-c.[144] mag-m. meph.[149] mez. mur-ac. nat-ar. nat-c. **NAT-M.** ***nit-ac.*** **OP.** petr. prun. ***puls.*** sars. ***sep.*** spig. stann. staph. stram. **SULPH.** ***syph.***[122] tab. ther.
Indifference; recovery, about his: ars.[1] aur-m-n.[162] ***calc.***
Indifference; religion, to his: anac. coloc. med.[179] sil.[137]
Indifference; reprimands, to all: ***merc.***[30]
Indifference; sadness, in: ***kali-ar.***[54] ***kali-br.***[54] ***plat.***[54]
Indifference; sexual desire diminished, with: ***kali-chl.***[54]
Indifference; stoical to what happens: ail.[54] myric.[25] op.[137]
Indifference; suffering, to: androc.[222] bac.[62] ***hell.*** **OP. STRAM.**
Indifference; suffering, to, others, of: anac.[10] lac-h.[229]
Indifference; superiority, with feeling of: ozone[227]
Indifference; surroundings, to: abel.[149] allox.[149] androc.[222] ars-i.[58] bac.[62] bufo[141] calc-s.[58] kali-p.[58] levo.[149] merc.[1] mez.[85] nat-sil.[58] phos.[58] phyt.[54] raja-s.[149] rumx.[54] sel.[54] sul-i.[58] thuj-l.[149]
Indifference; taciturn: bac.[62] bamb-a.[1184] calc.[10] ***hell.***[54] ***nit-s-d.***[54] plat.[10] staph.[10]
Indifference; typhoid, in: ail.[58] ***apis***[54] ***arn.*** chin. ***chin-s.***[54] ***colch.***[54] ***nit-s-d.***[54] ***ph-ac.*** ***verat.***[54]
Indifference; vexation with distress in stomach, after least: ***kali-bi.***[54]
Indifference; weather, in stormy: sang.[137] tub.[137]
Indifference; welfare of others, to: androc.[222] ars.[30] cand-a.[239] caust.[30] lach.[30] lap-mar-c.[194] nat-m.[30] ***nux-v.***[30] ozone[227] plat.[30] sep.[30] **SULPH.**
Indifference; well, to getting: ***calc.***[54]
Indifference; window, looks hours at: androc.[222] mez.[30]
Indifference; women, to: nat-m.[36]
Indifference; work aversion to: agar.[10] allox.[119] androc.[222] camph.[54] ign.[10] kali-m.[192] lach.[10] rhod.[54] squil.[10] staph.[10]
Jesting; alternating with, indifference: meny.[10]
Restlessness; alternating with, indifference: nat-m.[10]
Sadness; alternating with, indifference: bamb-a.[1184] sep.[137]
Sadness; indifference, with: ***plat.***[54]
Sensitive; want of sensitiveness: ant-c.[122] bell. ***bism.***[5] cann-i.[36] chin. con. cupr. cupr-acet.[36] cycl. daph. euphr. ***hydr-ac.***[30] ***hyos.***[5] ***lyc.***[30] ***op.***[5] ozone[227] ***ph-ac.*** phos. ran-b. rheum rhod. sabad.[5] sabin. ***sel.***[5] staph. stram.
Temperament; phlegmatic: agar.[163] aloe[54] alum.[163] ***am-c.***[163] ***am-m.***[54] ***ant-c.***[163] ant-t.[54] ***aran.***[163] asaf.[85] ***bad.***[163] bar-c.[163] ***bell.***[54] bov.[163] brom.[163] calad.[54] **CALC.**[54] ***caps.***[54] carb-an.[163] ***carb-v.***[163] ***chin.***[54] ***clem.***[54] cocc.[54] cupr.[163] cycl.[54] ***dulc.***[54] ferr.[163] ferr-p.[54] ***graph.***[163] hep.[54] ***hydr.***[163] kali-bi.[5] kali-c.[163] kali-chl.[163] kali-i.[163] ***kali-n.***[163] kreos.[54] ***lach.***[54] lyc.[163] mag-m.[163] mag-s.[163] mang.[163] ***med.***[163] ***merc.***[54] mez.[85] ***nat-c.***[54] ***nat-m.***[54] ***nat-n.***[163] ***nat-s.***[163] nit-ac.[163] petr.[163] ph-ac.[163] ***psor.***[163] **PULS.**[54] ***pyrog.***[163] rhus-t.[163] ***sabad.***[10] sabin.[163] sarr.[85] seneg.[54] ***sep.***[54] ***sil.***[163] spong.[163] stront-c.[163] sulph.[163] ***thuj.***[163] tub.[163] ***vario.***[163] verat.[163]
Unattractive, things seem: chin.
Unfeeling; family, with his: kali-i.[58]
Ungrateful: ars.[30] calc.[30] caust.[30] chin.[185] lach.[30] lyc.[30] nat-m.[30] nux-v.[30] **PLAT.**[30] puls.[109] staph.[30] ***sulph.***[122] tarent.[102]
Untidy; except in what he is performing: carc.[138]
Weeping; emotions, lack of emotions, about her: ozone[227]

ADAM. Sh, 6 - Felt really strong love for children. Looking at daughter had a feeling of a barrier being lifted or a cloud lifted from me. Felt I could really see her, that she was mine; of me but separate. 8, 6C, 02:XX:XX

AGN. Al, 1-,...he feels as if nothing existed around him; he is dissatisfied with himself all the time; he is incapable of attending to any business; the things around him are entirely indifferent to him;...

AIL. Al, 5 - Stoical indifference to whatever happens.

ANDROC. Sh, 29 - Could not care what others thought of her. (17)

Sh, 30 - Distant and staring. (20)
Sh, 34 - Much more untidy, the house was a mess and it didn't bother her. Made ineffectual efforts to tidy up and then lost interest. Desire to sit undisturbed and just look. (25)
Sh, 35 - Felt 'stoned', tried to express himself to a friend but could not. Behaved in a dreamy absent minded way. His friends thought that he had taken drugs. (29)
Sh, 38 - Things she would normally feel guilt about don't bother her, (cured symptom?). (7)

ANT-T. He, 6 - Apathy and indifference to everything, even death would have been welcome.

APIS. He, 66 - When asked if sick, he says: "Nothing is the matter".

ARG-N. He, 40 - Melancholy since an undeserved slight (scorn); fixed idea that he was neglected and despised by his family; his callings (job, work) became indifferent to him.

ARS. Ha, 1056 - Life appears to him naught (emptiness); he attaches no value (worth) to it. (insignificant, worthlessness)
Ha, 1057 - Uncommonly tranquil disposition; quite unconcerned about their approaching death, they neither hoped nor wished to recover.

BELL. Ha, 1390 - Excessive indifference, for hours; one might take her life, she would not stir. (move) (immobility)
He, 7 - Likes to brood in silence, supreme indifference, nothing makes an impression.

BRASS. Sh, 1 - General feeling of aloofness 08, 6C, 04:12:30
Sh, 3 - Am feeling light-headed (frivolous); do not feel in such contact with the ground; I have stumbled a few times 08, 6C, 01:23:30
Sh, 14 - Very irritable with no cause, snapping at the children for no reason; apathy, can't be bothered to do anything; restless, twitchy, can't settle to anything 3I, 00:04:00

CALC-A. Ha, 261 - Not without inclination to work, but indifferent to all external things; sunk in thought about the present and future.
Ha, 265-...very indifferent to the most important things; he did everything unwillingly (reluctant, averse) as if forced to do them.

CALC. Ha, 12 - Anxious about the present and the future, with deep reflection, at the same time indifferent to things outside...
Ha, 41 - Peevish, morose, very cross and most indifferent to the most important things; he also did everything repugnantly and as if by compulsion.
He, 34 - Does not care to get well, or to do anything to assist (aid) recovery.

CAMPH. He, 69 - An indifference whether the world (mankind) uses one well (suitable) or ill (depravity, wrong), everything is repulsive.(offensive)

CHOC. Sh, 319 - Felt emotionally numb and separated from things.[35], 30C, XX:XX:XX:
Sh, 322 - Have lost interest in my husband, feel totally indifferent. I have hardly spoken to him all weekend, with a desire to avoid him. Don't want to discuss or share anything with him.[15], 30C, 06:XX:XX

CIC. Al, 29 - He was indifferent to everything, and began to doubt whether he was really in the condition which he found himself.
Ha, 226 - He became indifferent to everything, and began to doubt whether this was really the condition in which he was.

CIMIC. He, 26 - Indifferent, taciturn, takes no interest in household matters.

CON. Al, 43-...a great guilt weighed upon him, with paralyzed feeling in all the limbs, indifference,..
He, 14 - Likes to wear his best clothes, (vanity) makes useless purchases, (squander) cares very little for things (indifferent), wastes or ruins them; does not want to work, prefers to play. (wanderer)
He, 35-...a great grief weighed upon him, with paralyzed feeling in all the limbs, indifference and taking no interest in anything.

CROT-H. He, 22 - Suspicion and snappishness (irritable), or quiet indifference.
He, 13 - Marked indifference, seems only half alive; utter apathy.

CUR. Al, 11 - Great despondency (grief) ; becomes reckless (careless) about himself.

CYCL. Al, 17 - Very fretful (irritable) the

whole day; disinclined to speak and insensible (indifferent), having very little feeling (emotion) in his body.

Ha, 201 - All day long he is peevish not disposed to talk, and insensible, so that he feels little (inadequate, incompetent) in his body.

CYPR. He, 2 - Profound indifference to everything, even to his studies, duties and common courtesies (kindness, compassion) of life.

EUPHR. Ha, 127 - Lazy, hypochondriacal; external objects had no charm (beauty), no life (animation) for him. (indifference)

FL-AC. He, 6 - Feeling of indifference towards those he loves best; has no objection to their presence but does not care to converse with them, yet if strangers or mere acquaintances come in will enter into animated conversation....

GERM. Sh, 100 - Cannot feel pleasure or sorrow. Everything is Chaos. Cannot restore my energy. Totally meaningless. Feels like an empty battery. Cannot take care of the kids as I should. 18, 30C, 183:XX:XX

Sh, 151-.... I feel I have no real contact with people, I have no emotion at all except for a feeling of isolation and a concern that people may not like me. I wish someone would cuddle me. By 10 o'clock I have a definite aversion to people, especially certain people- the stubborn or authoritarian kind. I become deeply involved in my own thoughts and can be very irritable and even angry when the thoughts are interrupted by people, but I don't show any signs of anger or irritation. The fate of other people leaves me cold, but I know this is not right. My mind is blank and I feel I could just sit and stare. I have no feelings, no emotions! I think a lot about my state of mind and try to understand it; it puzzles me. What is missing? Eating removes this thoughtful mood. By afternoon and evening I become gradually more involved with what I am doing but still feel isolated even when in the company of other people. I don't mind listening to people, but I contribute little to conversation. This state lasted for three days. 16, 30C, 04:XX:XX

Sh, 172 - Sad, indifferent and hopeless feeling. Want to cry but it won't come. 18, 30C, 00:14:00

HALI-L. Sh, 141 - The drama was clear; the good guy and bad guys. During the proving, I realized it all leads to the same thing. Withdraw. Actingwatching. A Chosen separation. Zen state of watching and witnessing, but I could see how it could become sociopathic. My kids were fighting and I grabbed them and spanked them. Normally, I would be wracked with guilt. It was lovely to be a parent without guilt for awhile. 09, 9C, XX:XX:XX

Sh, 142 - Good guys and bad guys. Drama of evil is set up by the bad guys. They always win, always a struggle to just keep going. That is where I came from. During the proving, I saw that even engaging in that struggle gives it power and meaning. If you stop and watch the game, eventually there won't be anyone playing anymore. Good and bad were still positions, but it was all the same game. 09, 9C, XX:XX:XX

Sh, 150 - Is this true calm or the calm of the dead? I'm not feeling so much, which is a relief because I was feeling so negative before. 09, 6C, 04:XX:XX

Sh, 153 - In retrospect, over the last few days, it seems as if the past and the future have collapsed into the present. The past was unimportant, and I don't concern myself over the future. 09, 6C, 08:XX:XX

Sh, 391 - Staff meeting was awful. Everyone feeling frustrated due to extra work, but I did not feel any blame. Normally I would have felt responsible, but this time I felt it was not my fault. 02, 30C, 01:10:XX -01:12:XX

Sh, 644 - The "fry an egg and eat it," repetitive, meaningless motion, reminds me of an extermination camp, of a killing machine; was about not caring; it's from the split or chasm. Not caring about anything, is part of what happens with the split. That's what evil is, that's really what it's about. 06, 6C, 01:00:XX

Sh, 645 - Caring equals oneness. A scary point about that acute phase yesterday—there was no caring. It didn't matter. Nothing mattered. I was alone and wanted to be that way. To have caring, there must be an attunement with the oneness of the universe. Is that where Hitler came from? The crack in the universe? 06, 6C, 01:09:00

HELL. Al, 7 - Sad mood, on account of his present condition (restriction, limitation), everything seems shallow (stupid, superficial) and has no incentive for him. (lost:motive, purpose, force, mission,) -(lost: depth, profundity, perception.)

Al,S-1 Happy carelessness about everything; feel indifferent to family.

Ha, 286 - Sad disposition respecting his present position, everything seems to him so insipid (tedious, boring,) and nothing interests him.

HYDROG. Sh, 174 - Emotionally cold and non-communicable with anger felt in stomach. 12, 6C, 17:XX:XX

Sh, 177 - Upset husband by telling him what I thought of the way he'd been behaving. I felt curiously uninvolved. Indifference to husband. Felt a little 'dead', uninvolved, wasn't really responding in any way — not in a good way or a bad way. Didn't feel cross, affectionate or anything. Very peculiar, like I was watching and its nothing to do with me. Like looking at somebody else, almost as if I wasn't there. Felt emotionally numb and unable to respond —as if I wasn't there. Like a living dead being alive and not being able to make the appropriate responses. Real total detachment. 08, 30C, 10:XX:XX

Sh, 180 - Indifference, despair and hopelessness—no way out. 32, 9C, 03:XX:XX

Sh, 184 - Feel despondent, indifferent, apathetic, separated from things and don't care. Deep sighing with sense of resignation. Can't be bothered to do things. 16, 30C, 02:XX:XX

IGN. He, 44-...;indifference to things she loved best ; sits alone and weeps, imagines things, a especially that she might go crazy; ..

IOD. Al, 31 - Mind feels tired, and does not care to work.

KALI-AR. He, 1 - Scolding (censorious) morose, retired, quarrelsome and discontented, jealous, indifferent to everything,...

KALI-BR. Al, 19 - Painful sadness, profound indifference, and almost disgust for life.

He, 31-...religious delusions and feeling of moral deficiency; ...profound indifference and almost disgust for life.

LAC-D. Al,N-1 - Depression of spirits; don't care to live (indifferent) ; question as to quietest and most certain way of hastening (accelerate) one's death.

He, 2 - Depression of spirits; don't care to live, question as to quietest and most certain way of hastening one's death.

LIL-T. He, 13-...indifference about everything being done for her.(help)

LYSS. Al, 39 - A strange oppression and indifference, as if he was unable to do anything if he forces himself; there is no power of mind.

Al,N-72 - An attack of mental depression and indifference quite (very) strange to him; feels as if he could do nothing; if he forces himself he lacks mental power.

He, 72 - An attack of mental depression and indifference quite strange to him; feels as if he could do nothing; if he forces himself he lacks mental power.

MERC. Al, 10 - Great seriousness, with much indifference all day; he was much offended if others laughed over a trifle, and yet was extremely indifferent to everything that took place about him.

Ha, 1241 - He wished to die, was indifferent to everything, even to what he took most delight in.

Ha, 1242 - All day long great seriousness with much indifference; he got angry when others laughed at a trifle, and at the same time was extremely indifferent to all about him.

Ha, 1243 - He is indifferent to everything in the world, has no desire to eat, and yet when he does eat he relishes (like) his food and can partake (eat) of what is required.(necessary)

He, 30 - Anxiety driving her to suicide ; thoughts of suicide; ...desire for death; great indifference even to those she formerly loved;...

MEZ. Al, 8 - Very sad; every trifle affects him disagreeably; indifferent to the whole world; has no desire for anything; disinclined to work.

Al, 14 - Indifferent to everything; he could scarcely compel himself to note the symptoms beyond brief annotations (as a sea-sickness)

Ha, 2-...everything seemed to him as if dead, and nothing made a vivid impression on him.

MYRIC. Al, 8-...;did not care about anything or for any friends; was perfectly wretched, beyond description.

NEON. Sh, 176 - Got up late in a horrible mood and reproached my partner again. I hurt him but I didn't care. I felt indifferent, malicious and vindictive, full of hate. 02, 6C, 05:22:10

Sh, 196 - I got nominated for a scholarship and I couldn't generate any excitement about it. I thought "I probably won't get it." 35, 6C, 02:XX:XX

Sh, 198 - Received a long letter from a patient today; haven't even read it, can't be bothered. Very unusual. In terms of indifference, I have felt disgusted with myself; one of these violent and malicious feelings. God, I feel so wretched. 02, 6C, 05:XX:XX

NUX-M. Al, 60 - State of mind similar to that of the opium-eater, entertaining no apprehension of the result, although aware of the presence of some danger.

He, 17 - The outer world had no existence for her; automatically she attended to her household duties, and on awaking from this condition she had not the slightest recollection of what she had done; ...

OP. Ha, 601 - Tranquil indifference to earthly things; she cared for nothing in comparison with ecstasies of the fantasy.

He, 22-... feeling of great strength; contempt of death;...indifference to joy and suffering.

PETR. Al, 28 - No desire to work; no pleasure in objects of which he was usually fond (loving), hence intolerable ennui.

PHOS. Ha, 82 - Indifferent to her child, whom at other times she dearly loved.

Ha, 12 - The world seemed dreadful to him; only weeping could relieve him, soon afterward apathy and indifference.

He, 31-...; indifference even towards dearest friends;... ; monomania de grandeur et de la richesse;...

He, 14 - Apathy; indifferent even to his own children;...

PIC-AC. Al, 6 - Great indifference; lack of will power to undertake anything.

PLAT. Ha, 39 - Indifference, cold (reserved), abstracted (separated) in company of friends,..

Ha, 40 - Indifference, he felt unconcerned (careless, insensible) as to whether his absent wife would die or not.

He, 10 - Cold, haughty, too well satisfied with one's self, and not at all anxious about the future. (presumptuous, egotistic, inexpugnable, safe)

PSOR. Al, 24-...only disagreeable things affect him, agreeable impressions he passes without noticing them.

PTEL. Al, 43 - Goes about his professional duties in a perfunctory (indifference) manner, very unlike (contradictory) his fiery (passionate) zeal with which he usually combats disease and his allopathic step-brethren (brotherhood).

PULS. Al, 5 - He wishes now for this, now for that employment, but when given to him he will have nothing to do with it.

RHUS-T. Ha, 950 - He could not be pleased, was indifferent to society.

SENEG. Al, 13 - Phlegmatic; inclines to quarrel and give offense.

SEP. Al, 24 - Feel very low-spirited, and don't care what becomes of me.

Al, 33 - Received news of the slight illness of a friend, which caused great mental depression (at another time it would not have made slightest impression); this condition grew on me until I became so nervous that I felt that unless I held on something, I should scream.

Al, 82 - Great indifference toward everything; no proper sense of life.

Al, 92 - One dose of the medicine takes away my ambition; I simply do not want to do anything, either work or play; it is even an exertion to think.

Ha, 59 - Great indifference to everything, no real vital feeling.

He, 38-...everything seems strange (unusual, unfamiliar) to her;...; it seems as if she could not understand (realize) anything and would have to learn anew everything she wished to do;...(lost: knowledge); greatest indifference to everything, the death of a near relative, or some happy occurrence, leaves her equally unaffected; no trace of her former love for friends or even for her child; aversion for social intercourse amounting to contempt;...

He, 3 - Felt all day as if he did not care what happened; ...

He, 6 - Great indifference to everything; no proper sense of life.

He, 22 - Great indifference to one's family, to those they love best.

SIL. He, 23-...believes she has swallowed pins, and asks those about her whether she has not done so; seeks for hours for lost pins; ...and careful examined her food for fear of pins; very indifferent to friends and former amusements;...

STAPH. Ha, 707 - Hypochondriacal humor; everything is indifferent to him; he would like to die.

Ha, 716 - She was all day long full of grief; she was afflicted (torment) to weeping about her circumstances (position), and she cared for nothing in the world.

Ha, 692 - The most attractive things made no impression on him.

Ha, 693 - Phlegmatic (indifferent), prostrate mind and sad disposition, unsympathetic, indifferent to all externals, yet not cross or exhausted.

He, 2 - Indifference, low-spirited, dullness of mind; after onanism.(masturbation)

SULPH. Ha, 51 - For hours he sits motionless and indolent, without any definite thoughts, though he has many things to attend to.

He, 32 - Melancholy mood; dwelling on religious or philosophic speculations; anxiety about soul's salvation; indifference about lot (destiny) of others.

SYPH. He, 11 - A far-away feeling, with apathy and indifference to future.

THUJ. Al, 51 - Remarkable indifference to the opposite sex. (sexual)

Al, 74 - Constant great despair changes at last to complete indifference.

TUB. Al,N-16 - Great anxiety for future, otherwise marked indifference.

UPA. Al, 4 - Melancholic; has to force the tears back; cold towards his friends, repelling everyone.

INDIGNATION

Ailments from; anger, indignation, with: ars.[5] ***aur.*** **COLOC.**[122] germ.[222] ip. lyc. m-p-a.[5] merc. mur-ac. nat-m. ***nux-v.*** plat. **STAPH.**[122]

Ailments from; honor, wounded: aur.[184] bamb-a.[1184] carc.[214] cham.[54] ign. ***nat-m.***[162] nat-s.[162] nux-v. pall.[144] plat.[137] ***staph.***[122] verat.[54]

Ailments from; indignation: acon.[10] ***ant-c.***[5] bell.[5] bry.[5] carb-v.[5] chin-s.[36] ***coloc.*** ferr.[38] ferr-p.[36] gels.[162] hecla.[234] hep.[5] ign.[171] ip. ***nat-m.*** ***nux-v.***[5] plat. **PULS.**[5] **STAPH.**[122]

Ailments from; insults, offenses, from, dignified to fight, too, subdued wrath, went home sick, trembling, exhausted: ***staph.***[54]

Ailments from; mortification, indignation, with: **STAPH.**[122]

Cheerfulness; alternating with, indignation, bursts of: aur. caps. croc. ign.

Delirium; indignant, in encephalitis: ***cocc.***[54]

Dreams; vexatious, wrong doings of others, over: dros.[54]

Grief; silent, indignation, with: ***coloc.***[54]

Hysteria; sick, after being insulted and subduing his wrath: ***staph.***[54]

Indignation: acon.[10] ambr. androc.[222] ***ars.*** aur. bry.[30] ***calc-p.*** caps. cham.[30] chin. cocc. ***coloc.*** croc. ferr-p.[36] gels.[162] germ.[222] graph.[1] ign. ip.[122] ***m-p-a.***[1] med.[149] nat-c. nat-m.[189] nitro-o.[36] nux-v.[30] oena.[36] psor.[106] sabad.[129] spig.[30] **STAPH.** sulph.[1] verat.[30]

Indignation; alternating with mildness: ***ars.***[36]

Indignation; dreams, at unpleasant: calc-p.

Indignation; emission, after: pip-m.[36]

Indignation; insults others: ozone[227]

Indignation; slandering, with: spig.[30]

Injustice, cannot support: calc.[189] calc-p.[108] carc.[233] caust.[162] chel.[188] coloc.[187] cupr.[210] dros.[156] hecla.[234] ign.[30] kali-i.[184] mag-m.[162] med.[193] merc.[210] nat-m.[189] nux-v.[1] phos.[193] plb.[201] sep.[93] ***staph.***[30] sulph.[184] verat.[111]

Irritability; indignation, with: staph.[1]

Mildness; alternating with, indignation: ars.[36]

Mirth; alternating with, indignation, bursts of: aur. caps. croc. ign.

Wildness; misdeeds of others, from: ***colch.***[36]

ARS. Al, 98 - Indignation in the morning when in bed; pushes the pillows about indignantly uncovers himself, sees no one, and does not want to be spoken to.

Al, 109 - Indignation, alternating with mildness; in her indignation she looks at nobody, and does not want to hear anything; she also cries.

Al, 94 - Very fretful, indignant, capricious; every word offends her, and makes her very angry, when she should answer.

CALC-P. Al, 14 - Violent, irritable, and snappish; it affects him most to hear that someone has done wrong; indignation rises in him...
Al, 15 - A communication in which some one is justly reproached concerning his conduct, affects him very disagreeably; he grows violent, and holds up his faults to himself.
Al, 16 - Unpleasant news makes him beside himself; sweat breaks out; inclined to indignation and anger.
CAMPH. Ha, 342 - The boy crawls into a corner and howls and weeps; he takes offense at everything one says to him, as if he thought he was being ordered (instructed) about, and he thinks he is insulted and affronted.
CAPS. Ha, 334 - He makes reproaches, and is indignant (angry) at the faults (errors) of others; he takes trifles ill and finds fault with them.
CHIN. Al, 39 - Fretful and irresolute; she is unable to accomplish her aim, and consequently is indignant. (angry)
CIC. Al, 26 - Contempt and scorn for mankind; he avoided them, abhorred their follies (stupidity) excessively, and his disposition seemed to tend towards misanthropy; he withdrew (retire) himself into solitude.
COCC. Ha, 554 - He is very indignant and annoyed at slight faults and fibs (lie, falsify) of others.
He, 39 - Angry and indignant form of delirium.
COLOC. He, 12 - Anger with indignation and extreme irritability; throws things out of his hands.
He, 13 - Indignation, with silent internal grief.
He, 14 - Affections from anger, with indignation, particularly vomiting and diarrhoea ...(ailments from)
GERM. Sh, 10 - Reacted very strongly to a very close friend. Something quite small sparked it off and I hung up the phone. Just felt I'd had enough. It's an issuefeeling that's been built up for months, but tonight I flipped inside. Only our third argument in years. I still feel indignant and angry 1 hour later, even after going and working in the garden. Won't answer her calls. 13, 30c, 06:08:30
Sh, 168 - Indignation. Think all falls on me. 21, 12C, 36:XX:XX.
GRAPH. Ha, 35 - Very peevish; everything vexes him and makes him indignant.(anger)
HYOS. He, 79 - After being harshly (severe) accused of theft (crime), continual delirium; fancies surrounded by objects of a terrifying nature; not a moment quiet, continual calling out that she saw the devil; denies herself guilty of theft (innocent, injustice), or that she has any concern with witches; ...
IOD. He, 15 - At night, especially when thinking of real or imaginary wrongs ...dares (try) to go home for fear of doing some dreadful (bad, wicked) deed (action); on one occasion was seized with an almost irresistible impulse to murder a woman who was acting as a guide (direct, conduct) for him, he having lost his way (direction);...must be constantly in action, in some laborious occupation. (lost; direction, correction, control)
NUX-V. Al, 4 - He is hasty; looked angrily at anyone who asked him a question without answering, as though he was obliged to restrain himself to avoid being insulting; he was in such an irritable and unrestrained mood that it seemed as though he would like to strike any one in the face who spoke a word to him.
Ha, 1270 - He is hasty (careless, rapid), looks malignantly (deadly) at any one who asks (asked) him anything, without answering, just as if he must control himself in order to avoid becoming coarse (rude), it seems as if he would like to strike any one in the face who speaks a word to him, so irritable and uncontrollable in his disposition.
STAPH. He, 11 - Great indignation about things done by others or by himself; grieves about consequences. (remorse)
He, 12 - Ailments from indignation and vexation, or reserved displeasure ;sleeplessness.
He, 14-...; was insulted (slandered, defamed, calumniated) being too dignified (reserved, lordly,) to fight (contest), subdued (control) his wrath(anger) and went home sick,.. (ailments, from offenses)

SULPH. Ha, 38 - He gets vexed about everything, takes every word ill and gets insulted (dishonored, degraded), he imagines he ought (must) to defend himself and gets angry.

Ha, 59 - A number of ideas from her past life, mostly disagreeable, causing indignation and mortification...come into her mind;...so that she cannot get rid of them, while she has nothing to do;...

INEXPUGNABLE

Delusions; building stones, appearance of: thuj.
- eternity, that he was in: cann-i.
- heart, live without, he can: ***nux-v.***[54]
- immortality, of: anh.[119]
- marble statue, he is a: cann-i.
- power over all disease, has: ***stram.***[54]
- statue, poses as: ***stram.***
- strong, he is: androc.[222] germ.[222] hydrog.[222]
- superhuman, is: cann-i. psil.[164]

Dreams; breath under water, she can: ozone[227]
- ➤ death, friend, of a, dear, which does not abate his mental exhilaration, looking at all with supernatural indifference: coff-t.[36]
- ➤ shed, being under a: merc-i-r.[36]

Indifference; stoical to what happens: ail.[54] myric.[25] op.[137]

Self-sufficient; help of others, needs no: calc.[189] mag-c.[214]

Self-sufficient; overly confident: ferr-ma.[10]

ADAM. Sh, 314 - Feeling of absolute power, invincible. 16, 12C, 14:14:00

Sh, 536 - With my eyes closed after meditating, to my right appeared a huge Tibetan deity. He appeared to know who I was. Felt it would be rude to ask his name. He said, "Do you want to know how powerful I am?" He was not friendly but powerful.... 16, 12C, 00:07:30

Sh, 541 - Feeling of absolute power, invincible.[16], 12C, 14:14:00

NEON. Sh, 24 - I feel invincible when upright. No wavering-like a laser. 20, 6C, 04:02:XX

OP. He, 22-... feeling of great strength; contempt of death;...indifference to joy and suffering.

PLAT. He, 10 - Cold, haughty, too well satisfied with one's self, and not at all anxious about the future. (presumptuous, egotistic, inexpugnable, safe)

STRAM. He, 102 - Mania with insomnia ; very talkative; thinks he has every imaginable disease; that he has power (powerful) over all disease; masturbates, fills his pockets with anything he can find (lack?), thinks he has snakes in him.

INFECTIOUS

Anger; worm complaints, in: ***carb-v.***[54] ***cina***[54]

Anxiety; pneumonia, in: ***ant-t.***[54] ***chel.***[54] squil.[54]

Anxiety; tuberculosis, in: agar.[54] ***chin-ar.***[54]

Anxiety; typhus, in: **ARS.**[54] **CALC.**[54] ***chin-s.***[54] **SPONG.**[54]

Anxiety; vaccination, after: ***thuj.***[54]

Aversion; wind, to: ozone[227]

Complaining; symptoms, about his numerous, in pneumonia: ***ant-t.***[54]

Death; conviction of, fever, after, epistaxis amel.: ***psor.***[54]

Delusions; breath is spoiled, his exhaled, cautions people not to inhale: lyss.[54]
- contaminates everything she touches: ars.
- die, about to, he is, tuberculosis, from: calc.[172] lac-c.[172] paull.[172] sep.[172] tarent.[172]
- die, tuberculosis, from: calc.[172] lac-c.[172] paull.[172] sep.[172] tarent.[172]
- disease, give, to others, that he will: ***chlol.***[54]
- disease, yellow fever, that he will have: camph.[54]
- tetanus must die of, with pain in right leg: ***mag-p.***[54]
- typhoid fever, he will have: nat-p.

Despair; recovery, ague, in: ***tarent.***[54]

Dreams; body, abdomen, cut, a big cut in, blood and pus, under which amounts of: ozone[227]
- ➤ cholera, of: linu-c.[36]
- ➤ death, dying, of, nervous fever, from: kali-chl.[36]
- ➤ diphtheria, of: bac.[62]
- ➤ disease, aids: bamb-a.[1184]
- ➤ disease, cholera: linu-c.
- ➤ disease, expectoration, purulent: hep.
- ➤ disease, fever: kali-chl. sulph.
- ➤ disease, hydrophobia: anan.
- ➤ disease, leper, being: paull.[36]
- ➤ disease, plague: ozone[227]
- ➤ disease, variola: anac.

➤ expectoration, purulent: hep.[1]
➤ fever, of: kali-chl.[10] sulph.
➤ feverish: euphr.[36] lachn.[36]
➤ funeral, people who had died of scarlatina, in trying to avoid wind blowing from procession toward him he awoke: form.[102]
➤ pus spitting: hep.[1]
➤ smallpox: anac.[10]
➤ vomiting, blood and pus: bamb-a.[1184]
➤ women, leprous: paull-p.[36]

Fear; brain, inflammation of, from dullness in head, amel. by epistaxis: psor.[54]
✦ choking, of, inflammation of throat, in: ***hep.***[54]
✦ cholera, of: arg-n.[172] ars.[30] jatr.[54] **LACH.**[122] **NIT-AC.** ph-ac.[54] verat.[30]
✦ cholera, of the, cramps in calves would set in, as if: ***jatr.***[54]
✦ cold, of taking: nat-c. sulph. syph.[193]
✦ consumption, of: ***calc.*** kali-c.[149] lac-c. paull. puls.[172] sep. tarent. ***tub.***[54]
✦ death, cholera asiatica, in: ***cupr.***[54] ***cupr-acet.***[54] **VERAT.**[54]
✦ death, diarrhea, in: ***ham.***[54]
✦ death, fever, during: calc. cocc. ip. mosch. ***nit-ac.*** **RUTA**
✦ death, heat, during: acon.[85] calc. cocc. ip. mosch. ***nit-ac.*** **RUTA**
✦ death, scarlatina, after: ***hell.***[54]
✦ death, smallpox, in: ***ph-ac.***[54]
✦ death, vexation, after, in cholera Asiatic: **ARS.**[54]
✦ diphtheria, of: bac.[62]
✦ disease, contagious, epidemic diseases, of: bar-c.[10] ***bor.*** bov.[36] bufo calad. **CALC.**[30] cur.[193] lach. nat-m.[185] sil.[193] **SULPH.**[193] syph.[193]
✦ disease; viral: nux-v.[172]
✦ exposure night in bed, of: mag-c.
✦ fever, going to bed, on: hura
✦ fever, of (while chilly): calc.[122] sulph.
✦ fever, typhus: cham.[54] nat-p.[172] tarent.
✦ fever, yellow: ***merc.***[54] ***sulph.***[54]
✦ heat, during: acon. ***ars.*** cham.[54] nux-m. spong.
✦ pneumonia, of: chel.
✦ smallpox, of: ***vac.***[54] ***vario.***[72]
✦ syphilis, of: ***hyos.*** merc.[30] syph.[162]
✦ tuberculosis, incipient, in: ***tub.***[54]
✦ tuberculosis, of: calc.[137]
✦ worm diseases, with: stann.[8]

Hydrophobia; bitten, after being: lyss.[54]
Indifference; condition does not seem dangerous to him, in typhus: colch.[54]
Indifference; typhoid, in: ail.[58] ***apis***[54] ***arn.*** chin. ***chin-s.***[54] ***colch.***[54] ***nit-s-d.***[54] ***ph-ac.*** ***verat.***[54]
Sadness; gonorrhea, in: ***hydr.***[54] ***merc.***[54] ***thuj.***[54]
Washing; always, hands, her: ars.[111] coca[122] cur.[162] ***lac-c.***[122] ***med.***[122] merc.[184] ***nat-m.***[162] plat.[126] psor.[111] sep.[162] sil.[185] ***sulph.***[162] syph. thuj.[162]
Washing; bathing, mania for: zea-i.[122]
Washing; cleanness, mania for: ars.[58] sep.[193] sil.[30] sulph.[30]

BOR. Al, 14 - Dread and fear of contagion.
Ha, 6 - Apprehension and fear of infection.
CALAD. He, 13 - Fear of catching scarlet fever when attending a case; a fear he never had before.
CALC. Al, 30 - Dread and anxiety of the future, with fear of consumption.
Ha, 25 - His heart is agitated with fear and anxiety for the future, with fear of consumption.(tuberculosis, ruin)
He, 53 - Fear: of death; of consumption (decay, waste, tuberculosis); of misfortune (disaster) ; of being alone. (lonely)
CAMPH. He, 21 - Very nervous; imagined various things; that he would get yellow fever.
CHEL. Al, 54 - Fear that pneumonia is coming on.
CHLOL. He, 3 - Fixed despair of recovery; believes he will give his imaginary disease (syphilis) to others.
CROT-H. He, 10 - Mania in zymotic (infectious) disease and when connected with puerperal or ovary-uterine disease.
LAC-C. Al,N-28 - Fear of disease; of consumption; of heart disease. (tuberculosis)
LACH. He, 55 - Nightly attacks of anxiety; afraid of chorea, gets cramps in calves from fear; nausea, heavy feeling in abdomen...
LYSS. Al,N-62 - He cautioned people around him not to inhale his exhaled air, it was spoiled (dirty), stinking (smelling) like rotten (putrefying) eggs, worse than cholera, and could injure. (contaminates, infects)
He, 62 - He cautioned people around him not to inhale his exhaled air, it was

spoiled, stinking like rotten eggs, worse than cholera, and could injure.
MUR-AC. Al, 637 - Dream that she had lice, which made her very much ashamed.(shame)
NAT-P. Al, 6 - Very despondent; imagined he was going to be sick, to have typhoid fever.
NIT-AC. He, 16 - Anxiety about his disease, with fear of death; morbid fear of cholera.
PSOR. He, 31 - Despairs recovery; thinks he will die; hopeless; especially after typhus...
SANG. He, 9-..."what will become of my condition, shall I have typhoid fever, inflammation of the brain, or shall I remain paralyzed?".
SEP. Al, 52 - She is filled with concern about her health; thinks she will have consumption and soon die.
Ha, 9 - She has none but troubled thoughts about her health, thinks she is getting the consumption (tuberculosis, degenerate, decomposition) and will die soon.
SULPH. Al, 60 - Fear that he would take cold in the open air; he did not know whether it was illusive or physical.
TARENT. Al, 57 - Fear of getting "typhus fever".
TUB. Al,N-45 - Insanity; acute or chronic, with a family history of tubercular affections.
Al,N-46 - When the best selected remedy fails to relieve or permanently cure in a marked tubercular diathesis, with a tubercular family history.

INJUSTICE

Ailments from; mortification, indignation, with: **STAPH.**[122]
Delusions; hell, suffers the torments of, without being able to explain: lyss.[54] ***merc.***[122]
- obscene, actions of which she had not been guilty, accuses herself of.: ***phos.***
- voices, hears, confess things she never did: lach.[58]
- witches, denies having anything to do with them, in delirium after being accused of theft: ***hyos.***[54]
- wrong, suffered, has: bac.[62] chin.[193] **HYOS.** lach. ***lyss.*** naja

Dreams; accusations, crime, wrongful of: choc.[222] clem.[10] hydrog.[222] sil.[58]
- defamatory: mosch.
- poisoned, about to be, while innocent of crime: chr-ac.[36]

Injustice, cannot support: calc.[189] calc-p.[108] carc.[233] caust.[162] chel.[188] coloc.[187] cupr.[210] dros.[156] hecla.[234] ign.[30] kali-i.[184] mag-m.[162] med.[193] merc.[210] nat-m.[189] nux-v.[1] phos.[193] plb.[201] sep.[93] ***staph.***[30] sulph.[184] verat.[111]
Sadness; blaming others, with: lil-t.[168]
Sadness; slight or treat, from an undeserved: arg-n.

ARG-N. He, 40 - Melancholy since an undeserved slight (scorn); fixed idea that he was neglected and despised by his family; his callings (job, work) became indifferent to him.
BAR-A. Al, 9 - Dread (fear). When walking in the street, she imagines that people were criticizing her, and judging her wrongfully which makes her anxious, so that she will not look up, will look (aversion) at no one, and sweats all over.
BAR-C. Ha, 4 - She suspected, that when walking in the street, men found fault (defect) with her, and judged her amiss (wrong), which made her anxious, so that she dared not look up, she looked at nobody, and perspired all over.
GERM. Sh, 153 - Thought nobody understood me and cared for what I felt. Felt it was unfair. I was presented with complaints about something others had done. Felt I was standing between two fighting parts. Felt awkward about it, embarrassed. Difficult to argue about such strong outburst. Thoughts about the day's arguing milling in my head all evening and night. 21, 12C, 32:XX.XX.
Sh, 168 - Indignation. Think all falls on me. 21, 12C, 36:XX:XX.
HYOS. Ha, 578 - He reproaches others, and complains of injustice that he imagines has been done him.
He, 66 - A gentle, lovable woman became extremely jealous of her husband, and although fully realizing that she did him injustice, she was so filled with grief that she found no rest day or night... (remorse)
He, 79 - After being harshly (severe) accused of theft (crime), continual delirium; fancies surrounded by objects of a terrifying nature; not a moment quiet, continual calling out that she saw the

devil; denies herself guilty of theft (innocent, injustice), or that she has any concern with witches; ...

LAM. Al, 2 - Extraordinary sadness; he thought he had been blamed for reverses (failure) for which he was blameless, and in consequence was obliged to suffer;...

LYSS. Al,N-23 - Imagine that they are being abused (injured, offended), and energetically defend themselves against attacks and insults, ...

He, 23 - Imagine that they are being abused (hurt, injured), and energetically defend themselves against attacks and insults, which in reality are products of their own fancy.

MANG. Ha, 329 - Embittered humor; he could not forget injustice done to him; he fostered (support) resentment for a long time.

STAPH. He, 6 - Hypochondriasis (depression);...;caused by unmerited insults (offenses, affronts, abuses) sexual excesses, or by persistently dwelling on sexual subjects.

He, 9 - Very sensitive to least impression; least word that seems wrong (offenses) hurts her very much.

He, 11 - Great indignation about things done by others or by himself; grieves about consequences. (remorse)

SULPH. Al, 87 - Embittered mood as if he had been injured.

Ha, 59 - A number of ideas from her past life, mostly disagreeable, causing indignation and mortification...come into her mind;...so that she cannot get rid of them, while she has nothing to do;...

ZINC. He, 43 - Great fear, as if persecuted by men or the devil, on account of crimes he has never done (injustice); is afraid of becoming imprisoned, or poisoned, or shot, or buried (inter) alive...[0] Delirium tremens.

INSANITY

Affectation; mania, in: ***stram.***[54]

Anxiety; control over senses is lost, with feeling that: acon.[210] gels.[210] manc.[210] ***merc.***[54] tarent.[210]

Anxiety; murdered someone, as if he had, mania, in: ***ars.***[54]

Brooding; law suit, over, by which he may gain or loose a million, and takes it in bad part if not allowed to read indictment for said lawsuit, a confused, irrational piece of work, on which he has been working all night, in insanity: ***nux-v.***[54]

Comprehension; easy, understands former mysterious things, in insanity: ***verat-v.***[54]

Concentration difficult; crazy feeling in the top of head, wild feeling in head with confusion of ideas: lil-t.

Confounding; objects and ideas: calc. cann-s. colch.[54] hyos. nux-v. phos.[189] plat. ***sulph.***

Confusion of mind; fits, in, almost to insanity: act-sp.[54]

Cursing; mania, in: ***hyos.***[54] lil-t.[100] ***nat-m.***[8] stram.[111] verat.[28]

Delirium: absin. acet-ac. ***acon.*** ***act-sp.*** aesc. ***aeth.*** aether[36] **AGAR.** agar-cps.[36] agar-pa.[36] agar-ph.[36] agn.[54] ail. alco.[36] alum.[54] am-c. amyg-am.[36] anac. anag.[54] anan. anh.[85] ant-c. ant-t. anthr. apis arg.[8] arn. **ARS.** ars-s-f.[58] **ARUM-T.** astac.[54] atro.[36] ***aur.*** aur-m.[54] ***bapt.*** bar-c. **BELL.** bism. bol-lu.[36] bomb-pr.[36] brom.[116] **BRY.** bufo cact. calad. ***calc.*** calc-caust.[10] calen.[54] ***camph.*** camph-br.[25] **CANN-I.** cann-s. ***canth.*** caps. carb-ac. carb-v. ***carbn-s.*** ***carl.***[36] caul.[54] ***cham.*** **CHEL.** chin. chin-ar. chin-s. chlf.[54] chlol.[25] chlor.[54] chloram.[149] chol. chr-ac.[54] ***cic.*** cic-m.[36] cimic. ***cina*** clem. coff. ***colch.*** coloc. ***con.*** convo-s.[119] cop. cor-r. croc.[58] **CROT-C.**[122] ***crot-h.*** ***cupr.*** ***cupr-acet.***[10] cupr-ar.[36] cypr.[25] cyt-l.[144] dat-f.[85] dat-m.[36] ***dig.*** diph.[102] dor. dubin.[36] ***dulc.*** eup-pur.[25] euph.[5] fagu.[36] ferr-p.[5] gall-ac.[85] ***gels.*** glon. graph. ham.[54] hell. hep. hipp. hippoz.[54] hydr.[54] **HYOS.** hyosin.[36] hyper. ign. iod. iodof.[85] ***ip.*** iris[54] iris-fl.[85] iris-foe.[36] jatr. juni-c.[36] kali-ar. kali-bi.[54] kali-br. kali-c. ***kali-chl.***[54] ***kali-i.***[54] kali-n. kali-p. kalm.[54] lac-c.[54] lacer.[36] **LACH.** lachn. lact. lat-k.[36] laur.[54] lept.[54] lil-t. lob. lol.[5] lup.[36] **LYC.** lycps.[25] lyss. mand.[119] ***meli.*** meny. ***merc.*** ***merc-c.***[122] merc-cy. merc-i-r.[5] merc-n.[36] merc-s.[36] merl. mez. ***mill.***[54] morph.[36] mosch.[5] mur-ac. mygal. naja nat-m. nat-s.[54] nicot.[36] **NIT-AC.** nit-s-d.[36] nitro-o.[36] ***nux-m.*** ***nux-v.*** ***oena.*** **OP.** oper.[102] orig.[25] ox-ac. paeon.[36] par. passi.[116] paull.[36] ***petr.*** ph-ac. ***phos.*** phyt. plat. ***plb.*** podo. psor. ***puls.*** pyre-p.[85] pyrog.[58] ran-b. ran-s. rheum rhod. **RHUS-T.** sabad. sabin. sal-ac. samb.

sang.[54] sant.[36] sapin.[36] sarr. **SEC.** sel.[5] sil. sin-n.[5] sol-n. spig.[5] stigm.[85] **STRAM.** stry. sul-ac. sul-h.[36] sulfa.[149] ***sulph.*** syph.[5] tab. tang.[36] tarax. tarent. tarent-c.[5] tax. ***ter.*** thea. trinit.[102] tub.[54] valer. vario.[54] **VERAT. VERAT-V.** verin.[36] vesp. vip. vip-a.[149] xan.[54] zea-i.[85] zinc. zinc-acet.[116] zinc-p.[58] zinc-s.[36]

Delirium tremens; angry rather than anxious, subjects not greatly exhausted: ***graph.***[54]

Delirium tremens; escape, attempts to: ***bell.***[116] stram.[116]

Delirium tremens; praying, with: aur.[162] **STRAM.**[54]

Delirium tremens; voices, heard continually on right side of occiput a loud voice, scolding, vituperating and accusing him of ungodliness, and also personifies voices: **STRAM.**[54]

Delirium; abandons her relatives: sec.

Delirium; accused of theft, after being harshly: ***hyos.***[54]

Delirium; addresses objects: stram.[5]

Delirium; alternating with, mental capacities heightened: lacer.[36]

Delirium; alternating with, sadness: tub.[102]

Delirium; anxious, approaching him, of everyone, shrinking from them: ***cupr.***[54]

Delirium; anxious, dog were attacking her, as if: **STRAM.**[54]

Delirium; anxious, men of: ***plat.***[54]

Delirium; asphyxia, with: ***ant-t.***[54]

Delirium; attacks people with knife: hyos.

Delirium; balance, losing: hyosin.[36]

Delirium; bellows like a calf: cupr.

Delirium; blessing, asks a: bell.[36]

Delirium; blood, from profuse loss of: arn.[5] ars.[5] bell.[5] ign.[5] lach.[5] lyc.[5] ph-ac.[5] phos.[5] sep.[5] squil.[5] sulph.[5] verat.[5]

Delirium; books, endeavored to grasp: atro.[36]

Delirium; busy: arum-t.[58] bapt. bell. ***bry.*** camph. ***hyos.*** kali-cy.[36] rhus-t. ***stram.*** sulph.

Delirium; calls for parents who are present trying to console: **STRAM.**[54]

Delirium; cheerful, alternating with, laughing, singing, whistling, crying etc.: stram.

Delirium; cheerful, gay, rage, changing to: ***bell.***[54]

Delirium; comical: ant-c.[85] ***hyos. stram.*** verat.

Delirium; crying, help, for: ***canth.*** stram.[54]

Delirium; dark, in: ***calc-ar. carb-v. cupr. stram.***

Delirium; death, talks about: ***acon.***[54]

Delirium; exaltation of strength, with: ***agar. aur.*** hyos. sec.[162] stram. tarent.[162]

Delirium; fatigue, study, over-exertion, from: ***lach.***[54]

Delirium; fear of men, with: bell. ***plat.***

Delirium; feces, swallows his own: verat.[60]

Delirium; frightful: ***acon.*** anac. ***atro.*** bar-c.[54] **BELL.** calc. canth. carb-v.[10] caust.[10] chin.[10] cic. colch. coloc. dig. hep.[30] ***hyos.*** lyc.[10] merc.[10] nat-m. nit-ac.[10] nux-v. ***op.*** phos.[58] ***plb.***[122] ***puls.*** rhod.[36] samb.[10] sec. sil. **STRAM.** sulph.[10] ***verat.*** zinc. zinc-p.[58]

Delirium; help, calling for: plat.

Delirium; home, wants to go: bell.[36] bry.[72] ***cupr-acet.***[54]

Delirium; hysterical, almost: bell. ***hyos.***[54] ign. tarent. verat.

Delirium; imperious: lyc.[36]

Delirium; indignant, in encephalitis: ***cocc.***[54]

Delirium; laughing: acon. apis[5] ***bell.*** colch. con. cupr.[5] ***hyos.*** hyosin.[36] ***ign.*** lach. lact. op. plb. sal-ac.[36] sec. sep. ***stram.*** sulph. thea. verat. zinc.

Delirium; light, with desire for: calc.[10]

Delirium; lively active, vivid, alternates in short periods with horrified fright, seeming to dread approach of some monster, appealing for help: stram.[54]

Delirium; loquacious, business of: ars.[36] bell.[111] **BRY.**[54] ***canth.***[111] dor.[54] **HYOS.**[54] op.[36] ***phos.***[111] **RHUS-T.**[111] stram.[36]

Delirium; loquacious, fire, of: ***calc.*** cupr.[162]

Delirium; loquacious, foreign countries, of: cann-i.

Delirium; loquacious, rhyme, in: thea.[36]

Delirium; maniacal, love, from disappointed: ***phos.***[54]

Delirium; mild: ***apis***[54] **BAPT.**[54] ***ph-ac.***[54] ***puls.***[54] rhus-t.[5] sec.[10] **STRAM.**[54] ***valer.***[54] ***vario.***[54] verat.[10]

Delirium; mild, roaring over fields or hard at work, he thinks he is: ***rhus-t.***[54]

Delirium; mortification, after: bell.[10] nux-v.[10] puls.[10]

Delirium; night, business of the day, of: bry.[54]

Delirium; quiet: **BRY.** calc-sil.[58] camph.[54] ***carb-v. chel.*** chin. chlf.[54] ***chlor.*** croc. cupr. cupr-acet.[58] **HYOS.** hyosin.[36] kali-p.[54] op. past.[36] ***ph-ac.*** phos. plb. rhus-t. sec. tab. valer. verat.

Delirium; quiet, alternating with restlessness and desire to run away: ***chlor.***[54]
Delirium; rabid: bell. canth. lyss. ***stram.***
Delirium; raging, raving: ***acon. act-sp. aeth.*** aether **AGAR.** agar-pa.[36] ail.[48] alco.[36] anac. ant-s. ***ant-t.*** apis[112] ***arg.***[54] arg-n. ars. ars-s-f.[58] atro.[54] **BELL.** bry. calc. ***camph.*** camph-br.[25] cann-i. cann-s.[5] **CANTH.** ***carbn-s.*** cham.[5] chel. chin. chin-s. cic. ***cimic.*** cina clem.[54] colch. coloc. cori-r.[36] ***cupr.*** cupr-acet.[36] dat-f.[36] dig. dulc. glon. graph. ***hell.*** hep. **HYOS.** hyper. jatr. juni-c.[36] ***kali-i.***[54] ***lach.***[5] lob. ***lol.***[5] **LYC.** ***merc.*** merc-cy. morph.[36] mosch. nat-m. **NIT-AC.** nux-m. nux-v.[36] ***oena.*** **OP.** par. phos. ***plb. puls.*** rheum **SEC.** ***sol-n.*** **STRAM.** sul-ac. sulph. ***tab.*** tarent. trach.[36] **VERAT.** verat-v.[54] vip. zinc. zinc-p.[58]
Delirium; raging, raving, alternating with, religious excitement: agar.[36]
Delirium; rambling: atro. ***bell.*** chlol.[36] ***chlor.***[54] hyos. ***nat-m.***[54] plb. sec.[54] ***sulph.***[54]
Delirium; refuses to take the medicine: agar-pr.[36] hyos.[162]
Delirium; religious: agar.[5] alco.[36] aur. lach. **VERAT.**[5]
Delirium; reproachful: hyos. lyc.
Delirium; restless: absin.[171] acon. ail.[58] ***ars.***[60] atro. bry.[116] **HYOS.**[54] iod.[116] merc-s.[54] phos.[36] plb. sant.[25] ***stram.***[54] sulph.[116] ***verat.***[54]
Delirium; romping, with, children: agar.
Delirium; sad: acon.[5] bell.[5] morph.[102] puls.[5]
Delirium; scolding: chr-ac.[54] hyos. merc. nit-ac.[137] stram. verat-v.[54]
Delirium; sexual excitement, with: **STRAM.**[54]
Delirium; shy, hides himself: **STRAM.**[54]
Delirium; silent: agar. sec.
Delirium; singing: agar.[116] cic.[116] lact.[36] stram.[36]
Delirium; sorrowful: acon. bell. dulc. lyc. puls.
Delirium; speeches, makes: lyss.[54]
Delirium; spits and licks it up or rubs it over the floor: merc.[36]
Delirium; strike, disposed to: **BELL.**[54]
Delirium; study, from excessive: hyos.[10] ***lach.***[54] nux-v.[10]
Delirium; threatening, with pain in face: ***kalm.***[54]
Delirium; throwing from windows: ***aeth.***[54] calc.[58] sil.[58]
Delirium; throwing from, height, a: **BELL.**[36]
Delirium; touch, with aversion to: merc.[36]
Delirium; vexation, from: bell.[10] **HYOS.**[54] plat.[10]
Delirium; violent: ***acon.*** aeth.[137] agar. alum.[54] ***apis*** **ARS.** atro. ***aur.***[54] **BELL.** camph. canth. chlf.[54] con. ***cupr.*** **HYOS.** ***lach. op.*** phos. plb. puls. ***sec.*** **STRAM.** verat. verat-v.[116] zinc. zinc-p.[58]
Delirium; water, jumping into: bell. sec.
Delirium; wedding, prepares for: ***hyos.***
Delirium; wild: atro.[116] **BELL.** ***bry.***[116] ***calen.***[54] camph. canth. chlol. colch. cupr. gall-ac.[36] ***gels.***[54] hydr-ac. ***hyos. kali-br.***[54] lach. nat-sal.[36] oena.[144] ***op.***[122] **PLB. STRAM.** ***valer.***[54] vario.[54] ***verat.***
Delirium; wild, stab and bite, attempts to: **STRAM.**[54]
Delirium; work, of his: bell.[5] **BRY.**[5] ***canth.***[5] ***phos.***[5] **RHUS-T.**[5]
Delirium; wraps up in fur during summer: hyos.
Delirium; wrongs, of fancied: hyos.
Delusions; asylum, insane, sent to: lach.[58]

- asylum, she will be sent to: cench.
- compass, fixing himself to correspond with points of, in insanity: hyos.[54]
- devils, erotic mania, in: orig.[54]
- devils, taken by, that he will be, mania, in religious: ***puls.***[54]
- insane, become, that she will: ***acon.*** act-sp.[162] agar.[139] ail.[139] alum.[5] ambr.[5] ars.[5] brom.[139] ***calc.***[5] cann-i. cann-s.[5] ***chel.*** chlor.[5] **CIMIC.** colch.[5] con.[58] cupr.[139] cycl.[139] ***eup-per.***[54] gels.[139] glon.[139] ham.[5] hydrog.[222] hyos.[139] ***ign.***[54] iod.[54] iris-t.[139] kali-bi.[123] ***kali-br.***[5] kali-p.[123] ***lac-c.***[5] lam.[36] lil-t. ***manc.*** med. merc. nat-m. nat-s.[139] nitro-o.[36] nux-v.[5] pall.[8] phys.[5] plat.[5] psor.[85] sil.[139] sulph.[139] ***syph.***[102] tanac. tarent.[36] vario.[123]
- insane, become, that she will, unless she got out of her body: lac-c.[54]
- insane, become, that she will, delivery, parturition, during: cimic.[54] coff.[54]
- insane, become, that she will, hold tightly upon herself, if she did not: lil-t.[54]
- insane, everyone but he himself, is: androc.[222]
- insane, he is: germ.[222] pall.[139] phys.[139] sulph.[139]
- insane, he is, half: sanic.[139]
- insane, people think her: **CALC.** germ.[222] hydrog.[222]

• maelstrom, carried down a psychical: cann-i.
• mind, going out of his, he is: ambr.[85] calc.[31] cot.[36] eup-per.[8] ham.[8] ***kali-br.***[8] ***lac-c.***[56] nit-ac.[85] ol-j.[139] paraf.[38] petr.[85] visc.[77]
• music, delirium, during: ***plb.***[54]
• persecuted, delirium in: ars.[30] calc.[30] hyos.[30] lach.[30] merc.[30] nat-m.[30] rhus-t.[30] stram.[30] verat.[30]
• sick, he is, mind and body, in: merc.[60]
• talking, insane irrationally: nit-ac.[1]
• visions, monsters, delirium, in: ***bell.***[54]
• wilderness, being in a: stram.[10]

Dementia; business, worry from: lil-t.[137]
Dementia; sadness, with: tarent.[58]
Desires; numerous, various things, insane: ars.[10] bry.[10] cham.[10] chin.[10] cina[10] coff.[10] dulc.[10] ign.[10] ip.[10] ***puls.***[10] rhus-t.[10]
Despair; insanity, as of incipient: ***med.***[54]
Despair; recovery, mania, in: ***verat.***[54]
Disgust; consciousness of his unnatural state mind: tarent.[54]
Dreams; animals, bulls, mad: ind.
➤ animals, dogs, mad dog: abrot. rumx.
➤ animals, dogs, mad dog, killing a: abrot.[85] rumx
➤ asylum of insane: lyss.[54]
➤ crazy, going: aloe apis ferr-p.[5]
➤ crazy, man, a: apis.[58]
➤ disease, insane, becoming: aloe ferr-p.
➤ killing, mad dog, a: rumx.
➤ monomania: acon.[10] ign.[10] puls.[10] stann.[10]

Escape; attempts to, delirium, during: alco.[36] bell.[36] ***cupr.***[54] dig.[36] merc.[36] oena.[36] phos.[36] sol-m.[85] ***stram.***[36] sul-ac.[36] verat.[36]
Exhilaration; delirium, followed by horrible: absin.[85]
Exhilaration; mania, in merry: ***stram.***[54]
Fear; approaching, others, of, delirium, in: cupr. stram. ***thuj.***
✦ death, delirious, from violent beating of carotid and temporal arteries: ***aur-m.***[54]
✦ death, impending, of, reason, and loss of: ***plat.***[54]
✦ death, reason, and loss of: ***plat.***[54]
✦ head, something wrong in her: bamb-a.[1184]
✦ insanity, fright, after: ***ign.***[54] ***stram.***[54]
✦ insanity, night: calc.[1] manc.[162] ***merc.*** phys.
✦ insanity, of losing his reason: acon. act-sp.[162] agar. ***alum.*** alum-p.[58] alum-sil.[58] ***alumn.***[36] ambr. **ANAC.**[185] antipyrin.[72] aq-mar.[149] arg.[102] arg-n. ars. ars-i. atro.[172] bov. bry. cact.[58] **CALC.**[122] ***calc-ar.***[122] calc-i.[58] calc-s. **CANN-I.** carb-an. carbn-s. carc.[207] caust.[172] ***chel.*** chlor. ***cimic.*** cupr. ***dig.*** ***eup-per.***[54] gels. ***graph.*** guare.[36] ***hell.***[184] hydrog.[222] ign. iod. kali-bi. ***kali-br.*** kali-c.[184] kali-p.[172] ***kali-s.***[8] ***lac-c.*** lach. lap-c-b.[194] lat-m.[119] laur. led.[172] levo.[149] lil-s.[36] ***lil-t.*** lyc.[172] lysim.[72] ***lyss.***[54] mag-c. **MANC.**[122] mang.[172] ***med.***[102] ***merc.*** merc-s.[172] merl. mosch. mur-ac.[144] ***nat-m.*** ***nux-v.*** ol-j.[54] ***phos.*** phys. pic-ac.[193] plat. prot.[136] psor.[56] **PULS.** rhod. ***sep.*** spong.[54] ***staph.***[30] ***stram.*** sul-i.[58] sulph. sumb.[8] syph. tarent. thuj. tub.[58] verat.[102]
✦ insanity, repose, if he wants to, must always move: ars.[58] iod.[58]
✦ mania, fright, after: ***ign.***[54] ***plat.***[54] ***stram.***[54]
✦ mania, in: bell.[60] cupr.[54] sec.[137] ***stram.***[54]
✦ poisoned; being, mania, in puerperal: ***verat-v.***[54]
✦ satiety of life, with, particularly in company, hysteric: ***lyc.***[54]
✦ self-control, of losing: alum.[214] ***arg-n.*** bamb-a.[1184] cann-i.[162] cupr.[210] ***cupr-acet.***[54] ***gels.*** germ.[222] ***merc.***[54] nux-v.[185] ozone[227] ***staph.*** sulph.[185] thea.[185] thuj.[184]

Haughty; mania, in: ***graph.***[54] ***lach.***[54] **PLAT.**[54] ***verat.***[54] ***verat-v.***[54]
Homesickness; mental derangement, in: manc.[54]
Insanity: absin. acon. aeth. aether[36] ***agar.*** ail. alco.[36] all-c. ***alum.*** alum-p.[58] alum-sil.[58] ***am-c.*** ambr.[111] ***anac.*** anag.[54] anan.[54] anh.[102] ant-c. ant-t. ***apis*** ***arg.*** arg-n. ***arn.*** **ARS.** ars-i. ars-s-f.[58] arum-t. atro.[116] ***aur.*** aur-ar.[58] aur-i.[58] aur-s.[58] bac.[62] bar-c. ***bar-m.*** **BELL.** berb.[5] bor.[58] bov. brom. bufo cact. calad. ***calc.*** calc-ar.[58] calc-i.[58] calc-s. calc-sil.[58] ***camph.*** cann-i. cann-s. ***canth.*** carb-an. carbn-s. ***caust.*** cench.[58] cere-b.[85] ***chel.***[54] chin-s. chlf.[54] chlol. chlor.[8] ***cic.*** ***cimic.*** ***cocc.*** coff. colch. coloc. ***con.*** cortiso.[119] ***croc.*** ***crot-c.*** crot-h. ***cupr.*** cur. ***cycl.*** dat-a.[25] dig. ***dulc.*** euph. fl-ac. gels.[116] germ.[222] ***glon.*** ***hell.*** ***hep.*** **HYOS.** ***ign.*** indg. iod. kali-ar. kali-bi.[36] ***kali-br.*** kali-c. ***kali-chl.*** kali-i. kali-ox. ***kali-p.*** ***lach.*** led. ***lil-t.*** lob.[36] ***lol.***[116] **LYC.** ***manc.*** mand.[119] med.[58] meli.[85] **MERC.** merc-c. mez. mosch.[116] murx.[116] naja nat-c. ***nat-m.*** nat-s. ***nux-m.*** **NUX-V.** oena. olnd. ***op.*** opun-a.[36] orig.[25] ***ox-ac.*** par. passi.[116] ph-ac. ***phos.*** phys. ***plat.*** plb. ***psor.*** ***puls.*** raph. rhod.

rhus-t. sabad. sec. seneg. sep. sil. sol-n.[116] squil. stann.[36] **STRAM.** stry.[36] ***sulph.*** syph.[111] **TARENT.** ter. thuj. thyr.[85] **VERAT.** verat-v. vip.[137] zinc. zinc-p.[58] zinc-val.[25]

Insanity; alternating with, depressive narcosis: apis[130] ***hyos.***[137]

Insanity; alternating with, sadness: tub.[102]

Insanity; anger, from: bell.[10] ***ign. lach.***[30] lyc.[10] op.[10] ***plat.***[122] staph.[30]

Insanity; black insanity with despair and weariness of life from fear of mortification or of loss of position: calc.[30] ign.[30] puls.[30] rhus-t.[30] staph.[30] sulph.[30] verat.[30]

Insanity; break pins, she will sit and: bell. calc.

Insanity; business, from failure in: ***cimic.***[54] ***lil-t.***[54]

Insanity; busy: **APIS** bell.[10] hyos.[58] ***iod.***[54] kali-br.

Insanity; capricious: raph.[54]

Insanity; character, of sombre: nat-sal.[36]

Insanity; company, with desire for light and: **STRAM.**[54]

Insanity; dancing, with: bell.[10] cic.[10] hyos.[10] ph-ac.[10]

Insanity; dictatorial: **LYC.**[10]

Insanity; dispute, to: camph.[60]

Insanity; domestic calamity, after: ***lach.***[54]

Insanity; dresses in his bests clothes: con.

Insanity; eats, dung or lapping up of saliva: merc.[5]

Insanity; eats, filth: ***camph.***[54] sulph.[10]

Insanity; eats, refuse, only: meli.

Insanity; emaciation, with: sulph.[60]

Insanity; ensue, feels as if it would: ***acon.***[5] ars.[5] ***calc.***[5] cimic.[5] colch.[5] ham.[5] ***lac-c.***[5] lil-t.[5] med.[5] ***merc.***[5] phys.[5] tarent.[5]

Insanity; envy, with: **LYC.**[30]

Insanity; erotic: ambr.[102] **APIS BAR-M.** bell.[10] bufo[107] calc-p.[36] camph.[85] ***cann-i.***[102] canth.[111] ferul.[102] gins.[102] grat.[102] ***hyos.*** kali-br. lil-t.[102] lyss. manc.[102] ***murx.***[102] ***nux-v.***[85] orig. ***phos. pic-ac.***[102] **PLAT.** ***puls.*** rob.[102] salx-n.[102] stann.[36] stram.[36] ***sulph. tarent.*** **VERAT.** zinc.[111]

Insanity; erotic, hysterical girl, in a: ***plat.***[54]

Insanity; erotic, jealousy, with: ***hyos.***[54]

Insanity; escape, desire to: ars.[10] ***bell.***[10] cupr.[10] dig.[10] nux-v.[10] ***op.***[30] stram.[30] verat.[10]

Insanity; fanatics, of: aur-ar.[58]

Insanity; feeling of: germ.[222] ***kali-br.***[54] ol-j.[54] spong.[54]

Insanity; females, of: ***acon.***[111] apis[130] ***bell.***[111] cimic.[137] ***orig.***[137] plat.[111] ***puls.***[111] stram.[111] verat.[111]

Insanity; females, self accusation, from: hell.[137]

Insanity; fortune, after gaining: bell.[30] ***caust.***[30] puls.[30] stram.[30] verat.[30]

Insanity; fortune, losing, after: calc.[30] ign.[30] rhus-t.[30] verat.[30]

Insanity; fright, from: **ARS.**[30] **BELL.**[30] ***ign.*** lach.[54] merc.[54] plat. sabad.[137] stram.[54]

Insanity; gluttony, with: chin.[30] **VERAT.**[30]

Insanity; gluttony, with, alternating with refusal to eat: hyos.[30] ip.[30] stram.[30] verat.[30]

Insanity; graveyards, visits: bell.[10] stram.[10]

Insanity; grief, from: **ARS.**[30] **BELL.**[30] ***cocc.***[54] ***plat.***[54]

Insanity; haughty: **HYOS.**[5] lach.[10] **LYC.**[5] ***stram.***[5] **VERAT.**[5]

Insanity; hemorrhage, after: carb-v. ***chin. cupr.*** kreos. ph-ac. ***sep.*** staph. verat.

Insanity; immobile as a statue: cham.[10] fl-ac.[58] hyos.[10]

Insanity; lamenting, moaning, only: bell.[10] hyos.[30] stram.[30]

Insanity; lascivious: ***hyos.***[5] tarent.[8] **VERAT.**[5]

Insanity; love, on account of unfortunate: tarent.[36]

Insanity; malicious, malignant: agar.[10] cann-s.[10] ***cupr.*** lyc.[10]

Insanity; masturbation, from: anan.[54] bufo ***cocc. hyos.*** op.[137] ***plb.***[54]

Insanity; mild: ***croc.***[5] ***verat.***[5]

Insanity; mortification, from: bell.[10] ***lach.***[30] **NUX-V.**[30] plat.[30] ***puls.***[10] ***staph.***[30]

Insanity; obsession, with: anac.[5] sulph.[5]

Insanity; obstinate in: ***dig.***[54] ***nux-v.***[54]

Insanity; orgasm, at height of: lac-c.[137]

Insanity; paralysis, with: ant-c.[102] ars.[102] aur.[102] bell.[8] ***cann-i.***[102] caust.[102] chlol.[8] crot-h.[137] hyos.[58] kali-br.[85] kali-i.[102] ***lach.***[122] lol.[77] merc-c.[102] nat-i.[102] nux-v.[102] op.[102] ***phos.***[85] phys.[102] plb.[102] stram.[102] sulph.[102] verat.[102]

Insanity; passes her feces on the floor: cupr.

Insanity; position, from fear to lose the: calc.[30] ign.[30] puls.[30] rhus-t.[30] staph.[30] sulph.[30] verat.[30]

Insanity; prayer at the tail of his horse, insists upon saying his: euph.

Insanity; prayer, raising hands and kneeling as in p.: ***ars.***[36]

Insanity; purchases, makes useless: con. ***nux-v.***[54]

Insanity; quarrelsome: hyos.[137] ***verat.***[8]
Insanity; rage: ars-s-f.[58] germ.[222] oena.[25] ***tarent.***[54]
Insanity; religious: anac.[58] ***ars.***[122] aur.[54] aur-ar.[58] bell.[116] croc.[116] ***hyos.***[116] ***kali-br.***[54] ***lach.***[58] lil-t.[58] lyc.[58] merc.[116] nat-c.[58] nux-v.[116] ***plat.***[54] ***puls.***[58] **STRAM.**[54] ***sulph.***[54] ***verat.***[10]
Insanity; reproaches others: **LYC.**[30]
Insanity; restlessness, with: ***ars.***[10] bell.[30] bry.[30] canth.[10] chin.[30] ***hyos.***[10] merc.[10] nux-v.[10] puls.[30] stram.[10] verat.[30]
Insanity; sadness: ars.[102] ***aur.***[102] bac.[56] bell.[30] calc.[30] caust.[102] cic.[102] hyos.[30] ***ign.***[10] ***kali-br.***[54] nux-v.[102] ***petr.***[30] ph-ac.[30] ***puls.***[102] rhus-t.[30] staph.[30] sulph.[30] verat.[30]
Insanity; secretive: dig.[1]
Insanity; self-accusation, from: hell.[137]
Insanity; shy: agar.[5]
Insanity; silent: verat.[10] ***verat-v.***[54]
Insanity; strength increased, with: agar. ***bell.*** canth. cori-r. hyos. ***plb.***[162] ***stram.*** **TARENT.**
Insanity; suicidal disposition, with: ars.[10] hyos.[10] naja[130] orig.[25] verat.[10]
Insanity; touched, will not be: ***thuj.***
Insanity; travel, with desire to: bell.[30] bry.[30] chin.[30] hyos.[30] nux-v.[30] puls.[30] stram.[30] tub.[58] verat.[30]
Insanity; wantonness, with: bell.[10] cupr. ***hyos.*** merc.[10] mez.[10] stram. verat.
Insanity; wedding preparations, of: hyos.[137]
Insanity; women, in: ***acon.***[111] apis[130] ***bell.***[111] cimic.[137] ***orig.***[137] plat.[111] ***puls.***[111] stram.[111] verat.[111]
Jealousy; insane: lach.[137]
Looking; about, shyly, in puerperal mania: ***puls.***[54]
Loquacity; exalted opinion of her own ideas and powers, with, in insanity: ***verat-v.***[54]
Mania, madness: absin. acon. acon-l.[36] aeth. aether[36] ***agar.***[5] ail. alco.[36] ***alum.*** alum-p.[58] ***anac.*** anag.[54] anan.[54] anh.[144] ant-c. ant-t.[5] ***apis arg. arn.*** **ARS.** ars-s-f.[58] ***arum-t.*** atro.[102] ***aur.*** aur-ar.[58] aur-i.[58] aur-s.[58] bapt.[102] bar-c. ***bar-m.*** **BELL.** ***brom.*** bry.[102] bufo cact. ***calad. calc.*** calc-i.[58] ***camph. cann-i. cann-s.***[5] ***canth.*** carbn-s.[58] carc.[207] caust.[5] cedr.[102] cham.[5] chel. ***chin.*** chin-s. chlol. cic. ***cimic.*** coca ***cocc.***[122] coff. colch. ***con.*** cori-r.[85] cortico.[119] croc.[5] crot-c. crot-h. ***cupr.*** cupr-acet.[102] ***cycl.*** dat-f.[85] dat-m.[85] der.[85] dig. dros.[5] dubin.[102] ferr-p.[58] gels.[5] glon. grat.[85] ***hell. hep.*** **HYOS.** hyosin.[85] ***ign.*** indg. ***iod.*** iodof.[85] iris-t.[85] kali-bi.[5] **KALI-BR.** kali-c.[5] **KALI-CHL.** kali-i. ***kali-p.*** kres.[144] ***lach.*** laur.[102] led. lil-t.[5] **LYC.** lyss.[85] ***manc.*** mand.[119] med.[5] **MERC.** merc-c. murx.[5] nat-m. nit-ac.[5] ***nux-m.*** **NUX-V.** oena. ***op.*** orig.[102] ***ox-ac.*** par.[85] passi.[102] petr.[5] ph-ac.[5] ***phos.*** pic-ac.[102] pisc.[102] ***plat.***[5] plb. ***psor.*** puls. raph. rhod. rhus-t.[5] ruta[5] sabad. sal-ac.[144] sec. senec.[85] seneg.[5] ***sep.*** sil.[85] sol-n.[85] spig-m.[102] spong.[102] staph.[85] **STRAM.** sul-h.[102] ***sulph. tarent.*** ter. thea.[85] thyr.[85] tub.[85] tub-k.[85] ust.[102] **VERAT.** verat-v. vip.[111] zinc.
Mania; abuses, violent outburst, abuses her child, parturition, after, puerperal: ***camph.***[54]
Mania; action, must be constantly in, in some laborious occupation: ***iod.***[54]
Mania; alternating with, sadness: arg.[149] ***con.***[54] cyt-l.[149] kres.[149] ***nat-s.***[54] psor.[122] ***staph.***[54] stram.[1] sulfa.[149] tub.[102] verat.[72]
Mania; alternating with, silence and refusing to talk: verat.[102]
Mania; business, discouragement, from: ***lil-t.***[54]
Mania; business, failure, from: ***cimic.***[54]
Mania; capricious: raph.[36]
Mania; comical: **HYOS.**[54]
Mania; domestic calamity, after: ***lach.***[54]
Mania; heart, affected, with: cupr.[54]
Mania; held, wants to be: **ARS.**
Mania; indecent: ***op.***[54]
Mania; masturbation, after: anan.[54]
Mania; masturbation, eight or ten years duration, of: ***plb.***[54]
Mania; midnight, dancing, laughing, striking, with: cic.[30]
Mania; paralysis, with: crot-h.[54] ***nat-m.***[54] ***nux-v.***[54] ***phos.***[54] ***phys.***[54] sec.[54]
Mania; philosophical: ***sulph.***[58]
Mania; prayer, as in, raising hands and kneeling: ***ars.***[36]
Mania; praying: stram.[60] verat.[60]
Mania; rage, with: acon.[58] anac.[58] ant-t.[10] arg.[85] ***arn.***[5] ars.[58] ***bell.***[5] **BRY.**[5] camph.[54] cann-i.[116] ***canth.***[10] ***cic.***[5] con.[58] croc.[58] cupr.[58] cur.[8] ***dig.***[8] **HYOS.**[5] kali-c.[58] lach.[58] lyc.[5] merc.[58] ***nat-m.***[8] nux-v.[54] op.[5] phos.[58] plat.[58] plb.[10] puls.[58] sec.[58] sol-n.[10] **STRAM.**[5] tarent.[187] verat.[58]
Mania; sexual, abuse, from: lil-t.[54] ***phos.***[54]
Mania; sexual, increased desire, from: apis[122] **BAR-M.**[54] **PHOS.** ***tarent.***

Mania; sexual, men, in: apis[117] canth.[102] **PHOS.** ***tarent.***
Mania; singing, with: bell.[10] cann-i.[60] cic.[149] ***cocc.***[54] cupr.[60] hyos.[60] ***nux-m.***[54] ***plat.***[54] stram.[60] ***tarent.***[54] ***verat.***[10]
Mania; study, from too much: ***lach.***[60]
Mania; suicidal: ***ars.***[54] ***verat.***[54]
Mania; suicidal, sexual symptoms, with: ***aur.***[54]
Mania; tear clothing: nux-v.[30] ***tarent.***[54] ***verat.***[54]
Mania; tear, hair, own: bell.[10] canth.[30] stram.[30] tarent.[36] verat.[30]
Mania; tear, himself to pieces with nails: canth.[30] stram.[30] verat.[30]
Mania; tears: ***cupr.***[54]
Mania; vexation, after: bell.[10] hyos.[10] ign.[10] nux-v.[10] ph-ac.[10] ***plat.***[54] staph.[10]
Mania; wild: kali-br.[54] ph-ac.[10]
Monomania: ***absin.***[102] acon. anac.[36] anan. aur.[5] bell.[10] camph. carb-v. carc.[207] cham.[10] chin.[10] cic.[5] cocc.[10] con.[10] croc.[10] cupr.[10] dros.[10] hell. hyos.[10] ***ign.*** iod.[10] lach.[10] lap-c-b.[194] mag-c.[10] nux-m. oxyt.[102] plat.[10] puls. rhus-t.[10] ***sil.*** stram. sulph. tarent.[102] thuj. verat.[10]
Monomania; going out, dressing in a grotesque manner: anan.
Naked, wants to be, delirium, in: ***bell.*** **HYOS.** merc. ***phos.*** phyt. ***sec.*** ***stram.***[54]
Plans; fantastic, in insanity: ***nux-v.***[54]
Play; piano, upon the, for hours, in puerperal mania: ***plat.***[54]
Religious affections; mania: ***lach.***[54] ***plat.***[54] plb.[85] ***puls.***[54] ***stram.***[54] sulph.[85] **VERAT.**[54]
Religious affections; mania, pious look, with: ***stram.***[54]
Religious affections; mania, praying all the time: ***aur.***[54]
Rover about; senseless, insane: bell. bry.[30] canth. chin.[30] coff. hyos. ***nux-v.*** puls.[30] sabad. stram. verat.
Runs about; madman, like a, from anger: bufo[105]
Sadness; conscious of unnatural state of mind, because: tarent.[54]
Schizophrenia: anh.[119] aur.[54] carc.[140] halo.[149] kres.[149] levo.[149] psil.[149] sulfa.[149] thiop.[149] tub.[148] ven-m.[149]
Schizophrenia; catatonic: chlorpr.[149] cic.[149] convo-s.[149] cortico.[119] halo.[149] rauw.[119] reser.[149] thala.[149] thiop.[149]
Schizophrenia; hebephrenia: anh.[149] chlorpr.[149] halo.[149] kres.[149] reser.[149] thala.[149] thiop.[149] thuj-l.[149]
Schizophrenia; paranoid: ***bell.***[111] ***hyos.***[111] med.[122] ***nux-v.***[111] op.[111] rauw.[119] stram.[111] verat.[111]
Suicidal disposition; drowning, by, mania, in: sec.[54]
Suicidal disposition; mania, in, puerperal, with aversion to husband, baby and coition: agn.[171]
Suspiciousness; mania, in: ***lach.***[54]
Suspiciousness; mania, in, delivery, parturition, after, puerperal: ***verat-v.***[54]
Thoughts; terrible, taking possession of him, in mania: ***iod.***[54]
Unconsciousness; alternating with, erotic mania: apis[98]
Weeping; fear of losing reason, or that she might commit suicide, with: ***puls.***[54]
Weeping; rage, maniacal: ***plb.***[54]
Work; crazy, seems to drive him, in mental occupation, owing to the impotency of his mind: ind. ***kali-p.*** med.

ACON. He, 23 - Pains are so intolerable, they drive him crazy; he becomes very restless.
He, 35 - Sadness with solicitude; concerned about future; about her recovery or fears loss of reason. (insanity)
ACT-SP. He, 3 - Judgment perplexed; bewildering fits, almost to insanity.
ALUM. Ha, 21 - Apprehension of losing his thoughts, his reason.
He, 18 - Apprehensive of losing his reason.
AMBR. Al,N-11 - Fears of becoming insane.
He, 10 - Fear to become crazy.
ANDROC. Sh, 123 - In the evening he became manic, stalked the streets and visited many friends for a short time only, but could not relax or relate to them. Was pleased when he found his friends were not at home. Spoke nonsense and tried to squeeze a laugh out of anything. (29)
Sh, 155 - At night —brain revving away like crazy, thoughts racing through his head. Very interesting and exciting thoughts. Stayed awake til early morning, enjoying himself tremendously, and felt young again. (4)
APIS. He, 29 - Insanity, particularly nymphomania...
BAPT. He, 4 - Cannot confine (control) his mind; a sort of wild, wandering feeling.

BELL. Ha, 1433 - Fearful madness; he is afraid (fear) of an imaginary black dog, of the gallows. (hanging)
Ha, 1434 - Madness; he thinks that his living body is putrefying. (decay, degeneracy)
BRY. Ha, 766 - Raving (insanity) about business for an hour.
CALC. Al, 21 - Anxious at night as she would become insane, followed by shuddering chilliness for a few minutes, and a sensation as if the body were dashed (hit) to pieces.
Ha, 26 - She is afraid of losing her reason. (sanity)
Ha, 27 - She is afraid people may notice (observed) the confusion (disorder) in her head.
He, 52 - Fears she will lose her reason (insanity), or that people will observe her confusion of mind.
CANN-I. He, 26 - He was in constant fear he would become insane.
CHEL. Al, 74 - It seems as though she could not think, and would lose her reason. (after three hours)
He, 6 - Imagines she cannot think and will lose her reason.(impediment)
He, 18 - Anxiety: allowing no rest at any employment (business) ; as if she had committed a crime; fear of getting crazy (insanity), with restlessness and heat.
CHLOL. Al, 3 - A horrible state of mind, fears he will go crazy, fears he cannot make a living.(subsistence)
CHLOR. Al, 4-...he is afraid of becoming insane; thinks it is impossible to get through it. (obstruction, impediment)
He, 3 - A horrible state of mind, fears he will go crazy, fears he cannot make a living.(subsistence)
CHOC. Sh, 179 - Apprehensive about the shift in consciousness and nervous someone would notice. It is reminiscent of L.S.D., the 'shifting edges', before the full blown trip arrives — an uneasiness and unsureness about which way things will go. A desire to hide in case things go to pieces. 15, 30C, 00:00:50
CIMIC. He, 5 - Thinks she is going crazy.
He, 24 - Fears she will become crazy, with headache on vertex.
COCC. He, 39 - Angry and indignant form of delirium.
COT. Al, 2 - Awoke, early in the morning, in a state in which she felt as if she were going out of her mind. (insanity)
CUPR. Ha, 23 - Fits of insanity, imagines he is a military commander.
Ha, 24 - Fits of insanity, he imagines (delirium) he has green herbs for sale.
Ha, 25 - Fits of insanity, he imagines he is repairing old chairs. (humility) (reparation, restitution)
Ha, 27 - Fits of insanity, he spits into people's faces, and laughs heartily (soberly) over it.
He, 6 - Craziness (insanity); attacks with savage malice (evil), with proud (arrogant) bearing (posture),...
He, 10 - Mania with biting, beating, and tearing things to pieces; insane foolish gestures of imitation and mimicry; full of insane spiteful (cruelty, brutality) tricks (deceitful, false), ..unhappy, despairing...miserable look...
He, 18 - Unconquerable sadness, constant restlessness, as if some misfortune were approaching; fears he will lose his reason.
CUR. Al, 1 - Paroxysm of insanity impelling him to attack himself; he strikes, scratches, and tears himself with a sort of relish, (enjoy) and without feeling any pain.
DIG. He, 11 - Melancholic, despondent, and constantly tortured by fear of death or loss of reason.
EUP-PER. He, 1 - Feels at night as if he was going out of his mind.(insanity)
EUPH. He, 3 - Temporary attacks of craziness, insists upon saying his prayers at the tail of his horse; knows his freaks (abnormality) and wants to be by himself and in silence.
FL-AC. He, 7 - Aversion to his own family, bordering on insanity.
GERM. Sh, 4 - Desperately angry. So intense that I could barely control it. I made noises like an animal, pushed my arms up and down - instead of hitting my children, which helped. Want to just leave the house and the kids. Felt completely mad, afraid of what the neighbors heard and thought. Very bad conscience afterwards, but no relief - didn't get the anger out. There are a lot of feelings inside that don't come out. 18, 30C, 02:09:00
HALI-L. Sh, 306 - When I'm focused I bring

it all in, in the present, There. like meditating, or seeing God. When I'm unfocussed it's like I'll go into the abyss, and won't come back, go crazy. 08, 30C, 31:XX:XX

Sh, 435 - I was feeling very self-destructive. I wanted to do crappy things to myself. The border's breaking loose. I know I have a part of me that does this. It's just rising up. Screw it all, the futility of it all; the futility of working toward the positive, of caring for my health, of doing good things. What for? My big fear is that I'm really crazy, that I'm making all this up, that I'm just crazy (i.e., that the remedy is a placebo). 06, 6C, 11:XX:XX

Sh, 640 - A lot of agitation and irritability on the surface. Underneath there was a crevice, a crack... in my soul or the universe. Dread or anticipation of what else could happen if this process went on. If the process went on, it could lead to complete insanity, completely being out of touch with reality. 06, 6C, 01:00:XX

Sh, 651 - When I'm focused, I bring it all in, in the present. There, like meditating, or seeing God. When I'm unfocussed, it's like I'll go into the abyss, and won't come back; go crazy. 08, 30C, 31:XX:XX

Sh, 662 - I can't stand it any longer. Spiraled and spiraled and spiraled. Feel like I'm going mad, like there's no escaping out of this. Pull, pull, like a hypoglycemic who hasn't eaten, and just wants to scream and yell. While I was in the shower I just wanted to kill. Feel like I'm going to lose it. Going stir crazy;...02, 30C, 11:XX:XX

Sh, 663 - In a total frenzy, like steaming horses that had escaped, running down the road. Very hard to keep any control, to be patient in traffic, or the grocery store. Couldn't handle it any longer. Put lip balm with camphor on, every ten minutes, and would feel calm momentarily. Finally got some tiger balm at a friend's house and used it two times. I was instantly calmer. Came back to being me. 02, 30C, 11:XX:XX

Sh, 664 - Feel deflated, calmer and flatter. The feeling of going mad goes back to when I was drinking 15 years ago. That feeling of not being able to decide what to do. Today feeling flat, exhausted; a wonderful day outside, unable to enjoy it. Feeling unenergized, although glad the craziness is gone. I felt I was on speed with emotions. I'm glad I antidoted that thing; feel like an empty balloon. It could have gotten down to a dangerous place. Reminded me of going mad; like the energy it gave me. Felt hooked on the remedy. 02, 30C, 12:XX:XX

HAM. He, 5 - Felt as if he was going out of his mind.

HELL. He, 11 - Psychical conditions occupying a place between melancholia and mania, and in conditions where true depression and weakness is present, in which the patient is governed by a fixed idea.

He, 12 - An old woman having been accused of theft by the women around, took it so much to heart that she hanged herself. This suicide produced a profound effect upon the women of the village. One after another accused herself of having caused the death of the old woman by their insinuations; they wept and howled, ran about day and night wringing their hands and despairing of salvation on account of their sin (error); they became quite irrepressible and deranged (disordered) In this way twenty -four or twenty five women were affected, every fresh case being followed by another. Hysterical mania.

HYDROG. Sh, 11 - I felt I had gone mad, possessed, hysterical laughter, singing and a feeling of non-reality, as if in a dream, out of the body — like my mind went out of the window. High one minute and then low. People asked if I was on speed. After seven hours, in the evening (7:30p.m.), the feeling changed to an angry mood and very irritable with a dry furry mouth,...l. 24, 30C, 00:00:45

Sh, 12 - Driving home I felt odd, as if I was hardly in my body. Feel like my body's working on automatic but I'm not really there. Driving along I kept forgetting where I was. Now I feel I'm really more "absent" than normal and feel quite afraid of losing my mind or having an accident. I feel my connection with the physical world is very loose, as though my soul was separated from my body. I have thoughts that this is a bit like dying — not unpleasant. 10, 200C, 13:02:XX

Sh, 27 - There is a very fine line at this time between enlightenment and insanity —a split consciousness. The dark side is horrendous, but the positive side of the proving has been well worth it. The positive aspects are beautiful. Its a shame we need to come down. I guess the price of going into the heavens is a trip to hell. 16, 30C, XX:XX:XX

Sh, 194 - Fear I may lose my mind, or even die. Fear about the proving. Feel I could bash the car so I have to make a real effort. 10, 200C, 12:XX:XX

Sh, 255 - Very worried that people don't like me and can't cope with me —that they will think I am insane. I think maybe I am insane. This is frightening me. 16, 30C, 25:XX:XX

Sh, 256 - Thought someone was telling someone else that I was mad and asking what should be done about it. 16, 30C, 25:XX:XX

HYOS. Al, 9 - Madness as if possessed by a devil.

Ha, 535 - In his mania, he acts as if he must drive away peacocks with his hands.(conduct)

Ha, 545 - Ridiculously solemn acts in improper clothing, mixed with fury. (In a priest's cassock, put on over nothing but a shirt, and in fur boots, he wishes to go to church, in order to preach and perform clerical offices there, and furiously attacks those who try to prevent him.)

He, 72 - He lies in bed nude and chatters; walks about insane, naked, wrapped in a skin during summer heat.

IGN. He, 44-...;indifference to things she loved best ; sits alone and weeps, imagines things, a especially that she might go crazy; ..

IND. Al, 4 - Felt almost crazed when attempting to study...

IOD. Ha, 17 - Restless moving about; she runs about incessantly and does not get to sit down, nor does she sleep at night, so that she has to be considered as crazy.

He, 3 - Must keep in motion day and night (restlessness), brain felt as if it was stirred (agitation) up, felt as if going crazy.

KALI-BR. He, 22 - Feels as if he would go out of his mind.

He, 23-...constantly brooding over loss of a daughter; almost crazy; ... (child)

He, 38 - Much concerned (anxiety) about health; complains without cause;...uncontrollable sensation of fear and anxiety, thinks she is becoming deranged (insanity) ; change of life.

He, 39-...fear and apprehension that she is losing her mind (insanity);...makes her utterly (completely) miserable to be looked at or spoken to; fear to see people; always depressed and lowspirited;...

He, 33 - Great despondency, with insanity, a feeling of moral deficiency, or a religious delusion, from anemia.

He, 30 - Great despondency; "feel as if they should go out of their minds."

LAC-C. Al,N-39 - Wakes distressed, and obliged to rise and occupy herself in some manner; fears she will be crazy.

He, 8 - Sensation as if she was going deranged, when sitting still and thinking; sometimes she has most horrible sights presented to her mental vision (not always snakes), feels horribly afraid that they will take objective form and show themselves to her natural eye.

He, 13 - Woke at daylight feeling that she is a loathsome (repulsive), horrible mass of disease (while the breasts were affected); could not bear to look at any portion of her body (loathing, himself), not even hands, as it intensified feeling of disgust and horror; could not bear to have any part of her body touch another, had to keep even fingers apart; felt that if she could not in some way get out of her body, she should soon become crazy .

He, 14-..;sometimes imagines heart or breathing are going to stop, or otherwise frightens himself, and this makes heart beat violently; occasionally very depressed, and fancies he is going out of his mind. (insanity)

He, 21 - Sits and looks under chairs, table, sofa and everything in room, expecting yet dreading (fear) to see some terrible monster creep forth and feeling all the time, that if it does, it will drive her raving mad; she is not afraid in dark, it is only in light where she can imagine that she can see them.

He, 32 - Wakes distressed, and obliged to rise and occupy herself in some manner; fears she will be crazy.

LACH. Al, 25 - Towards evening very unusual almost crazy jealousy, as foolish as it is irresistible.

LAM. Al, 5-...,(fixed ideas) so that at last she becomes sad about it, and thinks she shall lose her reason.

LIL-T. Al, 15 - Apprehensive as from impending disease or calamity (misfortune); fears insanity; fears heart disease; fears she is incurable; often with moderate or sub acute uterine or ovarian inflammation.

Al, 16 - Worse on going to bed; can't go to sleep; wild (tumultuous, uncontrollable) feeling in the head as though I should go crazy (insane) and no one would take care of me (forsaken, helpless); thoughts of suicide; how much opium would put me to sleep forever, and who would find my body, and who would care; ... (friendless, abandoned, deserted)

Al, 17-... and expressed to her sister great fear of insanity.(through the proving)

Al, 3 - A sense as if she were going to be crazy, if she did not hang on to herself, and hold tight.

He, 6 - Crazy feeling on top of head; wild feeling in head, with confusion of ideas.

He, 7 - Dementia produced by business discouragements and sexual excesses.

LYSS. Al,N-77 - Lyssophobia; fear of becoming mad. (hydrophobia)

Al,N-78 - Feels as if he cannot physically endure his fears much longer, and shall be compelled to go into an insane asylum.

He, 78 - Feels he cannot physically endure his fears much longer, and shall be compelled to go into an insane asylum.

MANC. He, 3 - Fear of getting crazy; of evil spirits; of being taken (possessed) by the devil.

MED. Al-N, 38-...;desire for rest and dread (fear) of change;...wild crazy feeling in brain...

Al,N-44 - The impatience, excitement, wild feelings; the unreal, dazed condition; the gloom (sadness) and fear in the dark;... are marked evidence of functional derangement of the nervous system.

Al,N-50 - It is always anticipating, fearing evil will happen, loss of reason or suicide.

Al,N-23 - Wild desperate feeling, as of incipient insanity.

He, 22 - Wild and desperate feeling, as of incipient insanity.

MERC. Ha, 1222 - Restlessness, he cannot remain quiet in any place; he can neither stand nor lie, and is as if mad, or as if he had committed a great crime.

Ha, 1236 - He thinks he is losing his reason,(intelligence, capacity) that he is going to die ; with illusions of imagination, e.g. he sees water flowing where there is none (in the morning). (water-[1] origin, genesis)

He, 28 - Anxiety and restless change of place; ebullitions, sweat; apprehensive, imaginary fears; fears he will lose his mind;...(sanity).

He, 14 - Believes he is losing his reason, thinks he is dying, with illusions of fantasy; sees water running where there is none.

MOSCH. Al, 19 - She sits in thought, strikes her hands together, makes various gestures, so that others fear she will lose her reason,...

NAJA. Al, 3-...having an axe in his hand,...he suddenly split his head in two; he had become insane.

NAT-M. Al, 71 - Fear of insanity.

Ha, 24 - Anxious about becoming insane.

Ha, 93 - Loss of memory; he could not recall anything about yesterday and was afraid he had lost his mind.

He, 35 - Fear of loss of reason.(sanity)

NIT-AC. Ha, 15 - Apprehensiveness, with stitches above the heart, and a fancy as if he was talking deliriously, with coldness of the body and a tendency to fall down.

NUX-V. He, 4 - Cannot read or calculate, for she loses the connection of ideas; thinks she will lose her reason.

PH-AC. Ha, 42 - In the evening, while sitting down, nothing but numbers appeared before his eyes, he felt stupid and ill in the head, and at last very hot.

PHYS. He, 3-...feels as if she must lose her mind and become insane or despondent;...;thinks she is a castaway (repudiated, discarded, rejected, forsaken);....fears she is crazy or will certainly lose her mind;...

PLB. Al, 20 - He was at time delirious, very restless, and manifested great concern (care) for his affairs.

Al, 38 - Begged and prayed to be released from the strait-waistcoat, "for", he said, "I am not mad; but the idea of being forcibly restrained is enough to drive me crazy".

PSOR. Al,N-46 - Attacks of fear; fear of fire, of being alone, of apoplexy, of becoming insane.

PULS. He, 21 - Continuous crying with great melancholy and fear of losing her reason, or that she might commit suicide.

SPONG. He, 11 - Crazy feeling, head feels blown up.

STRAM. Al, 23 - Violent delirium; whith was alternately mirthful, furious or dolorous (sad), directed to some imaginary source of pleasure or repugnance, and accompanied which corresponding gesticulations.

Ha, 507 - He fears he is losing his senses. (sanity)

He, 71 - Fears; he will lose his senses (insanity); his lips will grow together; to suffocate; of falling; everything is falling on her.

SULPH. Al, 3824 - The first three nights he rose from bed in a somnambulistic way, as if unconscious; cried, "My head, my head! I am crazy!" grasped his forehead; ...

Ha, 61 - Great inclination to philosophic and religious ravings.(insanity)

He, 13 - A little girl with religious insanity, takes passages of Scripture literally and acts upon them. (fanatical) (virtuous, noble, elevated)

He, 3-...feels as if crazy; does not know whether she has done what she intended (planned) or whether objects seen are really there, or whether she only imagines them to be, until she has touched them;...

SUMB. He, 2 - Happy disposition with continued smiling; expression idiotic; fear of becoming insane.

SYPH. Al,N-8 - Feeling as if going insane, or about to be paralyzed.

He, 10 - Feeling as if going insane, or about be paralyzed.

TARENT. Al, 2 - Insanity on account of an unfortunate love.

Al, 18 - Fourteen days after taking the medicine, the happy mood reached the borders of mania; the disposition to joke and laugh was extreme.

THUJ. Al, 1 - She herself desires, with anxiety and despair, to be taken to an insane asylum, (imprisonment, confining) and there to be treated very harshly and strictly, (penalized), so that her fixed ideas may be subdued and banished (purified); she knows very well that she does wrong (conscience) and thinks all sorts of bad thoughts (immoral), but she will not take the trouble to banish such thoughts; therewith she indistinctly gives to understand that she is constantly obliged to think of taking her own life, but feels the sinfulness (wicked) of it, in order to avoid it, desires the strict restraint of the asylum;...

Al, 2 - She fancies that she has intentionally represented herself as insane (feigning) in the presence of others in order to palliate a wrong supposed to have been done (penitence, remorse), and that now she is punished, therefore, by real insanity.

TUB. Al,N-11 - Felt positively ugly (repulsive, spiteful); personal aversions became almost a mania.

Al,N-45 - Insanity; acute or chronic, with a family history of tubercular affections.

INTEGRATION

Delusions; bed, covered the whole bed, she: pyrog.[139]
- body, covered whole, bed: pyrog
- body, covered whole, earth: cann-i.
- bones in fragments and cannot fit pieces together: phos.[54]
- connected, everything is: ozone[227]
- connected, feels connected to ground through feet: germ.[222]
- depending, everything is depending on them: lil-t.[168]
- eternity, mingled with present: anh.[119]

Dreams; person, creeps into another: ozone[227]

Ecstasy; sublime: crot-h.[36]

Ecstasy; sublime, impression, as after: lach.[36]

Heavenly sensation: arg.[54] calc-ar.[54] crot-h.[36]

Integrity, sensation of: nat-m.[189] nux-v.[189] plat.[162]

Love; nature, for: carc.[162] lap-c-b.[194]

Merging of self with one's environment: anh.[119]

Religious affections; happy to join her Redeemer, felt, in facial erysipelas: ***plat.***[54]

Unification; higher consciousness with: hydrog.[222]

ADAM. Sh, 303 - I feel connected with my children, that a barrier I've erected due to the fear of losing them has gone. 8, 6C, 20:XX:XX

CHOC. Sh, 74 - I saw a rat. We stood looking at each other. I felt we both recognised each other. It was very exciting.

Sh, 128 - The separation that I have always felt seems to be gone and I feel much more part of what's around.

Sh, 135 - The earth has taken on a new meaning. Before it was just there, now it has everything. A desire to be in contact with the earth.

Sh, 182 - This remedy is making me look more deeply into things. Found myself looking into a flower, plugging into its inner substance. 35, 30C, 05:XX:XX

Sh, 306 - Her usual sensation of left right body split has been much more defined. Later on during the proving this "split" became more balanced than usual and felt much more integrated, (curative).13, 12C, 02:XX:XX

Sh, 315 - Been on the move all day — painted a room blue. While lying in the bath looking out the window, the sky is the most glorious, vibrant blue —it seems like the most beautiful colour I've ever seen. Almost wept for the beauty of it. Suddenly, while I'm lying in the bath, the colour blue seems very important — seems very potent. It has the same quality and intensity that I remember colours having on L.S.D. I am very moved by this blue. I wanted to dissolve into it.15, 30C, 03:05:XX

GERM. Sh, 131 - Suddenly aware of my feet standing on the ground and feeling very connected to the ground through my feet. Rooted to the spot. Wanted to stay that way. Good feelings. Feet feeling at one with the ground. 04, 6C, 00.13.30.

Sh, 26 - Feel more aware and connected looking at the sun trees and sky colors. 04, 6C, 01.00.00.

Sh, 154 - When outside and looking at people thought to myself I know them. People were friendlier to me. Thought I could start a conversation with strangers . 07, 30C, 00.06.00.

Sh, 159 - People seem friendlier in the streets in London. Felt like I'd made some sort of contact -people smile at me and were chatty. 13, 30C, 02:XX:XX

Sh, 148 - The last days I have had moments when I have felt I have been united to the world and people - to humanity. Have felt more love and reconciliation towards myself and other people. Started to be more conscious about the environment and what I can do to our mutual benefit. Something is happening within me. I wish to get more contact with my feelings. 18, 30C, 64:XX:XX

HALI-L. Sh, 84 - Sensitive to energy. A lot of synchronicity going on. At a seminar, the teacher talked about the same topic I wrote a paper on. I met people from the same town I grew up in. When I wanted to get on to another subject, someone else would bring it up. I'd just answer the teacher's questions and it would be right. 08, 30C, 12:XX:XX

Sh, 605 - The remedy accelerated the personas out of me, and along with them, all these other problems. It forced me to look at all of it. Then my "I" came out! Has happened before but this was much more magnified. With the remedy, none of the fragmented personalities were willing to get behind the wheel and drive. It was like being driven, without going anywhere. Then, I slowly started seeing that these personas were just rationalizations that just didn't suffice. It helped me to come out to face them. With the remedy, I quickly pulled them together. 18, 30C, 35:XX:XX

Sh, 642 - I read prayers for safety before bed because I was afraid of what might happen when I went to sleep. When I came to the phrase "God is One" I realized that was the crux of it— the universe was cracked or split instead of one. Saying that prayer feels healing. Oneness is about caring; the split is about not caring. It's evil in a way. 06, 6C, 01:00:XX

Sh, 645 - Caring equals oneness. A scary point about that acute phase yesterday— there was no caring. It didn't matter. Nothing mattered. I was alone and wanted to be that way. To have caring, there must be an attunement with the oneness of the universe. Is that where Hitler came from? The crack in the universe? 06, 6C, 01:09:00

Sh, 676 - The remedy worked very directly on my will. Fragmentation is the denial of will. Integration is the use of will. All separate states under a unified country. 18, 30C, 35:XX:XX

HYDROG. Sh, 15 - I felt in the presence of a totally pure energy, like meeting God and feeling totally unworthy or like meeting a lover and feeling unworthy — realizing all the mistakes of a lifetime. This pure energy was around for some time protecting me. I feel this unification cleared out lifetimes of symptomatology for me. The joining with this energy was as if a male energy joined with me sexually, but with no desire, pleasure or pain involved. This unification with the male energy lasted quite a few days — I'm not used to seeing myself as a man. The morning after this unifying with the higher presence, I collapsed in emotional overflow. All my grief and pain came out. I was doubled upon the floor and went into a deep state of catharsis. It is not possible to describe where I went as there are no concepts applicable. I felt overflowing love for humanity and wanted to give everything away. My mind turned to the Buddha. It was like seeing the complete picture instead of fragmented bits. (These primary effects lasted about 28 days, then changing to a paranoia state). 16, 30C, 07.XX.XX

Sh, 26 - Felt inspired that the potential within is so great and we have a possibility of becoming whole and suddenly it comes crashing down into a sort of mundane realization —that the physical world would never reach the potential possible — like losing a dream. This is really bringing me down. 16, 30C, 08:XX:XX

Sh, 98 - It seems as if all the days became one. 16, 30C, XX:XX:XX

Sh, 100 - I was having problems assimilating the notion of time, outside time seemed beyond description. I Couldn't differentiate between backwards and forwards in time. Felt I had got stuck in time. 16, 30C, 10:XX:XX

IRID. Sh-7 - Abnormal mental awareness, very conscious of nature, everything seemed very vivid, very lovely. Profound feeling. F22

Sh, 18 - Sitting still and staring into space, feeling very defined and contained in my body again, as if in an invisible capsule. Warm in my own air and lack of thoughts inside. This state tends to happen when I'm in a warmish place, don't think it could happen outside. People's chatter washes over me, I don't notice them or their talk. Body feels exactly like when you've just woken up and don't want to move. E7

Sh, 20 - Skin to skin, started stroking arms, arms to face, hands to arms to face, then down body acutely aware of boundaries of body. Q1

Sh, 21 - The edges of my body felt very defined as if surrounded by warm skin or air. Very pleasant. The edges very clear, especially the back and top of arms, my neck and my back as if I've just woken in my own little capsule of warmth. E11

Sh, 22 - I feel whole and connected to everything, yet at the same time I feel I unreal, my boundaries don't feel the same. I1

Sh, 41 - Bumped into people I hadn't seen for ages, some for maybe six years. D24

Sh, 40 - Hairdresser cut my hair. I felt quite close to her though I don't really know her. Had these feelings of being closer to people. D11

Sh, 57 - On the bus a woman turned to me and said, "Your eyes are the same as my daughter's." Baby like me. I knew we had met before, knew that I knew her. She knew me as well. A wonderful moment. Q7

Sh, 67 - Sensation of movement in face as if head, face and skin full of magnetism. Sense of alignment. Q2

NEON. 5 - I've always really liked odd numbers. I suddenly felt the capacity to be even. Even numbers were much more attractive. It felt like I'd never known even numbers and now I did. Half was missing. Now, it was like a new toy of evenness. Before I had gaps and I was jumping; now I could move smoothly. It's like there was too big a gap at the synapses. Now there was no gap between the source and the action. 20, 6C, 01:01:17

Sh, 6 - Occasional thoughts about numbers: I had always felt comfortable with odd numbers. Now, being both gave a whole other dimension. To have had half missing for so long! What is different? From 3 to 1, slight tension. From 2 to 1, effortless natural progression. I had many thoughts on potency. It was important to chose the potency precisely, not to be so random in choosing a 9, 12, 15 etc. 20, 6C, 02:01:02

Sh, 8 - I had thoughts of odd and even numbers. I felt I had always jumped up from 3 to 1. That made me too high. I now feel that I need to work my way down, 1-2-3. In the past, it was easier for me to go up than come down. Now I feel that I can go down or either way. 20, 6C, 06:03:XX

Sh, 11 - Doing research on Uranus, I found that the planet has a tilt. For 42 years one side is in the dark and then comes into the light for 42 years. Interesting that I am now 43. Uranus feels very near, like a friend. The quasars are much further out and it was a real stretch for me to go so far. 20, 6C, XX:XX:XX

Sh, 21 - Walking was effortless, light and free, with a sensation of walking uniformly. I feel so different in my body. I am all in the now, especially in lower legs and feet. At last, I touch the earth. 20, 6C, 03:01:00

Sh, 34 - I feel more stable now that my feet touch the earth while still having my head touching the heavens. 20, 6C, 04:XX:XX

Sh, 53 - While lying awake in bed last night I heard a dinging sound, like glass or the sound of icicles tapping against each other. I looked but couldn't locate it. I tried to ignore it but the sound increased. I got up, went to the bedroom window and looked over the back garden. It was a fantastic cold, clear night. With a thrill of excitement I watched all the stars in the sky above and I just knew that the noise I'd heard was the stars trying to communicate with me. The noise seemed to last for ages. The thrill lasted for as long as I stood by the window. When I went back to bed I felt wonderful. The noise stopped. 02, 6C, 06:XX:XX

Sh, 54 - I just long for some clear nights, so I can see my stars. If I could reconnect, then everything would be all right. 02, 6C, 11:XX:XX

Sh, 57 - Felt wonderful. Kept going outside during the night, between midnight and 3 am. At last the sky was clear, moon brilliant, stars familiar, air cold. I felt so much a part of everything again. 20, 6C, 06:19:XX

Sh, 163 - My head above the eyes cleared. It felt like a very wide opening from the top of my head outward. I felt a total synchronicity. I didn't have to get to a thought, bring it up, act. I was observing the mechanics of thought instead of needing them. It was effortless. While I felt I wasn't having thoughts, I was still doing everything I usually do. Everything was more beautiful. There was total order in space, more stable. This was a contrast for me. I usually feel chaotic. 20, 6C, XX:XX:XX

INTOLERANCE

Ailments from; intolerance: nux-v.[36]

Contradiction; intolerant of: acon. aesc.[102] alco.[36] aloe alum. alum-sil.[58] am-c. anac.[162] ***ant-c.***[102] arn.[102] ars. asaf.[102] asar.[102] aster. **AUR.** bell.[102] ***bry.*** cact. calc-p. cann-i. cann-s.[85] canth.[102] ***caps.***[102] carbn-s.[36] carc.[122] cham.[88] chin.[102] ***cina***[98] ***cocc.*** ***colch.***[102] coloc.[102] con. echi. ***ferr.*** flav.[149] gall-ac.[162] glon.[102] grat. hecla.[234] hell.[36] ***helon.*** hep.[102] hura hyos.[5] ictod.[10] **IGN.** kali-i.[163] lach.[102] lact.[85] **LYC.** med.[122] merc. mez.[102] morph.[102] mur-ac.[102] ***nat-c.***[122] ***nat-m.***[102] nicc. nit-ac.[5] nuph.[36] nux-v. olnd. ***op.***[54] pall.[102] petr. phos.[102] plan. ***plat.***[102] prot.[136] puls.[102] sars.[102] **SEP.** ***sil.*** ***staph.***[102] stram. ***sulph.***[54] syph.[36] tarent. thuj. thyr.[102] til. tub.[212] ***verat.***[30]

Contradiction; intolerant of, shudders, blood boils with prickling: elaps[54]

Contradiction; intolerant of, throw themselves angrily on the floor and cannot get their breath when in the least opposed: thuj.[8]

Intolerance: ars.[30] bar-c.[30] caust.[30] choc.[222] con.[30] lac-h.[229] merc.[36] psor.[122]

Intolerance; annoyance: ferr-p.[36]

Intolerance; interruption, of: cham.[36] cocc.[36] germ.[222]

Intolerance; spoken to, of being: cham.[36]

Intolerance; vexation of: ferr-p.[36]

Intolerance; wind, of: caust.[60] ***cham.***[60] lach.[60] sel.[137]

ANDROC. Sh, 101 - Can't avoid shouting at people she was intolerant of, could not hide her feelings. More impatient with others and herself. (7)

CHOC. Sh, 328 - Humourless, intolerant -almost cruel. Scalded a child's hand out of anger, and nothing would make him apologise.[35], 30C, XX:XX:XX:

Sh, 331 - I became selfish, impatient and intolerant. Behaved in a strange way -hard and quarrelsome -snapping at people. Could not stand people wasting time or being inefficient, I wanted things done immediately.[35], 30C, XX:XX:XX:

INVADED

Delusions; animals, ants, bed seems full of: plb.
- animals, bed, on: ars.[10] colch. ***plb.***[122] stram. valer.
- animals, black, on walls and furniture, sees: bell. stram.[162]
- animals, snakes, in and around her: abel.[162] ail.[58] anh.[119] bell. calc. gels.[111] ***hyos. lac-c.*** lach. lachn.[111] op. phyt.[30] ***stram.***[8] tub.[56]
- baby, two in bed: petr.
- bed, evening, some one would get into and no room in it, or as if some one had sold it: nux-v.
- bed, occupied by another person: petr.[102]
- bed, someone, in with him: anac. apis ***bapt.*** carb-v. graph.[116] nux-v. ***op.***[54] ***petr.***[54] ***puls.*** rhus-t. sec. stram. valer.
- bed, someone, in with him, two persons in bed with her: cycl. petr.[162]
- bed, someone, tries to take away the bed clothes: bell.
- bed, strange boy prevents sleep: apis[54]
- bells, hears, door bell: thea.
- couriers, three are coming: sep.[1]
- dead, corpse, tall yellow c. trying to share bed with him and promptly ejected: bell.
- door, someone was coming in at the (at night): con.
- enemy, under the bed, is: am-m.
- entering, someone is (at night): con.[36]
- furniture is persons, night on waking: nat-p.
- house, people, full of: ars. cann-i. con. lach. lyc. merc. nat-m. nux-v. sil. stram.
- lying, near him, someone: petr.
- man, bed, on, at night: merc.
- man, huge drunk man coming toward her, who lies down beside her, she begs him to retire, falls into convulsions and turns over on her abdomen: cic.[54]
- people, entering the house at night: con.
- person, another in the room: anac.[1] brom.[111] cann-i. con.[111] hyos.[139] lyc.[5]
- policeman, come into house, he sees: ars.[58] hyos. kali-br.
- room, sees people bedside in: atro. con.
- room, sees people, entering, on: lyc.
- rowdies, brawlers, will break in if she is alone: elaps.[139]
- soldier, sees, bed, on his: lact.
- strangers, room, seem to be in the: bry.[10] ***tarent. thuj.***
- strangers, sees, every night since six weeks, causing fear, had to leave bed, a old woman: ***stram.***[54]
- strangers, snatching at her: ***bell.***[54]
- thieves, dream, after a, and will not believe the contrary until search is made: nat-m. sanic.[85]
- thieves, house, and space under bed are full of that: ***ars.***
- thieves, house, in: ars. cann-i. con.[30] ***cupr-acet.***[54] ***lach.*** merc. ***nat-m.*** sil. sol-t-ae.
- thieves, jump out of window, therefore wants to: ***lach.***[54]
- train or car in his ear: ***stram.***[54]
- vagina, living things creep into (at night): merc.
- window should be closed: lyss.[54]
- women, bedside, by: med.[54]
- women, his mothers house is invaded by lewd: kali-br.

Dreams; animals, toad in bed: allox.[119]
- ➤ another person lying in bed with him: petr.
- ➤ dead, bodies, bed, in, are put in bed with her: ozone[227]
- ➤ lying, bed, in, with another person: petr.[58]
- ➤ lying, someone is lying under him: nit-ac.[1]
- ➤ robbers, breaking into house and trying to kill her: mag-c.[36]
- ➤ robbers, house, want to go into: ozone[227]
- ➤ toilet, is sitting on the, the door opens constantly: ozone[227]

Fear; death, noise of door moving, from, in dark: ozone[227]
- ✦ door, bell ringing, on hearing: lyc.[137]

✦ door, closed, lest the d. should be: lac-d.[122]
✦ door, opening the: cic.[111] con.[111] lyc.[111]
✦ invaded, of being: lap-gr-m.[194]
✦ noise, from, door, at: ***aur.*** cic. ***lyc.***
✦ robbers, waking on: merc.[10] nat-m.[10] sil.[10]
Searching; thieves, for, at night: ars.

ADAM. Sh, 129 - Irritability about intrusion of space by my house guest. I felt hemmed in. 11, 30C, 07.XX.XX
Sh, 223 - Anger with aggressive attitude, short tempered and intolerant. I lashed out verbally when my partner invaded my space. I knew it was out of proportion at the time. 7, 6C, 30:00:XX
APIS. He, 19 - A strange boy lying in bed with him prevents (restrict) sleep.
ARS. Ha, 34 - He sees nothing but worms and bugs crawling about on his bed, from which he desires to run away (escape) and of which he throws out whole hands full.
Ha, 35 - He sees nothing but rogues in his room, and therefore always creeps under the bed.
Ha, 36 - His whole house, also under his bed, is full of rogues, which causes a cold sweat to break out, which runs down cold over his body.
Ha, 37 - In the night he runs all about the house, looking for thieves.
AUR. Ha, 348 - A noise before the door made him anxious; he feared lest some one would come in; like anthropophobia.
Ha, 14 - Anxiousness; even a noise before the door makes him anxious; he is afraid some one might come in; as if afraid of men.
BELL. Al,S-2552-...the yellow corpse of a tall man, shrouded (dressed, clothes) in white, tried to share the patient's bed with him, and the unwelcome visitor was promptly ejected. A crimson serpent came from the foot of the bed, with the design of fastening upon the patient's neck...
Ha, 1339 - Raves (delirious) about wolves being in the room; at the same time full pulse.
He, 18 - When closing eyes, though not asleep, patient sees fierce (wild), wicked looking large animals with horns and bushy (scabrous) heads; room seemed to be full of strange men passing in and out, who would snatch (take hold) at her as they passed, which frightened her very much, she thought the men wanted to take her away from home ; she then saw children sitting on low benches (seat) in rows (line) as in a school-room. (purity)
CANTH. Al, 16 - Visions at night, when half awake; she heard soft steps in the room, then knocking under the bed, and the bed was raised up.
CHAM. He, 14-..., vows there is some dreadful beast under his bed or in the room, and will not be appeased (calm) until the gas is lit and the room is searched.
CIC. He, 9 - She thinks she sees coming towards her a huge drunken man, who lies down alongside of her, she begs him to retire...
CON. Ha, 14 - He imagines that somebody has come in at the door by night.
HALI-L. Sh, 567 - Had to leave my house to study elsewhere, due to an unpleasant visitor at home. Someone I can't stand being around came to visit my partner and see our puppies. He wouldn't ask her to leave. I didn't want to engage with her, because there is no way you can win. If I had said, "It's time to go, now," then I am the ogre. There are no boundaries. 13, 30C, 00:06:00
Sh, 598 - Calmness continued, with the exception of seeing ants in my house. They had invaded my house, and I was irritated that I had to kill them and clean them up. I don't like to kill anything. My heart was racing and my face was sweaty while doing this. 03, 12C, 00:XX:XX
HYDROG. Sh, 243 - Fear that someone was trying to find out if I was home so that they could come and rape and murder me. 16, 30C, XX:XX:XX
HYOS. Al, 5-...suspicious of those about him; he became delirious, saw policeman coming into the house; heard them speaking about the hall;...
IRID. Sh, 82 - Last three Fridays, since proving began, have gone to bed very early. Really exhausted. Realized that part of the going to bed is to be by myself — needed space in bed, alone and quiet. Rare for me to go to bed and leave daughters up watching TV. Could hear it and felt it

invading my space. G26
Sh, 83 - It feels like my personality has been invaded, taken over. I7

KALI-BR. Al, 3 - Decidedly insane; had delusions that lewd women had got into his mother's house; that he was pursued by the police; that his wife was threatened by members of the family; that he had thousands of dollars in gold sewed up in his clothing; (rich, wealth)

LYC. Al, 50 - In the evening on entering a room he is attacked with fear, as though he saw some one; even during the day he believes that he hears some one in the room.
Ha, 27 - He is afraid (fear) in the evening, on entering a room, as if he saw somebody; by day also he sometimes imagines he hears somebody in the room.

LYSS. Al,N-28 - Complains bitterly that a fire has been lighted and that the stove is smoking, although there is no fire; another continually directed a window to be closed, which was not opened. (fear suffocation?)

MAG-C. Al, 959 - Dream of thieves who broke into the house and tried to kill her.

MED. He, 19 - One night saw large (big) people in room; large rats running; felt a delicate hand smoothing her head from front to back. (caressed)

MERC-I-F. Al, 1 - While in bed, he imagined that a man was in his room who intended to perforate his throat with a gimlet;...

NUX-V. Al, 1 - Anxious delirious fantasies, in the evening in bed, in the ninth hour, as if some one would get into his bed,(base, foundation) and there was no room (space) in it; or as if some one had sold his bed etc.

OP. He, 20-...declares he is not alone in bed; ..desire to escape; says a regiment of horsemen are upon his bed and that he fears to be trodden upon (run over, crushed); when told that horses are very careful, answered that he feared he would be crushed by the wagons that followed them.

PHOS. Al, 12-...; wherever he turned his eyes he saw faces; they swarmed (crowded, surrounded) by him in long panoramic succession; they leered (look lecherous) at him over the footboard of the bed; they squinted (look) at him though the windows, or came trooping (crowd) in when the doors were left ajar (open) (invade);..he fancied he was some one else, ...

PLAT. Ha, 15 - At odds (quarreling) with all the world, everything is too close (near, intimate) for her, with inclination to weep. (persecution)

SIL. Al, 21 - He woke with great anxiety about midnight, could not move in spite of every effort, and imagined that thieves were breaking in; on rising he became quiet, after lying down the anxiety returned.

STRAM. He, 63 - An old lady had a vision every night since six weeks, in which many persons, all strangers, came into her room and to her bedside, causing her such fear that she had to leave bed.

TARENT. Al, 12-...Hallucinations (delirium) sees strangers (aliens) in the room.

VERAT. He, 13 - After severe illness, aversion to husband and children; desire to leave house: hallucinations, room appeared full of people, crowding in, there was no longer room...

INVERSION

Delusions; bed, turning, is: nux-v.[139] plb.[139] puls.[139] sin-n.[139]
- bed, turning, is, circle, in a: con.[139] sol-n.[139]
- body, head, circle, going around in a: bry.[139] tub.[139]
- body, heart, turning around, is: aur.
- dimensions of things reversed (turned): camph-br.[102]
- directions seem to be reversed: camph-br.[102]
- hearing, of, sounds, are coming from left side when they really come from the right: ***nat-c.***[122]
- lying, upside down: calc.[1] calc-acet.[1]
- side, left and right side are not the same: bamb-a.[1184]

Dreams; actors, turning black, green and yellow: sol-t-ae.[36]
➤ body, brain revolving upwards from frontal sinus to occiput: phys.[36]
➤ turning around: lact.[10]

ADAM. Sh, 8 - Watched past emotions float away in reverse order. 16, 12C, 00:00:20

NEON. Sh, 88 - I remembered the incidences in dreams in the reverse order in which they happened—very unusual for me. 20, 6C, 01:01:55

Sh, 93 - I was confused about my watch. I couldn't tell which way was up on the clock face. 20, 6C, 00:01:50

IRRESOLUTION

Irresolution; evening, obstacles from: ferr-p.[36]

Irresolution; impulsive though, when decision is made: m-arct.[85]

Irresolution; marry, to, avarice, from: lyc.[148]

Restlessness; internal, indecision to do something, with: bamb-a.[1184]

ACT-SP. He, 17 - Irresolution, inconstancy and caprice.

ALUM. Al, 44 - Great absence of mind and irresolution.(undecided)

Ha, 39 - Great absent-mindedness and irresolution.

AM-C. Ha, 9 - Many afternoons she is seized with weakness and timidity, so that she cannot control herself and knew not what to do;...

ANAC. Ha, 37 - He can only think when a subject is suggested to him; he does not of himself think of anything; he cannot independently determine anything.

APIS. Al, 23 - It seems to her as if she did not know what to do, as if she had no volition (desire) of her own, her head feels stupid.

ARS. Ha, 1044 - Recurring fits of irresolution; he wishes something and when one attempts (try) to gratify his wish the merest trifle will alter his resolution, and he wishes it no longer.

Ha, 40 - Lack determination (indetermination); he desires something, and when the endeavor (try) is made to fulfill his desire; the merest trifle will change his determination and he is not willing to have it so.

BAR-A. Al, 13 - He wavers for a long time between opposite resolutions.(irresolute, indecision)

Al, 14 - During the day she resolves to undertake a certain matter in the evening, but scarcely is the time come when she repents it, and is undecided whether she shall do it or not.

Al, 15 - Extreme irresolution ; he proposes a short journey, but as soon as he makes preparation he changes his mind, and is inclined to remain at home.

BAR-C. Al, 16 - Great irresolution about small things; he wants to drink the cup of coffee, then again not, does not know what he shall do.

Ha, 12 - The greatest irresolution; he proposes to himself a brief journey, and as soon as he is to make his preparation, he is sorry for it and prefers to stay at home.

Ha, 13 - Long wavering between opposing resolutions.

Ha, 14 - During the day she determines to attend (take care) to some particular matter; but scarcely (just) has the time come, when she is sorry (give up) for it, and she knows not for irresolution what to do to leave undone.

BUFO-S. Al, 7 - He is unable to act with decision (doubtful) ; he forms projects and does not accomplish (succeed) them.

CHAM. Ha, 465 - Very anxious; nothing she does seems to her to be right; she is irresolute; ...(indecisive)

CON. Ha, 367 - Peevish disposition; he knows not what to occupy himself with, the times appears to pass too slowly.

Ha, 20 - Peevish mood, he does not know what to do with himself, the time passes too slow for him.

CUPR. Al, 13 - Irresolute; satisfied with nothing; this only lasts as long as he is fretful.

CUR. He, 1 - Indecision, no longer (more) wishes to think and act for herself.

DIG. He, 12 - Desponding (sad) and irresolute.(indecisive)

FERR-MA. Al-S, 4 - Irresolute; he considers for a long time before commencing anything .

GRAPH. Al, 43 - Extreme hesitation (doubtful); she is unable to make up her mind about anything.

Al, 45 - She was usually very quick to resolve, but soon after taking was very slow of thought and resolution.

Ha, 25 - Though usually quick to decide, she, soon after taking the medicine, becomes slow of recollection (memory) and resolution.(determination)

GRAT. Al, 16 - Irresolute; no persistence in work.

He, 1 - Irresolute (wavering); want of perseverance. (determination)
HYDROG. Sh, 64 - Irresolution about what she is going to do with her life. 14, 15C, 04:XX:XX
Sh, 131 - Marked tendency to panic at little things that go wrong or small decisions to be made. 08, 30C, 00:XX:XX
HYOS. He, 13 - Does not know whether or not to take what is offered.
IGN. Ha, 770 - Fickle, impatient, irresolute, quarrelsome.
He, 36 - Anxiety as though something terrible had happened cannot speak because of it; hurry, fearfulness, terror, alternating with irresolution and inertness.
KALI-C. Ha, 20 - Irresolution.
LED. Al, 11 - Morose mood, with much uneasiness and irresolution; he is unable to reflect constantly upon anything, or work with a quiet mind.
LIL-T. Al, 45 - She can't think; acts without thought; keeps walking fast as though by instinct; feels hurried, but doesn't know why; is forgetful, can't decide for herself; must depend on others.
LYC. Al, 127 - Indecision and loss of confidence.
LYSS. Al, 36 - Undecided about little things.
He, 84 - Indecision even in small matters.
MERC. He, 29 - Anxiety and apprehension; did not know what to do ; it seemed as though he had committed a crime ; without heat; also with a feeling that he had not control over his senses.
MEZ. Al, 38 - It becomes difficult for him to make a resolution.
Ha, 17 - He finds it difficult to come to a determination.
He, 4 - Irresolute (undecided); mind easily confused, unable to recollect; thinking is difficult.
NAJA. Al, 12 - Sadness or serious disposition; sadness and irresolution.
NAT-C. Ha, 23 - Restlessness and unsteadiness (inconstant); he knew not what he wanted, nor what he should do or leave undone.
Ha, 24 - Sensation of irresolution, in the morning.
NAT-M. Al, 132 - Irresolute at work; he could not see his way clearly.
Ha, 90 - Irresolution in doing mental work; he cannot easily find his way.
He, 2 - Absent minded or distracted while talking; does not know what he ought (have to) say; awkward in talking; easily makes mistakes.
NUX-M. Al, 24 - Variable mood; at one time he wishes to do something, but when he is about to accomplish it changes his mind.
He, 25 - Fickle (capricious); irresolute and wavering in his undertakings.
NUX-V. Al, 68 - Irresolution; constant fickleness in his plans.
Al, 69 - Dawdles (delay) and is irresolute.
Ha, 1256 - Anxious solicitude (care) and irresolution.
Ha, 1288 - Irresolution, constant hesitation in his intentions.
PETR. Ha, 8 - The greatest irresolution.
Ha, 9 - Lack of determination.(resolution)
He, 6 - Excitable, irritable with inclination to be angry and to scold; anxious and irresolute.
PULS. Al, 44 - Shuns business, is irresolute, with sighing respiration and a feeling as if he were beside himself.
He, 9 - Shuns business; irresolute; sighing respiration; feels as if he were beside himself.
SANT. Al, 6-...irresolution and want of confidence in my own powers as to render me quite unfit for work of any kind;
TAB. Al, 19 - Low spirits, want of resolution and general hypochondriasis.
Al, 45 - He was incapacitated for business of any kind, weak irresolute, and despondent.
TARAX. Al, 4 - Without occupation he is quite gloomy; does not know what to do, and cannot make up his mind to do anything.
Al, 6 - Irresolution and dread of work, though it progresses well as soon as he undertakes it.
He, 3 - Undecided, shunning (avoid) labor, but after beginning, works well.
TARENT. Al, 76-...changeable mind, tears, singing, and irresoluteness.(In a woman, twenty-six years old, who complained of violent sexual appetite.)
YUC. Al, 6-4 p.m. irresolute, changing mind once in fifteen minutes; don't know what to do; can't keep easy.

ISOLATION

Ascetic: diosm.[72]
Autism, mutinism: agra.[137] kali-br.[187] lyc.[137] tub.[187]
Delusions; coating around him, has a white: ozone[227]
- detached: hydrog.[222] lap-gr-m.[194]
- division between himself and others: hydrog.[222] nat-c.[58]
- faces, every ones face in a glass except his own: anac.[85]
- family, does not belong to her own: plat.
- far off: med.[139]
- hearing, of, sounds, distant, are: coca[25] lac-c.[137] sabal.[137]
- hearing, talk seems distant: aran.[149]
- hole, views the world through a: androc.[222]
- island, is on a distant, enjoying the tranquillity : phos.
- mind, going out of his, he is: ambr.[85] calc.[31] cot.[36] eup-per.[8] ham.[8] ***kali-br.***[8] ***lac-c.***[56] nit-ac.[85] ol-j.[139] paraf.[38] petr.[85] visc.[77]
- places, none in the world, she has: germ.[222] ***plat.***[54]
- separated, world, from the, that he is: ***anac.*** androc.[222] ***anh.***[119] carc.[227] choc.[222] germ.[222] **HYDROG.** thiop.[149] ven-m.[149]
- stranger, he is a: germ.[222] nat-m.[111] valer.
- strangers, amongst: aster.[137]
- world, she has her own little, in which things are clear, the outside is uncertain: camph.[54]

Desires; cavity, to be in: elaps.[36]
Detached: androc.[222] choc.[222] germ.[222] lac-h.[229]
Detached; ego, from: lac-h.[229]
Discontented; life, cut off from: bamb-a.[1184]
Dreams; clothes, wearing many layers of: hydrog.[222]
➤ separating from people: ozone[227]
Estranged; climacteric period, in: ***aster.***[122] cycl.[122] hipp.[122] ***lach.***[122] ***lil-t.***[122] ***puls.***[122] ***sep.***[122] ***sulph.***[122] ther.[122] ***verat.***[122]
Estranged; convulsions, during: cimic.[54]
Estranged; family, from her: am-c.[30] anac. arn.[85] ars. choc.[222] con. hep. hydrog.[222] lap-c-b.[194] ***nat-c.*** ***nat-m.*** nat-s. ***nit-ac.*** nux-v.[30] phos. plat. psor.[58] ***sep.*** staph.[30]
Estranged; flies her own children: lyc.
Estranged; forgetful of relatives and friends: lap-c-b.[194] lyss.[54]
Estranged; friends, from: hydrog.[222] nat-c.[58]
Estranged; ignores his relatives: bell.[5] hyos.[5] merc.[5] verat.[5]
Estranged; society, from: anac. choc.[222] lap-c-b.[194]
Estranged; strangers, being kind with, but not with his family and entourage: lyc.[30] nux-v.[30] puls.[30] verat.[30]
Estranged; wife, from his: ars. nat-c.[58] plat. staph.
Far away; as if, with apathy and indifference to the future: med.[137] syph.[54]
Fear; introversion, of: carc.[207]
Forsaken; feeling, isolation, sensation of: allox.[119] ***anac.*** ***androc.*** ***anh.***[119] ***arg-n.*** arist-cl.[149] camph. cann-i. cann-s.[36] choc.[222] coca cortico.[144] germ.[222] hura ***hydrog.*** lac-h.[229] lap-mar-c.[194] merc.[187] op.[231] ozone[227] pip-m.[231] plat. psil.[231] puls.[193] sac-alb.[210] stram. tab.[231]
Forsaken; feeling, isolation, sensation of, talking, on, people do not hear him: cortico.[119]
Haughty; weaning, over: grat.[137]
Indifference; family, to his: carb-v.[58] hell.[36] lap-gr-m.[194] nat-p.[58] nit-ac.[116] **PHOS.**[122] **SEP.**[122]
Indifference; relations, to: acon.[58] bac.[62] ***fl-ac.*** **HELL.** hep. hydrog.[222] kali-p.[58] lap-gr-m.[194] nat-c. nat-p.[58] **PHOS.**[122] plat. **SEP.**[122] ***syph.***[122]
Memory; active, past events, remembered as belonging to someone else, or as matter read: ail.[54]
Sadness; sits in corner and does not want to have anything to do with the world: ***hipp.***[54]
Weeping; emotions, lack of emotions, about her: ozone[227]

ADAM. Sh, 6 - Felt really strong love for children. Looking at daughter had a feeling of a barrier being lifted or a cloud lifted from me. Felt I could really see her, that she was mine; of me but separate. 8, 6C, 02:XX:XX

Sh, 119 - Feel drawn in on myself; don't find it easy to extend outwards. 8, 6C, 04:XX:XX

Sh, 150 - Felt separate from friends today, which was unusual. I felt outside them. I was quiet. Definitely unusual. 5, 30C, 00:06:50

Sh, 151 - The "cloud" feeling has left me with a sense of detachedness and separateness. 7, 6C, 04:08:00
Sh, 152 - I feel the separateness of me from the world, not my spirit from my body, the whole of me, I can't touch the world. 7, 6C, 04:08:00
Sh, 153 - I feel very irritated, I need to maintain separateness to keep the grumpiness to myself. 7, 6C, 04:08:00
Sh, 155 - I am feeling disconnected from what is going on in my relationship. It's hard to understand why she couldn't take my overall viewpoint. She seems stuck. I cut off and disconnected from her. 7, 6C, 14:00:XX
Sh, 157 - I am allowing myself to be detached and not fighting it. 7, 6C, 04:19:00
Sh, 158 - I feel detached and not sexual. I could bite my partner as a signal I loved her, not in a loving or hungry way. My partner said, "He is looking at me like a piece of steak, he wants to eat me. He looks like a cave man. He wants to nibble me." 7, 6C, 03:22:30
Sh, 159 - I felt detached during coition. 7, 6C, 13:23:00
Sh, 163 - A distant feeling, as if I'm not totally here, with need to blink left eye as if to clear it. 8, 6C, 20:00:00
Sh, 165 - I feel like I'm looking at the world through half-closed eyes, like slits. 7, 6C, 09:00:XX
Sh, 170 - Husband's description: "You are like Alice in Wonderland in an unreal world." 10, 6C, XX:XX:XX
Sh, 182 - Feel disconnected and distanced from everything. It's like keeping something in reserve, more observing. 7, 6C, 06:22:30
Sh, 183 - I couldn't get involved in the conversation at family supper. I didn't feel the need to. I spent most of the evening being there, but observing. It was a strange experience but I felt very calm and present. 7, 6C, 12:22:00
Sh, 184 - I didn't have any competitive feeling. All my senses went out and I didn't feel the need to get involved, so spent the evening observing and feeling. 7, 6C, 12:22:00
Sh, 185 - Feeling detached from things, observing again, not touching the world. 7, 6C, 44:00:XX

AIL. He, 1 - Past events are forgotten, remembered as belonging to someone else, or as matters read.

ANAC. He, 46 - Estrangement (separation) from individuals and society, with fear of future.
He, 66 - He is separated (divided, disconnect, estranged) from the whole world and has so little confidence in himself that he despairs of being able to do that which is required of him.

ANDROC. Sh, 19 - Feeling of separateness, usual sense of urgency gone. (15)
Sh, 24 - I feel entirely alone, that I am viewing the world through one hole, for it all seems just a picture, and the rest of the world share a different view finder together. I don't want to join theirs though. (7)
Sh, 25 - Felt disconnected from the human race, as if everyone were another species. Directionless. (7)
Sh, 26 - Totally detached —not from self but from surroundings. (10)
Sh, 30 - Distant and staring. (20)
Sh, 31 - Felt remote and ineffectual, a dreamy state. Felt more like a spectator than a participant. (25)
Sh, 35 - Felt 'stoned', tried to express himself to a friend but could not. Behaved in a dreamy absent minded way. His friends thought that he had taken drugs. (29)
Sh, 57 - In the evening felt very lonely and desolate, although not alone. She felt separated, detached, disconnected and unreal. (7)
Sh, 60 - Felt tense and absolutely alone, but sure that the rest of the world was mad, not her. She felt defiant with others and would not be manipulated. (7)
Sh, 63 - Desired company but could not be bothered to see anyone, felt lonely as if he didn't belong. (21)
Sh, 121 - When talking to friends felt 'paranoid', suspicious and guilty, when asked questions, he became hot and sweaty. He felt it was a game of who was cleverer, and tried to lie to and outwit his friend, though this gave no satisfaction.

His friends reported that he seemed unusually distant and cool. (29)

AUR. Ha, 340 - He sits apart (separated), all by himself in a corner, wrapt up in himself, as if in the deepest melancholy, when left undisturbed; but the slightest contradiction excites the greatest heat and anger,...

BRASS. Sh, 1 - General feeling of aloofness 08, 6C, 04:12:30

Sh, 2 - Feeling of aloofness still present, feeling of separation from others not so noticeable when with the children 08, 6C, 05:00:00

Sh, 3 - Am feeling light-headed (frivolous); do not feel in such contact with the ground; I have stumbled a few times 08, 6C, 01:23:30

Sh, 4 - Still feeling spaced out but centered, notice it most when sitting still. 08, 6C, 03:03:00

Sh, 13 - My wife was very emotional saying she would be happier if I left, yet my reaction was how inconvenient. I did not become emotionally involved. Also a friend at work asked me if I was alright as he thought I'd not been quite with it recently. The proving experience was generally pleasant for me, and I felt low coming back to my old self, rather like going away on holiday and coming back to a messy house and all the things you have to do. Prover's wife said he'd been unbearable all that week, Rremote and not with us at allS. It was his tendency anyway, but it had been exaggerated. 08, 6C, 10:00:00

CAMPH. Al, 46-...The external world existed for me no longer. (solitude) My thoughts were gone; one single fearful one remained; I imagined myself transferred to another world (estranged, alienated); for me all else was extinguished...

CANN-I. Al, 57 - Strange feeling of isolation (solitude) from all around him, with great sense of loneliness (isolation), though surrounded by his friends.

CANN-S. He, 5 - Voices including her own, seem to come from a distance; her own voice seems strange, as if it was somebody else speaking.

CARB-AN. Ha, 32 - The objects on the street seem to him changed, e.g., farther apart and brighter (vivid, brilliant) than usual, as an empty, abandoned city.

CAUST. Ha, 61 - A sort of absent-mindedness; while doing one thing, he always felt as if he had to do something else, more importance, (duty) and yet he knew not what ; he reflected about it, and yet thought nothing. (lost: signification, value, purpose)

He, 24 - Chilly, with sad mood and apprehension of the future < in evening.

CHOC. Sh, 208 - Felt rejected and oversensitive. Hid away from the world, felt my life would fall apart. 35, 30C, XX:XX:XX:

Sh, 210 - Felt totally isolated and averse to company. Estranged himself from his family and friends and stopped all communication with them for a long period. Did not reply to letters and left no address. He seemed to hide away and literally disappear. The state of Isolation resulted from feeling that "I didn't exist as a human being". This behaviour was in strong contrast to his normal sociable disposition. 35, 30C, XX:XX:XX:

Sh, 211 - Feeling like I don't belong in a crowd. Conscious of all social and economic pressures on people nowadays and was glad to get home.[41], 6C, 01:XX:XX

Sh, 308 - I feel both more present and more distant. 29, 200C, 02:XX:XX

Sh, 309 - A feeling of intoxication with double sensations. Colours are stronger and hearing is sharpened but at the same time feel absent and removed.[29], 200C, 00:XX:XX

Sh, 319 - Felt emotionally numb and separated from things.[35], 30C, XX:XX:XX:

Sh, 329 - Felt anger at life, I wasn't getting anywhere. The world appeared a cruel place to me, and I felt I had no place in the scheme of things.[35], 30C, XX:XX:XX:

COB. Al, 4 - Low-spirited; thinks too little of himself.

CROT-C. Al, 4 - Another attack of mental alienation; she hears voices, which she follows (obey); with copious tears.

GERM. Sh, 103 - Felt closed in. My every movement and thought controlled. Didn't know where to go for help. Felt like a coward . Felt afraid of violence. I don't know who I am. 04, 6C, XX:XX:XX

Sh, 11 - Feeling detached when involved in

a row with husband. No guilt that I'm not pleasing him . 04, 6C, 09:XX:XX

Sh, 110 - I don't like to be me. Want to be different. Have a distant feeling to myself yet long for physical contact, a boyfriend. Not able to do something about it. 18, 30c, 02:10:00

Sh, 142 - Observe the world as being shabby. I feel separated from people and places. I feel an intense yearning for the feminine. 08, 12C, 08:04:50

Sh, 136 - Feeling lonely like an alien freak. 08, 12C, 22:00:00

Sh, 151-.... I feel I have no real contact with people, I have no emotion at all except for a feeling of isolation and a concern that people may not like me. I wish someone would cuddle me. By 10 o'clock I have a definite aversion to people, especially certain people- the stubborn or authoritarian kind. I become deeply involved in my own thoughts and can be very irritable and even angry when the thoughts are interrupted by people, but I don't show any signs of anger or irritation. The fate of other people leaves me cold, but I know this is not right. My mind is blank and I feel I could just sit and stare. I have no feelings, no emotions! I think a lot about my state of mind and try to understand it; it puzzles me. What is missing? Eating removes this thoughtful mood. By afternoon and evening I become gradually more involved with what I am doing but still feel isolated even when in the company of other people. I don't mind listening to people, but I contribute little to conversation. This state lasted for three days. 16, 30C, 04:XX:XX

Sh, 144 - I have an intense feeling of estrangement and isolation, with a desire to start my life again. 08, 12C, 11:06:50

Sh, 143 - I Don't belong. I don't feel at home any place. Strong desire for finding a place to stay, to make a home for me and my kids. 18, 30C, 30:XX:XX

Sh, 149 - Feel lonely. I nearly always feel special -always on the sideoutside of others. Either better or smaller than others. 18, 30C, 46:XX:XX

Sh, 121 - Very strong longing for excitement and some love adventure. I planned to go out, but though I probably would be disappointed, so I stayed at home and was depressed instead. Feel like drinking - to get away from myself and everything. 18, 30C, 04:00:00

Sh, 27 - Felt very quiet and calm. Almost detached. More patient and less irritable. 11, 12C, 00:04:05

Sh, 37 - Difficult to concentrate, staring out of the window. Must find something to eat. Inefficient. I am feeling very far away. 18, 30C, 04:00:00

HALI-L. Sh, 96 - Feeling spacey and disoriented, stoned, far away from reality; am I making this up? I'm aware of my body, my breasts going up and down with my breath. I'm relaxed and sleepy. Time is very slowed down. I'm in the moment. Am I hot or cold? I don't know, I think it's kind of warm heat I'm feeling. Who is writing this anyway? 06, 6C, 00:00:05

Sh, 384 - There is some kind of barrier or buffer. Everything's kind of distant, like being wrapped in cotton wool. There's a distance between me and everything outside. Things weren't up close. Something between me and everything else. 07, 30C, 04:00:30

Sh, 386 - I feel removed and everything is in slow motion and I couldn't really contact reality. I felt like I was compensating for the lack of motion. (On this page of her journal she has doodled a picture of a slanted cube with vertical bars on it. It looks like an animal cage leaning to the right.) 01, 30C, 15:XX:XX

Sh, 403 - For three weeks I was in a depression, unlike anything I have felt for a long time. Deep sense of low self-worth. Feeling invisible, uncared for and envious. I was lethargic, couldn't do anything. My practice dropped, patients just didn't show up. I felt I sunk as low as I needed to go, unmotivated. Felt unappreciative of all I have. Unappreciative of my life which I usually adore. Anger, dissatisfaction with life, isolating. I wasn't seeing anyone not even my husband, exhaustive. Had no dreams during the depression —unusual. I am emerging from it now. 01, 30C, 30:XX:XX-50:XX:XX

Sh, 428 - Realizing we haven't had any fun as a family in forever. Haven't had any fun myself either. Like a caged animal, snarling. I'm in a pressure cooker. Can't even imagine what would get me out of this mood, what actually would be fun. Don't want to do anything, or talk to anyone. Like a porcupine or sea urchin. "Don't tread on me." 09, 6C, 30:XX:XX

Sh, 623 - I don't meet people like my girlfriends do. I walk around the world not seeing people look my way. Being unrecognized. It's like I'm not there. No one misses me when I'm gone. It's really uncomfortable. I never cared before. Now I want to be recognized, but I'm not. 08, 30C, 03:XX:XX

Sh, 927 - I've felt lonely over the last three to four days. This morning I realized how great the girls were and burst into tears — emotional, but separate. 20, 30C, 14:XX:XX

HIPP. He, 1 - Melancholy; a young man sits in the corner and does not want to have anything to do with the world. (alienated)

HYDROG. Sh, 12 - Driving home I felt odd, as if I was hardly in my body. Feel like my body's working on automatic but I'm not really there. Driving along I kept forgetting where I was. Now I feel I'm really more "absent" than normal and feel quite afraid of losing my mind or having an accident. I feel my connection with the physical world is very loose, as though my soul was separated from my body. I have thoughts that this is a bit like dying —not unpleasant. 10, 200C, 13:02:XX

Sh, 20 - Distortion of reality —that other places seemed a million times more real than the real world. Everything seemed a long way away. 16, 30C, 04:XX:XX

Sh, 144 - Feeling I want to isolate myself — want to be alone. 12, 6C, 27:XX:XX

Sh, 172 - Felt distant and detached. 32, 9C, 04:XX:XX

Sh, 174 - Emotionally cold and non-communicable with anger felt in stomach. 12, 6C, 17:XX:XX

Sh, 175 - At the family celebration, I could not feel that I belonged. 12, 6C, 34:XX:XX

Sh, 176 - Feel distant and separated from things and they feel unreal. 16, 30C, 01:XX:XX

Sh, 177 - Upset husband by telling him what I thought of the way he'd been behaving. I felt curiously uninvolved. Indifference to husband. Felt a little 'dead', uninvolved, wasn't really responding in any way — not in a good way or a bad way. Didn't feel cross, affectionate or anything. Very peculiar, like I was watching and its nothing to do with me. Like looking at somebody else, almost as if I wasn't there. Felt emotionally numb and unable to respond —as if I wasn't there. Like a living dead being alive and not being able to make the appropriate responses. Real total detachment. 08, 30C, 10:XX:XX

Sh, 184 - Feel despondent, indifferent, apathetic, separated from things and don't care. Deep sighing with sense of resignation. Can't be bothered to do things. 16, 30C, 02:XX:XX

Sh, 189 - As if in a dream, not there, difficult to stay with it all while driving home — very conscious of the blackbirds flying across the motorway. Better taking a nap and fresh air from opening the window. Concomitant to finger abscess. 02, 6C, 54:XX:XX

Sh, 248 - While sitting in a restaurant, felt progressively more cut off from friends at the table. I began to feel detached and paranoid. I felt disliked by people. They seemed to look at me menacingly. I became concerned that my lecture this afternoon had created conflict, mayhem and destruction, that my friends in the audience did not like me any more. I became aware of a dull ache in my sacrum making me want to shift backwards and forwards. At the same time, the people round the table seemed further away and smaller, as if I had moved four feet back from the table. I felt very uncomfortable and wanted to get out. I put my head down and rushed out without saying goodbye, feeling a sense of relief at getting away (all very unusual for me). Outside, I felt relief and my mind cleared and I walked home alone. 22, 12C, 04:XX:XX

Sh, 254 - When shopping, felt people did not accept me as belonging to the community. Felt isolated in the shop. Feeling unacceptable, 'as if I was a marked person' —but later felt better on my own. 12, 6C, 19:XX:XX

Sh, 258 - Felt cut off from people and suspicious. 22, 12C, 06:XX:XX

HYOS. He, 57 - Delirium tremens:...averse to light and company; visions as if persecuted preceded by an epileptic attack;... seeks to escape from men by whom he imagines himself surrounded and who are trying to capture him; does not recognize his wife who is standing by his side, but imagines he sees her under a distant bed.

IRID. Sh-2 - Felt similar to being in water or asleep, as if almost asleep or in a trance, aware, but floating in inner self, uncommunicative; like a near death experience, inner self is primary and separate. E1

Sh, 5 - I want to be a home-bird this week. I don't want to go out at all. D9

Sh-9 - Partner said, "I've never seen you so still. You look like a stone Buddha. Your speech is irritating, you can barely get to the end of your sentences." E1

Sh, 13 - Would like to sit down and go to sleep. Want to go and hibernate, go to bed. Feel happy to sit and stare at a blank wall and reduce input. A3

Sh, 15 - Don't feel like reading paper or working on the train. Very unusual; just want to look out of window at the snow. E2

Sh, 26 - Felt detached in company, reticent to speak my mind. Sat and listened but didn't speak at the moments I usually would. Felt "sidelined," watching what's going on, rather than being a part of it. Felt detachment and self-doubt. I didn't speak because didn't feel I would be able to answer them (subject matter was my area of expertise). B9

Sh, 29 - Feel like not talking at all. A far-away-from-others-deep-in-me feeling. E1

Sh, 30 - Feel as if I am the only person. E3

Sh, 36 - Went to a 40th birthday celebration. One very good friend said I didn't seem to be there. They seemed like strangers to me. I was looking at the situation, which needed jollying up, but was unable to do anything about it because I felt distanced from them. It felt strange as if I'd gone out with people I didn't want to be with. H3

Sh, 37 - I kept distancing myself from people, more than I normally do. For example, if I was in a group of people then I would be stood apart from the rest of the group or sat on my own at a distance. The remedy heightened my separation and isolation from people. I24

Sh, 74 - No desire to touch, make love to husband all week in spite of easy, relaxed week. I feel detached from him, as if this is a problem within me. B20

Sh, 127 - Bright cold day. My attention was taken by the light reflected off the wet road. The brightness meant I wasn't seeing the tree or road at all. It added to the feeling of detachment. B3

Sh, 151 - I feel slow and down and far away. E.1

LYC. He, 9 - Absent minded; supposes to be in two places at a time.

NAT-C. Al, 22 - His fancy is mostly busy with apprehensions of the future; he often makes plans for half an hour at a time as if it would go wrong with him, wherewith he seeks to be alone for several days together.

He, 4 - Aversion to mankind and society; estrangement (separation, alienation) from individuals and society; even from her husband and family.

NAT-M. Al, 62 - Woke at 2A.M. in perspiration, and with a distressing anxiety, as though he were shut up (lock) in a dark cellar; this sensation only disappeared on perceiving light through the window.(confined, restricted, incarcerated)

NEON. Sh, 89 - Husband comments that I seem "far away and long ago." He hasn't seen me this "gone" in a long time. 06, 12C, 00:04:55

NUX-M. He, 6 - Never accomplishes what he undertakes, but remains standing in one place, absent-minded...

PHOS. Ha, 89 - Delirious fantasies, while slumbering (sleep) and when awake, as if she was on a distant island (isolation, segregation), as if she had a large business, was a distinguished (important, rank) lady, etc.

PLAT. Ha, 15 - At odds (quarreling) with all the world, everything is too close (near, intimate) for her, with inclination to weep. (persecution)

Ha, 39 - Indifference, cold (reserved), abstracted (separated) in company of friends,..

Ha, 41 - She feels as if she did not at all belong to her family (stranger); after a short absence everything appears to be quite changed. (unfamiliar)

He, 8 - Arrogant, reserved, absent-minded.

He, 25 - Out of sorts (irritated) with the whole world; everything seems too narrow (restricted, confined, near) ; weeping mood.

He, 29-...thought she had no place in the world; life was wearisome (boring), but had great dread of death, which she believed near at hand.

He, 39 - It seems to her as if she does not belong to her own family; ...

PULS. Al, 25 - It seems so quiet (silent) in her head and everything feels so empty that she seems alone in the house and in the world; she will speak to no one, just as if her surroundings did not exist (estrange), and she paid attention to no one. (left, solitary)

Ha, 1143 - Her head is so quiet and all about her is so empty as if she were alone (solitude, loneliness) in the house and in the world; she does not wish to talk to any one, just as if all around her were no concern (relation) of hers and she belonged to nobody. (lonely, missed)

SEP. Al, 82 - Great indifference toward everything; no proper sense of life.

STRAM. He, 32 - After getting out of bed, vertigo and loss of thought; everything hovers dimly and distantly before his memory, there seems to be a veil before his eyes.

SYPH. He, 11 - A far-away feeling, with apathy and indifference to future.

THUJ. Al, 5 - She has a decided sensation that her soul is separated from her body (split), and in such a condition hears and feels everything as from distance.

VALER. Al, 11 - Anxious, hypochondriac feeling, as if the objects around him had been estranged from him; the room appears to him desolate (isolated), he does not feel at home in the room, he is impelled to leave it.

JEALOUSY

Ailments from; jealousy: ***apis***[54] **HYOS.**[5] ***ign.***[5] ***lach.***[5] **NUX-V.**[122] ***ph-ac.***[5] ***phos.***[162] **PULS.**[122] staph.[102]

Ailments from; love disappointed, jealousy, anger and incoherent talk, with: hyos. nat-m.[122]

Ailments from; love disappointed, jealousy, anger and incoherent talk, with: hyos. nat-m.[122]

Anger; jealousy, with: ***lach.***[54]

Delirium; jealousy, from: **HYOS.**[54] lach.[162]

Delusions; jealousy, lovers concealed behind stove wife has: ***stram.***[54]

- jealousy, with: ***lach.***[10] stram.[54]

Dreams; jealousy: androc.[222] bamb-a.[1184] lyc.[30]

Grief; jealousy, with: ***hyos.***[54]

Insanity; erotic, jealousy, with: ***hyos.***[54]

Jealousy: am-s.[209] anac.[5] anan. ***apis*** ars.[30] bamb-a.[1184] bar-c.[188] bar-s.[209] calc.[193] calc-p. ***calc-s.*** camph. ***cench.*** cham.[31] cocain.[72] cocc.[193] coff. coloc.[58] crot-c.[214] ferr-s.[209] gall-ac. gels.[171] **<u>HYOS.</u>**[122] ign. ilx-a.[120] ip.[54] kali-acet.[54] kali-ar.[54] kali-c.[122] kali-s.[209] **<u>LACH.</u>**[122] lil-t.[5] ***lyc.***[54] mag-s.[209] ***med.***[122] morg-g.[136] nat-m.[30] nat-s.[209] ***nux-m.***[122] **<u>NUX-V.</u>**[122] op. ph-ac. phos.[162] **PLAT.**[30] ***puls.*** raph. sac-alb.[210] sep.[30] ***staph.***[122] ***stram.*** sul-ac.[209] sulph.[187] thuj.[58] verat.[30] vip.[1212]

Jealousy; accuses wife of being faithless: ***stram.***[54]

Jealousy; animals and objects, of: caust.[30] hyos.[30] lach.[30] nux-v.[30]

Jealousy; brutal, kind man becoming: calc.[30] lach.[30] nux-v.[30] sulph.[30]

Jealousy; children, between: ars.[30] calc-s.[187] carc.[179] nat-m.[30] nux-v.[30] sep.[30]

Jealousy; children, in, when a new baby takes the attention of the family away: ***hyos.***[8] ign.[8]

Jealousy; crime, to a: hyos.[30] lach.[30]

Jealousy; drunkenness, during: ***hyos.***[30] lach.[30] nux-v.[30] puls.[30] staph.[30]

Jealousy; foolish as it is irresistible, as: ***lach.***

Jealousy; happy, seeing others: hell.[137]

Jealousy; images, with frightful, tendency to mock, satire and ridiculous ideas: ***lach.***

Jealousy; impotence, with: calad.[30] nux-v.[30]

Jealousy; insane: lach.[137]

Jealousy; insult, driving to: ***nux-v.***[54]

Jealousy; irrational: cocain.[137]

Jealousy; kill, driving to: **HYOS.**[54] lach.[108]

Jealousy; loquacity, with: lach.[30] mag-c.[30] petr.[30]

Jealousy; love disappointment, in: ***hyos.***[54]

Jealousy; men, between: ars.[30] lach.[30] puls.[30] verat.[30]
Jealousy; murder, with attempt to: **HYOS.**[54]
Jealousy; neglect, accuses husband of: ***stram.***[54]
Jealousy; others getting all attention: ozone[227]
Jealousy; people around, of: op.[36]
Jealousy; quarrels, reproaches, scolds, with: gall-ac.[36] ***lach.***[54] ***nux-v.***[54]
Jealousy; rage, with: **HYOS.**[54]
Jealousy; revenge, desires to take: hyos.[30]
Jealousy; sadness, with: ***kali-ar.***[54]
Jealousy; saying and making what he wouldn't say and make: bell.[30] lach.[30] sulph.[30]
Jealousy; sexual excitement, with: calc.[30] caust.[30] chin.[30] con.[30] hyos.[54] nux-v.[30] phos.[30]
Jealousy; strikes his wife: lach.[30] nux-v.[30]
Jealousy; tearing the hair: lach.[30]
Jealousy; value or appreciate anything, desires that others shall not: ***ip.***[54]
Jealousy; weeping, with: caust.[30] nux-v.[30] petr.[30]
Jealousy; women, between: ars.[30] nat-m.[30] nux-v.[30] sep.[30]
Jealousy; women, in: ***apis***[54]
Mocking; jealousy, with: ***lach.***[54]
Quarrelsomeness; jealousy, from: ***cench. hyos.***[10] ***lach.*** nux-v.
Quarrelsomeness; jealousy, from, unchaste expressions, with: ***nux-v.***[54]
Sadness; jealousy, with: ***kali-ar.***[54]

ADAM. Sh, 214 - I am fidgety and angry and very jealous of people. I feel cold and empty and very angry, almost cruel. 20, 1M, 02:XX:XX

ANAN. Al, 8 - Ungovernable jealousy; everything causes jealousy.

APIS. He, 77 - All her ideas turn around jealousy, very talkative (loquacity), sometimes disgusting salacious. (lascivious)

He, 76 - Jealousy.(in women)

He, 81 - Ailments from fright, rage, vexation, jealousy, or hearing bad news.

HALI-L. Sh, 581 - At a meeting for parents and children, I am very critical of my daughter and myself, comparing her to other kids, myself to other moms. Cringe when she sits with her mouth open, pulling on her hair and twisting it into braids. Want to warn her, don't do that! She looks to me like she's bossing someone. Compare myself to other woman who has perfectly put together hair, clothes, nails, boots, bracelets. Very angry and jealous. Make excuses for myself and tear her down inside. 09, 6C, 14:00:XX

HYOS. He, 62 - Jealousy: with rage and delirium; with attempt (try) to murder.

He, 64 - Serious illness (ailments) from jealousy and grief about faithless lover;...

He, 65 - Violent and threatening...; mind nearly deranged; disturbed by unfounded jealousy.

He, 66 - A gentle, lovable woman became extremely jealous of her husband, and although fully realizing that she did him injustice, she was so filled with grief that she found no rest day or night... (remorse)

He, 63 - Erotic mania accompanied by jealousy.

IGN. He, 50 - Jealousy, disappointed love.

KALI-AR. He, 1 - Scolding (censorious) morose, retired, quarrelsome and discontented, jealous, indifferent to everything,...

LACH. Al, 25 - Towards evening very unusual almost crazy jealousy, as foolish as it is irresistible.

He, 26 - Jealousy, with frightful images, great tendency to mock, to satire and ridiculous ideas.

He, 51 - Proud; jealous, suspicious; developing into mania.

He, 59 - Ailments from fright (fear), disappointed love or jealousy.

He, 60 - After a jealous quarrel, she put both hands to her chest and cried out "Oh! my heart!" then fell down and was in an asphyctic state for nearly twenty-four hours;...

He, 19 - Insane jealousy.

NUX-V. Ha, 1267 - Scolding, reproaches, abuse, jealous invectives (accusation), mixed with indelicate expressions -then soon howling and loud weeping.

He, 17 - He quarrels, reproaches, scolds, insults, from jealousy, mingled with unchaste (obscene) expressions; ...

OP. Al, 137 - Appeared jealous and afraid (fear) of people around.

STRAM. He, 56 - Believes to be in his grave; shrives,(confess) prays, asks to be killed (justified); accuses his wife of infidelity; scolds (cursing), strikes at everybody who wishes to restrain him; thinks they are dogs and barks at them to make himself understood.

He, 103 - Had many strange fancies, such as imagining his wife had lovers concealed (hidden) behind stove; ...afterward had a fit that looked so much like apoplexy that he was bled.(blood)

JUSTICE

Anxiety; business, lawsuit, as if engaged in a: ***nit-ac.***[60]

Anxiety; lawsuit or dispute, as if he was engaged in: ***nit-ac.***[54]

Brooding; law suit, over, by which he may gain or loose a million, and takes it in bad part if not allowed to read indictment for said lawsuit, a confused, irrational piece of work, on which he has been working all night, in insanity: ***nux-v.***[54]

Delusions; attacks and insults, defend themselves against imaginary: lyss.[54].
- called before court, on account of wicked actions during climacteric period: ***zinc.***[54]
- lawsuit, being engaged in a: ***nit-ac.***[36]

Dreams; court, stands before: bamb-a.[1184]
- ➤ crimes, answer, for which he is held to: nat-m.[36]
- ➤ crimes, witnessed: carbn-s.[36]

ACT-SP. He, 3 - Judgment perplexed; bewildering fits, almost to insanity.

CALC-P. Al, 15 - A communication in which some one is justly reproached concerning his conduct, affects him very disagreeably; he grows violent, and holds up his faults to himself.

CIC. Al, 27 - Want of confidence in mankind; with misanthropy; he forsook society, remained alone and reflected upon their errors and about himself.

COFF-T. Al, 12 - The power of judgment is increased.

DROS. Al, 1 - Joyful, good courage: he had no fear of evil, because he was conscious of having done right. (moral, virtuous, honest, fearless)

Ha, 287 - Happy steadfast (confiding) disposition; he dreaded no evil, because he was conscious of having acted honorably.

FL-AC. Al, 9 - Satisfaction, he desires no better state of things; all is right.

GLON. Al, 14 - Recalls old grievances...; he was constantly thinking of persons who had offended him, with determination to justify (excuse, defend) his own conduct.

HALI-L. Sh, 185 - I have a higher energy and things happen. I think of something and immediately someone hands it to me. The power is greater so I have to make sure the goals are right. Have to be in perfect order because goals will happen. 08, 30C, 12:XX:XX

Sh, 187 - I want more from school. Ethics and education are very important. I want things done to a very high standard. To be methodical and well thought out. Want higher quality. 08, 30C, 25:XX:XX

Sh, 517 - Dread of upcoming legal battle. 09, 6C, 15:XX:XX

Sh, 527 - I was paying attention to the obituaries at this time. Noticed people dying in the newspaper. I would get very angry and frustrated. For a short time, was looking at death notices on a daily basis, during the last week or so of the proving. My anger towards death. How unfair. I don't want it. I shouldn't have to have it. There should never be a day where the morning is taken from me. 18, 30C, 35:XX:XX

Sh, 528 - Noticed in the paper all cancer related deaths, particularly prostate, mostly men between 40-60. Seemed to be men who were very loved. Seemed most unfair. Fear that if I drank too much coffee I would get a headache, and the thought was cancer related. 18, 30C, 35:XX:XX

Sh, 615 - Don't have the guts to tell partner to stick it out a little longer, that it might work out. Feel totally devastated, but have a lot of energy to deal with it, to stick up for my rights. Felt quite centered, as if I can take care of it. Feels like being on a roller coaster, up and down, in and out. Partner wants to be friends, but not sexual. Feeling emotionally abused. 02, 30C, 09:XX:XX

Sh, 938 - I feel so heavy and earthbound, stuck with human desires that are not my own. Why don't I fit? Where is the truth and justice they talk about? Why do humans lie and deceive? I feel a big thing about truth and justice. "Why don't these people just tell me the truth?" It feels like a game, not telling me what they really want and need. 20, 30C, 15:XX:XX

Sh, 946 - Inner vision: I was a male Indian. I thought, "I'm not a brave. I don't deserve this feather". 20, 30C, 15:XX:XX

HYOS. Ha, 578 - He reproaches others, and complains of injustice that he imagines has been done him.

IGN. Ha, 792 - Delicate disposition (character), with very clear consciousness (justice, judgment, equity)

MERC. Al, 36 - Quarrels with everything; would above all have everything right; quarrelsome.

NAT-M. Al, 119 - The patient's mind was much weakened by disease and poison; her moral perceptions, her once keen (sharp) sense of honor, and of right and wrong, seemed blunted (dull); she was in turns vehement (angry) and passionate, and moody and silent.

NIT-AC. Ha, 16 - Anxiety, as if he was engaged in a disquieting lawsuit or contest. (conflict, debate, competition)

He, 15 - Anxiety as if he was engaged in a lawsuit or dispute, causing uneasiness.

NUX-V. Al, 88 - Clear consciousness of his existence; fine, strong, correct feeling of right and wrong.

Ha, 1301 - Clear consciousness of his existence; delicate, strong proper (accurate, correct, exact) feeling of right and wrong. (sapience) (justice)

He, 37-...betraying (play false, feigning) great moral and physical languor (indifference),..launches into high-flying, fantastic plans, fancies himself rich (rank, position) and wants to make presents of thousands (squanders, waste), and makes large useless purchases; does not consider himself ill; ...,and takes in bad part if not allowed to read indictment (accusation) for said lawsuit, a confused irrational piece of work...

He, 37-...brooding all night long over a lawsuit by which he may gain or lose a million (megalomania) ; ..replies reluctantly and slowly to physician's questions, and takes it in bad part (offenses) if not allowed to read indictment (accusation) for said lawsuit, a confused irrational piece of work, on which he has been working all night.

ZINC. He, 46-...; believed herself to be called before court (judged) on account of her wicked (immoral) actions; ....;believe the devil is after her;...(persecution)

KNOWLEDGE

Ailments from; literary, scientific failure: calc.[30] ign.[30] lyc.[30] nux-v.[30] puls.[30] sulph.[30]

Anxiety; hypochondriacal, mania to read medical books: **CALC.**[30] ***nux-v.***[30] ***puls.***[30] staph.[30] sulph.[30]

Aversion; literary persons: sulph.[137]

Comprehension; easy, understands former mysterious things, in insanity: ***verat-v.***[54]

Comprehension; ritualistic: anh.[212] ars.[187] con.[187] cupr.[210] iod.[187] lyss.[187] pin-s.[120] rhus-t.[187] tub.[187]

Conscientious about trifles; pedant, too much: plat.[30] puls.[30] sil.[30]

Delirium; alternating with, mental capacities heightened: lacer.[36]

Delirium; books, endeavored to grasp: atro.[36]

Delirium; study, from excessive: hyos.[10] ***lach.***[54] nux-v.[10]

Delusions; discoveries, makes: nitro-o.[36]

- disease, she has some organic disease nobody understands: ***lil-t.***[8]
- disease, unrecognized, has an: raph.
- knowledge, he possesses infinite: cann-i. psil.[164] verat-v.[171]
- newspapers, he sees: atro.
- read, it seems wrong to: lach.[36]
- understands everything: verat-v.[171]
- visions, telling him about what they are: psil.[164]

Dreams; complicated and containing its explanation, dream: asc-t.[36]

➤ computers, of: choc.[222]

➤ dead, bodies, dissecting: cench.[58] chel.[36] iris ped.[36] sang.

➤ doctor drawing a uterus and ovaries on a board: ozone[227]

➤ fruit, unknown, which he desires to taste: jac-c.[36]

➤ intellectual: all-s.[36] anac.[1] ars.[36] bufo-s.[36] carb-ac.[36] carb-an.[1] cinnb.[36] coloc.[36] ferr.[36] fl-ac.[36] guai.[36] ign.[36] ind.[36] kali-n.[10] lyc.[36] nat-p.[36] phos.[36] sabin.[36] ***senec.***[36] sil.[36] stram.[1] thuj.[36] ust.[36]

➤ inventions, full of: apis kali-n.[10] lach. sabin.

➤ literary matters: ign.[5]
➤ proving remedy: merc.[36] pip-m.[36]
➤ scientific: carb-an.[1] carb-v.[10] guai.[1] ***ign.***[10] m-arct.[10] spong.[10]

Forgetfulness; connection of consecutive thoughts, of, after apoplexy: ***op.***[54]

Haughty; intelligent, but very: lach.[30] nux-v.[30] ***plat.***[30] verat.[30]

Inquisitive: agar. ambr.[58] aur.[111] carb-v.[30] choc.[222] hyos.[30] lach. laur.[111] lyc.[30] puls. sep.[30] sulph.[30] verat.[30]

Inquisitive; supernatural or spiritual matters, about: calc.[162]

Intellectual: **ACON.**[111] ***anac.***[111] aur.[36] ***bapt.***[111] **BAR-C.**[111] **BELL.**[111] ***cann-i.***[111] carc.[207] ***cocc.***[111] germ.[222] **HELL.**[111] **HYOS.**[111] ***ign.***[111] **LACH.**[111] ***laur.***[111] **LYC.**[111] ***merc.***[111] ***nat-c.***[111] nat-m.[162] ***nux-v.***[111] **OP.**[111] **PH-AC.**[111] **PHOS.**[111] ***plat.***[111] ***puls.***[111] ***rhus-t.***[111] **SEP.**[111] sil.[162] **STRAM.**[111] sulph.[111] **VERAT.**[111] viol-o.[10]

Learning; desire for: graph.[10] gymne.[36] hyos.[10] lach.[10] ***lyc.***[54] mez.[10] nat-m.[10] op.[36] ***rhus-t.***[10] sulph.[10]

Literature, desires: nux-v.[30] **PULS.**[30]

Memory; active: acon. acon-f.[36] ***agar. aloe*** alum. anac. ang. anh.[119] ant-c. arn. ars. ars-s-f.[58] asaf. ***aur.*** aur-ar.[58] bad. bapt.[36] **BELL.** bov. brom. calc-p. camph. cann-i. cann-s. caps. carb-v. carc.[207] chin. cimic. cob. coc-c. coca cocc. **COFF.** coff-t.[36] croc. cub. cupr. cycl. dig. fl-ac. ***gels.*** glon. grat. **HYOS.** iber.[36] kali-p. lac-ac.[36] **LACH.** lyss. manc. meph. nat-m.[185] nat-p. ***nux-m. nux-v.*** **OP.** ox-ac. ***phos.*** phys. pip-m. plat. plb. puls. raph. rhus-t. senec.[54] seneg. sil. spig. ***stry. sul-ac.*** sulph. ter. thuj. valer. verat. verb. viol-o. zinc. zing.[36] ziz.

Memory; weakness, fear, from: ***anac.***[54] ***cupr.***[54]

Reading; desire for: alum.[193] anth.[36] carc.[166] cocc.[193]

Reading; desire for, biographies or autobiographies: thuj.[222]

Reading; desire for, medical books: ***calc.***[30] ***nux-v.***[30] ***puls.***[30] staph.[30] sulph.[30]

Suicidal disposition; easiest way, asks questions as to quietest and: ***lac-d.***[54]

Talk; sciences, of: cann-i.[36]

Thoughts; brilliancy: op.[36] thea.[36]

Thoughts; intrude and crowd around each other, closing eyes, on, a mass of subjects, some scientific, cross each other: spong.[54]

ABROT. He, 2 - No capacity for thinking, as if all bodily and mental power were gone.

ADAM. Sh, 292 - It's crystal clear! Clarifying female roles. Clarification of issues. Realization —anger and depression in the past, had to do with conditioning, not saying what I wanted, not having my needs met. 10, 6C, 47:XX:XX

AETH. Al, 30 - Loss of comprehension (understanding); a kind of stupefaction, as if there was a barrier (obstruction) between his organs of sense and external objects. (disconnection, interruption)

AGAR. Al, 29 - Taken in moderation it excites the intellect and inspires cheerfulness and courage.

ALUM. Al, 24 - He is apprehensive of losing his thoughts, and his understanding.
Ha, 52 - Everything is easy to him, the powers of his understanding and of his body seem excited.

ANAC. Ha, 37 - He can only think when a subject is suggested to him; he does not of himself think of anything; he cannot independently determine anything.
Ha, 33 - Increased, greater keenness (acutely) of memory; even the least circumstances of times long past come back to him, without cause; he would also be now able to easily learn by heart...

APIS. Al, 23 - It seems to her as if she did not know what to do, as if she had no volition (desire) of her own, her head feels stupid.

ARG-M. He, 4 - Imagines things about the military which he never liked; long forgotten old songs come into his mind.

ARG-N. He, 5 - In conversation, forgetting what he wanted to say, he looked around as if expecting some one to help (aid) him out.

ARN. Al, 31 - Excessive inclination to perform many and long literary labors, without possessing the strength which is required to terminate them without injuring health.

BELL. He, 4 - Memory lively; remembers things long gone by.

CALC-P. Al, 19 - He has a clearer oversight (observation), and more distinct views of many things.

CALC. Ha, 65 - Great weakness of the

imaginative (creative) faculty; with a very slight exertion in speaking, he felt as if his brain was paralyzed, ...;he could not think, nor recollect what was spoken of, with muddled (confused) feeling in the head.(lost: imagination, thoughts)

He, 96 - The slight effort of talking gave him sensation as if brain would be paralyzed (disable), mostly in occiput.

CAMPH. He, 11 - Though he could remember the name of everything, when he looked at it, yet it was not without investigating its nature that he could discover its use. (dissociation; memory x vision x knowledge)

He, 18-...one evening he went to the piano with closed eyes and played with great precision what at other times he could not have done without his notes; several times he wrote letters in an acquired (learned) language more correctly than in a waking state;...(clairvoyance)

CANN-I. Al, 24 - He seemed possessed with the idea that he did not know whether he himself existed, or whether men generally existed, or for what purpose (intention, mission, aim) he existed.(existence x nonexistence)

Al, 34 - All around and within seems to be a great mystery, and is terrifying.

Al, 58 - He imagines that he is possessed of infinite knowledge and power of vision, and then that he is Christ come to restore the world to perfect peace. (redemption, savior, rescuer)

CAPS. Ha, 177 - Vivid dreams about scientific subjects; straining of the thinking faculty when dreaming; he composed literary essays in thought and spoke aloud.

CARB-AC. He, 12 - Entire disinclination to study; what he had accomplished seemed very trifling. (unimportant)

CARB-AN. Ha, 177 - Vivid dreams about scientific (precise, accurate) subjects; straining (efforts) of the thinking faculty when dreaming; he composed literary essays in thought and spoke aloud.

CAUST. Ha, 61 - A sort of absent-mindedness; while doing one thing, he always felt as if he had to do something else, more importance, (duty) and yet he knew not what ; he reflected about it, and yet thought nothing. (lost: signification, value, purpose)

CHIN. Ha, 1105 - What formerly appeared to him in a bright genial light, seems now to be lusterless (lifeless), unworthy (inutile), and shallow (superficial, stupid)

CHOC. Sh, 90 - Concentration very sharp, as if my survival depended on it. I felt very focused. (During a lecture) My understanding was sharper. Normally I have many things going on in my head — too scattered — but in the last few days, narrower attention.

Sh, 122 - While looking out of the window, I realised I had the capacity to see from above and below at the same time —not a dividing in two from bottom to top, but a knowledge of both sides at once.

Sh, 218 - Had a deep conversation with a friend and felt more mature, as if being detached, is helping me to understand her more.[35], 30C, 04:XX:XX

COFF-T. Al, 12 - The power of judgment is increased.

COFF. He, 1 - Memory active, easy comprehension; increased power to think.

CYCL. Al, 28-...he constantly feels as though he had just suffered from an overwhelming (remarkable) affliction; only when he becomes excited is his mind somewhat clearer, and then he acts like one who has just awakened from slumber (sleep), and only half understands what is going on about him.

CYPR. He, 2 - Profound indifference to everything, even to his studies, duties and common courtesies (kindness, compassion) of life.

FORM. Al, 4 - During the day remarkably happy and able to study; everything seemed easy to be accomplished.

GELS. Al, 20 - The sensorial modification consisted of a mistiness (fog, cloudiness) within the brain, not much affecting the lucidity (precision) of thought, but somewhat confusing the perceptions, so that I experienced some difficulty in attending to the physical details connected with my practice.(lost, connections)

He, 27 - Mental exertions cause a sense of helplessness (disability) from brain-weakness; inability to attend to anything requiring thought.

GERM. Sh, 21 - Contemplative, like nice things, sees beauty in stones and nature. Good at instinctive understanding, compassionate. 16, 30C, 01:XX:XX

GLON. Al, 15 - My intellect returned almost immediately, and I remember saying, " This has nothing to do with homeopathy, but with a very powerful poison."

HALI-L. Sh, 577 - Children are an obstacle to enlightenment. 09, 6C, 05:XX:XX

Sh, 952 - Today felt ordinary. It felt like my head cleared. Like it's open again. It felt like it was blasted open from the sky coming downwards, like a thunderbolt — hot, sharp, and sudden — through the vertex while I was talking to someone. I just understood what's been happening the last couple of weeks, even the breast dreams. There was just clarity and I could see how I'd been in the wrong shape all these years. 20, 30C, 17:XX:XX

HURA. Al, 28 - Impatience, anger; she bites her hands, and gets into passion because her ideas come too slowly.

HYDROG. Sh, 19 - The general impression is that the prover entered a larger totalitydimension in terms of space and time, whereupon all previous or smaller totalities became trivial and alien. A conflict of understanding and behaviour arose. 16, 30C, XX:XX:XX

Sh, 28 - I felt an incredible clarity before and now I feel it may all have been a illusion. I am uncertain, don't know how I am anymore. I don't recognize what is happening. It's as if I have made a step into the unknown. I feel I'm in an unknown area without protection. Fear is the biggest limitation. 16, 30C, 05:XX:XX

IND. Al, 4 - Felt almost crazed when attempting to study...

IP. Ha, 218 - Repugnance to literary work; thoughts fail him.

IRID. Sh, 118 - Thoughts: Wind is breath of the spirit; love is the greatest of all messages between heaven and earth. Yes, go to heaven, but return to the world transformed by the light of experience, transcend and return; Metals —immortality; need knowledge of their names; Iridescence, oil mother of pearl metal, rainbow, seven plus seven, cosmic joke, messages in other languages —language of angels?; Seven heavens, seven earths. I adore these territories, not so much new as forgotten. Q20

LACH. Al, 22 - Sudden doubts (indecision) arise about truths (veracity) of which he had hitherto (before) been convinced (converted), in the afternoon.

Al, 23 - It frequently seems to him wrong to read long at a time, although the subject interests him.

Al, 43 - He is impelled to productive work in the evening, although he had been much fatigued during the day ... writes with the greatest freedom and increased vigor about everything he knows;...

Al, 44 - Increased power of originality in all mental work, increased activity of fancy; scenes and occurrences throng to him in an unusual amount.

Al, 45 - No sooner does one idea occur to him then a number of others follow in succession while he is writing down, so that he is unable to finish the record.

He, 5 - Quick comprehension; mental activity, with almost prophetical (oracular, predictive) perception; ecstasy; a kind of trance.

He, 54 - A girl, after excessive study, uses exalted language; exceedingly particular about language she uses, often correcting after using a word, and substituting another of very similar meaning, talking about being under influence of a superior power. (possessed) 0 Mania.

LIL-T. Al, 45 - She can't think; acts without thought; keeps walking fast as though by instinct; feels hurried, but doesn't know why; is forgetful, can't decide for herself; must depend on others.

He, 4 - Believes her disease to be incurable; that she has some organic disease that nobody understands. (misunderstanding, misjudged)

LYSS. Al, 6 - Exhilarated, felt as if he had received joyful intelligence, all day.

Al,N-14 - Is astonished (surprised) in his dream at the readiness with which he can express himself in elegant Latin.

MERC. Ha, 1237 - With absence of thought, (discernment, knowledge),he feels as if he had done something bad.

MEZ. Al, 47 - He looked out of the window for hours without thought, and without knowing what he was looking at.

He, 5 - No rest when alone; wants to be in company ...unable to repeat what has been learned by heart; looks through window for hours, without being conscious of objects around; knows not what she is about; forgets what she is about to utter (talk); looks ill humored, pale, wretched, fallen away; ......expecting some very unpleasant news.

NAT-AR. Al, 22-...mind not fit for study ...

NAT-M. Al, 119 - The patient's mind was much weakened by disease and poison; her moral perceptions, her once keen (sharp) sense of honor, and of right and wrong, seemed blunted (dull); she was in turns vehement (angry) and passionate, and moody and silent.

Al, 132 - Irresolute at work; he could not see his way clearly.

He, 2 - Absent minded or distracted while talking; does not know what he ought (have to) say; awkward in talking; easily makes mistakes.

NEON. Sh, 11 - Doing research on Uranus, I found that the planet has a tilt. For 42 years one side is in the dark and then comes into the light for 42 years. Interesting that I am now 43. Uranus feels very near, like a friend. The quasars are much further out and it was a real stretch for me to go so far. 20, 6C, XX:XX:XX

NUX-M. Al, 49 - It became difficult to recall to mind things learned shortly before; for many such things the mind seemed paralyzed for many days together.

NUX-V. Al, 73 - Dread of that kind of literary work at which one must think and employ the ideas, ...

Ha, 1294 - Something, he knows not what, hinders (opposed, obstructed) him, specially in scientific occupations.

Ha, 1301 - Clear consciousness of his existence; delicate, strong proper (accurate, correct, exact) feeling of right and wrong. (sapience) (justice)

Ha, 1296 - In the morning, dread of those literary occupations in which he must think for himself and unfold ideas from his own mind in order either to commit them to writing or to express them orally; but reading and learning by heart are not distasteful to him.

He, 4 - Cannot read or calculate, for she loses the connection of ideas; thinks she will lose her reason.

He, 19-...; imagines himself surrounded by persons who carry on all sorts of pranks (joke, jest), or ply (covering) him whith questions which he thinks he is compelled (forced) to answer (proved, questioned, interrogated);..; answers questions rationally and is conscious of his condition; ...appears to be haunted (obsessed) by a great fear.

He, 39 - Mania puerperalis...constantly complaining, criticizing or explaining, ... as soon she recognized physician she spoke of imperfection of medical knowledge and declared it an error that one could not live without a heart, inasmuch as she felt very well without one, it having come away with the afterbirth to which it had grown fast, the nurse having separated the two before her eyes; complains of her husband, says he wishes to convince her she is sick, ... nymphomania,... frequently sips at a bowl of warm sugar-water, declaring it will form her a new heart; .(health, healing)...(expert)

He, 30 - Ailments after continued mental exertion; indisposition to it, particularly to that form which involves elaboration and connection of subjective ideas independently of external objects.

OX-AC. Al, 32 - Greater presence of mind; the relations of the world seem to be clearer to him.

PH-AC. Ha, 40 - While reading, a thousand other thoughts crowd into his mind (dispersion) ; he could not comprehend anything, what he read was dark to him, and he forgot everything at once, with difficulty in recollecting what he had known a long time already. (lost: memory, concentration, comprehension, knowledge)

RAPH. Al, 16 - Her condition troubles her, and for a moment cannot believe it to be owing to the medicine; she forgets it entirely, and believes she has a disease which is not recognized. (unknown, undiscovered)

RHUS-T. Ha, 974 - He can restrain the rush of ideas at his will, follow out uninterruptedly any train of thought he chooses, without being troubled with other thoughts.

SEP. Al, 100-...seems as if my mind were hedged (enclose) in, as if it were circumscribed,...(encircle, confined)

Al, 101 - Dullness of comprehension; inability to collect or express his thoughts; constantly building air-castles or running on future events.

Al, 31-...I cannot recall things which I know very well; the thoughts will not come...

He, 38-...everything seems strange (unusual, unfamiliar) to her;...; it seems as if she could not understand (realize) anything and would have to learn anew everything she wished to do;...(lost: knowledge); greatest indifference to everything, the death of a near relative, or some happy occurrence, leaves her equally unaffected; no trace of her former love for friends or even for her child; aversion for social intercourse amounting to contempt;...

VERAT-V. He, 6 - Loquacity, with exaltation of ideas, or an exalted opinion of her own ideas and powers; everything seems clear to her; now clearly understands former mysterious things; wants no medicine, as that will restore her to former condition;...

VIOL-O. Al, 10 - He seems able to recognize only half an idea; he puts it in the proper place but cannot hold to it; he makes great effort to grasp (understand) the other half, but at the same moment half of another incomplete idea presses upon him, and so on; thoughts chase one another, but he always has only half a thought ...

LACK

Affection; absorbs: puls.[146]

Affection; children craving for: carc.[207]

Ailments from; death, child, of a: calc.[58] caust.[30] ***gels.***[54] **IGN.**[54] ***kali-br.***[54] lach.[30] nat-m.[85] nux-v.[30] ph-ac.[30] plat.[85] staph.[30] sulph.[30]

Ailments from; death, one death after another: ambr.[58]

Ailments from; death, parents or friends, of: ambr.[58] ars.[184] calc.[58] **CAUST.**[30] <u>**IGN.**</u>[122] kali-br.[137] 0nat-m.[184] nit-ac.[54] nux-v.[30] plat.[85] staph.[30]

Anger; absent persons while thinking of them: ***aur.*** kali-c. kali-cy.[36] lyc.

Anguish; loss of his friend, from: calc.[172] ign.[172] **NIT-AC.**[54]

Blackmail, emotional, says "you don't love me" when refused: puls.[189] tub.[189]

Brooding; constantly over loss of a child: ***gels.***[54] ***kali-br.***[54]

Caressed; propensity for being: cann-i.[36] carc.[140] germ.[222] lap-mar-c.[194] puls.[102] ***sac-alb.***[210]

Carried; desires to be, caressed and: acon.[122] kreos.[5] puls.[5]

Company, desire for; angina pectoris, in: ***aur-m.***[54]

Company, desire for; children that are rejected, in: carc.[207]

Company, desire for; friend, of a: lap-gr-m.[194] plb..

Company, desire for; heart, in organic disease of the: ***apis***[54]

Company; desire for: acon.[30] act-sp. aeth. all-s. androc.[222] ant-t. ***apis*** **ARG-N. ARS.** ars-h.[54] asaf. aur-m. bell. **BISM.** bov. brom. bry. bufo cadm-s. ***calc.*** calc-ar.[58] calc-p. ***camph.*** cann-s.[5] carb-v. carc.[193] caust. cench. choc.[222] ***clem.*** coca[25] coloc. ***con.*** cot.[36] crot-c.[5] crot-h. cyna.[149] der. dros. dys-co.[136] ***elaps*** fl-ac.[102] foll.[1201] gaert.[136] ***gels.*** hep. hydrog.[222] **HYOS.** ***ign. kali-ar.*** kali-br. **KALI-C.** ***kali-p.*** **LAC-C.** lac-h.[229] lach.[5] lap-c-b.[194] lap-gr-m.[194] ***lil-t.*** lith-c.[25] **LYC.** manc. merc. ***mez.*** mut.[136] naja[98] **NAT-C.**[5] nit-ac.[116] ***nux-v. pall.*** ph-ac.[102] <u>**PHOS.**</u>[122] plb. ***puls.*** rad-br.[102] ran-b. rat. sac-alb.[210] ***sep.*** sil.[102] skat.[102] ***stram. stry.*** sulph.[30] syph.[54] tab. tarent. thymol.[102] verat. verb. zinc. zinc-p.[58]

Conversation; desire for: ars.[36] chen-a.[36] narcot.[36]

Delusions; calls, absent peoples, for: hyos.
- dead, child was, her: ***kali-bi.***[54] kali-br.
- dead, corpse, husband: calc-sil.[58] plb.
- friend, affection of, has lost the: ***aur.*** hura hydrog.[222] hyos.[58]
- home, at, when not: cann-i. hyos.
- home, away from, must go there: ***bry.***[102] calc-p.[102] cimic.[102] hyos.[102] ***op.***[102]
- places, none in the world, she has: germ.[222] ***plat.***[54]
- want, had come to: cann-i.

Desires; anxious, full of, in hysteria: ***cast.***[54]

Desires; present, things not: bry.[5] calc-sil.[58] puls.[5] rheum[5]

Despair; death, separate him from his children, death will: bamb-a.[1184]

Despair; sexual craving, from: aster.[54]
Dreams; danger, want, and: am-c.[54]
➤ distant, acquaintances: fl-ac. plb. sel.
➤ distant, beloved one: plb.[36]
➤ family, own, losing his: choc.[222]
➤ friends, loses friend in the city, cannot find her: ozone[227]
➤ looking for someone and failing to find him: carc.[119]
➤ loss, disheartening: ***meph.***[36]
➤ loss, sensation of a, with: ozone[227]
➤ want, of: am-c.[36]
Escape; attempts to, visit his daughter, wants to: ars.
Excitement; absent persons, about: aur.
Fear; misfortune, of, losing something of great value: sec.[172]
Forgotten something, feels constantly as if he had: arg-n.[162] calc.[122] caust. cham.[162] ***iod.*** mill.[36] ***tub.***[162]
Forsaken; feeling, friendless, feels: arg-n.[58] ***lach.***[8] pip-n.[2103]
Grief; losing persons or objects, after: **IGN.**[54]
Hatred; persons, of, absent, amel. on seeing: fl-ac.
Irritability; absent persons, with: aur. fl-ac. kali-cy. lyc.
Sadness; children, want of, from: aur.[91]
Sympathy; compassion, desire, for: alco.[36] anac.[54] androc.[222] asaf.[111] **BELL.**[5] **CAMPH.**[5] carc.[146] caust.[36] cic.[5] germ.[222] <u>**HELL.**</u>[5] nat-c.[36] nat-m.[91] ***olnd.***[54] ozone[227] <u>**PHOS.**</u>[122] puls.[5] rhod.[36] sac-alb.[210] ***sep.***[36] thuj.[36] ***tub.***[189]
Thoughts; vanishing, sermon, during a: anag.[36]
Weeping; constant, wants: ail.[58]
Weeping; homesickness, as from: ph-ac.[36]
Weeping; need, about a fancied: chin.
Weeping; need, past, about: nat-m.[60]

AGAR. Al, 15 - The father had fantasies; seemed to see his dead sister in heaven.
ANAC. Ha, 26 - His thoughts leaves him.(empty)
Ha, 29-...he has a lack of ideas, and loses subject quickly and without perceiving it.
Ha, 38 - Everything intellectual is hard for him, as in a dearth (lack) of ideas.
ANDROC. Sh, 65 - Desired comfort and sympathy. (29)
BRASS. Sh, 10 - A very pleasant lack of thoughts; finding it harder to apply myself to the work I'm doing. Very difficult to describe the sensation, unable to find the right words, hard to explain things 08, 6C, 02:03:00
BRY. He, 14 - Desire to get out of bed and go home.
CAMPH. Al, 46-... My misery was boundless; time itself was no more; in short, I suffered such fearful anguish as no fancy can comprehend. What soul could paint to itself my everlasting (eternal) dwelling as the Evil One (devil), alone in a vast universe, without faith or hope, and my heart forever broken by unimaginable tortures? (miserable, timeless, endless, solitude, forsaken, faithless, hopeless)
Al, 46-.... As I lay stretched on my couch, as the evil demon, and suffered all the anguish of a condemned and God-forsaken soul, ...I was forever deprived of the Divine protection, and of every consolation and every hope. Nothing remained to me but the conviction of my everlasting damnation...
CHAM. Al, 13 - Piteous moaning of a child because he cannot have what he wants. (contrariety)
CHIN. Ha, 1103 - She falls time to time into a lachrymose humour, without external cause, from some self-made, trivial whim (caprice), e.q. from some imaginary want (lack, need), such as that she cannot eat enough...
He, 16-...;wants to destroy himself, but lacks courage.
COFF. He, 7 - Delirium tremens: unsteady running about; imagines he is not at home,...
DROS. Ha, 278 - Anxiety in solitude (alone) he wished to have someone always near him, could not bear to be without companions (friends, company), and was quieter when he had someone to speak to; but when they again left him in solitude, he was all the more anxious, until he fell asleep; on awaking the anxiety returned.
GELS. He, 6 - After losing son, inclined to brood over her loss; at times becomes unconscious, or, rather, "rapt"; in imagination thinks herself at the grave; smothered pressure on chest after the spell.
He, 28 - Great lack of courage.
He, 33 - Effects (ailments from) of grief;

cannot cry; when thinking of his symptoms (disease), also when spoken to of his loss ; >from diverting talk; oppression and palpitation of heart; feels a sense of peril (danger, harm, risk) ; face flushed; sleeplessness; subdued (subjugate, yielding) manner; ...

GERM. Sh, 111 - If I were me, nobody would like me -so I try to be what I think others expect me to be. I don't think I can be loved with all the parts of me which are ugly and bad. Lonely feelings. Longing for love and understanding. Feel I am so unfriendly to myself. 18, 30C, 04:00:00

Sh, 151-.... I feel I have no real contact with people, I have no emotion at all except for a feeling of isolation and a concern that people may not like me. I wish someone would cuddle me. By 10 o'clock I have a definite aversion to people, especially certain people- the stubborn or authoritarian kind. I become deeply involved in my own thoughts and can be very irritable and even angry when the thoughts are interrupted by people, but I don't show any signs of anger or irritation. The fate of other people leaves me cold, but I know this is not right. My mind is blank and I feel I could just sit and stare. I have no feelings, no emotions! I think a lot about my state of mind and try to understand it; it puzzles me. What is missing? Eating removes this thoughtful mood. By afternoon and evening I become gradually more involved with what I am doing but still feel isolated even when in the company of other people. I don't mind listening to people, but I contribute little to conversation. This state lasted for three days. 16, 30C, 04:XX:XX

Sh, 163 - Felt lack of romance in my life. Desired romantic love, to be loved. 05, 6C, 41:XX:XX

Sh, 200 - Constant need for cuddles without sexual desire. 16, 30C, 07:04:00

Sh, 150 - I only want to cry. Don't know what to do. Feel terrible and lonely. Cannot describe how I feel. Want attention, but don't dare to ask for it. Soon there is no more energy left. 18, 30C, 182:XX:XX

HALI-L. Sh, 25 - While listening to a patient grieve, had a return of increased awareness of right eye, especially the socket. I had a strong image of how my mother's right eye was knocked out when she was hit by a truck and killed 30 years ago. Feel a very strong sense of connection with her. Telling this to my proving supervisor later, I realized I had never said this to anyone. This was an aspect of her death I had suppressed. It had always been so horrifying to me I couldn't deal with it. I cried gently with lots of tears. Feeling very sad and some remorse that I couldn't have been with my mother when she died. Felt very calm with all of this. 03, 12C, 18:XX:XX

IGN. He, 26 - Great grief after losing persons or objects very dear.

IRID. Sh, 344 - Feels like I have lost something, feels like I am grieving. It is a bit of a swine really. I11

KALI-BR. He, 23-...constantly brooding over loss of a daughter; almost crazy; ... (child)

KALI-C. Al, 7 - Sad, lonely (solitary) ; she seeks society in order to enliven (animate) herself.

KALI-FCY. Al, 1 - Feeling of sadness and some disposition to tears, caused by an impression that he was soon to die and leave his friends; disposition to take a sad view of the beauties of autumn; the apprehension of approaching sickness and death can be overcome by reason, but soon returns.

LAC-D. Al,N-4 - Imagines that all her friends will die and that she must go to a convent. (purification, solitude)

LYSS. Al,N-45 - Wrote to doctor: I am waiting with impatience that you give me and my young ones something to eat.

MEZ. Al, 47 - He looked out of the window for hours without thought, and without knowing what he was looking at.

NAT-C. Al, 53 - Sensation of loss of will power, in the morning on waking.

Al, DREAM, 1102-..;of marrying two women, of parties, walks, entertainments, and excursions on horseback, afterwards they were frequently anxious, of going astray (lost),of murders, having his ears cut off; also vexatious dreams; he would take a journey and could not get away from the place,(immobilization) and when has reached the first station was obliged to turn back, on account of something he had forgotten.

NAT-M. Al, 45 - If she only thinks of a want (need, lack) long since past, tears come into her eyes.

Ha, 97 - Lack of memory, so that he thought his mother (present continually) had died, because he did not remember to have seen her.

NIT-AC. He, 17 - After continued loss of sleep, long-lasting anxiety, over-exertions of mind and body from nursing the sick, great anguish of mind from loss of his dearest friend.

PLB. Al, 127 - Longing (deprived, wanting) for a distant friend, in the evening...

RHUS-T. Ha, 953 - Melancholy, sad, and anxious, as if about to hear of a calamity,(misfortune, disaster) or as if she were solitary (lonely, alone) and all around her were dead (lifeless, extinct) and silent (quiet) ; or as if she had bid farewell (separation) to an intimate friend ; worst in the room, diminished by walking in a open air.

SIL. He, 9 - Longing for his relations and home.

STRAM. Ha, 559 - She fancies she sees a number of people who are not present, and she grasps at them.

LASCIVIOUS

Ailments from; abuse: ambr.[1189] aur-m.[198] calc-p.[198] hyos.[198] lyc.[198] nat-m.[198] staph.[198]

Ailments from; debauchery: agar.[58] ***anan.*** ant-c.[54] arg-n.[5] calad.[162] carb-v.[5] chin.[102] dig.[85] fl-ac.[122] lach.[111] **NUX-V.**[5] pic-ac.[122] sel.[137] sep.[122] spig.[54] stram.[137] sul-ac.[111]

Ailments from; debauchery, as after: clem.[36] conin.[36] kreos.[36] lact.[36] lyc.[36] nux-v.[1] op.[36] ox-ac.[36]

Ailments from; sexual, abuse: ambr.[1189] ***anac.***[102] arg-n.[102] aur.[102] aur-m.[137] calc-p.[137] 0caust.[137] chin.[102] cupr.[210] foll.[1201] hyos.[137] lil-t.[54] lyc.[193] nat-m.[102] nux-v.[102] orig.[187] ***ph-ac.***[54] ***phos.***[54] sep.[162] staph.[103] stram.[187] ***ust.***[8]

Ailments from; sexual, excesses: agar. agn.[122] alum. ***alum-p.***[122] **APIS**[5] arg-n.[122] arn.[85] ars. asaf. aur. aur-ar.[58] bell-p.[102] ***bov.*** calad. **CALC.** calc-p.[122] calc-sil.[58] carb-an.[5] ***carb-v.*** **CHIN.**[122] chin-ar. cocc. ***con.*** dig.[122] ***iod.*** kali-br.[5] ***kali-c.*** kali-p. kali-s. kali-sil.[58] lil-t. **LYC.** mag-m. ***merc.*** ***nat-c.*** nat-m. nat-p.[58] nit-ac. **NUX-V.** ol-an.[5] onos.[122] petr. **PH-AC.** **PHOS.** plat.[122] plb.[122] psor.[56] ***puls.*** sabal.[137] samb.[85] sec.[122] sel. **SEP.** ***sil.*** spig. **STAPH.** sulph. symph.[122] thuj. upa.[122] zinc. zinc-p.[58]

Amativeness: agn.[5] ant-c.[54] calc.[30] **CANTH.**[54] ***caust.***[30] ***con.***[54] ***hyos.***[54] ign.[10] kali-br.[122] ***lach.***[54] **LYC.**[54] ***merc.***[54] nat-m.[30] ph-ac.[30] ***phos.***[54] ***plat.***[30] sulph.[30] ***ust.***[54] verat.[30]

Amativeness; fits, in: acon.[60] ant-c.[60] hyos.[60] op.[60] stram.[60] verat.[60]

Amorous; disposition: acon.[5] agar. agn.[5] ***anan.***[162] androc.[222] **ANT-C.**[5] apis[5] ***bell.***[5] ***bufo***[5] calad.[5] **CALC.**[5] ***calc-p.***[5] camph.[5] cann-i.[116] **CANN-S.**[5] **CANTH.**[5] **CARB-V.**[5] **CAUST.**[30] **CHIN.**[5] coff.[5] ***coloc.***[5] ***con.***[5] croc.[5] dulc.[5] fl-ac.[5] ***graph.***[30] ***hyos.***[10] **IGN.**[5] ***iod.***[54] kali-br.[122] kali-c.[5] ***lach.***[54] lil-t.[5] **LYC.**[54] meny.[5] ***merc.***[54] ***mosch.***[5] ***murx.***[5] nat-c.[5] **NAT-M.**[5] nit-ac.[58] nux-m.[5] **NUX-V.**[5] ***op.***[5] orig.[137] ph-ac.[30] **PHOS.**[5] pic-ac.[5] **PLAT.**[5] plb.[5] plb-acet.[30] **PULS.**[5] rhus-t.[5] ruta[5] **SABIN.** sanic.[5] sars.[5] sel.[116] senec.[111] ***sep.***[5] **SIL.**[5] squil.[137] ***stann.***[5] ***staph.***[5] **STRAM.**[5] sulph.[122] thuj.[5] ***ust.***[54] **VERAT.**[5] verb.[5] zinc.[5]

Anxiety; coition, as if during, with palpitation and voluptuous sensation: plat.[54]

Anxiety; duty, as if he had not done his, religious, produced by lascivious impulses: ***orig.***[54]

Anxiety; lascivious impulses, from, on account of disinclination of religious duties in a married woman, mother of a family: ***orig.***[54]

Delusions; devils, erotic mania, in: orig.[54]

• lascivious: ambr.[10] bell.[10] calc.[10] sil.[10] ***stram.***[10] verb.[54]

• obscene: stram.

• women, his mothers house is invaded by lewd: kali-br.

Dementia; sexual excess, from: lil-t.[137]

Dreams; amorous, perverse: ind.[85]

➤ coition, desire for coition, of: sel.[36]

➤ indecent behavior of men and women: cench.[58]

➤ lewd, lascivious, voluptuous: acon.[36] adren.[56] am-c.[36] am-m.[36] ambr.[1] anag.[8] ant-c.[36] aran.[192] arg-n.[36] arn.[1] ars.[102] astac.[36] bism.[8] bor.[36] cact.[8] cahin.[36] ***calc.***[54] ***camph.***[54] ***cann-i.***[102] cann-s.[5] canth.[5] carb-ac.[36] carb-v.[36] cere-b.[36] clem.[8] cob.[36] colch.[36] coloc.[1] ***con.***[54] cop.[36] cycl.[36] dig.[8]

dios.[36] dros.[5] ery-a.[36] euph.[36] form.[5] ***graph.***[54] grat.[36] ham.[102] hipp.[36] hura[36] hydr.[36] hyos.[1] ign.[1] ind.[36] inul.[36] ***kali-br.***[8] kali-c.[36] kali-p.[36] lach.[36] lact.[36] lil-t.[36] linu-c.[36] lyc.[36] m-arct.[1] m-p-a.[1] meny.[1] merc-i-r.[36] merc-s.[36] nat-m.[36] ***nat-p.***[8] nit-ac.[36] nuph.[25] nux-v.[5] nym.[36] op.[1] orig.[36] ox-ac.[36] oxyt.[77] paraf.[77] petr.[36] ph-ac.[5] phos.[5] phys.[1] pic-ac.[36] plan.[36] ***plat.***[36] psor.[56] ptel.[36] puls.[1] raph.[36] rhod.[36] rhus-v.[36] sabad.[36] salx-n.[102] samb.[1] sars.[36] sel.[8] senec.[36] sep.[36] sil.[36] sin-n.[36] sol-t-ae.[36] spig.[1] spira.[36] spirae.[36] stann.[1] staph.[5] ***sulph.***[36] thuj.[1] thymol.[102] trom.[36] ust.[102] verat-v.[102] vinc.[36] ***viol-t.***[8] x-ray[56] yuc.[36]

➤ nakedness, about, running around naked: rumx.[36]

➤ water, people, bathing, swimming pool of hotel, in, naked: ozone[227]

➤ wedding, women, with two: nat-c.[10]

➤ women, naked indecently, she is, and spreads her legs: ozone[227]

Dress; indecently: aq-mar.[231] hell.[5] hyos.[5] sec.[122] ***stram.***[5]

Ecstasy, amorous, delirium, during: thea.[36]

Ecstasy, amorous, sleep, during: phos.

Ecstasy; sensitivity of female sexual organs, with: coff.[54]

Egotism; self-esteem, nymphomania, in: ***agar.***[54]

Excitement; lascivious, with painful nocturnal erections: ***merc.***[54]

Excitement; nymphomania, is: aster.[54]

Excitement; sexual, intense: foll.[149] pall.[137] tarent.[102] vip.[1212]

Fancies; lascivious: alum.[30] am-c. ***ambr.*** anac. androc.[222] arund. aur. bell. ***calad.***[54] ***calc.*** camph.[54] ***canth.***[10] carb-v. caust.[30] ***chin.*** cod.[54] ***con.***[10] cop.[54] dig. ***graph.*** hipp. ***hyos.***[162] ign. ***kali-br.***[54] ***lach.***[10] lil-t. ***lyc.*** lyss.[54] nat-c.[54] ***nat-m.***[10] ***nuph.***[36] nux-v.[30] ***op.*** ***orig.***[54] orig-v.[25] petr.[30] phos.[135] plat.[30] psor.[30] sang. ***sel.***[10] sep.[10] ***sil.***[54] sin-n.[54] staph.[30] stram.[10] tarent.[58] thuj. ***ust.***[54] ***verat.***[162] verb. yuc.[36] ***zinc.***[54]

Fancies; lascivious, erections, with, daytime: sin-n.[54]

Fancies; lascivious, erections, with, sleep, during, and impotence after waking: ***op.***[54]

Fancies; lascivious, frequent, involuntary: sil.[1]

Fancies; lascivious, impotency, with: calad.[58] ***chin.***[54] lach.[137] ***op.***[54] ***sel.***[54]

Fancies; lascivious, lying down, while: thuj.[36]

Fancies; lascivious, sleepiness, during: lyc.[193]

Fancies; lascivious, sweets, with desire for: ***chin.***[54]

Fear; coition, for, after too much indulgence: lyc.[172]

Hypochondriasis; sexual, abuse, after: ***ph-ac.***[54]

Hysteria; lascivious: agn.[54] mosch. ***plat.*** ***tarent.***

Hysteria; sexual excesses, after: agar. anac. con. lach. ***ph-ac.*** sep.

Imbecility; sexual, abuse, after: ***phos.***[54]

Indifference; exposure of her person, to: ***hyos.*** ***phos.*** ***phyt.*** ***sec.*** stram. verat.

Indifference; naked, to remain: **HYOS.**[122]

Insanity; dancing, with, and stripping himself: ***bell.***[122]

Insanity; erotic: ambr.[102] **APIS BAR-M.** bell.[10] bufo[107] calc-p.[36] camph.[85] ***cann-i.***[102] canth.[111] ferul.[102] gins.[102] grat.[102] ***hyos.*** kali-br. lil-t.[102] lyss. manc.[102] ***murx.***[102] ***nux-v.***[85] orig. ***phos.*** ***pic-ac.***[102] **PLAT.** ***puls.*** rob.[102] salx-n.[102] stann.[36] stram.[36] ***sulph.*** ***tarent.*** **VERAT.** zinc.[111]

Insanity; erotic, hysterical girl, in a: ***plat.***[54]

Insanity; erotic, jealousy, with: ***hyos.***[54]

Insanity; lascivious: ***hyos.***[5] tarent.[8] **VERAT.**[5]

Insanity; sexual excesses, from: anan.[54] ***apis***[130] ***lach.***[30] lil-t.[54] ***phos.***[54] staph.[30]

Insanity; wantonness, with: bell.[10] cupr. ***hyos.*** merc.[10] mez.[10] stram. verat.

Irritability; sexual, excesses, from: ol-an.[116]

Lasciviousness; animal, as if she were completely, mental power dormant: lach.[54]

Lasciviousness; convulsions, before: ***lach.***[54]

Lasciviousness; dreaming, after: sil.[10]

Lasciviousness; eating, after, with feeling of weakness in parts: lyss.[54]

Lasciviousness; emotions, with violent: cop.[54]

Lasciviousness; erections, with: op.[54] sin-n.[54]

Lasciviousness; erections, with, afternoon: lyss.[54]

Lasciviousness; erections, with, painful: lyss.[54]

Lasciviousness; erections, with, painful, night: ***merc.***[54]

Lasciviousness; erections, without: ambr.[5] calad.[5] caps.[5] **IGN.**[54] meny.[5] **SEL.**[5]

Lasciviousness; impotence, with: calad.[58] ***chin.***[54] ***op.***[54] ***sel.***[54]

Lasciviousness; lustfulness: ***acon.***[54] act-sp.[162] agar. agn.[137] aloe alum.[30] ***ambr.*** anac.[102] androc.[222] ant-c.[85] ant-i.[54] ***apis*** arund. aster.[54] aur. bell.[30] bor. bov.[36] ***bufo***[11] ***calad. calc.*** calc-p.[116] calc-s. calc-sil.[58] camph.[36] ***cann-i.***[116] cann-s.[116] ***canth. carb-v.*** carl.[36] ***caust.***[30] cedr.[85] cere-s.[36] ***chin.*** coc-c. cod.[36] ***con.*** cop. croc.[116] ***dig. fl-ac. graph.*** hydrog.[222] **HYOS.** hyper. ign. kali-br.[122] **LACH. LIL-T.** lyc. lyss. m-arct.[36] merc. mosch. ***murx.***[102] nat-c.[36] nat-m. nit-ac. nuph.[36] nux-m.[36] nux-v.[85] op. **ORIG.** ph-ac.[30] **PHOS. PIC-AC. PLAT.** plb.[116] ***puls.*** raja-s.[149] raph. ***sabin.***[116] salx-n.[72] sars.[36] ***sel. sep. sil.*** spig. squil.[137] stann.[36] **STAPH.** ***stram.*** sulph.[30] ***tarent.*** tere-ch.[149] tub.[122] ust.[116] ***verat.*** zinc.

Lasciviousness; ogling, women on the street: calad.[137] fl-ac.[137]

Lasciviousness; painful urging in penis, with, as after excessive coition: lyss.[54]

Lasciviousness; rage, with: ***hyos.***[54]

Lasciviousness; religious: ***plat.***[54]

Lasciviousness; rest, no: ***orig.***[54]

Lasciviousness; uncovers sexual parts: **HYOS.**[54]

Lasciviousness; voluptuous ideas, pleasure only in: bell.

Lasciviousness; women at every touch: ***murx.***[116]

Laughing; sexual excitement, with: stram.[137]

Lewdness, obscene: agn. alum.[30] anac.[102] androc.[222] apis bell. bufo[112] calc.[30] ***camph. canth.*** carb-v.[30] ***caust.***[30] chin.[30] con.[30] ***cub.*** fl-ac.[111] ***hyos. lach.*** lil-t.[36] lyc.[30] lyss. merc.[30] nat-m.[30] nux-v. op. orig.[30] ***phos. pic-ac. plat.***[122] puls.[30] raph.[36] rob. staph.[30] stram. sulph.[30] tarent. verat.

Lewdness; man searching for little girls: caust.[30] phos.[30] plat.[30] verat.[30]

Lewdness; talk: apis[130] aur. ***bell.*** bufo[112] ***calc.***[30] camph. chlf.[36] cub. ***hyos. lil-t.*** nux-m.[10] ***nux-v.*** phos. plat. ***stram.*** tub.[102] verat.

Libertinism: act-sp.[54] alum.[30] arn.[10] bar-c.[10] bell.[30] calc.[30] ***canth.***[30] carb-v.[30] ***caust.***[30] chin.[30] con.[30] fl-ac.[122] hyos.[30] lyc.[30] **MED.**[185] merc.[30] nat-m.[30] ***nux-v.*** orig.[30] ph-ac.[30] ***phos.***[30] pic-ac. ***plat.*** puls.[30] raph.[36] sep.[122] spong.[10] ***staph.*** stram.[30] sulph.[30] verat.[30]

Love; anal coition with a woman: caust.[30] plat.[30]

Love; married man or coachman, with: ign.[58] ***nat-m.***[122]

Love; own sex, men: med.[162] nat-m.[162] orig.[162] phos.[162] ***plat.***[30] puls.[162] sep.[162] staph.[162]

Love; own sex, with one of her, homosexuality, tribadism: anh.[144] calc.[30] calc-p. hydrog.[222] hyos.[185] hypoth.[149] ***lach.*** lyc.[148] nat-m. phos. **PLAT.**[122] puls.[122] ***sulph.*** syph.[85] thiop.[149]

Love; own sex, women: fl-ac.[162] med.[162] phos.[162] puls.[162] sulph.[162]

Love; perversity, animals, with, sodomy: ***plat.***[162]

Mania; indecent: ***op.***[54]

Mania; sexual in men: apis[117] canth.[102] **PHOS.** ***tarent.***

Mania; sexual, abuse, from: lil-t.[54] ***phos.***[54]

Mania; sexual, increased desire, from: apis[122] **BAR-M.**[54] **PHOS.** ***tarent.***

Mania; sexual, men, in: apis[117] canth.[102] **PHOS.** ***tarent.***

Mania; sexual, women in: **APIS**[54] canth.[102] **PHOS.**[122] raph.[36] ***tarent.***[122]

Memory; weakness, sexual excesses, from: agn.[102] anac.[102] arg-n.[102] aur.[102] calad. **CALC.**[54] chin.[102] **DIG.**[54] kali-br.[72] ***nat-ar.*** nat-m.[102] nux-v.[102] ***ph-ac.***[102] **PHOS.**[54] **STAPH.**[54]

Moral affections; perversions: ***anac.***[5] **BELL.**[5] bufo[5] **HYOS.**[5] nux-v.[5] ***op.***[5] ph-ac.[5] ***plat.***[5] **STRAM.**[5] tarent.[5] **VERAT.**[5]

Morose; erotomania, in: ***orig.***[54] ***plat.***[54]

Morose; sexual excesses, from: **STAPH.**[54]

Naked, wants to be, delirium, in: ***bell.*** **HYOS.** merc. ***phos.*** phyt. ***sec. stram.***[54]

Necromania: **AGAR.**[185]

Nymphomania: agar. ambr. androc.[222] anh.[149] ***ant-c. apis*** ars.[31] asaf.[54] aster.[149] aur-m-n.[85] ***bar-m. bell.*** calad. calc. ***calc-p.*** camph. camph-br.[25] ***cann-i. cann-s. canth.*** carb-v. cedr. ***chin.*** chlol.[25] chlor.[5] coca[98] cocc.[31] ***coff.*** con.[31] ***croc.***[5] cyna.[149] ***dig.*** dulc. ***ferul.***[102] ***fl-ac.*** gins.[102] graph. **GRAT. HYOS.** ign.[116] iod.[31] ***kali-br.*** kali-p. **LACH.** ***lil-t. lyc.*** manc.[116] ***merc.*** mosch. ***murx.*** nat-c. nat-m. ***nux-v.*** op. **ORIG.** orig-v.[25] ozone[227] ph-ac.[85] ***phos.*** pic-ac.[102] **PLAT.** plb. psil.[149] ***puls. raph.*** rob. ***sabad.*** sabin. salx-n.[85] sil. stann.[111] ***staph.*** **STRAM.** stry.[102] sulph. sumb.[111] ***tarent.*** thuj.[31] valer.[102] ***verat. zinc.*** zinc-pic.[85]

Nymphomania; climacteric period, at: lach.[102] manc.[102] ***murx.***[102]
Nymphomania; coition agg.: ***tarent.***[54]
Nymphomania; delivery, parturition, after, puerperal: bell.[10] ***chin.*** coca[83] kali-br. ***plat.*** verat. zinc.[54]
Nymphomania; girl young, in a: ***orig.***[54] raph.[85]
Nymphomania; loquacity, with: ***verat.***[54]
Nymphomania; menses, after: kali-br.[25] sul-ac.[116]
Nymphomania; menses, before: calc.[116] calc-p. kali-c.[116] ***phos.*** stram. ***verat.***
Nymphomania; menses, during: calc.[116] coca[83] ***hyos.*** kali-br. kali-c.[116] ***phos.***[54] ***plat.*** ***sec.*** stram. ***verat.***
Nymphomania; menses, suppressed: ant-c. canth. chin. cocc. hyos. ***murx.*** phos. ***plat.*** sil. stram. sulph. verat. zinc
Nymphomania; metrorrhagia, during: mosch. murx. plat. sabin.[85] sec.
Nymphomania; mirth, with: ***plat.***[54]
Prostration; sexual excesses, after: sel.[58]
Restlessness; lascivious thoughts, from: graph.[36]
Rover about; naked: hyos.
Sadness; sexual excesses, from: agar.[116] agn.[102] aur.[102] ***cimic.***[102] con.[116] ***lil-t.***[102] nux-v.[102] pic-ac.[102] plat.[102] sep.[102] spong.[137]
Satyriasis: agar.[5] agn.[5] anac.[149] androc.[222] ***apis***[130] bar-m.[85] camph.[36] cann-i.[36] canna[83] **CANTH.**[5] coca[83] con.[5] cyna.[149] ***fl-ac.***[54] ***gels.***[8] **GRAPH.**[5] grat.[54] hyos.[5] ***kali-br.***[54] kali-c.[5] **LYC.**[5] ***lyss.***[54] med.[187] **MERC.**[5] ***nat-m.***[5] **NUX-V.**[5] pen.[36] **PHOS.**[5] ***pic-ac.***[54] **PLAT.**[5] psor.[36] salx-n.[85] saroth.[149] **SIL.**[5] ***stram.***[5] ***sulph.***[5] thymol.[149] ust.[116] ***verat.***[5] zinc.[5] zinc-pic.[85]
Satyriasis; stallion, in a: ***lyss.***[8]
Shameless: alco.[36] ***anac.***[5] bell. ***bufo***[5] calc. camph.[5] cann-s.[5] canth. chlf.[46] cub. cupr. hell. <u>**HYOS.**</u>[122] lyc.[30] merc-c. mosch. ***murx.***[5] nat-m. nux-m. nux-v. ***op.***[5] **PHOS.** phyt. ***plat.***[5] sabin.[5] **SEC.** ***staph.***[193] ***stram.*** ***tarent.*** ***tub.***[122] ***verat.***
Shameless; exposes the person: **HYOS.** ***phos.*** phyt. ***sec.*** stram.[5] ***tarent.*** verat.[122]
Singing; obscene songs: alco.[36] canth.[58] ***hyos.*** op. raja-s.[149] stram. verat.[58]
Singing; obscene songs, nymphomania, in: ***stram.***[54]
Stupefaction; debauchery, as after: psor.[122]
Suicidal disposition; erotomania, in: orig.[137]
Thoughts; sexual, day and night: chin.[10] dig.[10]
Unconsciousness; alternating with, erotic mania: apis[98]
Violence; nymphomania, in: ***verat.***[54]
Weeping; easily, erotomania, in: ***plat.***[54]
Work; impossible, sexual excesses, after: ph-ac.[116] pic-ac.[116] ***sel.***[116]

ACT-SP. He, 7 - Inclined to debauchery.(seduction, lewdness)
AMBR. Al, 2 - Lewd fancies, even when dreaming; the mind and the sexual organs, however, do not feel excited by them.
Ha, 477 - The imagination is occupied with many lascivious ideas, even in dreams, and yet the disposition and the sexual organs are but little excited by them.
APIS. He, 29 - Insanity, particularly nymphomania...
He, 77 - All her ideas turn around jealousy, very talkative (loquacity), sometimes disgusting salacious. (lascivious)
ASTER. He, 17 - Nervous agitation, with erotic thoughts and sexual desire.
BAR-M. He, 4 - In every form of mania, as soon as the sexual desire is increased. (lascivious)
BELL. Ha, 1351 - Chattering (talk) lascivious.
He, 62 - Loud laughter, wild abandon, singing, whistling, lascivious conversation.
CALAD. He, 15 - Lascivious ideas. Gleet Impotence.
CALC. He, 71 - Voluptuous (sensual), lascivious fancies.
CANTH. He, 17 - Great amativeness, amorous frenzy.
He, 18 - Unbounded frantic sexual desire. Mania.
DIG. He, 7 - Lascivious fancies day and night.
HIPP. Al, 1 - Lascivious fancies in the forenoon.
HYOS. Ha, 67 - Amativeness; nymphomania; erotomania.(sexual)
He, 68 - Onanism since childhood; has always been greatly attracted by opposite sex and prematurely busied himself with thoughts of marriage;... secretly wrote his love affairs; mania,...one idea rapidly follow another, all in some away concern-

ing love, masturbates at every opportunity...(satyriasis)

He, 46 - Sings amorous and obscene songs.

He, 69 - Lascivious mania, uncovers body, especially sexual parts; sings amorous songs.

KALI-BR. Al, 3 - Decidedly insane; had delusions that lewd women had got into his mother's house; that he was pursued by the police; that his wife was threatened by members of the family; that he had thousands of dollars in gold sewed up in his clothing; (rich, wealth)

LACH. He, 33-...want of self control; lascivious; felt as if she was clear (pure) animal right through, whilst of all mental power was dormant; sensation as if hands of stronger power, as if charmed (enchanted), and as if could not break the spell (charm). (possessed, wildness)

He, 47 - Amorousness; amativeness.

LIL-T. Al, 351 - The sexual desire, dormant hitherto, was so strongly aroused that the prover said, "I am afraid of myself, I seem possessed of a demon."

He, 9 - Disposed to curse, to strike, to think of obscene things; as these mental states came, uterine irritation abated.(reduced)

NEON. Sh, 203 - Had thoughts of sex over 2 days; mentally planned scenarios of a clandestine meeting with an old boyfriend (more in the evening). 08, 30C, 00:00:20

PHOS. Al, 1-..this delirium, which preceded death, was erotic, with indications of great, excitement of the sexual system...

Ha, 27-....Talks in a vehement, (impetuous) commanding (dictatorial) tone; spits at nurse, lifts up her clothes (naked) and kisses hotly all who come near her;...

He, 28-...;erotic with indications of great excitement of sexual system; ... fancied he was in several pieces and could not get the fragments properly adjusted.(disconnection, fragmentation, split, disconnected, divided)

He, 29 - Crazy deliria in a young woman who was strictly moral and unhappy in her love; accused herself of the most obscene (immoral, wicked) actions, of which she never was guilty; ....

PLAT. He, 37-...depressed condition of physical powers; ...fear of approaching death; ... aversion to coition and yet dreams of intense lasciviousness,...

He, 40 - Disturbed state of mind; religious, with taciturnity, haughtiness, voluptuousness (sensual) and cruelty.

He, 42 - Mania; with great pride; fault-finding; unchaste (sensual) talk; ...(chaste = moral, pure)

RAPH. Al, 1 - Feeling of aversion towards all women; she is provoked by seeing women going and coming about her; their approach threw her into a fury; the mere contact with a woman's dress caused intolerable distress;...She is attracted to all men without distinction (nymphomania) ; when she gives her hand to a man, she feels great agitation,...When left alone for a hour in the evening, she gave herself a very deep wound in the lips with a penknife, in hopes to put an end to this condition (hurt, punishes). Moral feeling was completely extinct, the physical nature alone ruled and threw her into a frightful state (wild). From morning to noon she would not have been able to resist the advances even of a man for whom she had not the least friendly feeling; from noon to 6 p.m. she could not have held out against any man whatsoever; from 8 to 11 the demands of sense were so importunate as to silence the voice of shame and reason; ... and would have thrown herself into the arms of the first man she met...she was still unable to control her impulses;...

ROB. Al, 11 - Strong disposition to be obscene, to gormandize (gluttony, voracity), and for all kinds of orgies.

SEL. He, 8 - Lascivious thoughts with impotence.

STAPH. He, 6 - Hypochondriasis (depression);...;caused by unmerited insults (offenses, affronts, abuses) sexual excesses, or by persistently dwelling on sexual subjects.

STRAM. He, 111 - Nymphomania; with diaphragmitis; violent attacks, even to rage; exalted sexual passion.

He, 119 - His thoughts ran upon obscene things, frequently put his hands to erect penis; sought to bite or to catch flies.

TARENT. Al, 76-...changeable mind, tears, singing, and irresoluteness.(In a woman, twenty-six years old, who complained of violent sexual appetite.)

VERAT. He, 21 - Mania; with desire to cut and tear everything, especially clothes; with lewdness and lascivious talk; religious or amorous; de grandeur.

He, 22 - Nymphomania, with violence and destructiveness; had been disappointed in love; melancholia; ...great desire for sexual intercourse; void (empty) of shame; obscenity; ....

He, 50 - Religious melancholy or nymphomania, with desire to embrace everybody even inanimate objects;...[0]Puerperal mania.

LIAR

Delusions; lie, all she said is a: lac-c.

Liar: alco. androc.[222] arg-n.[122] bell.[30] calc.[30] carb-v.[30] caust.[30] coca[36] con.[30] lyc.[30] med.[212] merc.[30] **MORPH.**[122] nat-m.[30] nux-v.[85] **OP.**[122] phos.[189] puls.[30] sil.[30] staph.[30] sulph.[30] ***syph.***[122] **VERAT.**[122]

Liar; charlatan and: calc.[30] nat-m.[30] puls.[30]

Liar; deny obstinately that they have been bitten: lyss.[54]

Liar; describes some symptoms truly, misrepresents others: ***cupr-acet.***[54]

Liar; lie, believes all she says is a: ***lac-c.***

Liar; makes wrong statements to herself, because she does not know what to say next, begins all right but does not know how to finish: ***med.***[54]

Liar; never speaks the truth, does not know what she is saying: alco.[122] arg-n.[122] ***morph.***[122] **OP.**[122] ***syph.***[122] ***verat.***[122]

Mood; repulsive, food, saying one who does not work should not eat, but driven by hunger he tried to procure it secretly: ***arg-n.***[54]

Truth; thinks she does not tell the: macrin.[36]

Truth; want of: ferr.[30] iod.[30] mag-c.[30] nux-v.[30] sep.[30] sulph.[30]

ANDROC. Sh, 121 - When talking to friends felt 'paranoid', suspicious and guilty, when asked questions, he became hot and sweaty. He felt it was a game of who was cleverer, and tried to lie to and outwit his friend, though this gave no satisfaction. His friends reported that he seemed unusually distant and cool. (29)

BUFO. Al, 25 - Defiance (disobedience, challenger), duplicity (hypocrisy), spitefulness.(cruelty)

COCC. Al, 27 - Very much affected and offended by slight obliquities (immorality) and untruths (falsehood) of others.

Ha, 554 - He is very indignant and annoyed at slight faults and fibs (lie, falsify) of others.

GERM. Sh, 158 - Some persistent feelings coming up. Feel envious of a colleague who I feel manages so well. When I compare with myself I feel worthless and nothing. I feel like talking badly about her to my friends and I do this, even though she is not present. It takes a lot of my attention and energy. 21, 12C, 67:XX:XX.

LAC-C. Al,N -8 - Is impressed with the idea that all she says is a lie; it seems to be very difficult to speak the truth (liar, dissimulator), but continually distrusts things (suspicious); when reading anything she rapidly changes the meaning, omitting or adding things. (mischievous)

He, 6 - Is impressed with idea that all she says is a lie. (false)

MACRO. Al, 6 - Suspicious of everybody; thinks she has not told the truth (veracity) in regard to himself. (secretive, pretend)

TARENT. Al, 55 - Fear, which could not be stopped, in a young lady; questioned about it, she tried to find a cause, and leaves others to think there is one; but really there was none.

VERAT. He, 5 - Never speaks the truth; does not know herself what she is saying.

LIBERTY

Delusions; animals, birds, sees: bell. kali-c. lac-c.

- animals, pigeons flying in room which he tries to catch: ***kali-c.***[54]
- bird, he is a, runs about, chirping and twittering, until he faints: lyss.[54]
- birds, sees: bell. kali-c. lac-c.
- body, back, opens and wings are forming: choc.[222]
- fly, he can: camph.[139] lil-t.[139] tub.[139]
- flying, away, what he holds in his hands: coloc.[5] dulc.[5] **STAPH.**[5]
- flying, out of his skin: thuj.[5]
- goose, he is a: con.
- wings, her body is borne upon wings, after laughing: thuj.[54]

Dreams; animals, birds, of, large, black: choc.[222]

➤ animals, birds, of, singing: com.[36]
➤ animals, horses, running: atro. indg. lipp.[36]
➤ fights, galley slave, with: elaps[36]
➤ flying, apparatus, whose wings will not work: apis[36]
➤ flying, lighted street, along: convo-d.[36]
➤ flying, people: hydrog.[222]
➤ flying, tops of houses, over: xan.[54]
➤ mother, flying around the world: hydrog.[222]
➤ nakedness, about: androc.[222] cench.[58] erech.[36] kali-p.[58] rumx.
➤ prisoner, release of prisoners: hura.[36]

Fear; alone, of being, starts with a loud cry as if a bird flew towards the window: kali-c.[172]

Fly, desire to: choc.[222]

Freedom remarkable, in doing what he had to do: op.[36] ozone[227]

Independent: bell.[30] calc.[162] cupr.[210] nux-v.[30] sulph.[30]

ADAM. Sh, 283 - My husband has commented that I am talking more and cuddling less, and I realize I do not feel so dependent on him, I feel more of an individual. 12, 30C, 07.:XX:XX.

Sh, 292 - It's crystal clear! Clarifying female roles. Clarification of issues. Realization — anger and depression in the past, had to do with conditioning, not saying what I wanted, not having my needs met. 10, 6C, 47:XX:XX

Sh, 306 - Determined to help children recognize and free themselves from family patterns and to be themselves. 10, 6C, 34:XX:XX

Sh, 556 - Feel bright, free and beautiful, more feminine, more fertile and voluptuous. 16, 12C, 24:XX:XX

ARS. Ha, 1038 - When he is alone he is beset by thoughts about disease and other thoughts of an indifferent character, of which he cannot get rid.

He, 25 - Mania...sees a man who has hanged himself beckoning (call) him to cut him loose (rescue, deliverance, free, saving) on failing to accomplish this he attempts to hang himself (punish, penalize);...finally kneels down and lifts his hands in supplication.(forgiveness, absolution)

BELL. Al, 81 - He imagines he sees birds flying off through the chimney, and wishes to follow them by the same route. (desire: fly, liberty, freedom)

Al, 174 - He escaped, under some pretext, into the open field.(run away)

Al,S-2559 - Seems to see birds flying past and wishes to follow them.

Ha, 1436 - He makes an excuse (pretext) and runs out into the open fields.

CAMPH. Al, 46-...I feel a tendency to self contemplation; outer things vanish, and I behold myself in spirit freed from matter.

Al, 46-...I am alone. I feel a tendency to self contemplation; outer things vanished, and I behold myself in spirit freed from matter...

CANN-I. Al, 32 - He thinks he can fly through the air like the birds.

Al, 33 - Said "he had been transported to heaven (paradise)"...

Al, 42 - The soul seemed to be separated from the body, and to look down upon it, and view all the motions of the vital processes, and to be able to pass and repass though the solid walls of the room, and to view the landscape (view) beyond.

CARB-V. Ha, 37 - Freedom of spirit, lightness and general good health (curative...)

CHOC. Sh, 8 - I felt like being outside, roaming around without any possessions, to have the freedom to go where I want to go when the feeling took me. I felt very restricted.

Sh, 44 - Dream —coming out of the station a huge black bird the size of a dog with black long soft feathers like those of an ostrich, and a very big beak. It took my left hand in his beak. There were two gypsies there and they stood in front of me and opened their hands and I saw that they held a gold metal flat fish which I saw as a fortune telling object.

Sh, 50 - Panic feeling of being trapped and enclosed —worse when curtains are closed and the light blocked out. Strong desire to be outside and moving, to be in the bright and warm sunlight. Kept having to move my feet, which I felt I wanted to move.

Sh, 103 - On looking at a bird in a cage, felt it should be out.

Sh, 139 - Meditation is much smoother —an effortless zooming in. I feel much more comfortable in the world. Before I always wanted to get out. During meditation, felt a floating feeling, felt an opening and upwards movement in my back, as if wings were forming and I was just light.

Sh, 150 - People keep stopping me and saying they don't recognise me. I still have a silly grin on my face. Laugh more —so much joy inside and a sense of freedom very different to before the proving. Dogs seem to like me more and babies seem to like me more, and this was noticed by others too.

Sh, 314 - Talking about flying. I would like to be a bird or a bat or in a plane.01A, 30C, 00:12:XX

CON. Al, 6 - Delirious and stupid; they threw themselves into the water, thinking they were geese; for three years they remained partly paralytic, suffering from much pain.

FL-AC. Al, 1 - Great disposition, when alone, to repulsive fantastic imaginations, particularly in regard to persons with whom he stands in near relations, or with whom he is connected (united, joined); it seems, for example, as though he must get rid (discard, repudiate, reject) of all the servants, children must go out of house, a betrothal must be broken off, a marriage should be dissolved. (broke; vows)

HALI-L. Sh, 534 - The thing about the proving, I see now, was the intense trapped feeling. I felt trapped by people and situations. People who are being weird. Before, I would just let things slide, or roll off of me, like water off a duck's back. During the proving, I needed to break out, a screeching feeling. I had to speak out to change the situation. I had to stop letting things slide. 13, 30C, 7 months

Sh, 691 - Do fish, as well as birds, pair for life? I don't think so—a free for all. 20, 30C, 00:01:14

Sh, 900 - It was or is ? As if I'm not really used to domestic duties. I can't really do anything for any other, just hopefully glimpses of illumination. All on own—with everything. Just to give—Does it really help? Doesn't it make others expect, or more needy? They lose freedom—independence. 20, 30C, 10:XX:XX

HURA. Al, 700 - Dream about children and the release (liberty) of prisoners.

IRID. Sh, 54 - Getting dressed, didn't want to put clothes on, wanted the freedom of nakedness, chose clothes for their lack of restriction. G 6

Sh, 79 - Had this longing to find real wilderness. Britain is too full, nothing is really alive anymore except people. The world really feels too oppressed with people and roofs. I kept saying to partner, "Why do we live in this dreary, ugly place, where people know nothing about freedom, and certainly nothing about discovery or mystery, just tarmac and roofs." It struck me that the world was too small for me, and thought "That's got to be something about the remedy, something around pressure." E5

Sh, 81 - Feel hemmed in by ex-partner's needs, feel I'm being fitted into the little spaces in his life. Can no longer shrug and say, "Well this is how it is." G5

Sh, 82 - Last three Fridays, since proving began, have gone to bed very early. Really exhausted. Realized that part of the going to bed is to be by myself —needed space in bed, alone and quiet. Rare for me to go to bed and leave daughters up watching TV. Could hear it and felt it invading my space. G26

Sh, 101 - Went into pet shop. There was a budgie chirping in a cage. I was so upset. "Oh God, I want to let this bird out." I felt it was crying to be let out. Took me all my control not to let it out or shout at the man to do it. Then thought, "This is silly. It would get hurt, he'll think I'm mad." I slunk out of the shop thinking I'd really let that bird down. Distracted and nearly in tears. Walked round town in a daze, should I go back and ask him to at least open the door, knew that wasn't on. It might get out of the shop and die. Felt a real coward. Set up a train of thought —condor in bird garden —a notice justifying its captivity —it only flies for food —it's quite happy to be there because food comes to it. Weeping as I write this. Birds in cages can't lean on the air currents and be blown away. G6

Sh, 102 - Just before sleep, image came into head from nowhere. Sitting on an air current as if it was a soft comfy settee foam cushion. Started to move over a landscape, took me high up, trees, towns, like the flying sequence from The Snowman. The air was so supportive, like floating on water. It had real substance but unlike water it was bouncy. There was no way I was going to fall. I was sitting back, not floating, tummy down. Felt like a child bouncing on the air. Fun —at the same time sense of awe, experiencing something for the first time. No sense of danger — trust. Floatiness experienced before with cannabis but then I was anxious, "Would I get back into body?" With this I was still in my body —no separation. G44

Sh, 106 - Mental image: I am inside an egg —a bird, wet feathers, at the point it is smashing through its shell, bursting out; a chick, wet crumpled and hot, shell flying all over. The relief —getting to the air, refreshing, cool. Inside it was humid, stifling. Stretching vast wings, enjoying feeling the air dry them out. G5

Sh, 109 - Sensation as if wings 3 —4 p.m. Q5

Sh, 110 - Meditating, vision of an angel, face and wings. Q6

Sh, 112 - Sensation as if winged ankles, while wind blowing through house. Thought, "back to earth." Q17

Sh, 113 - Feel as if growing wings in back. SENSATION AS IF body wanting to change form, mainly in chest, face, back. Q4

KALI-C. Al, 25 - She is frightened with a loud cry, by an imaginary apparition (as for example, of a bird flying to the window).

Ha, 26 - She is frightened by an imaginary appearance (e.g. as if a bird was flying toward the window) and she utters a loud scream.

He, 5 - Imagines seeing birds flying in room; he tries to catch them. (seize)

LACH. Al, 43 - He is impelled to productive work in the evening, although he had been much fatigued during the day ... writes with the greatest freedom and increased vigor about everything he knows;...

LYSS. Al,N-26 - Thinks he is a dog or a bird, and runs up and down chirping and twittering...(liberty?)

He, 26 - Thinks he is a dog or a bird, and runs up and down, chirping and twittering, until he falls down fainting.

NEON. Sh, 21 - Walking was effortless, light and free, with a sensation of walking uniformly. I feel so different in my body. I am all in the now, especially in lower legs and feet. At last, I touch the earth. 20, 6C, 03:01:00

Sh, 60 - During the proving the prover separated from her partner of 13 years. She had attempted this several times previously, unsuccessfully. I asked her what had changed: "Somehow I had a very profound realization that this is my own life time. My usual feelings of guilt shifted and I was able to take responsibility for my own life. There was a sudden clarity. During the proving I wore my glasses more and had dreams of windows. As though there had been a shift of focus to my own needs." 02, 6C, XX:XX:XX

PHOS. Ha, 76 - Freedom (liberty) of spirit,... everything seems brighter (luminous, vivid) to him.

PLAT. He, 46-...;suffers unspeakable pangs (anxiety) of conscience in consequence of a faux (fault, mistake, embarrassing mistake?) pass when thirty-two years old; says she has brought disgrace upon her family, and that she has incurred the penalty of damnation; (doomed) in order to do penance (penitence) gave away whatever she could lay her hands upon, (redemption) so that she had to be constantly watched; after her confessor asserted that she could not hope for pardon or heaven (condemnable), she seemed in absolute despair ; bemoaned her misery throughout the night, wringing her hands and beseeching (implore) that she might be delivered (free) from the hell of her conscience; twice attempted self-destruction (suicide);...wished to live and do penance (penitence, purgation, purification) in order to mitigate her eternal punishment.

PLB. Al, 38 - Begged and prayed to be released from the strait-waistcoat, "for", he said, "I am not mad; but the idea of being forcibly restrained is enough to drive me crazy".

PULS. Al, 47 - He cannot at all get rid of a

thought that he once grasped.

RHUS-T. Ha, 973 - When she had disagreeable thoughts in her head she could not get rid of them.

STICT. Al, 1 - She got very lively (active), told her father she felt as if she would like to strike out, only for fun; she would like it just for fun of it. After awhile she lay down on the lounge, and began, to use a common expression, to kick up her heels; her mother reproaching, said, " Bella, do behave, that is not ladylike"; when child responded: " Ma, I cannot help it; I feel exactly as if I want to fly away"...

SULPH. Al, 8 - Numerous morbid ideas, extremely disagreeable, causing rancor, though with also joyous thoughts (and melodies) mostly from the past, take possession of her they throng one upon another so that she cannot free herself from them during the day, with neglect of business,...

Al, 10 - Vexatious and morbid ideas of the past arise from the most indifferent thoughts, and from every occurrence in life, which continue to be united with new vexations, so that she cannot free herself from them, together with a courageous mood which is ready for great resolution.

Ha, 58-..She thinks of nothing but anxious, annoying and dejecting thoughts, which she cannot get rid of; this makes her apprehensive and peevish unto tears.

LIFELESS

Delusions; soda water, being a bottle of: arg-n.[91] cann-i.[36]

Dreams; houses, cold, liveless, nearly threatening: ozone[227]

Sensitive; want of sensitiveness, stone, feels like a dead, insensitive: ozone[227]

ACON. Al, 71 - Dejected, as if she had no life in her. (lifeless)

Ha, 505 - Morose, as though she had no life in her. (animation)

ANAC. Ha, 37 - He can only think when a subject is suggested to him; he does not of himself think of anything; he cannot independently determine anything.

ARS. Ha, 1056 - Life appears to him naught (emptiness); he attaches no value (worth) to it. (insignificant, worthlessness)

CAMPH. Al, 46-... The sight increased my despair poor nature extinguished; the sky transparent and lifeless; the earth was still in the dim, dead light. I could not bear it. The sense of touch was gone, and my eyes protruded from their sockets.

CANN-I. Al, 69 - He seems to himself to be transformed into a vegetable existence, as a huge fern, and to be surrounded by clouds of music and perfume.

CHOC. Sh, 62 - The blackness of the trees is bothering me. They seem dark and leafless.

CROT-H. He, 13 - Marked indifference, seems only half alive; utter apathy.

CYCL. Al, 17 - Very fretful (irritable) the whole day; disinclined to speak and insensible (indifferent), having very little feeling (emotion) in his body.

EUPHR. Ha, 127 - Lazy, hypochondriacal; external objects had no charm (beauty), no life (animation) for him. (indifference)

MEZ. Ha, 2-...everything seemed to him as if dead, and nothing made a vivid impression on him.

He, 10-...; everything seems to him dead (lifeless, inert) and nothing makes a vivid impression upon his mind.

MUR-AC. Al, 5 - Sad absorbed in herself, as if there were no life (inert, lifeless) in her during menses.

Al, 15 - The brightness (lively, vivid) of his disposition constantly diminished, until in the evening he became very fretful (irritable).

Al, 6 - During the menses she is sad, taciturn, as if she had no life.

Ha, 2 - Sad and introverted, as if she had no life in her, during the menses.

PULS. Al, 25 - It seems so quiet (silent) in her head and everything feels so empty that she seems alone in the house and in the world; she will speak to no one, just as if her surroundings did not exist (estrange), and she paid attention to no one. (left, solitary)

RHUS-T. Al, 5 - Melancholy, ill-humor, and anxiety, as if a misfortune (disgrace) would happen, or as if she were alone (solitary), and all about her were dead (lifeless, inert) and still (silent, quiet), or as if she had been forsaken by a near friend; worse in the house, relieved by walking in the open air.

Ha, 953 - Melancholy, sad, and anxious, as if about to hear of a calamity, (misfortune, disaster) or as if she were solitary (lonely, alone) and all around her were dead (lifeless, extinct) and silent (quiet) ; or as if she had bid farewell (separation) to an intimate friend ; worst in the room, diminished by walking in a open air.

SEP. Al, 82 - Great indifference toward everything; no proper sense of life.

Ha, 59 - Great indifference to everything, no real vital feeling.

He, 6 - Great indifference to everything; no proper sense of life.

STAPH. Ha, 695 - As if dead (decease, lifeless, inert) in mind and sad, but not to weeping.

STRAM. Al, 122 - For some days the patient was affected with hallucinations and thought that one side of him was alive, while the other side was buried.

Ha, 519 - He speaks to absent persons as though they were present, and addresses(talk) lifeless objects (e.g. chess-men) by the names of those persons, but does not notice any of those around him.

TAB. Al, 2 - He went to sleep in the cabin, which was full of large packages of tobacco, ...His inability to move was not accompanied by any pain or uneasiness but he felt as if the principle of life had entirely departed from his frame.(body)

LIGHT

Cheerfulness; lightness, with feeling of: petr.[10]

Company, aversion to; dizzy, faint in a crowd, or where many gas lights are burning (in agoraphobia): ***nux-v.***[54]

Delirium; light, with desire for: calc.[10]

Delusions; air, he is hovering in, like a spirit: asar. lac-c.[58] lach.[58] psil.[164]

• body, immaterial, is: anh.[119]

• body, lighter than air, is: asar.[149] lach. lap-c-b.[194] ***op.*** thuj. visc.[149] xan.[85]

• body, lighter than air, is, embrace, after: agn.[36]

• body, lighter than air, is, masturbation, from, or hysterical subjects, in: gels.[137]

• clear, everything is too: ambr.[10]

• elevated in air: nitro-o.[36] phos.[139] rhus-t.[139] sil.[139]

• floating in air: ***acon.*** agar.[162] ***ambr.***[162] anh.[119] ***arg.***[162] arn.[193] asar. bell.[116] bry.[139] calc.[85] calc-ar.[58] camph. cand-a.[239] cann-i. canth. chlf.[36] cocain.[139] cocc.[137] coff.[137] dat-a.[36] euon.[122] euon-a.[85] germ.[222] hura hyos.[85] hyper.[102] jug-r.[85] kali-br. ***lac-c.***[72] ***lach.*** lact.[85] lat-k.[102] m-aust.[85] manc.[139] mosch.[139] nat-ar.[102] nat-m.[137] ***nux-m. op.***[137] ozone[227] passi.[85] pen.[85] ph-ac.[85] phos. phys.[85] pip-m.[139] rhus-g.[102] sep.[48] spig.[162] ***stach.***[116] ***stict.***[72] stram.[137] stroph.[85] ***tarent.***[85] tell.[85] tep.[139] ter.[5] thuj.[137] ***valer.*** visc.[149] xan.[85] zinc-i.[137]

• light, full of: anh.[119]

• light, incorporeal, immaterial, he is: agar.[116] ***asar.***[116] camph.[139] cann-i.[116] chin.[8] ***coff.***[116] ***croc.***[116] ***dat-a.***[25] dig.[1] eup-pur.[36] gels.[139] hyper.[102] lac-c.[116] lach.[139] lact.[116] lat-k.[102] manc.[139] mez.[116] nat-ar.[102] op.[116] phos.[116] puls.[36] rhus-g.[102] ***stict.***[116] stram.[116] tep.[139] thuj.[116] valer.[116] zinc.[116]

• light, incorporeal, immaterial, he is, walking while: spig.[137] thuj.[139]

• light, penetrates through body: cann-i.[36]

• light, there is too much in room (on falling to sleep): ambr.

• visions, sees them in the light not in the dark: lac-c.[108]

• weight, has no: cann-i. germ.[222] hyos.[85] op.

Dreams; body, cheek burnt by the light: mag-c.[36]

➤ illuminations: crot-c.

➤ light: coff.[5]

Euphoria; lightness, feeling of, as after an anesthesia by chlorethylene, with: asar.[149]

Excitement; violent, brought on by current of air, bright light, sight of any shining object, slightest touch, even by conversation in vicinity of a patient: lyss.[54]

Fear; alone, of being, light and company, wants: bism.[172] rad-br.[172] stram.[172]

✦ dawn, of the return of: kali-i.

Hysteria; light and noise agg.: ***stict.***[54]

Insanity; company, with desire for light and: **STRAM.**[54]

Light; bright light agg.: colch.[5]

Light; daylight agg.: acon.[10] arn.[10] ars.[10] bell.[10] calc.[10] cham.[10] chin.[10] coff.[10] hell.[10] hep.[10] hyos.[10] ign.[10] lyc.[10] merc.[10] nux-v.[10] ph-ac.[10] phos.[10] puls.[10] rhus-t.[10] sep.[10] sil.[10] stram.[10] sulph.[10]

Light; desire for: ***acon. am-m.*** asar.[149] **BELL.** ***calc.*** cann-s.[111] carb-an.[111] gaert.[136] **GELS.** grin.[111] lac-c. nat-m. phos.[111] plb.[111] ruta

sanic.[111] **STRAM.** ***stront-c.***[162] valer.
Light; shuns light: achy.[149] ambr. androc.[222] bell.[58] **CON.** hyos. plat.[193] stram.[58] tarent.[5] zinc.
Light; shuns light, brilliant objects: bufo[130]
Light; stained glass agg.: ant-c.[137] nat-s.[137]
Lightness, feeling of: agar.[36] ars.[36] asar.[10] buni-o.[149] cann-i.[36] cere-s.[36] cham.[36] chin-s.[36] cic.[36] coff.[10] dig.[36] eup-per.[36] fuc.[36] gamb.[36] gels.[36] germ.[222] gins.[36] hydr.[36] hyos.[36] jatr.[36] ***kali-br.***[8] kali-cy.[36] merc-c.[36] nat-m.[10] nitro-o.[36] ol-an.[36] ozone[227] petr.[10] ph-ac.[36] phos.[36] rhus-t.[36] sars.[36] stram.[10] tab.[36]
Longing; for, sunshine, light and society, for: grin. stram.
Reserved; light, with aversion to: con.[10]
Sensitive; light, to: ***acon.*** androc.[222] aquil.[102] ***ars.*** aur.[116] bad.[1] **BELL.**[122] buth-aust.[119] ***colch.*** con.[10] ***kali-p.*** lac-c. nat-m.[162] **NUX-V. PHOS.** sang.[116] stram.[58] tarent.[214]

ADAM. Sh, 43 - Feeling alone and tall and capable, like a beacon beaming out rays of light to all and sundry. 2, 12C, XX:XX:XX
Sh, 107 - Wearing light things instead of dark. Want light next to my skin. Desire for yellow silk underwear. 16, 12C, 26:XX:XX
Sh, 243 - Anger at people putting lights on instead of opening curtains. 16, 12C, 18:XX:XX
ANDROC. Sh, 83 - Woke at night to urinate. On going upstairs, all colours seemed incredibly bright and the walls were pulsating —in towards him and out again. This felt similar to an L.S.D. experience years ago. Did not know what to do, was stricken with panic. Terrified, he raced back to bed where he felt hot, so uncovered, then cold so covered, then hot, he uncovered and sat up and immediately felt better — no panic. As soon as he lay down he began to panic. Became afraid in the light and felt better in the dark with the lights off. He wanted to call someone for help, and felt angry about the proving. He then got up and walked around for a few minutes, got back to bed, and fell asleep. (2)
Sh, 118 - Irritability, worse for noise and bright lights. (17)
ANT-C. He, 22 - Sentimental mood in the moonlight, particularly ecstatic love.
ARS. Ha, 1049 - Discontented with everything, finds fault with everything; everything is too strong and too irritating, all conversation, all noise, and all light.
CANN-I. Al, 65 - Hallucinations which lead the patient to imagine that he is on horseback, is hunting, that he sees blue water, that he is swimming, or that he is captain of a vessel, that he is traveling, that he has no weight.(lightness)
CARB-V. Ha, 37 - Freedom of spirit, lightness and general good health (curative...)
CHIN. Ha, 1105 - What formerly appeared to him in a bright genial light, seems now to be lusterless (lifeless), unworthy (inutile), and shallow (superficial, stupid)
CHOC. Sh, 15 - I see plants in the house differently, very aware of them and want to give them more light.
Sh, 50 - Panic feeling of being trapped and enclosed —worse when curtains are closed and the light blocked out. Strong desire to be outside and moving, to be in the bright and warm sunlight. Kept having to move my feet, which I felt I wanted to move.
COT. Al, 1-...a feeling as if there was no foot. The head felt exceeding light, as if there were no solid head, and she could not articulate for some time, although she endeavored to do so....
GERM. Sh, 132 - Feeling of being pushed backwards, floating backwards in space, as if weightless. 10, 9C, 00:00:10
HALI-L. Sh, 12 - Returning home after dropping kids off at school, I feel light, my legs feel springy, the weight on my feet more forward, feel like I am floating around the house. Still calm. 09, 6C, 03:XX:XX
Sh, 20 - See the beginnings of rainbows in the sky. On second glance nothing is there. A sense of a rainbow starting to form, squinting I see faint pink & blue. Also see wavy motion in the sky, like a ripple of wind, like five lines of horizontal smoke but nothing is there. Periodically I see colors and motion. It is movement without an object. It occurs in the daytime, looking out from inside or when outside looking into the sky. pleasant sensation. 03, 12C, 02:XX:XX
Sh, 21 - Preoccupied with right eye aware-

ness. Staring at the rainbow colors on the beveling of a stained glass window. Excited to discover what might occur with my right eye. 03, 12C, 03:XX:XX

Sh, 22 - Sense of a rainbow at the edge of my right eye when looking outside, but there's nothing there. Noticed phenomenon of seeing color in the sky and having a second look and no color there. Now eager and expectant to see or sense it again. 03, 12C, 03:XX:XX

Sh, 26 - My eyes feel wide open when they are not. Unusual that I'm feeling the width and depth of the wide openness. I feel as if my eyes are taking in a lot of light. Repositories of light. 18, 30C, 00:11:30

Sh, 27 - Eyes feel like receptors to light the way a satellite dish is a receptor for stellar signals or microwaves, as if they are meant to capture light or receive it. Odd feeling. Sensitive to light but at the same time wide open to it, as if it is meant to be. 18, 30C, 03:XX:XX

Sh, 29 - I kept seeing deep purple light — amazingly deep. Watched the sun rise over the house —I had a desire for symmetry in the sky. I felt there should be two suns. Strange because it's been so hot. An image of light radiating towards me — white lightfull spectrum. 20, 30C, XX:XX:XX

Sh, 30 - After I looked at the sun, I saw four suns in a ring connected to each other, and another one above with strings of light. One had two lesser ones. 20, 30C, XX:XX:XX

Sh, 676 - The remedy worked very directly on my will. Fragmentation is the denial of will. Integration is the use of will. All separate states under a unified country. 18, 30C, 35:XX:XX

Sh, 812 - My bones feel lighter than the outside of me. I don't like this fat anymore. 20, 30C, 04:XX:XX

Sh, 966 - I'm so slow and heavy on earth and so light and swift in the air. 20, 30C, 19:XX:XX

HYDROG. Sh, 8 - I felt slightly high, removed from reality, yet very alert, clear and calm. Very aware of the colour of the sky, the light, birds singing, flowers —like a pastoral ideal. Feeling of expansiveness, mentally cool, airy and light. 28, 200C, 00:04:XX

HYOS. He, 57 - Delirium tremens:... averse to light and company; visions as if persecuted preceded by an epileptic attack;... seeks to escape from men by whom he imagines himself surrounded and who are trying to capture him; does not recognize his wife who is standing by his side, but imagines he sees her under a distant bed.

IRID. Sh, 103 - Felt light and young, found things fun and amusing. Walking effortlessly, easy, as if not touching the ground. Q1

Sh, 125 - Attracted to men with pale skins, appear even more beautiful, luminosity, light shining forth. Q5

LAC-C. He, 21 - Sits and looks under chairs, table, sofa and everything in room, expecting yet dreading (fear) to see some terrible monster creep forth and feeling all the time, that if it does, it will drive her raving mad; she is not afraid in dark, it is only in light where she can imagine that she can see them.

LYSS. Al,N-129 - Hyperesthesia, current of air, bright light, sight of any shining object, slightest touch, even conversation in vicinity of patient, may throw him into a most violent agitation and bring on severe convulsions.

MAG-C. Al, 951 - Frightful dream, that she burnt her cheek by the light.

NAT-M. Al, 62 - Woke at 2A.M. in perspiration, and with a distressing anxiety, as though he were shut up (lock) in a dark cellar; this sensation only disappeared on perceiving light through the window.(confined, restricted, incarcerated)

NEON. Sh, 1 - I was overwhelmingly agitated, amazed, confused, and upset about a neon tube discarded across the road. I couldn't believe that people could use these things. Where would the dustmen throw it? I thought, "It's the worst kind of light possible." I could not believe people would want it. 20, 6C, 00:03:05

Sh, 2 - I took a deep breath of relief as I saw the dustmen come for the neon strip light. 20, 6C, 00:04:30

Sh, 21 - Walking was effortless, light and free, with a sensation of walking uniformly. I feel so different in my body. I am all in the now, especially in lower legs and feet. At last, I touch the earth. 20, 6C,

03:01:00
Sh, 58 - Image of being inside my iris and looking through. That is, I see a large iris and I was looking through it. From the center of it light was radiating out. 20, 6C, 07:XX:XX
Sh, 69 - Recognized a change in awareness -a vaguely stoned,unreal feeling. Giggly, childish, grinning. Felt light. 05, 12C, 05:05:XX

NUX-V. Ha, 1272 - Over-sensitiveness to impressions of the senses; he cannot bear strong odors and bright light.

OP. Al, 43 - In walking I was hardly sensible that my feet touched the ground; it seemed as if I slid (floating) along the ground impelled by some invisible agent, and that my blood was composed of some ethereal fluid which rendered my body lighter than air.

STRAM. Al, 48 - She is all the time inconsolable; much affected by trifles; makes much fuss about trifles; disposed to weep, and sometimes also very easily vexed; now and then neglects her duties; now and then thinks she is not fitted for her position ; after the fall equinox...; she wants light and company.
He, 101 - Mania for light and company, cannot bear to be alone.
He, 107-...heard continually, on r. side of occiput, a loud voice, scolding, vituperating and accusing him of ungodliness (impious, sinful, irreligious, godless, profane); ....prayed expecting, with great anxiety, the flash of lightning which was to kill him;...(redemption, regeneration, salvation)

VALER. He, 11 - Feels light as if flying in air.

LOATHING

Amusement, averse to: androc.[222] bar-c. ***hep.***[54] ***ign.***[54] lil-t. meny. olnd. sulph.
Anger; work, aversion: bov.[10] m-aust.[10]
Answer; aversion to: ***agar.*** alum. alum-p.[58] am-c. am-m. ambr. anac. ***ant-c.***[102] ant-t.[102] apom.[36] arg-m.[58] ***arn.*** ars. ars-i. ars-s-f.[58] atro. ***aur.***[122] bell. ***bry.***[102] cact. calc-s. calc-sil.[58] carb-an.[102] carbn-h. carc.[138] caust. ***cham.***[102] chin. chin-s. chlol.[36] cimic. cocc. coff. ***coloc.*** con. cupr. euphr. ***gels.***[102] germ.[222] **GLON.** hell.[5] **HYOS.** ign.[102] iod. juni-c.[36] kali-ar. ***kali-p.*** lil-t. lyss. mag-m. **MANC.**[122] medus.[168] merc. mosch. mur-ac.[102] naja[98] ***nat-m.*** nat-s.[102] **NUX-V.**[122] op. oxyt.[102] petr.[1] **PH-AC.**[122] ***phos.***[122] ***puls.*** rhus-t. sabad. sars.[102] ***sec.*** sil.[102] spong. ***stann.*** stram. ***stry. sul-ac. sulph.*** tab. tarent. verat. vib.
Answer; aversion to, sings, talks, but will not answer questions: agar.
Anxiety; company, shuns, even his doctor: iod.[85]
Anxiety; weariness of life, with: ant-c.[116] ***aur.***[10] bell.[10] caust.[10] chin.[10] dros.[10] hep.[10] kali-p.[54] ***lach.***[54] ***lyc.***[54] merc.[116] ***nit-ac.***[54] ***nux-v.***[10] ***plat.***[10] ***puls.***[10] rhus-t.[10] sil.[116] spong.[10] staph.[10]
Aversion; approached, of being: arn.[162] aur. bry.[162] caj. canth.[85] cina[83] hell. helon. hipp. ***iod.*** lil-t. ***lyc.***[122] sanic.[85] sulph.
Aversion; family members, to: am-c.[5] am-m.[5] aran.[192] aur.[5] ***calc.*** calc-s.[108] cit-ac.[65] con.[5] ***crot-h. fl-ac.*** hep.[5] iod.[137] kali-c.[122] kali-p.[5] lyc.[5] ***merc.***[5] ***nat-c.*** nat-m.[30] ***phos.***[5] plat.[5] plb.[162] senec.[137] ***sep.***
Aversion; family members, to, female: am-c.[5]
Aversion; family, talks pleasantly to others: fl-ac.[137]
Aversion; flowers, smell of: graph.[36]
Aversion; friends, to: anac.[60] aur-m.[162] cedr. coloc.[137] ferr. fl-ac.[58] kali-m.[192] ***led.*** pitu-a.[164]
Aversion; herself, to: crot-h.[111] fl-ac.[111] iod.[111] kali-p.[111] lac-c.[122] lyc.[111] phos.[111] pitu-a.[164] plat.[111] senec.[111] sep.[111] spirae.[36]
Aversion; husband, and children: ***glon.***[54] verat.[54]
Aversion; husband, to: agn.[171] bamb-a.[1184] choc.[222] ***glon.*** kali-c.[122] kali-p. ***nat-c.*** nat-m. pitu-a.[164] **SEP.** thuj.[137] verat.
Aversion; interference: bar-c.[127] calc-p.[127] cham.[127] cina[122] nat-m.[127] sanic.[127] sil.[127] sulph.[127]
Aversion; interference, resents: cham.[127] nat-m.[127] sulph.[127]
Aversion; literary persons: sulph.[137]
Aversion; men, shuns the foolishness of: cic.
Aversion; men, to: hypoth.[149] **PULS.** raph.[54]
Aversion; mother, to: thuj.[137]
Aversion; noise, to: ferr.[36] kali-m.[192] raph.[36] zinc.[36]
Aversion; parents, to: fl-ac.[30]
Aversion; persons, to, all: absin.[36] calc.[30] chin.[30] germ.[222] ***merc-acet.***[30] ***nux-v.***[30] phos.[1] ***staph.***[30] ***sulph.***[30]

Aversion; persons, to, certain: am-c.[10] ***am-m.*** ***aur.***[122] **CALC.**[122] calc-p.[184] carc.[207] caust.[30] crot-h. fl-ac.[10] germ.[222] hep.[137] lap-c-b.[194] ***merc.***[30] **NAT-C.** nat-m.[30] nit-ac.[30] sel. sep.[162] stann.
Aversion; persons, to, certain, who do not agree with him: calc-s.[137]
Aversion; persons, to, those around: ars.
Aversion; persons, to, unaccountable dislikes: puls.[70]
Aversion; sex: hydrog.[222] raph.[122]
Aversion; sex, her own, to: raph.
Aversion; sex, opposite to, religious aversion: lyc. ***puls.*** sulph.
Aversion; sex, opposite, to: am-c.[10] nat-m.[36] puls.[162] staph.[5]
Aversion; society: anac.[60] bell.[36] caust.[30] cic.[1] clem.[38] coca[38] con.[1] graph.[30] ***kali-c.***[36] lyc.[1] nat-c.[137] stann.[1] syph.[137]
Aversion; society, shuns the foolishness of: cic.
Aversion; visits, to: bell.[36] ferr.[36]
Aversion; water to: am-c.[5] ***hyos.***[137] ***lyss.***[162] ***nux-v.***[137] ***stram.***[137]
Aversion; water to, thinking of it agg.: ham.[137]
Aversion; water to, thirst, with: hell.[137]
Aversion; water to, touch of it, cannot bear: am-c.[137]
Aversion; wife, to his: ars.[137] ***fl-ac.***[122] nat-s.[137] plat.[137] staph.[137]
Aversion; wind, to: ozone[227]
Aversion; women, to: am-c. bapt. con.[30] ***dios.*** ign.[36] ***lach.*** **LYC.**[30] mag-c.[36] nat-m. ***puls.*** raph.[36] sulph.
Aversion; women, to, homosexuality, with: phos.[162] ***plat.***[30] puls.[162] staph.[162]
Aversion; women, to, looks upon them as evil beings and is afraid their presence is injurious to his soul: ***puls.***[54]
Aversion; women, to, mannish: fl-ac.[122]
Aversion; women, to, sex, of her own: raph.
Black and somber, everything that is, aversion to: ant-t.[54] rob. stram. ***tarent.***
Business; averse to: acon-l.[122] agar. aloe[130] am-c. anac. androc.[222] arg-n.[137] arn.[5] ars. ars-h. asar.[54] aur-m. bapt.[137] ***brom.*** calc.[58] carb-v.[137] chel.[137] ***chin.***[137] chin-s. cimic. ***con.*** cop. cycl.[137] fl-ac. graph. ham.[137] hipp. kali-ar. kali-bi. kali-br. kali-c. kali-i. kali-s. lac-ac. ***lach.*** laur. lil-t. lyc.[1] mag-s. nat-ar.[58] nat-c.[30] **NAT-M.**[137] nux-v.[36] opun-a.[36] ***ph-ac.***[122] ***phos.***[137] ***phyt.*** psor.[137] ***puls.*** rhod.[58] rhus-t.[30] **SEP.** stann.[58] ***stram.***[5] ***sulph.***[58] syph.[58] ther.[54]
Cares; full of, company, with aversion to: con.[10] nat-m.[10]
Caressed; aversion to being: chin.[193] ***cina*** cupr.[210] ign.[193] nit-ac.[1] sac-alb.[210]
Casting off of people against her will: **PLAT.**[36]
Cheerfulness; alternating with, aversion to work: spong.
Cheerfulness; alternating with, sympathy, want of: merc
Children; aversion to: **CHOC.**[222] helon.[231] lyc.[137] medus.[231] plat. raph.[36] sep.[162] xan.[231]
Children; aversion, her own: glon. ***lyc.*** nux-v.[162] phos.[137] plat. sep.[162] verat.
Children; aversion, her own, daughter, in a woman: raph
Company, aversion to; agg.: absin.[36] achy.[149] acon. agar.[5] allox.[119] ***aloe*** **ALUM.**[122] alum-p.[58] alum-sil.[58] alumn.[36] am-m.[5] ***ambr.*** **ANAC.** anan. androc.[222] ant-c. ant-t. arag.[102] ***arg-n.***[5] arist-cl.[149] arn.[58] ars.[5] ***ars-met.***[54] atro. ***aur.*** aur-i.[58] ***aur-s.*** bamb-a.[1184] **BAR-C.** bar-i.[58] bar-m. bar-s.[58] ***bell.*** bov.[5] ***bry.*** bufo bufo-s. ***cact.*** cadm-s.[144] calc. calc-i.[58] ***calc-p.*** calc-s. camph.[5] cand-a.[239] cann-i. caps.[102] **CARB-AN.** ***carb-v.*** carbn-s. carc.[154] cedr. cench.[58] **CHAM.** ***chin.*** choc.[222] **<u>CIC.</u>**[122] cimic. cinnb. clem. coca ***coloc.*** ***con.*** convo-s.[149] cop. cortico.[119] ***cupr.*** cur. cycl.[58] ***dig.***[122] dios. elaps eug. euphr.[54] ***ferr.*** ferr-i. ferr-p. fl-ac. **GELS.** graph. grat. ham. ***hell.*** helon. ***hep.*** ***hipp.*** hydr. hydrog.[222] ***hyos.*** **IGN.** ***iod.*** jug-c. kali-bi. kali-br. kali-c. kali-i.[5] kali-m.[192] kali-p. kali-s. ***lac-d.*** lac-h.[229] ***lach.*** lap-c-b.[194] lap-gr-m.[194] lap-mar-c.[194] ***led.*** lil-t.[111] luna[228] ***lyc.*** ***m-aust.***[5] mag-c.[5] mag-m. mang. meny. meph.[149] moly.[149] murx.[10] ***nat-c.*** **<u>NAT-M.</u>**[122] nat-p. nat-s.[58] nicc. **NUX-V.** op.[5] ***oxyt.*** ozone[227] ***pall.***[5] pana.[36] petr. ph-ac.[54] phos. pic-ac. ***plat.*** ***plb.***[5] prot.[136] psor. ptel. ***puls.*** ***rhus-t.*** sabal.[144] sanic.[85] sapin.[36] sec. ***sel.*** ***sep.*** sieg.[144] ***stann.*** **STAPH.**[5] stram.[5] sul-ac. sul-i.[58] sulfonam. ***sulph.*** syph.[122] tanac.[25] ***tarent.***[122] tep. thala.[149] thiop.[149] ***thuj.*** til. trinit.[102] ust. ***verat.***[54] wye.[85] x-ray[115]
Company, aversion to; alone, agg. when alone and amel. in company: alum-sil.[58] bism.[10] hep.[10] ph-ac.[10] ran-b.[10]
Company, aversion to; alone, amel. when:

allox.[119] alum-sil.[162] ambr. arag.[102] ***bar-c.*** bell.[10] bov. carb-an. choc.[222] coca[15] con. convo-s.[119] cortico.[119] cycl. ferr. ferr-p. germ.[222] halo.[149] hell. hydrog.[222] ign.[102] ipom.[119] iris[152] lac-h.[229] lap-mar-c.[194] ***lyc.*** mag-c.[5] mag-s. meny.[36] ***nat-c. nat-m. oxyt.***[54] ozone[227] petr. ph-ac.[58] phos. plat.[10] ***plb.*** rauw.[119] **SEP.** stann. staph. stram. sulph. trio.[149] visc.[119]

Company, aversion to; alone, dreads being, yet: ars.[5] bufo ***clem. con.*** elaps kali-br. lyc. **NAT-C.**[122] nat-m.[5] ***sep.*** stram.[5] tarent.[5]

Company, aversion to; alternating with bursts of pleasantry and sarcasm: rad-br.[122] rhus-t.

Company, aversion to; avoids the sight of people: acon. ars.[30] calc.[122] **CIC.** ***cupr.*** cur.[122] ferr. ***gels.*** germ.[222] hydrog.[222] ***iod. lac-d.***[122] ***led. nat-c.*** psor.[185] ***sep. thuj.***

Company, aversion to; avoids the sight of people, lies with closed eyes, and: sep.

Company, aversion to; avoids the sight of people, shuts herself up: cur.

Company, aversion to; bear anybody, cannot: merc.[10] nux-v.[10] staph.[10] ***sulph.***[10]

Company, aversion to; country away from people, wants to get into the: androc.[222] calc. calc-p.[58] elaps merc.[137] sep.[137]

Company, aversion to; dizzy, faint in a crowd, or where many gas lights are burning (in agoraphobia): ***nux-v.***[54]

Company, aversion to; friends, meeting of, whom he imagines he has offended, to: ars.

Company, aversion to; friends, meeting them amel.: alum.[162]

Company, aversion to; friends, of intimate: bell. cham.[54] coloc. ***ferr.*** hep.[85] ***iod. nat-c. sel.***

Company, aversion to; loathing at company: bell.[30] ign.[30] lyc.[30] nux-v.[30] sep.[30] staph.[30]

Company, aversion to; presence of, strangers, to: **AMBR.**[122] ***bar-c. bry.*** bufo ***carb-v.*** **CIC.** cina[58] ***con. helon.***[163] ***iod. lach.***[8] lyc. nat-c.[58] petr. ***sep. stram.*** tarent.[193] ***thuj.***

Company, aversion to; solitude, fond of: **ACON.**[5] alum.[10] **AMBR.**[5] ***ant-c.***[8] ***ars.***[8] **AUR.**[5] bamb-a.[1184] bar-c.[1] ***bell.***[5] cact.[25] calc.[10] calc-p.[5] camph.[5] carb-an.[5] ***cham.***[8] chin.[1] cic.[1] coca[25] con.[5] cycl.[5] dig.[5] dios.[25] eug.[10] graph.[10] helon.[25] **IGN.**[5] led.[5] lyc.[5] m-aust.[10] mag-m.[10] meny.[5] nat-c.[5] ***nat-m.***[5] ***nux-v.***[5] op.[10] ozone[227] petr.[5] **PLAT.**[5] ptel.[25] **PULS.**[5] ***rhus-t.***[5] sep.[10] seq-s.[230] stann.[5] staph.[10] sulph.[10] tub.[189] verat.[10]

Company, aversion to; solitude, fond of, desires to practice masturbation: ***bufo*** ust.

Company, aversion to; solitude, fond of; fancy, to indulge her: ***lach.***

Company, aversion to; unpredictable, thinks people are: ozone[227]

Conversation; aversion to: ***ambr.***[30] ***ars.***[36] ars-s-f.[58] asim.[36] atro.[36] bell.[36] caj.[36] calc.[58] ***carb-an.***[36] carc.[140] ***cham.***[85] chel.[58] choc.[222] echi.[111] elaps[36] ferr.[36] gels.[36] germ.[222] ham.[36] hell.[36] kalm.[36] murx.[36] myric.[36] nat-s.[36] ox-ac.[58] plb.[36] ***ptel.***[54] tarent.[36] thea.[36] ziz.[36]

Conversation; aversion to, sadness, after: ziz.[36]

Darkness; aversion to: carb-v.[102] sanic.[122]

Death; desires, sadness, without, with disgust of life: rhus-t.[54]

Delirium; touch, with aversion to: merc.[36]

Delusions; baby, odious looks: puls.[54]

- company, people are averse to her: androc.[222]
- figures, old repulsive persons, which fill her with fear, in hysteria: ***kali-c.***[54]
- images, sleep, during, hateful (afternoon): lyc.
- insane, become, that she will, unless she got out of her body: lac-c.[54]
- repulsive fantastic, imaginations: ***fl-ac.***
- strange, familiar things seem horrible: plat.

Dirtiness; aversion to, especially of the hands: syph.[212]

Discouraged; business, aversion to: puls.[10]

Disgust: aloe[5] arn.[10] ars. asar.[162] aur.[10] caj.[25] camph.[10] caps.[10] caust.[10] cimx. coloc. con.[10] ***croc.***[10] dulc.[1] germ.[222] ***hep.***[10] ip.[10] ***kali-c.***[10] kali-i.[10] lac-c.[54] ***laur.***[10] led.[10] mag-c.[10] mag-m.[10] ***merc.*** mez. nux-v.[10] orig.[25] petr.[10] phos. plb.[10] **PULS.** samb.[10] sars.[10] sil.[10] spong.[10] ***stram.***[162] **SULPH.** syph.[122] tarent.[54] thea.[10] thlaspi[25] thuj.[10]

Disgust; consciousness of his unnatural state mind: tarent.[54]

Disgust; everything, with: arn.[10] aur.[10] caust.[10] con.[10] ip.[10] kali-i.[10] ***laur.***[10] ***led.***[10] mag-c.[10] mag-m.[10] ***merc.***[10] nux-v.[10] petr.[10] phos.[10] ***puls.***[10] samb.[10] sars.[10] spong.[10] thea.[10] ***thuj.***[10]

Disgust; exhilaration, of others, at: m-aust.[10]

Disgust; himself, with: germ.[222] lap-gr-m.[194]
Disgust; himself, with; courage to live, has none: ***merc.***[54]
Disgust; laughing of others, at: ambr.[10]
Disgust; medicine bottle, on sight of the: visc.[119]
Disgust; odor of his own, body: lac-c.[137] pyrog.[137] ***sulph.***[54]
Disgust; odor of his own, stool: ambr.[1189]
Disgust; society, with the follies, of: cic.[1]
Dreams; abortion, efforts and plans: ign.[36]
➤ amorous, pollutions, with, sticky, profuse, fluid emission, with aversion to coition: ***plat.***[54]
➤ animals, vermin: alum.[5] am-c. bell.[5] bov.[10] chel. colch. gamb. kali-c.[10] lac-c. mag-s. mur-ac. ***nux-v.*** ped.[85] phos. ran-s.[10] sep. sil.[5]
➤ disease, loathsome: anac.
➤ disgusting: alet.[5] aloe alumn. am-c. anac. arist-m.[36] bor.[36] cast-v. chel. ***chin.*** chin-b.[54] chr-ac.[54] con. eupi.[36] hydrog.[222] inul. kali-n.[1] ***kreos.*** ***lach.***[5] mag-m. mag-s.[10] merc.[5] mur-ac. nat-m. ***nux-v.***[122] ozone[227] phos. plan.[36] ***puls.*** rheum[36] sil.[1] sulph. zinc
➤ excrements, smeared with excrements, being: iod.[10] zinc.[36].
➤ stool: aloe androc.[222] cast-v. psor. sars. zinc.
➤ wedding, midnight, after, of marrying one she did not like: mag-c.[36]
Dress; aversion to, in sadness: ***con.***[54]
Duty; aversion to domestic: cench.[58] cit-l.[54] sul-i.[58]
Fancies; repulsive: fl-ac.[36] sel.[36]
Fancies; repulsive, when alone: fl-ac. sel. tarent.
Fear; alone, of being, disinclined to meet even agreeable company: clem.[172]
✦ death, weary of life: ***kali-p.***[54] ***nit-ac.***[54] ***plat.***[54] ***rhus-t.***[54]
✦ satiety of life, with, particularly in company, hysteric: ***lyc.***[54]
✦ visions of old repulsive persons, from, in hysteria: ***kali-c.***[54]
Foolish; behavior, grotesque: agar.[36] cact.[36] cori-r.[36]
Hatred; persons, of, repels everyone: aloe[54]
Hatred; sex, to opposite: sep.[137]
House; aversion to being kept in: lyc.[36]
Ideas; disgusting: sang.[54]
Indifference; work aversion to: agar.[10] allox.[119] androc.[222] camph.[54] ign.[10] kali-m.[192] lach.[10] rhod.[54] squil.[10] staph.[10]
Indolence; housework, aversion to her usual: bamb-a.[1184] cench.[58] ***cit-ac.*** cit-l.[54] sep.[137] sul-i.[58]
Laughing; alternating with, loathing of life: ***aur.***
Light; shuns light: achy.[149] ambr. androc.[222] bell.[58] **CON.** hyos. plat.[193] stram.[58] tarent.[5] zinc.
Light; shuns light, brilliant objects: bufo[130]
Loathing; general: acon. alum. ang. ant-t. arg.[149] ***arg-n.*** arn. asar. bamb-a.[1184] bell. benz-ac. bufo ***calc.*** canth. carbn-o.[36] cham. chel. hep.[30] hyos. ip.[30] jatr. kali-bi. kali-c. kali-chl.[10] laur. mag-m. merc. mez.[30] myric. paull.[36] phel. phyt. plat. ***plb.***[30] ***puls.*** raph. rat. sapin.[36] sec. seneg. stram. sumb. tarent. thea.
Loathing; general, business, his: ars-h.
Loathing; general, fear of death, during: cop.[36]
Loathing; life, of: act-sp. agn. alum. alum-p.[58] alum-sil.[58] am-c. ***ambr.*** **ANT-C.** ant-t. **ARS.** ars-s-f.[58] **AUR.** aur-ar.[58] ***aur-m.*** aur-s. bell. berb. bov. ***calc.*** calc-ar.[58] calc-s. calc-sil.[58] carb-an. ***carb-v.*** caust. **CHIN.** ***chin-ar.*** cic.[149] cop. dros. gels.[184] grat. hep. hydr.[102] hydro-c.[149] hyos. kali-bi. kali-br. kali-chl.[58] ***kali-p.*** kreos. lac-c.[102] lac-d.[102] ***lach.*** laur. led. ***lyc.*** med.[179] **MERC.** mez. naja[98] nat-ar. nat-c. **NAT-M.** ***nat-s.*** nat-sil.[58] ***nit-ac.*** ***nux-v.*** op. orig.[25] ***ph-ac.***[30] **PHOS.** ***plat.*** plb. podo. ***puls.*** ***rhus-t.*** ***rhus-v.*** ruta sac-alb.[210] sec. ***sep.*** ***sil.*** spig. ***spong.*** staph. stram. sul-ac. ***sulph.*** tab.[102] ***ter.*** thlaspi[25] **THUJ.** tub.[58] ***valer.***[122] verat.[102] zinc. ***zinc-p.***[58] ziz.
Loathing; life, of, restrain herself, must, to prevent doing herself injury: **NAT-S.**
Loathing; talking: anac. dios.
Loathing; work, at: anac.[102] arg-n. arn. bar-c.[54] calc. carb-ac.[54] chin.[30] cob.[54] con.[30] croc.[30] hyos. ***kali-bi.***[54] kali-c. lach.[30] ***lil-t.***[54] merc.[30] nat-m. nit-ac.[1] petr. ***puls.*** ran-b. ***sil.*** stann.[58] sulph. tab. tarax. ther.[36] tub.[102]
Marriage; aversion to: puls.[58]
Marriage; aversion to, enjoying society of men, while: pic-ac.[36]
Marriage; aversion to, women, in: ***lach.***[54]
Marriage; idea, seemed unendurable idea of: ***lach.*** ***med.***[122] nux-v.[187] pic-ac. puls. staph.[30]
Medicine; drugs, averse to: aesc.[36]
Mood; repulsive: acon. alum. am-c.[5] ambr.

anac.[185] ant-c. arn. ars. aur. bell. camph. caps. carb-ac.[36] caust. con. croc. ferr.[10] ***hep.*** ign. ip. kali-c. lact. laur. led. lyc. mag-c. mag-m. ***merc.*** nit-ac. nux-v. ozone[227] petr. phos. plat.[5] plb. ***psor.***[122] ***puls.*** samb. sars. sep.[30] sil. spong. sulph. thuj. upa.[85]

Mood; repulsive, asks for, for what he: arn.[5] bry.[185] cham.[5] dulc.[102] kreos.[102] puls.[5] staph.[144]

Mood; repulsive, food, saying one who does not work should not eat, but driven by hunger he tried to procure it secretly: ***arg-n.***[54]

Mood; repulsive, medicine, to take the: ***arn.***[122] calad.[137] cimic.[58] hyos. ***kali-p.***[54] **LACH.**[122] ***stram.***[54] tub.[160] ***verat-v.***[54] visc.[119]

Mood; repulsive, medicine, to take the, religious insanity, in: ***kali-p.***[54]

Mood; repulsive, treatment, every: bell.[30] caust.[30] lach.[30] plat.[30]

Mood; repulsive, treatment, every, sick, in spite of being very: ars.[30] caust.[30] nux-v.[30]

Music; aversion to: **ACON.**[122] alum.[30] bufo[54] carc.[144] caust.[36] cham.[36] hep.[30] merc.[10] nit-ac.[30] ***nux-v.***[5] ph-ac.[60] sabin.[5] sep.[144] tab.[60] viol-o.[36]

Music; aversion to, joyous, to, but immediately affected by saddest: mang.[54]

Music; aversion to, violin especially: viol-o.[36]

Quiet disposition; noise, intolerant to: con.[10]

Rage; women, approaching, in a woman: raph.[36]

Religious affections; horror of the opposite sex: lyc. nat-m.[193] ***plat.***[54] ***puls.*** sulph.

Reproaches; aversion to: carc.[187]

Reserved; light, with aversion to: con.[10]

Responsibility, aversion to: lac-h.[229] lap-mar-c.[194] lyc.[109] ***med.***[122] phos.[62]

Sadness; aversion to see her children from sadness: ***con.***[54]

Sadness; aversion, children to whom he is devotedly attached become burdensome: **KALI-I.**[54]

Sadness; company, aversion to, desire for solitude: alum.[10] aur.[10] bamb-a.[1184] ***con.***[116] cupr.[10] ***helon.***[116] ***led.***[54] murx.[10] nat-c.[10] nat-m.[116] rhus-t.[10] sep.[193]

Sadness; food, with aversion of: ***plat.***[54]

Sadness; men, with aversion to: stann.[54]

Sadness; work, aversion to, with: berb.[10] bov.[10] croto-t.[10] dros.[10] laur.[10] mez.[10] prun.[10] zinc.[10]

Sensitive; noise, aversion to: asar.[137] bor.[137] con.[137] ferr.[36] kali-c.[137] op.[137] raph.[36] zinc.[36]

Shining objects; aversion to, cannot bear: bufo[22]

Spoken to; averse to being: agar. am-c. anh.[144] ant-c.[5] ant-t. arn. ***ars.*** ***ars-i.*** ars-s-f.[58] aur. aur-ar.[58] aur-s.[58] bar-s.[58] bry.[58] caj. calc-s.[58] calc-sil.[30] camph. ***carbn-s.*** **CHAM.** ***cina***[98] con. cur.[5] cyn-d.[149] elaps fago. ***gels.*** ***graph.*** ham. hell. helon. ***hipp.*** hist.[144] ***hyos.*** ign. **IOD.**[122] kali-p. kalm. kreos.[164] lil-t. lyc.[58] mag-m. myric. nat-m. ***nat-s.*** nit-ac.[30] nux-v. op.[5] ***ph-ac.***[5] pitu-a.[164] plan. plat. plb.[5] puls.[5] puls-n. rhus-t. sanic.[102] sep.[5] sil. sin-n.[5] staph. stram. ***sulph.*** ***tarent.*** tep. teucr. thuj.[102] verat. zinc.

Spoken to; averse to being, alone, wants to be let: ant-t.[122] arn.[58] aur. caj. gels.[171] hell. helon. hipp. hydrog.[222] ***iod.*** lil-t. luna[29] nat-m.[91] stram.[36] ***sulph.***

Suicidal disposition; mania, in, puerperal, with aversion to husband, baby and coition: agn.[171]

Talk; indisposed, abortion, in threatening: nit-ac.[26]

Talk; indisposed, convulsions, during: plb.[36] sul-ac.[36]

Talk; indisposed, eating after: aloe arg-n. ferr-ma. mez. plb.

Talk; indisposed, foreign language which at other times he speaks fluently: pall.[54]

Thoughts; disgusting thoughts with nausea: sang.

Touched; aversion of being: ***acon.*** ***agar.*** **ANT-C.** ***ant-t.*** **ARN.**[122] ars. asar.[149] ***bell.*** ***bry.*** bufo calc. camph. cand-a.[239] canth.[85] carc.[207] **CHAM.** ***chin.*** cimic.[137] ***cina*** cocc. ***coff.*** colch. con.[111] cupr. gels.[116] hell.[58] hep.[137] hydrog.[222] ign.[111] iod. **KALI-C.** kali-fcy.[198] ***kali-i.*** ***lach.*** lyc.[111] mag-c. mag-m.[162] ***med.*** merc. mez. nit-ac.[102] nux-m.[36] nux-v. ozone[227] plb. sanic. ***sil.*** stram. **TARENT.** ***thuj.*** ***tub.***[36] verat. vip.[144]

Touched; aversion of being, cannot bear anyone to lie close to or touch him: sanic.[85]

Touched; aversion of being, caressed: ***cina*** nit-ac.[1]

Walk; aversion to: zinc.[85]

Washing; aversion to: lap-mar-c.[194] phys.[60]

Weary of life: agn. aloe[5] alum.[5] am-c. ambr. ant-c. ant-t.[5] apis aran-ix.[144] **ARS.** **AUR.** aur-ar.[58] ***aur-m.***[54] ***bell.*** berb. bov.

buth-aust.[144] calc. calc-ar.[58] calc-sil.[58] carb-v. caust. **CHIN.** chin-ar. con.[30] dros.[5] euph-c.[116] grat. hep. hipp. hydro-c.[149] hyos. kali-bi.[54] ***kali-br.***[54] kali-chl.[10] ***kali-p.*** kreos. ***lac-d.***[54] lach. laur. led. lyc. merc. mez. mur-ac. naja[5] nat-c. ***nat-m.*** **NAT-S.**[5] nat-sil.[58] nep.[144] ***nit-ac.*** ***nux-v.*** op.[5] ***ph-ac.***[30] **PHOS.** phyt. pic-ac.[5] pitu-p. plat. plb. psor.[5] ***puls.*** ***rhus-t.*** rhus-v. rib-ac.[149] ruta sec.[5] sep. ***sil.*** spig.[5] spong. staph. stram. sul-ac. sulph. ***ter.***[54] thuj. tub.[58] tub-r.[149] valer. verat. xan.[111] zinc.[54] ziz.[54]

Weary of life; company, particularly in: ***lyc.***[54]

Weary of life; fear of death, but: ***kali-p.***[54] ***nit-ac.***[54] ***plat.***[54] ***rhus-t.***[54]

Weary of life; future, from solicitude about: ***lach.***[54]

Weary of life; mortification, after: ***puls.***[54]

Weary of life; sadness, with: aur.[1] ***kali-br.***[54] ***sulph.***[54]

Work; aversion to mental, anger after: **NUX-V.**[54]

Work; aversion to mental, hypochondriasis, in: ***ip.***[54]

Work; aversion to mental, masturbation, after: ***dig.***[54]

Work; aversion to mental, sadness, in: ***arg-n.***[54]

Work; aversion to mental, thinks it will do him harm, he: ***arg-n.***[54]

Work; aversion to mental, wants to leave everything as soon as it is commenced: ***lac-c.***[54]

ADAM. Sh, 160 - Disliked being touched and uninterested in any sexual relationship. Began to be repulsed by boyfriend. 20, 1M, XX:XX:XX

Sh, 190 - Very unhappy with my body, I want to escape from it, to run away from myself. I want to go from me. 20, 1M, 08:XX:XX

Sh, 191 - I feel like vomiting out all my insides. I want to get rid of everything inside me I physically feel like vomiting all my stomach and even all my breath. I want everything to get out of me. 20, 1M, 07:XX:XX

Sh, 194 - Felt ugly, miserable and generally fed up with myself during menses, more intensely than I usually would at this time. 8, 6C, 17:XX:XX

Sh, 277 - Exceptionally strong desire to leave my marriage and children, to live a clear unmuddled life alone. 2, 12C, 74:XX:XX-160:XX:XX

AESC. Al, 1 - Great repugnance to the drug.(medicine)

AGAR. Ha, 17 - Disgust for all work which occupies the mind, ...

ALOE. Al, 21 - Irritable, he cannot endure the visit of many people, they are repugnant to him.

He, 3 - life is a burden. (load)

ANTH. Al, 5 - Dislike to go out of doors.

APIS. He, 77 - All her ideas turn around jealousy, very talkative (loquacity), sometimes disgusting salacious. (lascivious)

ARN. Ha, 619 - Uncommonly peevish, everything is repugnant to her; everything annoys her.

ARS. Al-S, 2893 - The whole head sick, the heart faint, she awoke in the morning wretched, her life a burden (load) weariness the day's portion, and each succeeding day like its predecessor, unless (except) physic (laxative) helped her with its little aid.

He, 48 - Averse to meeting acquaintances, (friends) because he imagines he has formerly offended them, though knows not how.

AUR-M. Al, 5 - Disgust for life; inclination to suicide.

BAPT. He, 16 - Aversion... to hear conversation about sickness or injuries; feeble mind. (impressionable) 0Spasmodic stricture of esophagus.

BELL. Al, 161 - In walking in the open air, she is overwhelmed with tearful anguish; she is weary of life, and inclines to drown herself.

Ha, 1395 - He wishes for solitude and quiet; all noise and visits from others are repugnant to him.

BOR. Ha, 20 - Disinclination to work, he only does what he has to do, as if compulsorily.

BROM. Al, 1 - He becomes averse to his business; it seems as though he must relinquish (quit) it.

He, 6 - Aversion to any kind of work, even reading; takes no interest in household duties.

CACT. Al, 6 - Decided repugnance to take

any more medicine.

CALC-A. Al, 10-...;he performed all his work with aversion and as if compelled (drive) to do so. (compulsive, obsessive)

CALC. Al, 4 - Repugnance, aversion, disgust for most persons.

Ha, 41 - Peevish, morose, very cross and most indifferent to the most important things; he also did everything repugnantly and as if by compulsion.

Ha, 45 - Everything is repugnant (offensive) to her, with much crossness.

Ha, 56 - Aversion, dislike and repugnance to most men.

CAMPH. Al, 40 - Afraid of the mirrors in the room, lest he should see himself in them; so excessive was this fear at times in the night that he would have got up and broken the mirrors, only that he was still more afraid to get up alone in the dark;...

Ha, 341 - All external things are repugnant to him, and excite in him a repellent (repulsive) crossness.

He, 69 - An indifference whether the world (mankind) uses one well (suitable) or ill (depravity, wrong), everything is repulsive.(offensive)

CARB-AC. He, 12 - Entire disinclination to study; what he had accomplished seemed very trifling. (unimportant)

CAUST. Al, 28 - Fear and anxiety, so that she does not wish to live. (death)

CHOC. Sh, 213 - Unsociable —averse company and conversation.[15], 30C, 04:XX:XX

Sh, 322 - Have lost interest in my husband, feel totally indifferent. I have hardly spoken to him all weekend, with a desire to avoid him. Don't want to discuss or share anything with him.[15], 30C, 06:XX:XX

CIC. Al, 26 - Contempt and scorn for mankind; he avoided them, abhorred their follies (stupidity) excessively, and his disposition seemed to tend towards misanthropy; he withdrew (retire) himself into solitude.

Ha, 237 - Depreciation and contempt of mankind; he fled (desert) his fellow-creatures, was in the highest degree disgusted with their follies (stupidity), and his disposition seemed to change into misanthropy; he withdrew into solitude.

He, 36 - Mistrust and shunning (avoid) of men; despises others.

CON. He, 18 - He is averse to being near people, and to the talk of those passing him (misanthropy); is inclined to seize hold of and abuse them. (insult, offend, curse)

COP. Al, 2 - Disgust (loathing) with life, and at the same time fear of death.

DIOS. Al, 1 - Desire to be alone; do not enjoy society (misanthropy); am usually quite fond of the society of ladies, but they now seem repulsive,...

FERR. Al, 20 - Excited by the slightest opposition; ... even her children's caresses increased her bad temper; she was often rude to those about her, because she hated to see or talk to them, and wanted them to leave her in solitude, which alone was pleasing to her.

FL-AC. Al, 1 - Great disposition, when alone, to repulsive fantastic imaginations, particularly in regard to persons with whom he stands in near relations, or with whom he is connected (united, joined); it seems, for example, as though he must get rid (discard, repudiate, reject) of all the servants, children must go out of house, a betrothal must be broken off, a marriage should be dissolved. (broke; vows)

He, 7 - Aversion to his own family, bordering on insanity.

GELS. He, 18 - Desires to be quiet, does not wish to speak, nor have any one near her for company, even if the person be silent.

GERM. Sh, 112 - Don't see why I am here. I can't bear it. I go mad. I hate myself. I want to beat myself and I do it. Tear my hair. Stop when it hurts too much. It is like hell !!! 18, 30C, 20:XX:XX

Sh, 99 - Came in contact with very much hate and disgust within, and it made a deep impression on me. I have to be reconciled with those parts of me. I think that power can be used in a different way - not so destructive. I am no person. Feel I have no power when I meet people. Sometimes I feel I disappear. I am not in my body. My hands feel gone. My feet are cold; I don't like them. Yet I feel I have great power inside, especially I feel it when I get angry or when I sing. 18, 30C, 46:XX:XX

Sh, 138 - Feeling of revulsion for many

people especially young parents with children, while wandering through town. Feel people are stuck in their lives. What a waste. 10, 9C, 00:05:00

Sh, 151-.... I feel I have no real contact with people, I have no emotion at all except for a feeling of isolation and a concern that people may not like me. I wish someone would cuddle me. By 10 o'clock I have a definite aversion to people, especially certain people- the stubborn or authoritarian kind. I become deeply involved in my own thoughts and can be very irritable and even angry when the thoughts are interrupted by people, but I don't show any signs of anger or irritation. The fate of other people leaves me cold, but I know this is not right. My mind is blank and I feel I could just sit and stare. I have no feelings, no emotions! I think a lot about my state of mind and try to understand it; it puzzles me. What is missing? Eating removes this thoughtful mood. By afternoon and evening I become gradually more involved with what I am doing but still feel isolated even when in the company of other people. I don't mind listening to people, but I contribute little to conversation. This state lasted for three days. 16, 30C, 04:XX:XX

Sh, 152 - Aversion to people. Abrupt when obliged to speak. Had a consultation at 10 o'clock and really messed it up. I wish everybody would just go away and leave me alone. No contact. 16, 30C, 07:04:00

GLON. He, 2 - Recognized no one; repulsed her husband and children; raved, screamed, and wished to rush from house; jumped out of bed, but fell because her knees gave way.

HALI-L. Sh, 331 - Don't like people and they don't like me. Feel over exposed. 16, 10C, 33:XX:XX

Sh, 333 - Aversion to going out of the house. 16, 10C, 07:XX:XX

HEP. Ha, 7 - Contrary mood; he does not like to look at his folks. (relatives)

He, 10 - Repulsive (offensive) mood, with desire to be left alone.

HIPP. Al, 8 - Ill-humored, weary of life, even to suicide, in both provings.

HYDROG. Sh, 147 - Aversion to being touched. 24, 30C, 01:XX:XX

Sh, 274 - Developed an aversion to the idea of sex —confused about sexual issues and identity. Became aware of being bi-sexual or homosexual (in a man). "I want to find out who I am. I should know at 23. I used to know. What am I sexually?" Very confused. This led to suicidal depression. 24, 30C, 100:XX:XX

HYOS. He, 85-...repelled with rage and seeming disgust his mother, of whom, in natural state, he was dotingly (loving) fond, did not know her, said she was not his mama;...0Maniacal fury.

IOD. He, 9 - Fear and anxiety shuns (avoid) even the doctor.

IP. Ha, 218 - Repugnance to literary work; thoughts fail him.

Ha, 219 - Sullen unsociable moroseness, that makes him disdain (reject) everything.

Ha, 216 - Everything is repugnant to him.

IRID. Sh, 74 - No desire to touch, make love to husband all week in spite of easy, relaxed week. I feel detached from him, as if this is a problem within me. B20

KALI-BI. He, 2 - Misanthropy and ill humor, even to disgust of life.

KALI-C. Ha, 11 - Anxiety and dislike company.

KALI-I. Al, 12 - He dreads to return of dawn (morning), and the most trivial details of daily life seem insupportable to him.

LAC-AC. He, 2 - Averse to business or what formerly was pleasant to do; lazy (indolent); dislikes to read or think; finds fault, is sarcastic, exacting. (exigent, severe)

LAC-C. Al,N-43 - Intense ugliness (repulsiveness, offensiveness) and hatefulness (odiousness, repellently); writes to her best friends all sorts of mean(vulgar) and contemptible things.

He, 13 - Woke at daylight feeling that she is a loathsome (repulsive), horrible mass of disease (while the breasts were affected); could not bear to look at any portion of her body (loathing, himself), not even hands, as it intensified feeling of disgust and horror; could not bear to have any part of her body touch another, had to keep even fingers apart; felt that if she could not in some way get out of her body, she should soon become crazy .

He, 24 - When paroxysms of intense nervousness (anxiety) come on, feels like tearing off her clothes; takes off her rings;

cannot bear anything to touch her, ...
He, 40 - Feels weak, and nerves so thoroughly out of order, that she cannot bear one finger touch another.
He, 20 - No desire to live.
LACH. He, 34-...repugnance to society and dislike to talk; solicitude about future, whith disgust of life; inclination to doubt everything; mistrusts (suspicious) and misconstrues (misjudge) ...0 Melancholia.
He, 44 - Satiety (loathing?) of life with longing (desiring) for death.
He, 31 - Disinclined to his own proper work; complains of trifles.
He, 32 - Aversion of women to marry.
He, 43 - Weary of life, looks at everything from dark side;...
LIM. Al, 3 - The great disinclination to work, and inability to accomplish much, which he had experienced since the sea-bath, disappeared completely during the day, and gave place to mental quiet and steadiness, with constancy and perseverance in performing very irksome duties.
MAG-M. Ha, 16 - Joyless and passive, whatever she looks at is repugnant (disgusting, offensive) to her, she answers very unwillingly,..
MEZ. Al, 36 - Quiet and contemplative; weary of life, and longing for death.
Al, 8 - Very sad; every trifle affects him disagreeably; indifferent to the whole world; has no desire for anything; disinclined to work.
Al, 23 - Very irritable mood; very averse to everything; desire to run away.
Ha, 8 - Introverted, tired of life and longing for death.
NAT-M. Ha, 22 - Hypochondriac, even to being tired of life.
NAT-S. He, 4 - Satiety (weary) of life; must use all self-control to prevent shooting himself.
NEON. Sh, 198 - Received a long letter from a patient today; haven't even read it, can't be bothered. Very unusual. In terms of indifference, I have felt disgusted with myself; one of these violent and malicious feelings. God, I feel so wretched. 02, 6C, 05:XX:XX
NIT-AC. Al, 62 - Discontented, despising (scorn) life.
Ha, 28 - Discontented despising life.
NUX-V. Al, 21 - Great aversion to fluids, which were swallowed with great difficulty and often not at all.
PHOS. He, 19 - Weary of life; full of gloomy (dark) forebodings.
PIC-AC. Al, 1 - While enjoying the society of gentlemen, the idea of marriage (wedding) seemed unendurable.
PLAT. Al, 11 - Contemptuous, pitiful looking down upon people usually venerated, with a kind of casting (reject, discard) them off in paroxysms, against her will.
He, 12 - Dislikes her children; calls them too little.
He, 23 - Satiety of life, with taciturnity and fear of death.
PULS. Al, 10 - Everything disgusts him; he seems averse to everything.
Ha, 1142 - Everything disgusts him; everything is repugnant to him.
He, 25 - Weary of life; thinks with pleasure of drowning. (suicide, water)
He, 47-...; pangs (pain, anxiety) of conscience about religion and female sex; violent palpitation in the presence of women; abhors (detests, aversion) and hates the sex; must go out of their way for fear of injuring them; looks upon them as evil beings and is afraid (fear; temptation, seduction); considers their presence injurious (insulted, offended) to his soul; ... (sexual loathing)
He, 36 - Mistrust; envy; covetousness (avidity); dislike to people.
He, 52 - After mortification, sad gloomy (melancholy) and weary (disgusted) of life;...thinks of drowning with great pleasure;...
RAPH. Al, 1 - Feeling of aversion towards all women; she is provoked by seeing women going and coming about her; their approach threw her into a fury; the mere contact with a woman's dress caused intolerable distress;...She is attracted to all men without distinction (nymphomania) ; when she gives her hand to a man, she feels great agitation,...When left alone for a hour in the evening, she gave herself a very deep wound in the lips with a penknife, in hopes to put an end to this condition (hurt, punishes). Moral feeling

was completely extinct, the physical nature alone ruled and threw her into a frightful state (wild). From morning to noon she would not have been able to resist the advances even of a man for whom she had not the least friendly feeling; from noon to 6 p.m. she could not have held out against any man whatsoever; from 8 to 11 the demands of sense were so importunate as to silence the voice of shame and reason; ... and would have thrown herself into the arms of the first man she met...she was still unable to control her impulses;...

RHUS-T. Al, 9 - Satiety (surfeit) of life, with desire to die without sadness.
Ha, 957 - Without sadness, as if tired of life, with desire to die.

RHUS-V. Al, 1 - Great sadness, no desire to live, everything seems gloomy.

SABIN. Al, 5-...music was intolerable, it penetrated marrow and bone,...feeling of weakness, debility.

SEP. Al, 36 - The greatest loathing of life; it seemed to him as if he could not endure so miserable an existence any longer, and as if he would pine away (longing, wanting) if he did not kill himself. (pine = intense longing or grief)
Al, 20 - Internal loathing of life.
Ha, 31 - Extreme loathing of life (existence he felt as if he could not any longer bear this miserable (wretched, unhappy) existence, and as if he would pine away (ruined) unless he made away with himself.-(suicidal)
He, 19 - Aversion to one's occupation (work) and family.

SIL. Ha, 16 - Internal surfeit (satiety) of life.

SPIRAE. Al, 1 - At 1 A.M. he was attacked with remorse over a long-past slight indiscretion (mistake, wrong), with most fearful qualms (anxiety) of conscience and loathing of himself; ....

STANN. Ha, 649 - Aversion from and dread (fear) of people.
Ha, 3 - Aversion and distaste for human society.

STAPH. Al, 15 - Anxious thoughts and events in the past came to him as if the past were present before him, which caused anxiety...then it became black before his eyes; he did not know whether the images were real or illusory, then everything seemed different, and he lost all desire to live.

STRAM. Al, 23 - Violent delirium; whith was alternately mirthful, furious or dolorous (sad), directed to some imaginary source of pleasure or repugnance, and accompanied which corresponding gesticulations.

SULPH. Ha, 5 - Sad pusillanimous, full of weariness (fatigue) of life.
He, 34-...; profound melancholy; considers herself disgraced (dishonor, degradation) ; speaks of dying, finds life insupportable;...
He, 21 - Satiety of life, longing for death.

THUJ. Al, 62 - Averse to everything; anxious and solicitous about the future.

TUB. Al,N-11 - Felt positively ugly (repulsive, spiteful); personal aversions became almost a mania.

VERAT. He, 13 - After severe illness, aversion to husband and children; desire to leave house: hallucinations, room appeared full of people, crowding in, there was no longer room...

BUFO-S. Al, 1 - Aversion to work, with unfitness for it, ...

LOST

Absent-mindedness; waking, on; does not know where he is or what to answer: ***nux-m.***[54]

Anxiety; conscience, unpardonable sin, feels she has done the, and will be eternally lost: ***chel.***[54].

Confusion of mind; location, about: cic.[58] ***glon.***[137] ***nux-m.***[137] ozone[227] ***petr.***[137]

Confusion of mind; loses his way in well-known streets: agar.[163] ***arg-n.***[163] bell.[163] ***bov.***[163] bry.[163] cann-i.[163] carb-v.[163] caust.[163] germ.[222] **GLON.** kali-chl.[163] lach.[163] lyc.[163] meli.[163] ***merc.*** nat-m.[163] ***nux-m.*** nux-v.[30] ozone[227] ***petr.*** phos.[163] plb.[36] psil.[164] psor.[163] puls.[30] ran-b. stram.[163] sulph.[163] thuj. verat.[163]

Delusions; bed, looks for it in yard, during pregnancy: puls.[54]
- doomed, soul cannot be saved, cries and rages: ***ign.***[54].
- house, place, not in right (while walking in the street after headache): glon.
- lost: cot.[139]

- lost, everything is: ign.[144]
- lost, salvation for: ars.[58] ***aur.*** hell.[58] hura plb.
- lost, salvation, waking, on: aesc.
- lost, salvation, despised, and, in erotomania: ***orig.***[54].
- lost, salvation, predestination, from: ***lach.***[30]
- lost, salvation, world, to the, beyond hope: ***arg-n.***[54]
- lost, way, his: aesc.[102]
- seeks something: stram.[139]
- strange, streets, loses his way in, the houses seem strange: ***glon.***[54].
- time, space, and, lost or confused: anh.[102] bor.[5] ***cann-i.***[102] caust.[5] cic.[102] ***glon.***[102] lach.[102] nux-m.[5]

Despair; lost, thinks everything is: aur.[10] ign.[10]

Dreams; children, about, lost in crowd: bamb-a.[1184]

➤ destination, not reaching her: cadm.[144]
➤ forest, going astray in a forest: mag-m.[10] sep.[10]
➤ friends, loses friend in the city, cannot find her: ozone[227]
➤ house, looses his way in his: mag-c.[1]
➤ houses, find house where he wants to go, cannot: ozone[227]
➤ journey, separated from party and had to walk a long distance and arrived at station in time to see train start: ***lac-c.***[54]
➤ lost, city, in an unknown: ozone[227]
➤ lost, forest, as in a: am-m. ind. mag-c. mag-m. mag-s. sep.
➤ lost, home, at: choc.[222] mag-c.[1]
➤ lost, mountains, in the: ind.[36]
➤ misfortune, street, cannot find the right: ozone[227]
➤ mother, taking the wrong road: ozone[227]
➤ road absent, they cannot go on: ozone[227]
➤ train, stop, does not, where he thinks it will: ozone[227]
➤ train, trying to catch a: hydrog.[222]
➤ unsuccessful efforts to, finding way in his own house: mag-c.
➤ unsuccessful efforts to, reach a distant place: croc. plat.
➤ way, loosing: nat-c.[1]

Fear; destination, of being unable to reach his: lyc.

Forgetfulness; going, of where he is: cench.[122] ***merc.***[30]

Forgetfulness; streets, of well-known: cann-i.[102] ***crot-h.***[54] germ.[222] **GLON.** hydrog.[222] lach.[102] ***nux-m. petr.*** plb.[201]

Recognize; does not, house, his own: cic.[58] meli. merc. psor.

Recognize; does not, streets, well known: arg-n.[116] cann-i. **GLON.** lach. **NUX-M. PETR.** plat.[116]

Stupefaction; knows not where he is: merc. plb.[201] ran-b. thuj.

Unconsciousness; dream; as in, does not know where he is: atro.[36] cic.[58] cortico.[119] ***glon.*** merc. ***nux-m. petr.*** plat.[116] ran-b.

ANDROC. Sh, 77 - While cooking dinner, she remembered a ring she had lost and began searching for it in a very disorganised fashion, completely forgetting what she had previously been doing. (25)

ARG-N. He, 19 - He wept and assured every one that he has lost beyond hope for this world; that no one could delude him in that respect, and no one could reason him out of it.

ATRO. Al, 21 - Keep his eyes closed, ..."Oh, I shall lose my train."
Al, 22 - Expostulates with those who try to lead him to bed; says he will lose the train, that all things are packed up, and that he must start immediately.

AUR. Ha, 21 - Crying and wailing (lamenting); she thinks that she is irretrievably lost.

BAR-C. Al, 5 - Sad and fearful; he has all kinds of sad thoughts about his future state, and thinks that he is lost entirely; in the evening.

BELL. He, 74 - Picking at bedclothes as if looking for something lost, with confused muttering.

CALAD. He, 3 - Opens her eyes and asks, "Where am I? what do you all want around me?" A few moments after Calad. 0typhus.

CANN-I. Al, 35 - Despair, and fear of being eternally lost.

CANN-S. He, 1 - Seems to be in a dream, as if things were not real; feels as if she did not know where she was; objects seem strange; feels at times as if she was somebody else;...

CHEL. He, 17 - Restlessness and uneasiness

of conscience; feels that she has committed the unpardonable sin (crime, transgression), and that she will be eternally lost.

COT. Al, 11 - Feels silly (ridiculous) and lost.

Al, 14 - After taking the medicine, she feels lost; cannot collect herself; forgets what she is doing and saying; difficulty in expressing herself.

GERM. Sh, 94 - Did not know which way to go on a well known route. 05, 6C, 08:XX:XX

Sh, 39 - Concentration difficult. I lost my pen. I am careful, afraid of doing or saying something silly. 16, 30C, 00:06:00

GLON. Al, 19 - Confusion of ideas so great that he could not tell where he was.

Al, 21 - As he returned home through the streets, after the headache, everything seemed strange to him, not as familiar as usual; he was obliged to look about him every few moments to convince himself of being in the right street; it seemed to him as if the houses were not in their right places, on the same route that he had passed over at least four times a day for years.

He, 4 - Well-known street seem strange; way home too long.

He, 5 - Loses his way in the known streets.

He, 7 - Loss of location (locating); commencement about ten years ago; loses himself, even when walking in streets that he has traveled in for years;...

He, 3 - She could not remember which side of the street her house was on.

GUAI. Al, 5 - Loss of ideas; he stands in one place, and looks in front of him without thought,...

HALI-L. Sh, 222 - Increased sensitivity to the shopping mall environment. It seems destructive, unpleasant. I feel over stimulated, easily distracted, not knowing what I wanted. Feeling ungrounded and out of body; walking but not seeing, aimless, without a mind of my own. 09, 6C, 04:XX:XX

Sh, 223 - Don't feel I have any direction. Usually I have a direction though I might not know where it is going to lead. Now I feel lost, like I have no ground under me. I have no idea. 08, 30C, 28:XX:XX

Sh, 324 - Don't feel I have any direction. Usually I have a direction though I might not know where it is going to lead. Now I feel lost, like I have no ground under me. I have no idea. 08, 30C, 28:XX:XX

Sh, 599 - Recall a detail I'd forgotten before—like the mist parting. Looked through my desk again and found the missing package. Recalled losing something earlier this week, probably thrown out. No one else saw it except me. The strangest feeling to remember having seen something, remembered the color of the paper, and the picture, and the wording, and yet not be able to confirm its existence with anyone. Beginning to doubt if it was really real, and yet I know it was. 09, 6C, 11:04:40

HYDROG. Sh, 12 - Driving home I felt odd, as if I was hardly in my body. Feel like my body's working on automatic but I'm not really there. Driving along I kept forgetting where I was. Now I feel I'm really more "absent" than normal and feel quite afraid of losing my mind or having an accident. I feel my connection with the physical world is very loose, as though my soul was separated from my body. I have thoughts that this is a bit like dying —not unpleasant. 10, 200C, 13:02:XX

Sh, 18 - Sometimes I think there isn't much of me left anymore —as if I left myself behind ages ago. 16, 30C, XX:XX:XX

Sh, 21 - I feel I have moved into a different state of consciousness and there aren't any guiding posts or means of navigation —a bit like being lost in space. 16, 30C, 06:XX:XX

Sh, 63-"Oh God, what shall I do? Where do things go from here? What way shall I go? Feel I'm cracking up". Emotional confusion. Try to find a path to be happy, but unsure of what I'm doing. 24, 30C, 100:XX:XX

Sh, 75 - Tendency to lose things and blamed myself. Became frantic searching for them. Tore open a friend's bag to find paper and wouldn't have cared if the bag had ripped. 22, 12C, 04:XX:XX

HYOS. He, 11 - Thinks he is in the wrong place.

IOD. He, 15 - At night, especially when thinking of real or imaginary wrongs ...dares (try) to go home for fear of doing some dreadful (bad, wicked) deed (action); on one occasion was seized with an almost irresistible impulse to murder a woman who was acting as a guide (direct, conduct) for him, he having lost his way (direction);...must be constantly in action, in some laborious occupation. (lost; direction, correction, control)

He, 1 - Feeling as of having forgotten something and does not know what.

KREOS. Al, 10 - When she undertakes to accomplish anything and has gone ten or twelve steps, she remains standing, and does not know what she had intended (planned) to do.

MAG-C. Al, 947 - Anxious dream as if he was unable to find his way in his own house.

MAG-M. Al, 710 - Dream that she became confused in a forest, and for a long time could not find her way.

NAT-C. Al, DREAM, 1102-..;of marrying two women, of parties, walks, entertainments, and excursions on horseback, afterwards they were frequently anxious, of going astray (lost),of murders, having his ears cut off; also vexatious dreams; he would take a journey and could not get away from the place,(immobilization) and when has reached the first station was obliged to turn back, on account of something he had forgotten.

NAT-M. Ha, 90 - Irresolution in doing mental work; he cannot easily find his way.

NEON. Sh, 77 - I don't quite seem to know where my body is in space, tripping and falling. 06, 12C, 00:05:00

Sh, 79 - Heard the sound of my foot move but was not aware of it moving. I did not know where I was. 20, 6C, 00:06:30

NIT-AC. Ha, 2 - Dejected, as if desponding and as if lost in thoughts.

NUX-M. Al, 56-...he went to the theater, which was at some distance; the way seemed to have no end (endless, interminable); ... Although he was, at times, quite unconscious, his limbs did not fail to their service; he went straight on, without recognizing the streets that crossed his way; he was concerned about the time, he feared to come too late..., fancy and reality battle (fight) with each other.

He, 15 - Surroundings seemed changed; fanciful, dreamy images; does not recognize the known street.

PALL. He, 1 - Extremely fatigued in evening; feels mentally gone; is averse to speaking a foreign language which at other times he speaks fluently; it is too much of an exertion, he is tired of it. (lack of communication)

PETR. He, 3 - Did not know where she was in the street.

PLB. He, 16 - Mental disturbance of eight or ten years' duration in a man addicted to masturbation; has several times attempted suicide; has been in seclusion (solitude); greatest dejection and despair;...; believes himself lost (condemned) ; has the sounds of hell constantly in his ears; hears voices and sees shadows of demons, great disposition to make away (suicide) with himself or do himself some bodily injury;

PULS. He, 46 - Dark suspicious and reserved manner; disturbed look on face; sleepless; looks for her bed in the yard (lost?); hides in a corner to escape from a little gray man who wanted to pull out her leg;...

SANG. He, 11 - It seems to her ...she is in a railroad car and begs others to hold her.

TUB. Al,N-38 - Soporous, dazed condition; unable to find the right way (lost); is confused; surroundings appear strange.

LOVE

Affectionate; love for everyone about him, during and after fainting: hura[60]

Ailments from; celibacy, being unmarried, continence: ***agn.***[8] apis[130] calc.[137] ***cann-i.***[137] con.[102] fl-ac.[137] lyc.[137] phos.[111] plat.[137] sep.[187]

Ailments from; love disappointed, drowsiness, with: **PH-AC.**[54]

Ailments from; love disappointed, emotional and mental symptoms from: ant-c.[8] ***aur.***[8] bell.[30] calc-p.[31] caust.[30] ***cimic.***[8] dig.[91] ***hyos.***[8] **IGN.**[8] ***lach.***[8] ***nat-m.***[54] ***ph-ac.***[8] ***phos.***[8] staph.[137] ***verat.***[8]

Ailments from; love disappointed, grief, with silent: **IGN. NAT-M. PH-AC.** phos.

Ailments from; love disappointed, jealousy, anger and incoherent talk, with: hyos. nat-m.[122]

Ailments from; love disappointed, laugh,

with inclination to: hyos.[54]
Ailments from; love disappointed, rage, with: hyos.[56]
Ailments from; love disappointed, sadness, with: ***aur.***[54] bell.[30] ***hyos.***[54] **IGN.**[54] ***nat-m.***[54]
Ailments from; love, disappointed, unhappy: ***acon.***[5] am-c.[5] androc.[222] ant-c. **AUR.**[5] ***bell.***[30] ***bufo***[117] cact.[5] ***calc-p. caust.***[5] ***cimic. coff.*** com.[5] ***con.***[116] dig.[85] ***hell.*** **HYOS.** **IGN.**[122] iod.[85] kali-c. ***kali-p.***[5] ***lach.*** **NAT-M.** nux-m. nux-v. orig.[187] ozone[227] **PH-AC.** phos.[5] pitu-a.[164] psor.[185] ***sac-alb.***[210] sep. seq-s.[230] **STAPH.**[122] stram.[37] sulph.[122] tarent. til.[36] verat.[54]
Amorous; fits, in: acon.[5] ant-c.[5] hyos.[5] op.[5] stram.[5] verat.[5]
Anxiety; health, loved persons, of: carc.[193] hep.[30] merc.[30]
Blackmail, emotional, says "you don't love me" when refused: puls.[189] tub.[189]
Brooding; disappointment, love: ***ph-ac.***[54]
Delirium; maniacal, love, from disappointed: ***phos.***[54]
Delirium; wedding, prepares for: ***hyos.***
Delusions; betrothal, engagement, must be broken: fl-ac.
- married, he is: ign.
- married, is going to be: hyos.
- wedding, of a: alum.[5] hyos.[5] mag-m.[5] nat-c.[5]

Despair; love, from disappointed: caust.[30] ***hyos.***[54]
Dreams; love, fallen in: bamb-a.[1184]
➤ romantic: am-c. ***kali-c.***[54]
➤ wedding: alum. bamb-a.[1184] chel. mag-c. mag-m.[1] mag-s. nat-c. nat-s.
➤ wedding, women, with two: nat-c.[10]
Ecstasy, amorous: ant-c.[1] op. pic-ac.
Forsaken; feeling, beloved by his parents, wife, friends, feels of not being: ***ars.***[30] calc.[30] lyc.[30] ***mag-c.***[122] sep.[30] sil.[30] sulph.[30]
Grief; silent, love, with disappointed: **IGN.**[54]
Insanity; love, on account of unfortunate: tarent.[36]
Irresolution; marry, to: carb-v.[30] ign.[30] lach.[30] nat-m.[30] nux-v.[30] phos.[30] plat.[30] sil.[30] staph.[30] verat.[30]
Jealousy; love disappointment, in: ***hyos.***[54]
Kill; sudden impulse to, husband, her beloved: ***merc. nux-v. plat.***
Laughing; love, from disappointed: ***hyos.***[54]
Love; animals, for: aeth.[162] calc-p.[184] carc.[193] med.[162] nat-m.[185] phos.[193] psor.[185]
Love; animals, for, cats, for: ***sulph.***[162]
Love; animals, for, pet, his: nat-m.[189]
Love; animals, for, suffering: nuph.[36]
Love; children, for: ***ars.***[10] ***hep.***[10] phos.[10] plat.[10] sep.[10]
Love; everybody around him, for, during and after fainting: hura[36]
Love; exalted: ant-c.[5] hyos.[5]
Love; falling in love easily: ign.[85]
Love; family, for: coff.[8] coff-t.[36]
Love; herself, towards: germ.[222]
Love; love-sick: ***ant-c.*** germ.[222] hydrog.[222] pip-m.[144] til.
Love; nature, for: carc.[162] lap-c-b.[194]
Love; overflowing, for humanity: germ.[222] hydrog.[222]
Love; own sex, men: med.[162] nat-m.[162] orig.[162] phos.[162] ***plat.***[30] puls.[162] sep.[162] staph.[162]
Love; perversity: hura[36] ind.[85] kali-n.[36] nux-v.[85] plat.[85]
Malicious; loved ones, to: germ.[222] sep.[58]
Marriage; idea, seemed unendurable idea of: ***lach. med.***[122] nux-v.[187] pic-ac. puls. staph.[30]
Rage; love, after disappointed: ***hyos.***[54]
Sadness; love, from disappointed: ***aur.***[54] bell.[30] dig.[137] ***hyos.***[54] **IGN.**[54] ***nat-m.***[54]
Sentimental; moonlight in, ecstatic love: **ANT-C.**
Suicidal disposition; drowning, by, love, from disappointed: ***hyos.***[54]
Suicidal disposition; love, from disappointed: ant-c.[188] ***aur.***[54] bell.[137] caust.[137] ***hyos.***[54] staph.[137]
Suicidal disposition; love, from disappointed, weeping, with: ***aur.***[54]
Weeping; love, from unrequited: ***ign.***[54]

ACON. Ha, 521 - Lucid vision: he says, now my beloved (70 miles away) must have sung the difficult passage (of Beethoven) that I was just singing.
He, 2 - Clairvoyance; conscious that his beloved, miles away, was singing a certain piece.

ANT-C. Ha, 18 - Continuous state of enthusiastic love and ecstatic longing for an ideal woman, which quite filled his fantasy;... (perfection, utopian)
Ha, 23 - Ecstasy and exalted love, with great anxiety about his fate (destiny, doom), and inclination to shoot himself;...
Ha, 28 - Consequences of (ailments from)

disappointed love.
He, 22 - Sentimental mood in the moonlight, particularly ecstatic love.
AUR. Ha, 3 - He believes that he has lost the love of others, and this mortifies him even to tears.
He, 59 - Disappointed love, with weeping and inclination to commit suicide.
He, 79 - Ailments from grief, disappointed love.
CALC-P. He, 19 - Ailments from grief, disappointed love.
CALC-S. Al, 7 - Excessive, bitter melancholy, with distressing apprehensions of evil to loved ones.
CIMIC. He, 34 - Mind disturbed by disappointed love, business failures.
COFF. He, 8 - Great loquacity, brain feels clear and is active, he feels strong enough to do anything, feels impelled to push things; veneration for the Supreme Being and love for family; benevolence excited.
He, 33 - Ailments from excessive joy, excessive laughing and playing; from disappointed love; from anger, from vexations with vehemence or fright...
FL-AC. He, 6 - Feeling of indifference towards those he loves best; has no objection to their presence but does not care to converse with them, yet if strangers or mere acquaintances come in will enter into animated conversation....
GERM. Sh, 111 - If I were me, nobody would like me - so I try to be what I think others expect me to be. I don't think I can be loved with all the parts of me which are ugly and bad. Lonely feelings. Longing for love and understanding. Feel I am so unfriendly to myself. 18, 30C, 04:00:00
Sh, 163 - Felt lack of romance in my life. Desired romantic love, to be loved. 05, 6C, 41:XX:XX
Sh, 121 - Very strong longing for excitement and some love adventure. I planned to go out, but though I probably would be disappointed, so I stayed at home and was depressed instead. Feel like drinking - to get away from myself and everything. 18, 30C, 04:00:00
HALI-L. Sh, 14 - Delusion—Small white animal, sweet and cuddly, has been living in a chair in my living room. 16, 10C, 04:XX:XX
Sh, 208 - Daughter home sick. I'm enjoying just hanging around with her being. "Mom." Realize I still don't feel like her mom. I'm not Mom; I'm just me. But to them, I'm Mom. Does my mom feel the same? 09, 6C, 23:XX:XX
Sh, 211 - I allowed my mother to mother me for the first time. It was a wonderful visit. For the first time ever I was allowing myself to be vulnerable and allowed her to love me. I had never felt I was the child with her before. These thoughts were foreign to me. 01, 30C, 21:XX:XX
Sh, 215 - Made up a meditation before going to bed. Felt both parents at the bedside. I am being totally held and loved by my father, wrapped up in blankets like I'm a baby. He is adoring me, cooing over me with my mother looking on. This calms my nerves and the sad feeling moves outward. This feels the same as swimming to me. The water on my skin calms my nerves. 08, 30C, 23:XX:XX
HURA. Al, 7 - During and after the fainting spell (trance), disposed to love everybody, especially those about him; he often thinks of death, but does not fear it; he feels as though he could die without regret.(fearless)
HYDROG. Sh, 13 - Falling in love on a very deep level. 16, 30C, XX:XX:XX
Sh, 14 - I felt so much love I didn't know how to focus it. Its like being in another state of consciousness. No one can come near and its frightening me. 16, 30C, 25:XX:XX
Sh, 15 - I felt in the presence of a totally pure energy, like meeting God and feeling totally unworthy or like meeting a lover and feeling unworthy —realizing all the mistakes of a lifetime. This pure energy was around for some time protecting me. I feel this unification cleared out lifetimes of symptomatology for me. The joining with this energy was as if a male energy joined with me sexually, but with no desire, pleasure or pain involved. This unification with the male energy lasted quite a few days — I'm not used to seeing myself as a man. The morning after this unifying with the higher presence, I collapsed in emotional overflow. All my grief and pain came out. I was doubled upon the floor and went into a deep state

of catharsis. It is not possible to describe where I went as there are no concepts applicable. I felt overflowing love for humanity and wanted to give everything away. My mind turned to the Buddha. It was like seeing the complete picture instead of fragmented bits. (These primary effects lasted about 28 days, then changing to a paranoia state). 16, 30C, 07.XX.XX

HYOS. He, 64 - Serious illness (ailments) from jealousy and grief about faithless lover;...

He, 68 - Onanism since childhood; has always been greatly attracted by opposite sex and prematurely busied himself with thoughts of marriage;... secretly wrote his love affairs; mania,...one idea rapidly follow another, all in some away concerning love, masturbates at every opportunity...(satyriasis)

He, 74 - Disappointed love followed by: epilepsy, melancholy, rage, or inclination to laugh at everything; despair and propensity to drown himself. (ailments from)

He, 46 - Sings amorous and obscene songs.

He, 69 - Lascivious mania, uncovers body, especially sexual parts; sings amorous songs.

He, 85-...repelled with rage and seeming disgust his mother, of whom, in natural state, he was dotingly (loving) fond, did not know her, said she was not his mama;...0Maniacal fury.

IGN. He, 37 - Tears wept inwardly, the pain and penalty (forfeit) of unrequited (unrecompensed) love; desires solitude so that one may nourish inward grief;...

He, 44-...;indifference to things she loved best ; sits alone and weeps, imagines things, a especially that she might go crazy; ..

He, 62 - Ill effects (ailments) from hearing bad news; from vexation with reserved displeasure ; from grief, or suppressed mental sufferings; of shame and disappointed love.

He, 24 - Melancholy after disappointed love, always combined with spinal symptoms.

He, 27 - Unhappy love with silent grief.

He, 50 - Jealousy, disappointed love.

IRID. Sh-7 - Abnormal mental awareness, very conscious of nature, everything seemed very vivid, very lovely. Profound feeling. F22

Sh, 59 - Woke from a dream about wedding, feeling of unease, remembered my own wedding day, got a letter of proposal from former lover. Went ahead despite. What did I do? Q7

Sh, 118 - Thoughts: Wind is breath of the spirit; love is the greatest of all messages between heaven and earth. Yes, go to heaven, but return to the world transformed by the light of experience, transcend and return; Metals —immortality; need knowledge of their names; Iridescence, oil mother of pearl metal, rainbow, seven plus seven, cosmic joke, messages in other languages —language of angels?; Seven heavens, seven earths. I adore these territories, not so much new as forgotten. Q20

LACH. He, 59 - Ailments from fright (fear), disappointed love or jealousy.

LYC. He, 28 - Amativeness or amorousness.

MAG-C. Al, 933 - Dream that she has to marry one she did not like, which she violently resisted;...

MERC. He, 30 - Anxiety driving her to suicide ; thoughts of suicide; ...desire for death; great indifference even to those she formerly loved;...

NAT-C. Al, DREAM, 1102-..;of marrying two women, of parties, walks, entertainments, and excursions on horseback, afterwards they were frequently anxious, of going astray (lost),of murders, having his ears cut off; also vexatious dreams; he would take a journey and could not get away from the place,(immobilization) and when has reached the first station was obliged to turn back, on account of something he had forgotten.

NEON. Sh, 35 - Feel like I have been kissed by heaven. 10, 6C, 07:01:XX

Sh, 38 - I have always felt comfortable with the division between the dark and the light. What I now need is the division of heavens and oceans. Thoughts about my love for the Pacific Ocean. 20, 6C, 06:XX:XX

OX-AC. Al, 19 - Philoprogenitiveness, greater love of his children, in one in whom this feeling was always predominating; a decidedly expressed and clearly distinguishable symptom, it being not traceable to any other cause. (love creation of child)

PH-AC. He, 11 - Ailments from care, grief, sorrow, chagrin, homesickness; or disappointed love;...

PHOS. Ha, 82 - Indifferent to her child, whom at other times she dearly loved.

He, 29 - Crazy deliria in a young woman who was strictly moral and unhappy in her love; accused herself of the most obscene (immoral, wicked) actions, of which she never was guilty; ....

PIC-AC. Al, 1 - While enjoying the society of gentlemen, the idea of marriage (wedding) seemed unendurable.

PLAT. Ha, 25-...felt like embracing everybody and could have laughed over the most sad things.

He, 2 - Inclination to embrace everybody. (contact)

He, 44 - Talks almost continually about fanciful things or such as have really occurred; of faithless love; of her teacher and old school days; ...

PULS. He, 39 - Children are extremely affectionate, which they manifest by kissing and caressing.

ROB. Al, 10 - Love and excited passions, leading him to the grossest (obscene, rude) excesses, even to homicide.

SEP. He, 38-...everything seems strange (unusual, unfamiliar) to her;...; it seems as if she could not understand (realize) anything and would have to learn anew everything she wished to do;...(lost: knowledge); greatest indifference to everything, the death of a near relative, or some happy occurrence, leaves her equally unaffected; no trace of her former love for friends or even for her child; aversion for social intercourse amounting to contempt;...

He, 22 - Great indifference to one's family, to those they love best.

TARENT. Al, 2 - Insanity on account of an unfortunate love.

TIL. Al, 2 - Lovesick (passion, fervor); all his thoughts centered upon an ideal woman; in this revery he was possessed by a sweet melancholy...

VERAT. He, 22 - Nymphomania, with violence and destructiveness; had been disappointed in love; melancholia; ...great desire for sexual intercourse; void (empty) of shame; obscenity; ....

He, 50 - Religious melancholy or nymphomania, with desire to embrace everybody even inanimate objects;...[0]Puerperal mania.

MAGIC

Delusions; beautiful, images, presenting themselves to her as if by charm: bell.[54]

- charmed and cannot break the spell: ***lach.***[54]
- enchantment, of: coff-t.[36]
- fairies, searching for: lap-mar-c.[194]
- gnome, he is a: cann-i.[36]
- magician, is a: bell.
- power over all disease, has: ***stram.***[54]
- witches, denies having anything to do with them, in delirium after being accused of theft: ***hyos.***[54]

Dreams; fairytale, as in a: ozone[227]

- ➤ magic: sol-t-ae.[36]
- ➤ mandala: androc.[222]
- ➤ pursued, witch, by a, creeps from under the door like a haze: ozone[227]

Mystical: camph.[36] pyrus[36]

MANIA

Dreams; monomania: acon.[10] ign.[10] puls.[10] stann.[10]

Mania; masturbation, eight or ten years duration, of: ***plb.***[54]

Mania; violence, with deeds of: ars.[10] ***bell.***[10] hyos.[10] ***plat.***[54] sec.[10] stram.[10]

Monomania: ***absin.***[102] acon. anac.[36] anan. aur.[5] bell.[10] camph. carb-v. carc.[207] cham.[10] chin.[10] cic.[5] cocc.[10] con.[10] croc.[10] cupr.[10] dros.[10] hell. hyos.[10] ***ign.*** iod.[10] lach.[10] lap-c-b.[194] mag-c.[10] nux-m. oxyt.[102] plat.[10] puls. rhus-t.[10] ***sil.*** stram. sulph. tarent.[102] thuj. verat.[10]

Talk; nothing but, one subject: ***arg-n.*** cann-i. cocain.[5] lap-c-b.[194] lyc. med.[137] petr. stram.

Thoughts; circles, moving in: cann-i.[36] choc.[222]

Thoughts; monotony of: anh.[144] chlol.[36]

ANAN. He, 8 - Monomania for doing same thing and frequenting same places.

APIS. He, 28 - Manias (insanity) especially

proceeding from a sexual cause in women.

AUR. He, 18 - Religious mania; prays all the time.

BAR-M. He, 4 - In every form of mania, as soon as the sexual desire is increased. (lascivious)

CAMPH. He, 16 - Monomania, with horrible visions and torturing ideas about religion, which he cannot shake off, although he is conscious that they are morbid.; is< at night.

CANN-I. Al, 23 - He seemed to have the one idea that he should die and soon be dissected.

HELL. He, 11 - Psychical conditions occupying a place between melancholia and mania, and in conditions where true depression and weakness is present, in which the patient is governed by a fixed idea.

He, 9 - Mania demoniac; sees evil (harmful) spirits at night.

HYOS. Al, 85 - Excessive fear of death, becoming a monomania,...

He, 63 - Erotic mania accompanied by jealousy.

LACH. He, 17 - Religious monomania, fear of being damned (condemned to eternal punishment).

He, 51 - Proud; jealous, suspicious; developing into mania.

LAM. Al, 5-...,(fixed ideas) so that at last she becomes sad about it, and thinks she shall lose her reason.

PHOS. He, 31-...; indifference even towards dearest friends;... ; monomania de grandeur et de la richesse;...

He, 25 - Amativeness; erotic mania.

PLAT. He, 42 - Mania; with great pride; fault-finding; unchaste (sensual) talk; ...(chaste = moral, pure)

PSOR. Al,N-44 - Mania of self-destruction.

PULS. He, 40 - Religious mania; sees the devil coming to take her; the world on fire during night; fear, rage in spells, or weeping... (captured, possessed)

STRAM. He, 101 - Mania for light and company, cannot bear to be alone.

SULPH. He, 13 - A little girl with religious insanity, takes passages of Scripture literally and acts upon them. (fanatical) (virtuous, noble, elevated)

MASOCHISM

Borrows trouble, always finds trouble: acet-ac.[58] apis[58] bar-c.[137] calc.[137] sang.[137]

Cheerfulness; death, while thinking of: aur.

Complaining; symptoms, about his numerous, in pneumonia: ***ant-t.***[54]

Death; desires, alternating with laughing: aur.[10]

Death; thoughts of, joy, give him: aur.[54]

Desires; unpleasant things, to think about: kiss.[36]

Dwells; grieve therefore, to: nat-m.[30]

Grief; hunting for something to grieve oneself: lil-t.

Hydrophobia; frequently speaks with a remarkably quick and sharp articulation of the impending result: lyss.[54]

Love; sadomasochistic: anac.[187]

Masochism: nat-c.[185] nat-m.[185] tub.[185]

Masochism; sexual: lach.[185] nat-m.[185] tub.[185]

Mortification; mortifies herself: cob.[102]

Sadness; enjoys: ign.[137] nat-m.[137]

Suicidal disposition; drowning, by, thinks with pleasure of: ***puls.***[54]

MEDITATION

Absorbed; alternating with frivolity: arg-n.

Absorbed; become of him, as to what would: nat-m.

Absorbed; buried in thought: acon. aloe alum. am-c.[5] am-m. ambr.[5] androc.[222] anh.[119] ant-c. ***arn.*** asar.[5] bar-c.[30] bell. bov. bruc.[10] bufo[170] calc. cann-i. cann-s.[5] canth. ***caps.*** carb-an.[137] ***carl.*** caust. cham. chel.[5] chin. cic. clem. ***cocc.*** con. cupr. cycl. dig.[5] elaps euphr.[10] grat. guai.[10] ham. **HELL.** hydrog.[222] hyos.[5] ign. indg.[10] iod.[5] ip. kali-c.[5] kiss.[36] kreos.[10] lach.[5] lap-c-b.[194] **LAUR.**[5] lil-t. mag-c.[5] mag-m.[10] mang. merc. **MEZ.** mosch. mur-ac. nat-c. ***nat-m.*** nat-p. nit-ac. **NUX-M.** ***nux-v.***[5] ol-an. ***onos. op.*** **PETR.**[5] phel. phos. plat.[5] plb.[5] ***puls.*** ran-b.[5] rheum ***rhus-t.***[5] sabad. sars. sel.[85] sep.[5] spig. stann. staph.[5] stram. stront-c.[10] **SULPH.** thuj.[5] verat.[5] viol-o.[5] vip.[10]

Absorbed; future, about: spig.[1]

Absorbed; strange, pregnancy, during: lyss.[137]

Abstraction of mind: acon.[1] acon-l.[122] agn.[10] ***alum.***[122] am-c.[10] aml-n. ang.[10] ***arn.***[10] bell.[1] berb.[10] bov.[10] bufo[170] camph. ***cann-i.*** caps.[10] carb-ac. carc.[207] caust. ***cham.***[10] choc.[222] cic. colch.[10] con. cortico.[149] ***croc.***[10]

cycl. elaps ***graph.***[10] guai. ***hell.*** hydrog.[222] ***hyos.*** ictod.[10] kali-c.[10] ***kreos.*** lap-c-b.[194] laur. ***lyc. lyss.***[122] mag-c.[10] mang.[10] ***merc.***[10] ***mez.***[122] nat-c.[10] ***nat-m.*** **NUX-M.** nux-v.[10] ***oena. ol-an.***[10] olnd.[10] ***onos.*** op. ph-ac. ***phos.***[122] plat. plb.[10] psil.[164] ran-b.[122] sabad. sars.[10] sec. sil. spong.[10] stann.[10] stram. sul-ac.[10] ***sulph.*** thuj.[10] ***tub.***[122] verb.[10] vesp. ***visc.***

Ailments from; meditation: arg.[5] olnd.[5] ran-b.[5]

Anxiety; meditation, from: acon.[60] ars.[60] calc.[60] camph.[60] cham.[60] nux-v.[60] puls.[60] rhus-t.[60] sec.[60] verat.[60]

Desires; muse: ham.[36] lil-t.[36]

Dreams; meditation, with: acon.[5] ***anac.***[5] arn.[5] ***bry.***[5] camph.[5] carb-an.[5] graph.[5] **IGN.**[5] ***lach.***[5] **NUX-V.**[5] puls.[5] rhus-t.[5] ***sabad.***[5] ***sabin.***[5] ***thuj.***[5]

Meditation: acon.[5] am-m. ant-c. aur. bar-c.[162] berb.[54] calc-s.[58] ***cann-i.***[102] cann-s. canth. **CARB-AN.** cham.[10] chin. choc.[222] cic. clem. cocc. coff.[102] con. cycl. eug. euph.[54] germ.[222] guai.[10] ham. hell. ***hyos.*** ign. ip. kali-n. kreos.[10] ***lach.*** led.[116] lyss.[54] manc. mang.[10] meny.[54] mez. mur-ac. naja[5] nat-c. ol-an.[54] phel. phos. plan.[25] plb. ran-b. rhus-t. sabad. senec.[25] sep. spig. staph. ***sulph.*** thuj.

Meditation; deep, profound: acon.[5] cocc.[10] **SEP.**[5] staph.[5]

Plans; reflects upon their execution: ***chin.***[54]

Reflecting: ***act-sp.***[111] aur.[36] bar-c.[10] berb.[54] ***carb-an.***[54] chin.[10] eug.[54] euph.[54] germ.[222] graph.[10] lyss.[54] m-arct.[10] meny.[54] mur-ac.[10] nux-v.[10] ol-an.[54] ***phos.***[54] sil.[10] sulph.[10] thuj.[10]

Reflecting; sadness, in: ***cocc.***[54]

Reflecting; sadness, in, deep: ***plat.***[54]

Sit; inclination to, corner, in: agar.[38] alco.[10] aur.[1] bar-c.[47] bar-m.[8] bell.[30] con.[58] fl-ac.[58] ***hep.***[8] hipp.[85] hyos.[58] lap-gr-m.[194] merc.[47] nat-m.[127] puls.[58] stram.[36] sulph.[58] verat.[1]

Sit; meditates: calc-s. carb-an.[187] cocc.[54] just.[97] lach.[36] sulph.[58]

Sit; meditates, misfortune, imaginary, over: calc-s.[58] lil-t.[137]

Thoughts; profound: androc.[222] bamb-a.[1184] bell. calc-ar.[36] cocc.[5] cycl. grat. kres.[144] lach.[60] mur-ac.

Thoughts; profound, future, about his: cycl. spig.

Thoughts; thoughtful: acon. alco.[36] aloe[36] alum.[36] am-m. arn. bamb-a.[1184] bar-c. bart.[36] bell. bor.[36] brom. calc. cann-s. canth. ***carb-an.*** cham. chin. cic. clem. ***cocc.*** cycl. euph. euphr. grat. guai.[10] ***hep.***[30] hyos. ***ign.*** ip. kali-n.[36] kreos.[10] ***lach.*** lyc. mag-m. manc. mang. mez. nat-c. nit-ac. nux-v. orig.[25] ***phos.*** plan.[36] plb. ***puls.***[30] ran-b. rhus-t. sabad. ***sep.*** spig. ***staph.*** stront-c. sulph. thea. thuj. til. viol-o.

Thoughts; thoughtful, errors of others, about the: cic.[36]

ALOE. Al, 2 - Before taking it, the disposition is apprehensive, speculative, amorous, after taking it, quiet ...reflective, more self sufficient,...

ALUM.Ha, 39 - Great absent-mindedness and irresolution.

ANAC. Ha, 7 - Anxious apprehension and deep thoughts, on meditating over his present and his future fate. (destiny)

ANT-C. Ha, 7 - Anxious meditation, during the day, about himself, his present and future fate. (doom, destine).

BELL. He, 7 - Likes to brood in silence, supreme indifference, nothing makes an impression.

CALC. Ha, 12 - Anxious about the present and the future, with deep reflection, at the same time indifferent to things outside...
He, 5 - Buried in deep thought; anxiety about present and future.(destine)

CAMPH. Al, 46-...I feel a tendency to self contemplation; outer things vanish, and I behold myself in spirit freed from matter.
Al, 46-...I am alone. I feel a tendency to self contemplation; outer things vanished, and I behold myself in spirit freed from matter...

CARB-AN. Al, 1 - Desire to be alone ; she is sad and reflective (thoughtful); avoids all conversation.

CHOC. Sh, 139 - Meditation is much smoother —an effortless zooming in. I feel much more comfortable in the world. Before I always wanted to get out. During meditation, felt a floating feeling, felt an opening and upwards movement in my back, as if wings were forming and I was just light.

CON. Al, 38 - Sunk in deep thought; he apprehensively considered the present and

the future, and sought (wanted) to be alone.
Ha, 365 - Sunk in deep thought, he cogitated timorously about the present and the future and sought (wants) solitude.
Ha, 8 - Lost in deep meditation, he anxiously thought over the present and the future, and sought solitude.
He, 10 - Buried in thought; apprehensive (anxiety) respecting the present or future.
CYCL. Ha, 194 - Sunk in deep thought (meditation), he sought (desire) solitude and thought about his future fate (destine, doom).
Ha, 195 - Deep thought about the present and future, so that he almost wept.
He, 4 - Absorbed in deep thought, seeks solitude, thinks about his future.
HELL. Ha, 287 - Wrapped (envelop) up in his own thoughts, silent humour, all the afternoon.
He, 20 - After typhoid, ...sits quietly in bed and seems lost in brooding;...constantly seeks (try) to escape, ...;without a word quietly climbs out of the window, and if she succeeds in escaping goes in direction of river; finally threw herself into privy (toilet), from which she was rescued.
IGN. He, 6 - Brooding over imaginary or real troubles; is wrappd in thought.
IRID. Sh, 110 - Meditating, vision of an angel, face and wings. Q6
JAMB. He, 1 - Constantly desirous of sitting alone and reflecting.
LED. Al, 11 - Morose mood, with much uneasiness and irresolution; he is unable to reflect constantly upon anything, or work with a quiet mind.
Ha, 336 - All day long great seriousness(gravity); he regarded everything that happened to him in a serious and thoughtful (meditative) manner.
MAG-C. Al, 929 - Dream of very small horses, that she exerted herself to reflect upon, after midnight.
MANG. Ha, 324 - Cross reflective, silently reserved, wrapped up in himself, with discomfort in the whole body, ...
MEZ. Al, 36 - Quiet and contemplative; weary of life, and longing for death.
MOSCH. Al, 19 - She sits in thought, strikes her hands together, makes various gestures, so that others fear she will lose her reason,...
MUR-AC. Al, 10 - Anxious thoughtfulness; he cannot free himself from the slightest trouble.
Al, 21 - Deep reflection, and quiet absorption in himself, as if something disagreeable were impending, though with desire to work.
Ha, 269 - Sunk in profound thought, as if something disagreeable were about to happen,...
Ha, 4 - Deep reflection, and quiet introversion, as if something unpleasant was impending,...
NAT-M. Al, 66 - Lost for hours in thought as to what would become of him.
Ha, 9 - For hours, immersed in thoughts, as to what would become of him.
NUX-V. He, 20 - Desire to talk about one's condition, with anxious reflections about it.
SPIG. Ha, 658 - Profound reflection about his future fate. (destiny)
STANN. Al, 7 - Quite absorbed in himself, solicitous for the future.
STAPH. Ha, 700 - All day long peevish and cross; he did not know what to do for ill-humor, and was extremely pensive.
SULPH. Ha, 61 - Great inclination to philosophic and religious ravings.(insanity)
He, 50 - Irritable mood; easily excited and always absorbed in himself.
THEA. Al, 20 - Nocturnal fright; sinister thoughts; invincible propensity to analyze his life, to look at it on the dark side, and to resolve it into its most hopeless realities.
THUJ. Ha, 628 - Prolonged thoughtfulness about the merest trifle.

MENACED

Delusions; bed, someone, stands at the foot menacing, someone: chlol.
- life, threatened, is: kali-br.
- people threatening her, screams horrible: ars-met.[54]
- people, threatening her, screams horrible: ars-met.[54]
- runs, away, has to run: ars-met.[139]
- sword hanging over head: am-m.

Dreams; bullying: peti.[36]

➤ houses, cold, liveless, nearly threatening: ozone[227]
➤ knives, threatened with, he is: ozone[227]
➤ rape, threats of rape: cench.[58] sep.
➤ stabbed, swordsmen threatened to stab him: op.[36]
➤ threats of rape: sep.[36]

Fearlessness; danger menaced him, as if, but without fear: fl-ac.[54]

Restlessness; suffocation, with threatening: gels.[85]

ADAM. Sh, 379 - Tearful and vulnerable. A situation I would normally cope with seemed threatening. 8, 6C, 01:20:00

AESC. Al, 9-...he had a feeling as if death was impending (imminent); but this was followed by an exalted condition of brain and nervous system...

ALUM. Ha, 18 - Restlessness in the evening, as if evil was imminent.
He, 19 - Uneasy evenings as from impending evil.

ARS-MET. He, 4 - Fearful visions of spectres (ghosts) in bright daylight; she sees threatening people after her,...

ASTER. He, 9 - It seems as if some misfortune was impending, as if bad news was about to arrive...

AUR-M. Al, 4 - Sad mood as though a great misfortune impending.
He, 7 - Sadness as when homesick; sad as though a great misfortune impended.

CAMPH. He, 61 - Felt a vague sense of impending danger to life,...

CAUST. Ha, 7 - Anxious, restlessness mood, as if something disagreeable (difficult) was impending (imminent), which keeps him from working.
He, 33 - Anxious uneasy mood, as if something unpleasant impended (threaten, frighten); this unfits (incompetent) him for every kind of work.(lost: competence)

CHIN-S. Al, 20-...; felt a gloom (darkness) come over me, as if some evil were impending; relieved by a specific trust in the Almighty;...(divine) (faithful, confiding, devoted)
He, 9 - Recurrence of feeling of impending evil.

CHLOL. Al, 5 - Became delirious, and hurled (throw) a hot-water bottle at an imaginary figure which stood menacing her at the foot of the bed.

CHOC. Sh, 121 - I met a dog this morning and felt that I understood it now and it wasn't a threat, whereas earlier I had been uncertain and wary.
Sh, 191 - I Since the being bitten by the dogs have developed a strong fear of dogs, and have been chased by one dog and growled at by another. This is coupled with a general fear of something happening. These fears are new to me and were better again after the proving. 27, 100C, 05:XX:XX

FL-AC. Al, 13 - Sensation as if dangers did menace (threaten) him, but without being afraid;...
He, 12 - Sensation as if danger menaced (threatened) him, but without fear. (fearless)

GRAPH. He, 13 - It frequently seemed to him as though his end was near, or the greatest misfortunes were impending.

HYDROG. Sh, 248 - While sitting in a restaurant, felt progressively more cut off from friends at the table. I began to feel detached and paranoid. I felt disliked by people. They seemed to look at me menacingly. I became concerned that my lecture this afternoon had created conflict, mayhem and destruction, that my friends in the audience did not like me any more. I became aware of a dull ache in my sacrum making me want to shift backwards and forwards. At the same time, the people round the table seemed further away and smaller, as if I had moved four feet back from the table. I felt very uncomfortable and wanted to get out. I put my head down and rushed out without saying goodbye, feeling a sense of relief at getting away (all very unusual for me). Outside, I felt relief and my mind cleared and I walked home alone. 22, 12C, 04:XX:XX

HYOS. Al, 80 - Anxiety, soon after dinner, as though a sad occurrence impended.

KALI-BR. Al, 3 - Decidedly insane; had delusions that lewd women had got into his mother's house; that he was pursued by the police; that his wife was threatened by members of the family; that he had thousands of dollars in gold sewed up in his clothing; (rich, wealth)

KALI-I. Al, 11 - Very apprehensive and lachrymose, as if some evil were impending, ...

Ha, 8 - Whining; apprehensive as from threatened accident.

LACH. Al, 19 - So great apprehensiveness while riding in the open air that it seemed to him some great evil (hurtful, injurious) was impending (imminent), like an evil foreboding; it torments him for more than an hour.

LIL-T. Al, 15 - Apprehensive as from impending disease or calamity (misfortune); fears insanity; fears heart disease; fears she is incurable; often with moderate or sub acute uterine or ovarian inflammation.

LIPP. Al, 2 - Feeling of great apprehension, while riding in a carriage; a kind of anxiety in the heart, as of impending misfortune, together with a kind of homesickness.

MACRO. Al, 4 - Fear of impending danger.

MAG-C. Ha, 1 - Trembling anguish and fear, as if evil was threatening (menacing, endangering); it passes off in the evening in bed.

MAG-M. Ha, 20-....when she raised her head up she seemed to see great clouds and rocks above her, ...

MED. Al,N-41 - Constant state of anguish. Always a feeling of impending danger, but knows not what. There is no cause for such feelings, as she is not obliged to do anything when disinclined; is so situated that nothing need cause her trouble.

MENY. Al, 8 - Apprehensive sensation about the heart, as of impending evil, and as if he had to endure some hardship. (adversity, privation, suffering)

MUR-AC. Al, 21 - Deep reflection, and quiet absorption in himself, as if something disagreeable were impending, though with desire to work.

Ha, 4 - Deep reflection, and quiet introversion, as if something unpleasant was impending,...

NAT-AR. Al, 3 - Feeling as something was impending, which caused him to move about.

NAT-C. Al,DREAM, 1111 - Dream of a flood (current, inundate), and threatening danger.

NICC. Al, 6 - Apprehensive and despondent, as if some misfortune were impending.

OP. Al, 16-...started up in a fright on account of fancied swordsmen (rival, competitor) who threatened to stab him; became angry if any one argued him or thought him delirious; however, he blamed (reproaches) himself while in delirium for his folly.

PHEL. Al, 9 - Sad mood and fear the whole day, as from impending misfortune; she wept, and was prone to think upon sad subjects.

PHOS. Al, 104 - Anxiety, as from impending misfortune.

He, 34-...full of fear, especially at piano; constantly on lookout (look carefully) for something to happen; ...sexual dreams and violent sexual excitement.

PLB. Al, 60-...; he hears everywhere threatening voices, officers come to arrest him, to seize his furniture (movables), (confiscated, expropriated) and to expel (eject) him from his lodgings (home) (expulsion, exiled) ; the voices come from the pillow, the mattress (bed); they enter by the window, where he sees people, and they consult about him with closed doors (secretive) ; ...

Al, 63 - The patient imagined that he was constantly followed (persecuted), and that he heard voices coming from the chimney... ; this man after a few days wished to leave the hospital and go home, because he was convinced that there were fiends in the building that pursued him and sought (want) his life.

PULS. Ha, 1115 - Anxiety, as if threatened with apoplexy, in the evening after lying down, ...

RHUS-T. He, 22-... great restlessness and anguish as if she had committed a crime or as if she thought some terrible calamity impended; these feelings drove her from one place to another; could not rest quietly at night in bed; was robbed of sleep and all desire to live;...

RUMX. Al, 4 - Depression, as if some evil was impending.

SPONG. Ha, 382 - Anxious as if misfortune (disaster) threatened (endangered) him and he had a foreboding of it.

STRAM. Al, 53-...throw the hands about the head as if attempting to ward off some threatening evil;...escape from the imaginary object ...

Al, 63-...I was assailed (attacked) by imaginary spectres, in the most hideous forms and menacing attitudes; and what was still to my torment my bed was suspended and tantalized (charmed) like a feather (plumage) between two floors.
He, 77 - Patient had a constant vision of an executioner(hangman, lynches) standing before him in spite of which he was lively, talkative, laughed and joked about his hallucination, yet it seemed to him a reality.
SULPH. He, 47 - Anxiety;...as if some great misfortune were impending (threatening);...
VERAT. Ha, 691 - Anxiety as though he anticipated (expected) misfortune, as if threatened with some calamity.(disaster)

MENACING

Company, desire for; treats them outrageously, yet: ***kali-c.***
Complaining; threatening, and: tarent.
Cursing; strong and violent expressions: pall.[54]
Cursing; threatening destruction and death: tarent.[54]
Delirium; threatening, with pain in face: ***kalm.***[54]
Dreams; threats: anac.[149] ars. sep.
Insanity; threatens destruction and death: ***tarent.***
Kill; threatens to k, wife and children: ***hep.***[54]
Kill; threatens to k.: ***hep.*** meli.[85] ***tarent.***
Kill; threatens to k., approach, those who: meli.[85]
Rage; menacing: agar.[54]
Talk; threatening: tarent.[36]
Thoughts; vanishing, threatening: croc.[36] merc.[36]
Threatening: agar.[10] choc.[222] ***hep.*** meli.[137] ***stram.*** **TARENT.** ***tub.***[122] valer.[36]
Threatening; kill, threatens to: ***hep.***[122] ***tarent.***[54]
Threatening; words of destruction: tarent.[36]

AGAR. Al, 3 - Fearless, menacing, mischievous (rude) frenzy; also, frenzy which causes the patient to assail and injure himself, with great exertion of power.
Ha, 23 - Fearless, threatening, destructive frenzy, also such as turns against itself and injures itself, combined with great exertion of strength.
CANN-I. Al, 66 - Illusion that he was a pump-log, through which a stream of hot water was playing, and threatening his friend with a wetting.
GERM. Sh, 9 - Carried out a threat to fold son's homework which creased it, but I didn't feel guilty. 04, 6C, 01.06.00
HEP. He, 8-...threatened to murder wife and children, attempted to set house on fire, and was with difficulty controlled; ... (pyromaniac) 0Scabies.
He, 23 - Wrathful irritability, even to the most extreme violence, threatening to end in murder and arson.(firing pyromania)
HYDROG. Sh, 240 - I feel life is a serious thing. When putting children to bed, I felt serious and uncompromising. I wanted them to do exactly as I said and, if not, threatened to hit them. 32, 9C, 03:XX:XX
HYOS. He, 65 - Violent and threatening...; mind nearly deranged; disturbed by unfounded jealousy.
LYSS. Al, 18-...caught myself saying to nephew, in severe tone, " If you do that again" etc., when he was not really in fault.
Al,N-58 - Ordered her husband to go away(forsakes), as she wanted to bite him, and joining (associated) act to threat(menace), she bit herself in arm.
OP. Al, 39-...threatened alternately self-destruction and injury to others.
OPUN-V. Al, 5 - Fit of swearing (cursing) at evening after coming home; praying in the morning, swearing (cursing) on disappointment in plans; fit of rage, on thwarting (frustrating) of plans.
STRAM. He, 99 - Acute mania; tears his clothing;... threatens to use knife on those about him.
He, 100-...threatens to knock everybody down, to break furniture, to throw himself out of window.
TARENT. Al, 1-...threatening words of destruction and death; she believes she is insulted; ...
He, 14 - Paroxysms of insanity; restlessness of legs; threatening words of destruction and death.

MILDNESS

Delirium; mild: ***apis***[54] **BAPT.**[54] ***ph-ac.***[54] ***puls.***[54] rhus-t.[5] sec.[10] **STRAM.**[54] ***valer.***[54] ***vario.***[54] verat.[10]
Dreams; friendly, being: ped.[36]
➤ voice, gentle, calling, six am.: rhus-t.[36]
Hysteria; mild, gentle, yielding, although whimsical and introverted: ***ign.***[54]
Indignation; alternating with mildness: ***ars.***[36]
Insanity; mild: ***croc.***[5] ***verat.***[5]
Irritability; alternating with, tenderness: croc.[10] plat.
Mildness: ***acon.*** aln.[85] alum.[85] alumn.[102] ambr. amph.[36] anac. apis[107] **ARN. ARS.** ***ars-i.*** asar. aur. bell. **BOR.** bov. ***cact. calad. calc.*** calc-sil.[58] ***cann-i.*** caps. carb-an. **CARC.**[185] cast.[10] caust. cedr. chel. chim-m.[54] chin.[111] cic. ***cina*** clem. **COCC.** ***croc. cupr.*** cycl. euph. euphr. hell. hydr.[10] hypoth.[149] ***ign. indg.*** iod. kali-c. kali-cy.[36] kali-p. lac-c.[122] laur.[10] ***lil-t. lyc. m-p-a.***[5] mag-m.[5] manc.[36] mang. mosch. mur-ac. murx.[102] nat-ar. nat-c. **NAT-M.** ***nit-ac. nux-v.***[5] op. ph-ac. ***phos.*** plb. **PULS. RHUS-T.** ***sep.*** **SIL.** ***spong.*** stann. staph.[111] ***stram. sulph.*** sumb.[36] ***thuj.*** tub.[104] ***verat.*** viol-o. zinc.
Mildness; alternating with, anger: kali-c.[30]
Mildness; alternating with, hardness: croc.[10]
Mildness; alternating with, indignation: ars.[36]
Mildness; alternating with, obstinacy: ***cupr.***[54]
Mildness; alternating with, rage: croc.[10]
Mildness; alternating with, sadness: plat.[10]
Mildness; complaining, bears suffering, even outrage without: ***ign.***[54]
Mildness; violence, masking the: carc.[207]
Obstinate; alternating with mildness: cupr.[85]
Obstinate; amiable, tries to appear: ***pall.***[54]
Political: choc.[222] sulph.[5]
Restlessness; mild, amiable, refined, sensitive, intellectual: chim-m.[54]
Sadness; mild persons, in: cocc.[10] con.[10] hell.[10] ign.[10] ***lyc.***[54] petr.[10] ph-ac.[10] ***puls.***[54] sil.[10] sulph.[10] verat.[10]
Talk; sleep, in, gentle voice, all night in a: ***camph.***[54]

ARS. Al, 109 - Indignation, alternating with mildness; in her indignation she looks at nobody, and does not want to hear anything; she also cries.

BAPT. He, 17 - A sensation as if some person touched him gently while dozing.(sleep)

CROC. Al, 28 - Vacillating (hesitate), peevish mood; the slightest cause excites his anger, for which, next moment, he is sorry (remorse), which however, soon returns, because his calmness frets (disturbs) him and prevents (stop) his exposing his feelings (oppressed); usually he changes a hard word which he has on his tongue to a mild one, but the latter seems too mild, and now chooses a more severe word, ...(sorry, guilty, by anger, mildness, x harsh, rude)

IGN. Ha, 793 - Sensitive disposition, delicate conscientiousness (careful, scrupulous)
Ha, 792 - Delicate disposition (character), with very clear consciousness (justice, judgment, equity)
He, 49 - Mild disposition; bears suffering, even outrage (offenses), without complaining.

IOD. Al, 8 - Disposition mild, scrupulous (careful) and timid (irresolute), with blunted (dull) sensibilities.

LYC. He, 20 - Melancholy: has doubts about her salvation; before catamenia; in mild (pacific) characters.

PALL. He, 14 - She tries to appear as amiable as possible, but is obstinate.

PULS. Ha, 18 - Mild, bashful, gentle, yielding disposition.
He, 23 - Disposition mild and gentle, never cross.

SUMB. Al, 8-...fond (love) of the society of women; ...sympathy with suffering seems robbed of its pain...nervous excitement and heat, especially in head from listening (hearing) to a disputation, ...humor depressed with despair of future...melancholy despondency, as if ill-treated by everyone purposely... mildness, amiability

TAB. Al, 42 - Evenness and mildness of temper, notwithstanding he felt very uneasy about his health.

MISANTHROPY

Ailments from; alone, being, fear of people, yet: ars.[5] bufo[5] ***clem.***[5] ***con.***[5] tarent.[5]
Aversion; persons, to, all: absin.[36] calc.[30]

chin.[30] germ.[222] *merc-acet.*[30] *nux-v.*[30] phos.[1] *staph.*[30] *sulph.*[30]

Aversion; society: anac.[60] bell.[36] caust.[30] cic.[1] clem.[38] coca[38] con.[1] graph.[30] *kali-c.*[36] lyc.[1] nat-c.[137] stann.[1] syph.[137]

Aversion; society, shuns the foolishness of: cic.

Company, aversion to; solitude, fond of: **ACON.**[5] alum.[10] **AMBR.**[5] *ant-c.*[8] *ars.*[8] **AUR.**[5] bamb-a.[1184] bar-c.[1] *bell.*[5] cact.[25] calc.[10] calc-p.[5] camph.[5] carb-an.[5] *cham.*[8] chin.[1] cic.[1] coca[25] con.[5] cycl.[5] dig.[5] dios.[25] eug.[10] graph.[10] helon.[25] **IGN.**[5] led.[5] lyc.[5] m-aust.[10] mag-m.[10] meny.[5] nat-c.[5] *nat-m.*[5] *nux-v.*[5] op.[10] ozone[227] petr.[5] **PLAT.**[5] ptel.[25] **PULS.**[5] *rhus-t.*[5] sep.[10] seq-s.[230] stann.[5] staph.[10] sulph.[10] tub.[189] verat.[10]

Company, aversion to; unpredictable, thinks people are: ozone[227]

Company, desire for; alone, while, yet fear of people: ars.[5] bufo[5] clem.[5] con.[5] tarent.[5]

Company, desire for; dislike to society, with: *con.*[54]

Disgust; society, with the follies, of: cic.[1]

Escape; attempts to, society, from: cic.[1]

Estranged; society, from: anac. choc.[222] lap-c-b.[194]

Fear; people, of, anthropophobia: acet-ac. *acon.* aloe alum. alum-p.[58] am-m. ambr. *anac.* *anh.*[144] *arist-cl.*[144] ars. ars-i. ars-s-f.[58] *aur.* aur-ar.[58] aur-i.[58] aur-s.[58] bar-acet.[36] *bar-c.* bar-i.[58] bar-m.[172] bar-s.[58] bell. bufo[5] bufo-s. calc. calc-i.[58] camph.[58] carb-an. *carb-v.* carbn-s. *caust.*[30] chin. **CIC.**[122] clem.[5] cocc.[137] *con.* crot-h. croto-t. cupr. dios. dys-co.[136] ferr. ferr-ar. ferr-p. fl-ac.[5] gels.[102] graph. hep. hydrc.[36] **HYOS.** ign. *iod.* *kali-ar.* kali-bi. kali-br. *kali-c.* kali-p. kali-s. lach. *led.* **LYC.** *m-aust.*[5] meli.[102] merc. morg-g.[136] *nat-ar.* **NAT-C.** *nat-m.* nat-s.[58] phos. *plat.* plb.[201] *puls.* rhus-g.[36] **RHUS-T.** sel. sep. sil.[5] stann. staph.[5] stram.[172] sul-i.[58] sulph. tab. tarent.[5] til.

✦ people, of, children, in: **BAR-C.** *lyc.*

✦ people, of, indisposition to meet: *kali-br.*[54] kali-p.[102]

Hatred; fellow beings, for: *led.*[54]

Hypochondriasis; dread of society, with: anan.[36]

Misanthropy: acon. all-c. *am-m.* *ambr.* *anac.* ant-c. ars.[102] *aur.* bar-c. bell. *calc.* cic. clem.[5] con. cop. crot-h. cupr. cur.[36] grat. guai. hydrc. *hyos.* iod. kali-bi. kali-c.[30] lach. *led.* *lyc.* mag-m.[149] merc. **NAT-C.**[122] nat-m. nit-ac. pall.[102] *phos.* plat. *puls.* rhus-g.[36] rhus-t. sep.[102] *stann.* staph.[30] stram.[5] sulph. tab.

Moral affections; antisocial: aesc.[120] anac.[137] ilx-a.[120] lap-gr-m.[194] sac-alb.[210] syph.[137]

AETH. Al,S-11 - Disposition becomes retiring (reserved) and tearful, as in nostalgia.

ALOE. He, 9 - Restlessness and fear; fear of men.

ANAN. Al, 4 - Hypochondria, with dread (fear) of society (people); he seeks solitude and obscurity; does not want to see or hear anything.

He, 3 - Hypochondriasis and dread of society.

ANDROC. Sh, 24 - I feel entirely alone, that I am viewing the world through one hole, for it all seems just a picture, and the rest of the world share a different view finder together. I don't want to join theirs though. (7)

Sh, 25 - Felt disconnected from the human race, as if everyone were another species. Directionless. (7)

Sh, 150 - Speech slurred, answered with difficulty, was indisposed to talk and averse to company. (16)

ARN. Al, 27 - Sullen (morose) insolence and imperiousness. (dictatorial)

AUR. Ha, 348 - A noise before the door made him anxious; he feared lest some one would come in; like anthropophobia.

He, 40 - Melancholic mood, disposed to shun people; if meeting some one it gives him a nervous trembling and has to weep.

BAR-M. He, 6 - Dejection and dread of men.

BELL. Ha, 1395 - He wishes for solitude and quiet; all noise and visits from others are repugnant to him.

CACT. Al, 3 - Loves solitude; he avoids those around him who wish to comfort him.

CALC. Al, 4 - Repugnance, aversion, disgust for most persons.

CAMPH. He, 69 - An indifference whether the world (mankind) uses one well (suitable) or ill (depravity, wrong), everything is repulsive.(offensive)

CARB-AN. Ha, 6 - Inclination to solitude (isolation), sad and introverted (egotistic), she always only wishes to be alone, and she shuns every conversation.

CEDR. Al, 5 - Dread of friends.(in females, particularly)

CHOC. Sh, 208 - Felt rejected and oversensitive. Hid away from the world, felt my life would fall apart. 35, 30C, XX:XX:XX:

Sh, 210 - Felt totally isolated and averse to company. Estranged himself from his family and friends and stopped all communication with them for a long period. Did not reply to letters and left no address. He seemed to hide away and literally disappear. The state of Isolation resulted from feeling that "I didn't exist as a human being". This behaviour was in strong contrast to his normal sociable disposition. 35, 30C, XX:XX:XX:

Sh, 227 - The phone rings and I think 'How typical, how thoughtless, to ring at this moment'. It feels like an intrusion. I stay polite, but am thinking 'Oh tell the truth or shut up'. 1, 30C, 00:XX:XX

CIC. Al, 26 - Contempt and scorn for mankind; he avoided them, abhorred their follies (stupidity) excessively, and his disposition seemed to tend towards misanthropy; he withdrew (retire) himself into solitude.

Al, 27 - Want of confidence in mankind; with misanthropy; he forsook society, remained alone and reflected upon their errors and about himself.

Ha, 237 - Depreciation and contempt of mankind; he fled (desert) his fellow-creatures, was in the highest degree disgusted with their follies (stupidity), and his disposition seemed to change into misanthropy; he withdrew into solitude.

Ha, 238 - Want of trust (mistrust, skepticism) in people and anthrophoby,(misanthropy) he fled (escape) from them remained solitary, and thought seriously about their errors and about himself.

He, 18 - Fondness (desire) for solitude; great disregard and dislike for society of others.

He, 34 - Is afraid (fear) of society, and wants to be alone.

He, 36 - Mistrust and shunning (avoid) of men; despises others.

COCC. He, 22 - Great sorrowfulness, with constant inclination to sit in a corner buried in thought.

CON. He, 17 - Dislike to society and yet a dread to be alone. (solitude)

He, 18 - He is averse to being near people, and to the talk of those passing him (misanthropy); is inclined to seize hold of and abuse them. (insult, offend, curse)

CUPR. Ha, 1 - Melancholy; she shuns the sight of men, seeks and loves (desire) solitude, and troubles herself about her imminent death (impending), which she supposes to be unavoidable.

DIOS. Al, 1 - Desire to be alone; do not enjoy society (misanthropy); am usually quite fond of the society of ladies, but they now seem repulsive,...

DROS. Al, 14 - Taciturn, quiet, and anxious; he was constantly in dread (fear) of hearing something unpleasant.

ELAPS. Al, 11 - Depression of spirits; desires to be in a deep cavern, where he can see no one.

FERR. Al, 20 - Excited by the slightest opposition; ... even her children's caresses increased her bad temper; she was often rude to those about her, because she hated to see or talk to them, and wanted them to leave her in solitude, which alone was pleasing to her.

Al, 4 - Constant desire for solitude; horror of conversation, noise, visits, and even the society of her cherished friends.

GERM. Sh, 151-.... I feel I have no real contact with people, I have no emotion at all except for a feeling of isolation and a concern that people may not like me. I wish someone would cuddle me. By 10 o'clock I have a definite aversion to people, especially certain people- the stubborn or authoritarian kind. I become deeply involved in my own thoughts and can be very irritable and even angry when the thoughts are interrupted by people, but I don't show any signs of anger or irritation. The fate of other people leaves me cold, but I know this is not right. My mind is blank and I feel I could just sit and stare. I have no feelings, no emotions! I think a lot about my state of mind and try to understand it; it puzzles me. What is missing? Eating removes this thoughtful mood. By afternoon and evening I become gradually more involved with what I am doing but still feel isolated even when in the company of other people. I don't mind listening to people, but I contribute little to conversation. This state lasted for three days. 16, 30C, 04:XX:XX

Sh, 152 - Aversion to people. Abrupt when obliged to speak. Had a consultation at 10 o'clock and really messed it up. I wish everybody would just go away and leave me alone. No contact. 16, 30C, 07:04:00

GRAT. Al, 8 - Fretful, irritated by every contradiction, angry outbreaks, misanthropic, whith solicitude about his own health.

HELON. Al, 4-.... could not endure the least contradiction or receive any suggestions in regard to any subject (fixed ideas) ;... what I most desired was to be left alone, reserved to myself the privilege of finding fault (imperfection) with everything around me;....

HEP. He, 10 - Repulsive (offensive) mood, with desire to be left alone.

HIPP. He, 1 - Melancholy; a young man sits in the corner and does not want to have anything to do with the world. (alienated)

HYDROG. Sh, 248 - While sitting in a restaurant, felt progressively more cut off from friends at the table. I began to feel detached and paranoid. I felt disliked by people. They seemed to look at me menacingly. I became concerned that my lecture this afternoon had created conflict, mayhem and destruction, that my friends in the audience did not like me any more. I became aware of a dull ache in my sacrum making me want to shift backwards and forwards. At the same time, the people round the table seemed further away and smaller, as if I had moved four feet back from the table. I felt very uncomfortable and wanted to get out. I put my head down and rushed out without saying goodbye, feeling a sense of relief at getting away (all very unusual for me). Outside, I felt relief and my mind cleared and I walked home alone. 22, 12C, 04:XX:XX

IP. Ha, 219 - Sullen unsociable moroseness, that makes him disdain (reject) everything.

Ha, 222 - Moroseness: he considers himself unfortunate.(unlucky, unsuccessful)

KALI-BI. He, 2 - Misanthropy and ill humor, even to disgust of life.

KALI-BR. He, 39-...fear and apprehension that she is losing her mind (insanity);...makes her utterly (completely) miserable to be looked at or spoken to; fear to see people; always depressed and lowspirited;...

He, 4-...constant worry, fears to see people or to be spoken to;...failure of mental and bodily strength;...constantly busy, tying his shoes, fumbling in his pockets, picking threads, etc.

KALI-C. Al, 20 - Apprehensiveness and aversion to society.

LACH. He, 34-...repugnance to society and dislike to talk; solicitude about future, whith disgust of life; inclination to doubt everything; mistrusts (suspicious) and misconstrues (misjudge) ...0 Melancholia.

LED. Al, 12 - Discontented all day with his companions, which at last amounts to misanthropy.

Ha, 329 - All day long; discontented with his fellow-creatures (friend, relations), which at last amounted to misanthropy.

He, 4 - Discontented; morose; hates his fellow beings.

LYC. He, 14 - Dread (fear) of men ; of solitude, irritability and melancholy.

He, 25 - Anthropophobia (in children); fear of phantoms in evening, with anguish.

He, 35 - Misanthropic; flies even from his own children.

MUR-AC. He, 2 - Taciturn, introverted and quiet; anxious care about future.

NAT-C. Al, 22 - His fancy is mostly busy with apprehensions of the future; he often makes plans for half an hour at a time as if it would go wrong with him, wherewith he seeks to be alone for several days together.

Al, 30 - He shuns (avoid) mankind.

Al, 29 - Anthropophobia and fearfulness.

Ha, 10 - His fancy is mostly anxiously occupied with the future; he paints to himself what misfortunes might happen to him; and he seeks solitude for several days.

Ha, 3 - Dread of men and timidity.

He, 4 - Aversion to mankind and society; estrangement (separation, alienation) from individuals and society; even from her husband and family.

NAT-M. He, 13 - Taciturnity; offended at every word (easily); avoids company;

hates persons because they have offended him; spleen.
He, 34 - A pregnant woman saw a man who had a disfiguring nasal cancer; this haunted (obsessed) her, and she was sure her child would be marked; she was melancholy, avoided society, wept continually.
NIT-AC. He, 8 - Taciturn, disinclined to communicate anything; moody in morning.
PLAT. He, 41 - Delirium, with fear of men (people); often changing, with overestimation (haughty) of oneself.
PULS. He, 36 - Mistrust; envy; covetousness (avidity); dislike to people.
RHUS-T. Ha, 950 - He could not be pleased, was indifferent to society.
SEL. He, 9 - Dread of society.
SEP. Ha, 17 - Dread of men.
He, 38- ...everything seems strange (unusual, unfamiliar) to her;...; it seems as if she could not understand (realize) anything and would have to learn anew everything she wished to do;...(lost: knowledge); greatest indifference to everything, the death of a near relative, or some happy occurrence, leaves her equally unaffected; no trace of her former love for friends or even for her child; aversion for social intercourse amounting to contempt;...
STANN. Ha, 649 - Aversion from and dread (fear) of people.
Ha, 3 - Aversion and distaste for human society.
THUJ. He, 29 - Feels as if she cannot exist any longer; quiet, shunning everybody.

MISERABLE

Ailments from; sympathy: ars.[137] ***bell.***[137] cact.[5] ***calc.***[137] coff.[5] con.[137] hell.[5] **IGN.**[137] kali-s.[137] ***nat-m.***[5] ***plat.***[137] sabal.[5] sep.[137] ***sil.***[137] sulph.[5] syph.[5]
Cheerfulness; simulates hilarity, while feels wretched: apis.[58]
Confidence, want of self; nobody, feels as if he is: agn.[36]
Delusions; disgraced, she is: kali-s.[214] mag-s.[214] nat-s.[214] nux-v.[37] plat.[214] rob.[36] staph.[214] sulph.
- faces, supplicating: germ.[222]
- insignificant, he is: bamb-a.[1184]
- worthless, he is: aur.[137] thuj.[187]
- wretched, she looks (when looking in a mirror): lap-c-b.[194] ***nat-m.***

Despair; existence, about miserable: ***sep.***[122]
Fear; pitied, of being: chin.[30] nat-m.[162]
Happy; seeing others, agg.: hell.[137] helon.[137]
Irritability; consolation agg.: ***bell. cact.*** calc. ***calc-p.*** calc-sil.[58] carc.[207] chin. hell. **IGN.** kali-c. kali-sil.[58] lil-t. lyc. merc. **NAT-M.** ***nit-ac.*** nux-v. ***plat.*** sabal.[122] **SEP. SIL.** staph.
Mirth; simulates hilarity while he feels wretched: apis[58]
Pathetic: stram.[36]
Pities herself: agar. androc.[222] bamb-a.[1184] **CALC.**[30] cand-a.[239] germ.[222] hydrog.[222] lap-gr-m.[194] nit-ac. ***staph.***[30]
Pities herself, pains, from: bamb-a.[1184]
Pities herself; sick, desire to show being: tarent.[36]
Sadness; sympathy agg.: con.[137]
Self-deprecation: ***naja***[5]
Suicidal disposition; despair, about his miserable existence: ***sep.***[54]
Talk; pathetic: lyss.[54]
Weeping; children, pitied, if he believes he is: nat-m.[70]
Weeping; children, pities herself: puls.[189]
Weeping; children, pitifully when awake: cina[56]
Weeping; meeting people, when: ***aur.***
Weeping; piteous: cham.[36] stram.[36]
Weeping; pitied, if believes he is: ***nat-m.***
Weeping; pities himself: graph.[184] puls.[189]
Weeping; telling of her illness, when: aster.[231] bry.[122] carc.[122] ign.[162] ***kali-c. med. nat-m.***[189] prot.[136] **PULS. SEP.**
Weeping; thought of others grief at her own death: lap-c-b.[194]
Weeping; weak mind, about her: ***stram.***[54]

ADAM. Sh, 194 - Felt ugly, miserable and generally fed up with myself during menses, more intensely than I usually would at this time. 8, 6C, 17:XX:XX
AESC. Al, 8 - Feels miserably cross.
AGAR. Al, 37 - An impulse to laugh overcame him in bed, owing to an indescribably mixed sensation of happiness and misery.(duality)
ARS. Al-S, 2893 - The whole head sick, the heart faint, she awoke in the morning wretched, her life a burden (load) weari-

ness the day's portion, and each succeeding day like its predecessor, unless (except) physic (laxative) helped her with its little aid.

BELL. Al, 58-... Passed a restless night, her sleep, she says, being disturbed by "miserable phantoms"...

CAMPH. Al, 32 - Indescribable wretchedness. (unhappiness)

He, 60 - Indescribable wretchedness.

CERE-B. Al, 11 - Arose feeling miserable.

CIMIC. Al, 3 - Miserable, dejected (sad) feeling.

He, 20 - Miserable dejected feeling; anxious weeping.

CUPR. He, 10 - Mania with biting, beating, and tearing things to pieces; insane foolish gestures of imitation and mimicry; full of insane spiteful (cruelty, brutality) tricks (deceitful, false), ..unhappy, despairing...miserable look...

GERM. Sh, 108 - Hopeless, helpless, gloom and doom. Weeping and self pity. 14, 30C, 23:00:00.

GRAPH. He, 9 - Feels miserable, unhappy.

HELON. Al, 2 - Reaction (from feeling of general wellness) began, and for a fortnight I was in a mental hell; it was the most profound mental depression I have ever known; I was plunged into the most abject despair.

HYDROG. Sh, 15 - I felt in the presence of a totally pure energy, like meeting God and feeling totally unworthy or like meeting a lover and feeling unworthy — realizing all the mistakes of a lifetime. This pure energy was around for some time protecting me. I feel this unification cleared out lifetimes of symptomatology for me. The joining with this energy was as if a male energy joined with me sexually, but with no desire, pleasure or pain involved. This unification with the male energy lasted quite a few days — I'm not used to seeing myself as a man. The morning after this unifying with the higher presence, I collapsed in emotional overflow. All my grief and pain came out. I was doubled upon the floor and went into a deep state of catharsis. It is not possible to describe where I went as there are no concepts applicable. I felt overflowing love for humanity and wanted to give everything away. My mind turned to the Buddha. It was like seeing the complete picture instead of fragmented bits. (These primary effects lasted about 28 days, then changing to a paranoia state). 16, 30C, 07.XX.XX

Sh, 234 - Developed a self pitying, very tearful depression through the morning. I was unable to communicate any of these feelings and this led to a fierce row with girlfriend. 04, 12C, 30:XX:XX

Sh, 235 - Feel a bit depressed and frustrated by present circumstances. Feel like the unappreciated victim. 04, 12C, 14:XX:XX

Sh, 242 - Felt vulnerable to criticism —felt people were getting at me. Felt people were not taking notice of poor little me —over-reacting —upset and hurt. 02, 6C, XX:XX:XX

KALI-BR. He, 39-...fear and apprehension that she is losing her mind (insanity);...makes her utterly (completely) miserable to be looked at or spoken to; fear to see people; always depressed and lowspirited;...

LYC. Al, 32 - She became very miserable...

LYSS. Al,N-22 - Believe that they are reduced to their present wretched (miserable) condition by the instrumentality (aid) of those about them.

Al,N-88 - Very cross, so much... he took offense at veriest trifles, scolding his wife and children, felt wretched, ...

He, 22 - Believe that they are reduced to their present wretched condition by the instrumentality (aid) of those about them.

He, 88 - Very cross, so much so that his children expressed great surprise; he took offense at veriest trifles, scolded his wife and children, felt wretched, ...

MACRO. Al, 2 - She feels miserable; words cannot express how badly she feels.

MEZ. He, 5 - No rest when alone; wants to be in company ...unable to repeat what has been learned by heart; looks through window for hours, without being conscious of objects around; knows not what she is about; forgets what she is about to utter (talk); looks ill humored, pale, wretched, fallen away; ......expecting some very unpleasant news.

MURX. Al, 4 - It made me miserable; I was so low-spirited that I gave up everything; I had no strength left.

MYRIC. Al, 6 - Miserable dejected (unhappy) feeling all day.
Al, 8-...;did not care about anything or for any friends; was perfectly wretched, beyond description.

NAJA. Al, 14 - Felt melancholy; began to form images of possible wrongs (mistaken) and misfortunes, over which the mind broods; very wretched at times;... a slight cause sets him in a perfect agony of mental suffering on another's behalf (welfare);...makes himself imaginary troubles and wrongs, and frets (bother) over them for two hours...
He, 3 - Melancholy; began to form images of possible wrongs (evils) and misfortunes over which the mind broods; very wretched (miserable) at times.

NAT-M. Al, 64 - She often looks into the mirror, and imagines that she looks wretched. (miserable, unhappy)
Al, 18 - If one only looked at him, he was obliged to weep.
Ha, 14 - From the looks of everyone, he concludes that people pity (compassion, sympathy) him for his misfortune, and he weeps.(miserable)
Ha, 15 - He had to weep as soon as anyone merely looked at him. (pitied)
Ha, 26 - She often looks into the looking-glass, (mirror) and thinks she looks wretched (miserable, contemptible).

NEON. Sh, 198 - Received a long letter from a patient today; haven't even read it, can't be bothered. Very unusual. In terms of indifference, I have felt disgusted with myself; one of these violent and malicious feelings. God, I feel so wretched. 02, 6C, 05:XX:XX

OP. Al, 187 - The memory and mental powers generally became greatly impaired, attended by a miserable depression of spirits.

PLAT. He, 46-...;suffers unspeakable pangs (anxiety) of conscience in consequence of a faux (fault, mistake, embarrassing mistake?) pass when thirty-two years old; says she has brought disgrace upon her family, and that she has incurred the penalty of damnation; (doomed) in order to do penance (penitence) gave away whatever she could lay her hands upon, (redemption) so that she had to be constantly watched; after her confessor asserted that she could not hope for pardon or heaven (condemnable), she seemed in absolute despair ; bemoaned her misery throughout the night, wringing her hands and beseeching (implore) that she might be delivered (free) from the hell of her conscience; twice attempted self-destruction (suicide);...wished to live and do penance (penitence, purgation, purification) in order to mitigate her eternal punishment.

PULS. He, 16-...easily moved to tears or laughter; well one hour, miserable (unhappy) the next.

ROB. Al, 3 - Moral agitation, great restlessness; he is always under the impression that he will be disgraced.

SARS. Al, 7 - The soul is affected inordinately by the pains; the mind is depressed the mood dull; he feels wretchedly, and moans involuntarily.

SCROPH-N. Al, 2 - A miserable and sluggish (inactive, lethargic) feeling of the mind when moving about.

SEP. Al, 36 - The greatest loathing of life; it seemed to him as if he could not endure so miserable an existence any longer, and as if he would pine away (longing, wanting) if he did not kill himself. (pine = intense longing or grief)
Al, 112 - Memory so poor I cannot remember the least thing, and it makes me feel very miserable.
Ha, 31 - Extreme loathing of life (existence he felt as if he could not any longer bear this miserable (wretched, unhappy) existence, and as if he would pine away (ruined) unless he made away with himself.-(suicidal)
He, 28 - Propensity to suicide from despair about his miserable (wretched, unfortunate) existence.

SOL-T-AE. Al, 5 - She is much concerned (care, anxiety) about her future, destiny, which she fancies will be wretched.(miserable)

STANN. He, 6 - A woman, age 39, pregnant in fourth month;...inability to do anything as she cannot muster sufficient courage,...great palpitation of heart and anxiety, especially if she has to give directions in her domestic affairs; thinking

makes her feel wretched, ...(unable, incapable)
SULPH. Ha, 4 - Often during the day, attacks lasting for several minutes, when she feels herself utterly (completely) miserable, without any cause, like melancholy; she desires to die.

MISFORTUNE

Absorbed; misfortune, imagines: calc-s.[122]
Ailments from; misfortune of others: coloc.[1]
Ailments from; shock, mental: ***acet-ac.***[5] **ACON.** ***am-c.***[5] ambr.[58] apis[58] ***arn.***[5] both-a.[3070] ***camph.***[5] carc.[207] cham.[5] cic.[5] coca[83] ***coff.***[5] ***gels.***[5] hecla.[234] hep.[5] hyos.[5] hyper.[5] iod.[85] kali-p.[85] ***merc.***[5] nat-m.[5] ***nux-v.***[8] op.[5] ph-ac.[102] ***pic-ac.***[54] plat.[58] puls.[5] sec.[5] stront-c.[5] sulph.[5] ***verat.***[5]
Anguish; horrible things, after hearing: calc.[30]
Anticipation; impending evil, sensation of: merc.[137]
Anticipation; unusual ordeal, of any: **GELS.**[54]
Anxiety; chest, heart, region of, evil was going to happen, as if something: meny.[137]
Anxiety; heart, evil was going to happen, as if something: meny.[137]
Borrows trouble, always finds trouble: acet-ac.[58] apis[58] bar-c.[137] calc.[137] sang.[137]
Company, desire for; happen, as if something horrible might: ***elaps***[54]
Delusions; destruction of all near her, impending: ***kali-br.***[54]
- fire, world is on: ***hep.*** ***puls.***[54] verat.[58]
- happen, something terrible is going to: fl-ac.[36] ***lyss.*** onos.[144] pall.[85]
- happened anything, of having: calc.[30] nux-v.[30] ***staph.***[30] sulph.[30]
- happened, that something dreadful had: ***med.***[179]
- happy is his own house, he will never be: ars.
- misfortune, inconsolable over fancied: alum.[102] calc-s.[58] ***verat.***
- pursued, tormented by a frightful scene of some mournful event of the past, and: spong.[54]
- ruined, he is: calc.[30] **IGN.**[30] verat.[30]
- strange, everything is, terrible, and: cic.[137] ***plat.***[54]
- troubles, great troubles have come over him: cycl.[139]
- troubles, impending, of: am-c.[139]

Dreams; children, about, something had happened to: hydrog.[222] kali-n.[36]
➤ disaster: sars.
➤ events, painful: osm.[54]
➤ evil impending, child, to a: ozone[227]
➤ evil, impending: cimic.[102]
➤ misfortune: alum. ***am-m.*** anac. ant-c. ***arn.*** ***ars.*** ars-s-f.[58] aur-m.[36] bamb-a.[1184] bar-c. bar-m. bar-s.[58] ***bell.*** cann-s. carb-an. ***cham.*** ***chin.*** chin-ar. clem. cocc. croc. **GRAPH.** guai. ign. iod.[10] ***kali-ar.*** ***kali-c.*** kali-chl.[58] kali-n. kali-p. kali-s. kreos.[10] laur. led. **LYC.** ***mag-c.*** mag-m.[10] mang. ***merc.*** mur-ac. nat-s.[10] nicc.[10] **NUX-V.** op. ozone[227] petr.[5] ph-ac. ***phos.*** **PULS.** ran-b. rhus-t. rhus-v.[10] sars. sel. spong. stann. staph. ***sul-ac.*** ***sulph.*** tarent. **THUJ.** verat. verb. zinc. zinc-p.[58]
➤ misfortune, car, function anymore, does not, brakes: bamb-a.[1184]
➤ misfortune, car, function anymore, does not, while driving: ozone[227]
➤ misfortune, impending: aur.[36] tarent.[36]
➤ misfortune, key, has taken the wrong: ozone[227]
➤ misfortune, others, of: cann-s.[36] mag-c.[36]
➤ misfortune, shower head falls out of her hand: ozone[227]
➤ misfortune, street, cannot find the right: ozone[227]
➤ unfortunate events: cocc.[36] sulph.[36]

Excitement; horrible things, after hearing: ***calc.*** ***chin.***[122] cic.[58] cocc. gels. ign. ***lach.*** nat-c. nux-v. ***teucr.*** ***zinc.***
Fancies; misfortune, all his efforts would miscarry: merc.[36]
Fancies; misfortune, evening: naja[36]
Fear; destruction to all near her, of impending: ***kali-br.***[54]
✦ disable, being: **ARS.**[162] mag-m.[162] psor.[162]
✦ disgrace, of: rob.[172]
✦ evil, of: acon. agar. alum. am-c. ambr.[5] anac. ant-c. ***arg-n.*** arn. ***ars.*** ars-i. ars-s-f. asaf.[5] aster. aur. aur-ar.[58] aur-i.[58] ***aur-m.***[54] aur-s.[58] bar-c. bar-i.[58] bar-m. bar-s.[58] bell.[1] bry. calad. **CALC.** calc-acet.[36] calc-p.[5] calc-s. camph.[5] caps.[5] carb-an. ***carb-v.*** carc.[207] cast. ***caust.*** cham.[5] ***chin.*** chin-ar. **CHIN-S.** cina clem.[36] ***cocc.*** ***coff.*** colch. croc.[5] crot-h.[5] cupr.[5] cycl. dig. dros. dulc. euph. ferr. ferr-ar. ferr-p. graph. hell. hep.[5] hydr-ac.[10] hyos. ***iod.*** ***kali-ar.***

kali-br.[172] kali-c. kali-chl.[58] **KALI-I.**[122] kali-p. kalm. ***lach.*** lap-c-b.[194] ***laur.*** ***lil-t.*** lyc.[30] ***lyss.*** m-arct.[10] mag-c. ***mag-s.***[10] ***manc.***[54] med.[179] meny. merc. mosch. mur-ac. nat-ar. ***nat-c.*** ***nat-m.*** nat-s.[58] nicc.[54] nit-ac. nux-v. ***onos.*** ***pall.*** petr. ***phos.*** **PSOR.** puls. rad-br.[119] rauw.[119] rhus-t. ruta sabad.[5] sabin. sec. ***sep.*** sil.[5] spig. spong. squil. ***stann.***[30] ***staph.***[122] stram.[54] stront-c. sul-ac. sulph. tarent. thuj. tub.[172] verat

✦ evil, of, overwhelms her: bar-c.[54]

✦ evil, of, sadness and weeping, with: **KALI-I.**[54]

✦ happen, had happened, as if something: med.[54]

✦ happen, something will: acet-ac.[58] acon.[102] act-sp.[162] alum. alum-p.[58] am-c.[139] aml-n.[36] anac.[58] androc.[222] anth.[36] apis[58] arn.[58] ***ars.*** bac.[62] bar-c.[58] bufo cact. ***calc.*** calc-s.[108] calen.[122] cand-a.[239] ***carb-v.*** carc.[207] **CAUST.** chel.[58] choc.[222] cocc.[58] coloc.[162] corn-a.[85] croto-t. cupr.[172] dig.[58] elaps fl-ac. gels. graph. hydrog.[222] ign.[58] ***iod.*** ***kali-ar.*** ***kali-br.*** kali-c.[58] kali-p. kalm.[36] ***lac-c.***[54] lap-gr-m.[194] lap-mar-c.[194] lappa[139] ***lil-t.*** lyc. lyss.[36] mag-c. ***manc.***[184] mang. **MED.**[122] meny.[85] merc.[58] mez.[58] morg.[136] mosch.[36] nat-ar. ***nat-m.*** ***nat-p.*** nicc. **NUX-V.**[30] ***onos.*** ***pall.***[54] ***ph-ac.*** **PHOS.** pic-ac.[162] pitu-a.[164] **PLAT.**[54] plb.[58] prot.[136] pyrus[58] rat.[36] sang.[137] sanic.[162] scut.[72] sep.[172] spong.[58] still.[102] stry. sul-i.[58] sulph.[172] syph.[193] tab. tarent.[58] thea. **TUB.**[122] xan.

✦ happen, something will, alone, when, amel. by conversation: rat.

✦ happen, something will, family, to, or to him: ars.[172] calc.[172] calc-s.[36] caust.[172] phos.[172] psor.[172] sep.[172] tub.[36]

✦ happen, something will, home, before he got: ***zing.***[54]

✦ happen, something will, husband will not return home: ars.[172] bar-c.[172] caust.[172] ***plat.*** sep.[172]

✦ happen, something will, morning, sinister and vague, something: nabal.[36]

✦ happen, something will, sad: aesc.[36] ***calc.***[54] ***phos.***[36] **STILL.**[36]

✦ happen, something will, terrible, horrible: aml-n.[139] ***calc.***[54] ***calen.***[162] carc.[207] elaps[139] fl-ac.[54] ***ign.***[54] lap-c-b.[194] lappa[139] **LYSS.**[162] mang.[172] med.[139] onos.[139] pall.[54] psor.[36] pyrus[139] ***scut.***[102] ***sep.***[36] thea.[139]

✦ misfortune, of: acon. agar. alco.[36] alum. alum-p.[58] alumn.[36] am-c. aml-n.[54] ***anac.*** ant-c. arn. ars.[116] ars-i.[58] aster. atro. bamb-a.[1184] bar-c.[10] ***bry.***[111] bufo cact. calad. ***calc.*** calc-f. calc-i.[58] calc-s. carbn-s. cast.[10] ***caust.***[5] ***cham.***[5] chin.[5] **CHIN-S.** cic. cimic.[137] ***clem.*** colch. croto-t. cupr. cycl. dig. digin.[36] dros. ferr. ferr-ar.[58] ferr-p. fl-ac. gins. glon. ***graph.*** hell.[1] ***hep.***[5] hura hydr-ac. ign.[8] ***iod.*** ip.[10] kali-c.[137] kali-i. kali-m.[137] lach. laur.[10] lil-t. lipp.[36] lyss. mag-c. mag-s. mang.[10] **MED.**[122] meny. ***merc.***[10] merc-c. mez. mur-ac.[1] naja[36] ***nat-c.***[122] nat-m. nat-p. nat-s. nicc. **NUX-V.**[122] ***petr.***[5] phel. phos. plat.[137] **PSOR.** ***puls.*** rhus-t. rumx. sabin.[10] sanic.[144] sec.[172] sil.[5] spong.[10] stram. sul-i.[58] sulph. tab. tarent. thuj.[137] valer. verat.[10] vichy-g.[36] vinc. zinc.[36]

✦ misfortune, of, losing something of great value: sec.[172]

✦ occurrence will end seriously, every little: iod.[85]

✦ ordeal, of an: ***arg-n.***[5] arn.[5] ars.[172] carb-v.[172] ***gels.***[5] kali-br.[5] ***lyss.***[5] ***stroph.***[111] thuj.[172]

✦ sleep, to go, lest, something should happen: sabal.[85]

✦ thinking of, when, disagreeable things: phos.

✦ thinking of, when, sad things: rhus-t.

✦ wrong, of something, indescribable: ***kali-br.***[54]

Howling; future trouble, about: lyc.[36]

Inconsolable; misfortune, over a fancied: **VERAT.**

Insanity; domestic calamity, after: ***lach.***[54]

Joy; misfortune of others, at the: anac.[185] ars. cupr.[171]

Lamenting; misfortune, over his imagined: alum-p.[58]

Laughing; misfortune, at: apis.

Mania; domestic calamity, after: ***lach.***[54]

Pessimist: agav-t.[149] ars.[30] aur.[58] bar-c.[30] calc.[1] carb-an.[36] caust.[30] cecr.[149] cic.[58] ferr-p.[36] gad.[36] germ.[222] graph.[36] halo.[149] hyos.[30] lach.[30] morph.[36] nat-c.[36] nat-m.[36] nit-ac.[36] ***nux-v.***[30] op.[36] pers.[149] ***psor.***[122] sec.[36] sep.[30] stann.[149] thuj.[36] vip-a.[149] wies.[36]

Prophesying; disagreeable events, of: med.[122]

Sadness; brooding over imaginary wrongs and misfortunes, by: naja[130]

Sadness; fear, with, evil, of impending: ***aur.***[54] **KALI-I.**[54]

Sadness; misfortune, as if from: ***calc.*** chin-s. cycl. ph-ac. phel. phos. puls. rhus-t. staph. sulph.
Sadness; misfortune, as if from, impending: ***chin-s.***[36] phel.[36] vichy-g.[36]
Sit; meditates, misfortune, imaginary, over: calc-s.[58] lil-t.[137]
Sympathetic; misfortune of others, greatly affected by: coloc.[137]
Talk; misfortune, about: ***verat.***[54]
Thoughts; persistent, evil, of: androc.[222] ***lach.***
Weeping; children, misfortune, on hearing of: caust.[109]
Weeping; evil impended, as if: kali-i.[36]

ACON. Al, 63 - Dread of some accident happening.
Al, 47 - Anxiety as though a great misfortune would happen to him.
Ha, 541 - Fear of some misfortune happening to him.
AGAR. Al, 45 - Anxiety, as though something unpleasant were going to happen to her.
Ha, 3 - Anxious forebodings (anticipation), as if she were about to experience something disagreeable.
ALUM. Al, 11 - She is constantly possessed by bad thoughts which oblige her to weep; at the same time she feels apprehensive and uneasy, as if something evil were to happen to her; everything she only looks at, fills her with sadness.
Ha, 7-...anxiety as if something bad would happen (misfortune) to her; whatever she looks at, fills her with sadness.
Ha, 18 - Restlessness in the evening, as if evil was imminent.
He, 19 - Uneasy evenings as from impending evil.
AM-C. Al, 11 - Sad, low-spirited, apprehensive of evil...
Ha, 7 - Sad, dejected, feeling as if a misfortune was imminent,..
AML-N. Al, 1 - Anxiety, as if something might happen; must have fresh air.
He, 11 - Cannot sit still for fear of something dreadful happening.
ANAC. Al, 15 - The future appears dangerous to him, as if nothing but misfortune and danger were reserved for him; want of confidence in his strength (vigor, force) and despondency.
Al, 1 - Illusions of fancy; he imagines he has his name called by the voice of his far-distant mother and sister, accompanied by an apprehension of misfortune and anxiety.
Ha, 4 - Internal anguish, which did not allow him to rest, he troubled himself about every trifle, as if it would cause great injure, with solicitude about the future.
Ha, 8 - The future seems to him very dangerous, as if nothing were imminent but misfortune and danger; distrust in his own power, and despondency.
Ha, 45 - Delusions of fancy, he thought his name was called by the voice of his (far distant) mother and sister; at the same time an apprehension and anguish foreboding misfortune.
Ha, 2 - Anguish and apprehension as of imminent misfortune.
He, 62 - Internal anxiety, which did not leave him any peace; he felt solicitous (careful) on account of every trifle, as if it would lead to some great trouble (misfortune); with apprehension (fear) of future.
He, 61 - Anxiety and feeling of impending misfortune.
ANDROC. Sh, 79 - Fear —as if something terrible would happen. (10)
ANTH. Al, 1 - Very low spirits; feeling as if something were about to happen; as if would like to get alone, and unburden (relieve) himself by crying ...
Al, 4 - Feeling as if something was about to happen to him.
APIS. Al, 2 - Laughs at every misfortune.
Al, 3-... He laughed at the greatest misfortune, as he would at a great comedy. (mockery)
ARN. Al, 16 - Apprehension of future evils.
Ha, 637 - Fears; anxious dread of coming evil.
ARS. Ha, 1036 - In the evening, in bed, anxious sad fancies, e.g. that something bad (misfortune) must have happened to his relatives.
He, 8 - Gloomy (dark) forebodings (premonition) while lying in bed, in evening, fears something may have happened to his relatives.
ASTER. Al, 6 - Feeling of excessive anguish...it seems as if some misfortune

was impending, as if he was going to hear bad news ...

Al, 7-...it seems as if some misfortune was about to happen to him, and that, should it actually (really) come upon him, he would weep, rather than brace (encourage) himself to meet it, or become angry.

He, 9 - It seems as if some misfortune was impending, as if bad news was about to arrive...

ATRO. Al, 33 - Mentally either very sad, depressed in constant anxiety and restlessness, fearful of misfortune, or angry and inclined to be alone, seldom lively.

AUR-M. Al, 4 - Sad mood as though a great misfortune impending.

He, 7 - Sadness as when homesick; sad as though a great misfortune impended.

BAR-C. He, 27 - She is suddenly overwhelmed with an evil apprehension; she imagines, for instance, that a beloved friend has suddenly fallen sick and is dying.

BRASS. Sh, 8 - Feeling of impending disaster, still cannot settle to anything 3I, 00:08:00

BUFO. Al, 12 - He is anxious about the state of his health; is afraid he will die or that some other misfortune will happen to him.

CACT. He, 15 - Indescribable fear that something terrible is going to happen to him.

CALC-A. Al, 7 - Apprehensive, sad mood, as though he were awaiting some depressing news.

Ha, 263 - Anxious disposition as if something evil had happened or he had to fear reproaches (censures); at the same time, however, persistent inclination to work. (industrious)

CALC-S. Al, 7 - Excessive, bitter melancholy, with distressing apprehensions of evil to loved ones.

CALC. Al, 16 - Sorrowful and peevish; she looked upon everything from the worst side, and imagined everything evil.

Al, 25 - Frightened apprehensive mood, as if some misfortune were about to happen to him, or some one else, which he could in no way overcome.

Ha, 22 - Timid and restless, as if evil (harmful, misfortune) was impending (imminent) over her.

Ha, 23 - Fearful, anxious forebodings, as if evil would befall (happen) him or some one else, and as if he could in no way evade it.

Ha, 29 - Despairing (hopeless) mood with fear of sickness (disease) and misery, with forebodings of sad events. (misfortune)

He, 8 - Mind full of concern about imaginary things that might happen to her. 0 Chlorosis.

He, 50 - Apprehensive (fearful, worried) mood ; as if some misfortune was about to happen; about his health (vigour) ; that he might have an organic disease of the heart.

He, 51 - Fear, that something sad or terrible will happen.

He, 53 - Fear: of death; of consumption (decay, waste, tuberculosis); of misfortune (disaster) ; of being alone. (lonely)

CANN-S. Ha, 303 - Dreams of misfortunes happening to others.

CARB-V. Ha, 9 - He felt like weeping, everything seemed to him dreadful (fearful), and he felt in despair.

CAUST. Al, 24 - Anxious apprehension lest something evil should happen, with urging to stool.

Ha, 6 - Anxiety the whole day, as if he had done something wrong, or to fear it, or as if a misfortune had happened.

Ha, 14 - Great apprehensions (forebodings) as to whatever happens.

CHAM. Al, 15 - Very depressed mood, with anxiety and oppression, as of impending evil.

CHIN-S. Al, 16 - Great anxiety, amounting to an apprehension, as if some evil would happen.

Al, 20-...; felt a gloom (darkness) come over me, as if some evil were impending; relieved by a specific trust in the Almighty;...(divine) (faithful, confiding, devoted)

He, 9 - Recurrence of feeling of impending evil.

CHOC. Sh, 191 - I Since the being bitten by the dogs have developed a strong fear of dogs, and have been chased by one dog and growled at by another. This is coupled with a general fear of something happening. These fears are new to me and were better again after the proving. 27, 100C, 05:XX:XX

CLEM. Al, 13 - Buried in sad thought and in dread (fear) of impending misfortune.
Al, 17 - Anxious uneasiness, as though some evil would befall him.
Al, 14 - He seemed oppressed by some grief or sorrow, or the shadow of impending misfortune.
COFF-T. He, 3 - Full of apprehension of terrible things happening.
CON. Al, 1277 - Dreams of wretched (miserable) diseases.
He, 28 - Solicitude (anxiety) concerning the future; great concern (cares) about any little thing that may happen.
CROT-T. He, 2 - Feeling of anxiety, as thought some personal misfortune would befall him.
CUPR. He, 18 - Unconquerable sadness, constant restlessness, as if some misfortune were approaching; fears he will lose his reason.
CYCL. Al, 16 - Fretful and sad; has no desire to work ; she feels a great anxiety, as if some great misfortune were impending.
DIRC. Al, 1 - Uneasy and sensation as if something unpleasant were to happen.
Al, 2 - In day time was constantly expecting some bad news; everything seemed worry and annoy.
DROS. Ha, 273 - Silent and reserved, with anxiety he always feared he was about to learn (discover) something disagreeable.
Ha, 275 - He is sad and dejected about the ills (evil) of life, which people cause one another and himself, respecting which he is anxious and concerned;...(ethical)
ELAPS. Al, 13 - Fearfulness, dread (fear) of being alone, as though something would happen, or as though rowdies (revolution, rebellious) would break in.
He, 5 - Fear of being left alone, as if something horrible might happen; horror of rain.
ELAT. He, 3 - Fear of some approaching disaster.
FERR. Al, 14 - Anxiety as if something evil had happened to her.
FL-AC. Al, 12 - During the tottering (tremble) sensation he has a decided though not anxious expectation, as if there was to happen something awful (horrible), but he feels no anxiety.
He, 13 - Felt certain (inevitable) that something dreadful would happen,...
GLON. Al, 8 - Feeling of impending misfortune, with a sensation in the chest.
GRAPH. Ha, 19 - Great anguish in the evening, as if a misfortune had happened,...
Ha, 20 - He often feels as if his end was near (death), or as if the greatest misfortune impended over him.
He, 13 - It frequently seemed to him as though his end was near, or the greatest misfortunes were impending.
HALI-L. Sh, 507 - Having some trouble speaking. Using the wrong words, or lacking words at times. Just keep it simple. Husband told the kids. We all laughed. I guess that's what you can say for adversity. If it happens enough you learn to get used to it. If it's not too hard. Began thinking about one of my kids dying—that would be too hard. I don't want to do that to find out. 09, 6C, 16:XX:XX
HELL. Ha, 278 - Restless and anxious, as if anticipating misfortune.
HURA. Al, 1 - Much excited and oppressed as if by some great misfortune.
HYDROG. Sh, 195 - Apprehensive, panicky, with cold sweat on palms. Feel extremely vulnerable emotionally —like an egg that has just broken. Frightened, anything can happen. 16, 30C, 05:XX:XX
Sh, 198 - Growing irritability. Anger below the surface if something is on the floor in my way or if something goes wrong. 12, 6C, 05:00:30
HYOS. Al, 80 - Anxiety, soon after dinner, as though a sad occurrence impended.
IGN. He, 36 - Anxiety as though something terrible had happened cannot speak because of it; hurry, fearfulness, terror, alternating with irresolution and inertness.
He, 39 - Anxiety and disquiet as if she had done something wrong, or as if some great misfortune were about to happen, this so overpowers her that she can with difficulty refrain from weeping;...
IOD. Al, 21 - He fears that from every trifle some misfortune would arise.
Ha, 21 - He is afraid at every trifle, that one or another mishap (accident) may rise from it.
He, 8 - Fear of evil with over carefulness.
IRID. Sh, 204 - All day, woke with sense of foreboding as if something bad was going

to happen. Feeling quite shaky, butterflies in tummy, a bit nauseous. I14

KALI-BR. He, 29-... dread of impending destruction of all near her.

KALI-C. Al, 14 - Sad presentiments of the future.

KALI-I. Al, 11 - Very apprehensive and lachrymose, as if some evil were impending, ...

He, 6 - Very great irritability and unwonted harshness of demeanor (behavior); his children, to whom he is devoted and attached, become burdensome to him; very passionate and spiteful temper;...constant apprehension of impending evil.

KALM. Al, 1 - A feeling of anxiety; feel as though something dreadful (calamitous) was going to happen to me.

LAUR. He, 6 - Fear and anxiety about imaginary evils;
despondency.(desperation)

LIL-T. Al, 15 - Apprehensive as from impending disease or calamity (misfortune); fears insanity; fears heart disease; fears she is incurable; often with moderate or sub acute uterine or ovarian inflammation.

Al, 19 - Apprehension of some calamity or serious disease very much increased.

LIPP. Al, 2 - Feeling of great apprehension, while riding in a carriage; a kind of anxiety in the heart, as of impending misfortune, together with a kind of homesickness.

LYC. Ha, 18 - He weeps and cries, at first, about the past, then about the coming evils.

LYSS. Al, 12 - Feeling as if I had heard, or was about to hear something bad...

Al, 15 - He cannot prevent ideas of something awful (terrible) about to happen, or as if he would do something awful (bad).

Al, 16 - An indescribable idea, which I could not shake off, (fixed idea) of something dreadful (calamitous) about to happen to me; all day feeling as if some great misfortune were about to occur.

Al, 13 - Mind much depressed; felt as if something disagreeable was about to happen.

Al,N-7 - Thoughts of something terrible going to happen come into his mind against his will; feels impelled to do reckless (impulsive) things, such as throwing child, which he carries in his arms, through the window, and the like.

Al,N-121 - Mortifying news affects him very much.

Al,N-8 - Could not get rid of the indescribable tormenting feeling that something terrible was going to happen to him.

He, 7 - Thoughts of something terrible going to happen come into his mind against his will; feels impelled to do reckless (impulsive, precipitated) things, such as throwing child, which he carries in his arms, through the window, and the like.

MAG-C. Al, 13 - Tremulous anxiety and fright, as if she apprehended some misfortune, disappearing in the evening in bed.

Al, 948 - Anxious dreams of the misfortune of relatives.

Ha, 1 - Trembling anguish and fear, as if evil was threatening (menacing, endangering); it passes off in the evening in bed.

MAG-S. Al, 4 - Anxious as if conscious of some evil...

Al, 5 - Apprehensive (fear), fearful, very gloomy; she thought some misfortune would happen to her;...

MED. Al,N-47 - It feels the evil coming to it, and the bad news before it arrives (clairvoyance), of course it is selfish, and it is easily hurt by a harsh (rude) word.

Al,N-50 - It is always anticipating, fearing evil will happen, loss of reason or suicide.

He, 33 - Woke at an early hour with a frightened sensation, as if something dreadful had happened;... as if she must do something to rid her mind of this torture.

MENY. Al, 8 - Apprehensive sensation about the heart, as of impending evil, and as if he had to endure some hardship. (adversity, privation, suffering)

Ha, 285 - Anxious feeling about the heart, as if something bad were about to happen, and he had to undergo (experience) a calamity. (cataclysm, disaster)

He, 2 - Anxiety about heart, as if some evil was going to happen.

MERC. Ha, 1235 - Anxiety that could drive him far away, as if he had committed a crime or some misfortune were about to happen to him.-(transgression)

Ha, 1249 - All day long depression of

spirits combined with anxiety; he always thought he was going to hear of something disagreeable.

He, 34 - Inexpressive pain of soul and body, anxious restlessness, as if some evil impended ...; disgusted (revolt) with himself, has not courage (cowardice) to live; constant suspicion (distrust), considering everybody his enemy.

MEZ. Ha, 4 - Apprehensiveness in the scrobiculus cordis, as if he expected something disagreeable.

He, 5 - No rest when alone; wants to be in company ...unable to repeat what has been learned by heart; looks through window for hours, without being conscious of objects around; knows not what she is about; forgets what she is about to utter (talk); looks ill humored, pale, wretched, fallen away; ......expecting some very unpleasant news.

MOSCH. Al, 7 - Anxiety, as if something were about to happen.

MUR-AC. Al, 21 - Deep reflection, and quiet absorption in himself, as if something disagreeable were impending, though with desire to work.

Ha, 269 - Sunk in profound thought, as if something disagreeable were about to happen,...

Ha, 4 - Deep reflection, and quiet introversion, as if something unpleasant was impending,...

Ha, 5 - Anxious apprehension; he cannot get over the slightest misfortune.

NAJA. Al, 14 - Felt melancholy; began to form images of possible wrongs (mistaken) and misfortunes, over which the mind broods; very wretched at times;... a slight cause sets him in a perfect agony of mental suffering on another's behalf (welfare);...makes himself imaginary troubles and wrongs, and frets (bother) over them for two hours...

He, 3 - Melancholy; began to form images of possible wrongs (evils) and misfortunes over which the mind broods; very wretched (miserable) at times.

NAT-C. Ha, 10 - His fancy is mostly anxiously occupied with the future; he paints to himself what misfortunes might happen to him; and he seeks solitude for several days.

He, 6 - Intolerable melancholy and apprehension; she is wholly occupied with sad thoughts.

NAT-M. Al, 70 - In the evening it seemed as though he became paralyzed from a fright (terrify) ; afterwards he seemed horrified, and apprehended some misfortune.

Ha, 14 - From the looks of everyone, he concludes that people pity (compassion, sympathy) him for his misfortune, and he weeps.(miserable)

He, 33 - Brain fag (weakness), with sleeplessness, gloomy (dark) forebodings, exhaustion after talking, embarrassment (confusion) of brain.

NAT-P. Al, 9 - Apprehensive (fear) of some approaching evil.

NAT-S. Al, 6 - Great fear, with dread of a misfortune.

NICC. Al, 6 - Apprehensive and despondent, as if some misfortune were impending.

He, 1 - Low-spirited, tearful; fears something evil will happen.

NUX-V. Ha, 1235-...anxiety and anxious solicitude (care), as if something important were to be feared (afraid).

PALL. He, 6 - Apprehension (fear) as if something horrible would happen.

PHEL. Al, 9 - Sad mood and fear the whole day, as from impending misfortune; she wept, and was prone to think upon sad subjects.

PHOS. Al, 69 - Sadness and melancholic, as if some misfortune had happened.

Al, 86-...; a feeling of dread (fear), as if awaiting something terrible, yet unable to resist or move (terrifying, scaring), overcame me; sometimes it seemed as if I was beginning to bloat (inhalant, inflate, vanity?), and then I could hear a multitude of voices saying in high glee, "Fill him up a little more and he will burst," (blow up) followed by demoniacal laughter, which made the cold chills run over me... I imagined myself an aurora borealis, and could distinctly hear voices shouting, "Beautiful! Oh, was not that splendid?"...

Al, 104 - Anxiety, as from impending misfortune.

Ha, 5 - Sad and melancholy, as if some accident had happened to his beloved ones.

Ha, 21 - Apprehensiveness, like the foreboding (anticipation) of misfortune.
He, 7 - Anxious: filled with gloomy (dark) forebodings; as if about to die; about termination (conclude) of her illness (disease); and restless ; at twilight; when alone; about future; during a thunderstorm; ..
He, 19 - Weary of life; full of gloomy (dark) forebodings.

PULS. He, 42-...full of anxiety, forebodings of impending (imminent, destined) disaster; ...

RHUS-T. Al, 5 - Melancholy, ill-humor, and anxiety, as if a misfortune (disgrace) would happen, or as if she were alone (solitary), and all about her were dead (lifeless, inert) and still (silent, quiet), or as if she had been forsaken by a near friend; worse in the house, relieved by walking in the open air.
Al, 33 - He is frightened (afraid, fear) by a trifle (insignificance) (on falling asleep) as if he had dreaded (worry) the greatest misfortune.
Ha, 946 - He is frightened (afraid, fearful) (on going to sleep) at a trifle, as if he had to fear the greatest calamity (disaster, misfortune) from it.
Ha, 953 - Melancholy, sad, and anxious, as if about to hear of a calamity,(misfortune, disaster) or as if she were solitary (lonely, alone) and all around her were dead (lifeless, extinct) and silent (quiet) ; or as if she had bid farewell (separation) to an intimate friend ; worst in the room, diminished by walking in a open air.
He, 22-... great restlessness and anguish as if she had committed a crime or as if she thought some terrible calamity impended; these feelings drove her from one place to another; could not rest quietly at night in bed; was robbed of sleep and all desire to live;...
He, 23 - Restlessness and anxiety about heart as if she had committed a crime or as if some great misfortune was in store (reserved) for her, is driven from one place to another; deprived of sleep and all desire to live; ...

SABIN. Al, 1 - Great anxiety, as if he apprehended some evil.

SAMB-C. Al, 1-...an indefinable fear as if the horse (a very gentle animal) might run away, or the wagon break at any moment; a dread of some undefined danger.

SEC. Al,N-18 - Anticipated misfortunes, as though about to lose something of great value.(estimate)

SEP. He, 21 - Anxiety; with fear, flushes of heat over face; about real or imaginary evils...

SPONG. Al, 5 - Anxiety as if a misfortune would befall him, which he seemed to foresee. (predict, prophesy)
Ha, 382 - Anxious as if misfortune (disaster) threatened (endangered) him and he had a foreboding of it.
He, 25 - He is anxious as if some misfortune would occur of which he has a presentiment.
He, 21 - She is very timid, and is especially pursued and incessantly tormented by a frightful scene of some mournful (unhappy) event of the past.

STANN. Ha, 659 - Calm, collected disposition: he was reconciled to his fate (destiny) and was perfectly contented with his lot. (destiny, doom)

STAPH. Ha, 708 - Sad, he apprehends (perceive) the worst consequences from slight (trivial) things and cannot calm himself.

STRAM. Al, 207 - His whole conduct and countenance was like that of a child severely frightened and apprehending some terrible calamity.

STRY. Al, 31 - A fear of something about to occur.

SULPH. Al, 45 - Anxious disposition I could not free myself from the anticipation of some great misfortune, though I had no ground for such fear,...
He, 47 - Anxiety;...as if some great misfortune were impending (threatening);...

TAB. Al, 30 - Uneasiness and anxiety in the afternoon, as if some misfortune would occur.
Al, 35 - Great apprehension with oppression of the chest, and a very despondent, sad mood, as if apprehended some misfortune,...

TARENT. Al, 34 - Lamentation, with oppressive pain in the heart, as if a misfortune had befallen her.
Al, 35 - Weeping, with oppression and pain

in the heart, as from misfortune;...
Al, 65-...great haste in whatever I undertook, from a constant fear that something would happen to prevent my finishing it;...fear that something would fall on me (doom, disgrace);...fear of striking it against some imaginary object which appeared to be suspended....(hurt)
Al, 65-... Great fear of an imaginary impending calamity (cataclysm, catastrophe) great desire of be alone, fear of being alone...
Al, 46 - Sadness, lamentation, as if a misfortune had befallen him;...
THUJ. Al, 49 - Sudden rising of dark thoughts (pessimism) causing uneasiness, apprehension (foreboding) of misfortune, with fancied scruples of conscience, ...
VERAT. Al, 45 - Anxiety as if he dread a misfortune, as if some evil were impending.
Ha, 688 - She is inconsolable (unhappy) about an imaginary misfortune, ...
Ha, 691 - Anxiety as though he anticipated (expected) misfortune, as if threatened with some calamity.(disaster)
He, 6 - She is inconsolable over a fancied misfortune,...
He, 29-...prays says it is a secret (secretive, mysterious) and a misfortune; ...saying she must strengthen (encourage) herself, ...imagines herself in heaven (elevated, sublime, noble) talking with God.
ZINC. Al, 24 - Anxious mood, as from a misfortune.
He, 13 - Anxious mood as from a misfortune.

MONEY

Ailments from; financial loss: ***arn.***[122] ars.[8] aur.[58] calc.[30] ign.[30] mez.[58] nat-m.[30] nux-v.[30] puls.[193] ***rhus-t.***[30] ***sars.***[8] stann.[30] verat.[30]
Ambition; much, money, for: ars.[30] calc.[30] lyc.[30] nux-v.[30] sulph.[30]
Anxiety; money matters, about: aur.[172] bac.[62] bry.[162] calc-f.[36] calc-sil.[58] cand-a.[239] choc.[222] ign.[172] kali-p.[172]
Brooding; law suit, over, by which he may gain or loose a million, and takes it in bad part if not allowed to read indictment for said lawsuit, a confused, irrational piece of work, on which he has been working all night, in insanity: ***nux-v.***[54]
Cares; full of, money, about: bamb-a.[1184] ozone[227]
Delusions; ciphers, sees: ***ph-ac.*** phos. sulph.
• distinguish, squanders money, proud of his position: ***verat.***[54]
• money, counting, he is: alum. bell. cycl. mag-c. zinc.
• money, sewed up in clothing, is: kali-br.
• money, talks of: calc. carbn-s. kali-br.[25]
• squanders money: ***verat.***[54]
Dreams; lottery, investing in, of: mag-c.[36]
➤ lottery, seeing the numbers he had taken: nat-s.[10]
➤ money: alum. bamb-a.[1184] ***cycl.*** hydrog.[222] mag-c. mag-m. phos. polym.[111] puls. zinc.[5] zinc-o.[10]
➤ money, counterfeit: zinc-o.
➤ money, disputing about money: chin.
➤ money, gold, of: ***cycl.*** puls.
➤ money, left behind without, he is: ozone[227]
➤ money, robbery, he found the money of a: bac.[226]
➤ money, stolen from her: ozone[227]
➤ quarrels, money, about: chin.
➤ shooting, someone, who owes him money: ozone[227]
➤ stealing, money: lap-mar-c.[194]
Gestures; makes, plays, buttons of his clothing, counting money, as if: calc.[30] nux-v.[30] staph.[30]
Grief; financial loss: arn.[137] aur.[137]
Indifference; money-making, to: chin.[30] kali-c.[30] merc.[30] nat-c.[30] sep.[30]
Kleptomania; steals, money: calc. puls.
Play; gambling, passion for: ars.[30] bell.[36] calc.[30] caust.[30] chin.[30] lyc.[30] mag-c.[30] mag-m.[30] merc.[30] nux-v.[30] staph.[30] sulph.[30] verat.[30]
Play; passion, making money, for, lotteries: mag-m.[30] merc.[30] staph.[30]
Play; passion, making money, to: bell.[36] calc.[30] lyc.[30] mag-m.[30] ***merc.***[30] ***nat-c.***[30] plat.[30] puls.[30] staph.[30] sulph.[30]
Play; passion, making money, to, staking money: calc.[30] mag-c.[30] merc.[30]
Play; passion, making money, to, stock market: mag-m.[30] merc.[30] staph.[30] ther.[231]
Squanders; money: bac.[162] verat.
Squanders; order, from want of: lyc.[30] plat.[58] sil.[30]
Talk; money, about: ars.[189] sulph.[189]

ADAM. Sh, 213 - Furious cold anger when money stolen from me. 2, 12C, 73:XX:XX

Sh, 357 - I have a great desire to feed huge nourishing meals to my family; to spend money in the achievement of their dreams. 2, 12C, 26:XX:XX

ARS. He, 58 - Melancholy; after financial losses; cannot be consoled; thinks he will have to die (sentenced), with his family, from starvation (hunger); sleepless nights; walks about wringing his hands, with moaning and groaning.

BELL. Al, 35-...she acts as if she were washing or counting money, or as if she were drinking.

Ha, 1366 - Ridiculous grimaces; ...acts as if she were washing, at another as if counting money, ...

BRY. He, 27 - She fears not to have wherewithal (money, funds) to live.

CALC-F. Al,S-1-...tendency to look on the dark side of things, with much depression of spirits. Feeling of anxiety about money matters, or thought would come to want (lack), or would soon be "running astern" (reversed, failure) financially...disposition to set a higher value on money than natural to him (avarice?, poverty?).

He, 2 - Depression of spirits and disposition to set a higher value on money than natural to him. (avarice?)

He, 3 - Feeling of anxiety about money matters; thought he would come to want (poverty) or would soon be "running astern" financially (entirely without occasion)

CARBN-S. Al-S, 754 - Hallucinations (delirium) of vision and hearing, he seemed to see splendid spectacles of carriages, with magnificent objects, talked of the emperor, of money, and of grandeur, often incoherently.

CHOC. Sh, 195 - No need to worry about money as usually do. 41, 6C, 00:XX:XX

CUPR-A. Al, 2 - Attacks of mania; he fancies that he is a military officer; a fancy that he is selling green vegetables; a fancy that he is repairing old chairs...he spits in the faces of the attendants, and laughs heartily at it.

CUPR. Ha, 24 - Fits of insanity, he imagines (delirium) he has green herbs for sale.

FORM. Al, 7 - Sudden and unexpected return of sense of mortification and grief, with vivid recollection of circumstances long since passed, which had caused great mortification and pain, and which had rendered several years of his life unhappy; this was caused by the transactions (doing) of a near relative; this grief continues...

HALI-L. Sh, 411 - The way I'm feeling today is aggravated and slightly depressed; mostly aggravated about financial things. Reflecting on a bigger picture now, need to do something about it. More on my mind than before. It has to do with my position and place in life; where I am at this particular point in life. Am I pleased? Am I happy? Am I disgruntled? Of course I'm disgruntled. A switch happened. I wasn't looking so detrimentally on my feelings about position and place. The remedy lightened everything, seasoned it, not as bland as I thought. Now things are bland—not spiced up or happy. 18, 30C, 03:11:XX

Sh, 569 - About 5:00 p.m. felt an irascibility again about people not paying me, but now it feels like an easily moving type of rage, not suppressed. 13, 30C, 01:11:XX

Sh, 691 - Do fish, as well as birds, pair for life? I don't think so—a free for all. 20, 30C, 00:01:14

Sh, 887 - I called Daughter a parasite last night, because of money. 20, 30C, 10:XX:XX

HYDROG. Sh, 130 - Anxiety about money and fear of poverty. 24, 30C, 100:XX:XX

KALI-BR. Al, 3 - Decidedly insane; had delusions that lewd women had got into his mother's house; that he was pursued by the police; that his wife was threatened by members of the family; that he had thousands of dollars in gold sewed up in his clothing; (rich, wealth)

MAG-C. Al, 927 - A pleasant dream of receiving money.

Al, 928 - Dream that she invested money in a lottery.

VERAT. He, 11 - Thinks himself distinguished (classify) ; squanders (futile) his money; proud (haughty) of his position.

MORTIFICATION

Absorbed; misfortune, imagines: calc-s.[122]

Absorbed; sadness, indulges in: *cocc.*[54]

Ailments from; bad news, mortifying, affects him very much: lyss.[54]

Ailments from; mortification, anger, during: **COLOC.**[122]
Ailments from; mortification, humiliation, chagrin: acon.[5] aloe[83] alum.[10] am-m.[137] ambr.[1189] ***anac.***[8] ***apoc.***[8] ***arg-n. ars.***[5] ***aur. aur-m.*** bell. ***bry. calc.***[8] camph.[1] carb-an.[5] carb-v.[10] caust.[5] **CHAM.**[5] ***chin.***[8] chin-b.[8] ***cocc.***[5] **COLOC.**[122] con.[103] cycl.[102] form.[36] gels.[5] graph.[37] grat.[5] **IGN.** ip.[5] ***lach.***[10] **LYC.** ***lyss.*** m-p-a.[10] merc. ***mur-ac.***[54] **NAT-M.** nit-ac.[5] ***nux-v.***[5] ***op.*** **PALL.** petr.[10] **PH-AC.** phel.[111] phos.[10] plat. ***puls.*** ran-b.[36] rham-p.[5] rhus-t. ***seneg. sep.***[54] ***sil.***[163] **STAPH.**[122] stram. ***sulph.*** verat. zinc.[5]
Ailments from; mortification, humiliation, chagrin, emotional or mental ailments from: anac.[8] ***apoc.***[8] ***aur.***[8] bell.[5] ***coloc.***[8] con.[103] cur.[11] ***ign.***[8] lach.[30] lyc.[58] lyss.[56] nat-m.[10] ***nux-v.***[10] pall.[116] plat.[30] ***puls.***[8] ran-b.[36] ***staph.***[54] verat.[30] zinc.[10]
Ailments from; mortification, indignation, with: **STAPH.**[122]
Anger; past events, about: calc. carb-an. sars.[54] sep. sulph.[54]
Anger; past events, about, arise from most indifferent thoughts and from every occurrence in life, unite with new vexations, cannot free herself from them: sulph.[54]
Anger; vexations, thinking about former: ***calc. carb-an.*** lyc.[1] sars.[54] sep. sulph.[54]
Anxiety; thoughts, from, disagreeable: phos.[1] sep.[1]
Brooding; condition, illness, over one's: aur.[114] kali-p.[58] ***ph-ac.***[1]
Brooding; constantly over loss of a child: ***gels.***[54] ***kali-br.***[54]
Brooding; disappointment, love: ***ph-ac.***[54]
Brooding; disappointment, over: **BELL.**[122] ***ph-ac.***[54]
Brooding; forbidden things, over: ***plb.***[54]
Brooding; unpleasant things: kiss.[36]
Complaining; mortification, from: ***staph.***[54]
Delirium; mortification, after: bell.[10] nux-v.[10] puls.[10]
Delusions; mortification, after: ***aur.***[116] bell.[10] nux-v.[10] ***puls.***[10]
- past anxious thoughts and things are present: staph.[1]
- pursued, tormented by a frightful scene of some mournful event of the past, and: spong.[54]
- troubles, broods over imaginary: ***ign.***[54] ***naja***[117]

Desires; unpleasant things, to think about: kiss.[36]
Dreams; anxious, mortification, after: ***puls.***
➤ mortification: asar.[54] ign.[54] mosch.[54] rheum[54] staph.[54]
Dullness; mortification, after: ***staph.***
Dwells on past disagreeable occurrences: am-c. arg-n. asar.[149] calc.[10] ***cham. chin.*** cob-n.[119] ***cocc. con.*** cop. form. glon. goss.[122] hep. hydrog.[222] hyos.[111] ***ign.***[54] kali-c.[108] ***kali-p.***[54] kiss.[36] lil-t.[58] luna[228] lyc. meny. mez. **NAT-M.** nit-ac. op.[30] opun-a.[36] phos.[111] ***plat.*** psor.[111] rhus-t. sars.[54] ***sep.*** spong.[1] staph.[30] ***sulph.*** syph.[122] thuj.[5] verat.[116] visc.[119]
Dwells; disappointments, on: ***ph-ac.***[54]
Dwells; grief from past offenses: calc.[30] staph.[30]
Dwells; grieve therefore, to: nat-m.[30]
Dwells; health, his broken: aur-m.[58]
Dwells; on past disagreeable occurrences, recalls old grievances: glon. sars.[54] sulph.[54]
Dwells; on past disagreeable occurrences, thinking of everything which others have done to displease him, lies awake all night to lay plans to talk to them about it, but forgets it in the morning: am-c.[58]
Dwells; unpleasant, disagreeable things: ***ambr. benz-ac.*** kreos.
Embittered, offenses, from slight: ang.[36]
Fear; thoughts, of his own: androc.[222] camph.
Grief; hunting for something to grieve oneself: lil-t.
Hatred; morbid ideas, from: sulph.[54]
Insanity; black insanity with despair and weariness of life from fear of mortification or of loss of position: calc.[30] ign.[30] puls.[30] rhus-t.[30] staph.[30] sulph.[30] verat.[30]
Insanity; mortification, from: bell.[10] ***lach.***[30] **NUX-V.**[30] plat.[30] ***puls.***[10] ***staph.***[30]
Masochism: nat-c.[185] nat-m.[185] tub.[185]
Masochism; sexual: lach.[185] nat-m.[185] tub.[185]
Memory; weakness, mortification, form: ***anac.***[54]
Moaning; offense happened long ago, for trifling: ***cham.***[54]
Mortification; emissions, after: **STAPH.**[54]
Mortification; mortifies herself: cob.[102]
Mortification; profound, throwing away what he may have in his hand: staph.[1]
Prostration; grief, from long: **IGN.**[54] kali-br.[137]

Religious affections; night tortured by religious ideas: camph.[54] lil-t.[58]
Sadness; dwell constantly over her condition, inclination to: ***sulph.***[54]
Sadness; grief, after: am-m.[54] ***aur.***[54] ***ign.***[8] ***nat-m.***[54] ***ph-ac.***[54]
Sadness; mortification, after: ***ign.***[54] ***puls.***[54]
Self-torture: acon.[111] ***ars.***[111] bell.[111] ***lil-t.***[111] plb.[111] tarent.[111] tub.[111]
Sit; wrapped in deep, sad thoughts and notices nothing, as if: alum-sil.[58] ***ambr.***[122] aur. cench.[58] cham.[1] cimic.[58] ***cocc.*** con.[58] elaps ***hipp.*** ***ign.***[54] ozone[227] plat.[137] psor.[137] ***puls.*** ***stram.***[54] ***verat.***
Suicidal disposition; shooting, by, night, at, obliged to get out of bed because he cannot put off the idea: ant-c.[36]
Talk; indisposed, mortification, after: ***ign.***[54]
Talk; sufferings, troubles, constantly of his: arg-n.[5] asaf.[137] ***mag-p.***[5] ***nux-v.***[5] zinc.[137]
Thinking; ailments, complaints, of, constantly to his: ***ham.***[122]
Thinking; disagreeable things agg., of: phos.[5]
Thinking; sad things agg, of: rhus-t.
Thoughts; himself, become of him, what would: nat-m.[137]
Thoughts; persistent, unpleasant subjects, haunted by: ***ambr.*** asar.[149] caust. ***cocc.***[54] graph. kali-c. **NAT-M.** petr.[1] rhus-t.
Thoughts; persons who had offended him, of: glon.[36]
Thoughts; suffering, of his own: sabal.[137]
Thoughts; tormenting, past disagreeable events, about: am-c.[1] spong.[1]
Torments; himself: acon.[111] ars.[111] bell.[111] ***lil-t.***[111] nat-m.[36] plb.[111] tarent.[111] tub.[111]
Weary of life; mortification, after: ***puls.***[54]
Weeping; mortification, after: coff.[58] coloc. pall.[116] puls.
Weeping; need, past, about: nat-m.[60]
Weeping; past events, thinking of: lyc.[1] ***nat-m.***

ACON. He, 8 - Ideas haunt (obsess) him, cannot get rid of them.
AGAR. Ha, 5 - The mind is restless and troubled; he was always solely occupied with his present and his future condition.
ALUM. Ha, 6 - Fancy paints to itself nothing but disagreeable, sad pictures.
ANAC. Ha, 7 - Anxious apprehension and deep thoughts, on meditating over his present and his future fate. (destiny)
ARS. Ha, 1038 - When he is alone he is beset by thoughts about disease and other thoughts of an indifferent character, of which he cannot get rid.
He, 7 - When alone, he falls to thinking about disease and other things, which he can scarcely keep out of his mind.
He, 58 - Melancholy; after financial losses; cannot be consoled; thinks he will have to die (sentenced), with his family, from starvation (hunger); sleepless nights; walks about wringing his hands, with moaning and groaning.
AUR. Ha, 344 - Discontented with all circumstances; he imagines that he finds everywhere some obstacle (impediment, restriction) in the way; at one time he thinks that this is owing to an unlucky (unfortunate) fate (destiny), at another that he himself is to blame (censured) for it ; when the latter was the case he was particularly mortified and dejected.
Ha, 3 - He believes that he has lost the love of others, and this mortifies him even to tears.
Ha, 4 - Discontented with all conditions; he thinks that he everywhere finds an impediment, caused now by an opposing fate,(destiny) then again by himself, which latter mortifies him and renders him dejected.(sad)
Ha, 28 - Excessively disposed to take offense; even the least thing seeming offensive to him, affected him deeply and caused resentment.
He, 80 - Ailments from fright, anger, contradiction, mortification, or vexation with dread, fear, reserved displeasure, or vehemence.
BRY. He, 47 - Bad effects from mortification, violence and anger.
CALC. Ha, 46 - Troubled and cross, she looked at the worst side of things, and sought (pursued) out all the evil.
CAMPH. He, 16 - Monomania, with horrible visions and torturing ideas about religion, which he cannot shake off, although he is conscious that they are morbid.; is< at night.
CARB-AN. Ha, 7 - Morose thoughts and ill-humor, not to be driven away, concerning things present and past, even to weeping.

CHAM. Al, 58 - He cannot stop talking about old vexatious (unpleasant) circumstances.

Ha, 470 - Cannot cease talking about old vexatious things.

CLEM. Al, 13 - Buried in sad thought and in dread (fear) of impending misfortune.

COCC. Al, 11 - Thoughts directed to an unpleasant object; she is absorbed in herself, and notices nothing about her.

COP. Al, 9 - Absurd recriminations about trifling and long -past occurrences.

CROC. Al, 2 - Suddenly there arises before her fancy a concern (care) which she attended a long time since, as vividly as if were she listening to it;...

CUR. Al, 10 - Brooding sadness, frequent weeping, with desire for solitude.

DROS. Ha, 281 - He takes insults very resentfully, not without vexation.

FORM. Al, 7 - Sudden and unexpected return of sense of mortification and grief, with vivid recollection of circumstances long since passed, which had caused great mortification and pain, and which had rendered several years of his life unhappy; this was caused by the transactions (doing) of a near relative; this grief continues...

GLON. Al, 14 - Recalls old grievances...; he was constantly thinking of persons who had offended him, with determination to justify (excuse, defend) his own conduct.

GRAPH. Al, 22 - At night, after lying down, thoughts full of care, from which she could not free herself, ...

HEP. Al, 5 - She remembers everything that has been unpleasant during her life.

Ha, 12 - She thinks about everything disagreeable that happened to her in her lifetime.

IGN. Ha, 791 - Thinks against his will of annoying, vexatious things, and dwells on them.

He, 2-...;sees everything as if through a fog (obscurity) ; sits quietly, with a vacant gaze (expression), always thinking of the mortification endured,... prefers to be alone; thinking of the past mortification...0Melancholy after mortification.

He, 11-...believes herself married (connected) and pregnant; is tormented by remorse of imagined crimes; seeks constantly to escape to drown (suicide) herself; ...;is only quiet when lying undisturbed and brooding over her troubles, which she rehearses (tell) in a doleful (unhappy) tone ;..." I am neglecting my duty, breaking my vow" (promise, engagement)...;conscientious scruples after eating.

He, 22 - Melancholia from suppressed mental sufferings, with much sighing; desire to be alone (solitude) so as to give way to her real or imaginary grief; weeps bitterly.

He, 37 - Tears wept inwardly, the pain and penalty (forfeit) of unrequited (unrecompensed) love; desires solitude so that one may nourish inward grief;...

He, 62 - Ill effects (ailments) from hearing bad news; from vexation with reserved displeasure ; from grief, or suppressed mental sufferings; of shame and disappointed love.

KALI-BR. Al, 5 - She had the erroneous idea that she was deserted by all her friends, and as a consequence she passed all her waking moments, which are not many in tears;...delusion that her child was dead, had taken fixed possession of her mind;...she declared that she saw it dead (corpse) before her, and when it was brought to her, she refused to acknowledge that it was hers, or had any resemblance to the one she imagined was dead.

He, 23-...constantly brooding over loss of a daughter; almost crazy; ... (child)

KREOS. He, 11 - Seeks for unpleasant things and broods over them.

LACH. Al, 28 - At times, can only think for a long time of some fancied worry.

LAM. Al, 2 - Extraordinary sadness; he thought he had been blamed for reverses (failure) for which he was blameless, and in consequence was obliged to suffer;...

LYC. Al, 91 - She is overpowered (defeat) by many unpleasant recollections (memory), about which she becomes vexed; even at night on waking.

Ha, 47 - She thinks of a number of disagreeable occurrences in former(past) times, which vex her, even at night, when she wakes up.

He, 39 - Ailments from fright, anger,

mortification, or vexation, with reserved displeasure.

LYSS. Al,N-121 - Mortifying news affects him very much.

MANG. Ha, 329 - Embittered humor; he could not forget injustice done to him; he fostered (support) resentment for a long time.

MENY. Ha, 290 - Melancholy humor; his thoughts are disposed to dwell on past sad disagreeable things.

MERC. He, 44 - Ailments from mortification; from insults; from egotism.

He, 49 - Ailments from mortification; from insults; from egotism.

MUR-AC. Al, 10 - Anxious thoughtfulness; he cannot free himself from the slightest trouble.

NAJA. Al, 14 - Felt melancholy; began to form images of possible wrongs (mistaken) and misfortunes, over which the mind broods; very wretched at times;... a slight cause sets him in a perfect agony of mental suffering on another's behalf (welfare);...makes himself imaginary troubles and wrongs, and frets (bother) over them for two hours...

NAT-C. Al, 11 - Intolerable melancholy and apprehension; she was wholly occupied whith sad thoughts.

Ha, 5 - Great melancholy and apprehensiveness; only occupied with sad thoughts.

NAT-M. Al, 47 - Full of grief; he tormented himself; he seemed to prefer disagreeable thoughts, which prostrated him very much.

Ha, 4 - Melancholy mood; he cannot remove from his thoughts injuries (insults) he has inflicted on others, or which have been inflicted on him, which depressed him so much that he had no pleasure in anything. (remorse)

Ha, 8 - He sorrowfully torments (torture) himself, by continually looking for disagreeable ideas, which weakens him.

Ha, 10 - In his thought he constantly recalls former disagreeable occurrences, so as to worry himself by thinking about them.

Ha, 13 - If she merely thinks of troubles past, tears come into her eyes.

Ha, 12 - When alone, she calls up disagreeable thoughts and has to weep.

Ha, 64 - Injuries which he had inflicted on others, or which others had done to him, always dwelled in his thoughts; he could not get rid of them, and this annoyed him, so that he had no pleasure in anything.

He, 21 - Gloomy thoughts, recalls (remember),insults long since suffered; likes to dwell upon past unpleasant occurrences.

He, 48 - Consequences (ailments) of fright, anger, vexation, mortification, or reserved displeasure.

He, 6 - Tries to recollect past disagreeable occurrences for the purpose of thinking on them and indulging (suffer) the grief which it causes.

NIT-AC. Al, 60 - Could scarcely free himself from sad thoughts.

Al, 33 - Depressed, as if despondent and as if in deep thought.

Ha, 12 - She falls to thinking over an anxious occurrence long past, and cannot rid herself of it, almost like as if in a waking dream; from time to time she, as it were, awakes from it startled, but is always absorbed in these ideas, without being able, in spite of strenuous efforts of thinking of anything else.

Ha, 4 - He cannot get rid of his sad thoughts.

He, 14 - Often anxious about his illness; constantly thinks about his past troubles; mind weak and wandering.

NUX-V. Ha, 1248 - Wrapped up in sorrow and care.

He, 33 - Mental disturbance, patient tortured with fixed idea.

PH-AC. Ha, 5 - Continually brooding over his disease.

PSOR. Al, 24-...only disagreeable things affect him, agreeable impressions he passes without noticing them.

PULS. He, 50 - After slight emotions, difficult breathing; bad effects from fright, mortification or excessive joy.(ailments from)

He, 52 - After mortification, sad gloomy (melancholy) and weary (disgusted) of life;...thinks of drowning with great pleasure;...

RAN-B. Al, 7 - The objects of his feelings, for instance, chagrin, occupy his mind long after the occurrence took place; one sees that he is thinking of those things; he talks to himself, gesticulates in his anger...

RHUS-T. Al, 31 - Fear and despair on account of sad thoughts, which she could not get rid of.

Ha, 973 - When she had disagreeable thoughts in her head she could not get rid of them.

He, 12 - Fear and despair on account of sad thoughts, which she could not get rid of. (fixed ideas)

SEP. Al, 95 - The recollection of past unpleasant circumstances puts him in an extreme ill-humor.

Ha, 42 - The remembrance of past trouble puts him into extreme ill humor.

Ha, 43 - Vexatious occurrences from past times keep recurring of themselves, which makes him so irritated ...

Ha, 11 - If he only thinks of his past troubles, his pulse is quickened and his breath fails him.

He, 29 - Fear to starve,(hunger) is peevish, and feels mortified (disgraced), easily frightened and full of evil forebodings.

SPONG. Ha, 381 - She is timorous (fearful) and particularly pursued and incessantly plagued (disturbed, bothered) by a frightful picture out of a melancholic past.

STAPH. Al, 15 - Anxious thoughts and events in the past came to him as if the past were present before him, which caused anxiety...then it became black before his eyes; he did not know whether the images were real or illusory, then everything seemed different, and he lost all desire to live.

Ha, 703 - Anxious thoughts and things long past come before him as if they were actually present and stood before him, which causes anxiety and the sweat of anguish -Then blackness comes before his eyes; he knows not if what he sees is true (real) or deception (false, unreal), then he regards (suppose) everything as something different to what it is (strange), and he loses all wish to live. (lost; discernment, perception)

SULPH. Al, 8 - Numerous morbid ideas, extremely disagreeable, causing rancor, though with also joyous thoughts (and melodies) mostly from the past, take possession of her they throng one upon another so that she cannot free herself from them during the day, with neglect of business,...

Al, 10 - Vexatious and morbid ideas of the past arise from the most indifferent thoughts, and from every occurrence in life, which continue to be united with new vexations, so that she cannot free herself from them, together with a courageous mood which is ready for great resolution.

Ha, 59 - A number of ideas from her past life, mostly disagreeable, causing indignation and mortification...come into her mind;...so that she cannot get rid of them, while she has nothing to do;...

Ha, 60 - Indifferent things and such things as naturally occur in life are attended in her mind with annoying, mortifying ideas from her past, which continually connect themselves with recent annoyances of which she cannot rid herself. This attended (accompanied) with a resoluteness of mind, which is ready for great resolves.(determination)

Ha, 58-..She thinks of nothing but anxious, annoying and dejecting thoughts, which she cannot get rid of; this makes her apprehensive and peevish unto tears.

He, 33 - Sleepless, disgusted with life, fears the future, where she sees nothing but misery (wretchedness, poverty) and suffering (misfortune). 0 Melancholia.

He, 8 - Numerous morbid ideas, extremely disagreeable, causing rancor; neglect of business;...

He, 29-...is filled with anxious, despondent (sad) thoughts, from which she cannot free herself, they make her suspicious, peevish and lachrymose.

He, 43 - Vexations and morbid ideas of past arise from most indifferent thoughts, and from every occurrence in life, which continue to be united with new vexations, so that she cannot free herself from them.

THEA. Al, 20 - Nocturnal fright; sinister thoughts; invincible propensity to analyze his life, to look at it on the dark side, and to resolve it into its most hopeless realities.

MOTHER

Aversion; mother, to: thuj.[137]

Clinging; children of, take the hand of mother, will always: ***bism.***[85] gels.[116] kali-c.[56] lil-t.[56] lyc.[56] phos.[162]

Delusions; calls, him with name, the absent mother or sister: anac.[10]
• dead, mother is, his: lach. nat-m.[1]
• murdered, mother had been, her: nux-v.
• women, his mothers house is invaded by lewd: kali-br.
Dreams; body, arm, hurt, mother's arm: chin.[36]
➤ dead, people, of, mother: mag-s.[36]
➤ death of, mother: chin.[36] mur-ac.[36]
➤ disease, sick people, mother, his: cast-eq.[36]
➤ drowning, mother had been drowned, that her: nicc. rauw.[119]
➤ house, mothers, her: ozone[227]
➤ mother: hydrog.[222]
➤ mother, flying around the world: hydrog.[222]
➤ mother, swinging on a pendulum, with: hydrog.[222]
➤ mother, taking the wrong road: ozone[227]
➤ water, falling into, mother: nicc.
Excitement; curses his mother, throws food or medicine across room: ***hydr.***[54]
Fear; killing, of, mother, her: der.[162]

ANAC. Al, 1 - Illusions of fancy; he imagines he has his name called by the voice of his far-distant mother and sister, accompanied by an apprehension of misfortune and anxiety.
Ha, 45 - Delusions of fancy, he thought his name was called by the voice of his (far distant) mother and sister; at the same time an apprehension and anguish foreboding misfortune.
He, 24 - Imagines he hears voice of mother or sister, who are far away.
ANDROC. Sh, 58-. Felt more love for her mother, friends and husband. (7)
CHIN. Al, DREAM-1110 - Dreamed that some one had stabbed his brother, and then called for his mother; that his mother was dead, and then he cried; that his mother's arms was hurt;...
HALI-L. Sh, 25 - While listening to a patient grieve, had a return of increased awareness of right eye, especially the socket. I had a strong image of how my mother's right eye was knocked out when she was hit by a truck and killed 30 years ago. Feel a very strong sense of connection with her. Telling this to my proving supervisor later, I realized I had never said this to anyone. This was an aspect of her death I had suppressed. It had always been so horrifying to me I couldn't deal with it. I cried gently with lots of tears. Feeling very sad and some remorse that I couldn't have been with my mother when she died. Felt very calm with all of this. 03, 12C, 18:XX:XX
KALI-BR. Al, 3 - Decidedly insane; had delusions that lewd women had got into his mother's house; that he was pursued by the police; that his wife was threatened by members of the family; that he had thousands of dollars in gold sewed up in his clothing; (rich, wealth)
MAG-C. Al, 956 - Dream that her mother had died, at which she woke, and believed that she was still weeping.
NAT-M. Ha, 97 - Lack of memory, so that he thought his mother (present continually) had died, because he did not remember to have seen her.
NUX-V. Al, 3 - Rushed into the room, exclaiming that her mother had been murdered.
STRAM. He, 59-...clings to her mother with as much desperation as if she were going to be thrown from a precipice.

MOVEMENT

Activity; desire for: aur.[85] calc.[85] hyper.[36] led.[36] menth.[85] merc.[85] naja[36] nat-s.[36] nux-v.[85] ozone[227] rhus-t.[36] sul-ac.[85] sulph.[85] sumb.[36] tub.[85]
Activity; desire for, exercise, physical: **BELL.**[36] cann-i.[36] coca[36] crot-c.[36] erech.[36] eucal.[36] orig.[36] phos.[36] ziz.[36]
Activity; hyperactive: agav-t.[149] chin.[47] cob-n.[149] gaert.[136] hyos.[5] ign.[10] lach.[155] lil-t.[36] op.[5] sep.[162] spig.[5] spong.[5] tarent.[187] verat.[5] verb.[5]
Activity; increased excessively: anag.[54] ang.[54] ant-c.[54] ars-s-r.[54] ***bell.***[54] canth.[54] carb-ac.[54] chlor.[54] ***cinnb.***[54] **COFF.**[54] ***coff-t.***[54] hyper.[54] ***op.***[54] ***phos.***[54] phys.[54] zing
Anguish; driving from place to place: **ARS.** ***rhus-t.***[54]
Anguish; motion, amel. from: des-ac.[149]
Anguish; restlessness, with: **ACON.**[137] ***ars.***[137] aur.[172] bell.[54]
Anxiety; motion, from, agg.: acon. aloe berb. bor. cocc.[54] **DIG.**[54] ***hyos.***[54] kali-i.[58] ***lach.***[54] mag-c. mang.[58] nat-c. nicc. rheum stann. stram.[54]

Anxiety; motion, from, airplane, of: **BOR.**[122]
Anxiety; motion, from, cable-railway, of: **BOR.**[122]
Anxiety; motion, from, downward: **BOR.** coff-t.[54] ***gels.*** sanic.
Anxiety; motion, from, elevator, of: **BOR.**[122]
Anxiety; motion, from, heart disease, in: **DIG.**[54]
Anxiety; music, from, church bells: lyss.[122]
Confusion of mind; motion, from, agg.: acon. ambr. bell. bry. calc-p. cob. ign. indg. kalm.[58] lob. mosch. nat-c. nux-v. phos. ***puls.*** tab.
Delusions; bed, headboard was swaying: lac-c.[54]
- bed, motion, in, on waking: clem.[139] lac-c
- bed, turning, is, circle, in a: con.[139] sol-n.[139]
- bird, he is a, runs about, chirping and twittering, until he faints: lyss.[54]
- blood, rushed through like roar of many waters: alumn.[58] cann-i.
- body, brain, moving, is: cycl.[139]
- body, brain, wobbling: ars.[139] cycl.[139] spira.[139]
- body, heart, turning around, is: aur.
- elevated, carried to an elevation: oena.
- fluids go right through him: arg-n.[85]
- hammock, swinging in a, above the treetops: coff-t.[139]
- head, pendulum, seems an inverted oscillating: cann-i.
- hearing, of, objects moving: ph-ac.[1]
- house, movable, is: cann-i.
- images, ever-changing: carbn-o.
- images, moving up and down, sees: zinc.[1]
- images, running, sees: nit-ac.[1]
- motion, all parts being in (during rest): anac.[102] canth.[102] kreos.[36] ***op.***[102] stram.[102]
- motion, bed and ground, of, on waking: clem.[36]
- motion, chair and table in different directions, m. of (while sitting): chlf.[36]
- motion, up and down, m. of: lach.[122] plb.[122] ***spong.***[122]
- move, things, near him and invisible, are moving: canth.[5] carb-v.[5] ph-ac. phos.[10]
- objects, motion, in: ***anh.***[119] carb-ac.[139] cic.[36] kali-cy.[139] mosch.[139] nat-sal.[139] nux-v.[139] phos.[5] sep.[139] thuj.[139]
- running, up and down: ambr.[122]
- saw, he was a huge, darting up and down: cann-i.
- smaller, objects appear in motion: anh.[119]
- spinning, is: hyos. stram.
- sun, reeling, is: cann-i.[36]
- walk, cannot walk, must run or hop: apis. hell.
- water, flowing, sees: ***merc.***

Desires; strength, feats of: coca[36]
Dreams; exertion, from: apis[98] ***ars.*** atro.[36] bapt.[102] brom.[54] ***bry.***[102] dicha.[144] med.[54] nat-m.[102] nux-v.[102] phos.[102] puls.[102] rhus-t. sel.[102] staph.[102]
- ➤ gymnastics: bell.[36] hydrog.[222]
- ➤ mother, swinging on a pendulum, with: hydrog.[222]
- ➤ playing base ball: atro.[36]
- ➤ running, cross country: bac.[226]
- ➤ running, vainly: croc.[10] ind.[36]
- ➤ spinning: lachn.[36] sars.

Fancies; sudden transition: cann-i.[54]
Fear; heart, cease beating, unless, not moving: coca[162] dig.[102]
- ✦ heart, cease to beating, unless constantly on the move, h. will: ***gels.***
- ✦ insanity, repose, if he wants to, must always move: ars.[58] iod.[58]
- ✦ motion, downward: **BOR.**[122] calc.[58] coca[117] cupr.[122] gels. hyper.[102] lac-c.[122] lil-t.[122] ***sanic.***[102] sil.[137] zinc.[137]
- ✦ motion, of: ***bry.***[102] calad.[102] ***gels.***[54] mag-p.[102]
- ✦ suffocation, motion, on, with dyspnea: ***spig.***[54]

Hurry; everybody moves too slowly: med.[58]
Hurry; movements, fast enough, cannot do things: aur. **SUL-AC.**
Hurry; movements, is: acon. arg-n.[137] ars. ars-s-f.[58] atro.[36] ***bell.*** camph. cann-i. coca coff. con. gins. ***hyos.*** kali-c. meny. merc. merl. **STRAM. SUL-AC.** ***sulph.*** **TARENT.** ***thuj.*** viol-t.
Impulse; run, to, convulsive paroxysms came on, when: agar-st.[36]
Impulse; run, to, dromomania: acon.[5] all-s.[36] androc.[222] bell.[5] bufo[5] calc.[161] cann-i.[36] canth.[5] dig.[1] glon.[36] **HYOS.**[5] ***iod.*** mez.[36] ***nux-v.***[5] orig.[5] phys.[36] **STRAM.**[5] tarent.[36] **TUB.**[122] **VERAT.**[5]
Mania; action, must be constantly in, in some laborious occupation: ***iod.***[54]
Restlessness; anxious, driving from place to place: ***tab.***[122]
Restlessness; drives him from place to place: acon.[10] ***am-c.***[10] ***ars.***[122] aur.[10] ***bell.***[10] bism.[10]

calc-p.[122] canth.[10] carb-v.[10] ***cedr.***[122] cench.[58] cimic.[149] crot-h.[10] ***cupr.***[116] dros.[10] graph.[10] ***hist.***[149] hyos.[10] iod.[10] kali-i.[58] kres.[144] lac-h.[229] ***lach.***[10] lyss.[54] meny.[10] merc.[10] nat-c.[10] nux-v.[10] plat.[10] prun.[10] puls.[10] sep.[10] sol-m.[10] spig.[10] stann.[10] staph.[10] ***tab.***[10] tarax.[10] tarent.[58] thlaspi[111] verat.[10]

Restlessness; move, must constantly: ***apis***[117] ***ars.***[122] ***bell.***[10] canth.[58] caust.[148] cench.[58] cham.[60] cimic.[116] coff.[26] cupr.[60] hep.[109] ign.[10] ***iod.***[122] ***kali-br.***[122] ***kreos.***[122] lap-gr-m.[194] ***led.***[162] manc.[122] ***puls.***[60] **RHUS-T.**[122] sac-alb.[210] sanic.[85] sol-n.[25] sul-i.[58] thlaspi[107] trom.[122] viol-o.[45]

Walk; must: acon.[36] ambr.[56] aur.[111] calc.[111] ***cham.***[5] dig.[111] ***dios.***[111] ign.[5] iod.[111] murx.[111] op.[111] paeon.[111] ruta[107] stront-c.[111] tarent.[111]

ACON. Al, 49 - Anxiety which does not allow him to remain in one place, he must constantly walk about. (restlessness)

Al, 23 - Excessive restlessness, all movements and actions are performed with great haste and hurry.

Al, 22 - Restlessness, uninterrupted, unpleasant; he must now sit, now stand, now walk, he does not know what is the matter.

He, 31 - Restlessness, agony, internal anxiety; does everything in great haste (rapidity); must move about or change position often.

ALOE. Al, 17 - Great anxiety, timorousness, restlessness, dread (fear) of death, and great anguish, so that she cannot stay anywhere.(restlessness)

ANG. Ha, 292 - No confidence in himself to undertake and carry through voluntary movements.

ARG-N. Ha, 16 - Anxiety that compels him to walk quickly.

He, 25 - Impulsive, must walk very fast; frequent turns of anxiety.

ARS. Al, 56 - Anguish and despair driving from one place to another for relief.

Ha, 1019 - Anxiety, trembling and quaking, with cold sweat in the face.

Ha, 1008 - He can find no rest in any place, continually changes his position in bed, will get out of one bed and into another, and lie now here, now there.

ASTER. Al, 5 - Melancholy, alternating with almost intolerable cerebral excitement; she is inclined to give herself up to mental or bodily work, to walk, or engage in a violent exercise;...

AUR-M. He, 13 - Insurmountable mental or bodily restlessness; he has to spend hours in street and in open air. 0 Angina pectoris.

AUR. Ha, 345 - An urging to activity, bodily as well as mental; when he did anything, he thought he did not do it quick enough, and that he had a great deal (much) more to do; he could not live to his liking. (desire, aspiration)

Ha, 346 - Remorse about his idleness (indolence), and yet he cannot work at anything; it drives him out of the house, he must always moving.

Ha, 6 - Great anxiety springing from the region of the heart, and which drives him from one place to another, so that he cannot long remain in a place. (restlessness)

Ha, 11 - Restlessness and hurried impulse to bodily and mental activity; he can not work fast enough; he could not act so as to satisfy himself.

Ha, 12 - He is driven to constant activity, and is sorry for his inaction, although he cannot do anything.

He, 55 - Great anguish coming from precordial region, and driving him from place to place, so that he can remain nowhere.

BAR-C. Ha, 11 - Anxious and fearful; a little noise on the street seems to him at once like fire alarm, and he is frightened by it, so that it darts (move quickly) through all his limbs.

BELL. Al, 121 - Inclination to violent exercise and rapid travelling.

Ha, 1329 - Great restlessness, she cannot remain long seated in one place; she is driven all about.

BOR. Ha, 5 - The child is timid while being dandled; when it is rocked up and down in the arms it makes a very frightened face...(fear, touch, caresses)

Ha, 21 - He fritters away the afternoon, without getting to any real work, goes from one work to another, from one room to another, without remaining in one thing.

He, 3 - The child becomes anxious when dancing; if one rocks it in arms it has an anxious expression of face during downward motion.

BRY. Al, 13 - Anxiety in the whole body, which compelled him to do something constantly, and wherever he went he found no rest.

He, 25 - Anxiety in whole body compelled him to do something constantly, wherever he went he found no rest.

CHOC. Sh, 50 - Panic feeling of being trapped and enclosed —worse when curtains are closed and the light blocked out. Strong desire to be outside and moving, to be in the bright and warm sunlight. Kept having to move my feet, which I felt I wanted to move.

ELAT. He, 2 - Irresistible propensity to wander from home, even in the night, and range (distance) in woods.(forest)

EUCAL. He, 2 - Irresistible desire to move about, with a feeling of buoyancy (happiness) and increased strength.

GELS. He, 13 - Confusion; when attempting to move, the muscles refuse to obey the will; head giddy.

GERM. Sh, 177 - Twice while driving I had an illusion -part of a stationery car on the right moved through my field of vision. 02, 6C, 01:XX:XX

HALI-L. Sh, 376 - Lethargic, spaced out. It feel like I don't have the impetus to move. Inertia. I just want to sleep, but there's this tension inside. 06, 6C, 00:11:00

HYOS. He, 50 - Tendency to action: wants to kill somebody or himself.

IOD. Ha, 17 - Restless moving about; she runs about incessantly and does not get to sit down, nor does she sleep at night, so that she has to be considered as crazy.

Ha, 18 - Restlessness, which keeps the body in constant activity.

He, 3 - Must keep in motion day and night (restlessness), brain felt as if it was stirred (agitation) up, felt as if going crazy.

He, 4 - Restless, inclined to move about not permitting to sit or sleep; thought she could tear everything to pieces.

He, 15 - At night, especially when thinking of real or imaginary wrongs ...dares (try) to go home for fear of doing some dreadful (bad, wicked) deed (action); on one occasion was seized with an almost irresistible impulse to murder a woman who was acting as a guide (direct, conduct) for him, he having lost his way (direction);...must be constantly in action, in some laborious occupation. (lost; direction, correction, control)

IRID. Sh-4 - This remedy makes me feel settled in one place, planted. No desire to move. E1

JAMB. He, 2 - Nothing seemed right, when sitting, he wanted to lie; when lying, he wanted to rise again.

LYSS. He, 40 - A strong and uncontrollable impulse to do certain acts; to spring at and to bite any moving object that came within reach; ...

He, 64 - Disinclination to change position of head; two distinct trains of thought existing at one time in her mind, the idea that she is unable to move her head (when lying down) with the positive conviction that she has only to make up her mind that she will do it to achieve it.

MERC. Ha, 1222 - Restlessness, he cannot remain quiet in any place; he can neither stand nor lie, and is as if mad, or as if he had committed a great crime.

Ha, 1231 - He has no rest, and must go hither and thither, and cannot remain long in one place.

Ha, 1235 - Anxiety that could drive him far away, as if he had committed a crime or some misfortune were about to happen to him.-(transgression)

Ha, 1227 - Much anxiety and ebullition in the blood at night, and shooting in the blood vessels.

NAT-AR. Al, 3 - Feeling as something was impending, which caused him to move about.

NAT-C. Al, 18 - Anxiety and hasty (fast) restlessness all day; he could not keep the limbs still, especially the arms; obliged to stretch them; it seemed as though they would be torn (cut) asunder. (in two divided).

NIT-AC. Ha, 18 - In the evening, he feels apprehensive; he cannot sit still, but has to walk about.

Ha, 42 - Peevishness with sadness and a crabbed (irritable) humor with restlessness, so that she knows not where to turn (drive)

PH-AC. Ha, 8 - Sad serious, disheartened

(depressed), only while walking in the open air, increasing the longer he walks; at home it gradually passed of and he became more serene.

RHUS-T. Al, 1382 DREAM-...it seemed to her that the head was hanging out of the bed and the blood was streaming (flow) into it, so that she could hear it flow; together with the appearance of a horrible image which she was obliged to accompany.

Ha, 953 - Melancholy, sad, and anxious, as if about to hear of a calamity, (misfortune, disaster) or as if she were solitary (lonely, alone) and all around her were dead (lifeless, extinct) and silent (quiet) ; or as if she had bid farewell (separation) to an intimate friend ; worst in the room, diminished by walking in a open air.

Ha, 960 - On account of inward (inside) uneasiness (agitation) she could not sit still, but must rock (shake) herself to and fro on her chair, and move all the limbs a little.

He, 22-... great restlessness and anguish as if she had committed a crime or as if she thought some terrible calamity impended; these feelings drove her from one place to another; could not rest quietly at night in bed; was robbed of sleep and all desire to live;...

He, 23 - Restlessness and anxiety about heart as if she had committed a crime or as if some great misfortune was in store (reserved) for her, is driven from one place to another; deprived of sleep and all desire to live; ...

SCROPH-N. Al, 2 - A miserable and sluggish (inactive, lethargic) feeling of the mind when moving about.

STAPH. Ha, 704 - Great inward anxiety, so that he cannot remain in one place, but he says nothing about it.(restlessness)

MURDERED

Delusions; animals, devouring him: ***hyos.***
- animals, dogs, biting and tearing flesh off his chest: stram.
- choked, he will be: ozone[227] phos.[5]
- execute him, people want to: ***op.***[54]
- murder, conspiring to murder him, others are: ars. hydrog.[222] plb. tab.[139]
- murdered, he is being: sulph.[139]
- murdered, he will be: absin.[102] am-m. ars.[58] ***bell. calc.*** camph.[36] cann-i.[58] hep.[30] ***hyos.*** ign. kali-br.[102] kali-c. lact. lyc. mag-c. merc. merc-i-f.[58] ***op.*** phos. plb.[102] ***rhus-t.*** staph.[116] ***stram.*** verat. zinc.
- murdered, killed, roasted and eaten: stram.
- murdered, mother had been, her: nux-v.
- murdered, persons are bribed to murder him: cann-i.
- murdered, sees someone: calc.
- murderer, everyone around him is a: ***plb.***
- pursued, murderers, robbers, by: alco.
- roasted, he will be: stram.[5]
- stab him, some one will: **OP.**[10]

Dreams; children, about, murdered, being: thea.[36]
- ➤ cutting, knife, of being cut with a, to pieces: lil-s.[36]
- ➤ disease, wounded by shot: lob.[54]
- ➤ murder: am-m. androc.[222] ***arn.*** aur-s.[58] bamb-a.[1184] bell. calad. calc. calc-sil.[58] cand-a.[239] carb-an. carc.[119] cast. chel. choc.[222] crot-h.[58] guai. hura hydrog.[222] ign. kali-i. kali-m.[192] kali-s.[58] kalm. kiss.[36] ***kreos.*** lach. lact. led. lyc. ***m-arct.***[10] mag-m. mand.[144] merc. merc-c. naja nat-ar. nat-c. ***nat-m.*** nat-sil.[58] nicc. ol-an. ***petr.*** puls. rhus-t. rhus-v.[10] rumx. sanic. saroth.[119] sedi.[36] sel.[149] ***sil.*** sol-a.[36] spong. ***staph.*** sulph. thea.[85] thuj. ven-m.[149] zinc.
- ➤ murder, blow on the head, after: ***nat-m.***[54]
- ➤ murder, murdered men, seeing: rumx.
- ➤ murdered, of being: am-m. cast.[36] chel. chr-ac.[54] guai. ign. kali-i. ***kreos.***[54] ***lach.*** lact. lyc. mag-m.[36] merc. merc-acet.[10] merc-c.[36] phos.[10] sil. staph.[1] xan.[111] zinc.
- ➤ robbers, breaking into house and trying to kill her: mag-c.[36]
- ➤ robbers, trying to kill him: merc-acet.[36]
- ➤ scalped, of being: xan.[111]
- ➤ stabbed, acquaintance was: lil-s.[36]
- ➤ stabbed, being: chin. guai. lil-s.[36] nat-c. op.
- ➤ stabbed, brother was: chin.[36]
- ➤ stabbed, fear of being stabbed: lach.
- ➤ stabbed, swordsmen threatened to stab him: op.[36]
- ➤ strangle, being: phos. sil. zinc.
- ➤ strangled, morning, in, fear lest the man who strangled her would return: zinc.[54]
- ➤ wounded, of being, shot, by: lob.[54]

Fear; animals, devoured him or her: hyos.[1] stram.

✦ death, kill him, that those in the house might: ***cimic.***[54]
✦ murdered, of being: absin. ars.[172] caps.[172] ***cimic.*** op. phos. ***plat.***[30] plb. rhus-t.[5] staph.[5] stram. tab.[137]
✦ roasted, to be: stram.[10]
✦ strangled, to be: **PLAT.**[122]
Killed, desire to be: ***ars.*** bell. coff-t. ***phyt.***[54] stram.
Killed; desire to be, stabbing heart, by (after midnight): ***ars.***[36]
Pleasure; waking from a dream of murder, on: thea.
Praying; killed, to be: bell.[30]
Talk; nothing but, murder, fire and rats: ***calc.*** calc-sil.[58]

ABSIN. Al,S-9 - Fear of assassination.
ARS. Al-S, 2879 - Became very nervous, agitated, and delirious, suspecting people were about the house plotting (conspiracy, betrayed) against his life, jumps out of the bed suddenly and reaches after imaginary objects, and stares wildly and suspiciously around him,...
BELL. Al, 162 - She begs the bystanders to kill her.
CALC. He, 28 - She thinks and talks of nothing but murder, fire, rats, etc.
He, 21 - Mania-a-potu, with delirious talk about fire, rats, mice and murder.
CAMPH. Al, 46-...I shriek and call for help, because it seems that a murderer stands at my bed side...
CANN-I. Al, 31 - Imagines men are bribed (suborn) to kill him.
CHIN. Al, DREAM-1110 - Dreamed that some one had stabbed his brother, and then called for his mother; that his mother was dead, and then he cried; that his mother's arms was hurt;...
CIMIC. He, 10 - Fear of death; fears those in house will kill him (murdered, by parents); saw wires encasing (lock, imprisoned) him; visions of rats and of strange objects.
COFF-T. He, 5 - Begs that someone might end her life. (salvation, redemption) (murdered)
GUAI. Ha, 125 - Dreams as if she would be stabbed with knives.
HYDROG. Sh, 243 - Fear that someone was trying to find out if I was home so that they could come and rape and murder me. 16, 30C, XX:XX:XX
MAG-C. Al, 959 - Dream of thieves who broke into the house and tried to kill her.
Al, 816 - Dream that some one came to murder her; that she jumped from a window,...
MERC-I-F. Al, 1 - While in bed, he imagined that a man was in his room who intended to perforate his throat with a gimlet;...
NAT-C. Al, DREAM, 1102-..;of marrying two women, of parties, walks, entertainments, and excursions on horseback, afterwards they were frequently anxious, of going astray (lost),of murders, having his ears cut off; also vexatious dreams; he would take a journey and could not get away from the place,(immobilization) and when has reached the first station was obliged to turn back, on account of something he had forgotten.
NUX-V. Al, 3 - Rushed into the room, exclaiming that her mother had been murdered.
OP. Al, 16-...started up in a fright on account of fancied swordsmen (rival, competitor) who threatened to stab him; became angry if any one argued him or thought him delirious; however, he blamed (reproaches) himself while in delirium for his folly.
Ha, 638 - He chattered all sorts of unconnected stuff and pointed with his fingers to imaginary masked people approaching him; ...he started at imaginary swordsmen, who might kill him ; ...
He, 21-...in old, emaciated persons; sees animals coming towards him; people want to hurt him, execute him ; creeping under covers or jumping out of bed; in "old sinners" (criminals) whose long lives of excess have thoroughly destroyed their constitutions; ...; believe themselves to be murderers or criminals to be executed; want to run away (escape) ;...
PLB. Al, 23-...His delirium turned chiefly upon the idea that his life was in danger from assassination or poisoning, and that every one about him was a murderer...
Al, 63 - The patient imagined that he was constantly followed (persecuted), and that he heard voices coming from the chimney... ; this man after a few days wished to leave the hospital and go home, because he was convinced that there were fiends in

the building that pursued him and sought (want) his life.
Al, 65 - Often getting out of bed and wishing to go home; sometimes not recognizing his family; thought they were conspiring to kill him.
He, 13 - Thought his life was in danger from assassination or poison and every one about him was a murderer.
STRAM. Ha, 548 - Nonsensical idea, as though he were killed, roasted, and being devoured.
He, 57 - Strange absurd ideas; thinks herself tall, double or lying crosswise; one half of body cut off (divided); bed is full of creases (wrinkle) (disorganization); that he was killed roasted and being eaten.
He, 77 - Patient had a constant vision of an executioner(hangman, lynches) standing before him in spite of which he was lively, talkative, laughed and joked about his hallucination, yet it seemed to him a reality.
SULPH. Al, 3813 - At night uncomfortable dreams of murders.
ZINC. He, 43 - Great fear, as if persecuted by men or the devil, on account of crimes he has never done (injustice); is afraid of becoming imprisoned, or poisoned, or shot, or buried (inter) alive...[0] Delirium tremens.

MUSIC

Anger; alternating with, singing: croc.[10]
Answer; aversion to, sings, talks, but will not answer questions: agar.
Anxiety; chest, playing piano, while: ***nat-c.***
Anxiety; dancing, when: ***bor.***[36]
Anxiety; music, from: bufo[58] dig. ***nat-c.***
Anxiety; playing piano, while: ***nat-c.***
Carried; music, as if by: anh.[119]
Cheerfulness; dancing, laughing, singing, with: bell.[10] hyos.[10] ***nat-m.***[10] nitro-o.[36] plat.[10] ***stram.***[10] tab.[10]
Cheerfulness; heart disease, laughs, sings and dances: ***nat-m.***[54]
Cheerfulness; music, from: ***croc.***[10]
Dancing; amel.: cann-s.[5] carc.[119] caust.[5] **IGN.**[5] nat-m.[5] **SEP.**[5] sil.[5] stann.[5] tarent.[214]
Dancing; desire for: acon. aether[36] ***agar.***[102] apis ***bell.*** cann-i. **CARC.**[122] chlol. ***cic. cocc.*** con. ***croc.*** croto-t. grat. ***hyos.*** ign.[5] lach.[146] merc. nat-m. nitro-o.[36] ozone[227] ph-ac. pip-m.[36] plat. rob. sant.[36] sep. sil.[5] stict.[122] ***stram.*** tab. **TARENT.**
Dancing; desire for, fetus, of, to music: carc.[147]
Dancing; desire for, grotesque: agar. ***cic.***
Dancing; desire for, night, in churchyard: cic.[36] stram.[36]
Dancing; desire for, rhythm, with strong sensation of: carc.[146] sep.[146]
Dancing; desire for, singing, and, inclination for: agar.[160]
Dancing; desire for; wild: androc.[222] ***bell.*** camph. tarent.
Delirium; cheerful, alternating with, laughing, singing, whistling, crying etc.: stram.
Delirium; music, from hearing: plb.[54]
Delirium; singing: agar.[116] cic.[116] lact.[36] stram.[36]
Delusions; animals, bed, on, dancing: con.
- choir, on hearing music he is in a cathedral: cann-i.
- churchyard, dancing in, he is: cic.[36] stram.
- dancing, he is: agar.[139] ars-s-f.[139] puls.[139]
- dancing, he was, all night: clem.[139] sabin.[139]
- dancing, satyrs and nodding mandarins: cann-i.
- hearing, of, music, all kinds of, when closing eyes, in puerperal fever: ***puls.***[54]
- music, delightful: lach. plb. puls.
- music, delirium, during: ***plb.***[54]
- music, evening, hears the music heard in the day: lyc.
- music, hears: anh.[144] **CANN-I.** croc. ign.[1] ***lach.*** lyc. merc.[122] nat-c.[122] plb. puls. sal-ac. sarr.[36] ***stram.*** thuj.
- music, melody, a: ign.[1] sulph.[36]
- music, sweetest and sublimest melody: cann-i. ***lach.***
- music, sweetest, primitive music seemed: psil.[164]
- music, unearthly: aether cann-s.[122]
- satyrs, vision of dancing: cann-i.
- singing, to be: cann-i.

Dream, as if in a; singing in ears, with: cann-i.[54]
Dreams; animals, birds, of, singing: com.[36]
➤ balls, being at: mag-c.[36] mag-s.[36]
➤ dancing: gamb. mag-c. mag-m. mag-s. zing.
➤ dancing, man, in an old: zing.[54]
➤ figures, grotesque, dancing before her: narcot.[36]

➤ monks, about, singing and dancing: ozone[227]
➤ music: canth.[5] carb-v.[5] mag-s.[10] sarr. sulph.[5]
➤ piano, playing, in public: lap-mar-c.[194]
➤ praying, public meeting with great applause, in: ars-h.[54]
➤ singing political songs, in presence of spies: asc-t.[5]
➤ unsuccessful efforts to, dress for a ball: mag-c. mag-s.
Dullness; alternating with, singing: spong.[10]
Excitement; dancing, singing and weeping, with: tarent.[58]
Excitement; evening, music, from: sumb.[36]
Excitement; music, from: carc.[207] ***kreos.*** pall.[54] sumb. ***tarent.***
Excitement; music, from, one hour after profuse and general perspiration: tarent.[54]
Excitement; singing, after sad: ***con.***[54]
Fear; music, from: ***acon.***[102] ***ambr.***[102] bar-c.[172] bufo[98] cocc.[172] dig. ***nat-c.*** nat-s.[58] nit-ac.[172] nux-v.[102] phos.[172] ***sabin.***[102] sulph.[172] tarent.[102] thuj.[102]
✦ piano, when playing: ***kali-br.***[54] ***phos.***
✦ sadness, with, music agg.: ***dig.***[36]
Forsaken; feeling, sighing, with: lith-c.[60]
Hysteria; music amel.: **TARENT.**
Ideas; gay and musical: sulph.[60]
Indifference; music, to, loves, which she: ***carb-v.*** caust.[10]
Insanity; dancing, with, and stripping himself: ***bell.***[122]
Insanity; dancing, with: bell.[10] cic.[10] hyos.[10] ph-ac.[10]
Irritability; music, during: anac.[116] ***calc.***[116] caust. ***mang.*** nat-c.[116] nat-m.[58] nux-v.[116] sep.[116] tarent.[122] viol-o.[116] zinc.[116]
Irritability; music, during, piano, of: anac.[116] ***sep.***[116] zinc.[116]
Irritability; music, during, saddest: ***mang.***[36]
Irritability; music, give music lessons, cannot: ***kali-br.***[54]
Mania; midnight, dancing, laughing, striking, with: cic.[30]
Mania; singing, with: bell.[10] cann-i.[60] cic.[149] ***cocc.***[54] cupr.[60] hyos.[60] ***nux-m.***[54] ***plat.***[54] stram.[60] ***tarent.***[54] ***verat.***[10]
Memory; active, music, for: croc.[10] lyc.[60]
Memory; weakness, music, for: ign.[58] lyc.[30] staph.[30] sulfa.[149]
Moaning; alternating with, dancing: bell.[10]
Moaning; alternating with, songs, gambols: bell.[36]
Morose; alternating with, singing: croc.[10]
Morose; music, agg., sad: ***mang.***[36]
Morose; music, amel.: mang.[10]
Music; agg.: **ACON.**[5] all-c.[137] ambr.[5] anac.[116] ant-c. bry.[5] bufo[117] cact.[122] calc.[116] ***carc.***[122] caust.[122] cham.[5] coff.[5] cop. croc.[137] ***dig.***[5] graph.[5] ***ign.***[5] ***kali-br.***[8] kali-n. kreos.[36] lyc.[5] mang.[36] merc.[122] nat-c. nat-m.[155] nat-p.[122] nat-s.[5] **NUX-V.**[1] phos.[155] plb.[137] ***sabal.***[137] sabin.[5] sumb.[36] tarent.[5] ***thuj.***[5] viol-o.[5] zinc.[116]
Music; agg. piano playing: all-c.[137] anac.[116] cham.[122] cop.[36] ***kali-br.***[8] ***nat-c.***[8] nat-s.[137] ***phos.***[8] sep.[5] zinc.[116]
Music; agreeable, is: cann-i.[36] ign.[1] tarent.[116]
Music; amel.: am-m.[122] ambr.[1189] androc.[222] anh.[119] **AUR.**[5] carc.[193] cupr.[193] hydrog.[222] merc.[193] nat-m.[5] sul-ac.[5] sumb.[5] <u>**TARENT.**</u>[122] ***thuj.***[5] tub.[5]
Music; amel. rhythmical: tarent.[231]
Music; amel. sad: mang.[1]
Music; aversion to: **ACON.**[122] alum.[30] bufo[54] carc.[144] caust.[36] cham.[36] hep.[30] merc.[10] nit-ac.[30] ***nux-v.***[5] ph-ac.[60] sabin.[5] sep.[144] tab.[60] viol-o.[36]
Music; aversion to, joyous, to, but immediately affected by saddest: mang.[54]
Music; aversion to, violin especially: viol-o.[36]
Music; carried by, sensation of being: anh.[119]
Music; desires: bamb-a.[1184] ***carc.***[187] staph.[30]
Music; desires, playing piano: chlf.[36] kali-n.[209] ***plat.***[54]
Music; desires, sad, melancholic: ozone[227]
Music; drums produce euphoria: anh.[119]
Play; piano, upon the, for hours, in puerperal mania: ***plat.***[54]
Quarrelsomeness; alternating with, singing: croc.
Religious affections; songs: raja-s.[149]
Restlessness; anxious, thunderstorm, especially during, music agg.: ***nat-c.***[54]
Restlessness; music, from: nat-c. sabin.[102] tarent.
Restlessness; noises and singing in ears, with: ***coff.***[54]
Sadness; music, from: ***acon.*** ***ambr.***[102] ars.[171] bor.[58] calc-p.[198] cham. ***dig.*** ***graph.*** ***kreos.*** lyc. ***nat-c.*** nat-m.[58] nat-p. ***nat-s.*** nux-v. ph-ac.[1065] phos. ***sabin.*** sep. tarent. thuj. tub.[1065]
Sadness; whistling and singing, with: merc-i-f.[54]
Sensitive; music, bird songs: choc.[222]

Sensitive; music, continues to hear the music he heard during day in the evening: lyc.[85]
Sensitive; music, every note causes stitches in ear, violent pains in head: ph-ac.[85]
Sensitive; music, piano: anac.[116] nat-c.[10] sep.[10] zinc.[116]
Sensitive; music, sacred m, to: lyss.[54] thuj.[122]
Sensitive; music, to: ***acon.*** aloe[117] ***ambr.*** anac.[116] androc.[222] aur.[46] bry.[5] bufo cact. ***calc.***[116] carb-an. ***carc.***[119] caust. ***cham.*** choc.[222] coff. cop.[122] croc.[5] cupr.[5] dig. ***graph.*** ign.[5] ip.[155] ***kreos.*** ***lyc.*** merc. **NAT-C.** ***nat-m.*** nat-p. ***nat-s.*** **NUX-V.** pall.[116] ***ph-ac.*** phos. psil.[164] puls.[5] ***sabal.***[137] ***sabin.*** **SEP.** stann. sulph.[122] ***tab.***[122] ***tarent.*** thuj. tub.[85] tub-k.[85] viol-o. zinc. zinc-p.[58]
Sensitive; music, violin: ***viol-o.***[5]
Sensitive; noise, music, amel: **AUR.** carc.[207] **TARENT.**
Sensitive; singing, to: lyss.[54] nux-v.
Sensitive; singing, to, involuntary joins in on hearing anyone sing: croc.[85]
Sighing; alternating with, dancing and jumping: bell.[36]
Singing: acon. agar. alco.[36] anan.[36] apis aur.[10] ***bell.*** cann-i. cann-s. caps. ***carbn-s.*** chin.[30] chlf. ***cic.*** ***cocc.*** cot.[36] ***croc.*** cupr. cupr-acet.[36] der. eup-pur.[8] ferr-p.[111] gels. hydr. hydrog.[222] ***hyos.*** ***hyper.***[8] kali-br.[36] kali-c. ***lach.*** lachn. lact. lap-mar-c.[194] lob-c. lyc. lyss. ***m-arct.***[10] mag-c. manc. merc-i-f. merl. mez. nat-c. nat-m. nux-m. op. ozone[227] peti.[36] ph-ac. phos. ***plat.*** plb.[36] psil.[164] sant.[85] sars. sep. ***spong.*** ***stram.*** sulo-ac. sulph.[5] tab. tarent. ***teucr.*** ther. ***verat.***
Singing; alternating with, anger and quarrelsomeness: croc.
Singing; alternating with, hatred of work: spong.
Singing; alternating with, vexation: agar. croc.
Singing; Latin paternosters: ***stram.***[54]
Singing; obscene songs: alco.[36] canth.[58] ***hyos.*** op. raja-s.[149] stram. verat.[58]
Singing; obscene songs, nymphomania, in: ***stram.***[54]
Singing; sadness, after: merc-i-f.[54]
Singing; singing, dancing and weeping: tarent.[58]
Singing; touches things constantly: bell.[54]
Suicidal disposition; music, from listening to: nat-c.[58]
Talk; alternating with singing: ***gels.***[54]
Thoughts; persistent, music, about, night: **PULS.**[122]
Thoughts; persistent, music, evening: ign.
Thoughts; persistent, music, song since four p.m.: myris.[36]
Trance; plays on piano with closed eyes, writes letters in an acquired language: ***camph.***[54]
Unconsciousness; music, from: cann-i. sumb.
Weeping; alternating with, dancing: bell.[10]
Weeping; children, music, from: thuj.[127]
Weeping; music, bells, of: ant-c. cop.[122]
Weeping; music, church music: ***thuj.***[184]
Weeping; music, from: acon.[5] all-c.[137] ***ambr.***[5] ant-c.[1] bor.[58] calc-p.[198] ***carc.***[193] cop.[36] croc.[111] dig. **GRAPH.** ign.[116] kali-n. kali-p.[102] ***kreos.*** ***mang.***[54] ***nat-c.*** nat-m.[122] nat-s. nux-v. tarent.[102] ***thuj.***
Weeping; music, organ, on hearing: **GRAPH.**[122]
Weeping; music, piano, of: all-c.[137] cop. ***nat-c.*** ***nat-s.***
Weeping; singing, while: hura

ACON. Ha, 521 - Lucid vision: he says, now my beloved (70 miles away) must have sung the difficult passage (of Beethoven) that I was just singing.
He, 2 - Clairvoyance; conscious that his beloved, miles away, was singing a certain piece.
ADAM. Sh, 100 - Sensitive to music that I know and like —very nostalgic. 20, 1M, 11:XX:XX
ANDROC. Sh, 140 - Very sensitive to music. During a black mood, almost any sort of music will shake me out of it. (7)
Sh, 141 - Danced all night in a frenzy, could not keep still, and was frustrated when the music finished. (29)
ARG-M. He, 4 - Imagines things about the military which he never liked; long forgotten old songs come into his mind.
BELL. Ha, 1361 - She bursts out in loud laughter, sings, and touches things near her.
He, 62 - Loud laughter, wild abandon, singing, whistling, lascivious conversation.
BRASS. Sh, 11 - I began to feel a little depressed; I'm definitely not in a party mood, desire to be still and quiet, maybe

listen to classical music, Bach, Chopin, something well composed and not Beethoven 08, 6C, 05:08:30

CAMPH. Al, 19 - Stripped naked, he danced wildly about, and attempted to jump out of the window.

He, 18-...one evening he went to the piano with closed eyes and played with great precision what at other times he could not have done without his notes; several times he wrote letters in an acquired (learned) language more correctly than in a waking state;...(clairvoyance)

CANN-I. Al, 36 - The sun seemed reeling (moving) from his place, and the clouds danced around him like a chorus.

Al, 69 - He seems to himself to be transformed into a vegetable existence, as a huge fern, and to be surrounded by clouds of music and perfume.

He, 15-...he is gradually swelling, his body becomes larger and larger; that someone calls him; that he hears numberless bells ringing most sweetly; imagines he hears music; shuts his eyes, and is lost for some time in the most delicious thoughts and dreams.

CAPS. Al, 18 - He is in a contented mood, is jocose, and sings, and still he becomes angry from the slightest causes.

He, 7 - He is in a content mood, is jocose, and sings, and still he becomes angry from the slightest cause.

CHOC. Sh, 104 - Rather than hearing the usual music I listen to, I wanted to hear a blackbird sing. The outdoors seems very familiar and my hands get excited at the thought of it.

Sh, 412 - Much more sensitive to music — especially happy music. It gives me incredible pleasure.01A, 30C, XX:XX:XX

CON. Al, 10 - The husband, who had been somewhat addicted to liquor, saw all sorts of animals dancing upon the bed, and "picked straws" a little.

CROC. Al, 5 - If any one happens to sing a single musical note, she begins involuntarily to sing, and then is obliged to laugh at herself; she however, soon sings in spite of her determination to stop. (sympathy)

CUR. Al, 3 - Fits of ecstasy at night, as if caused by hearing music.

DIG. Ha, 11 - Anxious apprehension (fear) of a sad kind, with great dejection, extremely aggravated by music.

GERM. Sh, 99 - Came in contact with very much hate and disgust within, and it made a deep impression on me. I have to be reconciled with those parts of me. I think that power can be used in a different way - not so destructive. I am no person. Feel I have no power when I meet people. Sometimes I feel I disappear. I am not in my body. My hands feel gone. My feet are cold; I don't like them. Yet I feel I have great power inside, especially I feel it when I get angry or when I sing. 18, 30C, 46:XX:XX

Sh, 69 - Want to sit alone in front of fire listening to music by myself. Fed up with people everywhere I go irritating me. Want to be looked after. 09, 9C, 01:11:00.

Sh, 182 - Engaged in my work and my music with fierce intensity. 08, 12C, 14:12:00

HURA. Al, 20 - Unusual inclination to weep, even when singing, followed by a suffocative feeling...

HYDR. Al, 4 - In high spirits; everything looked bright; felt happy, and wanted to sing.

HYDROG. Sh, 11 - I felt I had gone mad, possessed, hysterical laughter, singing and a feeling of non-reality, as if in a dream, out of the body — like my mind went out of the window. High one minute and then low. People asked if I was on speed. After seven hours, in the evening (7:30p.m.), the feeling changed to an angry mood and very irritable with a dry furry mouth,...l. 24, 30C, 00:00:45

Sh, 105 - I felt better when driving the car fast with company and loud music. 24, 30C, 03:XX:XX

Sh, 272 - Sudden thoughts of making love while cuddling child and listening to old song —very vivid. 08, 30C, 00:00:XX

HYOS. Al, 58 - He sings amorous and obscene songs.

He, 46 - Sings amorous and obscene songs.

He, 69 - Lascivious mania, uncovers body, especially sexual parts; sings amorous songs.

He, 41 - Comical alienation of mind; ludicrous actions like monkeys; makes ridiculous gestures like a dancing clown;...

IRID. sh, 48 - Desire to touch backs of hands on face. Enjoy touch on skin. Old memories of gentleness, delightfully feminine. Wearing bright pink (unusual!) and stroking my legs. Enjoying my skin, touching bottom, stroking it. Dancing erotically at 8.00 a.m. (one hour after remedy). Particularly joyous. Q1

Sh, 49 - Skin felt very alive, tactile, fingertips felt "awake." Feathers felt amazing. Skin to skin; very aware of contact of surfaces. More erotic dancing, morning. Q2

KALI-BR. Al, 25 - At times he cried most bitterly, yet twelve hours previously he was singing and dancing, saying he was "the happiest man alive".

MAG-C. Al, 931 - Dream that she was at a ball (dance) where they did not dance enough; also at first she could not get ready (fitted) with her dress.

Al, 964 - Dream of funeral; she was obliged to dress the hair of the company; also of balls and marriages.

MANG. Ha, 327 - Ill-humored, so that the most joyful music does not cheer (joy) him, but he feels as if refreshed by the most melancholy music.

NAT-C. He, 9 - Restlessness, with attacks of anxiety, especially during a thunderstorm; < from music.

NEON. Sh, 123 - Immediately after taking the remedy, everything stopped. I become very subdued and depressed. It felt like a void. No joy in birds singing. "How can I lift it?" 20, 6C, 00:00:00

NUX-V. Ha, 1273 - He cannot bear any noise or speaking; music and singing affect him strongly.

PHOS. He, 34-...full of fear, especially at piano; constantly on lookout (look carefully) for something to happen; ...sexual dreams and violent sexual excitement.

SABIN. Al, 5-...music was intolerable, it penetrated marrow and bone,...feeling of weakness, debility.

STRAM. Ha, 524 - He dances at night in the churchyard.

He, 68 - Hears dancing, music, sees men and hears them talk in foreign tongues.

He, 112 - Religious mania; pious (divine) looks, praying; restless nights; inspired talking, singing; despairs of her salvation.

SULPH. Al, 8 - Numerous morbid ideas, extremely disagreeable, causing rancor, though with also joyous thoughts (and melodies) mostly from the past, take possession of her they throng one upon another so that she cannot free herself from them during the day, with neglect of business,...

MUTILATED

Delusions; body, arms, cut off, are: bapt.[122]
- body, fingers, cut of: mosch.
- body, heart, has no: ozone[227]
- body, heart, has no, muscle, only feels a thin: ozone[227]
- body, legs, cut off, are: bapt.[122] bar-c. halo.[149] stram. tarent.
- body, one half cut off: ***stram.***[54]
- body, parts, absent: cocain.[137] cot.[102]
- body, parts, take away: ***bapt.***[122] daph.[122]
- body, toes cut of: mosch.
- cut through, he is: ***stram.***
- cut, two, in: ***bell.***[30] plat. stram.[30]
- dead, corpse, mutilated: ant-c. arn. con. mag-m. merc. nux-v. sep
- dissected, he will be: cann-i.
- head, rising up, tearing neck: bamb-a.[1184]
- headless: asar. calc-i. cocc.[8] cot.[139] nit-ac. nux-v.[10]
- mutilated bodies, find, will: lap-mar-c.[194]
- mutilated bodies, sees: ant-c. arn. con. mag-m. merc. ***nux-v.*** sep.
- penis, sees cut off penis on the grass: lap-mar-c.[194]
- rags, body torn into: phyt.[137]

Dreams; amputating a man's leg: atro.[36]
- ➤ body, arm, amputated: lob.[54]
- ➤ body, ears cut of, having: nat-c.
- ➤ body, face cut away, having one side of face: mag-m.[36]
- ➤ body, hands cut to pieces, being: sol-t-ae.[36]
- ➤ body, head, cut of: androc.[222] hura[36] nicc.[36]
- ➤ body, penis breaking off: kali-n.[36]
- ➤ body, penis, glands penis breaking off: kreos.[10]
- ➤ body, teeth, pulled out, being: cench.[58] nat-m.
- ➤ body, toe cut of: nat-s.[10]
- ➤ cutting, knife, of being cut with a, to pieces: lil-s.[36]
- ➤ cutting, seeing a person cut up: merc-s.[8] sulph.
- ➤ cutting, woman, of cutting a woman up for salting: calc-f.

➤ dead, bodies, arms cut off, with: hura[36]
➤ decapitation of people: ozone[227]
➤ heads: glon.[36] jac-c.[36]
➤ heads, picking up half roasted, which opened its eyes and spoke angrily, of: jac-c.[36]
➤ misfortune, woman has legs amputated because of him: ozone[227]
➤ mutilation: androc.[222] ant-c. arn.[10] con. hura m-arct.[10] mag-c. mag-m.[1] merc. ***nux-v.***
➤ scalped, of being: xan.[111]

Mutilating his body, inclination to: agar.[102] ars. bell.[102] hyos.[102] med.[212] stram.[102]

CON. Al, 1276 - Dreams of physical mutilation.

COT. Al, 1-...a feeling as if there was no foot. The head felt exceeding light, as if there were no solid head, and she could not articulate for some time, although she endeavored to do so....

HURA. Al, 709 - Restless night; dream about crimes, dead bodies (corpse), and children lying with their heads half cut off, while others were being decapitated.

MAG-M. Al, 715 - Dream that someone cut away one side of her face; that a skin was being taken from a dead body and the like.

NAT-C. Al, 18 - Anxiety and hasty (fast) restlessness all day; he could not keep the limbs still, especially the arms; obliged to stretch them; it seemed as though they would be torn (cut) asunder. (in two divided).

Al, DREAM, 1102-..;of marrying two women, of parties, walks, entertainments, and excursions on horseback, afterwards they were frequently anxious, of going astray (lost),of murders, having his ears cut off; also vexatious dreams; he would take a journey and could not get away from the place,(immobilization) and when has reached the first station was obliged to turn back, on account of something he had forgotten.

PULS. He, 46 - Dark suspicious and reserved manner; disturbed look on face; sleepless; looks for her bed in the yard (lost?); hides in a corner to escape from a little gray man who wanted to pull out her leg;...

STRAM. Ha, 360 - Sensation in the arms and legs as if the limbs were completely severed (separated, detached, cut of) from the body.

Ha, 361 - Sensation as if every portion of the limbs were completely severed in the joints from the other parts and could not be joined together again.

Ha, 363 - He feels his hands and feet as if separated in the joints, and he is inconsolable on account of this sensation.

He, 57 - Strange absurd ideas; thinks herself tall, double or lying crosswise; one half of body cut off (divided); bed is full of creases (wrinkle) (disorganization); that he was killed roasted and being eaten.

NAIVE

Childish behavior: acon. aeth.[137] ***agar.***[5] alco.[36] aloe[130] alum. ambr.[137] anac. ***apis arg-n.*** arn.[193] ars.[5] **<u>BAR-C.</u>**[122] ***bar-m.*** bell.[5] bov.[162] bufo calad. calc.[189] carb-an. carb-v. ***carbn-s.*** chlol. **CIC.** con.[137] ***croc.*** crot-c. germ.[222] ***hell.***[137] hyos.[5] ***ign.*** kali-br. kres.[144] lach.[137] lyc.[137] ***nat-c.***[137] ***nux-m.*** nux-v.[5] ***op.*** par. ***ph-ac.***[137] phos.[189] pic-ac.[137] plb.[137] puls. rhus-t. seneg. sep.[137] sil.[137] ***stram.*** sulfa.[114] sulph.[137] thyr.[137] tub.[193] verat.[137] viol-o.

Confiding: bar-c.[30] ***bell.***[30] hydrc. kres.[144] mur-ac. op.[36] ***puls.***[30] spig. staph.[30]

Delusions; born into the world and was overwhelmed with wonder at the novelty of his surroundings, feels as if newly: cori-r.[58]

Giggling: androc.[222] bamb-a.[1184] bufo[58] calc-s.[209] cann-i. choc.[222] germ.[222] hyosin.[36] kali-f.[209] nat-m.[162] stry.[36]

Obstinate; simpleton, as a: lyc.[30] plat.[30] verat.[30]

NATURE

Anxiety; environment, for: carc.[196]

Aversion; flowers, smell of: graph.[36]

Cares; full of, nature, for, animals, plants: lap-c-b.[194]

Charmed with description of beauties of nature: coff.[36]

Company, aversion to; country away from people, wants to get into the: androc.[222] calc. calc-p.[58] elaps merc.[137] sep.[137]

Country, desire for, to go into the: androc.[222] choc.[222] elaps[36] hydrog.[222]

Delirium; mild, roaring over fields or hard at work, he thinks he is: ***rhus-t.***[54]

Delusions; companions are half men, half plants: cann-i.
- flowers, of gigantic: cann-i.[36]
- roaming in the fields: rhus-t.
- room, hall in a garden, a bower, is a: calc.[1]
- trees are people in fantastic costume (afternoon, while riding): bell.
- wilderness, being in a: stram.[10]

Dreams; country: asc-t.[36]
- ➤ country beautiful: ol-an.[36] rumx.[36]
- ➤ flowers: mag-c. nat-s.
- ➤ forest, going astray in a forest: mag-m.[10] sep.[10]
- ➤ forest, of a: canth. com.[36] mag-m. sep.
- ➤ fruit, gathering in garden: mag-c.[36]
- ➤ fruit, hanging from trees in Winter: cast-eq.[36]
- ➤ gardens: com.[36] nat-s.[10] phel.[10]
- ➤ lost, forest, as in a: am-m. ind. mag-c. mag-m. mag-s. sep.
- ➤ lost, mountains, in the: ind.[36]
- ➤ men, green and covered with moss, living in water, changing into dogs: sol-t-ae.[36]
- ➤ mowing grain and clover, people: glon.[36]
- ➤ running, cross country: bac.[226]
- ➤ trees, of, growing on fences without ground under them: lyc.[54]
- ➤ vegetables: androc.[222]
- ➤ walking, woods, in: canth.[36]
- ➤ woodland: com.[36]

Longing; for, sunshine, light and society, for: grin. stram.

Love; nature, for: carc.[162] lap-c-b.[194]

Play; desire to, grass, in the: elaps.

Sadness; flowers, from smell of: hyos.

Sensitive; nature, to: carc.[227]

Sensitive; odors, to, flowers: all-c. chin. **GRAPH.** hyos. ***lac-c.*** lyc. **NUX-V. PHOS.** sabad.[137] sang.

Wander, desires to, home, from, and ranges in woods: ***elat.***[54]

ANDROC. Sh, 180 - Desire to be out in the country, intense desire to be on the rocks. Desire to feel the rocks, to stick hand beneath the rocks, to crawl into or behind rocks. (Clinical)

AUR-M. He, 6 - Everything is disagreeable, dreary (lugubrious, desolate, deserted), even nature around.

BELL. Al, 174 - He escaped, under some pretext, into the open field.(run away)
Ha, 1436 - He makes an excuse (pretext) and runs out into the open fields.

CALC. Al, 54 - Loss of consciousness, with illusion as regards place; it seems as if the room were a bower.

CAMPH. Al, 46-... The sight increased my despair poor nature extinguished; the sky transparent and lifeless; the earth was still in the dim, dead light. I could not bear it. The sense of touch was gone, and my eyes protruded from their sockets.

CHOC. Sh, 14 - Angry about being in city. When I look, I want to see far distances and sky, not houses. Went to estate agents to look at country houses.
Sh, 15 - I see plants in the house differently, very aware of them and want to give them more light.
Sh, 104 - Rather than hearing the usual music I listen to, I wanted to hear a blackbird sing. The outdoors seems very familiar and my hands get excited at the thought of it.
Sh, 130 - I feel slightly less like a hedgehog today, but the picture is still in my mind. Human things seem so trivial —so much energy wasted when you are human. Nature is so efficient. It never wastes a seed and we just spend energy every-where.
Sh, 135 - The earth has taken on a new meaning. Before it was just there, now it has everything. A desire to be in contact with the earth.
Sh, 182 - This remedy is making me look more deeply into things. Found myself looking into a flower, plugging into its inner substance. 35, 30C, 05:XX:XX

COFF. Al, 1 - Lively fancies; full of plans for the future; contrary to his custom is very much charmed by the beauties of nature,...
He, 24-...fear of fresh air and of least noise...

ELAPS. Al, 5 - Desire to go into to the country, and play about in the grass. (nature)

ELAT. He, 2 - Irresistible propensity to wander from home, even in the night, and range (distance) in woods.(forest)

FL-AC. Al, 8 - All nature seems to smile in the morning.

GERM. Sh, 26 - Feel more aware and connected looking at the sun trees and sky colors. 04, 6C, 01.00.00.

Sh, 21 - Contemplative, like nice things, sees beauty in stones and nature. Good at instinctive understanding, compassionate. 16, 30C, 01:XX:XX

Sh, 148 - The last days I have had moments when I have felt I have been united to the world and people - to humanity. Have felt more love and reconciliation towards myself and other people. Started to be more conscious about the environment and what I can do to our mutual benefit. Something is happening within me. I wish to get more contact with my feelings. 18, 30C, 64:XX:XX

HALI-L. Sh, 227 - Pictures of the mountains make me homesick. Deeper than homesick. Feeling low, remembering the freedom of going to them. Missing mountains and the outdoors. 02, 30C, 07:01:XX

Sh, 977 - Tears come easily, just on looking at an exhibition of wildlife —sobbing. It was beautiful and lit from the back. It was so beautiful I couldn't contain it. There were pictures of a bald eagle and of a hedgehog right next to each other. 20, 30C, 20:XX:XX

HYDROG. Sh, 8 - I felt slightly high, removed from reality, yet very alert, clear and calm. Very aware of the colour of the sky, the light, birds singing, flowers —like a pastoral ideal. Feeling of expansiveness, mentally cool, airy and light. 28, 200C, 00:04:XX

Sh, 294 - Spirits uplifted by wonderful weather. Felt strong, positive and adventurous. 04, 12C, 32:XX:XX

IRID. Sh, 76 - Twice now I have overtaken cars going up the hill out of town which were going only marginally slower than me. Had to get past them, urgency to get to the top out of the valley. G7

Sh, 77 - A sudden, very deep desire for wilderness, space and air and height. E15

Sh, 79 - Had this longing to find real wilderness. Britain is too full, nothing is really alive anymore except people. The world really feels too oppressed with people and roofs. I kept saying to partner, "Why do we live in this dreary, ugly place, where people know nothing about freedom, and certainly nothing about discovery or mystery, just tarmac and roofs." It struck me that the world was too small for me, and thought "That's got to be something about the remedy, something around pressure." E5

Sh, 87 - Somerset countryside not big enough. E14

KALI-FCY. Al, 1 - Feeling of sadness and some disposition to tears, caused by an impression that he was soon to die and leave his friends; disposition to take a sad view of the beauties of autumn; the apprehension of approaching sickness and death can be overcome by reason, but soon returns.

MAG-C. Al, 926 - Dream of gathering fruit in a garden.

Al, 932 - Dream of flowers, clothes, and other things; she had to make up the clothes, but had no inclination to do it, and besides did not understand how; she also saw many foreign plants, but during this she became soaked (wet) with rain.

MAG-M. Al, 710 - Dream that she became confused in a forest, and for a long time could not find her way.

NAT-M. He, 11-, ...uttered the most atrocious blasphemes, swore (blaspheme, curse) against God (divine) and the elements (environment), and after raging for awhile became exhausted,...

NEON. Sh, 38 - I have always felt comfortable with the division between the dark and the light. What I now need is the division of heavens and oceans. Thoughts about my love for the Pacific Ocean. 20, 6C, 06:XX:XX

Sh, 54 - I just long for some clear nights, so I can see my stars. If I could reconnect, then everything would be all right. 02, 6C, 11:XX:XX

RHUS-T. He, 5 - Low, mild delirium, thinks he is roaming (wander, travel) over fields, or hard at work.

NEGLIGENCE

Absent-mindedness; standing in one place, never accomplishes what he undertakes: med.[162] ***nux-m.***[54]

Anxiety; duty, as if had not done his: ars.[36] puls.[172]

Anxiety; duty, as if he had not done his, religious, produced by lascivious impulses: ***orig.***[54]

Anxiety; lascivious impulses, from, on account of disinclination of religious duties in a married woman, mother of a family: ***orig.***[54]
Business; averse to: acon-l.[122] agar. aloe[130] am-c. anac. androc.[222] arg-n.[137] arn.[5] ars. ars-h. asar.[54] aur-m. bapt.[137] ***brom.*** calc.[58] carb-v.[137] chel.[137] ***chin.***[137] chin-s. cimic. ***con.*** cop. cycl.[137] fl-ac. graph. ham.[137] hipp. kali-ar. kali-bi. kali-br. kali-c. kali-i. kali-s. lac-ac. ***lach.*** laur. lil-t. lyc.[1] mag-s. nat-ar.[58] nat-c.[30] **NAT-M.**[137] nux-v.[36] opun-a.[36] ***ph-ac.***[122] ***phos.***[137] ***phyt.*** psor.[137] ***puls.*** rhod.[58] rhus-t.[30] **SEP.** stann.[58] ***stram.***[5] ***sulph.***[58] syph.[58] ther.[54]
Business; neglects his: opun-a.[36] ptel.[144] ***sulph.***[36]
Carefree: ham.[5] laur.[5] op.[5] phos.[5] tarax.[5] zinc.[5]
Delusions; neglected his duty, he has: ars.[36] **AUR.** cur.[137] cycl. hell.[58] hyos. ign. ***lyc.*** naja[36] nat-ar. ptel.[36] puls.
- neglected, duty, his, deserves reproach: aur.[54] germ.[222]
- neglected, duty, his, headache, during: naja[36]
- neglected, duty, his, perfunctory manner, performed in: ptel.[36]
- neglected, friends, his: ***aur.***[58]
- reproach, has neglect duty and deserves: ***aur.***
- sick, he is, work, and for this reason will not: calc.[30] caust.[30] nux-v.[30] sep.[30]
- vow, breaking her: ign.

Dereliction, sensation of: bar-c.[10] carb-an.[10] nat-c.[10] plat.[10] stram.[10]
Dreams; business, neglected: hyper. myris. sil. stann.
- ➤ children, about, neglecting her: bamb-a.[1184]
- ➤ clothing, did not wish to make up: mag-c.[36]
- ➤ conversations, ending, never, forgetting people that are waiting for her: ozone[227]

Duty; want of sense of: alum.[30] ambr.[30] anac.[30] ars.[30] **CALC.**[36] cench.[58] coloc.[30] hep.[30] lach.[30] merc.[30] nat-m.[30] ptel.[36] sil.[30] sulph.[30]
Fear; duty, neglect her, to: aur.[30]
Forgetfulness; watch, to wind his: fl-ac.
Grief; neglected duty, over: cycl.[102]
Handle things anymore, cannot, responsible for everything, does not want to be: bamb-a.[1184]
Handle things anymore, cannot, support, looks for: bamb-a.[1184]
Handle things anymore, cannot, weight, wants to throw off the: bamb-a.[1184]
Heedless; business, about: myris.[36]
Heedless; talking and writing, in: carl.[36]
Indifference; business affairs, to: aesc.[162] agar. ***arg-n. arn.***[10] bamb-a.[1184] ***fl-ac.*** ham.[122] ***kali-bi.*** kali-p.[58] myris. nat-ar. ***ph-ac.*** phys. phyt.[58] psil.[164] ***ptel. puls.*** rhus-t.[162] ***sep. stram. sulph.***
Indifference; conscience, to the dictates of: cann-i. caust.[30] con.[30] graph.[30] petr.[30]
Indifference; important, things, to: calc. fl-ac.
Indifference; work aversion to: agar.[10] allox.[119] androc.[222] camph.[54] ign.[10] kali-m.[192] lach.[10] rhod.[54] squil.[10] staph.[10]
Indolence; difficulties, in face of: cocc.[54]
Indolence; housework, aversion to her usual: bamb-a.[1184] cench.[58] ***cit-ac.*** cit-l.[54] sep.[137] sul-i.[58]
Late, always too: calc.[30] cand-a.[239] plat.[30] puls.[30] sil.[30]
Neglects; children, her: aur-ar.[58]
Neglects; everything: am-c.[30] bar-c.[30] caust.[30] tell.[36]
Neglects; household, the: aur-ar.[58] sul-i.[58]
Neglects; important things: alum.[30] con.[30] kali-m.[192]
Persists in nothing: alum.[111] asaf.[137] aur.[1] bar-c.[10] calc.[189] grat.[54] lac-c. lach. lyc.[36] nux-v.[155] plan. ***sil.***[111] stann.[1] sulph.[111]
Postponing everything to next day: androc.[222] apis[117] bamb-a.[1184] calc.[189] hydrog.[222] ***med.***[54] ***nat-m.***[30] nux-v.[30] ozone[227] plat.[30] sil.[30] stram.[108]
Reproaches; accomplished enough, because he had not: ars.[54]
Responsibility, aversion to: lac-h.[229] lap-mar-c.[194] lyc.[109] ***med.***[122] phos.[62]
Responsibility; wants to give up her: sep.[187]
Restlessness; duty, as if he had not done his: ***puls.***[54]
Sadness; conscience, of, as if he had committed a bad action, or not done his duty: cycl.[54]
Sadness; disease, about, incurable, of heart, which makes him reckless: ***phos.***[54]
Time; fritters away his: bamb-a.[1184] bor.[10] cocc. croto-t.[10] lach.[10] ***nat-c.***[10] nat-m.[10] nux-v. stann.[10] staph.[30] ***sulph.***[10] tab.[30]
Undertakes; many things, perseveres in

nothing: ***acon.*** alum.[30] androc.[222] ant-c.[102] apis[83] bism.[1] bor.[1] canth.[85] cortico.[119] graph.[30] grat.[137] ign.[58] ***lac-c. lach.*** **LIL-T.**[36] lyc.[36] med.[179] ***nux-m.***[54] petr.[30] phos.[189] pin-s.[36] plan. sanic.[108] stann.[30] sulph.[81] verat.[1]

Unreliable; promises, in his: bell.[30] calc.[30] con.[30] lyc.[30] merc.[30] op.[30] sil.[30] sulph.[30]

Unsympathetic; unscrupulous, idleness, from: con.[54]

AIL. Al, 4 - Recklessness (careless) in regard (respect) to present and future.

ARS. Ha, 53 - Dissatisfied all day and extremely vexed at himself; he thought he had not worked enough and reproached himself most bitterly.

AUR. Ha, 346 - Remorse about his idleness (indolence), and yet he cannot work at anything; it drives him out of the house, he must always moving.

Ha, 347 - Always very restless and undecided (doubtful) -thought he was neglecting something for which he must incur (obtain) reproach - ...he seemed to carry about this restlessness with him in his inmost (deepest) parts ; this condition deprived him of all perseverance, all energy.

Ha, 13 - Restless and undecided, without perceptible ebullition of the blood; he always thinks he is neglecting something for which he will be reproached; he seems to carry with him this internal restlessness, and it took from him all perseverance and energy.

CALC-P. He, 11 - Does not want to do what he has to do.

CALC. He, 34 - Does not care to get well, or to do anything to assist (aid) recovery.

CON. He, 14 - Likes to wear his best clothes, (vanity) makes useless purchases, (squander) cares very little for things (indifferent), wastes or ruins them; does not want to work, prefers to play. (wanderer)

He, 33 - Timid, cannot be persuaded to work ; want of proper will. (lack of: resolution) (vagabond)

CUPR. Ha, 10 - Indisposition to work, and yet idleness is a burden to him.

CUR. Al, 11 - Great despondency (grief) ; becomes reckless (careless) about himself.

CYCL. Al, 10 - Internal grief and anxiety of conscience, as though he had not done his duty, or had committed a crime.

Ha, 196 - Inward grief and anxiety of conscience, as if he had not done his duty or had committed a crime.

Ha, 197 - Excessive sadness, as if he had done something bad and had neglected his duty.

He, 12 - Great sadness, as if he had committed a bad action or not done his duty.

HALI-L. Sh, 171 - Made a decision to play cards with my friend at work even though a guard who has been hassling me was nearby. She makes me uncomfortable. Decided not to let that person's presence get in the way of my life. Did it very confidently. Very confident! Confidence to accept and to go about my business without making detours. 18, 30C, 03:02:00

Sh, 389 - Hadn't studied for exams; normally would be extremely anxious. This time totally centered, hunkered down into hips, knew I didn't know the material. It was a nice exam. Enjoyed it. Feel no anxiety regarding exams. 02, 30C, 05:XX:XX

HAM. Al, 14 - I became impatient, and resolved not to take anymore of the medicine; felt as if I did not care whether I attended (guard) to my practice or not; did not want any one to call at the office for medicine.

HELL. Al,S-1 Happy carelessness about everything; feel indifferent to family.

IGN. He, 11-...believes herself married (connected) and pregnant; is tormented by remorse of imagined crimes; seeks constantly to escape to drown (suicide) herself; ...;is only quiet when lying undisturbed and brooding over her troubles, which she rehearses (tell) in a doleful (unhappy) tone ;..." I am neglecting my duty, breaking my vow" (promise, engagement)...;conscientious scruples after eating.

MED. Al,N-40 - Always wakens tired in the morning; hates to do anything that must be done (duty), even nice things; gets nervous and excited about riding and driving as soon the time is fixed.

NAJA. Al, 13-...I felt that everything that was done was done in a wrong way, and could not be rectified (corrected, revised);

if I felt that I had some duty to perform (execute), I had at the same time a strong impulse not to do it, and I am extremely restless in consequence; I seemed to have an increased perception of what I ought to do, but, at the same time, an unaccountable inclination not to do it, to which I was irresistibly compelled to yield "I couldn't help it, didn't know why, but couldn't do it."

NAT-C. Al, 56 - He has no desire to do anything, and can keep at nothing long.

NEON. Sh, 169 - Averse to doing practical jobs and put them off. I have not panicked as usual because I haven't done them. 10, 6C, 01:XX:XX

PTEL. Al, 21 - Able to examine the papers, but inclined to hurry with it, and in selecting the remedy, inclined to follow Fred Humphrey's rule, "First impressions are the best". (hastily, rapidly, quickly) (heedless)

PULS. Ha, 1120 - Restless state of the disposition, as if did not do his duty properly.

Ha, 1122 - Neglect of his business, hesitancy (indecision), sobbing (cry) respiration and loss of composure.(calm, serenity)

Ha, 1123 - Sometimes he wants to do one thing, sometimes another, and when he is given something to do, he will not do it.

He, 9 - Shuns business; irresolute; sighing respiration; feels as if he were beside himself.

SPIG. Al, 8 - Anxious forebodings, therewith inclination to a peevish indolent mood.

STANN. Al, 21 - Indolent and irritable, with heat in the face; would do everything, but really does nothing.

STRAM. Al, 48 - She is all the time inconsolable; much affected by trifles; makes much fuss about trifles; disposed to weep, and sometimes also very easily vexed; now and then neglects her duties; now and then thinks she is not fitted for her position ; after the fall equinox...; she wants light and company.

He, 177-...sometimes vexed; neglects her duties, thinks she is not fitted for her position;...

SULPH. Al, 8 - Numerous morbid ideas, extremely disagreeable, causing rancor, though with also joyous thoughts (and melodies) mostly from the past, take possession of her they throng one upon another so that she cannot free herself from them during the day, with neglect of business,...

Al, 94 - He sits for hours immovable and indolent, without definite thought, though he has much to accomplish.

Ha, 51 - For hours he sits motionless and indolent, without any definite thoughts, though he has many things to attend to.

He, 8 - Numerous morbid ideas, extremely disagreeable, causing rancor; neglect of business;...

TELL. Al, 3 - He forgets and neglects (ignores, indifference) much; also the writing down, and even the observing of symptoms ...when thinking of the one, or of any business, he forgets everything else, and on account of this he neglects much that is necessary.

NEWS

Ailments from; bad news: acon.[102] aln.[85] alum.[8] alumn.[85] ambr.[1189] ***apis arn.***[122] ars.[102] art-v.[85] aur.[102] aur-m.[122] bapt.[91] ***bry.***[102] **CALC.** calc-p. calc-s.[108] carc.[185] caust.[102] ***cham.***[102] chin. cic.[36] cinnb. cocc.[102] colch.[102] ***coloc.***[102] cupr. dig.[58] dros. form. **GELS.**[122] grat.[102] hist.[144] hyos.[102] ***ign.*** kali-c. kali-p. lac-v.[56] lach. ***lyc.***[122] lyss. manc.[162] ***med.*** mez.[8] nat-c. ***nat-m.*** nat-p. ***nit-ac.***[122] ***nux-v.***[102] paeon. ***pall.*** ph-ac.[85] phos. podo.[8] puls. sabin.[58] sep.[102] ***sil.***[122] ***staph.***[102] stram. ***sulph.*** tarent.[36] teucr.[58] zinc.[54]

Ailments from; bad news, mortifying, affects him very much: lyss.[54]

Anger; bad news: calc-p.[36]

Anxiety; news, as if he would hear unpleasant: dros.[36]

Beside oneself; news, after unpleasant: calc-p.[54]

Delusions; newspapers, he sees: atro.
- unpleasant, news, he is expecting: mez.[139]

Dullness; bad news, from: calc-p.

Excitement; bad news, after: ***apis calc.*** calc-p. chin. cinnb. cupr. form. **GELS.** ***ign.*** kali-c. kali-p. lach. nat-c. nat-m. phos. puls. stram. ***sulph.***

Fear; bad news, about to arrive, tears afford relieve, hysteric, as if: ***aster.***[8]

- ✦ bad news, of hearing: apis[162] aster.[54] calc.[1] ***calc-p.*** dirc.[36] dros. gels.[172] kali-c.[172] ***lyss.***[54] nat-m.[172] nat-p.
- ✦ bad news, of hearing, day time: dirc.[36]
- ✦ bad news, of hearing, weak afterwards: calc-p.[54]

Indifference; important, news, to: ars-h.[54]
News, unpleasant, he feels like after: alum.[54]
Sadness; bad news, after: calc-p. pall.[54] puls.
Weeping; sad, news, at: carb-v.[36] ph-ac.[122]
Wildness; bad news, from: calc-p.

ALUMN. Al, 9 - Excitability of feeling, as when one is agitated by unpleasant news.
He, 3 - Feels like after unpleasant news.
He, 6 - Unpleasant (bad) news excites and causes nervous tremors.
APIS. He, 81 - Ailments from fright, rage, vexation, jealousy, or hearing bad news.
ASTER. Al, 6 - Feeling of excessive anguish...it seems as if some misfortune was impending, as if he was going to hear bad news ...
He, 9 - It seems as if some misfortune was impending, as if bad news was about to arrive...
CALC-A. Al, 7 - Apprehensive, sad mood, as though he were awaiting some depressing news.
Ha, 264 - Very sad humor, as if he had to expect (anticipation) bad news.
CALC-P. Al, 16 - Unpleasant news makes him beside himself; sweat breaks out; inclined to indignation and anger.
He, 18 - Unpleasant news brings him beside himself; sweat breaks out.
CALC. Ha, 24 - Anxious, sad mood, as if he had to expect sad news.
COCC. He, 545 - He dreads any sudden surprise.
COFF. He, 23 - Fright from sudden pleasant surprises.
He, 35 - Affections after sudden emotions, particularly pleasant surprises.(ailments from)
DIRC. Al, 2 - In day time was constantly expecting some bad news; everything seemed worry and annoy.
DROS. Ha, 269 - Anxiety with feeling of heat quickly running all over the body, but especially all over the face, as though he were about to receive bad news ...rigor all over the body, without heat and without thirst.
GELS. He, 29 - Every exciting news causes diarrhea ; bad effects from fright and fear. (ailments from)
He, 30 - Bad effects (ailments) from suddenly hearing bad news; from fright(fear); diarrhea, abortion etc.
He, 32 - Complaints: (ailments) from exciting or bad news; sudden emotions; the anticipation of any unusual ordeal (difficulty) ; general depression from heat of sun or summer.
IGN. He, 62 - Ill effects (ailments) from hearing bad news; from vexation with reserved displeasure ; from grief, or suppressed mental sufferings; of shame and disappointed love.
LYSS. Al, 12 - Feeling as if I had heard, or was about to hear something bad...
Al,N-121 - Mortifying news affects him very much.
Al,N-75 - He feels as if he had heard unpleasant news, or would soon hear it; until 4 p.m.
MANG. Ha, 326 - Persistent restlessness of disposition, just as if he were going to hear some bad news.
Ha, 2 - Constant restlessness, as if he apprehended some sad news.
MED. Al,N-47 - It feels the evil coming to it, and the bad news before it arrives (clairvoyance), of course it is selfish, and it is easily hurt by a harsh (rude) word.
He, 32 - Everything startles her, news coming to her seems to touch her heart before she hears it.
MEZ. He, 5 - No rest when alone; wants to be in company ...unable to repeat what has been learned by heart; looks through window for hours, without being conscious of objects around; knows not what she is about; forgets what she is about to utter (talk); looks ill humored, pale, wretched, fallen away; ......expecting some very unpleasant news.
NAT-P. Al, 7 - Felt anxious about home (homesickness?); had misgivings (worry) ; feared bad news.
PAEON. He, 1 - Anxious, afraid (fear) to talk with any one; much affected by bad news, after pinching in belly.
PALL. He, 15 - Depressing news makes all her symptoms worse.
PHOS. Al, 94 - Anxiety; oppressed, as if I

had heard unpleasant (bad) news.
Al, 100 - She is made anxious by a disagreeable event, mingled with fear and vexation, and inclined to weep.
PULS. Al, 28 - He sinks into a condition of sadness and despondency from disagreeable news.
Ha, 1131 - On hearing some disagreeable news he became affected with sadness and despondency.
He, 51 - Sinks into a condition of sadness and despondency (grief) from disagreeable news.(ailments from)
SEP. Al, 33 - Received news of the slight illness of a friend, which caused great mental depression (at another time it would not have made slightest impression); this condition grew on me until I became so nervous that I felt that unless I held on something, I should scream.

NOISE

Anger; noise, at: bamb-a.[1184] hep.[30] ip.[36]
Anxiety; church bells, from hearing: ***lyss.***
Anxiety; fire were breaking out, as if, morning, on being awakened by noise in the street: tet.[36]
Anxiety; music, from, church bells: lyss.[122]
Anxiety; waking, on, something under the bed making a noise, from: ars.[172] bell.
Aversion; noise, to: ferr.[36] kali-m.[192] raph.[36] zinc.[36]
Cares; full of, noise, by, or interruption in business: ***lyc.***[54]
Complaining; noise, about too much: ign.[1]
Delusions; bed, someone, under it, knocking: bell.[5] calc. canth. colch.[5]
- bells, hears: ars.[36] cann-i. med.[185] ph-ac. thea. verat.[185]
- bells, hears, door bell: thea.
- blood, rushed through like roar of many waters: alumn.[58] cann-i.
- fire, every noise is a cry of fire, she thinks and she trembles: bar-c.
- growling as of a bear, hears: mag-m.
- hearing, of, objects moving: ph-ac.[1]
- hearing, of, someone approaches his bed: carb-v.[54]
- hearing, of, sounds, are coming from left side when they really come from the right: ***nat-c.***[122]
- hearing, of, sounds, color, are like: anh.[119]
- hearing, of, sounds, distant, are: coca[25] lac-c.[137] sabal.[137]
- hearing, of, sounds, double, whistling, are: med.[8]
- hearing, of, tone, comes from another world: **CARB-AN.**[54]
- noise, hears: anh.[144] bell. calc. canth.[5] carb-v. cham. cocain.[102] coff.[58] colch. con. hyos. mag-m. naja[98] ph-ac.[5] sulph.[1] verat.[10]
- noise, hears, bed, under: bell.[1]
- noise, hears, clattering above the bed when going to sleep: calc.
- noise, hears, knocking at the door: ant-c.[1]
- noise, hears, making a, delusions with: verat.[10]
- people, noise, making: puls.[122]
- sounds, listens to imaginary: hyos.
- wind sighing in chimney sounds like the hum of a vast wheel, and reverberates like a peal of thunder on a grand organ: cann-i.

Dreams; noise: atro.[36] cere-b.[36] lyc.[36] stann.[36]
➤ sound in the brain, as if beating on a metal that was swinging freely, amel. gradually after waking, five am: phel.[36]
➤ wind raised him in bed, and a storm howled through right side of upper part of head, before midnight: mill.[36]

Excitement; water poured out, from hearing: **LYSS. STRAM.**
Fear; death, noise of door moving, from, in dark: ozone[227]
✦ door, bell ringing, on hearing: lyc.[137]
✦ everything, constant of, ringing of a door bell, even at: ***lyc.***[54]
✦ noise, from: acon.[102] agar. aloe alum. ***ant-c. asar.***[102] ***aur.*** bar-c. ***bell.***[102] ***bor.*** calad.[102] cann-s. caps. carc.[227] ***caust. cham.***[102] chel. chin.[30] cic. ***cocc.*** coff. ferr.[102] gaert.[136] hipp. hura ign.[102] kali-c.[102] kali-s.[127] ***lyc.***[122] mag-m.[102] med.[102] mosch. nat-c. ***nat-s.*** nit-ac.[102] nux-v. petr. ***phos.***[102] pip-n.[172] puls. sabad. sep.[172] **SIL.** sulph.[30] tab. tanac.[102] tarent.[102] ***ther.***[102] zinc.[102]
✦ noise, from, door, at: ***aur.*** cic. ***lyc.***
✦ noise, from, night, emission, after: aloe[54]
✦ noise, from, rushing water, of: bell.[172] canth.[172] hyos.[58] **LYSS. STRAM.** sulph.[172]
✦ noise, from, street, in: bar-c. ***caust.***
✦ noise, from, sudden, of: ***bor. cocc.*** lap-c-b.[194]
✦ noise, night: bar-c. ***caust. nat-s.***
✦ telephone, of: visc.[119]

Frightened; easily, waking, in a fright from least noise: nux-v.

Hysteria; light and noise agg.: ***stict.***[54]

Irritability; noise, from: allox.[119] androc.[222] ant-t. ars. bad.[1] bell. caust. cinnb. cocc. ***ferr.*** iod. ip. kali-c. nat-c.[58] nat-m.[58] ozone[227] phos. pip-m. plect. ptel. puls-n. seq-s.[230] trio.[149] ven-m.[149]

Irritability; noise, from, crackling of newspapers, even from: ***asar.***[116] ***ferr.*** lyc.[58] nat-c.[58]

Noise; inclined to make a: acon.[137] **BELL.**[5] cham.[137] cic.[137] merc.[36] op.[36] verat.[36]

Quiet disposition; noise, intolerant to: con.[10]

Rage; noise, from least: ***zinc.***[54]

Reserved; noise, with sensitivity to: con.[10]

Restlessness; noises and singing in ears, with: ***coff.***[54]

Sadness; noise, from: ant-c. nat-c.[58] phos.

Sadness; sound of bells and sight of his surroundings, agg. by: ant-c.[36]

Sensitive; noise, aversion to: asar.[137] bor.[137] con.[137] ferr.[36] kali-c.[137] op.[137] raph.[36] zinc.[36]

Sensitive; noise, birds, of: bamb-a.[1184]

Sensitive; noise, car, traveling on the street: nit-ac.[58]

Sensitive; noise, crackling of paper, to: ***asar.***[116] bor. calad. ferr. lyc.[58] ***nat-c.*** nat-s.[137] tarax.[1] ther.[103] zinc.

Sensitive; noise, music, amel: **AUR.** carc.[207] **TARENT.**

Sensitive; noise, others eat apples, hawk or blow their noses, cannot bear to hear: lyss.[54]

Sensitive; noise, painful sensitiveness to: am-c.[54] arn.[54] ***coff.***[54] ***con.***[54] ***nux-v.***[122] ***sang.***[54] seneg.[54] ***sil.***[54] ***spig.***[54]

Sensitive; noise, penetrating: ***asar.***[111] bar-c.[111] chin.[111] cocc.[111] con.[111] ferr.[111] iod.[111] lept.[111] lil-t.[111] lyc.[111] manc.[111] mur-ac.[111] sabin.[111] ***ther.***[111]

Sensitive; noise, slightest: acon. aloe alum-sil.[58] ant-c. arg-n. ars.[54] **ASAR.**[122] bar-c. ***bell.***[54] ***bor.*** bufo[98] chin.[31] cinnb. ***cocc.***[54] **COFF.**[122] ***ferr.*** lach.[58] ***lyc.*** nat-c.[58] nat-s. nux-m.[171] **NUX-V.** **OP.** petr.[193] ***phos.*** ***sabin.*** ***sep.***[122] **SIL.** **THER.**[122] uva.[162] xan.[85]

Sensitive; noise, striking of clocks, ringing of bells, to: **ASAR.**[122] **COFF.**[122] dros.[122] **THER.**[122]

Sensitive; noise, sudden: **BOR.**[5] calad.[137] cocc.[137] lap-c-b.[194] nat-c.[137] nat-m.[137]

Sensitive; noise, to: achy.[149] **ACON.** agar.[163] allox.[119] aloe alum. alum-p.[58] alum-sil.[58] am-c. ambr. anac.[5] androc.[222] ***ang.***[5] anh.[119] ant-c. ant-t. apis aquil.[102] aran-ix.[119] ***arg-n.*** ***arn.*** ***ars.*** ***ars-i.*** ***asaf.***[171] **ASAR.** ***aur.*** aur-ar.[58] aur-i.[58] aur-m.[58] bad.[1] bamb-a.[1184] bapt. ***bar-c.*** bar-i.[58] **BELL.** **BOR.** ***bry.*** bufo buth-aust.[119] cact. ***calad.***[72] ***calc.*** calc-f.[119] calc-sil.[58] camph. cand-a.[239] cann-i.[36] cann-s. caps. carb-an. ***carb-v.*** ***carbn-s.*** carc.[140] card-m. ***caust.*** ***cham.*** chel. **CHIN.** chin-ar.[36] chin-b.[54] chlol.[54] chol.[54] cic. cimic. cinnb. ***cocc.*** **COFF.** colch. **CON.** convo-s.[119] cop.[36] crot-h.[54] cupr.[5] cyn-d.[149] ***ferr.*** ***ferr-ar.*** ***ferr-p.*** ***fl-ac.*** foll.[149] gaert.[136] gels. glon.[102] ***hell.*** hep.[85] hura hyos. ***ign.*** ***iod.***[122] ***ip.*** ipom.[119] just.[144] kali-ar. **KALI-C.** kali-i. ***kali-p.*** kali-s. kali-sil.[58] lac-ac.[54] ***lac-c.*** ***lach.*** ***lachn.***[54] ***lat-m.***[119] lept.[5] ***lyc.*** lycpr.[102] ***lyss.*** mag-c.[5] ***mag-m.*** mag-p.[58] manc. ***mand.***[119] mang. ***med.*** meny.[137] ***merc.*** mosch. ***mur-ac.***[36] nat-ar. ***nat-c.*** ***nat-m.*** nat-p. ***nat-s.*** nat-sil.[58] **NIT-AC.** ***nux-m.***[54] **NUX-V.** onos.[102] **OP.** ox-ac. palo.[149] petr.[5] ph-ac. phel.[116] ***phos.*** pitu-a.[164] plan.[36] ***plat.*** plb.[5] ptel. ***puls.*** raph.[36] rhus-t. sabad. sabin.[163] ***sang.***[8] sec.[54] seneg.[5] **SEP.** **SIL.** ***spig.*** stann. staph.[58] stram.[5] stry.[36] sulfonam.[149] sulph.[5] syph.[122] tanac. tarent.[102] **THER.** thuj.[163] **TUB.**[122] v-a-b.[149] valer.[5] verat.[5] verat-v.[25] viol-o.[5] visc.[119] xan.[198] yuc.[36] **ZINC.** **ZINC-P.**[122]

Sensitive; noise, water splashing: brom.[137] **LYSS.** **NIT-AC.** stram.

Starting; noise, from: acon.[122] act-sp.[111] adax.[96] aloe alum. ang.[1] ant-c. apis ars. asar.[149] aur. bar-acet.[36] ***bar-c.*** **BOR.** bufo calad. ***calc.*** camph. cann-s. carb-v. carc.[146] card-b.[36] ***caust.*** chel. ***cic.*** ***cocc.*** ***con.*** cub. hipp. hura kali-ar. **KALI-C.**[122] ***kali-i.*** ***kali-p.*** kali-s.[127] kali-sil.[58] ***lach.*** lap-gr-m.[194] ***lyc.*** lyss. mag-c. ***med.*** ***merc.*** mosch. ***nat-ar.*** **NAT-C.** **NAT-M.** **NAT-P.** **NAT-S.** ***nat-sil.***[58] nit-ac. **NUX-V.** ***op.*** ox-ac. prot.[136] ptel. puls.[127] rhus-t. sabad. sabin. **SIL.** spong. ***sul-ac.***[184] sulph. tab. tarent.[214] ther.[116] viol-o.[45] xan.[111]

Weeping; bells, sound of: ant-c. cop.[122]

Weeping; noise, at: aeth. ign. kreos. ***lach.***

Wildness; sounds, on hearing any, as striking of clock, etc., dances about, must be held: verat.[54]

ACON. Ha, 523 - The slightest noise is intolerable to him.

ADAM. Sh, 221 - I felt angry on waking, noise of people upstairs sounds like elephants. I want to kill them. I wanted to complain to them. 7, 6C, 03:06:00

ANDROC. Sh, 108 - Incredibly sensitive to noise, can't bear it, hundreds of thoughts pop in and out of my brain, thoughts of 'why are we here?', deep philosophical issues. Everyday things disappear from my mind. Am free from pressing, nagging responsibilities —just a black thunder sits within me, and I feel afraid of what I might do next. my eyes are staring and full of hate — just looking at the children sends them frantic. I have no control over my emotions. Then after 8:00 p.m., deadness resumes and I feel .k., but the end of myself as I usually am. (7)

Sh, 118 - Irritability, worse for noise and bright lights. (17)

ARS. Al, 109 - Indignation, alternating with mildness; in her indignation she looks at nobody, and does not want to hear anything; she also cries.

Ha, 1032 - Mania; first headache, horrible anxiety, noise before the ears, as from a number of large bells, and when he opened the eyes, he always saw a man who had (formerly) hung himself (suicidal, justified) on the ground-floor of the house, who incessantly beckoned (call) him to cut him down (help); he ran thither (there) with a knife, but, as he could not cut him down, (rescue) he became overwhelmed (beaten) with despair (remorse?) and wished (as his friends assured him) to hang himself (punish); but being prevented (stop) from doing so, he became so restless that he could hardly be kept in bed,... and he knelt down and raised his hands in a supplicating manner.

Ha, 1049 - Discontented with everything, finds fault with everything; everything is too strong and too irritating, all conversation, all noise, and all light.

AUR. Ha, 348 - A noise before the door made him anxious; he feared lest some one would come in; like anthropophobia.

Ha, 14 - Anxiousness; even a noise before the door makes him anxious; he is afraid some one might come in; as if afraid of men.

BAR-A. Al, 8 - Solicitous (careful) and fearful. The slightest noise in the street seems to him like a fire alarm, and he is frightened thereat, so that he starts in every limb.

BAR-C. Ha, 11 - Anxious and fearful; a little noise on the street seems to him at once like fire alarm, and he is frightened by it, so that it darts (move quickly) through all his limbs.

BELL. Ha, 1395 - He wishes for solitude and quiet; all noise and visits from others are repugnant to him.

Ha, 1400 - Great irritability and acuteness of the senses; everything tastes and smells stronger; the sense of touch, the sight, and the rearing are more acute,...

BUFO. Al, 14 - Very easily frightened; a bird or insect flying by causes a start.

CALC. Al, 1 - Illusion of fancy when going to sleep, as if she heard noises and clattering (noise) about her bed, which caused shuddering (tremor).

CANN-I. Al, 29 - Looks under beds and tables, unlocks and relocks doors, for the fancies he hears strange noises, and that thieves are in the house.

He, 15-...he is gradually swelling, his body becomes larger and larger; that someone calls him; that he hears numberless bells ringing most sweetly; imagines he hears music; shuts his eyes, and is lost for some time in the most delicious thoughts and dreams.

CANTH. Al, 16 - Visions at night, when half awake; she heard soft steps in the room, then knocking under the bed, and the bed was raised up.

CAUST. Ha, 20 - Extreme anxious timidity; she is so much afraid (fear) of a dog near her, which did not harm (hurt, injure) her at all,...every noise in the street made her afraid, and when she saw boys climbing she was very uneasy lest they might get hurt. (care, others)

CHEL. Al, 53 - Becomes frightened at the slightest noise, as if he had not a good conscience.

COCC. Ha, 548 - He cannot bear any interruption in conversation, nor any noise.

He, 18 - Intolerance of noise or any disturbing influence.

He, 9-...cannot bear least noise or contradiction.

COFF. He, 24-...fear of fresh air and of least noise...

FERR. Al, 4 - Constant desire for solitude; horror of conversation, noise, visits, and even the society of her cherished friends.

GERM. Sh, 187 - Head jumped inside when there was a sudden noise. 07, 30C, 00.09.30

HALI-L. Sh, 726 - Then I heard a milkman clinking bottles. I felt the sound in my upper arm bones. My upper arm bones felt hollow, and the sound resonated in them. Bone felt and sounded hollow. 20, 30C, 01:00:34

Sh, 923 - Any sudden noise was like painful shocks through my body, like my body being blasted. 20, 30C, 13:XX:XX

Sh, 943 - Excited by the sounds of beaks clicking together, even empty pistachio nut cases clicking together in the palm of my hand excited me. 20, 30C, 15:XX:XX

IGN. He, 28 - Senseless (illogical) staring at one object, with sighing and moaning; remorse about imaginary crimes, intolerance to noise; great inclination to have fixed ideas.

IRID. Sh, 68 - Woke up thinking my alarm clock was a hedgehog. I wondered what the spiky sound was. I10

Sh, 309 - I have found that voices are sounding really loud. I have turned the television down again, as I wish I could turn the children down and off. I feel really irritated around them. I feel better on my own. J4

KALI-C. Al, 25 - She is frightened with a loud cry, by an imaginary apparition (as for example, of a bird flying to the window).

LYC. Al, 50 - In the evening on entering a room he is attacked with fear, as though he saw some one; even during the day he believes that he hears some one in the room.

He, 24 - Easily frightened (afraid) and starts up; feels frightened at everything, even ringing of door bell.

LYSS. Al,N-79-...terror ...by endeavoring to take a drink of water, ...attacks...induced by running of water,...

Al,N-116 - Attacks of nervous headache become awful and insupportable if he hears water run out of a hydrant.

Al,N-118 - When he hears water poured out, or if he hears it run, or if he sees it, he becomes very irritable, nervous;...

Al,N-129 - Hyperesthesia, current of air, bright light, sight of any shining object, slightest touch, even conversation in vicinity of patient, may throw him into a most violent agitation and bring on severe convulsions.

MAG-M. Ha, 20 - Fanciful (fantastic) delusions: As if while she was reading in a book, another person was reading after her, and compelled her to read more quickly, with humming and buzzing (murmur) around her...(faster)

NAT-C. Al, 28 - He is very timid, and starts at the slightest noise.

NUX-V. Ha, 1273 - He cannot bear any noise or speaking; music and singing affect him strongly.

He, 10-...every harmless word offends, every little noise frightens, anxious and beside themselves, cannot bear even the least suitable medicine. (contrary)

PETR. Al, 10 - Anxiety at a noise of a crowd of many people.

PH-AC. Ha, 41 - Illusion of the senses, as if he heard the clock strike or as if lofty (tall, elevated) things lying out of his horizon were moving near him.

PLB. He, 16 - Mental disturbance of eight or ten years' duration in a man addicted to masturbation; has several times attempted suicide; has been in seclusion (solitude); greatest dejection and despair;...; believes himself lost (condemned) ; has the sounds of hell constantly in his ears; hears voices and sees shadows of demons, great disposition to make away (suicide) with himself or do himself some bodily injury;

SIL. Ha, 11 - Sensitive to noise, which makes him apprehensive.

Ha, 12 - Loud talking is oppressive to him.

TAB. Al, 41 - From having been one of the most healthy and fearless of men, he had become sick all over, and was timid as a girl; he could not even present a petition in Congress, much less say a word concerning it; ...by any ordinary noise, he was startled or thrown into tremulousness, and afraid to be alone at night.

THEA. Al, 11 - The sound of the "night bell" made me terribly nervous.

VERAT. Ha, 664 - Cursing and making a

noise all night, and complains of being stupid, with headache and flow of saliva.

NOSTALGIA

Ailments from; homesickness: ***caps.*** carc.[233] ***clem.*** eup-pur.[102] hell.[102] ***ign.***[102] mag-m.[102] **PH-AC.**[54] senec.[102]

Anxiety; evening, family, about his, which he left behind while on a journey: ***petr.***[54]

Delusions; companions, companions of his youth, is with the: aether.

Dreams; acquaintances, distant: choc.[222] fl-ac. plat.[36] plb. sel.

➤ dead, people, of, friends long deceased: arg-n. cedr.[36] coca[36] con.[1] ferr. nat-c.

➤ dead, people, of, friends, talking with deceased: lepi.[36]

➤ friends, old: ant-c.[1] bamb-a.[1184] ferr. lap-gr-m.[194] ozone[227] rumx.

➤ people, seen for years, not, twenty years: calad.[54] calc-ar.[54]

➤ schoolmate, meeting of old: ant-c.[10] ferr.[36]

➤ youth, time of: **SIL.**[36]

Talk; sleep, in, village, of a far distant: merc.[36]

Thoughts; past, of the, journeys: sol-t-ae.[36]

ADAM. Sh, 100 - Sensitive to music that I know and like —very nostalgic. 20, 1M, 11:XX:XX

Sh, 295 - On sniffing the remedy, I had an immediate vision and feeling of the place where I feel most at ease and comfortable (a cottage in the woods). A feeling of being at home. 1, 12C, 00:00:01

Sh, 296 - Thinking a lot about a cottage in Hampshire that I'd wanted to buy and feeling sad that I hadn't. Feeling that it would have been so blissful to be alone there, and be creative in the garden. No sound except birds, just to relax and be alone. 1, 12C, 01:XX:XX

Sh, 297 - I didn't want to go away to teach. Wanted to be at home. Feel happy at home with children. 2, 12C, 05:XX:XX

Sh, 309 - Vision: during meditation, image of deceased mother. Sobbed at the loss of her friendship and love. Later felt good — something had lifted. 5, 30C, 15:06:20

Sh, 393 - Remember old days, dwelling on past, especially about when my friend who died was still alive. I can't seem to let him go, I don't ever want to accept that he has gone, though I know I should because it will free his spirit, yet I love him too much to accept his death and allow his soul to go. 20, 1M, 06:XX:XX

AETH. Al,S-11 - Disposition becomes retiring (reserved) and tearful, as in nostalgia.

ANAC. Al, 1 - Illusions of fancy; he imagines he has his name called by the voice of his far-distant mother and sister, accompanied by an apprehension of misfortune and anxiety.

AUR. He, 29 - He gets excited in his thoughts about some absent persons.

CARB-AN. He, 13 - Homesick.

CARL. Al, 5 - Mood very much depressed, like an excessive homesickness; at last violent weeping.(second day) (after four glasses)

CHLOL. Al, 17-...a feeling as if he were now in one country and now in another, and with an anxious desire to go home.(abroad)

EUP-PUR. He, 7-... feeling like homesickness, though occupying her own home and surrounded by her own family,...

FERR. Al, 769 - Rested well, but dreamed a great deal of meeting with old schoolmates, of student life, etc.

GERM. Sh, 143 - I Don't belong. I don't feel at home any place. Strong desire for finding a place to stay, to make a home for me and my kids. 18, 30C, 30:XX:XX

HALI-L. Sh, 155 - Thoughts in the morning of our house when we lived in Japan. I can remember certain details so vividly. The carpet, kitchen, bath; the back door we never used, and the back yard I only went into three times. A feeling of longing for the past. 09, 6C, 08:14:XX

KALI-P. He, 17 - Homesickness, morbid activity of memory, haunted (obsessed) by visions of past, and longing after them.

NAT-M. Al, 45 - If she only thinks of a want (need, lack) long since past, tears come into her eyes.

PLAT. He, 44 - Talks almost continually about fanciful things or such as have really occurred; of faithless love; of her teacher and old school days; ...

PLB. Al, 66 - Hallucinations of mind, she seemed to see her dead husband and child in a tree out of the window.

SIL. He, 9 - Longing for his relations and home.

OBSERVED

Ailments from; looked at, being: ambr.[5] ***ant-c.*** ant-t. **ARS.** calc.[5] ***cham. chin. cina*** hell.[5] ***iod.*** lyc.[5] mag-c. merc.[116] nat-m. nux-v. rhus-t. stram. sulph.

Anger; looked at, when: ant-c.[127] ant-t.[47] ***cham.***[102] chin.[91] ***cina***[98] gels.[102] ***iod.***[8] ***nux-v.***[102] sanic.[102] ***sil.***[102]

Company, aversion to; avoids the sight of people: acon. ars.[30] calc.[122] **CIC.** ***cupr.*** cur.[122] ferr. ***gels.*** germ.[222] hydrog.[222] ***iod. lac-d.***[122] ***led. nat-c.*** psor.[185] ***sep. thuj.***

Company, aversion to; avoids the sight of people, lies with closed eyes, and: sep.

Company, aversion to; avoids the sight of people, shuts herself up: cur.

Company, desire for; wants to be watched constantly: gall-ac.[85]

Delusions; confusion, others will observe her: ***calc.***

- faces, looking out of every corner: phos.[139]
- faces, wherever he turns his eyes, or looking out from corns: aur. med. ***phos.***
- present, someone is: hyos. lyc. thuj.
- room, sees people bedside in: atro. con.
- spied on, being: aq-mar.[231] lach.[30] med.[56]
- strangers, looking over shoulder: brom.
- trees are people in fantastic costume (afternoon, while riding): bell.
- watched, she is being: aq-mar. **ARS.** ***bar-c. calc.***[5] choc.[222] ***hyos.*** med.[108] meli. rhus-t
- watched, that she is being, night: med.[85]

Dreams; spied, of being: aq-mar.[231]

Fear; observed, of her condition being: aq-mar.[231] atro. bamb-a.[1184] **CALC.** chel. choc.[222] germ.[222] lap-c-b.[194] lap-mar-c.[194]

Howling; looked at, when: ant-t.[47]

Hysteria; looked, at, when: plb.[137]

Looked at; cannot bear to be: ambr.[5] ***ant-c. ant-t.*** **ARS.** bamb-a.[1184] calc.[5] ***cham. chin. cina*** cupr.[210] gels.[102] hell.[36] ***iod.*** kali-br.[54] mag-c. merc.[5] ***nat-m.***[122] nux-v. puls.[137] rhus-t. sanic.[102] sil.[5] stram. sulph. tarent.[5] thuj.[102] ***tub.***[122]

Looked at; cannot bear to be, faces the wall if anybody talks to him: nat-m.[70]

Looked at; cannot bear to be, sadness, with: ***kali-br.***[54]

Morose; looked at, on being: ant-c.[10] ars.[10] cham.[10]

Shrieking; looked at, when: ***iod.***[8]

Weeping; children, looked at, when: ant-c.[8] ant-t.[58] brom.[47]

Weeping; looked at, when: ant-c.[122] ant-t.[141] kiss.[122] ***nat-m. tarent.***[54]

ADAM. Sh, 181 - I realized I am observing a lot and have a feeling of being observed. The observer bit is female aspect, and the male bit is a critical voice. 7, 6C, 06:06:00

ANT-T. Al, 17 - He rubs his eyes with his hands as if in a stupid sleep, and wakes in a very ill-humor e.g., if one looked at him he began to howl.

BAR-C. He, 12 - Walking in street she imagines men are laughing at her, criticizing to disadvantage; this makes her so timid that she dare (venture) not look up or at anybody, and she perspires over whole body.

BELL. Al, 48 - Very delirious; she would persist that there were very horrid monsters all over the room, staring at her.

CALC. Ha, 27 - She is afraid people may notice (observed) the confusion (disorder) in her head.

He, 15 - Imagines someone is walking beside her (persecution); that something hanging over back of chair is a person sitting there, etc.

He, 52 - Fears she will lose her reason (insanity), or that people will observe her confusion of mind.

CANN-I. Al, 25-...Now demoniac shapes clutched (grasp) at him from the darkness, cloaked (covered) from head to foot in inky (black) palls (mantle), glaring (staring, looking) at him with fiery eyes from beneath their cowls(mantle)....

Al, 41 - Felt as if he was a third person looking at himself and his friend.

CHLOL. He, 7-...inclined to wander and hide herself, avoiding shrewdly (astute) the vigilance of her friends...

CHOC. Sh, 188 - While walking outside, became anxious in a self-conscious way, anxious and vulnerable as if being watched or observed by something or someone -the attention was on me - anxiety that something would happen. Immediately afterwards I was attacked by four dogs and bitten on the calf. 27, 100C, 01:XX:XX

GERM. Sh, 156 - At night on closing the eyes I have a vision of a pair of eyes looking at me, then suddenly I saw the face very clearly. The face had an asking expression. 16, 30C, 07:04:00

HYOS. He, 78 - Groundless suspicion of being watched (observed, spied) by members of family with whom he had some slight misunderstanding (dispute); to avoid being recognized by them, clothed himself differently every day,...watching his relations suspiciously and imagining he might be poisoned;... (disguise, camouflage)

IGN. He, 31 - A peculiar trembling of hands disturbs her very much in writing, most when she has to write in any one's presence (public), gets worse as soon as she fancies any one might notice it. (observed)

MED. He, 17 - Thinks some one is behind her, (pursued) hear whispering; sees faces that peer (observe) at her from behind bed and furniture.(spied)

He, 18 - Persons come in, look at her (observed), whisper, and say "come". (spied, called)

MERC. Ha, 1127 - She dreams that people are before the window, and on being woke up thereby be cannot persuaded that they were not there. (observed)

NAT-M. Al, 18 - If one only looked at him, he was obliged to weep.

PHOS. Al, 12-...; wherever he turned his eyes he saw faces; they swarmed (crowded, surrounded) by him in long panoramic succession; they leered (look lecherous) at him over the footboard of the bed; they squinted (look) at him though the windows, or came trooping (crowd) in when the doors were left ajar (open) (invade);..he fancied he was some one else, ...

Al, 111 - Horrible fearfulness, late in the evening, as if a horrible face were looking out from every corner.

Ha, 31 - Dreadful fearfulness, late in the evening, as if a horrid face was looking out of every corner.

He, 8 - Fear and dread: in evening; of death; as if something were creeping out of every corner; late in evening as if a horrible face were looking out of every corner.

RHUS-T. He, 24-...a week later she told her mother to not look at her (observed) ; seemed to be distrustful (suspicious) and did not wish to see any one; she came running in from the street and said people were looking at her; ....; cries without cause, imagines people are finding fault (misconduct, criticized, censured) with her because she is earning (succeed, prosper, reach) nothing, acts in a childish manner;...

OBSTINATE

Fanaticism; philosophical: sulph.[60]

Firmness: lach.[36] squil.[36]

Firmness; morning: ferr-p.[36]

Gestures; makes, decided: fl-ac.[36]

Haughty; stiff and pretentious: ***lyc.***[54]

Ideas; fixed: acon.[5] aeth.[60] alum.[5] anac.[5] arg-n.[5] **ARS.**[5] aur.[5] benz-ac.[54] bry.[5] **CANN-I.**[54] **CANN-S.**[5] canth.[5] ***carb-v.***[54] cham.[1] chin.[85] cic.[5] coca[5] ***cocc.***[5] cupr.[5] **EUPHR.**[5] foll.[149] glon.[5] graph.[5] **HELL.**[5] **HYOS.**[5] **IGN.**[5] ***iod.***[5] lach.[5] lyss.[5] **MERC.**[5] **NAT-M.**[5] ***nit-ac.***[5] ***nux-v.***[54] **OP.**[5] petr.[60] ph-ac.[5] plat.[5] ***psor.***[5] ***puls.***[5] ***rhus-t.***[5] ***sabad.***[5] sil.[5] stann.[54] **STRAM.**[5] sulph.[5] ***thuj.***[5] **VERAT.**[5]

Insanity; obstinate in: ***dig.***[54] ***nux-v.***[54]

Irritability; obstinate, and: nit-ac.[1]

Mildness; alternating with, obstinacy: ***cupr.***[54]

Monomania: ***absin.***[102] acon. anac.[36] anan. aur.[5] bell.[10] camph. carb-v. carc.[207] cham.[10] chin.[10] cic.[5] cocc.[10] con.[10] croc.[10] cupr.[10] dros.[10] hell. hyos.[10] ***ign.*** iod.[10] lach.[10] lap-c-b.[194] mag-c.[10] nux-m. oxyt.[102] plat.[10] puls. rhus-t.[10] ***sil.*** stram. sulph. tarent.[102] thuj. verat.[10]

Narrow-minded: alum.[30] am-c.[30] bar-c.[30] con.[30]

Obstinate: abrot.[5] ***acon.*** act-sp. ***agar.*** alco.[36] aloe **ALUM.** alum-p.[58] alum-sil.[58] alumn. am-c. ambr.[1189] **ANAC.** androc.[222] ***ant-c.***[5] ant-t. apis <u>**ARG-N.**</u>[122] arn. ***ars.*** ars-s-f.[58] arum-t.[5] aur. aur-ar.[58] aur-s.[58] bac.[62] bar-acet.[36] **BAR-C.**[193] **BELL.** bry. **CALC.** calc-ar.[58] calc-f.[193] calc-p.[10] ***calc-s.***[122] camph. canth. ***caps.*** carb-an. carb-v. carbn-s.[36] carc.[119] caust. **CHAM.** chel. ***chin.*** chin-s. ***cina*** coca[54] coloc.[116] croc. ***crot-h.***[54] cupr.[10] cycl. dig. dros. ferr. ferr-ar. ferr-p. guai. hecla.[234] hell.[58] ***hep.*** hura hydrog.[222] hyos. ***ign.*** ip. ***kali-c.*** kali-chl.[58] kali-i. ***kali-p.*** kali-s. kali-sil.[58]

kalm. kreos. lach. ***lyc. mag-m.*** menis.[36] merc. mosch.[58] mur-ac. nat-c.[1] nat-m.[184] ***nit-ac.*** **NUX-V.** ***pall.*** petr.[116] ***ph-ac.*** phel.[10] phos. plat.[30] plb. ***psor.*** puls.[155] rhus-t.[10] sanic. sec. sep.[58] ***sil. spong. staph.***[102] stram. ***sulph.*** syph.[122] **TARENT.** thuj. tub.[5] verat.[30] viol-t. zinc. zinc-p.[58]

Obstinate; alternating with mildness: cupr.[85]

Obstinate; amiable, tries to appear: ***pall.***[54]

Obstinate; children, annoy those about them, with eruption: ***psor.***[54]

Obstinate; children, fat, inclined to grow: **CALC.**

Obstinate; children, masturbation, boys after: aur.[116]

Obstinate; declares there is nothing the matter with him: apis **ARN.**

Obstinate; execution of matured plans, in: dros.[36]

Obstinate; pertinacity: acon.[5] ars.[5] bamb-a.[1184] bry.[5] caps. cupr.[210] dig.[5] dros. guare.[36] lim.[36] lyc.[5] nat-c.[5] nit-ac.[5] nux-v.[5] phos.[5] plb.[201] stram. sulph.[5]

Obstinate; pertinacity, duties, in performing irksome: lim.[36]

Obstinate; purpose, but difficulty in way of carrying out its: ***phys.***[54]

Obstinate; queerest objection, against whatever was proposed, he had the: **ARG-N.**

Obstinate; resists wishes of others: alum.[36] **NUX-V.**[54]

Obstinate; simpleton, as a: lyc.[30] plat.[30] verat.[30]

Partial; prejudged: ars.[30] lach.[30]

Positiveness: androc.[222] ars.[30] camph. ***caust.***[122] choc.[222] ferr. hep.[179] hydrog.[222] lac-h.[229] ***lach.***[122] ***merc.***[58] nux-v.[30] ozone[227] sep.[30]

Prejudices, traditional: ars.[30] calc.[30] carb-v.[30] lach.[30] lyc.[30] plat.[30] verat.[30]

Religious affections; bible, want to read all day the: ***calc.***[122] stram.[122]

Religious affections; fanaticism: aur-ar.[58] med.[162] plb.[85] puls.[58] rat.[162] rob. sel. stram.[85] sulph. thuj.

Religious affections; narrow-minded in religious questions: hyos.[30] puls.[30] ***stram.***[30]

Restlessness; zealous: **NUX-V.**[54]

Rigidity: calc-sil.[185] cocc.[58] cupr.[210] nit-ac.[185] plb.[201]

Rooted people: bamb-a.[1184] calc-p.[198]

Sadness; alternating with, positiveness: ozone[227]

Seriousness, earnestness: aeth. ***alum.*** alum-p.[58] am-c. ***am-m.*** ambr. anac. ang. ant-c. arg. **ARS.**[122] ars-s-f.[58] asar.[162] aur. bamb-a.[1184] bar-c. bart.[36] bell. bor. bov.[5] bry.[10] cact.[36] calc. cann-s. caust. cham. chel.[10] chin. cic.[10] ***cina cocc.*** coff. con. cupr.[8] cycl. dros.[10] **EUPH.**[5] euphr. ferr. ferr-ar. graph.[10] grat. hydrog.[222] hyos.[5] ign. iod. ip.[10] lach.[116] ***led.*** lyc. lyss.[36] m-arct.[10] mang.[10] ***merc.*** mur-ac. naja nat-c. nat-m.[187] nat-p. nux-m. nux-v.[10] olnd. op. orig.[36] ph-ac. plat. plb. puls. rhus-t. seneg. ***sep.***[5] sil.[162] spig. staph. stram.[171] ***sul-ac.*** sulph. thuj. til. valer.[36] verat.

Shrieking; obstinate: ***cham.***[116]

Suggestions, will not receive: helon.

Talk; convincing: op.[36]

Talk; repetition of same phrases: coff-t.[36] euph.[171] germ.[222] kres.[144] lach.[122] lap-c-b.[194] plat.[5]

Thoughts; circles, moving in: cann-i.[36] choc.[222]

Thoughts; persistent, desires, of: bry.[30] ign.[30] puls.[30]

Thoughts; persistent, garment made the previous day, about a: aeth.

Unmanageable: aether[36] alco.[36] am-c.[1] atro.[36] bell.[36] petr.[36] stram.[36]

Yielding; alternating with obstinacy: cupr.[137]

ANAC. He, 29 - Has the fixed idea that her husband is not her husband, her child not her child; now she fondles (caress) them and again pushes them away. (reject, repudiate)

ANAN. He, 8 - Monomania for doing same thing and frequenting same places.

ANDROC. Sh, 72 - My mind is concentrated on one objective and I push aside all distracting influences. A mental 'tunnel vision'. (12)

ANG. He, 8 - Thinks about one project and nothing else, with great activity of mind.

ARN. Al, 28 - Obstinate and headstrong resistance to other people's opinions.
Ha, 633 - Stiff-necked obstinacy.

ARS. He, 104 - Obstinacy, avarice, inclined to malice and satire.

CALC. He, 70 - Excessive mischievousness, with obstinacy.

CHOC. Sh, 205 - Though Previously lazy,

became intensely obsessed with work for a long period of time. Put all my energy into work. 35, 30C, XX:XX:XX:

CUR. Al, 9 - Melancholy, egotistical, envious, obstinate...

DIG. He, 10 - Profound melancholy,...great fear of future; insane obstinacy and disobedience, with desire to escape.

DROS. Ha, 284 - Obstinate prosecution of resolutions he had formed.

He, 7 - Self-willed (inflexible); obstinate; insists upon carrying out his plans.(determination)

FERR. Al, 21 - Violence, quarrelsomeness; insists that he is right.

Ha, 291 - Violence, quarrelsomeness (litigious, combative), positiveness (obstinate, emphatic, resolute)

HELL. He, 11 - Psychical conditions occupying a place between melancholia and mania, and in conditions where true depression and weakness is present, in which the patient is governed by a fixed idea.

HELON. He, 5 - Irritable; cannot endure the least contradiction or receive suggestions in relation to any subject.

HEP. He, 22 - Temper obstinate and cross, a ferocious spleen (irascible) which would lead to cold blooded murder even among those habitually gay and benevolent.

He, 20 - Violent, passionate fretfulness; she spoke with such volubility that one could not always get a chance to reason with her, and she would not listen to the most just remarks.

HYDROG. Sh, 240 - I feel life is a serious thing. When putting children to bed, I felt serious and uncompromising. I wanted them to do exactly as I said and, if not, threatened to hit them. 32, 9C, 03:XX:XX

IGN. Al, 32 - He is discontented, morose, and obstinate towards evening; no one can do anything right or please him.

Al, 3 - A fixed idea, which he pursues in his thoughts, or expatiates (talk) upon with great earnestness and exhaustiveness in conversation (after two hours).

Ha, 768 - Towards evening he is discontented, sulky, stubborn (obstinate), no one can do anything right, anything to please him.

He, 28 - Senseless (illogical) staring at one object, with sighing and moaning; remorse about imaginary crimes, intolerance to noise; great inclination to have fixed ideas.

IRID. Sh, 327 - Had a massive argument with friend. For first time in my life really stood my ground. Went hot. Said, "This is my point and I am sticking to it." Burst into floods of tears. It was as though a volcano had erupted. Anger and grief were coming out. My friend had done this on purpose. I got on high horse. We parted friends and sorted it all out. I4

KALI-C. Al, 44 - Disagreeable mood; he is obstinate and frequently does not himself know what he wishes.

Ha, 32 - Contrary disposition; he is self-willed (obstinate) and often does not know himself what he wishes. (indecision)

LACH. Al, 33 - Unusually contentious (hostile) and obstinate, so that he quarrels with everything about him.

Al, 30 - Impatient; desires positive answers when this is not practicable.

LYC. Al, 94 - Indolent, obstinate (inflexible), rebellious (revolutionary, dissident), passionate, wrathful. (angry)

Ha, 48 - He has trouble to conceal (mask, hide) his internal obstinacy and vexation. (dissimulated)

He, 17-...imperiousness(domineering, despotic) ; speaks with an air of command (ordering, domination) ; manner stiff (severe, obstinate) and pretentious;...

He, 32 - Obstinate, defiant (contrary), arbitrary (capricious?); seeks disputes.

LYSS. Al,N-42 - Deny, with great obstinacy, that they have ever been bitten.

NIT-AC. He, 19-...headstrong (obstinate); trembling while quarreling; fits of rage with curses and maledictions; inveterate ill-will, unmoved by apologies.

NUX-V. Ha, 1269 - He obstinately opposes what others wish.

He, 12 - Inclined to find fault and scold (reprove); morose; stubborn; (obstinate) an insane desire when alone with her husband, whom she adores, to kill him.

He, 16 - Ill-humored, resists obstinately the wishes of others.

PALL. He, 14 - She tries to appear as amiable as possible, but is obstinate.

PLB. He, 15-...; despair of her salvation...; fixed idea that could only obtain peace and safety though absolution by a priest of the papal church, although she had been a zealous Protestant; ....brooded over any forbidden thing; would steal (leave) from house in servant's cloak (coat, camouflage) and bonnet (hat) to obtain stimulants (drugs), but from the moment their prohibition was withdrawn (retired) ceased to have any desire for them; after being permitted to visit a priest and converse with him ceased to talk and think of the church. (desire; redemption, absolution)

PSOR. Al,N-10 - Intolerable self-willed (obstinate), annoys those about him; a boy suffering from an eruption.

SIL. Al, 17 - Self-willed.
Ha, 26 - The child becomes self-willed, obstinate and headstrong.

SULPH. Ha, 53 - He is so peevish and obstinate, that he will not give an answer to anybody, he cannot bear to have anyone around him, and cannot get quickly enough what he wants.
Ha, 55-...cannot do anything to please herself, is obstinate and unyielding (rigorous), without herself knowing why.
He, 13 - A little girl with religious insanity, takes passages of Scripture literally and acts upon them. (fanatical) (virtuous, noble, elevated)

THUJ. Al, 1 - She herself desires, with anxiety and despair, to be taken to an insane asylum, (imprisonment, confining) and there to be treated very harshly and strictly, (penalized), so that her fixed ideas may be subdued and banished (purified); she knows very well that she does wrong (conscience) and thinks all sorts of bad thoughts (immoral), but she will not take the trouble to banish such thoughts; therewith she indistinctly gives to understand that she is constantly obliged to think of taking her own life, but feels the sinfulness (wicked) of it, in order to avoid it, desires the strict restraint of the asylum;...
Al, 16 - The child is excessively obstinate; on the slightest contradiction it throws itself in the ground in rage and loses its breath.

OBSTRUCTED

Anger; interruption, from: androc.[222] cench.[58] ***cham.*** cocc. germ.[222] graph.[1] ***hell.***[54] lac-h.[229] lap-mar-c.[194] ***nux-v.***

Anxiety; work, preventing work: aloe[60] mosch.[36]

Aversion; interference: bar-c.[127] calc-p.[127] cham.[127] cina[122] nat-m.[127] sanic.[127] sil.[127] sulph.[127]

Aversion; interference, resents: cham.[127] nat-m.[127] sulph.[127]

Cares; full of, noise, by, or interruption in business: ***lyc.***[54]

Concentration, difficult; dark before eyes on attempting: arg-n.

Delusions; body, brain, fog in: sulph.[139]
- body, goiter, that he cannot see over when sitting down: zinc.
- body, threads, inside is made of (afternoon on lying): nux-v.[36]
- clouds, sees, fancy, before the: hep. mag-m. rhus-t.
- corners of houses project so that he fears he will run against then while walking in the street: ***arg-n.***
- deaf and dumb: verat.
- disease, deaf, dumb and has cancer, is: verat.
- fluid, surrounded by ethereal, resisting passage: cann-i
- hear, he cannot: hyos.[10] mosch. verat.
- images, sleep, preventing: alum. ambr.[58] arg-n. lyc. op. tab.
- obstacles, in his way, caused partly by contrary fate, partly by himself: aur.[36]
- obstacles, wants them to be removed, in his sleep: cham.[60]
- people, front of him, in: con.[5]
- runs, against something: arg.[139]
- swallow, cannot: lyss.[54]
- think, she cannot: ***chel.***[54] onos.[139].
- work, hindered, is: ***chin.***

Development: mental, arrested: agki-p.[149] aur.[127] bac.[62] bar-c.[127] calc-p.[47] chap.[149] nitro-o.[146] per.[149] syph.[149] thuj.[127]

Dreams; bicycling difficult: visc.[119]
➤ blind, that he was: phys.
➤ body, ears, lump in: cinnb.[36]
➤ body, throat, stoppage of the throat: kreos.[36]
➤ bound, with chain across mouth, being: bapt.[36]

➤ coition, stranger coming in prevented the act: nat-p.[36]
➤ confused, streets, snow, obstructed by piles of: ozone[227]
➤ disease, stoppage, throat: kreos.
➤ disease, strangury: chr-ac.
➤ disease, suffocation: arn. chel.[193] ign.[162] iris kali-bi. kali-c.[1] sang.[193] xan.[85]
➤ drinking, impossible: arist-m.[36]
➤ journey, difficulties, with: am-m.[36] calc-p.[36] echi.[111] mag-s.[36] merc.[36] mez.[36] nat-c.[36]
➤ nightmare, inability to see, as if he could not escape from: cot.[36]
➤ unsuccessful efforts to, talk, large tongue which extended out of her mouth and up her nose, on account of: tab.[36]
➤ unsuccessful, efforts to, reach a distant place, to: croc. plat.
➤ urinate, that he must, followed by seminal emission, of which he knew nothing: merc-i-f.[54]
➤ urinating, desire for, bottle, in a, but could not on account of a crowd: am-br.[36]

Dullness; alone, when: ph-ac.
Dullness; coition, after: bar-c.[5] bov.[5] calc.[5] ***sep.***
Dullness; company, in: plat.
Dullness; condition, could not think of her: chel.
Dullness; fog, as envelop in a: petr.[122]
Dullness; impotency, with: ph-ac.[58]
Dullness; masturbation, after: ***agn.***[102] calc-p.[102] canth.[102] caust.[102] dam.[102] ***gels.***[54] nux-v.[102] **OP.**[102] ph-ac.[58] phos.[102] pic-ac.[102] **STAPH.**[54]
Dullness; mortification, after: ***staph.***
Expressing, oneself; difficult: crot-h.[137] kali-br.[25] lil-t.[36] thuj.[5]
Expressing, oneself; impossible: bell.[10] cann-i.[10] haem.[10] lyc.[10] ***nux-v.***[10] phys.[36] puls.[10] sep.[36] thuj.[10]
Fear; blind, of becoming: arge.[149] atro.[172] ***nux-v.***[54] ***sulph.***[54]
✦ vision, of losing his: euphr.[36] ***nux-v.***[54]
Interruption, agg. mental symptoms: colch.[5] culx.[58] staph.[5] verat.[5]
Interruption; aversion to: bar-c.[127] calc-p.[127] cham.[127] cina[122] nat-m.[127] sanic.[127] sil.[127] sulph.[127]
Intolerance; hindrance, of: ferr-p.[36]
Intolerance; interruption, of: cham.[36] cocc.[36] germ.[222]
Irresolution; evening, obstacles from: ferr-p.[36]
Sadness; difficulties, facing: ***cocc.***[54]
Sadness; imaginary obstacles, from: aur.[54]
Talk; sleep, in, obstacles being removed: cham.[1]
Weeping; children, interfered with, when: nat-m.[127]

ACON. Al, 55 - Flickering (spark, flash) before vision makes him anxious on street, he thinks he constantly jostles (press)the passers by.
Al, 14 - Excessive disagreeable restlessness; without occasion for hurrying, he is in the greatest haste, every obstacle that delays his rapid pace is excessively annoying; he knocks against some people who do not get out of his way fast enough, and runs in breathless haste up the steps;...
He, 40 - Thrice he became blind and affirmed that death was at hand.

ADAM. Sh, 4 - The cloud is lifting from neck and shoulders but it is still over eyes and forehead. I feel as if I'm waking up. 7, 6C, 10:11:00
Sh, 6 - Felt really strong love for children. Looking at daughter had a feeling of a barrier being lifted or a cloud lifted from me. Felt I could really see her, that she was mine; of me but separate. 8, 6C, 02:XX:XX
Sh, 39 - Drove (without a map) 120 miles to see a jewelry exhibition. Bought a wonderful book on minerals. Spent ages looking at the gems, but they all seemed too cloudy, except the Leopard stone. 2, 12C, 100:XX:XX

AETH. Al, 30 - Loss of comprehension (understanding); a kind of stupefaction, as if there was a barrier (obstruction) between his organs of sense and external objects. (disconnection, interruption)

ALUM. Ha, 55 - A numb (insensibility) feeling in the head as if his consciousness was outside of his body; when he says anything, he feels as if another person had said it; and when he sees anything, as if another person had seen it, or as if he could transfer himself into another, and only then could see. (transmigration)
Ha, 54 - Numb (paralyzed) feeling in the head, with a fear that he would become unconscious.

He, 16 - Low-spirited, trifling things appeared insurmountable. (impossible)

ANDROC. Sh, 111 - Short tempered in afternoon, easily excited to anger, worse from being interrupted. (12)

Sh, 114 - Intolerant of interruption and questions. (12)

ANG. Al, 15-,...prevented by the intrusion upon his mind of a rather agreeable project which he almost believes to be real and feasible, and which exclusively absorbs all his attention; it is a sort of waking dream.

ARN. Al, 39-...;one feels as if one were prevented (suspend) from doing something which is extremely necessary, accompanied by a total want of disposition for any kind of work.

Ha, 620 - Restlessness of body and mind, as if he was prevented (obstructed) doing something necessary, whith complete indisposition for occupation.

ATRO. Al, 24 - I imagined I had to go off by a railway train, which started at ten in the morning, and that the hour was approaching, whilst I had nothing ready for the journey; and I believed that I wished to dress and to pack my things, but was thwarted (stopped) and prevented by the people about me. At length I was persuaded, that it was too late to catch the train, and agreed to wait till evening.

AUR. Ha, 344 - Discontented with all circumstances; he imagines that he finds everywhere some obstacle (impediment, restriction) in the way; at one time he thinks that this is owing to an unlucky (unfortunate) fate (destiny), at another that he himself is to blame (censured) for it ; when the latter was the case he was particularly mortified and dejected.

Ha, 4 - Discontented with all conditions; he thinks that he everywhere finds an impediment, caused now by an opposing fate,(destiny) then again by himself, which latter mortifies him and renders him dejected.(sad)

BELL. Ha, 1372 - He walks lifting his feet high, as if he must step over things in his path, like a drunken person.

BOV. Al, 9 - Anguish; she felt as if enveloped in a black vapor. (cloud, fog)

BRASS. Sh, 7 - Twice this week I have had my view obstructed by someone sitting in front of me, each time I have had to move twice. 06, 30C, 04:00:00

BRY. Ha, 777 - Cross; imagined she could not finish her work (obstruction) ; she always took hold (continued) of the wrong thing and constantly wished to take something else ; then a pressing aching headache in the forehead.

Al, 39 - Imagination very sluggish (slow); it is impossible to make any plan for the future, even for the next day; the judgment (discernment), however, is unimpaired .

CALC. Al, 25 - Frightened apprehensive mood, as if some misfortune were about to happen to him, or some one else, which he could in no way overcome.

Ha, 65 - Great weakness of the imaginative (creative) faculty; with a very slight exertion in speaking, he felt as if his brain was paralyzed, ...;he could not think, nor recollect what was spoken of, with muddled (confused) feeling in the head.(lost: imagination, thoughts)

CAUST. Ha, 7 - Anxious, restlessness mood, as if something disagreeable (difficult) was impending (imminent), which keeps him from working.

CHEL. Al, 74 - It seems as though she could not think, and would lose her reason. (after three hours)

CHIN. Al, 47 - Discontent; he considers himself unhappy and thinks he is hindered (obstructed) and tormented by everyone. (after five hours)

CIMIC. He, 1 - Sensation as if a heavy black cloud (smoke) had settled (descent) all over her, and enveloped (surrounded, wrap) her head, so that all was darkness and confusion, while, at the same time, it weighed (heavy) like lead (metal) on her head.

CROT-T. He, 5 - Feeling as though one cannot think outside of himself, "feels all pent up" (restricted, limited, confined, circumscribed) inside, and no chance for thoughts to flow out; as if hide-bound.(obstinate)

CYCL. Al, 28-...he constantly feels as though he had just suffered from an overwhelming (remarkable) affliction; only when he becomes excited is his mind somewhat clearer, and then he acts like one who has just awakened from slumber (sleep), and only half understands what is going on about him.

DIG. Al, 43 - Intellectual faculties seemed to be affected, as if I had taken more wine than usual.

GELS. Al, 20 - The sensorial modification consisted of a mistiness (fog, cloudiness) within the brain, not much affecting the lucidity (precision) of thought, but somewhat confusing the perceptions, so that I experienced some difficulty in attending to the physical details connected with my practice.(lost, connections)

GERM. Sh, 151-.... I feel I have no real contact with people, I have no emotion at all except for a feeling of isolation and a concern that people may not like me. I wish someone would cuddle me. By 10 o'clock I have a definite aversion to people, especially certain people- the stubborn or authoritarian kind. I become deeply involved in my own thoughts and can be very irritable and even angry when the thoughts are interrupted by people, but I don't show any signs of anger or irritation. The fate of other people leaves me cold, but I know this is not right. My mind is blank and I feel I could just sit and stare. I have no feelings, no emotions! I think a lot about my state of mind and try to understand it; it puzzles me. What is missing? Eating removes this thoughtful mood. By afternoon and evening I become gradually more involved with what I am doing but still feel isolated even when in the company of other people. I don't mind listening to people, but I contribute little to conversation. This state lasted for three days. 16, 30C, 04:XX:XX

GRAPH. Al, 27 - Extreme apprehensiveness, so that she did not know how to overcome (succeed) it, disappearing after weeping.

He, 12 - Extreme apprehensiveness, so that she did not know how to overcome it.

HALI-L. Sh, 384 - There is some kind of barrier or buffer. Everything's kind of distant, like being wrapped in cotton wool. There's a distance between me and everything outside. Things weren't up close. Something between me and everything else. 07, 30C, 04:00:30

Sh, 577 - Children are an obstacle to enlightenment. 09, 6C, 05:XX:XX

Sh, 618 - I was trying to connect with husband. He starts sharing with me about his seminar. Daughter was calling me, "Mom, Mom.... Dinner on the table." There was this glass wall between us that neither one of us could traverse. 01, 30C, 03:09:30

Sh, 934 - As I woke, I decided I should be a nun. Strange. I feel like I've got my wings clipped when I think about men. 20, 30C, 15:XX:XX

HURA. Al, 28 - Impatience, anger; she bites her hands, and gets into passion because her ideas come too slowly.

HYDR. Al, 26-...forget, for a few seconds, what was wanted, which makes me very angry and feel like damning (swearing) and cursing (blaspheme) everything and anybody who bothered me the least.

HYDROG. Sh, 145 - Feel that I could get on with everything alright if those around me would either leave me alone or help constructively. 04, 12C, 19:XX:XX

Sh, 198 - Growing irritability. Anger below the surface if something is on the floor in my way or if something goes wrong. 12, 6C, 05:00:30

IGN. Ha, 753 - Extreme anxiety, which prevents (restrain) speaking.

Ha, 757 - He imagines he cannot get on (succeed), cannot walk.

He, 2-...;sees everything as if through a fog (obscurity) ; sits quietly, with a vacant gaze (expression), always thinking of the mortification endured,... prefers to be alone; thinking of the past mortification... 0Melancholy after mortification.

IOD. Al, 8 - Disposition mild, scrupulous (careful) and timid (irresolute), with blunted (dull) sensibilities.

KALI-BR. Al, 16 - A consciousness that the currents or sources of psychical force are hampered...(obstructed) sometimes makes an intellectual patient who is moderately bromized, reason himself into depression....

LACH. Al, 66 - It became extremely difficult for him to listen to others, though his hearing was not impaired; The words just spoken seemed obliterated.

LIL-T. Al, 32 - Perceptive and reflexive

faculties seem benumbed (confused), whereas at first she was overactive and seemed to be two individuals.

Al, 45 - She can't think; acts without thought; keeps walking fast as though by instinct; feels hurried, but doesn't know why; is forgetful, can't decide for herself; must depend on others.

MAG-C. Al, 946 - Dream that she made a long journey, and at last could go no farther (distance), at which she became very anxious. (limited, restricted)

MAG-M. Al, 711 - An anxious dream; she was lying in a strange house, where rubbish (garbage) was constantly falling upon her; she tried to cry out and could not, because there was too great heaviness on the chest.

MEZ. He, 4 - Irresolute (undecided); mind easily confused, unable to recollect; thinking is difficult.

MUR-AC. Ha, 5 - Anxious apprehension; he cannot get over the slightest misfortune.

NAT-AR. Al, 15 - Requires an effort to attend to accustomed duties; feels dull; tries to write, but it requires an effort to form each word.

NAT-C. Al, DREAM, 1102-..;of marrying two women, of parties, walks, entertainments, and excursions on horseback, afterwards they were frequently anxious, of going astray (lost),of murders, having his ears cut off; also vexatious dreams; he would take a journey and could not get away from the place,(immobilization) and when has reached the first station was obliged to turn back, on account of something he had forgotten.

NAT-M. Al, 119 - The patient's mind was much weakened by disease and poison; her moral perceptions, her once keen (sharp) sense of honor, and of right and wrong, seemed blunted (dull); she was in turns vehement (angry) and passionate, and moody and silent.

NUX-V. Ha, 1294 - Something, he knows not what, hinders (opposed, obstructed) him, specially in scientific occupations.

Ha, 1254 - She cannot get over the smallest evil.

OP. He, 7 - Drunkenness, with stupor; as if from smoke in brain;..

SEP. Al, 100-...seems as if my mind were hedged (enclose) in, as if it were circumscribed,...(encircle, confined)

STANN. Al, 20 - Fruitlessly busy, as if a rush of ideas prevented him from completing his work at a certain time; all sorts of things occur to him to be done.

Ha, 639 - Busy uselessness (inefficiency): he exerts (use) himself to get a necessary task (duty) done at the appointed hour, and cannot accomplish it, as though prevented (interrupted) by an over-crowding of thoughts, during which one thing and another occur to him which he wishes to do...

Ha, 10 - He is ineffectually (inefficiently) busied, as if he was prevented (obstructed) by super abundance of ideas from finishing his work at a certain time; he thinks of a number of things which he ought yet to attend to.

STAPH. Al, 15 - Anxious thoughts and events in the past came to him as if the past were present before him, which caused anxiety...then it became black before his eyes; he did not know whether the images were real or illusory, then everything seemed different, and he lost all desire to live.

Ha, 703 - Anxious thoughts and things long past come before him as if they were actually present and stood before him, which causes anxiety and the sweat of anguish - Then blackness comes before his eyes; he knows not if what he sees is true (real) or deception (false, unreal), then he regards (suppose) everything as something different to what it is (strange), and he loses all wish to live. (lost; discernment, perception)

STRAM. He, 32 - After getting out of bed, vertigo and loss of thought; everything hovers dimly and distantly before his memory, there seems to be a veil before his eyes.

TARENT. Al, 65-...great haste in whatever I undertook, from a constant fear that something would happen to prevent my finishing it;...fear that something would fall on me (doom, disgrace);...fear of striking it against some imaginary object which appeared to be suspended....(hurt)

THUJ. Al, 34 - While talking, she is unable to go on in spite of every effort; she begins to weep bitterly, and says she can no longer think or live.

VERAT. Al, 12 - He thinks that he is dumb and blind, and has a cancer.

Ha, 673 - He asserts (declare) that he is deaf and blind (obstructed) and that he has got cancer.

ZINC. Ha, 47 - Illusion of fancy, when holding down her head, as if she had a large goitre, which prevented her looking beyond it.

OFFENDED

Ailments from; admonition: agar.[5] ***bell.*** calc.[10] carc.[193] coloc.[137] germ.[222] ***ign.***[137] kali-c.[5] nit-ac.[5] ***nux-v.***[30] op.[137] ***plat.*** staph.[137] tarent.[137]

Ailments from; anger, indignation, with: ars.[5] ***aur.*** **COLOC.**[122] germ.[222] ip. lyc. m-p-a.[5] merc. mur-ac. nat-m. ***nux-v.*** plat. **STAPH.**[122]

Ailments from; honor, wounded: aur.[184] bamb-a.[1184] carc.[214] cham.[54] ign. ***nat-m.***[162] nat-s.[162] nux-v. pall.[144] plat.[137] ***staph.***[122] verat.[54]

Ailments from; indignation: acon.[10] ***ant-c.***[5] bell.[5] bry.[5] carb-v.[5] chin-s.[36] ***coloc.*** ferr.[38] ferr-p.[36] gels.[162] hecla.[234] hep.[5] ign.[171] ip. ***nat-m.*** ***nux-v.***[5] plat. **PULS.**[5] **STAPH.**[122]

Ailments from; insults, offenses, from: ang.[1] calc.[1] ***cham.***[1] cocc.[1] dros.[1] glon.[8] gran.[36] ***ign.***[22] ***merc.***[8] ***nat-m.***[36] nit-ac.[60] ***op.***[8] seneg.[5] ***staph.***[54] stram.[58] sulph.[1]

Ailments from; insults, offenses, from, dignified to fight, too, subdued wrath, went home sick, trembling, exhausted: ***staph.***[54]

Ailments from; mortification, indignation, with: **STAPH.**[122]

Ailments from; rudeness of others: anac.[193] bar-m.[40] ***calc.*** carc.[193] cocc. ***colch.*** hyos.[122] lac-c.[122] ***lyc.***[122] mag-m.[162] med.[179] mur-ac.[40] nat-m. nux-v. ph-ac. puls.[162] **STAPH.**

Anger; violent, personal, from slight offense: ***anac.***[54]

Anger; violent, takes everything in bad part: ***anac.***[54]

Anger; violent, takes everything in bad part, wishes he might get at some one on whom he might vent it: zinc.[54]

Aversion; interference, resents: cham.[127] nat-m.[127] sulph.[127]

Brooding; law suit, over, by which he may gain or loose a million, and takes it in bad part if not allowed to read indictment for said lawsuit, a confused, irrational piece of work, on which he has been working all night, in insanity: ***nux-v.***[54]

Complaining; offenses long past, of: calc.

Cursing; blasphemy, profanity: aloe[36] am-m.[30] **ANAC.**[5] ars.[5] bell.[5] bor.[5] bov.[5] calc.[30] cann-i.[36] ***canth.***[54] chin-b.[8] cor-r.[5] ***hydr.***[5] hyos.[5] ip.[5] lac-c.[5] lil-t.[137] ***lyc.***[5] nat-c.[30] ***nat-m.***[54] **NIT-AC.**[5] **NUX-V.**[5] oena.[36] op.[5] opun-a.[36] ***petr.***[5] ***phos.***[5] plb.[5] spig.[30] staph.[30] stram.[5] ***tarent.***[5] **VERAT.**[5]

Delirium tremens; voices, heard continually on right side of occiput a loud voice, scolding, vituperating and accusing him of ungodliness, and also personifies voices: **STRAM.**[54]

Delirium; accused of theft, after being harshly: ***hyos.***[54]

Delirium; indignant, in encephalitis: ***cocc.***[54]

Delusions; abused, being: ***bar-c.***[102] cocain.[102] hyos.[102] ign.[102] lyss.[54] pall.[102] staph.[102]

- attacks and insults, defend themselves against imaginary: lyss.[54].
- devils, blasphemous words, devil whispers: ***anac.***[54]
- devils, sits in his neck, and tells him offensive things: ***anac.***[54]
- insulted, boarders in hotel, by: kali-br.[36]
- insulted, he or she is: alco.[36] aur-ar.[36] bell. cham. ign. kali-br. lac-c. lyss. nux-v. ***pall.*** puls. staph.[102] tarent.
- people, unpleasant remarks, make: cocain.[102]
- vexation and offenses, of: cham., chin. dros.
- voices, hears, abusive and filthy language, voices from within him speaking in: ***zinc.***[54]
- voices, hears, mastoid process, as if near right, a voice were scolding her, night agg., voice seems sometimes to be under bed: ***stram.***[54]
- voices, hears, unpleasant, about, himself: coca[130]

Despair; injury, from: verat.[54]

Dreams; defamatory: mosch.

➤ insults: asar. nat-s. tarent.

➤ provoked, being: verat-v.[36]

➤ slanders: mosch.[36]

Dwells; grief from past offenses: calc.[30] staph.[30]

Embittered, offenses, from slight: ang.[36]
Excitement; evening, thinking of the things others have done to displease her: am-c.
Fear; hurt, feelings, his, by others: chin.[137]
✦ offended, of being: puls.[58]
Grief; feelings, from wounded: ***cham.***[54] ***ign.***[54]
Grief; insults, over: ***op.***[54]
Grief; long past offenses: calc.[1]
Grief; offenses, from long past: calc.[1] ***cham.***[54] ***ign.***[54] ***op.***[54] ***staph.***[30]
Hatred; bitter feelings for slight offenses, has: ang.
Hatred; persons, of, offended him, who had: agar.[60] am-c.[60] anac.[60] ***aur.*** calc.[30] cic.[60] lach.[60] led.[60] mang. med.[212] ***merc.***[30] ***nat-m.*** nit-ac. nux-v.[30] ph-ac.[60] sep.[122] stann.[60] staph.[30] sulph.
Hatred; persons, of, offended him, who had, unmoved by apologies: **NIT-AC.**
Haughty; wounded, wishes to be flattered: **PALL.**[54]
Hypochondriasis; insults, from: ***staph.***[54]
Hysteria; reprimands, after: ign.[189] nat-m.[162]
Hysteria; sick, after being insulted and subduing his wrath: ***staph.***[54]
Indignation: acon.[10] ambr. androc.[222] ***ars.*** aur. bry.[30] ***calc-p.*** caps. cham.[30] chin. cocc. ***coloc.*** croc. ferr-p.[36] gels.[162] germ.[222] graph.[1] ign. ip.[122] ***m-p-a.***[1] med.[149] nat-c. nat-m.[189] nitro-o.[36] nux-v.[30] oena.[36] psor.[106] sabad.[129] spig.[30] **STAPH.** sulph.[1] verat.[30]
Irritability; insults, from: canth.
Irritability; offenses, from: canth.[36]
Irritability; takes everything in bad part: alum.[85] anac.[137] bov. caps.[137] caust. cocc.[137] ***croc.*** mag-s.[85] nat-m. nux-v.[137] ***pall.*** puls. staph.[137] verat.[137]
Jesting; aversion to: ***acon.*** am-c. ang. apis ars. bor. bov. caps. carb-an. ***cina*** cocc. cycl. ***merc.***[122] nat-m. nux-v. puls. sabin. sil. spig. staph.[30] sulph. thuj.
Jesting; joke, cannot take a: ***acon.***[54] ang.[54] caps.[30] **IOD.**[30] lyc.[30] merc.[30] nat-m.[1] nux-v.[30] puls.[30] spig.[60] sulph.[30] viol-t.[60]
Kill; sudden impulse to, offense, for a slight: ***hep. merc. nux-v.***
Malicious; insults, long after: nit-ac.[60]
Mildness; complaining, bears suffering, even outrage without: ***ign.***[54]
Moaning; honor, effects of wounded: ***nux-v.***[54]
Moaning; offense happened long ago, for trifling: ***cham.***[54]
Mocking; others at him, thinks: ign.[30] nux-v.[30] ph-ac.[30] sep.[30]
Offended; criticism, takes advice as: lil-t.[168]
Offended; easily: ***acon.***[122] agar. ***alum.*** alum-sil.[162] am-br.[162] anac. ang. ant-c.[137] ant-t.[58] ***apis*** aq-mar.[231] arist-cl.[144] arn. **ARS.**[122] ars-s-f.[58] ***aur.*** aur-ar.[58] aur-s.[58] bamb-a.[1184] ***bell.***[10] bor. ***bov. bufo***[117] **CALC.**[122] calc-ar.[58] calc-s. camph. cann-s. ***caps.*** carb-an.[1] ***carb-v.*** carbn-s. **CARC.**[122] **CAUST.**[122] cench.[58] cham. ***chel.*** chin. chin-ar. cic.[54] cimic.[137] ***cina*** cinnb. ***cocc.*** coff.[36] ***coloc. croc.*** cupr.[104] ***cycl.*** dros. germ.[222] ***graph.*** hell.[8] hyos.[122] ign.[56] **IOD.**[122] kali-n.[10] ***lach.***[122] lap-c-b.[194] lap-gr-m.[194] lap-mar-c.[194] lil-t.[58] **LYC.**[122] lyss. mag-s.[10] med.[179] merc. morg-g.[136] nat-c.[10] ***nat-m.*** nit-ac.[36] **NUX-V.** ***pall. petr.*** phos. ***plat.*** prot.[193] ***puls.*** rad-br.[144] ran-b. samars.[111] sanic.[137] ***sars. sep. sil.***[10] ***spig.*** stann.[10] **STAPH.**[122] stram. sul-ac.[5] ***sulph. syph.***[56] tarent.[47] teucr.[36] thuj.[10] **TUB.**[122] ***verat.*** viol-t.[122] ***zinc.*** zinc-p.[58]
Offended; jokes, by: nat-m.[36]
Rage; insults, after: sang. stram.
Reproaches; others, imaginary insult, for: aur-ar.[58]
Sadness; harsh word, from a seemingly: med.[54]
Sadness; insult, as if from: ***cocc.***
Sensitive; laughed at, to being: calc.[127]
Sensitive; others say about her, what: stann.[137] staph.[102]
Sensitive; rudeness, to: bar-m.[162] ***calc.*** carc.[193] cocc. ***colch.*** mag-m.[162] med.[179] mur-ac.[162] nat-m. nux-v. ozone[227] ph-ac. puls.[187] stann.[187] **STAPH.**
Sighing; honor, effects of wounded: ***nux-v.***[54]
Somnambulism; honor, from wounded: ign.[137]
Talk; others agg., of, about her: ***bar-c.***[137] hyos.[137] ign.[137] pall.[137] stann.[137] staph.[137]
Thoughts; persons who had offended him, of: glon.[36]
Throws; things, persons, at, offend, who: **STAPH.**[122]
Weeping; offense, former: caust.[30] ign.[30] lach.[30] staph.[30]
Weeping; offense, from: ***stram.***[54]
Weeping; offense, imaginary, at least: cham.[1]

ADAM. Sh, 199 - The downside was that I also experienced hurt more keenly and felt mortally wounded more often than is good for me, in situations that I would normally have shrugged off. And when I felt bad, I felt rotten. 18, 30C, XX:XX:XX

Sh, 200 - I felt like I had been treated badly, a mixture of insult and humiliation. 15, 12C, 01:09:45

Sh, 203 - Insulted. The worst insult is being told I've become like my father. 7, 6C, 05:17:00

Sh, 204 - I feel overwhelmingly hard done by (mistreated) and need to feel heard and understood. 7, 6C, 13:00:XX

Sh, 205 - Get angry when criticized, yet easily critical of others.[20], 1M, 06:XX:XX

ANDROC. Sh, 96 - Increased irritability, a "how dare you!" feeling. Felt like tearing offenders to pieces with his bare hands. He felt an enormous surge of violent emotions at trifles, and had to exercise great control to stop outbursts of violence and impulses to hurt someone. Felt that "everyone were creeps", could not be bothered with anyone. (2)

ACON. Ha, 526 - He takes every joke in bad part.

He, 47 - Vexed at trifles; takes every joke in bad part.

ALUM. Al, 3 - He takes everything in the worse sense, and weeps and howls for hours.

Al, 32 - She is excessively peevish, and everything is offensive to her; she desires nothing but to quarrel and make a fuss,...

Ha, 33 - She is extremely peevish, and everything is offensive to her; she only wishes to scold (criticize) and to raise a fuss (trouble) in the afternoon.

ANAC. Ha, 15 - Very peevish and out of humor, with great sensitiveness to all offenses.

Ha, 18 - Extremely passionate at a slight offense, breaking out into violence.

Ha, 16 - He takes everything ill and becomes violent.

He, 25 - Has a devil in his ear whispering blasphemous words.

He, 30 - Hallucination; delirium a demon sits on his neck and tells him most offensive things.

ANG. Al, 10 - Discouragement; dissatisfaction with his situation; he does not bear a joke; slight offenses fill him with bitterness.

He, 3 - Ill-humored, oversensitive to jokes, slight offenses fill him with bitterness.

He, 4 - The slightest offense, a mere trifle, irritates.

ARS. Al, 94 - Very fretful, indignant, capricious; every word offends her, and makes her very angry, when she should answer.

Ha, 58 - Very peevish and sensitive; the least thing insults him and angers him.

He, 101 - The least thing offends him, and moves him to anger.

He, 59 - Very peevish and passionate, capricious, she takes every word ill and is cross when she has to answer.

AUR. Ha, 337 - Very much given to feel offended; the slightest thing which he thought offensive affected him deeply, and caused him to resent it.

Ha, 28 - Excessively disposed to take offense; even the least thing seeming offensive to him, affected him deeply and caused resentment.

BOR. Ha, 15 - Passionate, cross, takes offense easily.

BOV. Al, 10 - Great sensitiveness; became easily offended at everything.

CALC-P. Al, 15 - A communication in which some one is justly reproached concerning his conduct, affects him very disagreeably; he grows violent, and holds up his faults to himself.

CALC. Al, 9 - Cries and complains about the long-past offenses.

Ha, 9 - Grief and complains over insults long past.

He, 86 - Easily offended; takes everything amiss.

CAMPH. Ha, 342 - The boy crawls into a corner and howls and weeps; he takes offense at everything one says to him, as if he thought he was being ordered (instructed) about, and he thinks he is insulted and affronted.

He, 73 - Dogmatical, easily offended.

CAPS. Al, 1 - He makes reproaches and becomes angry at the faults of others; he becomes offended at trifles and finds fault.

Al, 2 - Even in the midst of joking he becomes offended at the slightest trifles.

Ha, 334 - He makes reproaches, and is indignant (angry) at the faults (errors) of others; he takes trifles ill and finds fault with them.

Ha, 335 - In the midst (center) of joking he takes the slightest trifle in bad part.

He, 14 - Peevish, irritable angry; easily offended, takes everything in bad part.

CARL. Al, 16 - Very much disposed to take everything in bad part and to be critical.(especially after three weeks and later)

CAUST. Ha, 39 - Unbounded inclination to take things ill.(insulted)

He, 58 - Irritable temper, disposition to take everything in bad part.

CHAM. Ha, 469 - Howling (scream) on account of a slight, even an imaginary insult, which indeed, occurred long ago. (past)

Ha, 471 - Suspicion that he may have been insulted.

He, 70 - Bad effects of having feelings wounded. (ailments from)

He, 16 - Moaning on account of a very trifling offense, which had happened a long time ago.

CINA. He, 8 - Great earnestness (serious) and sensitiveness; he is offended at slightest joke.

COCC. Al, 9 - Constant sad thoughts, as though he had suffered an insult.

Al, 10 - She is absorbed in the saddest thoughts, and affronts (indignity) sink deep into her heart.

Al, 26 - She is offended at the slightest circumstance, often to weeping, with contraction of the pupils: after weeping loss of appetite.

Al, 27 - Very much affected and offended by slight obliquities (immorality) and untruths (falsehood) of others.

Ha, 521 - He is sunk in saddest thoughts, and insults he has received he takes deeply to heart.

Ha, 524 - Continual sad thoughts, just as if he had received insults.

Ha, 547 - Great sensitiveness of disposition; everything offends him.

Ha, 554 - He is very indignant and annoyed at slight faults and fibs (lie, falsify) of others.

Ha, 551 - Easily annoyed; he takes everything in bad part.

He, 24 - Melancholy and sad; indulges in sad reveries (daydream); is sensitive to insults, slights (despises) and disappointment.

COFF. Al, 4 - He is able to hear many annoying things spoken of, without being affected or becoming offended thereby (curative action).

COLCH. He, 15 - Ailments from grief of misbehavior of others.

COLOC. He, 11 - Morose mood; becomes offended at everything.

CON. Ha, 10 - The propinquity (proximity) and the talk of people passing by is very offensive to him, and he feels impelled to assault and maltreat them.

CUR. Al, 4 - Everything he sees appears foul and nasty. (dirty, dishonest, offensive, injurious, indecent)

CYCL. Al, 13 - Ill-humored, morose mood; he could easily take offense at every trifle and get very much exercised about it.

Ha, 193 - Peevish, morose disposition; he easily takes every trifle in bad part, and gets angry over it.

He, 20 - Ill humored, morose mood; could easily take offense at every trifle.

DROS. Al, 14 - Taciturn, quiet, and anxious; he was constantly in dread (fear) of hearing something unpleasant.

Al, 15 - He is very much affected by offenses, with some vexation.

Al, 266 - Vivid frightful dreams about being maltreated (insulted, injured).

Ha, 281 - He takes insults very resentfully, not without vexation.

GERM. Sh, 8 - Weeping. Feeling very offended towards father who had objected because I had bought something expensive for myself. Felt anger because of my reaction, but also curiosity to find out why I reacted. Feel anxiety about all my responsibilities. Everything feels like too much. 21, 12C, 26:XX:XX.

Sh, 120 - Easily led of others opinion, and provoked. Sensitive to others attempts at restricting me. Feel like a teenager, but I don't dare to protest. I just feel it inside. 18, 30C, 04:00:00

Sh, 146 - Slightest criticism and I am broken hearted. Almost started to cry among all the people, very doubtful about relationships. It kills my confidence. Deep sigh. 21, 12C, 41:XX:XX

Sh, 145 - I am easily offended by being told that I look strange. 08, 12C, 18:06:10

Sh, 168 - Indignation. Think all falls on me. 21, 12C, 36:XX:XX.

GLON. Al, 14 - Recalls old grievances...; he was constantly thinking of persons who had offended him, with determination to justify (excuse, defend) his own conduct.

He, 8 - Long forgotten old offenses come back to him.

GRAN. Al, 10 - Inclined to get angry at offenses.

GRAPH. Al, 23 - He awoke at 2 a. m. with restless mood; everything that could injure him happened, and made him anxious, so that frequently he did not know where he should turn,...

He, 22 - Extremely fretful; everything angers and offends him.

HALI-L. Sh, 561 - Felt insulted and taunted by a bitchy patient all day. 16, 10C, 02:XX:XX

Sh, 572 - Dwell on past disagreeable occurrences. Hold a grudge. 16, 10C, 33:XX:XX

HYDROG. Sh, 253 - I was defensive and angry. I thought my friend didn't understand me. I had to apologise. I felt vulnerable and deeply hurt by her. 16, 30C, 05:XX:XX

HYOS. Al, 94 - He reproaches others, and complains of a supposed injury done him.

He, 16 - Fears: being left alone (solitude, deserted); poison, or being bitten (hurt); being poisoned or sold; being betrayed, or injured; wishes to run away. (escape)

He, 79 - After being harshly (severe) accused of theft (crime), continual delirium; fancies surrounded by objects of a terrifying nature; not a moment quiet, continual calling out that she saw the devil; denies herself guilty of theft (innocent, injustice), or that she has any concern with witches; ...

IGN. He, 49 - Mild disposition; bears suffering, even outrage (offenses), without complaining.

KALI-BR. Al, 6-...she fancied that the boarders in the hotel insulted her, and imagined that the weekly bills of the landlord (owner) were evidences of a conspiracy which had been got up against her father; ... while standing on the guards of the boat ...declared she had seen her brother fall overboard;...

KALI-CY. Al, 5 - At 7 p.m., while walking out of doors, feelings of crossness; carries on a kind of conversation within himself, as if quarreling with someone whith whom he had previously disagreed; thinks what he will reply in case certain things are said to him.

KALI-I. He, 6 - Very great irritability and unwonted harshness of demeanor (behavior); his children, to whom he is devoted and attached, become burdensome to him; very passionate and spiteful temper;...constant apprehension of impending evil.

LAC-C. Al,N-11 - Thinks that she is looked down upon (despised) by every one, that she is of no importance in life, and feels insulted thereat. (unimportant, worthless)

He, 36 - Feels insulted because she thinks she is looked down (scorn, despised) upon by everyone.

LACH. Al, 32 - Becomes easily peevish and mistrustful; believes himself intentionally injured (hurt, prejudice) by all his environments, and attaches the most hateful significance to the most innocent occurrences.

LYSS. Al, 28 - Very cross, so much that my children expressed great surprise; took offense at the merest trifles; scolded (censorious) my wife and children; ....

Al, 30 - Offended at everything; gives offensive answers.

Al,N-23 - Imagine that they are being abused (injured, offended), and energetically defend themselves against attacks and insults, ...

Al,N-88 - Very cross, so much... he took offense at veriest trifles, scolding his wife and children, felt wretched, ...

Al,N-124 - Every offense she feels very much.

He, 23 - Imagine that they are being abused (hurt, injured), and energetically defend themselves against attacks and insults, which in reality are products of their own fancy.

He, 88 - Very cross, so much so that his children expressed great surprise; he took offense at veriest trifles, scolded his wife and children, felt wretched, ...

MANG. Ha, 14 - Embittered humor; irreconcilable and long-continued resentment against those who injure him.

MED. Al,N-47 - It feels the evil coming to it, and the bad news before it arrives (clairvoyance), of course it is selfish, and it is easily hurt by a harsh (rude) word.

NEON. Sh, 175 - I've been in a rotten mood all day, dwelling on past offenses. I just can't let go, it's making me angry. I feel like I hate that bastard; it's not an emotion I've had before. Now I feel vindictive, really awful; I feel that if I ever found out that he had been lying to me again I would say to him, "I'll kill you," "I'll slit your throat." These violent feelings were much eased when alone. 02, 6C, 04:22:40

MERC. Al, 10 - Great seriousness, with much indifference all day; he was much offended if others laughed over a trifle, and yet was extremely indifferent to everything that took place about him.

Ha, 1242 - All day long great seriousness with much indifference; he got angry when others laughed at a trifle, and at the same time was extremely indifferent to all about him.

He, 44 - Ailments from mortification; from insults; from egotism.

He, 49 - Ailments from mortification; from insults; from egotism.

MEZ. Al, 32 - Is inclined to get angry with others about trifling and perfectly harmless things; everything vexes him, and he wants to say all kinds of annoying and vexatious things.

NAT-M. Al, 97 - She takes everything in bad part, and weeps and cries much.

Al, 103 - Hatred of people who had insulted him.

Al, 109 - Offended by a joke.

Ha, 4 - Melancholy mood; he cannot remove from his thoughts injuries (insults) he has inflicted on others, or which have been inflicted on him, which depressed him so much that he had no pleasure in anything. (remorse)

Ha, 68 - Hatred (rancor, resentment) against persons, who had formerly offended him.

Ha, 11 - She takes everything in bad part, and weeps and cries.

Ha, 57 - Offended by a joke.

Ha, 64 - Injuries which he had inflicted on others, or which others had done to him, always dwelled in his thoughts; he could not get rid of them, and this annoyed him, so that he had no pleasure in anything.

He, 13 - Taciturnity; offended at every word (easily); avoids company; hates persons because they have offended him; spleen.

He, 21 - Gloomy thoughts, recalls (remember),insults long since suffered; likes to dwell upon past unpleasant occurrences.

NUX-V. Ha, 1263 - He is peevish solicitous, takes everything amiss (erroneous), and readily breaks out into scolding and abuse.

He, 10-...every harmless word offends, every little noise frightens, anxious and beside themselves, cannot bear even the least suitable medicine. (contrary)

He, 19-...; imagines himself surrounded by persons who carry on all sorts of pranks (joke, jest), or ply (covering) him whith questions which he thinks he is compelled (forced) to answer (proved, questioned, interrogated);..; answers questions rationally and is conscious of his condition; ...appears to be haunted (obsessed) by a great fear.

He, 37-...betraying (play false, feigning) great moral and physical languor (indifference),..launches into high-flying, fantastic plans, fancies himself rich (rank, position) and wants to make presents of thousands (squanders, waste), and makes large useless purchases; does not consider himself ill; ...,and takes in bad part if not allowed to read indictment (accusation) for said lawsuit, a confused irrational piece of work...

He, 37-...brooding all night long over a lawsuit by which he may gain or lose a million (megalomania) ; ..replies reluctantly and slowly to physician's questions, and takes it in bad part (offenses) if not allowed to read indictment (accusation) for said lawsuit, a confused irrational piece of work, on which he has been working all night.

OP. He, 30 - Grief over insults is followed by convulsions.

OPUN-V. Al, 6 - In the afternoon, fit of petulance, angry at near relatives, swearing mood, not at all pleased, cannot get over the thought of injuries done by friends.

PALL. He, 8 - Imagines herself neglected

(scorned, despised); wounded pride.

PETR. Al, 8 - Violent irritable, offended at trifles.

He, 7 - Violent irritable, offended at trifles.

PH-AC. Ha, 25 - At a slight offense, he is, as it were, beside himself and passionate.

PHOS. Al, 136 - Felt exceedingly petulant (irritable, contemptuous) all day; nothing went right; felt as dissatisfied with myself as with others; seemed as if everybody said or did something to provoke me.

Ha, 17 - Apprehension, as if she was grieved about something, frequently recurring.

PLAT. Ha, 33 - Very cross and irritated at harmless matters and words; so that she at times would have liked to have beaten herself and friends.

PULS. Al, 32 - Extremely morose, will not answer, takes everything in bad part, in the evening towards sundown.

Ha, 1133 - Cross, takes in bad part what others say.

He, 47-...; pangs (pain, anxiety) of conscience about religion and female sex; violent palpitation in the presence of women; abhors (detests, aversion) and hates the sex; must go out of their way for fear of injuring them; looks upon them as evil beings and is afraid (fear; temptation, seduction); considers their presence injurious (insulted, offended) to his soul; ... (sexual loathing)

RAN-B. Al, 3 - Ill humored, and disposed to quarrel and scold the first forenoon; in the evening is desponding, apprehensive, sensitive, discontented; on the second day he again inclines to be provoked by innocent jests of his friends, etc.;...

SARS. Al, 19 - Every word may offend him.

Ha, 16 - Readily insulted by a word.

SEP. Ha, 34 - Very readily offended.

He, 34 - Greatest irritability from slightest causes; very easily offended.

He, 23 - Is easily offended and inclined to be vehement.(intense)

SIL. Ha, 18 - Capricious and disposed to take things ill.

SPIG. Al, 15 - Earnestness; he is vexed if one jokes in the least with him.

Ha, 665 - Serious humor, he gets cross if the slightest joke is attempted on him.

He, 6 - Easily irritated or offended.

STAPH. He, 6 - Hypochondriasis (depression);...;caused by unmerited insults (offenses, affronts, abuses) sexual excesses, or by persistently dwelling on sexual subjects.

He, 9 - Very sensitive to least impression; least word that seems wrong (offenses) hurts her very much.

He, 11 - Great indignation about things done by others or by himself; grieves about consequences. (remorse)

He, 14-...; was insulted (slandered, defamed, calumniated) being too dignified (reserved, lordly,) to fight (contest), subdued (control) his wrath(anger) and went home sick,.. (ailments, from offenses)

STRAM. He, 93 - Mania; thinks he is lying on his sepulchre (tomb); confessing, praying, wants to be killed (redemption, salvation, regeneration); laughs as if tickled (excited); wants to be kissed; accuses his wife of being faithless (betrayed); scolding (censure) beating in a rage, will not be taken hold of by attendants (suspicious?) ; takes them for dogs (contemptuous), and barks at them; talking in Jewish jargon; (rank?, stranger?) supposes his house to be surrounded by carts (vehicle), Jews (Judaism) and geese, offending him, ... -(strange, foreign, alien)

He, 107-...heard continually, on r. side of occiput, a loud voice, scolding, vituperating and accusing him of ungodliness (impious, sinful, irreligious, godless, profane); ....prayed expecting, with great anxiety, the flash of lightning which was to kill him;...(redemption, regeneration, salvation)

He, 171 - Crying mood, with inclination to give offense and to feel offended.

SULPH. Al, 84 - He is vexed at everything, gets angry and out of humor at every word, thinks he must be defended (protect) and becomes exasperated.

Al, 87 - Embittered mood as if he had been injured.

Ha, 38 - He gets vexed about everything, takes every word ill and gets insulted (dishonored, degraded), he imagines he ought (must) to defend himself and gets angry.

Ha, 56 - The mind is embittered, as if he had been insulted.

TARENT. Al, 1-...threatening words of destruction and death; she believes she is insulted; ...
THUJ. Al, 91 - Morose, quarrels about a harmless joke.
VERAT. He, 56 - Consequences (ailments from) of injured pride or honor.

OFFENSIVE

Abrupt, harsh: ***calc.***[122] cham.[58] germ.[222] hecla.[234] hep.[30] lil-t.[58] luna[228] lyc.[30] med.[137] ***nat-m.***[122] nit-ac.[30] nux-v.[122] ***plat.***[122] **PULS.**[122] rauw.[119] sil.[30] sulph.[30] ***tarent.***
Abrupt; affectionate, yet: aur-m.[162] lyc.[30] nux-v.[30] **PULS.**[30]
Abusive, insulting: ***abies-n.***[162] ***acon.***[10] alco.[36] am-c. am-m. ***anac.*** arn.[36] ars.[30] atro.[36] ***aur.***[5] ***bell.*** bor. bufo[141] camph.[5] canth.[10] caust. cere-s.[102] **CHAM.**[5] chin.[185] cic.[30] ***con.***[5] cor-r.[10] croc.[5] cupr-ar.[54] der.[36] dulc. elae.[36] gall-ac.[36] hep.[58] hist.[144] ***hyos. ign.*** ip. ***kali-ar.***[54] kali-i.[58] ***lac-c.***[102] lach.[30] lap-gr-m.[194] lil-t.[102] **LYC.**[5] ***lyss.*** m-aust.[10] mag-c.[144] med.[212] merc.[10] mosch. nat-c.[5] nit-ac. ***nux-v.*** ozone[227] pall.[5] ***petr.*** plat.[137] plb. raja-s.[149] ran-b. sarr.[36] ***seneg. sep.*** sil.[5] spong. staph.[5] ***stram.***[5] sulph.[137] syph.[122] ***tarent.***[137] ***tub.***[122] ***verat.*** viol-t.
Abusive; calling names and scolding, if irritated: **VERAT.**[54]
Abusive; children insulting parents: am-m.[30] cham.[162] hyos.[30] lach.[176] lyc.[30] nat-m.[30] ***plat.***[30]
Abusive; exhausted, until: mosch.[5] nat-c.[5]
Abusive; family and children, to: kali-i.[137]
Abusive; friends, even to his best: gall-ac.[36]
Abusive; husband insults wife, children, and: lyss.[36]
Abusive; husband insults wife, in front of children or vice versa: anac.[30] ars.[30] lach.[30] nux-v.[30] verat.[30]
Abusive; husband, to: thuj.[137]
Abusive; indecent language, in puerperal mania: ***camph.***[54]
Abusive; opposed, when: hydr.[36]
Abusive; scolds until the lips are blue and eyes stared and she falls down fainting: ***mosch.***
Answer; abruptly, shortly, curtly: ars. ars-h. cham.[58] ***cic.*** coff. gels. ***hyos.*** jatr. mur-ac. nux-v.[162] ***ph-ac.*** phos. plb. rhus-t. sec. sin-n.[58] ***stann. sulph. tarent.***
Answer; civil, cannot give: **CHAM.**[54]
Answer; offensive: lyss.[36]
Answer; violently, as if angry: rhus-t.[60]
Censorious; scolding, with: ars.[30] merc.[30]
Company, aversion to; friends, meeting of, whom he imagines he has offended, to: ars.
Company, desire for; treats them outrageously, yet: ***kali-c.***
Contrary; spiteful, just to be: tub.[162]
Cursing; curses, desire to curse: acon.[188] alco.[36] aloe am-c. am-m.[30] ambr.[162] **ANAC.** arn.[54] ***ars.*** bamb-a.[1184] ***bell.***[122] bor. bov. bufo[170] calc.[30] ***camph.***[8] cand-a.[239] cann-i. canth. caust.[30] cere-b.[77] cere-s.[102] chin-b.[8] chlf.[46] cimx.[100] coloc.[121] ***con.***[102] cor-r. cub.[36] cupr.[5] cupr-s.[36] dulc.[102] euon-a.[77] gall-ac. hydr.[36] ***hyos.*** ip. ***lac-c.*** lac-h.[229] ***lil-t. lyc.*** lyss. med.[212] ***mosch.***[102] nat-c.[30] ***nat-m.***[122] **NIT-AC.** ***nux-v.*** oena. op.[30] opun-a. pall. petr. phos.[122] plb. puls. sanic.[85] sep.[189] skat.[72] spig.[30] staph.[30] stram. tarent.[122] trich-d.[77] ***tub.*** valer.[79] ***verat.***
Cursing; disappointment in plans, on: opun-a.[36]
Cursing; herself, to: merc.[122]
Cursing; laughing, with, convulsive, spasmodic: oena.[36]
Cursing; laughing, with, immoderate: stram.[155]
Cursing; mania, in: ***hyos.***[54] lil-t.[100] ***nat-m.***[8] stram.[111] verat.[28]
Cursing; mother, throws food or medicine across room, curses his: ***hydr.***[8]
Cursing; rage, after: ***arn.***[54]
Cursing; strong and violent expressions: pall.[54]
Cursing; threatening destruction and death: tarent.[54]
Cursing; trifles, about: bor.[1] ozone[227] verat.[85]
Delirium; scolding: chr-ac.[54] hyos. merc. nit-ac.[137] stram. verat-v.[54]
Delusions; cursing, with: anac.[102] nit-ac.[162] verat.[10]
- friend, offended: ars.
- insulting, with: lyc.[10]
- offended, people, he has: **ARS.**[122] cere-b.[77] **HYOS.**[30] nit-ac.[30]
- people, sees, insults them, and: ***lyc.***[54]
- whispering, blasphemic: anac.[85]

Desires; vexatious things, to say: mez.[36]
Despair; rage, cursing and imprecations: **NIT-AC.**[30]
Discouraged; cursing, with: nit-ac.[10]

Dreams; cursing: caj.[36]
➤ intriguing character, that he has an: lach.
➤ scolding: am-c.[54]
Excitement; anger, with inclination to, and to scold: ***petr.***[54]
Excitement; curses his mother, throws food or medicine across room: ***hydr.***[54]
Fear; offending his associates, of: tus-f.[36]
Harshness, rough: anac.[162] ars.[30] **CAUST.**[30] ***graph.***[30] hep.[30] ***kali-i.***[54] lach.[30] lyss.[54] ***m-aust.***[5] med.[122] nat-m.[30] nit-ac.[30] nux-v.[30] pitu-a.[164] ***sep.***[122] ***staph.***[122] sulph.[30] tarent.[162]
Harshness; affectionate, yet: lyc.[30] nux-v.[30] **PULS.**[30]
Harshness; sadness, in: **KALI-I.**[54]
Hatred; persons, of, owner of dog that bit her, with inclination to utter maledictions which shock her: lyss.[54]
Hurt other peoples feelings, inclination to: chin.[102]
Impolite: aran-ix.[149] ***hep.***[30] lyc.[30] ***merc.***[30] plat.[30]
Impulse; rash: bell.[30] ***hyos.***[30] nux-v.[122] staph.[122] ***stram.***[30] verat.[30]
Indignation; insults others: ozone[227]
Indignation; slandering, with: spig.[30]
Indiscretion: acon. alum.[30] arn.[30] ***bar-c.***[30] bov.[30] bry. calad. calc.[30] camph. caps. caust.[30] con.[30] croc.[10] germ.[222] graph.[30] hyos. ign. kali-c.[149] laur. meny. ***merc.***[30] nat-m. ***nux-v.*** op.[30] plat.[30] puls. spong.[30] staph.[30] stram. verat.[30]
Insolence, impertinence: acon.[148] ***anac.***[102] arn.[1] ars.[102] bell. bufo calc.[30] ***canth.*** ***cham.***[102] chin.[102] cupr.[102] ***graph. hyos.*** ign.[10] ***lac-c.*** lach.[30] lap-gr-m.[194] lil-t.[137] **LYC.** lyss. med.[137] ***nat-m.***[30] nit-ac. ***nux-v.*** pall. par.[137] ***petr.*** phos. **PLAT.** ***psor.*** sac-alb.[85] spong.[36] staph.[30] ***stram.***[122] sulph.[137] tarent.[102] ***tub.***[122] **VERAT.**[122]
Insolence; acts, in: stram.[30] verat.[30]
Irritability; outrageously: gall-ac.[36] hep.[85]
Jealousy; accuses wife of being faithless: ***stram.***[54]
Jealousy; insult, driving to: ***nux-v.***[54]
Jealousy; neglect, accuses husband of: ***stram.***[54]
Jealousy; quarrels, reproaches, scolds, with: gall-ac.[36] ***lach.***[54] ***nux-v.***[54]
Malicious; insulting: hyos.[10] merc.[10]
Mania; abuses everyone: ***camph.***[54] ***stram.***[54] ***tarent.***[54]
Quarrelsomeness, scolding: acon. agar. alco.[36] aloe[5] alum. am-c. ambr. ***anac.*** anan. androc.[222] ang.[5] anh.[116] ant-t. ***arn. ars.*** ars-s-f.[58] **ASAF.**[5] asar.[149] aster. atro.[36] **AUR.** aur-ar.[58] aur-s.[58] bamb-a.[1184] bar-c. ***bell.*** bor. ***bov. brom. bry.*** bufo cael.[149] calc. calc-s. ***camph.*** cand-a.[239] cann-s.[10] canth. caps. carb-an.[10] carb-v.[10] ***caust.*** cench. ***cham.*** chap.[149] chel. chin. choc.[222] cocc.[10] coff.[5] colch.[5] ***con.*** cor-r. ***croc.*** crot-h. culx.[58] ***cupr.*** cycl.[10] cyn-d.[149] dig. ***dulc.*** elaps ferr. ferr-acet.[10] ferr-ar. fl-ac. germ.[222] gran.[10] graph.[10] hell.[10] ***hep.***[58] hipp. hir.[144] ***hist.***[119] hydrog.[222] **HYOS.**[122] ictod.[10] **IGN.** iod.[10] ip. kali-ar. kali-bi.[5] ***kali-c.*** kali-chl.[5] kali-i. kali-p.[58] ***lach.*** lap-gr-m.[194] lap-mar-c.[194] led.[10] lepi. ***lyc.*** lyss. m-aust.[10] mag-c.[144] mag-s.[119] mang.[10] med.[189] meph.[149] ***merc.*** merl. mez. ***mosch.*** mur-ac.[10] nat-ar. ***nat-c.*** ***nat-m.*** nat-s. nicc. ***nit-ac. nit-s-d.***[10] **NUX-V.** olnd. op.[5] ozone[227] pall. **PETR.** ***ph-ac. phos. plat.*** plb. prot.[136] ***psor.*** puls.[30] ***ran-b.*** rat. reser.[149] rheum **RHUS-T.**[5] rib-ac.[149] ruta sabad.[10] sac-alb.[36] seneg. ***sep. sil.***[5] spong. stann. ***staph. stram.*** stront-c. sul-ac. sulfonam.[149] **SULPH.** **TARENT.**[122] thea. ***thuj.*** til. tub.[36] tub-k.[70] upa.[85] ***verat. verat-v.*** viol-t. wye.[85] zinc.
Quarrelsomeness; jealousy, from, unchaste expressions, with: ***nux-v.***[54]
Rage; cursing, with: alco.[36] anac.[116] lac-c.[56] mosch.[58] ***nit-ac.***[10] tub.[189] verat.[10]
Reproaches; others, imaginary insult, for: aur-ar.[58]
Reverence; lack of: anac. coloc. verat.[30]
Rudeness: ambr. ***anac.***[5] androc.[222] ant-c.[5] aran-ix.[149] arn. aur. aur-s.[36] bar-c.[5] bell. bufo canth. ***cham.***[5] ***chin.***[54] eug. ferr.[36] gall-ac. graph. hell. ***hyos.*** ign.[5] ***lac-c.*** lach.[5] lap-gr-m.[194] **LYC.** lyss. med.[137] nat-m.[5] nit-ac. nux-m. ***nux-v.*** op. pall. par. petr.[5] phos. **PLAT.**[5] ***psor.***[5] rauw.[119] sieg.[144] spong.[5] ***stram.*** **VERAT.**
Rudeness; children, of naughty: ***ant-c.***[5] carc.[207] cham.[5] ***chin.***[54] cina[5] dulc.[5] ***merc.***[5] rheum[5] staph.[5]
Rudeness; employees to the chiefs, of: lyc.[30] nat-m.[30]
Rudeness; women, in: ***cham.***[116]
Runs about; against people, in walking: cann-i.[36]
Slander, disposition to: am-c. anac. ars. bell. bor. caust.[30] cor-r.[10] guai.[10] helon.[30] hyos. ip. lach.[30] lyc. merc.[10] nit-ac. ***nux-v.*** par.[116] petr. sep. spig.[30] stram. **VERAT.**[122]

Slander; disposition to sneak: ars.[30] lach.[30] nat-c.[30]
Slander; disposition to, denounce, and: ars.[30] lach.[30] nat-c.[30] nat-m.[30]
Slander; disposition to, hypocritical, and: phos.[30] sep.[30]
Spit, desire to; faces of people, in: ars. **BELL.** bufo[170] ***calc.*** cann-i. cann-s.[10] ***cupr.*** cupr-acet.[36] hyos. merc. phos. plb. ***stram. verat.***
Suspiciousness; insulting: merc.[10]
Talk; abrupt: ars.[36] cham.[5] lyss.[54] mur-ac.[36] plb.[36] sul-ac.[36] **TARENT.**[36]
Talk; abrupt, snappish: **CHAM.**[54]
Talk; offensive, inclination to: lyss.[36]
Talk; sharply: cham.[54] hyper.[36]
Teasing: aran-ix.[149] arn.[30] caust.[30] graph.[102] nux-v.[30] tub.[189]
Teasing; laugh at reprimands: graph.[102]
Truth, tells the plain: alum.[30] bov.[30] choc.[222] hyos.[30] verat.[30]
Truth; tell the truth to everyone, has to: ozone[227]

ADAM. Sh, 178 - I see myself as being too intrusive with people. 7, 6C, 14:00:XX
Sh, 180 - Generally fairly severe mood, very straightforward and will say what is needed to be said. Quite strict and harsh, yet not tactless or mean. 20, 1M, XX:XX:XX
Sh, 212 - Sharp and brusque with people. 8, 6C, 04:XX:XX
Sh, 215 - I feel very angry and extremely intolerant, cold and hard and I hate myself for feeling these harsh unkind feelings. 20, 1M, 02:XX:XX
Sh, 216 - Feel harder, more rebellious. I will do what I want. Inconsiderate and unsympathetic. Unfeeling in relationship and sexually. 22, 200C, 01:XX:XX
Sh, 234 - Swearing and cursing. A lot to do, finding it hard to set priorities in my work and the needs of my family. 10, 6C, 19:XX:XX
Sh, 278 - Felt I would create irreparable damage if I said how I feel. Thought I would say the most awful things that the kids would never recover from. Supreme effort to keep silent. Didn't want to be here. The kids were a hassle. I felt old and tired. Desire to get away from the fighting. 16, 12C, 17:XX:XX

ALOE. Al, 25 - Ill-humor; peevish (angry) about himself, so that he insults and blasphemes; worse afternoons.
ANAC. He, 40 - Uses profane language, swears, thinks himself a demon.
ANDROC. Sh, 102 - Assertive, impatient, aggressive. Felt resentful and abused. Had no control over her temper. Bellowed and lashed out at everyone. In the evening, furious for no apparent reason. Wanted to kill her husband and children, banged doors and threw things. By bed-time, she felt fine but the intensity of her evil thoughts was very frightening. (7)
Sh, 103 - Had a very caustic conversation with someone she hardly knew. Enjoyed her rudeness and was surprised by it. (7)
Sh, 116 - Impatient, snappy, shouting, felt trapped and despairing. Growled at her children. (12)
Sh, 126 - Great hostility to those around him, which manifested in brooding and stinging observations and comments directed at his friends. (29)
ARN. Al, 27 - Sullen (morose) insolence and imperiousness. (dictatorial)
Ha, 634 - Surly insolence and imperiousness. (domineering)
ARS. He, 48 - Averse to meeting acquaintances, (friends) because he imagines he has formerly offended them, though knows not how.
He, 76 - Anxiety like that of one who has committed murder; driven from place to place; avoids meeting persons, thinking that he has offended them.
BELL. Ha, 1364 - Unrestrainedly and exuberantly merry, inclined to scold (criticize) without cause, and to insult (affront, offend) in a laughing humor.
CHAM. He, 58 - Insulting, cross and uncivil temper.
CHIN. Ha, 1110 - Extremely disposed to be vexed, and to take every occasion to get cross; afterwards quarrelsome and disposed to vex others, and to make reproaches and give annoyance(irritation) to others.
CHOC. Sh, 7 - In the evening, felt angry with bristling down my back. Irritable with the kids, shouted a lot, slammed doors. Feeling very uncomfortable with my daughter near me. I made a huge issue

over something small which I would normally leave. I wanted to leave and walk out of the door on them. Felt very unsympathetic to the children. "You either go, or go to bed". Couldn't cuddle the children and took longer to say "Its all right". I thought that their father should look after them instead of me (very unusual). The feeling I can't be where I want to be because of them. I want to be roaming outside without my possessions. Left kids alone in the house for the first time. I was surprised at how easily I let them go. My daughter liked it very much.

Sh, 303 - I'm ready to speak my mind —I don't care if people cease to like me.[15], 30C, 20:XX:XX

Sh, 324 - Still snapping and resentful generally.[15], 30C, 36:XX:XX

Sh, 327 - My humour has taken a sarcastic turn, mocking people, a bit aggressive in a joking way.[35], 30C, 00:03:XX

Sh, 331 - I became selfish, impatient and intolerant. Behaved in a strange way -hard and quarrelsome -snapping at people. Could not stand people wasting time or being inefficient, I wanted things done immediately.[35], 30C, XX:XX:XX:

CON. Ha, 10 - The propinquity (proximity) and the talk of people passing by is very offensive to him, and he feels impelled to assault and maltreat them.

He, 18 - He is averse to being near people, and to the talk of those passing him (misanthropy); is inclined to seize hold of and abuse them. (insult, offend, curse)

He, 38 - Very much excited, passionate, domineering (dictatorial), quarrelsome, scolds (censorious) and will not bear contradiction.

CROC. Al, 28 - Vacillating (hesitate), peevish mood; the slightest cause excites his anger, for which, next moment, he is sorry (remorse), which however, soon returns, because his calmness frets (disturbs) him and prevents (stop) his exposing his feelings (oppressed); usually he changes a hard word which he has on his tongue to a mild one, but the latter seems too mild, and now chooses a more severe word, ...(sorry, guilty, by anger, mildness, x harsh, rude)

Al, 29 - He takes everything in anger and suddenly repents (apologize) of having injured (offend) others.

He, 13 - He takes everything in anger and suddenly repents (sorry) of having injured (offensive) others.

DER. Al, 6 - He is disposed to strike, and inveighs against his dearest friends.

FL-AC. Al, 15 - During the fourth week very irritable towards people, even to the greatest hatred, which he does not hesitate to give vent to in words, but as soon as he sees them everything is forgotten, and he has an entirely different opinion of them.

GERM. Sh, 139 - Feel angry hostile and tearful easily. Someone says that I have behaved as if I am from another planet. 08, 12C, 30:00:00

Sh, 152 - Aversion to people. Abrupt when obliged to speak. Had a consultation at 10 o'clock and really messed it up. I wish everybody would just go away and leave me alone. No contact. 16, 30C, 07:04:00

GRAN. Al, 11 - Inclined to criticize and blame.

HALI-L. Sh, 338 - Getting curt with people. Abrupt in conversation, cutting things off sooner. 09, 6C, 14:17:XX

Sh, 349 - I said I was moody. It wasn't as qualitative as she wanted, and she was asking for more details and I yelled, " A stupid five year old would understand what I was saying." I became sarcastic and very belligerent. I thought I was being simplistic and clear. I gave what I had to give. I was in a depressed state, lost my good feeling and was angry at being asked to explain the depression. She asked me what do you mean and I said, "XXXX off. If you don't understand that, too bad. Do you understand that?! Do you know the English language?" 18, 30C, 04:14:00

Sh, 607 - An urge to destroy my relationship, scream at people. It felt very destructive. 13, 30C, 04:06:30

HYDR. Al, 26-...forget, for a few seconds, what was wanted, which makes me very angry and feel like damning (swearing) and cursing (blaspheme) everything and anybody who bothered me the least.

HYDROG. Sh, 207 - Stormy and acrimonious (hash) row (fight) with girlfriend. Quarrelling continued throughout the day. Cried a lot —generally feeling rough with loss of appetite — heart pounding and sunk feeling in abdomen though I can't eat. 04, 12C, 01:00:30

Sh, 210 - I was shouting down the phone, but dead quiet with friends. I thought "Why are they talking? They haven't anything to say". I was very sarcastic. 24, 30C, 01:XX:XX

Sh, 241 - I'm afraid to go out because I think I frighten people. 16, 30C, XX:XX:XX

Sh, 248 - While sitting in a restaurant, felt progressively more cut off from friends at the table. I began to feel detached and paranoid. I felt disliked by people. They seemed to look at me menacingly. I became concerned that my lecture this afternoon had created conflict, mayhem and destruction, that my friends in the audience did not like me any more. I became aware of a dull ache in my sacrum making me want to shift backwards and forwards. At the same time, the people round the table seemed further away and smaller, as if I had moved four feet back from the table. I felt very uncomfortable and wanted to get out. I put my head down and rushed out without saying goodbye, feeling a sense of relief at getting away (all very unusual for me). Outside, I felt relief and my mind cleared and I walked home alone. 22, 12C, 04:XX:XX

Sh, 250 - I think I'm dangerous to people and they can't cope with me. 16, 30C, XX:XX:XX

HYOS. He, 34 - Scolds (censorious); raves; abuses those about him.

IRID. Sh, 325 - Stroppy —felt more frustrated, did not want to communicate at all, shouting and abusive. N7

LAC-C. He, 37 - Intense ugliness (repulsiveness, hideousness) and hatefulness (offensiveness); writes to her best friends all sorts of mean and contemptible things. (disdainful)

LIL-T. Al, 25 - While attending a lecture (speech), desire to hit the lecturer, and in the evening desirous of swearing and damning the fire and things generally, and to think and speak obscene things; disposed to strike and hit persons; as these feelings came, the uterine pains passed away.

He, 9 - Disposed to curse, to strike, to think of obscene things; as these mental states came, uterine irritation abated.(reduced)

LYC. Al, 97 - As if out of her mind, she seeks quarrels, makes unfounded reproaches, is most exceedingly violent, and strikes those whom she thus insults.

Ha, 60 - As if insane she seeks for quarrels, makes ungrounded reproaches abuses (insulting) most violently and beats the person whom she abuses.

LYSS. Al, 30 - Offended at everything; gives offensive answers.

Al-N, 37 - Inclined to use insulting language, scold his friends, beat and abuse those near him.

Al,N-88 - Very cross, so much... he took offense at veriest trifles, scolding his wife and children, felt wretched, ...

He, 88 - Very cross, so much so that his children expressed great surprise; he took offense at veriest trifles, scolded his wife and children, felt wretched, ...

MERC. Ha, 1256 - All day long sulky and distrustful (suspicious); he almost insulted those about him, and regarded them all as his greatest enemies.(opponent, rival)

Ha, 1263 - Mania; she throws off the clothes at night, tears the straw about, and scolds; by day she leaps (jump) up high like a petulant extravagant person...she talks and scolds much to herself,...spits frequently and spreads the saliva out with her feet, and licks some of it up again; she often licks cowdung (excrements) and the mud of ponds (lake); she often takes little stones in her mouth, without swallowing them, and at the same time complains that they are cutting her bowels; much clotted blood passes with her motion; ...

He, 37 - Morose and mistrustful; treated his associates almost insultingly, looked upon every one as his worst enemy.

MEZ. Al, 32 - Is inclined to get angry with others about trifling and perfectly harmless things; everything vexes him, and he wants to say all kinds of annoying and vexatious things.

He, 11 - Inclined to get angry with others about trifles; everything vexes him, he wants to say annoying and vexatious things; is soon sorry for it.

MOSCH. He, 3 - Scolding; keeps it up till

her lips turn blue, eyes stare, and she falls down fainting.

NAT-M. Al, 93 - Ill-humored does not want to go into society for fear of vexing others; feels that he could easily give offense.

Ha, 4 - Melancholy mood; he cannot remove from his thoughts injuries (insults) he has inflicted on others, or which have been inflicted on him, which depressed him so much that he had no pleasure in anything. (remorse)

Ha, 58 - Apt to be peevish and abrupt; he does not endure opposition.

Ha, 64 - Injuries which he had inflicted on others, or which others had done to him, always dwelled in his thoughts; he could not get rid of them, and this annoyed him, so that he had no pleasure in anything.

He, 11-, ...uttered the most atrocious blasphemes, swore (blaspheme, curse) against God (divine) and the elements (environment), and after raging for awhile became exhausted,...

NEON. Sh, 177 - I feel like writing a letter to Jeremy and reproaching him about the proving. I just realized that I want to reproach people. I reproach my partner as well. 02, 6C, 05:XX:XX

NIT-AC. Al, 2 - Attacks of rage and despair, with curses and imprecations.(blasphemy)

Ha, 48 - Passionateness, venting itself in abuse. (insult)

He, 19-...headstrong (obstinate); trembling while quarreling; fits of rage with curses and maledictions; inveterate ill-will, unmoved by apologies.

NUX-V. Al, 4 - He is hasty; looked angrily at anyone who asked him a question without answering, as though he was obliged to restrain himself to avoid being insulting; he was in such an irritable and unrestrained mood that it seemed as though he would like to strike any one in the face who spoke a word to him.

Ha, 1253 - Pains are not borne without loud whining and lamenting, mixed with reproaches and scolding.

Ha, 1263 - He is peevish solicitous, takes everything amiss (erroneous), and readily breaks out into scolding and abuse.

Ha, 1267 - Scolding, reproaches, abuse, jealous invectives (accusation), mixed with indelicate expressions -then soon howling and loud weeping.

He, 12 - Inclined to find fault and scold (reprove); morose; stubborn; (obstinate) an insane desire when alone with her husband, whom she adores, to kill him.

He, 17 - He quarrels, reproaches, scolds, insults, from jealousy, mingled with unchaste (obscene) expressions; ...

OPUN-V. Al, 5 - Fit of swearing (cursing) at evening after coming home; praying in the morning, swearing (cursing) on disappointment in plans; fit of rage, on thwarting (frustrating) of plans.

Al, 6 - In the afternoon, fit of petulance, angry at near relatives, swearing mood, not at all pleased, cannot get over the thought of injuries done by friends.

PALL. He, 12 - Greatly inclined to use strong and violent expressions.

PETR. He, 6 - Excitable, irritable with inclination to be angry and to scold; anxious and irresolute.

PLAT. Ha, 37 - During the caprice of contempt, suddenly a voracious hunger...

RAN-B. Al, 2 - Vexed and inclined to be angry; quarrels and scolds when the slightest cause is offered (after two hours).

Al, 3 - Ill humored, and disposed to quarrel and scold the first forenoon; in the evening is desponding, apprehensive, sensitive, discontented; on the second day he again inclines to be provoked by innocent jests of his friends, etc.;...

SENEG. Al, 13 - Phlegmatic; inclines to quarrel and give offense.

SEP. Al, 34 - Feel very much depressed, at 7 A.M.; feel like quarreling with everybody; became very much excited about a mere trifle, and said some very sharp things. (feeling ashamed of it at the same time)

STRAM. He, 56 - Believes to be in his grave; shrives,(confess) prays, asks to be killed (justified); accuses his wife of infidelity; scolds (cursing), strikes at everybody who wishes to restrain him; thinks they are dogs and barks at them to make himself understood.

He, 92 - Mania:... complains that a dog is biting and tearing flesh off his chest; merry exaltation; with pride (haughty) and affectation; runs about, complains of violent headache; ...;steals from his roommates...; disposition to scold persons whom he otherwise loved.

He, 171 - Crying mood, with inclination to give offense and to feel offended.
SULPH. Ha, 57 - His mood is quarrelsome and contentious (hostile) about everything.
TARENT. He, 16 - Attacks of hystero-mania... hits and abuses everyone, destroys whatever she can lay hold of,...mocks aged people with their old age, ...
VERAT. Ha, 664 - Cursing and making a noise all night, and complains of being stupid, with headache and flow of saliva.
He, 24 - Disposed to silence, or to talk about faults of others; if irritated scolding and calling names.
VIOL-T. He, 5 - Very sensitive and inclined to scold.

OFFICER

Delusions; army passed him in the street, a silent, while walking: cann-i.[36]
- figures, marching in the air (evening while half asleep): nat-c.
- general, he is a: cupr.
- military, about: arg.[54]
- officer, he is an: agar. bell. cann-i. ***cupr.*** cupr-acet.[36]
- people, sees, connected with the law who will seize him, causing great anxiety, cries like a child: ***cupr-acet.***[54]
- policeman, calls on him, officers: ***cupr.***[162]
- policeman, come into house, he sees: ars.[58] hyos. kali-br.
- policeman, physician is a: bell.
- pursued, police, by: alco.[36] ars.[58] bell. ***cupr. hyos. kali-br.*** meli. phos. plb. zinc.
- pursued, soldiers, by: absin. bell. bry. nat-c.[30] plb.
- soldier, he is a, (at night): chel.[36]
- soldier, sees: bar-c. ***bell.*** bry. nat-c.[10] op.
- soldier, sees, bed, on his: lact.
- soldier, sees, capture him, that will: bell.[10]
- soldier, sees, cutting him down (amel. on getting cool): bry.
- soldier, sees, in half asleep: nat-c.[1]
- soldier, sees, march silently past: cann-i.
- soldier, sees, surrounded by: nat-c.[30]
- soldiers, sees: bar-c. ***bell.*** bry. nat-c.[10] op.

Dreams; armies, rising from their graves: ptel.[36]
- ➤ fights, generals, with six or seven black, who garroted him and bound him with ropes, causing agony of mind: coca[36]
- ➤ grave, armies rising from their graves: ptel.[36]
- ➤ police, calling for, waking him in last part of night: frax.[36]
- ➤ pursued, police, by: lap-mar-c.[194]
- ➤ pursued, soldiers, by: mag-s.
- ➤ shooting, shot, soldier is shot, a: am-m.[58]
- ➤ soldier, being a: chel.[36]
- ➤ soldiers: bry.[10] chel. mang.[1] nat-c.[10] ozone[227] ptel.[25]
- ➤ soldiers, being pursued by a: mag-s.
- ➤ soldiers, seeing a soldier shot: am-m.

ABSIN. Al,S-6 - Terrifying hallucinations, he sees all kinds of animals, cats and rats of all colors, grotesque animals, fancies that he is pursued by soldiers.
AGAR. Al, 9 - Delirium; he imagines himself a military (martial) officer, commanding (dominant) at a drill (training) and directing the various maneuvers.
ARG-M. He, 4 - Imagines things about the military which he never liked; long forgotten old songs come into his mind.
BELL. He, 106 - Anxiety and fear of imaginary objects and hallucinations, ghosts, soldiers which come to take them away (arrest), black animals, rats dogs, wolves, etc.
He, 105 - Anxiety and fear of imaginary objects and hallucinations, ghosts, soldiers which come to take them away, black animals, rats, dogs, wolves, etc.
BRY. Al, 5-...a delirious frightful fantasy, as of soldiers cutting him down, that he was on the point of escaping;..
CANN-I. Al, 65 - Hallucinations which lead the patient to imagine that he is on horseback, is hunting, that he sees blue water, that he is swimming, or that he is captain of a vessel, that he is traveling, that he has no weight.(lightness)
CHEL. Al, 51 - Anxious about death and being a soldier (warrior, disputant), at night.
CUPR-A. Al, 2 - Attacks of mania; he fancies that he is a military officer; a fancy that he is selling green vegetables; a fancy that he is repairing old chairs...he spits in the faces of the attendants, and laughs heartily at it.
He, 4 - Fixed idea that he sees persons

connected with the law who are about to seize him (imprisoned),...at times sees thieves in the room, spirits, and various other immaterial objects;...

CUPR. Ha, 23 - Fits of insanity, imagines he is a military commander.

GERM. Sh, 128 - Afraid of the police of being caught and unveiled. 18, 30C, 02:10:00

HYOS. Al, 5-...suspicious of those about him; he became delirious, saw policeman coming into the house; heard them speaking about the hall;...

He, 60-... wants to run away for fear of being persecuted by police;...

KALI-BR. Al, 3 - Decidedly insane; had delusions that lewd women had got into his mother's house; that he was pursued by the police; that his wife was threatened by members of the family; that he had thousands of dollars in gold sewed up in his clothing; (rich, wealth)

Al, 4 - He imagined that he had been specially singled out (select) for divine vengeance... deploring his sad fate (destiny),...he informed me that he had been accused of robbing a friend, and that the officers were in search of him....

NAT-C. Al, DREAM, 1117 - Illusions of fantasy, in the evening, while half asleep; she sees figures, visions of soldiers marching in the air;..

OP. He, 20-...declares he is not alone in bed; ..desire to escape; says a regiment of horsemen are upon his bed and that he fears to be trodden upon (run over, crushed); when told that horses are very careful, answered that he feared he would be crushed by the wagons that followed them.

PLB. Al, 59-...;he fancied that a cavalry regiment was about to fall upon him (attacked); or that he was in the presence of his employer, who was finding fault with him.

Al, 60-...; he hears everywhere threatening voices, officers come to arrest him, to seize his furniture (movables), (confiscated, expropriated) and to expel (eject) him from his lodgings (home) (expulsion, exiled) ; the voices come from the pillow, the mattress (bed); they enter by the window, where he sees people, and they consult about him with closed doors (secretive) ; ...

OLD

Delusions; beautiful, old ragged woman is: psil.[164]
- bed, old ragged woman is: psil.[164]
- chairs, he is repairing old: cupr. cupr-acet.[36]
- crippled old man, that he is: hydrog.[222]
- figures, old repulsive persons, which fill her with fear, in hysteria: ***kali-c.***[54]
- man, old men with long beards and distorted faces, sees: laur.
- old, being: hydrog.[222] lap-c-b.[194]
- old, he looks: mag-m.[187]
- women, old and wrinkle, of: calc-sil. cann-i.

Dreams; body, hair, falling out: mag-c.
- ➤ dancing, man, in an old: zing.[54]
- ➤ ghosts, woman, of old: eupi.[36]
- ➤ old gentleman ran away from wife, suspected of having married another: sep.[36]

Dreams; old, things: androc.[222]

Fear; age, of people their own: cortico.[119]
- ✦ old, of getting: lap-mar-c.[194]
- ✦ visions of old repulsive persons, from, in hysteria: ***kali-c.***[54]

Forsaken; feeling, old people, in: aur.[193] psor.[193]

ADAM. Sh, 431 - I feel old and creaky. 7, 6C, 08:00:XX

Sh, 432 - This remedy is prematurely aging me. I feel the youthful bounce has gone. 7, 6C, 21:00:XX

HALI-L. Sh, 1 - Vision on waking of orange-red colored circles on my abdomen like the skin on an orange when it gets old and dry. 08, 30C, 00:07:00

Sh, 6 - Feeling old, really old. 02, 30C, 07:01:XX

HYDROG. Sh, 103 - Feel like a crippled old man. 38, 200C, 18:XX:XX

Sh, 104 - Don't want to move at all —want to be still and warm and lie around in a heap all day. like what it must feel to be old. I do feel old. 16, 30C, 02:XX:XX

IRID. Sh, 75 - While watching TV felt feelings of attraction to older men. I would not normally be attracted to older men. I6

OPPRESSION

Anguish; oppression with: ***calc.***[54] ***cann-i.***[54] ***op.***[54] verat.[54]

Anxiety; chest, compression in, as from: merc.[36]

Anxiety; constrictive, in the house, amel. in open air: carl.[36]

Anxiety; oppressive: acon.[60] alum.[60] am-m.[60] ant-t.[60] ***arn.***[60] ***ars.***[60] ***bell.***[60] calad.[60] calc.[60] ***canth.***[60] **CARB-V.**[54] ***caust.***[60] cham.[60] chel.[60] chin.[60] cina[60] cocc.[60] dig.[60] euph.[60] ***graph.***[60] iod.[60] lact.[60] meny.[60] ***merc.***[60] ***mur-ac.***[60] ***ph-ac.***[54] ***psor.***[54] rhus-t.[60] sep.[60] sil.[60] spig.[60] stront-c.[60] sul-ac.[60] sulph.[1] verat.[60] zinc.[60]

Anxiety; sudden, oppression of chest, with, driving from place to place: ***tab.***[54]

Delusions; clothes, tight, too: apis[8] arg.[36] ars-met.[54] benz-ac.[54] chin.[1] glon.[36] paraf.[77] thuj.[36]

- room, close and hot, is, oppressing: plan.
- soul, something presses on her: bamb-a.[1184]

Dreams; animals, dogs, many young dogs, fastening themselves tightly, in constant succession on various parts of his body: lyc.[36]

➤ body, chest, being pressed: am-m.[36]

➤ suffocation, being in danger of, from some one lying on chest: kali-bi.[36]

Restlessness; abdomen, constricted, as if everything in, was: mosch.[60]

Sadness; heart sensations, from, oppression: ***caust.***[54]

Sadness; pressure about chest and heart, from: asaf.[36] graph.

Shrieking; oppression of chest, during: tarent.[36]

Weeping; evening, oppression of chest, with: ***ran-b.***[54]

Weeping; evening, oppression of chest, with, solitude, with desire for: ***rhus-t.***[54]

ACON. Ha, 514 - Palpitation of the heart with great anxiety, oppression of the breathing and great weariness (lassitude) in all limbs...

He, 37 - Fears to go where is any excitement (tumult) or many people (crowd); thinks she is jostling (pressing) against everyone she meets (oppressed); countenance (expression) expressive of timidity; constant dread (fear) lest she stagger (vacillated) and fall.

AETH. He, 15 - Anxiousness sensation as if a heavy load was lying on chest.

ALUM. Al, 16 - Oppressive anxiety, attended with emptiness and confusion of the head...

He, 23 - Anguish, oppressive and vague fearfulness, or uneasiness as if he had committed a crime.

ALUMN. Al, 2-...felt very much oppressed, anxious, and heavy, like a stone on the chest, with inclination to take a long breath.

AM-C. Ha, 10 - Severe compression of the heart, he knows not how to help himself.

ANAC. Ha, 36 - His mind is very much oppressed, as if a cold in the head were coming on.

BAR-M. He, 7 - Sense of oppressive anxiety, accompanied by the illusory notion that he is walking on his knees, without legs. (inferiority, dwarf?)

BELL. Al, 161 - In walking in the open air, she is overwhelmed with tearful anguish; she is weary of life, and inclines to drown herself.

CALC. Al, 7 - Loneliness is very oppressive, with coldness of the face, hands, and feet.

CARB-V. Al, 12 - Anxiety in the evening after lying down, as from oppression of the chest, ...,a sensation as if the heart would be pressed downward; objects about her seem to become constantly narrower and smaller,...

Ha, 706 - Anxious as if oppressed, for several days.

Ha, 3 - Inexpressibly weighed down with anguish, every afternoon from four to six o'clock.

CHAM. Al, 15 - Very depressed mood, with anxiety and oppression, as of impending evil.

CLEM. Al, 14 - He seemed oppressed by some grief or sorrow, or the shadow of impending misfortune.

CROT-H. He, 15 - Oppression as if brain had been intoxicated by carbonic acid, or by degraded or non-oxygenated blood.

FERR. He, 9 - Mind in highest degree oppressed; despondent (sad); great solicitude (cares) about those belonging to him (relatives, family), with constant thoughts of death.

GELS. He, 33 - Effects (ailments from) of

grief; cannot cry; when thinking of his symptoms (disease), also when spoken to of his loss ; >from diverting talk; oppression and palpitation of heart; feels a sense of peril (danger, harm, risk) ; face flushed; sleeplessness; subdued (subjugate, yielding) manner; ...

GERM. Sh, 191 - Feeling in a rather poetical mood. I feel I can almost capture the essence of the feeling I have been going through: it's an eructation! As if a marble lands somewhere, chest, stomach, brain and sucks to it all the matter around it in a radius of 3-4 cm and packs it tighter and tighter. It gets hard and brittle, then suddenly it grows with a zoomy feeling, steadily becoming less dense and suddenly it bursts and spreads a cloud of relief. I think the remedy is Champagne. 16, 30C, 03:14:00

GRAPH. Ha, 17 - Great anguish, so that she trembles all over, for several minutes.

HURA. Al, 1 - Much excited and oppressed as if by some great misfortune.

IOD. Ha, 6-...oppressive sensation in the throat and chest, as when one is about to weep.

Ha, 15 - Oppression, and tightness of the chest.

LYC. Ha, 19 - Great oppression in the scrobiculus cordis from vexation.

LYSS. Al, 39 - A strange oppression and indifference, as if he was unable to do anything if he forces himself; there is no power of mind.

MAG-M. Al, 711 - An anxious dream; she was lying in a strange house, where rubbish (garbage) was constantly falling upon her; she tried to cry out and could not, because there was too great heaviness on the chest.

NIT-AC. Al, 30 - Anxious oppression, like nightmare, as if some one were lying under him and holding him fast with the arms about his abdomen, so that he could not free himself, immediately after falling asleep. (constriction, immobilization)

PETR. He, 12 - Sensation as if there were a cold stone in heart.(indifferent, careless)

PHOS. Al, 94 - Anxiety; oppressed, as if I had heard unpleasant (bad) news.

SARS. Ha, 3 - The soul is extraordinarily affected by the pains, the spirit is oppressed, the mind troubled; he feels unhappy and groans involuntarily.

SEP. Al, 38 - He feels oppressed in sultry weather, but becomes more cheerful when it thunders and lightens.

SIL. Ha, 12 - Loud talking is oppressive to him.

SPIG. Al, 3 - Lively contented, and trustful mood, alternating with palpitation and anxious oppression of the chest.

TAB. Al, 35 - Great apprehension with oppression of the chest, and a very despondent, sad mood, as if apprehended some misfortune,...

TARENT. Al, 34 - Lamentation, with oppressive pain in the heart, as if a misfortune had befallen her.

Al, 35 - Weeping, with oppression and pain in the heart, as from misfortune;...

ORDEALS

Ailments from; fright or fear, ordeal, of an: **ARG-N.**[5] **GELS.**[5]

Anticipation; examination, before: ***aeth.***[122] anac.[85] arg-n.[127] carb-v.[137] carc.[207] cupr.[122] ***gels.***[122] hydrog.[222] nux-v.[122] pic-ac.[122] sil.[58] thuj.[137]

Anticipation; unusual ordeal, of any: **GELS.**[54]

Fear; examination, before: ***aeth.***[122] anac.[85] arg-n.[172] ars.[172] carb-v.[172] carc.[140] ***gels.***[122] kali-p.[172] lyc.[112] med.[172] ph-ac.[172] pic-ac.[102] sil.[58] thuj.[172]

ANDROC. Sh, 84 - Overwhelmed by terror, panic and fear, like a psychic attack. Then specifically became fear of being psychically tested as if confronted by something absolutely horrible, as in a "cult initiation ordeal". He felt so scared he had to shut the door, with a feeling that something would appear from behind it if he left it open. (4)

ORGANIZATION

Death; presentiment of, rejoices and gives directions about funeral: stram.[54]

Death; presentiment of, near, seems, and must settle affairs: petr.[137]

Delusions; bed, creases, is full of: ***stram.***[54]

- body, scattered about bed, tossed about to get the pieces together: ***bapt.*** caj.[102] daph.[102] petr. ***phos.*** pyrog.[58] stram.[102]

- bones in fragments and cannot fit pieces together: phos.[54]
- child, sitting on low benches in rows as in a schoolroom: bell.[8]
- compass, fixing himself to correspond with points of, in insanity: hyos.[54]
- disorder, objects appear in: glon.[122] op.[36]
- funeral, preparations are made for: ***lach.***[54]
- lying crosswise: stram.
- wheelwright, he is a, and starts to bore holes: stram.[54]

Dreams; wedding, preparing: ozone[227]
Fear; death, farewell messages, prepares: ***lyc.***[54]
Rest; cannot, when things are not in proper place: anac. ***ars.*** carc.[102] sep.[193] sulph.[58]
Sensitive; disorder, to: ars.[137]
Squanders; order, from want of: lyc.[30] plat.[58] sil.[30]

ABSIN. Al, 4 - Very tranquil as if brain were rounded (spherical) and symmetrical.(balanced, regular, organized)

ADAM. Sh, 49 - Great desire to get my affairs in order, making phone calls without putting it off. Tidier mind. Better with homework, etc. I made a list of about 10 phone calls I had been putting off and then made each one. Paid all my outstanding bills, balanced my books, returned two questionnaires, prioritized work outstanding for school—in short, cleared my desk, and all in one day. 18, 30C, 09:XX:XX

Sh, 51 - Wanted to clean windows and wash clothes, enjoyed the cleaning. Most unusual. 12, 30C, 01.XX:XX

Sh, 58 - Watching the infinite variety created from simple building blocks. Only subtly energy creating difference. 16, 12C, 28:XX:XX

Sh, 169 - I realize that the remedy was, for me, about structure. With the cloud lifted I have got back a sense of structure which I had lost. This morning I know who I am and what I am doing. 7, 6C, 11:08:00

AGAR. Al, 9 - Delirium; he imagines himself a military (martial) officer, commanding (dominant) at a drill (training) and directing the various maneuvers.

AM-C. Ha, 37 - She cannot well arrange her ideas.

ANDROC. Sh, 34 - Much more untidy, the house was a mess and it didn't bother her. Made ineffectual efforts to tidy up and then lost interest. Desire to sit undisturbed and just look. (25)

Sh, 50 - Did the shopping in a very disorganised way, started one thing, forgot it, then started something else. (25)

GELS. He, 10 - Unconnected (disconnection, separation) ideas, cannot follow any idea for any length of time; if he attempts to think consecutively (step by step), he is attacked by a painful, vacant feeling of the mind.

HALI-L. Sh, 143 - Organized. I feel if I could get things neat and organized the world would be perfect, but I can never get to that point, because there will be a flow. Trying to get things organized at home, which is like trying to get my eyes focused . Other times I just stared out the window, unfocussed. I either feel totally in flow with the universe, or floating aimlessly down a river. When I'm unfocussed, it's like a place where you can get lost, as if you're going to lose it. When I'm focused, I bring it all in, in the present, There. like meditating, or seeing God. When I'm unfocussed it's like I'll go into the abyss, and won't come back, go crazy. 08, 30C, 31:XX:XX

Sh, 182 - Not doing enough. Feel somewhat critical of myself. Not getting anything done. Want to be in a structured, organized place and can't get there. I'd like to be really busy. I have more ideas in my head than I can do. I need to get active again, structure things, and set goals. 08, 30C, 03:XX:XX

Sh, 183 - I feel good, charged. Had a surge of energy. Feel very industrious. Organizing things, cleaning out my room. Organizing stuff to give away to charity. 01, 30C, 00:01:00

Sh, 184 - Totally in gear. Cleaned and organized my whole house. Wanted everything in order. If everything is in order then life will be great. It will go well. 08, 30C, 08:XX:XX

Sh, 186 - I've never been this clean for this long. I want to use up everything, all the leftovers. Everything has to be done and clean. Very methodically using up old things, like old jars of beans. I want everything to be in order and neat. 08, 30C, 22:XX:XX

Sh, 189 - Mad at a friend. Was at his house organizing stuff for him. I had the system organized and then he brought a whole other set of things and dumped them in. I was so furious, I left and got a headache from being angry. 08, 30C, 41:XX:XX

Sh, 190 - Something is changing like the feeling of a door opening. Wanting to get on with what I am doing in general. Cleaning up loose ends, and clutter and getting on top of daily details. More matter of fact. 11, 30C, 15:XX:XX

HAM. Al, 18 - Quick perception of anything out of shape or disproportioned.

HYDROG. Sh, 37 - Have given up my normal planning and making lists. I used to organise all the time (curative). 08, 30C, 09:XX:XX

Sh, 38 - Decided to clean the kitchen floor and to move my things into the new study for the first time —both unusual. 02, 6C, 00:03:XX

Sh, 160 - Wrote a letter to my son, 'to be opened after my death', not morbid, nor do I feel a premonition of death. Its something I've always meant to do —a sort of resolving. Wept with emotion as I wrote it. 12, 6C, 25:XX:XX

HYOS. He, 78-...fixing himself to correspond with the points of the compass and looking through his fingers; tracing the pattern of carpet with his feet and twisting his legs till he nearly fell down;...(direction)

IRID. Sh, 97 - Had a big clearout in the cellar (note: on the same day I was constipated!) .Enjoyed this spring cleaning and throwing loads of stuff away. I was making space for ex-partner to store stuff he still has in house which is suffocating me. I need the space to breathe. Feeling that if he doesn't put his things into the space in the cellar I shall explode. Generally not as lax about things, giving people the "hard word." G11 suffocation, organization

LYC. Al, 43 - Anxious thoughts, as if she were about to die, for which she even prepared by thinking of her farewell messages, in the morning...

He, 26 - Anxious thoughts, as if about to die, for which she prepares farewell (departure, adieu) messages.

MED. Al,N-44 - The impatience, excitement, wild feelings; the unreal, dazed condition; the gloom (sadness) and fear in the dark;... are marked evidence of functional derangement of the nervous system.

He, 20 - Is sure that she is worse, knows she is not going to live, cannot see any improvement, even when it is pointed out (antagonism); has no fear of death, speaks calmly about it, and gives directions as to the disposition of her affairs.

MERC. Ha, 1234 - Anxiety and apprehension in the blood, he knew not how to compose (control) himself; he felt as if he had committed a crime, without heat, also at the same time as if he was not quite master,(commander). of his senses all day. (lost: mastering, commander)

Ha, 1262 - He is silly, acts like a buffoon, ...he lit (burning) his fire, laid swords across one another, and put candles in one corner of the room, in the other boots (shoe),all this quite gravely...(serious)

NAT-C. Al, DREAM, 1117 - Illusions of fantasy, in the evening, while half asleep; she sees figures, visions of soldiers marching in the air;..

OX-AC. Al, 32 - Greater presence of mind; the relations of the world seem to be clearer to him.

PETR. He, 4 - Delirium; thinks another person lies alongside (close) of him, or that one limb is double.

PH-AC. Ha, 34 - He cannot get his ideas into their proper connection.

PHOS. Al, 12-...; wherever he turned his eyes he saw faces; they swarmed (crowded, surrounded) by him in long panoramic succession; they leered (look lecherous) at him over the footboard of the bed; they squinted (look) at him though the windows, or came trooping (crowd) in when the doors were left ajar (open) (invade);..he fancied he was some one else, ...

Al, 38 - Told those about him repeatedly that he could not possibly recover, and gave some disjointed directions about his business affairs.

He, 22-...uneasy about one's health; paroxysms of anguish, when alone or in a stormy weather, with timorous disposition; told those about him repeatedly that he could not possibly recover, and gave some disjointed (incoherent) directions about his business affairs.

RHUS-T. Ha, 974 - He can restrain the rush of ideas at his will, follow out uninterruptedly any train of thought he chooses, without being troubled with other thoughts.

STRAM. Ha, 549 - He thinks he is dying, and that he will not live over the evening, he rejoices that he is dying, and gives directions about his funeral, otherwise he is rational and does not feel particularly ill.

He, 40 - Aberration of mind; one carries home all sorts of wood in order to manufacture brandy (cognac) (busy, manufacturing) ; another placed two axes across each other in order to split wood in this way; a third burrowed in ground like a pig with his mouth (animal); a fourth alleged he was a wheelwright and began to bore holes; a fifth ran into forge to catch fish, which he saw swimming there; a lacemaker threw about her bobbins incessantly, and threw everything into confusion; another girl ran about the room and cried out that all evil spirits were pursuing her.(restoration, restitution)

He, 57 - Strange absurd ideas; thinks herself tall, double or lying crosswise; one half of body cut off (divided); bed is full of creases (wrinkle) (disorganization); that he was killed roasted and being eaten.

He, 65-"There", he replied, "A long train of bedbugs, and after them a procession of beetles and here come crawling over me a host (crowd) of cockroaches"; sank back in alarm, then suddenly said:" I believe I know they are not really bugs, but, except once in a while, they seem real to me. (organization, association, union)

He, 55 - He thinks that he is dying and that he will not live over night, rejoices (celebrate) and gives directions about his funeral.

TARENT. He, 15 - Suddenly sprang (escape) away from her attendants and swept (clean) ornaments from mantelpiece (an ornamental facing around fireplace); said she was sorry, but could not help it; very mischievous and destructive, ...

VIOL-O. He, 7 - Disconnected (separated) thoughts thronged (crowd) one upon the other, he was able to grasp none of them;...

OTHERS

Ailments from; misfortune of others: coloc.[1]

Anxiety; anticipating, relatives, for his: carc.[193]

Anxiety; children, about his: acet-ac. ars.[31] germ.[222] ph-ac.[30] phos.[31] rhus-t.[30] sep.[172] sulph.[31]

Anxiety; family, about his: acet-ac.[54] aeth.[193] ***ars.***[10] calc-sil.[58] carb-an.[184] carc.[140] ***caust.***[30] cupr.[210] germ.[222] hep.[1] lach.[30] petr.[54] phos.[10] **RHUS-T.**[10] ***spig.***[30] sulph.[10] zinc.[30]

Anxiety; friends at home, about: bar-c. ***phos.*** phys. puls.[172] ***sulph.***

Anxiety; health, loved persons, of: carc.[193] hep.[30] merc.[30]

Anxiety; health, relatives: ***ars.***[162] bar-c.[162] cand-a.[239] carb-v.[172] caust.[172] cocc.[36] **HEP.**[30] merc.[30] nat-c.[172] ***phos.***[162] puls.[172]

Anxiety; health, relatives, little concerned about his own: cocc.[54]

Anxiety; others, for: ***acon.*** androc.[222] ***arg-n.***[162] ***ars.*** aur. bar-c. ***calc-p.***[162] calc-s.[36] carb-v.[172] ***carc.***[193] caust.[10] chel.[162] cocc. cupr.[210] ***dulc.***[162] ***ferr.***[54] fl-ac.[162] germ.[222] hep.[1] ***manc.***[184] merc.[10] naja[36] nat-c.[172] ***nux-v.***[30] perh.[149] ph-ac.[30] ***phos. staph.***[30] ***sulph.***

Anxiety; others, losing their protectors or familiar relations, for: bar-c.[162]

Anxiety; others, loved persons, for: aeth.[184] sac-alb.[210]

Cares; full of, others, about: ars.[5] ***caust.***[30] cocc.[5] ***ign.***[5] lach.[30] lap-c-b.[194] sulph.[10] zinc.[30]

Complaining; others, of: hep.[137] ruta[130] sep.[54]

Cruelty; bear, cannot, done to other children: calc.[122]

Death; thoughts of, belonging to him, for those, with anxiety: ***ferr.***[54]

Delusions; accidents, of relatives: phos.[1]

- brother fell overboard in her sight: kali-br.
- calls, him with name, the absent mother or sister: anac.[10]
- calls, someone: anac. ant-c. bell.[111] cann-i. dros. hyos.[185] kali-c. med.[185] plat.[10] ***plb.*** ruta[10] stram.[185] thuj. verat.[185]
- division between himself and others: hydrog.[222] nat-c.[58]
- fire, neighbor's house on (morning, waking in a fright): hep.

• sick, members of the family are: hep.
• sick, someone else is: gels.[111]
Despair; others and oneself: ***arg-n.***[54] aur.[54]
Despair; others, about: ***aur.***
Discontented; others, with: cham.[127] hep.[137] ruta[130]
Discontented; wrong, everything another does is: ***cham.***[54]
Dreams; body, arm, hurt, mother's arm: chin.[36]
➤ cares, amel. when seeing the person worrying about: tarent.[36]
➤ cares, patients, for his: bac.[62]
➤ daughter, struck by paralysis, had been: nat-s.[36]
➤ misfortune, others, of: cann-s.[36] mag-c.[36]
Envy; qualities of others, at: ars.[122] calc.[122] lach.[122] lyc.[122] puls.[122] sulph.[122]
Fear; accidents, friends, to: ars.[172]
✦ accidents, loved ones, to: phos.[1]
✦ accidents, of, child, of: ars.[172]
✦ accidents, others, to: osm.[36]
✦ broken the arm of her child, that she has, in gastroenteritis during pregnancy: lyc.[172]
✦ disease, child, to: ars.[172]
✦ family matters, about: calc-sil.[58]
✦ friend has met with accident, that a: ars. ***caust.***[184]
✦ happen, something will, family, to, or to him: ars.[172] calc.[172] calc-s.[36] caust.[172] phos.[172] psor.[172] sep.[172] tub.[36]
✦ happen, something will, husband will not return home: ars.[172] bar-c.[172] caust.[172] ***plat.*** sep.[172]
Inconsolable; anxiety about his family, from, which he left behind while going on a short journey: ***petr.***[54]
Indifference; neighbors, towards: phos.[10] ***sep.***[10]
Indifference; opinion of others, to: androc.[222]
Indifference; others, about lot of: lap-mar-c.[194] plat.[185] sabad.[185] sulph.
Indifference; persons, to all: kali-m.[192] mez.[36]
Indifference; suffering, to, others, of: anac.[10] lac-h.[229]
Indifference; welfare of others, to: androc.[222] ars.[30] cand-a.[239] caust.[30] lach.[30] lap-mar-c.[194] nat-m.[30] ***nux-v.***[30] ozone[227] plat.[30] sep.[30] **SULPH.**
Joy; misfortune of others, at the: anac.[185] ars. cupr.[171]
Lamenting; others, about: merc.
Longing; for, good opinion of others: ***pall.***
Obstinate; resists wishes of others: alum.[36] **NUX-V.**[54]
Responsibility; strong, social: stront-c.[188]
Sadness; family, for his: ars.[10] hep.[10] rhus-t.[10]
Sadness; others, for: cocc.[10] sulph.[10]
Sympathetic; misfortune of others, greatly affected by: coloc.[137]
Thoughts; accidents, of, having happened to others: osm.[36]
Thoughts; persistent, injury to others, of doing: osm.[54]
Thoughts; thoughtful, errors of others, about the: cic.[36]

ACET-AC. He, 6 - Anxiety; grieves about his sickness and his children.

ANAC. Al, 1 - Illusions of fancy; he imagines he has his name called by the voice of his far-distant mother and sister, accompanied by an apprehension of misfortune and anxiety.

ANDROC. Sh, 176 - Fear of driving, especially fear of hurting someone else in an accident. (Clinical)

ARS. Ha, 1032 - Mania; first headache, horrible anxiety, noise before the ears, as from a number of large bells, and when he opened the eyes, he always saw a man who had (formerly) hung himself (suicidal, justified) on the ground-floor of the house, who incessantly beckoned (call) him to cut him down (help); he ran thither (there) with a knife, but, as he could not cut him down, (rescue) he became overwhelmed (beaten) with despair (remorse?) and wished (as his friends assured him) to hang himself (punish); but being prevented (stop) from doing so, he became so restless that he could hardly be kept in bed,... and he knelt down and raised his hands in a supplicating manner.

Ha, 1036 - In the evening, in bed, anxious sad fancies, e.g. that something bad (misfortune) must have happened to his relatives.

Ha, 3 - Sad, sorrowful ideas, in the evenings in bed, as if some misfortune (disaster, accident) might have happened to one's relatives.

He, 8 - Gloomy (dark) forebodings (premonition) while lying in bed, in evening, fears something may have happened to his relatives.

He, 10 - Fixed idea that he and his family will die of starvation. (hunger, privation, want)

BAR-A. Al, 10 - An evil, fearful suspicion suddenly takes possession of her, as if, for example, a loved friend had been taken suddenly deathly ill.

BAR-C. Ha, 7 - An evil fearful foreboding comes suddenly upon his soul, as if, e.g. a beloved friend might suddenly have fallen fatally ill.

He, 27 - She is suddenly overwhelmed with an evil apprehension; she imagines, for instance, that a beloved friend has suddenly fallen sick and is dying.

CALC-S. Al, 7 - Excessive, bitter melancholy, with distressing apprehensions of evil to loved ones.

CANN-S. Ha, 303 - Dreams of misfortunes happening to others.

CARL. Al, 4 - His nerves are so much affected that the sorrows of others cause him to weep easily.

CAUST. Al, 11 - Excessively sympathetic; she is beside herself, with weeping and sobbing and cannot be contented when listening to accounts of the hardships (misfortune, difficulty) of others.

Ha, 4 - Excessively compassionate (sympathetic); at the relations of others and of the cruelties inflicted upon them, she is beside herself for weeping and sobbing, and cannot content herself.

Ha, 20 - Extreme anxious timidity; she is so much afraid (fear) of a dog near her, which did not harm (hurt, injure) her at all,...every noise in the street made her afraid, and when she saw boys climbing she was very uneasy lest they might get hurt. (care, others)

He, 54 - Excessive sympathy for others.

CERE-B. Al, 4 - Felt a desire to give something quite necessary to myself to another. (altruism, helpful, sympathetic)

CHIN. Al, DREAM-1110 - Dreamed that some one had stabbed his brother, and then called for his mother; that his mother was dead, and then he cried; that his mother's arms was hurt;...

CHLOL. He, 3 - Fixed despair of recovery; believes he will give his imaginary disease (syphilis) to others.

CHOC. Sh, 145 - My fears around the kids —that they would die, etc. and that they were my total responsibility, like parasites —have gone and I know feel total trust that they will be o.k.

CIC. Ha, 232 - When others were gay he was sad.

He, 36 - Mistrust and shunning (avoid) of men; despises others.

COCC. Ha, 531 - Serious, and though caring little about his own health, he is very anxious about the illnesses of others.

CROC. Al, 29 - He takes everything in anger and suddenly repents (apologize) of having injured (offend) others.

CUPR. Ha, 5 - A kind of timidity; he felt as if he had to step softly, in order not to hurt himself, nor to disturb his room-mates. (friend) (cautious, prudent, gentle, delicate)

DROS. Ha, 275 - He is sad and dejected about the ills (evil) of life, which people cause one another and himself, respecting which he is anxious and concerned;...(ethical)

FERR. He, 9 - Mind in highest degree oppressed; despondent (sad); great solicitude (cares) about those belonging to him (relatives, family), with constant thoughts of death.

FL-AC. He, 6 - Feeling of indifference towards those he loves best; has no objection to their presence but does not care to converse with them, yet if strangers or mere acquaintances come in will enter into animated conversation....

HEP. Al, 1 - Ghostly image of one who was dead, in the morning, in bed, after waking and while conscious, which frightened him; it also seemed as though he saw his neighbor's house burning, which also frightened him.

Al, 10 - Fearful concerning sickness in the family, especially when walking alone in the open air.

Ha, 5 - Fear about the illness of his family, especially while walking in the open air.

IP. Ha, 221 - Sulky humor, that despises (scorn, intolerant, antipathy) everything, and he desires that others also should not esteem or care for anything.

LAC-D. He, 5 - Imagines that all her friends will die and that she must go to a convent. (purification, salvation)

LYC. Al, 96 - Quarrelsome rage, partly at herself partly at others.
Ha, 56 - Angry fury, partly against himself, and partly against others.
LYSS. Al,N-62 - He cautioned people around him not to inhale his exhaled air, it was spoiled (dirty), stinking (smelling) like rotten (putrefying) eggs, worse than cholera, and could injure. (contaminates, infects)
MAG-C. Al, 948 - Anxious dreams of the misfortune of relatives.
Al, 953 - Dream that she was sadly disturbed in company, where especially her grandmother was taken with spasms, and at last had apoplexy.
Al, 955 - Dream that she was weeping about the death of a near relative.
NAJA. Al, 14 - Felt melancholy; began to form images of possible wrongs (mistaken) and misfortunes, over which the mind broods; very wretched at times;... a slight cause sets him in a perfect agony of mental suffering on another's behalf (welfare);...makes himself imaginary troubles and wrongs, and frets (bother) over them for two hours...
NAT-M. Ha, 4 - Melancholy mood; he cannot remove from his thoughts injuries (insults) he has inflicted on others, or which have been inflicted on him, which depressed him so much that he had no pleasure in anything. (remorse)
NAT-P. Al, 10 - Awakens; fears his child, who has a trifling ailment (disease), is dead; he goes to her room to relieve the otherwise ineffaceable (perpetual) impression.
OSM. Al, 5 - Thoughts of accidents having happened to others, by a blow, a fall, or being dashed (crushed, hit, knock) to pieces; gradually these thoughts grow upon him, as if he were to do the same injuries to others.
PETR. He, 13 - Towards evening anxiety and apprehension about his family which he left behind while going on a short journey; the anxiety increases until he becomes inconsolable.
PHOS. Ha, 5 - Sad and melancholy, as if some accident had happened to his beloved ones.
PHYS. Al, 3 - Felt great anxiety about friends at home; could not get them out of mind.
PLB. Al, 53-...; he fancied one of the patients called to him, ran headlong (hurry) to help him, ...
RUTA. He, 2 - Dissatisfied with himself and others.
SEP. Al, 33 - Received news of the slight illness of a friend, which caused great mental depression (at another time it would not have made slightest impression); this condition grew on me until I became so nervous that I felt that unless I held on something, I should scream.
He, 38-...everything seems strange (unusual, unfamiliar) to her;...; it seems as if she could not understand (realize) anything and would have to learn anew everything she wished to do;...(lost: knowledge); greatest indifference to everything, the death of a near relative, or some happy occurrence, leaves her equally unaffected; no trace of her former love for friends or even for her child; aversion for social intercourse amounting to contempt;...
SULPH. Al, 56 - She is apprehensive for others, and anxious.
Ha, 25 - She is apprehensive for others, with anxiety.
He, 32 - Melancholy mood; dwelling on religious or philosophic speculations; anxiety about soul's salvation; indifference about lot (destiny) of others.
VERAT. Al, 62 - He seeks out faults in others and contemplates (examine, inspect) them. (critical)
Ha, 706 - He searches for faults in others and taunts (ridicule, mockery) them with them.

PARALYSIS

Anger; paralyzed, felt as: calc-p.[54] ***cist.***[54]
Anguish; evening, paralyzing, impossible to call and move, with heat in head: cob-n.[144]
Anguish; night, paralyzing, impossible to call and move, with heat in head: cob-n.[144]
Anxiety; paralyzed, as if: am-m.[54] cob-n.[119]
Confusion of mind; identity, paralysis, in: alum.[54]
Delusions; body, arms, stiff, very: bamb-a.[1184]
- body, legs, stiff, as if: nux-v.[137]
- body, mouth, open, cannot, lower jaw stiff and painful: lyss.[54]

- crippled old man, that he is: hydrog.[222]
- lazy to move, she is too: eucal.[139]
- marble statue, he is a: cann-i.
- move, he cannot: hom.[85]
- paralyzed, being: agar.[139] cist.[139] con.[139] cycl.[139] sac-alb.[139] ***sang.***[171] syph.[85]
- paralyzed, will be: syph.[139]
- swallow, cannot: lyss.[54]

Dreams; body, arm, paralyzed: nicc.[36]
➤ body, mouth, opening impossible: agar.[54]
➤ daughter, struck by paralysis, had been: nat-s.[36]
➤ disease, lethargy: graph.[1] op.[10]
➤ nightmare, inability to see, as if he could not escape from: cot.[36]
➤ paralyzing: pitu-a.[164]
➤ unsuccessful efforts to, open the mouth, to: agar.
➤ unsuccessful efforts to, running, of: croc. ind.
➤ walking, unable of, is: arist-m.[36]

Fear; catalepsy, of: art-v.[172]
✦ death, paralysis, in: ***caust.***[54]
✦ paralysis, of: ***anac.*** arn. asaf. bapt.[85] bell. kali-p.[172] syph.

Grief; paralytic state of body and mind, from: phys.[137]

Helplessness; feeling, of paralyzed, from sensation of being: ***sang.***[171]

Insanity; immobile as a statue: cham.[10] fl-ac.[58] hyos.[10]

Insanity; paralysis, with: ant-c.[102] ars.[102] aur.[102] bell.[8] ***cann-i.***[102] caust.[102] chlol.[8] crot-h.[137] hyos.[58] kali-br.[85] kali-i.[102] ***lach.***[122] lol.[77] merc-c.[102] nat-i.[102] nux-v.[102] op.[102] ***phos.***[85] phys.[102] plb.[102] stram.[102] sulph.[102] verat.[102]

Mania; paralysis, with: crot-h.[54] ***nat-m.***[54] ***nux-v.***[54] ***phos.***[54] ***phys.***[54] sec.[54]

Schizophrenia; catatonic: chlorpr.[149] cic.[149] convo-s.[149] cortico.[119] halo.[149] rauw.[119] reser.[149] thala.[149] thiop.[149]

Weeping; paralysis, in: ***caust.***[54]

AM-C. Al, 22 - At night, attack of great anxiety, as if she had to die, ... she was unable to move her eyes or to speak,...

ANAC. He, 59 - Fear of paralysis.

ASAF. He, 9 - Fear paralysis or softening of brain.

CALC. Ha, 65 - Great weakness of the imaginative (creative) faculty; with a very slight exertion in speaking, he felt as if his brain was paralyzed, ...;he could not think, nor recollect what was spoken of, with muddled (confused) feeling in the head.(lost: imagination, thoughts)
He, 96 - The slight effort of talking gave him sensation as if brain would be paralyzed (disable), mostly in occiput.

CARBN-O. Al, 7 - Frightful anxiety, and instinctive impulse to seek change of air, while he felt powerless to overcome the paralysis of his muscles and move from where he sat.

CHAM. Ha, 488 - She sits stiffly (rigid, petrified) on a chair like a statue, and seems to take no notice of anything about her.

CIST. He, 3 - Bad effects of vexation; feels as if paralyzed.

CON. Al, 6 - Delirious and stupid; they threw themselves into the water, thinking they were geese; for three years they remained partly paralytic, suffering from much pain.
Al, 43-...a great guilt weighed upon him, with paralyzed feeling in all the limbs, indifference,..
Ha, 18 - Very morose; ...as if a great guilt weighed him down; at the same time a sensation of paralysis in all the limbs; ...
He, 35-...a great grief weighed upon him, with paralyzed feeling in all the limbs, indifference and taking no interest in anything.

COT. Al, 1-...a feeling as if there was no foot. The head felt exceeding light, as if there were no solid head, and she could not articulate for some time, although she endeavored to do so....

HYDROG. Sh, 103 - Feel like a crippled old man. 38, 200C, 18:XX:XX

HYOS. Ha, 489 - Bereft (deprived) of all his senses, he sits in bed immovable, like a statue.

IGN. Al, 2 - He fancies that he is unable (incapable, powerless) to proceed (progress, advance), that he cannot walk.
Ha, 757 - He imagines he cannot get on (succeed), cannot walk.

LIL-T. He, 12 - Listless, inert, yet does not want to sit still (quiet); restless, yet does not want to walk; hurried manner, desire to do something, yet feels no ambition; feeling as of imperative duties and utter (complete) inability (incapacity, incompetence) to perform them; sexual excitement.

LYSS. Al,N-64 - Disinclination to change position of head; two distinct trains of thought existing at one time in her mind, the idea that she was unable to move her head (when lying down) with the positive conviction that she has only to make up her mind that she will do it to achieve it.

He, 64 - Disinclination to change position of head; two distinct trains of thought existing at one time in her mind, the idea that she is unable to move her head (when lying down) with the positive conviction that she has only to make up her mind that she will do it to achieve it.

NAT-C. Al, DREAM, 1102-..;of marrying two women, of parties, walks, entertainments, and excursions on horseback, afterwards they were frequently anxious, of going astray (lost),of murders, having his ears cut off; also vexatious dreams; he would take a journey and could not get away from the place,(immobilization) and when has reached the first station was obliged to turn back, on account of something he had forgotten.

NAT-M. Al, 70 - In the evening it seemed as though he became paralyzed from a fright (terrify) ; afterwards he seemed horrified, and apprehended some misfortune.

Al, 5 - Great excitement, followed by falling asleep and deadness of the limbs.

Ha, 54 - In the evening, he was, as it were, paralyzed by a fright, then he became horrified and apprehensive.

He, 51 - After violent fits of passion, paralysis.

NUX-M. Al, 49 - It became difficult to recall to mind things learned shortly before; for many such things the mind seemed paralyzed for many days together.

PHOS. Al, 86-...; a feeling of dread (fear), as if awaiting something terrible, yet unable to resist or move (terrifying, scaring), overcame me; sometimes it seemed as if I was beginning to bloat (inhalant, inflate, vanity?), and then I could hear a multitude of voices saying in high glee, "Fill him up a little more and he will burst," (blow up) followed by demoniacal laughter, which made the cold chills run over me... I imagined myself an aurora borealis, and could distinctly hear voices shouting, "Beautiful! Oh, was not that splendid?"...

SANG. He, 8 - Sensation as if paralyzed and unable to move while lying on her back, ...

He, 9-..."what will become of my condition, shall I have typhoid fever, inflammation of the brain, or shall I remain paralyzed?".

SEC. Al,N-13 - Paralytic mental diseases; treats his relations contemptuously and sarcastically.

He, 12 - Paralytic mental diseases; treats his relations contemptuously and sarcastically;...

SIL. Al, 21 - He woke with great anxiety about midnight, could not move in spite of every effort, and imagined that thieves were breaking in; on rising he became quiet, after lying down the anxiety returned.

SYPH. Al,N-8 - Feeling as if going insane, or about to be paralyzed.

He, 10 - Feeling as if going insane, or about be paralyzed.

TAB. Al, 2 - He went to sleep in the cabin, which was full of large packages of tobacco, ...His inability to move was not accompanied by any pain or uneasiness but he felt as if the principle of life had entirely departed from his frame.(body)

THUJ. Al, 9 - While half awake...cannot move a limb (paralyzed), with a sensation as though the whole body were as heavy as lead (heaviness), then she tries to call for help; can utter no sound, and lies with open eyes ...

PASSIONATE

Affectionate: acon. alum.[30] anac. ant-c. ***ars.***[10] bar-c.[30] bor. bry.[30] calc-p.[146] carb-an. carb-v. carc.[146] caust.[30] choc.[222] coff. ***croc.*** graph.[30] hura hydr.[36] ***ign.*** lach.[30] lyc.[30] murx.[102] ***nat-m.*** nit-ac.[30] ***nux-v.***[122] op.[36] ox-ac. par. ph-ac.[30] ***phos.***[122] plat. ***puls.*** seneg. sil.[122] staph.[30] stram.[36] thea.[36] verat.

Ailments from; vehemence: ***aur.***[54] coff.[54]

Anger; violent, personal, from slight offense: ***anac.***[54]

Ardent: alum.[30] androc.[222] caust.[30] nux-v. stann.[30] sulph.[30]

Cheerfulness; alternating with, passion, burst of: ***aur.*** caps. croc. ign. stram.

Desires; uncontrollable: alco.[36]

Dreams; feverish: euphr.[36] lachn.[36]

➤ passion, outburst of: mag-c.[5]
Impulsive: acon.[102] alum.[58] anac.[109] ant-c.[102] **ARG-N.** ***ars. aur.*** camph. caust.[36] cere-b.[36] cham.[102] choc.[222] ***cic.*** coloc.[102] croc.[111] cupr.[111] gins. hep.[58] **IGN.**[111] iod.[58] ip.[102] lach.[58] lap-mar-c.[194] med.[102] merc. nat-m.[172] nux-v. phos.[101] **PULS.**[111] rheum[98] rhus-t. sep.[102] staph. stram.[101] sulph.[102] tarent.[137] thea.
Lasciviousness; emotions, with violent: cop.[54]
Love; exalted: ant-c.[5] hyos.[5]
Love; falling in love easily: ign.[85]
Love; love-sick: ***ant-c.*** germ.[222] hydrog.[222] pip-m.[144] til.
Passionate: ***alco.***[36] **ANAC.**[5] ars.[36] ***aur.***[5] **BAR-C.**[5] **BELL.**[5] **BRY.**[5] calc.[30] cann-i.[36] canth.[36] carb-ac.[25] **CARB-V.**[5] carbn-s.[36] carc.[187] caust.[30] coff.[5] con.[54] croc.[5] cupr.[25] hep.[54] hura[36] hyos.[36] ign.[5] **IP.**[5] ***kali-c.***[54] **KALI-I.**[36] laur.[36] led.[5] **NAT-C.**[30] nat-m.[5] nat-s.[5] **NUX-V.**[5] olnd.[5] ***petr.***[5] ph-ac.[5] phos.[36] plat.[30] ***psor.***[54] ***sabad.***[5] seneg.[5] **SEP.**[5] ***stann.***[5] stram.[36] **SULPH.**[5] sumb.[36] tarent.[36] ***thuj.***[54]
Passionate; trifle, at every: nat-m.[36] ph-ac.[36] phos.[36] sumb.[36]
Sentimental: acon. ***agn.***[102] alco.[10] am-c.[102] am-m.[102] ambr.[116] androc.[222] **ANT-C.**[122] ars. ***aur.***[102] berb.[36] cact.[102] calc. ***calc-p.*** canth. carb-an.[102] carc.[162] cast. caust.[30] chin. chin-ar. cimic.[102] ***cocc. coff.*** con. crot-h.[5] ***cupr. cycl.***[102] dig.[8] ***graph.***[102] hydr-ac. ***iber.***[102] **IGN.** ***ind.***[102] joan.[97] kali-p.[102] kreos.[5] lach. laur.[10] lil-t.[102] lyc. manc. mur-ac.[102] naja[98] nat-c.[102] ***nat-m.***[162] ***nat-s.***[102] nit-ac.[10] nux-v. ph-ac.[102] ***phos.*** plat. plb.[30] ***psor.*** puls.[5] rhus-t.[102] sabad. sabin.[116] sec.[102] ***sel.***[102] ***sep.***[102] ***stann.***[102] staph. ***sulph.*** thuj.[102] tub.[187] zinc.[102]
Sentimental; ecstasy, with: ***coff.***[54]
Sentimental; girls: cocc.[102] tub.[65]
Sentimental; moonlight in, ecstatic love: **ANT-C.**
Sentimental; twilight, in: ant-c.[137]
Sentimental; young persons, in: ant-c.[85] ign.[85]
Temperament; choleric, ardent, disposed to anger, spite or deception, always irritable and impatient: **NUX-V.**[54]
Temperament; sanguine: ***acon.***[54] arn.[85] ars.[54] aur.[54] ***calc.***[54] ***cham.***[54] ***chin-s.***[54] ***coff.***[85] **FERR.**[54] glon.[85] **HYOS.**[54] ***ign.***[54] led.[85] murx.[54] ***nit-ac.***[54] ***nux-v.***[54] **PHOS.**[54] plat.[54] ruta[83] sac-alb.[36]
Unconsciousness; emotion, after: ***acon.*** am-c. camph. ***caust. cham.*** **COFF. IGN. LACH.** mosch.[116] nux-m. ***op. ph-ac.*** phos.[189] verat.

ANAC. Ha, 18 - Extremely passionate at a slight offense, breaking out into violence.
Ha, 17 - Passionate and contrary.
ANDROC. Sh, 96 - Increased irritability, a "how dare you!" feeling. Felt like tearing offenders to pieces with his bare hands. He felt an enormous surge of violent emotions at trifles, and had to exercise great control to stop outbursts of violence and impulses to hurt someone. Felt that "everyone were creeps", could not be bothered with anyone. (2)
Sh, 97 - Very strong liking and disliking to people —very intense —ranging from immense sexual attraction to extreme hatred. Spoke with hatred and maliciousness about colleagues. (4)
Sh, 129 - It seemed as though he was a different person, very similar to the way he had been in adolescence, but in a much more powerful manner. These emotions were so intense he wanted to rip his chest apart to let them out. He lost all control over his emotions, which seemed to come from a deep and distant part of himself, a darker side. He desired to continue the proving for the rest of his life. (29)
ANT-C. He, 24 - Sentimental or distrustful mood.
ARS. He, 59 - Very peevish and passionate, capricious, she takes every word ill and is cross when she has to answer.
AUR. He, 80 - Ailments from fright, anger, contradiction, mortification, or vexation with dread, fear, reserved displeasure, or vehemence.
BAR-C. He, 24 - Extremely contrary, irritable humor, passionate about trifles .
BOR. Ha, 15 - Passionate, cross, takes offense easily.
CHEL. He, 25 - Is vexed (anger, irritated) about every trifle and has violent attacks of passionate outbursts of temper.
CON. He, 38 - Very much excited, passionate, domineering (dictatorial), quarrelsome, scolds (censorious) and will not bear contradiction.

GERM. Sh, 8 - Weeping. Feeling very offended towards father who had objected because I had bought something expensive for myself. Felt anger because of my reaction, but also curiosity to find out why I reacted. Feel anxiety about all my responsibilities. Everything feels like too much. 21, 12C, 26:XX:XX.

HEP. Ha, 289 - The slightest thing put him into a violent passion, he could have murdered any one without hesitation.

He, 20 - Violent, passionate fretfulness; she spoke with such volubility that one could not always get a chance to reason with her, and she would not listen to the most just remarks.

HYDROG. Sh, 13 - Falling in love on a very deep level. 16, 30C, XX:XX:XX

Sh, 14 - I felt so much love I didn't know how to focus it. Its like being in another state of consciousness. No one can come near and its frightening me. 16, 30C, 25:XX:XX

HYOS. He, 76 - After a fit of passion, melancholia,... appetite gone;...

He, 77 - After a fit of passion and sudden fear, became so melancholy and timorous as to hide himself in every corner,...

IRID. Sh, 320 - Full of anger, like fire burning away inside me. Less tolerant with people. Normally I would say it's okay, but I haven't, and I feel very strong like I could chop any one down who got in the way. Feel very emotional. I would burst into tears if someone said the wrong thing. Similar to the feeling I used to have at school when I was being bullied, a defiant, "I'll show you one day!" type of feeling. I5

Sh, 327 - Had a massive argument with friend. For first time in my life really stood my ground. Went hot. Said, "This is my point and I am sticking to it." Burst into floods of tears. It was as though a volcano had erupted. Anger and grief were coming out. My friend had done this on purpose. I got on high horse. We parted friends and sorted it all out. I4

KALI-C. Ha, 49 - Changeful mood, now good and quiet, then passionate and angry about trifles; often hopeful, often despondent.

KALI-I. He, 6 - Very great irritability and unwonted harshness of demeanor (behavior); his children, to whom he is devoted and attached, become burdensome to him; very passionate and spiteful temper;...constant apprehension of impending evil.

LED. Ha, 335 - Passionate: he easily gives way to angry expressions.

LYC. Al, 94 - Indolent, obstinate (inflexible), rebellious (revolutionary, dissident), passionate, wrathful. (angry)

MEZ. Ha, 16 - Violent boiling over with passion about trifles, for which he is soon sorry.

NAT-C. Ha, 52 - Passionate; disposed to quarrel and fight, and cannot bear any contradiction.

NAT-M. Al, 119 - The patient's mind was much weakened by disease and poison; her moral perceptions, her once keen (sharp) sense of honor, and of right and wrong, seemed blunted (dull); she was in turns vehement (angry) and passionate, and moody and silent.

He, 42 - Quarrelsome fretfulness, gets into passion about trifles; passionate vehemence.

He, 51 - After violent fits of passion, paralysis.

NIT-AC. Ha, 47 - He is inclined to be passionate and contentious.(quarrelsome)

Ha, 48 - Passionateness, venting itself in abuse. (insult)

Ha, 49 - He gets violently excited about trifles, all the day, and has then to laugh at himself.

OLND. Al, 6 - He immediately became overheated; he became passionate, though he immediately repented (sorry) of it.

PH-AC. Ha, 25 - At a slight offense, he is, as it were, beside himself and passionate.

PTEL. Al, 43 - Goes about his professional duties in a perfunctory (indifference) manner, very unlike (contradictory) his fiery (passionate) zeal with which he usually combats disease and his allopathic step-brethren (brotherhood).

ROB. Al, 10 - Love and excited passions, leading him to the grossest (obscene, rude) excesses, even to homicide.

STANN. Ha, 655 - In the first three days he is rather calm and his vexation quickly passes off, does not fly into a passion, is rather quickly sensitive; the fourth day he is disposed to stormy anger and to fly into a passion...

STRAM. He, 111 - Nymphomania; with diaphragmitis; violent attacks, even to rage; exalted sexual passion.

PAST

Adolescent, felt he was again: androc.[222]

Ailments from; disappointment, deception, old: **NAT-M.**[122]

Ailments from; fright or fear, long lasting: carc.[207]

Anger; past events, about: calc. carb-an. sars.[54] sep. sulph.[54]

Anger; past events, about, arise from most indifferent thoughts and from every occurrence in life, unite with new vexations, cannot free herself from them: sulph.[54]

Anger; vexations, thinking about former: ***calc. carb-an.*** lyc.[1] sars.[54] sep. sulph.[54]

Complaining; offenses long past, of: calc.

Delusions; animals, ichthyosaurus, seeing an: cann-i.[36]

- images, ever-changing, past to present: mur-ac.
- life, symbols of, all past events revolve rapidly in wheels: cann-i.
- past anxious thoughts and things are present: staph.[1]
- past, of events long: atro. hyos.[58] op.[10]
- persecuted, that he is, tormented by some frightful scene of some mournful event of the past, and: spong.[54]
- pursued, tormented by a frightful scene of some mournful event of the past, and: spong.[54]
- things done today occur a week ago: ***med.***[54]
- visions, horrible, events, of past: spong.[36]

Dreams; boyfriend, of, old: hydrog.[222]

- ➤ childhood, about: ozone[227]
- ➤ childhood, about, past events mixed with present events: ozone[227]
- ➤ dead, people, of, relatives, long ago deceased: ferr.[36] sars.[36]
- ➤ events, long past, forgotten: acon.[36] am-c. anac.[10] androc.[222] bov.[10] calad. calc.[10] cere-b.[36] chin.[36] ferr. ferr-i. hydrog.[222] nat-c.[10] pull-g.[181] sel. senec. **SIL.** spig. sulph.[36] sumb.[36]
- ➤ friends, old: ant-c.[1] bamb-a.[1184] ferr. lap-gr-m.[194] ozone[227] rumx.
- ➤ historic: acon.[5] am-c. ant-t. brom.[5] caust. ***cham.*** cic.[5] croc. graph.[5] hell. hyos.[10] m-arct.[10] **M-P-A.**[5] ***mag-c.*** merc. ***phos.*** sel. ***sil.*** stram.
- ➤ houses, like the house of her youth: ozone[227]
- ➤ old, things: androc.[222]
- ➤ people, seen for years, not: hydrog.[222]
- ➤ people, seen for years, not, twenty years: calad.[54] calc-ar.[54]
- ➤ remorse, past mistakes, for: nat-m.[36]
- ➤ schoolmate, meeting of old: ant-c.[10] ferr.[36]
- ➤ youth, time of: **SIL.**[36]

Dwells on past disagreeable occurrences: am-c. arg-n. asar.[149] calc.[10] ***cham. chin.*** cob-n.[119] ***cocc. con.*** cop. form. glon. goss.[122] hep. hydrog.[222] hyos.[111] ***ign.***[54] kali-c.[108] ***kali-p.***[54] kiss.[36] lil-t.[58] luna[228] lyc. meny. mez. **NAT-M.** nit-ac. op.[30] opun-a.[36] phos.[111] ***plat.*** psor.[111] rhus-t. sars.[54] ***sep.*** spong.[1] staph.[30] ***sulph.*** syph.[122] thuj.[5] verat.[116] visc.[119]

Dwells; grief from past offenses: calc.[30] staph.[30]

Dwells; on past disagreeable occurrences, recalls old grievances: glon. sars.[54] sulph.[54]

Exhilaration; recall things long forgotten, can: ***gels.***

Grief; long past offenses: calc.[1]

Grief; offenses, from long past: calc.[1] ***cham.***[54] ***ign.***[54] ***op.***[54] ***staph.***[30]

Grief; past events, about: ***plat.***[54]

Irritability; grief, from, long: carc.[207]

Memory; active, past events, for: anh.[119] bell.[36] elaps[36] form.[36] ***hyos.***[10] seneg.[10]

Memory; active, past events, remembered as belonging to someone else, or as matter read: ail.[54]

Memory; active, recollection, involuntary: fl-ac.[5] ***hyos.***[5] nat-m.[5] seneg.[2]

Moaning; offense happened long ago, for trifling: ***cham.***[54]

Prostration; grief, from long: **IGN.**[54] kali-br.[137]

Reading; desire for, biographies or autobiographies: thuj.[222]

Remorse; indiscretion, over past: spira.[36]

Sadness; past or finished events, over: psil.[164]

Thoughts; morbid, past, of: sulph.[54]

Thoughts; past, of the: atro.[36] cann-i.[36] meny.[36] nat-m.[36] sulph.[54]

Thoughts; past, of the, journeys: sol-t-ae.[36]
Thoughts; tormenting, past disagreeable events, about: am-c.[1] spong.[1]
Weeping; need, past, about: nat-m.[60]
Weeping; offense, former: caust.[30] ign.[30] lach.[30] staph.[30]
Weeping; past events, thinking of: lyc.[1] ***nat-m.***
Weeping; vexation, from, old: caust.[30] cham.[10] ign.[30] lach.[30] lyc.[10] nat-m.[10] staph.[30]

ADAM. Sh, 8 - Watched past emotions float away in reverse order. 16, 12C, 00:00:20
Sh, 121 - Wanting to be alone with own thoughts. Guilt over past event: daughter's back injury that occurred 22 years ago as result of my taking her to a horse riding lesson. 5, 30C, 20:XX:XX
AIL. He, 1 - Past events are forgotten, remembered as belonging to someone else, or as matters read.
ALUM. He, 4 - Inability to recollect things or follow up a train of thought.
AM-C. Al, 16 - The recollection of past disagreeable occurrences torments him.
Ha, 5 - Thoughts of previous annoyances torment him.
ANAC. Ha, 33 - Increased, greater keenness (acutely) of memory; even the least circumstances of times long past come back to him, without cause; he would also be now able to easily learn by heart...
ARG-M. He, 4 - Imagines things about the military which he never liked; long forgotten old songs come into his mind.
ARS. Al, 78 - Anxiety and fear; he sees a absent acquaintance (friend) lying dead upon the sofa, and has great dread of him.
BAR-C. He, 16 - Inclined to make fruitless exertions of memory; tries to recollect past events.
BELL. He, 4 - Memory lively; remembers things long gone by.
CALC. Al, 9 - Cries and complains about the long-past offenses.
Ha, 9 - Grief and complains over insults long past.
Ha, 55 - Thoughts of former vexations irritate him to anger.
CANTH. Al, 14 - He talked deliriously when lying, sitting and walking, disconnectedly of his business and of people who had long since been dead.
CARB-AN. Al, 28 - Sullen (unsociable, silent) mood and ill-humor about present and past events; this cannot be overcome ; it even amounts to weeping.
Ha, 7 - Morose thoughts and ill-humor, not to be driven away, concerning things present and past, even to weeping.
CHAM. Al, 58 - He cannot stop talking about old vexatious (unpleasant) circumstances.
Ha, 469 - Howling (scream) on account of a slight, even an imaginary insult, which indeed, occurred long ago. (past)
Ha, 470 - Cannot cease talking about old vexatious things.
He, 16 - Moaning on account of a very trifling offense, which had happened a long time ago.
CHOC. Sh, 45 - When I woke from the dream, I had a little panic, an unusual childhood memory came back in which I remembered having read as a child about being covered in clay, baked and eaten. The thought came to me of the spines on my back covered in clay and baked and eaten like a hedgehog.
COP. Al, 9 - Absurd recriminations about trifling and long -past occurrences.
CROC. Al, 2 - Suddenly there arises before her fancy a concern (care) which she attended a long time since, as vividly as if were she listening to it;...
CUR. Al, 12 - Regrets (remorse) from the past.
CYCL. Ha, 202 - Towards evening there suddenly occurs a strange happy feeling and lively fancy, which conjures (remember) up agreeable pictures.
FERR. Al, 764 - Did not sleep well, as sleep was much disturbed by dreams of old friends.
Al, 769 - Rested well, but dreamed a great deal of meeting with old schoolmates, of student life, etc.
FORM. Al, 7 - Sudden and unexpected return of sense of mortification and grief, with vivid recollection of circumstances long since passed, which had caused great mortification and pain, and which had rendered several years of his life unhappy; this was caused by the transactions (doing) of a near relative; this grief continues...

GLON. Al, 14 - Recalls old grievances...; he was constantly thinking of persons who had offended him, with determination to justify (excuse, defend) his own conduct.
He, 8 - Long forgotten old offenses come back to him.
GRAPH. Ha, 46 - Only obscure remembrance, even of what has just passed.
HALI-L. Sh, 216 - Had an extreme emotional shift about my Dad and what he did to me in the past. Cried and cried and cried. Went into a deep place of far past stuff that I've rarely talked about. Surprised, because I didn't think I had anything to say. Went to co-counseling feeling happy and suddenly started crying. I was focused while I was crying. I had to tell everything and not stop until I was done, even though it went overtime. A part of me was above myself crying, watching me crying. 08, 30C, 21:XX:XX
Sh, 572 - Dwell on past disagreeable occurrences. Hold a grudge. 16, 10C, 33:XX:XX
HEP. Ha, 12 - She thinks about everything disagreeable that happened to her in her lifetime.
HYDROG. Sh, 18 - Sometimes I think there isn't much of me left anymore —as if I left myself behind ages ago. 16, 30C, XX:XX:XX
Sh, 236 - Dwells on past disagreeable occurrences. 16, 30C, XX:XX:XX
Sh, 261 - Almost the impression that I am pregnant —many old sensations and emotions from previous pregnancies recurred. Like having another person inside of me. All physical symptoms of pregnancy. Went for a test. 08, 30C, 01:XX:XX
HYOS. Al, 139 - He remembers persons and occurrences which he does not try to recollect.
IRID. sh, 48 - Desire to touch backs of hands on face. Enjoy touch on skin. Old memories of gentleness, delightfully feminine. Wearing bright pink (unusual!) and stroking my legs. Enjoying my skin, touching bottom, stroking it. Dancing erotically at 8.00 a.m. (one hour after remedy). Particularly joyous. Q1
Sh, 55 - Memories and associations of giving birth, and of being born. Warm nakedness. Marriage? Old memories of marriage and wedding day. Gently erotic and sensual. Q1
Sh, 59 - Woke from a dream about wedding, feeling of unease, remembered my own wedding day, got a letter of proposal from former lover. Went ahead despite. What did I do? Q7
KALI-P. He, 17 - Homesickness, morbid activity of memory, haunted (obsessed) by visions of past, and longing after them.
LYC. Al, 10 - He cries and howls, at first about past and then about future troubles.
Al, 91 - She is overpowered (defeat) by many unpleasant recollections (memory), about which she becomes vexed; even at night on waking.
Ha, 18 - He weeps and cries, at first, about the past, then about the coming evils.
Ha, 47 - She thinks of a number of disagreeable occurrences in former(past) times, which vex her, even at night, when she wakes up.
MED. Al,N-59 - Time moves so slowly that things done an hour ago appear to have occurred a year since; asked the time of day, and in five minutes insisted that half an hour had elapsed and could not believe it had till she had seen the watch.
MENY. Ha, 290 - Melancholy humor; his thoughts are disposed to dwell on past sad disagreeable things.
MEZ. He, 4 - Irresolute (undecided); mind easily confused, unable to recollect; thinking is difficult.
NAT-M. Al, 45 - If she only thinks of a want (need, lack) long since past, tears come into her eyes.
Al, 2761 - In a dream he reproached himself for past mistakes, full of restlessness and anxiety.
Ha, 10 - In his thought he constantly recalls former disagreeable occurrences, so as to worry himself by thinking about them.
Ha, 13 - If she merely thinks of troubles past, tears come into her eyes.
He, 21 - Gloomy thoughts, recalls (remember),insults long since suffered; likes to dwell upon past unpleasant occurrences.
He, 6 - Tries to recollect past disagreeable occurrences for the purpose of thinking on them and indulging (suffer) the grief which it causes.

NEON. Sh, 13 - Thoughts of twos and water. Saw images of Noah's ark. 20, 6C, 08:01:30
Sh, 46 - Had the strong thought, "my connection with the past is dissolving" at 2.15 pm. 05, 12C, 05:05:35
Sh, 91 - I'm finding it hard to judge how long ago recent events were. Can't seem to judge time in the past. Can't think back through the days. It's as if I've lost the thread with the past that connects all past days together. It has dissolved. I seem to be more in the moment and less hurried. I usually look at my watch often, but today I forgot I had put it on, and kept asking a friend the time. Was surprised when I discovered I'd been wearing it all day. Very unusual. 05, 12C, 05:XX:XX

NIT-AC. Ha, 12 - She falls to thinking over an anxious occurrence long past, and cannot rid herself of it, almost like as if in a waking dream; from time to time she, as it were, awakes from it startled, but is always absorbed in these ideas, without being able, in spite of strenuous efforts of thinking of anything else.
He, 14 - Often anxious about his illness; constantly thinks about his past troubles; mind weak and wandering.

PH-AC. Ha, 40 - While reading, a thousand other thoughts crowd into his mind (dispersion) ; he could not comprehend anything, what he read was dark to him, and he forgot everything at once, with difficulty in recollecting what he had known a long time already. (lost: memory, concentration, comprehension, knowledge)

PLAT. He, 44 - Talks almost continually about fanciful things or such as have really occurred; of faithless love; of her teacher and old school days; ...

SCROPH-N. Al, 1 - Desponding (sad), much troubled (worried) about the past, and very apprehensive of the future, which passed off after a few days, and left the intellect clear.

SENEG. Al, 14 - He recollects (remember) suddenly, without any cause, unimportant regions (places) which he had long seen ago, and which had never made a deep impression upon him.

SEP. Al, 3 - Attacks of anger over past times come on involuntarily, through which he becomes so excited that he does not know what to do, accompanied by anxiety, palpitation of the heart, and sweat of the whole body.
Al, 95 - The recollection of past unpleasant circumstances puts him in an extreme ill-humor.
Ha, 42 - The remembrance of past trouble puts him into extreme ill humor.
Ha, 43 - Vexatious occurrences from past times keep recurring of themselves, which makes him so irritated ...
Ha, 11 - If he only thinks of his past troubles, his pulse is quickened and his breath fails him.
Ha, 28 - Restless and lacking serenity, for many days; occupied with sad memories, and anxious, she has not the patience to stay long in place.

SPIRAE. Al, 1 - At 1 A.M. he was attacked with remorse over a long-past slight indiscretion (mistake, wrong), with most fearful qualms (anxiety) of conscience and loathing of himself; ....

SPONG. Al, 6 - She is very fearful, and tormented by a frightful image of a past sad event.
Ha, 381 - She is timorous (fearful) and particularly pursued and incessantly plagued (disturbed, bothered) by a frightful picture out of a melancholic past.
He, 21 - She is very timid, and is especially pursued and incessantly tormented by a frightful scene of some mournful (unhappy) event of the past.

STAPH. Al, 15 - Anxious thoughts and events in the past came to him as if the past were present before him, which caused anxiety...then it became black before his eyes; he did not know whether the images were real or illusory, then everything seemed different, and he lost all desire to live.
Ha, 703 - Anxious thoughts and things long past come before him as if they were actually present and stood before him, which causes anxiety and the sweat of anguish - Then blackness comes before his eyes; he knows not if what he sees is true (real) or deception (false, unreal), then he regards (suppose) everything as something different to what it is (strange), and he loses all wish to live. (lost; discernment, perception)

SULPH. Al, 8 - Numerous morbid ideas, extremely disagreeable, causing rancor, though with also joyous thoughts (and melodies) mostly from the past, take possession of her they throng one upon another so that she cannot free herself from them during the day, with neglect of business,...

Ha, 59 - A number of ideas from her past life, mostly disagreeable, causing indignation and mortification...come into her mind;...so that she cannot get rid of them, while she has nothing to do;...

Ha, 60 - Indifferent things and such things as naturally occur in life are attended in her mind with annoying, mortifying ideas from her past, which continually connect themselves with recent annoyances of which she cannot rid herself. This attended (accompanied) with a resoluteness of mind, which is ready for great resolves.(determination)

He, 43 - Vexations and morbid ideas of past arise from most indifferent thoughts, and from every occurrence in life, which continue to be united with new vexations, so that she cannot free herself from them.

PEACE

Comfort; sensation of: absin.[36] acon.[36] agar.[5] ars.[5] aur.[36] chlf.[36] chlor.[36] coca[5] dat-a.[36] gast.[36] kali-br.[36] mec.[36] nat-p.[5] op.[5] phos.[36] pic-ac.[5] scut.[25]

Delusions; obtain peace and safety through absolution from a priest of Papal church, although a zealous protestant, that she can only: ***plb.***[54]

Dreams; peaceful: nux-m.[36] spig.[36]

Longing; for, repose and tranquillity, for: nux-v. sulph.[1]

Quiet; wants to be: agn.[58] ars.[36] ***bac.***[62] bamb-a.[1184] bell. **BRY.**[122] cadm-s.[122] calc-p.[58] cand-a.[239] cann-i. chin.[36] choc.[222] coca colch.[137] cupr-s. dios. eryt-j.[36] euph. fago.[25] **GELS.** lap-mar-c.[194] lil-t.[25] nux-v.[10] ozone[227] prot.[136] ptel.[25] sal-ac. seq-s.[230] tanac.[25] verat-v.[25]

Quiet; wants to be, desires repose and tranquillity: bell.[30] con.[1] nux-v. sulph.[30]

Quiet; wants to be, walking in open air: arn. bor. calc-p. ph-ac.[10] sabin.

Quietude, stillness, sensation of, when she sits still: adax.[96] dat-a.[25] scut.[25]

Reconciled to fate, forenoon: aloe[36]

Rest; desire for: ***aesc.***[116] alum.[116] ***anac.***[116] arn.[116] bell.[54] brom.[116] **BRY.**[122] clem.[36] coca[36] ***colch.***[54] eug.[171] haem.[36] kali-bi.[36] lach.[116] lyc.[116] morph.[36] nux-v.[116] op.[116] ***ph-ac.***[116] sabad.[116] ***stann.***[116] vesp.[54]

ADAM. Sh, 296 - Thinking a lot about a cottage in Hampshire that I'd wanted to buy and feeling sad that I hadn't. Feeling that it would have been so blissful to be alone there, and be creative in the garden. No sound except birds, just to relax and be alone. 1, 12C, 01:XX:XX

ALOE. Al, 11 - In the afternoon, he is disposed to become reconciled (pacify) where he would not otherwise have been so.

ANAC. He, 62 - Internal anxiety, which did not leave him any peace; he felt solicitous (careful) on account of every trifle, as if it would lead to some great trouble (misfortune); with apprehension (fear) of future.

ARG-M. He, 13 - Great serenity, a heavenly sensation of peace.

ARS. Ha, 1057 - Uncommonly tranquil disposition; quite unconcerned about their approaching death, they neither hoped nor wished to recover.

Ha, 71 - During the first minutes great tranquillity of soul and serenity; but after half a hour excessive restlessness and anxiety; he imagines that the effects of the poison would be dreadful and desires to remain alive.(in a despondent suicide).

BELL. Al, 156 - By day great anxiety; she has no peace anywhere; it seems to her as if she must flee away.(escape)

Ha, 1395 - He wishes for solitude and quiet; all noise and visits from others are repugnant to him.

He, 108 - By day great anxiety; has no peace anywhere; it seemed to her as if she must fly away.

CANN-I. Al, 58 - He imagines that he is possessed of infinite knowledge and power of vision, and then that he is Christ come to restore the world to perfect peace. (redemption, savior, rescuer)

He, 14-... visions of a great sublimity (splendor) usually follow visions of a quiet, relaxing and recreating nature.

CHOC. Sh, 418 - Feel affectionate and quiet

in evening, less restless than usual.[11], 6C, 00:XX:XX
CLEM. Al, 19-...dreading to be alone, tired of living, full of thoughts of death, with fear that it would be speedy, longing however, for the repose of death; this mood was soon followed by apprehension, weeping, and homesickness, ...
FERR. Al, 6 - Temper more equable (regular) all through the proving.
GERM. Sh, 27 - Felt very quiet and calm. Almost detached. More patient and less irritable. 11, 12C, 00:04:05
LED. Ha, 338 - Calm and happy disposition with love for work and self-contented.
MUR-AC. Ha, 279 - Very tranquil, calm and free from care.
NEON. Sh, 36 - Now I felt no resistance, a harmony between heaven and earth. 20, 6C, XX:XX:XX
NUX-M. Al, 27 - As soon as she lay down felt a sinking sensation, as though she were going to die, with no fear, however, being perfectly at ease (peace) in mind,...
RHUS-T. Ha,(curative) 975 - He can master (leading, chief) his thoughts and think calmly (tranquillity) of any subject he will and as long as he likes, and at his pleasure take up some other topic, with tranquil, slow inspiration.
SULPH. Ha, 30 - He greatly feels the need of tranquillity of spirit, as his spirit is ever active.

PENITENCE

Begging, pray for him, to, and not to leave him alone: lyss.[54]
Delusions; convent, she will have to go to a: lac-d.
- doomed, expiated her sins and those of her family, to: ***lil-t.***[54].
- faces, supplicating: germ.[222]
- hell, gate of, obliged to confess his sins at: agar.
- hell, suffers the torments of, without being able to explain: lyss.[54] ***merc.***[122]
- martyrdom: carc.[207] nat-c.[162]
- mushroom, he is commanded to fall on his knees and confess his sins and rip up his bowels by a: agar.
- obtain peace and safety through absolution from a priest of Papal church, although a zealous protestant, that she can only: ***plb.***[54]
- starve, he must: kali-chl.[72]
- voices, hears, confess things she never did: lach.[58]

Despair; religious, constant prayer: ***puls.***[54]
Discouraged; praying, with: puls.[10]
Dreams; praying: ars-h.
➤ remorse, pleading for mercy at bar of judgment: aether[36]
Fear; poverty, spending, in case he is short of money in future, fear of: ***nux-v.***[30] stann.[30]
Insanity; prayer, raising hands and kneeling as in p.: ***ars.***[36]
Mania; prayer, as in, raising hands and kneeling: ***ars.***[36]
Mania; praying: stram.[60] verat.[60]
Praying; aloud, in sadness: ***plat.***[54]
Praying; begged others to pray for him: lyss.[54]
Praying; fervent: alum.[30] **SEP.**[30]
Praying; killed, to be: bell.[30]
Praying; kneeling and: ***ars.*** nat-s. ***stram.*** verat.
Praying; quietly, for her soul: arn.[54] ars.[54]
Praying; seeks relief in constant: ***puls.***[54]
Praying; sleep, during: stann.[54]
Praying; timidly, during sleep: stann.[54]
Praying; wanted people to join her in, with slight erysipelas of face: ***plat.***[54]
Religious affections; mania, praying all the time: ***aur.***[54]
Religious affections; penance, desires to do, wishes to live, in order to mitigate her eternal punishment, in sadness: ***plat.***[54]
Religious affections; sadness, gave away everything she could lay her hands on, in order to do penance: ***plat.***[54]
Talk; sleep, in, confess themselves loud, they: bell.[30] **HYOS.**[30] stram.[30]

AGAR. Al, 8-...called for his hatchet; had to be confined alternated with religious excitement.
Al, 14 - He imagines himself at a gate of the hell and that the mushroom commands him to fall on his knees and confess his sins, which he does. (forgiveness, absolution)
ARS. He, 25 - Mania...sees a man who has hanged himself beckoning (call) him to cut him loose (rescue, deliverance, free, saving) on failing to accomplish this he attempts to hang himself (punish, penalize);...finally kneels down and lifts

his hands in supplication.(forgiveness, absolution)

CAMPH. Al, 46-...And yet I confessed this every morning, and no heavy sin rests upon my conscience. And then came doubts about my doctrinal views, for I had never been of strong faith...

LAC-D. Al,N-4 - Imagines that all her friends will die and that she must go to a convent. (purification, solitude)

He, 5 - Imagines that all her friends will die and that she must go to a convent. (purification, salvation)

LIL-T. He, 16 - Doubts her salvation; thinks she is doomed to expiate her sins and those of her family; ... (redemption, salvation) (sacrifice)

LYSS. Al,N-11-...presentiment of impending death begged them to pray for him and not to leave him alone. (absolution, redemption)

PLAT. He, 36 - While suffering from a slight erysipelas faciei, took leave (quit, abandon) of her children, exhorted her husband to join (unite, combine) church, wanted people to join her in prayer (beg), felt happy to join her Redeemer.

He, 46-...;suffers unspeakable pangs (anxiety) of conscience in consequence of a faux (fault, mistake, embarrassing mistake?) pass when thirty-two years old; says she has brought disgrace upon her family, and that she has incurred the penalty of damnation; (doomed) in order to do penance (penitence) gave away whatever she could lay her hands upon, (redemption) so that she had to be constantly watched; after her confessor asserted that she could not hope for pardon or heaven (condemnable), she seemed in absolute despair ; bemoaned her misery throughout the night, wringing her hands and beseeching (implore) that she might be delivered (free) from the hell of her conscience; twice attempted self-destruction (suicide);...wished to live and do penance (penitence, purgation, purification) in order to mitigate her eternal punishment.

PLB. He, 15-...; despair of her salvation...; fixed idea that could only obtain peace and safety though absolution by a priest of the papal church, although she had been a zealous Protestant; ....brooded over any forbidden thing; would steal (leave) from house in servant's cloak (coat, camouflage) and bonnet (hat) to obtain stimulants (drugs), but from the moment their prohibition was withdrawn (retired) ceased to have any desire for them; after being permitted to visit a priest and converse with him ceased to talk and think of the church. (desire; redemption, absolution)

STRAM. He, 107-...heard continually, on r. side of occiput, a loud voice, scolding, vituperating and accusing him of ungodliness (impious, sinful, irreligious, godless, profane); ....prayed expecting, with great anxiety, the flash of lightning which was to kill him;...(redemption, regeneration, salvation)

THUJ. Al, 2 - She fancies that she has intentionally represented herself as insane (feigning) in the presence of others in order to palliate a wrong supposed to have been done (penitence, remorse), and that now she is punished, therefore, by real insanity.

Al, 7 - She constantly longs for the offices of the church in order to banish her sinful thoughts of suicide. (redemption, salvation)

PERFECTION

Admiration; things that are not admirable at all, for: sulph.[85]

Charmed with description of beauties of nature: coff.[36]

Comprehension; easy, quick perception for things out of shape or proportion: ham.[36]

Delusions; beautiful, atmosphere, in: dat-a.[36]

- beautiful, images, presenting themselves to her as if by charm: bell.[54]
- beautiful, landscape: ***coff. lach.***
- beautiful, old ragged woman is: psil.[164]
- beautiful, things look: bell.[5] eug.[36] germ.[222] hydrog.[222] olnd.[5] ***sulph.***[5] tab.[5]
- beautiful, wonderful: anh.[119] **BELL.** ***cann-i.*** coca ***lach. sulph.***
- cylinder, being a: cann-i
- paradise, he sees: coff.
- pleasing, accomplished, feels himself: phos.[1]
- sphere, he is a: cann-i.

- visions, sublimity, of great, follows those of quiet relaxing and recreating nature: ***cann-i.***[54]

Desires; beautiful things, finery: dat-a.[25] lil-t.[137] sulph.[137]
Desires; woman, ideal: ant-c.[36]
Dream, as if in a; beautiful: absin.[54]
Dreams; cities, beautiful: bamb-a.[1184]
➤ excelling in mental work: acon. anac. arn. ***bry.*** camph. carb-an. graph. ***ign.*** lach. ***nux-v.*** puls. rhus-t. sabad. ***sabin. thuj.***
➤ perfection: androc.[222]
➤ splendor: stann.[10]
➤ wonderful: bamb-a.[1184] chin-s.[36] op.[36] paeon.[36] ph-ac.[36]
Ecstasy; ideal had appeared to a poetic painter, as if an: jatr.[36]
Exhilaration; blissful: ***op.***[10]
Heavenly sensation: arg.[54] calc-ar.[54] crot-h.[36]
Idealistic: ***caust.***[162] ***ign.***[162] lyc.[30] ***plat.***[162]
Thoughts; rapid, quick perception of anything out of shape or disproportional: ham.[36]

ABSIN. Al, 4 - Very tranquil as if brain were rounded (spherical) and symmetrical.(balanced, regular, organized)
ADAM. Sh, 29-"Perfect" and "ideal" — someone commented I was using these words a lot. 8, 6C, 20:XX:XX
Sh, 40 - Overwhelmed by beauty of Sumatran tiger on TV, especially his eyes. 16, 12C, 01:XX:XX
Sh, 56 - Everything seems to complement everything else; balance and harmony, and order and form in the universe. 16, 12C, 26:XX:XX
ANT-C. Ha, 18 - Continuous state of enthusiastic love and ecstatic longing for an ideal woman, which quite filled his fantasy;... (perfection, utopian)
ARG-M. He, 13 - Great serenity, a heavenly sensation of peace.
CAMPH. He, 18-...one evening he went to the piano with closed eyes and played with great precision what at other times he could not have done without his notes; several times he wrote letters in an acquired (learned) language more correctly than in a waking state;...(clairvoyance)
He, 19 - It was to him as if he moved in his own little world, in which all things were clear (pure, perfect) and defined; outside of which uncertain (doubtful) and undefined. (obscure) (purity x impurity)
CANN-I. Al, 33 - Said "he had been transported to heaven (paradise)"...
Al, 58 - He imagines that he is possessed of infinite knowledge and power of vision, and then that he is Christ come to restore the world to perfect peace. (redemption, savior, rescuer)
CHOC. Sh, 86 - On seeing a bristly carpet, started laughing excitedly —had a familiar feeling, like meeting a friend. The texture of the carpet was very spiky like a Hedgehog. Told friend that they should come and see it. It's such a wonderful carpet!
Sh, 130 - I feel slightly less like a hedgehog today, but the picture is still in my mind. Human things seem so trivial —so much energy wasted when you are human. Nature is so efficient. It never wastes a seed and we just spend energy everywhere.
Sh, 149 - Hearing and smell still acute — nature seems wonderful. Saw nine magpies and they seemed much bigger than before.
Sh, 315 - Been on the move all day — painted a room blue. While lying in the bath looking out the window, the sky is the most glorious, vibrant blue — it seems like the most beautiful colour I've ever seen. Almost wept for the beauty of it. Suddenly, while I'm lying in the bath, the colour blue seems very important — seems very potent. It has the same quality and intensity that I remember colours having on L.S.D. I am very moved by this blue. I wanted to dissolve into it.[15], 30C, 03:05:XX
FL-AC. Al, 5 - Feeling of perfect happiness within (inside) and without.(outside)
Al, 9 - Satisfaction, he desires no better state of things; all is right.
GERM. Sh, 21 - Contemplative, like nice things, sees beauty in stones and nature. Good at instinctive understanding, compassionate. 16, 30C, 01:XX:XX
HALI-L. Sh, 187 - I want more from school. Ethics and education are very important. I want things done to a very high standard. To be methodical and well thought out. Want higher quality. 08, 30C, 25:XX:XX

Sh, 679 - Sun rose over house, felt there should be two suns. Desire for symmetry in the sky. 20, 30C, 00:00:20

Sh, 901 - Sensation of such harmonious balance when on the wing, Such power in these almost weightless wings. Sensation of deep warmth echoing the sun. 20, 30C, 10:XX:XX

HAM. Al, 18 - Quick perception of anything out of shape or disproportioned.

HYDROG. Sh, 27 - There is a very fine line at this time between enlightenment and insanity —a split consciousness. The dark side is horrendous, but the positive side of the proving has been well worth it. The positive aspects are beautiful. Its a shame we need to come down. I guess the price of going into the heavens is a trip to hell. 16, 30C, XX:XX:XX

Sh, 165 - I thought I could see energy moving around in the air. Colours looked bright and everything looked beautiful. 16, 30C, 25:XX:XX

IRID. Sh, 67 - Sensation of movement in face as if head, face and skin full of magnetism. Sense of alignment. Q2

JAMB. He, 4 - Sudden great change in him after micturition, everything seems more beautiful and bright, sky and trees more joyous and clear; but after quarter of an hour everything became gloomy again.

JATR. Al, 3 - An ecstasy, as if an ideal had appeared to a poetic painter, or like that which sometimes comes to a dying person, ...a feeling of lovely warmth and ethereal lightness...

KALI-BR. Al, 25 - At times he cried most bitterly, yet twelve hours previously he was singing and dancing, saying he was "the happiest man alive".

LACH. He, 54 - A girl, after excessive study, uses exalted language; exceedingly particular about language she uses, often correcting after using a word, and substituting another of very similar meaning, talking about being under influence of a superior power. (possessed) 0 Mania.

NEON. Sh, 39 - During the night, in a semi-sleep state, I had many thoughts of the second day of creation. I was aware that my form and weight were appropriate. 20, 6C, 03:XX:XX

Sh, 182 - Had an explosion for not being the perfect person. I was really pissed off at the situation. I felt out of control, helpless, and lashed out with vehemence and anger at the situation and myself. I'm in the "Valley of Discontent" and want to get out of Sacramento. 31, 12C, 16:XX:XX

NUX-V. Ha, 1301 - Clear consciousness of his existence; delicate, strong proper (accurate, correct, exact) feeling of right and wrong. (sapience) (justice)

He, 39 - Mania puerperalis...constantly complaining, criticizing or explaining, ... as soon she recognized physician she spoke of imperfection of medical knowledge and declared it an error that one could not live without a heart, inasmuch as she felt very well without one, it having come away with the afterbirth to which it had grown fast, the nurse having separated the two before her eyes; complains of her husband, says he wishes to convince her she is sick, ... nymphomania,... frequently sips at a bowl of warm sugar-water, declaring it will form her a new heart; .(health, healing)...(expert)

OLND. Al, 15 - While studying he had constantly other thoughts; he found himself dreaming of the future, and busying himself with beautiful images concerning it.

OP. Al, 45 - Sensation as if he had been taken to heaven; vivid, lovely fantasies float before his vision like a waking dream, which the slumber (sleep) drives away.

Al, 19-...each possessing some imaginary bliss (happiness) which " the dull (dark) reality of life" could never give....they are wrapped in an elysium, (heaven) from which they are only to be awakened by the miserable reaction which must, sooner or later recall them to existence.

Al, 19-...; all the actors are happy, and each retires home in a total state of irrationality, but likewise in the entire and full enjoyment of happiness not to be procured by reason. Disregarding the ridicule of those they meet, who divert themselves by making them talk absurdly, each imagines looks and feels himself possessed of whatever he wishes...

STRAM. Al, 45-...seemed to forget

herself...seemed to sit like a perfect idiot (fool),...

TIL. Al, 2 - Lovesick (passion, fervor); all his thoughts centered upon an ideal woman; in this revery he was possessed by a sweet melancholy...

PERSECUTION

Ailments from; looked at, being: ambr.[5] ***ant-c.*** ant-t. **ARS.** calc.[5] ***cham. chin. cina*** hell.[5] ***iod.*** lyc.[5] mag-c. merc.[116] nat-m. nux-v. rhus-t. stram. sulph.

Anxiety; pursued, as if: anac.[172] crot-h.[172] ***cupr-acet.***[54] hyos.[116] kali-br.[116] lach.[172] stram.[172] ***zinc.***[54]

Anxiety; pursued, as if, enemies, by: dros.[36]

Anxiety; pursued, as if, walking, when: ***anac.***

Anxiety; walking, while, people behind him might beat him, as if: alum.[122]

Anxiety; walking, while, pursued, as if: anac.[60]

Chases; imaginary objects: stram.

Chases; persons: cur.

Delusions; animals, bed, under the: cham.[54]

- animals, corners, coming out of: stram.[116]
- animals, dogs, swarm about him: bell. ***calc.***[54] stram.
- animals, running over her: cycl.[36]
- arrested, is about to be: arn. ars. ***bell.***[122] cupr. kali-br. meli. plb. ruta[36] tab.[85] ***zinc.***
- assaulted, is going to be: abel.[149] androc.[222] tarent.
- corner, figures coming out of, sees: stram.[116]
- corner, people coming out of, sees: stram.[54]
- corner, something coming out of: ***phos.*** stram.[162]
- dark, objects and figures, sees: cimic.[116]
- devils, after her: ***hyos. manc. zinc.***[54]
- devils, after her, climacteric period, during: zinc.[54]
- devils, persons are, all: **PLAT.** plb.[54]
- enemy, wait for an, lying in: alco.[36]
- faces, diabolical, get rid of them, cannot: ambr.
- faces, looking out of every corner: phos.[139]
- faces, wherever he turns his eyes, or looking out from corns: aur. med. ***phos.***
- figures, large black, about to jump on him: mosch.
- figures, strange accompany him, one on his right, the other on his left: ***anac.***[54]
- footsteps, hears, behind him: crot-c. ***med.***
- hearing, of, someone approaches his bed: carb-v.[54]
- images, all over: bry.[58] merc. ***sil.***
- images, side, at his: stram.
- jumped upon the ground before her, all sorts of things: brom. ther.[137]
- man, same man walking after him that he sees walking before him: euph.
- masks, sees: bell. kali-c. ***op.***
- noise, hears: anh.[144] bell. calc. canth.[5] carb-v. cham. cocain.[102] coff.[58] colch. con. hyos. mag-m. naja[98] ph-ac.[5] sulph.[1] verat.[10]
- noise, hears, bed, under: bell.[1]
- people, behind him, ascending from cellar, when: ozone[227]
- people, behind him, someone is: adax.[96] anac. bell.[5] brom. calc. casc. cench. crot-c. crot-h.[137] lach. led.[137] mag-m.[149] med. naja[36] ozone[227] psil.[164] ruta sac-l.[111] sanic.[137] sil. staph. tub.[137]
- people, behind him, whispering: med.[137]
- people, beside him, are: anac. apis ***ars.*** atro.[36] bell. calc. camph. carb-v. cench. nux-v. petr. thuj. valer.
- people, beside him, strange: ***thuj.***[54]
- people, closing eyes, see p. on: ars. ***bell.*** bry. **CHIN.** nat-m.
- people, coming out of corners: ***stram.***[54]
- people, sees: anac.[5] ***ars.*** atro. ***bell.*** brom.[5] ***bry. calc.*** chin. con. ***hyos.*** kali-c. lyc. lyss. mag-c.[5] mag-s. med. merc.[5] nat-m. op. petr.[58] plb. ***puls.*** rheum sep. ***stram.*** sulph. thuj. valer. verat.
- people, sees, connected with the law who will seize him, causing great anxiety, cries like a child: ***cupr-acet.***[54]
- people, sees, day and evening (on entering the room): lyc.[36]
- persecuted, delirium in: ars.[30] calc.[30] hyos.[30] lach.[30] merc.[30] nat-m.[30] rhus-t.[30] stram.[30] verat.[30]
- persecuted, that he is: abrot.[108] absin.[30] allox.[149] ***anac.***[5] androc.[222] ars.[5] aur.[5] bell.[5] brom.[127] calc.[30] cann-i.[187] ***cench.***[122] **CHIN.** choc.[222] ***cocain.***[102] con.[5] crot-h.[30] cupr.[30] cycl. **DROS.** hell.[30] hydrog.[222] hyos. ***ign.***[30] iodof.[171] kali-br. ***lach.***[30] lyc.[30] manc.[187] med.[108] meli.[30] merc.[30] nat-c.[30] nat-m.[30] nux-v.[30] op.[5] plb.[30] puls.[30] rhus-t.[5] sil.[30] spong.[54] staph.[5] stram. stry.[30] ***sulph.***[30]

syph.[30] thyr.[5] verat.[30] verat-v.[5] ***zinc.***[54]
- persecuted, that he is, everyone, by: ***cycl.***[54]
- persecuted, that he is, backward, and looks: staph.[30]
- persecuted, that he is, tormented by some frightful scene of some mournful event of the past, and: spong.[54]
- person, another in the room, waking, on: mag-p.[137]
- policeman, calls on him, officers: ***cupr.***[162]
- policeman, come into house, he sees: ars.[58] hyos. kali-br.
- policeman, physician is a: bell.
- present, someone is: hyos. lyc. thuj.
- pursued by enemies: absin. ***anac.***[102] ars. aur. ***bell. chin.*** cic. ***cocain.***[102] con. crot-h. cupr. cycl.[162] dros. hell. ***hyos.*** kali-br. ***lach.*** lepi. lyc. med.[108] meli. merc. nat-c. nux-v.[102] plb. ***puls.*** rhus-t. sil. stram. stry. zinc.
- pursued, by fiends (Allen, 63): plb.
- pursued, ghosts, by: lepi plat. stram.
- pursued, he is: absin. ***anac.***[122] ars. aur.[5] bell. bry. choc.[222] con.[5] cycl.[162] ***hyos.***[5] ***kali-br.*** lach.[58] med.[122] merc.[139] plb. rhus-t. sil.[30] staph. stram. thuj.[58] verat-v.[5]
- pursued, horrid thing, by some: anac.
- pursued, murderers, robbers, by: alco.
- pursued, phantom in a churchyard, by: lepi.[85]
- pursued, police, by: alco.[36] ars.[58] bell. ***cupr. hyos. kali-br.*** meli. phos. plb. zinc.
- pursued, robbing a friend, for: kali-br.[36]
- pursued, satan, by: vip.[1212]
- pursued, soldiers, by: absin. bell. bry. nat-c.[30] plb.
- pursued, spirits, evil, are pursuing him, runs around room, cries out: stram.[54]
- pursued, tormented by a frightful scene of some mournful event of the past, and: spong.[54]
- runs, backward, is chased and runs: sep.[139]
- soldier, sees, surrounded by: nat-c.[30]
- spectres, sees, behind him: lach.[85]
- strangers, looking over shoulder: brom.
- strangers, surrounded by: androc.[222] nit-ac.[30] ***puls.***[30]
- talking, persons near who are talking, about midnight: sep.
- thieves, robbers, sees: alum. ars. aur. bell. cupr. cupr-acet.[54] kali-c. kali-sil.[58] mag-c. mag-m. merc. nat-c. ***nat-m.*** petr. phos. sanic.[85] sil. sol-t-ae.[36] verat. zinc.
- thieves, sees, night: ***ars.***
- trees are people in fantastic costume (afternoon, while riding): bell.
- visions, eyes anxiously fixed sideways on one point where she imagines she sees a terrible hostile figure: ***stram.***[54]
- visions, horrible, behind him: ***lach.***[54]
- visions, horrible, beside him: ***stram.***[10]
- visions, leave the room, attempts to, as if frightened by visions behind him: ***lach.***[54]
- voices, hears: abrot. acon.[111] agar. anac. anh.[119] antipyrin.[102] ars.[102] aster. bell. benz-ac. calc.[5] calc-sil.[58] cann-i. ***cann-s.***[5] canth.[5] carb-v.[5] carbn-s. cench. **CHAM.**[122] chlol. coca ***coff.*** con.[5] ***crot-c.*** crot-h. ***cupr-acet.***[54] dros.[5] ***elaps*** germ.[222] hyos. ign.[5] ***kali-br.*** lac-c. lach. lyc. mag-m.[5] manc. med. nat-m. nit-ac.[5] petr. ph-ac.[5] ***phos.*** plb. rhus-t.[36] sol-n. stram. verat.[5] ***zinc.***[54]
- voices, hears, mastoid process, as if near right, a voice were scolding her, night agg., voice seems sometimes to be under bed: ***stram.***[54]
- walk, he sees the same one walking after him that he sees walking before him: euph.
- walk, someone walks behind him: anac.[149] calc.[137] crot-c. mag-m.[149] med.[122] ***staph.***[1]
- walk, someone walks behind him, dark, in the: ferr. sanic.
- watched, she is being: aq-mar. **ARS.** ***bar-c. calc.***[5] choc.[222] ***hyos.*** med.[108] meli. rhus-t
- watched, that she is being, night: med.[85]
- wrong, he has done, people are therefore against her: lil-t.[168]

Dreams; animals, bulls, chased by: ind. tarent.
- ➤ animals, cats, pursuing him: ***nux-v.*** sil. verat.
- ➤ animals, crocodiles, pursued by, and driving them away by sneezing: sedi.[36]
- ➤ animals, dogs, large dog following him: sil.
- ➤ animals, dogs, pursued by: ***nux-v.*** ozone[227] sil. verat.
- ➤ animals, horses, pursuing him: allox.[119] alum.
- ➤ animals, oxen, pursuing him: eupi. hipp.[36] tet.[36]

➤ animals, pursued by: allox.[119] alum. cench.[58] eupi. hipp.[36] hydr.[36] ind. led.[36] nux-v. sil. ***sulph.*** tarent. tet.[36] verat.
➤ animals, pursued by, wild: allox.[119] alum. cench.[58] eupi. hipp.[36] ind. led.[36] nux-v. sil. ***sulph.*** tet.[36] verat.
➤ ghosts, pursued, by: sil.
➤ giants, pursued by: bell.
➤ men, running, after: nicc.[36]
➤ police, calling for, waking him in last part of night: frax.[36]
➤ pursued, being: allox.[119] androc.[222] arg. atro. bell. con.[10] hir.[149] hydr.[36] kreos. mag-s.[10] nux-m. nux-v. ped.[36] ph-ac. sep. ***sil. sulph.*** verat. xan.[111] ***zinc.***
➤ pursued, enemies, by: con.
➤ pursued, ghosts, by: sil.
➤ pursued, giants, by: bell.
➤ pursued, man, red skinned, to harm her with his arrows: pitu-a.[164]
➤ pursued, police, by: lap-mar-c.[194]
➤ pursued, robbers, by: mag-m
➤ pursued, run backwards, must: sep.[58]
➤ pursued, soldiers, by: mag-s.
➤ pursued, witch, by a, creeps from under the door like a haze: ozone[227]
➤ rape, pursued for the purpose of: ***cench.***[122] kreos.
➤ running, after someone: cadm.[119]
➤ soldiers, being pursued by a: mag-s.
➤ strangled, morning, in, fear lest the man who strangled her would return: zinc.[54]

Escape; attempts to, run away, to, wants, and hide as she insists that everyone is looking at her: meli.[85]

Fear; arrested, of being: ars.[137] bell.[172] meli.[85] plb.[137] ruta[162] tab.[137] zinc.[72]
✦ behind him, someone is: anac. brom. crot-c. lach. **MED.** merc.[162] phel.[162] staph.[172]
✦ called by his name, being: sulph.[172]
✦ enemies, pursuing: bell.[172] sil.[172]
✦ looked at: aq-mar.[231] ars.[193] bar-c.[193] calc.[172] meli.[193] rhus-t.[193]
✦ persecution, of: bell.[172] dros.[172] hyos.[5] ***zinc.***[54]
✦ pursuit, of: hyos.[5]

Hysteria; looked, at, when: plb.[137]

Impulse; run, to, followed, thinks he is: anac.[109]

Insanity; persecution mania: **ARS.**[30] calc.[30] caust.[30] lach.[30] sulfonam.[149] verat.[30]

Sadness; persecutions of others, by: ***dros.***[54]

Schizophrenia; paranoid: ***bell.***[111] ***hyos.***[111] med.[122] ***nux-v.***[111] op.[111] rauw.[119] stram.[111] verat.[111]

Searching; thieves, dreamt of them, after having: nat-m.

Suspiciousness; looks on all sides: kali-br.[137]

ABSIN. Al,S-5 - Terrifying hallucination of persons pursuing him.
Al,S-6 - Terrifying hallucinations, he sees all kinds of animals, cats and rats of all colors, grotesque animals, fancies that he is pursued by soldiers.
Al,S-7 - Hallucination of vision and of hearing, that is pursued by imaginary enemies; hallucinations of various kinds, of naked women, etc.

ADAM. Sh, 195 - Bad paranoia, that people hate me, anyone just walking down the street hates me. I think they will hit me. 20, 1M, 07:XX:XX

ANAC. Al, 11 - When walking he felt anxious, as if some one were pursuing him; he suspected everything around him.
Ha, 5 - In walking and in standing, uneasiness, as if someone were coming behind him (persecuted); everything around him seemed to him suspicious.
Ha, 6 - Timorous in all his actions; he views everything more anxiously and timidly, always thinks of being surrounded by enemies, then he becomes hot, his blood seems to boil in his chest.
He, 28 - Fixed ideas: that mind and body are separated ; about redemption (salvation) of soul and about the devil; that a stranger is constantly by his side (pursued); that strange forms accompany him, one to his right and one to his left.
He, 56 - When walking he left anxious, as if some one were pursuing him; he suspected everything around him.

ANDROC. Sh, 84 - Overwhelmed by terror, panic and fear, like a psychic attack. Then specifically became fear of being psychically tested as if confronted by something absolutely horrible, as in a "cult initiation ordeal". He felt so scared he had to shut the door, with a feeling that something would appear from behind it if he left it open. (4)
Sh, 121 - When talking to friends felt 'paranoid', suspicious and guilty, when

asked questions, he became hot and sweaty. He felt it was a game of who was cleverer, and tried to lie to and outwit his friend, though this gave no satisfaction. His friends reported that he seemed unusually distant and cool. (29)

Sh, 123 - In the evening he became manic, stalked the streets and visited many friends for a short time only, but could not relax or relate to them. Was pleased when he found his friends were not at home. Spoke nonsense and tried to squeeze a laugh out of anything. (29)

ARS-MET. He, 4 - Fearful visions of spectres (ghosts) in bright daylight; she sees threatening people after her,...

ARS. Al, 90 - He sees vermin and bugs crawl about his bed, from which he wants to escape, and constantly throws away whole handfuls of them.

He, 17 - He sees all kinds of vermin (insects) on his bed, throws handfuls of them away, and tries to escape from them.

BROM. He, 2 - In the evening when alone, felt as if he would see something if he should turn around; as if some one was back of him.

He, 3 - Expects to see something jump around floor.

CALC. He, 15 - Imagines someone is walking beside her (persecution); that something hanging over back of chair is a person sitting there, etc.

He, 18 - Mental aberration with horrid visions before eyes and cardiac anxiety; he despairs of his salvation (pardon, rescue) and wants to stab himself.

CHIN. He, 10 - Fixed idea that he is unhappy, persecuted by enemies.

He, 11 - She thinks she is very unfortunate and constantly harassed (molested, tormented) by enemies.

CHLOL. He, 7-...inclined to wander and hide herself, avoiding shrewdly (astute) the vigilance of her friends...

CHOC. Sh, 193 - Husband wants to go out for a walk. I don't want to go. I feel paranoid that someone will see me and think 'on drugs' and arrest me or cart me off to an institution. 15, 30C, 00:02:00

CROT-C. Al, 3-... hears a strange voice to her left, and behind her; she follows it, throws herself against closed doors, and scratches them with her nails...She cries out: " He is in the den, but the lions will not eat him"

Al, 8 - He fancies he hears some one walking behind him.

CYCL. He, 17-...fear of death, or an illusion of being deserted or persecuted by every one.

DROS. Al, 11 - Anxiety as if his enemies allowed him no rest, but persecuted and pursued him.

Al, 4 - He is depressed by the persecutions of others on all sides, and also discouraged and solicitous about the future.

Ha, 274 - Anxiety, as if his enemies would not leave him quiet, envied (competition, rivalry, opposition, spite) and persecuted him.

He, 2 - Depressed by persecutions of others on all sides, and also discouraged and solicitous about future.

EUPH. He, 4 - Imagines he sees the same man walking after him that he sees walking before him.

GERM. Sh, 134 - Felt uncomfortable if any one stood close to me. Felt uneasy and paranoid in class. Feel as if done something wrong. 10, 9C, 06:06:00

HYDROG. Sh, 244 - Paranoid feeling with cold perspiration. 16, 30C, XX:XX:XX

Sh, 245 - Feel I can't trust anyone — 'paranoia'. 24, 30C, 100:XX:XX

Sh, 246 - I felt mistrust, suspicion and paranoia. 16, 30C, Letter

Sh, 248 - While sitting in a restaurant, felt progressively more cut off from friends at the table. I began to feel detached and paranoid. I felt disliked by people. They seemed to look at me menacingly. I became concerned that my lecture this afternoon had created conflict, mayhem and destruction, that my friends in the audience did not like me any more. I became aware of a dull ache in my sacrum making me want to shift backwards and forwards. At the same time, the people round the table seemed further away and smaller, as if I had moved four feet back from the table. I felt very uncomfortable and wanted to get out. I put my head down and rushed out without saying goodbye, feeling a sense of relief at getting away (all very unusual for me). Outside, I felt relief and my mind cleared and I walked home alone. 22, 12C, 04:XX:XX

HYOS. He, 59-...constantly pointing to serpents (snakes) which she saw creeping up towards her...

He, 60-... wants to run away for fear of being persecuted by police;...

He, 57 - Delirium tremens:...averse to light and company; visions as if persecuted preceded by an epileptic attack;... seeks to escape from men by whom he imagines himself surrounded and who are trying to capture him; does not recognize his wife who is standing by his side, but imagines he sees her under a distant bed.

KALI-BR. Al, 2 - General delirium, with hallucinations; delusions about persecution and violence.

Al, 3 - Decidedly insane; had delusions that lewd women had got into his mother's house; that he was pursued by the police; that his wife was threatened by members of the family; that he had thousands of dollars in gold sewed up in his clothing; (rich, wealth)

Al, 4 - He imagined that he had been specially singled out (select) for divine vengeance... deploring his sad fate (destiny),...he informed me that he had been accused of robbing a friend, and that the officers were in search of him....

He, 17 - Delirium with delusions; thinks he is pursued (hunt); will be poisoned; is selected (designated) for divine vengeance (revenge); that her child is dead, etc.

LAC-C. He, 15 - Sensation or delusion as if surrounded by myriads of snakes, some running like lightning up and down inside the skin ; some that are inside feel long and thin; fears to put her feet on floor, lest she should tread (walk) on them and make them squirm (shake) and wind (round) around her legs; is afraid to look behind her, for fear that she will see snakes there, does not dream of them and is seldom troubled with them after dark; on going to bed she was afraid to shut her eyes for fear that a large snake, the size of her arm, would hit her in the face.

LACH. Al, 32 - Becomes easily peevish and mistrustful; believes himself intentionally injured (hurt, prejudice) by all his environments, and attaches the most hateful significance to the most innocent occurrences.

He, 8 - Thinks: she is somebody else in the hands (seized) of a stronger power; (supremacy, superiority).or that she is dead, and preparations are made for funeral (cortege) or that she is nearly dead and wishes some one would help her off; herself pursued by enemies, or fears medicine is poison; there are robbers in house and wants to jump out the window; herself under super-human control; visions real, he will die. (helplessness, desire; aid, comfort, salvation)

He, 9 - Imagines he is followed (pursued) by enemies who are trying to harm (hurt, injure) him; attempts to leave room as if frightened by visions behind him.

He, 21-...imagines he is followed by enemies who are trying to harm him; attempts to leave room as if frightened by visions behind him.

LEPI. Al, 1 - She fancies herself alone in a graveyard, pursued by a ghost, and screams so that her voice is lost next day; yet nobody hears her. (helpless)

MAG-M. Al, 714 - Frightful dreams; that she was pursued by robbers; that she burned her hand by washing ...

MED. He, 17 - Thinks some one is behind her, (pursued) hear whispering; sees faces that peer (observe) at her from behind bed and furniture.(spied)

MERC. Ha, 1127 - She dreams that people are before the window, and on being woke up thereby be cannot persuaded that they were not there. (observed)

NEON. Sh, 40 - Twice thought I heard someone at the door but when I checked there was no one there. Thought there might have been a noise which suggested somebody was there. This happened twice during the proving. 05, 12C, 01:06:20

Sh, 41 - Twice at 5.45 am I was awakened by hearing a doorbell -leapt out of bed to open the door but no one was there.09, 12C, 17:XX:XX

PHOS. Al, 12-...; wherever he turned his eyes he saw faces; they swarmed (crowded, surrounded) by him in long panoramic succession; they leered (look lecherous) at him over the footboard of the bed; they squinted (look) at him though the windows, or came trooping (crowd) in when the doors were left ajar (open) (invade);..he fancied he was some one else, ...

Al, 111 - Horrible fearfulness, late in the evening, as if a horrible face were looking out from every corner.

Ha, 31 - Dreadful fearfulness, late in the evening, as if a horrid face was looking out of every corner.

He, 8 - Fear and dread: in evening; of death; as if something were creeping out of every corner; late in evening as if a horrible face were looking out of every corner.

PLB. Al, 63 - The patient imagined that he was constantly followed (persecuted), and that he heard voices coming from the chimney... ; this man after a few days wished to leave the hospital and go home, because he was convinced that there were fiends in the building that pursued him and sought (want) his life.

PULS. He, 46 - Dark suspicious and reserved manner; disturbed look on face; sleepless; looks for her bed in the yard (lost?); hides in a corner to escape from a little gray man who wanted to pull out her leg;...

SPONG. He, 21 - She is very timid, and is especially pursued and incessantly tormented by a frightful scene of some mournful (unhappy) event of the past.

STAPH. Ha, 697 - When he walks quickly he feels as if some one were following him; this caused anxiety and fear, and he must always look about him.

STRAM. Al, 53-...throw the hands about the head as if attempting to ward off some threatening evil;...escape from the imaginary object ...

Ha, 562 - His surroundings appear to him quite strange; (unfamiliar) although in the first minutes he knows that he is surrounded by his friends, he forgets this in the second minute, and imagines he is quite alone (solitary, deserted) in a desert (wildness), and is afraid (fearful) ; figures of beasts suddenly spring out of the ground at his side, so that he moves to the other side, where, however, other similar figures pursue him, and he runs forward.

He, 40 - Aberration of mind; one carries home all sorts of wood in order to manufacture brandy (cognac) (busy, manufacturing) ; another placed two axes across each other in order to split wood in this way; a third burrowed in ground like a pig with his mouth (animal); a fourth alleged he was a wheelwright and began to bore holes; a fifth ran into forge to catch fish, which he saw swimming there; a lacemaker threw about her bobbins incessantly, and threw everything into confusion; another girl ran about the room and cried out that all evil spirits were pursuing her.(restoration, restitution)

He, 63 - An old lady had a vision every night since six weeks, in which many persons, all strangers, came into her room and to her bedside, causing her such fear that she had to leave bed.

STRY. Al, 3 - Shouted out, "They are coming for me".

SULPH. Al, 3780 - At night, very vivid anxious dreams, as if was pursued by wild beasts.

THYR. Al,N-4-"All progressed cases of myxedema ... delusions ...suspicion, and persecution".

Al,N-5 - Delirium of persecution (three cases observed, one fatal, the result of taking Thyro in tablets to reduce obesity).

VERAT. He, 26 - Chases (pursue, hunt) his family out of house ; declares the sun travels around the earth (geocentric); fear of death, restlessness, despair...

ZINC. He, 43 - Great fear, as if persecuted by men or the devil, on account of crimes he has never done (injustice); is afraid of becoming imprisoned, or poisoned, or shot, or buried (inter) alive...[0] Delirium tremens.

He, 46-...; believed herself to be called before court (judged) on account of her wicked (immoral) actions; ....;believe the devil is after her;...(persecution)

PESSIMISM

Delusions; troubles, trifle, every, leads to big trouble: anac.[139]

• unpleasant, news, he is expecting: mez.[139]

Imbecility; negativism: hell.[122] ign.[122]

Pessimist: agav-t.[149] ars.[30] aur.[58] bar-c.[30] calc.[1] carb-an.[36] caust.[30] cecr.[149] cic.[58] ferr-p.[36] gad.[36] germ.[222] graph.[36] halo.[149] hyos.[30]

lach.[30] morph.[36] nat-c.[36] nat-m.[36] nit-ac.[36] ***nux-v.***[30] op.[36] pers.[149] ***psor.***[122] sec.[36] sep.[30] stann.[149] thuj.[36] vip-a.[149] wies.[36]

Thoughts; morbid: carc.[207] op.[36] opun-a.[36] plb.[36]

Thoughts; obscurity of: aesc.[36] bell.[36] cann-i.[36] coff.[36] dig.[36] graph.[36] kali-br.[36] op.[36] rhus-t.[36] sapin.[36] thea.[36] upa.[36]

AESC. Al, 6 - Gloomy (dark) forebodings.

ALUM. Al, 11 - She is constantly possessed by bad thoughts which oblige her to weep; at the same time she feels apprehensive and uneasy, as if something evil were to happen to her; everything she only looks at, fills her with sadness.

Al, 7 - The person imagines only disagreeable, sad images.

Ha, 7-...anxiety as if something bad would happen (misfortune) to her; whatever she looks at, fills her with sadness.

Ha, 10 - She looks at everything in the worst light, and weeps and cries for hours.

ANAC. Al, 16 - Anxiety in all his actions; everything appears to him more terrible; he imagine himself surrounded with enemies; then he feels warm and the blood seems to boil within him.

He, 49 - Sadness; looks on dark side of everything.

AUR. Ha, 342 - Peevish (irritable) dejection; (sadness) he thinks nothing will succeed (prosper) with him.

Ha, 19 - Dispirited and despondent; he thinks that everything goes awkwardly (incapacity, unfit) with him, and nothing will succeed with him.

He, 8 - Looks on dark side, weeps, prays, thinks she is not fit for this world, longs for death, strong inclination to commit suicide; desperate, desires to jump from a height.

BAR-C. Al, 5 - Sad and fearful; he has all kinds of sad thoughts about his future state, and thinks that he is lost entirely; in the evening.

CALC-F. Al,S-1-...tendency to look on the dark side of things, with much depression of spirits. Feeling of anxiety about money matters, or thought would come to want (lack), or would soon be "running astern" (reversed, failure) financially...disposition to set a higher value on money than natural to him (avarice?, poverty?).

He, 1 - All day an unusual tendency to look on the dark side of things; with much depression of spirits.

CALC. Al, 16 - Sorrowful and peevish; she looked upon everything from the worst side, and imagined everything evil.

Al, 18 - Despairing mood, with dread of disease and suffering, with foreboding of sad events.

Ha, 46 - Troubled and cross, she looked at the worst side of things, and sought (pursued) out all the evil.

CAUST. He, 30 - Melancholy; she looks upon the dark side of everything. O Amenorrhoea. 0 Menorrhagia.

CHEL. Al, 27 - Extremely depressed; full of sad thoughts about the present and future, even to weeping; he had no rest of any kind.

Ha, 154 - Extraordinarily depressed, full of gloomy (dark) thoughts about the present and future, causing him to weep;...

FERR. He, 8 - Mental depression, gloomy (dark) foreboding thoughts.

FL-AC. Al, 18 - In the evening he is very discontented; he looks at everything in the worst light; ...

KALI-BR. Al, 11-...gloomy ideas relative to his present and future condition, if an opinion could be formed from the signs of distress, such as weeping, moaning, and wringing his hands,...

KALI-P. He, 5 - Anxiety, nervous dread without special cause, gloomy moods, fancies, taking dark views of things, dark forebodings.

LACH. He, 43 - Weary of life, looks at everything from dark side;...

MED. He, 20 - Is sure that she is worse, knows she is not going to live, cannot see any improvement, even when it is pointed out (antagonism); has no fear of death, speaks calmly about it, and gives directions as to the disposition of her affairs.

NAT-C. He, 6 - Intolerable melancholy and apprehension; she is wholly occupied with sad thoughts.

NAT-M. He, 33 - Brain fag (weakness), with sleeplessness, gloomy (dark) forebodings, exhaustion after talking, embarrassment (confusion) of brain.

NAT-S. Al, 4 - Lachrymose; thinks only of sad things.
PHOS. Al, 71 - Filled whith gloomy forebodings.
Ha, 62 - Very irritable mood, she takes every word ill and becomes pusillanimous (coward) from it.
He, 7 - Anxious: filled with gloomy (dark) forebodings; as if about to die; about termination (conclude) of her illness (disease); and restless ; at twilight; when alone; about future; during a thunderstorm; ..
He, 19 - Weary of life; full of gloomy (dark) forebodings.
POLYG-H. He, 2 - Gloomy (dark) views of life, dislike of change (evolution, transformation) and excessive dread (fear) of death.
PSOR. Al,N-14 - Anxious, full of fear, melancholic; evil forebodings.
He, 13 - Anxious, full of fear, melancholic; evil forebodings.
SAPIN. Al, 5 - Quite ill-natured and inclined to view matters in a disagreeable light; did not seem able to feel settled (decided) enough to know what to do; the crossness became so intense, that I felt myself getting very unreasonable, especially as to food, which seemed all wrong in some way;...
SEP. Al, 29 - Dark forebodings about his disease in regard to the future.
Al, 30 - All her troubles appear to her mind in a very gloomy light, so that she is fearful.
Ha, 10 - All her troubles present themselves in a very sad light to her mind, so that she is despondent.(sad, depressed)
He, 13 - Dark forebodings about his disease in regard to the future.
He, 29 - Fear to starve,(hunger) is peevish, and feels mortified (disgraced), easily frightened and full of evil forebodings.
SIL. He, 14 - Gloomy, feels as if she would die.
STAPH. Al, 6 - Sad; he fears the worst results from slight causes, and cannot quiet himself.
Ha, 708 - Sad, he apprehends (perceive) the worst consequences from slight (trivial) things and cannot calm himself.
STRAM. He, 175 - Sad; apprehends evil consequences from trifling things.
SULPH. Al, 8 - Numerous morbid ideas, extremely disagreeable, causing rancor, though with also joyous thoughts (and melodies) mostly from the past, take possession of her they throng one upon another so that she cannot free herself from them during the day, with neglect of business,...
He, 33 - Sleepless, disgusted with life, fears the future, where she sees nothing but misery (wretchedness, poverty) and suffering (misfortune). 0 Melancholia.
THEA. Al, 20 - Nocturnal fright; sinister thoughts; invincible propensity to analyze his life, to look at it on the dark side, and to resolve it into its most hopeless realities.
THUJ. Al, 49 - Sudden rising of dark thoughts (pessimism) causing uneasiness, apprehension (foreboding) of misfortune, with fancied scruples of conscience, ...

PHILOSOPHY

Fanaticism; philosophical: sulph.[60]
Mania; philosophical: ***sulph.***[58]
Philosophy; ability for: anac.[30] halo.[149] hep.[30] hydrog.[222] lach.[30] nit-ac.[30] ***sulph.***[58]
Religious affections; speculations, dwells on: **SULPH.**[54]
Theorizing; philosophic, mind dwells on: hydrog.[222] **SULPH.**[54]

ANDROC. Sh, 108 - Incredibly sensitive to noise, can't bear it, hundreds of thoughts pop in and out of my brain, thoughts of 'why are we here?', deep philosophical issues. Everyday things disappear from my mind. Am free from pressing, nagging responsibilities —just a black thunder sits within me, and I feel afraid of what I might do next. my eyes are staring and full of hate — just looking at the children sends them frantic. I have no control over my emotions. Then after 8:00 p.m., deadness resumes and I feel .k., but the end of myself as I usually am. (7)
CHOC. Sh, 180 - I felt that I was making exceptionally profound statements about life. 35, 30C, 03:XX:XX
Sh, 181 - Attitude good, feel calm and philosophical about things[45], 30C, 02:XX:XX

Sh, 183 - Thoughts of what's in all this for me? What am I getting out of this? Wondering about his life and why I continue with it. 45, 30C, 23:XX:XX

HYDROG. Sh, 265 - Greatly increased tendency to theorize and philosophise, especially concerning esoteric matters. 16, 30C, 05:XX:XX

SULPH. Ha, 61 - Great inclination to philosophic and religious ravings.(insanity)

He, 9 - Rack (torture) their brains about metaphysical subtleties (nuances).

He, 32 - Melancholy mood; dwelling on religious or philosophic speculations; anxiety about soul's salvation; indifference about lot (destiny) of others.

PLANNING

Doubtful, plans, about realizing her: bamb-a.[1184]

Dreams; business, projects: camph.[36]

➤ plans: psor.[36] sulph.[198]

➤ plans, tomorrow: naja[85]

➤ projects: anac.[10] bufo[5] camph.[10] rhus-t.[10]

➤ projects, coming true (in the dreams): rhus-t.[10]

Obstinate; execution of matured plans, in: dros.[36]

Plans; bold: agar.[36]

Plans; fantastic, in insanity: ***nux-v.***[54]

Plans; future, for the: ***coff.***[54]

Plans; gigantic: op.

Plans; many: anac. ang. arg-n. ***chin. chin-s. coff.*** hydrog.[222] nux-v. olnd. op. sep. ***sulph.*** tab.[5] visc.[149]

Plans; reflects upon their execution: ***chin.***[54]

Plans; revengeful: agar.

AGAR. Al, 4 - He is intoxicated with fearless frenzy; forming bold (courageous, brave) and revengeful projects.

Al, 9 - Delirium; he imagines himself a military (martial) officer, commanding (dominant) at a drill (training) and directing the various maneuvers.

ANAC. Al, 28 - Extreme excitement of the fancy, with a number of projects, in the evening...

ANG. Al, 14-...internal uneasiness, such as is experienced by those who anticipate some great pleasure, or also owing to all sorts of plans crowding upon his mind.

Al, 15-,...prevented by the intrusion upon his mind of a rather agreeable project which he almost believes to be real and feasible, and which exclusively absorbs all his attention; it is a sort of waking dream.

He, 8 - Thinks about one project and nothing else, with great activity of mind.

BAR-C. Ha, 12 - The greatest irresolution; he proposes to himself a brief journey, and as soon as he is to make his preparation, he is sorry for it and prefers to stay at home.

BRY. Al, 39 - Imagination very sluggish (slow); it is impossible to make any plan for the future, even for the next day; the judgment (discernment), however, is unimpaired .

BUFO-S. Al, 7 - He is unable to act with decision (doubtful) ; he forms projects and does not accomplish (succeed) them.

CHIN. Al, 56 - A large number of projects.

Ha, 1135 - He makes a number of grand (great) plans for the future.

Ha, 1136 - He makes many plans, and thinks over their accomplishment (execution, success), many ideas force themselves upon him at once.

Ha, 1137 - He has many ideas, undertakes (begin, try) to carry out (achieve, perform, execute) all sorts of things, builds castles in air.(fanciful)

Ha, 1138 - He has a number of plans in his head which he greatly desires to carry into execution (progress), in the evening.

He, 55 - He has many ideas, a variety of things occupy his mind; he builds castles in the air (after a few hours).

COFF-T. Al, 15 - It gives rise to a need of creative activity, a vivacity of thought, a versatility and ardor of desire, more favorable to the exaggerated expression of ideas previously formed, than to the quiet examination of new conceptions.

COFF. Al, 1 - Lively fancies; full of plans for the future; contrary to his custom is very much charmed by the beauties of nature,...

He, 5 - Lively fancies; full of plans for the future.

DROS. He, 7 - Self-willed (inflexible); obstinate; insists upon carrying out his plans.(determination)

GERM. Sh, 176 - Woke up and could not relax. Thought about how to solve problems, found a plan at last. 21, 12C, 34:XX:XX.

HALI-L. Sh, 182 - Not doing enough. Feel somewhat critical of myself. Not getting anything done. Want to be in a structured, organized place and can't get there. I'd like to be really busy. I have more ideas in my head than I can do. I need to get active again, structure things, and set goals. 08, 30C, 03:XX:XX

LACH. Al, 5 - A kind of ecstasy, as after sublime impressions, or excessive joy, throughout the day; he constantly wishes to talk and do much, and even more seems to be at his command.(control, domination)

NAT-C. Al, 22 - His fancy is mostly busy with apprehensions of the future; he often makes plans for half an hour at a time as if it would go wrong with him, wherewith he seeks to be alone for several days together.

NUX-V. He, 37-...betraying (play false, feigning) great moral and physical languor (indifference),..launches into high-flying, fantastic plans, fancies himself rich (rank, position) and wants to make presents of thousands (squanders, waste), and makes large useless purchases; does not consider himself ill; ...,and takes in bad part if not allowed to read indictment (accusation) for said lawsuit, a confused irrational piece of work...

OP. Al, 148-...his mind to be not only clear and active, but filled with gigantic schemes and theories, the realization of which seems to him quite natural and easy; his faculties are remarkably keen (sharp)...

OPUN-V. Al, 5 - Fit of swearing (cursing) at evening after coming home; praying in the morning, swearing (cursing) on disappointment in plans; fit of rage, on thwarting (frustrating) of plans.

SEP. Al, 101 - Dullness of comprehension; inability to collect or express his thoughts; constantly building air-castles or running on future events.

TAB. Al, 51 - Exalted action of the brain; copious flow of ideas; ...leaving me in the morning worn-out and sick, I would conceive and elaborate about twenty undertakings, of which probably not one would ever come to light.

PLEASURE

Ailments from; excitement, general symptoms from, sudden, pleasant: **COFF.**[54]

Ailments from; joy, excessive: ***acon.*** ars.[163] aur.[163] ***bad.***[5] caust. chin.[163] ***chin-ar.***[163] **COFF.**[5] croc. cycl. helon.[116] ***manc.***[122] merc.[163] nat-c. ***op. ped.***[122] plat.[163] ***puls.*** tarent.[36] valer.[163] verat.[30]

Ailments from; surprises, pleasant: chin.[1] **COFF.** ferr.[116] merc.[5] ***op.***[30] verat.[30]

Amusement, averse to: androc.[222] bar-c. ***hep.***[54] ***ign.***[54] lil-t. meny. olnd. sulph.

Amusement; desire for: cann-i.[25] coca[25] ***lach.*** pip-m. sumb.[25]

Anger; alternating with, cheerfulness: ant-t.[10] aur. cann-s.[10] caps. caust.[10] cocc.[10] croc. ign. nat-m.[10] op.[10] seneg.[10] spong.[10] stram. zinc.[10]

Anger; alternating with, jesting: caps.[10] cocc.[10] ign.[10]

Anger; alternating with, laughing: croc.[10] ***plat.***[54] stram.[10]

Animation agg.: ***coff.***[122] ***hyos.***[122] ***lach.***[122] ***par.***[122] ***sabad.***[122] ***valer.***[122]

Anxiety; pleasurable events, over formerly anticipated: bell.[36]

Aversion; faces, to laughing: m-aust.[85]

Blissful feeling: androc.[222] coff.[1] **OP.**[5]

Cheerfulness; alternating with, aversion to work: spong.

Cheerfulness; alternating with, impatience: tell.[149]

Cheerfulness; alternating with, indifference: tarent.[36]

Cheerfulness; alternating with, indignation, bursts of: aur. caps. croc. ign.

Cheerfulness; alternating with, vexation: ant-t.[10] bor.[5] caust.[10] cocc.[10] cortiso.[119] croc.[10] nat-m.[10] spong.[10]

Cheerfulness; coition, after: nat-m.

Cheerfulness; company, in: bov.

Cheerfulness; death, while thinking of: aur.

Cheerfulness; evening, grief, changes to: calc-s.[36]

Cheerfulness; evening, sad in morning, and: nux-v.[30]

Cheerfulness; fearful, but: ***nat-c.***[137]

Cheerfulness; lightness, with feeling of: petr.[10]

Cheerfulness; morbidly: aur-s.[58]

Cheerfulness; never: hep.[30] nit-ac.[30]

Cheerfulness; pollutions, after: pip-m.[58]

Cheerfulness; spirituality, followed by fading of: lach.[54]
Cheerfulness; thunders and at lightnings, when it: bell-p.[193] calc.[184] ***carc.***[122] caust.[185] lyc.[148] ***sep.***
Cheerfulness; work, during manual: ang.[54]
Death; desires, alternating with laughing: aur.[10]
Death; presentiment of, rejoices and gives directions about funeral: stram.[54]
Death; thoughts of, joy, give him: aur.[54]
Delirium; cheerful, alternating with, laughing, singing, whistling, crying etc.: stram.
Delirium; cheerful, gay, rage, changing to: ***bell.***[54]
Delirium; laughing: acon. apis[5] ***bell.*** colch. con. cupr.[5] ***hyos.*** hyosin.[36] ***ign.*** lach. lact. op. plb. sal-ac.[36] sec. sep. ***stram.*** sulph. thea. verat. zinc.
Delirium; romping, with, children: agar.
Delusions; beautiful, things look: bell.[5] eug.[36] germ.[222] hydrog.[222] olnd.[5] ***sulph.***[5] tab.[5]
- body, sweets, is made of: merc.
- delightful: aeth.[36] nitro-o.[36]
- heaven, is in: cann-i. hydrog.[222] op. ***verat.***[54]
- images, pleasant: bell.[54] cann-i. cycl. ***lach.***
- island, is on a distant, enjoying the tranquillity : phos.
- laughter, with: op.[10] sep.[10] ***stram.***[10] ***verat.***[10]
- ludicrous: calc.[10] cann-i. cann-s. hyos.[10] nat-m. ***nux-m.*** plat.[1] stram. sulph.[10] tarent.
- ludicrous, antics: ***bell.***[10] cic.[10]
- masks, laughing, sees (at night in bed): ***bell.***[54]
- music, delightful: lach. plb. puls.
- music, sweetest and sublimest melody: cann-i. ***lach.***
- music, unearthly: aether cann-s.[122]
- paradise, he sees: coff.
- pleasing: atro. cann-i. nitro-o.[36] op. psil.[164] stram.
- pleasing, morning after sleep: bell.
- sweets, body is made of: merc.[137]
- toys, objects seemed as attractive as: cic.
- toys, playing with: atro.
- visions, beautiful: bell. ***cann-i.*** coca lac-c. lach. olnd. **OP.** psil.[164]
- visions, wonderful: calc. camph. cann-i. lach. psil.[164]
- water, nectar, water is delicious, when drinking: cann-i.
- wings, her body is borne upon wings, after laughing: thuj.[54]

Desires; drugs, recreation: androc.[222]
Desires; merriment, for: chin.[36]
Disgust; exhilaration, of others, at: m-aust.[10]
Dream, as if in a; delicious: ***cann-i.***[54]
Dreams; animals, playing with: gran.[36]
- ➤ anxious, pleasant, partly: dros.[54]
- ➤ carousing: ars.[10] calc.[10] carb-an.[10] carb-v.[10] cham.[10] chin.[10] con.[10] graph. kali-c. kali-n.[10] led.[10] lyc. mur-ac.[10] nat-c. nat-m. nit-ac. nux-v. petr. sep.[10] sil. spong.[10] sulph. zinc.
- ➤ children, became a three year old, and rejoiced much: mag-c.[36]
- ➤ circus, of: hydrog.[222]
- ➤ comical: choc.[222] ***glon.*** lach.[10] ***sulph.***
- ➤ ecstatic: cann-i.[36]
- ➤ entertainment: nat-c.[36]
- ➤ happy, she is, but does not notice it: ozone[227]
- ➤ joke, relating a: coca[36]
- ➤ ludicrous: bell. cod.[36] glon. grat.[36] iber.[36] jug-c. lach. merc-c. merc-i-r.[36] mez. mygal. phos. sedi.[36] sol-t-ae. ***sulph.***
- ➤ parties, giving surprise to friend: pip-m.[36]
- ➤ parties, of pleasure: crot-c.[36] hura[36] nat-c.[36] phel.[36]
- ➤ quarrels, changing suddenly to happy conversation with another person: ferr-p.[85]
- ➤ romantic: am-c. ***kali-c.***[54]
- ➤ water, skating in Summer with water up to thighs, of seeing people: ped.[36]

Ecstasy: **ACON.** aether[36] ***agar.*** agn. am-c. androc.[222] ang. ***anh.***[119] ***ant-c.*** apis[5] arn. astra-e.[149] bell. berb.[116] bry. camph. cann-i. **CANN-S.**[5] canth.[5] carbn-h. cast.[116] cham. ***cic.*** coca[36] ***cocc.*** ***coff.*** croc.[5] crot-h. cupr. cupr-am-s.[36] cur. cypr. ery-a.[36] fl-ac.[36] hyos. ***ign.***[5] iod.[36] jatr. keroso.[85] kres.[149] ***lach.*** lyss.[54] nitro-o.[36] nux-m. olnd. ***op.*** ph-ac. **PHOS.** plat. plb. sel.[5] sil.[5] stann.[5] staph.[5] stram. sulph.[111] sumb.[36] thea. valer. ***verat.***[5]
Ecstasy, amorous, delirium, during: thea.[36]
Ecstasy, amorous, sleep, during: phos.
Ecstasy; alternating with sadness: senec.
Ecstasy; ideal had appeared to a poetic painter, as if an: jatr.[36]

Ecstasy; joy, as after excessive: lach.[36]
Ecstasy; periodical, twice a day, seems to be dying: ***cic.***[54]
Ecstasy; sensitivity of female sexual organs, with: coff.[54]
Euphoria; alternating with, despair: ozone[227]
Euphoria; alternating with, indifference: ozone[227]
Euphoria; alternating with, quarrel: thyr.[149]
Euphoria; alternating with, sadness: asar.[149] cortiso.[149] hydro-c.[149] mand.[149]
Euphoria; lightness, feeling of, as after an anesthesia by chlorethylene, with: asar.[149]
Euphoria; working, when: dicha.[149]
Excitement; hope, as in joyous: ***aur.***[54] choc.[222]
Exhilaration; blissful: ***op.***[10]
Exhilaration; coition, after: bor.
Exhilaration; laugh at merest trifles, with disposition to: **CANN-I.**[54]
Exhilaration; mania, in merry: ***stram.***[54]
Exhilaration; recall things long forgotten, can: ***gels.***
Fear; death, alternate laughing and weeping, with (after anger): ***plat.***[54]
✦ surprises, from pleasant: ***coff.***
Foolish; behavior, happiness and pride: **SULPH.**
Foolish; behavior, hilarity, with riotous, and subsequent angry savageness, or tearful sorrow: op.[54]
Heavenly sensation: arg.[54] calc-ar.[54] crot-h.[36]
Ideas; gay and musical: sulph.[60]
Indifference; agreeable things, to: ambr. anac. apis[58] cina corn. merc.[30] op. rhod. staph. stram.
Indifference; happiness, to: ars-i.[58]
Indifference; pleasure: alum. anac. androc.[222] ***apis***[170] ***arg-n. ars.*** ars-i.[58] calc-ar.[58] cench.[58] ***cham.*** chin-ar.[58] ***chin-s.*** cocc. croc. ferr-p. germ.[222] graph. **HELL.** hep. hura ip. kali-ar. kali-c. kali-chl.[58] kali-sil.[58] mag-c.[144] mag-m. meph.[149] mez. mur-ac. nat-ar. nat-c. **NAT-M.** ***nit-ac.*** **OP.** petr. prun. ***puls.*** sars. ***sep.*** spig. stann. staph. stram. **SULPH.** ***syph.***[122] tab. ther.
Jesting; erotic: bell.[30] ***calc.***[30] hyos.[30] nux-v.[30]
Jesting; fun of somebody, making: ***lach.***[30]
Jesting; trifles with everything: alum.[30] con.[30]
Joy; alternating with, sadness: stram.[102]
Joy; death, when thinking of: aur.[54]
Joy; misfortune of others, at the: anac.[185] ars. cupr.[171]
Lasciviousness; voluptuous ideas, pleasure only in: bell.
Laughing; alternating with, anguish, fear of death: ***plat.***[54]
Laughing; alternating with, loathing of life: ***aur.***
Laughing; alternating with, vexation, ill-humor: croc. sanic. stram.
Laughing; alternating with, violence: aur.[10] croc. stram.
Laughing; contemptuous: alum.
Laughing; love, from disappointed: ***hyos.***[54]
Laughing; misfortune, at: apis.
Laughing; mocking: tarent.[36]
Laughing; overwork, after: ***cupr.***[54]
Laughing; wildly: atro.[36] calc. cann-i.[25]
Mania; comical: **HYOS.**[54]
Mirth; alternating with, indignation, bursts of: aur. caps. croc. ign.
Mirth; alternating with, sadness: cann-i. caust. croc. ferr. hell. indol.[77] m-arct.[1] med.[58] nat-c. nit-ac. petr. ***phos.*** plat. ptel.[36] sep. tarent. zinc.
Music; aversion to, joyous, to, but immediately affected by saddest: mang.[54]
Music; carried by, sensation of being: anh.[119]
Play; desire to, grass, in the: elaps.
Play; dirty trick on others or their teachers, schoolboys p. a: lach.[30] zinc.[30]
Pleasure; seeking: lap-mar-c.[194]
Pleasure; waking from a dream of murder, on: thea.
Rage; laughing, with: ***stram.***[10]
Revelry, feasting: agar.[5] ambr.[5] ang.[5] ant-c.[5] ip.[30] kali-c.[30] ***lach.***[5] ***nat-c.***[30] **NUX-V.**[5] sel.[5] sulph.[5]
Sadness; alternating with, exuberance: aster.[149] coff.[137] ferr.[10] ign.[109] meph.[149] mit.[72] nid.[149] onop.[149] petr.[10] plat.[10] senec.[137]
Sadness; enjoys: ign.[137] nat-m.[137]
Sadness; happy, on seeing others: cic.[36] hell.[1] helon.
Sentimental; ecstasy, with: ***coff.***[54]
Sentimental; moonlight in, ecstatic love: **ANT-C.**
Smiling; alone, when: bar-c.[53]
Smiling; convulsions, during: ***bell.***[10]
Smiling; sardonic: bell.
Talk; ecstatic: aether[36] agar.[1]
Thoughts; keenness of perception of the ludicrous: cann-i.[36]
Thoughts; persistent, humorous: nux-m.
Weary of life; alternating with cheerfulness: bor.[10]

ABROT. He, 4 - Excited, loquacious, feels like shouting.

ACON-F. Al, 3 - In the intervals of relief from distressing symptoms, he laughed and joked about his very comical condition;...(proper disease)

AGAR. Al, 37 - An impulse to laugh overcame him in bed, owing to an indescribably mixed sensation of happiness and misery.(duality)

Ha, 27 - Extravagant fancy, rapture (ecstasy), prophesying, making verses.

Ha, 28 - Quiet, equable (tranquil), sociable, active, and glad of having done his duty.

ALOE. Al, 5 - Merry, self-contented; fraternized with the whole world.

ALUM. Ha, 35 - He laughs contemptuously at everything.

ANAC. Ha, 3 - Anxiety and apprehension in the evening, after cheerfulness during the day.

Ha, 25 - He is compelled to laugh, while engaged in very serious matters, ...;in laughable matters he can keep serious. (contrary)

Ha, 24 - He laughs, when he ought to be serious.

ANDROC. Sh, 45 - Incredible upsurge of energy —laughing, felt very high, then low, then high again. (4, 29)

Sh, 113 - Argumentative. Pursued conflict almost with relish. (12)

Sh, 153 - Words and thoughts tripped over themselves, but he laughed and enjoyed himself. (29)

Sh, 155 - At night —brain revving away like crazy, thoughts racing through his head. Very interesting and exciting thoughts. Stayed awake til early morning, enjoying himself tremendously, and felt young again. (4)

ANG. Al, 14-...internal uneasiness, such as is experienced by those who anticipate some great pleasure, or also owing to all sorts of plans crowding upon his mind.

Al, 15-,...prevented by the intrusion upon his mind of a rather agreeable project which he almost believes to be real and feasible, and which exclusively absorbs all his attention; it is a sort of waking dream.

ANT-C. Ha, 18 - Continuous state of enthusiastic love and ecstatic longing for an ideal woman, which quite filled his fantasy;... (perfection, utopian)

Ha, 23 - Ecstasy and exalted love, with great anxiety about his fate (destiny, doom), and inclination to shoot himself;...

He, 22 - Sentimental mood in the moonlight, particularly ecstatic love.

ANT-T. He, 41 - Gaiety, wild mirthfulness, with subsequent ill humor and anxiety for future.

APIS. Al, 2 - Laughs at every misfortune.

Al, 3-... He laughed at the greatest misfortune, as he would at a great comedy. (mockery)

He, 11 - Lets everything fall out of her hand, or breaks things and laughs over it.

He, 53 - Eccentric cheerfulness, despondency, or hopelessness.

ARS-MET. He, 6 - She would very much like to die, or fall asleep (sleep), never to awaken.

ATRO. Al, 3-...the mind would become filled with strange and fanciful ideas ...fits of wild, uncontrollable laughter...I fancied myself afflicted with epilepsy, and was constantly fearful lest others should discover my unfortunate condition; ...

AUR. Ha, 334 - Trembling agitation of the nerves as if under the influence of some joyous hope.(faith, optimism)

Ha, 356 - Melancholy; he imagines he is unfitted (incompetent, unqualified) for the world ; he is filled (full) with intense delight when he thinks of death, so that he longs to die. (punishment)

Ha, 5 - Melancholy; he imagines that he is not fitted for the world, he therefore longs for death, of which he thinks with the most intense delight.

He, 12 - Thinking of death, gives him intense joy.

BELL. Al, 57-...ludicrous and fantastic spectacles were always uppermost in my mind...my mind was in a state of delightful exhilaration.

Al, 134 - Great mirthfulness (happy) after supper; the vital powers were increased to an extraordinary degree for a quarter of an hour, after which came drowsiness.

Al, 167 - Events which had been previously anticipated with pleasure appeared to him in an anxious light; he thought them fearful and dreadful.

Al, 34 - He took a piece of bread for a stone, and threw it far away, laughing violently and running about the room.
Ha, 1324 - Events which hitherto he had hoped for with pleasure, now appear to him in an anxious light; they appear to him frightful and horrible. (attractive x horrible, terrible)
Ha, 1364 - Unrestrainedly and exuberantly merry, inclined to scold (criticize) without cause, and to insult (affront, offend) in a laughing humor.
Ha, 1357 - Involuntary, almost loud laughter, without having any laughable thoughts.
Ha, 1361 - She bursts out in loud laughter, sings, and touches things near her.
Ha, 1365 - Excessive gaiety (happiness) after supper, the vital powers extraordinarily increased for a quarter of a hour, followed by drowsiness.
He, 80 - The boy ran around room laughing immoderately, desired neither food nor drink; a piece of bread, which he took to be a stone, he threw far from him;...
He, 62 - Loud laughter, wild abandon, singing, whistling, lascivious conversation.

BRASS. Sh, 10 - A very pleasant lack of thoughts; finding it harder to apply myself to the work I'm doing. Very difficult to describe the sensation, unable to find the right words, hard to explain things 08, 6C, 02:03:00

CACT. Al, 7 - Was affected with impulses to do something facetious (comical), which were repelled. (rejected)

CANN-I. Al, 33 - Said "he had been transported to heaven (paradise)"...
Al, 40 - Had a feeling of duality. One of his minds would be thinking of something, while the other would laugh at it...
Al, 69 - He seems to himself to be transformed into a vegetable existence, as a huge fern, and to be surrounded by clouds of music and perfume.
He, 22 - Uncontrollable laughter, till the face becomes purple, and back and loins ache.
He, 14-... visions of a great sublimity (splendor) usually follow visions of a quiet, relaxing and recreating nature.
He, 15-...he is gradually swelling, his body becomes larger and larger; that someone calls him; that he hears numberless bells ringing most sweetly; imagines he hears music; shuts his eyes, and is lost for some time in the most delicious thoughts and dreams.

CAPS. Al, 18 - He is in a contented mood, is jocose, and sings, and still he becomes angry from the slightest causes.
He, 7 - He is in a content mood, is jocose, and sings, and still he becomes angry from the slightest cause.

CARB-V. Al, 2 - Immoderately jovial (sociable, friendly), though easily put out of humor.(irritable)

CARBN-O. Al, 11 - After supper, felt buoyant (happy) and in good humor, an effect never produced by tea; this mental sensation soon passed over into an irritable and sarcastic one, so that I sharply criticized an article in a medical journal, which a few hours ago I hardly thought worth that trouble, and threw away in disgust a book of reference as flat and superficial, which I highly sluggish.(inactive)

CERE-B. Al, 8 - A grateful feeling of dependence (need, faith, relation) on a divine spirit was experienced. (reverence, veneration, praise)

CHIN. Ha, 1134 - Liking for work, reading, writing, and thinking; particularly well disposed and industrious.

CHLOL. He, 10 - Gorgeous (superb, beautiful) visions of arches, tapestry (decoration) and colors pass before the eyes when shut, or open in the dark.

CHOC. Sh, 150 - People keep stopping me and saying they don't recognise me. I still have a silly grin on my face. Laugh more —so much joy inside and a sense of freedom very different to before the proving. Dogs seem to like me more and babies seem to like me more, and this was noticed by others too.
Sh, 315 - Been on the move all day — painted a room blue. While lying in the bath looking out the window, the sky is the most glorious, vibrant blue —it seems like the most beautiful colour I've ever seen. Almost wept for the beauty of it. Suddenly, while I'm lying in the bath, the colour blue seems very important — seems very potent. It has the same quality

and intensity that I remember colours having on L.S.D. I am very moved by this blue. I wanted to dissolve into it.[15], 30C, 03:05:XX

Sh, 412 - Much more sensitive to music — especially happy music. It gives me incredible pleasure.[01]A, 30C, XX:XX:XX

CIC. Ha, 240 - He felt like a child of seven or eight years old, objects were very dear and attractive to him, as toys are to a child. (purity)

Ha, 241 - Tranquillity of mind; he was extremely satisfied with his position, and with himself, and very cheerful.

COCC. Ha, 550 - Everything angers and vexes him; after a few hours he becomes lively and disposed to make jokes.

COFF. Al, 1 - Lively fancies; full of plans for the future; contrary to his custom is very much charmed by the beauties of nature,...

He, 23 - Fright from sudden pleasant surprises.

He, 33 - Ailments from excessive joy, excessive laughing and playing; from disappointed love; from anger, from vexations with vehemence or fright...

He, 35 - Affections after sudden emotions, particularly pleasant surprises.(ailments from)

CON. Al, 15 - Tendency to laugh, with loss of vital energy.

He, 14 - Likes to wear his best clothes, (vanity) makes useless purchases, (squander) cares very little for things (indifferent), wastes or ruins them; does not want to work, prefers to play. (wanderer)

CROC. Al, 10 - Immoderate laughter, as if he would die.

Al, 11 - Sardonic (sarcastic, satirical) laughter, and attacks of morbid jollity.

Al, 14 - Very lively (happy) mood, witty, jocose, excessively talkative.(loquacious)

Al, 18 - Irresistible inclination to joke and laugh, with great prostration, and great dilatation of the pupils.

He, 12 - Vexation, contradicted by bursts of laughter.

CUPR-A. Al, 2 - Attacks of mania; he fancies that he is a military officer; a fancy that he is selling green vegetables; a fancy that he is repairing old chairs...he spits in the faces of the attendants, and laughs heartily at it.

CUPR. Ha, 27 - Fits of insanity, he spits into people's faces, and laughs heartily (soberly) over it.

CUR. Al, 1 - Paroxysm of insanity impelling him to attack himself; he strikes, scratches, and tears himself with a sort of relish, (enjoy) and without feeling any pain.

Al, 3 - Fits of ecstasy at night, as if caused by hearing music.

CYCL. Al, 19 - Sometimes he is very ill-humored and fretful, but suddenly he feels again a strange joyous sensation,...

Ha, 202 - Towards evening there suddenly occurs a strange happy feeling and lively fancy, which conjures (remember) up agreeable pictures.

DROS. Ha, 287 - Happy steadfast (confiding) disposition; he dreaded no evil, because he was conscious of having acted honorably.

ELAPS. Al, 5 - Desire to go into to the country, and play about in the grass. (nature)

EUCAL. He, 2 - Irresistible desire to move about, with a feeling of buoyancy (happiness) and increased strength.

FERR. Al, 20 - Excited by the slightest opposition; ... even her children's caresses increased her bad temper; she was often rude to those about her, because she hated to see or talk to them, and wanted them to leave her in solitude, which alone was pleasing to her.

FL-AC. Al, 5 - Feeling of perfect happiness within (inside) and without.(outside)

Al, 8 - All nature seems to smile in the morning.

FORM. Al, 4 - During the day remarkably happy and able to study; everything seemed easy to be accomplished.

GERM. Sh, 131 - Suddenly aware of my feet standing on the ground and feeling very connected to the ground through my feet. Rooted to the spot. Wanted to stay that way. Good feelings. Feet feeling at one with the ground. 04, 6C, 00.[13].[30].

Sh, 21 - Contemplative, like nice things, sees beauty in stones and nature. Good at instinctive understanding, compassionate. 16, 30C, 01:XX:XX

GRAPH. Ha, 7 - Very much disposed to grieve and to weep, in the evening; while in the morning, contrary to her wont, she laughs (smile) at every trifle.

HALI-L. Sh, 794 - A very pleasurable sensation, walking around with the top half of body naked, and feeling the skin under my arms. Great pleasure with naked of softness of underarm against side of body. 20, 30C, 04:01:36

Sh, 901 - Sensation of such harmonious balance when on the wing, Such power in these almost weightless wings. Sensation of deep warmth echoing the sun. 20, 30C, 10:XX:XX

HELL. Al, 10 - He becomes melancholy on beholding (observe) a cheerful person, and then, for the first time, feels very unhappy.

HEP. He, 9 - Malicious (vindictive, malevolent) mood; feels as if he could murder someone whith pleasure.

HYDR. Al, 4 - In high spirits; everything looked bright; felt happy, and wanted to sing.

HYDROG. Sh, 220 - Laughter wicked and voice seemed low. 24, 30C, 02:XX:XX

Sh, 294 - Spirits uplifted by wonderful weather. Felt strong, positive and adventurous. 04, 12C, 32:XX:XX

HYOS. Al, 48 - Laughed and said he was exceedingly well.

IRID. Sh, 55 - Memories and associations of giving birth, and of being born. Warm nakedness. Marriage? Old memories of marriage and wedding day. Gently erotic and sensual. Q1

Sh, 57 - On the bus a woman turned to me and said, "Your eyes are the same as my daughter's." Baby like me. I knew we had met before, knew that I knew her. She knew me as well. A wonderful moment. Q7

Sh, 58 - Felt child-like, innocent, happy as though seeing things from a child's perspective. Sat watching a milk tanker, it looks just like a child's toy. Felt like I could pick it up and brrrm brrrm it up the lane. I9

Sh, 103 - Felt light and young, found things fun and amusing. Walking effortlessly, easy, as if not touching the ground. Q1

Sh, 106 - Mental image: I am inside an egg —a bird, wet feathers, at the point it is smashing through its shell, bursting out; a chick, wet crumpled and hot, shell flying all over. The relief —getting to the air, refreshing, cool. Inside it was humid, stifling. Stretching vast wings, enjoying feeling the air dry them out. G5

IRIS. Al, 3 - Despondency; thinks he is going to be very sick, then a disposition to laugh at his fears, which, however, soon return.

JAMB. He, 4 - Sudden great change in him after micturition, everything seems more beautiful and bright, sky and trees more joyous and clear; but after quarter of an hour everything became gloomy again.

JATR. Al, 3 - An ecstasy, as if an ideal had appeared to a poetic painter, or like that which sometimes comes to a dying person, ...a feeling of lovely warmth and ethereal lightness...

KALI-BR. Al, 25 - At times he cried most bitterly, yet twelve hours previously he was singing and dancing, saying he was "the happiest man alive".

KALI-C. Ha, 5 - Sad, she feels lonesome (solitary, lonely); she seeks for company to cheer her up.

KALI-CY. Al, 3 - Had occasion to get angry, but could not; felt more like laughing instead.

LACH. Al, 5 - A kind of ecstasy, as after sublime impressions, or excessive joy, throughout the day; he constantly wishes to talk and do much, and even more seems to be at his command.(control, domination)

Al, 15 - The more cause for fretfulness, the greater inclination for humour, jest, satire, and humorous fancies.

LED. Ha, 338 - Calm and happy disposition with love for work and self-contented.

LYC. Al, 12 - If one looks at her to say anything serious she is obliged to laugh.

Ha, 68 - After being anxious, there is a great inclination to laugh about trifles, for several hours, and then weeping for half an hour without cause.

LYSS. Al, 6 - Exhilarated, felt as if he had received joyful intelligence, all day.

He, 10 - They appreciate the formidable (terrible) character of the disease and speak frequently with a remarkable (unusual) quick and sharp articulation of the impending fatal results.

MAG-C. Al, 923 - Dream that she had become a child three years old, which rejoiced her very much. (youngish)

MANC. Al, 4 - Disposed to take everything in good part (first day).

MANG. Ha, 327 - Ill-humored, so that the most joyful music does not cheer (joy) him, but he feels as if refreshed by the most melancholy music.

MUR-AC. Al, 2 - Joyous trustful (hopeful) mood.

NAT-C. Al, DREAM, 1102-..;of marrying two women, of parties, walks, entertainments, and excursions on horseback, afterwards they were frequently anxious, of going astray (lost),of murders, having his ears cut off; also vexatious dreams; he would take a journey and could not get away from the place,(immobilization) and when has reached the first station was obliged to turn back, on account of something he had forgotten.

NAT-M. Al, 12 - She laughed so immoderately at something not ludicrous, that she could not be quieted, and tears come into her eyes, so that she looked as though she had been weeping.

NEON. Sh, 35 - Feel like I have been kissed by heaven. 10, 6C, 07:01:XX

Sh, 52 - Thoughts of rivers and oceans and being very happy by them. 20, 6C, 08:XX:XX

NIT-AC. Ha, 49 - He gets violently excited about trifles, all the day, and has then to laugh at himself.

NUX-M. He, 24 - Fitful mood, changing from deepest sorrow to most frolicsome (happy) behavior; now grave (serious), now gay.

OLND. Al, 15 - While studying he had constantly other thoughts; he found himself dreaming of the future, and busying himself with beautiful images concerning it.

OP. Al, 45 - Sensation as if he had been taken to heaven; vivid, lovely fantasies float before his vision like a waking dream, which the slumber (sleep) drives away.

Al, 19-...each possessing some imaginary bliss (happiness) which " the dull (dark) reality of life" could never give....they are wrapped in an elysium, (heaven) from which they are only to be awakened by the miserable reaction which must, sooner or later recall them to existence.

Al, 19-...; all the actors are happy, and each retires home in a total state of irrationality, but likewise in the entire and full enjoyment of happiness not to be procured by reason. Disregarding the ridicule of those they meet, who divert themselves by making them talk absurdly, each imagines looks and feels himself possessed of whatever he wishes...

Ha, 601 - Tranquil indifference to earthly things; she cared for nothing in comparison with ecstasies of the fantasy.

Ha, 621 - Feeling of courage and merriment (joy), so that he is as if he would carry out what was required with energy, without repugnance or fear, with a peculiar feeling of voluptuousness...(sensuality)

He, 22-... feeling of great strength; contempt of death;...indifference to joy and suffering.

PHOS. Ha, 78 - She has to laugh against her will, while she is sad.

He, 1 - Excited imagination; zoomagnetic (animal magnetism) condition; ecstasy; clairvoyance.

PLAT. Ha, 25-...felt like embracing everybody and could have laughed over the most sad things.

He, 3 - Attacks of cheerfulness; increased feeling of strength.

He, 17 - After anger alternate laughing and weeping, with great anguish and fear of death.

PSOR. Al, 24-...only disagreeable things affect him, agreeable impressions he passes without noticing them.

Al, 5 - He pictures the future in the brightest colors.

PULS. He, 25 - Weary of life; thinks with pleasure of drowning. (suicide, water)

He, 50 - After slight emotions, difficult breathing; bad effects from fright, mortification or excessive joy.(ailments from)

He, 52 - After mortification, sad gloomy (melancholy) and weary (disgusted) of life;...thinks of drowning with great pleasure;...

PYROG. Al,N-9 - Increased buoyancy (happy) of spirits, although he felt ill.

ROB. Al, 11 - Strong disposition to be obscene, to gormandize (gluttony, voracity), and for all kinds of orgies.

Al, 13 - Hypochondriac grief; he seeks

pleasures and tries to divert his mind, without succeeding.

SEP. Al, 38 - He feels oppressed in sultry weather, but becomes more cheerful when it thunders and lightens.

Al, 92 - One dose of the medicine takes away my ambition; I simply do not want to do anything, either work or play; it is even an exertion to think.

SIL. He, 23-...believes she has swallowed pins, and asks those about her whether she has not done so; seeks for hours for lost pins; ...and careful examined her food for fear of pins; very indifferent to friends and former amusements;...

STAPH. Al, 1 - He was joyous, enjoyed society, and was good-humored.

STICT. Al, 1 - She got very lively (active), told her father she felt as if she would like to strike out, only for fun; she would like it just for fun of it. After awhile she lay down on the lounge, and began, to use a common expression, to kick up her heels; her mother reproaching, said, " Bella, do behave, that is not ladylike"; when child responded: " Ma, I cannot help it; I feel exactly as if I want to fly away"...

STRAM. Al, 23 - Violent delirium; whith was alternately mirthful, furious or dolorous (sad), directed to some imaginary source of pleasure or repugnance, and accompanied which corresponding gesticulations.

Ha, 549 - He thinks he is dying, and that he will not live over the evening, he rejoices that he is dying, and gives directions about his funeral, otherwise he is rational and does not feel particularly ill.

He, 77 - Patient had a constant vision of an executioner(hangman, lynches) standing before him in spite of which he was lively, talkative, laughed and joked about his hallucination, yet it seemed to him a reality.

He, 92 - Mania:... complains that a dog is biting and tearing flesh off his chest; merry exaltation; with pride (haughty) and affectation; runs about, complains of violent headache; ...;steals from his roommates...; disposition to scold persons whom he otherwise loved.

SULPH. Al, 3784 - At night, vivid dreams of a comic character, with loud laughter, ...

SUMB. Al, 2 - More cheerful in humor and more disposed for intellectual occupation; he felt in the happy enthusiastic state of mind that accompanies the consciousness of having performed a noble (generous, virtuous) deed; this sort of medicinal intoxication went away in a few hours.

He, 2 - Happy disposition with continued smiling; expression idiotic; fear of becoming insane.

TARENT. Al, 18 - Fourteen days after taking the medicine, the happy mood reached the borders of mania; the disposition to joke and laugh was extreme.

THEA. Al, 3 - Delirium with great ecstasy; the patient laughed incessantly talked constantly in rhyme, showed us that he felt extraordinarily well.

THUJ. Al, 10-,...; his whole existence consists of only extremes, wherewith he is always irresistibly inclined to agreeable (pleasing) exciting, heating drinks, but without intoxication; these happy and exalted reveries constantly increase from day to day, overstepping (exceed) all bounds and becoming a joyful, dizzy intoxication, with entire extinction of reason.(torpid)(ludicrous)

Al, 11 - He often dreamed in a clear day, with open eyes...; in this he especially reveled in a overpowering selfishness, himself the central point about which everything must turn, with an intoxicated feeling of the most joyous self-satisfaction, ... (egotism)

POETRY

Day-dreaming; poetical, about the future: olnd.[60]

Delirium; loquacious, rhyme, in: thea.[36]

Dream, as if in a; future, poetical: olnd.

Dreams; poetical: ars-h.[54] bufo-s. lach. nat-m.[10] olnd.[10] til.

Ecstasy; ideal had appeared to a poetic painter, as if an: jatr.[36]

Mood; poetical: germ.[222]

Prophesying; rhyming: agar.[102]

Talk; verses, in: nat-c.[137]

Verses, makes: agar. am-c.[30] ***ant-c.*** cann-i. carb-v.[30] chin.[30] coff.[30] lach.[30] lyc.[30] nat-m.[30] staph.[30] stram. thea.

Verses; makes, sleep, on falling asleep: nat-m.[1]

Weeping; poetry, at soothing: lach.

AGAR. Ha, 27 - Extravagant fancy, rapture (ecstasy), prophesying, making verses.
ANT-C. He, 26 - Irresistible desire to talk in rhymes or verses. (poetry)
GERM. Sh, 191 - Feeling in a rather poetical mood. I feel I can almost capture the essence of the feeling I have been going through: it's an eructation! As if a marble lands somewhere, chest, stomach, brain and sucks to it all the matter around it in a radius of 3-4 cm and packs it tighter and tighter. It gets hard and brittle, then suddenly it grows with a zoomy feeling, steadily becoming less dense and suddenly it bursts and spreads a cloud of relief. I think the remedy is Champagne. 16, 30C, 03:14:00
JATR. Al, 3 - An ecstasy, as if an ideal had appeared to a poetic painter, or like that which sometimes comes to a dying person, ...a feeling of lovely warmth and ethereal lightness...
THEA. Al, 3 - Delirium with great ecstasy; the patient laughed incessantly talked constantly in rhyme, showed us that he felt extraordinarily well.

POINTED

Anger; stabbed any one, so that he could have: anac.[10] chin. **HEP.** merc. mosch.[10] nux-v. stront-c.[10] zinc.[10] zinc-acet.[10]
Blood or a knife, cannot look at: **ALUM.** nux-m.[137] plat.[137] sac-alb.[210]
Break things, desire to, pins: **BELL.**
Delirium; attacks people with knife: hyos.
Delirium; wild, stab and bite, attempts to: **STRAM.**[54]
Delusions; animals, hedgehogs, sees: choc.[222]
• man, room, in the, intending to perforate his throat with a gimlet: merc-i-f.
• murder, family with a hatchet, that she will: jab.
• pins, needles, about: merc. **NUX-M.**[162] ***sil.*** spig.
• pins, swallows: ***sil.***[54]
• stab him, some one will: **OP.**[10]
• stabbed a person who passed on the street, he had: ***bell.***
• sword hanging over head: am-m.
• umbrella was a knife: androc.[222]

Dreams; body, muscles pierced with arrows: bomb-pr.[36]
➤ cutting, knife, of being cut with a: frax.[36] guai. nat-s.[36]
➤ cutting, knife, of being cut with a, to pieces: lil-s.[36]
➤ cutting, woman, of cutting a woman up for salting: calc-f.
➤ dead, bodies, digging knife into wounds of: elaps[36]
➤ knives: am-m.[5] guai. lach. nat-c. ozone[227]
➤ knives, keeping them ready for use: lach.[36]
➤ knives, threatened with, he is: ozone[227]
➤ murdering, Arab, an, with four stabs in chest: ozone[227]
➤ needles: androc.[222]
➤ pins, of: merc.
➤ pursued, man, red skinned, to harm her with his arrows: pitu-a.[164]
➤ stab others, will: lach.[10]
➤ stab, antagonist, his: nat-c.[36] ozone[227]
➤ stab, friend, his: allox.[119]
➤ stabbed, acquaintance was: lil-s.[36]
➤ stabbed, antagonist in chest, with large knife, his: nat-c.[36]
➤ stabbed, being: chin. guai. lil-s.[36] nat-c. op.
➤ stabbed, brother was: chin.[36]
➤ stabbed, fear of being stabbed: lach.
➤ stabbed, swordsmen threatened to stab him: op.[36]
➤ swallowing pins: merc.[10]
Fear; injured, of being, sewing, when: sep.[172]
✦ killing, of, knife, with a: ars. der. ***nux-v.***
✦ knives, of: alum.[111] ars.[111] chin.[111] hyos.[111] lac-c.[54] lyss.[111] merc.[162] nux-v.[137]
✦ knives, of, thinks how horrible it would be if a sharp pain like a knife should go through her, on lying down: lac-c.[54]
✦ pins, hunts for pointed things, although afraid of them: sil.[85]
✦ pins, pointed, sharp things, of: alum.[5] apis[107] ars.[5] bov.[5] lac-f.[122] merc.[5] nat-m.[122] plat.[5] **SIL.**[122] **SPIG.**[122]
✦ suicide, knife, with a: merc.[162]
Impulse; stab his flesh with the knife he holds, to: ***lyss.***.
Insanity; break pins, she will sit and: bell. calc.
Kill; desire to, knife, at sight of a: ***alum.*** ars.[172] ***merc.***[30] nux-v.[30] plat.
Kill; desire to, knife, at sight of a knife or a gun: ***alum.***
Kill; desire to, knife, with a: ***alum.*** ars.[1]

chin.[54] ***hep.***[54] ***hyos.***[30] **LYC.**[30] lyss.[5] ***merc.***[54] ***nux-v.***[54] plat. ***stram.***[54]

Kill; sudden impulse to, husband, her beloved, menses, particularly during, implores him to hide his razor: ***merc.***[54]

Killed; desire to be, stabbing heart, by (after midnight): ***ars.***[36]

Restlessness; cutting himself while shaving: calad.[54]

Sensitive; steel points directed toward her: apis nat-m.[122] **SIL.**[122] **SPIG.**[122]

Sits; breaks pins, and: **BELL.** calc.[58]

Suicidal disposition; knife, razor with a: acon.[30] alum.[122] ***stram.***[54]

Suicidal disposition; knife, with a: alum. ***ars.*** bell. ***calc.*** hyos.[30] ***merc.*** nux-v.[137] stram.

Suicidal disposition; knife, with a, cutting his throat: alum.[171]

Suicidal disposition; seeing blood or a knife, she has horrid, thoughts of killing herself, though she abhors the idea: ***alum.***

Suicidal disposition; seeing, an open window or knives: arg-n. camph. chin. ***merc.***

Suicidal disposition; seeing, blood or a knife, shaving, when: alum.[122]

Suicidal disposition; seeing, open windows or knife: arg-n. camph. chin. ***merc.***

Thoughts; frightful, seeing blood, or a knife, on: ***alum.***

ADAM. Sh, 374 - Joyless, desired death. Looked at a pair of scissors and thought of suicide. 16, 12C, 17:XX:XX

Sh, 376 - Cried with despair. Nothing I do is right. Rocking from side to side sobbing. Desire to stab with a knife or scissors. Felt very different from other humans. Long, late phone call ameliorates. 16, 12C, 43:XX:XX

ALUM. Ha, 22 - She cannot see blood nor a knife without horrible thoughts pressing in upon her, as if she should, e. g. commit suicide; though she has the greatest horror of it.

He, 9 - Mania to kill himself with a sharp weapon.

He, 10 - Seeing blood on a knife, she has horrid ideas of killing herself, though she abhors the idea.

ANDROC. Sh, 40 - She dreamt that she had murdered her grandfather by poking a knitting needle through his eyes while he slept. Though she felt no remorse, she wanted to be punished but no-one would accept her guilt. Was told by her friends that she had responsibilities and could not go to jail and the police refused to prosecute. Was frightened by the dream. (7)

Sh, 124 - In the street, he felt aggressive and very strong, that his umbrella was a knife, and desired to smash people up. (29)

ARS. Al, 6 - After midnight, a frequent desire to kill himself, by stabbing his heart through and through.

Al, 85 - He is anxious and trembling, and is afraid he shall not be able to prevent himself from killing a person with a knife.

Ha, 1027 - Trembling, anxious, he is afraid (fear) that he cannot refrain (restrain) from killing some one with a sharp knife.

Ha, 1032 - Mania; first headache, horrible anxiety, noise before the ears, as from a number of large bells, and when he opened the eyes, he always saw a man who had (formerly) hung himself (suicidal, justified) on the ground-floor of the house, who incessantly beckoned (call) him to cut him down (help); he ran thither (there) with a knife, but, as he could not cut him down, (rescue) he became overwhelmed (beaten) with despair (remorse?) and wished (as his friends assured him) to hang himself (punish); but being prevented (stop) from doing so, he became so restless that he could hardly be kept in bed,... and he knelt down and raised his hands in a supplicating manner.

ART-V. He, 11 - Picking (gathering) of bedcovers, making a fold (wrap) of skin on back of her mother's hand, saying that it will not come off (disconnected), wants a knife to cut it off. (stab, wound)

BELL. He, 102 - Became fearful when persons approached him in street, and when they had passed, he insisted on it that he had stabbed them.

CALC. He, 18 - Mental aberration with horrid visions before eyes and cardiac anxiety; he despairs of his salvation (pardon, rescue) and wants to stab himself.

CHIN. Al, DREAM-1110 - Dreamed that some one had stabbed his brother, and then called for his mother; that his mother was dead, and then he cried; that his mother's arms was hurt;...

Al, 35 - Ill-humor, amounting to the most violent wrath (fury), so that he could have stabbed any one.
Ha, 1093-...;he jumps out of the bed and wants to make away whith himself (suicide), and yet he fears to go near and open window or to approach a knife.
DER. Al, 5 - He is afraid of killing some one with a knife.
GUAI. Ha, 125 - Dreams as if she would be stabbed with knives.
HALI-L. Sh, 588 - I was in a gallows humor, cruel but funny. My friends had never seen that side of me before. Like I was on speed. I had no control. They asked me not to cut up vegetables, not to use a knife. I was waving the knife around. I threw the knife at a potato. 02, 30C, XX:XX:XX
HYOS. Ha, 562 - Extreme fury: he rushes at people with knives.
LAC-C. He, 17 - On lying down either by day or night begins to think how horrible it would be if a very sharp pain, like a knife, should go through her, and thought of it causes great mental distress.
LAC-F. Al,N-5 - Mental illusion that the corners of furniture, or any pointed object near her, were about to run into eyes;...
LYSS. Al, 32 - Thought came into his mind to attack others in a mean way; to cut others with a knife he holds; to throw water he has in a tumbler into another's face.
Al,N-34-....to stab his flesh with the knife he is holding, and the like.
MERC-I-F. Al, 1 - While in bed, he imagined that a man was in his room who intended to perforate his throat with a gimlet;...
MERC. He, 20 - After suppression of foot sweat, whenever he sees an open window or cutting instruments breaks into a sweat, with great heat of head, and is seized with an almost uncontrollable desire to commit suicide.
NAT-C. Al, 1114 - Dream of a quarrel, in which he stabbed his antagonist (enemy) in the chest with a large knife.
NEON. Sh, 175 - I've been in a rotten mood all day, dwelling on past offenses. I just can't let go, it's making me angry. I feel like I hate that bastard; it's not an emotion I've had before. Now I feel vindictive, really awful; I feel that if I ever found out that he had been lying to me again I would say to him, "I'll kill you," "I'll slit your throat." These violent feelings were much eased when alone. 02, 6C, 04:22:40
NUX-V. He, 38 - Three months ago mental shock, since then fears to be alone,...fears as if she would choke (suffocation)...fears to be alone, fear of knives and the like, (similar) lest she should kill herself or others...
OP. Al, 16-...started up in a fright on account of fancied swordsmen (rival, competitor) who threatened to stab him; became angry if any one argued him or thought him delirious; however, he blamed (reproaches) himself while in delirium for his folly.
Ha, 638 - He chattered all sorts of unconnected stuff and pointed with his fingers to imaginary masked people approaching him; ...he started at imaginary swordsmen, who might kill him ; ...
SIL. He, 23-...believes she has swallowed pins, and asks those about her whether she has not done so; seeks for hours for lost pins; ...and careful examined her food for fear of pins; very indifferent to friends and former amusements;...
SPIG. He, 5 - Afraid (fear) of pointed things, pins, etc.
STRAM. He, 81-...attempts to stab and bite;...with sexual excitement; fear as if a dog were attacking him;...
He, 99 - Acute mania; tears his clothing;... threatens to use knife on those about him.
He, 114-...seeing rats and cats in room,...wanted a razor;...
THEA. Al, 4 - Sensation as if impelled by some uncontrollable power to commit suicide, to jump out of window, to put her baby in the boiler with the clothes, to cut its throat while cutting bread, to throw it downstairs (in a woman who kept a pot of tea boiling on the stove and drank several bowlfuls every day; cured with tea cm, Finckle)

POISONED

Anguish; eating, after: ***asaf.***[54] sep.[54]
Anguish; eating, while: hyos.[85] sep.
Anxiety; eating before: mez. ran-b.
Anxiety; eating while: ***carb-v.*** kali-sil.[58] mag-c. merc.[58] mez. ran-b.[85] sabad. ***sep.***

Anxiety; food, about: lac-h.[229]
Delirium; refuses to take the medicine: agar-pr.[36] hyos.[162]
Delusions; animals, scorpions, sees: op.
• animals, snakes, black: arg-n.[5] cund.[111]
• animals, snakes, crawling up her leg, feels a: ail.[122]
• animals, snakes, white: gels.[5] ign.[111]
• animals, spiders: ***lac-c.***
• eat, she must not: kali-chl.[58]
• poison, of: cocc.[5]
• poisoned, about to be, that he is: carc.[207] ***hyos.***[10] kali-br. lach.[102] plb. ***rhus-t.*** verat-v.[102]
• poisoned, has been, delivery, after: verat-v.[85]
• poisoned, has been, drugged: lap-mar-c.[194]
• poisoned, has been, he: agar.[139] ang.[139] bufo[139] caj.[85] carb-ac.[139] chin-s.[139] chlor.[139] cic.[139] cimic. cocc.[139] cor-r.[139] croc.[139] culx.[58] cur.[139] euph.[139] ferr.[139] gels.[139] glon.[139] hydr.[139] hydrog.[222] ***hyos.*** iodof.[139] jug-r.[139] kali-br.[139] kali-c.[139] kali-i.[139] ***lach.***[116] lact.[139] lap-mar-c.[194] lil-t.[139] lina.[139] lyc.[139] m-aust.[139] mag-p.[139] med.[139] merl.[139] mez.[139] mill.[139] nicc.[139] nux-m.[139] nux-v.[139] olnd.[139] op.[139] petr.[139] ph-ac.[139] phos.[139] pip-m.[139] plat-m. psor.[139] ptel.[139] puls.[139] ran-b.[139] raph.[139] rat.[139] rheum[139] rhod.[139] rhus-t.[102] sabad.[139] sec.[139] sep.[139] sol-n.[139] spig.[139] squil.[139] staph.[139] stram.[37] sul-ac.[139] sulph.[139] tab.[139] tarax.[139] thuj.[139] valer.[139] verat-v.[102] zinc.[139]
• poisoned, medicine is: cimic.[58] hyos.[58] lach. rhus-t.[172]
• snow, polluted by industry, poisonous: ozone[227]

Desires; poison, another portion of: op.[36]
Discomfort; eating, after: bar-acet.[36] bry.[36] clem.[36] olnd.[36] ph-ac.[36] zinc.[36]
Disgust; medicine bottle, on sight of the: visc.[119]
Dreams; animals, poisonous: tarent.[36]
➤ animals, snakes: alum. ***arg-n.*** bov. carc.[193] cench.[58] colch.[36] daph.[102] grat. indol.[77] iris kali-c. kalm.[54] ***lac-c.*** lach.[122] merl.[36] op.[102] ozone[227] pitu-a.[164] ptel. ran-b.[54] ***ran-s.*** rat. sep. sil. sol-n. sphing.[36] tab. teucr.[111] tub.[56]
➤ animals, snakes, bed, in: ***lac-c.***[54]
➤ animals, snakes, bitten by, of being: bov. cench.[58] med.[212] ozone[227]
➤ animals, snakes, horrifying: ***arg-n.***[36]
➤ animals, snakes, killing snakes: ptel.[25]
➤ animals, spiders: cinnb. convo-d.[231] crot-c. sars.[1] ven-m.[149]
➤ animals, spiders, black, creeping into corner of mouth: ozone[227]
➤ animals, spiders, hairy, very, which tried to climb on him: crot-c.[36]
➤ gasmasks, people wearing: ozone[227]
➤ poison, that he has taken: ***kreos.***
➤ poisoned, about to be, while innocent of crime: chr-ac.[36]
➤ poisoned, by herself: kali-n.[36]
➤ poisoned, of being: chr-ac.[36] kali-n.[36] ***kreos.*** nat-m. oci.
➤ snow, polluted by industry, poisonous: ozone[227]
➤ water, poisoned: ozone[227]
➤ water, wading in, serpents, in which are, of which he is afraid: alum.

Fear; animals, scorpions: abel.[149] op.[30]
✦ animals, snakes, of: abel.[149] arg-n.[172] bell.[162] calc.[183] calc-s.[196] carc.[207] elaps[152] hep.[162] ign.[187] lac-c.[162] ***lach.***[122] nat-m.[212] puls.[212] ruta[152] sep.[172] spig.[162] sulph.[162] syph.[162]

Dreams; animals, spiders, of: abel.[149] calc.[162] carc.[210] lac-c.[185] mag-m.[166] nat-m.[162] phos.[155] stram.[172] tarent.[185]
✦ animals, venomous, of, at night: abel.[149]
✦ drink, offered, what is: hyos.[172]
✦ drink, thirst, during: tarent.[36]
✦ drink, to: ars.[8] malar.[56] plb.[36]
✦ eating, after e., food: asaf.[5] canth. carb-v.[5] caust.[58] chin.[172] hyos.[5] kali-c.[5] lach. mag-m. nit-ac.[5] nux-v.[5] onos.[172] petr.[172] phel. tab. thuj.[5] viol-t.[5]
✦ eating, agg., while: bran.[36] caust. grat. op. puls. tarent.
✦ eating, agg., while, hungry: grat. iod.[58]
✦ eating, agg., while, offered, what is: hyos.[172]
✦ food, after: canth. caust. mag-m. phel. tab.
✦ food, for her: grat.[60] op.[36]
✦ medicine, bear any kind of, of not being able to: all-s.[54]
✦ medicine, taking too much, fear of: all-s. iber.
✦ poisoned, has been: euph.[1] glon.
✦ poisoned, night: ars-met.
✦ poisoned; being: all-s. anac.[5] apis arge.[149] ***ars.***[184] ars-met. bapt.[5] ***bell.*** bry. cimic. dros.[172] euph.[1] glon. ***hyos.*** ign.[30] ***kali-bi.***[54] ***kali-br. lach.*** lyss.[172] nat-m.[122] ph-ac.[30] phos. plb. ***rhus-t. verat.***[54] verat-v.

✦ poisoned; being, camphor, with spirits of: ***apis***[54]
✦ poisoned; being, mania, in puerperal: ***verat-v.***[54]
✦ poisoned; being, night: ars-met.
Hypochondriasis; eating, after: anac.[54] chin.[54] ***nat-c.***[54] ***nux-v.***[10] zinc.[10]
Irritability; medicine, at thought to take the: mim-p.[149]
Medicine; drugs, averse to: aesc.[36]
Mood; repulsive, medicine, to take the: ***arn.***[122] calad.[137] cimic.[58] hyos. ***kali-p.***[54] **LACH.**[122] ***stram.***[54] tub.[160] ***verat-v.***[54] visc.[119]
Mood; repulsive, medicine, to take the, religious insanity, in: ***kali-p.***[54]
Rage; eat, when something to, was offered: ars.[54]
Rage; medicine, from forcible administration of: ***bell.***[36]
Rebels against poultice: bor.[1] bry.[1] ***calc.***[1] carb-v.[1] ***cham.***[1] ***lyc.***[1] merc.[1] mur-ac.[1] nit-ac.[1] nux-v.[1] phos.[1] puls.[1] rhus-t.[1] sep.[1] spig.[1] staph.[1] ***sulph.***[1]
Refuses; medicine, to take the: ***arn.***[122] ***cimic.***[54] hyos. ***kali-p.***[54] **LACH.**[122] ***stram.***[54] ***verat-v.***[54] visc.[119]
Suicidal disposition; poison, by: ars.[30] ***bell.***[30] ign.[54] lil-t. op.[36] puls.[30]

AESC. Al, 1 - Great repugnance to the drug.(medicine)
ALL-S. Al, 4 - Dread (fear) of being poisoned.
He, 3 - Sadness when alone; moral uneasiness; afraid of never getting well; fear of not being able to bear any kind of medicine; fear of being poisoned...
APIS. He, 61 - Will not take spirits of camphor, fears she will be poisoned.
ARS-MET. He, 11 - Afraid (fear) she will be poisoned.
ARS. Ha, 1065-...extreme anxiety, restlessness; he had a great dread (fear) of the effects of the poison and desired to life.
ASAF. He, 17 - If he thinks of having taken drug, it brings on faintness. (medicine)
CACT. Al, 6 - Decided repugnance to take any more medicine.
CALAD. He, 8 - So averse to the medicine, that it required a desperate effort to overcome it.
CERE-B. Al, 6 - Reluctance (doubt) to take medicine.
CIMIC. He, 15 - Declares she has been poisoned.
He, 29 - Suspicious of everything, would not take medicine if she knew it.
CROT-H. He, 15 - Oppression as if brain had been intoxicated by carbonic acid, or by degraded or non-oxygenated blood.
EUPH. Al, 4 - Anxiety as if he had taken poison.(venom)
Ha, 2 - Anxiety as if he had swallowed poison.
GLON. Al, 13-...fear she had been poisoned, and that no one would catch her taking any more.
Al, 15 - My intellect returned almost immediately, and I remember saying, " This has nothing to do with homeopathy, but with a very powerful poison."
He, 15 - Fear; throat feels swollen; chest as if screwed together; apprehensive of approaching death; fears she has been poisoned.
HAM. Al, 15 - Was afraid to risk (danger) another dose (medicine); his mind was in a fearful condition.
HYDROG. Sh, 251 - A spark of a paranoid thought —"maybe I'm being poisoned". 10, 200C, 00:00:00
HYOS. Al, 86 - He complained that he had been poisoned.
Ha, 573 - He complains that he has been poisoned.
He, 14 - Dread of drinks; of water.
He, 16 - Fears: being left alone (solitude, deserted); poison, or being bitten (hurt); being poisoned or sold; being betrayed, or injured; wishes to run away. (escape)
He, 78 - Groundless suspicion of being watched (observed, spied) by members of family with whom he had some slight misunderstanding (dispute); to avoid being recognized by them, clothed himself differently every day,...watching his relations suspiciously and imagining he might be poisoned;... (disguise, camouflage)
He, 84-...constant talking, particularly on religious subjects; believes himself poisoned, or that there is a stinking odor from his mouth;...
He, 87-...; refused medicine, and cunningly (skill) evaded all stratagems to give it; escaped from room, ...

He, 17 - Complains of having been poisoned.
IBER. Al, 1 - Frightened mood; fears she has taken too much of the drug; in the evening.(medicine)
Al, 2 - Feels frightened; ...as if she had taken a dangerous dose.(medicine)
KALI-BR. He, 17 - Delirium with delusions; thinks he is pursued (hunt); will be poisoned; is selected (designated) for divine vengeance (revenge); that her child is dead, etc.
LACH. He, 8 - Thinks: she is somebody else in the hands (seized) of a stronger power; (supremacy, superiority).or that she is dead, and preparations are made for funeral (cortege) or that she is nearly dead and wishes some one would help her off; herself pursued by enemies, or fears medicine is poison; there are robbers in house and wants to jump out the window; herself under super-human control; visions real, he will die. (helplessness, desire; aid, comfort, salvation)
He, 41 - Dread (fear) of death, fears to go to bed ; fears of being poisoned.
MERC. Al, 1......she puts small stones into her mouth without swallowing them, and complains that they cut her intestines; ...
NAT-M. Al, 119 - The patient's mind was much weakened by disease and poison; her moral perceptions, her once keen (sharp) sense of honor, and of right and wrong, seemed blunted (dull); she was in turns vehement (angry) and passionate, and moody and silent.
PIP-N. Al,S-4 - Hypochondriac, with fear of being poisoned.
PLB. Al, 23-...His delirium turned chiefly upon the idea that his life was in danger from assassination or poisoning, and that every one about him was a murderer...
Al, 75-..imagined he was going to be poisoned; that his bed was full of ants.
He, 13 - Thought his life was in danger from assassination or poison and every one about him was a murderer.
RHUS-T. Al, 32 - He thought an enemy want to poison him.
Ha, 965 - He imagines an enemy seeks to poison him.
He, 13 - Fear: that he will die; with anxiousness and sighing; of being poisoned.
SARS. He, 6 - Thinking about the food he has been eating makes him sick. (indigestion)
VERAT-V. He, 4 - Puerperal mania: silent, suspicious; will not see physician, he seems to terrify her; fears being poisoned;...
ZINC. He, 43 - Great fear, as if persecuted by men or the devil, on account of crimes he has never done (injustice); is afraid of becoming imprisoned, or poisoned, or shot, or buried (inter) alive...[0] Delirium tremens.

POSITION

Ailments from; position, job, loss of: ***ign.***[30] ***nux-v.***[8] pers.[149] ***plat.***[30] staph.[30]
Ailments from; reversal of fortune: ambr.[116] con.[116] dig.[116] lach.[116] stann.[116] staph.[116]
Anxiety; money matters, about: aur.[172] bac.[62] bry.[162] calc-f.[36] calc-sil.[58] cand-a.[239] choc.[222] ign.[172] kali-p.[172]
Avarice; anxiety about future, from: ***nux-v.***[30] ***ph-ac.***[30] stann.[30]
Boaster; squander through ostentation: calc.[30] nux-v.[30] plat.[30] puls.[30]
Change; desire for, position: pip-m.[102]
Delusions; distinguish, squanders money, proud of his position: ***verat.***[54]
• fortune, he was going to lose his: psor. staph.
• money, talks of: calc. carbn-s. kali-br.[25]
• position, she is not fitted for her: stram.[54]
• rank, he is a person of: cupr. phos. ***stram.***[54] verat.
• wealth, of: agn. alco. bell. calc. cann-i. kali-br. nit-ac.[5] phos.[102] ***plat.***[102] ***pyrog.*** ***sulph.*** verat.
Desires; beautiful things, finery: dat-a.[25] lil-t.[137] sulph.[137]
Desires; grandeur, for: cur.[36]
Desires; servants: lap-mar-c.[194]
Despair; social position, of: calc.[30] ign.[30] puls.[30] rhus-t.[30] sep.[30] staph.[30] sulph.[30] **VERAT.**
Dignity: caj.[25] calc.[36] guare.[25] nat-c.[188] nat-m.[187] staph.[188]
Dreams; beggars: mag-c.[10]
Fear; position, to lose his lucrative: calc.[30] ign.[30] puls.[30] rhus-t.[30] sep.[30] staph.[30] sulph.[30] verat.[30]
✦ social position, about his: chel.[172] cub.[36] sep.[30] staph.[30] verat.

Grief; financial loss: arn.[137] aur.[137]
Insanity; black insanity with despair and weariness of life from fear of mortification or of loss of position: calc.[30] ign.[30] puls.[30] rhus-t.[30] staph.[30] sulph.[30] verat.[30]
Insanity; fortune, losing, after: calc.[30] ign.[30] rhus-t.[30] verat.[30]
Insanity; position, from fear to lose the: calc.[30] ign.[30] puls.[30] rhus-t.[30] staph.[30] sulph.[30] verat.[30]
Sadness; loss, after financial: arn.[137] ars.[54] aur.[137] mez.[137] psor.[137]
Sadness; thinking, position, of his: hell.[30]
Social; position, concerning about: aeth.[193] ***agar.***[193] alum.[193] bell.[193] calc.[193] cann-i.[193] coca[137] cupr.[193] ign.[193] lyc.[193] lyss.[193] nux-v.[193] pall.[137] phos.[193] plat.[193] puls.[193] rhus-t.[193] sep.[193] staph.[193] sulph.[193] **VERAT.**[193]

AGAR. Al, 46 - His mind is uneasy and anxious; he was constantly concerned only about himself, his present and future condition.

ALOE. Al, 9 - Contented with his station (position, rank) in life; it involuntarily occurs to him, that he is really much better off than many other people.

ARS. He, 58 - Melancholy; after financial losses; cannot be consoled; thinks he will have to die (sentenced), with his family, from starvation (hunger); sleepless nights; walks about wringing his hands, with moaning and groaning.

AUR. Ha, 331 - Cheerful humor; he was always disposed to converse with others and was quite contented with his position.(rank)

BELL. Al, 203-..;he imagined himself rich, owner of a large house, etc. (great person)

BISM. Al, 3 - He is morose and discontented with his condition (health, position) and complains about it.
He, 11 - Ill humor; he is morose and discontented with his condition (position), and complains about it.

BRY. He, 27 - She fears not to have wherewithal (money, funds) to live.

CIC. Ha, 241 - Tranquillity of mind; he was extremely satisfied with his position, and with himself, and very cheerful.

HALI-L. Sh, 55 - I usually relate to people who make a lot less money than me. I had an argument with a friend who is in a high class about money. Am thinking about taking a job that would put me in a high class, but don't know if I would want to work with those kind of people—downtown people into their careers who make hundreds of thousands. They make me nervous. Afraid they will snub me. So much to do with worth. What am I worth? 08, 30C, 42:XX:XX
Sh, 56 - Lately thinking over my worth and friendships. Who are my friends and where am I wasting my time. What is my position in society in relationship to career, how friends view me and relationships with men? I find myself going back to having older friends and finding them to be true to me. 08, 30C, 42:XX:XX
Sh, 411 - The way I'm feeling today is aggravated and slightly depressed; mostly aggravated about financial things. Reflecting on a bigger picture now, need to do something about it. More on my mind than before. It has to do with my position and place in life; where I am at this particular point in life. Am I pleased? Am I happy? Am I disgruntled? Of course I'm disgruntled. A switch happened. I wasn't looking so detrimentally on my feelings about position and place. The remedy lightened everything, seasoned it, not as bland as I thought. Now things are bland—not spiced up or happy. 18, 30C, 03:11:XX

HELL. Ha, 286 - Sad disposition respecting his present position, everything seems to him so insipid (tedious, boring,) and nothing interests him.

KALI-BR. Al, 3 - Decidedly insane; had delusions that lewd women had got into his mother's house; that he was pursued by the police; that his wife was threatened by members of the family; that he had thousands of dollars in gold sewed up in his clothing; (rich, wealth)

MENY. Al, 2 - Quiet mood; contented with his circumstances. (chances)
Ha, 286 - Cross, ill-humored and discontented with himself and his position (rank); anxiety drives him from one place to another.(restlessness)
Ha, 295 - Tranquil disposition; he was contented with his position.

MERC. Ha, 1248 - Without cause he is very

discontented with himself and his position.
He, 35 - Grief, with fear at night: disposition to quarrel; complaining of relations and surroundings. (living conditions)
MEZ. Al, 10 - Great discontent with himself and his surroundings (living, conditions, position) for several weeks...
NUX-V. He, 26 - Melancholic in consequence of losing his position (rank),...the least contradiction puts him out entirely...(ailments from)
He, 37-...betraying (play false, feigning) great moral and physical languor (indifference),..launches into high-flying, fantastic plans, fancies himself rich (rank, position) and wants to make presents of thousands (squanders, waste), and makes large useless purchases; does not consider himself ill; ...,and takes in bad part if not allowed to read indictment (accusation) for said lawsuit, a confused irrational piece of work...
PHOS. Ha, 89 - Delirious fantasies, while slumbering (sleep) and when awake, as if she was on a distant island (isolation, segregation), as if she had a large business, was a distinguished (important, rank) lady, etc.
STAPH. He, 15-...; firmly believed he would lose his fortune, constantly told his wife to be careful that they did not starve; thinks his wife will run away from him (deserted) (lost: position, rank), ... amuses himself by throwing into the fire any article near at hand, regardless of value; at times more violent, strikes at any one coming near him, ...tells his wife he will try not kill any one;...
STRAM. Al, 48 - She is all the time inconsolable; much affected by trifles; makes much fuss about trifles; disposed to weep, and sometimes also very easily vexed; now and then neglects her duties; now and then thinks she is not fitted for her position ; after the fall equinox...; she wants light and company.
He, 61 - Thinks she is not fitted for her position.
He, 98 - Mania; affects (pretend) being a distinguished (label) person, of high rank (position, nobility) ; is full of fear.
He, 177-...sometimes vexed; neglects her duties, thinks she is not fitted for her position;...
VERAT. Al, 4 - He imagines that he is a prince (noble) and behaves in a very haughty manner. (proud, arrogant)
Ha, 672 - He pretends (simulate, feigning) he is a prince, and gives himself airs (affectation, pretentious) accordingly.
He, 11 - Thinks himself distinguished (classify) ; squanders (futile) his money; proud (haughty) of his position.
He, 52 - Despair about his position in society, feels very unlucky.

POSTPONING

Postponing everything to next day, business seems so long lasting, or as if it never could be accomplished: med.[54]
Work; aversion to mental, wants to leave everything as soon as it is commenced: ***lac-c.***[54]

HALI-L. Sh, 318 - Procrastinated doing grocery shopping. Debated which day to go, and which store. Decided much later to go to neither place, and just pick up what I absolutely needed. 03, 12C, 15:XX:XX
MED. He, 2 - Dullness of memory and desire to procrastinate (delay), because business seemed so long lasting (permanent), or as if it never could be accomplished. (postponing)
NUX-V. Al, 69 - Dawdles (delay) and is irresolute.
STANN. Al, 21 - Indolent and irritable, with heat in the face; would do everything, but really does nothing.

POVERTY

Ailments from; financial loss: ***arn.***[122] ars.[8] aur.[58] calc.[30] ign.[30] mez.[58] nat-m.[30] nux-v.[30] puls.[193] ***rhus-t.***[30] ***sars.***[8] stann.[30] verat.[30]
Cares; full of, money, about: bamb-a.[1184] ozone[227]
Delusions; clothes, rags, clad in: ***cann-i.***
- family, get along without her, cannot: lil-t.[168]
- fasting: brom.[36] euphr.[36] iod.[36]
- fortune, he was going to lose his: psor. staph.
- poor, he is: bamb-a.[1184] bell. bry.[185] calc-f. hep. mez. nux-v. psor.[58] ***sep.*** stram. valer.

• starve, family will: ars. calc-sil.[58] ***sep.*** staph.
• starved, being: naja[36]
• want, had come to: cann-i.
• want, will come to: calc-f. chlor.[139] sulph.

Despair; social position, of: calc.[30] ign.[30] puls.[30] rhus-t.[30] sep.[30] staph.[30] sulph.[30] **VERAT.**

Dreams; beggars: mag-c.[10]
➤ danger, want, and: am-c.[54]
➤ misery: ozone[227]
➤ money, left behind without, he is: ozone[227]
➤ thirstily, being: dros. mag-c. **NAT-M.** viol-o.[45]
➤ want, of: am-c.[36]

Fear; death, hunger from: calc.[122]
✦ death, starvation, from: ars.[137]
✦ family, to bring up his: ***staph.***[162]
✦ fasting, of: kreos.
✦ poverty, of: ambr. ars.[137] **BRY.** ***calc. calc-f.*** calc-s.[108] calc-sil.[58] cand-a.[239] chlor. graph.[184] hydrog.[222] kali-c.[122] meli. nux-v. ***psor.*** puls. ***sep.*** staph.[172] sulph.
✦ poverty, prosperous, although: psor.[137]
✦ poverty, spending, in case he is short of money in future, fear of: ***nux-v.***[30] stann.[30]
✦ social position, about his: chel.[172] cub.[36] sep.[30] staph.[30] verat.
✦ starving, of: ars.[172] ***bry.***[54] calc. kali-m.[61] ***sep.***[54] sulph.

ARS. He, 10 - Fixed idea that he and his family will die of starvation. (hunger, privation, want)
He, 58 - Melancholy; after financial losses; cannot be consoled; thinks he will have to die (sentenced), with his family, from starvation (hunger); sleepless nights; walks about wringing his hands, with moaning and groaning.

BRY. He, 27 - She fears not to have wherewithal (money, funds) to live.

CALC-F. Al,S-1-...tendency to look on the dark side of things, with much depression of spirits. Feeling of anxiety about money matters, or thought would come to want (lack), or would soon be "running astern" (reversed, failure) financially...disposition to set a higher value on money than natural to him (avarice?, poverty?).
He, 3 - Feeling of anxiety about money matters; thought he would come to want (poverty) or would soon be "running astern" financially (entirely without occasion)

CALC. Ha, 29 - Despairing (hopeless) mood with fear of sickness (disease) and misery, with forebodings of sad events. (misfortune)

CHIN. Ha, 1103 - She falls time to time into a lachrymose humour, without external cause, from some self-made, trivial whim (caprice), e.q. from some imaginary want (lack, need), such as that she cannot eat enough...

CHLOL. Al, 3 - A horrible state of mind, fears he will go crazy, fears he cannot make a living.(subsistence)

CHLOR. He, 3 - A horrible state of mind, fears he will go crazy, fears he cannot make a living.(subsistence)

HYDROG. Sh, 130 - Anxiety about money and fear of poverty. 24, 30C, 100:XX:XX

LYSS. Al,N-46 - After fainting (weak) spell he wrote on paper: I am forsaken by all; even the birds of heaven, they do not look at me (despised), do not fed me if hungry (helplessness) ; I hunger with the young ones and am thirsty with their she ones (starving); my nest (house) is made out of dirt (soiled), not gotten by my own exertions (efforts), but by driving them out of their nests (home) and sitting there with the females and the young.

MAG-C. Al, 969 - Dream...he quarreled with a beggar.

SULPH. He, 33 - Sleepless, disgusted with life, fears the future, where she sees nothing but misery (wretchedness, poverty) and suffering (misfortune). 0 Melancholia.

PUNISHED

Dreams; remorse, God was punishing her for her sins, that: aether[36]
➤ remorse, pleading for mercy at bar of judgment: aether[36]
➤ whipped, getting: ptel.[36]

Fear; punished, of being: plb.[201]
✦ punished, of being, child: camph.[54]
✦ punishment, after, in children, if brought to bed too soon get convulsions in sleep: ***ign.***[54]

Grief; punishment, after: ***ign.***[54]

Mood; repulsive, food, saying one who does not work should not eat, but driven by hunger he tried to procure it secretly: ***arg-n.***[54]
Sadness; punishment, after: ***ign.***[54]

ANDROC. Sh, 40 - She dreamt that she had murdered her grandfather by poking a knitting needle through his eyes while he slept. Though she felt no remorse, she wanted to be punished but no-one would accept her guilt. Was told by her friends that she had responsibilities and could not go to jail and the police refused to prosecute. Was frightened by the dream. (7)
ARG-N. He, 17 - Refused food, saying one who does not work should not eat (punishment); but driven by hunger he tried to secretly procure it.
CAMPH. Al, 27 - The child creeps (crawl) into a corner, howls and cries; everything that is said to him is taken as if one were ordering him, and he were considered naughty (disobedient) and should be punished.
He, 53-...everything that is said is taken as if one was ordering him, and he was considered naughty (disobedient) and would be punished.
GERM. Sh, 180 - Woke up early 3.30 am. had strong feeling, like a visualization. I picture myself lying on floor in fetal position and being shot in the head like a horse or a dog. Almost welcomed it. Then thought my children still need me. A very strong feeling of failure accompanied this. I felt I did not deserve to live. Better crying next day when talking to husband. This feeling of depression carried on for several nights. As soon as I wake up in the early morning, my mind is active and a feeling of inadequacy comes on strongly. 05, 6C, 28:XX:XX
Sh, 116 - Blaming myself for having taken too many doses. Was afraid that I would not get the symptoms out strongly enough. Maybe I spoiled the whole proving. Still accusing myself. I felt it does not matter how much I suffer - it's what other think of me that is important. I think that I ought to suffer a good deal. 18, 30C, 01:08:15
Sh, 102 - Everything is my fault -I asked for 'drubbing' (beating) and I have got it. The kids are afraid of me, and I feel insecure about what I'm able to do. I called my sister -the only person I could talk to - but she was not at home. With an enormous effort, with heart palpitations, pain in the stomach, trembling and aggravation of headache I rang another prover. But I didn't get through -it was occupied. 18, 30C, XX:XX:XX
Sh, 123 - Don't understand anything, the meaning of life. Feel also strength somewhere inside. I wish a change could happen, I ought to bring myself together and change. It is silly of me to go on like this. I despise myself. I am hard to myself, but I don't deserve anything else. I think other people are silly too. 18, 30C, 06:XX:XX
Sh, 112 - Don't see why I am here. I can't bear it. I go mad. I hate myself. I want to beat myself and I do it. Tear my hair. Stop when it hurts too much. It is like hell !!! 18, 30C, 20:XX:XX

PURE

Adolescent, felt he was again: androc.[222]
Delusions; body, immaterial, is: anh.[119]
- child, he is again a, acts like a, and: ***cic.***
- childish fantasies, has: lyc.
- divine, he is: cann-i. glon.[116] stram.
- heaven, is in: cann-i. hydrog.[222] op. ***verat.***[54]
- pure, that she is: stram.[122]

Dreams; girl, that he is a: apis.
➤ water, poured upon him, is: ox-ac.
Naive: aesc.[120] ***bell.***[30] bov.[5] cic.[30] stram.[30]
Naive; intelligent, but very: ***chin.***[30] hyos.[30] ***stram.***[30] ***sulph.***[30] verat.[30]

ADAM. Sh, 36 - White frost this morning. At last some purity in this world. Every ice crystal sparkled like jewels. 16, 12C, 27:XX:XX
Sh, 37 - Great joy at the beauty of the snow, especially at night, reflecting light. Sparkled like jewels, purity. After the snow, joy at seeing greens again, appeared brighter and clearer than before the snow. 16, 12C, 67:XX:XX

Sh, 47 - Need air—fresh, cold, clean. I feel stuffy inside. This feeling is related to the feeling of food being dirty. 20, 1M, 06:XX:XX

BELL. He, 18 - When closing eyes, though not asleep, patient sees fierce (wild), wicked looking large animals with horns and bushy (scabrous) heads; room seemed to be full of strange men passing in and out, who would snatch (take hold) at her as they passed, which frightened her very much, she thought the men wanted to take her away from home ; she then saw children sitting on low benches (seat) in rows (line) as in a school-room. (purity)

CAMPH. He, 19 - It was to him as if he moved in his own little world, in which all things were clear (pure, perfect) and defined; outside of which uncertain (doubtful) and undefined. (obscure) (purity x impurity)

CANTH. Al, 22-...; she feels as if newly (recently) born;... (innocent, naive, pure)

CIC. Ha, 240 - He felt like a child of seven or eight years old, objects were very dear and attractive to him, as toys are to a child. (purity)

He, 7 - He thinks himself a young child. (purity, juvenile, infant)

HURA. Al, 3 - Every paroxysm of pain excites a nervous laugh, with moanings like those of a sick child.

IRID. Sh, 58 - Felt child-like, innocent, happy as though seeing things from a child's perspective. Sat watching a milk tanker, it looks just like a child's toy. Felt like I could pick it up and brrrm brrrm it up the lane. I9

MAG-C. Al, 923 - Dream that she had become a child three years old, which rejoiced her very much. (youngish)

RELIGIOUS

Ailments from; domination by others, religious: foll.[1179]

Ailments from; excitement, religious: stram.[48] sulph.[48] verat.[48]

Anxiety; conscience, women and religion, about: puls.[54]

Anxiety; duty, as if he had not done his, religious, produced by lascivious impulses: ***orig.***[54]

Anxiety; lascivious impulses, from, on account of disinclination of religious duties in a married woman, mother of a family: ***orig.***[54]

Anxiety; salvation, about: aq-mar.[149] **ARS.** ars-s-f.[58] ***aur.*** aur-ar.[58] aur-s.[58] ***calc.*** ***calc-ar.***[122] calc-s. ***camph.*** cann-i. carbn-s. chel. ***graph.*** hura ign. kali-p. **LACH.** **LIL-T.** ***lyc. med. mez.*** nat-m. nux-v.[30] ph-ac.[30] plat. plb.[58] podo.[58] ***psor. puls.*** **STAPH.**[30] ***stram. sulph. thuj.*** **VERAT.**

Anxiety; salvation, hell, of: ***plat.***[54]

Anxiety; salvation, scrupulous as to their religious practices, too: ars.[30] ign.[30] lyc.[30] nux-v.[30] ph-ac.[30] puls.[30] **STAPH.**[30] **SULPH.**[30]

Aversion; sex, opposite to, religious aversion: lyc. ***puls.*** sulph.

Aversion; women, to, looks upon them as evil beings and is afraid their presence is injurious to his soul: ***puls.***[54]

Begging, entreating supplicating: ars. aur.[5] bell.[5] kali-c.[5] plat.[5] puls.[5] stram.

Begging, pray for him, to, and not to leave him alone: lyss.[54]

Blissful feeling: androc.[222] coff.[1] **OP.**[5]

Cheerfulness; spirituality, followed by fading of: lach.[54]

Consolation; amel. religious: raph.[85]

Conversation; desire for, sublime, to hear: ham.[36]

Cruelty; religiousness, with: ***plat.***[54]

Delirium tremens; praying, with: aur.[162] **STRAM.**[54]

Delirium; blessing, asks a: bell.[36]

Delirium; raging, raving, alternating with, religious excitement: agar.[36]

Delirium; religious: agar.[5] alco.[36] aur. lach. **VERAT.**[5]

Delusions; angels, seeing: aether[36] cann-i.[36] stram.[58]

- choir, on hearing music he is in a cathedral: cann-i.
- Christ, himself to be: cann-i. verat.[58]
- convent, she will have to go to a: lac-d.
- devils, taken by, that he will be, mania, in religious: ***puls.***[54]
- divine, he is: cann-i. glon.[116] stram.
- God, communication with, he is in: psil.[164] stram. verat.
- God, he is, then he is devil: **STRAM.**[54]
- God, presence of God, that he is in the: hydrog.[222]
- God, sees: aether.[36]

- hearing, tone, comes from another world: **CARB-AN.**[54]
- heaven, is in: cann-i. hydrog.[222] op. ***verat.***[54]
- martyrdom: carc.[207] nat-c.[162]
- mesmerized by her absent pastor, she is: meli.
- obtain peace and safety through absolution from a priest of Papal church, although a zealous protestant, that she can only: ***plb.***[54]
- possessed, God and the devil, alternately by: psil.[164]
- religious: alum-sil.[162] ***anac.***[54] ***ars.***[116] aur.[116] bell.[116] croc.[116] ***hyos.***[116] ***kali-br.***[54] lach.[10] lyc.[116] med.[54] merc.[116] nux-v.[116] plat.[116] ***puls.***[116] ***stram.***[10] ***sulph.***[116] ***verat.***[10]
- religious, redemption and devil, about: ***anac.***[54]
- sinned away his day of grace, unpardonable: ars.[58] aur.[58] kali-p.[58] med.[54] plb.[58] podo.[58] psor.[58] puls.[58] stram.[85] sulph.[58]
- vengeance, thinks he is singled out for Divine: **KALI-BR.**
- Virgin Mary, she is: cann-i.
- visions, strikes at them and holds up the cross: ***puls.***[122]
- visions, sublimity, of great, follows those of quiet relaxing and recreating nature: ***cann-i.***[54]

Despair; religious: ***arg-n.*** **ARS. AUR.** aur-ar.[58] aur-i.[58] aur-s.[58] ***calc.*** calc-ar.[58] calc-i.[58] ***camph. chel.*** cycl.[116] hell. hura ign. ***kali-p.*** **LACH. LIL-T.** ***lyc.*** med. ***mez.*** nat-m. ozone[227] plat. plb. podo. ***psor.*** **PULS.**[122] ***stram. sulph. thuj.*** **VERAT.**

Despair; religious, alternating with sexual excitement: ***lil-t.***

Despair; religious, constant prayer: ***puls.***[54]

Despair; religious, suicidal tendency, with: verat.[54]

Discouraged; praying, with: puls.[10]

Doubtful; soul's welfare, of: **ARS. AUR.** bell. calc. chel. croc. cycl.[5] dig. hyos. **LACH.** ***lil-t.*** lyc. nux-v. **PULS.** sel. stram. ***sulph.***[5] ***verat.***

Dreams; churches: asc-t. coc-c. lyss. ozone[227] zing.

- ➤ crimes, discovered by priest: nat-s.[36]
- ➤ escape, Buddhist monastery, from: lap-mar-c.[194]
- ➤ fire, cathedral on: kali-c.[36]
- ➤ prayer meeting, of being conducted to, by unknown woman, it then changed into a restaurant: pip-m.[36]
- ➤ praying: ars-h.
- ➤ preaching: allox.[119] anac. ant-t.
- ➤ preaching, has to preach: anac.[1]
- ➤ preaching, stuck, and get: ant-t.[36]
- ➤ prude, being: **TUB.**[122]
- ➤ religious: hydrog.[222] kali-m.[192] sol-t-ae.[36] ***sulph.***[10]
- ➤ resurrection: allox.[149]
- ➤ sacred place, of: ozone[227]
- ➤ wedding, procession passing her, of: nat-s.[36]
- ➤ wedding, repeated, has to be, since only one half of the body has been married: bamb-a.[1184]

Dullness; fanaticism, with pious: ***thuj.***[54]

Eccentricity; religious: puls.[30] sel.[10] stram.[30] sulph.[10] verat.[30]

Ecstasy; sublime: crot-h.[36]

Ecstasy; sublime, impression, as after: lach.[36]

Excitement; religious: agar.[36] ***aur.*** plb.[8] stram. sulph. verat.

Fanaticism: aur-ar.[58] bell.[137] carc.[207] caust. con.[137] cupr.[210] lap-c-b.[194] puls.[58] rob. sel. sulph. ***thuj.*** valer.[111]

Fear; faith, to lose his religious: coloc.[162] merc.[162] nux-v.[162] staph.[162] ***sulph.***[162]

Haughty; religiousness, with: ***plat.***[54]

Indifference; religion, to his: anac. coloc. med.[179] sil.[137]

Inquisitive; supernatural or spiritual matters, about: calc.[162]

Insanity; fanatics, of: aur-ar.[58]

Insanity; prayer at the tail of his horse, insists upon saying his: euph.

Insanity; prayer, raising hands and kneeling as in p.: ***ars.***[36]

Insanity; religious: anac.[58] ***ars.***[122] aur.[54] aur-ar.[58] bell.[116] croc.[116] ***hyos.***[116] ***kali-br.***[54] ***lach.***[58] lil-t.[58] lyc.[58] merc.[116] nat-c.[58] nux-v.[116] ***plat.***[54] ***puls.***[58] **STRAM.**[54] ***sulph.***[54] ***verat.***[10]

Lasciviousness; religious: ***plat.***[54]

Loquacity; devout, mostly: ***stram.***[54]

Loquacity; religious subjects, about: ***verat.***[36]

Mania; prayer, as in, raising hands and kneeling: ***ars.***[36]

Mania; praying: stram.[60] verat.[60]

Mood; repulsive, medicine, to take the, religious insanity, in: ***kali-p.***[54]

Morose; religiousness, with: ***plat.***[54]

Mystical: camph.[36] pyrus[36]

Praying: ***alum.***[30] ***anac.***[103] arn. ***ars.*** **AUR.** ***bell.*** cere-b. cere-s.[36] euph. hyos. lyss.[54] manc.[30] mygal.[47] nat-s. op. opun-a.[36] plat. **PULS.** rhus-t.[30] **SEP.**[30] **STRAM.**[122] sul-ac. sulo-ac.[36] sulph.[58] **VERAT.**

Praying; aloud, in sadness: ***plat.***[54]

Praying; begged others to pray for him: lyss.[54]

Praying; fervent: alum.[30] **SEP.**[30]

Praying; killed, to be: bell.[30]

Praying; kneeling and: ***ars.*** nat-s. ***stram.*** verat.

Praying; quietly, for her soul: arn.[54] ars.[54]

Praying; seeks relief in constant: ***puls.***[54]

Praying; sleep, during: stann.[54]

Praying; timidly, during sleep: stann.[54]

Praying; wanted people to join her in, with slight erysipelas of face: ***plat.***[54]

Precocity; religious: calc.[58]

Rage; alternating with; religious excitement: agar.

Religious affections: ***alum.***[122] alum-sil.[58] am-c. anac.[58] aq-mar.[149] ***arg-n.*** ***ars.*** ars-s-f.[58] ***aur.*** bar-c. ***bell.*** ***calc.*** camph. ***carb-v.*** carbn-s. caust. ***cham.*** ***chel.*** cina coff. con. croc. cycl. dig. ferr. ferr-ar. ***graph.*** hura hydrog.[222] **HYOS.** hyper.[36] ***ign.*** kali-br. ***kali-p.*** **LACH.** **LIL-T.** ***lyc.*** ***med.*** ***meli.*** merc. ***mez.*** nat-c.[58] nat-m. nux-v. ph-ac.[30] ***plat.*** ***psor.*** ***puls.*** ***rhus-t.***[122] rob. ruta sabad. sel. **SEP.**[122] sil. stann. staph.[30] **STRAM.**[122] **SULPH.** tarax.[36] thuj. **VERAT.** **ZINC.**

Religious affections, sadness, remorse, from: aur.[30] con.[30]

Religious affections; alternating with sexual excitement: lil-t. ***plat.***

Religious affections; bible, want to read all day the: ***calc.***[122] stram.[122]

Religious affections; children, in: ***ars.*** ***calc.*** ***lach.*** ***stram.***[122] ***sulph.***

Religious affections; eternal bliss, believes herself unworthy of, because she is unable to perform her duties: stram.[54]

Religious affections; fanaticism: aur-ar.[58] med.[162] plb.[85] puls.[58] rat.[162] rob. sel. stram.[85] sulph. thuj.

Religious affections; happy to join her Redeemer, felt, in facial erysipelas: ***plat.***[54]

Religious affections; horror of the opposite sex: lyc. nat-m.[193] ***plat.***[54] ***puls.*** sulph.

Religious affections; mania: ***lach.***[54] ***plat.***[54] plb.[85] ***puls.***[54] ***stram.***[54] sulph.[85] **VERAT.**[54]

Religious affections; mania, pious look, with: ***stram.***[54]

Religious affections; mania, praying all the time: ***aur.***[54]

Religious affections; narrow-minded in religious questions: hyos.[30] puls.[30] ***stram.***[30]

Religious affections; night tortured by religious ideas: camph.[54] lil-t.[58]

Religious affections; penance, desires to do, wishes to live, in order to mitigate her eternal punishment, in sadness: ***plat.***[54]

Religious affections; preoccupations: achy.[149]

Religious affections; puberty, in: ***ars.***[122] ***calc.***[122] ***lach.***[122] ***sulph.***[122]

Religious affections; sadness: ars.[5] aur.[5] bac.[62] bell.[10] con.[30] croc.[10] graph.[60] ***kali-br.***[54] ***kali-p.***[54] ***lach.***[10] lil-t.[58] lyc.[10] ***meli.***[54] mez.[58] ***plat.***[54] plb.[102] psor.[102] puls.[10] sel.[10] sil.[58] ***stram.***[10] ***sulph.***[10] ***verat.***[10]

Religious affections; sadness, doubt about salvation, with: ***lyc.***[54]

Religious affections; sadness, gave away everything she could lay her hands on, in order to do penance: ***plat.***[54]

Religious affections; songs: raja-s.[149]

Religious affections; speculations, dwells on: **SULPH.**[54]

Religious affections; spiritual improvement, desires: ***cinnb.***[36]

Religious affections; taciturnity, haughtiness, voluptuousness, cruelty, r. a with: ***plat.***[54]

Religious affections; talking on religious subjects: ***hyos.***[54] stram.[60] ***verat.***[60]

Religious; affections, sadness, four months standing, of: ***meli.***[54]

Sensitive; music, sacred m, to: lyss.[54] thuj.[122]

Singing; Latin paternosters: ***stram.***[54]

Suicidal disposition; despair, from, religious: verat.[54]

Tears; things, clothing, nightdress and bed clothes, sadness, in religious: ***kali-p.***[54]

Thoughts; vanishing, sermon, during a: anag.[36]

Veneration: anac.[10] ars.[10] aur.[10] bell.[10] cic.[30] coff. croc.[10] hyos.[10] lach.[10] lyc.[10] puls.[10] stram.[10] sulph.[10] verat.[10]

Veneration; Supreme Being, for: coff.[36]

Weeping; music, church music: ***thuj.***[184]

Weeping; thoughts, religious: ***kali-p.***[54]

AGAR. Al, 8-...called for his hatchet; had to be confined alternated with religious excitement.

Al, 14 - He imagines himself at a gate of the hell and that the mushroom commands him to fall on his knees and confess his sins, which he does. (forgiveness, absolution)

ANAC. He, 28 - Fixed ideas: that mind and body are separated ; about redemption (salvation) of soul and about the devil; that a stranger is constantly by his side (pursued); that strange forms accompany him, one to his right and one to his left.

ARN. He, 27 - Prays quietly for her soul. (salvation)

ARS. Ha, 1032 - Mania; first headache, horrible anxiety, noise before the ears, as from a number of large bells, and when he opened the eyes, he always saw a man who had (formerly) hung himself (suicidal, justified) on the ground-floor of the house, who incessantly beckoned (call) him to cut him down (help); he ran thither (there) with a knife, but, as he could not cut him down, (rescue) he became overwhelmed (beaten) with despair (remorse?) and wished (as his friends assured him) to hang himself (punish); but being prevented (stop) from doing so, he became so restless that he could hardly be kept in bed,... and he knelt down and raised his hands in a supplicating manner.

He, 25 - Mania...sees a man who has hanged himself beckoning (call) him to cut him loose (rescue, deliverance, free, saving) on failing to accomplish this he attempts to hang himself (punish, penalize);...finally kneels down and lifts his hands in supplication.(forgiveness, absolution)

He, 61 - Religious melancholy; hopelessness, despair.

AUR. He, 8 - Looks on dark side, weeps, prays, thinks she is not fit for this world, longs for death, strong inclination to commit suicide; desperate, desires to jump from a height.

He, 18 - Religious mania; prays all the time.

CALC. He, 55 - Concern (anxiety, care) about spiritual welfare.(salvation)

CAMPH. Al, 46-...I sat up in bed, but all about me had indeed disappeared. I was alone in the great universe, the last of all things. My ideas of the world, God and religion, now seemed to me to have existed only in my imagination; the earth upon which yesterday I lived and moved, had run its appointed course, and I was the final and solitary fragment of the whole creation...(meaningless, unimportant, neglected, forsaken, loneliness, deserted) (godless)

Al, 46-... Faith and hope were gone. There was here no longer any God, or rather the Infinite himself, like all his works, had ceased to be... (hopeless, faithless, godless, privation, want, destitution)

Al, 46-...And yet I confessed this every morning, and no heavy sin rests upon my conscience. And then came doubts about my doctrinal views, for I had never been of strong faith...

He, 16 - Monomania, with horrible visions and torturing ideas about religion, which he cannot shake off, although he is conscious that they are morbid.; is< at night.

CERE-B. Al, 8 - A grateful feeling of dependence (need, faith, relation) on a divine spirit was experienced. (reverence, veneration, praise)

CHIN-S. Al, 20-...; felt a gloom (darkness) come over me, as if some evil were impending; relieved by a specific trust in the Almighty;...(divine) (faithful, confiding, devoted)

CHOC. Sh, 185 - Religious like feeling. 45, 30C, 00:00:10

COFF-T. Al, 6 - Veneration for Supreme Being.

COFF. He, 8 - Great loquacity, brain feels clear and is active, he feels strong enough to do anything, feels impelled to push things; veneration for the Supreme Being and love for family; benevolence excited.

CUPR-A. He, 10 - Awoke suddenly from sleep...and wished to escape...thinks she is about to die and desires to see the pastor;...

EUPH. He, 3 - Temporary attacks of craziness, insists upon saying his prayers at the tail of his horse; knows his freaks (abnormality) and wants to be by himself and in silence.

GRAPH. He, 15 - Solicitude (anxiety) concerning spiritual welfare.

HALI-L. Sh, 306 - When I'm focused I bring it all in, in the present, There. like meditating, or seeing God. When I'm unfocussed it's like I'll go into the abyss, and won't come back, go crazy. 08, 30C, 31:XX:XX

Sh, 803 - I feel like a sexual nun. 20, 30C, 04:XX:XX

Sh, 934 - As I woke, I decided I should be a nun. Strange. I feel like I've got my wings clipped when I think about men. 20, 30C, 15:XX:XX

HELL. Al, 15 - Dread of death (in a sufferer from religious melancholy).

Al, 19 - Dread of death.(in a sufferer from religious melancholy)

He, 12 - An old woman having been accused of theft by the women around, took it so much to heart that she hanged herself. This suicide produced a profound effect upon the women of the village. One after another accused herself of having caused the death of the old woman by their insinuations; they wept and howled, ran about day and night wringing their hands and despairing of salvation on account of their sin (error); they became quite irrepressible and deranged (disordered) In this way twenty - four or twenty five women were affected, every fresh case being followed by another. Hysterical mania.

HURA. Al, 23 - Anxiety about his salvation, during the nervous attack.

HYDROG. Sh, 8 - I felt slightly high, removed from reality, yet very alert, clear and calm. Very aware of the colour of the sky, the light, birds singing, flowers — like a pastoral ideal. Feeling of expansiveness, mentally cool, airy and light. 28, 200C, 00:04:XX

Sh, 15 - I felt in the presence of a totally pure energy, like meeting God and feeling totally unworthy or like meeting a lover and feeling unworthy — realizing all the mistakes of a lifetime. This pure energy was around for some time protecting me. I feel this unification cleared out lifetimes of symptomatology for me. The joining with this energy was as if a male energy joined with me sexually, but with no desire, pleasure or pain involved. This unification with the male energy lasted quite a few days — I'm not used to seeing myself as a man. The morning after this unifying with the higher presence, I collapsed in emotional overflow. All my grief and pain came out. I was doubled upon the floor and went into a deep state of catharsis. It is not possible to describe where I went as there are no concepts applicable. I felt overflowing love for humanity and wanted to give everything away. My mind turned to the Buddha. It was like seeing the complete picture instead of fragmented bits. (These primary effects lasted about 28 days, then changing to a paranoia state). 16, 30C, 07.XX.XX

Sh, 27 - There is a very fine line at this time between enlightenment and insanity — a split consciousness. The dark side is horrendous, but the positive side of the proving has been well worth it. The positive aspects are beautiful. Its a shame we need to come down. I guess the price of going into the heavens is a trip to hell. 16, 30C, XX:XX:XX

Sh, 33 - About two months after beginning the proving, developed an extreme range of mental symptoms that he had never had before. These included severe depression with strong alternations of moods, & high then low &, with suicidal tendency, desire to jump from a high building or cut wrist, confusion of identity (especially concerning sex and homosexuality) and became more religious. He moved away from his parents home (which he had never before been able t o do) and shut himself away in a small flat. This condition lasted for another six or seven months and was finally antidoted by Phosphorus 200. Before that, he had tried to anti-dote it with acupuncture, to no avail. 24, 30C, 60:XX:XX

Sh, 263 - Turned to Christianity in which he had never had interest before. 24, 30C, 100:XX:XX

HYOS. Ha, 545 - Ridiculously solemn acts in improper clothing, mixed with fury. (In a priest's cassock, put on over nothing but a shirt, and in fur boots, he wishes to go to church, in order to preach and perform clerical offices there, and furiously attacks those who try to prevent him.)

He, 84-...constant talking, particularly on religious subjects; believes himself poisoned, or that there is a stinking odor from his mouth;...

IGN. He, 10 - Spasms and insanity after fright; imagines her soul cannot be saved (rescued), and cries very much; ...(lost, sentenced)

IRID. Sh, 110 - Meditating, vision of an angel, face and wings. Q6

KALI-BR. He, 10 - Imagines he is singled out as an object of divine wrath (fury, rage); extreme drowsiness.

He, 17 - Delirium with delusions; thinks he is pursued (hunt); will be poisoned; is selected (designated) for divine vengeance (revenge); that her child is dead, etc.

He, 31-...religious delusions and feeling of moral deficiency; ...profound indifference and almost disgust for life.

He, 33 - Great despondency, with insanity, a feeling of moral deficiency, or a religious delusion, from anemia.

LAC-D. Al,N-4 - Imagines that all her friends will die and that she must go to a convent. (purification, solitude)

He, 5 - Imagines that all her friends will die and that she must go to a convent. (purification, salvation)

LACH. He, 17 - Religious monomania, fear of being damned (condemned to eternal punishment).

LIL-T. He, 5 - Tormented about her salvation.

He, 16 - Doubts her salvation; thinks she is doomed to expiate her sins and those of her family; ... (redemption, salvation) (sacrifice)

LYC. He, 20 - Melancholy: has doubts about her salvation; before catamenia; in mild (pacific) characters.

LYSS. Al,N-11-...presentiment of impending death begged them to pray for him and not to leave him alone. (absolution, redemption)

MED. Al,N-52 - Feeling of desperation; did not care if he went to heaven or hell.

He, 37 - Feeling of desperation, did not care if he went to heaven or hell.

MELI. He, 8 - Religious melancholy of four months' standing; ...

MEZ. He, 8 - Despairs of eternal salvation.

OP. Al, 19-...each possessing some imaginary bliss (happiness) which " the dull (dark) reality of life" could never give....they are wrapped in an elysium, (heaven) from which they are only to be awakened by the miserable reaction which must, sooner or later recall them to existence.

OPUN-V. Al, 5 - Fit of swearing (cursing) at evening after coming home; praying in the morning, swearing (cursing) on disappointment in plans; fit of rage, on thwarting (frustrating) of plans.

Al, 4 - In a few minutes, desire to be at prayer; go there, and in a minute or two desire to go out and "tidy" up; soon went out on an errand downstairs, then come up and go again to prayer.

PLAT. He, 36 - While suffering from a slight erysipelas faciei, took leave (quit, abandon) of her children, exhorted her husband to join (unite, combine) church, wanted people to join her in prayer (beg), felt happy to join her Redeemer.

He, 46-...;suffers unspeakable pangs (anxiety) of conscience in consequence of a faux (fault, mistake, embarrassing mistake?) pass when thirty-two years old; says she has brought disgrace upon her family, and that she has incurred the penalty of damnation; (doomed) in order to do penance (penitence) gave away whatever she could lay her hands upon, (redemption) so that she had to be constantly watched; after her confessor asserted that she could not hope for pardon or heaven (condemnable), she seemed in absolute despair ; bemoaned her misery throughout the night, wringing her hands and beseeching (implore) that she might be delivered (free) from the hell of her conscience; twice attempted self-destruction (suicide);...wished to live and do penance (penitence, purgation, purification) in order to mitigate her eternal punishment.

He, 40 - Disturbed state of mind; religious, with taciturnity, haughtiness, voluptuousness (sensual) and cruelty.

PLB. He, 15-...; despair of her salvation...; fixed idea that could only obtain peace and safety though absolution by a priest of the papal church, although she had been a zealous Protestant; ....brooded over any forbidden thing; would steal (leave) from house in servant's cloak (coat, camouflage) and bonnet (hat) to obtain stimulants (drugs), but from the moment their prohibition was withdrawn (retired) ceased to have any desire for them; after being permitted to visit a priest and converse with him ceased to talk and think of the church. (desire; redemption, absolution)

PULS. He, 40 - Religious mania; sees the devil coming to take her; the world on fire during night; fear, rage in spells, or weeping... (captured, possessed)

He, 47-...; pangs (pain, anxiety) of conscience about religion and female sex; violent palpitation in the presence of women; abhors (detests, aversion) and hates the sex; must go out of their way for fear of injuring them; looks upon them as evil beings and is afraid (fear; temptation, seduction); considers their presence injurious (insulted, offended) to his soul; ... (sexual loathing)

He, 48-...despaired of her soul's salvation; did not believe she would be restored to health ; ...

He, 43 - Sleepless nights on account of great fear and anxious restlessness; despairs of her salvation and seeks aid in constant prayer;...

ROB. Al, 9 - Bacchanalian (love to be drunken), erotic, or religious madness.

STRAM. He, 49 - After spasms she fell into a trance, says she is under influence(seized) of spirits, and has had conversation with spirits, communications from God; delivers emphatic sermons, prophecies. (missionary)

He, 56 - Believes to be in his grave; shrives,(confess) prays, asks to be killed (justified); accuses his wife of infidelity; scolds (cursing), strikes at everybody who wishes to restrain him; thinks they are dogs and barks at them to make himself understood.

He, 93 - Mania; thinks he is lying on his sepulchre (tomb); confessing, praying, wants to be killed (redemption, salvation, regeneration); laughs as if tickled (excited); wants to be kissed; accuses his wife of being faithless (betrayed); scolding (censure) beating in a rage, will not be taken hold of by attendants (suspicious?) ; takes them for dogs (contemptuous), and barks at them; talking in Jewish jargon; (rank?, stranger?) supposes his house to be surrounded by carts (vehicle), Jews (Judaism) and geese, offending him, ... -(strange, foreign, alien)

He, 87 - After a dreadful shock, occasioned by death of his brother, who fell dead in his arms,...struck all at around him...spoke at one time in Hungarian, and then in Wallachian language; sang Latin paternosters, declared he was God, and then that he was the devil;...

He, 112 - Religious mania; pious (divine) looks, praying; restless nights; inspired talking, singing; despairs of her salvation.

He, 122 - Excessive loquacity each time during menses; tears and prayers and earnest (ardent) supplications.

He, 117 - Ceaseless talking mostly devout; very earnestly beseeching. (supplicating)

He, 172 - Downcast and full of anguish, believes herself unworthy of eternal bliss, because she is unable to perform her duties.

SULPH. Ha, 61 - Great inclination to philosophic and religious ravings.(insanity)

He, 13 - A little girl with religious insanity, takes passages of Scripture literally and acts upon them. (fanatical) (virtuous, noble, elevated)

He, 32 - Melancholy mood; dwelling on religious or philosophic speculations; anxiety about soul's salvation; indifference about lot (destiny) of others.

THUJ. Al, 1 - She herself desires, with anxiety and despair, to be taken to an insane asylum, (imprisonment, confining) and there to be treated very harshly and strictly, (penalized), so that her fixed ideas may be subdued and banished (purified); she knows very well that she does wrong (conscience) and thinks all sorts of bad thoughts (immoral), but she will not take the trouble to banish such thoughts; therewith she indistinctly gives to understand that she is constantly obliged to think of taking her own life, but feels the sinfulness (wicked) of it, in order to avoid it, desires the strict restraint of the asylum;...

Al, 4 - She fancies that she has committed a sin.(wrong)

Al, 7 - She constantly longs for the offices of the church in order to banish her sinful thoughts of suicide. (redemption, salvation)

VERAT. Al, 2 - Slight delirium; ...he prattles about religious subjects and about vows to be performed, prays, believes that he is not in his own house.
He, 10 - Suicidal tendency from religious despair.
He, 16-... prattles about religious subjects and about vows (promise) to be performed, prays, believes that he is not in his own house.
He, 29-...prays says it is a secret (secretive, mysterious) and a misfortune; ...saying she must strengthen (encourage) herself, ...imagines herself in heaven (elevated, sublime, noble) talking with God.
He, 53 - Despair of her salvation;...
He, 21 - Mania; with desire to cut and tear everything, especially clothes; with lewdness and lascivious talk; religious or amorous; de grandeur.
He, 28 - Talks much on religious subjects; praying; is overconscientious.
He, 50 - Religious melancholy or nymphomania, with desire to embrace everybody even inanimate objects;...[0]Puerperal mania.

REMORSE

Delusions; disgraced, family or his absent friends, he disgraced his: sarr.[36]
• disgraced, family, she disgraced her: ***plat.***[8]
• neglected, duty, his, deserves reproach: aur.[54] germ.[222]
Dreams; misfortune, woman has legs amputated because of him: ozone[227]
➤ remorse, God was punishing her for her sins, that: aether[36]
➤ remorse, of: aether[36] arn.[36] ars.[1] elaps[36] fl-ac.[36] hyper.[36] lach.[10] led.[10] nat-c.[10] nat-m.[36] sanic.
➤ remorse, past mistakes, for: nat-m.[36]
➤ remorse, pleading for mercy at bar of judgment: aether[36]
➤ remorse, repudiated by God, of being: hyper.[36]
➤ repentance: ars.[36]
➤ reproaches himself: nat-m.[1]
Inconsolable; actions, over all her, which she thinks are evil: sulph.[1]
Inconsolable; heat, with, would rather die on the spot: spong.[54]
Insanity; females, self accusation, from: hell.[137]
Irritability; alternating with, remorse: mez.[10]
Mood; repulsive, food, saying one who does not work should not eat, but driven by hunger he tried to procure it secretly: ***arg-n.***[54]
Praying; killed, to be: bell.[30]
Religious affections, sadness, remorse, from: aur.[30] con.[30]
Remorse: achy.[149] agn.[58] alum. alum-sil.[58] am-c. anac.[5] androc.[222] ***ars.*** ars-s-f.[58] ***aur.*** aur-ar.[58] ***bell.*** cact.[5] ***calc.***[122] calc-p.[5] cand-a.[239] ***carb-an.***[5] carb-v. carc.[138] caust. cham. chel. chin-b.[54] cina clem.[5] ***cocc.*** **COFF.** con. croc.[88] ***cupr.*** cycl. ***dig.*** ferr. ferr-ar. germ.[222] graph. hell.[187] ***hyos. ign.*** kali-br.[5] lach. ***lil-t.***[187] lyss.[56] ***med.*** merc. mez.[30] nat-c. nat-m. nit-ac. nux-v. olnd.[5] ***ph-ac.***[5] phos.[5] plat. psor.[122] ***puls.*** rheum[5] ruta sabad. sec.[5] sel. ***sep.***[187] ***sil.*** spirae.[36] stram. stront-c. sulph. ***verat.*** vinc.[36] ***zinc.***
Remorse; fury, after attacks of, makes earnest apologies: lyss.[54]
Remorse; indiscretion, over past: spira.[36]
Remorse; masturbation, after: staph.[92]
Remorse; repents quickly: croc. olnd. sulph.[30]
Remorse; repents quickly, apologies, making earnest: lyss.[54]
Remorse; trifles: ***sil.***

ADAM. Sh, 238 - Quickly felt remorse after anger. 8, 6C, 04:XX:XX
ANDROC. Sh, 115 - When reflecting on her anger and arguments, was filled with remorse, although at the time she believed she was being perfectly reasonable. (12)
GERM. Sh, 6 - Difficult to accept my own feelings, accusing myself for letting them out, especially anger. Felt a rage, had to use all my power to control it. Lost my patience because of something my son did. I got angry with him, but at the same time despised myself for not having patience with him. I did not want to report this, because I feel unveiled - now everybody can see what awful person I am. I go completely mad of all my thoughts; can't bear it anymore. Inside me everything is chaos. Feel no power. 18, 30C, 18:XX:XX
Sh, 116 - Blaming myself for having taken too many doses. Was afraid that I would not get the symptoms out strongly enough. Maybe I spoiled the whole proving. Still accusing myself. I felt it

does not matter how much I suffer - it's what other think of me that is important. I think that I ought to suffer a good deal. 18, 30C, 01:08:15

RESENTMENT

Ailments from; admonition: agar.[5] ***bell.*** calc.[10] carc.[193] coloc.[137] germ.[222] ***ign.***[137] kali-c.[5] nit-ac.[5] ***nux-v.***[30] op.[137] ***plat.*** staph.[137] tarent.[137]
Ailments from; insults, offenses, from: ang.[1] calc.[1] ***cham.***[1] cocc.[1] dros.[1] glon.[8] gran.[36] ***ign.***[22] ***merc.***[8] ***nat-m.***[36] nit-ac.[60] ***op.***[8] seneg.[5] ***staph.***[54] stram.[58] sulph.[1]
Anger; past events, about: calc. carb-an. sars.[54] sep. sulph.[54]
Anger; temper tantrums: acon.[8] aur.[162] bell.[189] bor.[127] calc.[189] carc.[207] cere-s.[85] cham.[127] chel.[54] cina[148] cocc.[5] cupr.[116] hep.[189] hyos.[8] lach.[189] luna[228] lyss.[54] nat-m.[162] ***nux-v.***[5] olnd.[5] phos.[70] prot.[136] puls.[70] sac-alb.[210] sil.[70] ***staph.***[85] stront-c.[137] sulph.[189] tarent.[189] tell.[54] thuj.[8] thyr.[5] tub.[5]
Anger; temper tantrums, falls on the floor kicking and screaming: nat-m.[162]
Anger; temper tantrums, opposed, when at the least: thuj.[8]
Anger; temper tantrums, reprimands, after: nat-m.[162]
Anger; temper tantrums, throw themselves on the floor during, cannot get their breath: thuj.[8]
Anger; vexations, thinking about former: ***calc. carb-an.*** lyc.[1] sars.[54] sep. sulph.[54]
Complaining; offenses long past, of: calc.
Dwells on past disagreeable occurrences: am-c. arg-n. asar.[149] calc.[10] ***cham. chin.*** cob-n.[119] ***cocc. con.*** cop. form. glon. goss.[122] hep. hydrog.[222] hyos.[111] ***ign.***[54] kali-c.[108] ***kali-p.***[54] kiss.[36] lil-t.[58] luna[228] lyc. meny. mez. **NAT-M.** nit-ac. op.[30] opun-a.[36] phos.[111] ***plat.*** psor.[111] rhus-t. sars.[54] ***sep.*** spong.[1] staph.[30] ***sulph.*** syph.[122] thuj.[5] verat.[116] visc.[119]
Dwells; grief from past offenses: calc.[30] staph.[30]
Dwells; on past disagreeable occurrences, thinking of everything which others have done to displease him, lies awake all night to lay plans to talk to them about it, but forgets it in the morning: am-c.[58]
Excitement; evening, thinking of the things others have done to displease her: am-c.
Grief; long past offenses: calc.[1]
Hatred; bitter feelings for slight offenses, has: ang.
Hatred; persons, of, offended him, who had: agar.[60] am-c.[60] anac.[60] ***aur.*** calc.[30] cic.[60] lach.[60] led.[60] mang. med.[212] ***merc.***[30] ***nat-m.*** nit-ac. nux-v.[30] ph-ac.[60] sep.[122] stann.[60] staph.[30] sulph.
Hatred; persons, of, offended him, who had, unmoved by apologies: **NIT-AC.**
Hatred; persons, of, owner of dog that bit her, with inclination to utter maledictions which shock her: lyss.[54]
Hysteria; reprimands, after: ign.[189] nat-m.[162]
Insanity; malicious, malignant: agar.[10] cann-s.[10] ***cupr.*** lyc.[10]
Malicious; insults, long after: nit-ac.[60]
Moaning; honor, effects of wounded: ***nux-v.***[54]
Moaning; offense happened long ago, for trifling: ***cham.***[54]
Somnambulism; strike sleepers, from vengeance, to: **NAT-M.**[30] nit-ac.[30]
Thoughts; persons who had offended him, of: glon.[36]
Weeping; offense, former: caust.[30] ign.[30] lach.[30] staph.[30]
Weeping; vexation, from, old: caust.[30] cham.[10] ign.[30] lach.[30] lyc.[10] nat-m.[10] staph.[30]

ADAM. Sh, 228 - Resentful towards others. 20, 1M, 10:XX:XX
Sh, 229 - Feeling very angry towards others and hate people. I want to be alone and away from people who upset me. I hate feeling angry and resentful, a lot of it is directed to myself. 20, 1M, XX:XX:XX
Sh, 262 - Resentful, feeling aware of being used by husband and family; having to fit into their demands rather than have a life of my own. 8, 6C, 17:XX:XX
ANDROC. Sh, 102 - Assertive, impatient, aggressive. Felt resentful and abused. Had no control over her temper. Bellowed and lashed out at everyone. In the evening, furious for no apparent reason. Wanted to kill her husband and children, banged doors and threw things. By bed-time, she felt fine but the intensity of her evil thoughts was very frightening. (7)
AUR. Ha, 337 - Very much given to feel offended; the slightest thing which he

thought offensive affected him deeply, and caused him to resent it.
Ha, 28 - Excessively disposed to take offense; even the least thing seeming offensive to him, affected him deeply and caused resentment.
CHAM. He, 16 - Moaning on account of a very trifling offense, which had happened a long time ago.
CHOC. Sh, 324 - Still snapping and resentful generally.[15], 30C, 36:XX:XX
DROS. Ha, 281 - He takes insults very resentfully, not without vexation.
HALI-L. Sh, 110 - In the evening I felt very different in relating in bed with my husband. It hasn't been nice for a long time because of my long-standing resentment towards him. It was as if there was no history between us, relating more in the moment. It was nice to be cuddling without feeling pressured by him or myself. We were communicating. 09, 6C, 01:05:25
Sh, 170 - More self confident and self accepting than in the past. Questioning the times I'm not confident, and what to do about it. Instead of viewing it in a paranoid way, I'm treating it in a more matter of fact way. My feelings changed about certain people at work who have bothered me. Bouncing back quicker. Before, hours and hours would pass thinking about it. 18, 30C, 01:13:30
Sh, 572 - Dwell on past disagreeable occurrences. Hold a grudge. 16, 10C, 33:XX:XX
HYDROG. Sh, 114 - I feel quite resentful about having to hurry. 08, 30C, 09:XX:XX
MANG. Ha, 329 - Embittered humor; he could not forget injustice done to him; he fostered (support) resentment for a long time.
Ha, 14 - Embittered humor; irreconcilable and long-continued resentment against those who injure him.
NAT-M. Ha, 68 - Hatred (rancor, resentment) against persons, who had formerly offended him.
He, 43 - Hateful and vindictive nature.
NEON. Sh, 175 - I've been in a rotten mood all day, dwelling on past offenses. I just can't let go, it's making me angry. I feel like I hate that bastard; it's not an emotion I've had before. Now I feel vindictive, really awful; I feel that if I ever found out that he had been lying to me again I would say to him, "I'll kill you," "I'll slit your throat." These violent feelings were much eased when alone. 02, 6C, 04:22:40
NIT-AC. Al, 5 - Long-continued rancor, insensible to apologies and excuses.
Ha, 51 - Long-continued rancor; insensible to apology and excuses.
He, 19-...headstrong (obstinate); trembling while quarreling; fits of rage with curses and maledictions; inveterate ill-will, unmoved by apologies.
SULPH. Al, 8 - Numerous morbid ideas, extremely disagreeable, causing rancor, though with also joyous thoughts (and melodies) mostly from the past, take possession of her they throng one upon another so that she cannot free herself from them during the day, with neglect of business,...
He, 8 - Numerous morbid ideas, extremely disagreeable, causing rancor; neglect of business;...

RESERVED

Affection; demonstrate, cannot: nat-m.[189] sep.[137]
Ailments from; grief, cry, cannot: aeth.[162] am-m.[85] apis[36] carc.[146] crot-c.[36] ***gels.*** ign.[36] kali-fcy.[198] **NAT-M.** nux-v.[5] op.[36] puls.[36]
Ailments from; love disappointed, grief, with silent: **IGN. NAT-M. PH-AC.** phos.
Anger; introversion, with: lap-gr-m.[194]
Cares; full of, quietly: ***coff.***[54]
Censorious; find fault or is silent, disposed to: hydrog.[222] ***verat.***
Delirium; quiet: **BRY.** calc-sil.[58] camph.[54] ***carb-v. chel.*** chin. chlf.[54] ***chlor.*** croc. cupr. cupr-acet.[58] **HYOS.** hyosin.[36] kali-p.[54] op. past.[36] ***ph-ac.*** phos. plb. rhus-t. sec. tab. valer. verat.
Delusions; sensations, misrepresents his: bell.
• sorrow, everyone he meets has a secret: cann-i.
Discouraged; quiet, and: lyc.[10]
Excitement; alternating with, taciturn, afternoon: thiop.[149]
Expressing, oneself; difficult: crot-h.[137] kali-br.[25] lil-t.[36] thuj.[5]

Expressing, oneself; impossible: bell.[10] cann-i.[10] haem.[10] lyc.[10] ***nux-v.***[10] phys.[36] puls.[10] sep.[36] thuj.[10]
Fear; introversion, of: carc.[207]
✦ taciturn, after: ***ign.***[54]
Haughty; introverted, and: lap-gr-m.[194]
Hysteria; mild, gentle, yielding, although whimsical and introverted: ***ign.***[54]
Indifference; taciturn: bac.[62] bamb-a.[1184] calc.[10] ***hell.***[54] ***nit-s-d.***[54] plat.[10] staph.[10]
Insanity; character, of sombre: nat-sal.[36]
Insanity; secretive: dig.[1]
Introspection: **ACON.**[5] alum. am-m.[5] ***ambr.***[5] ***anh.***[119] arg.[149] arn.[5] ***aur.*** bamb-a.[1184] bell. bism.[5] bov. cann-i.[36] canth.[5] caps.[5] carb-an. carc.[214] carl.[36] caust. cham. ***chin.***[122] choc.[222] cic.[36] clem. **COCC.** cycl. dig. dros.[5] euph. euphr.[5] germ.[222] hell. hyos.[5] **IGN.** ***indg.***[54] ***ip.*** lil-t.[58] lyc.[5] mag-m. med.[56] meny.[5] mez. morg.[136] mur-ac. nux-v. ol-an.[36] olnd.[5] op.[5] ozone[227] phel.[36] plb.[5] **PULS.** ***rheum***[5] sabad.[5] sars. ***sep.***[54] stann. staph.[5] stram.[5] ***sulph.*** verat.[5] ***viol-t.***[5]
Introverted: ambr.[187] arist-cl.[161] aur.[193] carc.[193] ***cham.***[8] chin.[187] ***cocc.***[137] con.[193] cupr.[193] ***ign.***[8] ***indg.***[8] kali-c.[193] lach.[187] lap-gr-m.[194] lyc.[187] ***med.***[162] ***merc.***[162] ***mur-ac.***[8] nat-c.[193] nat-m.[187] nat-s.[193] ol-an.[137] ozone[227] psor.[185] ***puls.***[137] sep.[187] ***staph.***[162] thuj.[193]
Irritability; silent: puls.[1]
Irritability; taciturn: am-c.[10] ars.[10] calc.[54] coloc.[10] puls.[10] sulph.[10]
Jesting; alternating with, taciturnity: plat.[10]
Laughing; alternating with, taciturnity: plat.[10]
Loquacity; alternating with, silence: bell.[1] buth-aust.[144] cimic.[122] ign.[36]
Mania; alternating with, silence and refusing to talk: verat.[102]
Quarrelsomeness; alternating with, sadness, silent: ***con.***
Quiet disposition; masturbation, in: ***hyos.***[54]
Religious affections; taciturnity, haughtiness, voluptuousness, cruelty, r. a with: ***plat.***[54]
Reserved: acon.[10] aeth. agar.[10] alco.[36] alum. alum-p.[58] am-br.[162] am-c.[10] am-m.[10] ambr.[10] anac.[10] ant-t.[10] aq-mar.[231] arg-n. arn.[30] ars. asar.[162] aur. aur-ar.[58] bell. bism. bor.[10] cact.[116] ***calc.*** cand-a.[239] canth.[10] caps. carb-an. carc.[146] caust. cham. chin. cic.[10] cina[10] clem. cocc.[10] coloc. con.[10] cupr.[10] cycl. dig.[10] dros. euph. euphr. fl-ac.[58] graph.[10] grat. guai.[10] ***hell.*** hep.[10] hydrog.[222] ***hyos. ign.*** indg. ip. kalm.[10] lach. led.[10] lyc. mag-c. mag-m.[10] ***mang.*** meny.[5] merc.[10] mez.[10] ***mur-ac.*** nat-c.[10] nat-m. nit-ac. nux-m.[10] nux-v. olnd. op. petr. ph-ac. **PHOS.**[122] pitu-a.[164] ***plat.*** plb. ***puls.*** rheum sabad. sabin. sars.[10] sep.[10] sil.[58] spig.[10] spong. squil.[10] ***stann. staph.***[137] stront-c.[10] sul-ac.[10] sulph.[10] thuj.[10] verat. viol-o.[2] viol-t.[10]
Reserved; displeasure: aur.[137] ign.[137] ip.[137] nat-m.[137] ***staph.***[137]
Reserved; light, with aversion to: con.[10]
Reserved; noise, with sensitivity to: con.[10]
Sadness; talk, indisposed to: **ARG-N.**[54] ***ars.***[10] bar-c.[10] ***cact.***[116] ign.[30] mag-c.[54] nit-ac.[10] ph-ac.[30] ***puls.***[54] stann.[54] tarent.[192] verat.[116]
Secretive; eating, while: lac-h.[229]
Self-sufficient; help of others, needs no: calc.[189] mag-c.[214]
Sit; still, silent: alum.[1] alum-p.[58] alum-sil.[58] arn. aur. aur-s.[58] bar-c.[58] bar-i.[58] bar-m.[58] brom. calc-sil.[58] carbn-s.[58] cham. chin-ar. choc.[222] cimic.[58] coca[25] ***cocc.*** con.[1] elaps fl-ac.[58] ***gels.*** ham.[36] hell. ***hep.*** **HIPP.** hyos.[58] ***ign.***[54] kali-acet.[58] kali-chl.[58] kali-sil.[58] lyc.[58] mag-p.[78] nat-p.[58] ***nux-v.***[54] ol-an.[85] ***pic-ac.***[122] ***plat.*** **PULS.** ***sep.*** stram. thala.[149] **VERAT.**[122] zinc-p.[58]
Suicidal disposition; prepares himself silently: **AUR.**[122]
Suspiciousness; reserved, and, during pregnancy: ***puls.***[54]
Sympathy; compassion, bars all sympathy of friends: arg.[58]
Sympathy; compassion, desire, for, vexed by, but: camph.[54] nat-m.[58]
Talk; indisposed, alternating with, jesting: plat.[10]
Talk; indisposed, alternating with, laughing: plat.[10]
Talk; indisposed, alternating with, quarrelsomeness: ***con.***
Talk; indisposed, alternating with, violence: aur-ar.[58]
Talk; indisposed, anger, during: croc.[36]
Talk; indisposed, closed sensation in throat, with: nat-p.[36]
Talk; indisposed, company, in: arg.[58] hydrog.[222]
Talk; indisposed, condition, about her: chel.[36]

Talk; indisposed, die, as if he would: ***mur-ac.***[54]
Talk; indisposed, foreign language which at other times he speaks fluently: pall.[54]
Talk; indisposed, grief, during: peti.[36]
Talk; indisposed, illness or injuries, about: **BAPT.**[54]
Talk; indisposed, mortification, after: ***ign.***[54]
Talk; indisposed, sadness, in: **ARG-N.**[54] ***ars.***[10] bar-c.[10] ***cact.***[116] clem.[1] ign.[30] mag-c.[54] nit-ac.[10] ph-ac.[30] ***puls.***[54] stann.[54] verat.[116]
Talk; indisposed, sexual abuse, after: **STAPH.**[54]
Talk; indisposed, sufferings, over his: ign.[5]
Talk; intend, says what she does not: germ.[222] nat-m.[36]
Unfriendly humor: am-c. mag-m. plat. rauw.[119]

ADAM. Sh, 134 - I am behaving differently with strangers, containing myself, letting them make the first move. 7, 6C, 07:21:30
Sh, 135 - I am less grumpy during the day. People are saying I am holding back, different, not so open. 7, 6C, 07:21:30
Sh, 182 - Feel disconnected and distanced from everything. It's like keeping something in reserve, more observing. 7, 6C, 06:22:30
AETH. Al, 15 - The disposition becomes retiring (reserved) and tearful, as in nostalgia.
Al,S-11 - Disposition becomes retiring (reserved) and tearful, as in nostalgia.
ALOE. Al, 40-...wrap up in himself (introspection), as after a sickness or a fit of anger, which still gnaws (bite) internally, which one cannot express.
AM-C. He, 5 - Gloomy, depressed, with feeling of impending trouble,...
ANDROC. Sh, 61 - Felt constrained and had a gloomy approach to everything, averse company, desire to be alone. I feel people will not want to talk or be with me. (28)
Sh, 99 - Felt angry, did not want to speak to anyone, in the evening with friends he felt very lively, self-confident and forceful, rather biting at times. (4)
AUR. He, 80 - Ailments from fright, anger, contradiction, mortification, or vexation with dread, fear, reserved displeasure, or vehemence.
BRASS. Sh, 1 - General feeling of aloofness 08, 6C, 04:12:30
Sh, 2 - Feeling of aloofness still present, feeling of separation from others not so noticeable when with the children 08, 6C, 05:00:00
Sh, 13 - My wife was very emotional saying she would be happier if I left, yet my reaction was how inconvenient. I did not become emotionally involved. Also a friend at work asked me if I was alright as he thought I'd not been quite with it recently. The proving experience was generally pleasant for me, and I felt low coming back to my old self, rather like going away on holiday and coming back to a messy house and all the things you have to do. Prover's wife said he'd been unbearable all that week, Rremote and not with us at allS. It was his tendency anyway, but it had been exaggerated. 08, 6C, 10:00:00
Sh, 16 - Prefer to be silent, not talk. There is much I could say but who really wants to listen 08, 6C, 05:00:00
CARB-AN. Ha, 6 - Inclination to solitude (isolation), sad and introverted (egotistic), she always only wishes to be alone, and she shuns every conversation.
CHAM. Al, 6 - Earnest (serious) and taciturn mood; reconciled to his fate (destiny), about which he is deeply affected (later action).
Ha, 491 - Serious reservedness; calm submission to his profoundly felt fate (destiny).
CHOC. Sh, 210 - Felt totally isolated and averse to company. Estranged himself from his family and friends and stopped all communication with them for a long period. Did not reply to letters and left no address. He seemed to hide away and literally disappear. The state of Isolation resulted from feeling that "I didn't exist as a human being". This behaviour was in strong contrast to his normal sociable disposition. 35, 30C, XX:XX:XX:
CIMIC. He, 26 - Indifferent, taciturn, takes no interest in household matters.
CIMX. He, 4 - Sensation as if he would creep (slide) into himself, and on that account could not sufficiently crouch (bend, incline) together.

CROT-T. He, 5 - Feeling as though one cannot think outside of himself, "feels all pent up" (restricted, limited, confined, circumscribed) inside, and no chance for thoughts to flow out; as if hide-bound.(obstinate)

DROS. Al, 14 - Taciturn, quiet, and anxious; he was constantly in dread (fear) of hearing something unpleasant.

Ha, 273 - Silent and reserved, with anxiety he always feared he was about to learn (discover) something disagreeable.

HALI-L. Sh, 341 - Can't be bothered to write symptoms down because they seem so minor. Feel this is too private. 02, 30C, 04:XX:XX

HELL. Ha, 287 - Wrapped (envelop) up in his own thoughts, silent humour, all the afternoon.

HELON. Al, 4-.... could not endure the least contradiction or receive any suggestions in regard to any subject (fixed ideas) ;... what I most desired was to be left alone, reserved to myself the privilege of finding fault (imperfection) with everything around me;....

HYDROG. Sh, 174 - Emotionally cold and non-communicable with anger felt in stomach. 12, 6C, 17:XX:XX

Sh, 210 - I was shouting down the phone, but dead quiet with friends. I thought "Why are they talking? They haven't anything to say". I was very sarcastic. 24, 30C, 01:XX:XX

Sh, 231 - Silent, morose and introverted, with headache. 12, 6C, 05:06:45

Sh, 234 - Developed a self pitying, very tearful depression through the morning. I was unable to communicate any of these feelings and this led to a fierce row with girlfriend. 04, 12C, 30:XX:XX

IGN. He, 14 - Inclined to be very secretive (taciturn) and passive.(yielding)

He, 62 - Ill effects (ailments) from hearing bad news; from vexation with reserved displeasure ; from grief, or suppressed mental sufferings; of shame and disappointed love.

IP. He, 13 - Ailments from vexation (worry) and reserved displeasure.

IRID. Sh, 39 - I am less reserved than normal, more confident; but my boundaries have altered. I get less drawn into other people's emotional problems, less sympathetic. I26

KALI-AR. He, 1 - Scolding (censorious) morose, retired, quarrelsome and discontented, jealous, indifferent to everything,...

LYC. He, 39 - Ailments from fright, anger, mortification, or vexation, with reserved displeasure.

MANG. Ha, 324 - Cross reflective, silently reserved, wrapped up in himself, with discomfort in the whole body, ...

MED. Al,N-48 - It is also introspective, self-accusative, remorseful. Time moves slowly to it, therefore it is hurried.

MENY. Al, 3 - Quiet, reserved, contented with himself all day.

MEZ. Ha, 8 - Introverted, tired of life and longing for death.

MUR-AC. Al, 5 - Sad absorbed in herself, as if there were no life (inert, lifeless) in her during menses.

Ha, 266 - Silent reserve, with anxious concern about the present and future.

Ha, 2 - Sad and introverted, as if she had no life in her, during the menses.

Ha, 4 - Deep reflection, and quiet introversion, as if something unpleasant was impending,...

He, 2 - Taciturn, introverted and quiet; anxious care about future.

NAT-M. He, 48 - Consequences (ailments) of fright, anger, vexation, mortification, or reserved displeasure.

NUX-M. Al, 48 - He never accomplishes what she undertakes, but remains standing in one place, absent minded; he appears quite changed to his companions.

PLAT. He, 8 - Arrogant, reserved, absent-minded.

He, 23 - Satiety of life, with taciturnity and fear of death.

PULS. He, 46 - Dark suspicious and reserved manner; disturbed look on face; sleepless; looks for her bed in the yard (lost?); hides in a corner to escape from a little gray man who wanted to pull out her leg;...

STANN. Ha, 648 - Silent reserved disposition; he thought about the present and the future and was much concerned (care) about the latter.

Ha, 16 - The mind is quiet, introverted, solicitous (anxiety) about the future.

STAPH. Ha, 691 - Serious, silent, occupied with himself, he speaks but little.
Ha, 693 - Phlegmatic (indifferent), prostrate mind and sad disposition, unsympathetic, indifferent to all externals, yet not cross or exhausted.
He, 12 - Ailments from indignation and vexation, or reserved displeasure ;sleeplessness.
He, 14-...; was insulted (slandered, defamed, calumniated) being too dignified (reserved, lordly,) to fight (contest), subdued (control) his wrath(anger) and went home sick,.. (ailments, from offenses)
TARENT. He, 2 - Great taciturnity and irritability; desire to strike himself and others.
VERAT-V. He, 4 - Puerperal mania: silent, suspicious; will not see physician, he seems to terrify her; fears being poisoned;...
VERAT. He, 24 - Disposed to silence, or to talk about faults of others; if irritated scolding and calling names.

RESTLESS

Activity: acon.[5] acon-f.[36] agar.[36] agav-t.[149] aloe[5] amn-l.[119] anag.[54] ang.[5] ant-c.[8] ***apis***[5] arag.[85] arg-cy.[54] arist-cl.[161] arn.[5] ars.[5] ars-s-f.[54] ars-s-r.[54] aur.[5] aur-ar.[58] aur-s.[58] ***ba-tn.***[136] bad.[36] bar-c.[5] bell.[5] ***brom.***[5] bry.[5] ***calc.***[5] camph.[36] cann-i.[36] cann-s.[5] canth.[36] caps.[5] carb-ac.[36] carbn-o.[36] carbn-s.[36] chin.[5] chlor.[54] choc.[222] cic.[149] cimic.[5] ***cinnb.***[54] clem.[36] cob-n.[149] coca[36] cocain.[72] ***cocc.***[5] **COFF.**[5] coff-t.[36] cortiso.[149] ***cycl.***[5] dig.[5] eaux[36] eucal.[36] euphr.[5] fl-ac.[5] flor-p.[149] form.[36] fuc.[36] gaert.[136] galv.[10] gamb.[10] gels.[36] germ.[222] ***helon.***[5] hura[36] ***hyos.***[5] hyper.[54] iber.[36] ***ign.***[5] **IOD.**[5] ip.[5] iris[36] ***kali-br.***[5] kali-s.[58] lac-h.[229] **LACH.**[5] laur.[5] lil-t.[36] lycps.[8] m-p-a.[1] mag-c.[5] mag-m.[5] manc.[36] mesm.[5] mez.[36] ***morg.***[136] morph.[36] mosch.[10] mur-ac.[36] naja[36] nat-ar.[58] nat-c.[5] nep.[144] nitro-o.[36] nux-v.[5] **OP.**[5] ox-ac.[60] penic.[149] **PHOS.**[5] ***phys.***[36] pic-ac.[5] pip-m.[36] plb.[5] puls.[5] raph.[36] reser.[149] sarr.[36] scut.[114] ***sep.***[5] sil.[36] spig.[36] **STANN.**[5] staph.[5] stram.[5] stry.[36] sul-ac.[5] sulph.[5] sumb.[36] tarent.[5] thea.[36] **VALER.**[5] verat.[5] viol-o.[5] visc.[119] wies.[36] zinc-fcy.[36] zing.[36]
Activity; ceaseless: bar-c.[30] lach.[30] verat.[30]
Activity; desire for, exercise, physical: **BELL.**[36] cann-i.[36] coca[36] crot-c.[36] erech.[36] eucal.[36] orig.[36] phos.[36] ziz.[36]
Activity; hyperactive: agav-t.[149] chin.[47] cob-n.[149] gaert.[136] hyos.[5] ign.[10] lach.[155] lil-t.[36] op.[5] sep.[162] spig.[5] spong.[5] tarent.[187] verat.[5] verb.[5]
Activity; increased excessively: anag.[54] ang.[54] ant-c.[54] ars-s-r.[54] ***bell.***[54] canth.[54] carb-ac.[54] chlor.[54] ***cinnb.***[54] **COFF.**[54] ***coff-t.***[54] hyper.[54] ***op.***[54] ***phos.***[54] phys.[54] zing
Activity; night: ***agar.***[58] dig.[30] hydrog.[222] ***lach.***[36] nitro-o.[36] sin-n.[36] stann.[1158]
Activity; restless: dig.[36] ign.[30] lach.[30] lycps.[36] nux-v.[10] verat.[10] viol-o.[137]
Ailments from; anxiety: aur.[58] calc.[122] calc-p. cimic.[8] hyos.[10] kali-p.[58] lyc.[36] nit-ac.[36] ph-ac.[10] samb.[8] **SIL.**[54] staph.[36]
Ailments from; excitement, general symptoms from: acet-ac. **ACON.**[5] agar.[85] ***ambr.***[5] anac.[58] ***arg-n. arn.*** ars.[85] asaf.[116] aster. ***aur. bell.***[10] bry.[10] ***calc.*** calc-ar. calc-p. **CAPS.** ***caust.*** **CHAM.**[5] cimic.[122] ***cist. cob.*** **COCC.**[5] coch. cod.[85] **COFF.** coff-t.[85] **COLL.** coloc.[163] ***con.*** convo-s.[119] croc.[163] ***cupr.***[8] cypr.[85] dys-co.[136] epip.[85] ferr.[85] **GELS.** ***glon.*** goss.[122] hyos.[5] **IGN.**[5] ***kali-br.*** kali-c.[5] ***kali-p.*** kreos. lach.[10] lyc. lycps.[163] ***lyss.*** m-p-a.[1] med. merc.[163] morg-g.[136] nat-c. ***nat-m.*** nat-p.[163] nit-ac. nux-m. ***nux-v. op.***[163] ***pall.*** petr.[102] **PH-AC.** ***phos.*** phys.[85] plat.[5] prot.[136] ***psor.*** **PULS.** sac-alb.[85] samb.[85] scut.[77] sel.[5] ***sep.***[122] stann.[85] **STAPH.** stram.[163] ***sumb.***[163] ***tarent.***[122] thuj.[163] **TUB.**[122] valer.[163] ***verat.*** vesp.[58] ***zinc.***
Ailments from; excitement, general symptoms from, long lasting: petr.[137]
Anger; activity, with great physical: ***plat.***[54]
Anguish; driving from place to place: **ARS.** ***rhus-t.***[54]
Anguish; driving from place to place, restlessness, with: **ACON.**[54] **ARS.**[54] ***ars-i.***[162] **BISM.**[54]
Anguish; restlessness, with: **ACON.**[137] ***ars.***[137] aur.[172] bell.[54]
Anxiety; bed, driving out of: ars.[1] ars-s-f.[172] bar-s.[172] bry.[10] carb-v. carbn-s.[10] caust.[10] ***cham.***[10] chin.[10] chin-s.[10] germ.[222] graph.[1] ***hep.***[10] hyos.[60] lyss.[54] nat-m.[10] nit-ac.[1] ***puls.***[54] ***rhus-t.***[1] sul-ac.[172]
Anxiety; chest, heart, region of, driving him from place to place: ars.[172] aur.[172]

Anxiety; conscience, no rest night or day, prevents lying down: ***phos.***[54]
Anxiety; conscience, of, no rest night or day, prevents lying down: ***phos.***[54]
Anxiety; driving from place to place: acon.[10] aeth.[10] alum.[10] am-c.[10] ambr.[10] anac.[10] ***ars.***[54] asaf.[10] aur.[116] bell.[10] bov.[10] bry.[58] calc.[10] calc-p.[60] camph.[10] caps.[10] carb-an.[10] carb-v.[10] caust.[10] ***cham.***[54] chin.[10] chin-s.[10] cimic.[60] coff.[10] croc.[60] crot-h.[10] dros.[10] ***graph.***[54] hell.[63] hep.[63] iod.[116] lact.[10] lam.[60] m-arct.[10] meny.[10] ***merc.***[10] nat-c.[10] nat-m.[10] nit-ac.[10] nux-v.[10] op.[10] ph-ac.[10] phos.[10] plat.[10] puls.[10] rhus-t.[10] ruta[10] sabad.[10] sep.[10] sil.[60] spig.[10] spong.[10] staph.[1] sul-i.[58] ***tab.***[60] valer.[10] verat.[10] zinc.[60]
Anxiety; fly away, as if she must, no peace anywhere: ***bell.***[54]
Anxiety; sudden, oppression of chest, with, driving from place to place: ***tab.***[54]
Delirium; quiet, alternating with restlessness and desire to run away: ***chlor.***[54]
Delirium; restless: absin.[171] acon. ail.[58] ***ars.***[60] atro. bry.[116] **HYOS.**[54] iod.[116] merc-s.[54] phos.[36] plb. sant.[25] ***stram.***[54] sulph.[116] ***verat.***[54]
Delusions; floating, bed, resting in is not: ***lach.*** stict.
Dreams; anxious, restless: ***ars.***[54] ***led.***[54]
➤ fights, fitful slumbers, in: phos.[36]
➤ striving and urging, anxious: rhus-t.[1]
Excitement; alone, when: ars.[10]
Excitement; alternating with indecision: cortiso.[149]
Excitement; alternating with, sadness: ambr.[58] aster.[36] colch.[149] ***con.*** cortiso.[149] eug.[102] ferr-p.[58] foll.[149] ox-ac.[58] petr.[60] phenob.[149] ***plb.***[54] rad-br.[149] rauw.[149] sul-ac.[10] thyr.[85] thyreotr.[149]
Excitement; alternating with, taciturn, afternoon: thiop.[149]
Excitement; anger, with inclination to, and to scold: ***petr.***[54]
Excitement; anticipating events, when: ***arg-n. gels.*** hydrog.[222] kali-br. med.
Excitement; bad news, after: ***apis calc.*** calc-p. chin. cinnb. cupr. form. **GELS.** ***ign.*** kali-c. kali-p. lach. nat-c. nat-m. phos. puls. stram. ***sulph.***
Excitement; bath, during: gast.[36]
Excitement; coition, after: ***calc.***
Excitement; contradiction, from slightest: ***ferr.***[54]
Excitement; conversation, from hearing: ***lyss.***
Excitement; curses his mother, throws food or medicine across room: ***hydr.***[54]
Excitement; dancing, singing and weeping, with: tarent.[58]
Excitement; debate, during: ***caust. nit-ac.***
Excitement; desire for: carc.[187] cot.[36] germ.[222]
Excitement; frantic: atro.[54] camph.[54] hyosin.[85] ***kali-i.***[54]
Excitement; frantic, hypochondriasis, in: ***arg-n.***[54]
Excitement; heart, organic disease of, in: ***apis***[54]
Excitement; hope, as in joyous: ***aur.***[54] choc.[222]
Excitement; horrible things, after hearing: ***calc. chin.***[122] cic.[58] cocc. gels. ign. ***lach.*** nat-c. nux-v. ***teucr. zinc.***
Excitement; hungry, when: kali-c.
Excitement; lascivious, with painful nocturnal erections: ***merc.***[54]
Excitement; mental work, from: ambr.[85] ind. kali-p. med. nat-p.[1] tub.
Excitement; religious: agar.[36] ***aur.*** plb.[8] stram. sulph. verat.
Excitement; sadness, after: ***cann-i.***[116] spig.
Excitement; sadness, before: nat-m.[85]
Excitement; unemployed, when: sulph.[10]
Excitement; water poured out, from hearing: **LYSS. STRAM.**
Fear; bed, of the, sit up and wander about the house as for them the nights are too long and restlessness comes with approaching day: syph.[172]
✦ driving him from place to place: acon.[10] aeth.[10] alum.[10] am-c.[10] ambr.[10] asaf.[10] aur.[116] bell.[10] bov.[10] bry.[58] calc-p.[60] camph.[10] caps.[10] carb-an.[10] carb-v.[10] caust.[10] chin.[10] chin-s.[10] cimic.[60] coff.[10] croc.[60] crot-h.[10] dros.[10] hep.[63] iod.[116] lact.[10] lam.[60] m-arct.[10] meny. ***merc.***[10] nat-c.[10] nat-m.[10] nit-ac.[10] nux-v.[10] op.[10] ph-ac.[10] phos.[10] plat.[10] puls.[10] rhus-t.[10] ruta[10] sabad.[10] sep.[10] sil.[60] spig.[10] spong.[10] staph.[10] sul-i.[58] ***tab.***[60] valer.[10] verat.[10] zinc.[60]
✦ driving him from place to place, dyspnea, in: ***acet-ac.***[54] acon-f.[36] ars.[60] astac.[54] bism.[54] ***carb-an.***[54] hydr-ac.[60] ***kalm.***[54] kreos.[60] ***lyc.***[54] ***phos.***[54] plat.[60] seneg.[60] **SPONG.**[54] viol-o.[54]
✦ injured, of being, stay in bed, would not: ***cupr-acet.***[54]
✦ jumps, out of bed from: ***ars.*** **BELL.**[54] stann.[54]

✦ suffocation, bed, drives him out of, at night: ***dig.***[54]
Home; desires to go, go out, and when there: ***bry.***[54] ***calc.***[54] **CALC-P.**[54] ***cupr-acet.***[54]
Impatience; runs about, never sits or sleeps at night: ***iod.***[54]
Impulse; run, to, dromomania: acon.[5] all-s.[36] androc.[222] bell.[5] bufo[5] calc.[161] cann-i.[36] canth.[5] dig.[1] glon.[36] **HYOS.**[5] ***iod.*** mez.[36] ***nux-v.***[5] orig.[5] phys.[36] **STRAM.**[5] tarent.[36] **TUB.**[122] **VERAT.**[5]
Indifference; alternating with, anxiety and restlessness: ant-t.[54] nat-m.
Insanity; restlessness, with: ***ars.***[10] bell.[30] bry.[30] canth.[10] chin.[30] ***hyos.***[10] merc.[10] nux-v.[10] puls.[30] stram.[10] verat.[30]
Irritability; restless: bism.[36] hyos.[54] mag-c.[54] ozone[227] sil.[54] staph.[1] valer.[54]
Lasciviousness; rest, no: ***orig.***[54]
Mania; action, must be constantly in, in some laborious occupation: ***iod.***[54]
Restlessness; abdomen, constricted, as if everything in, was: mosch.[60]
Restlessness; alone, when, agg.: all-s. mez. ***phos.***
Restlessness; alternating with, fainting: vip.[36]
Restlessness; alternating with, indifference: nat-m.[10]
Restlessness; alternating with, sadness: apis[5]
Restlessness; anger, from: ***cham.***[116] **COLOC.**[54]
Restlessness; angina pectoris, in: ***aur-m.***[54]
Restlessness; anxious, driving from place to place: ***tab.***[122]
Restlessness; anxious, has to do something: ***bry.***[54]
Restlessness; anxious, has to, walk rapidly: androc.[222] ***arg-n.*** **ARS.** cimic.[144] lil-t. sul-ac. **TARENT.**
Restlessness; anxious, megrim, in: aeth.[54]
Restlessness; anxious, rage, ending in: ***canth.***[54]
Restlessness; anxious, thunderstorm, especially during, music agg.: ***nat-c.***[54]
Restlessness; ardent: **NUX-V.**[54]
Restlessness; bashful, timid, ill at easy in society: ***coca***[54]
Restlessness; busy: acon.[10] ars.[127] ***aur.***[10] bell.[10] bry.[10] caps.[1] choc.[222] cocc.[1] dig.[10] hyos.[10] ***ign.***[1] ip.[10] ***lach.***[10] m-arct.[10] ***mosch.***[10] nat-c.[10] nux-v.[30] stann.[10] sul-ac.[10] ther.[123] verat.[1]
Restlessness; careful: **NUX-V.**[54]
Restlessness; cares, from: kali-br.[85]
Restlessness; coition, after: **CALC.** cop. dig. mez.[122] petr. ***sep.*** staph.[122]
Restlessness; company, in: androc.[222] ***carb-v.*** mez.[162] staph.[162]
Restlessness; conversation, from: ***ambr.***
Restlessness; crime, as if he had committed a: ***alum.***[54]
Restlessness; cutting himself while shaving: calad.[54]
Restlessness; drives him from place to place: acon.[10] ***am-c.***[10] ***ars.***[122] aur.[10] ***bell.***[10] bism.[10] ***calc-p.***[122] canth.[10] carb-v.[10] ***cedr.***[122] cench.[58] cimic.[149] crot-h.[10] ***cupr.***[116] dros.[10] graph.[10] ***hist.***[149] hyos.[10] iod.[10] kali-i.[58] kres.[144] lac-h.[229] ***lach.***[10] lyss.[54] meny.[10] merc.[10] nat-c.[10] nux-v.[10] plat.[10] prun.[10] puls.[10] sep.[10] sol-m.[10] spig.[10] stann.[10] staph.[10] ***tab.***[10] tarax.[10] tarent.[58] thlaspi[111] verat.[10]
Restlessness; duty, as if he had not done his: ***puls.***[54]
Restlessness; fainting, followed by: calc.
Restlessness; hemorrhage, during uterine: apis[54] op.[54] pyrog.[54]
Restlessness; hunger, with: abies-n.[72] iod.[187] kali-c.[148] nat-m.[36] podo.[8]
Restlessness; hypochondriacal: ars.[10] ***asaf.***[54] graph.[36] valer.[10]
Restlessness; hysterical: arg-n.[54] ***asaf.***[122] aur.[60] cast.[54] **GELS.**[54] **IGN.**[54] **MOSCH.**[54] plat.[54] valer.[60] viol-o.[54]
Restlessness; internal, beat about herself with hands and feet, as if he would: lyc.
Restlessness; internal, indecision to do something, with: bamb-a.[1184]
Restlessness; lascivious thoughts, from: graph.[36]
Restlessness; mild, amiable, refined, sensitive, intellectual: chim-m.[54]
Restlessness; move, must constantly: ***apis***[117] ***ars.***[122] ***bell.***[10] canth.[58] caust.[148] cench.[58] cham.[60] cimic.[116] coff.[26] cupr.[60] hep.[109] ign.[10] ***iod.***[122] ***kali-br.***[122] ***kreos.***[122] lap-gr-m.[194] ***led.***[162] manc.[122] ***puls.***[60] **RHUS-T.**[122] sac-alb.[210] sanic.[85] sol-n.[25] sul-i.[58] thlaspi[107] trom.[122] viol-o.[45]
Restlessness; music, from: nat-c. sabin.[102] tarent.
Restlessness; noises and singing in ears, with: ***coff.***[54]
Restlessness; rage, ending in a: canth.
Restlessness; rest, has none, at any employment: ***chel.***[54]

Restlessness; sadness, with: nux-v.[54] ***plat.***[54]
Restlessness; sensitive, hysterical people, anomalous functional disorders of the heart: sumb.[54]
Restlessness; sensitive, remains long impressed by even slight mechanical injuries: ***arn.***[54]
Restlessness; sexual excitement, in: ant-c.[10] cann-i.[102] ***canth.***[102] ***kali-br.***[102] kali-p.[85] ***raph.***[102] staph.[116]
Restlessness; storm, before: ***gels.***[54] ***psor.***
Restlessness; storm, during: gels. nat-c. ***nat-m. phos.*** psor.
Restlessness; suffocation, with threatening: gels.[85]
Restlessness; thunderstorm, before: psor.[122]
Restlessness; thunderstorm, during: nat-c.[60] nat-m.[60] phos.[1] rhod.[54]
Restlessness; thunderstorm, thunderbolt, after heavy, with terrific screams: ***gels.***[54]
Restlessness; timid: asar.[54] ***calc.***[54] **PULS.**[54] rhod.[54]
Restlessness; touch, on: nat-m.[189] oena.[60]
Restlessness; zealous: **NUX-V.**[54]
Shrieking; help, for, Springing up from bed: hep.[10] rhus-t.[10]
Stupor; alternating with, restlessness: ***acon.***[54] **ARS.**[36]
Suicidal disposition; thoughts, drive him out of bed: ***ant-c.***
Walk; must: acon.[36] ambr.[56] aur.[111] calc.[111] ***cham.***[5] dig.[111] ***dios.***[111] ign.[5] iod.[111] murx.[111] op.[111] paeon.[111] ruta[107] stront-c.[111] tarent.[111]
Walks more than is good for her: ars.[1]

ACON. Al, 49 - Anxiety which does not allow him to remain in one place, he must constantly walk about. (restlessness)
Al, 23 - Excessive restlessness, all movements and actions are performed with great haste and hurry.
Al, 14 - Excessive disagreeable restlessness; without occasion for hurrying, he is in the greatest haste, every obstacle that delays his rapid pace is excessively annoying; he knocks against some people who do not get out of his way fast enough, and runs in breathless haste up the steps;...
Al, 22 - Restlessness, uninterrupted, unpleasant; he must now sit, now stand, now walk, he does not know what is the matter.
He, 23 - Pains are so intolerable, they drive him crazy; he becomes very restless.
He, 31 - Restlessness, agony, internal anxiety; does everything in great haste (rapidity); must move about or change position often.
AGAR. Ha, 5 - The mind is restless and troubled; he was always solely occupied with his present and his future condition.
ALOE. Al, 17 - Great anxiety, timorousness, restlessness, dread (fear) of death, and great anguish, so that she cannot stay anywhere.(restlessness)
ALUM. Al, 17 - Anxiety with external heat and uneasiness as if she had done something bad.
ALUMN. Al, 9 - Excitability of feeling, as when one is agitated by unpleasant news.
AM-C. Ha, 11 - The mind is restless and feels uncanny. (mysterious, strange)
Ha, 12 - She finds no rest (restlessness), and prosper (realize, achieve) in nothing.
AML-N. He, 11 - Cannot sit still for fear of something dreadful happening.
ANAC. Ha, 4 - Internal anguish, which did not allow him to rest, he troubled himself about every trifle, as if it would cause great injure, with solicitude about the future.
ANDROC. Sh, 141 - Danced all night in a frenzy, could not keep still, and was frustrated when the music finished. (29)
Sh, 179 - Extreme anguish and restlessness, but at the same time felt like an observer of my condition, watching it all transpire without being able to change anything. Mind fixed on the physical anguish. It dominates my senses. (21)
ARG-N. He, 27 - If a time is set, becomes uneasy the day before; is worried and ready long before the time.(anticipation)
ARN. Ha, 620 - Restlessness of body and mind, as if he was prevented (obstructed) doing something necessary, whith complete indisposition for occupation.
ARS. Al, 70 - The anxiety and restlessness are indescribable; "Kill me", he cried, "or relieve my pains!".(help)
Ha, 1020 - Anxiety and restlessness in the whole body.
Ha, 1065-...extreme anxiety, restlessness; he had a great dread (fear) of the effects of the poison and desired to life.
Ha, 1008 - He can find no rest in any place,

continually changes his position in bed, will get out of one bed and into another, and lie now here, now there.

Ha, 71 - During the first minutes great tranquillity of soul and serenity; but after half a hour excessive restlessness and anxiety; he imagines that the effects of the poison would be dreadful and desires to remain alive.(in a despondent suicide).

He, 76 - Anxiety like that of one who has committed murder; driven from place to place; avoids meeting persons, thinking that he has offended them.

He, 77 - Terrible anxiety, flushing up; restless glance (look), no rest by day or night; inclination to commit suicide.

ASTER. Al, 5 - Melancholy, alternating with almost intolerable cerebral excitement; she is inclined to give herself up to mental or bodily work, to walk, or engage in a violent exercise;...

ATRO. Al, 33 - Mentally either very sad, depressed in constant anxiety and restlessness, fearful of misfortune, or angry and inclined to be alone, seldom lively.

AUR-M. He, 13 - Insurmountable mental or bodily restlessness; he has to spend hours in street and in open air. 0 Angina pectoris.

AUR. Ha, 345 - An urging to activity, bodily as well as mental; when he did anything, he thought he did not do it quick enough, and that he had a great deal (much) more to do; he could not live to his liking. (desire, aspiration)

Ha, 347 - Always very restless and undecided (doubtful) -thought he was neglecting something for which he must incur (obtain) reproach - ...he seemed to carry about this restlessness with him in his inmost (deepest) parts ; this condition deprived him of all perseverance, all energy.

Ha, 6 - Great anxiety springing from the region of the heart, and which drives him from one place to another, so that he cannot long remain in a place. (restlessness)

Ha, 11 - Restlessness and hurried impulse to bodily and mental activity; he can not work fast enough; he could not act so as to satisfy himself.

Ha, 12 - He is driven to constant activity, and is sorry for his inaction, although he cannot do anything.

Ha, 13 - Restless and undecided, without perceptible ebullition of the blood; he always thinks he is neglecting something for which he will be reproached; he seems to carry with him this internal restlessness, and it took from him all perseverance and energy.

He, 55 - Great anguish coming from precordial region, and driving him from place to place, so that he can remain nowhere.

BAR-A. Al, 6 - Great solicitude and anxious care.

BAR-C. Ha, 11 - Anxious and fearful; a little noise on the street seems to him at once like fire alarm, and he is frightened by it, so that it darts (move quickly) through all his limbs.

BELL. Ha, 1312 - By day great anxiety; she cannot rest (restlessness) anywhere; she feels as if she should run away.

Ha, 1329 - Great restlessness, she cannot remain long seated in one place; she is driven all about.

BRASS. Sh, 14 - Very irritable with no cause, snapping at the children for no reason; apathy, can't be bothered to do anything; restless, twitchy, can't settle to anything 3I, 00:04:00

BRY. Al, 13 - Anxiety in the whole body, which compelled him to do something constantly, and wherever he went he found no rest.

He, 46 - Restlessness: wants change; with fear of future; fear of death, which he thinks is near; with nocturnal heat.

He, 25 - Anxiety in whole body compelled him to do something constantly, wherever he went he found no rest.

CALC. Al, 22 - Anxious, restless, and busy mood; she is undertaking much things but accomplish nothing...

Ha, 22 - Timid and restless, as if evil (harmful, misfortune) was impending (imminent) over her.

CARBN-O. Al, 7 - Frightful anxiety, and instinctive impulse to seek change of air, while he felt powerless to overcome the paralysis of his muscles and move from where he sat.

CAUST. Ha, 7 - Anxious, restlessness mood, as if something disagreeable (difficult) was impending (imminent), which keeps him from working.

He, 33 - Anxious uneasy mood, as if something unpleasant impended (threaten, frighten); this unfits (incompetent) him for every kind of work.(lost: competence)
He, 17 - Great restlessness, which prompts him to run away.

CUPR. He, 18 - Unconquerable sadness, constant restlessness, as if some misfortune were approaching; fears he will lose his reason.

GERM. Sh, 15 - Wake feeling anxious, increasingly. Legs tremble and shake. I have to get out of bed. I am scared that a heart attack is imminent and cannot be prevented. It's to late to do anything. I walk from room to room, thirsty, chilly and in turmoil. Accompanied by a desire for stool and flatulence. 08, 12C, 80:00:00

GLON. He, 12 - Great mental agitation; attempts to run away; attempted to spring from window.

GRAPH. Al, 23 - He awoke at 2 a. m. with restless mood; everything that could injure him happened, and made him anxious, so that frequently he did not know where he should turn,...

HALI-L. Sh, 194 - Uptight, jittery, as from a lot of coffee. Inner agitation, tension. Anxious agitation welling up. 06, 6C, 05:13:00

HELL. Ha, 278 - Restless and anxious, as if anticipating misfortune.

HYDROG. Sh, 266 - While talking, restless, impatient and ill at ease, as if wanting to leave. 22, 12C, 06:XX:XX

HYOS. He, 79 - After being harshly (severe) accused of theft (crime), continual delirium; fancies surrounded by objects of a terrifying nature; not a moment quiet, continual calling out that she saw the devil; denies herself guilty of theft (innocent, injustice), or that she has any concern with witches; ...

IGN. Ha, 755 - Excessively busy: he restlessly sets about doing first one thing then another.
He, 39 - Anxiety and disquiet as if she had done something wrong, or as if some great misfortune were about to happen, this so overpowers her that she can with difficulty refrain from weeping;...

IOD. Ha, 17 - Restless moving about; she runs about incessantly and does not get to sit down, nor does she sleep at night, so that she has to be considered as crazy.
Ha, 18 - Restlessness, which keeps the body in constant activity.
He, 3 - Must keep in motion day and night (restlessness), brain felt as if it was stirred (agitation) up, felt as if going crazy.
He, 13 - Excessive kind of impatience, she is running about all the time and never sits down or sleeps at night.

JAMB. He, 2 - Nothing seemed right, when sitting, he wanted to lie; when lying, he wanted to rise again.

LED. Al, 11 - Morose mood, with much uneasiness and irresolution; he is unable to reflect constantly upon anything, or work with a quiet mind.

LIL-T. He, 12 - Listless, inert, yet does not want to sit still (quiet); restless, yet does not want to walk; hurried manner, desire to do something, yet feels no ambition; feeling as of imperative duties and utter (complete) inability (incapacity, incompetence) to perform them; sexual excitement.

LYC. Al, 113 - Excited, busy mood in the evening, without perseverance, changing from one subject to another, with difficulty of fixing the thoughts, and greater difficulty in accomplishing anything; while reading fell asleep...

LYSS. Al,N-129 - Hyperesthesia, current of air, bright light, sight of any shining object, slightest touch, even conversation in vicinity of patient, may throw him into a most violent agitation and bring on severe convulsions.

MANG. Ha, 326 - Persistent restlessness of disposition, just as if he were going to hear some bad news.
Ha, 330 - Great restlessness of body and disposition, as if something bothered him.
Ha, 2 - Constant restlessness, as if he apprehended some sad news.
Ha, 3 - Great restlessness of body and mind, as if something was tormenting him.

MENY. Ha, 286 - Cross, ill-humored and discontented with himself and his position (rank); anxiety drives him from one place to another.(restlessness)

MERC. Ha, 1222 - Restlessness, he cannot remain quiet in any place; he can neither stand nor lie, and is as if mad, or as if he had committed a great crime.

Ha, 1231 - He has no rest, and must go hither and thither, and cannot remain long in one place.

Ha, 1234 - Anxiety and apprehension in the blood, he knew not how to compose (control) himself; he felt as if he had committed a crime, without heat, also at the same time as if he was not quite master,(commander). of his senses all day. (lost: mastering, commander)

Ha, 1235 - Anxiety that could drive him far away, as if he had committed a crime or some misfortune were about to happen to him.-(transgression)

He, 16 - Great restlessness as if he had committed a great crime; ...considers everybody his enemy;...great inclination when walking to take people by the nose;...(desire: conduct, direct, guide)

He, 28 - Anxiety and restless change of place; ebullitions, sweat; apprehensive, imaginary fears; fears he will lose his mind;...(sanity).

He, 38 - Great restlessness, must constantly change her place; fear, with desire to escape, as if she had committed some crime.

MEZ. Ha, 7 - Restless when alone, he wishes to be in company.

He, 5 - No rest when alone; wants to be in company ...unable to repeat what has been learned by heart; looks through window for hours, without being conscious of objects around; knows not what she is about; forgets what she is about to utter (talk); looks ill humored, pale, wretched, fallen away; ......expecting some very unpleasant news.

MUR-AC. Ha, 267-...anxiety and restlessness in the upper extremities (as if in the blood vessels)...

NAJA. Al, 13-...I felt that everything that was done was done in a wrong way, and could not be rectified (corrected, revised); if I felt that I had some duty to perform (execute), I had at the same time a strong impulse not to do it, and I am extremely restless in consequence; I seemed to have an increased perception of what I ought to do, but, at the same time, an unaccountable inclination not to do it, to which I was irresistibly compelled to yield "I couldn't help it, didn't know why, but couldn't do it."

NAT-C. Al, 17 - Anxiety and restlessness; he thought he could do nothing properly.(rightly, correctly)

Al, 18 - Anxiety and hasty (fast) restlessness all day; he could not keep the limbs still, especially the arms; obliged to stretch them; it seemed as though they would be torn (cut) asunder. (in two divided).

Ha, 23 - Restlessness and unsteadiness (inconstant); he knew not what he wanted, nor what he should do or leave undone.

He, 9 - Restlessness, with attacks of anxiety, especially during a thunderstorm; < from music.

NAT-M. Al, 2761 - In a dream he reproached himself for past mistakes, full of restlessness and anxiety.

NIT-AC. Ha, 18 - In the evening, he feels apprehensive; he cannot sit still, but has to walk about.

Ha, 42 - Peevishness with sadness and a crabbed (irritable) humor with restlessness, so that she knows not where to turn (drive)

NUX-V. Al, 39 - Great anxiety; he had to rise from any place and wished rather (first) to die.

Ha, 1237 - Great anxiety; he cannot rest in any place, (restlessness) and would rather die.

PETR. He, 5 - Since confinement two weeks ago when in bed, in dark room, at night, delusion that there is another baby (small, tiny) in bed which requires attention also that she has a third leg which would not remain quiet.

PH-AC. Ha, 668 - Inward restlessness hinders (delay) him in his work.

PHOS. Al, 101 - Anxiety all night without heat, as if he had murdered some one, with constant tossing about.

Al, 107 - Anxiety and internal restlessness, without grounds (reason) therefor.

He, 7 - Anxious: filled with gloomy (dark) forebodings; as if about to die; about termination (conclude) of her illness (disease); and restless ; at twilight; when alone; about future; during a thunderstorm; ..

PLAT. Ha, 11 - Great restlessness of mind,

so that she knows not where to stay (indecision), with gloominess (melancholy) which spoils even what should be most enjoyable; she imagines she is not fit (unfit, incapable) for this world, is tired (weary) of life, but has a great horror of the death she believes to be approaching.

PULS. He, 43 - Sleepless nights on account of great fear and anxious restlessness; despairs of her salvation and seeks aid in constant prayer;...

RHUS-T. Ha, 960 - On account of inward (inside) uneasiness (agitation) she could not sit still, but must rock (shake) herself to and fro on her chair, and move all the limbs a little.

Ha, 961 - Very restless disposition, and anxiety and anguish, so that she had always a clutching (grasp) at the heart, with dyspnea.

Ha,(curative) 975 - He can master (leading, chief) his thoughts and think calmly (tranquillity) of any subject he will and as long as he likes, and at his pleasure take up some other topic, with tranquil, slow inspiration.

He, 22-... great restlessness and anguish as if she had committed a crime or as if she thought some terrible calamity impended; these feelings drove her from one place to another; could not rest quietly at night in bed; was robbed of sleep and all desire to live;...

He, 23 - Restlessness and anxiety about heart as if she had committed a crime or as if some great misfortune was in store (reserved) for her, is driven from one place to another; deprived of sleep and all desire to live; ...

ROB. Al, 3 - Moral agitation, great restlessness; he is always under the impression that he will be disgraced.

SEC. Al, 20 - She was conscious, but the room (space) presented to her the impression of water excessively agitated on its surface. She could compare it only to the "foaming of a troubled sea" (storm, tempest)

SEP. Al, 3 - Attacks of anger over past times come on involuntarily, through which he becomes so excited that he does not know what to do, accompanied by anxiety, palpitation of the heart, and sweat of the whole body.

Ha, 27 - Great internal restlessness, for many days, with hastiness (hurried); he wants to be done with his work even as he begins it.

Ha, 28 - Restless and lacking serenity, for many days; occupied with sad memories, and anxious, she has not the patience to stay long in place.

SPIG. He, 3 - Restless and anxious; solicitude about the future.

STANN. Ha, 8 - Restless and distracted, no perseverance in her work (at once).

STAPH. Ha, 704 - Great inward anxiety, so that he cannot remain in one place, but he says nothing about it.(restlessness)

SULPH. Ha, 30 - He greatly feels the need of tranquillity of spirit, as his spirit is ever active.

TARENT. Al, 65-...great haste in whatever I undertook, from a constant fear that something would happen to prevent my finishing it;...fear that something would fall on me (doom, disgrace);...fear of striking it against some imaginary object which appeared to be suspended....(hurt)

He, 14 - Paroxysms of insanity; restlessness of legs; threatening words of destruction and death.

TELL. Al, 2 - Her disposition is particularly quiet, being otherwise very lively, anxious and full of care.

VERAT. Ha, 713 - Busy restlessness; he undertakes many things, but becomes always tired of them, nothing succeeds with him.

REVENGEFUL

Delusions; vengeance, thinks he is singled out for Divine: **KALI-BR.**

• vindictive: agar.[10]

Dreams; vengeance, of talking: lach.[36]

Hatred; revenge, and: ***agar.***[5] aloe[5] am-c.[30] am-m.[5] ***anac.***[5] ***aur.***[5] calc.[5] cic.[5] fl-ac.[5] hep.[5] hydr.[5] lach.[58] led.[5] mang.[5] med.[212] mygal.[5] **NAT-M.**[5] **NIT-AC.**[5] op.[5] ***ph-ac.***[30] phos.[5] stann.[5] **SULPH.**[5] vip.[1212]

Insanity; malicious, malignant: agar.[10] cann-s.[10] ***cupr.*** lyc.[10]

Jealousy; revenge, desires to take: hyos.[30]

Malicious, spiteful, vindictive: abrot. ***acon.*** agar. alco.[36] aloe am-c. am-m. ambr. <u>**ANAC.**</u>[122] androc.[222] arn. **ARS.**[122] ars-s-f.[58] ***aur.*** aur-ar.[58] bar-c. ***bell.*** berb. ***bor.*** bry.[85]

bufo ***calc.*** calc-s. cand-a.[239] cann-s. canth. caps. carb-an. caust. cham.[111] chin. choc.[222] cic. clem. coca[30] cocc. coloc. com. con. croc. ***cupr.*** cycl.[10] cyna.[149] fl-ac.[30] gall-ac.[162] glon. guai. haem.[36] ***hep.*** hydr. ***hyos.*** ign. ilx-a.[120] ip.[10] kali-c.[10] kali-i. ***lac-c.*** lac-h.[229] ***lach.*** lap-c-b.[194] lap-mar-c.[194] ***led.*** levo.[149] ***lyc.*** mang. med.[189] merc. mosch. ***nat-c.***[122] **NAT-M.**[122] nicc. ***nit-ac.*** **NUX-V.** op. opun-a.[36] ozone[227] par. ped.[36] petr. ***ph-ac.***[30] phos. pitu-a.[164] plat. puls.[30] ran-b.[10] ***sac-alb.***[210] sarr.[36] sec. sep.[58] sol-m.[10] spong.[10] squil. stann. ***staph.***[30] **STRAM.** stront-c. sulph. syph.[122] tarent.[111] thuj.[5] **TUB.**[122] tus-f.[36] verat. zinc. zinc-p.[58]

Plans; revengeful: agar.

Somnambulism; strike sleepers, from vengeance, to: **NAT-M.**[30] nit-ac.[30]

AGAR. Al, 4 - He is intoxicated with fearless frenzy; forming bold (courageous, brave) and revengeful projects.

Ha, 20 - Drunken fearless frenzy with bold (courageous), vengeful determinations.

ALOE. He, 12 - An easily excited, angry, revengeful state of mind, could not brook opposition (contradiction), wanted to destroy object of wrath, relief from tea or milk stimulants;...

HALI-L. Sh, 431 - The first thing that happened was I became very depressed and fearful. I was weak and couldn't resolve my issues. I became a laughable matter. The next thing I knew, I became embittered at all those I thought were laughing at me. During the last week of the proving, the vindictive side of reacting to that depression came out. 18, 30C, 7:XX:XX

Sh, 670 - When I was alone in my apartment with the lights on, I manifested many fragmented personalities, probably around five or six. Never did before like this. What was different was nobody was in the room to make a chain reaction. I was alone. Needed no provocation to make a change, or experience a change. I talk outloud, and talk to the person in a number of different ways. Fearful Joe, Vindictive Joe, One That's Just Like Someone Else Joe — each will act out in a number of different ways. 18, 30C, 35:XX:XX

KALI-I. He, 6 - Very great irritability and unwonted harshness of demeanor (behavior); his children, to whom he is devoted and attached, become burdensome to him; very passionate and spiteful temper;...constant apprehension of impending evil.

NAT-M. He, 43 - Hateful and vindictive nature.

NEON. Sh, 175 - I've been in a rotten mood all day, dwelling on past offenses. I just can't let go, it's making me angry. I feel like I hate that bastard; it's not an emotion I've had before. Now I feel vindictive, really awful; I feel that if I ever found out that he had been lying to me again I would say to him, "I'll kill you," "I'll slit your throat." These violent feelings were much eased when alone. 02, 6C, 04:22:40

Sh, 176 - Got up late in a horrible mood and reproached my partner again. I hurt him but I didn't care. I felt indifferent, malicious and vindictive, full of hate. 02, 6C, 05:22:10

OPUN-V. Al, 8 - Very vindictive at night.

REVOLUTIONARY

Anarchist: ***arg-n.*** caust.[30] ***merc.***

Anarchist; revolutionary: caust.[179] kali-c.[179] **MERC.**[30] sep.[179]

Delusions; hearing, of, drums which proclaim his execution, chides father for taking part in revolutions: verat.[54]

- rowdies, brawlers, will break in if she is alone: elaps.[139]

Discontented; revolutionary: **MERC.**[30]

Dreams; revolution: hura[36] merc.[36]

➤ riots: bry. con. guai. indg. kali-c. kali-n.[10] lyc. m-aust.[10] merc.[10] nat-c. nat-m. ped.[36] phos. puls. sars.[10] stann.

➤ rowdy, feeling disposed to act like a: caj.[36]

➤ singing political songs, in presence of spies: asc-t.[5]

ADAM. Sh, 216 - Feel harder, more rebellious. I will do what I want. Inconsiderate and unsympathetic. Unfeeling in relationship and sexually. 22, 200C, 01:XX:XX

ELAPS. Al, 13 - Fearfulness, dread (fear) of being alone, as though something would happen, or as though rowdies (revolution, rebellious) would break in.

MERC. Ha, 1125 - Anxious dreams; of being

bitten by dog, of getting up a revolution (revolutionary, revolting, radical) after midnight.

VERAT. He, 48 - A crippled girl...; chides (censure) her father for taking part in revolution; thinks she hears drum (timpani) which proclaims his execution; this is followed by silent brooding and occasional starts;...

RIDICULOUS

Delirium; comical: ant-c.[85] ***hyos. stram.*** verat.

Delusions; faces, ridiculous: cann-i.

Dreams; ridiculous: mez.[1] mygal.[8] tanac.[25]

Foolish; behavior, grotesque: agar.[36] cact.[36] cori-r.[36]

Foolish; behavior, monkeys, like: **HYOS.**[54]

Ideas; ridiculous: cann-i. hydrog.[222] kali-p. **LACH.** ***stram.***

Jealousy; foolish as it is irresistible, as: ***lach.***

Jealousy; images, with frightful, tendency to mock, satire and ridiculous ideas: ***lach.***

Jesting; ridiculous or foolish: androc.[222] bell. ***cic.*** croc. hyos. ***stram.*** tanac. ***verat.***

Laughing; actions, at his own, stand or walk, at an attempt to: agar.[54]

Ludicrous, things seem: calc.[10] cann-i. cann-s. hyos.[10] nat-m. ***nux-m.*** plat.[1] stram. sulph.[10] tarent.

Talk; ridiculous: bell.[36] par.[36]

BELL. Ha, 1366 - Ridiculous grimaces; ...acts as if she were washing, at another as if counting money, ...

COT. Al, 11 - Feels silly (ridiculous) and lost.

CROC. Al, 5 - If any one happens to sing a single musical note, she begins involuntarily to sing, and then is obliged to laugh at herself; she however, soon sings in spite of her determination to stop. (sympathy)

HALI-L. Sh, 2 - Looking in the mirror is weird. Feel ugly. Very pale. I feel I look ugly, pale, big body and butt. Throughout the whole day I kept catching myself in the mirror and felt this all day. 01, 30C, 01:XX:XX

HYDROG. Sh, 219 - Things seem ridiculous and amusing, ordinary things like birds. Laughing at them. Everything seemed so absurd or futile. 16, 30C, 02:XX:XX

Sh, 222 - Feel that the things we do are on different levels. Some of them are on higher and more meaningful levels —the real me —and others are just a trivial game. Laughing at the absurdity of notions — everything seems ridiculous. 16, 30C, 09:XX:XX

HYOS. Al, 53 - They laughed aloud because all persons seemed ridiculous;...the old woman talked of future,...

Ha, 529 - Comical confusion of mind: they perform all sorts of ridiculous antics (jokes), like monkeys.

Ha, 533 - He gesticulates like a harlequin. (buffoon) (foot-note: "like an actor" -Hughes). (feigning)

Ha, 545 - Ridiculously solemn acts in improper clothing, mixed with fury. (In a priest's cassock, put on over nothing but a shirt, and in fur boots, he wishes to go to church, in order to preach and perform clerical offices there, and furiously attacks those who try to prevent him.)

He, 41 - Comical alienation of mind; ludicrous actions like monkeys; makes ridiculous gestures like a dancing clown;...

LACH. Al, 25 - Towards evening very unusual almost crazy jealousy, as foolish as it is irresistible.

He, 26 - Jealousy, with frightful images, great tendency to mock, to satire and ridiculous ideas.

MERC. Ha, 1262 - He is silly, acts like a buffoon, ...he lit (burning) his fire, laid swords across one another, and put candles in one corner of the room, in the other boots (shoe),all this quite gravely...(serious)

NAT-M. Al, 11 - Constant laughing; everything in the room looked so ridiculous.

NUX-M. Al, 32 - Many ridiculous or extravagant acts or expressions, like idiocy, while she seemed perfectly conscious, and at the next moment would appear chagrined at her conduct, and said she could not control her actions...

OP. Al, 19-...; all the actors are happy, and each retires home in a total state of irrationality, but likewise in the entire and full enjoyment of happiness not to be procured by reason. Disregarding the ridicule of those they meet, who divert themselves by making them talk absurdly, each imagines looks and feels himself possessed of whatever he wishes.

ROBBER

Delirium; accused of theft, after being harshly: ***hyos.***[54]
Delusions; pursued, robbing a friend, for: kali-br.[36]
- stolen, somebody thinks it: lach.[58]
- stolen, something, she has: lach.[58]
- thieves, accused of robbing, he has been: kali-br.
- thieves, dream, after a, and will not believe the contrary until search is made: nat-m. sanic.[85]
- thieves, dreams of robbers is frightened on waking, and thinks dream is true: verat.
- thieves, house, in: ars. cann-i. con.[30] ***cupr-acet.***[54] ***lach.*** merc. ***nat-m.*** sil. sol-t-ae.
- thieves, robbers, sees: alum. ars. aur. bell. cupr. cupr-acet.[54] kali-c. kali-sil.[58] mag-c. mag-m. merc. nat-c. ***nat-m.*** petr. phos. sanic.[85] sil. sol-t-ae.[36] verat. zinc.
- thieves, sees, night: ***ars.***
- voices, hears, steal and kill, that she must: lach.[58]
- witches, denies having anything to do with them, in delirium after being accused of theft: ***hyos.***[54]
- assaulted, is going to be: abel.[149] androc.[222] tarent.
- bed, evening, some one would get into and no room in it, or as if some one had sold it: nux-v.
- bed, someone, tries to take away the bed clothes: bell.
- dreams have been stolen or belong to another: choc.[222]
- pursued, murderers, robbers, by: alco.
- robbed, is going to be: bar-c.[30] bor.[30] caust.[30] sep.[30]
- sold, bed, someone has sold his: nux-v.
- thieves, house, and space under bed are full of that: ***ars.***
- thieves, jump out of window, therefore wants to: ***lach.***[54]

Dreams; animals, horses, stealing, his horse: aether[36]
➤ money, stolen from her: ozone[227]
➤ pursued, robbers, by: mag-m
➤ robbers, anxious, wakes frequently, with violent palpitation and screaming: ***zinc.***[54]
➤ robbers, breaking into house and trying to kill her: mag-c.[36]
➤ robbers, house, want to go into: ozone[227]
➤ robbers, laying snares for him: jac-c.[36]
➤ robbers, waking, with frightened, and a fixed idea that dream is true: verat.[54]
➤ stealing, someone is stealing his horse: aether.

Fear; door, closed, lest the d. should be: lac-d.[122]
✦ robbers, of: agar.[172] alum. anac.[58] ***arg-n.*** **ARS.**[122] aur. aur-s.[58] bell. cand-a.[239] ***con.*** elaps ***ign.*** kali-p.[122] ***lach.*** lyc.[212] mag-c. mag-m. ***merc.*** nat-c. ***nat-m. phos.*** sanic. sil. sol-t-ae. sulph. verat. ***zinc.*** zinc-p.[58]
✦ robbers, of, midnight, on waking: ars.[172] ***ign.*** nat-m.[1] sulph.
✦ robbers, waking on: merc.[10] nat-m.[10] sil.[10]

Dreams; animals, horses, stealing a horse: aether36
➤ robbers: allox.[119] **ALUM.** alum-p.[58] ***arn. aur.*** aur-s.[58] bamb-a.[1184] bell. calc-p. carb-v. cast. cench.[58] ferr-i. jac-c. ***kali-c.*** kali-s.[58] lil-s.[36] **MAG-C.** mag-m. mag-s. ***merc.*** merc-acet.[10] nat-c. **NAT-M.** ozone[227] petr. phel. phos. plb.[5] psil.[164] psor. ptel. rumx.[36] ***sanic.*** sel.[149] ***sil.*** sin-n. tub.[85] verat. ***zinc.***
➤ robbers, blow on the head, after: ***nat-m.***[54]
➤ robbers, detecting robbers: merc-i-r.
➤ robbers, fighting, with: ferr-i. jac-c.[36] mag-c. nat-c. psil.[164] sil.
➤ robbers, street robbers: bell.[54]
➤ robbers, trying to kill him: merc-acet.[36]
➤ robbery, of committing: hydrog.[222]
➤ robbing a bank: hydrog.[222]
➤ stealing, fruit: plb.
➤ stealing, money: lap-mar-c.[194]
➤ theft, committed, of having: alum. plb.

Fear; robbers, of, night: cupr.[172] lach.[30]
✦ robbers, of, waking, on: merc.[10] nat-m.[10] sil.[10]

Kleptomania: absin. ars. ***art-v.*** **BELL.**[30] bry. calc.[30] carb-v.[30] carc.[207] caust. cic.[102] ***cur.*** hyos.[102] kali-br.[198] kali-c. lach.[189] lyc. mand.[231] nat-m.[30] ***nux-v.*** oxyt.[102] plat.[102] puls. sep. sil.[30] staph. stram. ***sulph.***[122] syph.[5] tarent. thuj.[162]
Kleptomania; boy with epilepsy: ***art-v.***[54]
Kleptomania; goes about house in search of something, not knowing what, but if attracted by any object puts it in his pocket, or hides it in coat: ***staph.***[54]
Kleptomania; steals, dainties: mag-m. nat-c.
Kleptomania; steals, money: calc. puls.
Searching; thieves, dreamt of them, after having: nat-m.

Searching; thieves, for, at night: ars.

ADAM. Sh, 213 - Furious cold anger when money stolen from me. 2, 12C, 73:XX:XX
ARS. Al, 87 - He imagines that the whole house, and the space under the bed, are full of thieves, which causes, from fright, anxious cold sweat to break out over his body.
Al, 89 - He sees thieves in his room, and therefore hides himself under the bed.
Al, 86 - He runs through the whole house at night in search of thieves.
Ha, 37 - In the night he runs all about the house, looking for thieves.
He, 43 - Runs about house at night looking for thieves. (search)
He, 18 - He imagines that he sees burglars (robbers) in the room, and listens under the bed; he is bathed in cold sweat.
ART-V. He, 8 - Inclination to steal.(rob, kleptomania)
BELL. Al, 124 - Dread (fear) of solitude, of ghosts and thieves.
CANN-I. Al, 29 - Looks under beds and tables, unlocks and relocks doors, for the fancies he hears strange noises, and that thieves are in the house.
CON. Al, 40 - Fear of thieves.
Ha, 13 - Fear of thieves.
CUPR-A. He, 4 - Fixed idea that he sees persons connected with the law who are about to seize him (imprisoned),...at times sees thieves in the room, spirits, and various other immaterial objects;...
CUR. Al, 17 - Irascibility, wicked disposition; desires to lie in wait in order to assault others, and even to kill and rob them.
IGN. Al, 21 - Fear of thieves, on waking after midnight.
Ha, 760 - On waking, after midnight, has fears of thieves.
He, 34 - Fear of thieves, on waking after midnight.
KALI-BR. Al, 4 - He imagined that he had been specially singled out (select) for divine vengeance... deploring his sad fate (destiny),...he informed me that he had been accused of robbing a friend, and that the officers were in search of him....
LACH. He, 8 - Thinks: she is somebody else in the hands (seized) of a stronger power; (supremacy, superiority).or that she is dead, and preparations are made for funeral (cortege) or that she is nearly dead and wishes some one would help her off; herself pursued by enemies, or fears medicine is poison; there are robbers in house and wants to jump out the window; herself under super-human control; visions real, he will die. (helplessness, desire; aid, comfort, salvation)
MAG-C. Al, 958 - Anxious dream of a fight with robbers.
Al, 959 - Dream of thieves who broke into the house and tried to kill her.
MAG-M. Al, 714 - Frightful dreams; that she was pursued by robbers; that she burned her hand by washing ...
NAT-C. Al,DREAM, 1113 - Anxious, vivid, frightful dreams of thieves, from which he started up with loud cry, and when awake could scarcely realize that his fears were groundless.
NUX-V. Al, 1 - Anxious delirious fantasies, in the evening in bed, in the ninth hour, as if some one would get into his bed,(base, foundation) and there was no room (space) in it; or as if some one had sold his bed etc.
PLB. Al, 60-...; he hears everywhere threatening voices, officers come to arrest him, to seize his furniture (movables), (confiscated, expropriated) and to expel (eject) him from his lodgings (home) (expulsion, exiled) ; the voices come from the pillow, the mattress (bed); they enter by the window, where he sees people, and they consult about him with closed doors (secretive) ; ...
SIL. Al, 21 - He woke with great anxiety about midnight, could not move in spite of every effort, and imagined that thieves were breaking in; on rising he became quiet, after lying down the anxiety returned.
SOL-T-AE. Al, 1 - She rises in the night, imagining that thieves are hidden behind the curtains; but she not dare (risk) to look for them, and begs some one else to do so.
SULPH. Al, 3815 - At night, horrible dreams, with great palpitation or heart, and on awaking, sometimes rigor, sometimes heat and fear of robbers.
TARENT. Al, 56 - Fear and shaking; the

patient cannot find a suitable place where to hide himself; thinks he is going to be assaulted.

ZINC. Ha, 11 - Fear of thieves or of horrible phantoms, seen while waking as if in a feverish fancy.

He, 10 - Anxiety on account of thieves or horrible apparitions, while awake, like a feverish fancy.

ROTTEN

Delusions; body, brain, decaying, is: crot-h.[72]
- body, brain, dissolving: calc.[139]
- body, mouth, stinking odor from: ***hyos.***[54]
- body, putrefy, will: ***ars.*** bell.
- body, shrunken, like the dead, is: ***sabad.***
- body, withering, is: sabad.[58]
- breath is spoiled, his exhaled, cautions people not to inhale: lyss.[54]
- fermenting, everything is: nux-m.[139]
- world, shabby, is: germ.[222]

Dreams; animals, oxen, putrid: hura[36]
➤ body, penis, prepuce sloughed off: linu-c.
➤ dead, bodies, smell of dead: calc. crot-h.[58]
➤ excrements, large amounts: hydrog.[222]
➤ excrements, soiling himself with excrements: aloe cast-v. iod. sars.[58] zinc.
➤ excrements, wading in excrements: iod.[10]
➤ water, putrid: arg-n.

Fear; putrefy, body will: bell.
Sensitive; odors, to, filthy: ***sulph.***[58]
Sensitive; odors, to, foul things: par.[137]
Sensitive; odors, to, foul things, remains for a long time: dios.[137]

ADAM. Sh, 199 - The downside was that I also experienced hurt more keenly and felt mortally wounded more often than is good for me, in situations that I would normally have shrugged off. And when I felt bad, I felt rotten. 18, 30C, XX:XX:XX

BELL. Ha, 1434 - Madness; he thinks that his living body is putrefying. (decay, degeneracy)

HALI-L. Sh, 596 - Drive through New Mexico. Long scary dirt road. Stop to look at a dead lamb by the side of the road and the stink of the carrion smelt good. I am intoxicated by the smell; I can't get enough of it. 16, 10C, 16:XX:XX

HYOS. He, 84-...constant talking, particularly on religious subjects; believes himself poisoned, or that there is a stinking odor from his mouth;...

LYSS. Al,N-62 - He cautioned people around him not to inhale his exhaled air, it was spoiled (dirty), stinking (smelling) like rotten (putrefying) eggs, worse than cholera, and could injure. (contaminates, infects)

He, 62 - He cautioned people around him not to inhale his exhaled air, it was spoiled, stinking like rotten eggs, worse than cholera, and could injure.

RUINED

Business; man, in worn out: ***coca***[54] kali-p.[85] **NUX-V.**[54] zinc-p.[137]

Delusions; annihilation, about to sink into: calc.[1] cann-i. carbn-h.
- body, abdomen, fallen in, his stomach devoured, his scrotum swollen: **SABAD.**
- body, brain, decaying, is: crot-h.[72]
- body, brain, dissolving: calc.[139]
- body, brain, dissolving: calc.[139]
- body, brain, softening: abrot. ***arg-n.***[8] cann-i.[58]
- body, dashed to pieces, being: calc.[36].
- body, disintegrating: ***lach.***[36] lap-mar-c.[194]
- body, liver comes out with blood of menses: ozone[227]
- body, pieces, in danger of coming in: thuj.[36]
- body, putrefy, will: ***ars.*** bell.
- body, scattered about bed, tossed about to get the pieces together: ***bapt.*** caj.[102] daph.[102] petr. ***phos.*** pyrog.[58] stram.[102]
- body, shrunken, like the dead, is: ***sabad.***
- body, sink down between the thighs, will: bell.
- body, spotted brown, is: bell.
- body, stomach, has corrosion of: acet-ac.[54] ign. sabad.
- body, withering, is: sabad.[58]
- decline, she is going into a: ***xan.***[54]
- falling, pieces, to: lac-c.[5] xan.[139]
- health, he has ruined his: bamb-a.[1184] chel.
- hollow, whole body is: aur. ***kali-c.*** nux-v. pall.
- melting away, he or she is, agg. from change, amel. in recumbent position: sumb.
- room, falling to pieces, is: cann-i.[139]
- ruined, he is: calc.[30] **IGN.**[30] verat.[30]
- ruined, will be: puls.[139]
- sinking, to be: bapt.[116] benz.[36] kali-c.[116] lyc.[1] lyss.[139]

• wasting away, he is: naja[36]
• world, shabby, is: germ.[222]
Dreams; blood, mangled remains, and: merc.[36]
➤ body, disfigured: sep.
➤ body, liver comes out with blood of menses: ozone[227]
➤ body, pieces, in: dict.[111]
➤ body, prepuce sloughed off: linu-c.
➤ body, teeth breaking off: kali-n. rauw.[119] sul-ac.[10] ther. thuj.
➤ body, teeth falling, filling is falling out: nux-v.[36]
➤ body, teeth, falling out: bamb-a.[1184] coca[36] cocc. convo-d.[36] nicc. nux-v. sul-ac.[10] tab.
➤ buildings, demolished: hura[36]
➤ cities, destroyed by fire: sol-t-ae.[36]
➤ cough, dry, chronic and consumptive: eupi.[36]
➤ disease, hair falling out: mag-c.
➤ emaciated, becoming: kali-n.[36] kreos.
➤ excrements, soiling himself with excrements: aloe cast-v. iod. sars.[58] zinc.
➤ helpless feeling, as if the end of the world: hydrog.[222]
➤ nightmare, left side from neck to knee were jerking up and down like a mass of jelly, as if, this motion extending into chest and centering at heart: gels.[36]
➤ walking, ruins, among: hura[36] iod.[36]
Fear; age, of people their own: cortico.[119]
✦ biting, of, lest teeth would fall out: nit-ac.[172]
✦ brain, of softening of: abrot. ***arg-n.***[8] asaf. calc-sil.[58]
✦ chlorosis, in: ***calc.***[122]
✦ health, ruined her, that she has: calc.[122] chel. staph.[122]
✦ old, of getting: lap-mar-c.[194]
✦ osteoporosis: calc.[185]
✦ putrefy, body will: bell.
✦ stress, of breaking down under: lyc.[102]
Home; desires to go, old, deteriorated people: cic.[193]

ABROT. He, 3 - Thinks her brain is softening. (dissolving)
ADAM. Sh, 423 - Extreme weakness, painful cough, weak chest. Feels like TB or wasting disease. 22, 200C, 01:XX:XX
Sh, 424 - Mind alive but body feels wrecked. 7, 6C, 23:10:00
Sh, 431 - I feel old and creaky. 7, 6C, 08:00:XX
Sh, 520 - Thoughts of creativity and destruction. One does not exist without the other. 16, 12C, 30:XX:XX
ALOE. Al, 40-...wrap up in himself (introspection), as after a sickness or a fit of anger, which still gnaws (bite) internally, which one cannot express.
ARG-N. He, 14 - Thinks he has softening of brain, or some other incurable affection (disease), which almost drives him to despair.
CALC. Ha, 25 - His heart is agitated with fear and anxiety for the future, with fear of consumption.(tuberculosis, ruin)
CAMPH. Al, 46-... The sight increased my despair poor nature extinguished; the sky transparent and lifeless; the earth was still in the dim, dead light. I could not bear it. The sense of touch was gone, and my eyes protruded from their sockets.
CHEL. Al, 24 - Sad mood; she fears that she has ruined her health by the proving.
CON. He, 14 - Likes to wear his best clothes, (vanity) makes useless purchases, (squander) cares very little for things (indifferent), wastes or ruins them; does not want to work, prefers to play. (wanderer)
CROT-H. He, 15 - Oppression as if brain had been intoxicated by carbonic acid, or by degraded or non-oxygenated blood.
HALI-L. Sh, 435 - I was feeling very self-destructive. I wanted to do crappy things to myself. The border's breaking loose. I know I have a part of me that does this. It's just rising up. Screw it all, the futility of it all; the futility of working toward the positive, of caring for my health, of doing good things. What for? My big fear is that I'm really crazy, that I'm making all this up, that I'm just crazy (i.e., that the remedy is a placebo). 06, 6C, 11:XX:XX
HEP. Ha, 296 - In the evening a frightful anxiety for two hours; he thought he must be ruined (lost, failed), and was sad to that degree that he could have killed himself.
LYSS. Al,N-80 - Felt as if she was going to die, as if she was going to sink away.(decline)
He, 80 - Felt as if she was going to die; as if she was going to sink away.
MAG-C. Al, 935 - Dream of her hair falling out, which made her very sad.

PLAT. He, 46-...;suffers unspeakable pangs (anxiety) of conscience in consequence of a faux (fault, mistake, embarrassing mistake?) pass when thirty-two years old; says she has brought disgrace upon her family, and that she has incurred the penalty of damnation; (doomed) in order to do penance (penitence) gave away whatever she could lay her hands upon, (redemption) so that she had to be constantly watched; after her confessor asserted that she could not hope for pardon or heaven (condemnable), she seemed in absolute despair ; bemoaned her misery throughout the night, wringing her hands and beseeching (implore) that she might be delivered (free) from the hell of her conscience; twice attempted self-destruction (suicide);...wished to live and do penance (penitence, purgation, purification) in order to mitigate her eternal punishment.

PULS. Ha, 1113 - Anxiety, thinks he will be ruined.(decay, perdition)

SABAD. Al, 2 - He imagines all sorts of strange things about his own body, for instance, that it had shrunk (dry, wrinkled) like that of dead persons (corpse), that his stomach was corroded (degeneracy, decomposition), that the scrotum was swollen (enlarged), etc.;...

Al, 3 - Imagines: himself sick; parts shrunken (small wrinkled) ; that she is pregnant (important?), when she is merely swollen from flatus; that she has some horrible throat disease which will end fatally. (incurable)

SEP. Ha, 9 - She has none but troubled thoughts about her health, thinks she is getting the consumption (tuberculosis, degenerate, decomposition) and will die soon.

Ha, 31 - Extreme loathing of life (existence he felt as if he could not any longer bear this miserable (wretched, unhappy) existence, and as if he would pine away (ruined) unless he made away with himself.-(suicidal)

STRAM. He, 102 - Mania with insomnia ; very talkative; thinks he has every imaginable disease; that he has power (powerful) over all disease; masturbates, fills his pockets with anything he can find (lack?), thinks he has snakes in him.

SULPH. Ha, 63 - Insanity; she spoils (ruin) her things and throws them away, imagining she has an abundance of everything; at the same time she becomes emaciated, like a skeleton.-(wealthy, rich X miserable, poor, destitute)

He, 46 - Great anxiety, fear lest she should come to ruin (destruction); ..tried to run away...

THUJ. He, 9 - Sensation as if whole body were thin and delicate, (weak, fragile, frail) and could not resist least attack (illness); as if continuity of body would be dissolved.

RUN OVER

Fear; approaching, vehicles, of: anth. hydr-ac. lyss.[122] phos.

- ✦ cars, vehicles in the streets, of: hydr-ac.[102]
- ✦ crossing, streets: acon.[85] ferr-p.[172] gaert.[136] hydr-ac.[137] kali-p.[172] plat.[137]
- ✦ run over, of being (on going out): anth.[172] hydr-ac. lyss. op.[8] phos.
- ✦ walking, of, across busy street: ***acon.*** carc.[162] crot-h.[5] hydr-ac.[102] kali-p.[172] plat.[102] psor.[162]

Frightened; easily, locomotive, as if about to be run over by a: phos.[36]

Suicidal disposition; car, throw himself in front of a: ozone[227]

Suicidal disposition; run over, to be: alum.[116] ars.[116] aur.[116] kali-br.[5] lach.[30] pitu-a.[164]

ANTH. Al, 6 - On going out of doors, in evening, felt nervous, and exceedingly afraid of being run over.

CHOC. Sh, 189 - While outside became very weary of cars and people. Felt open and vulnerable. Fear of accidents, cars, or of someone leaping into the road and punching me. This anxiety was worse out of doors. 27, 100C, 01:XX:XX

HYDR-AC. He, 3 - Could not remain in middle of road when he saw a vehicle approaching him even at a considerable distance,... (run over)

OP. Al, 29 - A half intoxicated and excited condition, so that I came near being run over by a carriage, and at another time of running into a horse, though I had seen it coming from some distance.

He, 20-...declares he is not alone in bed; ..desire to escape; says a regiment of horsemen are upon his bed and that he fears to be trodden upon (run over, crushed); when told that horses are very careful, answered that he feared he would be crushed by the wagons that followed them.

PHOS. Al, 115 - Frightened feeling, as if I was about to be run over by a locomotive. (crushed, smash)

SADISM

Anger; laughing, bursts of, with: ***croc.***[54]
Break things, desire to, laughs over it: ***apis***[54]
Break things, desire to, possession, parents most prized: tub.[189]
Cheerfulness; alternating with, vandalism: spong.[184]
Cheerfulness; morbidly: aur-s.[58]
Cruelty, animals to: **ARS.**[162] ***bell.*** calc.[193] med.[162]
Cruelty, brutality, inhumanity: abrot. absin. alco.[36] **ANAC.**[122] androc.[222] ***ars.***[30] ***aur.*** bell.[102] bry.[102] canth.[102] carc.[207] chin.[5] choc.[222] croc. cur. **HEP.**[30] ***hyos.***[30] ***kali-i.***[58] kali-p.[5] ***lach.***[122] lap-mar-c.[194] med.[137] nicc.[30] ***nit-ac.***[102] nux-v. op. ***plat.*** sabad.[10] sel.[30] squil.[10] staph.[102] ***stram.***[102] tarent.[102] verat.[102]
Cruelty; religiousness, with: ***plat.***[54]
Cursing; laughing, with, convulsive, spasmodic: oena.[36]
Cursing; laughing, with, immoderate: stram.[155]
Cut, mutilate, slit others, desire to: lyss. verat.[58]
Delusions; injury, inflict, will, on someone: lap-c-b.[194]
Dreams; cruelty: ***ign.***[10] lil-t.[36] nat-m. nux-v. sel. sil. stann.
➤ cruelty, anger, without: lil-t.[36]
➤ cutting, trying to cut off finger of acquaintance: nicc.[36]
➤ dead, bodies, digging knife into wounds of: elaps[36]
Joy; misfortune of others, at the: anac.[185] ars. cupr.[171]
Laughing; misfortune, at: apis.
Love; perversity: hura[36] ind.[85] kali-n.[36] nux-v.[85] plat.[85]
Love; sadistic: thiop.[149]
Love; sadomasochistic: anac.[187]
Malicious; injure someone, desire to: androc.[222] levo.[149] osm.[36]
Malicious; laughing: cupr.[10] lap-mar-c.[194]
Mania; destructive efforts, sudden foxlike, requiring utmost vigilance, followed by laughter and apologies: ***tarent.***[54]
Mischievous: ***agar.*** aloe **ANAC.** arn. ***ars.*** bar-c. bufo ***calc.*** calc-ar.[58] **CANN-I.** cann-s.[137] **CHAM.**[85] ***cupr.*** dam.[85] hep.[109] ***hyos.*** ign.[189] ***lach.*** ***merc.*** **NUX-V.** puls.[85] spong.[10] **STANN.**[30] ***stram.*** ***tarent.*** tub.[189] ***verat.***
Mischievous; play tricks with their elders: phos.[189]
Pleasure; waking from a dream of murder, on: thea.
Smiling; sad things, about: plat.[30]
Striking; animals, at: med.[193]
Striking; desire to strike: alum.[122] androc.[222] bell. bufo carbn-s. der.[36] elaps hydr. **HYOS.** lil-t. nat-c. **NUX-V.**[122] ***staph.***
Talk; misfortune, about: ***verat.***[54]
Talk; nothing but, murder, fire and rats: ***calc.*** calc-sil.[58]

ABROT. He, 12 - Exceedingly peevish, feels as if she would like to do something cruel (sadistic, torture); no humanity.

ANDROC. Sh, 103 - Had a very caustic conversation with someone she hardly knew. Enjoyed her rudeness and was surprised by it. (7)

CHOC. Sh, 328 - Humourless, intolerant -almost cruel. Scalded a child's hand out of anger, and nothing would make him apologise.[35], 30C, XX:XX:XX:

CUPR. Ha, 27 - Fits of insanity, he spits into people's faces, and laughs heartily (soberly) over it.

HEP. He, 9 - Malicious (vindictive, malevolent) mood; feels as if he could murder someone whith pleasure.

LYSS. Al,N-10 - They appreciate the formidable character of the disease and speak frequently with a remarkable quick and sharp articulation of the impending fatal results.

He, 10 - They appreciate the formidable (terrible) character of the disease and speak frequently with a remarkable (unusual) quick and sharp articulation of the impending fatal results.

STICT. Al, 1 - She got very lively (active), told her father she felt as if she would like to strike out, only for fun; she would like it just for fun of it. After awhile she lay down on the lounge, and began, to use a common expression, to kick up her heels; her mother reproaching, said, " Bella, do behave, that is not ladylike"; when child responded: " Ma, I cannot help it; I feel exactly as if I want to fly away"...

SADNESS

Absorbed; sadness, indulges in: ***cocc.***[54]
Ailments from; excitement, general symptoms from, depressing: gels.[85] nat-m.[5]
Ailments from; love disappointed, sadness, with: ***aur.***[54] bell.[30] ***hyos.***[54] **IGN.**[54] ***nat-m.***[54]
Anger; alternating with, sadness: ambr.[10] coff.[10] sumb.[116] zinc.[10]
Anguish; sadness, in: ***arg-n.***[54] crot-h.[54]
Anxiety; future, sadness, with: ***sulph.***[54]
Anxiety; riding, while, hypochondriasis, in: ***arg-n.***[54]
Anxiety; thoughts, from, sad: alum.[1] clem.[1] cocc.[85] rhus-t.[1]
Brooding; corner, brooding or moping in a: aur.[5] aur-s.[58] bar-c.[5] bar-i.[58] bell.[5] camph.[5] cocc.[54] con.[58] cupr.[5] hyos.[5] ph-ac.[5] **VERAT.**[5]
Brooding; imaginary troubles, over, sadness, with: naja[54]
Cheerfulness; alternating with, sadness: abrot.[122] acon. agar. androc.[222] aran.[149] arg.[149] asar. ***aur.***[54] bell.[30] calc-s.[54] cann-i. cann-s.[5] canth. carb-an. caust. cench.[122] ***chin.*** chlf.[46] cimic. clem. coc-c.[58] coff.[30] croc. crot-h.[36] cupr.[54] cycl.[85] ferr. fl-ac. gels. ***graph.***[10] hell. hyos.[30] ign. iod. ***kali-chl.*** lach.[58] lap-c-b.[194] lapa.[36] lyc. ***m-arct.***[10] med. nat-c. ***nat-m.*** nid.[149] nit-ac. ***nux-m.*** ***nux-v.***[54] onop.[149] op.[10] ozone[227] petr. ***phos.*** plat. psor. senec. sep. spig. staph.[30] ***stram.***[10] sulfa.[149] sulfon.[102] tarent. thyr.[85] tub.[102] zinc. ziz.
Cheerfulness; appears, but looks down when on street: ***dios.***[54]
Cheerfulness; evening, sad in morning, and: nux-v.[30]
Cheerfulness; followed by, sadness: gels. graph. meph.[149] ***nux-m.***[54] petr. plat. ziz.
Cheerfulness; sadness, with: **BELL.**[162] **COFF.**[162] **HYOS.**[162] petr.[5] **STAPH.**[162] **STRAM.**[162] zinc.[162]
Childish behavior, sadness, in: ***kali-br.***[54]
Complaining; sadness, in: ***plat.***[54]
Confusion of mind; sadness, in: ***kali-br.***[54]
Consolation; agg. sad and weeping mood, with: **NAT-M.**[54]
Conversation; aversion to, sadness, after: ziz.[36]
Cowardice; sadness, with: ***sulph.***[54]
Death; desires, hypochondriasis, with: ***aur.***[54]
Death; thoughts of, sadness, with: **GRAPH.**[54] vinc.[54]
Delirium; alternating with, sadness: tub.[102]
Delirium; sad: acon.[5] bell.[5] morph.[102] puls.[5]
Delusions; painful, with sadness: ***kali-br.***[54]
- persecuted, that he is, tormented by some frightful scene of some mournful event of the past, and: spong.[54]
- sadness, with: alum. ambr.[137] ***aur.***[116] **KALI-BR.**[54] murx.[10] nux-v.[10] plat.[10]
- sadness, with, half awake at night, while: nux-v.

Dementia; sadness, with: tarent.[58]
Despair; sad thoughts, on account of: rhus-t.[54]
Dreams; amorous, sadness, during: ***aur.***[54]
➤ frightful, hypochondriasis, in: ***arg-n.***[54]
➤ frightful, sadness, in: ***naja***[54]
➤ sad: alum.[5] ant-c.[5] ***ars.*** asar.[5] asc-t. aur. aur-m.[54] bamb-a.[1184] cann-i. caps. carb-an. carbn-s. cast.[10] caust. chin.[5] croto-t.[10] graph. guare. ign. junc.[36] laur. lepi.[122] lob.[25] lyc. mag-c. manc. mosch.[5] mur-ac. nat-c.[10] ***nat-m.*** nit-ac. ***nux-v.*** op. ozone[227] paeon. paull.[36] peti.[36] phos. plan. ***puls.*** rat.[10] ***rheum*** rhus-t.[5] ruta[5] spong. stront-c. tarent. ust. zinc.
➤ water, looking at water flowing, but became sad on looking at sky: tarent.[36]
➤ weeping, frightful or sad: ***puls.***[54]
Dress; aversion to, in sadness: ***con.***[54]
Eccentricity; alternating with, sadness: petr.[36] stram.[54]
Ecstasy; alternating with sadness: senec.
Elated; alternating with sadness: caust.[198] senec.[36] ***sul-ac.***[209] visc.[119]
Euphoria; alternating with, sadness: asar.[149] cortiso.[149] hydro-c.[149] mand.[149]
Excitement; alternating with, sadness: ambr.[58] aster.[36] colch.[149] ***con.*** cortiso.[149] eug.[102] ferr-p.[58] foll.[149] ox-ac.[58] petr.[60] phenob.[149] ***plb.***[54] rad-br.[149] rauw.[149] sul-ac.[10] thyr.[85] thyreotr.[149]
Excitement; cerebral, alternating with, sadness: astac.[36]
Excitement; sadness, after: ***cann-i.***[116] spig.
Excitement; sadness, before: nat-m.[85]

Excitement; singing, after sad: ***con.***[54]

Exhilaration; alternating with, sadness lasting twelve hours, then sadness for several days: ziz.[54]

Exhilaration; sadness, after: thlaspi[25] ziz.[36]

Exhilaration; sadness, followed by: myric.[54]

Exuberance; alternating with, sadness: petr.[10]

Fancies; hypochondriasis, in: ***arg-n.***[54] stram.[36]

Fear; alternating with, sadness: zinc.[5]

✦ death, sadness with: cupr.[137] ***plat.***[54] vinc.[54]

✦ evil, of, sadness and weeping, with: **KALI-I.**[54]

✦ room, seemed gloomy and unpleasant: **PLAT.**[54]

✦ sadness, of: **LYC.**[54]

✦ sadness, with: am-m.[5] cic.[5] croc.[5] ***crot-h.***[54] ***dig.***[36] hep.[5] ***kali-br.***[54] kali-c.[5] **KALI-I.**[54] lyc.[5] ***nat-m.***[54] plat.[54] ***plb.***[54] rhus-t.[54] tab. vinc.[54]

✦ sadness, with, music agg.: ***dig.***[36]

✦ thinking of, when, sad things: rhus-t.

Frightened; easily, alternating with sadness: zinc.[10]

Harshness; sadness, in: **KALI-I.**[54]

Hopefulness; alternating with, sadness: acon. kali-c.[10] raph. sulfon.[72]

Horrible things sad stories, affected her profoundly: ars.[122] ***aur.***[122] ***aur-m.***[122] benz-ac.[58] **CALC.**[122] calc-s.[108] cand-a.[239] carb-v.[193] carc.[146] ***caust.***[122] cench.[58] chin.[162] **CIC.** coca[153] cocc. con.[122] ferr.[122] gels. ***hep.***[122] ign. **IOD.**[122] ***kali-c.***[184] ***lach.*** lap-c-b.[194] lap-mar-c.[194] ***lyc.***[122] manc.[162] nat-c. nat-m.[162] ***nit-ac.***[122] ***nux-v.*** op.[163] ozone[227] ***phos.***[122] plat.[137] prot.[193] ***puls.***[122] ***sep.***[122] ***sil.***[122] staph.[1] ***sulph.***[122] ***teucr.*** ***zinc.***

Horrible things sad stories, affected her profoundly, thoughts, her own, during labor: plat.[54]

Hypochondriasis: abies-n.[85] ***acon.***[5] agn.[5] alf.[102] aloe[5] alum.[5] ***ambr.***[5] anac.[5] anag.[54] anan.[54] ***ant-t.***[54] arg.[149] arg-n.[5] ***arn.***[5] ***ars.***[5] arum-m.[54] ***asaf.***[5] **AUR.**[5] ***aur-m.***[54] aur-s.[10] aven.[102] aza.[149] bamb-a.[1184] ***bell.***[5] **BENZ-AC.**[54] bism.[5] both-l.[3070] bran.[10] brom.[5] bry.[5] **CACT.**[54] **CALC.**[5] ***cann-s.***[5] canth.[5] ***caps.***[122] carc.[207] card-m.[25] caust.[5] ***cham.***[5] chin.[5] ***cimic.***[102] coca[25] cocc.[5] coff.[5] ***colch.***[54] **CON.**[5] croc.[5] cupr.[5] ***cycl.***[5] dig.[5] esp-g.[149] euphr.[5] ferr.[5] ferr-p.[58] gels.[5] gran.[10] **GRAPH.**[5] ***grat.***[54] ***hell.***[5] helon.[102] hep.[5] hydr-ac.[102] ***hyos.***[54] **IGN.**[5] iod.[5] ***ip.***[54] kali-br.[102] kali-c.[5] kali-chl.[10] kali-hp.[25] kali-p.[5] **LACH.**[5] lath.[102] ***lil-t.***[54] ***lyc.***[5] lycps.[85] mag-c.[144] **MAG-M.**[5] merc.[5] merc-d.[5] ***mez.***[5] ***mill.***[54] ***mosch.***[5] murx.[54] ***nat-c.***[5] **NAT-M.**[5] nep.[144] nit-ac.[5] nux-m.[5] **NUX-V.**[5] ***ol-an.***[5] op.[5] ***petr.***[5] ***ph-ac.***[5] ***phos.***[5] ***plat.***[5] plb.[5] podo.[5] ***puls.***[5] ***rhus-t.***[5] sabad.[5] sabin.[5] sac-alb.[85] ***sel.***[5] seneg.[5] ***sep.***[5] sin-n.[54] ***spong.***[5] ***stann.***[5] ***staph.***[5] stram.[5] sul-ac.[5] ***sulph.***[5] sumb.[102] tab.[5] tarent.[102] ***ter.***[54] thuj.[102] v-a-b.[149] **VALER.**[5] ***verat.***[5] vib-t.[85] ***viol-o.***[5] **ZINC.**[5] zinc-o.[102] zinc-val.[85] ***zing.***[54] ziz.[102]

Hypochondriasis; dread of society, with: anan.[36]

Hypochondriasis; epistaxis amel.: kali-chl.[116]

Hypochondriasis; inert, takes no interest in his surroundings: euphr.[54]

Hypochondriasis; morose: con.[10] graph.[10] grat.[10] m-arct.[10] ***mosch.***[54] petr.[10] phos.[10] **PULS.**[54] sabin.[10] sulph.[10]

Hypochondriasis; sullen mood, with: anac.[54]

Hypochondriasis; suppression of eruptions, after: **SULPH.**[54]

Hypochondriasis; timid, fearful: cocc.[54]

Hypochondriasis; weeping, with: am-c.[10] calc.[10] kali-c.[10] mez.[54] plat.[10] ***puls.***[10] stram.[10] viol-o.[10]

Hysteria; sexual, suppression of s. excitement, from, low spirited, anxiety and sadness: **CON.**[54]

Ideas; sad and joyless: ***psor.***[54]

Impatience; sadness, in: ***kali-c.***[54]

Indifference; sadness, in: ***kali-ar.***[54] ***kali-br.***[54] ***plat.***[54]

Indolence; sad, making him, with feeling of deep-seated inward trouble: sabin.[54]

Indolence; sadness, from: berb.[10] bov.[10] croto-t.[10] dor.[10] laur.[10] mez.[10] prun.[10] zinc.[10]

Insanity; alternating with, sadness: tub.[102]

Insanity; character, of sombre: nat-sal.[36]

Insanity; sadness: ars.[102] ***aur.***[102] bac.[56] bell.[30] calc.[30] caust.[102] cic.[102] hyos.[30] ***ign.***[10] ***kali-br.***[54] nux-v.[102] ***petr.***[30] ph-ac.[30] ***puls.***[102] rhus-t.[30] staph.[30] sulph.[30] verat.[30]

Irritability; hypochondriasis, in: grat.[54] ***puls.***[54]

Irritability; music, during, saddest: ***mang.***[36]

Irritability; sadness, with: ant-c.[10] asar.[54] aur.[10] bac.[62] bov.[10] dig.[10] kali-br.[54] ***kali-c.***[54] **KALI-I.**[54] lyc.[10] ***nat-m.***[54] nit-ac.[10] plat.[10]

polyg.[54] ptel.[111] sal-ac.[54] sep.[10] sul-ac.[10] ***sulph.***[54] tarent.[192] ziz.[54]
Jealousy; sadness, with: ***kali-ar.***[54]
Joy; alternating with, sadness: stram.[102]
Joyless: hydro-c.[2147] mag-m.[5] sars.[5]
Kill; desire to, hysterical sadness, with: ***merc.***[54]
Lamenting; sadness, in: ***puls.***[54]
Laughing; alternating with, sadness: androc.[222] canth. caust. nat-c. nid.[149] ***phos.*** stram. zinc.
Laughing; sad, when: lap-c-b.[194] ***phos.***[54]
Looked at; cannot bear to be, sadness, with: ***kali-br.***[54]
Loquacity; alternating with, sadness: arg.[149]
Malicious; sadness, in: **KALI-I.**[54]
Mania; alternating with, sadness: arg.[149] ***con.***[54] cyt-l.[149] kres.[149] ***nat-s.***[54] psor.[122] ***staph.***[54] stram.[1] sulfa.[149] tub.[102] verat.[72]
Memory; weakness, sadness, with: ***arg-n.***[54]
Mildness; alternating with, sadness: plat.[10]
Mirth; alternating with, sadness: cann-i. caust. croc. ferr. hell. indol.[77] m-arct.[1] med.[58] nat-c. nit-ac. petr. ***phos.*** plat. ptel.[36] sep. tarent. zinc.
Moral affections; want of moral feeling, sadness, with: ***kali-br.***[54]
Morose; music, agg., sad: ***mang.***[36]
Morose; sadness, with: **ARG-N.**[54] ***kali-ar.***[54] mag-c.[54] ***puls.***[54]
Music; amel. sad: mang.[1]
Music; aversion to, joyous, to, but immediately affected by saddest: mang.[54]
Music; desires, sad, melancholic: ozone[227]
Praying; aloud, in sadness: ***plat.***[54]
Quarrelsomeness; alternating with, sadness, silent: ***con.***
Quarrelsomeness; sadness, in: ***kali-ar.***[54]
Quiet disposition; sadness, in: ***kali-ar.***[54]
Quiet disposition; suffering, with much apparent, and sadness: ziz.[54]
Reflecting; sadness, in: ***cocc.***[54]
Reflecting; sadness, in, deep: ***plat.***[54]
Religious affections, sadness, remorse, from: aur.[30] con.[30]
Religious affections; sadness: ars.[5] aur.[5] bac.[62] bell.[10] con.[30] croc.[10] graph.[60] ***kali-br.***[54] ***kali-p.***[54] ***lach.***[10] lil-t.[58] lyc.[10] ***meli.***[54] mez.[58] ***plat.***[54] plb.[102] psor.[102] puls.[10] sel.[10] sil.[58] ***stram.***[10] ***sulph.***[10] ***verat.***[10]
Religious affections; sadness, doubt about salvation, with: ***lyc.***[54]
Religious affections; sadness, gave away everything she could lay her hands on, in order to do penance: ***plat.***[54]
Religious; affections, sadness, four months standing, of: ***meli.***[54]
Restlessness; alternating with, sadness: apis[5]
Restlessness; anxious, megrim, in: aeth.[54]
Restlessness; sadness, with: nux-v.[54] ***plat.***[54]
Sadness, despondency, depression, melancholy: ***abies-n.*** abrot. acal. acet-ac. achy.[149] **ACON.** acon-f.[36] act-sp. adlu.[149] adon.[116] ***aesc.*** aeth.[10] aether[36] agar. agav-t.[149] ***agn.*** ail. alco.[36] alf.[102] all-c. all-s.[36] allox.[119] aloe ***alum.*** ***alum-sil.***[58] alumn. am-br.[116] ***am-c.*** ***am-m.*** ***ambr.*** ***aml-n.***[54] ammc. amph.[36] ***anac.*** anag.[54] anan. androc.[222] ang.[1] anh.[149] ***ant-c.*** ant-o.[85] ***ant-t.***[54] anthr.[36] apis apoc. aq-mar.[149] arag.[102] aran. aran-ix.[119] ***arg.*** ***arg-n.*** ***arist-cl.***[119] ***arn.*** **ARS.** **ARS-I.** ars-met.[54] ars-s-r.[54] arum-d.[36] arum-m.[54] arum-t. ***asaf.*** asar. asc-t.[54] astac.[54] aster. astra-e.[149] atro.[36] **AUR.** aur-i.[58] **AUR-M.** ***aur-s.***[122] aza.[149] ***ba-tn.***[136] bac.[62] ***bamb-a.***[1184] bapt. bar-acet.[36] ***bar-c.*** bar-i.[58] ***bar-m.*** ***bell.*** benz-ac. berb. bol. bor.[36] both-a.[139] bov. bran.[10] ***brom.*** ***bry.*** ***bufo*** bufo-s.[36] buni-o.[149] but-ac.[102] cac.[85] ***cact.*** cadm-s.[144] caj.[36] calad. **CALC.** calc-acet.[36] **CALC-AR.** ***calc-f.*** **CALC-I.**[58] ***calc-p.*** **CALC-S.** ***calc-sil.***[58] ***camph.*** camph-br.[85] cann-i. ***cann-s.*** ***canth.*** ***caps.*** carb-ac.[36] **CARB-AN.** ***carb-v.*** carbn-o.[36] **CARBN-S.** carc.[85] card-m. carl. cass.[36] cast. **CAUST.** cecr.[149] cedr.[36] cench.[58] **CHAM.** ***chel.*** chim.[36] **CHIN.** ***chin-ar.*** chin-b.[54] ***chin-s.*** ***chlol.***[54] chlor.[36] chloram.[149] chlorpr.[149] choc.[222] chr-ac.[54] ***cic.*** **CIMIC.** ***cina*** cinnb. ***clem.*** cob. cob-n.[119] coc-c.[58] coca ***cocc.*** coch. cod.[25] ***coff.*** ***colch.*** ***coloc.*** ***con.*** conch.[10] convo-d.[36] convo-s.[119] cop.[54] ***corn.*** cortico.[119] cortiso.[149] cot.[36] ***croc.*** **CROT-C.** ***crot-h.*** croto-t. cund.[36] ***cupr.*** ***cupr-acet.***[10] cupr-ar.[36] ***cur.*** ***cycl.*** cypr.[85] cyt-l.[119] ***daph.***[10] der.[36] ***dig.*** ***dios.***[54] dirc.[85] ***dros.*** ***dulc.*** dys-co.[136] echi. elae.[36] elaps elat.[85] ergot.[149] erig.[36] ery-a.[54] esp-g.[149] eug. euon.[102] eup-per. eup-pur. euph. euphr. fago.[36] fagu.[36] **FERR.** ***ferr-ar.*** **FERR-I.** ferr-m.[54] ***ferr-p.*** ferul.[36] fic.[144] fl-ac. flav.[149] flor-p.[149] foll.[1201] form.[36] frax.[122] gad.[36] gaert.[136] gamb. **GELS.** germ.[222] glon. goss.[122] gran.[10] **GRAPH.** ***grat.*** guai. guat.[149] haem. halo.[149] ham. **HELL.** ***helon.*** ***hep.*** **HIPP.** hir.[144] hist.[119] ***hura*** ***hydr.*** hydr-ac.[10] hydrc.

hydro-c. hydrog.[222] **HYOS.**[122] hyper. hypoth.[149] iber.[36] **IGN.** ind. ***indg.*** indol.[102] **IOD.** ***ip.*** iris iris-t.[36] jac-c.[36] jug-c.[54] kali-acet.[36] ***kali-ar.*** kali-bi. **KALI-BR.** ***kali-c.*** kali-chl. kali-fcy.[36] kali-hp.[25] ***kali-i.*** kali-n. **KALI-P.** kali-s. kalm. kreos. kres.[144] kurch.[192] **LAC-C.** ***lac-d.*** **LACH.** lachn. lact. lam. lap-c-b.[194] lapa.[36] lat-m.[119] lath.[85] ***laur.*** ***lec.*** led.[1] lepi.[36] **LEPT.** lil-s.[36] **LIL-T.** lipp.[36] lith-c.[5] lob. lob-c.[54] ***lob-s.***[54] luf-op.[144] luna[228] lup.[10] **LYC.** lycps. lyss.[36] m-arct.[10] m-aust.[10] macrin.[36] mag-c. mag-f.[144] mag-m. mag-p.[116] mag-s. **MANC.** ***mand.***[119] ***mang.*** med. meli.[85] menis.[36] meny. meph.[149] **MERC.** ***merc-aur.***[5] ***merc-c.*** ***merc-i-f.***[36] ***merc-i-r.*** merl. methys.[149] **MEZ.** ***mill.***[54] mit.[36] moly.[149] ***morg.***[136] morg-g.[136] morph.[58] mosch. ***mur-ac.*** **MURX.** ***mygal.*** myric. nabal.[36] ***naja*** **NAT-AR.** nat-br.[36] **NAT-C.** nat-f.[149] nat-hchls.[36] **NAT-M.** nat-n.[116] ***nat-p.*** **NAT-S.** nat-sal.[85] nep.[149] nicc. **NIT-AC.** nux-m. ***nux-v.*** oena.[36] ***ol-an.*** olnd. onop.[149] **OP.**[122] orig.[36] ox-ac.[58] oxyt. ozone[227] palo.[149] parat.[149] paull.[36] ped.[85] pen.[36] penic.[149] perh.[149] peti.[36] ***petr.*** ***ph-ac.*** phel. phenob.[149] ***phos.*** ***phyt.*** pic-ac. picro.[36] pin-s.[36] pitu-a.[164] plan. **PLAT.** ***plb.*** plb-acet.[102] plect.[36] plumbg.[36] pneu.[149] podo. polyg.[54] polyp-p.[36] prot.[136] prun. psil.[149] **PSOR.** ptel. **PULS.** puls-n.[36] pyrus[36] rad-br.[102] ran-b.[36] ran-s. raph. rauw.[119] reser.[149] rham-f.[36] rheum rhod. **RHUS-T.** ***rhus-v.*** rib-ac.[149] rob. rumx. ***ruta*** sabad. ***sabin.***[122] sac-alb.[36] sal-ac.[54] sang. sanic. sant.[36] sapin.[36] sarcol-ac.[102] saroth.[149] sarr. sars. scut.[85] sec. **SEL.** senec. senec-j.[85] seneg. **SEP.** seq-s.[230] sieg.[144] ***sil.*** sol-c.[102] sol-o.[36] sol-t-ae.[36] ***spig.*** spira.[36] ***spong.*** squil.[10] **STANN.** stann-i.[116] ***staph.*** ***still.*** ***stram.*** stront-c. **STRY.**[122] ***sul-ac.*** ***sul-i.***[58] sulfa.[119] sulfonam.[149] **SULPH.** sumb.[36] syc-co.[136] ***syph.***[58] ***tab.*** tanac.[25] tarax.[111] ***tarent.***[122] tell. ***ter.***[122] tere-ch.[149] thal.[85] thea.[36] ther.[58] thiop.[149] thlaspi[25] **THUJ.** thymol.[119] thyreotr.[149] til. tinos.[97] tong.[10] tril. trinit.[102] trio.[149] tub.[5] tub-r.[149] upa.[36] 122 ust. v-a-b.[149] valer. vanad.[72] ven-m.[149] **VERAT.** ***verat-v.*** verb. verbe-u.[102] vesp.[36] vib. ***vinc.***[10] viol-o.[5] viol-t. ***vip.***[10] vip-a.[149] ***visc.*** wild.[36] wye.[58] x-ray[115] xan. yuc.[36] **ZINC.** **ZINC-P.**[58] zing. ziz.

Sadness; advice, if they cannot give: lil-t.[168]

Sadness; alone, when, agg.: aeth. all-s. allox.[119] **ARS.**[122] aur. bov. ***calc.*** con. ***dros.*** ferr. ***ferr-ar.*** hep.[10] kali-ar. kali-c. kali-n. lyc. m-aust.[10] mag-m.[10] ***mez.*** ***nat-m.*** phos. rat.[38] sil. ***stram.*** valer. zinc.

Sadness; alone, when, amel.: allox.[119] hydro-c.[2147]

Sadness; alternating with, anger: kali-fcy.[198] zinc.[10]

Sadness; alternating with, eccentricity: petr.[10]

Sadness; alternating with, energy, physical: ***aur.*** hir.[149]

Sadness; alternating with, exuberance: aster.[149] coff.[137] ferr.[10] ign.[109] meph.[149] mit.[72] nid.[149] onop.[149] petr.[10] plat.[10] senec.[137]

Sadness; alternating with, indifference: bamb-a.[1184] sep.[137]

Sadness; alternating with, positiveness: ozone[227]

Sadness; alternating with, quarrelsomeness: ***con.***[54] sulfonam.[149]

Sadness; alternating with, sexual excitement: lil-t.

Sadness; alternating with, tenderness: plat.[10]

Sadness; anger, after: apis ars. bell. foll.[1201] hydrog.[222] nux-v. petr.[1] phos. plat. puls. sep.

Sadness; anger, from: aur.[10] calc-p.[54] ign.[10] lyc.[10] nit-ac.[10] ***puls.***[54] spig.[10]

Sadness; angina, in: ***apis***[54]

Sadness; appearance, of: viol-o.[54]

Sadness; asthma, with, die, thinks he will: ars.[102] phos.[54] psor.[102] spong.[54]

Sadness; aversion to see her children from sadness: ***con.***[54]

Sadness; awkward and helpless manner, with: anac.[1]

Sadness; bad news, after: calc-p. pall.[54] puls.

Sadness; blaming others, with: lil-t.[168]

Sadness; brooding over imaginary wrongs and misfortunes, by: naja[130]

Sadness; business, when thinking of: mez.[58] ***puls.*** syph.[122]

Sadness; cardiac rheumatism, in: ***cact.***[54]

Sadness; cardialgia, in: ***kali-c.***[54]

Sadness; children, want of, from: aur.[91]

Sadness; coition, after: ***agar.***[116] calc. cedr.[54] con. ***nat-m.*** ph-ac.[144] sel.[116] ***sep.*** staph. sulph.[137]

Sadness; company, agg. in: agar.[60] euph. ***lyc.***[54]

Sadness; company, aversion to, desire for solitude: alum.[10] aur.[10] bamb-a.[1184] ***con.***[116] cupr.[10] ***helon.***[116] ***led.***[54] murx.[10] nat-c.[10] nat-m.[116] rhus-t.[10] sep.[193]
Sadness; company, desire for: stram.[10]
Sadness; conscience, of, as if he had committed a bad action, or not done his duty: cycl.[54]
Sadness; conscious of unnatural state of mind, because: tarent.[54]
Sadness; consoled, cannot be: ars.[54] nat-m.[189] nux-v.[189]
Sadness; continence, from: bell. **CON.** hyos. stram.
Sadness; criminal as if being the greatest: cycl.[60] sabad.[36]
Sadness; darkness: am-m.[116] ars.[116] calc. calc-sil.[58] camph. ***phos.*** plat. rhus-t. stram.
Sadness; despairing: ***agn.***[54] **HELL.**[54] ***plat.***[54] ***sars.***[54]
Sadness; difficulties, facing: ***cocc.***[54]
Sadness; disappointment, from: dig.[36] ign.[109]
Sadness; disease, about: alum.[36] cecr.[149] sin-n.[54] ***sulph.***[54] syph.[54]
Sadness; disease, about, incurable, of heart, which makes him reckless: ***phos.***[54]
Sadness; disease, about, sure he would not recover, in bronchial asthma: ***sin-n.***[54]
Sadness; disease, about, sure he, is going to die in twenty four hours: lac-d.[54]
Sadness; disease, as from, approaching: ph-ac.[36]
Sadness; disease, sure he, would not recover, in bronchial asthma: ***sin-n.***[54]
Sadness; diverted from thoughts of himself, desires to be: ***aur.***[54] camph.[54]
Sadness; domestic affairs, over: bar-c.[10] puls.[10] rhus-t.[10] ***sep.***[54] viol-t.[8]
Sadness; dwell constantly over her condition, inclination to: ***sulph.***[54]
Sadness; eating, after: alum. ***anac.*** ant-c.[85] arg-n. ***ars.*** asaf. bar-c. canth. caust. cham. ***chin.*** ***cinnb.*** con. graph.[111] hyos. iod. mosch. ***nat-c.*** **NUX-V.** ol-an. podo. ptel.[36] ***puls.*** til. zinc.
Sadness; eating, amel.: am-c. am-m. clem. kali-bi. mag-m. tarent.
Sadness; eating, desire for, with: ign.[193]
Sadness; emission, from: aur. carb-ac.[25] ***cypr.***[54] dig. dios. ***ery-a.***[54] ham. **KALI-BR.**[54] nat-c.[1] nat-p. **NUX-V.** ph-ac. ***puls.*** sang. sep.[54] ust.
Sadness; enjoys: ign.[137] nat-m.[137]
Sadness; epilepsy, with: ***atro.***[54] ***indg.***[54] ***sulph.***[54] tarent.[54]
Sadness; epistaxis, after: puls.
Sadness; errors of diet, from: **NAT-C.**
Sadness; fainting, with: ars.[10] ***lach.***[54] mosch.[10]
Sadness; family, for his: ars.[10] hep.[10] rhus-t.[10]
Sadness; fate, bemoaning: ***kali-br.***[54]
Sadness; fault, as if in: tarent.[36]
Sadness; fear, from: cimic.[58] nux-m.[54] sec.[137] ***stram.***[54]
Sadness; fear, with, death, of: cupr.[137] ***plat.***[54]
Sadness; fear, with, evil, of impending: ***aur.***[54] **KALI-I.**[54]
Sadness; flowers, from smell of: hyos.
Sadness; food, with aversion of: ***plat.***[54]
Sadness; fright, after: ign.[172] ***nux-m.***[54] ***stram.***[54]
Sadness; gloomy: anac.[10] ant-c.[10] ars.[10] aur.[10] bov.[5] calc.[10] cupr.[5] graph.[5] lach.[10] merc.[10] nux-v.[10] sep.[5] sulph.[10]
Sadness; gonorrhea, in: ***hydr.***[54] ***merc.***[54] ***thuj.***[54]
Sadness; grief, with: alum.[54] ***ign.***[54] ***lyc.***[54]
Sadness; happy, on seeing others: cic.[36] hell.[1] helon.
Sadness; harsh word, from a seemingly: med.[54]
Sadness; health, about the: acon.[54] ***sep.***[36] staph.[54]
Sadness; heart sensations, from: asaf.[54] lyc.[1]
Sadness; heart sensations, from, oppression: ***caust.***[54]
Sadness; heaviness of, body, with: ***cedr.***[54] graph.[10]
Sadness; heaviness of, feet, with: graph.[10]
Sadness; heaviness of, legs, with: calc.[1]
Sadness; house, driving out of: laur.[10]
Sadness; house, entering, on: plat.[36] tarent.[36]
Sadness; house, in, agg.: ***plat.***[36] **RHUS-T.**[36]
Sadness; hunger, with canine: ***nat-m.***[54]
Sadness; hypochondriacal: ***arg-n.***[54] caust.[1] con.[36b]
Sadness; hysteria, in: ***bell.***[54] ***cast.***[54] ***cocc.***[54] ***mosch.***[54]
Sadness; hysteria, in, inclination to murder, with: ***merc.***[54]
Sadness; imaginary obstacles, from: aur.[54]
Sadness; impotence, with: ***aur.***[54] ***calad.***[54] ***gels.***[54] **KALI-BR.**[54] ***spong.***[54]
Sadness; indifference, with: ***plat.***[54]
Sadness; injuries, from: ***hyper.***[54]
Sadness; injuries, from, head, of the: arn. ***cic.*** con. ***nat-s.*** puls. rhus-t. sul-ac.[8] sulph.

Sadness; insult, as if from: ***cocc.***
Sadness; intolerable: **NAT-C.**[54]
Sadness; jealousy, with: ***kali-ar.***[54]
Sadness; loss, after financial: arn.[137] ars.[54] aur.[137] mez.[137] psor.[137]
Sadness; love, from disappointed: ***aur.***[54] bell.[30] dig.[137] ***hyos.***[54] **IGN.**[54] ***nat-m.***[54]
Sadness; masturbation, from: agar. ***aur.***[54] calad. cocc. ***con. gels.***[54] ham. ***nat-m.*** nat-p. nux-v. **PH-AC.** ***plat.*** sars. sil. staph. sulph.
Sadness; men, with aversion to: stann.[54]
Sadness; mild persons, in: cocc.[10] con.[10] hell.[10] ign.[10] ***lyc.***[54] petr.[10] ph-ac.[10] ***puls.***[54] sil.[10] sulph.[10] verat.[10]
Sadness; misfortune, as if from: ***calc.*** chin-s. cycl. ph-ac. phel. phos. puls. rhus-t. staph. sulph.
Sadness; misfortune, as if from, impending: ***chin-s.***[36] phel.[36] vichy-g.[36]
Sadness; mortification, after: ***ign.***[54] ***puls.***[54]
Sadness; music, from: ***acon. ambr.***[102] ars.[171] bor.[58] calc-p.[198] cham. ***dig. graph. kreos.*** lyc. ***nat-c.*** nat-m.[58] nat-p. ***nat-s.*** nux-v. ph-ac.[1065] phos. ***sabin.*** sep. tarent. thuj. tub.[1065]
Sadness; noise, from: ant-c. nat-c.[58] phos.
Sadness; others, for: cocc.[10] sulph.[10]
Sadness; overwork and excesses, by: ***coca***[11] ign.[109]
Sadness; pain, from, heart, in region of: both-a.[139] crot-h.[36]
Sadness; past or finished events, over: psil.[164]
Sadness; persecutions of others, by: ***dros.***[54]
Sadness; pollutions, from: agar.[54] aur. ***calad.***[54] ***con.***[54] ***cypr.***[54] dig. dios. ***ery-a.***[54] ferr-br.[116] ham. **KALI-BR.**[54] med.[54] ***nat-m.***[54] nat-p. **NUX-V.** ph-ac. ***puls.*** sang. sars.[54] ***sep.***[54] sulph.[54] ust.
Sadness; preoccupied: ***clem.***[54]
Sadness; pressure about chest and heart, from: asaf.[36] graph.
Sadness; punishment, after: ***ign.***[54]
Sadness; quarrel with husband, after: ***anac.***[54]
Sadness; quiet: ars.[30] ***hell.***[54] ign. nux-v. ph-ac.[30] puls.[30] ziz.[54]
Sadness; respiration, impeded: ant-c. caust.[5] lach. laur. ***lyc.***[54] sep. tab.
Sadness; sexual excesses, from: agar.[116] agn.[102] aur.[102] ***cimic.***[102] con.[116] ***lil-t.***[102] nux-v.[102] pic-ac.[102] plat.[102] sep.[102] spong.[137]
Sadness; sexual, excitement, after: tarent.
Sadness; sexual, excitement, suppressed: **CON.**[162]
Sadness; sexual, excitement, with: bell.[10] manc.[122] naja[85]
Sadness; sexual, organs, with distress about: naja[85]
Sadness; shock, as from: nitro-o.[36]
Sadness; silent: **ARG-N.**[54] ***ars.***[10] bar-c.[10] ***cact.***[116] ***hell.***[54] ***ign.***[54] mag-c.[54] nit-ac.[10] ph-ac.[30] ***puls.***[54] stann.[54] verat.[116]
Sadness; sits in corner and does not want to have anything to do with the world: ***hipp.***[54]
Sadness; sleep, never awake, would like to: ars-met.[54]
Sadness; slight or treat, from an undeserved: arg-n.
Sadness; smiling, with: coffin.[1] lyc.[1]
Sadness; sound of bells and sight of his surroundings, agg. by: ant-c.[36]
Sadness; spermatorrhea, in: ***cypr.***[54] ***ph-ac.***[54] ***ust.***[54]
Sadness; sterility, from: aur.[137]
Sadness; stories, from sad: **CIC.**
Sadness; suicidal disposition, with: alum.[30] **AUR.**[54] calc.[30] caust.[30] chin.[30] cimic.[54] con.[30] graph.[30] ***hep.***[54] hydrog.[222] ign.[30] med.[54] ***merc-aur.***[116] ***naja***[54] ***nat-m.***[30] ***nat-s.***[116] op.[36] orni.[144] ***psor.***[36] ran-b.[54] rumx.[54] sep.[30] ***spig.***[54] **STAPH.**[30] sulph.[30]
Sadness; superfluous feeling, with: ***naja***[11]
Sadness; sympathy agg.: con.[137]
Sadness; talk, indisposed to: **ARG-N.**[54] ***ars.***[10] bar-c.[10] ***cact.***[116] ign.[30] mag-c.[54] nit-ac.[10] ph-ac.[30] ***puls.***[54] stann.[54] tarent.[192] verat.[116]
Sadness; thinking, marriage, about, amel.: orig.[137]
Sadness; thinking, position, of his: hell.[30]
Sadness; thunderstorm amel: bell-p.[146] carc.[146] sep.
Sadness; timidity, with: ***crot-h.***[54] plb.[54]
Sadness; vexation, after: calc-p.[54] kali-bi. ***plat.***[54] ***puls.***[54]
Sadness; weather, cloudy, in: aloe[140] am-c. bac.[62] plat.[193] sep.[193]
Sadness; weather, wet, in: am-c.[171] ***elaps***[54] rhus-t.[122]
Sadness; whistling and singing, with: merc-i-f.[54]
Sadness; work, aversion to, with: berb.[10] bov.[10] croto-t.[10] dros.[10] laur.[10] mez.[10] prun.[10] zinc.[10]
Sadness; wrong way, as if having done everything in, during headache: ***naja***[36]
Shrieking; sadness, with: ***plat.***[54]

Singing; sadness, after: merc-i-f.[54]
Sit; wrapped in deep, sad thoughts and notices nothing, as if: alum-sil.[58] ***ambr.***[122] aur. cench.[58] cham.[1] cimic.[58] ***cocc.*** con.[58] elaps ***hipp. ign.***[54] ozone[227] plat.[137] psor.[137] ***puls. stram.***[54] ***verat.***
Starting; alternating with sadness and faintness of heart: zinc.[10]
Strength increased, mental; sensation, alternating with sadness and weeping: ozone[227]
Talk; indisposed, sadness, in: **ARG-N.**[54] ***ars.***[10] bar-c.[10] ***cact.***[116] clem.[1] ign.[30] mag-c.[54] nit-ac.[10] ph-ac.[30] ***puls.***[54] stann.[54] verat.[116]
Tears; things, clothing, nightdress and bed clothes, sadness, in religious: ***kali-p.***[54]
Thinking; sad things agg, of: rhus-t.
Timidity; alternating with, sadness: zinc.[10]
Tranquillity; sadness, with: ***ars.***[54]
Unconsciousness; alternating with, sadness: thyr.[102]
Unconsciousness; sadness, from: aur.[184] visc.[184]
Vivacious; evening, low spirited at noon, or vice versa: ***zinc.***[54]
Vivaciousness; alternating with, sadness: sep.[36]
Vivaciousness; sadness, followed by: gels.[85]
Weary of life; sadness, with: aur.[1] ***kali-br.***[54] ***sulph.***[54]
Weeping; hypochondriasis, in: ***arg-n.***[54] mez.[54]
Weeping; sad, news, at: carb-v.[36] ph-ac.[122]
Weeping; sad, thoughts: alum. carb-v. cina kali-c. ***lac-d.***[54] lap-gr-m.[194] lob.[54] phel. plat. stram.
Weeping; thoughts, religious: ***kali-p.***[54]
Whistling; sadness, after great: merc-i-f.[54]
Will; loss of, sadness, from: ***arg-n.***[54]
Work; aversion to mental, hypochondriasis, in: ***ip.***[54]
Work; aversion to mental, sadness, in: ***arg-n.***[54]

ACON. Al, 71 - Dejected, as if she had no life in her. (lifeless)
Al, 28 - Variable humour, at one time gay, at another dejected.
He, 35 - Sadness with solicitude; concerned about future; about her recovery or fears loss of reason. (insanity)
AETH. He, 14 - Great sadness when alone.
AGN. Al, 3 - She is very sad, and keeps repeating that she will soon die.
He, 3 - Low spirited, fears of approaching death.
He, 4 - Despairing sadness; keeps repeating that she will die, that there is no use doing anything.
ALL-S. He, 3 - Sadness when alone; moral uneasiness; afraid of never getting well; fear of not being able to bear any kind of medicine; fear of being poisoned...
ALUM. Al, 6 - Depressed and friendless; he wishes only to be left alone, in the forenoon.
Al, 11 - She is constantly possessed by bad thoughts which oblige her to weep; at the same time she feels apprehensive and uneasy, as if something evil were to happen to her; everything she only looks at, fills her with sadness.
Al, 7 - The person imagines only disagreeable, sad images.
Ha, 4 - Dejected (depressed, unhappy) as to his disease.
Ha, 7-...anxiety as if something bad would happen (misfortune) to her; whatever she looks at, fills her with sadness.
Ha, 6 - Fancy paints to itself nothing but disagreeable, sad pictures.
He, 16 - Low-spirited, trifling things appeared insurmountable. (impossible)
AM-C. Al, 11 - Sad, low-spirited, apprehensive of evil...
Al, 13 - Kind of sadness not usual with me; no inclination to go out.
Ha, 3 - Very lugubrious (sad), with thoughts of death.
Ha, 16 - Cloudy weather makes her very sad.
AM-M. Ha, 2 - Anxious and melancholy, as if internal grief or sorrow were gnawing in her heart.
AMBR. Al,N-8 - Great sadness; despondent, does not want to live.
Ha, 483 - Sad thoughts take possession of him, with sinking feeling about the heart; he is for a long time depressed in spirits.
ANAC. Ha, 10 - In the forenoon, extremely hypochondriac, discouraged and despondent, with awkward (unskillful), helpless manner; ...
He, 49 - Sadness; looks on dark side of everything.
ANDROC. Sh, 144 - Sadness and confusion, unable to see a solution to her problems.

Worse 6:00 p.m. onwards. (28)
Sh, 154 - Sighing —sighed deeply all day, as if trying to remove a sadness from his diaphragm. (29)
ANT-T. He, 30 - Depression of mind and fear that he will never get well.
ANTH. Al, 1 - Very low spirits; feeling as if something were about to happen; as if would like to get alone, and unburden (relieve) himself by crying ...
ARG-N. He, 35 - Sad; fear of apoplexy.
ARS. Ha, 45 - Super-sensitiveness and over-tenderness of mind; dejected, sad and lugubrious (unhappy), she is troubled and solicitous about the merest trifles.
He, 61 - Religious melancholy; hopelessness, despair.
ASAF. He, 5 - Anxious sadness and apprehensions (fear) of dying.
ATRO. Al, 33 - Mentally either very sad, depressed in constant anxiety and restlessness, fearful of misfortune, or angry and inclined to be alone, seldom lively.
Ha, 17 - Sad and morose, preferring solitude and a dark room to society of friends.
AUR. Ha, 340 - He sits apart (separated), all by himself in a corner, wrapt up in himself, as if in the deepest melancholy, when left undisturbed; but the slightest contradiction excites the greatest heat and anger,...
Ha, 344 - Discontented with all circumstances; he imagines that he finds everywhere some obstacle (impediment, restriction) in the way; at one time he thinks that this is owing to an unlucky (unfortunate) fate (destiny), at another that he himself is to blame (censured) for it ; when the latter was the case he was particularly mortified and dejected.
Ha, 355 - He is discontented with himself and depressed in spirits.
Ha, 4 - Discontented with all conditions; he thinks that he everywhere finds an impediment, caused now by an opposing fate,(destiny) then again by himself, which latter mortifies him and renders him dejected.(sad)
He, 79 - Ailments from grief, disappointed love.
BAR-C. Al, 9 - Extremely despondent and depressed; she believes that she must die; cries.
Al, 5 - Sad and fearful; he has all kinds of sad thoughts about his future state, and thinks that he is lost entirely; in the evening.
Ha, 6 - Sad and anxious; all manner of gloomy (sad) ideas as to his future fate (destiny) rise in his mind, and believes himself totally forsaken (deserted); in the evening.
BOV. He, 6 - Sad, depressed and desponding when alone.
BRASS. Sh, 11 - I began to feel a little depressed; I'm definitely not in a party mood, desire to be still and quiet, maybe listen to classical music, Bach, Chopin, something well composed and not Beethoven 08, 6C, 05:08:30
BRY. Ha, 779 - Morose; looking at everything with ill-will.
He, 20 - Great sense of insecurity, with mental depression.
CALC-A. Al, 7 - Apprehensive, sad mood, as though he were awaiting some depressing news.
Ha, 264 - Very sad humor, as if he had to expect (anticipation) bad news.
CALC-F. Al,S-1-...tendency to look on the dark side of things, with much depression of spirits. Feeling of anxiety about money matters, or thought would come to want (lack), or would soon be "running astern" (reversed, failure) financially...disposition to set a higher value on money than natural to him (avarice?, poverty?).
He, 1 - All day an unusual tendency to look on the dark side of things; with much depression of spirits.
CALC-S. Al, 7 - Excessive, bitter melancholy, with distressing apprehensions of evil to loved ones.
CALC. Ha, 2 - Melancholy, not really mournful (unhappy) feeling, about the heart, without cause, with a sort of voluptuous tremor all over the body.
Ha, 9 - Grief and complains over insults long past.
Ha, 30 - She despairs of her life and believes she has to die (punishment?) ; her heart is sad with weeping, and frequent attacks of sudden, general heat, as if she had hot water poured (flow) over her.
He, 51 - Fear, that something sad or terrible will happen.

He, 38 - Low-spirited and melancholy, with weeping and despair of life.

CARB-AN. Al, 1 - Desire to be alone ; she is sad and reflective (thoughtful); avoids all conversation.

Al, 10 - Discouraged and sad (unhappy); everything seems so sad and lonely that she desires to weep.

Ha, 1 - Extremely melancholy (depression, grief) mood, with a sensation of being deserted.

Ha, 5 - Pusillanimous (cowardice) and sad; everything seems to her so lonely (alone, deserted) and sad, that she would like to weep.

Ha, 7 - Morose thoughts and ill-humor, not to be driven away, concerning things present and past, even to weeping.

CARL. Al, 5 - Mood very much depressed, like an excessive homesickness; at last violent weeping.(second day) (after four glasses)

CAST. Al, 2 - Very melancholy and depressed, as if something evil would befall her, in the afternoon.

CAUST. Al, 9 - Sad, weeping mood, full of care, as if beside oneself.

Ha, 24 - Discontented with himself, of gloomy (melancholic) countenance.

He, 25 - Sorrowful thoughts during night, during day weeping, anxiety and misgiving (doubt) about the future.

He, 27 - Melancholy mood; sadness; hopelessness.

CHAM. Al, 15 - Very depressed mood, with anxiety and oppression, as of impending evil.

CHEL. Al, 25 - Sadness, even to weeping, and despondency (desperation) about the present and future.

Al, 27 - Extremely depressed; full of sad thoughts about the present and future, even to weeping; he had no rest of any kind.

Ha, 154 - Extraordinarily depressed, full of gloomy (dark) thoughts about the present and future, causing him to weep;...

Ha, 155 - Sad to weeping and depressed about the present and future.

CHIN. Ha, 1119 - Humour gloomy, no wish to live.

CIC. Ha, 228 - He thought with anxiety of the future and was always sad.

Ha, 229 - Anxiety; he was violently affected by sad stories.

He, 30 - Anxiety, excessively affected by sad stories.

CIMIC. Al, 3 - Miserable, dejected (sad) feeling.

He, 20 - Miserable dejected feeling; anxious weeping.

COB. Al, 4 - Low-spirited; thinks too little of himself.

COCC. Al, 9 - Constant sad thoughts, as though he had suffered an insult.

Al, 10 - She is absorbed in the saddest thoughts, and affronts (indignity) sink deep into her heart.

Ha, 521 - He is sunk in saddest thoughts, and insults he has received he takes deeply to heart.

Ha, 524 - Continual sad thoughts, just as if he had received insults.

He, 22 - Great sorrowfulness, with constant inclination to sit in a corner buried in thought.

He, 24 - Melancholy and sad; indulges in sad reveries (daydream); is sensitive to insults, slights (despises) and disappointment.

He, 25 - Melancholy and sadness, with weeping and constant profound absorption in sorrowful thoughts; great apprehensive anxiety of conscience, and feeling at heart as after committing a wicked deed (act), with desire to escape.

COLOC. He, 11 - Morose mood; becomes offended at everything.

CON. Ha, 18 - Very morose; ...as if a great guilt weighed him down; at the same time a sensation of paralysis in all the limbs; ...

CROT-C. Al, 18 - Her thoughts dwell on death; with great sadness.

CUPR. He, 18 - Unconquerable sadness, constant restlessness, as if some misfortune were approaching; fears he will lose his reason.

CUR. Al, 10 - Brooding sadness, frequent weeping, with desire for solitude.

He, 2 - Very much depressed about herself, desire only to shut herself up away from people.

CYCL. Ha, 197 - Excessive sadness, as if he had done something bad and had neglected his duty.

He, 12 - Great sadness, as if he had committed a bad action or not done his duty.

He, 20 - Ill humored, morose mood; could easily take offense at every trifle.

DIG. Al, 19 - Weeping sadness about many things which have disappointed him.

Al, 31 - Great irritability; everything especially sad things affected him very much, and the merest trifle can make him hopelessly despondent; lasting more than three months.

Ha, 14-..he is much affected by everything, but especially by sad things, and the least trifle can throw him into disconsolate despair.(sensitive)

He, 10 - Profound melancholy,...great fear of future; insane obstinacy and disobedience, with desire to escape.

He, 14 - Gloomy, peevish and distrustful.(suspicious)

DROS. Al, 4 - He is depressed by the persecutions of others on all sides, and also discouraged and solicitous about the future.

Ha, 275 - He is sad and dejected about the ills (evil) of life, which people cause one another and himself, respecting which he is anxious and concerned;...(ethical)

ELAPS. He, 3 - Depression of spirits, and desire for solitude.

FERR. Al, 12 - She never complained or wept and was always plunged (fall) in deep melancholy when no one was about her.

Ha, 290 - Low spirits (sad) as if from bowels being too relaxed.

He, 8 - Mental depression, gloomy (dark) foreboding thoughts.

He, 15 - Excited by slightest opposition; everything irritates or depresses her.

GELS. He, 32 - Complaints: (ailments) from exciting or bad news; sudden emotions; the anticipation of any unusual ordeal (difficulty) ; general depression from heat of sun or summer.

He, 33 - Effects (ailments from) of grief; cannot cry; when thinking of his symptoms (disease), also when spoken to of his loss ; >from diverting talk; oppression and palpitation of heart; feels a sense of peril (danger, harm, risk) ; face flushed; sleeplessness; subdued (subjugate, yielding) manner; ...

GERM. Sh, 121 - Very strong longing for excitement and some love adventure. I planned to go out, but though I probably would be disappointed, so I stayed at home and was depressed instead. Feel like drinking - to get away from myself and everything. 18, 30C, 04:00:00

Sh, 173 - Sadness from the pains. Not irritable, just gently sad. 05, 6C, 25:00:00

Sh, 108 - Hopeless, helpless, gloom and doom. Weeping and self pity. 14, 30C, 23:00:00.

Sh, 172 - Sad, indifferent and hopeless feeling. Want to cry but it won't come. 18, 30C, 00:14:00

Sh, 114 - Difficult to feel joy, pleasure. It is more safe to be sad, unhappy, to suffer. Because joy doesn't last. 18, 30C, 85:XX:XX

Sh, 169 - Depressed, wonder how I would manage economically. 21, 12C, 39:XX:XX

GRAPH. Al, 3 - Sadness, with thoughts of nothing but death.

He, 6 - Sadness, with thoughts of nothing but death.

HALI-L. Sh, 227 - Pictures of the mountains make me homesick. Deeper than homesick. Feeling low, remembering the freedom of going to them. Missing mountains and the outdoors. 02, 30C, 07:01:XX

Sh, 403 - For three weeks I was in a depression, unlike anything I have felt for a long time. Deep sense of low self-worth. Feeling invisible, uncared for and envious. I was lethargic, couldn't do anything. My practice dropped, patients just didn't show up. I felt I sunk as low as I needed to go, unmotivated. Felt unappreciative of all I have. Unappreciative of my life which I usually adore. Anger, dissatisfaction with life, isolating. I wasn't seeing anyone not even my husband, exhaustive. Had no dreams during the depression —unusual. I am emerging from it now. 01, 30C, 30:XX:XX-50:XX:XX

Sh, 412 - Somewhat apathetic with an undercurrent of depression. Neither here nor there. I was water. Moody as a rainy day, down, blue, depressed, easily aggravated. 18, 30C, 04:13:30

Sh, 416 - Feel really dull with the rain. I think I'm in a mild depression. I'm not visiting friends, just hanging around. No

goals, not doing things. 08, 30C, 03:XX:XX
Sh, 417 - Frustrated and depressed. Feeling lonely, friendless and unaccomplished. 18, 30C, 15:XX:XX
Sh, 431 - The first thing that happened was I became very depressed and fearful. I was weak and couldn't resolve my issues. I became a laughable matter. The next thing I knew, I became embittered at all those I thought were laughing at me. During the last week of the proving, the vindictive side of reacting to that depression came out. 18, 30C, 7:XX:XX

HELL. Al, 7 - Sad mood, on account of his present condition (restriction, limitation), everything seems shallow (stupid, superficial) and has no incentive for him. (lost:motive, purpose, force, mission,) -(lost: depth, profundity, perception.)
Al, 15 - Dread of death (in a sufferer from religious melancholy).
Al, 10 - He becomes melancholy on beholding (observe) a cheerful person, and then, for the first time, feels very unhappy.
Ha, 284 - On seeing a happy person he becomes melancholy and then only he feels very unhappy.
Ha, 286 - Sad disposition respecting his present position, everything seems to him so insipid (tedious, boring,) and nothing interests him.
He, 11 - Psychical conditions occupying a place between melancholia and mania, and in conditions where true depression and weakness is present, in which the patient is governed by a fixed idea.

HELON. Al, 2 - Reaction (from feeling of general wellness) began, and for a fortnight I was in a mental hell; it was the most profound mental depression I have ever known; I was plunged into the most abject despair.

HEP. Ha, 296 - In the evening a frightful anxiety for two hours; he thought he must be ruined (lost, failed), and was sad to that degree that he could have killed himself.
Ha, 4 - Fearful anguish, in the evening, for two hours; he thought he had to perish (die), and was sad even so that he could have committed suicide. (redemption, salvation)
He, 14 - Low spirited, even to thoughts of suicide.

HURA. Al, 10 - Sadness, melancholy; she thinks despondingly of the future.
Al, 12 - Flow of sad thoughts; she fancies she is about to lose a dear friend.
Al, 15 - Hypochondria, sadness, despair; he fancies he is repudiated and deserted by his relations. (rejected, refused)

HYDR. He, 5 - Depression of spirits, sure of death and desires it.

HYDROG. Sh, 32 - Depressed —like seeing a window open and unable to go through it. 16, 30C, 08:XX:XX
Sh, 33 - About two months after beginning the proving, developed an extreme range of mental symptoms that he had never had before. These included severe depression with strong alternations of moods, & high then low, & with suicidal tendency, desire to jump from a high building or cut wrist, confusion of identity (especially concerning sex and homosexuality) and became more religious. He moved away from his parents home (which he had never before been able t o do) and shut himself away in a small flat. This condition lasted for another six or seven months and was finally antidoted by Phosphorus 200. Before that, he had tried to anti-dote it with acupuncture, to no avail. 24, 30C, 60:XX:XX
Sh, 155 - In the afternoon (during the full moon) I felt low and depressed, insecure and vulnerable. Could not cope with work load and didn't want to be alone. 12, 6C, 39:XX:XX
Sh, 182 - A feeling of boredom and depression at 10:00p.m., whilst in company — very distressful. I didn't talk at all, friends thought something had greatly upset me. 24, 30C, 01:10:XX
Sh, 233 - Feel a blanket of depression over me. 08, 30C, 09:XX:XX
Sh, 234 - Developed a self pitying, very tearful depression through the morning. I was unable to communicate any of these feelings and this led to a fierce row with girlfriend. 04, 12C, 30:XX:XX
Sh, 235 - Feel a bit depressed and frustrated by present circumstances. Feel like the unappreciated victim. 04, 12C, 14:XX:XX
Sh, 274 - Developed an aversion to the idea of sex —confused about sexual issues and identity. Became aware of being bi-sexual

or homosexual (in a man). "I want to find out who I am. I should know at 23. I used to know. What am I sexually?" Very confused. This led to suicidal depression. 24, 30C, 100:XX:XX

HYOS. He, 74 - Disappointed love followed by: epilepsy, melancholy, rage, or inclination to laugh at everything; despair and propensity to drown himself. (ailments from)

He, 76 - After a fit of passion, melancholia,... appetite gone;...

He, 77 - After a fit of passion and sudden fear, became so melancholy and timorous as to hide himself in every corner,...

IGN. He, 2-...;sees everything as if through a fog (obscurity) ; sits quietly, with a vacant gaze (expression), always thinking of the mortification endured,... prefers to be alone; thinking of the past mortification...[0]Melancholy after mortification.

He, 22 - Melancholia from suppressed mental sufferings, with much sighing; desire to be alone (solitude) so as to give way to her real or imaginary grief; weeps bitterly.

He, 26 - Great grief after losing persons or objects very dear.

He, 37 - Tears wept inwardly, the pain and penalty (forfeit) of unrequited (unrecompensed) love; desires solitude so that one may nourish inward grief;...

He, 61 - Melancholia after great grief and domestic trouble; complete sleeplessness; suicidal thoughts and desire to escape.

He, 62 - Ill effects (ailments) from hearing bad news; from vexation with reserved displeasure ; from grief, or suppressed mental sufferings; of shame and disappointed love.

He, 30 - Became bilious, nervous, depressed, and would scarce move from the fire, for days together. Morbid grief

He, 55 - Anger, followed by quiet grief or sorrow.

KALI-BR. Al, 14 - Great mental depression, a feeling (sensation) of approaching death.

Al, 19 - Painful sadness, profound indifference, and almost disgust for life.

Al, 16 - A consciousness that the currents or sources of psychical force are hampered...(obstructed) sometimes makes an intellectual patient who is moderately bromized, reason himself into depression....

Al, 24 - The patient, who has been violently excited, glorying (adoration) in his imaginary power of body and mind, becomes desponding sullen, melancholic, and frequently lachrymose, often even despairing.

He, 39-...fear and apprehension that she is losing her mind (insanity);...makes her utterly (completely) miserable to be looked at or spoken to; fear to see people; always depressed and lowspirited;...

KALI-C. Al, 7 - Sad, lonely (solitary) ; she seeks society in order to enliven (animate) herself.

Al, 15 - At night after lying down, sad forebodings overtake him, on account of which he is unable to sleep.

Al, 4 - Very much depressed; she was obliged to weep much, because it was constantly in her thoughts that she must die.

Al, 21 - Apprehensiveness and great sadness.

KALI-FCY. Al, 1 - Feeling of sadness and some disposition to tears, caused by an impression that he was soon to die and leave his friends; disposition to take a sad view of the beauties of autumn; the apprehension of approaching sickness and death can be overcome by reason, but soon returns.

KALI-P. He, 15 - Profound hypochondria and melancholia, weariness of life and fear of death, suspiciousness...

KREOS. Al, 5 - Towards evening her spirits were much depressed, and she was doubtful whether she would ever be well again.

LAC-C. Al,N-33 - Depression of spirits, doubts her ability and success, thinks she will have heart disease and die of it.

He, 26 - Depression of spirits, doubts her ability (competence, aptitude) and success (prospering, progressing, achieving), thinks she will have heart disease and die of it.

He, 27 - Chronic "blue" condition; everything seems so dark that it can grow no darker.

LAC-D. Al,N-1 - Depression of spirits; don't care to live (indifferent) ; question as to quietest and most certain way of hastening (accelerate) one's death.

LACH. He, 39 - Weak and unhappy, particularly in morning, when she feels, on awaking, friendless and forsaken; ...(deserted) has had domestic troubles. 0 Melancholia

He, 35 - Feels extremely sad, unhappy and distressed in mind on waking in morning.

LAM. Al, 2 - Extraordinary sadness; he thought he had been blamed for reverses (failure) for which he was blameless, and in consequence was obliged to suffer;...

LAUR. He, 6 - Fear and anxiety about imaginary evils; despondency.(desperation)

LEPI. Al, 6 - Deep melancholy; with thoughts of sickness.

LIL-T. Al, 9 - Depression of spirits; constant inclination to weep, with fearfulness, and apprehension of suffering from some terrible internal disease, already seated.

LOB-S. He, 1 - Much depressed, tearful, unhappy.

He, 4 - Great depression of spirits; unhappy state of mind,...

LYC. Ha, 68 - After being anxious, there is a great inclination to laugh about trifles, for several hours, and then weeping for half an hour without cause.

He, 14 - Dread (fear) of men ; of solitude, irritability and melancholy.

LYSS. Al,N-72 - An attack of mental depression and indifference quite (very) strange to him; feels as if he could do nothing; if he forces himself he lacks mental power.

He, 72 - An attack of mental depression and indifference quite strange to him; feels as if he could do nothing; if he forces himself he lacks mental power.

MAG-M. Ha, 3 - Apprehensive and melancholic, lonely (isolated, abandoned) ; she is homesick and weeps.

He, 2 - Tearful, inclined to weep; sad and homesick.

MANG. Al, 3 - Constant uneasiness (restlessness), as if he apprehended something sad.

Ha, 327 - Ill-humored, so that the most joyful music does not cheer (joy) him, but he feels as if refreshed by the most melancholy music.

MED. He, 28 - Spirits in the depths, weighed down with heavy, solid gloom (sadness),> by torrents of tears.

MELI. He, 8 - Religious melancholy of four months' standing; ...

MERC. Ha, 1249 - All day long depression of spirits combined with anxiety; he always thought he was going to hear of something disagreeable.

He, 32 - Much wretchedness (miserable, unhappy) and dejection (sadness) of spirits, with diarrhea.

He, 33 - Hysterical melancholia, with inclination to murder.

MORPH. Al, 13 - Complete melancholy, so that he desired to commit suicide.

MUR-AC. Al, 4 - Sad, quiet, and discontented with his lot.(destiny)

Al, 6 - During the menses she is sad, taciturn, as if she had no life.

Ha, 2 - Sad and introverted, as if she had no life in her, during the menses.

MURX. Al, 2 - Great depression of spirits; it seemed to her that she was hopelessly ill.

Al, 4 - It made me miserable; I was so low-spirited that I gave up everything; I had no strength left.

He, 2 - Deep sadness at approach of menses, all her symptoms gave her great concern (care); seemed to her she was hopelessly ill; she gave up everything.

NAJA. Al, 9 - Considerable depression of spirits, and a feeling of inability to exertion of any kind, and a conviction that all is going wrong;...

Al, 10 - Great depression of spirits this morning; everything for two or three hours appeared to go wrong with me, and to be without remedy;...

Al, 11 - Great depression of mind, with the distress, about the generative organs. (sexual)

Al, 12 - Sadness or serious disposition; sadness and irresolution.

NAT-C. Al, 11 - Intolerable melancholy and apprehension; she was wholly occupied whith sad thoughts.

Ha, 5 - Great melancholy and apprehensiveness; only occupied with sad thoughts.

NAT-M. Al, 35 - Sad as if sick (suffering), in the afternoon.

Al, 42 - Melancholic depression, and sad apprehension, and disheartened (depress, discourage) all day, without definite cause,

with constant palpitation, without physical infirmity.
Al, 6 - She talked more than usual, but did not like so much to be talked to; when she had nothing to say, she became depressed and melancholy.
Al, 39 - Melancholy mood; she has preferred to be alone for several days past.
Ha, 5 - Melancholy dejection and sorrowful anxious despondency all day, without any known cause, with unceasing palpitation,...
He, 34 - A pregnant woman saw a man who had a disfiguring nasal cancer; this haunted (obsessed) her, and she was sure her child would be marked; she was melancholy, avoided society, wept continually.
NAT-P. Al, 6 - Very despondent; imagined he was going to be sick, to have typhoid fever.
NAT-S. Al, 4 - Lachrymose; thinks only of sad things.
NEON. Sh, 84 - Repeated prophetic notions of daily events before hearing of them, causing anxiety and discomfort; thoughts of a person not seen for months and found he had phoned a few days before, depression and sadness unexplained until heard of sad family news that had already happened. 10, 6C, 01:XX:XX
Sh, 123 - Immediately after taking the remedy, everything stopped. I become very subdued and depressed. It felt like a void. No joy in birds singing. "How can I lift it?" 20, 6C, 00:00:00
Sh, 193 - Feel sad and depressed while walking outside in the cold, clear, open air. I don't want to be outside, and walk with head down. On returning inside, I feel in suspended animation. Listless, low energy. Want to close my eyes, which are dry, with heavy, slightly numb lids. I don't feel like working and would just like to go to sleep or read a good book in bed under covers. I still feel chilly from 5 minute walk outside though I've been inside and dressed warmly for 5 minutes. 06, 12C, 00:01:00
NICC. He, 1 - Low-spirited, tearful; fears something evil will happen.
NIT-AC. Al, 33 - Depressed, as if despondent and as if in deep thought.
Ha, 2 - Dejected, as if desponding and as if lost in thoughts.
NUX-V. He, 26 - Melancholic in consequence of losing his position (rank),...the least contradiction puts him out entirely...(ailments from)
OP. Al, 187 - The memory and mental powers generally became greatly impaired, attended by a miserable depression of spirits.
PALL. He, 15 - Depressing news makes all her symptoms worse.
PETR. Ha, 1 - Sad and dispirited, with a sick (suffering) feeling owing (due) to weakness of the heart.
He, 11 - Melancholy mood, imagines but little time is left him to make his will.
PH-AC. Al, 12 - Sad, earnest, discouraged only when walking in the open air, the farther (great distance) he walks the more it increases; in the house it gradually disappears.
Al, 9 - Sad and solicitous concerning the future.
Al, 10 - Sadness and feeling of solitude, as if she would be sick.
Ha, 3 - Sad and full of solicitude (anxiety), afraid she might fall ill.
Ha, 8 - Sad serious, disheartened (depressed), only while walking in the open air, increasing the longer he walks; at home it gradually passed of and he became more serene.
He, 11 - Ailments from care, grief, sorrow, chagrin, homesickness; or disappointed love;...
PHEL. Al, 9 - Sad mood and fear the whole day, as from impending misfortune; she wept, and was prone to think upon sad subjects.
PHOS. Al, 69 - Sadness and melancholic, as if some misfortune had happened.
Al, 80 - Mental depression, and a most uncommon fearfulness or timidity, with a great sense of fatigue.
Ha, 5 - Sad and melancholy, as if some accident had happened to his beloved ones.
Ha, 43 - Depressed on account of his health.
Ha, 78 - She has to laugh against her will, while she is sad.
He, 21 - Dejection (sadness); thought he would die.
PLAT. Ha, 18 - Taciturnity and involuntary weeping, even after the most friendly

address (communication), so that she gets vexed (anger) about it herself.
He, 48 - Mental depression from onanism. (masturbation)
PLB. Al, 112 - He is very sad, has no desire to live, and has threatened to destroy himself, and is very fault-finding (severe, critical) with his friends.
Al, 114-...he imagined his disease incurable, and gave way to the gloomy thoughts which the fear of death excited, and to repinings (sadness) caused by the dread of his journey to Valencia.
PODO. He, 3 - Depression: imagines he is going to die or be very ill;...
PSOR. Al, 13 - She is so downhearted (unhappy) that she could commit suicide, then is full of phantasms.
Al, 14 - Very melancholy and despairing; he wishes to die in spite of his good luck.
Al,N-22 - Depressed in spirits and hopeless.
Al,N-14 - Anxious, full of fear, melancholic; evil forebodings.
Al,N-21 - Very depressed, sad, suicidal thoughts.
Al,N-27 - Is so downhearted she could commit suicide, then is so full of phantasms.
Al,N-32 - Melancholy after suppressed itch;...seeks solitude, despairs of recovery; ...
Al,N-25 - Much depression on account of an eruption on dorsum of hand which appears over night.
Al,N-28 - Great depression of mind during climaxes, with chronic abdominal disorders.
He, 21 - Very depressed, sad, suicidal thoughts.
He, 22 - Depressed in spirits and hopeless.
PTEL. Al, 2 - Depression of spirits, and a feeling of anxiety about some unknown thing, with the severe headache, in the afternoon.
PULS-N. Al, 3 - Great depression of spirits, in the afternoon; a kind of homesickness, with despondency.(grief)
PULS. Al, 28 - He sinks into a condition of sadness and despondency from disagreeable news.
Al, 32 - Extremely morose, will not answer, takes everything in bad part, in the evening towards sundown.
Ha, 1131 - On hearing some disagreeable news he became affected with sadness and despondency.
He, 21 - Continuous crying with great melancholy and fear of losing her reason, or that she might commit suicide.
He, 51 - Sinks into a condition of sadness and despondency (grief) from disagreeable news.(ailments from)
He, 52 - After mortification, sad gloomy (melancholy) and weary (disgusted) of life;...thinks of drowning with great pleasure;...
RAN-B. Al, 3 - Ill humored, and disposed to quarrel and scold the first forenoon; in the evening is desponding, apprehensive, sensitive, discontented; on the second day he again inclines to be provoked by innocent jests of his friends, etc.;...
RHUS-T. Al, 4 - Full of sad thoughts, anxious and fearful, wherewith she gradually lost strength, and was obliged to lie down for hours in order to regain vigor.
Ha, 953 - Melancholy, sad, and anxious, as if about to hear of a calamity,(misfortune, disaster) or as if she were solitary (lonely, alone) and all around her were dead (lifeless, extinct) and silent (quiet) ; or as if she had bid farewell (separation) to an intimate friend ; worst in the room, diminished by walking in a open air.
Ha, 964 - Full of sad thoughts, anxious and timorous (timid), during which she always lost her strength, (power) and must lie down for hours; in order to recover her strength. (inert, motionless)
Ha, 972 - From sad thoughts, which she could not get rid of, she became timorous and fainthearted.(coward, fearful)
Ha, 963 - Ill-humored, dejected, and as if in despair.
Ha, 952 - Sadness, making him prefer quiet solitude.
He, 12 - Fear and despair on account of sad thoughts, which she could not get rid of. (fixed ideas)
RHUS-V. Al, 1 - Great sadness, no desire to live, everything seems gloomy.
ROB. Al, 13 - Hypochondriac grief; he seeks pleasures and tries to divert his mind, without succeeding.
RUMX. Al, 4 - Depression, as if some evil was impending.
SABIN. He, 4 - Great tiredness and laziness,

with a feeling of deep-seated inward trouble, which makes him melancholy and sad.
SEC. Al, 36 - The greatest depression of mind and loss of strength, a very sick feeling.
SEP. Al, 22 - Sadness about her health.
Al, 24 - Feel very low-spirited, and don't care what becomes of me.
Al, 33 - Received news of the slight illness of a friend, which caused great mental depression (at another time it would not have made slightest impression); this condition grew on me until I became so nervous that I felt that unless I held on something, I should scream.
Al, 34 - Feel very much depressed, at 7 A.M.; feel like quarreling with everybody; became very much excited about a mere trifle, and said some very sharp things. (feeling ashamed of it at the same time)
Ha, 5 - Sad (despair) about her health.(vitality)
Ha, 10 - All her troubles present themselves in a very sad light to her mind, so that she is despondent.(sad, depressed)
He, 11 - Sad about her health and domestic affairs, discontented with everything.
SIL. Al, 11 - Gloominess; she felt as if she would die, and for the time lost her memory.
He, 8 - Overanxious about himself; low-spirited...
He, 13 - Desponding, melancholy, tired of life.
STAPH. Ha, 695 - As if dead (decease, lifeless, inert) in mind and sad, but not to weeping.
He, 4 - Sad distressing thoughts about one's illness.
He, 2 - Indifference, low-spirited, dullness of mind; after onanism.(masturbation)
STRAM. He, 172 - Downcast and full of anguish, believes herself unworthy of eternal bliss, because she is unable to perform her duties.
SULPH. Al, 41 - Frequently during the day she has attacks of melancholy, lasting a few minutes, when she feels extremely unhappy, without cause; she wishes to die.
Ha, 4 - Often during the day, attacks lasting for several minutes, when she feels herself utterly (completely) miserable, without any cause, like melancholy; she desires to die.
Ha, 5 - Sad pusillanimous, full of weariness (fatigue) of life.
Ha, 58-..She thinks of nothing but anxious, annoying and dejecting thoughts, which she cannot get rid of; this makes her apprehensive and peevish unto tears.
He, 31 - Depressed about her illness, and out of humor.
He, 32 - Melancholy mood; dwelling on religious or philosophic speculations; anxiety about soul's salvation; indifference about lot (destiny) of others.
He, 34-...; profound melancholy; considers herself disgraced (dishonor, degradation) ; speaks of dying, finds life insupportable;...
TAB. Al, 20 - Gloom, hypochondria, apprehensions of sudden death.
Al, 19 - Low spirits, want of resolution and general hypochondriasis.
TARENT. Al, 46 - Sadness, lamentation, as if a misfortune had befallen him;...
THUJ. He, 23 - Mental depression, after childbirth (puerperal), in consequence of being told that there had been a slight rupture (division, hurt) of perineum; grows quiet; thinks she must die;...wants to jumps the window; does not care for children or her relatives (careless) ;..(sensitive to disrupt, partition)
UST. He, 2 - Very sad, cries frequently; excessively prostrated from sexual abuse and loss of semen; sleep restless.
VERAT-V. He, 3 - From sudden cerebral congestion: quarrelsome delirium; great mental depression and fear of death;...
VERAT. He, 22 - Nymphomania, with violence and destructiveness; had been disappointed in love; melancholia; ...great desire for sexual intercourse; void (empty) of shame; obscenity; ....
VINC. He, 2 - Sadness, with fear of death.
ZINC. He, 29-...;sad, weeps frequently; despairs of her recovery;...

SALVATION

Anxiety; salvation, about: aq-mar.[149] **ARS.** ars-s-f.[58] ***aur.*** aur-ar.[58] aur-s.[58] ***calc.*** ***calc-ar.***[122] calc-s. ***camph.*** cann-i. carbn-s. chel. ***graph.*** hura ign. kali-p. **LACH.** **LIL-T.** ***lyc.*** ***med.*** ***mez.*** nat-m. nux-v.[30]

ph-ac.[30] plat. plb.[58] podo.[58] ***psor. puls.*** **STAPH.**[30] ***stram. sulph. thuj.*** **VERAT.**

Anxiety; salvation, faith, about loss of his: coloc.[30] merc.[30] nux-v.[30] staph.[30] sulph.[30]

Anxiety; salvation, hell, of: ***plat.***[54]

Anxiety; salvation, scrupulous as to their religious practices, too: ars.[30] ign.[30] lyc.[30] nux-v.[30] ph-ac.[30] puls.[30] **STAPH.**[30] **SULPH.**[30]

Begging, entreating supplicating: ars. aur.[5] bell.[5] kali-c.[5] plat.[5] puls.[5] stram.

Begging, pray for him, to, and not to leave him alone: lyss.[54]

Begging; relief, for: plb.[36]

Delirium; blessing, asks a: bell.[36]

Delusions; doomed, soul cannot be saved, cries and rages: ***ign.***[54].

- hanging, sees persons, beckoning him to cut them loose: ars.[54]
- lost, salvation for: ars.[58] ***aur.*** hell.[58] hura plb.
- martyrdom: carc.[207] nat-c.[162]
- obtain peace and safety through absolution from a priest of Papal church, although a zealous protestant, that she can only: ***plb.***[54]
- religious, redemption and devil, about: ***anac.***[54]

Despair; religious: ***arg-n.*** **ARS. AUR.** aur-ar.[58] aur-i.[58] aur-s.[58] ***calc.*** calc-ar.[58] calc-i.[58] ***camph. chel.*** cycl.[116] hell. hura ign. ***kali-p.*** **LACH. LIL-T.** ***lyc.*** med. ***mez.*** nat-m. ozone[227] plat. plb. podo. ***psor.*** **PULS.**[122] ***stram. sulph. thuj.*** **VERAT.**

Despair; salvation of soul, of eternal, after fright: stram.[54]

Doubtful; soul's welfare, of: **ARS. AUR.** bell. calc. chel. croc. cycl.[5] dig. hyos. **LACH.** ***lil-t.*** lyc. nux-v. **PULS.** sel. stram. ***sulph.***[5] ***verat.***

Insanity; prayer, raising hands and kneeling as in p.: ***ars.***[36]

Praying; begged others to pray for him: lyss.[54]

Praying; quietly, for her soul: arn.[54] ars.[54]

Praying; seeks relief in constant: ***puls.***[54]

Praying; sleep, during: stann.[54]

Praying; wanted people to join her in, with slight erysipelas of face: ***plat.***[54]

Religious affections; sadness, doubt about salvation, with: ***lyc.***[54]

AGAR. Al, 14 - He imagines himself at a gate of the hell and that the mushroom commands him to fall on his knees and confess his sins, which he does. (forgiveness, absolution)

ANAC. He, 28 - Fixed ideas: that mind and body are separated ; about redemption (salvation) of soul and about the devil; that a stranger is constantly by his side (pursued); that strange forms accompany him, one to his right and one to his left.

ARN. He, 27 - Prays quietly for her soul. (salvation)

ARS. Ha, 1032 - Mania; first headache, horrible anxiety, noise before the ears, as from a number of large bells, and when he opened the eyes, he always saw a man who had (formerly) hung himself (suicidal, justified) on the ground-floor of the house, who incessantly beckoned (call) him to cut him down (help); he ran thither (there) with a knife, but, as he could not cut him down, (rescue) he became overwhelmed (beaten) with despair (remorse?) and wished (as his friends assured him) to hang himself (punish); but being prevented (stop) from doing so, he became so restless that he could hardly be kept in bed,... and he knelt down and raised his hands in a supplicating manner.

He, 25 - Mania...sees a man who has hanged himself beckoning (call) him to cut him loose (rescue, deliverance, free, saving) on failing to accomplish this he attempts to hang himself (punish, penalize);...finally kneels down and lifts his hands in supplication.(forgiveness, absolution)

CALC. He, 18 - Mental aberration with horrid visions before eyes and cardiac anxiety; he despairs of his salvation (pardon, rescue) and wants to stab himself.

He, 55 - Concern (anxiety, care) about spiritual welfare.(salvation)

CANN-I. Al, 58 - He imagines that he is possessed of infinite knowledge and power of vision, and then that he is Christ come to restore the world to perfect peace. (redemption, savior, rescuer)

CLEM. He, 8 - Ailments from homesickness, or contrition (penitence, remorse) of spirit.

CUPR-A. He, 10 - Awoke suddenly from sleep...and wished to escape...thinks she is about to die and desires to see the pastor;...

EUPH. He, 3 - Temporary attacks of craziness, insists upon saying his prayers at the tail of his horse; knows his freaks (abnormality) and wants to be by himself and in silence.

GRAPH. He, 15 - Solicitude (anxiety) concerning spiritual welfare.

HELL. He, 12 - An old woman having been accused of theft by the women around, took it so much to heart that she hanged herself. This suicide produced a profound effect upon the women of the village. One after another accused herself of having caused the death of the old woman by their insinuations; they wept and howled, ran about day and night wringing their hands and despairing of salvation on account of their sin (error); they became quite irrepressible and deranged (disordered) In this way twenty -four or twenty five women were affected, every fresh case being followed by another. Hysterical mania.

HURA. Al, 23 - Anxiety about his salvation, during the nervous attack.

IGN. He, 10 - Spasms and insanity after fright; imagines her soul cannot be saved (rescued), and cries very much; ...(lost, sentenced)

LIL-T. He, 5 - Tormented about her salvation.

He, 16 - Doubts her salvation; thinks she is doomed to expiate her sins and those of her family; ... (redemption, salvation) (sacrifice)

LYC. He, 20 - Melancholy: has doubts about her salvation; before catamenia; in mild (pacific) characters.

LYSS. Al,N-11-...presentiment of impending death begged them to pray for him and not to leave him alone. (absolution, redemption)

MED. He, 37 - Feeling of desperation, did not care if he went to heaven or hell.

MEZ. He, 8 - Despairs of eternal salvation.

PLAT. He, 36 - While suffering from a slight erysipelas faciei, took leave (quit, abandon) of her children, exhorted her husband to join (unite, combine) church, wanted people to join her in prayer (beg), felt happy to join her Redeemer.

He, 46-...;suffers unspeakable pangs (anxiety) of conscience in consequence of a faux (fault, mistake, embarrassing mistake?) pass when thirty-two years old; says she has brought disgrace upon her family, and that she has incurred the penalty of damnation; (doomed) in order to do penance (penitence) gave away whatever she could lay her hands upon, (redemption) so that she had to be constantly watched; after her confessor asserted that she could not hope for pardon or heaven (condemnable), she seemed in absolute despair ; bemoaned her misery throughout the night, wringing her hands and beseeching (implore) that she might be delivered (free) from the hell of her conscience; twice attempted self-destruction (suicide);...wished to live and do penance (penitence, purgation, purification) in order to mitigate her eternal punishment.

PLB. He, 15-...; despair of her salvation...; fixed idea that could only obtain peace and safety though absolution by a priest of the papal church, although she had been a zealous Protestant; ....brooded over any forbidden thing; would steal (leave) from house in servant's cloak (coat, camouflage) and bonnet (hat) to obtain stimulants (drugs), but from the moment their prohibition was withdrawn (retired) ceased to have any desire for them; after being permitted to visit a priest and converse with him ceased to talk and think of the church. (desire; redemption, absolution)

PULS. He, 48-...despaired of her soul's salvation; did not believe she would be restored to health ; ...

He, 43 - Sleepless nights on account of great fear and anxious restlessness; despairs of her salvation and seeks aid in constant prayer;...

STRAM. Ha, 565 - Nowhere has he rest, is startled by dream-pictures, even when his eyes are open, which in the form of big dogs, cats and other horrible beasts, grow (expand) out of the ground at his side, and from which he jumps away to the side with signs of terror (fear), and knows not how to save (rescue, free) himself. (cornered, corralled)

He, 93 - Mania; thinks he is lying on his sepulchre (tomb); confessing, praying, wants to be killed (redemption, salvation, regeneration); laughs as if tickled (excited); wants to be kissed; accuses his wife of being faithless (betrayed); scolding (censure) beating in a rage, will not be taken hold of by attendants (suspicious?) ; takes them for dogs (contemptuous), and barks at them; talking in Jewish jargon; (rank?, stranger?) supposes his house to be surrounded by carts (vehicle), Jews (Judaism) and geese, offending him, ... -(strange, foreign, alien)

He, 107-...heard continually, on r. side of occiput, a loud voice, scolding, vituperating and accusing him of ungodliness (impious, sinful, irreligious, godless, profane); ....prayed expecting, with great anxiety, the flash of lightning which was to kill him;...(redemption, regeneration, salvation)

He, 112 - Religious mania; pious (divine) looks, praying; restless nights; inspired talking, singing; despairs of her salvation.

He, 122 - Excessive loquacity each time during menses; tears and prayers and earnest (ardent) supplications.

He, 117 - Ceaseless talking mostly devout; very earnestly beseeching. (supplicating)

SULPH. He, 32 - Melancholy mood; dwelling on religious or philosophic speculations; anxiety about soul's salvation; indifference about lot (destiny) of others.

THUJ. Al, 1 - She herself desires, with anxiety and despair, to be taken to an insane asylum, (imprisonment, confining) and there to be treated very harshly and strictly, (penalized), so that her fixed ideas may be subdued and banished (purified); she knows very well that she does wrong (conscience) and thinks all sorts of bad thoughts (immoral), but she will not take the trouble to banish such thoughts; therewith she indistinctly gives to understand that she is constantly obliged to think of taking her own life, but feels the sinfulness (wicked) of it, in order to avoid it, desires the strict restraint of the asylum;...

Al, 7 - She constantly longs for the offices of the church in order to banish her sinful thoughts of suicide. (redemption, salvation)

VERAT. He, 53 - Despair of her salvation;...

SARCASM

Ailments from; love disappointed, laugh, with inclination to: hyos.[54]

Company, aversion to; alternating with bursts of pleasantry and sarcasm: rad-br.[122] rhus-t.

Desires; satire: lach.[36]

Laughing; agg., others, of: ambr.[162]

Laughing; ludicrous, everything seems: hydrog.[222] hyos. lyc. ***nux-m.*** sabad.

Laughing; sardonic: amyg-am.[36] **BELL.** camph.[5] cann-i.[36] ***caust. colch.*** con. croc.[36] cupr.[210] hydr-ac.[5] hydrog.[222] ***hyos.*** ign. nux-m. ***oena.*** ozone[227] phyt.[5] plb. ran-b.[116] ran-s. ***sec.*** sol-n. ***stram.*** stry. tarent. verat. zinc. zinc-o.[10] zinc-p.[58]

Laughing; scornful: alum.[5]

Laughing; serious matters, over: ***anac.*** apis arg-n. asar.[198] bar-c.[198] bufo[58] cann-i. cast-eq. caust.[198] coff.[198] germ.[222] hydrog.[222] ign. lac-h.[229] lap-gr-m.[194] lil-t. lyc. ***nat-m.*** nux-m. phos.[1] ***plat.*** sil.[198] sulph. viol-o.[45]

Laughing; vexation, at: lyc.[116]

Ludicrous, things seem: calc.[10] cann-i. cann-s. hyos.[10] nat-m. ***nux-m.*** plat.[1] stram. sulph.[10] tarent.

Mocking; ridicule, passion to: acon. hyos. lach. nux-v. verat.

Mocking; sarcasm: androc.[222] anh.[144] ***ars.***[122] bry.[30] cann-i.[36] **CARB-V.**[30] carbn-o.[36] caust.[30] cham.[193] choc.[222] cinnb.[36] **GRAPH.**[30] hyper.[193] ign.[30] lac-ac.[54] ***lach.***[5] lyc.[155] nit-ac.[137] nux-v.[30] pall.[116] ***par.***[5] petr.[30] rad-br.[122] rhus-t. sac-l.[85] sec.[54] sep.[58] tarent.[137]

Mocking; sarcasm, satire, desire for: ars.[5] lac-ac.[54] ***lach.***[5] sec.[54] stann.[30]

Nipping at everyone: hyos.[36]

Reproaches; laughing at reproaches: ***graph.***[8]

Ridicule, mania to: acon. hyos. lach. nux-v. verat.

Smiling; sardonic: bell.

ACON-F. Al, 3 - In the intervals of relief from distressing symptoms, he laughed and joked about his very comical condition;...(proper disease)

ALUM. Ha, 35 - He laughs contemptuously at everything.

ANDROC. Sh, 98 - A colleague thought he was being very sarcastic. (4)

APIS. Al, 2 - Laughs at every misfortune.

Al, 3-... He laughed at the greatest misfortune, as he would at a great comedy. (mockery)

He, 11 - Lets everything fall out of her hand, or breaks things and laughs over it.

ARS. Ha, 60 - Inclined to sarcastic mocking.

He, 104 - Obstinacy, avarice, inclined to malice and satire.

CARBN-O. Al, 11 - After supper, felt buoyant (happy) and in good humor, an effect never produced by tea; this mental sensation soon passed over into an irritable and sarcastic one, so that I sharply criticized an article in a medical journal, which a few hours ago I hardly thought worth that trouble, and threw away in disgust a book of reference as flat and superficial, which I highly sluggish.(inactive)

CHOC. Sh, 327 - My humour has taken a sarcastic turn, mocking people, a bit aggressive in a joking way.[35], 30C, 00:03:XX

CROC. Al, 5 - If any one happens to sing a single musical note, she begins involuntarily to sing, and then is obliged to laugh at herself; she however, soon sings in spite of her determination to stop. (sympathy)

Al, 11 - Sardonic (sarcastic, satirical) laughter, and attacks of morbid jollity.

Al, 14 - Very lively (happy) mood, witty, jocose, excessively talkative.(loquacious)

HALI-L. Sh, 349 - I said I was moody. It wasn't as qualitative as she wanted, and she was asking for more details and I yelled, " A stupid five year old would understand what I was saying." I became sarcastic and very belligerent. I thought I was being simplistic and clear. I gave what I had to give. I was in a depressed state, lost my good feeling and was angry at being asked to explain the depression. She asked me what do you mean and I said, "XXXX off. If you don't understand that, too bad. Do you understand that?! Do you know the English language?" 18, 30C, 04:14:00

HYDROG. Sh, 210 - I was shouting down the phone, but dead quiet with friends. I thought "Why are they talking? They haven't anything to say". I was very sarcastic. 24, 30C, 01:XX:XX

Sh, 223 - Tried to talk to someone who is afraid of dying and I wanted to laugh. Thought I shouldn't talk to anybody in case I laugh. 16, 30C, 04:XX:XX

HYOS. He, 74 - Disappointed love followed by: epilepsy, melancholy, rage, or inclination to laugh at everything; despair and propensity to drown himself. (ailments from)

LAC-AC. He, 2 - Averse to business or what formerly was pleasant to do; lazy (indolent); dislikes to read or think; finds fault, is sarcastic, exacting. (exigent, severe)

LACH. Al, 15 - The more cause for fretfulness, the greater inclination for humour, jest, satire, and humorous fancies.

He, 26 - Jealousy, with frightful images, great tendency to mock, to satire and ridiculous ideas.

NAT-M. Al, 11 - Constant laughing; everything in the room looked so ridiculous.

SEC. Al,N-13 - Paralytic mental diseases; treats his relations contemptuously and sarcastically.

He, 12 - Paralytic mental diseases; treats his relations contemptuously and sarcastically;...

SEIZED

Carried; music, as if by: anh.[119]

Charmed with description of beauties of nature: coff.[36]

Delusions; beautiful, images, presenting themselves to her as if by charm: bell.[54]

- bewitched, he is: cann-i.
- body, brain, possesses stomach: acon.[102]
- body, nose, someone else's, has: lac-c.
- charmed and cannot break the spell: ***lach.***[54]
- controlled, every movement and thought is: germ.[222]
- devils, connected to, he is, arrogant towards those who strive to purity, light and love: ozone[227]
- devils, possessed of a devil, is: bor.[58] cann-i.[36] hyos. plat.[30] stram.[85]
- devils, possessed, everyone is: meli.
- devils, speaking in one ear, angel in the other, prompting to murder, or acts of benevolence, devil: ***anac.***[54]
- devils, taken by the devil, he will be: bell.[30] manc. ***puls.***[54]

- devils, taken by, that he will be, mania, in religious: ***puls.***[54]
- enchantment, of: coff-t.[36]
- incubus, being weighted down by: cere-b.[36]
- influence, is under a powerful: cere-b. foll.[1201] germ.[222] ***hyos. lach.*** ozone[227] psil.[164] ***stram.***[54] thuj.[139] verat.[162]
- mesmerized by her absent pastor, she is: meli.
- possessed, being: ***anac.***[122] bell. canth.[58] carb-v.[58] hydrog.[222] hyos. **MANC.** mand.[119] op.[5] plat.[5] psil.[164] sil.[5] stram.[30] ***sulph.***[5] verat.[5]
- possessed, God and the devil, alternately by: psil.[164]
- scream, says it is something within him that screams: ars.[54]
- seized, as if: canth. ***hyos.***[54] phos.[5]
- strangers, control of, under: aster. bry.
- superhuman, control, is under: agar. anac. carc.[207] ***lach. naja*** op.[102] plat.[102] psil.[164] ***thuj.***
- symptoms come from outside, his: bamb-a.[1184]
- voices, hears, command him to commit crime: lach.[58]
- voices, hears, follow, that he must: anac.[58] crot-c. lach.[58]
- voices, hears, steal and kill, that she must: lach.[58]
- wills, possessed of two: anac.[1] lach.[102]

Dreams; magnetic slumber, that he was in: ang.[36]
➤ person, creeps into another: ozone[227]
➤ witches: sol-t-ae.[36]

Fear; devil, of being taken by the: anac.[116] manc. puls.[172]

Insanity; obsession, with: anac.[5] sulph.[5]

Marriage; obsessed by idea of m. excited sexual girls are: bell.[30] ***caust.***[30] plat.[30] verat.[30]

Thoughts; intrude and crowd around each other, closing eyes, on, a mass of subjects, some scientific, cross each other: spong.[54]

Thoughts; intrude and crowd around each other, work, while at: mur-ac. ***sulph.***

Thoughts; morbid, prevent, he cannot: viol-o.[54]

Thoughts; persistent, thinks of nothing but murder, fire and rats: ***calc.***

Thoughts; persistent, unpleasant subjects, haunted by: ***ambr.*** asar.[149] caust. ***cocc.***[54] graph. kali-c. **NAT-M.** petr.[1] rhus-t.

Thoughts; sexual, day and night: chin.[10] dig.[10]

Thoughts; terrible, taking possession of him, in mania: ***iod.***[54]

Trance: ***acon.***[102] aml-n.[25] art-v.[102] camph.[5] camph-br.[102] ***cann-i.***[102] cham.[102] choc.[222] keroso.[36] **LACH.**[54] ***morph.***[102] ***mosch.***[102] nitro-o.[36] nux-m.[102] op.[5] sabad.[102] stram.[102] ter.[36]

Unconsciousness; trance, as in a: **LACH.** ***laur.*** tab.

Will; astonished of finding themselves not masters of their own acts: cann-i.[36]

ACON. He, 8 - Ideas haunt (obsess) him, cannot get rid of them.

ADAM. Sh, 1 - I felt as if a heavy, grey cloud with red specks descended down to my chest entering into me. 7, 6C, 02:00:XX
Sh, 244 - Anger with my attraction to P. He's a walker and I wanted to walk with him. I didn't want to be attracted but was, as if enchanted. 16, 12C, 18:XX:XX

AGAR. Al, 2 - He becomes so furious that he can hardly be restrained from ripping up his bowels, as he fancies the mushroom had ordered him to do.
Al, 8-...called for his hatchet; had to be confined alternated with religious excitement.
Al, 14 - He imagines himself at a gate of the hell and that the mushroom commands him to fall on his knees and confess his sins, which he does. (forgiveness, absolution)

AMBR. Ha, 478 - Distorted fancies, grimaces, satanic faces take possession of the mind, and he cannot get rid of them.

AML-N. He, 2 - A trancelike state, everything seeming unreal to her.
He, 13 - Haunted (obsessed) many times a day with an indescribable dread and sensation as of an oncoming fit, although it came on only once or twice a week.

ANAC. Al, 26 - Increased fancy; he constantly thinks of some new object to which the mind forcibly clings.(adhere)
He, 25 - Has a devil in his ear whispering blasphemous words.
He, 30 - Hallucination; delirium a demon sits on his neck and tells him most offensive things.
He, 40 - Uses profane language, swears, thinks himself a demon.

He, 69 - In one ear a devil, in the other an angel, prompts (incite) him to do murder or acts of benevolence. (homicidal, x helpfulness, kindness)

BELL. He, 33 - In evening he was seized with such violent delirium, that required three men to confine him;...

CAMPH. Al, 46-.... As I lay stretched on my couch, as the evil demon, and suffered all the anguish of a condemned and God-forsaken soul, ...I was forever deprived of the Divine protection, and of every consolation and every hope. Nothing remained to me but the conviction of my everlasting damnation...

Al, 46-...A fearful terror seized me, and I knew not whither to fly. I cried out aloud, "And so I am indeed dead; that hell I used to think about is no fiction, but a reality which I am doomed to experience forever...

CANN-I. Al, 25-...Now demoniac shapes clutched (grasp) at him from the darkness, cloaked (covered) from head to foot in inky (black) palls (mantle), glaring (staring, looking) at him with fiery eyes from beneath their cowls(mantle)....

Al, 58 - He imagines that he is possessed of infinite knowledge and power of vision, and then that he is Christ come to restore the world to perfect peace. (redemption, savior, rescuer)

COFF. Al, 1 - Lively fancies; full of plans for the future; contrary to his custom is very much charmed by the beauties of nature,...

CROT-C. Al, 3-... hears a strange voice to her left, and behind her; she follows it, throws herself against closed doors, and scratches them with her nails...She cries out: " He is in the den, but the lions will not eat him"

Al, 19 - Thoughts of death haunt (torment) her everywhere, especially when alone.

Al, 4 - Another attack of mental alienation; she hears voices, which she follows (obey); with copious tears.

GELS. He, 6 - After losing son, inclined to brood over her loss; at times becomes unconscious, or, rather, "rapt"; in imagination thinks herself at the grave; smothered pressure on chest after the spell.

GERM. Sh, 137 - Entertain myself with mischievous reflections and realize that these are more thoughts of an outsider. 08, 12C, 02:14:10

HURA. Al, 7 - During and after the fainting spell (trance), disposed to love everybody, especially those about him; he often thinks of death, but does not fear it; he feels as though he could die without regret.(fearless)

HYDROG. Sh, 11 - I felt I had gone mad, possessed, hysterical laughter, singing and a feeling of non-reality, as if in a dream, out of the body — like my mind went out of the window. High one minute and then low. People asked if I was on speed. After seven hours, in the evening (7:30p.m.), the feeling changed to an angry mood and very irritable with a dry furry mouth,...1. 24, 30C, 00:00:45

HYOS. Al, 9 - Madness as if possessed by a devil.

Ha, 541 - Mania, as if possessed by the devil.

He, 81-...attempts to escape from room; frightful hallucinations of figures coming to seize him, hens (chicken) bound (imprisoned) with chains,...

IOD. He, 15 - At night, especially when thinking of real or imaginary wrongs ...dares (try) to go home for fear of doing some dreadful (bad, wicked) deed (action); on one occasion was seized with an almost irresistible impulse to murder a woman who was acting as a guide (direct, conduct) for him, he having lost his way (direction);...must be constantly in action, in some laborious occupation. (lost; direction, correction, control)

IRID. Sh, 83 - It feels like my personality has been invaded, taken over. I7

KALI-BR. He, 11 - Imagines she is a devil; cannot sleep; fears to be alone.

KALI-P. He, 17 - Homesickness, morbid activity of memory, haunted (obsessed) by visions of past, and longing after them.

LACH. Al, 5 - A kind of ecstasy, as after sublime impressions, or excessive joy, throughout the day; he constantly wishes to talk and do much, and even more seems to be at his command.(control, domination)

He, 5 - Quick comprehension; mental activity, with almost prophetical (oracular, predictive) perception; ecstasy; a kind of trance.

He, 8 - Thinks: she is somebody else in the hands (seized) of a stronger power; (supremacy, superiority).or that she is dead, and preparations are made for funeral (cortege) or that she is nearly dead and wishes some one would help her off; herself pursued by enemies, or fears medicine is poison; there are robbers in house and wants to jump out the window; herself under super-human control; visions real, he will die. (helplessness, desire; aid, comfort, salvation)

He, 33-...want of self control; lascivious; felt as if she was clear (pure) animal right through, whilst of all mental power was dormant; sensation as if hands of stronger power, as if charmed (enchanted), and as if could not break the spell (charm). (possessed, wildness)

He, 45 - She is tormented by the idea that her better principles (ideals) might be overcome (beaten) by irresistible desire to suicide. (lost: moral) 0 Mania.

He, 54 - A girl, after excessive study, uses exalted language; exceedingly particular about language she uses, often correcting after using a word, and substituting another of very similar meaning, talking about being under influence of a superior power. (possessed) 0 Mania.

LIL-T. Al, 351 - The sexual desire, dormant hitherto, was so strongly aroused that the prover said, "I am afraid of myself, I seem possessed of a demon."

LYC. Al, 52 - Great fear of frightful images which her fancy conjures(charm) up, in the evening, and lachrymose during the day.

Al, 91 - She is overpowered (defeat) by many unpleasant recollections (memory), about which she becomes vexed; even at night on waking.

Al, 51 - In the evening, in the dark, he is seized with fear when a door that he wishes to open moves with difficulty.

LYSS. He, 15 - It seems to her as if two entirely different trains of thought influenced her at the same time.

MANC. He, 3 - Fear of getting crazy; of evil spirits; of being taken (possessed) by the devil.

He, 5-...about midnight attacks of fear and trembling; afraid of evil spirits, of being taken (possessed) hold of by the devil;...

MED. He, 18 - Persons come in, look at her (observed), whisper, and say "come". (spied, called)

MERC. He, 22 - Great desire to murder (homicidal) or committed suicide ...is fearful that she may commit some wrong and kill herself (punishment); something urges her to kill her husband, of whom she is very fond (loving), and she implores him to hide his razor (knife).

He, 20 - After suppression of foot sweat, whenever he sees an open window or cutting instruments breaks into a sweat, with great heat of head, and is seized with an almost uncontrollable desire to commit suicide.

NAT-M. He, 34 - A pregnant woman saw a man who had a disfiguring nasal cancer; this haunted (obsessed) her, and she was sure her child would be marked; she was melancholy, avoided society, wept continually.

He, 5 - Haunted with thoughts that something unpleasant will happen.

NEON. Sh, 37 - On walking in the fresh air I suddenly felt as if I was cruising along on an energy which was not of my own muscular power. It seemed as if it was coming from somewhere else. It seemed effortless and unreal. I felt as if I was passing everyone else. 02, 6C, 13:XX:XX

OP. Al, 37 - Conscious of being possessed (seized) of two persons (double) of another self besides his real self, the Opium man does things which the real self considers wrong, and it is not always sure which will conquer the other.

Al, 19-...each possessing some imaginary bliss (happiness) which " the dull (dark) reality of life" could never give....they are wrapped in an elysium, (heaven) from which they are only to be awakened by the miserable reaction which must, sooner or later recall them to existence.

PULS. He, 40 - Religious mania; sees the devil coming to take her; the world on fire during night; fear, rage in spells, or weeping... (captured, possessed)

RAN-B. Al, 1 - Fearfulness in the evening, she does not want to remain alone, she is afraid she may be haunted (seized) by ghosts.

RAPH. Al, 1 - Feeling of aversion towards all women; she is provoked by seeing women going and coming about her; their approach threw her into a fury; the mere contact with a woman's dress caused intolerable distress;...She is attracted to all men without distinction (nymphomania) ; when she gives her hand to a man, she feels great agitation,...When left alone for a hour in the evening, she gave herself a very deep wound in the lips with a penknife, in hopes to put an end to this condition (hurt, punishes). Moral feeling was completely extinct, the physical nature alone ruled and threw her into a frightful state (wild). From morning to noon she would not have been able to resist the advances even of a man for whom she had not the least friendly feeling; from noon to 6 p.m. she could not have held out against any man whatsoever; from 8 to 11 the demands of sense were so importunate as to silence the voice of shame and reason; ... and would have thrown herself into the arms of the first man she met...she was still unable to control her impulses;...

SIL. Ha, 6 - He is frequently seized by anguish, so that he cannot sit still.(silent)

SPONG. Ha, 381 - She is timorous (fearful) and particularly pursued and incessantly plagued (disturbed, bothered) by a frightful picture out of a melancholic past.

STRAM. He, 49 - After spasms she fell into a trance, says she is under influence(seized) of spirits, and has had conversation with spirits, communications from God; delivers emphatic sermons, prophecies. (missionary)

He, 53 - Hallucinations which terrify patient; sees ghosts, hears voices back his ear; sees strangers.

He, 69 - Hallucinations as if near r.mastoid process a voice were scolding (censured, reproved), her < at night, sometimes voice seemed to be under bed.

He, 47 - He is like one enchanted and beside himself.

He, 87 - After a dreadful shock, occasioned by death of his brother, who fell dead in his arms,...struck all at around him...spoke at one time in Hungarian, and then in Wallachian language; sang Latin paternosters, declared he was God, and then that he was the devil;...

He, 112 - Religious mania; pious (divine) looks, praying; restless nights; inspired talking, singing; despairs of her salvation.

THEA. Al, 4 - Sensation as if impelled by some uncontrollable power to commit suicide, to jump out of window, to put her baby in the boiler with the clothes, to cut its throat while cutting bread, to throw it downstairs (in a woman who kept a pot of tea boiling on the stove and drank several bowlfuls every day; cured with tea cm, Finckle)

THUJ. Al, 1 - She herself desires, with anxiety and despair, to be taken to an insane asylum, (imprisonment, confining) and there to be treated very harshly and strictly, (penalized), so that her fixed ideas may be subdued and banished (purified); she knows very well that she does wrong (conscience) and thinks all sorts of bad thoughts (immoral), but she will not take the trouble to banish such thoughts; therewith she indistinctly gives to understand that she is constantly obliged to think of taking her own life, but feels the sinfulness (wicked) of it, in order to avoid it, desires the strict restraint of the asylum;...

He, 10 - Fixed ideas: as if a strange person were at his side; as if soul and body were separated (split) ; that body, particularly limbs, are made of glass (frail) and will readily break (weakness); as if a living animal were in abdomen ;talks about being under the influence of a superior power. (possessed)

SENSITIVE

Ailments from; sensory impressions: tarent.[214]

Anguish; shock from injury, in: ***op.***[54]

Anxiety; cruelties, after hearing of: ***calc.***

Anxiety; hysterical: ***asaf.***[54] ***con.***[10] **THER.**[54]

Blood; wounds cannot look at: **NUX-V.**[122] staph.[122]

Cruelty; children cannot bear to see cruelty in cinema: calc.[122]

Delicacy, feeling of: ign.[5] nux-v.[5]

Delusions; spinal column is a barometer: cann-i.

Dreams; fights, suggested by reading: coca[36]

Excitement; music, from: carc.[207] ***kreos.*** pall.[54] sumb. ***tarent.***

Fear; cruelties, from report of, excite: calc.
✦ sensation, of making: med.[58]
✦ senses, with exalted state of, smell, taste, touch: lyss.[54]
✦ wounds, to see: calc.[30]
Horrible things sad stories, affected her profoundly: ars.[122] ***aur.***[122] ***aur-m.***[122] benz-ac.[58] **CALC.**[122] calc-s.[108] cand-a.[239] carb-v.[193] carc.[146] ***caust.***[122] cench.[58] chin.[162] **CIC.** coca[153] cocc. con.[122] ferr.[122] gels. ***hep.***[122] ign. **IOD.**[122] ***kali-c.***[184] ***lach.*** lap-c-b.[194] lap-mar-c.[194] ***lyc.***[122] manc.[162] nat-c. nat-m.[162] ***nit-ac.***[122] ***nux-v.*** op.[163] ozone[227] ***phos.***[122] plat.[137] prot.[193] ***puls.***[122] ***sep.***[122] ***sil.***[122] staph.[1] ***sulph.***[122] ***teucr. zinc.***
Horrible things sad stories, affected her profoundly, thoughts, her own, during labor: plat.[54]
Impressionable, susceptible: am-c.[30] ant-c.[54] aur.[30] bar-c.[30] calc.[30] ***canth.***[8] **CARC.**[122] chin.[30] ***cocc.***[85] coff.[72] croc.[5] graph.[85] **IOD.**[122] nitro-o.[36] nux-v.[30] phos.[54] puls.[30] **STAPH.**[30] tarent.[5] **TUB.**[122] ***verat.***[30] viol-o.[85] zinc.[30]
Impressionable; everything, by, unpleasantly: ***con.***[54]
Reserved; noise, with sensitivity to: con.[10]
Restlessness; mild, amiable, refined, sensitive, intellectual: chim-m.[54]
Sadness; shock, as from: nitro-o.[36]
Sadness; stories, from sad: **CIC.**
Senses; acute, birds, for: lap-mar-c.[194]
Sensitive; arts, drawing or literature, to: carc.[207]
Sensitive; aura of others, to: nabal.[102]
Sensitive; certain persons, to: am-m. aur. calc. carc.[207] crot-h. **NAT-C.** sel. stann.
Sensitive; colors, to: choc.[222] kali-c.[10] tarent.[144]
Sensitive; cruelties, when hearing of: **CALC.** hep.[162]
Sensitive; crying of children, to: caust. phos.
Sensitive; disharmony and quarrel, home, in: nat-m.[162]
Sensitive; disorder, to: ars.[137]
Sensitive; emotional: caust.[127] luna[228] paull.[54] seq-s.[239] thuj.[127]
Sensitive; external impressions, to all: anac.[60] arg.[58] arn. ars.[58] aur.[60] bac.[62] bell.[58] ***canth.***[8] caps.[58] carc.[227] cast.[54] cham.[58] choc.[222] clem. ***cocc.*** coff.[60] ***colch.*** gaert.[136] hep.[58] hydrog.[222] ***iod.***[122] just.[102] lac-c.[122] lach.[58] lap-c-b.[194] ***nit-ac. nux-v.*** ph-ac. ***phos.*** sanic.[85] ***staph.*** stry.[36] sul-i.[137]
Sensitive; laughed at, to being: calc.[127]
Sensitive; light, to: ***acon.*** androc.[222] aquil.[102] ***ars.*** aur.[116] bad.[1] **BELL.**[122] buth-aust.[119] ***colch.*** con.[10] ***kali-p.*** lac-c. nat-m.[162] **NUX-V. PHOS.** sang.[116] stram.[58] tarent.[214]
Sensitive; moral impressions, to: all-s. aster.[36] chin.[30] coff.[20] dig. hep.[20] hydrog.[222] ign. nuph.[25] nux-v.[30] plb.[36] psor. ***puls.***[30] staph.[30] upa.[36]
Sensitive; music, bird songs: choc.[222]
Sensitive; music, continues to hear the music he heard during day in the evening: lyc.[85]
Sensitive; music, every note causes stitches in ear, violent pains in head: ph-ac.[85]
Sensitive; music, piano: anac.[116] nat-c.[10] sep.[10] zinc.[116]
Sensitive; music, sacred m, to: lyss.[54] thuj.[122]
Sensitive; music, to: ***acon.*** aloe[117] ***ambr.*** anac.[116] androc.[222] aur.[46] bry.[5] bufo cact. ***calc.***[116] carb-an. ***carc.***[119] caust. ***cham.*** choc.[222] coff. cop.[122] croc.[5] cupr.[5] dig. ***graph.*** ign.[5] ip.[155] ***kreos. lyc.*** merc. **NAT-C.** ***nat-m.*** nat-p. ***nat-s.*** **NUX-V.** pall.[116] ***ph-ac.*** phos. psil.[164] puls.[5] ***sabal.***[137] ***sabin.*** **SEP.** stann. sulph.[122] ***tab.***[122] ***tarent.*** thuj. tub.[85] tub-k.[85] viol-o. zinc. zinc-p.[58]
Sensitive; music, violin: ***viol-o.***[5]
Sensitive; nature, to: carc.[227]
Sensitive; noise, aversion to: asar.[137] bor.[137] con.[137] ferr.[36] kali-c.[137] op.[137] raph.[36] zinc.[36]
Sensitive; noise, birds, of: bamb-a.[1184]
Sensitive; noise, car, traveling on the street: nit-ac.[58]
Sensitive; noise, crackling of paper, to: ***asar.***[116] bor. calad. ferr. lyc.[58] ***nat-c.*** nat-s.[137] tarax.[1] ther.[103] zinc.
Sensitive; noise, music, amel: **AUR.** carc.[207] **TARENT.**
Sensitive; noise, others eat apples, hawk or blow their noses, cannot bear to hear: lyss.[54]
Sensitive; noise, painful sensitiveness to: am-c.[54] arn.[54] ***coff.***[54] ***con.***[54] ***nux-v.***[122] ***sang.***[54] seneg.[54] ***sil.***[54] ***spig.***[54]
Sensitive; noise, penetrating: ***asar.***[111] bar-c.[111] chin.[111] cocc.[111] con.[111] ferr.[111] iod.[111] lept.[111] lil-t.[111] lyc.[111] manc.[111] mur-ac.[111] sabin.[111] ***ther.***[111]
Sensitive; noise, slightest: acon. aloe alum-sil.[58] ant-c. arg-n. ars.[54] **ASAR.**[122] bar-c. ***bell.***[54] ***bor.*** bufo[98] chin.[31] cinnb. ***cocc.***[54] **COFF.**[122] ***ferr.*** lach.[58] ***lyc.*** nat-c.[58]

nat-s. nux-m.[171] **NUX-V. OP.** petr.[193] ***phos. sabin. sep.***[122] **SIL. THER.**[122] uva.[162] xan.[85]
Sensitive; noise, striking of clocks, ringing of bells, to: **ASAR.**[122] **COFF.**[122] dros.[122] **THER.**[122]
Sensitive; noise, sudden: **BOR.**[5] calad.[137] cocc.[137] lap-c-b.[194] nat-c.[137] nat-m.[137]
Sensitive; noise, to: achy.[149] **ACON.** agar.[163] allox.[119] aloe alum. alum-p.[58] alum-sil.[58] am-c. ambr. anac.[5] androc.[222] ***ang.***[5] anh.[119] ant-c. ant-t. apis aquil.[102] aran-ix.[119] ***arg-n. arn. ars. ars-i. asaf.***[171] **ASAR.** ***aur.*** aur-ar.[58] aur-i.[58] aur-m.[58] bad.[1] bamb-a.[1184] bapt. ***bar-c.*** bar-i.[58] **BELL. BOR.** ***bry.*** bufo buth-aust.[119] cact. ***calad.***[72] ***calc.*** calc-f.[119] calc-sil.[58] camph. cand-a.[239] cann-i.[36] cann-s. caps. carb-an. ***carb-v. carbn-s.*** carc.[140] card-m. ***caust. cham.*** chel. **CHIN.** chin-ar.[36] chin-b.[54] chlol.[54] chol.[54] cic. cimic. cinnb. ***cocc.*** **COFF.** colch. **CON.** convo-s.[119] cop.[36] crot-h.[54] cupr.[5] cyn-d.[149] ***ferr. ferr-ar. ferr-p. fl-ac.*** foll.[149] gaert.[136] gels. glon.[102] ***hell.*** hep.[85] hura hyos. ***ign. iod.***[122] ***ip.*** ipom.[119] just.[144] kali-ar. **KALI-C.** kali-i. ***kali-p.*** kali-s. kali-sil.[58] lac-ac.[54] ***lac-c. lach. lachn.***[54] ***lat-m.***[119] lept.[5] ***lyc.*** lycpr.[102] ***lyss.*** mag-c.[5] ***mag-m.*** mag-p.[58] manc. ***mand.***[119] mang. ***med.*** meny.[137] ***merc.*** mosch. ***mur-ac.***[36] nat-ar. ***nat-c. nat-m.*** nat-p. ***nat-s.*** nat-sil.[58] **NIT-AC.** ***nux-m.***[54] **NUX-V.** onos.[102] **OP.** ox-ac. palo.[149] petr.[5] ph-ac. phel.[116] ***phos.*** pitu-a.[164] plan.[36] ***plat.*** plb.[5] ptel. ***puls.*** raph.[36] rhus-t. sabad. sabin.[163] ***sang.***[8] sec.[54] seneg.[5] **SEP. SIL.** ***spig.*** stann. staph.[58] stram.[5] stry.[36] sulfonam.[149] sulph.[5] syph.[122] tanac. tarent.[102] **THER.** thuj.[163] **TUB.**[122] v-a-b.[149] valer.[5] verat.[5] verat-v.[25] viol-o.[5] visc.[119] xan.[198] yuc.[36] **ZINC. ZINC-P.**[122]
Sensitive; noise, water splashing: brom.[137] **LYSS. NIT-AC.** stram.
Sensitive; odors, to: ***acon.***[163] agar.[163] all-c.[163] ambr.[1189] anac.[163] aran-ix.[119] ars.[5] aur.[5] bell.[5] calc.[163] calc-f.[119] carb-ac.[5] ***caust.***[30] cham.[30] ***chin.***[163] ***cocc.***[163] coff.[5] **COLCH.**[5] con.[163] dros.[5] eup-per.[5] graph.[5] hyper.[163] ign.[5] kali-chl.[163] lach.[58] lyc.[122] lyss.[85] mag-m.[163] mand.[144] merc.[30] ***merc-i-f.***[5] nux-m.[163] ***nux-v.***[5] op.[137] ph-ac.[163] phos.[5] plat.[163] plb.[163] puls.[163] sabad.[137] sang.[5] ***sel.***[163] **SEP.**[5] ***sil.***[163] stann.[5] staph.[58] stict.[163] ***sulph.***[58] ther.[5] vario.[5]
Sensitive; odors, to, dirty clothing: ***carb-an.***[137]
Sensitive; odors, to, filthy: ***sulph.***[58]
Sensitive; odors, to, flowers: all-c. chin. **GRAPH.** hyos. ***lac-c.*** lyc. **NUX-V. PHOS.** sabad.[137] sang.
Sensitive; odors, to, foul things: par.[137]
Sensitive; odors, to, foul things, remains for a long time: dios.[137]
Sensitive; others say about her, what: stann.[137] staph.[102]
Sensitive; people, to: cham.[127] ***hep.***[58] thuj.[127]
Sensitive; reprimands, criticism, reproaches, to: ars.[189] bamb-a.[1184] calc.[189] calc-sil.[58] cand-a.[239] caps.[85] ***carc.***[122] cina[130] foll.[1201] ign.[85] lap-mar-c.[194] ***med.***[122] nat-m.[189] nat-s.[146] nux-v.[189] ozone[227] puls.[189] ***sac-alb.***[210] staph.[70]
Sensitive; rudeness, to: bar-m.[162] ***calc.*** carc.[193] cocc. ***colch.*** mag-m.[162] med.[179] mur-ac.[162] nat-m. nux-v. ozone[227] ph-ac. puls.[187] stann.[187] **STAPH.**
Sensitive; sad stories, to: cic.
Sensitive; singing, to, involuntary joins in on hearing anyone sing: croc.[85]
Sensitive; steel points directed toward her: apis nat-m.[122] **SIL.**[122] **SPIG.**[122]
Sensitive; touch, to: abrot.[127] ***acon.***[116] arn.[171] ars.[58] ***bell.***[58] caps.[127] caust.[58] chin.[116] ***chin-ar.***[58] cina[58] coff.[58] foll.[149] hep.[109] kali-c.[171] ***lach.***[122] meny.[116] op.[30] phos.[58] ruta[161] spig.[171] staph.[58] tarent.[214] tell.[149]
Talk; unpleasant things of agg.: ***calc.*** cic. ign. ***teucr.***
Vulnerable, emotionally: am-m.[209] am-s.[209] anac.[187] ars.[187] bamb-a.[1184] calc.[198] calc-f.[214] calc-p.[198] carc.[227] ***caust.***[198] choc.[222] hep.[187] hydrog.[222] hyos.[198] lap-gr-m.[194] mag-p.[209] med.[198] merc.[187] ***nat-c.***[98] nat-m.[187] nat-p.[209] nat-s.[187] nat-sil.[198] ph-ac.[209] puls.[187]
Weeping; answering questions: **PULS.**[54]
Weeping; children, misfortune, on hearing of: caust.[109]
Weeping; emotions, slight, after: aster. con.[30] **CUPR.**[122] kreos. ***lach.***[116] lyc.[58] naja
Weeping; joyful or sad things, at: **PULS.**[54]

ADAM. Sh, 204 - I feel overwhelmingly hard done by (mistreated) and need to feel heard and understood. 7, 6C, 13:00:XX
ANAC. Ha, 15 - Very peevish and out of humor, with great sensitiveness to all offenses.
ANDROC. Sh, 147 - Sensitive to others' emotions. I feel I know how people are feeling. (25)

ANG. He, 3 - Ill-humored, oversensitive to jokes, slight offenses fill him with bitterness.

ANT-C. Al, 10-...the sound of the bells as well as the sight of that which surrounds him, moves him to tears;...

ARN. Ha, 625 - Over-excitability; she could easily laugh when there was no occasion for it, and when one said something annoying to her, she got angry ...

ARS. Ha, 45 - Super-sensitiveness and over-tenderness of mind; dejected, sad and lugubrious (unhappy), she is troubled and solicitous about the merest trifles.

Ha, 58 - Very peevish and sensitive; the least thing insults him and angers him.

BAPT. He, 16 - Aversion... to hear conversation about sickness or injuries; feeble mind. (impressionable) 0Spasmodic stricture of esophagus.

BELL. Ha, 1400 - Great irritability and acuteness of the senses; everything tastes and smells stronger; the sense of touch, the sight, and the rearing are more acute,...

BOV. Al, 10 - Great sensitiveness; became easily offended at everything.

CALC-P. Al, 15 - A communication in which some one is justly reproached concerning his conduct, affects him very disagreeably; he grows violent, and holds up his faults to himself.

CHOC. Sh, 38 - Sense of smell very acute. Hearing more acute, especially for deeper tones which have more resonance.

Sh, 110 - I really like my nose. It feels more useful in the dark.

Sh, 122 - While looking out of the window, I realised I had the capacity to see from above and below at the same time —not a dividing in two from bottom to top, but a knowledge of both sides at once.

Sh, 124 - I see things differently than before —everything more clear and three-dimensional —more real. Textures and shapes seem different- like a new way of seeing. I seem to have a fascination with certain objects and textures, like wood on doors or colours of hair. Sense of smell very acute. I can smell what people drink from the other side of the room and where to locate it.

Sh, 149 - Hearing and smell still acute — nature seems wonderful. Saw nine magpies and they seemed much bigger than before.

Sh, 208 - Felt rejected and oversensitive. Hid away from the world, felt my life would fall apart. 35, 30C, XX:XX:XX:

Sh, 309 - A feeling of intoxication with double sensations. Colours are stronger and hearing is sharpened but at the same time feel absent and removed.[29], 200C, 00:XX:XX

CIC. He, 30 - Anxiety, excessively affected by sad stories.

CINA. He, 8 - Great earnestness (serious) and sensitiveness; he is offended at slightest joke.

COCC. He, 24 - Melancholy and sad; indulges in sad reveries (daydream); is sensitive to insults, slights (despises) and disappointment.

DIG. Ha, 14-..he is much affected by everything, but especially by sad things, and the least trifle can throw him into disconsolate despair.(sensitive)

GERM. Sh, 120 - Easily led of others opinion, and provoked. Sensitive to others attempts at restricting me. Feel like a teenager, but I don't dare to protest. I just feel it inside. 18, 30C, 04:00:00

Sh, 146 - Slightest criticism and I am broken hearted. Almost started to cry among all the people, very doubtful about relationships. It kills my confidence. Deep sigh. 21, 12C, 41:XX:XX

HALI-L. Sh, 166 - Very sensitive to people. If I looked at them I would see their emotions written on them. I worked on one patient and felt his deep seated grief. Intense hypersensitivity to people. 13, 30C, 06:XX:XX

IGN. Ha, 793 - Sensitive disposition, delicate conscientiousness (careful, scrupulous)

LYC. He, 31 - Sensitive, irritable disposition; peevish and cross on getting awake; easily excited to anger; cannot endure slightest opposition, and is speedily beside herself.

LYSS. Al,N-121 - Mortifying news affects him very much.

Al,N-92 - Exalted state of smell, taste and touch, with a feeling of anxiety and a fear of being alone.

MED. He, 32 - Everything startles her, news coming to her seems to touch her heart before she hears it.

NAT-C. Al, 3 - Every event makes a strong impression upon her; a wavy trembling in the nerves, with a sensation of faintness.

NUX-V. Ha, 1272 - Over-sensitiveness to impressions of the senses; he cannot bear strong odors and bright light.

Ha, 1273 - He cannot bear any noise or speaking; music and singing affect him strongly.

He, 11 - Cannot bear reading or conversation; irritable and wishes to be alone.

PAEON. He, 1 - Anxious, afraid (fear) to talk with any one; much affected by bad news, after pinching in belly.

PHOS. Ha, 79 - In the evening, usually of so vivid an imagination that the mere representation of disagreeable things causes horror with her.

RAN-B. Al, 3 - Ill humored, and disposed to quarrel and scold the first forenoon; in the evening is desponding, apprehensive, sensitive, discontented; on the second day he again inclines to be provoked by innocent jests of his friends, etc.;...

SEP. Al, 33 - Received news of the slight illness of a friend, which caused great mental depression (at another time it would not have made slightest impression); this condition grew on me until I became so nervous that I felt that unless I held on something, I should scream.

SIL. Ha, 11 - Sensitive to noise, which makes him apprehensive.

Ha, 12 - Loud talking is oppressive to him.

SPIG. Ha, 666 - He is very cross and sensitive to everything that he thinks not good, for many hours.

STAPH. He, 9 - Very sensitive to least impression; least word that seems wrong (offenses) hurts her very much.

SEXUAL

Adulterous: calc.[30] canth.[30] caust.[30] fl-ac.[156] lach.[30] lap-mar-c.[194] phos.[30] plat.[30] puls.[30] staph.[30] verat.[30] vip.[1212]

Ailments from; abuse: ambr.[1189] aur-m.[198] calc-p.[198] hyos.[198] lyc.[198] nat-m.[198] staph.[198]

Ailments from; celibacy, being unmarried, continence: ***agn.***[8] apis[130] calc.[137] ***cann-i.***[137] con.[102] fl-ac.[137] lyc.[137] phos.[111] plat.[137] sep.[187]

Ailments from; debauchery: agar.[58] ***anan.*** ant-c.[54] arg-n.[5] calad.[162] carb-v.[5] chin.[102] dig.[85] fl-ac.[122] lach.[111] **NUX-V.**[5] pic-ac.[122] sel.[137] sep.[122] spig.[54] stram.[137] sul-ac.[111]

Ailments from; debauchery, as after: clem.[36] conin.[36] kreos.[36] lact.[36] lyc.[36] nux-v.[1] op.[36] ox-ac.[36]

Ailments from; excitement sexual: kali-br.[54] kali-p.[85] ***nat-m.***[54] ***plat.***[122] psor.[162] staph.[58]

Ailments from; excitement, sexual: kali-br.[54] kali-p.[85] ***nat-m.***[54] ***plat.***[122] psor.[162] staph.[58]

Ailments from; excitement: sexual suppressed: con.[85] cot.[72] kali-p.[85]

Ailments from; masturbation: agar.[58] agn. anan.[54] aur.[10] bar-c.[91] bell.[10] bufo[58] calad.[58] calc.[10] cann-i.[116] ***chin.***[54] cina[10] ***cocc.***[58] ***con.***[58] ***dig.***[54] ***gels.***[54] ***hyos.***[54] ***ign.***[8] kali-br.[116] lil-t. merc.[10] ***nat-m.***[58] ***nat-p.***[58] ***nux-v.***[10] ***op.***[8] ***orig.***[54] ph-ac.[10] ***phos.***[54] ***plat.***[8] ***plb.***[8] raph.[171] sars.[58] ***sil.***[58] ***staph.***[10] **SULPH.**[10] ***tarent.***[54]

Ailments from; sexual, abuse: ambr.[1189] ***anac.***[102] arg-n.[102] aur.[102] aur-m.[137] calc-p.[137] 0caust.[137] chin.[102] cupr.[210] foll.[1201] hyos.[137] lil-t.[54] lyc.[193] nat-m.[102] nux-v.[102] orig.[187] ***ph-ac.***[54] ***phos.***[54] sep.[162] staph.[103] stram.[187] ***ust.***[8]

Ailments from; sexual, abuse, raped, being: acon.[185] caust.[185] foll.[1201] ign.[185] sep.[185] staph.[185]

Ailments from; sexual, excesses: agar. agn.[122] alum. ***alum-p.***[122] **APIS**[5] arg-n.[122] arn.[85] ars. asaf. aur. aur-ar.[58] bell-p.[102] ***bov.*** calad. **CALC.** calc-p.[122] calc-sil.[58] carb-an.[5] ***carb-v.*** **CHIN.**[122] chin-ar. cocc. ***con.*** dig.[122] ***iod.*** kali-br.[5] ***kali-c.*** kali-p. kali-s. kali-sil.[58] lil-t. **LYC.** mag-m. ***merc.*** ***nat-c.*** nat-m. nat-p.[58] nit-ac. **NUX-V.** ol-an.[5] onos.[122] petr. **PH-AC.** **PHOS.** plat.[122] plb.[122] psor.[56] ***puls.*** sabal.[137] samb.[85] sec.[122] sel. **SEP.** ***sil.*** spig. **STAPH.** sulph. symph.[122] thuj. upa.[122] zinc. zinc-p.[58]

Amativeness: agn.[5] ant-c.[54] calc.[30] **CANTH.**[54] ***caust.***[30] ***con.***[54] ***hyos.***[54] ign.[10] kali-br.[122] ***lach.***[54] **LYC.**[54] ***merc.***[54] nat-m.[30] ph-ac.[30] ***phos.***[54] ***plat.***[30] sulph.[30] ***ust.***[54] verat.[30]

Amativeness; fits, in: acon.[60] ant-c.[60] hyos.[60] op.[60] stram.[60] verat.[60]

Amativeness; want of, men, in: con.[30] ***lyc.***[30]

Amativeness; want of, women, in: caust.[30] lyc.[30] sulph.[30]

Amorous; disposition: acon.[5] agar. agn.[5] ***anan.***[162] androc.[222] **ANT-C.**[5] apis[5] ***bell.***[5] ***bufo***[5] calad.[5] **CALC.**[5] ***calc-p.***[5] camph.[5] cann-i.[116] **CANN-S.**[5] **CANTH.**[5] **CARB-V.**[5]

CAUST.[30] **CHIN.**[5] coff.[5] ***coloc.***[5] ***con.***[5] croc.[5] dulc.[5] fl-ac.[5] ***graph.***[30] ***hyos.***[10] **IGN.**[5] ***iod.***[54] kali-br.[122] kali-c.[5] ***lach.***[54] lil-t.[5] **LYC.**[54] meny.[5] ***merc.***[54] ***mosch.***[5] ***murx.***[5] nat-c.[5] **NAT-M.**[5] nit-ac.[58] nux-m.[5] **NUX-V.**[5] ***op.***[5] orig.[137] ph-ac.[30] **PHOS.**[5] pic-ac.[5] **PLAT.**[5] plb.[5] plb-acet.[30] **PULS.**[5] rhus-t.[5] ruta[5] **SABIN.** sanic.[5] sars.[5] sel.[116] senec.[111] ***sep.***[5] **SIL.**[5] squil.[137] ***stann.***[5] ***staph.***[5] **STRAM.**[5] sulph.[122] thuj.[5] ***ust.***[54] **VERAT.**[5] verb.[5] zinc.[5]

Amorous; fits, in: acon.[5] ant-c.[5] hyos.[5] op.[5] stram.[5] verat.[5]

Anger; coition, after: ***calc.***[10] ***calc-ar.***[36]

Anxiety; coition, after: kali-c.[58] sep.

Anxiety; coition, as if during, with palpitation and voluptuous sensation: plat.[54]

Anxiety; coition, becoming, on: carb-ac.[36] lap-mar-c.[194] manc. nux-v.[36] psor.[162]

Anxiety; coition, during: kreos.[54]

Anxiety; conscience, masturbation, after: **PH-AC.**[54]

Anxiety; conscience, women and religion, about: puls.[54]

Anxiety; duty, as if he had not done his, religious, produced by lascivious impulses: ***orig.***[54]

Anxiety; emissions, after: carb-an. petr. ***phos.***[54]

Anxiety; lascivious impulses, from, on account of disinclination of religious duties in a married woman, mother of a family: ***orig.***[54]

Anxiety; masturbation, from: cann-i.[116] staph.[162]

Anxiety; pollutions, after: aloe carb-an. petr. ***phos.***[54]

Anxiety; spermatorrhea, in: ***phos.***[54]

Aversion; family members, to, female: am-c.[5]

Aversion; men, to: hypoth.[149] **PULS.** raph.[54]

Aversion; sex: hydrog.[222] raph.[122]

Aversion; sex, her own, to: raph.

Aversion; sex, opposite to, religious aversion: lyc. ***puls.*** sulph.

Aversion; sex, opposite, to: am-c.[10] nat-m.[36] puls.[162] staph.[5]

Aversion; women, to: am-c. bapt. con.[30] ***dios.*** ign.[36] ***lach.*** **LYC.**[30] mag-c.[36] nat-m. ***puls.*** raph.[36] sulph.

Aversion; women, to, homosexuality, with: phos.[162] ***plat.***[30] puls.[162] staph.[162]

Aversion; women, to, looks upon them as evil beings and is afraid their presence is injurious to his soul: ***puls.***[54]

Aversion; women, to, mannish: fl-ac.[122]

Aversion; women, to, sex, of her own: raph.

Bed; desires to remain in, sexual excitement, from: ***verat.***[54]

Cheerfulness; coition, after: nat-m.

Cheerfulness; emission, after: pip-m.

Cheerfulness; pollutions, after: pip-m.[58]

Children; aversion, her own, daughter, in a woman: raph

Children; desires to, have to beget: ox-ac.

Coition; after, mental symptoms after: bov.[5] **CALC.**[5] dig.[5] mez.[5] nat-m.[5] petr.[5] ph-ac.[5] ***sel.***[5] ***sep.***[5] sil.[5] staph.[5] thuj.[5]

Coition; amel. mental symptoms: tarent.[5]

Company, aversion to; solitude, fond of, desires to practice masturbation: ***bufo*** ust.

Concentration, difficult; emission, after: ***lil-t.***[54]

Concentration, difficult; masturbation, from: aven.[85]

Confusion of mind; coition, after: bov. calc. caust. mez. ***ph-ac.*** phos. rhod. sel. sep. staph.[162]

Confusion of mind; emissions, from: ***sel.*** sumb.[36]

Confusion of mind; identity, sexual: hydrog.[222]

Confusion of mind; masturbation, from: ***gels.***[54]

Day-dreaming; amorous: ant-c.[5] verb.[5]

Delirium; anxious, men of: ***plat.***[54]

Delirium; erotic: camph. cann-i. ***canth. hyos.***[102] kali-br. ***lach. phos. plat.***[162] ***sec.***[122] ***stram.*** tarent.[162] verat.[102]

Delirium; fear of men, with: bell. ***plat.***

Delirium; sexual excitement, with: **STRAM.**[54]

Delusions; body, lighter than air, is, masturbation, from, or hysterical subjects, in: gels.[137]

- devils, erotic mania, in: orig.[54]
- hell, chains, in erotomania: ***orig.***[54]
- lascivious: ambr.[10] bell.[10] calc.[10] sil.[10] ***stram.***[10] verb.[54]
- lost, salvation, despised, and, in erotomania: ***orig.***[54].
- man, bed, on, at night: merc.
- man, naked man in bed: ***puls.***
- naked, he is: stram. sulph.[139]
- obscene: stram.
- obscene, actions of which she had not been guilty, accuses herself of.: ***phos.***
- penis, sees cut off penis on the grass:

lap-mar-c.[194]
- sensual: verb.[54]
- vagina, living things creep into (at night): merc.
- voices, hears, abusive and filthy language, voices from within him speaking in: ***zinc.***[54]
- wedding, of a: alum.[5] hyos.[5] mag-m.[5] nat-c.[5]
- women, bedside, by: med.[54]
- women, evil, are, and will injure his soul: puls.
- women, his mothers house is invaded by lewd: kali-br.

Dementia; sexual excess, from: lil-t.[137]
Desires; captivating others: lap-mar-c.[194]
Desires; woman, ideal: ant-c.[36]
Despair; masturbation, in: ***op.***[54]
Despair; religious, alternating with sexual excitement: ***lil-t.***
Despair; sexual craving, from: aster.[54]
Discomfort; sexual desire, with: ant-c.[137]
Discontented; coition, after: ***calc.*** sel.[116]
Discouraged; coition, after: sep.
Dreams; abortion: m-arct.[5]

➤ amorous: acon. aesc. aether[36] agn. ***alum.*** alum-sil.[58] am-c. **AM-M.** ambr. anag.[54] androc.[222] ang. ***ant-c.*** aphis.[36] ***arg-n.*** arist-m.[149] arn. ars. ars-i. ars-s-f.[54] astac. aster. ***aur.*** aur-ar.[58] aur-i.[58] aur-s.[58] bamb-a.[1184] bar-c. bar-i.[58] ***bar-m.*** bell.[5] bism. bor. bov.[5] **BUFO**[171] cact. cahin. caj.[36] calad.[102] ***calc.*** calc-ar. calc-i.[58] calc-p. calc-sil.[58] ***camph. cann-i.*** cann-s. ***canth. carb-ac.*** carb-an. carb-v. carbn-s. carl. cast. caust. ***cench.***[122] cent.[36] chel. ***chin.***[5] ***cic.*** cinnb. clem. ***cob.*** cob-n.[119] coc-c. coca ***cocc.***[5] colch. coloc. ***con.*** cop. cycl. des-ac.[149] ***dig. dios.*** ery-a. euph. form. gall-ac.[36] gast.[36] ***gels.*** gins.[36] goss.[119] ***graph.*** grat. ham. hipp.[36] hura hydr. hydrog.[222] hyos. hyper. ***ign.*** ind. inul. iod. ***iris*** kali-ar. ***kali-br. kali-c.*** kali-chl. kali-cy.[36] kali-fcy.[36] kali-n. ***kali-p.***[58] ***kalm.*** kreos. lac-ac. **LACH.** lact.[36] led. ***lil-t.*** linu-c.[36] lith-c. ***lyc.*** lyss.[54] m-arct.[10] m-p-a.[1] ***mag-c.*** mag-m. mag-s. meny. merc. merc-c. merc-i-f. merc-i-r.[54] merc-s.[36] mez. mur-ac. myric. nat-ar. **NAT-C.** ***nat-m. nat-p.*** nicc.[10] nit-ac. nitro-o.[36] nux-m. **NUX-V.** olnd. **OP.** orig.[36] orig-v.[25] ox-ac. ozone[227] paeon. par. ped.[36] pen.[36] ***petr.*** **PH-AC.** ***phos.*** phys. pic-ac. pip-m. plan. ***plat.*** plb. polym.[111] psil.[164] ***psor.*** ptel.[25] ***puls.*** ran-b. raph. rauw.[144] rhod. rhus-v. ***sabad.*** sabin. salx-n.[102] samb. sanic.[111] sapin.[36] ***sars.*** sel. senec. ***sep.*** serp.[36] ***sil.*** sin-n. sol-t-ae. spig. spira.[36] spirae.[36] squil. stann. **STAPH.** stram. sul-ac. sul-i.[58] sulph. sumb. ***tarax. thuj.*** thymol.[119] trom. tub.[193] ust. v-a-b.[149] valer. ***verat.***[5] verat-v.[102] vinc. **VIOL-T.** x-ray[115] yuc.[36] zinc.[5] ***zinc-pic.***[5]

➤ amorous, coition, after: kali-c.[10]

➤ amorous, erections, with: aur.[10] cact.[54] camph.[122] ***cann-i.***[36] clem.[36] coloc.[10] dios.[25] kreos.[10] lac-ac.[54] led.[10] merc.[10] mur-ac.[1] ***nat-c.***[10] nat-m.[10] par.[10] ph-ac.[1] pic-ac.[122] plat.[1] plb.[10] ran-b.[10] rhod.[54] ***sars.***[54] sep.[36] sil.[10] sin-n.[54] ***spig.***[36] stann.[1] thuj.[10]

➤ amorous, erections, with, painful: cact.[54]

➤ amorous, erections, with, priapism, with: ***camph.***[54] ***pic-ac.***[54]

➤ amorous, excitement of sexual organs, with: ***op.***[54]

➤ amorous, looked into her eyes, after a man: ozone[227]

➤ amorous, morning: aloe colch. grat. lil-t. plb. ptel.[25] sabad. sil. sumb.

➤ amorous, orgasm, with: bamb-a.[1184]

➤ amorous, penis, with relaxed: sabad.[54]

➤ amorous, perverse: ind.[85]

➤ amorous, pollutions, with: ***alum.***[5] ambr.[102] ang.[10] ***ant-c.***[5] aphis.[10] arist-m.[36] arn.[5] ars.[5] ars-s-f.[54] aur.[5] bar-c.[5] bell.[5] bism.[5] bor.[5] bov.[5] cahin.[54] ***calad.***[102] ***calc.***[5] calc-acet.[36] calc-p.[36] ***camph.***[54] cann-i.[36] cann-s.[116] canth.[116] carb-ac.[36] carb-an.[5] caust.[10] chin.[5] ***cic.***[54] ***cob.***[36] coloc.[5] con.[102] cycl.[58] ***dig.***[5] dios.[54] euph.[10] ferr.[10] form.[36] ***gels.***[54] ***graph.***[54] grat.[5] ham.[5] hura[36] hydr.[36] indg.[36] iod.[58] ***iris***[36] ***kali-br.***[54] ***kali-c.***[5] kali-chl.[10] kali-s.[5] lach.[10] lact.[10] led.[5] ***lil-t.***[36] lipp.[36] lyc.[36] lyss.[36] merc-i-f.[54] merc-s.[36] myric.[36] ***nat-c.***[5] nat-m.[10] nat-p.[36] **NUX-V.**[5] ***olnd.***[5] op.[54] paeon.[36] par.[5] ***ph-ac.***[5] ***phos.***[5] ***pic-ac.***[54] plat.[122] plb.[5] ***puls.***[36] ran-b.[5] rhod.[5] sabad.[5] samb.[5] ***sars.***[5] sel.[54] senec.[36] ***sep.***[5] ***sil.*** sin-n.[36] ***spig.***[5] spira.[36] stann.[36] staph.[36] stram.[10] sul-ac.[26] sulph.[5] thuj.[10] thymol.[102] ust.[54] ***viol-t.***[5]

➤ amorous, pollutions, with, erections, with long continued: rhod.[54]

➤ amorous, pollutions, with, painful: ***sars.***[54]

➤ amorous, pollutions, with, profuse: cann-i.[54] ***kali-c.***[54] merc-i-f.[54] ***olnd.***[54]

➤ amorous, pollutions, with, sleep, as soon as he falls to: ***pic-ac.***[54]
➤ amorous, pollutions, with, sticky, profuse, fluid emission, with aversion to coition: ***plat.***[54]
➤ amorous, pollutions, with, two in one night: ***puls.***[54]
➤ amorous, pollutions, with, violent: ***kali-chl.***[54]
➤ amorous, pollutions, with, waking him, headache, with, dim sight, prostration and vertigo: ***sars.***[54]
➤ amorous, sadness, during: ***aur.***[54]
➤ amorous, weakness, with, in both sexes: plat.[54]
➤ animals, copulating: cench.[58]
➤ birth, of giving: lap-gr-m.[194]
➤ body, penis breaking off: kali-n.[36]
➤ body, penis, glands penis breaking off: kreos.[10]
➤ body, penis, prepuce sloughed off: linu-c.
➤ boyfriend, of, old: hydrog.[222]
➤ children, about, abused: ozone[227]
➤ coition of: am-c.[1] am-m.[1] bamb-a.[1184] bor.[1] corn-a.[85] ind.[36] lac-ac.[54] lyc.[1] nat-m.[47] nat-p.[36] ***plat.***[8] polym.[111] sil.[1] sul-ac.[1] sumb.[36] thuj.[1] ***zinc-pic.***[116]
➤ coition, desire for coition, of: sel.[36]
➤ coition, stranger coming in prevented the act: nat-p.[36]
➤ coition, unsuccessful: ind.[36]
➤ coition, unsuccessful, men, with, in men: ind.[36]
➤ coition, urinating during coition, and: kreos.[114] puls.[114]
➤ conversations, women, with: cedr.[10]
➤ dirt, linen, couple makes love in dirty linen: ozone[227]
➤ doctor drawing a uterus and ovaries on a board: ozone[227]
➤ drinking, emission, followed by: merc-i-f.[137]
➤ emission, which did not take place: thuj.[36]
➤ erections, of: kreos.[102]
➤ harassing: thuj.[36]
➤ incestuous: lap-mar-c.[194]
➤ indecent behavior of men and women: cench.[58]
➤ Indian, of, graceful, silent, following sensual forms: lap-mar-c.[194]
➤ lewd, lascivious, voluptuous: acon.[36] adren.[56] am-c.[36] am-m.[36] ambr.[1] anag.[8] ant-c.[36] aran.[192] arg-n.[36] arn.[1] ars.[102] astac.[36] bism.[8] bor.[36] cact.[8] cahin.[36] ***calc.***[54] ***camph.***[54] ***cann-i.***[102] cann-s.[5] canth.[5] carb-ac.[36] carb-v.[36] cere-b.[36] clem.[8] cob.[36] colch.[36] coloc.[1] ***con.***[54] cop.[36] cycl.[36] dig.[8] dios.[36] dros.[5] ery-a.[36] euph.[36] form.[5] ***graph.***[54] grat.[36] ham.[102] hipp.[36] hura[36] hydr.[36] hyos.[1] ign.[1] ind.[36] inul.[36] ***kali-br.***[8] kali-c.[36] kali-p.[36] lach.[36] lact.[36] lil-t.[36] linu-c.[36] lyc.[36] m-arct.[1] m-p-a.[1] meny.[1] merc-i-r.[36] merc-s.[36] nat-m.[36] ***nat-p.***[8] nit-ac.[36] nuph.[25] nux-v.[5] nym.[36] op.[1] orig.[36] ox-ac.[36] oxyt.[77] paraf.[77] petr.[36] ph-ac.[5] phos.[5] phys.[1] pic-ac.[36] plan.[36] ***plat.***[36] psor.[56] ptel.[36] puls.[1] raph.[36] rhod.[36] rhus-v.[36] sabad.[36] salx-n.[102] samb.[1] sars.[36] sel.[8] senec.[36] sep.[36] sil.[36] sin-n.[36] sol-t-ae.[36] spig.[1] spira.[36] spirae.[36] stann.[1] staph.[5] ***sulph.***[36] thuj.[1] thymol.[102] trom.[36] ust.[102] verat-v.[102] vinc.[36] ***viol-t.***[8] x-ray[56] yuc.[36]
➤ men: frax.[36] nicc. ***puls.***[36]
➤ men, caressing her back: ozone[227]
➤ men, naked: cench.[58] eupi. ***puls.***
➤ nakedness, about: androc.[222] cench.[58] erech.[36] kali-p.[58] rumx.
➤ nightmare, amorous dreams, during: nit-ac.[36]
➤ pollution which did not take place: cann-i.[25] dios.[25] thuj.[36]
➤ pregnant, of being: choc.[222] hydrog.[222] lap-gr-m.[194] pic-ac.
➤ rape: cand-a.[239] ***cench.***[58] kreos.[10] lap-gr-m.[194] petr. sep.[10]
➤ rape, pursued for the purpose of: ***cench.***[122] kreos.
➤ rape, seeing, of: ***cench.***
➤ rape, that he has committed: ***cench.*** kreos.[10] petr. sep.[10]
➤ rape, threats of rape: cench.[58] sep.
➤ threats of rape: sep.[36]
➤ unsuccessful efforts to, coition, in: ind.[36]
➤ urinate, that he must, followed by seminal emission, of which he knew nothing: merc-i-f.[54]
➤ vivid, emissions, with nocturnal: ***viol-t.***[54]
➤ vivid, erections, during: sulph.[36]
➤ vulgar scenes: chin-b.[54]
➤ women: ***dios.***[8] lach.[36] opun-a.[36]
➤ women, looking under their skirts: ozone[227]
➤ women, naked: androc.[222] ozone[227] ***staph.***[8]
➤ women, naked indecently, she is, and spreads her legs: ozone[227]

Dress; indecently: aq-mar.[231] hell.[5] hyos.[5] sec.[122] ***stram.***[5]

Dullness; coition, after: bar-c.[5] bov.[5] calc.[5] *sep.*
Dullness; emissions, pollutions, after: bov.[5] calc.[5] caust. ind.[36] **KALI-BR.**[54] nat-c.[5] ph-ac.[102] ran-b.[5] sabad.[5] sep.[5] sil.[5]
Dullness; emissions, pollutions, with: **KALI-BR.**[54]
Dullness; impotency, with: ph-ac.[58]
Dullness; masturbation, after: *agn.*[102] calc-p.[102] canth.[102] caust.[102] dam.[102] *gels.*[54] nux-v.[102] **OP.**[102] ph-ac.[58] phos.[102] pic-ac.[102] **STAPH.**[54]
Dullness; sexual excesses, after: *agn.*[102] *anac.*[102] arg-n.[102] aur.[102] chin.[102] nat-m.[102] nux-v.[102] *ph-ac.*[102] *sel.*[116] *staph.*[102]
Dwells; on past disagreeable occurrences, sexual matters, on: staph.[102]
Ecstasy, amorous: ant-c.[1] op. pic-ac.
Ecstasy, amorous, delirium, during: thea.[36]
Ecstasy, amorous, sleep, during: phos.
Ecstasy; sensitivity of female sexual organs, with: coff.[54]
Effeminate: calc.[30] lyc.[30] *plat.*[30] **PULS.**[162] sil.[30]
Egotism; self-esteem, nymphomania, in: *agar.*[54]
Excitement; coition, after: *calc.*
Excitement; lascivious, with painful nocturnal erections: *merc.*[54]
Excitement; nymphomania, is: aster.[54]
Excitement; sexual, children, in: aloe[36] bell.[149] *orig.*[54] plat.[58] verat.[149]
Excitement; sexual, intense: foll.[149] pall.[137] tarent.[102] vip.[1212]
Excitement; women, in: cedr.[85] con.[85] ign.[85]
Exhilaration; coition, after: bor.
Fancies; lascivious: alum.[30] am-c. *ambr.* anac. androc.[222] arund. aur. bell. *calad.*[54] *calc.* camph.[54] *canth.*[10] carb-v. caust.[30] *chin.* cod.[54] *con.*[10] cop.[54] dig. *graph.* hipp. *hyos.*[162] ign. *kali-br.*[54] *lach.*[10] lil-t. *lyc.* lyss.[54] nat-c.[54] *nat-m.*[10] *nuph.*[36] nux-v.[30] *op.* *orig.*[54] orig-v.[25] petr.[30] phos.[135] plat.[30] psor.[30] sang. *sel.*[10] sep.[10] *sil.*[54] sin-n.[54] staph.[30] stram.[10] tarent.[58] thuj. *ust.*[54] *verat.*[162] verb. yuc.[36] *zinc.*[54]
Fancies; lascivious, erections, with, daytime: sin-n.[54]
Fancies; lascivious, erections, with, sleep, during, and impotence after waking: *op.*[54]
Fancies; lascivious, frequent, involuntary: sil.[1]
Fancies; lascivious, impotency, with: calad.[58] *chin.*[54] lach.[137] *op.*[54] *sel.*[54]
Fancies; lascivious, sweets, with desire for: *chin.*[54]
Fear; coition, during, impotence, causing: *sin-n.*[54]
✦ coition, during, incontinence of urine, causing long lasting: *lyc.*[54]
✦ coition, for, after too much indulgence: lyc.[172]
✦ coition, thought of, in a woman, rape: arn.[162] *kreos.* ozone[227]
✦ emission, after an: aloe carb-an. petr.[137]
✦ friends, of, female: cedr.[25]
✦ homosexuality, of: hydr-ac.[102] manc.[162] *puls.*[162] *staph.*[162]
✦ impotence, of: nat-m.[172] onos.[172] pitu-p.[149]
✦ impotence, old people, in: phos.[172] stry.[172]
✦ men, girls, in: puls.[109]
✦ men, of: 0aloe 0aur. 0bar-c. bar-m. choc.[222] 0con. dios. hypoth.[149] ign. 0lach. lap-mar-c.[194] *led.* 0lyc. 0nat-c. 0nat-m. 0phos. *plat.* *puls.* raph. sep. 0stann. 0sulph.
✦ moral obliquity alternating with sexual, excitement: lil-t.
✦ noise, from, night, emission, after: aloe[54]
✦ sex, of opposite: kali-p.[172] puls.[172] sep.[172] staph.[172]
✦ women, of: puls. raph.[36] sep.[172] staph.[185]
✦ women, of, boys, in: puls.[70]
Forgetfulness; coition, after: *sec.*
Forgetfulness; masturbations, after: *dig.*[54] kali-br.[116] staph.[85]
Forgetfulness; pollutions, after: staph.[5]
Frightened; easily, pollutions, after: aloe[1]
Frightened; easily, spermatorrhea, in: *phos.*[54]
Gestures; grasping, genitals, children: *acon.*[54] bell.[122] **BUFO**[171] maland.[171] *merc.*[54] *stram.*[54] *zinc.*[54]
Gestures; makes, grasping, genitals: *acon.* bell. bufo canth. colch.[5] *hyos.* maland.[85] med.[85] *merc.* *puls.*[54] sep.[5] *stram.* tab.[5] thuj.[5] ust.[102] *zinc.*[5]
Hatred; men, of: bar-c. ign. led. lyc. phos. stann.
Hatred; sex, to opposite: sep.[137]
Hatred; women, of: *puls.* raph.[36]
Hypochondriasis; continence in unmarried men, from: con.[1]
Hypochondriasis; masturbation, after: *tarent.*[54]
Hypochondriasis; pollutions, after: anac.[5] sil.[5] staph.[5]
Hypochondriasis; sexual: *mosch.*[54]

Hypochondriasis; sexual, abstinence, from: **CON.**[54] mosch.[54]
Hypochondriasis; sexual, abuse, after: ***ph-ac.***[54]
Hypochondriasis; sexual, dwelling on sexual subjects: ***staph.***[54]
Hypochondriasis; sexual, excesses, from: anac.[10] calc.[10] chin.[10] **CON.**[54] nat-m.[10] nux-v.[10] ***ph-ac.***[54] sep.[10] **STAPH.**[54] sulph.[10]
Hysteria; coition amel.: con.[116]
Hysteria; coition, agg. at height of orgasm: lac-c.[137]
Hysteria; lascivious: agn.[54] mosch. ***plat. tarent.***
Hysteria; masturbation, with: raph.[171]
Hysteria; pollutions, after: anac.[5] sil.[5] staph.[5]
Hysteria; sexual excesses, after: agar. anac. con. lach. ***ph-ac.*** sep.
Hysteria; sexual, derangement of sexual functions, with: **NUX-M.**[54]
Hysteria; sexual, irritation, from excessive: ***orig.***[54]
Hysteria; sexual, suppression of s. excitement, from: ***brom.***[162] **CON.**[54]
Hysteria; sexual, suppression of s. excitement, from, low spirited, anxiety and sadness: **CON.**[54]
Idiocy; masturbation, after: ***op.***[54] ***orig.***[54]
Idiocy; masturbation, with: bufo[117] med.[122] orig.[122]
Imbecility; masturbation, after: tarent.[36]
Imbecility; sexual, abuse, after: ***phos.***[54]
Imbecility; sexual, excitement, with: ***bell.***[122] ***hep.***[122] ***hyos.***[122] ***phos.***[122] ***staph.***[122] ***stram.***[122]
Indifference; coition, after: ***calc.***[137]
Indifference; coition, after, menses, before: sep.[26]
Indifference; coition, during: lyss.[36]
Indifference; masturbation, after: **STAPH.**
Indifference; opposite sex, to: ***puls.***[162] **SEP.**[162] thuj.
Indifference; sexual desire diminished, with: ***kali-chl.***[54]
Indifference; women, to: nat-m.[36]
Indignation; emission, after: pip-m.[36]
Indolence; coition, after: nat-c.[10]
Indolence; emissions, after: ***dios.***[54] nat-c.[1] sep.
Indolence; masturbation, after: ***dig.***[54] ***gels.***[54]
Industrious; coition, after: calc-p.
Insanity; dancing, with, and stripping himself: ***bell.***[122]
Insanity; erotic: ambr.[102] **APIS BAR-M.** bell.[10] bufo[107] calc-p.[36] camph.[85] ***cann-i.***[102] canth.[111] ferul.[102] gins.[102] grat.[102] ***hyos.*** kali-br. lil-t.[102] lyss. manc.[102] ***murx.***[102] ***nux-v.***[85] orig. ***phos. pic-ac.***[102] **PLAT.** ***puls.*** rob.[102] salx-n.[102] stann.[36] stram.[36] ***sulph. tarent.*** **VERAT.** zinc.[111]
Insanity; erotic, hysterical girl, in a: ***plat.***[54]
Insanity; erotic, jealousy, with: ***hyos.***[54]
Insanity; females, of: ***acon.***[111] apis[130] ***bell.***[111] cimic.[137] ***orig.***[137] plat.[111] ***puls.***[111] stram.[111] verat.[111]
Insanity; lascivious: ***hyos.***[5] tarent.[8] **VERAT.**[5]
Insanity; masturbation, from: anan.[54] bufo ***cocc. hyos.*** op.[137] ***plb.***[54]
Insanity; orgasm, at height of: lac-c.[137]
Insanity; sexual excesses, from: anan.[54] ***apis***[130] ***lach.***[30] lil-t.[54] ***phos.***[54] staph.[30]
Insanity; wantonness, with: bell.[10] cupr. ***hyos.*** merc.[10] mez.[10] stram. verat.
Insanity; women, in: ***acon.***[111] apis[130] ***bell.***[111] cimic.[137] ***orig.***[137] plat.[111] ***puls.***[111] stram.[111] verat.[111]
Irritability; coition, after, agg.: agar. aster.[8] bov. calad. **CALC.** calc-s. calc-sil.[58] ***chin.*** dig. graph. ***kali-c.*** kali-p. ***kali-sil.***[58] mag-m. ***nat-c.*** nat-m. nat-sil.[58] nit-ac. nux-v. ***petr.*** ph-ac. ***phos. sel.***[122] **SEP. SIL.** staph. thuj.[111]
Irritability; coition, after, agg., easy and lighthearted at first, later ill humored: ***nat-m.***[54]
Irritability; coition, after, agg., weakness, with: calc.[102]
Irritability; coition, amel.: tarent.[122]
Irritability; emission, after: coff. dig. gels.[60] ***lil-t.*** nat-c. ***nux-v.*** sang.[122] sel. **STAPH.** ***thuj.***[54] ust.
Irritability; emission, during: ***aur.***[102] calad.[102] ***calc.***[102] ***chin.***[102] ***cimic.***[102] clem.[36] ***con.***[102] dios.[102] kali-br.[102] ***nux-v.***[102] ph-ac.[102] phos.[102] ***sel.***[102] ***staph.***[102]
Irritability; impotency, with: ***pic-ac.***[54]
Irritability; masturbation, after: ***hyos.***[54]
Irritability; orgasm, after: ang.[36]
Irritability; sexual, appetite, from loss: sabal.[137]
Irritability; sexual, excesses, from: ol-an.[116]
Irritability; sexual, excitement, from dreams and orgasm, in a woman: ***nux-v.***[54]
Irritability; sexual, excitement, from, amel.: tarent.[36]
Irritability; sexual, weakness, with: ***pic-ac.***
Jealousy; impotence, with: calad.[30] nux-v.[30]

Jealousy; men, between: ars.[30] lach.[30] puls.[30] verat.[30]

Jealousy; sexual excitement, with: calc.[30] caust.[30] chin.[30] con.[30] hyos.[54] nux-v.[30] phos.[30]

Jealousy; women, between: ars.[30] nat-m.[30] nux-v.[30] sep.[30]

Jesting; erotic: bell.[30] ***calc.***[30] hyos.[30] nux-v.[30]

Kill; sudden impulse to, woman, a, almost irresistible: ***iod.***[54]

Lasciviousness; animal, as if she were completely, mental power dormant: lach.[54]

Lasciviousness; eating, after, with feeling of weakness in parts: lyss.[54]

Lasciviousness; emotions, with violent: cop.[54]

Lasciviousness; erections, with: op.[54] sin-n.[54]

Lasciviousness; erections, with, painful: lyss.[54]

Lasciviousness; erections, without: ambr.[5] calad.[5] caps.[5] **IGN.**[54] meny.[5] **SEL.**[5]

Lasciviousness; impotence, with: calad.[58] ***chin.***[54] ***op.***[54] ***sel.***[54]

Lasciviousness; lustfulness: ***acon.***[54] act-sp.[162] agar. agn.[137] aloe alum.[30] ***ambr.*** anac.[102] androc.[222] ant-c.[85] ant-i.[54] ***apis*** arund. aster.[54] aur. bell.[30] bor. bov.[36] ***bufo***[11] ***calad. calc.*** calc-p.[116] calc-s. calc-sil.[58] camph.[36] ***cann-i.***[116] cann-s.[116] ***canth. carb-v.*** carl.[36] ***caust.***[30] cedr.[85] cere-s.[36] ***chin.*** coc-c. cod.[36] ***con.*** cop. croc.[116] ***dig. fl-ac. graph.*** hydrog.[222] **HYOS.** hyper. ign. kali-br.[122] **LACH. LIL-T.** lyc. lyss. m-arct.[36] merc. mosch. ***murx.***[102] nat-c.[36] nat-m. nit-ac. nuph.[36] nux-m.[36] nux-v.[85] op. **ORIG.** ph-ac.[30] **PHOS. PIC-AC. PLAT.** plb.[116] ***puls.*** raja-s.[149] raph. ***sabin.***[116] salx-n.[72] sars.[36] ***sel. sep. sil.*** spig. squil.[137] stann.[36] **STAPH.** ***stram.*** sulph.[30] ***tarent.*** tere-ch.[149] tub.[122] ust.[116] ***verat.*** zinc.

Lasciviousness; ogling, women on the street: calad.[137] fl-ac.[137]

Lasciviousness; painful urging in penis, with, as after excessive coition: lyss.[54]

Lasciviousness; rage, with: ***hyos.***[54]

Lasciviousness; religious: ***plat.***[54]

Lasciviousness; rest, no: ***orig.***[54]

Lasciviousness; uncovers sexual parts: **HYOS.**[54]

Lasciviousness; voluptuous ideas, pleasure only in: bell.

Lasciviousness; women at every touch: ***murx.***[116]

Laughing; sexual excitement, with: stram.[137]

Lewdness, obscene: agn. alum.[30] anac.[102] androc.[222] apis bell. bufo[112] calc.[30] ***camph. canth.*** carb-v.[30] ***caust.***[30] chin.[30] con.[30] ***cub.*** fl-ac.[111] ***hyos. lach.*** lil-t.[36] lyc.[30] lyss. merc.[30] nat-m.[30] nux-v. op. orig.[30] ***phos. pic-ac. plat.***[122] puls.[30] raph.[36] rob. staph.[30] stram. sulph.[30] tarent. verat.

Lewdness; man searching for little girls: caust.[30] phos.[30] plat.[30] verat.[30]

Lewdness; talk: apis[130] aur. ***bell.*** bufo[112] ***calc.***[30] camph. chlf.[36] cub. ***hyos. lil-t.*** nux-m.[10] ***nux-v.*** phos. plat. ***stram.*** tub.[102] verat.

Libertinism: act-sp.[54] alum.[30] arn.[10] bar-c.[10] bell.[30] calc.[30] ***canth.***[30] carb-v.[30] ***caust.***[30] chin.[30] con.[30] fl-ac.[122] hyos.[30] lyc.[30] **MED.**[185] merc.[30] nat-m.[30] ***nux-v.*** orig.[30] ph-ac.[30] ***phos.***[30] pic-ac. ***plat.*** puls.[30] raph.[36] sep.[122] spong.[10] ***staph.*** stram.[30] sulph.[30] verat.[30]

Love; anal coition with a woman: caust.[30] plat.[30]

Love; married man or coachman, with: ign.[58] ***nat-m.***[122]

Love; own sex, aversion of neck band, with: lach.[148]

Love; own sex, loquacity, with: lach.[148]

Love; own sex, men: med.[162] nat-m.[162] orig.[162] phos.[162] ***plat.***[30] puls.[162] sep.[162] staph.[162]

Love; own sex, with one of her, homosexuality, tribadism: anh.[144] calc.[30] calc-p. hydrog.[222] hyos.[185] hypoth.[149] ***lach.*** lyc.[148] nat-m. phos. **PLAT.**[122] puls.[122] ***sulph.*** syph.[85] thiop.[149]

Love; own sex, women: fl-ac.[162] med.[162] phos.[162] puls.[162] sulph.[162]

Love; perversity, animals, with, sodomy: ***plat.***[162]

Love; sadomasochistic: anac.[187]

Mania; indecent: ***op.***[54]

Mania; masturbation, after: anan.[54]

Mania; masturbation, eight or ten years duration, of: ***plb.***[54]

Mania; sexual in men: apis[117] canth.[102] **PHOS.** ***tarent.***

Mania; sexual, abuse, from: lil-t.[54] ***phos.***[54]

Mania; sexual, increased desire, from: apis[122] **BAR-M.**[54] **PHOS.** ***tarent.***

Mania; sexual, men, in: apis[117] canth.[102] **PHOS.** ***tarent.***

Mania; sexual, women in: **APIS**[54] canth.[102] **PHOS.**[122] raph.[36] ***tarent.***[122]

Mania; suicidal, sexual symptoms, with: ***aur.***[54]

Mannish habits of girls: carb-v.[30] cimic.[144] cortiso.[144] ***nat-m.***[30] petr.[30] plat.[30]

Mannish habits of women: fl-ac.[122]

Marriage; aversion to: puls.[58]

Marriage; aversion to, enjoying society of men, while: pic-ac.[36]

Marriage; aversion to, women, in: ***lach.***[54]

Marriage; obsessed by idea of m. excited sexual girls are: bell.[30] ***caust.***[30] plat.[30] verat.[30]

Masochism; sexual: lach.[185] nat-m.[185] tub.[185]

Memory; active, suppression sexual desire, from: lach.

Memory; weakness, coition, after exhausting: ***sec.***[54]

Memory; weakness, impotence, with: **KALI-BR.**[54]

Memory; weakness, masturbation, after: ***dig.***[54] ***gels.***[54] ***phos.***[54]

Memory; weakness, sexual excesses, from: agn.[102] anac.[102] arg-n.[102] aur.[102] calad. **CALC.**[54] chin.[102] **DIG.**[54] kali-br.[72] ***nat-ar.*** nat-m.[102] nux-v.[102] ***ph-ac.***[102] **PHOS.**[54] **STAPH.**[54]

Mirth; emission, after an: pip-m.

Moaning; pollutions, after: hipp.[36]

Moral affections; perversions: ***anac.***[5] **BELL.**[5] bufo[5] **HYOS.**[5] nux-v.[5] ***op.***[5] ph-ac.[5] ***plat.***[5] **STRAM.**[5] tarent.[5] **VERAT.**[5]

Morose; coition, after: ang.[36] calc.[5] nat-c.[10] ***nat-m.***[36] petr.[5] ***sel.***[5] sil.[5]

Morose; erotomania, in: ***orig.***[54] ***plat.***[54]

Morose; pollutions, after: ***dig.***[54] nat-c.[5] ***thuj.***[54]

Morose; sexual excesses, from: **STAPH.**[54]

Mortification; emissions, after: **STAPH.**[54]

Naked, wants to be: bamb-a.[1184] ***bell.*** bufo[170] but-ac.[119] camph. cham. **HYOS.**[122] merc. merc-c. ***phos.*** phyt. ***sec. stram.*** tarent.[137] ***verat.***[122]

Naked, wants to be, delirium, in: ***bell.*** **HYOS.** merc. ***phos.*** phyt. ***sec. stram.***[54]

Necromania: **AGAR.**[185]

Nymphomania: agar. ambr. androc.[222] anh.[149] ***ant-c. apis*** ars.[31] asaf.[54] aster.[149] aur-m-n.[85] ***bar-m. bell.*** calad. calc. ***calc-p.*** camph. camph-br.[25] ***cann-i. cann-s. canth.*** carb-v. cedr. ***chin.*** chlol.[25] chlor.[5] coca[98] cocc.[31] ***coff.*** con.[31] ***croc.***[5] cyna.[149] ***dig.*** dulc. ***ferul.***[102] ***fl-ac.*** gins.[102] graph. **GRAT. HYOS.** ign.[116] iod.[31] ***kali-br.*** kali-p. **LACH.** ***lil-t. lyc.*** manc.[116] ***merc.*** mosch. ***murx.*** nat-c. nat-m. ***nux-v.*** op. **ORIG.** orig-v.[25] ozone[227] ph-ac.[85] ***phos.*** pic-ac.[102] **PLAT.** plb. psil.[149] ***puls. raph.*** rob. ***sabad.*** sabin. salx-n.[85] sil. stann.[111] ***staph.*** **STRAM.** stry.[102] sulph. sumb.[111] ***tarent.*** thuj.[31] valer.[102] ***verat. zinc.*** zinc-pic.[85]

Nymphomania; climacteric period, at: lach.[102] manc.[102] ***murx.***[102]

Nymphomania; coition agg.: ***tarent.***[54]

Nymphomania; delivery, parturition, after, puerperal: bell.[10] ***chin.*** coca[83] kali-br. ***plat.*** verat. zinc.[54]

Nymphomania; girl young, in a: ***orig.***[54] raph.[85]

Nymphomania; loquacity, with: ***verat.***[54]

Nymphomania; menses, after: kali-br.[25] sul-ac.[116]

Nymphomania; menses, before: calc.[116] calc-p. kali-c.[116] ***phos.*** stram. ***verat.***

Nymphomania; menses, during: calc.[116] coca[83] ***hyos.*** kali-br. kali-c.[116] ***phos.***[54] ***plat. sec.*** stram. ***verat.***

Nymphomania; menses, suppressed: ant-c. canth. chin. cocc. hyos. ***murx.*** phos. ***plat.*** sil. stram. sulph. verat. zinc

Nymphomania; metrorrhagia, during: mosch. murx. plat. sabin.[85] sec.

Obstinate; children, masturbation, boys after: aur.[116]

Precocity; sexual: chlorpr.[149] hyos.[187] lach.[187] orig.[187] parot.[100] supren.[100]

Prostration; coition, after: ***calc.***[122] coca[54] sep.[5]

Prostration; masturbation, after: orig-v.[25]

Prostration; sexual excesses, after: sel.[58]

Quiet disposition; masturbation, in: ***hyos.***[54]

Rage; amorous: **CANTH.**[54]

Rage; amorous, morning when rising: agn.[36]

Rage; women, approaching, in a woman: raph.[36]

Religious affections; alternating with sexual excitement: lil-t. ***plat.***

Religious affections; horror of the opposite sex: lyc. nat-m.[193] ***plat.***[54] ***puls.*** sulph.

Religious affections; taciturnity, haughtiness, voluptuousness, cruelty, r. a with: ***plat.***[54]

Remorse; masturbation, after: staph.[92]

Restlessness; coition, after: **CALC.** cop. dig. mez.[122] petr. ***sep.*** staph.[122]

Restlessness; coition, during: upa.[36]

Restlessness; lascivious thoughts, from: graph.[36]

Restlessness; sexual excitement, in: ant-c.[10] cann-i.[102] ***canth.***[102] ***kali-br.***[102] kali-p.[85] ***raph.***[102] staph.[116]

Sadness; alternating with, sexual excitement: lil-t.
Sadness; coition, after: ***agar.***[116] calc. cedr.[54] con. ***nat-m.*** ph-ac.[144] sel.[116] ***sep.*** staph. sulph.[137]
Sadness; continence, from: bell. **CON.** hyos. stram.
Sadness; emission, from: aur. carb-ac.[25] ***cypr.***[54] dig. dios. ***ery-a.***[54] ham. **KALI-BR.**[54] nat-c.[1] nat-p. **NUX-V.** ph-ac. ***puls.*** sang. sep.[54] ust.
Sadness; impotence, with: ***aur.***[54] ***calad.***[54] ***gels.***[54] **KALI-BR.**[54] ***spong.***[54]
Sadness; masturbation, from: agar. ***aur.***[54] calad. cocc. ***con. gels.***[54] ham. ***nat-m.*** nat-p. nux-v. **PH-AC.** ***plat.*** sars. sil. staph. sulph.
Sadness; men, with aversion to: stann.[54]
Sadness; pollutions, from: agar.[54] aur. ***calad.***[54] ***con.***[54] ***cypr.***[54] dig. dios. ***ery-a.***[54] ferr-br.[116] ham. **KALI-BR.**[54] med.[54] ***nat-m.***[54] nat-p. **NUX-V.** ph-ac. ***puls.*** sang. sars.[54] ***sep.***[54] sulph.[54] ust.
Sadness; sexual excesses, from: agar.[116] agn.[102] aur.[102] ***cimic.***[102] con.[116] ***lil-t.***[102] nux-v.[102] pic-ac.[102] plat.[102] sep.[102] spong.[137]
Sadness; sexual, excitement, after: tarent.
Sadness; sexual, excitement, suppressed: **CON.**[162]
Sadness; sexual, excitement, with: bell.[10] manc.[122] naja[85]
Sadness; sexual, organs, with distress about: naja[85]
Sadness; spermatorrhea, in: ***cypr.***[54] ***ph-ac.***[54] ***ust.***[54]
Sadness; sterility, from: aur.[137]
Satyriasis: agar.[5] agn.[5] anac.[149] androc.[222] ***apis***[130] bar-m.[85] camph.[36] cann-i.[36] canna[83] **CANTH.**[5] coca[83] con.[5] cyna.[149] ***fl-ac.***[54] ***gels.***[8] **GRAPH.**[5] grat.[54] hyos.[5] ***kali-br.***[54] kali-c.[5] **LYC.**[5] ***lyss.***[54] med.[187] **MERC.**[5] ***nat-m.***[5] **NUX-V.**[5] pen.[36] **PHOS.**[5] ***pic-ac.***[54] **PLAT.**[5] psor.[36] salx-n.[85] saroth.[149] **SIL.**[5] ***stram.***[5] ***sulph.***[5] thymol.[149] ust.[116] ***verat.***[5] zinc.[5] zinc-pic.[85]
Satyriasis; stallion, in a: ***lyss.***[8]
Sensitive; sensual impressions, to: ***am-c.*** ars. ars-i. ***aur.*** bar-c. berb.[36] calc. carc.[193] cast.[54] ***chin. coff.***[144] dig. ***graph.*** hep. iod. ***lyc.*** mag-c. ***nat-c. nit-ac.*** nux-v. petr.[122] ***phos. sep.*** sil. thuj. valer.[144] ***zinc.***
Sensual: bufo[187]
Shameless: alco.[36] ***anac.***[5] bell. ***bufo***[5] calc. camph.[5] cann-s.[5] canth. chlf.[46] cub. cupr. hell. <u>**HYOS.**</u>[122] lyc.[30] merc-c. mosch. ***murx.***[5] nat-m. nux-m. nux-v. ***op.***[5] **PHOS.** phyt. ***plat.***[5] sabin.[5] **SEC.** ***staph.***[193] ***stram. tarent. tub.***[122] ***verat.***
Shameless; exposes the person: **HYOS.** ***phos.*** phyt. ***sec.*** stram.[5] ***tarent.*** verat.[122]
Sighing; ejaculations, and: ***cimic.***[54]
Singing; obscene songs: alco.[36] canth.[58] ***hyos.*** op. raja-s.[149] stram. verat.[58]
Singing; obscene songs, nymphomania, in: ***stram.***[54]
Starting; coition, after: sep.[1]
Stupefaction; debauchery, as after: psor.[122]
Stupefaction; emissions, after: caust. lact.[85]
Stupor; sexual excitement, with: hyos.[162] ***orig.***[54] ***stram.***[54]
Suicidal disposition; erotomania, in: orig.[137]
Suicidal disposition; mania, in, puerperal, with aversion to husband, baby and coition: agn.[171]
Suicidal disposition; thoughts, spermatorrhea from masturbation, in: ***gels.***[54]
Talk; indisposed, sexual abuse, after: **STAPH.**[54]
Tears; himself, genitals, his: sec. tab.[5]
Thoughts; amorous: ant-c.[5] canth.[5] ***carb-an.***[5] ***chin.***[5] ***dig.***[5] graph.[5] lach.[5] plat.[5] sel.[5] ***staph.***[5] verb.[5]
Thoughts; marriage, of: orig.[36]
Thoughts; marriage, of, masturbation, in: ***hyos.***[54]
Thoughts; sexual: aloe ambr.[10] androc.[222] ***aq-mar.***[149] arund.[122] aster.[54] bamb-a.[1184] bell.[10] calc.[10] camph.[36] canth.[108] carb-v.[54] cod.[25] con. foll.[149] ***graph. hyper.***[54] ***kali-br.***[54] med.[162] nat-c.[10] ***nuph.***[54] orig.[122] orig-v.[25] ozone[227] ***phos.*** pic-ac. ***plat.*** salx-n.[102] saroth.[144] sel.[58] sep.[10] sil.[10] ***staph. stram.***[10] sulph.[116] tarent.[192] ust.[193]
Thoughts; sexual, day and night: chin.[10] dig.[10]
Thoughts; sexual, impotence, with: ***calad.***[54] ***sel.***[116]
Thoughts; sexual, intercourse, of lavish: staph.[109]
Thoughts; sexual, masturbation, with: ***hyos.***[54] ust.[116]
Thoughts; sexual, tormenting: aq-mar.[149] aster.[85] canth.[58] con. graph. ozone[227] ***staph.*** tarent.[192]
Thoughts; vanishing, coition, during: gels.[184]
Thoughts; vanishing, sexual excitement, during: arund.[162] orig.[162]

Unconsciousness; alternating with, erotic mania: apis[98]
Unconsciousness; coition, after: ***agar.*** asaf. ***dig.***
Unconsciousness; erotomania, in: apis[98] ***orig.***[54]
Unconsciousness; sexual excitement, with: ***orig.***[54] ***stram.***[54]
Violence; nymphomania, in: ***verat.***[54]
Vivaciousness; pollutions, after: pip-m.[36]
Weary of life; spermatorrhea, in: ***sil.***[54]
Weeping; easily, erotomania, in: ***plat.***[54]
Weeping; emission, after an: hipp.
Weeping; excitement, from, sexual: aster.[137] stram.[137]
Weeping; pollutions, after: manc. ***ust.***[54]
Work; aversion to mental, masturbation, after: ***dig.***[54]
Work; impossible, sexual excesses, after: ph-ac.[116] pic-ac.[116] ***sel.***[116]

ABSIN. Al,S-7 - Hallucination of vision and of hearing, that is pursued by imaginary enemies; hallucinations of various kinds, of naked women, etc.
ACT-SP. He, 7 - Inclined to debauchery.(seduction, lewdness)
ADAM. Sh, 158 - I feel detached and not sexual. I could bite my partner as a signal I loved her, not in a loving or hungry way. My partner said, "He is looking at me like a piece of steak, he wants to eat me. He looks like a cave man. He wants to nibble me." 7, 6C, 03:22:30
Sh, 159 - I felt detached during coition. 7, 6C, 13:23:00
Sh, 160 - Disliked being touched and uninterested in any sexual relationship. Began to be repulsed by boyfriend. 20, 1M, XX:XX:XX
Sh, 216 - Feel harder, more rebellious. I will do what I want. Inconsiderate and unsympathetic. Unfeeling in relationship and sexually. 22, 200C, 01:XX:XX
Sh, 244 - Anger with my attraction to P. He's a walker and I wanted to walk with him. I didn't want to be attracted but was, as if enchanted. 16, 12C, 18:XX:XX
Sh, 556 - Feel bright, free and beautiful, more feminine, more fertile and voluptuous. 16, 12C, 24:XX:XX
Sh, 557 - Males finding me attractive. I'm finding others more attractive. 16, 12C, 31:XX:XX
Sh, 555 - Feel feminine and beautiful. 16, 12C, 26:XX:XX
AGAR. He, 23 - Great selfishness. 0 Nymphomania.
ALOE. Al, 1 - Amorous (sexual) thoughts present themselves which are very annoying.
Al, 2 - Before taking it, the disposition is apprehensive, speculative, amorous, after taking it, quiet ...reflective, more self sufficient,...
AMBR. Al, 4 - Uncommonly long excitement.
Al, 2 - Lewd fancies, even when dreaming; the mind and the sexual organs, however, do not feel excited by them.
Ha, 477 - The imagination is occupied with many lascivious ideas, even in dreams, and yet the disposition and the sexual organs are but little excited by them.
ANDROC. Sh, 52 - Behaved as if drunk, swayed and slurred her words with increased sexual desire. (25)
Sh, 97 - Very strong liking and disliking to people —very intense —ranging from immense sexual attraction to extreme hatred. Spoke with hatred and maliciousness about colleagues. (4)
APIS. He, 28 - Manias (insanity) especially proceeding from a sexual cause in women.
He, 29 - Insanity, particularly nymphomania...
He, 77 - All her ideas turn around jealousy, very talkative (loquacity), sometimes disgusting salacious. (lascivious)
ARG-M. He, 19 - Fear of concussion (hurt, injure) as if he might run against something, with pain in testicles.
ASTER. He, 17 - Nervous agitation, with erotic thoughts and sexual desire.
AUR-M. He, 11 - Loss of energy; diminished virility; unrefreshing sleep.
AUR. He, 17 - Suicidal mania or melancholia, tedium vitae, with genital symptoms.(sexual)
BAR-M. He, 4 - In every form of mania, as soon as the sexual desire is increased. (lascivious)
BELL. Ha, 1351 - Chattering (talk) lascivious.
He, 62 - Loud laughter, wild abandon, singing, whistling, lascivious conversation.

BUFO. He, 1 - Desire for solitude, to practice masturbation.

CALAD. He, 15 - Lascivious ideas. 0Gleet 0Impotence.

CALC. Al, 15 - Melancholy, not exactly a sad feeling, about the heart, without cause, with a kind of voluptuous trembling of the body.

Ha, 56 - Aversion, dislike and repugnance to most men.

He, 71 - Voluptuous (sensual), lascivious fancies.

CANTH. He, 17 - Great amativeness, amorous frenzy.

He, 18 - Unbounded frantic sexual desire. 0 Mania.

CHOC. Sh, 40 - Became aware of a man's hair and had an intense desire to touch it, to make contact with it.

Sh, 41 - When hearing talk of babies, breasts aching with a sensation as if filling up with milk —an aching fullness. An image came to me where I found myself suckling young hairy babies, sometimes animals, especially hedgehogs.

Sh, 42 - Attracted to a man's beard. I could just feel his hair around the mouth.

Sh, 127 - Before this, I never felt very comfortable with men. Now I feel much more comfortable. I feel I've lost that extreme feeling of totally female identity. I feel like a female animal, but its not really in my awareness, it just is. Desire to curl up over a man's back. It felt right and comfortable.

Sh, 322 - Have lost interest in my husband, feel totally indifferent. I have hardly spoken to him all weekend, with a desire to avoid him. Don't want to discuss or share anything with him.15, 30C, 06:XX:XX

CON. He, 29 - Hypochondriasis and hysteria from suppression of, or too free indulgence in, sexual instinct,...(ailments from)

DIG. He, 7 - Lascivious fancies day and night.

DIOS. Al, 1 - Desire to be alone; do not enjoy society (misanthropy); am usually quite fond of the society of ladies, but they now seem repulsive,...

GERM. Sh, 110 - I don't like to be me. Want to be different. Have a distant feeling to myself yet long for physical contact, a boyfriend. Not able to do something about it. 18, 30c, 02:10:00

Sh, 142 - Observe the world as being shabby. I feel separated from people and places. I feel an intense yearning for the feminine. 08, 12C, 08:04:50

HALI-L. Sh, 13 - Increased sense of sensuality to the skin, pulling on jeans is a luxury, I feel like a kitten, soft, cuddly and warm. 09, 6C, 03:XX:XX

Sh, 606 - No more sense of sensuality, no more connection with my husband. I'm back in my head when it comes to relating to others. Damn it, it's gone. It slipped through my fingers. 09, 6C, 06:XX:XX

Sh, 614 - Full of energy in the morning. Run and walk in the sea, amazed at my high energy. Feel like I have to let out lack of sex. Want partner badly but mad at her and at myself for being so open. Feel speedy. 02, 30C, 08:03:XX

Sh, 791 - Desire to find a mate. I'm feeling sexual and just want a mate. 03:23:00

Sh, 802 - A guy told me I was hugging him like a nun. I didn't want my genitals to touch his. 20, 30C, 04:XX:XX

Sh, 803 - I feel like a sexual nun. 20, 30C, 04:XX:XX

Sh, 819 - Why am I mostly on my own? I'm not lonely with so much beauty but desire a mate -a parallel. Together, but still space in between. 05:01:XX

Sh, 877 - Inner vision—more images of courtingcopulating birds soaring together, playing with talons locked, plummeting, sounds of beaks, whooshing wind, magnificently exhilarating. 20, 30C, 09:XX:XX

Sh, 934 - As I woke, I decided I should be a nun. Strange. I feel like I've got my wings clipped when I think about men. 20, 30C, 15:XX:XX

HAM. Al, 9 - Regretful (sorry) in mind for having had emissions at night.

HIPP. Al, 1 - Lascivious fancies in the forenoon.

HYDROG. Sh, 15 - I felt in the presence of a totally pure energy, like meeting God and feeling totally unworthy or like meeting a lover and feeling unworthy — realizing all the mistakes of a lifetime. This pure energy was around for some time protecting me. I feel this unification cleared out lifetimes of symptomatology for me. The joining with this energy was as if a male energy joined with me sexually, but with no desire, pleasure or pain involved. This unification with the male energy lasted quite a few days — I'm not used to seeing myself as a man. The morning after this unifying with the higher presence, I collapsed in emotional overflow. All my grief and pain came out. I was doubled upon the floor and went into a deep state of catharsis. It is not possible to describe where I went as there are no concepts applicable. I felt overflowing love for humanity and wanted to give everything away. My mind turned to the Buddha. It was like seeing the complete picture instead of fragmented bits. (These primary effects lasted about 28 days, then changing to a paranoia state). 16, 30C, 07.XX.XX

Sh, 33 - About two months after beginning the proving, developed an extreme range of mental symptoms that he had never had before. These included severe depression with strong alternations of moods, & high then low &, with suicidal tendency, desire to jump from a high building or cut wrist, confusion of identity (especially concerning sex and homosexuality) and became more religious. He moved away from his parents home (which he had never before been able t o do) and shut himself away in a small flat. This condition lasted for another six or seven months and was finally antidoted by Phosphorus 200. Before that, he had tried to anti-dote it with acupuncture, to no avail. 24, 30C, 60:XX:XX

Sh, 156 - Felt extremely ill at ease and embarrassed when spoken to by male hairdresser. 12, 6C, 23:XX:XX

Sh, 161 - I am aware of some ridiculous thoughts coming into my mind, odd unconnected sentences such as about killing a 13 year old girl. 12, 6C, 22:XX:XX

Sh, 243 - Fear that someone was trying to find out if I was home so that they could come and rape and murder me. 16, 30C, XX:XX:XX

Sh, 272 - Sudden thoughts of making love while cuddling child and listening to old song —very vivid. 08, 30C, 00:00:XX

Sh, 273 - Sexual desire for men (in a man). 24, 30C, 100:XX:XX (homosexuality)

Sh, 274 - Developed an aversion to the idea of sex —confused about sexual issues and identity. Became aware of being bi-sexual or homosexual (in a man). "I want to find out who I am. I should know at 23. I used to know. What am I sexually?" Very confused. This led to suicidal depression. 24, 30C, 100:XX:XX

Sh, 275 - Sexually totally closed when my girlfriend kissed me. I felt as if it was a sin. 24, 30C, 00:08:XX

Sh, 276 - Feelings of vulnerability and anxiety about being masculine, both in looks and in behaviourroles. Hope it doesn't get more. To counteract this, I have been stressing the feminine. I spent lots of money on silk clothing and spent a lot of time making myself up, curling hair, etc. People comment that I look softer, but I feel harder inside. I feel confused about my sexual identity. This is in contrast to my previous proving of the remedy, when people commented that my moustache disappeared and breasts grew. 12, 6C, 30:XX:XX (homosexuality)

Sh, 277 - I've been looking at other men in a sexual light. 08, 30C, 10:XX:XX

HYOS. Al, 58 - He sings amorous and obscene songs.

Ha, 67 - Amativeness; nymphomania; erotomania.(sexual)

He, 68 - Onanism since childhood; has always been greatly attracted by opposite sex and prematurely busied himself with thoughts of marriage;... secretly wrote his love affairs; mania,...one idea rapidly follow another, all in some away concerning love, masturbates at every opportunity...(satyriasis)

He, 46 - Sings amorous and obscene songs.

He, 63 - Erotic mania accompanied by jealousy.

He, 69 - Lascivious mania, uncovers body, especially sexual parts; sings amorous songs.

HYPER. He, 3 - Erotic ideas; brain excited, as after tea.

IOD. He, 14 - Consequences of amorousness.(passionate, libidinous)(ailments from)

IRID. sh, 48 - Desire to touch backs of hands on face. Enjoy touch on skin. Old memories of gentleness, delightfully feminine. Wearing bright pink (unusual!) and stroking my legs. Enjoying my skin, touching bottom, stroking it. Dancing erotically at 8.00 a.m. (one hour after remedy). Particularly joyous. Q1

Sh, 49 - Skin felt very alive, tactile, fingertips felt "awake." Feathers felt amazing. Skin to skin; very aware of contact of surfaces. More erotic dancing, morning. Q2

Sh, 55 - Memories and associations of giving birth, and of being born. Warm nakedness. Marriage? Old memories of marriage and wedding day. Gently erotic and sensual. Q1

Sh, 56 - Delight at seeing my own female form in mirror, desire to shave legs so they would be smooth. Highly sexual, more refined, dressed in best clothes today. Desire to dance naked in moonlight. Q6

Sh, 65 - Motivation difficult, Sensation as if trapped in magnetic fields. Curled up stroking body, especially legs, feet together, Feeling as if they were magnetic. Desire for a young man. Thought that the feminine form is rounded and curved due to magnetism; arcs due to magnetic forces. Q2

Sh, 71 - Feel more sexually stimulated. More aware of it. Sensitive to others' sexuality since proving. A9

Sh, 72 - Very sexual thoughts on waking (male prover). More sexual than I have been for several weeks. K5

Sh, 73 - I imagined being naked, not having sex, with female houseguest. (Male prover) K5

Sh, 74 - No desire to touch, make love to husband all week in spite of easy, relaxed week. I feel detached from him, as if this is a problem within me. B20

Sh, 75 - While watching TV felt feelings of attraction to older men. I would not normally be attracted to older men. I6

Sh, 125 - Attracted to men with pale skins, appear even more beautiful, luminosity, light shining forth. Q5

KALI-BR. Al, 3 - Decidedly insane; had delusions that lewd women had got into his mother's house; that he was pursued by the police; that his wife was threatened by members of the family; that he had thousands of dollars in gold sewed up in his clothing; (rich, wealth)

LACH. He, 33-...want of self control; lascivious; felt as if she was clear (pure) animal right through, whilst of all mental power was dormant; sensation as if hands of stronger power, as if charmed (enchanted), and as if could not break the spell (charm). (possessed, wildness)

He, 32 - Aversion of women to marry.

He, 47 - Amorousness; amativeness.

LIL-T. Al, 10 - Profound mental depression; to the prover "the heavens seemed brass and the earth iron;" an apprehension of moral obliquity weighed grievously upon her, for about ten days after the sexual excitement,...

Al, 30 - Constant hurried (precipitation) feeling as of imperative duties and utter inability to perform them; during the sexual excitement.

Al, 351 - The sexual desire, dormant hitherto, was so strongly aroused that the prover said, "I am afraid of myself, I seem possessed of a demon."

Al, 25 - While attending a lecture (speech), desire to hit the lecturer, and in the evening desirous of swearing and damning the fire and things generally, and to think and speak obscene things; disposed to strike and hit persons; as these feelings came, the uterine pains passed away.

He, 7 - Dementia produced by business discouragements and sexual excesses.

He, 8 - Disposition to weep, with pain in back; has to keep very busy to repress (control) sexual desire.

He, 12 - Listless, inert, yet does not want to sit still (quiet); restless, yet does not want to walk; hurried manner, desire to do something, yet feels no ambition; feeling as of imperative duties and utter (complete) inability (incapacity, incompetence) to perform them; sexual excitement.

He, 9 - Disposed to curse, to strike, to think of obscene things; as these mental states came, uterine irritation abated.(reduced)

LYC. He, 28 - Amativeness or amorousness.

MOSCH. He, 5 - Hypochondriacal complaints having their origin in sexual system.

MURX. He, 2 - Deep sadness at approach of menses, all her symptoms gave her great concern (care); seemed to her she was hopelessly ill; she gave up everything.

NAJA. Al, 11 - Great depression of mind, with the distress, about the generative organs. (sexual)

NEON. Sh, 203 - Had thoughts of sex over 2 days; mentally planned scenarios of a clandestine meeting with an old boyfriend (more in the evening). 08, 30C, 00:00:20

Sh, 204 - While dancing with a slightly known acquaintance felt sexually aroused; unusual for me. 08, 30C, 00:12:30

Sh, 205 - Sexy thoughts with increased desire; made love, felt nicely physical. 08, 30C, 00:00:40

NUX-V. He, 39 - Mania puerperalis...constantly complaining, criticizing or explaining, ... as soon she recognized physician she spoke of imperfection of medical knowledge and declared it an error that one could not live without a heart, inasmuch as she felt very well without one, it having come away with the afterbirth to which it had grown fast, the nurse having separated the two before her eyes; complains of her husband, says he wishes to convince her she is sick, ... nymphomania,... frequently sips at a bowl of warm sugar-water, declaring it will form her a new heart; .(health, healing)...(expert)

OP. Al, 70 - Sensation of courage with activity, as if he could forcibly accomplish whatever was required without dread or fear, with a peculiar sensation of lustiness. (strong)

Ha, 621 - Feeling of courage and merriment (joy), so that he is as if he would carry out what was required with energy, without repugnance or fear, with a peculiar feeling of voluptuousness...(sensuality)

OX-AC. Al, 19 - Philoprogenitiveness, greater love of his children, in one in whom this feeling was always predominating; a decidedly expressed and clearly distinguishable symptom, it being not traceable to any other cause. (love creation of child)

PH-AC. Ha, 47 - Muddled (confused) feeling of the head, as from excessive coitus, for three days.

PHOS. Al, 1-..this delirium, which preceded death, was erotic, with indications of great, excitement of the sexual system...

Ha, 27-....Talks in a vehement, (impetuous) commanding (dictatorial) tone; spits at nurse, lifts up her clothes (naked) and kisses hotly all who come near her;...

He, 28-...;erotic with indications of great excitement of sexual system; ... fancied he was in several pieces and could not get the fragments properly adjusted.(disconnection, fragmentation, split, disconnected, divided)

He, 29 - Crazy deliria in a young woman who was strictly moral and unhappy in her love; accused herself of the most obscene (immoral, wicked) actions, of which she never was guilty; ....

He, 25 - Amativeness; erotic mania.

He, 34-...full of fear, especially at piano; constantly on lookout (look carefully) for something to happen; ...sexual dreams and violent sexual excitement.

PIP-N. Al,S-3 - Amorous (passionate, ardent) thoughts and desires, with hypochondria.

PLAT. He, 37-...depressed condition of physical powers; ...fear of approaching death; ... aversion to coition and yet dreams of intense lasciviousness,...

He, 41 - Delirium, with fear of men (people); often changing, with overestimation (haughty) of oneself.

He, 40 - Disturbed state of mind; religious, with taciturnity, haughtiness, voluptuousness (sensual) and cruelty.

He, 42 - Mania; with great pride; fault-finding; unchaste (sensual) talk; ...(chaste = moral, pure)

He, 48 - Mental depression from onanism. (masturbation)

PLB. He, 16 - Mental disturbance of eight or ten years' duration in a man addicted to masturbation; has several times attempted suicide; has been in seclusion (solitude); greatest dejection and despair;...; believes himself lost (condemned) ; has the sounds of hell constantly in his ears; hears voices and sees shadows of demons, great disposition to make away (suicide) with himself or do himself some bodily injury;

PULS. He, 5 - Fancies a naked man is wrapped in her bedclothes; dreams of men.

He, 47-...; pangs (pain, anxiety) of conscience about religion and female sex; violent palpitation in the presence of women; abhors (detests, aversion) and hates the sex; must go out of their way for fear of injuring them; looks upon them as evil beings and is afraid (fear; temptation, seduction); considers their presence injurious (insulted, offended) to his soul; ... (sexual loathing)

RAPH. Al, 1 - Feeling of aversion towards all women; she is provoked by seeing women going and coming about her; their approach threw her into a fury; the mere contact with a woman's dress caused intolerable distress;...She is attracted to all men without distinction (nymphomania) ; when she gives her hand to a man, she feels great agitation,...When left alone for a hour in the evening, she gave herself a very deep wound in the lips with a penknife, in hopes to put an end to this condition (hurt, punishes). Moral feeling was completely extinct, the physical nature alone ruled and threw her into a frightful state (wild). From morning to noon she would not have been able to resist the advances even of a man for whom she had not the least friendly feeling; from noon to 6 p.m. she could not have held out against any man whatsoever; from 8 to 11 the demands of sense were so importunate as to silence the voice of shame and reason; ... and would have thrown herself into the arms of the first man she met...she was still unable to control her impulses;...

ROB. Al, 11 - Strong disposition to be obscene, to gormandize (gluttony, voracity), and for all kinds of orgies.

Al, 9 - Bacchanalian (love to be drunken), erotic, or religious madness.

SEL. He, 8 - Lascivious thoughts with impotence.

SEP. Ha, 17 - Dread of men.

SIN-N. He, 3 - From fright during coition, impotence.

SPONG. He, 29 - Nervous; despondent about loss of sexual power.

STANN. He, 1 - Sadness, with aversion to men and disinclination to talk.

STAPH. He, 6 - Hypochondriasis (depression);...;caused by unmerited insults (offenses, affronts, abuses) sexual excesses, or by persistently dwelling on sexual subjects.

He, 2 - Indifference, low-spirited, dullness of mind; after onanism.(masturbation)

STRAM. He, 102 - Mania with insomnia ; very talkative; thinks he has every imaginable disease; that he has power (powerful) over all disease; masturbates, fills his pockets with anything he can find (lack?), thinks he has snakes in him.

He, 11 - Stupor: weakened intellect; torpor and fits; extreme excitement of sexual parts,...

He, 51-...converses with spirits who approach his bed, lays hold of a stick and strikes about him,...great sexual excitement.

He, 81-...attempts to stab and bite;...with sexual excitement; fear as if a dog were attacking him;...

He, 111 - Nymphomania; with diaphragmitis; violent attacks, even to rage; exalted sexual passion.

He, 119 - His thoughts ran upon obscene things, frequently put his hands to erect penis; sought to bite or to catch flies.

SUMB. Al, 8- ...fond (love) of the society of women; ...sympathy with suffering seems robbed of its pain...nervous excitement and heat, especially in head from listening (hearing) to a disputation, ...humor depressed with despair of future...melancholy despondency, as if ill-treated by everyone purposely... mildness, amiability

TARENT. Al, 76-...changeable mind, tears, singing, and irresoluteness.(In a woman, twenty-six years old, who complained of violent sexual appetite.)

He, 5 - Mental chorea; hyperaemia and hyperesthesia of female sexual organs.

THUJ. Al, 51 - Remarkable indifference to the opposite sex. (sexual)

UST. He, 2 - Very sad, cries frequently; excessively prostrated from sexual abuse and loss of semen; sleep restless.

VERAT. Ha, 674 - She asserts that she has labour pains (pregnant).(important?)

Ha, 676 - She announces her imminent confinement.

He, 3 - Fancies herself pregnant, or that she will be delivered (liberation) soon; that she is in throes (spasms) of childbirth.(labor)

He, 19 - A woman, ...hopeless despair, ...brought on by sexual excitement.

He, 21 - Mania; with desire to cut and tear everything, especially clothes; with lewdness and lascivious talk; religious or

amorous; de grandeur.
He, 22 - Nymphomania, with violence and destructiveness; had been disappointed in love; melancholia; ...great desire for sexual intercourse; void (empty) of shame; obscenity; ....
He, 50 - Religious melancholy or nymphomania, with desire to embrace everybody even inanimate objects;...0Puerperal mania.
VERB. Al, 1 - Excited fantasies, especially of a sensual nature, for several days.

SHAME

Ailments from; looked at, being: ambr.[5] ***ant-c.*** ant-t. **ARS.** calc.[5] ***cham. chin. cina*** hell.[5] ***iod.*** lyc.[5] mag-c. merc.[116] nat-m. nux-v. rhus-t. stram. sulph.
Ailments from; mortification, humiliation, chagrin, emotional or mental ailments from: anac.[8] ***apoc.***[8] ***aur.***[8] bell.[5] ***coloc.***[8] con.[103] cur.[11] ***ign.***[8] lach.[30] lyc.[58] lyss.[56] nat-m.[10] ***nux-v.***[10] pall.[116] plat.[30] ***puls.***[8] ran-b.[36] ***staph.***[54] verat.[30] zinc.[10]
Ailments from; punishment: agar.[137] ambr.[5] con.[5] dam.[85] dig.[5] ign.[5] lach.[5] nat-m.[162] stann.[5] staph.[5] tarent.[85]
Ailments from; reproaches: agar.[5] **AMBR.**[162] bell.[162] cadm-s.[144] calc-sil.[58] carc.[144] cina[58] coloc. croc.[5] dys-co.[136] gels.[5] germ.[222] ***ign.*** med.[144] mosch.[58] **NAT-M.**[193] nit-ac.[10] nux-v.[189] **OP.**[122] ph-ac. ***plat.***[35] sac-alb.[210] ***staph. stram.***[54] tarent.[85]
Ailments from; reputation, from loss of: kali-br.[137] ***sulph.***
Ailments from; scorn, looked down upon by everyone, feels he is: ***lac-c.***[54]
Ailments from; shame: aur.[102] ***ign.***[54] nat-m.[102] **OP.**[54] ***staph.***[102]
Awkwardness; timidity, from: nat-c.[30] nat-m.[30] nux-v.[30] sil.[30] sulph.[30]
Children; covering their face with their hands, but looking through their fingers: bar-c.[122]
Company, aversion to; avoids the sight of people: acon. ars.[30] calc.[122] **CIC.** ***cupr.*** cur.[122] ferr. ***gels.*** germ.[222] hydrog.[222] ***iod.*** ***lac-d.***[122] ***led. nat-c.*** psor.[185] ***sep. thuj.***
Delirium; shy, hides himself: **STRAM.**[54]
Delusions; confusion, others will observe her: ***calc.***
• flatus, everyone notices his: zinc-p.[162]
• laughed at, criticized to disadvantage, makes her timid, and she dare not look up while walking in street: bar-c.[54]
• laughed at, hides behind furniture, therefore: ***bar-c.***[122]
• naked, he is: stram. sulph.[139]
• neglected, duty, his, deserves reproach: aur.[54] germ.[222]
Dreams; ashamed, dirty and sloppy house, because of her: ozone[227]
➤ ashamed, she is: ozone[227]
➤ body, hair, obliged to dress hair in company: mag-c.
➤ shameful: acon.[36] alum. am-c.[5] arn.[10] ***asar.***[5] con. erech.[36] hydrog.[222] led.[1] mag-m.[1] mosch.[5] mur-ac.[1] ozone[227] staph.[5] tub.[111]
➤ toilet, is sitting on the, the door opens constantly: ozone[227]
➤ urinating, desire for, bottle, in a, but could not on account of a crowd: am-br.[36]
Escape; attempts to, run away, to, wants, and hide as she insists that everyone is looking at her: meli.[85]
Faces the wall if anybody talks to him: nat-m.[70]
Fear; humiliated, of being: puls.[30] ***sep.***[30]
✦ looked at: aq-mar.[231] ars.[193] bar-c.[193] calc.[172] meli.[193] rhus-t.[193]
✦ observed, of her condition being: aq-mar.[231] atro. bamb-a.[1184] **CALC.** chel. choc.[222] germ.[222] lap-c-b.[194] lap-mar-c.[194]
✦ stool, escape, should, with flatus or urination: aloe[162] carb-v.[172] nat-m.[172] nat-p.[172] nat-s.[172] olnd.[172] ph-ac.[172] podo.[172] sulph.[172] verat.[172]
✦ stool, involuntary, of: ***phos.***[54] sep.[1]
Hide; desire to, children, strangers, from: bar-c.[85]
Hide; desire to, children, thinks all visitors laugh at it and hides behind furniture: ***bar-c.***
Humiliation, painful sense of: chin-b.[54]
Hysteria; covers face with handkerchief: ***hyos.***[54]
Hysteria; looked, at, when: plb.[137]
Looked at; cannot bear to be: ambr.[5] ***ant-c. ant-t.*** **ARS.** bamb-a.[1184] calc.[5] ***cham. chin. cina*** cupr.[210] gels.[102] hell.[36] ***iod.*** kali-br.[54] mag-c. merc.[5] ***nat-m.***[122] nux-v. puls.[137] rhus-t. sanic.[102] sil.[5] stram. sulph. tarent.[5] thuj.[102] ***tub.***[122]
Looked at; cannot bear to be, faces the wall if anybody talks to him: nat-m.[70]
Looked at; cannot bear to be, sadness, with: ***kali-br.***[54]

Looking; about, shyly, in puerperal mania: ***puls.***[54]
Restlessness; bashful, timid, ill at easy in society: ***coca***[54]
Sadness; appearance, of: viol-o.[54]
Somnambulism; honor, from wounded: ign.[137]
Thoughts; inmost, seem laid bare: cann-i.[36]
Timidity; bashful: aloe ***ambr.*** anac. aq-mar.[231] arg-n. ars-s-f.[58] aur. ***bar-c.*** bar-s.[58] bell. ***calc.*** calc-s.[58] calc-sil.[58] ***carb-an.*** carb-v. caust.[102] ***chin.*** **COCA** coff. con. ***cupr.*** dys-co.[136] graph.[102] hyos. ***ign.*** iod. kali-bi. kali-br.[25] kali-i.[137] ***kali-p.***[122] lil-t.[102] manc. mang. meli.[102] ***merc.***[54] mez. ***nat-c.*** nat-m.[189] nat-p.[58] nit-ac. nux-v. ***petr.*** phos. **PULS.** rhus-t.[137] sil.[102] staph.[85] ***stram.*** ***sulph.*** tab. tarent.[54] zinc.[58]
Timidity; bashful, blushing, with: ambr.[137] puls.[155]
Weeping; children, looked at, when: ant-c.[8] ant-t.[58] brom.[47]
Weeping; looked at, when: ant-c.[122] ant-t.[141] kiss.[122] ***nat-m. tarent.***[54]

ADAM. Sh, 554 - Image of reptilian dinosaur skins. Reached up and took his head off. Inside, a human was underneath dinosaur skin. The head was hanging down in shame. 16, 12C, 00:07:30
ARS. He, 48 - Averse to meeting acquaintances, (friends) because he imagines he has formerly offended them, though knows not how.
He, 76 - Anxiety like that of one who has committed murder; driven from place to place; avoids meeting persons, thinking that he has offended them.
ATRO. Al, 3-...the mind would become filled with strange and fanciful ideas ...fits of wild, uncontrollable laughter...I fancied myself afflicted with epilepsy, and was constantly fearful lest others should discover my unfortunate condition; ...
BAR-A. Al, 9 - Dread (fear). When walking in the street, she imagines that people were criticizing her, and judging her wrongfully which makes her anxious, so that she will not look up, will look (aversion) at no one, and sweats all over.
BAR-C. Ha, 4 - She suspected, that when walking in the street, men found fault (defect) with her, and judged her amiss (wrong), which made her anxious, so that she dared not look up, she looked at nobody, and perspired all over.
He, 12 - Walking in street she imagines men are laughing at her, criticizing to disadvantage; this makes her so timid that she dare (venture) not look up or at anybody, and she perspires over whole body.
CALC. Ha, 27 - She is afraid people may notice (observed) the confusion (disorder) in her head.
He, 52 - Fears she will lose her reason (insanity), or that people will observe her confusion of mind.
CHOC. Sh, 179 - Apprehensive about the shift in consciousness and nervous someone would notice. It is reminiscent of L.S.D., the 'shifting edges', before the full blown trip arrives — an uneasiness and unsureness about which way things will go. A desire to hide in case things go to pieces. 15, 30C, 00:00:50
COB. Al, 5 - Condemned, mean feeling, as though guilty of some deed (action) of which others knew; as if he could not look one in the face. (shame, dishonored)
CUPR. Al, 5 - Melancholy; she shuns the sight of people (observed), seeks and loves to be alone, and becomes anxious about her death, which she supposes imminent and inevitable.
Ha, 1 - Melancholy; she shuns the sight of men, seeks and loves (desire) solitude, and troubles herself about her imminent death (impending), which she supposes to be unavoidable.
GERM. Sh, 4 - Desperately angry. So intense that I could barely control it. I made noises like an animal, pushed my arms up and down - instead of hitting my children, which helped. Want to just leave the house and the kids. Felt completely mad, afraid of what the neighbors heard and thought. Very bad conscience afterwards, but no relief - didn't get the anger out. There are a lot of feelings inside that don't come out. 18, 30C, 02:09:00
Sh, 126 - I have a guilty feeling if I get too much attention. I am afraid of bothering others. 18, 30C, 13:XX:XX
Sh, 115 - Very much in doubt whether I should take any more tablets. Whatever I do, I feel that somebody will criticize me,

that I do something wrong. Difficult to make a decision. Afraid that other people will laugh at me or say, haven't you understood anything?" Crying. Don't want to get up. Don't want to bother the supervisor so early in the morning. I am a failure. 18, 30C, 01:06:30

IGN. Ha, 764 - Slight blame (censuring) or contradiction excites him to quarrel, and he is vexed at himself for doing so.

He, 62 - Ill effects (ailments) from hearing bad news; from vexation with reserved displeasure ; from grief, or suppressed mental sufferings; of shame and disappointed love.

He, 31 - A peculiar trembling of hands disturbs her very much in writing, most when she has to write in any one's presence (public), gets worse as soon as she fancies any one might notice it. (observed)

MAG-C. Al, 937 - Dream she had something contraband, and wanted to snatch (seize) it away from those looking at it, and lock it up.

MUR-AC. Al, 637 - Dream that she had lice, which made her very much ashamed.(shame)

NEON. Sh, 193 - Feel sad and depressed while walking outside in the cold, clear, open air. I don't want to be outside, and walk with head down. On returning inside, I feel in suspended animation. Listless, low energy. Want to close my eyes, which are dry, with heavy, slightly numb lids. I don't feel like working and would just like to go to sleep or read a good book in bed under covers. I still feel chilly from 5 minute walk outside though I've been inside and dressed warmly for 5 minutes. 06, 12C, 00:01:00

NUX-M. Al, 32 - Many ridiculous or extravagant acts or expressions, like idiocy, while she seemed perfectly conscious, and at the next moment would appear chagrined at her conduct, and said she could not control her actions...

RAPH. Al, 1 - Feeling of aversion towards all women; she is provoked by seeing women going and coming about her; their approach threw her into a fury; the mere contact with a woman's dress caused intolerable distress;...She is attracted to all men without distinction (nymphomania) ; when she gives her hand to a man, she feels great agitation,...When left alone for a hour in the evening, she gave herself a very deep wound in the lips with a penknife, in hopes to put an end to this condition (hurt, punishes). Moral feeling was completely extinct, the physical nature alone ruled and threw her into a frightful state (wild). From morning to noon she would not have been able to resist the advances even of a man for whom she had not the least friendly feeling; from noon to 6 p.m. she could not have held out against any man whatsoever; from 8 to 11 the demands of sense were so importunate as to silence the voice of shame and reason; ... and would have thrown herself into the arms of the first man she met...she was still unable to control her impulses;...

SEP. Al, 34 - Feel very much depressed, at 7 A.M.; feel like quarreling with everybody; became very much excited about a mere trifle, and said some very sharp things. (feeling ashamed of it at the same time)

SINKING

Anguish; sinking sensation, with: carb-an.[54]

Delusions; bed, sinking, is: bapt.[102] ***bell.*** ***benz.***[102] bry. calc-p. chin-s. dulc. kali-c. ***lach.*** lyc.[137] plb.[201] rhus-t. sac-alb. sec.[139]

- body, sink down between the thighs, will: bell.
- dragged from the lowest abyss of darkness (at night, on waking): thea.
- floor, sinking, is: lepi.[139]
- floor, soft like wool, is, while walking: xan.[139]
- gave way, everything under him: sanic.[139]
- gave way; ground under him: digin.[139] kali-br.[139] tep.[139]
- melting away, he or she is, agg. from change, amel. in recumbent position: sumb.
- sinking, floor, through: benz.[137] hyos.[137] phos.[137]
- sinking, to be: bapt.[116] benz.[36] kali-c.[116] lyc.[1] lyss.[139]

Dreams; accidents, boat foundering: alum. bamb-a.[1184] lyc. sil.

- ➤ boat being foundering: alum. lyc. sil.
- ➤ drowning, foundering boat, on a: alum. lyc.

➤ places, pushing through low: merc-i-r.[36]
➤ water, boat, foundering: alum. bamb-a.[1184] lyc. sil.

CANN-I. Al, 26 - The idea that he must die returned several times, and seemed to be particularly connected with the sinking and disappearance of the pulse. (blood, circulation)
CAUST. Al, 36 - Extreme irritability of mind; the slightest vexation affects her whole body, so that her knees sink under her.
CHAM. Ha, 458 - He feels a sinking in the precordium; he is beside himself with anxiety,...
COCC. Ha, 521 - He is sunk in saddest thoughts, and insults he has received he takes deeply to heart.
GERM. Sh, 187 - Head jumped inside when there was a sudden noise. 07, 30C, 00.[09].[30]
LYSS. Al,N-80 - Felt as if she was going to die, as if she was going to sink away.(decline)
He, 80 - Felt as if she was going to die; as if she was going to sink away.
NUX-M. Al, 27 - As soon as she lay down felt a sinking sensation, as though she were going to die, with no fear, however, being perfectly at ease (peace) in mind,...

SISTER

Delusions; calls, him with name, the absent mother or sister: anac.[10]
- dead, corpse, sister, of: agar.
- shopping with her sister: atro.
- talking, sister, with his dead: bell.[54] ***hyos.***[54]
- talking, sister, with his dead, churchyard, in: bell.[10]

Dreams; death of, sister, of distant: plat.[36]

AGAR. Al, 15 - The father had fantasies; seemed to see his dead sister in heaven.
ANAC. Al, 1 - Illusions of fancy; he imagines he has his name called by the voice of his far-distant mother and sister, accompanied by an apprehension of misfortune and anxiety.
Ha, 45 - Delusions of fancy, he thought his name was called by the voice of his (far distant) mother and sister; at the same time an apprehension and anguish foreboding misfortune.
He, 24 - Imagines he hears voice of mother or sister, who are far away.
HYOS. He, 83-...imagining that her deceased sister was sitting by her bedside, and talking with this imaginary person...
LIL-T. Al, 17-... and expressed to her sister great fear of insanity.(through the proving)

SMALL

Delusions; bed, large enough, not: sulph.[139]
- bed, small, too, to hold him: germ.[222] sulph.[137]
- body, brain, far from skull, as if too: staph.
- body, brain, smaller then skull: acon. glon.
- body, diminished: agar.
- body, diminished, left: lap-c-b.[194]
- body, head, skull diminished: chel.[137] glon.[137] grat.[137]
- body, legs, shortened: ambr.[137] coloc.[137] mez.[137] olnd.[137] phos.[137] sep.[137]
- body, mammae are too big or too small: bar-c.[162]
- body, nose, smaller: choc.[222]
- body, parts, short: lac-c.
- body, parts, smaller, scalp is: ***stict.***[54]
- body, skin is very thin: bamb-a.[1184]
- body, smaller, left side of body is: cinnam.
- diminished, all is: cann-i. cinnam. grat. hydrog.[222] lac-c. plat.[102] sabad. sulph.
- diminished, everything in room is, while she is tall and elevated: plat.
- diminished, objects: plat.[1] stram.[1]
- diminished, short, he is: lac-c.
- diminished, small, he is: choc.[222] grat.
- enlarged, objects are, diminished and, letters are: ***anh.***[122]
- enlarged, objects are, diminished, and: ***anh.***[122]
- images, increasing and decreasing, sees: nit-ac.[1]
- lower, surrounding objects are, he is much taller: staph.[85]
- room, small, is too: cycl.[139]
- room, smaller, is: germ.[222]
- smaller: agar.[137] cact.[137] calc.[137] cann-i. carb-v. cinnam. croc.[137] germ.[222] glon.[137] grat. kreos.[137] lac-c. phys. **PLAT.** sabad. staph.[30] ***stram.***[54] sulph. tab.[137] tarent.[137]
- smaller, he is: acon. agar. alum-sil.[58] ambr.[162] bar-c.[162] cact.[137] calc. carb-v.

croc.[137] glon.[137] hydrog.[222] kreos.[137] ozone[227] sabad. tab.[137] tarent.
• smaller, he is, epileptic fit, before: carb-v.
• smaller, objects appear in motion: anh.[119]
• smaller, things are: aur. berb.[137] carb-v.[137] cycl.[137] hyos.[116] merc-c.[137] nat-c.[122] ozone[227] ***plat.*** puls.[116] staph.[30] stram. thuj.[116]
• smaller, things grow smaller: agar.[5] cact.[5] camph. carb-v. nit-ac. plat.[10] stram.[10] tab.[5]
• soul, body is too small for, or that it is separated from: anac. cann-i. hydrog.[222] nit-ac.[102] sabad.[5] thuj.

Dreams; animals, elephant, small, very, the size of a dog: ozone[227]
➤ animals, horses, small, very: ozone[227]
➤ bed too small: ferr-i.[36]
➤ fire, small flames, with: cass.[36]
➤ things, small seem: ferr-i.[36]
➤ women, waking, on, saw a woman of pleasant face, dressed in gray, standing by bedside, wiping a tumbler, she backed miles away, becoming very small: med.[54]

Size; frame, of, seems lessened: phys.

CARB-V. Al, 12 - Anxiety in the evening after lying down, as from oppression of the chest, ...,a sensation as if the heart would be pressed downward; objects about her seem to become constantly narrower and smaller,...

CHOC. Sh, 52 - My right hand feels bigger and wider and I feel more powerful. But my wrists feel weaker and flatter. Sensation of opening of hands and tightness in the forearm.

Sh, 58 - My nose has been running in the cold, dripping. It feels smaller.

Sh, 134 - I felt small enough to get into a drawer in a desk full of rubbish and rout around under things, a kind of curiosity.

CYCL. He, 6-...love of (desire) solitude;....;sensation as if room was too small, with reluctance to go into open air;...

GERM. Sh, 130 - While standing felt my spirit step backwards. The kitchen seems smaller and lower down. 04, 6C, 00.10.00.

HALI-L. Sh, 8 - Delusions legs feel shorter by a foot while laying in bed. 09, 6C, 00:05:00

Sh, 796 - Head felt disproportionately small compared with side of shoulders and arms when washing hair. When I touched my head this morning, when washing my hair, it felt very small in relation to my arms and shoulders. It was a shock. 20, 30C, 04:02:30

HYDROG. Sh, 168 - Sensation of being smaller than normal, while making porridge. 10, 200C, 13:20:XX

IRID. Sh, 79 - Had this longing to find real wilderness. Britain is too full, nothing is really alive anymore except people. The world really feels too oppressed with people and roofs. I kept saying to partner, "Why do we live in this dreary, ugly place, where people know nothing about freedom, and certainly nothing about discovery or mystery, just tarmac and roofs." It struck me that the world was too small for me, and thought "That's got to be something about the remedy, something around pressure." E5

Sh, 91 - Felt very low again, like being covered by a heavy blanket. I felt weighed down by it. B3

LAC-C. Al,N-15 - Feels very short in morning; while walking; same in evening.

MAG-C. Al, 929 - Dream of very small horses, that she exerted herself to reflect upon, after midnight.

NAT-C. Al, 41-..;the room seems too small for him, and even in open air he walks without anything seeming right to him;... (confined, limited, restricted)

NEON. Sh, 16 - When I first put the remedy in my mouth I felt as if I had shrunk, particularly the legs. 02, 6C, 00:00:00

Sh, 17 - Legs felt shorter.20, 6C, 00:02:40

PLAT. Ha, 35 - Illusion of the imagination; on entering the room after walking for an hour, everything around her seemed very small and all persons physically and bodily inferior to her, but she herself great and lofty (distinguish, elevated) in body;...

PLB. Al, 69 - On first recovering consciousness the people in the ward (hospital) seemed to him as small as dolls (toy, little), and the opposite of the room seemed to be sunk (under, below) forty feet below his own level.

STRAM. Ha, 504 - He appears to himself large and tall, but surrounding objects appear small to him.

SOLITUDE

Ailments from; alone, being: aeth.[5] agar.[5] ant-t.[5] **APIS**[5] **ARS.**[5] asaf.[5] ***aur-m.***[8] bell.[5] ***bism.***[5] bov.[5] bufo[5] calc.[5] camph.[5] cedr.[5] clem.[5] **CON.**[5] **DROS.**[5] elaps[5] **FL-AC.**[5] gels.[5] **HEP.**[5] **HYOS.**[5] **KALI-C.**[5] ***lach.***[5] lil-t.[5] **LYC.**[5] **MERC.**[5] ***mez.***[5] nat-c.[5] nat-m.[5] ***ph-ac.***[5] **PHOS.**[5] plb.[5] ***ran-b.***[5] ***sep.***[5] ***sil.***[5] stann.[5] **STRAM.**[5] verat.[5] zinc.[5]

Ailments from; alone, being, fear of people, yet: ars.[5] bufo[5] ***clem.***[5] ***con.***[5] tarent.[5]

Anguish; alone, when: ***phos.***[54]

Anxiety; alone, as if, and all about were dead and still: ***rhus-t.***[54]

Anxiety; alone, watched, desires to be: gall-ac.[36]

Anxiety; alone, when: alco.[36] arg-n.[162] **ARS.** cadm-s. caust.[116] cortico.[119] cupr.[210] ***dros.*** gaert.[136] gall-ac.[36] hep.[10] ***kali-br.***[116] kali-c.[116] ***mez.*** morg.[136] nit-ac.[116] **PHOS.** rat. ***rhus-t.***[54] sep.[116] tab. zinc.

Anxiety; evening, alone, when: ***dros.***[54]

Anxiety; night, alone, when: tab.[36]

Begging, pray for him, to, and not to leave him alone: lyss.[54]

Cares; full of, alone, when: hep.[10]

Company desire for; alone, while, agg.: ***act-sp.***[162] aeth.[5] agar.[5] ambr. ant-t.[5] ***apis***[5] **ARS.** asaf.[5] bell.[5] bism.[5] bov. brom. bufo[5] cadm-s. calc. calc-s.[108] calc-sil.[58] ***camph.*** carc.[207] cedr.[5] clem.[5] con. ***dros.*** elaps ***fl-ac.***[5] foll.[1201] gaert.[136] **GALL-AC.**[198] gels.[5] **HEP.**[5] hydrog.[222] ***hyos.***[5] ***kali-c.*** lac-c.[58] lach.[5] lil-t.[5] ***lyc.*** ***merc.***[5] ***mez.*** nat-c.[5] nat-m.[5] ***pall.*** ph-ac.[5] **PHOS.**[122] plb.[5] puls.[160] ran-b.[5] rat. sep.[5] sil. stann.[5] ***stram.*** tab. trif-r.[102] zinc. zinc-p.[58]

Company, aversion to; alone, agg. when alone and amel. in company: alum-sil.[58] bism.[10] hep.[10] ph-ac.[10] ran-b.[10]

Company, aversion to; alone, amel. when: allox.[119] alum-sil.[162] ambr. arag.[102] ***bar-c.*** bell.[10] bov. carb-an. choc.[222] coca[15] con. convo-s.[119] cortico.[119] cycl. ferr. ferr-p. germ.[222] halo.[149] hell. hydrog.[222] ign.[102] ipom.[119] iris[152] lac-h.[229] lap-mar-c.[194] ***lyc.*** mag-c.[5] mag-s. meny.[36] ***nat-c.*** ***nat-m.*** ***oxyt.***[54] ozone[227] petr. ph-ac.[58] phos. plat.[10] ***plb.*** rauw.[119] **SEP.** stann. staph. stram. sulph. trio.[149] visc.[119]

Company, aversion to; alone, dreads being, yet: ars.[5] bufo ***clem.*** ***con.*** elaps kali-br. lyc. **NAT-C.**[122] nat-m.[5] ***sep.*** stram.[5] tarent.[5]

Company, aversion to; country away from people, wants to get into the: androc.[222] calc. calc-p.[58] elaps merc.[137] sep.[137]

Company, aversion to; solitude, fond of: **ACON.**[5] alum.[10] **AMBR.**[5] ***ant-c.***[8] ***ars.***[8] **AUR.**[5] bamb-a.[1184] bar-c.[1] ***bell.***[5] cact.[25] calc.[10] calc-p.[5] camph.[5] carb-an.[5] ***cham.***[8] chin.[1] cic.[1] coca[25] con.[5] cycl.[5] dig.[5] dios.[25] eug.[10] graph.[10] helon.[25] **IGN.**[5] led.[5] lyc.[5] m-aust.[10] mag-m.[10] meny.[5] nat-c.[5] ***nat-m.***[5] ***nux-v.***[5] op.[10] ozone[227] petr.[5] **PLAT.**[5] ptel.[25] **PULS.**[5] ***rhus-t.***[5] sep.[10] seq-s.[230] stann.[5] staph.[10] sulph.[10] tub.[189] verat.[10]

Company, aversion to; solitude, fond of, desires to practice masturbation: ***bufo*** ust.

Company, aversion to; solitude, fond of; fancy, to indulge her: ***lach.***

Company, desire for; alone, while, yet fear of people: ars.[5] bufo[5] clem.[5] con.[5] tarent.[5]

Darkness; desire for, lie down in the dark and not be talked to, to: aur.[162] aur-m.[162] bry.[162] tarent.

Death; thoughts of, alone, when: ***crot-c.***

Delusions; alone, always: puls. stram.

- alone, castaway, being a: germ.[222] ***phys.***[54]
- alone, graveyard, she is: lepi sep.
- alone, wilderness, being a. in a: stram.
- alone, world, she is a. in the: ***androc.*** bamb-a.[1184] camph. choc.[222] ***cycl.***[122] germ.[222] hura ***plat.*** ***puls.***
- asylum, insane, sent to: lach.[58]
- asylum, she will be sent to: cench.
- deserted, forsaken, is: **ARG-N.** ***aur.***[116] bamb-a.[1184] bar-c. camph. cann-i. carb-an. carb-v. chin. ***cycl.*** hura hyos. ***kali-br.*** lach.[139] lap-c-b.[194] lap-gr-m.[194] lap-mar-c.[194] lil-t. lyss. **MAG-C.**[185] nat-c. ozone[227] pall. ***plat.*** puls. rhus-t.[139] sac-alb.[210] sanic.[85] ***stram.***
- home, away from, is: acon. aster.[8] bell. **BRY.** calc. calc-p.[102] cic. cimic.[102] ***coff.*** germ.[222] ***hyos.*** lach. lap-c-b.[194] meli. merc.[15] ***nux-v.***[30] ***op.*** par.[10] plb.[5] puls.[122] ***rhus-t.*** valer. verat. vip.
- home, away from, must go there: ***bry.***[102] calc-p.[102] cimic.[102] hyos.[102] ***op.***[102]
- images, alone, when: fl-ac. lach.
- island, is on a distant, enjoying the tranquillity : phos.
- places, finds himself in strange and solitary, at night on waking: par.
- room, desolated, is: valer.[36]

• rowdies, brawlers, will break in if she is alone: elaps.[139]
• separated, world, from the, that he is: ***anac.*** androc.[222] ***anh.***[119] carc.[227] choc.[222] germ.[222] **HYDROG.** thiop.[149] ven-m.[149]
• town, he is in desert: carb-an.[10]

Desires; cavity, to be in: elaps.[36]
Desolate, room appears: valer.[36]
Dreams; desert, of: sil.[10]
➤ frightful, alone, when: kali-c.[58]
Dullness; alone, when: ph-ac.
Excitement; alone, when: ars.[10]
Fancies; exaltation of, alone, when: ars.[10]
Fancies; repulsive, when alone: fl-ac. sel. tarent.
Fear; alone, of being: act-sp. all-s. ant-t. ***apis*** **ARG-N.** ***arist-cl.***[119] **ARS.** ***ars-s-f.***[58] asaf. aur-ar.[58] bar-c.[127] bell. bism. bov.[10] brom. bry. bufo cadm-s. calc. calc-ar.[58] ***camph.*** carb-v.[184] carc.[207] ***clem. con.*** **CROT-C.** dros. dys-co.[136] ***elaps*** gall-ac.[36] ***gels.*** hep. **HYOS.** kali-ar. kali-br. **KALI-C.** ***kali-p. lac-c.*** lap-c-b.[194] lil-t.[172] **LYC.** ***lyss. manc.***[184] menis.[111] merc. mez. naja[98] nat-c.[116] nat-m.[212] nit-ac.[116] nux-v. **PHOS.** pitu-a.[164] plb. prot.[136] psor.[56] ***puls.*** rad-br.[85] ran-b. rat. sac-alb.[210] ***sep.*** sil.[53] ***stram.*** syc-co.[136] tab. tarent. tub.[212] valer.[137] verat. zinc.[85]
✦ alone, of being, child wants mother to hold her hand: bism.[172] kali-c.[172] lil-t.[172] lyc.[172] sac-alb.[210] stram.[172]
✦ alone, of being, company, with aversion to, yet fears to be alone: alum.[35] ars.[5] bufo ***clem. con.*** elaps gels.[111] kali-ar.[58] kali-br. kali-c.[56] lyc. morg.[136] **NAT-C.**[35] ***sep.*** stram.[5] tarent.[111]
✦ alone, of being, crime and cruelty would be committed, lest: kali-br.[172]
✦ alone, of being, darkness, in: camph.[54] kali-br.[137] kali-p.[172] puls.[212] rad-br.[102] valer.[137]
✦ alone, of being, desire of being alone, but,: con.[54] kali-c.[172] lyc.[172]
✦ alone, of being, die, lest he: ***arg-n.*** **ARS.**[122] ***ars-h.***[122] bell.[58] ***kali-c. phos.***
✦ alone, of being, disinclined to meet even agreeable company: clem.[172]
✦ alone, of being, evening: brom. dros. kali-c. puls. ran-b. tab.
✦ alone, of being, light and company, wants: bism.[172] rad-br.[172] stram.[172]
✦ alone, of being, night: arg-n.[162] ***camph.*** carb-v.[58] ***caust.*** gaert.[136] ***hell.***[122] ***med.***[162] **STRAM.**[122] tab.[36]
✦ alone, of being, starts with a loud cry as if a bird flew towards the window: kali-c.[172]
✦ alternating with, rage: bell.[10]
✦ alternating with, sadness: zinc.[5]
✦ bed, of the, alone when: ars.[172] ***camph.***[54] ***caust.***[54] xan.[111]
✦ death, alone, evening in bed: act-sp.[162] ***ars. caust.***[54] kali-c.
✦ death, alone, when: ***arg-n. arn.***[122] **ARS.** ars-h. bell. camph.[172] caust.[172] ***kali-ar.***[184] ***kali-c.***[122] menis.[111] ***phos.*** tub.[108]
✦ going out, alone: ars.[127] ign.[127] pitu-a.[164]
✦ happen, something will, alone, when, amel. by conversation: rat.
✦ out of doors, to go, darkness, in, alone: acon.[172]

Forsaken; feeling, isolation, sensation of: allox.[119] ***anac. androc. anh.***[119] ***arg-n.*** arist-cl.[149] camph. cann-i. cann-s.[36] choc.[222] coca cortico.[144] germ.[222] hura ***hydrog.*** lac-h.[229] lap-mar-c.[194] merc.[187] op.[231] ozone[227] pip-m.[231] plat. psil.[231] puls.[193] sac-alb.[210] stram. tab.[231]
Forsaken; feeling, thinks she is left alone in the world: plat.[60]
Hypochondriasis; alone: ars.[10]
Inconsolable; alone and darkness agg.: stram.
Injure; fears to be left alone, lest he should, himself: alum. arg-n. ars. ***cimic.***[54] ***merc. nat-s.*** sep.
Irritability; alone, when: cortico.[144] phos.
Irritability; alone, wishes to be: adax.[96] bry.[54] choc.[222] gels.[85] hydrog.[222] lac-h.[229]
Morose; thinking of his ailments when alone, on: **AUR-M.**[54]
Rage; alone, while: bufo.
Restlessness; alone, when, agg.: all-s. mez. ***phos.***
Sadness; alone, when, agg.: aeth. all-s. allox.[119] **ARS.**[122] aur. bov. ***calc.*** con. ***dros.*** ferr. ***ferr-ar.*** hep.[10] kali-ar. kali-c. kali-n. lyc. m-aust.[10] mag-m.[10] ***mez. nat-m.*** phos. rat.[38] sil. ***stram.*** valer. zinc.
Sadness; alone, when, amel.: allox.[119] hydro-c.[2147]
Sadness; company, aversion to, desire for solitude: alum.[10] aur.[10] bamb-a.[1184] ***con.***[116] cupr.[10] ***helon.***[116] ***led.***[54] murx.[10] nat-c.[10] nat-m.[116] rhus-t.[10] sep.[193]
Smiling; alone, when: bar-c.[53]
Spoken to; averse to being, alone, wants to be let: ant-t.[122] arn.[58] aur. caj. gels.[171] hell.

helon. hipp. hydrog.[222] ***iod.*** lil-t. luna[29] nat-m.[91] stram.[36] ***sulph.***
Suspiciousness; solitude, desire for: cic.[10] croto-t.[10]
Talk; desires to t. to someone: ***arg. arg-n.*** buth-aust.[144] ***cann-i.***[25] caust. eup-pur.[25] lachn.[25] lap-c-b.[194] lil-t. nux-m.[54] petr. phys.[25] ***stict.***[54] tarax.[54]
Thinking; ailments, of, alone, when left: ars.[54]
Thoughts; persistent, alone: ars. kali-c. zinc.
Thoughts; rush, alone, when: ars.[10]
Timidity; alone, when: sil.[58]
Unconsciousness; alone, when: ***ph-ac.***
Weeping; alone, when, agg.: ***con.*** ign.[162] lap-gr-m.[194] ***nat-m.*** ozone[227]
Weeping; evening, oppression of chest, with, solitude, with desire for: ***rhus-t.***[54]
Weeping; goes off alone and weeps as if she had no friends: bar-c.
Weeping; lonesome condition, over his: lith-c.[36]

ADAM. Sh, 43 - Feeling alone and tall and capable, like a beacon beaming out rays of light to all and sundry. 2, 12C, XX:XX:XX
Sh, 229 - Feeling very angry towards others and hate people. I want to be alone and away from people who upset me. I hate feeling angry and resentful, a lot of it is directed to myself. 20, 1M, XX:XX:XX
AETH. He, 14 - Great sadness when alone.
ALL-S. He, 3 - Sadness when alone; moral uneasiness; afraid of never getting well; fear of not being able to bear any kind of medicine; fear of being poisoned...
ALUM. Al, 6 - Depressed and friendless; he wishes only to be left alone, in the forenoon.
Ha, 1 - Dejected and joyless; he only desires to be left alone, forenoon.
ANAN. Al, 4 - Hypochondria, with dread (fear) of society (people); he seeks solitude and obscurity; does not want to see or hear anything.
ANDROC. Sh, 24 - I feel entirely alone, that I am viewing the world through one hole, for it all seems just a picture, and the rest of the world share a different view finder together. I don't want to join theirs though. (7)
Sh, 57 - In the evening felt very lonely and desolate, although not alone. She felt separated, detached, disconnected and unreal. (7)
Sh, 60 - Felt tense and absolutely alone, but sure that the rest of the world was mad, not her. She felt defiant with others and would not be manipulated. (7)
Sh, 61 - Felt constrained and had a gloomy approach to everything, averse company, desire to be alone. I feel people will not want to talk or be with me. (28)
Sh, 63 - Desired company but could not be bothered to see anyone, felt lonely as if he didn't belong. (21)
ANT-T. Al, 12 - Dreaded (fear) to be left alone even for a few moments, lest he " should be dreadfully nervous and not know what to do with himself."
He, 18 - Fear and dread of being alone.
ANTH. Al, 1 - Very low spirits; feeling as if something were about to happen; as if would like to get alone, and unburden (relieve) himself by crying ...
APIS. He, 49 - Cannot bear (endure) to be left alone.
ARG-N. He, 48 - Great nervousness and prostration (lassitude); fears to be alone because he thinks he will die ; is apprehensive of some serious disease, which almost drives him to despair.
ARS-H. He, 13 - Afraid (fear) of being alone he thinks he will die.
ARS. Al, 91-...she was afraid (fear) of solitude and death; the slightest cause was sufficient to put her into anger and rage, which especially occurred when one spoke of her complete recovery which she considered wholly impossible.
Al, 83 - Dread of death coming on suddenly when alone, or on going to bed.
Ha, 1038 - When he is alone he is beset by thoughts about disease and other thoughts of an indifferent character, of which he cannot get rid.
Ha, 42 - When he is alone he falls into thoughts about disease and other things, from which he can not easily tear himself away.
He, 7 - When alone, he falls to thinking about disease and other things, which he can scarcely keep out of his mind.
He, 62 - Fear of being left alone.
He, 63 - Dread (fear) of death when alone, or on going to bed.

ASAF. He, 10 - Dislike for solitude.

ATRO. Al, 33 - Mentally either very sad, depressed in constant anxiety and restlessness, fearful of misfortune, or angry and inclined to be alone, seldom lively.

Ha, 17 - Sad and morose, preferring solitude and a dark room to society of friends.

AUR-M. He, 2 - If left alone he thinks about nothing but his ailments,... ; desires company.

He, 6 - Everything is disagreeable, dreary (lugubrious, desolate, deserted), even nature around.

AUR. Ha, 340 - He sits apart (separated), all by himself in a corner, wrapt up in himself, as if in the deepest melancholy, when left undisturbed; but the slightest contradiction excites the greatest heat and anger,...

BELL. Al, 124 - Dread (fear) of solitude, of ghosts and thieves.

Ha, 1395 - He wishes for solitude and quiet; all noise and visits from others are repugnant to him.

BISM. Al, 1 - Solitude is unendurable.

Ha, 108 - Solitude (isolation) is intolerable to him.

He, 7 - Solitude is unbearable.

BOV. He, 6 - Sad, depressed and desponding when alone.

BRASS. Sh, 11 - I began to feel a little depressed; I'm definitely not in a party mood, desire to be still and quiet, maybe listen to classical music, Bach, Chopin, something well composed and not Beethoven 08, 6C, 05:08:30

BUFO. Al, 7 - Desires solitude, and yet is afraid of being left alone and dying forsaken.

He, 1 - Desire for solitude, to practice masturbation.

CACT. Al, 3 - Loves solitude; he avoids those around him who wish to comfort him.

CAJ. Al,S-60 - Want to walk in a low and a very dignified (nobility, honored, proud, refined) manner, and prefer to walk alone.

CALC. Al, 7 - Loneliness is very oppressive, with coldness of the face, hands, and feet.

Ha, 21 - Solitude is a burden (load) to him, with coldness of the face, of the hands and feet.

He, 53 - Fear: of death; of consumption (decay, waste, tuberculosis); of misfortune (disaster) ; of being alone. (lonely)

CAMPH. Al, 46-...The external world existed for me no longer. (solitude) My thoughts were gone; one single fearful one remained; I imagined myself transferred to another world (estranged, alienated); for me all else was extinguished...

Al, 46-...I sat up in bed, but all about me had indeed disappeared. I was alone in the great universe, the last of all things. My ideas of the world, God and religion, now seemed to me to have existed only in my imagination; the earth upon which yesterday I lived and moved, had run its appointed course, and I was the final and solitary fragment of the whole creation...(meaningless, unimportant, neglected, forsaken, loneliness, deserted) (godless)

Al, 46-... My misery was boundless; time itself was no more; in short, I suffered such fearful anguish as no fancy can comprehend. What soul could paint to itself my everlasting (eternal) dwelling as the Evil One (devil), alone in a vast universe, without faith or hope, and my heart forever broken by unimaginable tortures? (miserable, timeless, endless, solitude, forsaken, faithless, hopeless)

Al, 38 - Dread of being alone in the dark.

Al, 46-...I am alone. I feel a tendency to self contemplation; outer things vanished, and I behold myself in spirit freed from matter...

He, 62 - Dread of being alone in dark.

He, 72 - Palpitation; vexed by want of sympathy (compassion, aid), afraid to be alone a moment, fears death.

CANN-I. Al, 57 - Strange feeling of isolation (solitude) from all around him, with great sense of loneliness (isolation), though surrounded by his friends.

CARB-AN. Al, 1 - Desire to be alone ; she is sad and reflective (thoughtful); avoids all conversation.

Al, 10 - Discouraged and sad (unhappy); everything seems so sad and lonely that she desires to weep.

Al, 28 - Sullen (unsociable, silent) mood and ill-humor about present and past events; this cannot be overcome ; it even amounts to weeping.

Ha, 5 - Pusillanimous (cowardice) and sad; everything seems to her so lonely (alone, deserted) and sad, that she would like to weep.

Ha, 6 - Inclination to solitude (isolation), sad and introverted (egotistic), she always only wishes to be alone, and she shuns every conversation.

Ha, 32 - The objects on the street seem to him changed, e.g., farther apart and brighter (vivid, brilliant) than usual, as an empty, abandoned city.

CAUST. He, 37 - Full of timorous fancies, evenings; child fears to go to bed alone.

CHOC. Sh, 212 - Felt more desire to be alone and more able to live alone. 07, 100C, 19:XX:XX

Sh, 213 - Unsociable —averse company and conversation.[15], 30C, 04:XX:XX

Sh, 322 - Have lost interest in my husband, feel totally indifferent. I have hardly spoken to him all weekend, with a desire to avoid him. Don't want to discuss or share anything with him.[15], 30C, 06:XX:XX

CIC. Al, 26 - Contempt and scorn for mankind; he avoided them, abhorred their follies (stupidity) excessively, and his disposition seemed to tend towards misanthropy; he withdrew (retire) himself into solitude.

Al, 27 - Want of confidence in mankind; with misanthropy; he forsook society, remained alone and reflected upon their errors and about himself.

Ha, 237 - Depreciation and contempt of mankind; he fled (desert) his fellow-creatures, was in the highest degree disgusted with their follies (stupidity), and his disposition seemed to change into misanthropy; he withdrew into solitude.

Ha, 238 - Want of trust (mistrust, skepticism) in people and anthrophoby,(misanthropy) he fled (escape) from them remained solitary, and thought seriously about their errors and about himself.

He, 18 - Fondness (desire) for solitude; great disregard and dislike for society of others.

He, 34 - Is afraid (fear) of society, and wants to be alone.

CIMIC. He, 13 - Desire for solitude, or to wander from place to place.

CLEM. Al, 19-...dreading to be alone, tired of living, full of thoughts of death, with fear that it would be speedy, longing however, for the repose of death; this mood was soon followed by apprehension, weeping, and homesickness, ...

He, 5 - Fear of being alone, but disinclined to meet even agreeable company.

COCC. He, 22 - Great sorrowfulness, with constant inclination to sit in a corner buried in thought.

CON. Al, 39 - Dread (fear) of men of their approach, yet with dread of being alone.

Al, 38 - Sunk in deep thought; he apprehensively considered the present and the future, and sought (wanted) to be alone.

Ha, 365 - Sunk in deep thought, he cogitated timorously about the present and the future and sought (wants) solitude.

Ha, 8 - Lost in deep meditation, he anxiously thought over the present and the future, and sought solitude.

Ha, 9 - Shyness (timidity) at the approach of people, and yet also dread of being alone.

He, 17 - Dislike to society and yet a dread to be alone. (solitude)

CROT-C. Al, 19 - Thoughts of death haunt (torment) her everywhere, especially when alone.

CUPR. Al, 5 - Melancholy; she shuns the sight of people (observed), seeks and loves to be alone, and becomes anxious about her death, which she supposes imminent and inevitable.

Ha, 1 - Melancholy; she shuns the sight of men, seeks and loves (desire) solitude, and troubles herself about her imminent death (impending), which she supposes to be unavoidable.

Ha, 8 - Peevishness, he himself does not know what he wants, he wishes to be alone;...

CUR. Al, 10 - Brooding sadness, frequent weeping, with desire for solitude.

He, 2 - Very much depressed about herself, desire only to shut herself up away from people.

CYCL. Ha, 194 - Sunk in deep thought (meditation), he sought (desire) solitude and thought about his future fate (destine, doom).

He, 6-...love of (desire) solitude;....;sensation as if room was too small, with reluctance to go into open air;...

He, 4 - Absorbed in deep thought, seeks solitude, thinks about his future.

DER. Al, 4 - He dreads pain, and is averse to solitude with great anxiety.

DIG. Al, 9 - Great desire to be alone.

DIOS. Al, 1 - Desire to be alone; do not enjoy society (misanthropy); am usually quite fond of the society of ladies, but they now seem repulsive,...

DROS. Ha, 278 - Anxiety in solitude (alone) he wished to have someone always near him, could not bear to be without companions (friends, company), and was quieter when he had someone to speak to; but when they again left him in solitude, he was all the more anxious, until he fell asleep; on awaking the anxiety returned.

He, 3 - Anxiety: with flushes of heat; when alone (solitude), ...as if it would impel him to commit suicide by drowning. (water will purify?)

He, 4 - Dread (fear) of ghosts and of being alone.

ELAPS. Al, 11 - Depression of spirits; desires to be in a deep cavern, where he can see no one.

Al, 13 - Fearfulness, dread (fear) of being alone, as though something would happen, or as though rowdies (revolution, rebellious) would break in.

Al, 6 - Desire to be alone; she takes refuge for days together in a corner of the antechamber.

Al, 7 - She seeks a retired room to work in.

He, 5 - Fear of being left alone, as if something horrible might happen; horror of rain.

He, 3 - Depression of spirits, and desire for solitude.

EUPH. He, 3 - Temporary attacks of craziness, insists upon saying his prayers at the tail of his horse; knows his freaks (abnormality) and wants to be by himself and in silence.

FERR. Al, 20 - Excited by the slightest opposition; ... even her children's caresses increased her bad temper; she was often rude to those about her, because she hated to see or talk to them, and wanted them to leave her in solitude, which alone was pleasing to her.

Al, 4 - Constant desire for solitude; horror of conversation, noise, visits, and even the society of her cherished friends.

Al, 12 - She never complained or wept and was always plunged (fall) in deep melancholy when no one was about her.

FL-AC. Al, 15 - During the fourth week very irritable towards people, even to the greatest hatred, which he does not hesitate to give vent to in words, but as soon as he sees them everything is forgotten, and he has an entirely different opinion of them.

GELS. He, 18 - Desires to be quiet, does not wish to speak, nor have any one near her for company, even if the person be silent.

GERM. Sh, 111 - If I were me, nobody would like me -so I try to be what I think others expect me to be. I don't think I can be loved with all the parts of me which are ugly and bad. Lonely feelings. Longing for love and understanding. Feel I am so unfriendly to myself. 18, 30C, 04:00:00

Sh, 140 - Feel I am in an impossible situation. Nobody to talk to who understands me. I can't say things as they are because I have to take others feelings into consideration. I need comfort and encouragement, but no one can give me. Weeping. 18, 30C, 36:XX:XX

Sh, 141 - Painfully aware of the feelings of being an outcast. 08, 12C, 02:00:10

Sh, 136 - Feeling lonely like an alien freak. 08, 12C, 22:00:00

Sh, 151-.... I feel I have no real contact with people, I have no emotion at all except for a feeling of isolation and a concern that people may not like me. I wish someone would cuddle me. By 10 o'clock I have a definite aversion to people, especially certain people- the stubborn or authoritarian kind. I become deeply involved in my own thoughts and can be very irritable and even angry when the thoughts are interrupted by people, but I don't show any signs of anger or irritation. The fate of other people leaves me cold, but I know this is not right. My mind is blank and I feel I could just sit and stare. I have no feelings, no emotions! I think a lot about my state of mind and try to understand it; it puzzles me. What is missing? Eating removes this thoughtful mood. By afternoon and evening I become gradually more involved with what I am doing but still feel isolated even when in the company of other people. I don't mind listening to people, but I contribute little to conversation. This state lasted for three days. 16, 30C, 04:XX:XX

Sh, 149 - Feel lonely. I nearly always feel special -always on the sideoutside of others. Either better or smaller than others. 18, 30C, 46:XX:XX

Sh, 153 - Thought nobody understood me and cared for what I felt. Felt it was unfair. I was presented with complaints about something others had done. Felt I was standing between two fighting parts. Felt awkward about it, embarrassed. Difficult to argue about such strong outburst. Thoughts about the day's arguing milling in my head all evening and night. 21, 12C, 32:XX.XX.

Sh, 152 - Aversion to people. Abrupt when obliged to speak. Had a consultation at 10 o'clock and really messed it up. I wish everybody would just go away and leave me alone. No contact. 16, 30C, 07:04:00

Sh, 69 - Want to sit alone in front of fire listening to music by myself. Fed up with people everywhere I go irritating me. Want to be looked after. 09, 9C, 01:11:00.

Sh, 150 - I only want to cry. Don't know what to do. Feel terrible and lonely. Cannot describe how I feel. Want attention, but don't dare to ask for it. Soon there is no more energy left. 18, 30C, 182:XX:XX

GRAPH. Ha, 36 - He would like to be alone, every disturbance vexes him.

HALI-L. Sh, 213 - I wanted to do more mothering while I was being mothered and at the same time not mothering the son I do have. Feeling envy of all families who had more children. Constant state of desire for something other than what I had. If busy, I wanted to be not busy. If no one calls, I felt nobody cares about me. Could find no comfort anywhere and felt isolatedalone. 01, 30C,, 21:XX:XX

Sh, 401 - Worried feeling. Tearful but can't cry. Want to be with someone. Can't let it go that a friend yelled at me two days ago. I'm more sad than I should be. I don't want to be by myself. Want to cry but can't. Feel better with people and worse being alone. This is happening during my period; usually happens before menses. 08, 30C, 17:XX:XX

Sh, 625 - I find that I don't have a real friend. I have acquaintances, but not a friend. That has been bothering me. A new realization. The friends I have cultivated are caught up in their own lives, and they don't have time for me. This is different—now I have time to think about it. I'm seeing for myself. At times I'm extremely lonely. I like my own place but sometimes it's nice to have a friend. 18, 30C, 17:XX:XX

Sh, 927 - I've felt lonely over the last three to four days. This morning I realized how great the girls were and burst into tears — emotional, but separate. 20, 30C, 14:XX:XX

HELON. Al, 4-.... could not endure the least contradiction or receive any suggestions in regard to any subject (fixed ideas) ;... what I most desired was to be left alone, reserved to myself the privilege of finding fault (imperfection) with everything around me;....

HEP. Al, 16 - Irritable mood; everything that she undertook was wrong; she desired to be alone.

Al, 10 - Fearful concerning sickness in the family, especially when walking alone in the open air.

Ha, 9 - Irritable mood; whatever she started to do, was not satisfactory, she wished to be alone.

He, 10 - Repulsive (offensive) mood, with desire to be left alone.

HIPP. He, 1 - Melancholy; a young man sits in the corner and does not want to have anything to do with the world. (alienated)

HURA. Al, 16 - She fancies she is left alone (lonely, solitary, forsaken) in the world and is lost.

HYDROG. Sh, 144 - Feeling I want to isolate myself —want to be alone. 12, 6C, 27:XX:XX

Sh, 145 - Feel that I could get on with everything alright if those around me would either leave me alone or help constructively. 04, 12C, 19:XX:XX

Sh, 150 - Feeling weepy and vulnerable — want someone to "manage" things for me. Feel so fed up of having to do it all myself. 18, 200C, 26:XX:XX

Sh, 155 - In the afternoon (during the full moon) I felt low and depressed, insecure and vulnerable. Could not cope with work load and didn't want to be alone. 12, 6C, 39:XX:XX

Sh, 189 - As if in a dream, not there, difficult to stay with it all while driving home —very conscious of the blackbirds flying across the motorway. Better taking a nap and fresh air from opening the window. Concomitant to finger abscess. 02, 6C, 54:XX:XX

Sh, 254 - When shopping, felt people did not accept me as belonging to the community. Felt isolated in the shop. Feeling unacceptable, 'as if I was a marked person' —but later felt better on my own. 12, 6C, 19:XX:XX

HYOS. He, 16 - Fears: being left alone (solitude, deserted); poison, or being bitten (hurt); being poisoned or sold; being betrayed, or injured; wishes to run away. (escape)

IGN. He, 2-...;sees everything as if through a fog (obscurity) ; sits quietly, with a vacant gaze (expression), always thinking of the mortification endured,... prefers to be alone; thinking of the past mortification...0Melancholy after mortification.

He, 22 - Melancholia from suppressed mental sufferings, with much sighing; desire to be alone (solitude) so as to give way to her real or imaginary grief; weeps bitterly.

He, 35 - Fearfulness; does not like to talk; prefers to be alone.

He, 37 - Tears wept inwardly, the pain and penalty (forfeit) of unrequited (unrecompensed) love; desires solitude so that one may nourish inward grief;...

He, 44-...;indifference to things she loved best ; sits alone and weeps, imagines things, a especially that she might go crazy; ..

IP. Al, 12 - Ill-humored, quiet, retired in himself, scorning everything.

Ha, 219 - Sullen unsociable moroseness, that makes him disdain (reject) everything.

JAMB. He, 1 - Constantly desirous of sitting alone and reflecting.

KALI-BR. He, 11 - Imagines she is a devil; cannot sleep; fears to be alone.

KALI-C. Al, 7 - Sad, lonely (solitary) ; she seeks society in order to enliven (animate) herself.

Al, 2 - Dread of being alone.

Al, 20 - Apprehensiveness and aversion to society.

Ha, 5 - Sad, she feels lonesome (solitary, lonely); she seeks for company to cheer her up.

Ha, 23 - Fearful about being alone.

He, 11 - Fear of being alone; fears she will die.

KEROSE. Al, 1 - As you breathe the vapor you seem to float into a wavy maze (labyrinth, puzzle), with a sense of complete loneliness; there appears to be but one object in the universe, and that object is yourself; on recovery the first thing seen is deemed (judge, conclude) the next only existence in the universe; ...

LAC-C. He, 19 - Cannot bear to be left alone for an instant.

LAC-D. Al,N-4 - Imagines that all her friends will die and that she must go to a convent. (purification, solitude)

He, 5 - Imagines that all her friends will die and that she must go to a convent. (purification, salvation)

LED. Ha, 329 - All day long; discontented with his fellow-creatures (friend, relations), which at last amounted to misanthropy.

Ha, 333 - Cross: he retired into solitude, and almost weeping he longed for death.

LEPI. Al, 1 - She fancies herself alone in a graveyard, pursued by a ghost, and screams so that her voice is lost next day; yet nobody hears her. (helpless)

LIL-T. He, 10 - Aversion to being alone, and yet no dread felt.

LITH. He, 2 - Disposed to weep about lonesome condition.

LYC. Al, 6 - Desires to be alone.

Ha, 28 - She is afraid of being alone.

He, 14 - Dread (fear) of men ; of solitude, irritability and melancholy.

LYSS. Al,N-92 - Exalted state of smell, taste and touch, with a feeling of anxiety and a fear of being alone.

MAG-M. Ha, 3 - Apprehensive and melancholic, lonely (isolated, abandoned) ; she is homesick and weeps.

Ha, 18 - He hated to talk; he desired to follow his thought in solitude.

MERC. He, 27 - Fear of being alone.

MEZ. Al, 2 - No rest when alone; he desires company.

Ha, 7 - Restless when alone, he wishes to be in company.

He, 5 - No rest when alone; wants to be in company ...unable to repeat what has been learned by heart; looks through window for hours, without being conscious of objects around; knows not what she is about; forgets what she is about to utter (talk); looks ill humored, pale, wretched, fallen away; ......expecting some very unpleasant news.

NAT-C. Al, 22 - His fancy is mostly busy with apprehensions of the future; he often makes plans for half an hour at a time as if it would go wrong with him, wherewith he seeks to be alone for several days together.

Al, 24 - She does not know what to do, on account of apprehensiveness and ennui and thinks that she is quite lonely (alone, solitary, insulated) and forsaken, all day.

Al, 30 - He shuns (avoid) mankind.

Al, 29 - Anthropophobia and fearfulness.

Ha, 8 - Apprehensive and ennui (tedium, monotony), so that she cannot contain herself; she deems (believe), herself altogether (entirely) lonely (solitary) and forsaken.

Ha, 10 - His fancy is mostly anxiously occupied with the future; he paints to himself what misfortunes might happen to him; and he seeks solitude for several days.

He, 4 - Aversion to mankind and society; estrangement (separation, alienation) from individuals and society; even from her husband and family.

NAT-M. Al, 63 - When alone, she becomes uneasy (discontent) about herself, and must weep.

Al, 39 - Melancholy mood; she has preferred to be alone for several days past.

Al, 93 - Ill-humored does not want to go into society for fear of vexing others; feels that he could easily give offense.

Ha, 59 - He feels peevish and avoids company, because he foresees that he might easily annoy (bother, molest) others. (intrude)

Ha, 12 - When alone, she calls up disagreeable thoughts and has to weep.

He, 13 - Taciturnity; offended at every word (easily); avoids company; hates persons because they have offended him; spleen.

He, 34 - A pregnant woman saw a man who had a disfiguring nasal cancer; this haunted (obsessed) her, and she was sure her child would be marked; she was melancholy, avoided society, wept continually.

He, 15 - Whenever alone she wished to cry, she did not know why.

NEON. Sh, 165 - I felt alone and as if everyone perceived me as odd. I felt strange, like an outsider and could not connect on any level. 02, 6C, 22:XX:XX

Sh, 201 - Mental symptoms accompanying cystitis: I was very withdrawn, grouchy, wanted to be alone. Stayed in bed a lot and did a lot of mental work withdrawn from emotions. This is how I always was during my many past bouts of cystitis. 06, 12C, XX:XX:X

NICC. Al, 9 - Tremulous, fearful, with inclination to be alone all day.

NIT-AC. He, 8 - Taciturn, disinclined to communicate anything; moody in morning.

NUX-V. He, 38 - Three months ago mental shock, since then fears to be alone,...fears as if she would choke (suffocation)...fears to be alone, fear of knives and the like, (similar) lest she should kill herself or others...

He, 11 - Cannot bear reading or conversation; irritable and wishes to be alone.

PH-AC. Al, 10 - Sadness and feeling of solitude, as if she would be sick.

PHOS. Al, 96 - Great anxiety and irritability when alone.

Ha, 89 - Delirious fantasies, while slumbering (sleep) and when awake, as if she was on a distant island (isolation, segregation), as if she had a large business, was a distinguished (important, rank) lady, etc.

He, 22-...uneasy about one's health; paroxysms of anguish, when alone or in a stormy weather, with timorous disposition; told those about him repeatedly that

he could not possibly recover, and gave some disjointed (incoherent) directions about his business affairs.
He, 18 - Does not like to be alone.
PLAT. Ha, 2 - She imagines herself deserted (abandoned) and standing alone in the world.
Ha, 17 - Sad and sullen, she sits solitary, without speaking and she cannot ward off sleep; then inconsolable weeping, especially when she is addressed.
He, 28 - Thinks she is left entirely to herself and stands alone in the world. (loneliness)
PLB. Al, 118 - Much depressed, fearing to die if left alone.
He, 16 - Mental disturbance of eight or ten years' duration in a man addicted to masturbation; has several times attempted suicide; has been in seclusion (solitude); greatest dejection and despair;...; believes himself lost (condemned) ; has the sounds of hell constantly in his ears; hears voices and sees shadows of demons, great disposition to make away (suicide) with himself or do himself some bodily injury;
PSOR. Al,N-46 - Attacks of fear; fear of fire, of being alone, of apoplexy, of becoming insane.
Al,N-32 - Melancholy after suppressed itch;...seeks solitude, despairs of recovery; ...
He, 32 - Melancholy after suppressed itch;...seeks solitude, despair of recovery;...
PULS. Al, 25 - It seems so quiet (silent) in her head and everything feels so empty that she seems alone in the house and in the world; she will speak to no one, just as if her surroundings did not exist (estrange), and she paid attention to no one. (left, solitary)
Ha, 1143 - Her head is so quiet and all about her is so empty as if she were alone (solitude, loneliness) in the house and in the world; she does not wish to talk to any one, just as if all around her were no concern (relation) of hers and she belonged to nobody. (lonely, missed)
RAN-B. Al, 1 - Fearfulness in the evening, she does not want to remain alone, she is afraid she may be haunted (seized) by ghosts.
He, 4 - Afraid of ghosts; does not like to remain alone.
RHUS-T. Al, 5 - Melancholy, ill-humor, and anxiety, as if a misfortune (disgrace) would happen, or as if she were alone (solitary), and all about her were dead (lifeless, inert) and still (silent, quiet), or as if she had been forsaken by a near friend; worse in the house, relieved by walking in the open air.
Ha, 953 - Melancholy, sad, and anxious, as if about to hear of a calamity,(misfortune, disaster) or as if she were solitary (lonely, alone) and all around her were dead (lifeless, extinct) and silent (quiet) ; or as if she had bid farewell (separation) to an intimate friend ; worst in the room, diminished by walking in a open air.
Ha, 952 - Sadness, making him prefer quiet solitude.
SEP. Al, 39 - She wishes to be alone and lie with closed eyes.
Ha, 18 - She wishes to be by herself and to lie with closed eyes.
Ha, 19 - He must not be alone for a moment.
He, 20 - Dread of being alone.
STRAM. Al, 206 - Fear of being in the dark and a less extent of being alone, in the evening after sunset.
Ha, 562 - His surroundings appear to him quite strange; (unfamiliar) although in the first minutes he knows that he is surrounded by his friends, he forgets this in the second minute, and imagines he is quite alone (solitary, deserted) in a desert (wildness), and is afraid (fearful) ; figures of beasts suddenly spring out of the ground at his side, so that he moves to the other side, where, however, other similar figures pursue him, and he runs forward.
Ha, 564 - He always imagines he is alone (solitary, lonely) and is afraid.
He, 101 - Mania for light and company, cannot bear to be alone.
He, 113 - Hydrophobia; water, a mirror, or anything bright, excites convulsion...,afraid to be alone;...
He, 156 - Endeavors to escape, imagines he is alone all the time, and is afraid. (loneliness, isolation)
He, 58 - Imagines he is alone, and is frightened.
STRY. Al, 5 - A peculiar nervous erethism, almost resembling what I had seen in a

case of hydrophobia ...wandering when left to himself, and begged most piteously (miserable) that I would not hurt him...fear of being injured...
Al, 30 - He had a feeling of dread, and begged he might not be left alone.
SUL-AC. Al, 5 - He was roused (waken) with difficulty, and when roused, resisted fiercely, saying in a hoarse muffled (deaden) voice, "Let me alone, let me die".
TAB. Al, 28 - Anxiety of being alone at night.
TARENT. Al, 65-... Great fear of an imaginary impending calamity (cataclysm, catastrophe) great desire of be alone, fear of being alone...
VALER. Al, 11 - Anxious, hypochondriac feeling, as if the objects around him had been estranged from him; the room appears to him desolate (isolated), he does not feel at home in the room, he is impelled to leave it.

SQUANDERS

Avarice; alternating with squandering: calc.[30] lach.[30] merc.[30] sulph.[30]
Avarice; generosity towards strangers, as regards his family: carb-v.[30] hyos.[30] nat-m.[30] nux-v.[30]
Avarice; squandering on oneself, but: calc.[30] hyos.[30] lap-mar-c.[194] nux-v.[30] sep.[30]
Boaster; squander through ostentation: calc.[30] nux-v.[30] plat.[30] puls.[30]
Delusions; distinguish, squanders money, proud of his position: ***verat.***[54]
• squanders money: ***verat.***[54]
• wealth, makes useless purchases, and: ***nux-v.***[54]
Dreams; purchase, making: hura.[36]
➤ time lost, sense of: bamb-a.[1184]
Extravagance; economy, for want of: agar.[30] alum.[30] nux-v.[30] sulph.[30]
Extravagance; sometimes, sometimes miserly: lach.[30] merc.[30]
Extravagance; themselves, for, and miserly as regards others: calc.[30] caust.[30] nux-v.[30] sep.[30]
Extravagance; work, with hard: paull.[36]
Fear; extravagance, of: op.
Generous; too much: cere-b.[36] nux-v.[30] op.[36] staph.[30] sulph.[189]
Insanity; purchases, makes useless: con. ***nux-v.***[54]
Squanders: agar.[30] alum.[30] ***bell.***[30] calc.[30] caust.[30] con.[30] hep.[30] **MERC.**[30] ***nux-v.***[30] stram.[30] sulph.[30] ***syph.***[122]
Squanders; money: bac.[162] verat.
Squanders; order, from want of: lyc.[30] plat.[58] sil.[30]

CON. He, 14 - Likes to wear his best clothes, (vanity) makes useless purchases, (squander) cares very little for things (indifferent), wastes or ruins them; does not want to work, prefers to play. (wanderer)
NUX-V. He, 37-...betraying (play false, feigning) great moral and physical languor (indifference),..launches into high-flying, fantastic plans, fancies himself rich (rank, position) and wants to make presents of thousands (squanders, waste), and makes large useless purchases; does not consider himself ill; ...,and takes in bad part if not allowed to read indictment (accusation) for said lawsuit, a confused irrational piece of work...
SULPH. Ha, 63 - Insanity; she spoils (ruin) her things and throws them away, imagining she has an abundance of everything; at the same time she becomes emaciated, like a skeleton.-(wealthy, rich X miserable, poor, destitute)
VERAT. He, 11 - Thinks himself distinguished (classify) ; squanders (futile) his money; proud (haughty) of his position.

STAGNATION

Anxiety; congestion, heart in: nit-ac.[1]
Delusions; blood, ceased to flow, in vertigo: seneg.[139]
• blood, circulate well, does not: ***atro.***[36]
• body, heart, stops beating, when sitting: ***arg-n.***[54] gels.[162]
• heart or respiration is going to stop, or otherwise frightens herself causing heart to beat violently: ***lac-c.***[54]
Fear; heart, cease beating, unless, not moving: coca[162] dig.[102]
✦ heart, cease beating, will: both-a.[3070]
✦ heart, cease beating, will, lying down, on: lach.[137]
✦ heart, cease to beating, unless constantly on the move, h. will: ***gels.***
✦ stoppage of circulation, with sensation of, at night, in angina pectoris: ***lyc.***[54]
Thoughts; stagnation of: ***cann-s.***[10] chin.[10]

hyos.[36] iod.[10] lyc.[10] m-arct.[10] ph-ac.[10] seneg.[36] sulph.[10] thuj.[10]

ATRO. Al, 25 - Insisted repeatedly that her blood did not circulate, and that her feet must put into warm or she should die.
CANN-I. Al, 26 - The idea that he must die returned several times, and seemed to be particularly connected with the sinking and disappearance of the pulse. (blood, circulation)
CHOC. Sh, 109 - In the night, heart stops beating. All very still inside.
Sh, 192 - I woke up and could not feel the usual sensation of my heart bulging or beating through my ribs while lying on my left side. I felt shock and thought 'perhaps I'm dead'. Groped for pulse and was reassured to be able to feel it. 15, 30C, 02:02:XX
LAC-C. He, 14-..;sometimes imagines heart or breathing are going to stop, or otherwise frightens himself, and this makes heart beat violently; occasionally very depressed, and fancies he is going out of his mind. (insanity)

STARVING

Anorexia mentalis: arg-n.[172] ars.[30] calc.[30] carc.[108] chin.[30] ign.[30] kali-p.[172] lach.[30] levo.[149] merc.[30] ***nat-m.***[148] perh.[149] ph-ac.[30] puls.[162] rhus-t.[36] ***sac-alb.***[210] ***sep.***[148] staph.[30] **SULPH.**[30] tarent.[30] vanad.[209] verat.[30]
Anxiety; fasting, when: cina[162] **IOD.**[54] sulph.[172]
Anxiety; hungry, when: cina[36] ***iod. kali-c.***
Aversion; water to, thirst, with: hell.[137]
Cares; full of, eat, if he does not: ***cocc.***[54] **IOD.**[54]
Contemptuous; ravenous hunger and greed, hasty eating, c. with sudden: ***plat.***[36]
Delusions; eat, cannot: myric.[137]
- fasting: brom.[36] euphr.[36] iod.[36]
- fasting, afternoon: iod.[36]
- starve, family will: ars. calc-sil.[58] ***sep.*** staph.
- starve, he must: kali-chl.[72]
- starved, being: naja[36]
- want, had come to: cann-i.
- want, will come to: calc-f. chlor.[139] sulph.

Desires; forage for food, to: choc.[222]
Dreams; body, emaciated, becoming: kali-n.[36] kreos.[58]
➤ drinking, impossible: arist-m.[36]
➤ famine, being left in a dungeon to die of; escaping by crawling out: ped.[36]
➤ hunger: ***arg-n.*** bry. calc. ign.
➤ hunger, morning, waking him: arg-n.[54]
➤ thirstily, being: dros. mag-c. **NAT-M.** viol-o.[45]
➤ want, of: am-c.[36]

Eating; refuses to: anac.[137] apis[8] ars. bar-c.[137] bell. ***bor.***[54] caul.[122] caust. ***chin.***[5] cocc. ***croc.*** grat. **HYOS.** ***ign.*** kali-bi.[8] kali-br.[184] **KALI-CHL.** kali-p. lach.[58] op. paull.[54] **PH-AC.** ***phyt.*** plat. puls. ***rhus-t.***[8] sep. sulph.[193] **TARENT. VERAT. VIOL-O.** zinc-chr.[137]
Excitement; hungry, when: kali-c.
Fear; death, hunger from: calc.[122]
✦ death, starvation, from: ars.[137]
✦ eating, agg., while, hungry: grat. iod.[58]
✦ family, to bring up his: ***staph.***[162]
✦ fasting, of: kreos.
✦ starving, of: ars.[172] ***bry.***[54] calc. kali-m.[61] ***sep.***[54] sulph.

Indifference; eating, to: bac.[62] chin.[1] lac-h.[229] merc.[30] nat-c.[30] nat-m.[30] ***rhus-t.***[5] ***staph.***[30] valer.[5]
Indifference; emaciation and weakness, especially with: **PH-AC.**[54]
Insanity; eats, refuse, only: meli.
Insanity; emaciation, with: sulph.[60]
Insanity; gluttony, with, alternating with refusal to eat: hyos.[30] ip.[30] stram.[30] verat.[30]
Irritability; hungry, when: ***sac-alb.***[210]
Mood; repulsive, food, saying one who does not work should not eat, but driven by hunger he tried to procure it secretly: ***arg-n.***[54]
Restlessness; hunger, with: abies-n.[72] iod.[187] kali-c.[148] nat-m.[36] podo.[8]
Sadness; hunger, with canine: ***nat-m.***[54]
Somnambulism; fasting, from: lap-a.[102]
Suicidal disposition; starving, by: merc.[5]

ARG-N. He, 17 - Refused food, saying one who does not work should not eat (punishment); but driven by hunger he tried to secretly procure it.
ARS. He, 10 - Fixed idea that he and his family will die of starvation. (hunger, privation, want)
He, 58 - Melancholy; after financial losses; cannot be consoled; thinks he will have to die (sentenced), with his family, from

starvation (hunger); sleepless nights; walks about wringing his hands, with moaning and groaning.

CHIN. Ha, 1103 - She falls time to time into a lachrymose humour, without external cause, from some self-made, trivial whim (caprice), e.q. from some imaginary want (lack, need), such as that she cannot eat enough...

CHLOL. Al, 3 - A horrible state of mind, fears he will go crazy, fears he cannot make a living.(subsistence)

LYSS. Al,N-45 - Wrote to doctor: I am waiting with impatience that you give me and my young ones something to eat.
Al,N-46 - After fainting (weak) spell he wrote on paper: I am forsaken by all; even the birds of heaven, they do not look at me (despised), do not fed me if hungry (helplessness) ; I hunger with the young ones and am thirsty with their she ones (starving); my nest (house) is made out of dirt (soiled), not gotten by my own exertions (efforts), but by driving them out of their nests (home) and sitting there with the females and the young.

PLAT. Ha, 37 - During the caprice of contempt, suddenly a voracious hunger...

SEC. Al, 57 - The only expression that he gave utterance (say) to was a stupid kind of "I am hungry".

SEP. He, 29 - Fear to starve,(hunger) is peevish, and feels mortified (disgraced), easily frightened and full of evil forebodings.

STAPH. He, 15-...; firmly believed he would lose his fortune, constantly told his wife to be careful that they did not starve; thinks his wife will run away from him (deserted) (lost: position, rank), ... amuses himself by throwing into the fire any article near at hand, regardless of value; at times more violent, strikes at any one coming near him, ...tells his wife he will try not kill any one;...

SULPH. Al, 2 - Delirium; she destroys her things, throws them away, thinking that she has a superfluity (excess) of everything, wherewith she wastes(thin) to a skeleton.(wealth?)
Ha, 63 - Insanity; she spoils (ruin) her things and throws them away, imagining she has an abundance of everything; at the same time she becomes emaciated, like a skeleton.-(wealthy, rich X miserable, poor, destitute)

STORM

Anguish; weather, in stormy: ***phos.***[54]
Anxiety; night, storm, during: nat-m.[36]
Anxiety; thunderstorm, before: ***gels.***[54] ***nat-c.***[116] ***phos.***[116]
Anxiety; thunderstorm, during: caust.[116] gels. ***nat-c.*** nat-m. ***nit-ac.*** **<u>PHOS.</u>**[122] sep.
Anxiety; weather, during stormy: gels.[60] ***lyc.***[54] nat-c.[10] nat-m.[10] nit-ac.[36] phos.[10]
Aversion; wind, to: ozone[227]
Beside oneself; weather, from bad: am-c.[122]
Cheerfulness; thunders and at lightnings, when it: bell-p.[193] calc.[184] ***carc.***[122] caust.[185] lyc.[148] ***sep.***
Delusions; black, thunder sits within her: androc.[222]
- earthquake, of a: fl-ac.[139]
- head, cold breeze blows on: petr.
- rain, exposed to: kalm.[36]
- rain, he hears: calc.[30] chin.[30] ph-ac.[30] staph.[30] sulph.[30] verat.[30]
- rain; out in the rain, he had been, from having wet cloth on head: atro.
- rainstorm, she is in a terrible, complaining of being so cold, and that carriage has turned over and hurt her head: naja.[8]
- room, foam of a troubled sea, is the: sec.
- ship, on board of, in a storm: alco.
- wind sighing in chimney sounds like the hum of a vast wheel, and reverberates like a peal of thunder on a grand organ: cann-i.

Discontented; weather, in rainy: aloe.
Dreams; accidents, struck by lightning, being: ***arn.***
➤ earthquake: ozone[227] rat. sil.
➤ fire, lightning, from: euphr.[36]
➤ flood: aran.[192] mag-c. merc. nat-c. rumx. ***sil.***
➤ freezing, about: grat.
➤ lightning: ***arn.*** bell.[102] euphr. lach.[102] phel. phos.[102] spig.
➤ lightning, struck by lightning, being: ***arn.***
➤ Noah's ark: bamb-a.[1184]
➤ rain, of being soaked in: mag-c.
➤ rainbows spanning the sky: coff-t.[36]
➤ snow: art-v. bapt. hydrog.[222] ***kreos.*** ozone[227]
➤ snow, storms, of being out in: ***kreos.***

➤ snow, working in snow: bapt.
➤ soaked with rain, being: mag-c.
➤ storms: all-s. ***ars.*** jac-c. mag-c. ***sil.***
➤ storms, destroying palaces: jac-c.[36]
➤ storms, frightful: sil.[36]
➤ storms, sea, at: all-c. sil.
➤ storms, thunderstorm: ***arn. ars.*** euphr. nat-c. phel.[10] spig.[5]
➤ water, waves, of high: ***all-c.***[54] ozone[227]
➤ wind raised him in bed, and a storm howled through right side of upper part of head, before midnight: mill.[36]

Fear; lightning, of: bell.[5] cycl.[5] dig.[5] lach.[5] phos.[5] phys.[5] sil.[5]
✦ rain, of: calc.[162] cor-r.[172] elaps naja[72]
✦ thunderstorm, approach of, at: ***gels.***[54] nat-c.[116] ***phos.***[116] psor.[162] rhod.[162]
✦ thunderstorm, night, driving her out of bed: nat-m.[1]
✦ thunderstorm, of: bell.[162] ***bor.***[5] ***bry.***[122] ***calc.***[30] calc-p.[162] carc.[207] caust.[30] ***coloc.***[162] con.[162] cycl.[162] dig.[162] dys-co.[136] electr.[10] ***gels.***[122] ***graph.***[162] hep. lac-c.[162] lach. lyc.[5] merc.[30] ***nat-c. nat-m. nit-ac.*** **PHOS.**[122] psor.[102] ***rhod.*** rhus-t.[172] ***sep.*** sil.[102] **STAPH.**[162] stram.[70] sulph. tub.[186]
✦ thunderstorm, thunder, especially of: rhod.[100]
✦ wind, of: bar-m.[209] ***cham.*** mang.[209] thuj.[122]

Indifference; weather, in stormy: sang.[137] tub.[137]
Irritability; thunderstorm, before: nat-c.[116]
Irritability; weather, in rainy or cloudy: aloe. am-c.
Irritability; weather, stormy: am-c.[8]
Morose; thunderstorm: am-c.[54]
Morose; weather, bad, from: aloe[117] am-c.[30]
Restlessness; anxious, thunderstorm, especially during, music agg.: ***nat-c.***[54]
Restlessness; storm, before: ***gels.***[54] ***psor.***
Restlessness; storm, during: gels. nat-c. ***nat-m. phos.*** psor.
Restlessness; thunderstorm, before: psor.[122]
Restlessness; thunderstorm, during: nat-c.[60] nat-m.[60] phos.[1] rhod.[54]
Restlessness; thunderstorm, thunderbolt, after heavy, with terrific screams: ***gels.***[54]
Sadness; thunderstorm amel: bell-p.[146] carc.[146] sep.
Shrieking; thunderstorm, during: gels.
Thunderstorm, mind symptoms before: bry. hyper. ***nat-c.***[116] nat-m.[116] petr.[116] **RHOD.** zinc.[54]
Thunderstorm; during, agg.: bor.[5] bry. caust. hyper.[5] lach. nat-c. nat-m. nat-p.[137] nit-ac. petr. ***phos.*** psor.[137] ***rhod.*** sep. ***sil.*** syph.[137]
Thunderstorm; during, amel.: ***carc.***[149] lyc.[85] rhus-r.[137] sep.[122]

AM-C. Ha, 16 - Cloudy weather makes her very sad.

CHAM. Al, 20 - Great dread of wind.

ELAPS. Al, 14 - Excessive horror of rain.
He, 5 - Fear of being left alone, as if something horrible might happen; horror of rain.

HALI-L. Sh, 917 - Air very hot today. All day, desire to create a storm, but one is not forecast for two days. That night we had a storm. I wanted thunder and lightning. 20, 30C, 12:XX:XX
Sh, 951 - Phoned a friend to hear what I already knew. As I heard the words, I felt a sensation as if hit by a thunderbolt through the vertex, down to hit my heart then spread up and across my shoulders out to my hands. (Drawing shows hands like wing tips). 20, 30C, 17:XX:XX
Sh, 952 - Today felt ordinary. It felt like my head cleared. Like it's open again. It felt like it was blasted open from the sky coming downwards, like a thunderbolt — hot, sharp, and sudden — through the vertex while I was talking to someone. I just understood what's been happening the last couple of weeks, even the breast dreams. There was just clarity and I could see how I'd been in the wrong shape all these years. 20, 30C, 17:XX:XX
Sh, 953 - Memories triggered off by the sensation in my head back and feet. Twenty three years ago in the States, I fell off a wall and smashed lots of vertebrae together. I was told I would never walk again. At the time, I got an internal explosion in my head opposite to what happened yesterday with the lightning in my vertex. 20, 30C, 18:XX:XX

MAG-C. Al, 944 - Dream of a flood, which flowed across the market-place, from which she woke in fright.

NAJA. He, 5-...imagines she is in a terrible rainstorm, complains of being so cold (coldness), and that the carriage has turned over and hurt her head. (accident)

NAT-C. Al,DREAM, 1111 - Dream of a flood (current, inundate), and threatening danger.
Ha, 11 - Less anxious than usual during a thunderstorm.
He, 9 - Restlessness, with attacks of anxiety, especially during a thunderstorm; < from music.
NIT-AC. Al, 24 - More anxious than usual during a storm.
Ha, 19 - More apprehensive during a thunderstorm than usually.
PHOS. He, 7 - Anxious: filled with gloomy (dark) forebodings; as if about to die; about termination (conclude) of her illness (disease); and restless ; at twilight; when alone; about future; during a thunderstorm; ..
He, 22-...uneasy about one's health; paroxysms of anguish, when alone or in a stormy weather, with timorous disposition; told those about him repeatedly that he could not possibly recover, and gave some disjointed (incoherent) directions about his business affairs.
RHOD. He, 4 - Nervous persons who dread a storm and are particularly afraid of thunder.
SEC. Al, 20 - She was conscious, but the room (space) presented to her the impression of water excessively agitated on its surface. She could compare it only to the "foaming of a troubled sea" (storm, tempest)
SEP. Al, 38 - He feels oppressed in sultry weather, but becomes more cheerful when it thunders and lightens.

STRANGE

Absorbed; strange, pregnancy, during: lyss.[137]
Affectation: alum.[30] carb-v.[30] caust.[30] con.[30] graph.[30] hyos.[30] lyc.[30] mez.[1] nat-m.[30] 0pall.[185] petr.[30] plat.[30] ***stram.*** verat.[30]
Affectation; gestures and acts, in: hyos.[30] mez.[1] stram.[108] verat.[30]
Cheerfulness; eccentric: apis[54] **CANN-I.**[54]
Contemptuous; self, of, alternating with eccentricity: agn.[10]
Dancing; desire for, grotesque: agar. ***cic.***
Delusions; bed, strange objects in: cimic.[54]
- changed, everything is: arg-n. bar-m. carb-an. ***nux-m.***[111] ***plat.*** stram.[54]
- dimensions of things reversed (turned): camph-br.[102]
- disease, unrecognized, has an: raph.
- dresses in strange costumes: iodof.[85]
- figures, strange accompany him, one on his right, the other on his left: ***anac.***[54]
- home, changed, everything at h., has: arg-n.
- house, place, not in right (while walking in the street after headache): glon.
- living under ordinary relations, is not: cic.
- locality is transformed: bar-m.[54]
- mystery, everything around seems a terrifying: aether[36] androc.[222] cann-i.
- new, everything is: ***hell.*** stram.
- objects, appear different: germ.[222] nat-m.
- people, beside him, strange: ***thuj.***[54]
- places, finds himself in strange and solitary, at night on waking: par.
- places, wrong, in, but does not want to go home: hyos.
- something, else, objects are something: staph.
- strange, everything is: anac.[5] anh.[144] bac.[62] ***bar-m.*** camph.[36] cann-i.[36] cann-s.[5] carb-an. ***cic.***[122] ***croc.***[5] glon.[111] ***graph. hydrog.***[222] ***hyos.***[5] kali-p. ***med.***[137] ***nux-m. op.***[5] petr.[5] ***plat.*** plb.[5] sep.[54] staph. stram. tub. valer.[5] verat.[5]
- strange, everything is, disagreeable, and: valer.[137]
- strange, everything is, terrible, and: cic.[137] ***plat.***[54]
- strange, familiar places are: bac.[149] cic. hyos.[102] plat.[102] rhus-t. tub.[102]
- strange, familiar places are, stranger, he is a stranger: bac.[149]
- strange, familiar places are, stranger, headache, after: glon.
- strange, familiar things are: arg-n. atro. bar-m. bell. bov.[102] calc. ***cann-i. cann-s.***[54] carb-an. choc.[222] cic. ***cocc.***[122] croc. glon. ***graph.*** hydrog.[222] hyos. kali-ma.[162] kali-p.[111] lyss. mag-m. med. merc.[111] mosch. ***nux-m.***[122] op. petr.[162] phos.[111] ***plat.*** **PULS.**[122] ran-b.[111] rhus-t. staph. stram. sulph.[111] thuj.[122] tub.[111] valer. verat.
- strange, familiar things seem horrible: plat.
- strange, familiar things seem, ludicrous: cann-i. hyos. nux-m.
- strange, land, as if in a: bry. par. plat. verat.

- strange, objects seem: carbn-s.[36] cic.[1] ***cimic.***[54]
- strange, streets, loses his way in, the houses seem strange: ***glon.***[54].
- strange, symptoms, his, are: bamb-a.[1184]
- strange, thing inside her: ozone[227]
- strange, voice, her own and of others, is: ***cann-i.*** **CANN-S.** cic.[58]
- transferred to another, room: coloc.
- transferred to another, world: cann-i.
- unusual, everything is: germ.[222]
- voices, hears, his own, sounds strange and seems to reverberate like thunder: cann-i.

Dreams; acquaintances, strange things: plat.[1]
- ➤ anger, pupils, because he has square: ozone[227]
- ➤ changed, everything is: ozone[227]
- ➤ cities, strange: ozone[227]
- ➤ distant, things, strange, on closing eyes: plat.[1]
- ➤ eccentric: jac-c.[36]
- ➤ people, strange things, doing: hydrog.[222]
- ➤ reveling a perplexed situation when waking: ***acon.***[10]
- ➤ strange: acon.[36] ant-t.[36] bar-acet.[36] chin-s.[10] ***lach.***[10] lact.[10] nit-ac.[10] ph-ac.[10] sarr.[36] stram.[36]
- ➤ things, strange: plat.[1]

Eccentricity: aesc.[36] agn.[36] alco.[36] am-c.[10] ambr.[30] ang.[10] apis[8] arg-n.[54] ars-h.[54] ***asar.***[10] asc-t.[54] ***bell.***[54] bufo[141] calc.[189] ***cann-i.***[36] ***cina***[130] cocc.[137] coff.[54] coff-t.[36] ***coloc.***[137] cub.[54] cupr.[10] cupr-acet.[54] cupr-ar.[36] cycl.[54] form.[36] gamb.[137] hoit.[149] hyos.[36] iodof.[54] kali-c.[149] lac-ac.[36] **LACH.**[54] lact.[10] lyc.[137] lyss.[36] merc.[137] muru.[36] nat-m.[189] nitro-o.[36] nux-v.[137] ***op.***[36] petr.[10] ***plb.***[137] raja-s.[149] sang.[36] sep.[54] spig.[10] stram.[10] sul-ac.[10] sulph.[36] sumb.[36] ***tarent.***[54] teucr.[36] thea.[36] valer.[10] verat. verat-v.[54] verb.[10] zinc.[137]

Eccentricity; alternating with, sadness: petr.[36] stram.[54]

Eccentricity; alternating with, timidity: sul-ac.[10]

Eccentricity; dressing: ery-m.[36] hell.[30] sil.[30] sulph.[30]

Eccentricity; political: ars.[30] bell.[30] caust.[30] lach.[30] nux-v.[30]

Eccentricity; religious: puls.[30] sel.[10] stram.[30] sulph.[10] verat.[30]

Elegance; want of: am-c.[30] am-m.[30] caps.[30] nat-c.[30] nat-m.[30] nux-v.[30] sil.[30] sulph.[30]

Fancies; strange: germ.[222] **STRAM.**[36]

Fear; strange place, as if he was in a: bar-c.[172] carb-v.[172] caust.[172] cic.[54] cupr.[172] kali-p.[172] thuj.[172]
- ✦ surroundings, of strange: kali-s.[127] puls.[127]

Monomania; going out, dressing in a grotesque manner: anan.

Sadness; alternating with, eccentricity: petr.[10]

Spaced-out feeling: foll.[1201] **HYDROG.** lac-h.[229] luna[228]

Strange; crank: bell.[30] calc.[30] chin.[30] hell.[8] hyos.[30] ip.[30] ***lach.***[30] nat-m.[30] puls.[30] stram.[30] verat.[30]

Strange; crank, opinions and acts, in: calc.[30] sulph.[30] verat.[30]

Strange; things, impulse to do: arg-n.[58] cact. iod.[137] sep.[137]

Talk; strange: aether cham. gall-ac.

Tastelessness in dressing: ***calc.***[30] caust.[30] hell.[1] hyos.[1] lyc.[30] ***nat-m.***[30] nux-v.[30] sec.[1] staph.[30] stram.[1] sulph.[30]

Thoughts; strangeness: arg-n.[111] calc.[30] canth.[54] ***lyss.***[54] raph.[36] ***stram.***[54] sulph.[30] verat.[30]

ADAM. Sh, 246 - Cried with despair. Nothing I do is right. Rocking from side to side, sobbing. Desire to stab with a knife or scissors. Felt very different from other humans. Long, late phone call ameliorates. 16, 12C, 43:XX:XX

Sh, 376 - Cried with despair. Nothing I do is right. Rocking from side to side sobbing. Desire to stab with a knife or scissors. Felt very different from other humans. Long, late phone call ameliorates. 16, 12C, 43:XX:XX

AIL. He, 1 - Past events are forgotten, remembered as belonging to someone else, or as matters read.

AM-C. Ha, 11 - The mind is restless and feels uncanny. (mysterious, strange)

ANAC. He, 26 - Idea as if everything perceived had no reality, all things appear as in a dream.

He, 28 - Fixed ideas: that mind and body are separated ; about redemption (salvation) of soul and about the devil; that a stranger is constantly by his side (pursued); that strange forms accompany him, one to his right and one to his left.

ANDROC. Sh, 62 - A friend commented that

she "looked strange and not at all like herself". (7)

Sh, 129 - It seemed as though he was a different person, very similar to the way he had been in adolescence, but in a much more powerful manner. These emotions were so intense he wanted to rip his chest apart to let them out. He lost all control over his emotions, which seemed to come from a deep and distant part of himself, a darker side. He desired to continue the proving for the rest of his life. (29)

APIS. Al, 15 - She thought she must die, she felt so strangely.(strange)

He, 19 - A strange boy lying in bed with him prevents (restrict) sleep.

ARG-N. He, 18 - Feels as if everything at home had changed and that his mind is weak.

He, 59 - Against whatever was proposed he had the queerest objections. 0 Melancholia.

ATRO. Al, 3-...the mind would become filled with strange and fanciful ideas ...fits of wild, uncontrollable laughter...I fancied myself afflicted with epilepsy, and was constantly fearful lest others should discover my unfortunate condition; ...

BAR-M. He, 1 - The locality around him seems transformed.(strange, unfamiliar)

CACT. Al, 8 - Impulses to do something bordering, on the grotesque.(bizarre, strange)

CALC-A. Al, 5 - Anxious thoughts, which came and went, before going to sleep in the evening; with which the objects seemed like different (strange) objects; he dreaded (fear) the dark, and made an effort to look at the light; all of which was relieved after the passage of flatus.

CAMPH. Al, 46-..." I am death! No, I am not death! but indeed I must be dead!" And thus I flew round about myself like a top, with no other feeling than for the strong smell of the Camphor. The external world existed for me no longer....

Al, 46-...The external world existed for me no longer. (solitude) My thoughts were gone; one single fearful one remained; I imagined myself transferred to another world (estranged, alienated); for me all else was extinguished...

Al, 46-...I sat up in bed, but all about me had indeed disappeared. I was alone in the great universe, the last of all things. My ideas of the world, God and religion, now seemed to me to have existed only in my imagination; the earth upon which yesterday I lived and moved, had run its appointed course, and I was the final and solitary fragment of the whole creation...(meaningless, unimportant, neglected, forsaken, loneliness, deserted) (godless)

CANN-I. Al, 29 - Looks under beds and tables, unlocks and relocks doors, for the fancies he hears strange noises, and that thieves are in the house.

CANN-S. He, 1 - Seems to be in a dream, as if things were not real; feels as if she did not know where she was; objects seem strange; feels at times as if she was somebody else;...

He, 5 - Voices including her own, seem to come from a distance; her own voice seems strange, as if it was somebody else speaking.

CANTH. He, 6 - Strange ideas crowd on him against his will.

CARB-AN. Ha, 32 - The objects on the street seem to him changed, e.g., farther apart and brighter (vivid, brilliant) than usual, as an empty, abandoned city.

CHOC. Sh, 32 - When I look in the mirror, I don't recognise myself. I look different, especially around and over the eyes —my face doesn't seem familiar. The area around my forehead feels more congested and bigger.

Sh, 307 - Talking to a friend, noticed her mouth felt strange, almost as if she had two mouths, one on top of the other. No other part appeared double.[27], 100C, 00:22:15

CIC. Al, 9 - He did not believe that he was living under ordinary relations; everything seemed strange and almost fearful to him; it seemed as though he has awakened from an acute fever...

Al, 29 - He was indifferent to everything, and began to doubt whether he was really in the condition which he found himself.

Ha, 235-...; everything appeared to him strange and almost frightful; it was as if he woke up out of an acute fever and saw all sorts of figures, and yet he did not feel corporeally ill.

He, 8 - He imagined he was not living in his usual condition and circumstances; everything appears to him strange and almost terrible.
He, 10 - Feels as if he was in a strange place, which causes fear.
CIMIC. He, 7 - Imagines strange objects about bed, as rats, sheep, etc.
He, 10 - Fear of death; fears those in house will kill him (murdered, by parents); saw wires encasing (lock, imprisoned) him; visions of rats and of strange objects.
CROT-C. Al, 3-... hears a strange voice to her left, and behind her; she follows it, throws herself against closed doors, and scratches them with her nails...She cries out: " He is in the den, but the lions will not eat him"
CYCL. Al, 19 - Sometimes he is very ill-humored and fretful, but suddenly he feels again a strange joyous sensation,...
Ha, 202 - Towards evening there suddenly occurs a strange happy feeling and lively fancy, which conjures (remember) up agreeable pictures.
ERY-A. Al, 1 - Felt very queer (eccentric, inadequate) before completely dressed.
GERM. Sh, 144 - I have an intense feeling of estrangement and isolation, with a desire to start my life again. 08, 12C, 11:06:50
Sh, 145 - I am easily offended by being told that I look strange. 08, 12C, 18:06:10
GLON. Al, 21 - As he returned home through the streets, after the headache, everything seemed strange to him, not as familiar as usual; he was obliged to look about him every few moments to convince himself of being in the right street; it seemed to him as if the houses were not in their right places, on the same route that he had passed over at least four times a day for years.
He, 4 - Well-known street seem strange; way home too long.
HYDROG. Sh, 10 - I feel a bit unreal —like taking drugs —a weird spaced-outness. The top of my head feels very clear — seeing and hearing clear and remote, but from the sinus down, I feel muzzy and warm. 08, 30C, 00:01:XX
IRID. Sh, 36 - Went to a 40th birthday celebration. One very good friend said I didn't seem to be there. They seemed like strangers to me. I was looking at the situation, which needed jollying up, but was unable to do anything about it because I felt distanced from them. It felt strange as if I'd gone out with people I didn't want to be with. H3
Sh, 115 - Inner vision, rows upon rows of letters. Thought, "This looks Greek to me." Q8
LYSS. Al, 39 - A strange oppression and indifference, as if he was unable to do anything if he forces himself; there is no power of mind.
MAG-M. Al, 711 - An anxious dream; she was lying in a strange house, where rubbish (garbage) was constantly falling upon her; she tried to cry out and could not, because there was too great heaviness on the chest.
MAG-S. Al, 11-..while knitting she constantly saw strange persons about (surround) her, though she knew it was an illusion.
MED. He, 7 - Reads a letter and thinks the words look queer (inadequate) and are spelled wrong.
NEON. Sh, 65 - While looking at a star map, it looked unfamiliar, as if I had always been seeing the stars from the other side. 20, 6C, 08:09:XX
Sh, 165 - I felt alone and as if everyone perceived me as odd. I felt strange, like an outsider and could not connect on any level. 02, 6C, 22:XX:XX
NUX-M. He, 15 - Surroundings seemed changed; fanciful, dreamy images; does not recognize the known street.
PLAT. Ha, 41 - She feels as if she did not at all belong to her family (stranger); after a short absence everything appears to be quite changed. (unfamiliar)
He, 20 - Everything seems strange and horrible to her.
PULS. Al, 25 - It seems so quiet (silent) in her head and everything feels so empty that she seems alone in the house and in the world; she will speak to no one, just as if her surroundings did not exist (estrange), and she paid attention to no one. (left, solitary)
RAPH. Al, 16 - Her condition troubles her, and for a moment cannot believe it to be owing to the medicine; she forgets it

entirely, and believes she has a disease which is not recognized. (unknown, undiscovered)

SABAD. Al, 2 - He imagines all sorts of strange things about his own body, for instance, that it had shrunk (dry, wrinkled) like that of dead persons (corpse), that his stomach was corroded (degeneracy, decomposition), that the scrotum was swollen (enlarged), etc.;...

SEP. He, 38-...everything seems strange (unusual, unfamiliar) to her;...; it seems as if she could not understand (realize) anything and would have to learn anew everything she wished to do;...(lost: knowledge); greatest indifference to everything, the death of a near relative, or some happy occurrence, leaves her equally unaffected; no trace of her former love for friends or even for her child; aversion for social intercourse amounting to contempt;...

STAPH. Al, 15 - Anxious thoughts and events in the past came to him as if the past were present before him, which caused anxiety...then it became black before his eyes; he did not know whether the images were real or illusory, then everything seemed different, and he lost all desire to live.

STRAM. Ha, 562 - His surroundings appear to him quite strange; (unfamiliar) although in the first minutes he knows that he is surrounded by his friends, he forgets this in the second minute, and imagines he is quite alone (solitary, deserted) in a desert (wildness), and is afraid (fearful) ; figures of beasts suddenly spring out of the ground at his side, so that he moves to the other side, where, however, other similar figures pursue him, and he runs forward.

Ha, 503 - After waking all objects seem to him new (strange, unusual) even his friends as though he had never in his life seen them before.

He, 57 - Strange absurd ideas; thinks herself tall, double or lying crosswise; one half of body cut off (divided); bed is full of creases (wrinkle) (disorganization); that he was killed roasted and being eaten.

THUJ. He, 10 - Fixed ideas: as if a strange person were at his side; as if soul and body were separated (split) ; that body, particularly limbs, are made of glass (frail) and will readily break (weakness); as if a living animal were in abdomen ;talks about being under the influence of a superior power. (possessed)

TUB. Al,N-25 - Everything in the room seems strange, as though in a strange place.

Al,N-38 - Soporous, dazed condition; unable to find the right way (lost); is confused; surroundings appear strange.

VALER. Al, 11 - Anxious, hypochondriac feeling, as if the objects around him had been estranged from him; the room appears to him desolate (isolated), he does not feel at home in the room, he is impelled to leave it.

VERAT. Ha, 709 - He is too lively (energetic), eccentric, extravagant.(wasteful)

STRANGER

Anger; strangers, at: hep.[109]

Company, aversion to; presence of, strangers, to: **AMBR.**[122] ***bar-c. bry.*** bufo ***carb-v.*** **CIC.** cina[58] ***con. helon.***[163] ***iod. lach.***[8] lyc. nat-c.[58] petr. ***sep. stram.*** tarent.[193] ***thuj.***

Delusions; abroad, being: verat.[30]

- family, does not belong to her own: plat.
- friend, he had never seen them (after waking): stram.[54]
- home, away from, strangers, in midst of, in epilepsy: ***aster.***[54]
- man, talking in foreign languages: ***stram.***[54]
- people, seized them, sees a number of strangers and tries to: stram.[54]
- strange, familiar places are, stranger, he is a stranger: bac.[149]
- strange, land, as if in a: bry. par. plat. verat.
- stranger, he is a: germ.[222] nat-m.[111] valer.
- strangers, amongst: aster.[137]
- strangers, control of, under: aster. bry.
- strangers, friends appears as: bry. stram.
- strangers, looking over shoulder: brom.
- strangers, room, seem to be in the: bry.[10] ***tarent. thuj.***
- strangers, sees: anac.[58] cann-i. mag-s. nit-ac.[30] nux-v. ***puls.***[30] stram. ***thuj.***
- strangers, sees, every night since six weeks, causing fear, had to leave bed, a old woman: ***stram.***[54]
- strangers, sees, knitting while: mag-s.

• strangers, snatching at her: ***bell.***[54]
• strangers, surrounded by: androc.[222] nit-ac.[30] ***puls.***[30]
• voices, hears, strangers, of: bell.[30] ***cham.***[30]
Dreams; cities, strange: ozone[227]
➤ country, foreign: ind.[54] ozone[227] plat.[10] sil.[10]
➤ country, native country: ant-c.[1] lach.[36] mur-ac.[36]
➤ father is an Arab: ozone[227]
➤ gypsies, of: choc.[222]
➤ Indians, being among: jug-c.
➤ Latin, he admires his own skill in speaking: lyss.[36]
➤ murdering, Arab, an, with four stabs in chest: ozone[227]
➤ strangers, of: art-v.[54]
Embarrassment; strangers, in presence of: ambr.[5] bar-c.[5] ***dig.***[8] tarent.[5]
Excitement; stammers when talking to strangers: dig.
Fear; strangers, of: ambr. ***bar-c.*** bufo[130] ***carb-v.*** carc.[207] caust.[58] ***cupr.*** dys-co.[136] kali-p.[172] lach. lyc.[58] plb.[201] puls.[70] sil.[185] stram. ***thuj.*** tub.[70]
Hide; desire to, children, strangers, from: bar-c.[85]
Indifference; loved ones; to, strangers, but animated to: ***fl-ac.***[54]
Strangers: presence of, agg.: ***ambr. bar-c. bry.*** bufo carb-v.[137] caust.[5] cic.[58] cina[58] con. iod.[58] lyc. nat-m.[5] petr. phos.[5] ***sep. stram.*** tarent.[5] ***thuj.***
Talk; American accent, with: lap-c-b.[194]
Talk; foreign language, in: camph.[54] lach. m-arct.[1] nit-ac.[137] sol-n.[1] ***stram.***
Talk; indisposed, foreign language which at other times he speaks fluently: pall.[54]
Trance; plays on piano with closed eyes, writes letters in an acquired language: ***camph.***[54]

ADAM. Sh, 525 - Delusion I saw a man with a green face. I looked to see if his ears were pointed, but they were normal. Thought he might be a Vulcan. 16, 12C, 51:XX:XX
ANAC. He, 28 - Fixed ideas: that mind and body are separated ; about redemption (salvation) of soul and about the devil; that a stranger is constantly by his side (pursued); that strange forms accompany him, one to his right and one to his left.
APIS. He, 53 - Eccentric cheerfulness, despondency, or hopelessness.
ASTER. He, 2-...hallucinations as if away from home in midst (middle) of strangers; hears voices to which he replies.
BELL. He, 18 - When closing eyes, though not asleep, patient sees fierce (wild), wicked looking large animals with horns and bushy (scabrous) heads; room seemed to be full of strange men passing in and out, who would snatch (take hold) at her as they passed, which frightened her very much, she thought the men wanted to take her away from home ; she then saw children sitting on low benches (seat) in rows (line) as in a school-room. (purity)
CAMPH. Al, 46-...The external world existed for me no longer. (solitude) My thoughts were gone; one single fearful one remained; I imagined myself transferred to another world (estranged, alienated); for me all else was extinguished...
CHLOL. Al, 17-...a feeling as if he were now in one country and now in another, and with an anxious desire to go home.(abroad)
CHOC. Sh, 44 - Dream —coming out of the station a huge black bird the size of a dog with black long soft feathers like those of an ostrich, and a very big beak. It took my left hand in his beak. There were two gypsies there and they stood in front of me and opened their hands and I saw that they held a gold metal flat fish which I saw as a fortune telling object.
Sh, 211 - Feeling like I don't belong in a crowd. Conscious of all social and economic pressures on people nowadays and was glad to get home.[41], 6C, 01:XX:XX
GERM. Sh, 137 - Entertain myself with mischievous reflections and realize that these are more thoughts of an outsider. 08, 12C, 02:14:10
Sh, 136 - Feeling lonely like an alien freak. 08, 12C, 22:00:00
Sh, 139 - Feel angry hostile and tearful easily. Someone says that I have behaved as if I am from another planet. 08, 12C, 30:00:00
Sh, 149 - Feel lonely. I nearly always feel special -always on the sideoutside of others. Either better or smaller than others. 18, 30C, 46:XX:XX

Sh, 135 - I see a stranger who looks so familiar . 08, 12C, 11:04:20

LYSS. Al,N-14 - Is astonished (surprised) in his dream at the readiness with which he can express himself in elegant Latin.

MAG-C. Al, 932 - Dream of flowers, clothes, and other things; she had to make up the clothes, but had no inclination to do it, and besides did not understand how; she also saw many foreign plants, but during this she became soaked (wet) with rain.

MERC. Ha, 1130 - Frightful dreams, in which he started up; he imagined he was not in his own house, sat up in bed and spoke about a distant village.

NAT-C. Al, DREAM, 1102-..;of marrying two women, of parties, walks, entertainments, and excursions on horseback, afterwards they were frequently anxious, of going astray (lost),of murders, having his ears cut off; also vexatious dreams; he would take a journey and could not get away from the place,(immobilization) and when has reached the first station was obliged to turn back, on account of something he had forgotten.

He, 4 - Aversion to mankind and society; estrangement (separation, alienation) from individuals and society; even from her husband and family.

NEON. Sh, 164 - One of our visitors had gone out to buy a newspaper. When he came back I could not recognize him, although I've known him for 12 years. It took 30 seconds or more, not just a flash, thinking he was a total stranger. 02, 6C, 15:XX:XX

NUX-M. Al, 30 - While writing he omitted letters, wrote in different alphabets against his will and changed from one subject to another.

OP. He, 11 - Thinks he is not in his own house; imagines himself living in a locality three hours distant from his house; detains all passers-by and wishes to take them into his house; ...he does not recognize friends;... (estranged, alien)

PALL. He, 1 - Extremely fatigued in evening; feels mentally gone; is averse to speaking a foreign language which at other times he speaks fluently; it is too much of an exertion, he is tired of it. (lack of communication)

PLAT. Ha, 41 - She feels as if she did not at all belong to her family (stranger); after a short absence everything appears to be quite changed. (unfamiliar)

He, 25 - Out of sorts (irritated) with the whole world; everything seems too narrow (restricted, confined, near) ; weeping mood.

He, 39 - It seems to her as if she does not belong to her own family; ...

STRAM. He, 53 - Hallucinations which terrify patient; sees ghosts, hears voices back his ear; sees strangers.

He, 63 - An old lady had a vision every night since six weeks, in which many persons, all strangers, came into her room and to her bedside, causing her such fear that she had to leave bed.

He, 93 - Mania; thinks he is lying on his sepulchre (tomb); confessing, praying, wants to be killed (redemption, salvation, regeneration); laughs as if tickled (excited); wants to be kissed; accuses his wife of being faithless (betrayed); scolding (censure) beating in a rage, will not be taken hold of by attendants (suspicious?) ; takes them for dogs (contemptuous), and barks at them; talking in Jewish jargon; (rank?, stranger?) supposes his house to be surrounded by carts (vehicle), Jews (Judaism) and geese, offending him, ... -(strange, foreign, alien)

He, 29 - Talking in Jewish jargon.(clichÇ)

He, 68 - Hears dancing, music, sees men and hears them talk in foreign tongues.

He, 87 - After a dreadful shock, occasioned by death of his brother, who fell dead in his arms,...struck all at around him...spoke at one time in Hungarian, and then in Wallachian language; sang Latin paternosters, declared he was God, and then that he was the devil;...

He, 130 - Talks in a foreign tongue.

TARENT. Al, 12-...Hallucinations (delirium) sees strangers (aliens) in the room.

THUJ. He, 13 - Nervousness to such a degree that approach of a stranger gave her sudden twitches...

SUCCEED

Anxiety; success, from doubt about: aloe[36] ***lac-c.***[54]

Deeds; he could do great, as if: cocain.[162] hell.

Delusions; business, success, is a: phos.[1]
- succeed, he cannot; does everything wrong: anac. ***arg-n.*** arn.[114] ***aur.***[122] bamb-a.[1184] bapt.[58] bar-c.[162] gels.[114] naja[130] nat-c. nat-m.[114] ozone[227] phos.[114] sulph.[137]
- succeed, that he cannot, unfit for this world: ***aur.***[54]
- work, accomplish the, he cannot: bry.[36]
- work, advance fast enough, does not: gamb.[36]

Despair; work, over his: anac.[58]
Doubtful, plans, about realizing her: bamb-a.[1184]
Dreams; business, accomplish, cannot: mag-m. ***phos.*** sabad.
➤ projects, coming true (in the dreams): rhus-t.[10]
Fear; destination, of being unable to reach his: lyc.
✦ failure, of: act-sp.[162] aloe[36] arg-n.[5] arn.[5] carc.[193] cob-n.[144] cupr.[210] gels.[5] iod.[116] ***lac-c.***[54] lyc.[172] naja[141] nat-m.[5] phos.[5] plb.[201] ***sac-alb.***[210] sil.[58] sulph.[5]
✦ undertaking anything: ***arg-n. ars.*** kali-p.[172] ***lyc.*** sil.[58]
✦ undertaking, enterprise, a new: cupr.[210] lyc.[201] plb.[201] ***sil.***[54]
Persists in nothing: alum.[111] asaf.[137] aur.[1] bar-c.[10] calc.[189] grat.[54] lac-c. lach. lyc.[36] nux-v.[155] plan. ***sil.***[111] stann.[1] sulph.[111]
Succeeds, never: am-c. asar. aur. canth. merc.[1] mur-ac. nat-c. nat-s. nux-v. spong.[1]
Talk; sleep, in, obstacles being removed: cham.[1]
Thoughts; rush, business accomplished, evening of: sulph.[36]
Undertakes; lacks will power to undertake anything: androc.[222] phos. ***pic-ac.***
Undertakes; many things, perseveres in nothing: ***acon.*** alum.[30] androc.[222] ant-c.[102] apis[83] bism.[1] bor.[1] canth.[85] cortico.[119] graph.[30] grat.[137] ign.[58] ***lac-c. lach.*** **LIL-T.**[36] lyc.[36] med.[179] ***nux-m.***[54] petr.[30] phos.[189] pin-s.[36] plan. sanic.[108] stann.[30] sulph.[81] verat.[1]
Undertakes; nothing lest he fail: ***arg-n.*** nux-v.[36] sil.

ACT-SP. He, 16 - Desperation of success of every, even most trifling undertaking.
ALOE. Al, 20 - Little inclination to labor; discouraged, apprehensive about his success.
AM-C. Ha, 12 - She finds no rest (restlessness), and prosper (realize, achieve) in nothing.
ANAC. Ha, 9 - He is at odds (quarreling) with the whole world, and has so little confidence in himself that he despairs of being able to accomplish (succeed) what is demanded of him.
Ha, 20 - Indisposition to work; he is afraid to undertake anything, he has no pleasure in anything.
ANG. Ha, 298 - Cheerfulness and self-confidence that he can undertake anything with power.
ARG-N. Al, 6 - He fells very much affected bodily and mentally; he does not undertake anything lest he should not succeed.
He, 16 - Possessed of distressing idea that all his undertakings will and must fail.
He, 31 - Does not work, thinking it will do him harm or that he is not able to stand it.
ARN. Ha, 623 - Over-busy, inclination and disposition for great and continuous literary work with no power to do it without injury to the health.
ARS. He, 95 - Dissatisfied and angry with himself all day; thinks he has not accomplished enough, and reproaches himself bitterly.
AUR. Ha, 342 - Peevish (irritable) dejection; (sadness) he thinks nothing will succeed (prosper) with him.
Ha, 345 - An urging to activity, bodily as well as mental; when he did anything, he thought he did not do it quick enough, and that he had a great deal (much) more to do; he could not live to his liking. (desire, aspiration)
Ha, 12 - He is driven to constant activity, and is sorry for his inaction, although he cannot do anything.
Ha, 18 - Dispirited ill-humor; he thinks he cannot succeed in anything.
Ha, 19 - Dispirited and despondent; he thinks that everything goes awkwardly (incapacity, unfit) with him, and nothing will succeed with him.
He, 10 - Imagines he cannot succeed (perform, prosper) in anything, (failure) and he does everything wrong; he is in disunion whith himself.
BAR-A. Al, 14 - During the day she resolves to undertake a certain matter in the evening, but scarcely is the time come

when she repents it, and is undecided whether she shall do it or not.

BAR-C. Ha, 14 - During the day she determines to attend (take care) to some particular matter; but scarcely (just) has the time come, when she is sorry (give up) for it, and she knows not for irresolution what to do to leave undone.

BISM. Al, 5 - He commences one thing and then another, but keeps to one thing only a short time.

He, 10 - Unstable-minded; begin now this, again that, holds but short time to any one thing.

BOR. Ha, 21 - He fritters away the afternoon, without getting to any real work, goes from one work to another, from one room to another, without remaining in one thing.

BRY. Ha, 777 - Cross; imagined she could not finish her work (obstruction) ; she always took hold (continued) of the wrong thing and constantly wished to take something else ; then a pressing aching headache in the forehead.

Al, 25 - Fretful; she imagines that she cannot accomplish (realize) her work; constantly takes up the wrong piece, and always inclined to change and take another; ...

Al, 37 - Over-busy (industrious); she undertakes and works far too much.

Ha, 780 - Too busy; she wishes to undertake and to work at too many things.

BUFO-S. Al, 7 - He is unable to act with decision (doubtful) ; he forms projects and does not accomplish (succeed) them.

CACT. Al, 19 - Disposition to do deliberately (resolutely, carefully) whatever was undertaken.

CALAD. He, 4 - Very forgetful; he cannot remember if what he ought to have done and written during the day is really accomplished until he convinces himself of it.

CALC. Al, 22 - Anxious, restless, and busy mood; she is undertaking much things but accomplish nothing...

CANTH. He, 14 - Constantly attempting (try) to do something, but accomplishing nothing.

CARB-AC. He, 12 - Entire disinclination to study; what he had accomplished seemed very trifling. (unimportant)

CHAM. He, 32 - Very anxious; everything she undertakes is very unsatisfactory (disappointed) ; she is irresolute,...(indecision)

CHIN. Al, 39 - Fretful and irresolute; she is unable to accomplish her aim, and consequently is indignant. (angry)

Ha, 1136 - He makes many plans, and thinks over their accomplishment (execution, success), many ideas force themselves upon him at once.

Ha, 1137 - He has many ideas, undertakes (begin, try) to carry out (achieve, perform, execute) all sorts of things, builds castles in air.(fanciful)

Ha, 1138 - He has a number of plans in his head which he greatly desires to carry into execution (progress), in the evening.

Ha, 1134 - Liking for work, reading, writing, and thinking; particularly well disposed and industrious.

COCC. Ha, 532 - She dawdles (indolent); in business she cannot accomplish anything nor finish anything, with contracted pupils.

FORM. Al, 4 - During the day remarkably happy and able to study; everything seemed easy to be accomplished.

GRAT. Al, 16 - Irresolute; no persistence in work.

IGN. Al, 20 - Fearfulness timidity; she has no confidence in herself, gives up (desist) everything.

Ha, 759 - Fearfulness, cowardice cannot trust himself to do anything, considers all is lost .

Ha, 755 - Excessively busy: he restlessly sets about doing first one thing then another.

IP. Al, 11 - Ill-humored and vexed that his business does not proceed fast enough.

Ha, 224 - He is morose and vexed that his business is not performed quick enough. (time)

KALI-C. Ha, 51 - Lack of presence of mind; he cannot proceed right along in his business.

LAC-C. Al,N-33 - Depression of spirits, doubts her ability and success, thinks she will have heart disease and die of it.

He, 26 - Depression of spirits, doubts her ability (competence, aptitude) and success (prospering, progressing, achieving),

thinks she will have heart disease and die of it.
He, 29 - Fears she will become unable to perform (achieve, accomplish) her duties.(responsibility)
LACH. Al, 54 - Dilatory (slow); he cannot accomplish his business as usual.
He, 40 - He wishes to do a great deal; begins many things. (undertakes)
He, 30 - Undertakes many things, perseveres in nothing.
LIL-T. Al, 24-..a feeling of irritation and of something wrong in abdomen and pelvic organs (disease); feels hurried (fast) and yet incapable (incompetent), as if she had a great deal (busy) to do and cannot do it.
He, 12 - Listless, inert, yet does not want to sit still (quiet); restless, yet does not want to walk; hurried manner, desire to do something, yet feels no ambition; feeling as of imperative duties and utter (complete) inability (incapacity, incompetence) to perform them; sexual excitement.
LIM. Al, 3 - The great disinclination to work, and inability to accomplish much, which he had experienced since the sea-bath, disappeared completely during the day, and gave place to mental quiet and steadiness, with constancy and perseverance in performing very irksome duties.
LYC. Al, 113 - Excited, busy mood in the evening, without perseverance, changing from one subject to another, with difficulty of fixing the thoughts, and greater difficulty in accomplishing anything; while reading fell asleep...
MAG-C. Al, 22 - So fretful (irritable) that she does not know what she shall undertake...(begin)
MED. Al,N-40 - Always wakens tired in the morning; hates to do anything that must be done (duty), even nice things; gets nervous and excited about riding and driving as soon the time is fixed.
Al,N-41 - Constant state of anguish. Always a feeling of impending danger, but knows not what. There is no cause for such feelings, as she is not obliged to do anything when disinclined; is so situated that nothing need cause her trouble.
He, 2 - Dullness of memory and desire to procrastinate (delay), because business seemed so long lasting (permanent), or as if it never could be accomplished. (postponing)
MUR-AC. Ha, 8-...no work succeeds in his hands,...
NAT-AR. Al, 5 - Feel well; can study easily ; disposed to be reconciled to circumstances, favorable and unfavorable; feel like working hard; no undertaking too large for me.
Al, 15 - Requires an effort to attend to accustomed duties; feels dull; tries to write, but it requires an effort to form each word.
NAT-C. Al, 56 - He has no desire to do anything, and can keep at nothing long.
Ha, 13 - Anxious and restless, he thinks he cannot do anything right.
Ha, 23 - Restlessness and unsteadiness (inconstant); he knew not what he wanted, nor what he should do or leave undone.
NAT-S. Al, 12 - Nothing that she undertakes succeeds well, and she does not know why.
NUX-M. Al, 24 - Variable mood; at one time he wishes to do something, but when he is about to accomplish it changes his mind.
Al, 48 - He never accomplishes what she undertakes, but remains standing in one place, absent minded; he appears quite changed to his companions.
He, 25 - Fickle (capricious); irresolute and wavering in his undertakings.
NUX-V. Al, 71 - She wishes to accomplish much, but thinks it will not succeed.
Ha, 1289 - She wishes to do much, but thinks she will not succeed.
Ha, 1289 - She wishes to do much, but thinks she will not succeed.
He, 23 - Great anxiety of mind without particular cause; thinks she will not be able to get along (prosper) in life; caducity; (senility)...
OP. Al, 70 - Sensation of courage with activity, as if he could forcibly accomplish whatever was required without dread or fear, with a peculiar sensation of lustiness. (strong)
RHUS-T. Al, 40 - Impatient desire to accomplish several kinds of business, chiefly intellectual,...
He, 24-...a week later she told her mother to not look at her (observed) ; seemed to be

distrustful (suspicious) and did not wish to see any one; she came running in from the street and said people were looking at her; ....; cries without cause, imagines people are finding fault (misconduct, criticized, censured) with her because she is earning (succeed, prosper, reach) nothing, acts in a childish manner;...

SIL. Al, 40 - She could and would do nothing on account of ill-humor.

Ha, 14 - She could not and would not attend to anything.

SPONG. Al, 11 - She is dissatisfied with what she accomplishes; she cannot rightly help herself at work (helpless) (incompetent) ; she does not succeed.

Ha, 384 - She is not satisfied with her work; she cannot do her work properly, she is not successful with it.

He, 12 - Feels awkward (unskillful) about her work, which she cannot accomplish (succeed, prosper) satisfactorily.

STANN. Al, 20 - Fruitlessly busy, as if a rush of ideas prevented him from completing his work at a certain time; all sorts of things occur to him to be done.

Ha, 638 - Dawdling and irritable, whith heat of face; she wished to do all sorts of things and could accomplish nothing.

Ha, 639 - Busy uselessness (inefficiency): he exerts (use) himself to get a necessary task (duty) done at the appointed hour, and cannot accomplish it, as though prevented (interrupted) by an over-crowding of thoughts, during which one thing and another occur to him which he wishes to do...

Ha, 7 - Dawdling (indolent) and irritated, with heat in the face; she wanted to do a number of things, but accomplished (complete) nothing.

Ha, 10 - He is ineffectually (inefficiently) busied, as if he was prevented (obstructed) by super abundance of ideas from finishing his work at a certain time; he thinks of a number of things which he ought yet to attend to.

Ha, 8 - Restless and distracted, no perseverance in her work (at once).

SUL-AC. Al, 9 - Hasty (hurried, fast) mood; nothing that she does can be finished quickly enough, though she makes unusual effort.

Ha, 12 - Hastiness (fast) ; everything she does, she cannot accomplish fast enough; but it fatigues her exceedingly.

Ha, 16 - Vexed, peevish, impatient, at once when he does not succeed in his work.

He, 2 - Must do everything in a great hurry; nothing can be finished quickly enough.

SULPH. Al, 94 - He sits for hours immovable and indolent, without definite thought, though he has much to accomplish.

TAB. Al, 51 - Exalted action of the brain; copious flow of ideas; ...leaving me in the morning worn-out and sick, I would conceive and elaborate about twenty undertakings, of which probably not one would ever come to light.

TARAX. Al, 6 - Irresolution and dread of work, though it progresses well as soon as he undertakes it.

He, 3 - Undecided, shunning (avoid) labor, but after beginning, works well.

TARENT. Al, 52 - Worried (troubled) and greatly vexed (disturbing), with much weeping, as if one could not realize (accomplish, complete) something earnestly (ardently) desired.

THER. Al, 3 - Time appears to him to pass more rapidly, although he does very little.

VERAT. Ha, 713 - Busy restlessness; he undertakes many things, but becomes always tired of them, nothing succeeds with him.

He, 8 - Attempts (try) a great many things, but accomplishes (achieve) nothing.

SUFFOCATION

Anger; suffocative attack, with: ***cham.***[54]

Anger; temper tantrums, throw themselves on the floor during, cannot get their breath: thuj.[8]

Anguish; clothing too tight when walking in open air, as if: arg.[36]

Anguish; constricted, as if everything become: ***ars.***[36] chel.[25]

Anguish; oppression with: ***calc.***[54] ***cann-i.***[54] ***op.***[54] verat.[54]

Anxiety; asthma, with: ***arg-n.***[54] ars.[10] ***dig.***[54] hydr-ac.[10] kreos.[10] m-p-a.[10] plat.[10] seneg.[10]

Anxiety; breathing, preventing: acon.[1] ant-t.[5] ***arn.***[5] ars.[1] chlor.[36] croc.[5] eup-per.[25] lyc.[5] **NUX-V.**[5] puls.[5] rhus-t.[5] ***ruta***[5] ***stann.***[5] valer.[5] verat.[1] viol-o.[5]

Anxiety; clothing loosen, must, and open window: nux-v.[122] puls.[122] sulph.[1]
Anxiety; clothing, tight, as if too, walking out doors: arg.[54]
Anxiety; constriction of chest: alum.[54] ars.[36] ***cupr.***[54] gins.[36] ozone[227] ***spig.***[54] stann.[1]
Anxiety; dyspnea, in: ***acet-ac.***[54] acon-f.[36] ars.[60] astac.[54] bism.[54] ***carb-an.***[54] hydr-ac.[60] ***kalm.***[54] kreos.[60] ***lyc.***[54] ***phos.***[54] plat.[60] seneg.[60] **SPONG.**[54] viol-o.[54]
Anxiety; oppressive: acon.[60] alum.[60] am-m.[60] ant-t.[60] ***arn.***[60] ***ars.***[60] ***bell.***[60] calad.[60] calc.[60] ***canth.***[60] **CARB-V.**[54] ***caust.***[60] cham.[60] chel.[60] chin.[60] cina[60] cocc.[60] dig.[60] euph.[60] ***graph.***[60] iod.[60] lact.[60] meny.[60] ***merc.***[60] ***mur-ac.***[60] ***ph-ac.***[54] ***psor.***[54] rhus-t.[60] sep.[60] sil.[60] spig.[60] stront-c.[60] sul-ac.[60] sulph.[1] verat.[60] zinc.[60]
Anxiety; pressure, chest, on, from: ***acon.***[54] aur.[1] **CARB-V.**[54] coca[54] ***dig.***[54] ign.[162] lach.[162] ph-ac.[54] ***plat.***[54] ***psor.***[54] sabad.[54] **SULPH.** ***tab.***[54]
Anxiety; rolling on ground, with, and want of breath: bar-m.[8]
Anxiety; suffocation, with: ***ars.***[54]
Anxiety; suffocation, with, palpitation, and, wakes after midnight: **SPONG.**[54]
Anxiety; suffocation, with, spasms, with, before menses: puls.[54]
Anxiety; suffocation, with, suffocate at night, thinks he will: phos.[54]
Death; conviction of, dyspnea, in: lach.[54] ***mosch.***[54]
Delirium; asphyxia, with: ***ant-t.***[54]
Delusions; animals, snakes, crimson, or, fastening around his neck: bell.
• choked, he will be: ozone[227] phos.[5]
• choked, ice-cold hands, by: canth.
• choked, night on waking: cann-i. phos.[10] ***plat.***[30]
• clothes, tight, too: apis[8] arg.[36] ars-met.[54] benz-ac.[54] chin.[1] glon.[36] paraf.[77] thuj.[36]
• narrow, everything is too: guai. plat.
• room, close and hot, is, oppressing: plan.
• room, small, is too: cycl.[139]
• something comes from above which pressing chest: sep.[1]
• suffocated, she will be: ***stram.***[54]
Dreams; anxious, suffocated, as if: agar.[54]
➤ body, chest, being pressed: am-m.[36]
➤ body, throat, stoppage of the throat: kreos.[36]
➤ children, wanted to save asphyxiated: cass.[36]
➤ dead, bodies, sprang from dissecting table and seized throat: chel.[36]
➤ disease, stoppage, throat: kreos.
➤ disease, suffocation: arn. chel.[193] ign.[162] iris kali-bi. kali-c.[1] sang.[193] xan.[85]
➤ fights, generals, with six or seven black, who garroted him and bound him with ropes, causing agony of mind: coca[36]
➤ gasmasks, people wearing: ozone[227]
➤ meat, thrust into mouth: alum.[36]
➤ stone lying on him: kali-c.
➤ strangle, being: phos. sil. zinc.
➤ strangled, morning, in, fear lest the man who strangled her would return: zinc.[54]
➤ suffocation: arn. chel.[193] ign.[162] iris kali-bi. kali-c.[1] sang.[193] xan.[85]
➤ suffocation, being in danger of, from some one lying on chest: kali-bi.[36]
➤ suffocation, sheet of paper was coming down to smother him, from an immense: merc-i-r.[36]
➤ throat grows up: xan.[85]
Fear; breath, takes away: ***rhus-t.***[54] ***verat.***[54]
✦ choking, of: lyss.[187]
✦ choking, of, inflammation of throat, in: ***hep.***[54]
✦ death, suffocation, from: ***spong.***[54]
✦ lips will grow together, his: stram.[54]
✦ narrow place, claustrophobia: absin.[162] ***acon.*** ***ambr.*** aran.[149] aran-s.[122] ***arg-n.*** ars.[193] bry.[193] ***calc.***[162] carb-an.[193] carc.[207] caust.[193] chin-ar.[162] cimic.[137] cocc.[122] ***dys-co.***[136] ***ign.***[162] kali-ar.[162] kali-c.[193] ***lac-d.***[122] lach.[193] **LYC.**[30] lyss.[162] manc.[162] med.[193] merc-i-f.[193] morg.[136] morg-g.[136] nat-m.[189] nat-s.[193] nux-v.[122] plb.[54] psor.[162] **PULS.**[30] ruta[152] sep.[193] staph.[30] stram. succ.[122] sulph.[122] tab.[122] til.[36] valer.
✦ narrow place, trains and closed places, of: succ.[85]
✦ narrow place, vaults, churches and cellars, of: acon.[137] ***ars.***[116] ***calc.***[116] carb-an.[116] carc.[184] caust.[116] dulc.[137] nat-s.[137] puls.[116] sep.[116] stram.[116]
✦ respiration, of: bell.[8] osm.[36].
✦ strangled, to be: **PLAT.**[122]
✦ subways, of: **ACON.**[162]
✦ suffocation, asthma, with: ***phos.***[54]
✦ suffocation, bed, drives him out of, at night: ***dig.***[54]
✦ suffocation, closing eyes, on: carb-an.
✦ suffocation, dark, in the: aeth.[162]
✦ suffocation, goiter, in: ***merc-i-f.***[122]

✦ suffocation, heart disease, in: ***dig.***[122] lach.[162] ***spong.***[122]
✦ suffocation, lie down, cannot: ars.[172] dig.[172] sil.[172]
✦ suffocation, lying, while: carb-an. mosch.
✦ suffocation, motion, on, with dyspnea: ***spig.***[54]
✦ suffocation, mucus in, bronchi, from: arund.[54]
✦ suffocation, mucus in, throat, from: carb-an.[1]
✦ suffocation, night: agar. ***ant-t.***[122] arn. ars. aur-m.[122] cact. ***chin.***[122] ***dig.***[54] ip.[85] ***lyc.***[54] med.[122] ***puls.***[122] sil.[1] ***spong.***[54] ***sulph.***[122]
✦ suffocation, of: **ACON.**[122] acon-f.[85] am-br.[85] am-c.[144] amyg-am.[122] apis[5] ***ars.***[5] ***bry.***[30] carb-an. ***carb-v.***[5] ***dig.***[122] grin.[5] ***kali-i.***[116] lac-d.[58] lach.[5] lat-m.[102] ***lob.***[54] **LYSS.**[162] merc. mosch.[144] nux-v.[30] ***phos.*** rob. samb.[122] ***spig.***[54] ***spong.***[122] ***staph.***[8] ***stram.*** ***sulph.***[5]
✦ suffocation, palpitations, with, wakes after midnight: **SPONG.**[54]
✦ suffocation, sleeps, when he: bapt.[122]
✦ suffocation, walk about, must: am-br.[85]
✦ throat, sensation of swelling of, from: ***glon.*** nat-m.[1]
✦ toilet, in: ***lac-d.***[122]
✦ trains and closed places: acon.[162] arg-n.[172] bar-c.[30] cimic.[172] dys-co.[136] ferr.[30] nat-m.[172] puls.[30] succ.[85]
✦ tunnels, no light in carriage, with, may cause fainting: stram.[85]
✦ tunnels, of: acon.[162] arg-n.[162] cimic.[172] lyc.[162] nat-m.[172] **STRAM.**[122] succ.[172]

Restlessness; suffocation, with threatening: gels.[85]
Sadness; respiration, impeded: ant-c. caust.[5] lach. laur. ***lyc.***[54] sep. tab.
Suicidal disposition; despair, from, spells of asthma, during: ***rumx.***[54]
Talk; indisposed, closed sensation in throat, with: nat-p.[36]

ACON. He, 37 - Fears to go where is any excitement (tumult) or many people (crowd); thinks she is jostling (pressing) against everyone she meets (oppressed); countenance (expression) expressive of timidity; constant dread (fear) lest she stagger (vacillated) and fall.

APIS. Al, 12 - Dread (fear) of death, or sensation as if he should not be able to breathe again.

He, 59 - Dread of death or sensation as if he should not be able to breath again.

ARS. Al, 34 - Piteous (miserable) complainings (lamenting)... and excessive mental anguish took away his breath ...

Ha, 1021 - On account of increasing pains he appeared to lie at the last gasp (breath), with unspeakable anxiety.

Ha, 1026 - Piteous lamentations, that the most intolerable anxiety, with extremely disagreeable sensation in the whole abdomen, took away his breath and compelled him to curl (bend) himself together now here now there, then again to rise up and walk about.(dyspneia)

BELL. Al, 172 - She tries to strangle herself, and begs the bystanders to kill her, because she believes that she will certainly die.

Al,S-2552-...the yellow corpse of a tall man, shrouded (dressed, clothes) in white, tried to share the patient's bed with him, and the unwelcome visitor was promptly ejected. A crimson serpent came from the foot of the bed, with the design of fastening upon the patient's neck...

BOR. Ha, 4 - Very timid, in driving down a mountain (elevation); quite at variance with his customary bearing; he felt as if it would take his breath away.

GELS. He, 6 - After losing son, inclined to brood over her loss; at times becomes unconscious, or, rather, "rapt"; in imagination thinks herself at the grave; smothered pressure on chest after the spell.

GUAI. Ha, 131 - Whilst he lay asleep on his back, he dreamt that some one was lying on him; from anxiety he could not fetch his breath nor cry out; ...

HURA. Al, 20 - Unusual inclination to weep, even when singing, followed by a suffocative feeling...

IGN. He, 42 - A state of anguish in which she shrieks (scream) for help, with suffocating constriction of throat...

IRID. Sh, 80 - I felt all closed in like I couldn't move, I couldn't breathe. I felt oppressed by being in this room, there's no space. It's funny but I felt like that tonight when I was sitting outside. There were lots of clouds in the sky and it felt like they were coming down on me. Like the sky had been really close and the clouds in the sky were nearer to me; I noticed it because I was watching the moon waxing. It was like I hadn't really noticed the clouds at night before. J5

Sh, 97 - Had a big clearout in the cellar (note: on the same day I was constipated!) .Enjoyed this spring cleaning and throwing loads of stuff away. I was making space for ex-partner to store stuff he still has in house which is suffocating me. I need the space to breathe. Feeling that if he doesn't put his things into the space in the cellar I shall explode. Generally not as lax about things, giving people the "hard word." G[11] suffocation, organization

LACH. He, 60 - After a jealous quarrel, she put both hands to her chest and cried out "Oh! my heart!" then fell down and was in an asphyctic state for nearly twenty-four hours;...

NUX-V. He, 38 - Three months ago mental shock, since then fears to be alone,...fears as if she would choke (suffocation)...fears to be alone, fear of knives and the like, (similar) lest she should kill herself or others...

PSOR. He, 15 - Great fear of death; anxiety about heart and dyspnea,...

SPONG. He, 19 - She is very fretful and anxious about her condition, fears she will die of suffocation.

He, 24 - Terror and fear: of approaching death; that she will die of suffocation; with heart disease;...

STRAM. He, 71 - Fears; he will lose his senses (insanity); his lips will grow together; to suffocate; of falling; everything is falling on her.

THUJ. Al, 64 - Frightful anxiety, like death agony; a nameless internal ache, as if the soul were escaping from the body (split), with most terrible uneasiness, frightful orgasm of blood, at night, even to suffocation.

ZINC. He, 43 - Great fear, as if persecuted by men or the devil, on account of crimes he has never done (injustice); is afraid of becoming imprisoned, or poisoned, or shot, or buried (inter) alive...[0] Delirium tremens.

SUICIDAL

Anger; tear himself to pieces, could: sulph.[54]

Anguish; evening, suicidal thoughts, with: hep.[102]

Anguish; self-destruction, increasing to: aur.[172]

Anguish; suicide, attempts to commit: ***hep.***[54]

Anxiety; suicidal disposition, with: ***aur.*** bell.[10] carc.[214] caust. chin.[10] ***dros.*** hep. ***merc.*** nux-v. plat. ***puls. rhus-t.*** staph

Bed; jumps out of, wants to destroy himself but lacks courage: chin.

Death; desires, meditates on easiest way of self destruction: lac-d.[8]

Delirium; throwing from windows: ***aeth.***[54] calc.[58] sil.[58]

Delirium; throwing from, height, a: **BELL.**[36]

Delirium; water, jumping into: bell. sec.

Delusions; hang, wants to hang himself: ***ars.***[116]
- man, hung himself, saw, who: ars.
- mushroom, he is commanded to fall on his knees and confess his sins and rip up his bowels by a: agar.
- rags, body torn into: phyt.[137]
- suicide, driving to: ars.[10] hyos.[10] verat.[10]

Desires; poison, another portion of: op.[36]

Despair; religious, suicidal tendency, with: verat.[54]

Dreams; disease, injuries, self-inflicted: nicc.
- ➤ poison, that he has taken: ***kreos.***
- ➤ poisoned, by herself: kali-n.[36]
- ➤ suicide: hydrog.[222] naja polym.[111] rad-br.[144]
- ➤ window, jumping from: mag-m.

Fear; alone, of being, injure himself, and: ars. merc.[137] nat-s.[137]
- ✦ death, suicidal tendency, with: **NUX-V.**[54] ***plat.***[54]
- ✦ high places, throw himself down, lest he: arg-n.[172]
- ✦ impulses, of his own: alum.[111] androc.[222] germ.[222] osm.[36]
- ✦ suicide, knife, with a: merc.[162]
- ✦ suicide, of: ***alum.*** arg-n. ***ars.*** lach.[172] med.[179] ***merc. nat-s. nux-v.***[54] plat.[54] ***rhus-t.*** sep. tub.[172]

Hypochondriasis; suicide, leading to: alum.[30] aur.[30] calc.[30] caust.[30] chin.[30] con.[30] graph.[30] hep.[10] ***nat-m.***[30] sep.[30] **STAPH.**[30] sulph.[30]

Impatience; suicidal desperation, with: carb-v.[1]

Impulse; stab his flesh with the knife he holds, to: ***lyss.***.

Inconsolable; suicide, even to: **CHIN.**[54]

Injure; herself, himself, feels could, rage, out of: agar. germ.[222] lyss.[36]

Injure; satiety of life, must use self-control to prevent shooting himself: ***nat-s.***

Insanity; suicidal disposition, with: ars.[10] hyos.[10] naja[130] orig.[25] verat.[10]

Irritability; anxiety, with, suicide, with inclination to commit, afraid to die: **NUX-V.**[54]

Jumping; impulse to, height, from a: anac. ***arg-n.*** **AUR.** gels. lap-mar-c.[194] staph.

Jumping; impulse to, river, into: ***arg-n.*** sec. sil.

Jumping; impulse to, window, from: ***aeth.*** arg-n.[122] ars. **AUR.** bell. calc.[161] calc-sil.[58] camph. ***carbn-s.*** chin. crot-c. gels. ***glon.*** thea. thuj. verat.

Jumping; impulse to, window, from, dash herself down, or, during parturition: aur.[54]

Jumping; impulse to, window, from, pain makes her so despaired that she would like to: ***aur.***[54]

Kill; sudden impulse to, herself: iod.[137] meli.[137] merc.[58] ***nat-s.*** ***nux-v.***[54] rumx.[185] thea.[36] thuj.

Loathing; life, of, restrain herself, must, to prevent doing herself injury: **NAT-S.**

Mania; suicidal: ***ars.***[54] ***verat.***[54]

Mania; suicidal, sexual symptoms, with: ***aur.***[54]

Medicine; drugs, desire to swallow large doses of: cact.[36]

Rage; suicidal disposition, with: ant-t.[10] sec.[116] stram.[10]

Sadness; suicidal disposition, with: alum.[30] **AUR.**[54] calc.[30] caust.[30] chin.[30] cimic.[54] con.[30] graph.[30] ***hep.***[54] hydrog.[222] ign.[30] med.[54] ***merc-aur.***[116] ***naja***[54] ***nat-m.***[30] ***nat-s.***[116] op.[36] orni.[144] ***psor.***[36] ran-b.[54] rumx.[54] sep.[30] ***spig.***[54] **STAPH.**[30] sulph.[30]

Striking; knocking his head against wall, and things: apis ars. bac.[55] **BELL.**[122] con. hyos. mag-c. **MILL.**[122] ozone[227] ***phos.***[184] rhus-t. scut.[193] syph.[85] **TUB.**[122]

Suicidal disposition: alco.[36] ***alum.***[122] alum-p.[58] alum-sil.[58] am-c. ambr. ***anac.*** anan. anh.[144] ***ant-c.*** ***ant-t.*** arg-n. ***ars.*** asaf. **AUR.** aur-ar.[58] **AUR-M.** aur-m-n.[85] aur-s.[58] ***bell.***[122] berb.[10] bov.[10] buni-o.[149] ***calc.*** calc-sil.[58] camph.[1] ***caps.*** carb-v. carc.[144] caust. chel.[5] ***chin.*** chin-ar. cic. ***cimic.*** clem. crot-h. cur. der. dros. fuli.[102] gels. graph.[30] grat. hell. ***hep.*** hipp. hydr-ac.[10] hydrog.[222] ***hyos.*** ***ign.***[102] iod. ***iodof.***[116] kali-ar. ***kali-br.*** kali-chl.[10] kreos. ***lac-d.*** ***lach.*** lap-mar-c.[194] laur.[10] led.[10] lil-t. lyc.[58] med. meli. ***merc.*** ***merc-aur.***[102] mez. morg.[136] morph. naja nat-c.[10] ***nat-m.***[30] **NAT-S.** nit-ac. ***nux-m.*** ***nux-v.*** op.[30] orig. orni.[144] ozone[227] phos. plat. ***plb.*** **PSOR.**[122] ***puls.*** rauw.[119] reser.[149] rhus-t. rumx. ruta[10] sarr. sec. ***sep.*** sil. ***spig.*** spong.[10] staph.[30] ***stram.*** sul-ac.[10] sulph. tab. tarent. ter. thal.[85] thea. thlaspi[98] thuj. thuj-l.[149] tub.[111] ust.[102] verat. ***zinc.*** zinc-p.[58] ziz.[102]

Suicidal disposition; abortion, in threatening: aur.[26]

Suicidal disposition; anger driving to suicide: carb-v.[10]

Suicidal disposition; axe, with an: naja.

Suicidal disposition; cancer patients, in: carc.[85] scirr.[85]

Suicidal disposition; car, throw himself in front of a: ozone[227]

Suicidal disposition; children, in: aur.[161]

Suicidal disposition; courage, but lacks: alum. **CHIN.** nit-ac. **NUX-V.** ozone[227] phos. plat. rhus-t. ***sulph.***[54] tab.

Suicidal disposition; delivery, parturition, during: aur.[54]

Suicidal disposition; despair, about his miserable existence: ***sep.***[54]

Suicidal disposition; despair, from: ambr.[116] ant-c.[54] carb-v.[116] hyos.[116]

Suicidal disposition; despair, from, religious: verat.[54]

Suicidal disposition; despair, from, spells of asthma, during: ***rumx.***[54]

Suicidal disposition; drowning, by: ant-c. ***arg-n.***[122] ***aur.***[5] ***bell.*** ***dros.*** ***hell.*** hep.[116] ***hyos.*** ign. ***lach.*** nux-v.[30] ped.[122] ***puls.*** ***rhus-t.*** sec. ***sil.*** staph.[30] sulph. ***ust.***[184] verat.

Suicidal disposition; drowning, by, love, from disappointed: ***hyos.***[54]

Suicidal disposition; drowning, by, mania, in: sec.[54]

Suicidal disposition; drowning, by, seeks to escape, after menses: ***ign.***[54]

Suicidal disposition; drowning, by, thinks with pleasure of: ***puls.***[54]

Suicidal disposition; easiest way, asks questions as to quietest and: ***lac-d.***[54]

Suicidal disposition; erotomania, in: orig.[137]
Suicidal disposition; fear of death, with: alum.[54] **ARS.**[94] aur.[94] ***chin.***[30] hep.[94] kali-ar.[58] **NIT-AC.**[30] nux-v.[94] ***plat.***[54] rhus-t.[58] ***staph.***[30] tab.[36]
Suicidal disposition; fire, to set oneself on: ***ars.***[122] hep.[58]
Suicidal disposition; fright, after: ***ars.***[1] puls.[172]
Suicidal disposition; gas, by: ars.[30] nux-v.[30]
Suicidal disposition; hanging, by: **ARS.**[122] aur.[58] ***bell.***[122] carb-v.[30] hell.[58] nat-s. ter.
Suicidal disposition; homesickness, from: caps.[5]
Suicidal disposition; knife, razor with a: acon.[30] alum.[122] ***stram.***[54]
Suicidal disposition; knife, with a: alum. ***ars.*** bell. ***calc.*** hyos.[30] ***merc.*** nux-v.[137] stram.
Suicidal disposition; knife, with a, cutting his throat: alum.[171]
Suicidal disposition; love, from disappointed: ant-c.[188] ***aur.***[54] bell.[137] caust.[137] ***hyos.***[54] staph.[137]
Suicidal disposition; love, from disappointed, weeping, with: ***aur.***[54]
Suicidal disposition; mania, in, puerperal, with aversion to husband, baby and coition: agn.[171]
Suicidal disposition; music, from listening to: nat-c.[58]
Suicidal disposition; poison, by: ars.[30] ***bell.***[30] ign.[54] lil-t. op.[36] puls.[30]
Suicidal disposition; prepares himself silently: <u>**AUR.**</u>[122]
Suicidal disposition; run over, to be: alum.[116] ars.[116] aur.[116] kali-br.[5] lach.[30] pitu-a.[164]
Suicidal disposition; seeing blood or a knife, she has horrid, thoughts of killing herself, though she abhors the idea: ***alum.***
Suicidal disposition; seeing, an open window or knives: arg-n. camph. chin. ***merc.***
Suicidal disposition; seeing, blood or a knife, shaving, when: alum.[122]
Suicidal disposition; seeing, open windows or knife: arg-n. camph. chin. ***merc.***
Suicidal disposition; shooting, by: alum.[116] anac. ***ant-c.*** aur. calc.[30] carb-v. chin.[30] hep. med. nat-m.[30] nat-s. nit-ac.[162] nux-v. op.[30] puls. sep.[30] **STAPH.**[30] sulph.[30]
Suicidal disposition; shooting, by, must use all self control: ***nat-s.***[54]
Suicidal disposition; shooting, by, night, at, obliged to get out of bed because he cannot put off the idea: ant-c.[36]
Suicidal disposition; starving, by: merc.[5]
Suicidal disposition; talks always of suicide, but does not commit: <u>**NUX-V.**</u>[122]
Suicidal disposition; thoughts: agn.[58] alum. alum-p.[58] alum-sil.[58] ***anac.***[184] ***ant-c.*** arg-n. **AUR. AUR-S.**[58] but-ac.[102] ***caps.***[122] dros. fuli.[102] ***hep.*** hydrog.[222] ***ign.*** iris[152] kali-ar.[58] kali-br. lac-d.[58] lach.[58] lil-t. med.[171] ***merc.*** naja[141] **NAT-S.** nit-ac.[162] prot.[149] **PSOR.** ***puls. rhus-t.*** thuj. ***thuj-l.***[149] zinc-p.[58]
Suicidal disposition; thoughts, drive him out of bed: ***ant-c.***
Suicidal disposition; thoughts, spermatorrhea from masturbation, in: ***gels.***[54]
Suicidal disposition; throwing himself from, height, a: anac. ***arg-n.*** ars. **AUR. BELL.**[122] camph. crot-h. gels. glon.[5] hydrog.[222] hyos.[30] ign.[122] iod.[5] iodof.[116] lach.[5] ***lyss.***[162] ***nux-v.*** orig. sec.[30] ***sel.***[162] sil.[30] staph.[58] stram. ***sulph.***[54] x-ray[152]
Suicidal disposition; throwing, windows, from: ***aeth.*** arg-n.[122] ***ars.***[122] **AUR.** aur-ar.[58] bell. camph. ***carbn-s.*** chin. crot-c. gels. ***glon. iod.***[116] ***iodof.***[116] nux-v.[116] ***sulph.***[54] thea. thuj. verat.
Suicidal disposition; waking, on: lyc. med.[179] nat-c.
Tears; himself: ars. bell. cur. lach.[189] plb. sec. **STRAM.**
Thoughts; frightful, seeing blood, or a knife, on: ***alum.***
Weeping; fear of losing reason, or that she might commit suicide, with: ***puls.***[54]

ADAM. Sh, 246 - Cried with despair. Nothing I do is right. Rocking from side to side, sobbing. Desire to stab with a knife or scissors. Felt very different from other humans. Long, late phone call ameliorates. 16, 12C, 43:XX:XX
Sh, 374 - Joyless, desired death. Looked at a pair of scissors and thought of suicide. 16, 12C, 17:XX:XX
Sh, 376 - Cried with despair. Nothing I do is right. Rocking from side to side sobbing. Desire to stab with a knife or scissors. Felt very different from other humans. Long, late phone call ameliorates. 16, 12C, 43:XX:XX
AETH. Al, 9 - Delirium; he jumps out of window.
AGAR. Al, 2 - He becomes so furious that

he can hardly be restrained from ripping up his bowels, as he fancies the mushroom had ordered him to do.

Ha, 23 - Fearless, threatening, destructive frenzy, also such as turns against itself and injures itself, combined with great exertion of strength.

ALUM. Ha, 22 - She cannot see blood nor a knife without horrible thoughts pressing in upon her, as if she should, e. g. commit suicide; though she has the greatest horror of it.

He, 21 - Dread (fear) of death, with thoughts of suicide.

He, 9 - Mania to kill himself with a sharp weapon.

He, 10 - Seeing blood on a knife, she has horrid ideas of killing herself, though she abhors the idea.

ANT-C. Ha, 8 - Decided impulse to shoot himself, at night, but no inclination to any other kind of suicide; ...

Ha, 23 - Ecstasy and exalted love, with great anxiety about his fate (destiny, doom), and inclination to shoot himself;...

He, 20 - Is driven to despair, resolved to drown himself.

He, 6 - Inclined to suicide by shooting; at night he is obliged to get out of bed, because he cannot free himself of the idea.

ANT-T. Al, 2 - Suicidal mood; he raves (talk incoherently) and does not know what he is doing.

ARG-N. He, 20 - Thoughts about suicide.

He, 22 - On crossing a bridge, almost irresistible desire to jump into river; meeting some one prevented it.

He, 21 - Thinks about killing himself.

ARS. Al, 6 - After midnight, a frequent desire to kill himself, by stabbing his heart through and through.

Ha, 1032 - Mania; first headache, horrible anxiety, noise before the ears, as from a number of large bells, and when he opened the eyes, he always saw a man who had (formerly) hung himself (suicidal, justified) on the ground-floor of the house, who incessantly beckoned (call) him to cut him down (help); he ran thither (there) with a knife, but, as he could not cut him down, (rescue) he became overwhelmed (beaten) with despair (remorse?) and wished (as his friends assured him) to hang himself (punish); but being prevented (stop) from doing so, he became so restless that he could hardly be kept in bed,... and he knelt down and raised his hands in a supplicating manner.

Ha, 71 - During the first minutes great tranquillity of soul and serenity; but after half a hour excessive restlessness and anxiety; he imagines that the effects of the poison would be dreadful and desires to remain alive.(in a despondent suicide).

He, 25 - Mania...sees a man who has hanged himself beckoning (call) him to cut him loose (rescue, deliverance, free, saving) on failing to accomplish this he attempts to hang himself (punish, penalize);...finally kneels down and lifts his hands in supplication.(forgiveness, absolution)

He, 27 - Suicidal mania.

He, 77 - Terrible anxiety, flushing up; restless glance (look), no rest by day or night; inclination to commit suicide.

AUR-M. Al, 5 - Disgust for life; inclination to suicide.

He, 3 - Inclined to suicide; frequent weeping; aversion to occupation.

AUR. Ha, 10 - Great anguish, mounting even to suicide with spasmodic contraction in the abdomen.

He, 22 - Disposition to commit suicide.

He, 53 - Great anguish increasing unto self-destruction, with spasmodic contraction of abdomen.

He, 8 - Looks on dark side, weeps, prays, thinks she is not fit for this world, longs for death, strong inclination to commit suicide; desperate, desires to jump from a height.

He, 59 - Disappointed love, with weeping and inclination to commit suicide.

He, 17 - Suicidal mania or melancholia, tedium vitae, with genital symptoms.(sexual)

He, 43 - Is very unhappy; continued thought of suicide. 0Puerperal mania.

BELL. Al, 161 - In walking in the open air, she is overwhelmed with tearful anguish; she is weary of life, and inclines to drown herself.

Al, 96 - In his delirium he threw himself down from a height.

Al, 172 - She tries to strangle herself, and begs the bystanders to kill her, because she believes that she will certainly die.

Ha, 1381-...she is weary of life, and wishes to go into the water to drown herself.

Ha, 1390 - Excessive indifference, for hours; one might take her life, she would not stir. (move) (immobility)

Ha, 1437 - She tries to strangle herself, and begs those about her to kill her, for this time she must die. (redemption, regeneration, salvation)

Ha, 1439 - Throws herself down from a height.(in delirium)

Ha, 1440 - Throws herself into water. (drowning)

He, 53 - Weary of life, with desire to drown herself.

CACT. Al, 17 - Feeling of doing violence (injury) to myself.

Al, 4 - Felt decided impulses to swallow large and unwholesome portions of medicine.

CALC. He, 18 - Mental aberration with horrid visions before eyes and cardiac anxiety; he despairs of his salvation (pardon, rescue) and wants to stab himself.

CAMPH. Al, 46-...For a moment I resolved to throw myself from the window and sweep through the domain of my infernal kingdom, but a weak glimmer of reason held me back...

Al, 19 - Stripped naked, he danced wildly about, and attempted to jump out of the window.

He, 36 - Impulse to jump out the window.

He, 51 - Strips (undress) himself (naked), and tries to jump out of window.

CAPS. He, 4 - Haunted (obsessed) by a disposition to suicide.

CARB-V. Ha, 714 - Peevish, impatient and desperate, so much so that he would like to shoot himself.

Ha, 10 - Great disposition to weep, he wishes to shoot himself.

Ha, 21 - Peevish, impatient, desperate, so that he would like to shoot himself.

CHIN. Ha, 1093-...;he jumps out of the bed and wants to make away whith himself (suicide), and yet he fears to go near and open window or to approach a knife.

He, 16-...;wants to destroy himself, but lacks courage.

He, 27 - Inconsolable anxiety, even to suicide.

CIMIC. He, 21 - Mental depression, with suicidal mood; also after checked neuralgia.

CLEM. Al, 11 - Very sad humor with thoughts of suicide.

CROT-C. Al, 5 - She stands for ten minutes on the window-sill, and is arrested when on the point of throwing herself off.

CUR. Al, 13 - Disposition to suicide.

DER. Al, 2 - He desires death and will attempt (try) suicide.

DROS. Ha, 277 - Anxiety; ...,as if he were impelled to jump into the water in order to take his own life by drowning he was not impelled to any other mode of death.

He, 3 - Anxiety: with flushes of heat; when alone (solitude), ...as if it would impel him to commit suicide by drowning. (water will purify?)

GLON. He, 9 - Frantic; attempted to jump from the window.

HALI-L. Sh, 350-... "Considered committing suicide. Feeling that life has passed me by. Thinking about my mortality. Terrified of dying. My time has run out." ...[18], 30C, 05:XX:XX-[16]:XX:XX

Sh, 433 - Feel self-destructive, like eating greasy fatty junk food, not exercising, slowly kill myself that way. Why care? 06, 6C, 10:XX:XX

Sh, 436 - About suicide; I would never have entertained a thought to do something like this. The thought of suicide was destined to make me look beyond it. It wasn't a game. It was just part of a phase that was passing—the last rung of it. 18, 30C, 35:XX:XX

HELL. He, 12 - An old woman having been accused of theft by the women around, took it so much to heart that she hanged herself. This suicide produced a profound effect upon the women of the village. One after another accused herself of having caused the death of the old woman by their insinuations; they wept and howled, ran about day and night wringing their hands and despairing of salvation on account of their sin (error); they became quite irrepressible and deranged (disordered) In this way twenty - four or twenty five women were affected, every fresh case being followed by another. Hysterical mania.

He, 20 - After typhoid, ...sits quietly in bed and seems lost in brooding;...constantly seeks (try) to escape, ...;without a word quietly climbs out of the window, and if she succeeds in escaping goes in direction of river; finally threw herself into privy (toilet), from which she was rescued.

He, 19 - Tries to escape, to throw herself into the river.

HEP. Ha, 296 - In the evening a frightful anxiety for two hours; he thought he must be ruined (lost, failed), and was sad to that degree that he could have killed himself.

Ha, 4 - Fearful anguish, in the evening, for two hours; he thought he had to perish (die), and was sad even so that he could have committed suicide. (redemption, salvation)

He, 14 - Low spirited, even to thoughts of suicide.

He, 17 - Impelled by unaccountable attacks of internal anguish, which sometimes come on quite suddenly, to attempt suicide.

HIPP. Al, 8 - Ill-humored, weary of life, even to suicide, in both provings.

HYDROG. Sh, 33 - About two months after beginning the proving, developed an extreme range of mental symptoms that he had never had before. These included severe depression with strong alternations of moods, & high then low &, with suicidal tendency, desire to jump from a high building or cut wrist, confusion of identity (especially concerning sex and homosexuality) and became more religious. He moved away from his parents home (which he had never before been able t o do) and shut himself away in a small flat. This condition lasted for another six or seven months and was finally antidoted by Phosphorus 200. Before that, he had tried to anti-dote it with acupuncture, to no avail. 24, 30C, 60:XX:XX

Sh, 158 - Thoughts of death and suicide. 16, 30C, 25:XX:XX

Sh, 274 - Developed an aversion to the idea of sex —confused about sexual issues and identity. Became aware of being bi-sexual or homosexual (in a man). "I want to find out who I am. I should know at 23. I used to know. What am I sexually?" Very confused. This led to suicidal depression. 24, 30C, 100:XX:XX

HYOS. Al, 82 - In despair, he wishes to drown himself.

Ha, 579 - In despair he wishes to take his life, and throw himself into the water.(suicidal)

He, 50 - Tendency to action: wants to kill somebody or himself.

He, 74 - Disappointed love followed by: epilepsy, melancholy, rage, or inclination to laugh at everything; despair and propensity to drown himself. (ailments from)

IGN. He, 11-...believes herself married (connected) and pregnant; is tormented by remorse of imagined crimes; seeks constantly to escape to drown (suicide) herself; ...;is only quiet when lying undisturbed and brooding over her troubles, which she rehearses (tell) in a doleful (unhappy) tone ;..." I am neglecting my duty, breaking my vow" (promise, engagement)...;conscientious scruples after eating.

He, 61 - Melancholia after great grief and domestic trouble; complete sleeplessness; suicidal thoughts and desire to escape.

He, 41 - Altered appearance; made an unsuccessful attempt to end his most unendurable (intolerable) sufferings, by eating the phosphorus from matches; after business embarrassment.

KALI-BR. Al, 3-...his character also had undergone a radical change, from having been very frank and brave, he had become excessively timid, and suspicious of every trifling circumstance; ...several times he attempted to throw himself from a window and battered down a door with an axe, in order to escape from some imaginary danger;...

LAC-D. Al,N-1 - Depression of spirits; don't care to live (indifferent) ; question as to quietest and most certain way of hastening (accelerate) one's death.

He, 2 - Depression of spirits; don't care to live, question as to quietest and most certain way of hastening one's death.

LACH. He, 8 - Thinks: she is somebody else in the hands (seized) of a stronger power; (supremacy, superiority).or that she is dead, and preparations are made for funeral (cortege) or that she is nearly dead and wishes some one would help her off; herself pursued by enemies, or fears medicine is poison; there are robbers in house and wants to jump out the window; herself under super-human control; visions real, he will die. (helplessness, desire; aid, comfort, salvation)

He, 45 - She is tormented by the idea that her better principles (ideals) might be overcome (beaten) by irresistible desire to suicide. (lost: moral) 0 Mania.

He, 22 - She is tempted to commit suicide.

LIL-T. Al, 16 - Worse on going to bed; can't go to sleep; wild (tumultuous, uncontrollable) feeling in the head as though I should go crazy (insane) and no one would take care of me (forsaken, helpless); thoughts of suicide; how much opium would put me to sleep forever, and who would find my body, and who would care; ... (friendless, abandoned, deserted)

LYSS. Al,N-34-....to stab his flesh with the knife he is holding, and the like.

MED. Al,N-50 - It is always anticipating, fearing evil will happen, loss of reason or suicide.

Al,N-25 - Tendency to suicide, gets up in night and takes his pistol, but his wife prevents him.

He, 24 - Tendency to suicide, gets up in night and takes his pistol (gun), but his wife prevents him.

MERC. He, 22 - Great desire to murder (homicidal) or committed suicide ...is fearful that she may commit some wrong and kill herself (punishment); something urges her to kill her husband, of whom she is very fond (loving), and she implores him to hide his razor (knife).

He, 30 - Anxiety driving her to suicide ; thoughts of suicide; ...desire for death; great indifference even to those she formerly loved;...

He, 20 - After suppression of foot sweat, whenever he sees an open window or cutting instruments breaks into a sweat, with great heat of head, and is seized with an almost uncontrollable desire to commit suicide.

MORPH. Al, 13 - Complete melancholy, so that he desired to commit suicide.

NAJA. Al, 3-...having an axe in his hand,...he suddenly split his head in two; he had become insane.

NAT-S. He, 4 - Satiety (weary) of life; must use all self-control to prevent shooting himself.

NUX-V. Al, 6 - The usual pain seems intolerable; she would rather take her life.

Al, 5-(Suicide; she throws herself down from a height)

Ha, 1238 - After midnight very violent palpitation of the heart with extreme anxiety, which urges (impulse) him to commit suicide.

Ha, 1239 - She deems (believe) the pain she suffers intolerable and will rather take her own life.

Ha, 1241-(Suicide; she throws herself from a height.)

Ha, 1240 - Anxiety with impulse to commit suicide.

He, 38 - Three months ago mental shock, since then fears to be alone,...fears as if she would choke (suffocation)...fears to be alone, fear of knives and the like, (similar) lest she should kill herself or others...

He, 21 - Anxiety with irritability and inclination to commit suicide, but is afraid to die.

OP. Al, 39-...threatened alternately self-destruction and injury to others.

PHOS. Al, 40 - As the darkness of night began to enclose (surround) the earth, my peace was disturbed by the most frightful visions and thoughts; constant fear of death, with an almost uncontrollable desire to commit suicide.

PLAT. He, 46-...;suffers unspeakable pangs (anxiety) of conscience in consequence of a faux (fault, mistake, embarrassing mistake?) pass when thirty-two years old; says she has brought disgrace upon her family, and that she has incurred the penalty of damnation; (doomed) in order to do penance (penitence) gave away whatever she could lay her hands upon, (redemption) so that she had to be constantly watched; after her confessor asserted that she could not hope for pardon or heaven (condemnable), she seemed in absolute despair ; bemoaned her misery throughout the night, wringing her hands and beseeching (implore) that she might be delivered (free) from the hell of her conscience; twice attempted self-destruction (suicide);...wished to live and do penance (penitence, purgation, purification) in order to mitigate her eternal punishment.

PLB. Al, 112 - He is very sad, has no desire to live, and has threatened to destroy himself, and is very fault-finding (severe, critical) with his friends.

He, 16 - Mental disturbance of eight or ten years' duration in a man addicted to masturbation; has several times attempted suicide; has been in seclusion (solitude); greatest dejection and despair;...; believes himself lost (condemned) ; has the sounds of hell constantly in his ears; hears voices and sees shadows of demons, great disposition to make away (suicide) with himself or do himself some bodily injury;

PSOR. Al, 13 - She is so downhearted (unhappy) that she could commit suicide, then is full of phantasms.

Al,N-44 - Mania of self-destruction.

Al,N-21 - Very depressed, sad, suicidal thoughts.

Al,N-27 - Is so downhearted she could commit suicide, then is so full of phantasms.

He, 21 - Very depressed, sad, suicidal thoughts.

He, 27 - Is so downhearted she could committed suicide, then is full of phantasms.

PULS. Ha, 1114 - Anxiety in the region of the heart, with suicidal impulse, and feeling or inclination to vomit in the scrobiculus cordis.

He, 21 - Continuous crying with great melancholy and fear of losing her reason, or that she might commit suicide.

He, 25 - Weary of life; thinks with pleasure of drowning. (suicide, water)

He, 26 - Anxiety: thinks to die; does not know what to do; as if in a hot atmosphere; in region of heart; even to suicide;...

He, 27 - Anguish in region of heart, sometimes increasing to a desire for suicide.

He, 52 - After mortification, sad gloomy (melancholy) and weary (disgusted) of life;...thinks of drowning with great pleasure;...

RHUS-T. Ha, 970 - In the dusk, towards evening, anxiety and anguish, as if he would kill himself, for an hour.

He, 11 - Anxiety: while sitting was obliged to take hold (grasp, keep) of something because she did not think she could keep up (support) on account of the beating and drawing pains in limbs; and apprehension as if he wished to take his own life; with loss of strength (vigor, vitality) as if he would die.

He, 18 - Disgust of life: thoughts of suicide; wants to drown (immerse) himself; with fear of death: with desire to die, without sadness.

RUMX. He, 1 - Low-spirited: with serious expression of face; with suicidal mood.

SEC. Al, 10 - Raving (talk wildly), whith an attempt to jump into the water.

He, 4 - Mania; with inclination to bite; with inclination to drown.

SEP. Al, 36 - The greatest loathing of life; it seemed to him as if he could not endure so miserable an existence any longer, and as if he would pine away (longing, wanting) if he did not kill himself. (pine = intense longing or grief)

Ha, 31 - Extreme loathing of life (existence he felt as if he could not any longer bear this miserable (wretched, unhappy) existence, and as if he would pine away (ruined) unless he made away with himself.-(suicidal)

He, 28 - Propensity to suicide from despair about his miserable (wretched, unfortunate) existence.

SIL. He, 15 - Wishes to drown herself.

SPIG. Al, 17 - Extreme ill humor in the evening; he could kill himself, with chilliness of the body.

Ha, 664 - Great dejection, in the evening; he could have killed himself...

He, 4 - Gloomy suicidal mood.

STRAM. Ha, 547 - Furious endeavor to kill himself.

He, 155 - Disposition to suicide; wanted a razor (blade, knife) to cut his throat.

He, 100-...threatens to knock everybody down, to break furniture, to throw himself out of window.

SULPH. He, 35-...,strong impulsive tendency to suicide, by drowning or by

precipitating herself from window;...(high, water)
He, 37 - Great dejection,(grief), with thoughts of suicide; feels inferior (mediocre, lower) to everybody; can decide nothing;...

TER. He, 12 - Suicide by hanging, in two cases followed washing of laces in oil of turpentine and alcohol.

THEA. Al, 4 - Sensation as if impelled by some uncontrollable power to commit suicide, to jump out of window, to put her baby in the boiler with the clothes, to cut its throat while cutting bread, to throw it downstairs (in a woman who kept a pot of tea boiling on the stove and drank several bowlfuls every day; cured with tea cm, Finckle)

THUJ. Al, 1 - She herself desires, with anxiety and despair, to be taken to an insane asylum, (imprisonment, confining) and there to be treated very harshly and strictly, (penalized), so that her fixed ideas may be subdued and banished (purified); she knows very well that she does wrong (conscience) and thinks all sorts of bad thoughts (immoral), but she will not take the trouble to banish such thoughts; therewith she indistinctly gives to understand that she is constantly obliged to think of taking her own life, but feels the sinfulness (wicked) of it, in order to avoid it, desires the strict restraint of the asylum;...
Al, 7 - She constantly longs for the offices of the church in order to banish her sinful thoughts of suicide. (redemption, salvation)
He, 23 - Mental depression, after childbirth (puerperal), in consequence of being told that there had been a slight rupture (division, hurt) of perineum; grows quiet; thinks she must die;...wants to jumps the window; does not care for children or her relatives (careless) ;..(sensitive to disrupt, partition)

VALER. Al, 1 - Extremely delirious, attempting to get out of the window, ... imagined himself away from home, and beset (surrounded) with all sorts of danger, from which he was attempting to escape, although unable to walk without staggering from side to side.

VERAT. He, 10 - Suicidal tendency from religious despair.
He, 54 - Despair of his recovery; attempts suicide.

SUPERNATURAL

Comprehension; ritualistic: anh.[212] ars.[187] con.[187] cupr.[210] iod.[187] lyss.[187] pin-s.[120] rhus-t.[187] tub.[187]

Delusions; hearing, of, tone, comes from another world: **CARB-AN.**[54]
- hearing, tone, comes from another world: **CARB-AN.**[54]
- journey, traveling through worlds: aether bell.[72]
- light, incorporeal, immaterial, he is, walking while: spig.[137] thuj.[139]
- music, unearthly: aether cann-s.[122]
- paradise, he sees: coff.
- superhuman, control, is under: agar. anac. carc.[207] ***lach. naja*** op.[102] plat.[102] psil.[164] ***thuj.***
- superhuman, is: cann-i. psil.[164]
- transferred to another, world: cann-i.
- unearthly, of something: cann-i.[36]
- world, new world, he is moving in a: camph.[139]

Dreams; supernatural things: asc-t.[36]

Fear; superstitious: rhus-t.

Inquisitive; supernatural or spiritual matters, about: calc.[162]

Superstitious: agar.[187] arg-n.[162] bell.[5] carc.[207] ***con.*** kali-ar.[184] ***med.***[162] op.[5] phel.[231] rat.[162] rhus-t.[36] stram.[5] syph.[162] tub.[162] zinc.

HALI-L. Sh, 792 - Parallel universes—all happening somewhere else. Everything in home, food, etc.: carry in. I felt maybe I was in a parallel universe and it's all happening the same somewhere else. Not lonely. Just what happens. 20, 30C, 03:23:00

IRID. Sh, 118 - Thoughts: Wind is breath of the spirit; love is the greatest of all messages between heaven and earth. Yes, go to heaven, but return to the world transformed by the light of experience, transcend and return; Metals —immortality; need knowledge of their names; Iridescence, oil mother of pearl metal, rainbow, seven plus seven, cosmic joke, messages in other languages —language of angels?; Seven heavens, seven earths. I adore these territories, not so much new as forgotten. Q20

SUPPRESSED

Affection; demonstrate, cannot: nat-m.[189] sep.[137]
Ailments from; anger, grief, with silent: **ACON.**[5] alum. am-m.[116] ars. aur. aur-ar.[58] bell. **BRY.**[5] carc.[210] ***cham.***[5] ***chin.***[116] ***cocc. coloc. gels.***[5] hyos. **IGN. LYC.** nat-c. ***nat-m.*** nux-v. ***ph-ac.*** phos. plat. puls. **STAPH.** verat. ***zinc.***[5]
Ailments from; anger, suppressed: agar.[198] ***aur.***[54] bamb-a.[1184] ***cand-a.***[239] carc.[207] cham. germ.[222] gink.[149] hep.[5] ***ign.*** ilx-a.[120] **IP.**[54] lachn.[36] **LYC.**[54] lyss.[214] mag-p.[209] ***nat-m.***[54] sep. **STAPH.**[54] 0stram.[185]
Ailments from; celibacy, being unmarried, continence: ***agn.***[8] apis[130] calc.[137] ***cann-i.***[137] con.[102] fl-ac.[137] lyc.[137] phos.[111] plat.[137] sep.[187]
Ailments from; domination by others, a long history of: carc.[140] foll.[1179] lyc.[193] sep.[193]
Ailments from; domination by others, religious: foll.[1179]
Ailments from; excitation, sexual, suppressed: con.[85] cot.[72] kali-p.[85]
Ailments from; excitement, general symptoms from, suppressed: cot.[102] cupr.[162] kali-c.[162] lach.[155]
Ailments from; grief, cry, cannot: aeth.[162] am-m.[85] apis[36] carc.[146] crot-c.[36] ***gels.*** ign.[36] kali-fcy.[198] **NAT-M.** nux-v.[5] op.[36] puls.[36]
Ailments from; insults, offenses, from, dignified to fight, too, subdued wrath, went home sick, trembling, exhausted: ***staph.***[54]
Ailments from; love disappointed, grief, with silent: **IGN. NAT-M. PH-AC.** phos.
Anger; introversion, with: lap-gr-m.[194]
Anger; trembling, with, anger, with suppressed: aur.[54]
Anxiety; inexpressible, with fainting: ***dig.***[54]
Ascetic: diosm.[72]
Brooding; silence, in: bell.[54] ***verat.***[54]
Delirium; quiet: **BRY.** calc-sil.[58] camph.[54] ***carb-v. chel.*** chin. chlf.[54] ***chlor.*** croc. cupr. cupr-acet.[58] **HYOS.** hyosin.[36] kali-p.[54] op. past.[36] ***ph-ac.*** phos. plb. rhus-t. sec. tab. valer. verat.
Delirium; silent: agar. sec.
Delusions; sorrow, everyone he meets has a secret: cann-i.
Destructiveness; emotions, from suppressed: cand-a.[239]
Dreams; clothes, wearing many layers of: hydrog.[222]
➤ emotions, suppressing: hydrog.[222]
Emotions; controlled by the intellect, need to be: plb.[201] valer.[60] ***viol-o.***[122]
Ennui; silent: ***plb.***[30]
Grief; silent: am-m.[54] anthr.[162] apis[117] aq-mar.[231] aur-ar.[58] carc.[146] ***coff.***[54] coloc.[5] crot-c.[36] cycl.[58] ***gels.*** **IGN.** ***indg.***[8] ip.[122] kali-fcy.[198] lach.[5] lap-gr-m.[194] lyc.[5] **NAT-M.**[122] nux-v.[1] peti.[36] ph-ac.[137] ***puls.*** sal-ac.[54]
Grief; silent, anger, after: ***ign.***[54]
Grief; silent, indignation, with: ***coloc.***[54]
Grief; silent, love, with disappointed: **IGN.**[54]
Grief; silent, submissiveness, with: **PULS.**[54]
Grief; undemonstrative: cycl. ***ign.***
Homesickness; silent ill humor, with: nit-ac. ***ph-ac.***
Hysteria; mild, gentle, yielding, although whimsical and introverted: ***ign.***[54]
Hysteria; sexual, suppression of s. excitement, from: ***brom.***[162] **CON.**[54]
Hysteria; sexual, suppression of s. excitement, from, low spirited, anxiety and sadness: **CON.**[54]
Hysteria; sick, after being insulted and subduing his wrath: ***staph.***[54]
Insanity; secretive: dig.[1]
Insanity; silent: verat.[10] ***verat-v.***[54]
Irritability; anger, after suppressed: sep.[36]
Irritability; taciturn: am-c.[10] ars.[10] calc.[54] coloc.[10] puls.[10] sulph.[10]
Memory; active, suppression sexual desire, from: lach.
Mildness; complaining, bears suffering, even outrage without: ***ign.***[54]
Quarrelsomeness; alternating with, sadness, silent: ***con.***
Quiet disposition; masturbation, in: ***hyos.***[54]
Reserved; displeasure: aur.[137] ign.[137] ip.[137] nat-m.[137] ***staph.***[137]
Sadness; continence, from: bell. **CON.** hyos. stram.
Sadness; quiet: ars.[30] ***hell.***[54] ign. nux-v. ph-ac.[30] puls.[30] ziz.[54]
Sadness; sexual, excitement, suppressed: **CON.**[162]
Sadness; silent: **ARG-N.**[54] ***ars.***[10] bar-c.[10] ***cact.***[116] ***hell.***[54] ***ign.***[54] mag-c.[54] nit-ac.[10] ph-ac.[30] ***puls.***[54] stann.[54] verat.[116]

Self-control: mosch.[36] nat-c.[36] nat-s.[58]
Self-control, wants to control himself: anac.[137] arg.[137] caust.[58] germ.[222] kali-c.[162] lach.[54] lyc.[109] merc.[58] olnd.[137] sil.[54] staph.[137] tarent.[111]
Shrieking; must, feels as though she: ***anac.*** androc.[222] apis aur. ***calc.*** calc-p. cic. cina ***elaps*** hell. ***lil-t.*** nux-v. ***sep.*** sil. stann.
Sits; quite stiff: ***cham. hyos.*** kali-m.[137] puls. ***sep. stram.***
Somnambulism; emotions, from suppressed: ***zinc.***
Suppression of natural inclinations, desires: carc.[214]
Suppression; right hand, forced to write with the: staph.[162]
Suppression; will, by, in order to proper: sil.[162]
Sympathy; compassion, bars all sympathy of friends: arg.[58]
Sympathy; compassion, desire, for, vexed by, but: camph.[54] nat-m.[58]
Talk; formal: arn.[111] cham.[111] ign.[111] lach.[111]
Weeping; controlled: ign.[193] nat-m.[193]
Weeping; silence, in: cycl.[137] ***plat.***[54]

ADAM. Sh, 278 - Felt I would create irreparable damage if I said how I feel. Thought I would say the most awful things that the kids would never recover from. Supreme effort to keep silent. Didn't want to be here. The kids were a hassle. I felt old and tired. Desire to get away from the fighting. 16, 12C, 17:XX:XX

Sh, 292 - It's crystal clear! Clarifying female roles. Clarification of issues. Realization — anger and depression in the past, had to do with conditioning, not saying what I wanted, not having my needs met. 10, 6C, 47:XX:XX

ALOE. Al, 40-...wrap up in himself (introspection), as after a sickness or a fit of anger, which still gnaws (bite) internally, which one cannot express.

ANDROC. Sh, 61 - Felt constrained and had a gloomy approach to everything, averse company, desire to be alone. I feel people will not want to talk or be with me. (28)

AUR. He, 80 - Ailments from fright, anger, contradiction, mortification, or vexation with dread, fear, reserved displeasure, or vehemence.

CACT. Al, 7 - Was affected with impulses to do something facetious (comical), which were repelled. (rejected)

CHAM. He, 55 - In all her sufferings there is a vein of ill humor; she can hardly speak pleasantly; feels like scolding (censorious, offensive) about everything; she often gives vent to her ill humor in spite of all restraint.

CHIN. Al, 47 - Discontent; he considers himself unhappy and thinks he is hindered (obstructed) and tormented by everyone. (after five hours)

CHOC. Sh, 8 - I felt like being outside, roaming around without any possessions, to have the freedom to go where I want to go when the feeling took me. I felt very restricted.

Sh, 228 - Thoughts about the 'veneer of civilisation' that inhibits how we really feel and keeps us from displaying what we're like beneath the surface. It seems a legitimate layer, but so is the layer beneath it, and I feel amused and happy to meet it. This feeling continued for a few days, a very graphic picture of a veneer -a layer of learned social behaviour lifting and detaching from a basis that is thick, dark, solid, instinctual animal.15, 30C, 00:00:30

COLOC. He, 13 - Indignation, with silent internal grief.

CON. He, 29 - Hypochondriasis and hysteria from suppression of, or too free indulgence in, sexual instinct,...(ailments from)

CROT-T. He, 5 - Feeling as though one cannot think outside of himself, "feels all pent up" (restricted, limited, confined, circumscribed) inside, and no chance for thoughts to flow out; as if hide-bound.(obstinate)

FERR. Al, 12 - She never complained or wept and was always plunged (fall) in deep melancholy when no one was about her.

FL-AC. Al, 16 - Whilst (while) considering what might happen he gets into a most ungovernable anger, but only in his thoughts;..(lost relation; anger x action)

GERM. Sh, 124-. I was supposed to talk seriously, but started to laugh instead. I couldn't stop it, the laughter bubbled inside and had to come out. Laughing when supposed to talk seriously, nervous laughter, quite near weeping. Felt I held back something, tried to avoid an ugly noise - something which touched me deeply inside, something unveiling. 18, 30C, 07:XX:XX

HALI-L. Sh, 533 - Boxed in feeling with no way to express anger. Start taking it out on the kids, as if they are trying to break me, to get me. Better getting out, going away from home and family. 09, 6C, 20:XX:XX

HURA. Al, 1 - Much excited and oppressed as if by some great misfortune.

HYDROG. Sh, 275 - Sexually totally closed when my girlfriend kissed me. I felt as if it was a sin. 24, 30C, 00:08:XX

IGN. He, 14 - Inclined to be very secretive (taciturn) and passive.(yielding)

He, 22 - Melancholia from suppressed mental sufferings, with much sighing; desire to be alone (solitude) so as to give way to her real or imaginary grief; weeps bitterly.

He, 62 - Ill effects (ailments) from hearing bad news; from vexation with reserved displeasure ; from grief, or suppressed mental sufferings; of shame and disappointed love.

He, 49 - Mild disposition; bears suffering, even outrage (offenses), without complaining.

IP. He, 13 - Ailments from vexation (worry) and reserved displeasure.

LACHN. Al, 5 - Became much excited over a trifle; he had suppressed his anger, in the evening.

LIL-T. He, 8 - Disposition to weep, with pain in back; has to keep very busy to repress (control) sexual desire.

LYC. Ha, 48 - He has trouble to conceal (mask, hide) his internal obstinacy and vexation. (dissimulated)

He, 39 - Ailments from fright, anger, mortification, or vexation, with reserved displeasure.

NAT-M. He, 48 - Consequences (ailments) of fright, anger, vexation, mortification, or reserved displeasure.

NUX-M. He, 6 - Never accomplishes what he undertakes, but remains standing in one place, absent-minded...

NUX-V. Al, 4 - He is hasty; looked angrily at anyone who asked him a question without answering, as though he was obliged to restrain himself to avoid being insulting; he was in such an irritable and unrestrained mood that it seemed as though he would like to strike any one in the face who spoke a word to him.

Ha, 1270 - He is hasty (careless, rapid), looks malignantly (deadly) at any one who asks (asked) him anything, without answering, just as if he must control himself in order to avoid becoming coarse (rude), it seems as if he would like to strike any one in the face who speaks a word to him, so irritable and uncontrollable in his disposition.

PULS. He, 19 - Silent mood; inclined to silent grief with submissiveness.

RAPH. Al, 7-...dangerous fancies assail (attacks) her, but she restrains (suppress) herself from putting them into execution.

SEP. Al, 76 - Peevish mood, as after suppressed anger.

Ha, 37 - Sorrowful mood, as after secret vexation.

STAPH. He, 12 - Ailments from indignation and vexation, or reserved displeasure ;sleeplessness.

He, 14-...; was insulted (slandered, defamed, calumniated) being too dignified (reserved, lordly,) to fight (contest), subdued (control) his wrath(anger) and went home sick,.. (ailments, from offenses)

UPA. Al, 4 - Melancholic; has to force the tears back; cold towards his friends, repelling everyone.

SURROUNDED

Delusions; animals, dogs, swarm about him: bell. ***calc.***[54] stram.

- animals, snakes, in and around her: abel.[162] ail.[58] anh.[119] bell. calc. gels.[111] ***hyos. lac-c.*** lach. lachn.[111] op. phyt.[30] ***stram.***[8] tub.[56]
- animals, surrounded by hideous: ***crot-h.***[54]
- animals, swarmed about the room: bell.
- bed, surrounded by devils, is: op.[10]
- clouds, enveloped her, heavy black: arg-n.[102] ***cimic. lac-c.***[102] puls.[102]
- crowded with arms and legs: ***pyrog.***[122]
- enemy, surrounded by enemies: ***anac.*** cand-a.[239] carbn-s. ***crot-h.*** dros.[1] lap-mar-c.[194] ***merc.***

- faces, diabolical, crowd upon him: ***ambr.*** carb-an. caust. tarent.[58]
- fire, head is surrounded by: am-m.
- fluid, surrounded by ethereal, resisting passage: cann-i
- friend, surrounded by friends, shaking hands and calling them by name: ***hydr-ac.***[54]
- home, away from, strangers, in midst of, in epilepsy: ***aster.***[54]
- house, surrounded, is: stram.
- people in, sees, babies, full of white and colored: morph.[85]
- soldier, sees, surrounded by: nat-c.[30]
- spectres, sees, throng upon him: ***psor.***[54] verb.[54]
- strangers, amongst: aster.[137]
- strangers, surrounded by: androc.[222] nit-ac.[30] ***puls.***[30]
- surrounded by friends, is: bell. cann-i.
- walls, surrounded by high: cann-i.

Dreams; animals, dogs, many young dogs, fastening themselves tightly, in constant succession on various parts of his body: lyc.[36]

➤ encircled tightly, being: ruta.

Dullness; fog, as envelop in a: petr.[122]

Escape; attempts to, surrounded and captured from men, as if: ***hyos.***[54]

Striking; imaginary objects, at: ***bell.*** canth. **CINA**[5] cupr. ***hyos. kali-c.*** kreos.[5] lil-t.[5] lyc. mosch. nat-c. nux-v. op. phos. plat. ***stram.*** stront-c. verat.[5]

ANAC. Al, 16 - Anxiety in all his actions; everything appears to him more terrible; he imagine himself surrounded with enemies; then he feels warm and the blood seems to boil within him.

Ha, 6 - Timorous in all his actions; he views everything more anxiously and timidly, always thinks of being surrounded by enemies, then he becomes hot, his blood seems to boil in his chest.

ARS. Al, 87 - He imagines that the whole house, and the space under the bed, are full of thieves, which causes, from fright, anxious cold sweat to break out over his body.

BELL. Al, 82 - Delirious talk of dogs, as if they swarmed (crowd) about him.

Al, 86-...pointing with trembling fingers to swarms (crowd) of unclean (dirty) beasts wich she fancied were scrambling (mix) all over the walls, beds, table, etc. of the wards.

Ha, 1340 - Delirious talk about dogs surrounding him.

He, 30 - Delirium: with frightful figures and images before eyes; is afraid (fear) of imaginary things; sees monsters; talks of dogs as if they swarmed (crowded) about him; furious.

BOV. Al, 9 - Anguish; she felt as if enveloped in a black vapor. (cloud, fog)

CALAD. He, 3 - Opens her eyes and asks, "Where am I? what do you all want around me?" A few moments after Calad. 0typhus.

CALC. He, 22 - Mania; sees many curs (dogs) crowding (compress) around him, fights them off. (surrounded)

CANN-I. Al, 25-...He seemed to be walking in a vast arena, encircled by tremendous walls... (confined, limited)

Al, 36 - The sun seemed reeling (moving) from his place, and the clouds danced around him like a chorus.

Al, 69 - He seems to himself to be transformed into a vegetable existence, as a huge fern, and to be surrounded by clouds of music and perfume.

CARBN-S. Al-S, 753 - At one time during the night he seemed to be surrounded by enemies; persons were coming to harm him;...

CIMIC. He, 1 - Sensation as if a heavy black cloud (smoke) had settled (descent) all over her, and enveloped (surrounded, wrap) her head, so that all was darkness and confusion, while, at the same time, it weighed (heavy) like lead (metal) on her head.

CROT-H. He, 5-...imagines himself surrounded by enemies or hideous animals;...

CROT-T. He, 5 - Feeling as though one cannot think outside of himself, "feels all pent up" (restricted, limited, confined, circumscribed) inside, and no chance for thoughts to flow out; as if hide-bound.(obstinate)

HYOS. He, 79 - After being harshly (severe) accused of theft (crime), continual delirium; fancies surrounded by objects of a terrifying nature; not a moment quiet, continual calling out that she saw the devil; denies herself guilty of theft (innocent, injustice), or that she has any concern with witches; ...

He, 57 - Delirium tremens:...averse to light and company; visions as if persecuted preceded by an epileptic attack;... seeks to escape from men by whom he imagines himself surrounded and who are trying to capture him; does not recognize his wife who is standing by his side, but imagines he sees her under a distant bed.

LAC-C. He, 15 - Sensation or delusion as if surrounded by myriads of snakes, some running like lightning up and down inside the skin ; some that are inside feel long and thin; fears to put her feet on floor, lest she should tread (walk) on them and make them squirm (shake) and wind (round) around her legs; is afraid to look behind her, for fear that she will see snakes there, does not dream of them and is seldom troubled with them after dark; on going to bed she was afraid to shut her eyes for fear that a large snake, the size of her arm, would hit her in the face.

LYC. Ha, 25 - Great fear of phantoms, (ghosts) which crowd upon her fancy in the evening; during the day she is disposed to weep.

MAG-S. Al, 11-..while knitting she constantly saw strange persons about (surround) her, though she knew it was an illusion.

NUX-V. He, 19-...; imagines himself surrounded by persons who carry on all sorts of pranks (joke, jest), or ply (covering) him whith questions which he thinks he is compelled (forced) to answer (proved, questioned, interrogated);..; answers questions rationally and is conscious of his condition; ...appears to be haunted (obsessed) by a great fear.

OP. Ha, 637 - She was troubled when awake with the supposed sight of ghosts, devils and spectres, which she believed to be surrounding her bed...

PHOS. Al, 12-...; wherever he turned his eyes he saw faces; they swarmed (crowded, surrounded) by him in long panoramic succession; they leered (look lecherous) at him over the footboard of the bed; they squinted (look) at him though the windows, or came trooping (crowd) in when the doors were left ajar (open) (invade);..he fancied he was some one else, ...

Al, 40 - As the darkness of night began to enclose (surround) the earth, my peace was disturbed by the most frightful visions and thoughts; constant fear of death, with an almost uncontrollable desire to commit suicide.

PSOR. He, 27 - Is so downhearted she could committed suicide, then is full of phantasms.

STRAM. Ha, 562 - His surroundings appear to him quite strange; (unfamiliar) although in the first minutes he knows that he is surrounded by his friends, he forgets this in the second minute, and imagines he is quite alone (solitary, deserted) in a desert (wildness), and is afraid (fearful) ; figures of beasts suddenly spring out of the ground at his side, so that he moves to the other side, where, however, other similar figures pursue him, and he runs forward.

Ha, 551 - She sometimes cries out about cats, dogs and rabbits, which were approaching (pursuing) her from above, from the side and from the middle of the room.

Ha, 563 - As a rule he has more imaginary figures at his side than in front of him, they all inspire him with horror.

He, 66 - Woke suddenly in night and said there were snakes under and about her; looked wild, screamed and pointed to them.

He, 93 - Mania; thinks he is lying on his sepulchre (tomb); confessing, praying, wants to be killed (redemption, salvation, regeneration); laughs as if tickled (excited); wants to be kissed; accuses his wife of being faithless (betrayed); scolding (censure) beating in a rage, will not be taken hold of by attendants (suspicious?) ; takes them for dogs (contemptuous), and barks at them; talking in Jewish jargon; (rank?, stranger?) supposes his house to be surrounded by carts (vehicle), Jews (Judaism) and geese, offending him, ... -(strange, foreign, alien)

VALER. Al, 1 - Extremely delirious, attempting to get out of the window, ... imagined himself away from home, and beset (surrounded) with all sorts of danger, from which he was attempting to escape, although unable to walk without staggering from side to side.

SUSPICIOUS

Ailments from; jealousy: ***apis***[54] **HYOS.**[5] ***ign.***[5] ***lach.***[5] **NUX-V.**[122] ***ph-ac.***[5] ***phos.***[162] **PULS.**[122] staph.[102]
Anger; looked at, when: ant-c.[127] ant-t.[47] ***cham.***[102] chin.[91] ***cina***[98] gels.[102] ***iod.***[8] ***nux-v.***[102] sanic.[102] ***sil.***[102]
Anguish; eating, after: ***asaf.***[54] sep.[54]
Anguish; eating, while: hyos.[85] sep.
Anxiety; company, shuns, even his doctor: iod.[85]
Anxiety; eating before: mez. ran-b.
Anxiety; eating while: ***carb-v.*** kali-sil.[58] mag-c. merc.[58] mez. ran-b.[85] sabad. ***sep.***
Anxiety; waking, on, something under the bed making a noise, from: ars.[172] bell.
Aversion; parents, to: fl-ac.[30]
Children; watchful, they are on the look out for every gesture: phos.[122]
Company, aversion to; presence of, strangers, to: **AMBR.**[122] ***bar-c. bry.*** bufo ***carb-v.*** **CIC.** cina[58] ***con. helon.***[163] ***iod. lach.***[8] lyc. nat-c.[58] petr. ***sep. stram.*** tarent.[193] ***thuj.***
Delirium; refuses to take the medicine: agar-pr.[36] hyos.[162]
Delusions; animals, bed, under the: cham.[54]
- bed, someone, under it: am-m. ars. bell. calc. canth. colch.
- bed, someone, under it, knocking: bell.[5] calc. canth. colch.[5]
- betrayed, that she is: hydrog.[222]
- conspiracies against her father, the landlord's bills are: kali-br.
- conspiracies, against him, there are: ars. kali-br.[25] lach. plb. puls.[137]
- danger, family, from his: kali-br.
- deceived, is: bamb-a.[1184] dros.[1] ozone[227] ruta[130]
- devils, persons are, all: **PLAT.** plb.[54]
- devils, present, are: anac. cann-i. op. phos. **PLAT.**
- eat, she must not: kali-chl.[58]
- enemy, everyone is an: ***merc.*** plat. ***puls.***[54]
- enemy, surrounded by enemies: ***anac.*** cand-a.[239] carbn-s. ***crot-h.*** dros.[1] lap-mar-c.[194] ***merc.***
- enemy, under the bed, is: am-m.
- enemy, wait for an, lying in: alco.[36]
- footsteps, hears: canth. carb-v. crot-c. nat-p.
- footsteps, hears, next room, in: nat-p.
- furniture is persons, night on waking: nat-p.
- hated by others, he is: lach.[137] sanic.[144]
- inanimate objects are persons: bell. calc. nat-p. stram.
- injury, injured, surroundings, by his: **HYOS.**[122] ***lach. naja***[117]
- injury, receive, will, friends, from: lach.[58]
- insecure, everything is: bamb-a.[1184]
- jealousy, lovers concealed behind stove wife has: ***stram.***[54]
- murder, conspiring to murder him, others are: ars. hydrog.[222] plb. tab.[139]
- murderer, everyone around him is a: ***plb.***
- noise, hears: anh.[144] bell. calc. canth.[5] carb-v. cham. cocain.[102] coff.[58] colch. con. hyos. mag-m. naja[98] ph-ac.[5] sulph.[1] verat.[10]
- noise, hears, bed, under: bell.[1]
- noise, hears, clattering above the bed when going to sleep: calc.
- noise, hears, knocking at the door: ant-c.[1]
- person, something hanging over chair is a p. sitting there: calc.
- poisoned, about to be, that he is: carc.[207] ***hyos.***[10] kali-br. lach.[102] plb. ***rhus-t.*** verat-v.[102]
- poisoned, has been, he: agar.[139] ang.[139] bufo[139] caj.[85] carb-ac.[139] chin-s.[139] chlor.[139] cic.[139] cimic. cocc.[139] cor-r.[139] croc.[139] culx.[58] cur.[139] euph.[139] ferr.[139] gels.[139] glon.[139] hydr.[139] hydrog.[222] ***hyos.*** iodof.[139] jug-r.[139] kali-br.[139] kali-c.[139] kali-i.[139] ***lach.***[116] lact.[139] lap-mar-c.[194] lil-t.[139] lina.[139] lyc.[139] m-aust.[139] mag-p.[139] med.[139] merl.[139] mez.[139] mill.[139] nicc.[139] nux-m.[139] nux-v.[139] olnd.[139] op.[139] petr.[139] ph-ac.[139] phos.[139] pip-m.[139] plat-m. psor.[139] ptel.[139] puls.[139] ran-b.[139] raph.[139] rat.[139] rheum[139] rhod.[139] rhus-t.[102] sabad.[139] sec.[139] sep.[139] sol-n.[139] spig.[139] squil.[139] staph.[139] stram.[37] sul-ac.[139] sulph.[139] tab.[139] tarax.[139] thuj.[139] valer.[139] verat-v.[102] zinc.[139]
- poisoned, medicine is: cimic.[58] hyos.[58] lach. rhus-t.[172]
- policeman, physician is a: bell.
- present, someone is: hyos. lyc. thuj.
- pursued, he is: absin. ***anac.***[122] ars. aur.[5] bell. bry. choc.[222] con.[5] cycl.[162] ***hyos.***[5] ***kali-br.*** lach.[58] med.[122] merc.[139] plb. rhus-t. sil.[30] staph. stram. thuj.[58] verat-v.[5]

• robbed, is going to be: bar-c.[30] bor.[30] caust.[30] sep.[30]
• room, sees people, entering, on: lyc.
• servants, he must get rid of: fl-ac.
• spied on, being: aq-mar.[231] lach.[30] med.[56]
• strangers, friends appears as: bry. stram.
• strangers, looking over shoulder: brom.
• strangers, room, seem to be in the: bry.[10] ***tarent. thuj.***
• strangers, sees: anac.[58] cann-i. mag-s. nit-ac.[30] nux-v. ***puls.***[30] stram. ***thuj.***
• strangers, sees, knitting while: mag-s.
• strangers, snatching at her: ***bell.***[54]
• talking, friends talking about her: lach.[58]
• thieves, dream, after a, and will not believe the contrary until search is made: nat-m. sanic.[85]
• thieves, house, in: ars. cann-i. con.[30] ***cupr-acet.***[54] ***lach.*** merc. ***nat-m.*** sil. sol-t-ae.
• thieves, sees, night: ***ars.***
• wife is faithless: hyos. stram.
• women, evil, are, and will injure his soul: puls.

Dreams; betrayed, having been: sil.[1]
➤ conspiracies: mosch.[36] ped.[36]
➤ lying, someone is lying under him: nit-ac.[1]
➤ nightmare, room must be searched before appeased: ***cham.***[54]
➤ old gentleman ran away from wife, suspected of having married another: sep.[36]
➤ singing political songs, in presence of spies: asc-t.[5]

Dullness; suspiciousness, with: cham.[5] cic.[5]

Fear; betrayed, of being: hyos. lyss.[172]
✦ dentist, of going to: calc.[122] puls.[70] tub.[70]
✦ drink, offered, what is: hyos.[172]
✦ eating, after e., food: asaf.[5] canth. carb-v.[5] caust.[58] chin.[172] hyos.[5] kali-c.[5] lach. mag-m. nit-ac.[5] nux-v.[5] onos.[172] petr.[172] phel. tab. thuj.[5] viol-t.[5]
✦ eating, agg., while, offered, what is: hyos.[172]
✦ knaves, of: alum.[5] ars.[5] chin.[5] hyos.[5] lyss.[5]
✦ looking before her, when: sulph.
✦ men, of: 0aloe 0aur. 0bar-c. bar-m. choc.[222] 0con. dios. hypoth.[149] ign. 0lach. lap-mar-c.[194] ***led.*** 0lyc. 0nat-c. 0nat-m. 0phos. ***plat. puls.*** raph. sep. 0stann. 0sulph.
✦ poisoned, has been: euph.[1] glon.
✦ poisoned; being: all-s. anac.[5] apis arge.[149] ***ars.***[184] ars-met. bapt.[5] ***bell.*** bry. cimic. dros.[172] euph.[1] glon. ***hyos.*** ign.[30] ***kali-bi.***[54] ***kali-br. lach.*** lyss.[172] nat-m.[122] ph-ac.[30] phos. plb. ***rhus-t. verat.***[54] verat-v.
✦ room, entering, on: alum. lyc. plat. til. ***valer.***
✦ sold, of being: ***bell.***[60] bry.[60] ***hyos.*** lyss.[172] rhus-t.[60]
✦ strange place, as if he was in a: bar-c.[172] carb-v.[172] caust.[172] cic.[54] cupr.[172] kali-p.[172] thuj.[172]
✦ struck by those coming toward him, of being, walking behind him, by those: alum.[122]

Hide; desire to, children, strangers, from: bar-c.[85]

Hides things: bell. ***staph.***[8] tarent.[58]

Hypochondriasis; eating, after: anac.[54] chin.[54] ***nat-c.***[54] ***nux-v.***[10] zinc.[10]

Irritability; medicine, at thought to take the: mim-p.[149]

Irritability; suspicious: cham.[10] lyc.[10] merc.[10]

Looking; bed, about, as if to find something: ***ign.***[54]

Looking; sides, on all: kali-br.[137] stram.[5]

Medicine; drugs, averse to: aesc.[36]

Men; loss of confidence in: cic.[36]

Rage; eat, when something to, was offered: ars.[54]

Rage; medicine, from forcible administration of: ***bell.***[36]

Rebels against poultice: bor.[1] bry.[1] ***calc.***[1] carb-v.[1] ***cham.***[1] ***lyc.***[1] merc.[1] mur-ac.[1] nit-ac.[1] nux-v.[1] phos.[1] puls.[1] rhus-t.[1] sep.[1] spig.[1] staph.[1] ***sulph.***[1]

Refuses; medicine, to take the: ***arn.***[122] ***cimic.***[54] hyos. ***kali-p.***[54] **LACH.**[122] ***stram.***[54] ***verat-v.***[54] visc.[119]

Refuses; treatment, every: bell.[30] caust.[30] lach.[30] plat.[30]

Refuses; treatment, sick, in spite of being very: ars.[30] caust.[30] nux-v.[30]

Rejects everything offered to him: oena.[36] past.[36]

Striking; imaginary objects, at: ***bell.*** canth. **CINA**[5] cupr. ***hyos. kali-c.*** kreos.[5] lil-t.[5] lyc. mosch. nat-c. nux-v. op. phos. plat. ***stram.*** stront-c. verat.[5]

Suspiciousness, mistrustfulness: **ACON.** act-sp.[111] ambr. **ANAC.**[122] anan. androc.[222] ang. anh.[102] ant-c. apis[5] ***arn.*** **ARS.** ars-s-f.[58] ***aur.*** aur-s.[58] ***bapt.*** bar-acet.[10] **BAR-C.** ***bar-m. bar-s.***[58] ***bell. bor.*** **BRY.**

bufo[30] ***cact.*** cadm-s.[144] calc.[5] ***calc-p.*** calc-s. cand-a.[239] **CANN-I.** cann-s.[5] canth. caps.[58] carb-v.[5] carbn-s. carc.[207] **CAUST. CENCH.** cham. chin. chin-ar. **CIC.** ***cimic.*** coca ***cocc.*** con. ***crot-h. cupr.*** **DIG.** ***dros. dulc.***[184] eup-a.[25] graph. ***hell.*** hydrog.[222] ***hyos.*** ign.[5] ip. **KALI-AR.** kali-bi.[5] kali-br. ***kali-p.*** **LACH.** lap-gr-m.[194] lap-mar-c.[194] **LYC.**[122] ***lycps.***[54] macrin.[36] ***med.***[162] meli. meny. ***merc.*** mez. ***morph.***[116] mur-ac. ***nat-ar. nat-c.*** nat-p. nat-s.[58] ***nit-ac. nux-v. op.*** ph-ac.[36] ***phos.*** plat.[116] ***plb.*** psor.[185] **PULS. RHUS-T.** ruta sanic. sarr. **SEC.** sel. ***sep.*** seq-s.[230] sil. ***spig.***[30] ***stann. staph.***[122] still.[116] **STRAM.** ***sul-ac.*** sul-i. **SULPH.** syph.[122] thuj. thyr.[85] verat.[102] ***verat-v.*** viol-t.

Suspiciousness; everyone, to: cench.[58]

Suspiciousness; family, towards: ars-s-f.[58]

Suspiciousness; fear of company: ambr.[10] bar-c.[10] ***nat-c.***[10]

Suspiciousness; friends, to: ars-s-f.[58] kali-ar.[58]

Suspiciousness; insulting: merc.[10]

Suspiciousness; looks on all sides: kali-br.[137]

Suspiciousness; mania, in: ***lach.***[54]

Suspiciousness; mania, in, delivery, parturition, after, puerperal: ***verat-v.***[54]

Suspiciousness; reserved, and, during pregnancy: ***puls.***[54]

Suspiciousness; solitude, desire for: cic.[10] croto-t.[10]

Suspiciousness; talking about her, people are: ***bar-c.*** hyos.[137] ign.[137] pall.[137] staph.[137]

Watchfulness: ars.[36] eup-a.[25] stram.[36]

ADAM. 197 - Suspiciousconfusion that people are making a fool of me, laughing at me. 2, 12C, XX:XX:XX

Sh, 202 - Preoccupied with the past on waking, concerning betrayal of trust in relationships. 15, 12C, 07:XX:XX

AESC. Al, 1 - Great repugnance to the drug.(medicine)

ALL-S. He, 3 - Sadness when alone; moral uneasiness; afraid of never getting well; fear of not being able to bear any kind of medicine; fear of being poisoned...

ANAC. Al, 11 - When walking he felt anxious, as if some one were pursuing him; he suspected everything around him.

Ha, 5 - In walking and in standing, uneasiness, as if someone were coming behind him (persecuted); everything around him seemed to him suspicious.

He, 56 - When walking he left anxious, as if some one were pursuing him; he suspected everything around him.

ANAN. Al, 5 - Restless, suspicious, and very irritable character, or apathetic and as if besotted.(intoxicated)

ANDROC. Sh, 60 - Felt tense and absolutely alone, but sure that the rest of the world was mad, not her. She felt defiant with others and would not be manipulated. (7)

Sh, 121 - When talking to friends felt 'paranoid', suspicious and guilty, when asked questions, he became hot and sweaty. He felt it was a game of who was cleverer, and tried to lie to and outwit his friend, though this gave no satisfaction. His friends reported that he seemed unusually distant and cool. (29)

Sh, 122 - When his friends were talking, he became very suspicious and fearful, but had no fear of strangers or the police. (29)

Sh, 123 - In the evening he became manic, stalked the streets and visited many friends for a short time only, but could not relax or relate to them. Was pleased when he found his friends were not at home. Spoke nonsense and tried to squeeze a laugh out of anything. (29)

ANT-C. He, 24 - Sentimental or distrustful mood.

ARS. Al, 86 - He runs through the whole house at night in search of thieves.

Al-S, 2879 - Became very nervous, agitated, and delirious, suspecting people were about the house plotting (conspiracy, betrayed) against his life, jumps out of the bed suddenly and reaches after imaginary objects, and stares wildly and suspiciously around him,...

Ha, 36 - His whole house, also under his bed, is full of rogues, which causes a cold sweat to break out, which runs down cold over his body.

Ha, 37 - In the night he runs all about the house, looking for thieves.

He, 43 - Runs about house at night looking for thieves. (search)

He, 18 - He imagines that he sees burglars (robbers) in the room, and listens under the bed; he is bathed in cold sweat.

AUR. He, 72 - Contradiction excites wrath; distrust.

BAR-C. Ha, 4 - She suspected, that when

walking in the street, men found fault (defect) with her, and judged her amiss (wrong), which made her anxious, so that she dared not look up, she looked at nobody, and perspired all over.
BAR-M. He, 6 - Dejection and dread of men.
BELL. Ha, 1432 - Fearful mistrust.
Al, 165 - Cowardice, distrust, suspicion, inclination to run away.
He, 18 - When closing eyes, though not asleep, patient sees fierce (wild), wicked looking large animals with horns and bushy (scabrous) heads; room seemed to be full of strange men passing in and out, who would snatch (take hold) at her as they passed, which frightened her very much, she thought the men wanted to take her away from home ; she then saw children sitting on low benches (seat) in rows (line) as in a school-room. (purity)
He, 102 - Became fearful when persons approached him in street, and when they had passed, he insisted on it that he had stabbed them.
CACT. Al, 6 - Decided repugnance to take any more medicine.
CALAD. He, 8 - So averse to the medicine, that it required a desperate effort to overcome it.
CANN-I. Al, 29 - Looks under beds and tables, unlocks and relocks doors, for the fancies he hears strange noises, and that thieves are in the house.
CANTH. Al, 26 - Distrust of himself, like a hypochondriac.
CAUST. He, 61 - Very suspicious and distrustful.
CERE-B. Al, 6 - Reluctance (doubt) to take medicine.
CHAM. Al, 40 - Ill-humor; he suspects that he has been imposed upon.
Ha, 471 - Suspicion that he may have been insulted.
CIC. Al, 27 - Want of confidence in mankind; with misanthropy; he forsook society, remained alone and reflected upon their errors and about himself.
Ha, 238 - Want of trust (mistrust, skepticism) in people and anthrophoby,(misanthropy) he fled (escape) from them remained solitary, and thought seriously about their errors and about himself.
He, 36 - Mistrust and shunning (avoid) of men; despises others.
CIMIC. He, 10 - Fear of death; fears those in house will kill him (murdered, by parents); saw wires encasing (lock, imprisoned) him; visions of rats and of strange objects.
He, 15 - Declares she has been poisoned.
He, 29 - Suspicious of everything, would not take medicine if she knew it.
CON. Ha, 14 - He imagines that somebody has come in at the door by night.
CROT-H. He, 22 - Suspicion and snappishness (irritable), or quiet indifference.
DIG. He, 14 - Gloomy, peevish and distrustful.(suspicious)
DROS. Al, 12 - Restless mood and anxiety the whole day; full of distrust, as if he were dealing with none but false men.
Al, 13 - Extremely uneasy, sad mood the whole day; he imagines that he would be deceived by tricky, designing (tricky) men.
Ha, 271 - All day long, uneasiness of disposition and anxiety, full of mistrust (suspicious) as if he had to do with none but false (faithless) people.
Ha, 272 - Extremely uneasy, sad disposition, all day he imagined he was being deceived (deluded, defrauded) by spiteful (hateful), envious people.
He, 5 - Great mistrust.
FL-AC. Al, 1 - Great disposition, when alone, to repulsive fantastic imaginations, particularly in regard to persons with whom he stands in near relations, or with whom he is connected (united, joined); it seems, for example, as though he must get rid (discard, repudiate, reject) of all the servants, children must go out of house, a betrothal must be broken off, a marriage should be dissolved. (broke; vows)
GLON. Al, 13-...fear she had been poisoned, and that no one would catch her taking any more.
HYDROG. Sh, 245 - Feel I can't trust anyone —'paranoia'. 24, 30C, 100:XX:XX
Sh, 246 - I felt mistrust, suspicion and paranoia. 16, 30C, Letter
Sh, 247 - I feel people are playing games with me. Everything is out of balance. (prejudiced)16, 30C, XX:XX:XX
Sh, 248 - While sitting in a restaurant, felt

progressively more cut off from friends at the table. I began to feel detached and paranoid. I felt disliked by people. They seemed to look at me menacingly. I became concerned that my lecture this afternoon had created conflict, mayhem and destruction, that my friends in the audience did not like me any more. I became aware of a dull ache in my sacrum making me want to shift backwards and forwards. At the same time, the people round the table seemed further away and smaller, as if I had moved four feet back from the table. I felt very uncomfortable and wanted to get out. I put my head down and rushed out without saying goodbye, feeling a sense of relief at getting away (all very unusual for me). Outside, I felt relief and my mind cleared and I walked home alone. 22, 12C, 04:XX:XX

Sh, 251 - A spark of a paranoid thought — "maybe I'm being poisoned". 10, 200C, 00:00:00

Sh, 256 - Thought someone was telling someone else that I was mad and asking what should be done about it. 16, 30C, 25:XX:XX

Sh, 257 - Feeling suspicious all day. Anxious and conscious of vulnerability. (Asked husband to move out if he was thinking of being unfaithful). 12, 6C, 06:XX:XX

Sh, 258 - Felt cut off from people and suspicious. 22, 12C, 06:XX:XX

HYOS. Al, 5-...suspicious of those about him; he became delirious, saw policeman coming into the house; heard them speaking about the hall;...

He, 65 - Violent and threatening...; mind nearly deranged; disturbed by unfounded jealousy.

He, 78 - Groundless suspicion of being watched (observed, spied) by members of family with whom he had some slight misunderstanding (dispute); to avoid being recognized by them, clothed himself differently every day,...watching his relations suspiciously and imagining he might be poisoned;... (disguise, camouflage)

He, 87-...; refused medicine, and cunningly (skill) evaded all stratagems to give it; escaped from room, ...

He, 13 - Does not know whether or not to take what is offered.

He, 17 - Complains of having been poisoned.

He, 19 - Very suspicious.

IOD. He, 9 - Fear and anxiety shuns (avoid) even the doctor.

KALI-BR. Al, 3-...his character also had undergone a radical change, from having been very frank and brave, he had become excessively timid, and suspicious of every trifling circumstance; ...several times he attempted to throw himself from a window and battered down a door with an axe, in order to escape from some imaginary danger;...

He, 37 - Timid, suspicious, full of fear.

KALI-P. He, 3 - Delirium tremens; horrors of drunkards; fear, sleeplessness, ... and suspicion; rambling (incoherent) talk...

He, 4 - Says she is eternally and irretrievably damned;...food and medicine must be forcibly administered. 0 Melancholia religious.

He, 15 - Profound hypochondria and melancholia, weariness of life and fear of death, suspiciousness...

LAC-C. Al,N -8 - Is impressed with the idea that all she says is a lie; it seems to be very difficult to speak the truth (liar, dissimulator), but continually distrusts things (suspicious); when reading anything she rapidly changes the meaning, omitting or adding things. (mischievous)

LACH. Al, 32 - Becomes easily peevish and mistrustful; believes himself intentionally injured (hurt, prejudice) by all his environments, and attaches the most hateful significance to the most innocent occurrences.

He, 16 - Most extraordinary loquacity, making speeches in very select (finest, excellent) phrases (pretentious), but jumping off to most heterogeneous subjects; at the same time proud (haughty), full of mistrust. 0Mania.

He, 34-...repugnance to society and dislike to talk; solicitude about future, whith disgust of life; inclination to doubt everything; mistrusts (suspicious) and misconstrues (misjudge) ...0 Melancholia.

He, 41 - Dread (fear) of death, fears to go to bed ; fears of being poisoned.

He, 51 - Proud; jealous, suspicious; developing into mania.

LYC. Al, 40 - If people come near her, she is immediately attacked with anxiety at the pit of the stomach.

Al, 50 - In the evening on entering a room he is attacked with fear, as though he saw some one; even during the day he believes that he hears some one in the room.

Ha, 27 - He is afraid (fear) in the evening, on entering a room, as if he saw somebody; by day also he sometimes imagines he hears somebody in the room.

Ha, 34 - Distrustful, suspicious, inclined to take things ill.

Ha, 35 - Extremely distrustful and suspicious.

He, 36 - Distrustful, suspicious and fault (mistake) finding. (judgment)

LYSS. Al,N-28 - Complains bitterly that a fire has been lighted and that the stove is smoking, although there is no fire; another continually directed a window to be closed, which was not opened. (fear suffocation?)

MACRO. Al, 6 - Suspicious of everybody; thinks she has not told the truth (veracity) in regard to himself. (secretive, pretend)

MERC. Ha, 1256 - All day long sulky and distrustful (suspicious); he almost insulted those about him, and regarded them all as his greatest enemies.(opponent, rival)

Ha, 1127 - She dreams that people are before the window, and on being woke up thereby be cannot persuaded that they were not there. (observed)

Ha, 1253 - Very cross and intolerant, easily irritated, very suspicious.

He, 16 - Great restlessness as if he had committed a great crime; ...considers everybody his enemy;...great inclination when walking to take people by the nose;...(desire: conduct, direct, guide)

He, 34 - Inexpressive pain of soul and body, anxious restlessness, as if some evil impended ...; disgusted (revolt) with himself, has not courage (cowardice) to live; constant suspicion (distrust), considering everybody his enemy.

He, 37 - Morose and mistrustful; treated his associates almost insultingly, looked upon every one as his worst enemy.

NUX-V. Al, 45 - Anxiety, caused by a suspicious and apprehensive condition of mind, especially during the afternoon hours.

Ha, 1257 - Anxiety from suspicious and timorous (timidity) solicitude, especially in the hours after midnight.

He, 10-...every harmless word offends, every little noise frightens, anxious and beside themselves, cannot bear even the least suitable medicine. (contrary)

OP. Al, 137 - Appeared jealous and afraid (fear) of people around.

He, 12 - Said many disconnected things and pointed to masked people who seemed to approach him.

PHOS. Al, 12-...; wherever he turned his eyes he saw faces; they swarmed (crowded, surrounded) by him in long panoramic succession; they leered (look lecherous) at him over the footboard of the bed; they squinted (look) at him though the windows, or came trooping (crowd) in when the doors were left ajar (open) (invade);..he fancied he was some one else, ...

PLAT. Ha, 21 - She thinks all persons are demons.

PLB. Al, 23-...His delirium turned chiefly upon the idea that his life was in danger from assassination or poisoning, and that every one about him was a murderer...

Al, 63 - The patient imagined that he was constantly followed (persecuted), and that he heard voices coming from the chimney... ; this man after a few days wished to leave the hospital and go home, because he was convinced that there were fiends in the building that pursued him and sought (want) his life.

He, 13 - Thought his life was in danger from assassination or poison and every one about him was a murderer.

PULS. He, 47-...; pangs (pain, anxiety) of conscience about religion and female sex; violent palpitation in the presence of women; abhors (detests, aversion) and hates the sex; must go out of their way for fear of injuring them; looks upon them as evil beings and is afraid (fear; temptation, seduction); considers their presence injurious (insulted, offended) to his soul; ... (sexual loathing)

He, 53-...afraid of everybody; considers

every one her enemy, despairs of everything; ...;trusts no one;.. (suspicious)

He, 36 - Mistrust; envy; covetousness (avidity); dislike to people.

He, 46 - Dark suspicious and reserved manner; disturbed look on face; sleepless; looks for her bed in the yard (lost?); hides in a corner to escape from a little gray man who wanted to pull out her leg;...

RHUS-T. Al, 32 - He thought an enemy want to poison him.

Ha, 965 - He imagines an enemy seeks to poison him.

He, 24-...a week later she told her mother to not look at her (observed) ; seemed to be distrustful (suspicious) and did not wish to see any one; she came running in from the street and said people were looking at her; ....; cries without cause, imagines people are finding fault (misconduct, criticized, censured) with her because she is earning (succeed, prosper, reach) nothing, acts in a childish manner;...

RUTA. Al, 8 - Peevish and mistrustful (suspicious) all day; he no longer trusted his best friends, he thought that he was constantly deceived.(deluded)

Ha, 286 - All day long cross and suspicious; he would no longer trust (mistrust) his best friend, and imagined he was always being deceived.

SEL. Al, 4 - Dread of people and of his occupation, but overcoming this he is able to continue his work.

SIL. He, 23-...believes she has swallowed pins, and asks those about her whether she has not done so; seeks for hours for lost pins; ...and careful examined her food for fear of pins; very indifferent to friends and former amusements;...

STAPH. Ha, 697 - When he walks quickly he feels as if some one were following him; this caused anxiety and fear, and he must always look about him.

STRAM. He, 56 - Believes to be in his grave; shrives,(confess) prays, asks to be killed (justified); accuses his wife of infidelity; scolds (cursing), strikes at everybody who wishes to restrain him; thinks they are dogs and barks at them to make himself understood.

He, 93 - Mania; thinks he is lying on his sepulchre (tomb); confessing, praying, wants to be killed (redemption, salvation, regeneration); laughs as if tickled (excited); wants to be kissed; accuses his wife of being faithless (betrayed); scolding (censure) beating in a rage, will not be taken hold of by attendants (suspicious?) ; takes them for dogs (contemptuous), and barks at them; talking in Jewish jargon; (rank?, stranger?) supposes his house to be surrounded by carts (vehicle), Jews (Judaism) and geese, offending him, ... -(strange, foreign, alien)

He, 103 - Had many strange fancies, such as imagining his wife had lovers concealed (hidden) behind stove; ...afterward had a fit that looked so much like apoplexy that he was bled.(blood)

He, 163 - Cries out fearfully, hides face in pillow, is terrified by presence or approach of physician; after attack of typhoid.

SUL-AC. Al, 28 - Very fearful; extremely mistrustful.

Ha, 7 - Fearing many things, exceedingly suspicious.

SULPH. He, 29-...is filled with anxious, despondent (sad) thoughts, from which she cannot free herself, they make her suspicious, peevish and lachrymose.

THYR. Al,N-4-"All progressed cases of myxedema ... delusions ...suspicion, and persecution".

VERAT-V. He, 4 - Puerperal mania: silent, suspicious; will not see physician, he seems to terrify her; fears being poisoned;...

He, 6 - Loquacity, with exaltation of ideas, or an exalted opinion of her own ideas and powers; everything seems clear to her; now clearly understands former mysterious things; wants no medicine, as that will restore her to former condition;...

TALK

Anger; conversation, from: puls.[36] tarent-c.[36]

Anger; himself, with, spoken to, does not wish to be: elaps[54]

Anger; questioned, on being: coloc.[54]

Anger; spoken to, when: ***cham.***[54] ***elaps***[54] ***hell.***[54]

Anger; talk, indisposed to: am-m.[10] ***ign.***[10] hydrog.[222] nat-m.[10] petr.[10] puls.[10] stann.[10] stront-c.[144] sul-ac.[10] verat.[144]

Anger; voices of people, to: con. teucr. zinc.

Answer; aversion to: ***agar.*** alum. alum-p.[58] am-c. am-m. ambr. anac. ***ant-c.***[102] ant-t.[102] apom.[36] arg-m.[58] ***arn.*** ars. ars-i. ars-s-f.[58] atro. ***aur.***[122] bell. ***bry.***[102] cact. calc-s. calc-sil.[58] carb-an.[102] carbn-h. carc.[138] caust. ***cham.***[102] chin. chin-s. chlol.[36] cimic. cocc. coff. ***coloc.*** con. cupr. euphr. ***gels.***[102] germ.[222] **GLON.** hell.[5] **HYOS.** ign.[102] iod. juni-c.[36] kali-ar. ***kali-p.*** lil-t. lyss. mag-m. **MANC.**[122] medus.[168] merc. mosch. mur-ac.[102] naja[98] ***nat-m.*** nat-s.[102] **NUX-V.**[122] op. oxyt.[102] petr.[1] **PH-AC.**[122] ***phos.***[122] ***puls.*** rhus-t. sabad. sars.[102] ***sec.*** sil.[102] spong. ***stann.*** stram. ***stry.*** ***sul-ac.*** ***sulph.*** tab. tarent. verat. vib.

Answer; aversion to, sings, talks, but will not answer questions: agar.

Answer; questioned, when, says nothing, indifferent, does not answer: alum.[36] apom.[36] chlol.[36] cocc.[36] ***colch.***[162] hyos.[36] juni-c.[36] mosch.[36] op.[36] ozone[227] tarent.[58] thuj.[8] zinc.[171]

Answer; refuses to: ***agar.*** ambr. ***arn.*** ars. ***atro.***[36] bac.[62] bell. calc-sil.[58] ***camph.*** caust. ***chin.*** chin-ar. ***cimic.*** ***hell.*** ***hyos.*** kali-acet.[58] led. lyss. med.[162] nux-m. nux-v. petr. ph-ac. **PHOS.** sabad. sec. ***stram.*** ***sul-ac.*** **SULPH.** tab.[36] tarent. ***verat.*** ***verat-v.***[54]

Answer; violently, as if angry: rhus-t.[60]

Conversation; agg.: acon. alum. am-c. **AMBR.** arn.[58] aur. calc. cann-s. canth. carc.[140] chin. cocc. coff. dios. ferr. ***fl-ac.*** graph. helon.[137] **IGN.** iod. kali-c. lach.[58] lap-c-b.[194] lap-gr-m.[194] mag-m. mang. mez. **NAT-M.** nat-p. ***nux-m.*** ***nux-v.*** ph-ac. plat. psil.[164] puls. ***rhus-t.*** sars. sep. **SIL.**[122] spig. staph.[137] sulph. thuj.

Conversation; amel.: aeth.[54] ars.[58] eup-per.[102] lac-d.[137] lyss.[54]

Conversation; aversion to: ***ambr.***[30] ***ars.***[36] ars-s-f.[58] asim.[36] atro.[36] bell.[36] caj.[36] calc.[58] ***carb-an.***[36] carc.[140] ***cham.***[85] chel.[58] choc.[222] echi.[111] elaps[36] ferr.[36] gels.[36] germ.[222] ham.[36] hell.[36] kalm.[36] murx.[36] myric.[36] nat-s.[36] ox-ac.[58] plb.[36] ***ptel.***[54] tarent.[36] thea.[36] ziz.[36]

Conversation; aversion to, sadness, after: ziz.[36]

Conversation; desire for: ars.[36] chen-a.[36] narcot.[36]

Conversation; desire for, sublime, to hear: ham.[36]

Death; talks about: mosch.[58]

Delirium; addresses objects: stram.[5]

Delirium; death, talks about: ***acon.***[54]

Delirium; loquacious, business of: ars.[36] bell.[111] **BRY.**[54] ***canth.***[111] dor.[54] **HYOS.**[54] op.[36] ***phos.***[111] **RHUS-T.**[111] stram.[36]

Delirium; loquacious, fire, of: ***calc.*** cupr.[162]

Delirium; loquacious, foreign countries, of: cann-i.

Delirium; loquacious, rhyme, in: thea.[36]

Delirium; speeches, makes: lyss.[54]

Delusions; emperor, talked of: carbn-s.

- hearing, talk seems distant: aran.[149]
- loquacity, with: ***bell.***[10] hyos.[10] lach.[10] op.[10] rhus-t.[10] ***stram.***[10] ***verat.***[10]
- money, talks of: calc. carbn-s. kali-br.[25]
- people, sees, constantly speaks to them: ***verat.***[54]
- people, talks with absent: agar. amyg-am.[54] aur. bell. calc.[58] cham.[1] crot-c. dig. hyos. lach. op. ***stram.*** thuj. ***verat.***[54]
- people, talks with, dead: bell. **CALC-SIL.** canth. chol.[54] hell. ***hyos.*** nat-m. stram.
- says something, it seems to him as though somebody else has said it, when he: alum.
- spectres, sees, talking with, he is: nat-m.[30] nit-ac.[137] plat.[30]
- talking, dead people, with: bell. **CALC-SIL.** canth. hell. ***hyos.*** med.[58] nat-m. stram.
- talking, hears, he: elaps[36]
- talking, inanimate objects with names, t. to but observes no one standing by him: stram.[10]
- talking, insane irrationally: nit-ac.[1]
- talking, persons near who are talking, about midnight: sep.
- talking, rapidly, all around her are t.: ***sang.***[54]
- talking, sister, with his dead: bell.[54] ***hyos.***[54]
- talking, sister, with his dead, churchyard, in: bell.[10]
- talking, someone behind him, with: ***med.***[162]
- talking, spirits, with: bell.[10] **NAT-M.**[122] nit-ac.[137] ***plat.***[122] stram.
- talking, to another part of body, one part is: bapt. 58
- voices, hears, his own, sounds strange and seems to reverberate like thunder: cann-i.
- water, talking of, with: sep.[10]

• whispering, him anything, someone: anac.[137] med.[58]
Dictatorial; command, talking with air of: arn.[10] cupr.[10] ***lyc.***[10] ***phos.***[54]
Dreams; conversations, ending, never, forgetting people that are waiting for her: ozone[227]
➤ conversations, women, with: cedr.[10]
➤ dead, people, of, friends, talking with deceased: lepi.[36]
➤ dead, people, of, talking with: lepi.[36]
➤ interviews, social, with women: cedr.[36]
➤ Latin, he admires his own skill in speaking: lyss.[36]
➤ speech, giving: cham.[1] hydrog.[222]
➤ speech, making a long: arn.[10] cham.[10]
➤ unsuccessful efforts to, talk: mag-c.
➤ unsuccessful efforts to, talk, large tongue which extended out of her mouth and up her nose, on account of: tab.[36]
Dullness; conversation, from: sil. staph.
Egotism; self-esteem, speaking always about themselves in company: lach.[30] par.[10] staph.[30]
Eloquent: cann-s.[1] lachn.[22] op.[36]
Excitement; conversation, from hearing: ***lyss.***
Excitement; stammers when talking to strangers: dig.
Excitement; violent, brought on by current of air, bright light, sight of any shining object, slightest touch, even by conversation in vicinity of a patient: lyss.[54]
Expressing, oneself; difficult: crot-h.[137] kali-br.[25] lil-t.[36] thuj.[5]
Expressing, oneself; impossible: bell.[10] cann-i.[10] haem.[10] lyc.[10] ***nux-v.***[10] phys.[36] puls.[10] sep.[36] thuj.[10]
Fear; conversation, of: bar-s.[58]
✦ say something wrong, lest he should: bamb-a.[1184] germ.[222] ***lil-t.*** med.[85]
✦ speak, to: arg.[58] sep.
✦ speak; cannot: ***ign.***[54]
✦ spoken to, when: kali-br. sep.
✦ talk to someone, to: paeon.[54]
✦ talking, loud talking would kill her, that: meli.
✦ talking, of, on entering room, after walk: alumn.[36]
Heedless; talking and writing, in: carl.[36]
Home; talks of h.: bell. ***bry.***
Inquisitive; jumping from one subject to another: ***ambr.***[58]
Irritability; conversation, from: ***ambr.*** dros.[85] plect.[36] ptel.[54] puls.[60] tarent.[60]
Jealousy; loquacity, with: lach.[30] mag-c.[30] petr.[30]
Lewdness; talk: apis[130] aur. ***bell.*** bufo[112] ***calc.***[30] camph. chlf.[36] cub. ***hyos. lil-t.*** nux-m.[10] ***nux-v.*** phos. plat. ***stram.*** tub.[102] verat.
Loathing; talking: anac. dios.
Loquacity; alternating with, maliciousness: ars-s-f.[58]
Loquacity; alternating with, rage: stram.[10]
Loquacity; alternating with, sadness: arg.[149]
Loquacity; alternating with, silence: bell.[1] buth-aust.[144] cimic.[122] ign.[36]
Loquacity; busy: lach.[10] ther.[10]
Loquacity; devout, mostly: ***stram.***[54]
Loquacity; domineering: ozone[227]
Loquacity; escape, with desire to: crot-h.[102]
Loquacity; excited, heart disease, in: ***op.***[54]
Loquacity; health, about his: **NUX-V.**[122]
Loquacity; heedless: germ.[222] ***iod.***[54]
Loquacity; hoarseness, only kept in check by: ***lach.***[54]
Loquacity; open-hearted: anh.[116] bov.[30]
Loquacity; religious subjects, about: ***verat.***[36]
Loquacity; selected expressions, in: lach.[10]
Loquacity; self-satisfied: par.[10]
Loquacity; speeches, makes: arn. cham. ign.[5] ***lach.*** lachn.[102]
Love; own sex, loquacity, with: lach.[148]
Narrating her symptoms agg.: **CALC.** cic. ign. ***kali-c.***[163] ***med.***[163] ***puls. sep.***[163] teucr.
Nymphomania; loquacity, with: ***verat.***[54]
Religious affections; talking on religious subjects: ***hyos.***[54] stram.[60] ***verat.***[60]
Spoken to; averse to being: agar. am-c. anh.[144] ant-c.[5] ant-t. arn. ***ars. ars-i.*** ars-s-f.[58] aur. aur-ar.[58] aur-s.[58] bar-s.[58] bry.[58] caj. calc-s.[58] calc-sil.[30] camph. ***carbn-s.*** **CHAM.** ***cina***[98] con. cur.[5] cyn-d.[149] elaps fago. ***gels. graph.*** ham. hell. helon. ***hipp.*** hist.[144] ***hyos.*** ign. **IOD.**[122] kali-p. kalm. kreos.[164] lil-t. lyc.[58] mag-m. myric. nat-m. ***nat-s.*** nit-ac.[30] nux-v. op.[5] ***ph-ac.***[5] pitu-a.[164] plan. plat. plb.[5] puls.[5] puls-n. rhus-t. sanic.[102] sep.[5] sil. sin-n.[5] staph. stram. ***sulph. tarent.*** tep. teucr. thuj.[102] verat. zinc.
Spoken to; averse to being, alone, wants to be let: ant-t.[122] arn.[58] aur. caj. gels.[171] hell. helon. hipp. hydrog.[222] ***iod.*** lil-t. luna[29] nat-m.[91] stram.[36] ***sulph.***

Spoken to; being, agg.: ars.[5] **BELL.**[5] **CALC.**[5] **CHAM.**[5] chin.[5] **IGN.**[5] kalm.[5] **NAT-M.**[5] nux-v.[5] **PLAT.**[5] **SEP.**[5] **SIL.**[5] **STAPH.**[5]
Strange; crank, opinions and acts, in: calc.[30] sulph.[30] verat.[30]
Suicidal disposition; talks always of suicide, but does not commit: **NUX-V.**[122]
Talk; battles, about: bell. hyos.
Talk; bombast, worthless: crot-h.[30] ***lach.***[30] nux-v.[30] staph.[30]
Talk; calculations, loud, in dreams: sel.[36]
Talk; desires to t. to someone: ***arg. arg-n.*** buth-aust.[144] ***cann-i.***[25] caust. eup-pur.[25] lachn.[25] lap-c-b.[194] lil-t. nux-m.[54] petr. phys.[25] ***stict.***[54] tarax.[54]
Talk; dictatorial: ***lyc.***[54] ***phos.***[54]
Talk; foreign language, in: camph.[54] lach. m-arct.[1] nit-ac.[137] sol-n.[1] ***stram.***
Talk; indisposed, abortion, in threatening: nit-ac.[26]
Talk; indisposed, convulsions, during: plb.[36] sul-ac.[36]
Talk; indisposed, eating after: aloe arg-n. ferr-ma. mez. plb.
Talk; indisposed, foreign language which at other times he speaks fluently: pall.[54]
Talk; money, about: ars.[189] sulph.[189]
Talk; nothing but, murder, fire and rats: ***calc.*** calc-sil.[58]
Talk; others agg., of: ***acon.***[5] agar. alum. am-c. ambr.[122] androc.[222] ant-t.[58] **ARS.** aur. ***cact.*** cadm-s.[58] carb-an.[122] chin. ***cocc.*** colch. ***con.*** elaps ferr. ferr-ar. ***hell. helon.***[54] hydrog.[222] **HYOS.** ***kali-c.*** kalm. lap-c-b.[194] ***lyss.***[5] mag-m. mang. mez.[111] nat-ar. ***nat-c.*** nat-m.[122] ***nat-s. nit-ac.*** **NUX-V.** petr.[122] ***ph-ac.***[122] rhus-t. ***sep.*** sil. ***stram.*** teucr. verat. ***zinc.***
Talk; sleep, in, business, of: com. rhus-t. sulph.
Talk; sleep, in, confess themselves loud, they: bell.[30] **HYOS.**[30] stram.[30]
Talk; sleep, in, war, of: hyos.[1]
Talk; sufferings, troubles, constantly of his: arg-n.[5] asaf.[137] ***mag-p.***[5] ***nux-v.***[5] zinc.[137]
Timidity; public, talk to: cupr.[122] lach.[30] lyc.[122] med.[187] sil.[122]
Timidity; public, talk to, but capable to: lyc.[1]
Timidity; public, talk to, inapt to talk: ***carb-v.***[30] petr.[30]
Violence; talk of others, from: con.[30] mang.[10]

ABROT. He, 4 - Excited, loquacious, feels like shouting.
ACON. He, 21 - Delirium, with talk about death.
He, 39 - Fear of death; during pregnancy or confinement; with prolapsus uteri; with great loquacity or anxiety in region of heart.
ADAM. Sh, 140 - Does not like to talk. As if nothing needs to be said: it's all obvious so why talk about it. 2, 12C, 111:XX:XX
Sh, 144 - I don't want to be touched or talked to. 7, 6C, 04:08:00
AETH. He, 22 - After social talking, all symptoms disappear.
AGN. Al, 2 - He sometimes feels as if he were nobody (unimportant, insignificant, worthless), and would rather be dead than have that feeling; when possessed by that feeling he has no courage to undertake anything; and when free from it he feels exalted, would like to read like an orator, etc.
ALUM. He, 6 - Makes mistakes in speaking, using words not intended.
ANDROC. Sh, 150 - Speech slurred, answered with difficulty, was indisposed to talk and averse to company. (16)
ANT-C. He, 26 - Irresistible desire to talk in rhymes or verses. (poetry)
APIS. He, 77 - All her ideas turn around jealousy, very talkative (loquacity), sometimes disgusting salacious. (lascivious)
ARG-N. He, 23 - Often awakes his wife or child to have some one to talk to.
ARS. Ha, 1015 - Talks little, only complains of anxiety.
He, 59 - Very peevish and passionate, capricious, she takes every word ill and is cross when she has to answer.
AUR. Ha, 330 - All day long good humor; he was talkative and contented with himself.
Ha, 331 - Cheerful humor; he was always disposed to converse with others and was quite contented with his position.(rank)
BAPT. He, 8 - He thinks his legs are holding a conversation with each other. 0Gout.
He, 9 - He thinks his gouty toe is holding a confab (conversation, talk) with his gouty thumb.
BAR-C. He, 5 - Forgets what was just said, just done, or what he was going to do or get.

He, 15 - Mania; talks much and confusedly; wants to go out of house. 0during pregnancy.

BELL. Al, 82 - Delirious talk of dogs, as if they swarmed (crowd) about him.

Al, 109 - A tailor was poisoned with a belladona injection, and for fifteen hours, though speechless and insensible to external objects, went through all the customary operations of his trade with great vivacity and moved his lips as if in conversation.(busy)

Ha, 1351 - Chattering (talk) lascivious.

BRY. He, 16 - Irrational talk or prattle of his business.

He, 10 - Nightly delirium; delirious talk, especially about business.< after 3 a.m.

He, 12 - Talking of business of day in his delirium at night.

CALC. Ha, 65 - Great weakness of the imaginative (creative) faculty; with a very slight exertion in speaking, he felt as if his brain was paralyzed, ...;he could not think, nor recollect what was spoken of, with muddled (confused) feeling in the head.(lost: imagination, thoughts)

Ha, 62 - He is cheerful, and would like to be among men, to walk with them.

He, 21 - Mania-a-potu, with delirious talk about fire, rats, mice and murder.

CANN-I. Al, 59 - He believes there is creative power in his own word, and that he has only to speak, and it will be done.

CANTH. Al, 14 - He talked deliriously when lying, sitting and walking, disconnectedly of his business and of people who had long since been dead.

CARB-AN. Al, 1 - Desire to be alone ; she is sad and reflective (thoughtful); avoids all conversation.

Ha, 6 - Inclination to solitude (isolation), sad and introverted (egotistic), she always only wishes to be alone, and she shuns every conversation.

Ha, 177 - Vivid dreams about scientific (precise, accurate) subjects; straining (efforts) of the thinking faculty when dreaming; he composed literary essays in thought and spoke aloud.

CHAM. Al, 64 - He stammers (hesitate) uses wrong expressions, and corrects himself.

Ha, 470 - Cannot cease talking about old vexatious things.

He, 25 - Cannot endure being spoken to, or interrupted while speaking, ...

He, 59 - Great tendency to quarrel, to speak in an obstreperous (rude, vulgar) manner.

CHOC. Sh, 213 - Unsociable —averse company and conversation.[15], 30C, 04:XX:XX

COFF. He, 8 - Great loquacity, brain feels clear and is active, he feels strong enough to do anything, feels impelled to push things; veneration for the Supreme Being and love for family; benevolence excited.

COLCH. He, 5 - Says nothing unless questioned, his condition does not seem to him dangerous. 0Typhus.

CON. He, 18 - He is averse to being near people, and to the talk of those passing him (misanthropy); is inclined to seize hold of and abuse them. (insult, offend, curse)

COT. Al, 1-...a feeling as if there was no foot. The head felt exceeding light, as if there were no solid head, and she could not articulate for some time, although she endeavored to do so....

CROC. Al, 14 - Very lively (happy) mood, witty, jocose, excessively talkative.(loquacious)

CROT-C. Al, 9 - While in a clairvoyant state, he speaks to some one who does not answer.

CYCL. Al, 17 - Very fretful (irritable) the whole day; disinclined to speak and insensible (indifferent), having very little feeling (emotion) in his body.

Ha, 188 - He is always in a reverie (meditation, air castles), and not inclined to speak. (talk, aversion)

Ha, 201 - All day long he is peevish not disposed to talk, and insensible, so that he feels little (inadequate, incompetent) in his body.

DROS. Ha, 278 - Anxiety in solitude (alone) he wished to have someone always near him, could not bear to be without companions (friends, company), and was quieter when he had someone to speak to; but when they again left him in solitude, he was all the more anxious, until he fell asleep; on awaking the anxiety returned.

ELAPS. Al, 17 - Peevish in the afternoon, did not want to be spoken to, even fretful (irritable) about herself.

He, 2 - Imagines he hears some one talking.
He, 6 - Angry about one's self, does not wish to be spoken to.

FERR. Al, 20 - Excited by the slightest opposition; ... even her children's caresses increased her bad temper; she was often rude to those about her, because she hated to see or talk to them, and wanted them to leave her in solitude, which alone was pleasing to her.
Al, 4 - Constant desire for solitude; horror of conversation, noise, visits, and even the society of her cherished friends.

GELS. He, 31 - Nervous dread (fear) of appearing in public; singers and speakers.(talking?, acting?)
He, 18 - Desires to be quiet, does not wish to speak, nor have any one near her for company, even if the person be silent.

HALI-L. Sh, 336 - Changed work shift. Didn't want to go to work. Don't like being at work at all. Frustrated at lack of ability to communicate with patient I was assisting. 02, 30C, 10:XX:XX

HEP. He, 20 - Violent, passionate fretfulness; she spoke with such volubility that one could not always get a chance to reason with her, and she would not listen to the most just remarks.

HYOS. Al, 67 - He prattles and makes preparations for his wedding.
Al, 73 - In speaking, used very fine language, so that the usually quiet and indolent peasant (farmer) was scarcely recognized.
Ha, 525 - Chattering he prepares for a journey.
Ha, 526 - Chattering he makes preparation for a wedding.
He, 83-...imagining that her deceased sister was sitting by her bedside, and talking with this imaginary person...
He, 84-...constant talking, particularly on religious subjects; believes himself poisoned, or that there is a stinking odor from his mouth;...
He, 72 - He lies in bed nude and chatters; walks about insane, naked, wrapped in a skin during summer heat.

IGN. Al, 3 - A fixed idea, which he pursues in his thoughts, or expatiates (talk) upon with great earnestness and exhaustiveness in conversation (after two hours).
Ha, 753 - Extreme anxiety, which prevents (restrain) speaking.
Ha, 754-,... he cannot express himself in talking, write, or do anything as quickly as he wishes; ...he makes mistakes in speaking and writing, and does everything awkwardly...
He, 35 - Fearfulness; does not like to talk; prefers to be alone.
He, 36 - Anxiety as though something terrible had happened cannot speak because of it; hurry, fearfulness, terror, alternating with irresolution and inertness.

IOD. Al, 6 - Remarkably lively and talkative, no one else is able to get in a word.

IRID. Sh-9 - Partner said, "I've never seen you so still. You look like a stone Buddha. Your speech is irritating, you can barely get to the end of your sentences." E1
Sh, 19 - Still didn't feel much like talking. Feel very contained and self contained and my mind feels still. Unintellectual, unthinking, heavy. I wanted to be pre-verbal like the cat. Words too much effort. E1
Sh, 26 - Felt detached in company, reticent to speak my mind. Sat and listened but didn't speak at the moments I usually would. Felt "sidelined," watching what's going on, rather than being a part of it. Felt detachment and self-doubt. I didn't speak because didn't feel I would be able to answer them (subject matter was my area of expertise). B9
Sh, 43 - Overall felt better for animated conversation. O13
Sh, 117 - Attention wanders to messages that I hear in my head to pass onto people. QXX

KALI-BR. He, 4-...constant worry, fears to see people or to be spoken to;...failure of mental and bodily strength;...constantly busy, tying his shoes, fumbling in his pockets, picking threads, etc.

LACH. Al, 5 - A kind of ecstasy, as after sublime impressions, or excessive joy, throughout the day; he constantly wishes to talk and do much, and even more seems to be at his command.(control, domination)
Al, 11 - An unusual inclination to be communicative. (affectionate)
He, 16 - Most extraordinary loquacity, making speeches in very select (finest,

excellent) phrases (pretentious), but jumping off to most heterogeneous subjects; at the same time proud (haughty), full of mistrust. 0Mania.

He, 34-...repugnance to society and dislike to talk; solicitude about future, whith disgust of life; inclination to doubt everything; mistrusts (suspicious) and misconstrues (misjudge) ...0 Melancholia.

He, 24 - Inclination to be communicative; vivid imagination; extremely impatient at tedious and dry (arid) things.

He, 25 - Is morbidly talkative and gives a rambling (discursive) account of her ailments.

LIL-T. Al, 49 - She dreads saying anything to anybody, lest she should say something wrong, and yet she wants to walk.

LYC. He, 17-...imperiousness(domineering, despotic) ; speaks with an air of command (ordering, domination) ; manner stiff (severe, obstinate) and pretentious;...

LYSS. Al,N-129 - Hyperesthesia, current of air, bright light, sight of any shining object, slightest touch, even conversation in vicinity of patient, may throw him into a most violent agitation and bring on severe convulsions.

He, 33 - Makes speeches in delirium; thinks he is a man of great authority.

MAG-M. Ha, 18 - He hated to talk; he desired to follow his thought in solitude.

MED. He, 31 - Dread of saying the wrong thing when she has headache.

MERC. Al, 31 - Fretful all day; very much out of sorts and discontented with himself; he had no desire to talk or joke.

Ha, 1257 - During the whole day cross, as if at variance and dissatisfied with himself, and had no inclination for speaking and joking.

MEZ. He, 5 - No rest when alone; wants to be in company ...unable to repeat what has been learned by heart; looks through window for hours, without being conscious of objects around; knows not what she is about; forgets what she is about to utter (talk); looks ill humored, pale, wretched, fallen away; ......expecting some very unpleasant news.

MOSCH. He, 4 - Great dread (fear) of death, with paleness of face, fainting; talks only of approaching (nearing) death.

NAT-M. Al, 6 - She talked more than usual, but did not like so much to be talked to; when she had nothing to say, she became depressed and melancholy.

He, 2 - Absent minded or distracted while talking; does not know what he ought (have to) say; awkward in talking; easily makes mistakes.

NIT-AC. Ha, 15 - Apprehensiveness, with stitches above the heart, and a fancy as if he was talking deliriously, with coldness of the body and a tendency to fall down.

NUX-M. Al, 31 - The words he employed to express his sensations remarkable for the merit of being the opposite (contrary) to what he should have used;...

NUX-V. Ha, 1273 - He cannot bear any noise or speaking; music and singing affect him strongly.

He, 11 - Cannot bear reading or conversation; irritable and wishes to be alone.

He, 20 - Desire to talk about one's condition, with anxious reflections about it.

PAEON. He, 1 - Anxious, afraid (fear) to talk with any one; much affected by bad news, after pinching in belly.

PALL. He, 1 - Extremely fatigued in evening; feels mentally gone; is averse to speaking a foreign language which at other times he speaks fluently; it is too much of an exertion, he is tired of it. (lack of communication)

PETR. Ha, 10 - He does not know how to stop talking about a thing.

PH-AC. Ha, 13 - Hurried in talking; he cannot get anything fast enough.

PHOS. Ha, 27-....Talks in a vehement, (impetuous) commanding (dictatorial) tone; spits at nurse, lifts up her clothes (naked) and kisses hotly all who come near her;...

PLAT. He, 42 - Mania; with great pride; fault-finding; unchaste (sensual) talk; ...(chaste = moral, pure)

SIL. Ha, 36 - Even from little conversation, his head at once becomes muddled (confusion) and there is general exhaustion,...

He, 4 - Reading and writing fatigue, cannot bear to think.

STANN. He, 1 - Sadness, with aversion to men and disinclination to talk.

STAPH. Ha, 691 - Serious, silent, occupied with himself, he speaks but little.

STICT. He, 2 - Great desire to talk about anything and everything, does not care whether any one listens or not, she must talk; feels as if she cannot keep her tongue still.

STRAM. Ha, 499 - In this slumber he hears two persons talking but knows not who they are.

Ha, 519 - He speaks to absent persons as though they were present, and addresses(talk) lifeless objects (e.g. chess-men) by the names of those persons, but does not notice any of those around him.

He, 29 - Talking in Jewish jargon.(clichÇ)

He, 51-...converses with spirits who approach his bed, lays hold of a stick and strikes about him,...great sexual excitement.

He, 68 - Hears dancing, music, sees men and hears them talk in foreign tongues.

He, 122 - Excessive loquacity each time during menses; tears and prayers and earnest (ardent) supplications.

He, 117 - Ceaseless talking mostly devout; very earnestly beseeching. (supplicating)

He, 130 - Talks in a foreign tongue.

TAB. Al, 41 - From having been one of the most healthy and fearless of men, he had become sick all over, and was timid as a girl; he could not even present a petition in Congress, much less say a word concerning it; ...by any ordinary noise, he was startled or thrown into tremulousness, and afraid to be alone at night.

THEA. Al, 3 - Delirium with great ecstasy; the patient laughed incessantly talked constantly in rhyme, showed us that he felt extraordinarily well.

THUJ. Al, 34 - While talking, she is unable to go on in spite of every effort; she begins to weep bitterly, and says she can no longer think or live.

VERAT. Al, 2 - Slight delirium; ...he prattles about religious subjects and about vows to be performed, prays, believes that he is not in his own house.

He, 21 - Mania; with desire to cut and tear everything, especially clothes; with lewdness and lascivious talk; religious or amorous; de grandeur.

He, 24 - Disposed to silence, or to talk about faults of others; if irritated scolding and calling names.

He, 28 - Talks much on religious subjects; praying; is overconscientious.

TEAR

Anger; tear himself to pieces, could: sulph.[54]

Delusions; abundance, of, destroys clothing: ***sulph.***[54]

• head, rising up, tearing neck: bamb-a.[1184]

Destructiveness; clothing, of: ***bell. camph.*** hyos.[54] ***ign.*** nux-v.[30] plb.[111] ***stram. sulph.*** **TARENT.** ***verat.***

Jealousy; tearing the hair: lach.[30]

Mania; tear clothing: nux-v.[30] ***tarent.***[54] ***verat.***[54]

Mania; tear, hair, own: bell.[10] canth.[30] stram.[30] tarent.[36] verat.[30]

Mania; tear, himself to pieces with nails: canth.[30] stram.[30] verat.[30]

Mania; tears: ***cupr.***[54]

Rage; tears clothing: ***camph.***[54]

Shrieking; wild, with disposition to bite and tear: ***verat.***[54]

Tears; himself: ars. bell. cur. lach.[189] plb. sec. **STRAM.**

Tears; himself, genitals, his: sec. tab.[5]

Tears; himself, hair his, headache, during: bac.[55]

Tears; himself, hair, his: ***ars.***[137] bac.[55] ***bell. cupr.***[137] dig.[137] ***lil-t.*** med.[137] tarent. tub.[8] xan.[137]

Tears; himself, skin around nails: carc.[149]

Tears; things: agar.[102] **BELL.** bufo[98] ***camph.*** canth. ***cimx.***[102] cupr. gink.[149] hyos. ign. iod. ***kali-p. lil-t.***[102] merc. ***nux-v.***[122] ***oena.***[54] op. phos. prot.[136] <u>**STRAM.**</u>[122] sulph. tarent.[102] ***verat.***

Tears; things, books, his: tarent.[146]

Tears; things, buttons of her dress, agg. during menses: ***oena.***[54]

Tears; things, clothing: bell.[36] camph.[171] ***ign.***[54] ***stram.***[54] tarent.[58] verat.[58]

Tears; things, clothing, nightdress and bed clothes: ***bell.***[54]

Tears; things, clothing, nightdress and bed clothes, sadness, in religious: ***kali-p.***[54]

Tears; things, everything she can reach: op.[36]

Tears; things, pieces, to, everything: iod.[54]

Tears; things, pieces, to, intermittent, in: ***cimx.***[54]

Tears; things, pillow, with teeth: phos. **STRAM.**

AGAR. Al, 2 - He becomes so furious that

he can hardly be restrained from ripping up his bowels, as he fancies the mushroom had ordered him to do.

BELL. Ha, 1426 - Inclination to tear everything about her to pieces.

CUR. Al, 1 - Paroxysm of insanity impelling him to attack himself; he strikes, scratches, and tears himself with a sort of relish, (enjoy) and without feeling any pain.

GERM. Sh, 112 - Don't see why I am here. I can't bear it. I go mad. I hate myself. I want to beat myself and I do it. Tear my hair. Stop when it hurts too much. It is like hell !!! 18, 30C, 20:XX:XX

IOD. He, 4 - Restless, inclined to move about not permitting to sit or sleep; thought she could tear everything to pieces.

LAC-C. He, 24 - When paroxysms of intense nervousness (anxiety) come on, feels like tearing off her clothes; takes off her rings; cannot bear anything to touch her, ...

MERC. Ha, 1263 - Mania; she throws off the clothes at night, tears the straw about, and scolds; by day she leaps (jump) up high like a petulant extravagant person...she talks and scolds much to herself,...spits frequently and spreads the saliva out with her feet, and licks some of it up again; she often licks cowdung (excrements) and the mud of ponds (lake); she often takes little stones in her mouth, without swallowing them, and at the same time complains that they are cutting her bowels; much clotted blood passes with her motion; ...

STRAM. Ha, 520 - Loquacious madness; he complains of a dog biting and tearing the flesh off his chest.

Ha, 544 - Great desire to bite and tear everything with his teeth that comes near his mouth, even his own limbs.

He, 92 - Mania:... complains that a dog is biting and tearing flesh off his chest; merry exaltation; with pride (haughty) and affectation; runs about, complains of violent headache; ...;steals from his roommates...; disposition to scold persons whom he otherwise loved.

He, 99 - Acute mania; tears his clothing;... threatens to use knife on those about him.

SULPH. Al, 85 - He could tear himself to pieces from vexation.

He, 56 - He could tear himself to pieces with vexation.

VERAT. He, 21 - Mania; with desire to cut and tear everything, especially clothes; with lewdness and lascivious talk; religious or amorous; de grandeur.

TEDIUM

Ennui, boredom: acon.[137] agar.[137] ***alum.*** alumn. ambr.[10] amph.[36] androc.[222] ars.[58] aur. aur-m.[10] bamb-a.[1184] bar-c. bor. cahin. calc.[58] camph. canth.[10] carb-an.[10] cere-s.[36] chin. choc.[222] con. croc.[10] cupr. cur. cycl.[10] elaps ferr. germ.[222] graph.[137] hura hydr. hydrc. ***hydrog.***[222] ign. ip.[10] kali-bi. kali-i.[137] kali-n. kiss.[36] lac-h.[229] lach. laur. led.[5] ***lyc.*** mag-c.[10] mag-m. manc. **MERC.**[30] mez. mosch.[10] ***nat-c.*** nat-m.[10] nit-ac.[58] ***nux-v.*** ozone[227] paull.[36] petr. ph-ac.[109] phos.[189] pip-m. plat. plb. ran-b.[10] rhus-t. sec.[137] ***spig.***[30] spira.[36] sulph.[10] tarent. tub.[58] ven-m.[149] zinc

Ennui; homesickness, with: alum.[162] ***caps.***[122] ***clem.***[122]

Ennui; silent: ***plb.***[30]

Fear; satiety of life, with, particularly in company, hysteric: ***lyc.***[54]

Indifference; ennui, with: alum.[10] choc.[222] con.[10] ***kali-n.***[10] lach.[10] lyc.[10] ***nat-c.***[10] ***nux-v.***[10] petr.[10] ***plb.***[10] zinc.[10]

Morose; life, with satiety of: ***plat.***[54]

New, do anything, cannot: agar.[137]

wearisome: acon. aeth. allox.[119] alum. am-m. anac. ant-c. arg-n. arn. ars. asar. ***ba-sv.***[136] bell. bism. both-a.[139] bov. bry. calc. ***calc-s.*** cann-s. caps. carb-an. caust. cham. chin. clem. cocc. colch. coloc. con. cupr. cycl. dig. ***euon.*** graph. ***grat.*** guai. hep. ign. indg. ip. kali-c. kali-n.[1] kreos. lach. lap-gr-m.[194] led. lyc. ***mang.*** merc. mez. mur-ac. nat-c. nat-m. nat-s. nit-ac. nux-v. olnd. paull.[36] petr. ***ph-ac.*** phos. plat. puls. ran-b. rat. rheum rhus-t. sabin. samb. sars. sep. spong. squil. ***staph. stront-c.*** stry.[36] ***sul-ac.*** sulph. teucr. thuj. verb. viol-t. ***zinc.***

Weary of life; alternating with cheerfulness: bor.[10]

Weary of life; spermatorrhea, in: ***sil.***[54]

ALUM. He, 7 - Time passes too slowly; intolerable ennui; an hour seems half a day.

AUR. He, 17 - Suicidal mania or melancho-

lia, tedium vitae, with genital symptoms.(sexual)
CALC. Ha, 40 - As soon he is idle (unoccupied) and sits still, he becomes peevish and drowsy (tired), and everything goes against him.
CLEM. Al, 19-...dreading to be alone, tired of living, full of thoughts of death, with fear that it would be speedy, longing however, for the repose of death; this mood was soon followed by apprehension, weeping, and homesickness, ...
CON. Al, 46 - Fretful mood; he does not knows how he shall busy himself; the times passes too slowly. (tedium)
HELL. Al, 7 - Sad mood, on account of his present condition (restriction, limitation), everything seems shallow (stupid, superficial) and has no incentive for him. (lost:motive, purpose, force, mission,) -(lost: depth, profundity, perception.)
Ha, 286 - Sad disposition respecting his present position, everything seems to him so insipid (tedious, boring,) and nothing interests him.
HYDROG. Sh, 182 - A feeling of boredom and depression at 10:00p.m., whilst in company —very distressful. I didn't talk at all, friends thought something had greatly upset me. 24, 30C, 01:10:XX
LACH. He, 44 - Satiety (loathing?) of life with longing (desiring) for death.
He, 43 - Weary of life, looks at everything from dark side;...
NAT-C. Al, 24 - She does not know what to do, on account of apprehensiveness and ennui and thinks that she is quite lonely (alone, solitary, insulated) and forsaken, all day.
Ha, 8 - Apprehensive and ennui (tedium, monotony), so that she cannot contain herself; she deems (believe), herself altogether (entirely) lonely (solitary) and forsaken.
NAT-M. Ha, 22 - Hypochondriac, even to being tired of life.
NIT-AC. Al, 18 - Satiety of life with fear of death.
NUX-V. Ha, 1283 - Ennui; time seems to him intolerably long.
He, 6 - Ennui; the time seems intolerably long, passes slowly.
PETR. Al, 28 - No desire to work; no pleasure in objects of which he was usually fond (loving), hence intolerable ennui.
PLAT. He, 29-...thought she had no place in the world; life was wearisome (boring), but had great dread of death, which she believed near at hand.
SIL. He, 13 - Desponding, melancholy, tired of life.
SPONG. He, 6 - Fear of future, tired of life.(ennui)
SULPH. He, 21 - Satiety of life, longing for death.
ZINC. Ha, 13 - Apprehension and ennui; she seeks company.

THEORIZING

Fanaticism; philosophical: sulph.[60]
Religious affections; speculations, dwells on: **SULPH.**[54]
Theorizing: androc.[222] ang. apis[58] arg-n. ars. ***aur.*** **CANN-I.** ***chin.*** cocc.[102] ***coff.*** hydrog.[222] ***lach.***[122] lyc. nat-c.[36] nitro-o.[36] op.[36] puls.[58] sel. ***sep.*** sil. ***sulph. verat.***[30]
Theorizing; gigantic: ***cann-i.***[36] op.[36]
Theorizing; health, about: kali-c.[215]
Theorizing; philosophic, mind dwells on: hydrog.[222] **SULPH.**[54]
ALOE. Al, 2 - Before taking it, the disposition is apprehensive, speculative, amorous, after taking it, quiet ...reflective, more self sufficient,...
CHOC. Sh, 180 - I felt that I was making exceptionally profound statements about life. 35, 30C, 03:XX:XX
HYDROG. Sh, 265 - Greatly increased tendency to theorize and philosophise, especially concerning esoteric matters. 16, 30C, 05:XX:XX
OP. Al, 148-...his mind to be not only clear and active, but filled with gigantic schemes and theories, the realization of which seems to him quite natural and easy; his faculties are remarkably keen (sharp)...
SULPH. He, 9 - Rack (torture) their brains about metaphysical subtleties (nuances).
He, 32 - Melancholy mood; dwelling on religious or philosophic speculations; anxiety about soul's salvation; indifference about lot (destiny) of others.

TIME

Anxiety; church bells, from hearing: ***lyss.***
Anxiety; music, from, church bells: lyss.[122]

Anxiety; time is set, if a: alum.[162] ***arg-n.*** gels. med.
Death; presentiment of, predicts the time: **ACON.**[122] agn.[162] ***aloe***[54] alum.[122] ***arg-n.*** cench.[58] hell.[58] ***lac-d.***[54] thea.[122]
Delusions; afternoon, that it is always: lach. stann.
• bell over him, a transparent: ozone[227]
• bells, hears: ars.[36] cann-i. med.[185] ph-ac. thea. verat.[185]
• bells, hears ringing of, his funeral: aether.
• clock, hears strike of: ph-ac.
• die, about to, will, thinks there is but little time to make his: ***petr.***[54]
• die, time has come to: ars. bell. lach. med.[85] sabad. thuj.
• eternity, lived an, he has: aether[36]
• eternity, mingled with present: anh.[119]
• eternity, that he was in: cann-i.
• existence, begins at that moment, his: camph.[139]
• head, pendulum, seems an inverted oscillating: cann-i.
• hearing, of, wrist-watch, winding up of: ambr.[36]
• immortality, of: anh.[119]
• man, old men with long beards and distorted faces, sees: laur.
• old, he looks: mag-m.[187]
• places, being in different, at a time: anac.[5] brom.[5] cann-i. ***cench. lyc.*** plb. raph. ***sil.***
• places, two at the same time, of being in: anac.[5] brom.[5] cann-i. ***cench. lyc.*** plb. raph. ***sil***
• things done today occur a week ago: ***med.***[54]
• time, earlier, is: sulph.
• time, exaggeration of: **CANN-I.** cann-s. hydrog.[222] nux-m. onos.
• time, passes too, quickly: ***cocc.***[102] sulph. ***thea.***[36] ther.[102]
• time, passes too, slowly: ***alum.***[102] ambr.[102] anh.[102] ***arg-n.***[102] **CANN-I.** cann-s. cere-b.[36] con.[116] dirc.[36] germ.[222] med.[102] nux-m. nux-v.[102] onos. pall.[36]
• time, space, and, lost or confused: anh.[102] bor.[5] ***cann-i.***[102] caust.[5] cic.[102] ***glon.***[102] lach.[102] nux-m.[5]
• time, working against: nat-ar.[168]
• women, old and wrinkle, of: calc-sil. cann-i.
• wrist-watch, winding up of: ambr.[36]
Distance; exaggerated, is, time during sleepiness, and: nux-v.[10]
Dreams; time lost, sense of: bamb-a.[1184]
Fear; age, of people their own: cortico.[119]
✦ death, predicts the time: **ACON.** apis[162] ***arg-n.***
✦ visions of old repulsive persons, from, in hysteria: ***kali-c.***[54]
Forgetfulness; watch, to wind his: fl-ac.
Hurry; everybody moves too slowly: med.[58]
Hurry; everybody must hurry: arg-n.[102] cann-i.[102] ***lach.*** nat-p.[58] ***nux-m.***[102] **TARENT.**
Hurry; movements, fast enough, cannot do things: aur. **SUL-AC.**
Hurry; time, for the appointed, to arrive: **ARG-N.** carc.[138] cupr.[210]
Late, always too: calc.[30] cand-a.[239] plat.[30] puls.[30] sil.[30]
Memory; weakness, time, for: bamb-a.[1184] ***lach.***[10] merc.
Mistakes; makes, time, in: acon. alum. anac. ***anh.***[102] atro. bad. bamb-a.[1184] bor. bov.[116] camph. cand-a.[239] cann-i. cann-s.[5] cere-b. choc.[222] cic. cocc. con. croc. dirc. elaps fl-ac. germ.[222] glon. halo.[149] hura hydrog.[222] ***lach.*** med. merc.[137] nux-m. nux-v. op. ozone[227] pall. petr. plb. psor.[122] sulph. ther.
Prophesying; predicts the time of death: **ACON.** ***arg-n.***[122] thea.[122]
Punctuality, always on time: arg-n.[214] aur-ar.[214] kali-n.[222]
Sadness; disease, about, sure he, is going to die in twenty four hours: lac-d.[54]
Sadness; sound of bells and sight of his surroundings, agg. by: ant-c.[36]
Sensitive; noise, striking of clocks, ringing of bells, to: **ASAR.**[122] **COFF.**[122] dros.[122] **THER.**[122]
Time; asking the time, constantly: lap-mar-c.[194]
Time; far off sensation: med.[179]
Time; fritters away his: bamb-a.[1184] bor.[10] cocc. croto-t.[10] lach.[10] ***nat-c.***[10] nat-m.[10] nux-v. stann.[10] staph.[30] ***sulph.***[10] tab.[30]
Time; loss of conception of: anh.[85] hydrog.[222]
Time; passes too quickly, appears shorter: ***anh.***[119] atro. bamb-a.[1184] cand-a.[239] choc.[222] coca **COCC.** elaps hydrog.[222] lil-t.[25] op. psil.[149] sieg.[144] sulph. ***ther.*** thuj. visc.[119]
Time; passes too slowly, ages, a few seconds seem: cann-i.
Time; passes too slowly, appears longer: aloe

alum. ambr.[5] androc.[222] ***anh.***[102] aran-ix.[144] arg.[102] ***arg-n.*** bar-c. camph. **CANN-I.** ***cann-s.*** carc.[227] ***cench.*** cere-b.[36] con. dirc. germ.[222] **GLON.** hep.[30] lach. lap-c-b.[194] lyc. mag-m. ***med. merc.*** nat-c. nitro-o.[36] ***nux-m. nux-v.*** onos. ozone[227] pall. petr. plb.

Time; passes too slowly, night: nux-v.[36]

Time; passes too slowly, post-partum hemorrhage, in: ***cann-s.***[54]

Time; passes too slowly, way home too long: **GLON.**[54]

Weeping; bells, sound of: ant-c. cop.[122]

ACON. Al, 14 - Excessive disagreeable restlessness; without occasion for hurrying, he is in the greatest haste, every obstacle that delays his rapid pace is excessively annoying; he knocks against some people who do not get out of his way fast enough, and runs in breathless haste up the steps;...

Al, 59 - Feeling as if his last hour had come.

ADAM. Sh, 82 - Finding it difficult to treat, finding I'm there for my patients too much. Sensation as if there's no time to wait to let them finish their story. 7, 6C, 18:00:XX

Sh, 89 - Feeling of time passing slowly. I kept thinking it was earlier than it was. 8, 6C, 07:XX:XX

Sh, 95 - Great difference between the thought of how long it will take and actuality. Thought much longer than actuality. 16, 12C, 22:XX:XX

Sh, 226 - Angry at my daughter for ignoring that I want my time to do my things. 10, 6C, 17:XX:XX

ALUM. He, 7 - Time passes too slowly; intolerable ennui; an hour seems half a day.

ANAC. Ha, 47 - He mixes up the present with the future.

ANDROC. Sh, 92 - Time seemed to go slowly. (2, 25)

Sh, 93 - Felt that she was driving very slowly. Could not judge the speeds of cars coming towards her. While playing the flute, she had the sensation that she was playing very slowly. Felt disconnected from the music but able to play. (25)

ANT-C. Al, 10-...the sound of the bells as well as the sight of that which surrounds him, moves him to tears;...

ARG-N. He, 13 - Frequently settle (decide, fix) upon time he should die. (death)

He, 27 - If a time is set, becomes uneasy the day before; is worried and ready long before the time.(anticipation)

He, 42 - Fits of despondency and all kinds of fanciful (unreal) notions for example, that whilst walking along street he could not pass a given point without falling; frequently settled on the time he was to die.

ARS. Ha, 1032 - Mania; first headache, horrible anxiety, noise before the ears, as from a number of large bells, and when he opened the eyes, he always saw a man who had (formerly) hung himself (suicidal, justified) on the ground-floor of the house, who incessantly beckoned (call) him to cut him down (help); he ran thither (there) with a knife, but, as he could not cut him down, (rescue) he became overwhelmed (beaten) with despair (remorse?) and wished (as his friends assured him) to hang himself (punish); but being prevented (stop) from doing so, he became so restless that he could hardly be kept in bed,... and he knelt down and raised his hands in a supplicating manner.

ATRO. Al, 21 - Keep his eyes closed, ..."Oh, I shall lose my train."

Al, 22 - Expostulates with those who try to lead him to bed; says he will lose the train, that all things are packed up, and that he must start immediately.

Al, 24 - I imagined I had to go off by a railway train, which started at ten in the morning, and that the hour was approaching, whilst I had nothing ready for the journey; and I believed that I wished to dress and to pack my things, but was thwarted (stopped) and prevented by the people about me. At length I was persuaded, that it was too late to catch the train, and agreed to wait till evening.

AUR. Ha, 345 - An urging to activity, bodily as well as mental; when he did anything, he thought he did not do it quick enough, and that he had a great deal (much) more to do; he could not live to his liking. (desire, aspiration)

CAMPH. Al, 46-... My misery was boundless; time itself was no more; in short, I suffered such fearful anguish as no fancy can comprehend. What soul could paint to itself my everlasting (eternal) dwelling as the Evil One (devil), alone in a vast universe, without faith or hope, and my heart forever broken by unimaginable tortures? (miserable, timeless, endless, solitude, forsaken, faithless, hopeless)

CANN-I. Al, 44 - Extreme exaggerations of the duration of time and extent of space-a few seconds seem ages- the utterance (declaration) of a word seems as long as a whole drama, and a few rods are a distance which can never be passed it is so great.(distances)

Al, 48 - Attention principally occupied by an hallucination that time was indefinitely prolonged. (infinite)

He, 16 - Exaggeration of duration of time and extend of space; a few seconds seem ages; a few rods an immense distance.

CERE-B. Al, 2 - Desire to have the time all employed. (work)

CHAM. He, 49 - Great impatience, everything seems to go too slowly.

CHOC. Sh, 186 - It seems like ages ago I started the proving and I can hardly believe its only the fourth day. It seems like I'm going through a whole lifetime of emotions in a short time. 4, 6C, 05:XX:XX

CIC. Ha, 227 - He confounded the present with the past.

COCC. Ha, 523 - Time passes too rapidly with him, several hours appears to him as short as one hour.

Ha, 532 - She dawdles (indolent); in business she cannot accomplish anything nor finish anything, with contracted pupils.

CON. Al, 46 - Fretful mood; he does not knows how he shall busy himself; the times passes too slowly. (tedium)

Ha, 367 - Peevish disposition; he knows not what to occupy himself with, the times appears to pass too slowly.

Ha, 20 - Peevish mood, he does not know what to do with himself, the time passes too slow for him.

GERM. Sh, 181 - Ten minutes seemed like an hour. Time seemed to pass slowly. 06, 6C, 06.09.00

GRAPH. Ha, 25 - Though usually quick to decide, she, soon after taking the medicine, becomes slow of recollection (memory) and resolution.(determination)

HALI-L. Sh, 96 - Feeling spacey and disoriented, stoned, far away from reality; am I making this up? I'm aware of my body, my breasts going up and down with my breath. I'm relaxed and sleepy. Time is very slowed down. I'm in the moment. Am I hot or cold? I don't know, I think it's kind of warm heat I'm feeling. Who is writing this anyway? 06, 6C, 00:00:05

Sh, 97 - I get energy rushes like from a good meditation or a martial arts workout. I felt in the moment. Every moment is an eternity. Being very still, in the moment, every thing was really slow. Time had slowed down. 06, 6C, 00:01:00

Sh, 153 - In retrospect, over the last few days, it seems as if the past and the future have collapsed into the present. The past was unimportant, and I don't concern myself over the future. 09, 6C, 08:XX:XX

Sh, 156 - A person is late to meet me. This is unusual, as I am almost always late. I think, "This is why I am always late, so I don't have to wait. This is what it feels like for other people when I keep them waiting." I have sympathy for people whom I have kept waiting. 09, 6C, 10:06:40

Sh, 157 - Called into work a half an hour early, for an emergency. Went into automatic overwhelm. Felt a lot of responsibilities. I didn't have the time to do all the things I wanted to do. 01, 30C, 01:23:XX

Sh, 161 - I feel like I should write down, "Pandora's box," in my journal. I feel like something started and I don't know where the end is. It's an endless feeling. 06, 6C, 00:12:30

Sh, 163 - Sitting down watching things pass you by. Time is a factor. You only have a certain amount of time to get there. After a certain time you've blocked yourself from the opportunity to have made a move. 18, 30C, 17:XX:XX

Sh, 350-... "Considered committing suicide. Feeling that life has passed me by. Thinking about my mortality. Terrified of dying. My time has run out." ...18, 30C, 05:XX:XX-16:XX:XX

HYDROG. Sh, 19 - The general impression is that the prover entered a larger totalitydimension in terms of space and time, whereupon all previous or smaller totalities became trivial and alien. A conflict of understanding and behaviour arose. 16, 30C, XX:XX:XX

Sh, 93 - I can't believe its only a week ago I took the remedy. It seems like an aeon. 16, 30C, 08:XX:XX

Sh, 94 - Time sense seems warped. 12, 6C, 09:XX:XX

Sh, 95 - I looked at the clock. I think it was about an hour clock time. Time is different on this level, its moving very quickly. 16, 30C, Letter

Sh, 96 - Looking at my life from a distance and thinking probably only thirty or forty summers left to be around, and it looked like a short time and very unimportant. A lifetime is a very short space of time. 16, 30C, 02:XX:XX

Sh, 97 - My whole time scale has changed since taking the remedy, I've lost a lot of boundaries on time. Don't hurry, just do things in my own time. 08, 30C, 06:XX:XX

Sh, 98 - It seems as if all the days became one. 16, 30C, XX:XX:XX

Sh, 100 - I was having problems assimilating the notion of time, outside time seemed beyond description. I Couldn't differentiate between backwards and forwards in time. Felt I had got stuck in time. 16, 30C, 10:XX:XX

Sh, 104 - Don't want to move at all —want to be still and warm and lie around in a heap all day. like what it must feel to be old. I do feel old. 16, 30C, 02:XX:XX

HYOS. Ha, 582 - Impatient: he thought he should die when he had to wait for something of quite trivial nature.

IGN. Ha, 754-,... he cannot express himself in talking, write, or do anything as quickly as he wishes; ...he makes mistakes in speaking and writing, and does everything awkwardly...

IP. Al, 11 - Ill-humored and vexed that his business does not proceed fast enough.

Ha, 224 - He is morose and vexed that his business is not performed quick enough. (time)

IRID. Sh, 146 - Am realizing that time is passing very quickly. Thursday now, and Monday seems only yesterday. G18

Sh, 153 - Time seems to have gone extremely slowly; it feels like weeks have passed since proving started. Time either goes fast or slow, it feels a bit warped. E5

Sh, 155 - Very restless night, not insomnia, just kept rising into consciousness, thinking it had to be morning now. Knew I had to be up at 6.30 a.m., and the night seemed so long, I kept checking to see if the alarm was working. Even at 1.30 a.m., thought it was morning; shocked it was so early. Night seemed elastic. The night stretched and stretched and seemed so long. E7

MED. Al,N-40 - Always wakens tired in the morning; hates to do anything that must be done (duty), even nice things; gets nervous and excited about riding and driving as soon the time is fixed.

Al,N-48 - It is also introspective, self-accusative, remorseful. Time moves slowly to it, therefore it is hurried.

Al,N-59 - Time moves so slowly that things done an hour ago appear to have occurred a year since; asked the time of day, and in five minutes insisted that half an hour had elapsed and could not believe it had till she had seen the watch.

He, 2 - Dullness of memory and desire to procrastinate (delay), because business seemed so long lasting (permanent), or as if it never could be accomplished. (postponing)

He, 8 - Time moves too slowly.

He, 9 - Dazed (confused) feeling; a far (distant) sensation, as though things done to-day occurred a week ago.(time)

He, 25 - Is in a great hurry; when doing anything is in such a hurry that she gets fatigued.

MEZ. Al, 47 - He looked out of the window for hours without thought, and without knowing what he was looking at.

Ha, 23 - He would vacantly (empty) look through the windows for hours, without becoming conscious of what he saw, and without then thinking about anything.

NAT-C. Al, 22 - His fancy is mostly busy with apprehensions of the future; he often makes plans for half an hour at a time as if it would go wrong with him, wherewith he seeks to be alone for several days together.

NEON. Sh, 85 - Feel out of control, as if time is moving relentlessly and remorselessly forward and I'm stuck behind, unable to keep up. Panic, guilt, constant anxiety that I won't get it all done, including keeping up this journal. 10, 6C, 12:XX:XX

Sh, 91 - I'm finding it hard to judge how long ago recent events were. Can't seem to judge time in the past. Can't think back through the days. It's as if I've lost the thread with the past that connects all past days together. It has dissolved. I seem to be more in the moment and less hurried. I usually look at my watch often, but today I forgot I had put it on, and kept asking a friend the time. Was surprised when I discovered I'd been wearing it all day. Very unusual. 05, 12C, 05:XX:XX

Sh, 92 - I had a sense of timelessness and wanted to find the clock but could not. I had no reference points and thought that if I could find the time, it would be a reference point in the void. 20, 6C, 00:00:30

NUX-M. Al, 56-...he went to the theater, which was at some distance; the way seemed to have no end (endless, interminable); ... Although he was, at times, quite unconscious, his limbs did not fail to their service; he went straight on, without recognizing the streets that crossed his way; he was concerned about the time, he feared to come too late..., fancy and reality battle (fight) with each other.

NUX-V. Ha, 1283 - Ennui; time seems to him intolerably long.

He, 6 - Ennui; the time seems intolerably long, passes slowly.

PALL. He, 2 - Time seems longer to him, as if contained more; when he looks at the clock far less has been spent than he expected.

PETR. He, 11 - Melancholy mood, imagines but little time is left him to make his will.

PH-AC. Ha, 41 - Illusion of the senses, as if he heard the clock strike or as if lofty (tall, elevated) things lying out of his horizon were moving near him.

Ha, 13 - Hurried in talking; he cannot get anything fast enough.

PTEL. Al, 20 - In writing a letter, felt a curious and unusual disposition to hurry (run, hasten, speed) through with it as quickly as possible, hardly taking time to write the words.

STANN. Al, 20 - Fruitlessly busy, as if a rush of ideas prevented him from completing his work at a certain time; all sorts of things occur to him to be done.

SUL-AC. Al, 9 - Hasty (hurried, fast) mood; nothing that she does can be finished quickly enough, though she makes unusual effort.

Ha, 12 - Hastiness (fast) ; everything she does, she cannot accomplish fast enough; but it fatigues her exceedingly.

He, 2 - Must do everything in a great hurry; nothing can be finished quickly enough.

THEA. Al, 11 - The sound of the "night bell" made me terribly nervous.

THER. Al, 3 - Time appears to him to pass more rapidly, although he does very little.

TIMIDITY

Ailments from; anticipation, stage-fright: acon.[163] anac.[102] arg-n.[102] ***ars.***[163] bor.[163] calad.[163] calc-p.[163] carb-v.[163] carc.[207] cina[153] coff.[163] crot-c.[163] crot-h.[163] ***cypr.***[163] ***gels.***[102] hyos.[163] ign.[163] ***kali-br.***[163] kali-p.[163] lach.[30] ***lyc.***[163] lyss.[163] ***med.***[163] ***merc.***[163] nat-m.[163] nat-p.[163] nat-s.[163] ox-ac.[163] petr.[163] ***ph-ac.***[163] ***pic-ac.***[163] plb.[163] psor.[163] puls.[163] sep.[163] ***sil.***[163] ***stroph.***[163] sulph.[163] syph.[163] ***thuj.***[163] tub.[163] ***zinc.***[163]

Ailments from; anticipation, stage-fright singers and speakers, in: arg-n.[155] **GELS.**[54]

Anger; alternating with, timidity: ran-b.[10] zinc.[10]

Awkwardness; timidity, from: nat-c.[30] nat-m.[30] nux-v.[30] sil.[30] sulph.[30]

Cheerfulness; alternating with, timidity: m-arct.[10]

Children; covering their face with their hands, but looking through their fingers: bar-c.[122]

Courageous; alternating with, timidity: ***alum.***[30]

Delirium; shy, hides himself: **STRAM.**[54]

Delusions; laughed at, criticized to disadvantage, makes her timid, and she dare not look up while walking in street: bar-c.[54]

Desires; familiar surroundings: bar-c.[8]

Eccentricity; alternating with, timidity: sul-ac.[10]

Embarrassment: ***ambr.***[5] ***bar-c.***[5] carb-v.[5] chin.[36] ferr.[5] gels.[137] germ.[222] hydrog.[222] hyos.[60] ign.[5] kali-br.[137] ***merc.***[8] op.[137] phos.[5] sulph.[5]

Embarrassment; strangers, in presence of: ambr.[5] bar-c.[5] ***dig.***[8] tarent.[5]

Faces the wall if anybody talks to him: nat-m.[70]

Fear; conversation, of: bar-s.[58]
✦ looked at: aq-mar.[231] ars.[193] bar-c.[193] calc.[172] meli.[193] rhus-t.[193]
Hypochondriasis; timid, fearful: cocc.[54]
Indifference; alternating with, timidity: stram.[10]
Insanity; shy: agar.[5]
Irritability; alternating with, timidity: ran-b.[10] zinc.[10]
Praying; timidly, during sleep: stann.[54]
Restlessness; bashful, timid, ill at easy in society: ***coca***[54]
Restlessness; timid: asar.[54] ***calc.***[54] **PULS.**[54] rhod.[54]
Sadness; timidity, with: ***crot-h.***[54] plb.[54]
Talk; sleep, in, supplicates timidly: stann.[54]
Timidity: ***acon.*** aloe ***alum.*** alum-p.[58] alum-sil.[58] ***alumn.***[36] am-br.[162] am-c. am-caust.[36] ***am-m.*** ambr. anac. ang. ant-t.[10] arg-n.[5] arn. ***ars.*** ars-i. ars-s-f.[58] ***aur.*** aur-ar.[58] aur-i.[58] aur-s.[58] ***bac.***[62] **BAR-C.** bar-i.[58] bar-m.[58] bell. ***bor.*** bry. calad.[60] **CALC.** calc-ar.[58] **CALC-S.** calc-sil.[58] cand-a.[239] canth. carb-an. ***carb-v. carbn-s.*** carc.[119] carl.[36] ***caust.*** cham.[5] ***chin.*** chin-ar. cina[60] ***coca*** cocc. coff. ***con.*** cortico.[119] croc. ***crot-h.***[122] ***cupr.*** daph. dat-m.[85] dros.[5] dys-co.[136] elaps[231] ferr-p.[36] **GELS.** ***graph.*** hydr-ac.[10] hyos. ***ign.*** iod. ip. ***kali-ar.*** kali-bi.[36] kali-br. **KALI-C.** kali-i.[137] kali-n. ***kali-p.***[122] ***kali-s. kali-sil.***[58] lach.[5] laur. lil-t. **LYC.** ***m-arct.***[10] m-aust.[10] mag-c. ***mag-s.***[60] manc. med.[94] meli.[102] meny.[60] ***merc.*** mur-ac. naja[141] ***nat-ar.*** **NAT-C.** ***nat-m.*** nat-p. nat-s.[85] nicc.[60] ***nit-ac. nux-v.*** op. **PETR.** phel.[60] **PHOS.** plat. **PLB.** ptel.[25] **PULS.**[122] ran-b. ***rhus-t.*** ruta[10] sabad.[102] ***sac-alb.***[210] sec. **SEP.** **SIL.**[122] spig. ***spong.*** staph. ***stram. stront-c.***[60] sul-ac. sul-i.[58] **SULPH.** syc-co.[136] tab. tanac.[25] tart-ac.[60] tub.[94] verat. verb. zinc. zinc-p.[58]
Timidity; alone, when: sil.[58]
Timidity; alternating with, anger: zinc.[10]
Timidity; alternating with, assurance: ***alum.***
Timidity; alternating with, hope: kali-c.[10]
Timidity; alternating with, quarrelsomeness: ran-b.[10]
Timidity; alternating with, sadness: zinc.[10]
Timidity; bashful: aloe ***ambr.*** anac. aq-mar.[231] arg-n. ars-s-f.[58] aur. ***bar-c.*** bar-s.[58] bell. ***calc.*** calc-s.[58] calc-sil.[58] ***carb-an.*** carb-v. caust.[102] ***chin.*** **COCA** coff. con. ***cupr.*** dys-co.[136] graph.[102] hyos. ***ign.*** iod. kali-bi. kali-br.[25] kali-i.[137] ***kali-p.***[122] lil-t.[102] manc. mang. meli.[102] ***merc.***[54] mez. ***nat-c.*** nat-m.[189] nat-p.[58] nit-ac. nux-v. ***petr.*** phos. **PULS.** rhus-t.[137] sil.[102] staph.[85] ***stram. sulph.*** tab. tarent.[54] zinc.[58]
Timidity; bashful, awkward, and: ambr.[116] bar-c.[162] calc.[30] carb-v.[30] nat-c.[30] nat-m.[30] nux-v.[30] puls.[30] sil.[30] sulph.[30]
Timidity; bashful, blushing, with: ambr.[137] puls.[155]
Timidity; bashful, children: bov.[122] bufo[117] tub.[122]
Timidity; bed, about going to: acon. ars. bapt. camph. cann-i. ***caust.*** cench. lach. lyc. nat-c. squil.
Timidity; business, in transacting: op.[36]
Timidity; children, with other: ars.[146] ars-i.[146] calc-p.[146] cand-a.[239] carc.[146] phos.[146] sil.[146]
Timidity; fear, with: manc.[54] ***nux-v.***[54]
Timidity; fright, after: ***acon.***[36] merc.[54]
Timidity; public, about appearing in: aeth.[122] **AMBR.**[122] anac.[85] arg-n.[36] bamb-a.[1184] ***carb-v.*** chin.[30] cocc.[172] cortico.[119] dys-co.[104] **GELS.**[122] graph.[184] kali-p.[172] ***lyc.***[36] med.[187] ***ph-ac.***[36] **PLB.**[122] **SIL.** staph.[36] thuj.[198]
Timidity; public, talk to: cupr.[122] lach.[30] lyc.[122] med.[187] sil.[122]
Timidity; public, talk to, but capable to: lyc.[1]
Timidity; public, talk to, inapt to talk: ***carb-v.***[30] petr.[30]

ACON. He, 36 - Extreme timidity, especially after a fright; afraid (fear) in dark.
ALUM. He, 25 - Variable mood, at one time confident, at another timid.
AM-C. Ha, 9 - Many afternoons she is seized with weakness and timidity, so that she cannot control herself and knew not what to do;...
AMBR. He, 16 - Embarrassed (inhibit) manner in company.
ANAC. Ha, 6 - Timorous in all his actions; he views everything more anxiously and timidly, always thinks of being surrounded by enemies, then he becomes hot, his blood seems to boil in his chest.
BAR-C. Ha, 16 - Great timidity and cowardice.
CALC. Ha, 22 - Timid and restless, as if evil (harmful, misfortune) was impending (imminent) over her.
CAUST. Ha, 20 - Extreme anxious timidity; she is so much afraid (fear) of a dog near

her, which did not harm (hurt, injure) her at all,...every noise in the street made her afraid, and when she saw boys climbing she was very uneasy lest they might get hurt. (care, others)

CON. Ha, 9 - Shyness (timidity) at the approach of people, and yet also dread of being alone.

GERM. Sh, 126 - I have a guilty feeling if I get too much attention. I am afraid of bothering others. 18, 30C, 13:XX:XX

GRAPH. He, 19 - Extreme hesitation; she is unable to make up her mind about anything; timidity.

IGN. Al, 20 - Fearfulness timidity; she has no confidence in herself, gives up (desist) everything.

IOD. Al, 8 - Disposition mild, scrupulous (careful) and timid (irresolute), with blunted (dull) sensibilities.

KALI-BR. He, 37 - Timid, suspicious, full of fear.

KALI-C. Al, 22 - Faint-hearted and despondent to an excessive degree.

LYC. He, 29 - Want of self confidence; indecision; timidity; resignation.

NAT-C. Al, 28 - He is very timid, and starts at the slightest noise.

Ha, 3 - Dread of men and timidity.

PHOS. Al, 80 - Mental depression, and a most uncommon fearfulness or timidity, with a great sense of fatigue.

He, 9 - Mental depression and a most uncommon fearfulness or timidity with great sense of fatigue.

PULS. Ha, 18 - Mild, bashful, gentle, yielding disposition.

SIL. He, 16 - Yielding, faint-hearted, anxious mood.

SPONG. He, 21 - She is very timid, and is especially pursued and incessantly tormented by a frightful scene of some mournful (unhappy) event of the past.

TAB. Al, 41 - From having been one of the most healthy and fearless of men, he had become sick all over, and was timid as a girl; he could not even present a petition in Congress, much less say a word concerning it; ...by any ordinary noise, he was startled or thrown into tremulousness, and afraid to be alone at night.

TORMENTED

Delusions; hell, suffers the torments of, without being able to explain: lyss.[54] ***merc.***[122]

- persecuted, that he is, tormented by some frightful scene of some mournful event of the past, and: spong.[54]
- pursued, tormented by a frightful scene of some mournful event of the past, and: spong.[54]
- tormented, he is: ***aq-mar.***[149] ***chin.*** lyss.

Dreams; anxious, tormenting: aur-m.[54]

Thoughts; sexual, tormenting: aq-mar.[149] aster.[85] canth.[58] con. graph. ozone[227] ***staph.*** tarent.[192]

Thoughts; tormenting: acon.[54] alum. am-c. ambr.[1189] ant-c. arg-n. ***ars.*** ars-i.[58] astra-e.[149] calc-s.[58] caps.[58] carbn-s.[58] ***caust.*** con. graph.[10] guat.[149] kali-ar.[58] lac-ac. lac-c. ***lach.*** ***lyc.*** mez. **NAT-M.** ***nit-ac.*** nitro-o.[36] phos. plat.[54] ***rhus-t.*** sep. sul-i.[58] ***sulph.*** thea. tub.[58]

Thoughts; tormenting, past disagreeable events, about: am-c.[1] spong.[1]

AGAR. Ha, 5 - The mind is restless and troubled; he was always solely occupied with his present and his future condition.

ALOE. Al, 1 - Amorous (sexual) thoughts present themselves which are very annoying.

AM-C. Al, 16 - The recollection of past disagreeable occurrences torments him.

Ha, 5 - Thoughts of previous annoyances torment him.

ANAC. He, 62 - Internal anxiety, which did not leave him any peace; he felt solicitous (careful) on account of every trifle, as if it would lead to some great trouble (misfortune); with apprehension (fear) of future.

ARS. Ha, 1038 - When he is alone he is beset by thoughts about disease and other thoughts of an indifferent character, of which he cannot get rid.

He, 16 - Tormenting hallucination, as if there was one by his side who did that he was doing, eating, washing etc.

CHIN. Al, 47 - Discontent; he considers himself unhappy and thinks he is hindered (obstructed) and tormented by everyone. (after five hours)

Ha, 1113 - Discontented; he thinks himself unfortunate (unsuccessful), and fancies he is opposed (confronted, hostilised), and tormented (molested) by everybody.

He, 11 - She thinks she is very unfortunate and constantly harassed (molested, tormented) by enemies.

HALI-L. Sh, 172 - I have an inner sense of confidence. I feel good about the things I do. I am able to let my friend go and not torment myself about things which haven't working out. 08, 30C, 19:XX:XX

IGN. He, 11-...believes herself married (connected) and pregnant; is tormented by remorse of imagined crimes; seeks constantly to escape to drown (suicide) herself; ...;is only quiet when lying undisturbed and brooding over her troubles, which she rehearses (tell) in a doleful (unhappy) tone ;..." I am neglecting my duty, breaking my vow" (promise, engagement)...;conscientious scruples after eating.

LACH. Al, 19 - So great apprehensiveness while riding in the open air that it seemed to him some great evil (hurtful, injurious) was impending (imminent), like an evil foreboding; it torments him for more than an hour.

He, 45 - She is tormented by the idea that her better principles (ideals) might be overcome (beaten) by irresistible desire to suicide. (lost: moral) 0 Mania.

LIL-T. He, 5 - Tormented about her salvation.

LYC. Ha, 1 - Hypochondriac, tormenting mood; he feels unhappy.

LYSS. Al,N-50 - Declares amid violent sobs that she is suffering the torments of hell.

Al,N-8 - Could not get rid of the indescribable tormenting feeling that something terrible was going to happen to him.

He, 50 - Declares amid violent sobs that she is suffering the torments of hell.

MANG. Ha, 3 - Great restlessness of body and mind, as if something was tormenting him.

MUR-AC. Al, 10 - Anxious thoughtfulness; he cannot free himself from the slightest trouble.

NAT-M. Al, 47 - Full of grief; he tormented himself; he seemed to prefer disagreeable thoughts, which prostrated him very much.

Ha, 8 - He sorrowfully torments (torture) himself, by continually looking for disagreeable ideas, which weakens him.

Ha, 64 - Injuries which he had inflicted on others, or which others had done to him, always dwelled in his thoughts; he could not get rid of them, and this annoyed him, so that he had no pleasure in anything.

SPONG. Al, 6 - She is very fearful, and tormented by a frightful image of a past sad event.

Ha, 381 - She is timorous (fearful) and particularly pursued and incessantly plagued (disturbed, bothered) by a frightful picture out of a melancholic past.

He, 21 - She is very timid, and is especially pursued and incessantly tormented by a frightful scene of some mournful (unhappy) event of the past.

STRAM. Al, 63-...I was assailed (attacked) by imaginary spectres, in the most hideous forms and menacing attitudes; and what was still to my torment my bed was suspended and tantalized (charmed) like a feather (plumage) between two floors.

SULPH. Al, 8 - Numerous morbid ideas, extremely disagreeable, causing rancor, though with also joyous thoughts (and melodies) mostly from the past, take possession of her they throng one upon another so that she cannot free herself from them during the day, with neglect of business,...

He, 9 - Rack (torture) their brains about metaphysical subtleties (nuances).

He, 43 - Vexations and morbid ideas of past arise from most indifferent thoughts, and from every occurrence in life, which continue to be united with new vexations, so that she cannot free herself from them.

VERAT. He, 45-... he is tormented by fearful anxiety, wherewith forehead becomes covered with cold sweat and he becomes sick to vomiting.

TORTURED

Delusions; tortured, he is: ozone[227]
Dreams; anxious, racking his brain: kalm.[54]
Fear; torturing, of: ars-s-f.[54]
Religious affections; night tortured by religious ideas: camph.[54] lil-t.[58]
Self-torture: acon.[111] ***ars.***[111] bell.[111] ***lil-t.***[111] plb.[111] tarent.[111] tub.[111]

CAMPH. Al, 46-... My misery was boundless; time itself was no more; in short, I suffered such fearful anguish as no fancy can comprehend. What soul could paint to itself my everlasting (eternal) dwelling as the Evil One (devil), alone in a vast universe, without faith or hope, and my heart forever broken by unimaginable tortures? (miserable, timeless, endless, solitude, forsaken, faithless, hopeless)

He, 16 - Monomania, with horrible visions and torturing ideas about religion, which he cannot shake off, although he is conscious that they are morbid.; is< at night.

COP. Al, 9 - Absurd recriminations about trifling and long -past occurrences.

DIG. He, 11 - Melancholic, despondent, and constantly tortured by fear of death or loss of reason.

MED. He, 33 - Woke at an early hour with a frightened sensation, as if something dreadful had happened;... as if she must do something to rid her mind of this torture.

MERC. Ha, 1225 - Imagines he is enduring the tortures (torment) of hell, without being able to account for it (explain). -(lost understanding, judgment)

NIT-AC. Ha, 4 - He cannot get rid of his sad thoughts.

NUX-V. He, 33 - Mental disturbance, patient tortured with fixed idea.

RHUS-T. Ha, 973 - When she had disagreeable thoughts in her head she could not get rid of them.

STAPH. Ha, 716 - She was all day long full of grief; she was afflicted (torment) to weeping about her circumstances (position), and she cared for nothing in the world.

SULPH. Ha, 59 - A number of ideas from her past life, mostly disagreeable, causing indignation and mortification...come into her mind;...so that she cannot get rid of them, while she has nothing to do;...

Ha, 60 - Indifferent things and such things as naturally occur in life are attended in her mind with annoying, mortifying ideas from her past, which continually connect themselves with recent annoyances of which she cannot rid herself. This attended (accompanied) with a resoluteness of mind, which is ready for great resolves.(determination)

He, 29-...is filled with anxious, despondent (sad) thoughts, from which she cannot free herself, they make her suspicious, peevish and lachrymose.

TOUCH

Anger; caressing, from: chin. ***cina***[179] nit-ac.[193]

Anger; touched, when: ***ant-c.*** cham.[162] cina[47] iod. lach.[10] sanic.[137] **TARENT.**

Aversion; water to, touch of it, cannot bear: am-c.[137]

Caressed; agg. being: bell.[137] calc.[137] chin.[137] ign.[137] plat.[137]

Caressed; aversion to being: chin.[193] ***cina*** cupr.[210] ign.[193] nit-ac.[1] sac-alb.[210]

Caressed; caressing husband and child, then pushes away: ***anac.***[54]

Caressed; propensity for being: cann-i.[36] carc.[140] germ.[222] lap-mar-c.[194] puls.[102] ***sac-alb.***[210]

Carried; desires to be, caressed and: acon.[122] kreos.[5] puls.[5]

Delirium; touch, with aversion to: merc.[36]

Delusions; hand, delicate, smoothing her head: med.

- hand, passes over body: carb-v.[1]
- throat, someone with icy-cold hands took her by the: canth.
- touch everything: bell.
- touch, cannot, she: pall.[85]
- touch, rough, everything is too: par.[171]
- touch, sensory: acon. ***alum.*** anac. ant-t. arn. ars. ***asaf.*** asar. bar-c. ***bell.*** bism. bor. bov. bry. ***calc.*** cann-s. canth. caps. carbn-o.[72] caust. chel. coc-c. cocc. coloc. con. ***croc.*** dros. dulc. glon. graph. guai. hell. hep. hyos. ***ign.*** indg. iod. kali-c. kali-n. kreos. ***lach.*** laur. lyc. mag-c. mag-m. meny. merc. mosch. nat-c. nat-m. nux-v. olnd. op. ***par.*** ph-ac. phos. plat. ***plb. puls.*** ran-b. ran-s. rheum rhod. **RHUS-T.** ruta sabad. samb. seneg. sep. sil. ***spig.*** spong. squil. staph. ***stram.*** sul-ac. ***sulph.***[122] tarax. thuj. valer. verat. verb.
- touches her head, someone: **MED.**[162]

Dreams; men, caressing her back: ozone[227]

Excitement; violent, brought on by current of air, bright light, sight of any shining object, slightest touch, even by conversation in vicinity of a patient: lyss.[54]

Fear; approaching, of others: acet-ac. ***ambr.*** anac. ant-c.[162] <u>**ARN.**</u>[122] ars.[172] bar-c.[5] ***bell.*** cadm-s. cann-i. caust.[5] cham.[162] con. ***cupr. cupr-acet.***[54] graph.[146] ***ign.*** iod. ***lyc.*** nux-v.[54]

op. petr.[5] phos.[5] plb.[111] rhod.[122] sep.[5] ***stram.*** stry.[5] tarent.[5] ***thuj.*** valer.[172]
✦ approaching, others, of, children cannot bear to have anyone come near them: ambr.[172] ant-c.[162] arn.[172] bell.[172] ***cina cupr.*** ign.[172] kali-c.[172] lach.[172] stram.[172] thuj.[172]
✦ approaching, others, of, touched, lest he be: **ARN.**[122] ars.[172] chin.[172] coff.[172] colch.[5] kali-c.[172] lach.[172] mag-p.[172] rhod.[122] stram.[172] tell.[172] valer.[172]
✦ examination, medical: ant-t.[103] phos.[146] puls.[70] sanic.[141] tub.[70]
✦ jumps, touch, on: bell.
✦ senses, with exalted state of, smell, taste, touch: lyss.[54]
✦ touch, chest wall, on: stroph-s.[119]
✦ touch, of: ***acon.***[102] ang.[102] ant-c.[116] ant-t.[102] apis[98] **ARN.**[122] ars.[172] asar.[149] ***bell.***[102] calc-sil.[58] ***cham.***[102] ***chin.***[102] cina[98] coff. ***colch.***[102] con.[137] cupr.[137] ***hep.***[102] ign.[137] iod.[102] ***kali-c.***[122] lach. lyc.[137] mag-p.[102] nit-ac.[102] nux-m.[102] ***nux-v.***[54] ph-ac.[54] phos.[102] ***plb.***[102] sanic.[102] sep.[102] sieg.[144] ***spig.***[102] stram.[102] sulph.[102] ***tarent.***[102] tart-ac.[122] ***tell.***[122] thuj.[102] valer.[172]
✦ touch, others passing, by: acon.[137]

Frightened; easily, touch, from: ***kali-c.*** ruta[36]

Hydrophobia; spasms renewed by contact: ***bell.***[54]

Hydrophobia; touch, cannot bear: am-c.[137]

Hysteria; touch and pressure, intolerance of: ***tarent.***[54]

Insanity; touched, will not be: ***thuj.***

Irritability; touch, by: ***ant-c.***[54] lach.[10] tarent.[137]

Lasciviousness; women at every touch: ***murx.***[116]

Moaning; children, in, touched, when: ant-t.[72]

Rage; touch, renewed by: ***bell.*** lach.[116] ***op. stram.***

Restlessness; touch, on: nat-m.[189] oena.[60]

Sensitive; touch, to: abrot.[127] ***acon.***[116] arn.[171] ars.[58] ***bell.***[58] caps.[127] caust.[58] chin.[116] ***chin-ar.***[58] cina[58] coff.[58] foll.[149] hep.[109] kali-c.[171] ***lach.***[122] meny.[116] op.[30] phos.[58] ruta[161] spig.[171] staph.[58] tarent.[214] tell.[149]

Shrieking; touched, slightest, at, with pain: ***acon.***[54] colch.[100] cupr.[10] kali-c.[8] oci.[36] phos.[38] rhus-t.[54] verat.[37] zinc.[54]

Shrieking; touched, when: ***acon.***[54] ant-c.[116] ***ant-t.***[54] arn.[58] chel.[38] hep.[171] ***iod.***[8] kali-c.[111] mag-c.[144] ***merc.***[54] ruta[107] stram.[137] stry.[36]

Singing; touches things constantly: bell.[54]

Starting; touched, when: bamb-a.[1184] ***bell. cocc.*** coff.[47] coffin.[38] **KALI-C.** ***kali-p.*** kali-sil.[58] m-aust.[1] mag-c. prot.[136] ruta ***sil.*** stram.[85] stry.[47]

Touch things, impelled to: bell.[1] carc.[122] hyos.[36] lycps. ***merc.***[30] sac-alb.[210] sulph.[102] ***thuj.***[30]

Touch; impelled to, does not know if objects are really until she has touched them: sulph.[54]

Touched; agg. being, mental symptoms: canth.[5] cina[5] colch.[5]

Touched; aversion of being: ***acon. agar.*** **ANT-C.** ***ant-t.*** **ARN.**[122] ars. asar.[149] ***bell. bry.*** bufo calc. camph. cand-a.[239] canth.[85] carc.[207] **CHAM.** ***chin.*** cimic.[137] ***cina*** cocc. ***coff.*** colch. con.[111] cupr. gels.[116] hell.[58] hep.[137] hydrog.[222] ign.[111] iod. **KALI-C.** kali-fcy.[198] ***kali-i. lach.*** lyc.[111] mag-c. mag-m.[162] ***med.*** merc. mez. nit-ac.[102] nux-m.[36] nux-v. ozone[227] plb. sanic. ***sil.*** stram. **TARENT.** ***thuj. tub.***[36] verat. vip.[144]

Touched; aversion of being, cannot bear anyone to lie close to or touch him: sanic.[85]

Touched; aversion of being, caressed: ***cina*** nit-ac.[1]

Violence; touch, from: lach.[10]

Weeping; children, touched, when: ant-t.[102]

Weeping; touched, when: ant-c. ant-t. cina sil.[1] stram.[10]

Wildness; bright light, strong odors or touch, from: ***colch.***

ACON. Al, 55 - Flickering (spark, flash) before vision makes him anxious on street, he thinks he constantly jostles (press)the passers by.

ADAM. Sh, 108 - I feel like burying myself in grass and earth. I love touching and covering my hands with earth. I want to be enclosed and hidden in the earth. 20, 1M, 08:XX:XX
Sh, 144 - I don't want to be touched or talked to. 7, 6C, 04:08:00
Sh, 160 - Disliked being touched and uninterested in any sexual relationship. Began to be repulsed by boyfriend. 20, 1M, XX:XX:XX

ARN. He, 34 - Fears being struck (hit, hurt) by those coming towards him; fears even the possibility of being touched.

ARS-MET. He, 5 - Feels as if she had to run away (escape), far away, and as if she would hardly touch ground.

He, 5 - Feels as if she had to run away, far away, and as if she would hardly touch ground.

BAPT. He, 17 - A sensation as if some person touched him gently while dozing.(sleep)

BELL. Ha, 1361 - She bursts out in loud laughter, sings, and touches things near her.

Ha, 1400 - Great irritability and acuteness of the senses; everything tastes and smells stronger; the sense of touch, the sight, and the rearing are more acute,...

CAMPH. Al, 46-... The sight increased my despair poor nature extinguished; the sky transparent and lifeless; the earth was still in the dim, dead light. I could not bear it. The sense of touch was gone, and my eyes protruded from their sockets.

CANTH. Al, 17 - Visions...something took hold of her hand, and bent it several times up and down, then it seemed as if someone took her by the throat with ice-cold hands.

CHOC. Sh, 40 - Became aware of a man's hair and had an intense desire to touch it, to make contact with it.

GERM. Sh, 200 - Constant need for cuddles without sexual desire. 16, 30C, 07:04:00

HALI-L. Sh, 13 - Increased sense of sensuality to the skin, pulling on jeans is a luxury, I feel like a kitten, soft, cuddly and warm. 09, 6C, 03:XX:XX

Sh, 217 - Skin feels softer, a hardness is gone from it. Feels squishier, more pliable. It reminds me of my mother's skin, which gives me the creeps. Not wanting to be like my mother. 09, 6C, 02:XX:XX

Sh, 537 - While asleep in bed, my husband touched my leg and I started from sleep. Oversensitive to touch and sound. Aversion to being touched. I just wanted to be left alone. Too irritable. 06, 6C, 00:05:00

Sh, 794 - A very pleasurable sensation, walking around with the top half of body naked, and feeling the skin under my arms. Great pleasure with naked of softness of underarm against side of body. 20, 30C, 04:01:36

Sh, 802 - A guy told me I was hugging him like a nun. I didn't want my genitals to touch his. 20, 30C, 04:XX:XX

HYDROG. Sh, 147 - Aversion to being touched. 24, 30C, 01:XX:XX

Sh, 272 - Sudden thoughts of making love while cuddling child and listening to old song —very vivid. 08, 30C, 00:00:XX

IRID. sh, 48 - Desire to touch backs of hands on face. Enjoy touch on skin. Old memories of gentleness, delightfully feminine. Wearing bright pink (unusual!) and stroking my legs. Enjoying my skin, touching bottom, stroking it. Dancing erotically at 8.00 a.m. (one hour after remedy). Particularly joyous. Q1

Sh, 49 - Skin felt very alive, tactile, fingertips felt "awake." Feathers felt amazing. Skin to skin; very aware of contact of surfaces. More erotic dancing, morning. Q2

Sh, 50 - When a friend visited, she touched me a lot, and I noticed it. I've not touched people as much as I normally do. B4

Sh, 52 - Woke in white softness, like rabbit's fur. Q3

Sh, 56 - Delight at seeing my own female form in mirror, desire to shave legs so they would be smooth. Highly sexual, more refined, dressed in best clothes today. Desire to dance naked in moonlight. Q6

KALI-C. Ha, 25 - Readily frightened, especially by a slight touch of the body.

He, 16 - Very easily frightened; shrieks about imaginary appearances; starts when touched.

He, 17 - Is frightened and cries out whenever he is touched lightly on his feet.

LAC-C. He, 13 - Woke at daylight feeling that she is a loathsome (repulsive), horrible mass of disease (while the breasts were affected); could not bear to look at any portion of her body (loathing, himself), not even hands, as it intensified feeling of disgust and horror; could not bear to have any part of her body touch another, had to keep even fingers apart; felt that if she could not in some way get out of her body, she should soon become crazy .

He, 15 - Sensation or delusion as if surrounded by myriads of snakes, some running like lightning up and down inside the skin ; some that are inside feel long and thin; fears to put her feet on floor, lest she should tread (walk) on them and make them squirm (shake) and wind (round) around her legs; is afraid to look behind her, for fear that she will see snakes there, does not dream of them and is seldom troubled with them after dark; on going to bed she was afraid to shut her eyes for fear that a large snake, the size of her arm, would hit her in the face.

He, 24 - When paroxysms of intense nervousness (anxiety) come on, feels like tearing off her clothes; takes off her rings; cannot bear anything to touch her, ...

He, 25 - Had to keep her fingers apart from each other.

He, 40 - Feels weak, and nerves so thoroughly out of order, that she cannot bear one finger touch another.

LYSS. Al,N-129 - Hyperesthesia, current of air, bright light, sight of any shining object, slightest touch, even conversation in vicinity of patient, may throw him into a most violent agitation and bring on severe convulsions.

Al,N-92 - Exalted state of smell, taste and touch, with a feeling of anxiety and a fear of being alone.

MED. He, 19 - One night saw large (big) people in room; large rats running; felt a delicate hand smoothing her head from front to back. (caressed)

PLAT. He, 2 - Inclination to embrace everybody. (contact)

RAPH. Al, 1 - Feeling of aversion towards all women; she is provoked by seeing women going and coming about her; their approach threw her into a fury; the mere contact with a woman's dress caused intolerable distress;...She is attracted to all men without distinction (nymphomania) ; when she gives her hand to a man, she feels great agitation,...When left alone for a hour in the evening, she gave herself a very deep wound in the lips with a penknife, in hopes to put an end to this condition (hurt, punishes). Moral feeling was completely extinct, the physical nature alone ruled and threw her into a frightful state (wild). From morning to noon she would not have been able to resist the advances even of a man for whom she had not the least friendly feeling; from noon to 6 p.m. she could not have held out against any man whatsoever; from 8 to 11 the demands of sense were so importunate as to silence the voice of shame and reason; ... and would have thrown herself into the arms of the first man she met...she was still unable to control her impulses;...

SEP. He, 14 - Felt that unless he held on to something he should scream.

SULPH. He, 3-...feels as if crazy; does not know whether she has done what she intended (planned) or whether objects seen are really there, or whether she only imagines them to be, until she has touched them;...

TELL. He, 2 - Fear of being touched in sensitive places.

THUJ. He, 12 - Insane women will not be touched or approached.

TRANSMUTATION

Delusions; animals, persons are: bell.[162] hyos. stram.
- animals, persons are, unclean animals: bell.
- consciousness belongs to another: alum.
- double, lying on one side, she is one, and lying on the other side she is another person: pyrog.[139]
- hearing, of, his own voice seems changed: alum.[1]
- life, careering from live to: cann-i.[36]
- locality is transformed: bar-m.[54]
- person, existed in another person, she: pyrog.[139]
- says something, it seems to him as though somebody else has said it, when he: alum.
- sees anything, as if another person had seen it, or as if he could transfer himself into another and only then could see: alum.
- something, else, objects are something: staph.
- talking, someone else is, when he speaks: alum.[36] cann-s.[58]
- two dimensional objects are three dimensional: anh.[119]

Dreams; animals, horses, changing into dogs: zinc.
- ➤ changed, everything is: ozone[227]
- ➤ men, green and covered with moss, living in water, changing into dogs: sol-t-ae.[36]
- ➤ men, transforming into talking animals: sol-t-ae.[85]

- prayer meeting, of being conducted to, by unknown woman, it then changed into a restaurant: pip-m.[36]
- pub in a former sanatorium: ozone[227]
- women, animals, changed into: sol-t-ae.[36]

Memory; active, past events, remembered as belonging to someone else, or as matter read: ail.[54]

ADAM. Sh, 523 - Delusion animals are changing form, i.e. see a cat and when closer it's actually a dog. 16, 12C, 28:XX:XX

Sh, 554 - Image of reptilian dinosaur skins. Reached up and took his head off. Inside, a human was underneath dinosaur skin. The head was hanging down in shame. 16, 12C, 00:07:30

CHOC. Sh, 45 - When I woke from the dream, I had a little panic, an unusual childhood memory came back in which I remembered having read as a child about being covered in clay, baked and eaten. The thought came to me of the spines on my back covered in clay and baked and eaten like a hedgehog.

Sh, 57 - Keep getting a picture of the prickles of the start of the hairline of the hedgehog and am aware of this point in me —not discomfort, but keep pushing hair back and pulling my fingers backwards through my hair, thinking its nice that its not in my face. Keep getting pictures of faces of hedgehogs, (rather than the spiny bits) especially the nose, which seems so black and wet.

Sh, 96 - Everything seems right and in order now. I feel much better. Only survival matters, simpler. All the trivial affairs and worries of humans are irrelevant. The only things that matter are food and warmth. I need just enough to eat — red berries. On a walk I saw red berries and thought everything is there, no problem. I have no worries like humans have —no decision making —there isn't any choice.

Sh, 107 - A strange feeling of being an animal, yet having this thinking.

Sh, 114 - When I feel like a hedgehog, my heart is much faster, but when I feel the stillness, I don't feel my heart at all.

Sh, 117 - I thought how would an animal be if it had my body. What would they do with thought. I think I'm better off.

Sh, 120 - Felt as if I was hibernating — mouth sealed up perfectly and my tongue seems to fill all the space. I usually sleep with my mouth open as I cannot breathe through my nose, but now my mouth is perfectly sealed and nose free-flowing.

Sh, 139 - Meditation is much smoother —an effortless zooming in. I feel much more comfortable in the world. Before I always wanted to get out. During meditation, felt a floating feeling, felt an opening and upwards movement in my back, as if wings were forming and I was just light.

Sh, 153 - Since the proving, I know how it feels to be a animal or a plant. I know the feeling of daffodil, of flower, of hedgehog, of dog.

HALI-L. Sh, 690 - Seeing faces—I do sometimes anyway. These were human faces, broadened in the middle and the eyes went round the sides. They changed from human to birds to fish . Image of human face becoming alien looking as eyes became less central and changed to bird to fish then, as bird. 20, 30C, 00:01:14

Sh, 727 - Overwhelming images of very wrinkled skin on bony naked legs and buttocks of premature babies covered in meconium. Wiping meconium off, and then it changed to naked featherless young birds — necks and upper bits of the birds. They were sitting in meconium. 20, 30C, 01:00:40

Sh, 783 - On waking, my arms felt like wings. I was spread-eagled across the bed, front and back. Normally I would sleep on my side, but I can't get the right position on my arms. 20, 30C, 03:23:00

Sh, 852 - Feel twice as wide as high (line drawing of long outspread arms, tiny head, shorter spine, no legs, just feet). 20, 30C, 07:XX:XX

Sh, 901 - Sensation of such harmonious balance when on the wing, Such power in these almost weightless wings. Sensation of deep warmth echoing the sun. 20, 30C, 10:XX:XX

Sh, 958 - This morning, my bones in my arms felt different —lighter and less dense. 20, 30C, 18:XX:XX

Sh, 958 - This morning, my bones in my arms felt different —lighter and less dense. 20, 30C, 18:XX:XX

IRID. Sh, 19 - Still didn't feel much like talking. Feel very contained and self contained and my mind feels still. Unintellectual, unthinking, heavy. I wanted to be pre-verbal like the cat. Words too much effort. E1

Sh, 61 - I feel buzzy and vibrating, feels as if my hair is stood on end. I keep talking about being a dog. H1

Sh, 68 - Woke up thinking my alarm clock was a hedgehog. I wondered what the spiky sound was. I10

Sh, 84 - Morning getting dressed, didn't really want to put clothes on, felt I was taking the first gulp of air that the first breathing animal took as it came out of the water, bursting through the surface, lungs expanding. As with the egg image (day 5), the movement is forceful, BURSTING with great relief. G6

Sh, 88 - Forgot to race downhill again. Voice sounded deeper. My immediate reaction, "Oh God, I'm turning into a man." Felt I was overwhelming colleague so didn't ask if I really was. I seemed to take up a lot of space in the room so I drew back and left. G5

Sh, 99 - Sat at the bus stop. Felt like a really small, frightened rabbit, with a large shadow of this great bird hovering over ready to pounce. G8

Sh, 107 - On waking, hands joined by first fingers; hands fused to become wings; thumbs crossed in the form of a heart. Q2

Sh, 109 - Sensation as if wings 3 —4 p.m. Q5

Sh, 112 - Sensation as if winged ankles, while wind blowing through house. Thought, "back to earth." Q17

Sh, 113 - Feel as if growing wings in back. SENSATION AS IF body wanting to change form, mainly in chest, face, back. Q4

TRAVEL

Anxiety; evening, family, about his, which he left behind while on a journey: ***petr.***[54]

Anxiety; railroad, when about to journey by, amel. while in train: arg-n.[58] ars.

Anxiety; riding, while: ***arg-n.***[54] ***aur. bor. lach.***[122] psor. sep.

Anxiety; riding, while, closed carriage, in: bor.[172] cimic.[102] nat-m.[172] succ.[137]

Anxiety; riding, while, down hill: **BOR.** ***psor.***

Anxiety; riding, while, hypochondriasis, in: ***arg-n.***[54]

Anxiety; riding, while, rapidly: staph.[172]

Confusion of mind; country, as if now in one, now in another: chlol.[36]

Country, desire for, to go into the: androc.[222] choc.[222] elaps[36] hydrog.[222]

Delirium; rambling: atro. ***bell.*** chlol.[36] ***chlor.***[54] hyos. ***nat-m.***[54] plb. sec.[54] ***sulph.***[54]

Delusions; abroad, being: verat.[30]

- boat, owns a: lap-c-b.[194]
- clothes, fly away and become wandering stars, will (on undressing): cann-i
- journey, he is on a: bell. brom. cann-i. cann-s.[5] chin-ar.[139] crot-h. hyos. lach. mag-m. nat-c. op. sang. sil.
- journey, traveling through worlds: aether bell.[72]
- railway train, go off by, he was obliged to: atro.
- roaming in the fields: rhus-t.
- seasick, he is: der. magn-gr.[139] nitro-o.[36] tab.[139]
- ship, ocean, on, sees: lap-c-b.[194]
- ship, on board of, in a storm: alco.
- space, carried into, that he is, orbit, and compelled to describe a vast: cann-i.[36]
- space, carried into, that he is, while lying: cann-i.[58] coca germ.[222] ***lach.***
- space, he is in: germ.[222]

Dreams; animals, horses, riding: bamb-a.[1184] nat-c. ther.

- animals, horses, riding, stream, through a: chr-ac.[8]
- astray, going: mag-c.[10] mag-m.[10] nat-c.[1] sep.[10]
- cars, automobiles, of: choc.[222] ozone[227]
- country, foreign: ind.[54] ozone[227] plat.[10] sil.[10]
- country, native country: ant-c.[1] lach.[36] mur-ac.[36]
- driving, car, a: aq-mar.[231] choc.[222] hydrog.[222]
- flying, airplane, in: allox.[119] hydrog.[222]
- forest, going astray in a forest: mag-m.[10] sep.[10]
- journey: all-s.[54] am-c. am-m. anan. ***apis*** bamb-a.[1184] bart.[36] brom. bufo calc-f. ***calc-p. carb-ac.*** carc.[119] chel. chin-b. choc.[222] cortico.[119] ***crot-h.*** elaps hura hydr. hydrog.[222] hyper. ind. indg. joan.[102] **KALI-N.** lac-c. lac-d. ***lach.*** linu-c.[36] lipp.[36]

mag-c. mag-m. mag-s. merc. merc-c. merc-i-r. merc-s.[36] mez. ***nat-c.*** nat-m. ***op.*** ozone[227] pip-m.[36] psor. rauw.[119] ***rhus-t.*** rob.[36] sang. sel. ***sil.*** sin-a.[36] ther. ***tub.***[122]
➤ journey, airplane, by: ozone[227]
➤ journey, bus, by: ozone[227]
➤ journey, car, by: choc.[222] ***hydrog.***[222] ozone[227]
➤ journey, China, to: bamb-a.[1184]
➤ journey, countries, in foreign: ind.[54]
➤ journey, cruise around the world: bamb-a.[1184]
➤ journey, desert, to the: ozone[227]
➤ journey, difficulties, with: am-m.[36] calc-p.[36] echi.[111] mag-s.[36] merc.[36] mez.[36] nat-c.[36]
➤ journey, distant regions, in: ther.[54]
➤ journey, horseback, on: nat-c. ther.
➤ journey, island, to an: ozone[227]
➤ journey, long: nat-m.[1]
➤ journey, Peking, to: ozone[227]
➤ journey, perplexities, amid: merc-s.[54]
➤ journey, railroad, by: apis cortico.[119] ozone[227]
➤ journey, roaming over fields, of: **RHUS-T.**[54]
➤ journey, separated from party and had to walk a long distance and arrived at station in time to see train start: ***lac-c.***[54]
➤ journey, water, by: alum.[10] chin-b.[8] nat-s.[10] sang.[10] valer.[10]
➤ moped, driving one hundred kilometers an hour: ozone[227]
➤ mother, flying around the world: hydrog.[222]
➤ riding: chr-ac.[54] nat-c.[58] ther.[58]
➤ riding, carriage, in: bell.[36] indg.[36] nat-s.[10]
➤ roaming over fields: **RHUS-T.**
➤ ships: bamb-a.[1184]
➤ ships, wartime, in: hydrog.[222]
➤ sleigh-riders: sars.[36] tril.[36]
➤ stream, crossing a stream on horseback: chr-ac.[54]
➤ tent, erecting a large: hydrog.[222]
➤ thrown from a carriage, being: nat-s.[36]
➤ train, stop, does not, where he thinks it will: ozone[227]
➤ train, trying to catch a: hydrog.[222]
➤ unsuccessful, efforts to, reach a distant place, to: croc. plat.
➤ wagons: nux-v.[30] senec.[36]
➤ wandering: cench.[58] stram.[36] zing.[36]
➤ water, boat, rubberboat going up a mountain stream: ozone[227]
➤ water, led over, of being: eupi.[36]
➤ water, sailing: alum.[10] chin. hura nat-s. sang. senec. valer.[10] verat-v.
➤ water, sailing, dangerous sailing in a small boat: nat-m.[36]
➤ water, stream, crossing a, on horseback, and water froze: chr-ac.[36]

Fear; riding in a carriage, when: acon.[193] androc.[222] arg-n.[185] ***aur.***[193] ***bor.*** bry.[126] carc.[227] cimic.[172] cocc.[172] cupr.[210] gins.[122] ***lach.*** lipp.[36] pitu-a.[164] ***psor.*** sanic.[126] ***sep.***

Inconsolable; anxiety about his family, from, which he left behind while going on a short journey: ***petr.***[54]

Insanity; travel, with desire to: bell.[30] bry.[30] chin.[30] hyos.[30] nux-v.[30] puls.[30] stram.[30] tub.[58] verat.[30]

Irritability; travel goes too slow, when: cortiso.[119]

Riding in a carriage, averse to: psor.

Riding in a carriage; desires: psor.[122]

Thoughts; past, of the, journeys: sol-t-ae.[36]

Travel, desire to: am-c.[30] am-m.[30] anan. arag.[102] aur. bac.[149] bar-c.[30] bell.[30] bry.[102] calc.[58] **CALC-P.** ***carc.***[122] caust.[30] choc.[222] cimic. cur. elaps elat.[102] goss.[122] ***hipp.*** hydrog.[222] ***ign.***[184] ***iod.*** lach. lyss.[137] mag-c.[30] ***merc.***[122] merc-i-f.[214] plat.[184] sanic. thea.[30] <u>**TUB.**</u>[122] verat.[102]

Travel; amel.: carc.[183] ign.[162]

Travel; desires to, far away, almost uncontrollable: ***merc.***[54]

Travel; desires to, one place to another, from: bac.[149] calc-p.[176]

Wander, desires to: arag.[102] ***bry.***[102] ***calc-p.*** cench.[58] choc.[222] cimic. elat.[102] ***kali-br.***[54] lach.[102] lyss.[111] merc. sanic.[122] **TUB.**[122] verat. verat-v.[5]

Wander, desires to, home, from, and ranges in woods: ***elat.***[54]

ADAM. Sh, 128 - I really need to escape, booked trip to France. 7, 6C 14:00:xx
Sh, 434 - Before a journey, fear of not being able to get home. 8, 6C, 01:09:00

ANAN. Al, 14 - Ardent desire to travel.

ANDROC. Sh, 180 - Desire to be out in the country, intense desire to be on the rocks. Desire to feel the rocks, to stick hand beneath the rocks, to crawl into or behind rocks. (Clinical)

ATRO. Al, 22 - Expostulates with those who try to lead him to bed; says he will lose the train, that all things are packed up, and that he must start immediately.

Al, 24 - I imagined I had to go off by a railway train, which started at ten in the morning, and that the hour was approaching, whilst I had nothing ready for the journey; and I believed that I wished to dress and to pack my things, but was thwarted (stopped) and prevented by the people about me. At length I was persuaded, that it was too late to catch the train, and agreed to wait till evening.

BAR-A. Al, 15 - Extreme irresolution ; he proposes a short journey, but as soon as he makes preparation he changes his mind, and is inclined to remain at home.

BAR-C. Ha, 12 - The greatest irresolution; he proposes to himself a brief journey, and as soon as he is to make his preparation, he is sorry for it and prefers to stay at home.

BELL. Al, 121 - Inclination to violent exercise and rapid travelling.

He, 24 - Fixed ideas, thinks he is riding on an ox, uses a stick for a gun, growling and barking like a dog.

CANN-I. Al, 65 - Hallucinations which lead the patient to imagine that he is on horseback, is hunting, that he sees blue water, that he is swimming, or that he is captain of a vessel, that he is traveling, that he has no weight.(lightness)

CHLOL. Al, 17-...a feeling as if he were now in one country and now in another, and with an anxious desire to go home.(abroad)

CHOC. Sh, 14 - Angry about being in city. When I look, I want to see far distances and sky, not houses. Went to estate agents to look at country houses.

Sh, 420 - Urgency and strong desire to travel decreased since proving, (curative).[11], 6C, XX:XX:XX

CIMIC. He, 13 - Desire for solitude, or to wander from place to place.

CUR. Al, 6 - He would like to go travel in a great style.(luxury)

DER. Al, 1 - He fancies he is seasick. (nauseated)

ELAT. He, 2 - Irresistible propensity to wander from home, even in the night, and range (distance) in woods.(forest)

HALI-L. Sh, 305 - I could hear something on a railroad traveling from east to west across the States. I was above looking down. 20, 30C, XX:XX:XX

Sh, 993 - I was traveling around inside my head last night — Israel, the States, New Zealand and Scotland. All places I've never been, but all the same sort of terrain, like barren, down South, New Zealand. I was looking for a new home. 20, 30C, 31:XX:XX

HYOS. Ha, 525 - Chattering he prepares for a journey.

Ha, 544 - Naked and enveloped in a fur cloak, he senselessly wanders about to a great distance in the summer heat.

IRID. Sh, 114 - Felt I had been given the role of messenger, wasn't always in English. Q3

MAG-C. Al, 946 - Dream that she made a long journey, and at last could go no farther (distance), at which she became very anxious. (limited, restricted)

MERC. Ha, 1259 - An almost irresistible desire to travel (explore, wandering) away to a distance.

Ha, 1130 - Frightful dreams, in which he started up; he imagined he was not in his own house, sat up in bed and spoke about a distant village.

He, 19 - Homesickness (nostalgia, isolation), or desire to travel; wants to go abroad (absent, nomad); nightly anxiety and perspiration.(wander)

NAT-C. Al, DREAM, 1102-..;of marrying two women, of parties, walks, entertainments, and excursions on horseback, afterwards they were frequently anxious, of going astray (lost),of murders, having his ears cut off; also vexatious dreams; he would take a journey and could not get away from the place,(immobilization) and when has reached the first station was obliged to turn back, on account of something he had forgotten.

NIT-AC. Al, 17 - At once she is taken which peculiar anguish, runs to her physician, but he is not at home, hires a carriage to drive to the house where she expects to find him; during her ride all the anguish is gone; arrived at home she feels as bad as ever, and feels herself thus forced to drive about the whole day, till all the effects of the Nitric acid have passed off.

PETR. He, 13 - Towards evening anxiety and apprehension about his family which he left behind while going on a short journey; the anxiety increases until he becomes inconsolable.

PLAN. Al, 19 - Feeling great desire to be at home when abroad.

PLB. Al, 114-...he imagined his disease incurable, and gave way to the gloomy thoughts which the fear of death excited, and to repinings (sadness) caused by the dread of his journey to Valencia.

PSOR. Al, 9 - Unusual anxiety when riding in a carriage.

Al, 32 - Great disinclination to ride in a carriage; then at once she wants to ride all the time, even in bad weather.

RHUS-T. He, 5 - Low, mild delirium, thinks he is roaming (wander, travel) over fields, or hard at work.

SANG. He, 11 - It seems to her ...she is in a railroad car and begs others to hold her.

THUJ. Ha, 630 - Walking is performed with extreme ease; she feels as though her body were borne up by wings; she ran many miles in an uncommonly short time, and with unusual high spirits.

UGLY

Comprehension; easy, quick perception for things out of shape or proportion: ham.[36]

Dancing; desire for, grotesque: agar. ***cic.***

Delusions; animals, grotesque: absin.

- animals, surrounded by hideous: ***crot-h.***[54]
- body, deformed some parts is: acon.[162] sabad.[36]
- body, face distorted: lac-h.[229]
- faces, doctor is making faces at her, she looked black: puls.[54]
- faces, hideous: ***ambr. bell.*** **<u>CALC.</u>**[122] calc-sil. cann-i. carb-an. caust. cocc.[116] ***kali-c.***[54] lac-c. lyc.[10] merc. nux-v. **OP.** phos.[111] stram.[116] stry. sulph.[10] ***tarent.***
- faces, ridiculous: cann-i.
- faces, ugly faces seem pleasing: cann-i.
- figures, old repulsive persons, which fill her with fear, in hysteria: ***kali-c.***[54]
- frightens others, that she: hydrog.[222]
- grotesque: cann-i.[36] plb.[36] sulph.[5]
- grotesque, people appear: hyos.[36]
- images, distorted: ambr.[1] caust.[1] lac-c.[58]
- images, frightful: absin.[54] ***ambr.*** anac. arg-n. arn. ars. atro. bar-c. ***bell.*** bry.[1] **CALC.** calc-s. camph. ***carb-an. carb-v. caust.*** chin. chin-ar. cina[58] coca con. croc. gels. graph. ***hep.*** hyos. ign. kali-ar. ***kali-br.*** kali-c. ***kali-p.*** kali-sil.[58] ***lac-c. lach.*** lap-mar-c.[194] laur. lyc. mang. ***merc.*** mur-ac. nat-c. nat-p. nit-ac. nux-v. ***op.*** petr. ph-ac. ***phos.*** puls. rhod. rhus-t. samb. sars. sec. sil. spong. ***stram.*** sulph. tab. tarent.
- images, sleep, during, hateful (afternoon): lyc.
- man, old men with long beards and distorted faces, sees: laur.
- objects, crooked: glon.
- objects, deformed: anh.[119]
- pursued, horrid thing, by some: anac.
- strange, familiar things seem horrible: plat.
- ugly, is: thuj.[183] tub.[36]
- visions, horrible, afraid they will take objective form: ***lac-c.***[54]
- visions, horrible, eyes, when opening: calc.[102]
- women, old and wrinkle, of: calc-sil. cann-i.

Dreams; anger, pupils, because he has square: ozone[227]

- ➤ animals, horses, ugly: merl. phos.
- ➤ body, disfigured: sep.
- ➤ body, face, disfigured: sep.[1]
- ➤ figures, grotesque, dancing before her: narcot.[36]
- ➤ figures, horrid, presenting a bottle: merc-c.[36]
- ➤ ghosts, horrid: cham.[54]
- ➤ grimaces, horrible: op.[10]
- ➤ monstrous: arg-n.[85]
- ➤ waking, falling into a pit with grotesque figures: narcot.[36]

Fear; disfigured, of being: hep.[30]

- ✦ mirrors in room, of, see himself, lest he should: camph.[54]
- ✦ pregnancy, during, child would be deformed, that: acon.[172]
- ✦ visions of old repulsive persons, from, in hysteria: ***kali-c.***[54]

Foolish; behavior, grotesque: agar.[36] cact.[36] cori-r.[36]

Frightened; easily, hideous objects, cries as if being frightened by seeing: stram.[8]

Monomania; going out, dressing in a grotesque manner: anan.

Sadness; appearance, of: viol-o.[54]

Tastelessness in dressing: ***calc.***[30] caust.[30]

hell.[1] hyos.[1] lyc.[30] ***nat-m.***[30] nux-v.[30] sec.[1] staph.[30] stram.[1] sulph.[30]
Ugly behavior: bry.[137] bufo[107] ***cham.***[111] ***cina***[107] ***nux-v.***[111]

ABSIN. Al,S-6 - Terrifying hallucinations, he sees all kinds of animals, cats and rats of all colors, grotesque animals, fancies that he is pursued by soldiers.
ADAM. Sh, 194 - Felt ugly, miserable and generally fed up with myself during menses, more intensely than I usually would at this time. 8, 6C, 17:XX:XX
ARG-N. Al, 1-... visions and distorted (deform) faces hover before his imagination...
BELL. Al, 48 - Very delirious; she would persist that there were very horrid monsters all over the room, staring at her.
He, 20 - Imagines he sees ghosts, hideous (horrible) faces and various insects.
BENZ-AC. Al, 2-...If he saw any one who was deformed (disfigured) it made him shudder. (tremor)
CAUST. Ha, 19 - When she closes her eyes, she always sees frightful visages and distorted human faces before her.
GERM. Sh, 111 - If I were me, nobody would like me -so I try to be what I think others expect me to be. I don't think I can be loved with all the parts of me which are ugly and bad. Lonely feelings. Longing for love and understanding. Feel I am so unfriendly to myself. 18, 30C, 04:00:00
Sh, 136 - Feeling lonely like an alien freak. 08, 12C, 22:00:00
Sh, 124-. I was supposed to talk seriously, but started to laugh instead. I couldn't stop it, the laughter bubbled inside and had to come out. Laughing when supposed to talk seriously, nervous laughter, quite near weeping. Felt I held back something, tried to avoid an ugly noise -something which touched me deeply inside, something unveiling. 18, 30C, 07:XX:XX
HALI-L. Sh, 2 - Looking in the mirror is weird. Feel ugly. Very pale. I feel I look ugly, pale, big body and butt. Throughout the whole day I kept catching myself in the mirror and felt this all day. 01, 30C, 01:XX:XX
HYDROG. Sh, 241 - I'm afraid to go out because I think I frighten people. 16, 30C, XX:XX:XX
HYOS. Al, 28 - The people in the room seemed to assume grotesque appearances; ...
LAC-C. He, 13 - Woke at daylight feeling that she is a loathsome (repulsive), horrible mass of disease (while the breasts were affected); could not bear to look at any portion of her body (loathing, himself), not even hands, as it intensified feeling of disgust and horror; could not bear to have any part of her body touch another, had to keep even fingers apart; felt that if she could not in some way get out of her body, she should soon become crazy .
PHOS. Al, 111 - Horrible fearfulness, late in the evening, as if a horrible face were looking out from every corner.
Ha, 31 - Dreadful fearfulness, late in the evening, as if a horrid face was looking out of every corner.
He, 8 - Fear and dread: in evening; of death; as if something were creeping out of every corner; late in evening as if a horrible face were looking out of every corner.
PLAT. He, 20 - Everything seems strange and horrible to her.
SEP. Al, 2162 - Anxious dreams as if the body were disfigured.(distort, deface)
STRAM. Al, 63-...I was assailed (attacked) by imaginary spectres, in the most hideous forms and menacing attitudes; and what was still to my torment my bed was suspended and tantalized (charmed) like a feather (plumage) between two floors.
TUB. Al,N-11 - Felt positively ugly (repulsive, spiteful); personal aversions became almost a mania.

UNFIT

Anger; work, cannot: calc-p.[54]
Anxiety; work, preventing work: aloe[60] mosch.[36]
Business; incapacity for: agn. am-c.[30] ars.[30] caust.[58] chin-s.[36] ferr.[30] kali-bi. lyc.[30] mag-c.[30] mit.[36] nux-v.[30] sel.[58] sil.[30] sul-i. tab.[36]
Delusions; business, accomplished, can not be: med.[139]
- business, unfit for, that he is: ***croc.***
- disabled, she is: cit-v.
- do nothing, he can: lyss.[139]

• position, she is not fitted for her: stram.[54]
• sick, he is, work, and for this reason will not: calc.[30] caust.[30] nux-v.[30] sep.[30]
• succeed, that he cannot, unfit for this world: ***aur.***[54]
• unfit for, life: sep.[137]
• unfit for, work: cupr.[193] meph.[54]
• unfit for, world, the: ***aur.***[54]
• unworthy to live: nat-s.[137] plat.[137]
• work, accomplish the, he cannot: bry.[36]

Dreams; disease, sick people, help them, cannot: ozone[227]
➤ flying, apparatus, whose wings will not work: apis[36]
➤ friends, loses friend in the city, cannot find her: ozone[227]
➤ nightmare, inability to see, as if he could not escape from: cot.[36]
➤ shriek, unable to: am-m.[36] ars.[10] cast.[10] mag-m.[10] sil.[10] tab.[10]
➤ theater, but could not get dressed, which woke her, going to: mag-s.[36]
➤ unsuccessful efforts to, coition, in: ind.[36]
➤ unsuccessful efforts to, do various things: am-m. androc.[222] cadm.[149] calc. calc-f. cann-s.[10] carl. cham.[10] choc.[222] croc. dig. ign. mag-c. mag-s. mosch. mur-ac.[1] nat-c.[10] op. ozone[227] ph-ac. plat. polym.[111] stann.[10] tab. vanad.[209]
➤ unsuccessful efforts to, do various things, get cooking ready for brother and father: am-m.[36]
➤ unsuccessful efforts to, do various things, jumping long distance contest: ozone[227]
➤ unsuccessful efforts to, dress for a ball: mag-c. mag-s.
➤ unsuccessful efforts to, reach a distant place: croc. plat.
➤ unsuccessful efforts to, talk: mag-c.
➤ unsuccessful efforts to, talk, large tongue which extended out of her mouth and up her nose, on account of: tab.[36]
➤ unsuccessful efforts to, theater, for going to: mag-s.[54]
➤ walking, unable of, is: arist-m.[36]

Dress; unable to: merc.[36]

Fancies; lascivious, erections, with, sleep, during, and impotence after waking: ***op.***[54]

Fear; disable, being: **ARS.**[162] mag-m.[162] psor.[162]
✦ duty, being unable to do her: ***lac-c.***[54]
✦ medicine, bear any kind of, of not being able to: all-s.[54]
✦ occupation, of: lyc.[172] sel. sil.[172]
✦ piano, when playing: ***kali-br.***[54] ***phos.***
✦ undertaking, enterprise, a new: cupr.[210] lyc.[201] plb.[201] ***sil.***[54]
✦ work, become unfit for, to: cean.[54]

Handle things anymore, cannot, fast, when happening fast: arg.[209]

Handle things anymore, cannot, force himself to do something, has to: bamb-a.[1184]

Handle things anymore, cannot, housewives: bamb-a.[1184] sep.[187]

Handle things anymore, cannot, overwhelmed by stress: anh.[204] ***bamb-a.***[1184] bar-n.[209] calc.[198] calc-p.[198] caust.[198] cocc.[187] lac-eq.[204] med.[198] nat-n.[209] ph-ac.[188] sulph.[198]

Handle things anymore, cannot, responsible for everything, does not want to be: bamb-a.[1184]

Handle things anymore, cannot, support, looks for: bamb-a.[1184]

Helplessness; feeling of, mental exertion, from: gels.[8]

Helplessness; feeling of, weakness, from, in mental exertion: ***gels.***[54]

Helplessness; feeling, of paralyzed, from sensation of being: ***sang.***[171]

House-keeping, women inapt to: cit-l.[54] lyc.[30] nux-v.[30] pitu-a.[164] sil.[30] sulph.[30]

Hurry; movements, fast enough, cannot do things, angry, making him: sul-ac.[85]

Postponing everything to next day, business seems so long lasting, or as if it never could be accomplished: med.[54]

Religious affections; eternal bliss, believes herself unworthy of, because she is unable to perform her duties: stram.[54]

Reproaches; accomplished enough, because he had not: ars.[54]

Sadness; superfluous feeling, with: ***naja***[11]

Timidity; public, talk to, inapt to talk: ***carb-v.***[30] petr.[30]

Undertakes; lacks will power to undertake anything: androc.[222] phos. ***pic-ac.***

Unworthy; life, for, feels: ***nat-s.***[137] plat.[137]

Walk; room, about, cannot make up his mind to do anything: **KALI-BR.**[54]

Work; aversion to mental, anger after: **NUX-V.**[54]

Work; aversion to mental, masturbation, after: ***dig.***[54]

Work; crazy, seems to drive him, in mental

occupation, owing to the impotency of his mind: ind. ***kali-p.*** med.

ACT-SP. He, 6 - Great desire to work, though incapacity of it.
ADAM. Sh, 188 - Lack of confidence. I feel worthless. I haven't got a life. All that I have revolves around boyfriend. If something happened to him I'd be at a loss. No direction. 22, 200C, 01:XX:XX
Sh, 189 - Low self esteem. Felt I am not worthy or not pretty or not interesting enough for people. 20, 1M, XX:XX:XX
AGN. Al, 1-,...he feels as if nothing existed around him; he is dissatisfied with himself all the time; he is incapable of attending to any business; the things around him are entirely indifferent to him;...
ALL-S. Al, 6 - Fears of being unable to bear any medicine.
ALUM. Al, 9 - He believes he will not be able to recover his health.
He, 4 - Inability to recollect things or follow up a train of thought.
ANAC. Ha, 9 - He is at odds (quarreling) with the whole world, and has so little confidence in himself that he despairs of being able to accomplish (succeed) what is demanded of him.
Ha, 10 - In the forenoon, extremely hypochondriac, discouraged and despondent, with awkward (unskillful), helpless manner; ...
Ha, 20 - Indisposition to work; he is afraid to undertake anything, he has no pleasure in anything.
He, 66 - He is separated (divided, disconnect, estranged) from the whole world and has so little confidence in himself that he despairs of being able to do that which is required of him.
ANDROC. Sh, 81 - Felt out of control, his emotions took over. Felt terror, panic, fear and that he could not cope. (2)
ANG. He, 2 - No confidence in use of voluntary muscles; could not finish what he attempted.
APIS. He, 48 - Constantly busily engaged doing this or that, but do nothing right; young girls.
ARG-N. He, 10-...; does not work because he thinks it will do him harm (hurt), or that he is not able to stand it.
He, 31 - Does not work, thinking it will do him harm or that he is not able to stand it.
ARN. Al, 31 - Excessive inclination to perform many and long literary labors, without possessing the strength which is required to terminate them without injuring health.
Ha, 620 - Restlessness of body and mind, as if he was prevented (obstructed) doing something necessary, whith complete indisposition for occupation.
He, 46 - Sensation of being good for nothing. (incompetent, unable, incapable)
He, 49 - Inability to perform continued active work.
ARS. Ha, 1032 - Mania; first headache, horrible anxiety, noise before the ears, as from a number of large bells, and when he opened the eyes, he always saw a man who had (formerly) hung himself (suicidal, justified) on the ground-floor of the house, who incessantly beckoned (call) him to cut him down (help); he ran thither (there) with a knife, but, as he could not cut him down, (rescue) he became overwhelmed (beaten) with despair (remorse?) and wished (as his friends assured him) to hang himself (punish); but being prevented (stop) from doing so, he became so restless that he could hardly be kept in bed,... and he knelt down and raised his hands in a supplicating manner.
AUR. Ha, 346 - Remorse about his idleness (indolence), and yet he cannot work at anything; it drives him out of the house, he must always moving.
Ha, 356 - Melancholy; he imagines he is unfitted (incompetent, unqualified) for the world ; he is filled (full) with intense delight when he thinks of death, so that he longs to die. (punishment)
Ha, 5 - Melancholy; he imagines that he is not fitted for the world, he therefore longs for death, of which he thinks with the most intense delight.
Ha, 12 - He is driven to constant activity, and is sorry for his inaction, although he cannot do anything.
Ha, 18 - Dispirited ill-humor; he thinks he cannot succeed in anything.
He, 8 - Looks on dark side, weeps, prays, thinks she is not fit for this world, longs for death, strong inclination to commit

suicide; desperate, desires to jump from a height.

BRY. Ha, 777 - Cross; imagined she could not finish her work (obstruction) ; she always took hold (continued) of the wrong thing and constantly wished to take something else ; then a pressing aching headache in the forehead.

Al, 25 - Fretful; she imagines that she cannot accomplish (realize) her work; constantly takes up the wrong piece, and always inclined to change and take another; ...

Al, 39 - Imagination very sluggish (slow); it is impossible to make any plan for the future, even for the next day; the judgment (discernment), however, is unimpaired .

BUFO-S. Al, 7 - He is unable to act with decision (doubtful) ; he forms projects and does not accomplish (succeed) them.

CALC-P. Al, 13 - Grows very violent, if his opinion is differed from, or if contradicted, so that he is vexed not to have been able to control himself.

CARBN-O. Al, 7 - Frightful anxiety, and instinctive impulse to seek change of air, while he felt powerless to overcome the paralysis of his muscles and move from where he sat.

CAUST. He, 33 - Anxious uneasy mood, as if something unpleasant impended (threaten, frighten); this unfits (incompetent) him for every kind of work.(lost: competence)

CHEL. Al, 74 - It seems as though she could not think, and would lose her reason. (after three hours)

He, 6 - Imagines she cannot think and will lose her reason.(impediment)

CHIN. Al, 39 - Fretful and irresolute; she is unable to accomplish her aim, and consequently is indignant. (angry)

COCC. Ha, 532 - She dawdles (indolent); in business she cannot accomplish anything nor finish anything, with contracted pupils.

CROC. He, 3 - Greatly concerned about his life, believes that he will die, is no longer fit for business.

CYCL. Ha, 201 - All day long he is peevish not disposed to talk, and insensible, so that he feels little (inadequate, incompetent) in his body.

GELS. He, 27 - Mental exertions cause a sense of helplessness (disability) from brain-weakness; inability to attend to anything requiring thought.

GERM. Sh, 116 - Blaming myself for having taken too many doses. Was afraid that I would not get the symptoms out strongly enough. Maybe I spoiled the whole proving. Still accusing myself. I felt it does not matter how much I suffer - it's what other think of me that is important. I think that I ought to suffer a good deal. 18, 30C, 01:08:15

Sh, 99 - Came in contact with very much hate and disgust within, and it made a deep impression on me. I have to be reconciled with those parts of me. I think that power can be used in a different way - not so destructive. I am no person. Feel I have no power when I meet people. Sometimes I feel I disappear. I am not in my body. My hands feel gone. My feet are cold; I don't like them. Yet I feel I have great power inside, especially I feel it when I get angry or when I sing. 18, 30C, 46:XX:XX

Sh, 120 - Easily led of others opinion, and provoked. Sensitive to others attempts at restricting me. Feel like a teenager, but I don't dare to protest. I just feel it inside. 18, 30C, 04:00:00

GRAPH. Al, 43 - Extreme hesitation (doubtful); she is unable to make up her mind about anything.

He, 19 - Extreme hesitation; she is unable to make up her mind about anything; timidity.

HALI-L. Sh, 182 - Not doing enough. Feel somewhat critical of myself. Not getting anything done. Want to be in a structured, organized place and can't get there. I'd like to be really busy. I have more ideas in my head than I can do. I need to get active again, structure things, and set goals. 08, 30C, 03:XX:XX

Sh, 900 - It was or is ? As if I'm not really used to domestic duties. I can't really do anything for any other, just hopefully glimpses of illumination. All on own—with everything. Just to give—Does it really help? Doesn't it make others expect, or more needy? They lose freedom—independence. 20, 30C, 10:XX:XX

Sh, 938 - I feel so heavy and earthbound,

stuck with human desires that are not my own. Why don't I fit? Where is the truth and justice they talk about? Why do humans lie and deceive? I feel a big thing about truth and justice. "Why don't these people just tell me the truth?" It feels like a game, not telling me what they really want and need. 20, 30C, 15:XX:XX

HYDROG. Sh, 15 - I felt in the presence of a totally pure energy, like meeting God and feeling totally unworthy or like meeting a lover and feeling unworthy — realizing all the mistakes of a lifetime. This pure energy was around for some time protecting me. I feel this unification cleared out lifetimes of symptomatology for me. The joining with this energy was as if a male energy joined with me sexually, but with no desire, pleasure or pain involved. This unification with the male energy lasted quite a few days — I'm not used to seeing myself as a man. The morning after this unifying with the higher presence, I collapsed in emotional overflow. All my grief and pain came out. I was doubled upon the floor and went into a deep state of catharsis. It is not possible to describe where I went as there are no concepts applicable. I felt overflowing love for humanity and wanted to give everything away. My mind turned to the Buddha. It was like seeing the complete picture instead of fragmented bits. (These primary effects lasted about 28 days, then changing to a paranoia state). 16, 30C, 07.XX.XX

Sh, 30 - The whole environment I am in feels wrong now as if my life doesn't fit anymore. 16, 30C, 08:XX:XX

Sh, 32 - Depressed —like seeing a window open and unable to go through it. 16, 30C, 08:XX:XX

Sh, 152 - Feel helpless, as if I may need to be looked after because I don't feel I can do anything. 16, 30C, 00:00:30

Sh, 155 - In the afternoon (during the full moon) I felt low and depressed, insecure and vulnerable. Could not cope with work load and didn't want to be alone. 12, 6C, 39:XX:XX

IGN. Al, 2 - He fancies that he is unable (incapable, powerless) to proceed (progress, advance), that he cannot walk.

IOD. Al, 39 - Feels unfitted for everything.

Ha, 25 - He feels unable to do anything.

IP. Ha, 218 - Repugnance to literary work; thoughts fail him.

IRID. Sh, 197 - There's a slight element of confusion and a faint glimmer of not being able to cope. The feeling of not coping came on this afternoon. I've got lots to do and I've done nothing. I don't feel like doing anything but the concern is will I ever be able to focus my mind long enough to get anything done! M4

Sh, 198 - The class I was teaching did not go well and left me feeling upset. I did not perform well and I felt low after it. I identified myself as the problem. I began to doubt the work I'm doing was being valued. Wasn't myself. It was the thirteenth time I'd done similar material and it was as if I had never done it before. I tripped over words, couldn't concentrate on what I was doing. (Added at a later date: "This was like I was pregnant.") No one in class had noticed anything was wrong. It was more my own perception. B2

KALI-C. Ha, 51 - Lack of presence of mind; he cannot proceed right along in his business.

LAC-C. Al,N-36 - Fears she will become unable to perform her duties.

Al,N-33 - Depression of spirits, doubts her ability and success, thinks she will have heart disease and die of it.

He, 5 - Very restlessness; cannot concentrate her thoughts or mind to read; wants to leave everything as soon as it is commenced.

He, 26 - Depression of spirits, doubts her ability (competence, aptitude) and success (prospering, progressing, achieving), thinks she will have heart disease and die of it.

He, 29 - Fears she will become unable to perform (achieve, accomplish) her duties.(responsibility)

LACH. Al, 45 - No sooner does one idea occur to him then a number of others follow in succession while he is writing down, so that he is unable to finish the record.

LED. Al, 11 - Morose mood, with much uneasiness and irresolution; he is unable to reflect constantly upon anything, or work with a quiet mind.

LIL-T. Al, 24-..a feeling of irritation and of something wrong in abdomen and pelvic organs (disease); feels hurried (fast) and yet incapable (incompetent), as if she had a great deal (busy) to do and cannot do it.

Al, 30 - Constant hurried (precipitation) feeling as of imperative duties and utter inability to perform them; during the sexual excitement.

Al, 40-...I can see around me any number of things I must do, but cannot force myself to do anything.

Al, 45 - She can't think; acts without thought; keeps walking fast as though by instinct; feels hurried, but doesn't know why; is forgetful, can't decide for herself; must depend on others.

He, 12 - Listless, inert, yet does not want to sit still (quiet); restless, yet does not want to walk; hurried manner, desire to do something, yet feels no ambition; feeling as of imperative duties and utter (complete) inability (incapacity, incompetence) to perform them; sexual excitement.

LIM. Al, 3 - The great disinclination to work, and inability to accomplish much, which he had experienced since the sea-bath, disappeared completely during the day, and gave place to mental quiet and steadiness, with constancy and perseverance in performing very irksome duties.

LYC. Al, 128 - He is unable to do anything, cannot think; passes his time with trifles, without being able to make up his mind what to do.

Ha, 78 - He cannot do nor think anything; he spends his time in trifling, and is not able to resolve to do what he has to do.

LYSS. Al, 39 - A strange oppression and indifference, as if he was unable to do anything if he forces himself; there is no power of mind.

Al,N-72 - An attack of mental depression and indifference quite (very) strange to him; feels as if he could do nothing; if he forces himself he lacks mental power.

He, 64 - Disinclination to change position of head; two distinct trains of thought existing at one time in her mind, the idea that she is unable to move her head (when lying down) with the positive conviction that she has only to make up her mind that she will do it to achieve it.

He, 72 - An attack of mental depression and indifference quite strange to him; feels as if he could do nothing; if he forces himself he lacks mental power.

MAG-C. Al, 931 - Dream that she was at a ball (dance) where they did not dance enough; also at first she could not get ready (fitted) with her dress.

Al, 932 - Dream of flowers, clothes, and other things; she had to make up the clothes, but had no inclination to do it, and besides did not understand how; she also saw many foreign plants, but during this she became soaked (wet) with rain.

Al, 947 - Anxious dream as if he was unable to find his way in his own house.

MAG-M. Al, 709 - She becomes anxious in a dream about the work that she could not accomplish.

MED. He, 2 - Dullness of memory and desire to procrastinate (delay), because business seemed so long lasting (permanent), or as if it never could be accomplished. (postponing)

NAJA. Al, 9 - Considerable depression of spirits, and a feeling of inability to exertion of any kind, and a conviction that all is going wrong;...

NAT-AR. Al, 22-...mind not fit for study ...

NEON. Sh, 85 - Feel out of control, as if time is moving relentlessly and remorselessly forward and I'm stuck behind, unable to keep up. Panic, guilt, constant anxiety that I won't get it all done, including keeping up this journal. 10, 6C, 12:XX:XX

NUX-V. Ha, 1254 - She cannot get over the smallest evil.

He, 23 - Great anxiety of mind without particular cause; thinks she will not be able to get along (prosper) in life; caducity; (senility)...

He, 30 - Ailments after continued mental exertion; indisposition to it, particularly to that form which involves elaboration and connection of subjective ideas independently of external objects.

PLAT. Ha, 11 - Great restlessness of mind, so that she knows not where to stay (indecision), with gloominess (melancholy) which spoils even what should be most enjoyable; she imagines she is not fit (unfit, incapable) for this world, is tired (weary) of life, but has a great horror of the death she believes to be approaching.

SANT. Al, 6-...irresolution and want of confidence in my own powers as to render me quite unfit for work of any kind;

SIL. Al, 40 - She could and would do nothing on account of ill-humor.

He, 4 - Reading and writing fatigue, cannot bear to think.

He, 5 - Becomes confused, makes mistakes; she is unable to control himself.

SPONG. Al, 11 - She is dissatisfied with what she accomplishes; she cannot rightly help herself at work (helpless) (incompetent) ; she does not succeed.

Ha, 384 - She is not satisfied with her work; she cannot do her work properly, she is not successful with it.

He, 12 - Feels awkward (unskillful) about her work, which she cannot accomplish (succeed, prosper) satisfactorily.

STANN. Ha, 638 - Dawdling and irritable, whith heat of face; she wished to do all sorts of things and could accomplish nothing.

He, 6 - A woman, age 39, pregnant in fourth month;...inability to do anything as she cannot muster sufficient courage,...great palpitation of heart and anxiety, especially if she has to give directions in her domestic affairs; thinking makes her feel wretched, ...(unable, incapable)

STRAM. Al, 48 - She is all the time inconsolable; much affected by trifles; makes much fuss about trifles; disposed to weep, and sometimes also very easily vexed; now and then neglects her duties; now and then thinks she is not fitted for her position ; after the fall equinox...; she wants light and company.

He, 61 - Thinks she is not fitted for her position.

He, 172 - Downcast and full of anguish, believes herself unworthy of eternal bliss, because she is unable to perform her duties.

He, 177-...sometimes vexed; neglects her duties, thinks she is not fitted for her position;...

SUL-AC. He, 6-... unfit for work, would sit and weep whole day long;...

SULPH. Al, 42-...discontented with himself and all about him, which made him unfit for any serious occupations...whole evening he was absorbed in himself and unable to command his thoughts to read...

TAB. Al, 45 - He was incapacitated for business of any kind, weak irresolute, and despondent.

THUJ. Al, 3 - She feels and says that she is deranged (insane, disordered) and unfit (unsuitable) to life, as a punishment for a fault (penitence) which she cannot name, ...

Al, 34 - While talking, she is unable to go on in spite of every effort; she begins to weep bitterly, and says she can no longer think or live.

TUB. Al,N-38 - Soporous, dazed condition; unable to find the right way (lost); is confused; surroundings appear strange.

UNFORTUNATE

Ailments from; love, disappointed, unhappy: ***acon.***[5] am-c.[5] androc.[222] ant-c. **AUR.**[5] ***bell.***[30] ***bufo***[117] cact.[5] ***calc-p. caust.***[5] ***cimic. coff.*** com.[5] ***con.***[116] dig.[85] ***hell.*** **HYOS.** **<u>IGN.</u>**[122] iod.[85] kali-c. ***kali-p.***[5] ***lach.*** **NAT-M.** nux-m. nux-v. orig.[187] ozone[227] **PH-AC.** phos.[5] pitu-a.[164] psor.[185] ***sac-alb.***[210] sep. seq-s.[230] **<u>STAPH.</u>**[122] stram.[37] sulph.[122] tarent. til.[36] verat.[54]

Anxiety; unfortunate, as if he had been: caust.[36]

Confidence; thinks others have none, which makes her unhappy, and: ***aur.***

Delusions; disgraced, she is: kali-s.[214] mag-s.[214] nat-s.[214] nux-v.[37] plat.[214] rob.[36] staph.[214] sulph.
- happy is his own house, he will never be: ars.
- misfortune, inconsolable over fancied: alum.[102] calc-s.[58] ***verat.***
- pitied on account of his misfortune and he weeps, he is: nat-m.[1]
- unfortunate, he is: bry. caust.[36] ***chin.*** cub. graph.[30] hura ip. lyc. sep. staph.[30] verat.

Inconsolable; weeping from consolation, continuous: nat-c.[30]

Suicidal disposition; despair, about his miserable existence: ***sep.***[54]

Talk; sufferings, troubles, constantly of his: arg-n.[5] asaf.[137] ***mag-p.***[5] ***nux-v.***[5] zinc.[137]

Unfortunate, feels: bry. carb-v.[30] carc.[146] caust.[36] ***chel.***[10] ***chin.*** cub. ***graph.***[10] hell.[10] hura ip. kali-c.[10] ***lyc.***[122] merc.[36] rhus-t.[10] sars.[1] ***sep.***[36] ***staph.***[30] sulph.[10] ***tab.***[10] verat.
Weeping; bitterly: hep.[36] nat-m.[137]

ADAM. Sh, 190 - Very unhappy with my body, I want to escape from it, to run away from myself. I want to go from me. 20, 1M, 08:XX:XX
AGAR. Al, 37 - An impulse to laugh overcame him in bed, owing to an indescribably mixed sensation of happiness and misery.(duality)
ALUM. Al, 10 - He feels low-spirited on account of his disease.
ARS. Al, 34 - Piteous (miserable) complainings (lamenting)... and excessive mental anguish took away his breath ...
ATRO. Al, 3-...the mind would become filled with strange and fanciful ideas ...fits of wild, uncontrollable laughter...I fancied myself afflicted with epilepsy, and was constantly fearful lest others should discover my unfortunate condition; ...
AUR. Ha, 344 - Discontented with all circumstances; he imagines that he finds everywhere some obstacle (impediment, restriction) in the way; at one time he thinks that this is owing to an unlucky (unfortunate) fate (destiny), at another that he himself is to blame (censured) for it ; when the latter was the case he was particularly mortified and dejected.
He, 61 - Has no confidence in herself, thinks others have none; this makes her unhappy. (merit, value)
He, 43 - Is very unhappy; continued thought of suicide. 0Puerperal mania.
CALC. Ha, 2 - Melancholy, not really mournful (unhappy) feeling, about the heart, without cause, with a sort of voluptuous tremor all over the body.
CAMPH. Al, 32 - Indescribable wretchedness. (unhappiness)
Al, 46-... My misery was boundless; time itself was no more; in short, I suffered such fearful anguish as no fancy can comprehend. What soul could paint to itself my everlasting (eternal) dwelling as the Evil One (devil), alone in a vast universe, without faith or hope, and my heart forever broken by unimaginable tortures? (miserable, timeless, endless, solitude, forsaken, faithless, hopeless)
CANN-I. Al, 25... The stars seemed to look upon him with pitying (compassion) human aspect, and to bewail (lament) his condition.
CARB-V. Al, 7 - She desired death, she felt so unhappy.
Ha, 11 - She wishes to die, she feels so unhappy.
He, 13 - Feels unhappy with every little pain.
CAUST. Al, 12 - Anxiety the whole day, as if he had done something bad, or apprehended it, or as if he had been unfortunate (unsuccessful, umprosperous).
CERE-B. Al, 11 - Arose feeling miserable.
CHIN. Al, 47 - Discontent; he considers himself unhappy and thinks he is hindered (obstructed) and tormented by everyone. (after five hours)
Ha, 1113 - Discontented; he thinks himself unfortunate (unsuccessful), and fancies he is opposed (confronted, hostilised), and tormented (molested) by everybody.
He, 10 - Fixed idea that he is unhappy, persecuted by enemies.
He, 11 - She thinks she is very unfortunate and constantly harassed (molested, tormented) by enemies.
CON. He, 26 - Great unhappiness of mind, recurring every fourteen days.
CUPR. He, 10 - Mania with biting, beating, and tearing things to pieces; insane foolish gestures of imitation and mimicry; full of insane spiteful (cruelty, brutality) tricks (deceitful, false), ..unhappy, despairing...miserable look...
DIG. Ha, 420 - Lachrymose sadness about many things in which he has been unsuccessful.
DROS. Ha, 276 - He is dejected (unhappy) about the malice (rancor, hostility) of others on all hands, and at the same time disheartened (discouraged) and concerned about the future.(disgusted, revolted)
FORM. Al, 5-...sudden but momentary spells of unhappiness; everything looks dark.(obscure)
Al, 7 - Sudden and unexpected return of sense of mortification and grief, with vivid recollection of circumstances long since passed, which had caused great mortifica-

tion and pain, and which had rendered several years of his life unhappy; this was caused by the transactions (doing) of a near relative; this grief continues...

GERM. Sh, 114 - Difficult to feel joy, pleasure. It is more safe to be sad, unhappy, to suffer. Because joy doesn't last. 18, 30C, 85:XX:XX

GRAPH. He, 9 - Feels miserable, unhappy.

HELL. Al, 10 - He becomes melancholy on beholding (observe) a cheerful person, and then, for the first time, feels very unhappy.

Ha, 284 - On seeing a happy person he becomes melancholy and then only he feels very unhappy.

He, 24 - Dread of dying ; feels unhappy in presence of cheerful faces. (spite)

HURA. Al, 19 - Inclination to weep, chest constrict, as from emotion...the least thing disturbs her and makes her sad;...

IGN. He, 11-...believes herself married (connected) and pregnant; is tormented by remorse of imagined crimes; seeks constantly to escape to drown (suicide) herself; ...;is only quiet when lying undisturbed and brooding over her troubles, which she rehearses (tell) in a doleful (unhappy) tone ;..." I am neglecting my duty, breaking my vow" (promise, engagement)...;conscientious scruples after eating.

He, 27 - Unhappy love with silent grief.

IP. Al, 9 - Ill-humored; he thinks that he is very unhappy.

Ha, 222 - Moroseness: he considers himself unfortunate.(unlucky, unsuccessful)

KALI-BR. Al, 25 - At times he cried most bitterly, yet twelve hours previously he was singing and dancing, saying he was "the happiest man alive".

He, 39-...fear and apprehension that she is losing her mind (insanity);...makes her utterly (completely) miserable to be looked at or spoken to; fear to see people; always depressed and lowspirited;...

KALI-C. Ha, 31 - She is always in antagonism with herself; she knows not what she wants, and feels exceedingly unhappy.

LACH. He, 39 - Weak and unhappy, particularly in morning, when she feels, on awaking, friendless and forsaken; ...(deserted) has had domestic troubles. 0 Melancholia

He, 35 - Feels extremely sad, unhappy and distressed in mind on waking in morning.

LOB-S. He, 1 - Much depressed, tearful, unhappy.

He, 4 - Great depression of spirits; unhappy state of mind,...

LYC. Al, 32 - She became very miserable...

Al, 36 - Hypochondriac, complaining mood; he feels unhappy.

Ha, 1 - Hypochondriac, tormenting mood; he feels unhappy.

LYSS. He, 22 - Believe that they are reduced to their present wretched condition by the instrumentality (aid) of those about them.

MERC. He, 32 - Much wretchedness (miserable, unhappy) and dejection (sadness) of spirits, with diarrhea.

MEZ. He, 5 - No rest when alone; wants to be in company ...unable to repeat what has been learned by heart; looks through window for hours, without being conscious of objects around; knows not what she is about; forgets what she is about to utter (talk); looks ill humored, pale, wretched, fallen away; ......expecting some very unpleasant news.

MYRIC. Al, 6 - Miserable dejected (unhappy) feeling all day.

NAJA. Al, 14 - Felt melancholy; began to form images of possible wrongs (mistaken) and misfortunes, over which the mind broods; very wretched at times;... a slight cause sets him in a perfect agony of mental suffering on another's behalf (welfare);...makes himself imaginary troubles and wrongs, and frets (bother) over them for two hours...

NAT-C. Al, 22 - His fancy is mostly busy with apprehensions of the future; he often makes plans for half an hour at a time as if it would go wrong with him, wherewith he seeks to be alone for several days together.

NAT-M. Al, 44 - The more he was consoled, the more he was affected. (aggravate)

Al, 18 - If one only looked at him, he was obliged to weep.

Ha, 14 - From the looks of everyone, he concludes that people pity (compassion, sympathy) him for his misfortune, and he weeps.(miserable)

Ha, 15 - He had to weep as soon as anyone merely looked at him. (pitied)

Ha, 26 - She often looks into the looking-glass, (mirror) and thinks she looks wretched (miserable, contemptible).

PHOS. Al, 108 - Anxiously solicitous concerning the unfortunate termination of her illness.

Ha, 23 - Anxiously solicitous, about the unfortunate (unlucky) issue (subject) of her disease.

He, 29 - Crazy deliria in a young woman who was strictly moral and unhappy in her love; accused herself of the most obscene (immoral, wicked) actions, of which she never was guilty; ....

PLAT. Ha, 17 - Sad and sullen, she sits solitary, without speaking and she cannot ward off sleep; then inconsolable weeping, especially when she is addressed.

He, 46-...;suffers unspeakable pangs (anxiety) of conscience in consequence of a faux (fault, mistake, embarrassing mistake?) pass when thirty-two years old; says she has brought disgrace upon her family, and that she has incurred the penalty of damnation; (doomed) in order to do penance (penitence) gave away whatever she could lay her hands upon, (redemption) so that she had to be constantly watched; after her confessor asserted that she could not hope for pardon or heaven (condemnable), she seemed in absolute despair ; bemoaned her misery throughout the night, wringing her hands and beseeching (implore) that she might be delivered (free) from the hell of her conscience; twice attempted self-destruction (suicide);...wished to live and do penance (penitence, purgation, purification) in order to mitigate her eternal punishment.

RHUS-T. He, 14 - Fretful; general unhappiness of temper.

SARS. Al, 7 - The soul is affected inordinately by the pains; the mind is depressed the mood dull; he feels wretchedly, and moans involuntarily.

Ha, 3 - The soul is extraordinarily affected by the pains, the spirit is oppressed, the mind troubled; he feels unhappy and groans involuntarily.

SEP. Al, 28 - Gloominess (melancholy); she felt unfortunate, without cause.

Ha, 31 - Extreme loathing of life (existence he felt as if he could not any longer bear this miserable (wretched, unhappy) existence, and as if he would pine away (ruined) unless he made away with himself.-(suicidal)

Ha, 16 - Melancholy, she feels unhappy without cause.

He, 12 - Gloominess; she feels unfortunate (unhappy) without cause.

SOL-T-AE. Al, 5 - She is much concerned (care, anxiety) about her future, destiny, which she fancies will be wretched.(miserable)

SULPH. Al, 41 - Frequently during the day she has attacks of melancholy, lasting a few minutes, when she feels extremely unhappy, without cause; she wishes to die.

He, 33 - Sleepless, disgusted with life, fears the future, where she sees nothing but misery (wretchedness, poverty) and suffering (misfortune). 0 Melancholia.

He, 34-...; profound melancholy; considers herself disgraced (dishonor, degradation) ; speaks of dying, finds life insupportable;...

He, 36-..., feels extremely unhappy without cause, she wishes to die.

He, 37 - Great dejection,(grief), with thoughts of suicide; feels inferior (mediocre, lower) to everybody; can decide nothing;...

He, 39 - Too lazy (indolent) to rouse (animate) himself up, and too unhappy to live.

TARENT. Al, 2 - Insanity on account of an unfortunate love.

VERAT. He, 52 - Despair about his position in society, feels very unlucky.

UNION

Ailments from; celibacy, being unmarried, continence: ***agn.***[8] apis[130] calc.[137] ***cann-i.***[137] con.[102] fl-ac.[137] lyc.[137] phos.[111] plat.[137] sep.[187]

Delirium; wedding, prepares for: ***hyos.***

Delusions; betrothal, engagement, must be broken: fl-ac.

- marriage, must dissolve: fl-ac.
- married, he is: ign.
- married, is going to be: hyos.
- vow, breaking her: ign.
- vow, keep it, must: verat.[10]
- wedding, of a: alum.[5] hyos.[5] mag-m.[5] nat-c.[5]

Dreams; wedding: alum. bamb-a.[1184] chel. mag-c. mag-m.[1] mag-s. nat-c. nat-s.
➤ wedding, busy, at which she was: mag-s.[36]
➤ wedding, everyone is going to a, except her: hydrog.[222]
➤ wedding, midnight, after, of marrying one she did not like: mag-c.[36]
➤ wedding, preparing: ozone[227]
➤ wedding, procession passing her, of: nat-s.[36]
➤ wedding, repeated, has to be, since only one half of the body has been married: bamb-a.[1184]
➤ wedding, women, with two: nat-c.[10]
Fear; marriage: ***lach.***[5] nux-v.[187]
Insanity; wedding preparations, of: hyos.[137]
Irresolution; marry, to: carb-v.[30] ign.[30] lach.[30] nat-m.[30] nux-v.[30] phos.[30] plat.[30] sil.[30] staph.[30] verat.[30]
Irresolution; marry, to, avarice, from: lyc.[148]
Marriage; aversion to: puls.[58]
Marriage; aversion to, enjoying society of men, while: pic-ac.[36]
Marriage; aversion to, women, in: ***lach.***[54]
Marriage; idea, seemed unendurable idea of: ***lach. med.***[122] nux-v.[187] pic-ac. puls. staph.[30]
Marriage; obsessed by idea of m. excited sexual girls are: bell.[30] ***caust.***[30] plat.[30] verat.[30]
Sadness; thinking, marriage, about, amel.: orig.[137]
Thoughts; marriage, of: orig.[36]
Thoughts; marriage, of, masturbation, in: ***hyos.***[54]

ACON. He, 2 - Clairvoyance; conscious that his beloved, miles away, was singing a certain piece.

ADAM. Sh, 277 - Exceptionally strong desire to leave my marriage and children, to live a clear unmuddled life alone. 2, 12C, 74:XX:XX-160:XX:XX

ALOE. Al, 5 - Merry, self-contented; fraternized with the whole world.

ANT-C. Ha, 18 - Continuous state of enthusiastic love and ecstatic longing for an ideal woman, which quite filled his fantasy;... (perfection, utopian)

ART-V. He, 11 - Picking (gathering) of bedcovers, making a fold (wrap) of skin on back of her mother's hand, saying that it will not come off (disconnected), wants a knife to cut it off. (stab, wound)

CALC-P. He, 19 - Ailments from grief, disappointed love.

FL-AC. Al, 1 - Great disposition, when alone, to repulsive fantastic imaginations, particularly in regard to persons with whom he stands in near relations, or with whom he is connected (united, joined); it seems, for example, as though he must get rid (discard, repudiate, reject) of all the servants, children must go out of house, a betrothal must be broken off, a marriage should be dissolved. (broke; vows)
He, 6 - Feeling of indifference towards those he loves best; has no objection to their presence but does not care to converse with them, yet if strangers or mere acquaintances come in will enter into animated conversation....

GERM. Sh, 148 - The last days I have had moments when I have felt I have been united to the world and people -to humanity. Have felt more love and reconciliation towards myself and other people. Started to be more conscious about the environment and what I can do to our mutual benefit. Something is happening within me. I wish to get more contact with my feelings. 18, 30C, 64:XX:XX

HALI-L. Sh, 608 - Sad that there is a crack, a possibility my relationship might end. 02, 30C, 00:14:XX
Sh, 612 - Anxious all day. Feel my relationship is on the rocks as if partner is emotionally abusing me. 02, 30C, 05:XX:XX

HYDROG. Sh, 15 - I felt in the presence of a totally pure energy, like meeting God and feeling totally unworthy or like meeting a lover and feeling unworthy — realizing all the mistakes of a lifetime. This pure energy was around for some time protecting me. I feel this unification cleared out lifetimes of symptomatology for me. The joining with this energy was as if a male energy joined with me sexually, but with no desire, pleasure or pain involved. This unification with the male energy lasted quite a few days — I'm not used to seeing myself as a man. The morning after this unifying with the higher presence, I collapsed in emotional overflow. All my grief and pain came out. I was doubled upon the floor and went into a deep state of catharsis. It is not possible to describe where I went as there are no concepts applicable. I felt overflowing love for humanity and wanted to give everything away. My mind turned to the Buddha. It was like seeing the complete picture instead of fragmented bits. (These primary effects lasted about 28 days, then changing to a paranoia state). 16, 30C, 07.XX.XX

Sh, 16 - I felt I could see more deeply into people —beyond the roles they were playing. 16, 30C, XX:XX:XX

Sh, 26 - Felt inspired that the potential within is so great and we have a possibility of becoming whole and suddenly it comes crashing down into a sort of mundane realization —that the physical world would never reach the potential possible — like losing a dream. This is really bringing me down. 16, 30C, 08:XX:XX

HYOS. Al, 67 - He prattles and makes preparations for his wedding.

Ha, 526 - Chattering he makes preparation for a wedding.

He, 68 - Onanism since childhood; has always been greatly attracted by opposite sex and prematurely busied himself with thoughts of marriage;... secretly wrote his love affairs; mania,...one idea rapidly follow another, all in some away concerning love, masturbates at every opportunity...(satyriasis)

IGN. He, 11-...believes herself married (connected) and pregnant; is tormented by remorse of imagined crimes; seeks constantly to escape to drown (suicide) herself; ...;is only quiet when lying undisturbed and brooding over her troubles, which she rehearses (tell) in a doleful (unhappy) tone ;..." I am neglecting my duty, breaking my vow" (promise, engagement)...;conscientious scruples after eating.

IRID. Sh, 55 - Memories and associations of giving birth, and of being born. Warm nakedness. Marriage? Old memories of marriage and wedding day. Gently erotic and sensual. Q1

Sh, 59 - Woke from a dream about wedding, feeling of unease, remembered my own wedding day, got a letter of proposal from former lover. Went ahead despite. What did I do? Q7

LACH. He, 32 - Aversion of women to marry.

MAG-C. Al, 933 - Dream that she has to marry one she did not like, which she violently resisted;...

Al, 964 - Dream of funeral; she was obliged to dress the hair of the company; also of balls and marriages.

NAT-C. Al, DREAM, 1102-..;of marrying two women, of parties, walks, entertainments, and excursions on horseback, afterwards they were frequently anxious, of going astray (lost),of murders, having his ears cut off; also vexatious dreams; he would take a journey and could not get away from the place,(immobilization) and when has reached the first station was obliged to turn back, on account of something he had forgotten.

NEON. Sh, 4 - I have been living without a partner for 10 years, which I really enjoyed. Now I have an uncomfortable feeling of needing a partner. Usually I only want a partner because I have so much that I want to share it. This is a feeling of only being half and needing another. 20, 6C, 01:03:40

Sh, 60 - During the proving the prover separated from her partner of 13 years. She had attempted this several times previously, unsuccessfully. I asked her what had changed: "Somehow I had a very profound realization that this is my own life time. My usual feelings of guilt shifted and I was able to take responsibility for my own life. There was a sudden clarity. During the proving I wore my glasses more and had dreams of windows. As though there had been a shift of focus to my own needs." 02, 6C, XX:XX:XX

PIC-AC. Al, 1 - While enjoying the society of gentlemen, the idea of marriage (wedding) seemed unendurable.

PLAT. Ha, 25-...felt like embracing everybody and could have laughed over the most sad things.

He, 36 - While suffering from a slight erysipelas faciei, took leave (quit, abandon) of her children, exhorted her husband to join (unite, combine) church, wanted people to join her in prayer (beg), felt happy to join her Redeemer.

STRAM. He, 65-"There", he replied, "A long

train of bedbugs, and after them a procession of beetles and here come crawling over me a host (crowd) of cockroaches"; sank back in alarm, then suddenly said:" I believe I know they are not really bugs, but, except once in a while, they seem real to me. (organization, association, union)

TARENT. Al, 2 - Insanity on account of an unfortunate love.

TIL. Al, 2 - Lovesick (passion, fervor); all his thoughts centered upon an ideal woman; in this revery he was possessed by a sweet melancholy...

VERAT. He, 22 - Nymphomania, with violence and destructiveness; had been disappointed in love; melancholia; ...great desire for sexual intercourse; void (empty) of shame; obscenity; ....

UNREAL

Absent-mindedness; dreamy: ang.[10] arn.[10] ***cench.***[58] olnd.[10] sep.[122] staph.[122]

Absorbed; walking in a dream, as if, when spoken to: sulph.[36]

Confusion of mind; dream, as if in: ail.[116] ambr.[58] androc.[222] arn. bamb-a.[1184] bell. calc.[1] ***cann-i.*** cann-s. carb-an.[1] ***carb-v.*** cham. chin. cupr.[1] grat. guai. ign. ***lec.*** med.[40] meli. mez. nux-m.[162] ***phos.*** rhus-t. sep. spig. squil. sulph. thuj. zinc.

Confusion of mind; mixes subjective and objective: calc.[5] cann-s.[5] hyos.[5] nux-v.[5] plat.[5] ***sulph.***[5]

Confusion of mind; reality, cannot tell what is real and what is not: lap-c-b.[194]

Delusions; air, he is hovering in, like a spirit: asar. lac-c.[58] lach.[58] psil.[164]

- body, absent: germ.[222]
- body, immaterial, is: anh.[119]
- body, lighter than air, is: asar.[149] lach. lap-c-b.[194] ***op.*** thuj. visc.[149] xan.[85]
- body, no body, he has: psor.[139]
- body, nose, transparent, is: bell.
- dreaming when awake, imagines himself: bell.
- emptiness: ***calad.***[122] **COCC.**[122] ign.[122] ***kali-c.***[122] ***mur-ac.***[122] ***olnd.***[122] **PULS.**[122] sars.[122] **SEP.**[122] stann.[122] ***sulph.***[122] ***zing.***[122]
- existence, doubt if anything had: agn.
- existence, doubted his own: cann-i.
- existence, without form in vast space: cann-i.[36]
- friend, fantasy world of imaginary friends, lives in a: calc.[189]
- light, incorporeal, immaterial, he is: agar.[116] ***asar.***[116] camph.[139] cann-i.[116] chin.[8] ***coff.***[116] ***croc.***[116] ***dat-a.***[25] dig.[1] eup-pur.[36] gels.[139] hyper.[102] lac-c.[116] lach.[139] lact.[116] lat-k.[102] manc.[139] mez.[116] nat-ar.[102] op.[116] phos.[116] puls.[36] rhus-g.[102] ***stict.***[116] stram.[116] tep.[139] thuj.[116] valer.[116] zinc.[116]
- living under ordinary relations, is not: cic.
- meaningless, everything is: bamb-a.[1184]
- move, things, near him and invisible, are moving: canth.[5] carb-v.[5] ph-ac. phos.[10]
- objects, immaterial, in room: ***cupr-acet.***[54] lyss.[54]
- repulsive fantastic, imaginations: ***fl-ac.***
- sleeping, while awake, insists that he was: acon. alco.[36] ant-t.[139] rhus-t.[139] ter.[139] visc.[139]
- sounds, listens to imaginary: hyos.
- spirit, he is a: cann-i.
- strange, familiar things seem, ludicrous: cann-i. hyos. nux-m.
- surroundings, exist, do not: agn.[139] nux-m.[139] puls.[139]
- transparent, everything is: ***anh.***[119]
- transparent, he is: anh.[149] bell.[10] cann-i.
- unreal, everything is: ail. ***alum.*** aml-n.[54] ***anac.***[54] androc.[222] anh.[119] aran.[149] aran-ix.[144] cann-i. cann-s. cic.[116] ***cocc.***[111] con.[85] dat-a.[25] germ.[222] gink.[149] halo.[149] ***hydrog.***[222] lac-c. lap-c-b.[194] lil-t. ***med.*** psil.[164] rauw.[119] staph.
- unreal, everything seems, hemorrhage, in post partum: ***cann-s.***[54]
- unreal, felt, in company: psil.[164]
- unseen things: tarent.
- vanish, everything will: lyc.
- visions, real, are: ***lach.***[54]

Dream, as if in a: absin. acon. agar.[137] ail. alum. ***ambr.*** aml-n. ***anac.*** androc.[222] ang. anh.[119] ***ant-c.***[137] ***apis*** ***arg-n.***[5] arn. ars. atro. bamb-a.[1184] ***bell.*** bry.[5] buth-aust.[119] ***calc.*** cand-a.[239] ***cann-i.*** ***cann-s.*** carb-ac. carb-an. ***carb-v.*** ***cench.***[58] cham. chin.[5] coca[5] cocc.[1] **COFF.**[5] ***con.*** cupr. dat-a.[25] fago.[25] germ.[222] glon. ***hell.*** hep. hydrog.[222] ***hyos.*** lac-h.[229] ***lach.*** lap-c-b.[194] lil-t. ***med.***[122] merc. morph.[102] ***nat-m.*** **NUX-M.** nux-v.[5] oena. ol-an. olnd.[5] **OP.** ***ph-ac.*** ***phos.*** phys. plb.[201] puls.[5] rheum[117] sabad.[5] sep.[137] sil. squil. staph.[119] **STRAM.** ***sulph.*** thuj. valer. ***verat.*** ***visc.*** zinc.[111] zing.[5] ziz.[36]

Dream, as if in a; beautiful: absin.[54]
Dream, as if in a; delicious: ***cann-i.***[54]
Dream, as if in a; future, poetical: olnd.
Dream, as if in a; singing in ears, with: cann-i.[54]
Dreams; true, seem, on waking: am-m. anac.[10] ***arg.*** arn.[10] caps.[1] cina[58] hydrog.[222] hyos.[58] merc.[1] nat-c. nat-m. rad-br.[137] verat.
➤ vivid, recurred during day, as if really happened: anac.[54]
Dullness; world, the outer, has no existence for her: ***nux-m.***[54]
Escape; attempts to, dreams, in a world of: anh.[149]
Reality, flight from: anh.[119]
Touch; impelled to, does not know if objects are really until she has touched them: sulph.[54]
Unconsciousness; dream; as in a: ambr. anac. cann-i. carb-an. con. **NUX-M.** phos. rheum stram. valer. ***verat.***
Unconsciousness; dream; as in, does not know where he is: atro.[36] cic.[58] cortico.[119] ***glon.*** merc. ***nux-m. petr.*** plat.[116] ran-b.

ACON. He, 7 - Memory lively, or weak; what has just been done seems like a remote dream; cannot remember dates.
ADAM. Sh, 61 - Material objects appear to lack substance. I see molecules.[16], 12C, 34:XX:XX
Sh, 163 - A distant feeling, as if I'm not totally here, with need to blink left eye as if to clear it. 8, 6C, 20:00:00
Sh, 170 - Husband's description: "You are like Alice in Wonderland in an unreal world." 10, 6C, XX:XX:XX
AGN. Al, 1-,...he feels as if nothing existed around him; he is dissatisfied with himself all the time; he is incapable of attending to any business; the things around him are entirely indifferent to him;...
AMBR. Al, 21 - He is always as if he were in a dream.
AML-N. He, 1 - Mental confusion and dreamlike state.
He, 2 - A trancelike state, everything seeming unreal to her.
ANAC. He, 26 - Idea as if everything perceived had no reality, all things appear as in a dream.
He, 1 - Everything appears as in a dream.
ANDROC. Sh, 31 - Felt remote and ineffectual, a dreamy state. Felt more like a spectator than a participant. (25)
Sh, 57 - In the evening felt very lonely and desolate, although not alone. She felt separated, detached, disconnected and unreal. (7)
BAR-M. He, 1 - The locality around him seems transformed.(strange, unfamiliar)
CAMPH. Al, 46-..." I am death! No, I am not death! but indeed I must be dead!" And thus I flew round about myself like a top, with no other feeling than for the strong smell of the Camphor. The external world existed for me no longer....
Al, 46-...The external world existed for me no longer. (solitude) My thoughts were gone; one single fearful one remained; I imagined myself transferred to another world (estranged, alienated); for me all else was extinguished...
Al, 46-...I sat up in bed, but all about me had indeed disappeared. I was alone in the great universe, the last of all things. My ideas of the world, God and religion, now seemed to me to have existed only in my imagination; the earth upon which yesterday I lived and moved, had run its appointed course, and I was the final and solitary fragment of the whole creation...(meaningless, unimportant, neglected, forsaken, loneliness, deserted) (godless)
Al, 46-... Faith and hope were gone. There was here no longer any God, or rather the Infinite himself, like all his works, had ceased to be... (hopeless, faithless, godless, privation, want, destitution)
Al, 46-...I feel a tendency to self contemplation; outer things vanish, and I behold myself in spirit freed from matter.
Al, 46-...I am alone. I feel a tendency to self contemplation; outer things vanished, and I behold myself in spirit freed from matter...
CANN-I. Al, 24 - He seemed possessed with the idea that he did not know whether he himself existed, or whether men generally existed, or for what purpose (intention, mission, aim) he existed.(existence x nonexistence)
CANN-S. He, 1 - Seems to be in a dream, as if things were not real; feels as if she did not know where she was; objects seem

strange; feels at times as if she was somebody else;...

CIC. Al, 9 - He did not believe that he was living under ordinary relations; everything seemed strange and almost fearful to him; it seemed as though he has awakened from an acute fever...

Al, 29 - He was indifferent to everything, and began to doubt whether he was really in the condition which he found himself.

Ha, 226 - He became indifferent to everything, and began to doubt whether this was really the condition in which he was.

He, 8 - He imagined he was not living in his usual condition and circumstances; everything appears to him strange and almost terrible.

CYCL. Al, 28-...he constantly feels as though he had just suffered from an overwhelming (remarkable) affliction; only when he becomes excited is his mind somewhat clearer, and then he acts like one who has just awakened from slumber (sleep), and only half understands what is going on about him.

GERM. Sh, 129 - Felt not enough space in bed. It's a big bed. I felt spacy, out of focus, odd, slightly, not there. Maybe in a dream. 05, 6C, 06.00.00

Sh, 129 - I felt spacy, out of focus, odd, slightly, not there. Maybe in a dream. 05, 6C,

Sh, 178 - Generally a sense of unreality. A kind of fuzzy sensation around the periphery of where I imagined my brain to be in my head i.e. just below the surface. 02, 6C, 01:XX:XX

GLON. Al, 20 - When the effect (in head and arms), which she exactly described, ceased after five minutes, it seemed to her as if she awoke from a dream; ...

Al, 21 - As he returned home through the streets, after the headache, everything seemed strange to him, not as familiar as usual; he was obliged to look about him every few moments to convince himself of being in the right street; it seemed to him as if the houses were not in their right places, on the same route that he had passed over at least four times a day for years.

HALI-L. Sh, 599 - Recall a detail I'd forgotten before—like the mist parting. Looked through my desk again and found the missing package. Recalled losing something earlier this week, probably thrown out. No one else saw it except me. The strangest feeling to remember having seen something, remembered the color of the paper, and the picture, and the wording, and yet not be able to confirm its existence with anyone. Beginning to doubt if it was really real, and yet I know it was. 09, 6C, 11:04:40

HYDROG. Sh, 6 - Feeling of being out of reality. 24, 30C, 02:XX:XX

Sh, 8 - I felt slightly high, removed from reality, yet very alert, clear and calm. Very aware of the colour of the sky, the light, birds singing, flowers —like a pastoral ideal. Feeling of expansiveness, mentally cool, airy and light. 28, 200C, 00:04:XX

Sh, 10 - I feel a bit unreal —like taking drugs —a weird spaced-outness. The top of my head feels very clear —seeing and hearing clear and remote, but from the sinus down, I feel muzzy and warm. 08, 30C, 00:01:XX

Sh, 11 - I felt I had gone mad, possessed, hysterical laughter, singing and a feeling of non-reality, as if in a dream, out of the body — like my mind went out of the window. High one minute and then low. People asked if I was on speed. After seven hours, in the evening (7:30p.m.), the feeling changed to an angry mood and very irritable with a dry furry mouth,...l. 24, 30C, 00:00:45

Sh, 12 - Driving home I felt odd, as if I was hardly in my body. Feel like my body's working on automatic but I'm not really there. Driving along I kept forgetting where I was. Now I feel I'm really more "absent" than normal and feel quite afraid of losing my mind or having an accident. I feel my connection with the physical world is very loose, as though my soul was separated from my body. I have thoughts that this is a bit like dying —not unpleasant. 10, 200C, 13:02:XX

Sh, 20 - Distortion of reality —that other places seemed a million times more real than the real world. Everything seemed a long way away. 16, 30C, 04:XX:XX

Sh, 21 - I feel I have moved into a different state of consciousness and there aren't any guiding posts or means of navigation —a bit like being lost in space. 16, 30C, 06:XX:XX

Sh, 28 - I felt an incredible clarity before and now I feel it may all have been a illusion. I am uncertain, don't know how I am anymore. I don't recognize what is happening. It's as if I have made a step into the unknown. I feel I'm in an unknown area without protection. Fear is the biggest limitation. 16, 30C, 05:XX:XX

Sh, 176 - Feel distant and separated from things and they feel unreal. 16, 30C, 01:XX:XX

Sh, 189 - As if in a dream, not there, difficult to stay with it all while driving home —very conscious of the blackbirds flying across the motorway. Better taking a nap and fresh air from opening the window. Concomitant to finger abscess. 02, 6C, 54:XX:XX

Sh, 219 - Things seem ridiculous and amusing, ordinary things like birds. Laughing at them. Everything seemed so absurd or futile. 16, 30C, 02:XX:XX

IRID. Sh, 22 - I feel whole and connected to everything, yet at the same time I feel I unreal, my boundaries don't feel the same. I1

Sh, 25 - Feeling of being on the outside. F9

KALI-BR. Al, 44 - Felt as if everything that I feel, see or think, had been experienced before, as in a dream; this delusion is so strong that I could swear I dreamt it all.

LIL-T. Al, 47 - Everything seems unreal to me.

MED. Al,N-44 - The impatience, excitement, wild feelings; the unreal, dazed condition; the gloom (sadness) and fear in the dark;... are marked evidence of functional derangement of the nervous system.

Al,N-22 - Sensation as if all life was unreal, like a dream.

He, 21 - Sensation as if life was unreal, like a dream.

MEZ. He, 5 - No rest when alone; wants to be in company ...unable to repeat what has been learned by heart; looks through window for hours, without being conscious of objects around; knows not what she is about; forgets what she is about to utter (talk); looks ill humored, pale, wretched, fallen away; ......expecting some very unpleasant news.

NEON. Sh, 37 - On walking in the fresh air I suddenly felt as if I was cruising along on an energy which was not of my own muscular power. It seemed as if it was coming from somewhere else. It seemed effortless and unreal. I felt as if I was passing everyone else. 02, 6C, 13:XX:XX

Sh, 69 - Recognized a change in awareness -a vaguely stoned,unreal feeling. Giggly, childish, grinning. Felt light. 05, 12C, 05:05:XX

NUX-M. Al, 56-...he went to the theater, which was at some distance; the way seemed to have no end (endless, interminable); ... Although he was, at times, quite unconscious, his limbs did not fail to their service; he went straight on, without recognizing the streets that crossed his way; he was concerned about the time, he feared to come too late..., fancy and reality battle (fight) with each other.

He, 17 - The outer world had no existence for her; automatically she attended to her household duties, and on awaking from this condition she had not the slightest recollection of what she had done; ...

He, 15 - Surroundings seemed changed; fanciful, dreamy images; does not recognize the known street.

OP. Al, 43 - In walking I was hardly sensible that my feet touched the ground; it seemed as if I slid (floating) along the ground impelled by some invisible agent, and that my blood was composed of some ethereal fluid which rendered my body lighter than air.

Al, 45 - Sensation as if he had been taken to heaven; vivid, lovely fantasies float before his vision like a waking dream, which the slumber (sleep) drives away.

STAPH. Al, 15 - Anxious thoughts and events in the past came to him as if the past were present before him, which caused anxiety...then it became black before his eyes; he did not know whether the images were real or illusory, then everything seemed different, and he lost all desire to live.

Ha, 703 - Anxious thoughts and things long past come before him as if they were actually present and stood before him, which causes anxiety and the sweat of anguish -Then blackness comes before his eyes; he knows not if what he sees is true (real) or deception (false, unreal), then he regards (suppose) everything as something different to what it is (strange), and he loses all wish to live. (lost; discernment, perception)

Ha, 696 - He does not know if what is hovering before his imagination like something in his memory has actually taken place or whether he only dreamt it.

SULPH. He, 3-...feels as if crazy; does not know whether she has done what she intended (planned) or whether objects seen are really there, or whether she only imagines them to be, until she has touched them;...

VALER. Al, 11 - Anxious, hypochondriac feeling, as if the objects around him had been estranged from him; the room appears to him desolate (isolated), he does not feel at home in the room, he is impelled to leave it.

VERAT. He, 1 - Is conscious only as in a dream.

VANITY

Boaster, braggart: agn.[162] alco.[36] arn.[30] ars.[30] bell.[30] hydrog.[222] lach.[30] lil-t.[184] lyc.[162] med.[162] merc.[30] nat-m.[30] nux-v.[30] plat.[30] stram.[30] sulph.[189]
Boaster; belongings, toys, about his: sulph.[127]
Boaster; rich, wishes to be considered as: lach.[30] lyc.[30] verat.[30]
Boaster; squander through ostentation: calc.[30] nux-v.[30] plat.[30] puls.[30]
Business; talk of, exploits, their: agar.[36]
Coquettish, too much: bell.[30] lyc.[30] nux-v.[30] puls.[30] sulph.[30]
Delirium; presumptuous: lyc.[36]
Delusions; beautiful, rags seem, even: ***sulph.***
• beautiful, she is b. and wants to be: stram.[122]
• clothes, beautiful, they are: aeth. ***sulph.***
Desires; clothing, to wear his best: con.[137]
Desires; great things, to do: cocain.[137]
Desires; respect, due to him shown: ham.[137]
Desires; riches, abundant means: lap-mar-c.[194]
Dreams; boasting: asc-t.[36] m-p-a.[1]
➤ body, hair, obliged to dress hair in company: mag-c.
➤ glorification of oneself: saroth.[144]
Dress; best, at his: con.[137]
Egotism; self-esteem, nymphomania, in: ***agar.***[54]
Egotism; self-esteem, over-estimation of him self: cic.[137]
Egotism; self-esteem, speaking always about themselves in company: lach.[30] par.[10] staph.[30]
Finery, luxurious clothing, wants: aeth.[5] cur.[36] lil-t.[111] ***sulph.***[5]
Foppish, elegant, dandy: chin.[30] lach.[30] nux-v.[30] phos.[30] ***plat.***[30] verat.[30]
Frivolous: agar.[30] ***apis***[5] arg-n.[58] ***arn.***[122] bar-c. bell.[30] calad.[5] con.[30] lach.[30] **MERC.**[122] par. **PULS.**[5] sep.[10] sil.[30] spong. stram.[8] sulph.[30]
Haughty; clothing, likes to wear his best: ***con.***[54]
Imbecility; old rags are as fine as silk: **SULPH.**
Importance; feels his, pompous: alco.[36] arn.[5] bell.[5] calc.[137] cann-i.[36] cupr.[5] ferr.[60] ferr-ma.[36] glon.[5] hyos.[60] ***lyc.***[5] phos.[5] **PLAT.**[5] stram.[5] sulph.[5] ***verat.***[5]
Insanity; dresses in his bests clothes: con.
Loquacity; exalted opinion of her own ideas and powers, with, in insanity: ***verat-v.***[54]
Loquacity; self-satisfied: par.[10]
Respect, thinks he earns: ham.[36]
Self-deception: act-sp.[54]
Smiling; self-satisfied: anan.[36]
Talk; pleasure in his own talking: nat-m. par. stram. sulph.[189]
Untidy: am-c.[102] androc.[222] aur-ar.[58] caps.[102] carc.[207] lac-h.[229] ***psor.***[102] sil.[102] ***sulph.***[122]
Vanity: ***bell.***[30] lap-mar-c.[194] lil-t.[137] lyc.[30] ***merc.***[30] nux-v.[30] plat.[30] ***puls.***[30] sulph.[30] ***verat.***[137]

ACT-SP. He, 4 - Self-deception; self-satisfaction.

AGAR. Al, 16-.... reciting (enumerate) before the beauties of the tribe their exploits (adventures) in war or the chase.(hunting) Their physical strength is increased...(boasting)

CON. He, 14 - Likes to wear his best clothes, (vanity) makes useless purchases, (squander) cares very little for things (indifferent), wastes or ruins them; does not want to work, prefers to play. (wanderer)

HYDROG. Sh, 276 - Feelings of vulnerability and anxiety about being masculine, both in looks and in behaviourroles. Hope it doesn't get more. To counteract this, I have been stressing the feminine. I spent lots of money on silk clothing and spent a lot of time making myself up, curling hair, etc. People comment that I look softer, but I feel harder inside. I feel confused about my sexual identity. This is in contrast to my previous proving of the remedy, when people commented that my moustache disappeared and breasts grew. 12, 6C, 30:XX:XX (homosexuality)

IRID. Sh, 56 - Delight at seeing my own female form in mirror, desire to shave legs so they would be smooth. Highly sexual, more refined, dressed in best clothes today. Desire to dance naked in moonlight. Q6

KALI-BR. Al, 24 - The patient, who has been violently excited, glorying (adoration) in his imaginary power of body and mind, becomes desponding sullen, melancholic, and frequently lachrymose, often even despairing.

MAG-C. Al, 964 - Dream of funeral; she was obliged to dress the hair of the company; also of balls and marriages.

OPUN-V. Al, 4 - In a few minutes, desire to be at prayer; go there, and in a minute or two desire to go out and "tidy" up; soon went out on an errand downstairs, then come up and go again to prayer.

PLAT. He, 50 - Puerperal mania...assumed or seemed to feel herself a person of great superiority;...

SULPH. Al, 12 - She fancies that she has beautiful (refined) clothes; old rags look like fine things, a coat like a beautiful jacket, a cap like a beautiful hat.

Ha, 62 - She imagines that she has beautiful clothes, she takes old rags for beautiful clothes, she takes a coat for a jacket, a cap for a hat.

He, 11 - Foolish happiness and pride(haughtiness),thinks himself in possession of beautiful (attractive) things; even rags seem beautiful. (rank, position, distinction)

VERAT. Ha, 675 - She boasts (exult, triumph) that she is pregnant.

He, 11 - Thinks himself distinguished (classify) ; squanders (futile) his money; proud (haughty) of his position.

He, 56 - Consequences (ailments from) of injured pride or honor.

VEXATION

Abusive; opposed, when: hydr.[36]

Ailments from; anger, fright, shock, with: **ACON.** ***aur. bell.*** calc. cocc. coff.[54] cupr. **GELS.**[5] ***glon.***[5] **IGN.** nat-c. ***nux-v. op. petr. phos. plat. puls.*** samb. sep. **STRAM.**[5] sulph. zinc.

Ailments from; anger, vexation: **ACON.** agar. alum. alum-sil.[58] am-c. anac.[30] ***ant-c.***[5] ***ant-t. apis*** arg.[58] arn. ***ars.*** ars-s-f.[58] ***aur.*** aur-ar.[58] ***aur-m.*** aur-m-n.[85] bar-c.[5] ***bell. bry.*** cadm-s. calc. calc-ar. ***calc-p.*** calc-s. calc-sil.[58] camph.[85] ***cand-a.***[239] carc.[210] caust. **CHAM.** chin. cimic. cina[5] cist. **COCC.** ***coch.***[54] ***coff.*** colch.[102] **COLOC.** croc. cupr. ferr. ferr-p.[46] ***gels.*** graph.[58] grat.[102] hecla.[234] hyos. **IGN.** iod.[5] **IP.** kali-br.[85] ***kali-p. lach. lyc.*** m-p-a.[1] mag-c. mag-m. manc. merc.[5] mez. nat-ar.[58] nat-c. ***nat-m.*** nat-p. nat-s. ***nit-ac.***[163] nux-m. **NUX-V.** ol-an.[5] olnd.[5] **OP.** petr. ***ph-ac. phos.*** **PLAT.** ***puls.*** ran-b. rhus-t. sac-alb.[36] samb. scroph-n.[85] sec. sel. sep. sil. stann. **STAPH.**[122] stram. stront-c.[5] sulph. ***tarent.*** verat. vesp.[58] vinc.[85] zinc. zinc-p.[58]

Ailments from; contrariety: acon.[30] anac.[30] coff.[30] lach.[30] nux-v.[30]

Anger; happen, at what he thinks may: sol-m.[36]

Anger; past events, about, arise from most indifferent thoughts and from every occurrence in life, unite with new vexations, cannot free herself from them: sulph.[54]

Anger; vexations, thinking about former: ***calc. carb-an.*** lyc.[1] sars.[54] sep. sulph.[54]

Anxiety; chest, heart, region of, vexation, after: lyc.

Anxiety; stomach, vexation, after: **LYC.**

Anxiety; vexation, after: acon. ars.[172] bov.[10] lyc. phos. sep. staph. verat. zinc.[10]

Biting; everyone who disturbs him: hyos.[36]

Cheerfulness; alternating with, vexation: ant-t.[10] bor.[5] caust.[10] cocc.[10] cortiso.[119] croc.[10] nat-m.[10] spong.[10]

Confusion of mind; vexation, after: nux-v.

Delirium; vexation, from: bell.[10] **HYOS.**[54] plat.[10]

Delusions; vexation and offenses, of: cham., chin. dros.

• vexation, after: bell.[10] ***plat.***[10]

Dreams; accidents, annoying: ind.[54]

➤ business, vexatious: apis[36]

➤ daughter, vexed her, had: nat-s.[36]
➤ vexatious, wrong doings of others, over: dros.[54]
Dullness; chagrin, vexation; from: ign. lach.
Embittered, exasperated: ambr.[5] ang.[10] ars.[10] ign.[30] mang.[5] nit-ac.[5] puls.[30] seq-s.[230] sulph.[5] valer.[58]
Excitement; heart, vexation, trembling and fluttering, with, painful to shoulders, in valvular insufficiency: ***lith-c.***[54]
Fear; death, vexation, after, in cholera Asiatic: **ARS.**[54]
✦ vexation, after: ***ars.***[54] cham. coff.[54] lyc.[5] ***petr.***[54] verat.[5]
Indifference; alternating with, vexation: cham. chin.
Indifference; vexation with distress in stomach, after least: ***kali-bi.***[54]
Irritability; disturbance, from any: ant-t.[58] choc.[222] ferr-p.[60] graph.[10] lap-c-b.[194] op.[36]
Jesting; alternating with, vexation: cocc.[10]
Laughing; alternating with, vexation, ill-humor: croc. sanic. stram.
Laughing; vexation, at: lyc.[116]
Mania; vexation, after: bell.[10] hyos.[10] ign.[10] nux-v.[10] ph-ac.[10] ***plat.***[54] staph.[10]
Prostration; vexation, from: ***staph.***[116] zinc.[60]
Quarrelsomeness; vexation, with tearful: ***mosch.***[54]
Sadness; vexation, after: calc-p.[54] kali-bi. ***plat.***[54] ***puls.***[54]
Sighing; vexation, after: ***zinc.***[60]
Singing; alternating with, vexation: agar. croc.
Talk; vexatious things, desire to say, with quick repentance: mez.[36]
Vexation; lower limbs, felt in: nux-v.[122]
Violence; crossed, when: prot.[136] ***sil.***[54]
Weeping; disturbed at work, when: ***puls.***
Weeping; vexation, from: bell.[10] calad. cham. hydrog.[222] ign. m-aust.[10] nux-v. petr. sabin.[10] spong.[10] sulph. tarent. ***zinc.***
Weeping; vexation, from, old: caust.[30] cham.[10] ign.[30] lach.[30] lyc.[10] nat-m.[10] staph.[30]
Wildness; vexation, from: ph-ac.

VIOLENCE

Ailments from; anger; violence, with: **ACON.**[5] aur.[5] bell.[5] ***bry.***[5] **CHAM.**[5] ***coff.***[5] hyos.[5] lyc.[5] nat-m.[5] **NUX-V.**[5] phos.[5] sep.[5] sulph.[5] verat.[5] zinc.[5]
Ailments from; violence: ***aur.***[54] ***bry.***[54] coff.[54]
Anger; beating friends: plat.[30]
Anger; violent: **ACON.** aesc.[102] ambr.[10] **ANAC.** androc.[222] ***apis ars.*** **AUR.** aur-s.[58] bamb-a.[1184] bar-c. bell. bor.[10] ***bry.*** bufo cahin. ***calc.*** camph.[54] cann-s.[10] canth.[54] ***carb-v.*** carbn-s. carc.[207] ***caust.***[10] cere-s.[85] **CHAM.** ***chel.***[54] chin-b.[54] cimx.[85] cocc.[10] coff. ***croc.***[10] cupr.[54] cypr.[54] dros.[54] ferr. ferr-p. germ.[222] ***graph.*** grat. hecla.[234] **HEP.** hydrog.[222] ***hyos.***[122] ictod.[10] ign. iod.[122] ***kali-c.***[10] kali-chl.[10] kali-i. lach.[10] led.[10] ***lyc.*** lyss.[54] ***m-aust.***[10] mag-c.[85] mag-s.[10] med.[212] ***meli.***[54] mez.[10] mosch.[10] ***nat-m.*** nat-s.[10] **NIT-AC. NUX-V.** oena.[116] olnd.[10] ozone[227] pall. ***petr.*** ph-ac.[10] phos. pitu-a.[164] ***plat.***[10] prot.[136] puls.[54] seneg.[10] ***sep.***[122] sil.[10] ***stann.***[10] **STAPH.** stram.[10] stront-c.[10] sulph. **TARENT.** tell.[54] thyr.[5] tub.[5] tub-k.[70] verat. zinc. zinc-p.[58]
Anger; violent, personal, from slight offense: ***anac.***[54]
Anger; violent, takes everything in bad part: ***anac.***[54]
Anger; violent, takes everything in bad part, wishes he might get at some one on whom he might vent it: zinc.[54]
Attack others, desire to: hyos.[162] lyss.[36] stram.[162] tarent.[162]
Break things, desire to: androc.[222] ***apis*** bell.[58] carbn-s.[58] hura hyos.[30] ***nux-v.***[30] sang.[36] sol-t-ae.[36] staph.[30] ***stram.*** sulph.[30] tarent.[146] ***tub.*** verat.[30]
Break things, desire to, bright objects: lyss.[85]
Break things, desire to, chairs with remarkable celerity: ***stram.***[54]
Break things, desire to, laughs over it: ***apis***[54]
Break things, desire to, pins: **BELL.**
Break things, desire to, possession, parents most prized: tub.[189]
Cheerfulness; alternating with, vandalism: spong.[184]
Cheerfulness; alternating with, violence: aur. croc. stram.
Children; desires to, beat: chel.
Contradiction; intolerant of, restrain himself, has to, to keep from violence: aloe. sil.
Cursing; threatening destruction and death: tarent.[54]
Delirium; fierce: agar. ***bapt.***[54] bell. hyos. ***stram.***
Delirium; strike, disposed to: **BELL.**[54]
Delirium; violent: ***acon.*** aeth.[137] agar. alum.[54] ***apis*** **ARS.** atro. ***aur.***[54] **BELL.** camph. canth. chlf.[54] con. ***cupr.*** **HYOS.** ***lach. op.***

phos. plb. puls. ***sec.*** **STRAM.** verat. verat-v.[116] zinc. zinc-p.[58]
Delirium; wild, stab and bite, attempts to: **STRAM.**[54]
Delusions; injury, inflict, will, on someone: lap-c-b.[194]
• shoot with a stick, tries to: bell.[5] merc.
• violence, about: kali-br.
• violent: ***bell.***[10] hyos.[10] sec.[10] stram.[10]
Destructiveness: agar. anan. androc.[222] apis bac.[62] ***bell.*** bufo calc. ***camph.*** cand-a.[239] canth. carbn-s. carc.[207] chlol.[25] ***cimx.***[54] ***con.***[54] ***cupr.*** cur. fl-ac.[111] gall-ac.[162] hep.[58] hura ***hyos.*** iod.[54] kali-p.[193] lach. laur. lil-t.[102] med.[40] merc-i-f. mosch. nux-v.[5] oena.[54] op. phos. plat. plb. prot.[136] sec.[102] sol-t-ae. staph. **STRAM.**[122] stront-c. sulph. ***tarent. tub. verat.*** verat-v.[102]
Destructiveness; clothing, cuts them up: ***verat.***
Destructiveness; clothing, of: ***bell. camph.*** hyos.[54] ***ign.*** nux-v.[30] plb.[111] ***stram. sulph.*** **TARENT.** ***verat.***
Destructiveness; emotions, from suppressed: cand-a.[239]
Destructiveness; temptation, can scarcely resist, to throw lamp out of window: merc-i-f.[54]
Dreams; animals, dogs, mad dog, killing a: abrot.[85] rumx
➤ animals, mice, kill it, had to, and step on it: lap-mar-c.[194]
➤ animals, snakes, killing snakes: ptel.[25]
➤ brutality: cand-a.[239]
➤ children, about, beaten, had been: kali-c.[36] kali-n. nat-m.[36]
➤ cutting, trying to cut off finger of acquaintance: nicc.[36]
➤ dead, bodies, digging knife into wounds of: elaps[36]
➤ killing, mad dog, a: rumx.
➤ rape, seeing, of: ***cench.***
➤ rape, that he has committed: ***cench.*** kreos.[10] petr. sep.[10]
➤ terrorists, of: ozone[227]
➤ violence: androc.[222] apoc-a.[36] aran-ix.[144] arg-n.[58] aur.[36] bell.[58] cact.[58] lap-gr-m.[194] led. ven-m.[149]
Fear; violence, of: germ.[222]
Gestures; makes, violent: agar. ***bell. camph.*** cic-m.[36] ***hep. hyos.*** kali-br.[36] plb.[36] ***stram.***
Impulse; run, to, violence, and to: iod.[102]
Impulse; violence, to do: merc.[58]
Insanity; threatens destruction and death: ***tarent.***
Irritability; rage, violent, easily producing: bor.[127]
Jealousy; brutal, kind man becoming: calc.[30] lach.[30] nux-v.[30] sulph.[30]
Jealousy; crime, to a: hyos.[30] lach.[30]
Jealousy; strikes his wife: lach.[30] nux-v.[30]
Kicks: ***bell.*** carb-v. cham.[5] cina[99] gall-ac.[162] hyos.[1] ***lyc.*** med.[212] nux-v.[162] ozone[227] prot.[149] sac-alb.[210] sanic.[85] ***stram.*** stry. tarent. tub.[189] verat-v.
Laughing; alternating with, violence: aur.[10] croc. stram.
Mania; abuses, violent outburst, abuses her child, parturition, after, puerperal: ***camph.***[54]
Mania; destructive efforts, sudden foxlike, requiring utmost vigilance, followed by laughter and apologies: ***tarent.***[54]
Mania; midnight, dancing, laughing, striking, with: cic.[30]
Mania; violence, with deeds of: ars.[10] ***bell.***[10] hyos.[10] ***plat.***[54] sec.[10] stram.[10]
Mildness; violence, masking the: carc.[207]
Pull; desires to, teeth, one's: bell.
Pull; desires to, hair, ones, others, or: ***ars.***[5] bell. **CUPR.**[5] lil-t.[5] med.[5] mez.[5] tarent.[5] tub.[5] xan.[137]
Rage; beating others: hyos.[1]
Rage; striking, with: anac.[198] ***arg.***[8] ***bell.***[8] canth.[88] ***carb-v.***[8] cupr.[116] lap-mar-c.[194] lyc.[116] ***stram.***[8]
Rage; uncontrollable, can scarcely be restrained: cere-s.[36] ***hyos.***[54] stram.[54]
Striking: alum.[122] ambr.[162] anan.[36] androc.[222] ***arg.*** atro.[36] **BELL.** bov. bufo camph. ***canth.*** carb-v. carbn-s. ***cham.***[137] chel.[36] choc.[222] **CINA**[54] con.[30] ***croc.***[5] cub. ***cupr.*** der. elaps fl-ac.[127] gall-ac.[162] ***glon.*** hell. hep.[85] hydr. **HYOS.** ***ign. kali-c.*** kreos.[5] lach.[189] lap-mar-c.[194] lil-t. ***lyc.*** lyss. med.[212] mosch. nat-c. ***nux-v.*** phos. pitu-a.[164] plat. ***plb.*** prot.[136] sac-alb.[210] scut.[193] sieg.[144] ***staph. stram.*** stront-c. stry. syph.[56] **TARENT.** ter.[144] ***verat.*** visc.[119]
Striking; anger, from: anan.[36] arg.[214] bufo[36] cina[100] kurch.[192] lap-mar-c.[194] ***nat-c.***[30] tub.[187]
Striking; anger, from, friends his: plat.[30] tarent.[58]
Striking; animals, at: med.[193]
Striking; boy clawing his fathers face: **STRAM.**[54]

Striking; bystanders, at: **BELL.**[36] carbn-s.[36] chen-a.[36] hell.[8] ***hyos.***[36] lyc.[36]
Striking; bystanders, at, grows angry, and: ***lyc.***[54]
Striking; children, in: cand-a.[239] **CHAM.** chel.[36] **CINA** cur.[5] lyc.[85]
Striking; desire to strike: alum.[122] androc.[222] bell. bufo carbn-s. der.[36] elaps hydr. **HYOS.** lil-t. nat-c. **NUX-V.**[122] ***staph.***
Striking; knocking his head against wall, and things: apis ars. bac.[55] **BELL.**[122] con. hyos. mag-c. **MILL.**[122] ozone[227] ***phos.***[184] rhus-t. scut.[193] syph.[85] **TUB.**[122]
Striking; reprimanded, when: tub.[193]
Striking; tells his wife he will try not to kill anyone: ***staph.***[54]
Striking; wall, the: canth. con.[5] ***syph.***[56]
Talk; indisposed, alternating with, violence: aur-ar.[58]
Talk; violent: anac.[102] bell.[36] cann-i.[36] lach.[189] lyc.[109] ***nat-c.***[30] nit-ac.[102] stram.[58]
Tears; things: agar.[102] **BELL.** bufo[98] ***camph.*** canth. ***cimx.***[102] cupr. gink.[149] hyos. ign. iod. ***kali-p.*** ***lil-t.***[102] merc. ***nux-v.***[122] ***oena.***[54] op. phos. prot.[136] **STRAM.**[122] sulph. tarent.[102] ***verat.***
Tears; things, books, his: tarent.[146]
Threatening; words of destruction: tarent.[36]
Throw; things away: acon.[58] agar.[137] androc.[222] ars. bry. camph. cham. ***cina*** coff. coloc. dulc. ***kreos.*** lyss.[36] prot.[136] **STAPH.** stram.[54] tarent. thea. thuj.[137] tub.[111] tub-k.[70]
Throws; things, persons, at: agar. bell. lil-t.[58] lyss.[36] med.[212] tub.
Unconsciousness; alternating with, dangerous violence: absin.
Violence: abrot. absin.[54] acon. aesc. ***agar.***[5] agav-t.[149] alco.[36] alum.[54] am-c. am-m.[5] ambr. ***anac.*** ***androc.*** ang. ***ant-t.***[54] apis arn. ars. **AUR.** aur-ar.[58] aur-s.[58] bar-c. **BELL.** bor. ***bry.*** calc. calc-p. camph. cand-a.[239] canth. ***carb-v.*** ***carbn-s.*** caust. ***cham.*** chap.[149] chin.[5] chol.[25] **CIC.** cocc.[5] coff.[5] coloc. con.[5] corn. croc. cupr. cyna.[149] dros. dulc. ferr. gall-ac.[198] graph. grat.[10] **HEP.**[122] **HYOS.** ictod.[10] ign.[5] **IOD.**[5] kali-bi.[5] kali-c. kali-i.[5] ***kali-p.*** lach. ***led.*** lil-t.[58] ***lyc.*** ***m-arct.***[10] mag-s.[10] mang. med.[212] merc. merc-c.[111] merl. mez. mosch. nat-c. ***nat-m.*** nat-s.[10] nit-ac. nitro-o.[36] **NUX-V.** oena.[25] olnd. ox-ac.[111] ozone[227] ***petr.*** ph-ac.[1] ***phos.*** plat. plb.[5] prot.[136] ran-b. sabad. sac-alb.[36] seneg. ***sep.*** sil.[122] spig.[111] stann. staph.[30] **STRAM.** stront-c. ***sulph.*** syph.[149] ***tarent.*** teucr.[30] tub.[149] tub-k.[149] ***verat.*** verat-v.[5] ***visc.*** zinc.[5]
Violence; chases family out of house: ***verat.***[54]
Violence; crossed, when: prot.[136] ***sil.***[54]
Violence; deeds of, rage leading to: agar.[116] anac. ars.[30] bar-c. ***bell.*** bry.[30] calc.[30] ***camph.***[171] canth.[10] carc.[207] chin. cic.[122] cocc. con. croc.[10] cupr.[10] ***hep.*** hyos. ***ign.*** ***iod.***[122] iodof.[116] kali-ar.[58] lach. lil-t.[116] lyc. mosch. nat-c. nicc.[10] nit-ac.[47] ***nux-v.*** phos.[30] plat. stram. stront-c.[10] tarent. tub.[70] ***verat.***[116] zinc
Violence; friends, to his: kali-ar.[58]
Violence; nymphomania, in: ***verat.***[54]
Violence; observed, when he thinks he is not: tarent.[146]
Violence; reproached, when hearing another: calc-p.[36]
Violence; sick, when: bell.[85]
Violence; suddenly sprang away from attendants and swept everything from mantelpiece, said she was sorry, but could not help it: ***tarent.***[54]
Violence; talk of others, from: con.[30] mang.[10]
Violence; touch, from: lach.[10]
Weeping; anger, with, violent quarreling, even to extreme malice and rage: ***mosch.***[54]
Wildness; misdeeds of others, from: ***colch.***[36]

ADAM. Sh, 227 - Get very easily angry. Needed to assert myself and pick on someone who I neither know nor respect. My anger was very violent. 20, 1M, 10:XX:XX
AGAR. Al, 13 - She ran about the yard, romped (playing) with the children, threw them down, even hit them.
Ha, 23 - Fearless, threatening, destructive frenzy, also such as turns against itself and injures itself, combined with great exertion of strength.
Ha, 20 - Drunken fearless frenzy with bold (courageous), vengeful determinations.
ALOE. He, 12 - An easily excited, angry, revengeful state of mind, could not brook opposition (contradiction), wanted to destroy object of wrath, relief from tea or milk stimulants;...
ANAC. Ha, 18 - Extremely passionate at a slight offense, breaking out into violence.
Ha, 16 - He takes everything ill and becomes violent.

ANAN. Al, 6 - Disposition to anger, with desire to strike and destroy.

ANDROC. Sh, 96 - Increased irritability, a "how dare you!" feeling. Felt like tearing offenders to pieces with his bare hands. He felt an enormous surge of violent emotions at trifles, and had to exercise great control to stop outbursts of violence and impulses to hurt someone. Felt that "everyone were creeps", could not be bothered with anyone. (2)

Sh, 106 - Desire to break things. (7)

Sh, 109 - Black, horrible moods which don't last long, but are frightening in their violence. (7)

Sh, 124 - In the street, he felt aggressive and very strong, that his umbrella was a knife, and desired to smash people up. (29)

BELL. Ha, 1419 - Fury; he injures himself and others and strikes about him. (beat, hit)

Ha, 1422 - Along with burning heat of the body, with open, staring, and fixed eyes, such fury she must constantly be held fast in order to prevent her attacking others,...

He, 85-...patient must do everything violently; she wishes those around her to kill her. (salvation, redemption)

He, 33 - In evening he was seized with such violent delirium, that required three men to confine him;...

BRY. He, 47 - Bad effects from mortification, violence and anger.

BUFO. Al, 26 - Anger with desire to strike and destroy.

CALC-P. Al, 14 - Violent, irritable, and snappish; it affects him most to hear that someone has done wrong; indignation rises in him...

Al, 13 - Grows very violent, if his opinion is differed from, or if contradicted, so that he is vexed not to have been able to control himself.

Al, 15 - A communication in which some one is justly reproached concerning his conduct, affects him very disagreeably; he grows violent, and holds up his faults to himself.

CHEL. Al, 55 - Mood very irritable, daily outbreaks of anger without cause (causeless); feels as though she could beat the children, and trembles from rage because she has no reason for doing it.

CHIN. Al, 35 - Ill-humor, amounting to the most violent wrath (fury), so that he could have stabbed any one.

CHOC. Sh, 302 - Tonight my husband committed a large annoyance. I felt rage rise up in me — he jumped back and cowered! I wanted to beat some sensibility into him, stopping short of actually wanting to kill him, I felt: 'its not fair', 'how inconsiderate and thoughtless to an extreme degree'. However, my will intervened before I made a scene. Its as if I'm more aware of my 'shadow side' and really feeling it, but precisely because I'm more aware of it, I can step in with my will and curb my behaviour if it looks as if I'm likely to hurt someone else.[15], 30C, 03:XX:XX

CON. Ha, 10 - The propinquity (proximity) and the talk of people passing by is very offensive to him, and he feels impelled to assault and maltreat them.

CUPR. He, 6 - Craziness (insanity); attacks with savage malice (evil), with proud (arrogant) bearing (posture),...

He, 10 - Mania with biting, beating, and tearing things to pieces; insane foolish gestures of imitation and mimicry; full of insane spiteful (cruelty, brutality) tricks (deceitful, false), ..unhappy, despairing...miserable look...

DER. Al, 6 - He is disposed to strike, and inveighs against his dearest friends.

ELAPS. Al, 16 - Inclination to strike and pick a quarrel.

FERR. Al, 21 - Violence, quarrelsomeness; insists that he is right.

Ha, 291 - Violence, quarrelsomeness (litigious, combative), positiveness (obstinate, emphatic, resolute)

GERM. Sh, 103 - Felt closed in. My every movement and thought controlled. Didn't know where to go for help. Felt like a coward . Felt afraid of violence. I don't know who I am. 04, 6C, XX:XX:XX

Sh, 101 - I'm desperate. I want to die. Feel the power to kill. Feel like a wild animal locked in. It's strong, so intense. I hate so strong-feel a terrible disgust and I'm afraid of what I'm able to do. It's completely impossible to be in it and impossible to get out of it. 18, 30C, 190:XX:XX

HALI-L. Sh, 589 - I wanted to really hurt

somebody or something, no respect for the person, anyway that I could. There was another part of me that couldn't believe I was doing that. It was like a horror movie. I got to that place of no boundaries or responsibility to life. It didn't matter what I did. Indifferent. Like ice, no feeling. Just like if I killed someone there would be no regrets. Just the thought: This is what I have to do now. Desire to kill. It did not matter. Just do it. You've got to. I had no fear. I could do anything, whatever I was asked to do, I could do it then. I was a strong person. The me was the only thing that kept me from doing it. That's where I got scared. The last five days of the proving were in a black hole. I refused to write anything down. A god-like place or a devil-like place. Why do I have these things? Human things. 02, 30C, XX:XX:XX

Sh, 592 - Had a peculiar experience during the day. While playing with one of my dogs, I started to wonder what it would be like to crush her. Suddenly I thought how sensual it would be to crush its little head and rip its flesh. There was something very sensual about the idea of crushing flesh and bones of a soft creature that would not be able to fight me off. It was not a strong, powerful impulse, but there was something compelling about the idea. 04, 30C, 02:XX:XX

Sh, 594 - Yesterday and today, when I was playing with my puppy I felt like hurting her. Today while playing, the feeling was how much stronger I was than her and I could really hurt her. It's a strange feeling. I really love my puppy. This reminds me of when I was 20 years old and there was a child sitting on the steps. I felt I could crush her. I realized how strong I am. I'm not usually a psychopath. It's a feeling of violence. 04, 30C, 04:XX:XX

Sh, 610 - Want to stay in integrity with myself and not run after my lover. We talked about commitment and she got scared. I got angry. This is it. I told her I'm not going all over the place with you. Want you XX per cent here. Feel angry at her indecision and confusion. Feel I want to hit and shake her. Ran on the beach instead. 02, 30C, 02:09:XX

HEP. Ha, 289 - The slightest thing put him into a violent passion, he could have murdered any one without hesitation.

He, 22 - Temper obstinate and cross, a ferocious spleen (irascible) which would lead to cold blooded murder even among those habitually gay and benevolent.

He, 20 - Violent, passionate fretfulness; she spoke with such volubility that one could not always get a chance to reason with her, and she would not listen to the most just remarks.

He, 23 - Wrathful irritability, even to the most extreme violence, threatening to end in murder and arson.(firing pyromania)

HYDROG. Sh, 202 - The instant I woke I felt angry, felt like throwing the clock at the wall. Didn't feel like talking to anyone and felt a desire to kick the furniture —seemed the only way to let my anger out. 10, 200C, 16:XX:XX

HYOS. Ha, 562 - Extreme fury: he rushes at people with knives.

Ha, 545 - Ridiculously solemn acts in improper clothing, mixed with fury. (In a priest's cassock, put on over nothing but a shirt, and in fur boots, he wishes to go to church, in order to preach and perform clerical offices there, and furiously attacks those who try to prevent him.)

Ha, 559 - Fury; he tries to inflict injury on and hurt others.

Ha, 563 - He strikes and tries to murder those he meets.

He, 65 - Violent and threatening...; mind nearly deranged; disturbed by unfounded jealousy.

He, 54 - Tries to injure those around him; convulsions after trying to swallow.

KALI-BR. Al, 2 - General delirium, with hallucinations; delusions about persecution and violence.

LIL-T. Al, 25 - While attending a lecture (speech), desire to hit the lecturer, and in the evening desirous of swearing and damning the fire and things generally, and to think and speak obscene things; disposed to strike and hit persons; as these feelings came, the uterine pains passed away.

He, 9 - Disposed to curse, to strike, to think of obscene things; as these mental states came, uterine irritation abated.(reduced)

LYC. Al, 97 - As if out of her mind, she seeks quarrels, makes unfounded reproaches, is most exceedingly violent, and strikes those whom she thus insults.

Ha, 60 - As if insane she seeks for quarrels, makes ungrounded reproaches abuses (insulting) most violently and beats the person whom she abuses.

LYSS. Al, 32 - Thought came into his mind to attack others in a mean way; to cut others with a knife he holds; to throw water he has in a tumbler into another's face.

NAT-C. Al, 48 - He is angry, and inclined to fight and strike, and cannot tolerate contradiction,...

NEON. Sh, 175 - I've been in a rotten mood all day, dwelling on past offenses. I just can't let go, it's making me angry. I feel like I hate that bastard; it's not an emotion I've had before. Now I feel vindictive, really awful; I feel that if I ever found out that he had been lying to me again I would say to him, "I'll kill you," "I'll slit your throat." These violent feelings were much eased when alone. 02, 6C, 04:22:40

Sh, 198 - Received a long letter from a patient today; haven't even read it, can't be bothered. Very unusual. In terms of indifference, I have felt disgusted with myself; one of these violent and malicious feelings. God, I feel so wretched. 02, 6C, 05:XX:XX

NIT-AC. Ha, 6 - Inclined to be violent and to quarrel.

NUX-V. Al, 4 - He is hasty; looked angrily at anyone who asked him a question without answering, as though he was obliged to restrain himself to avoid being insulting; he was in such an irritable and unrestrained mood that it seemed as though he would like to strike any one in the face who spoke a word to him.

Ha, 1270 - He is hasty (careless, rapid), looks malignantly (deadly) at any one who asks (asked) him anything, without answering, just as if he must control himself in order to avoid becoming coarse (rude), it seems as if he would like to strike any one in the face who speaks a word to him, so irritable and uncontrollable in his disposition.

OP. Al, 39-...threatened alternately self-destruction and injury to others.

PALL. He, 12 - Greatly inclined to use strong and violent expressions.

PETR. Al, 8 - Violent irritable, offended at trifles.

He, 7 - Violent irritable, offended at trifles.

PLAT. Ha, 33 - Very cross and irritated at harmless matters and words; so that she at times would have liked to have beaten herself and friends.

He, 16 - Very peevish and easily excited; he could have beaten any one without provocation.

PULS. He, 47- ...; pangs (pain, anxiety) of conscience about religion and female sex; violent palpitation in the presence of women; abhors (detests, aversion) and hates the sex; must go out of their way for fear of injuring them; looks upon them as evil beings and is afraid (fear; temptation, seduction); considers their presence injurious (insulted, offended) to his soul; ... (sexual loathing)

ROB. Al, 10 - Love and excited passions, leading him to the grossest (obscene, rude) excesses, even to homicide.

SIL. He, 19 - When crossed has to restrain himself to keep from doing violence.

STAPH. He, 15-...; firmly believed he would lose his fortune, constantly told his wife to be careful that they did not starve; thinks his wife will run away from him (deserted) (lost: position, rank), ... amuses himself by throwing into the fire any article near at hand, regardless of value; at times more violent, strikes at any one coming near him, ...tells his wife he will try not kill any one;...

STRAM. He, 56 - Believes to be in his grave; shrives,(confess) prays, asks to be killed (justified); accuses his wife of infidelity; scolds (cursing), strikes at everybody who wishes to restrain him; thinks they are dogs and barks at them to make himself understood.

He, 51-...converses with spirits who approach his bed, lays hold of a stick and strikes about him,...great sexual excitement.

He, 81-...attempts to stab and bite;...with sexual excitement; fear as if a dog were attacking him;...

He, 100-...threatens to knock everybody down, to break furniture, to throw himself out of window.

He, 110-...frightful dreams about fighting and killing; takes offensive in imaginary quarrels, and attacks aggressor; runs against supposed object to attack it;...
SYPH. Al,N-5-... violent on being opposed, has tremors, seems on the verge of convulsions,...always washing her hands.
TARENT. Al, 1-...threatening words of destruction and death; she believes she is insulted; ...
Al, 16 - Great taciturnity and irritability; desire to strike himself and others.
He, 2 - Great taciturnity and irritability; desire to strike himself and others.
He, 12 - Sudden foxlike destructive efforts, requiring utmost vigilance to prevent damage;...
He, 14 - Paroxysms of insanity; restlessness of legs; threatening words of destruction and death.
He, 15 - Suddenly sprang (escape) away from her attendants and swept (clean) ornaments from mantelpiece (an ornamental facing around fireplace); said she was sorry, but could not help it; very mischievous and destructive, ...
He, 16 - Attacks of hystero-mania... hits and abuses everyone, destroys whatever she can lay hold of,...mocks aged people with their old age, ...
THYR. Al,N-1-...at times dangerous and homicidal, would put her arms round the necks of other patients so tightly as almost to strangle them (in this case the insanity was primary and the myxedema secondary; both conditions were removed). Evinced increased vivacity by quarreling with another patient about a trifling difference of opinion.
VERAT. He, 22 - Nymphomania, with violence and destructiveness; had been disappointed in love; melancholia; ...great desire for sexual intercourse; void (empty) of shame; obscenity; ....

VORACITY

Contemptuous; ravenous hunger and greed, hasty eating, c. with sudden: ***plat.***[36]
Desires; everything, for: sant.[36]
Desires; numerous, various things, refused when offered, food: rheum[5]
Drinks; more as she should: ars.[1]
Eats more than she should: aq-mar.[231] ars.[1]
Gourmand: calc.[30] chin.[30] ip.[30] mag-c.[30] merc.[30] nat-c.[30] **VERAT.**[30]
Greed; eating, in: abies-c.[137] acon.[163] agar.[5] all-c.[163] all-s.[85] ang.[5] ant-c.[85] ***ant-t.***[163] arg-n.[163] ***ars.***[163] ***asaf.***[163] bry.[85] ***calc.***[5] caps.[163] ***carb-v.***[163] caust.[30] cham.[163] **CHIN.**[5] chin-ar.[163] ***cina***[5] coff.[163] euph.[5] ferr.[163] fl-ac.[5] graph.[1] hell.[5] hep.[1] iod.[5] ***ip.***[163] ***kali-bi.***[163] kali-c.[1] lob.[163] **LYC.**[5] ***mag-c.***[30] ***merc.***[5] ***mur-ac.***[5] nat-c.[137] nat-m.[163] nat-p.[163] nat-s.[163] ***nux-m.***[5] ***nux-v.***[163] op.[36] petr.[5] phos.[1] plat.[5] ***puls.***[163] ***sec.***[5] ***sep.***[5] sil.[163] sol-n.[1] spong.[5] squil.[5] ***stann.***[5] staph.[5] ***sul-ac.***[163] sulph.[1] tarent.[163] thuj.[163] **VERAT.**[5] zinc.[5]
Hurry; drinking: anac.[102] ***ars.***[5] ***bell.***[54] bry.[54] cina[54] ***coff. hell.***[5] ***hep.*** ip.[5] lyc.[54] nat-m.[5] nit-ac.[5] nux-v.[5] ***sil.***[5] ***stram.***[54] sulph.[5] verat.[5] ***zinc.***[54]
Insanity; gluttony, with: chin.[30] **VERAT.**[30]
Insanity; gluttony, with, alternating with refusal to eat: hyos.[30] ip.[30] stram.[30] verat.[30]

ARS. Ha, 1045 - Her desire is greater then her need ; she eats and drinks more than is good for her; she walks further than she need do or can bear. (avidity)
He, 26 - Her desires are greater than her need; she eats and drinks more than is good for her, and walks farther (great distance) than she ought to do.
ROB. Al, 11 - Strong disposition to be obscene, to gormandize (gluttony, voracity), and for all kinds of orgies.

WALK

Anxiety; pursued, as if, walking, when: ***anac.***
Delusions; body, able to go out of b. and walk around, looking down upon: agar.[162] anh.[144] cann-i.[162] pyrus[36]
- water, wades, in he: ant-t.[10]

Dreams; mud, walking in: iod.
- ➤ unsuccessful efforts to, running, of: croc. ind.
- ➤ walking, floor, on hot: apis[36]
- ➤ walking, of: agar.[54] bell.[36] canth.[10] cench.[58] elaps[36] med. nat-c.[36] nat-s.[10] pall.[36] rhus-t.
- ➤ walking, roads, over dirty wet: apis[36]
- ➤ walking, unable of, is: arist-m.[36]
- ➤ walking, woods, in: canth.[36]
- ➤ water, wading in: ant-t.[10] merc-i-r. verat-v.[54]
- ➤ water, wading in, acquaintances, of

seeing: ped.[36]
➤ water, wading in, serpents, in which are, of which he is afraid: alum.
➤ water, walking in: merc-i-r.
➤ water, walking on, acquaintances: ped.[11]
Fear; death, walking while: ***dig.***
✦ walking, of: nat-m.
Hurry; walking, while: acon. **ARG-N.** canth. carb-an.[1] fl-ac.[5] iod. mosch. prun. sep.[5] stram. **SUL-AC.** sul-i.[58] ***sulph.*** **TARENT.** ***thuj.***
Kill; desire to, walking in open air and street, while: camph. hyos.[30]
Restlessness; anxious, has to, walk rapidly: androc.[222] ***arg-n.*** **ARS.** cimic.[144] lil-t. sul-ac. **TARENT.**
Walk; aversion to: zinc.[85]
Walk; circle, walks in a: bell.[36] ***stram.***[36] ***thuj.***[54]
Walk; self-sufficient impression of importance, walks along with a: ferr-ma.[36]
Walks more than is good for her: ars.[1]

WATER

Anxiety; bathing the feet, after: nat-c. sep.[172]
Aversion; water to: am-c.[5] ***hyos.***[137] ***lyss.***[162] ***nux-v.***[137] ***stram.***[137]
Aversion; water to, thinking of it agg.: ham.[137]
Aversion; water to, thirst, with: hell.[137]
Aversion; water to, touch of it, cannot bear: am-c.[137]
Delirium; water, jumping into: bell. sec.
Delusions; animals, fishes, sees: bell. ***stram.***
• animals, geese, threw themselves into water, thinking themselves to be: con.
• boat, owns a: lap-c-b.[194]
• body, brain, swimming, is: sol-n.[139]
• clothes, wet, is: calc.[137] guai.[137] lac-d.[137] lyc.[137] phos.[137] ran-b.[137] sanic.[137] sep.[137] verat-v.[137]
• floating, bed, swimming in: bell. stram.
• rain, exposed to: kalm.[36]
• rain; out in the rain, he had been, from having wet cloth on head: atro.
• room, foam of a troubled sea, is the: sec.
• seasick, he is: der. magn-gr.[139] nitro-o.[36] tab.[139]
• ship, ocean, on, sees: lap-c-b.[194]
• ship, on board of, in a storm: alco.
• soda water, being a bottle of: arg-n.[91] cann-i.[36]
• swimming, is: cann-i. rhus-t.
• water: alum.[5] am-m.[5] ***ant-t.***[5] ars.[5] bov.[5] dig.[5] ferr.[5] graph.[5] hep.[10] ign.[5] iod.[5] kali-c.[5] kali-n.[5] mag-c.[5] mag-m.[5] meph.[5] ***merc.***[5] nat-c.[5] ran-b.[5] sep.[5] sil.[5]
• water, disasters by: cann-i.
• water, flowing, sees: ***merc.***
• water, lake, a spoonful of water is a: agar.
• water, nectar, water is delicious, when drinking: cann-i.
• water, talking of, with: sep.[10]
• water, under water, he is: lap-c-b.[194]
• water, wades, in he: ant-t.[10]
Dreams; animals, fishes: arg-n.[36] chin-b. kali-c.[5] kali-m.[192] mag-c.[5]
➤ animals, fishes, big as a room: ozone[227]
➤ animals, fishes, gold metal: choc.[222]
➤ animals, fishes, swimming in water: chin-b.
➤ animals, horses, riding, stream, through a: chr-ac.[8]
➤ breath under water, she can: ozone[227]
➤ danger, drowning, of: bov.[36]
➤ disease, burning hands by washing: mag-m.
➤ drinking: ars.[102] dros. med. nat-m.[102] phos.[102]
➤ drowning, danger of: bov.[36]
➤ drowning, drowning man, of a: ***lyc.***[54] ***sil.*** sol-t-ae.
➤ drowning, foundering boat, on a: alum. lyc.
➤ falling, flood, into a: am-m.
➤ flood: aran.[192] mag-c. merc. nat-c. rumx. ***sil.***
➤ hydrophobia, of: anan.
➤ journey, water, by: alum.[10] chin-b.[8] nat-s.[10] sang.[10] valer.[10]
➤ jumping, river, in: polym.[111]
➤ men, green and covered with moss, living in water, changing into dogs: sol-t-ae.[36]
➤ murdering, drowning two people in pool: ozone[227]
➤ Noah's ark: bamb-a.[1184]
➤ rain, of being soaked in: mag-c.
➤ rowing: rhus-t.
➤ ships: bamb-a.[1184]
➤ ships, wartime, in: hydrog.[222]
➤ skating in the water: ped.[36]
➤ soaked with rain, being: mag-c.
➤ storms, sea, at: all-c. sil.
➤ stream: com.[58]
➤ stream, crossing a stream on horseback: chr-ac.[54]

➤ torches in the sea: ozone[227]
➤ vivid, burning thirst, of, unquenchable by beer: nat-m.[36]
➤ walking, roads, over dirty wet: apis[36]
➤ water: ***all-c.*** ***all-s.*** alum. **AM-M.** androc.[222] ant-t.[10] arg-n. arn.[58] ***ars.*** bamb-a.[1184] ***bell.*** bol.[36] bov. carb-v. chin. chr-ac.[36] com. ***dig.*** eupi. ***ferr.*** ***graph.*** hura hydrog.[222] ign. iod. ***kali-c.*** kali-n. kali-sil.[58] kalm. ***lyc.*** mag-c. mag-m. mag-s. ***meph.*** ***merc.*** merc-i-r. murx. nat-c. nat-m. nat-s. nicc. ox-ac. ozone[227] ran-b. rhus-t. sang. ***sil.*** sol-t-ae. sulph. tarent. valer. verat. ***verat-v.*** viol-o.[45] zinc.
➤ water, black: ***ars.*** lac-c.[193] ozone[227]
➤ water, black, tar, like: ozone[227]
➤ water, boat, foundering: alum. bamb-a.[1184] lyc. sil.
➤ water, boat, rubberboat going up a mountain stream: ozone[227]
➤ water, child bathing in boiling: mag-c.
➤ water, coming out of drain: bamb-a.[1184]
➤ water, danger from: ars. ars-met.[54] ***graph.*** kali-n. ***mag-c.*** mag-m.[1] merc. merc-acet.[10] nat-c.[1] sulph.
➤ water, daughter is in water and crying for help: nat-s.
➤ water, dirty, bathing impossible: ozone[227]
➤ water, drawing water from yellow looking marsh: hura[36]
➤ water, falling into: ***am-m.*** ***dig.*** eupi. ***ferr.*** ign. iod. mag-m. mag-s. merc. mez.[10] nicc. ph-ac.[1] plb.[10] puls.[10] sars.[10] sep.[10] sulph.[10] zinc.[10]
➤ water, falling into, child, her: eupi.
➤ water, falling into, daughter: iod.
➤ water, falling into, ice, through: ozone[227]
➤ water, falling into, mother: nicc.
➤ water, flood, of a: bamb-a.[1184] mag-c. merc. nat-c. ozone[227] rumx. ***sil.***
➤ water, led over, of being: eupi.[36]
➤ water, looking at water flowing, but became sad on looking at sky: tarent.[36]
➤ water, men, two, jumping into: mag-s.
➤ water, people, bathing: chin-b.
➤ water, people, bathing, boiling water, in: mag-c.[58]
➤ water, people, bathing, lake, in a: ozone[227]
➤ water, people, bathing, swimming pool of hotel, in, naked: ozone[227]
➤ water, people, swimming pool of hotel, walking on water: ozone[227]
➤ water, poisoned: ozone[227]
➤ water, putrid: arg-n.
➤ water, rowing on: rhus-t.
➤ water, running: nat-s.[102]
➤ water, sailing: alum.[10] chin. hura nat-s. sang. senec. valer.[10] verat-v.
➤ water, sailing, dangerous sailing in a small boat: nat-m.[36]
➤ water, sea, of: all-c. androc.[222] chin. chin-b.[8] choc.[222] hydrog.[222] murx.[10]
➤ water, skating in Summer with water up to thighs, of seeing people: ped.[36]
➤ water, stream, crossing a, on horseback, and water froze: chr-ac.[36]
➤ water, stream, of: com.
➤ water, swimming in: ***bell.*** chin-b.[54] hura iod. lyc. merc-i-r. ran-b. rhus-t. sol-t-ae. viol-o.[45]
➤ water, swimming in, dark green: hura[36]
➤ water, swimming in, get out, and cannot: sol-t-ae.[36]
➤ water, swimming in, warm: hura[36]
➤ water, wading in: ant-t.[10] merc-i-r. verat-v.[54]
➤ water, wading in, acquaintances, of seeing: ped.[36]
➤ water, wading in, serpents, in which are, of which he is afraid: alum.
➤ water, walking in: merc-i-r.
➤ water, walking on, acquaintances: ped.[11]
➤ water, waves, coming out of drain: bamb-a.[1184]
➤ water, waves, head, in, causing vertigo: bamb-a.[1184]
➤ water, waves, of high: ***all-c.***[54] ozone[227]
➤ water, waves, putting him on land, on his feet: ozone[227]
➤ water, yellow: hura.
➤ wells, let down into, of being: ***all-s.*** merc-c.
➤ wells, trying to get out of: all-c.[36]
➤ wood, being floated down and fearing damage: nat-s.[36]

Escape; attempts to, throw himself into the river, tries to: ***hell.***[54]

Excitement; bath, during: gast.[36]

Excitement; water poured out, from hearing: **LYSS. STRAM.**

Fear; bath, of: ant-c.[172] rhus-t.[172] sep.[172] spig.[172] sulph.[172]
✦ bed, of the, wetting: alum.[137]
✦ drink, to: ars.[8] malar.[56] plb.[36]
✦ drowned, of being: cann-i.
✦ falling, water, into: perh.[149]

✦ noise, from, rushing water, of: bell.[172] canth.[172] hyos.[58] **LYSS. STRAM.** sulph.[172]
✦ sea, of the: morbill.[162]
✦ walking, of, canal by a: ang.[137]
✦ water, fossets, of: lyss.[122]
✦ water, large bodies of: med.[212]
✦ water, of: acet-ac. agav-a.[102] anag.[102] ant-c.[102] ***bell.*** cann-i. canth. carc.[207] cocci-s.[102] cupr. fagu.[36] gels. **HYOS.** iod. jatr.[36] ***lach.*** laur.[102] lycps.[187] **LYSS.** med.[212] merc.[111] nux-v. perh.[149] phel.[36] ***phos.*** plb. ruta sabad. spirae.[102] **STRAM.** sulph.[58] tanac.[102] tarent. verat.[102] xan.[102]

Frightened; easily, liquids, at sight of: bell.[36]
Frightened; easily, night, starting up as if falling from a height into water: ph-ac.[36]
Hydrophobia: acet-ac. acon.[36] aconin.[36] agav-a.[72] agn.[172] anag.[77] anan.[85] ant-c.[5] anthr.[56] apis[5] aran.[47] arg-n. ars. ***aspar.***[8] ***bell.*** brom.[137] calc. camph.[5] cann-i. ***canth.*** carc.[207] cedr.[85] chlol. cocci-s.[72] crot-h. cupr. ***cur.*** fagu.[77] gels.[5] gent-c.[85] grin.[54] gua.[85] ho.[85] **HYDR-AC.**[5] ***hyos.*** hyper.[85] iod. jatr.[5] ***lach.*** laur.[1] **LYSS.**[122] mand.[72] merc. naja[51] nat-m.[54] nux-v.[5] phel.[58] phos. plb.[5] ran-s. ruta[5] sabad. scut.[85] spirae.[72] **STRAM.** stry.[36] sulph.[5] tanac.[102] tann-ac.[85] tarent.[5] ter. trach.[36] verat. xanth.[72]
Hydrophobia; bitten, after being: lyss.[54]
Hydrophobia; convulsions, during: canth.[54] lyss.[54]
Hydrophobia; frequently speaks with a remarkably quick and sharp articulation of the impending result: lyss.[54]
Hydrophobia; grief agg.: lyss.[54]
Hydrophobia; idea of fluids may cause a paroxysm, the mere: lyss.[54]
Hydrophobia; moaning and violent cries alternating with barking: canth.[85]
Hydrophobia; prophylactic: ***bell.***[137] canth.[137] hyos.[137] lyss.[137] stram.[137]
Hydrophobia; screams or howls in a high voice: ***stram.***[54]
Hydrophobia; spasms renewed by contact: ***bell.***[54]
Hydrophobia; symptoms resembling: cann-i.[36] **STRAM.**[36]
Hydrophobia; touch, cannot bear: am-c.[137]
Hydrophobia; water, could not hear mentioned without shudder of fear: ***lyss.***[54] phys.[137]
Irritability; weather, in rainy or cloudy: aloe. am-c.
Rage; water, at sight of: ***bell. canth.*** cupr. hyos. lach. merc.[10] ***stram.***
Sadness; weather, wet, in: am-c.[171] ***elaps***[54] rhus-t.[122]
Sensitive; noise, water splashing: brom.[137] **LYSS. NIT-AC.** stram.
Shining objects; agg. surface of water: **LYSS.**
Washing; aversion, children, in: am-c.[58] ant-c.[127] psor.[127] **SULPH.**[54] tub.[106]
Washing; desire for, cold water, in: meph.[60] phyt.[60]

ACON. Al, 46 - Anxiety only transiently relieved by drinking cold water.

ADAM. Sh, 429 - Fear something could happen if I had a bath. Want to keep dry. 7, 6C, 20:09:00

ANT-C. He, 20 - Is driven to despair, resolved to drown himself.

ARG-N. He, 22 - On crossing a bridge, almost irresistible desire to jump into river; meeting some one prevented it.

ARS-H. He, 23 - Thinking of water irritates him, as if he would have to vomit; it nauseates him.

BELL. Al, 127 - Aversion to all fluids (liquid, water) so that she demeaned (conduct) herself frightfully (fear) at the sight of them.

Al, 161 - In walking in the open air, she is overwhelmed with tearful anguish; she is weary of life, and inclines to drown herself.

Ha, 1381-...she is weary of life, and wishes to go into the water to drown herself.

Ha, 1440 - Throws herself into water. (drowning)

He, 53 - Weary of life, with desire to drown herself.

CALC. Al, 19 - She despaired of her life, and believed that she must die, with a most sad mood, and weeping, and frequent sudden attacks of general heat, as if hot water had been dashed over her.

Ha, 30 - She despairs of her life and believes she has to die (punishment?) ; her heart is sad with weeping, and frequent attacks of sudden, general heat, as if she had hot water poured (flow) over her.

CANN-I. Al, 65 - Hallucinations which lead the patient to imagine that he is on horseback, is hunting, that he sees blue water, that he is swimming, or that he is captain of a vessel, that he is traveling, that he has no weight.(lightness)

Al, 66 - Illusion that he was a pump-log, through which a stream of hot water was playing, and threatening his friend with a wetting.

CON. Al, 6 - Delirious and stupid; they threw themselves into the water, thinking they were geese; for three years they remained partly paralytic, suffering from much pain.

DROS. Ha, 277 - Anxiety; ...,as if he were impelled to jump into the water in order to take his own life by drowning he was not impelled to any other mode of death.

He, 3 - Anxiety: with flushes of heat; when alone (solitude), ...as if it would impel him to commit suicide by drowning. (water will purify?)

ELAPS. Al, 14 - Excessive horror of rain.

He, 5 - Fear of being left alone, as if something horrible might happen; horror of rain.

FERR. Al, 766 - Dreams he is in battle, that he has fallen into the water, etc.

Ha, 270 - Dreams that he is in battle, that he has fallen into the water...

HALI-L. Sh, 215 - Made up a meditation before going to bed. Felt both parents at the bedside. I am being totally held and loved by my father, wrapped up in blankets like I'm a baby. He is adoring me, cooing over me with my mother looking on. This calms my nerves and the sad feeling moves outward. This feels the same as swimming to me. The water on my skin calms my nerves. 08, 30C, 23:XX:XX

Sh, 416 - Feel really dull with the rain. I think I'm in a mild depression. I'm not visiting friends, just hanging around. No goals, not doing things. 08, 30C, 03:XX:XX

Sh, 520 - When the rain came down hard, there was a roaring from the creek outside. Awful sleep. I'd wake up with each roar, envisioning the water rising up, fearing the creek was backed up and would overflow its banks. I'd listen till the sound died down, then I could go back to sleep. 08, 30C, 06:XX:XX

HELL. He, 20 - After typhoid, ...sits quietly in bed and seems lost in brooding;...constantly seeks (try) to escape, ...;without a word quietly climbs out of the window, and if she succeeds in escaping goes in direction of river; finally threw herself into privy (toilet), from which she was rescued.

He, 19 - Tries to escape, to throw herself into the river.

HYOS. Al, 82 - In despair, he wishes to drown himself.

Al, 89 - Dread of water.

Ha, 579 - In despair he wishes to take his life, and throw himself into the water.(suicidal)

He, 14 - Dread of drinks; of water.

He, 74 - Disappointed love followed by: epilepsy, melancholy, rage, or inclination to laugh at everything; despair and propensity to drown himself. (ailments from)

IGN. He, 11-...believes herself married (connected) and pregnant; is tormented by remorse of imagined crimes; seeks constantly to escape to drown (suicide) herself; ...;is only quiet when lying undisturbed and brooding over her troubles, which she rehearses (tell) in a doleful (unhappy) tone ;..." I am neglecting my duty, breaking my vow" (promise, engagement)...;conscientious scruples after eating.

IRID. Sh-2 - Felt similar to being in water or asleep, as if almost asleep or in a trance, aware, but floating in inner self, uncommunicative; like a near death experience, inner self is primary and separate. E1

Sh, 70 - Felt cold water running through my arms and legs and out; though it didn't make me feel cold. D34

LYSS. Al,N-77 - Lyssophobia; fear of becoming mad. (hydrophobia)

Al,N-79-...terror ...by endeavoring to take a drink of water, ...attacks...induced by running of water,...

Al,N-116 - Attacks of nervous headache become awful and insupportable if he hears water run out of a hydrant.

Al,N-118 - When he hears water poured out, or if he hears it run, or if he sees it, he becomes very irritable, nervous;...

Al,N-127 - Thinking of fluids of any kind, even of blood, brings on convulsions.

MAG-C. Al, 932 - Dream of flowers, clothes, and other things; she had to make up the clothes, but had no inclination to do it, and besides did not understand how; she also saw many foreign plants, but during this she became soaked (wet) with rain.

Al, 943 - Dream of danger by water.

Al, 944 - Dream of a flood, which flowed across the market-place, from which she woke in fright.

Al, 945 - Anxious dream, that a child was bathing in boiling water. (purification?)

MAG-M. Al, 714 - Frightful dreams; that she was pursued by robbers; that she burned her hand by washing ...

MERC. Ha, 1236 - He thinks he is losing his reason,(intelligence, capacity) that he is going to die ; with illusions of imagination, e.g. he sees water flowing where there is none (in the morning). (water-[1] origin, genesis)

He, 14 - Believes he is losing his reason, thinks he is dying, with illusions of fantasy; sees water running where there is none.

NAT-C. Al,DREAM, 1111 - Dream of a flood (current, inundate), and threatening danger.

NEON. Sh, 50 - I have superbly fluid and graceful motions, as if I were moving in water instead of air. I have much pleasure in the right shoulder being free. 20, 6C, 05:XX:XX

Sh, 13 - Thoughts of twos and water. Saw images of Noah's ark. 20, 6C, 08:01:30

Sh, 48 - A phrase from a Lewis Carroll poem repeated itself over and over in my mind: "Come tell me aged man he cried, come tell me how you live. And his answer trickled through my brain like water through a sieve." I felt this was about dissolving, which related to my feeling in the proving. 05, 12C, 05:05:XX

Sh, 49 - I have lost the delusion, which I have always had, that I could walk on water. 20, 6C, 04:XX:XX

Sh, 51 - I have many thoughts of freezing. "Why would people want to deep freeze themselves? Why not freeze dry them?" 20, 6C, 05:XX:XX

Sh, 52 - Thoughts of rivers and oceans and being very happy by them. 20, 6C, 08:XX:XX

NUX-V. Al, 21 - Great aversion to fluids, which were swallowed with great difficulty and often not at all.

PULS. Ha, 1101 - Anxious heat as if hot water were thrown over him, with cold forehead.

He, 25 - Weary of life; thinks with pleasure of drowning. (suicide, water)

He, 52 - After mortification, sad gloomy (melancholy) and weary (disgusted) of life;...thinks of drowning with great pleasure;...

RHUS-T. He, 18 - Disgust of life: thoughts of suicide; wants to drown (immerse) himself; with fear of death: with desire to die, without sadness.

SEC. Al, 10 - Raving (talk wildly), whith an attempt to jump into the water.

Al, 20 - She was conscious, but the room (space) presented to her the impression of water excessively agitated on its surface. She could compare it only to the "foaming of a troubled sea" (storm, tempest)

He, 4 - Mania; with inclination to bite; with inclination to drown.

SIL. He, 15 - Wishes to drown herself.

STRAM. He, 113 - Hydrophobia; water, a mirror, or anything bright, excites convulsion...,afraid to be alone;...

SULPH. He, 35-...,strong impulsive tendency to suicide, by drowning or by precipitating herself from window;...(high, water)

He, 51 - Dread of being washed.

WEALTH

Ailments from; reversal of fortune: ambr.[116] con.[116] dig.[116] lach.[116] stann.[116] staph.[116]

Ambition; much, money, for: ars.[30] calc.[30] lyc.[30] nux-v.[30] sulph.[30]

Avarice; collects carefully the debris of his fortune: stann.[30] staph.[30]

Delusions; castles and palaces, sees: plb.

- fortune, he was going to lose his: psor. staph.
- squanders money: ***verat.***[54]
- visions, grandeur, of magnificent: cann-i.[54] carbn-s. coff.
- wealth, makes useless purchases, and: ***nux-v.***[54]
- wealth, of: agn. alco. bell. calc. cann-i. kali-br. nit-ac.[5] phos.[102] ***plat.***[102] ***pyrog.*** ***sulph.*** verat.

Desires; riches, abundant means: lap-mar-c.[194]

Desires; servants: lap-mar-c.[194]
Dreams; animals, fishes, gold metal: choc.[222]
➤ buildings, admirable: graph.[30]
➤ houses, crystal and marble, built of: ozone[227]
➤ money, gold, of: ***cycl.*** puls.
➤ storms, destroying palaces: jac-c.[36]
Finery, luxurious clothing, wants: aeth.[5] cur.[36] lil-t.[111] ***sulph.***[5]
Insanity; fortune, after gaining: bell.[30] ***caust.***[30] puls.[30] stram.[30] verat.[30]
Insanity; fortune, losing, after: calc.[30] ign.[30] rhus-t.[30] verat.[30]

ADAM. Sh, 359 - Feeling a sense of wealth of prosperity of a beneficent universe. 32SA, 200C, XX:XX:XX

BELL. Al, 203-..;he imagined himself rich, owner of a large house, etc. (great person)

CANN-I. Al, 61 - Then he possesses the wealth of the world, and with a benevolence equal to his wealth, showers riches on all the needy around him.
Al, 63 - His body seemed to him become transparent, and he imagined he saw within his breast the hashish he had eaten in the form of an emerald, from which issued millions of little sparks.

CARBN-S. Al-S, 754 - Hallucinations (delirium) of vision and hearing, he seemed to see splendid spectacles of carriages, with magnificent objects, talked of the emperor, of money, and of grandeur, often incoherently.

CHLOL. He, 10 - Gorgeous (superb, beautiful) visions of arches, tapestry (decoration) and colors pass before the eyes when shut, or open in the dark.

CHOC. Sh, 44 - Dream — coming out of the station a huge black bird the size of a dog with black long soft feathers like those of an ostrich, and a very big beak. It took my left hand in his beak. There were two gypsies there and they stood in front of me and opened their hands and I saw that they held a gold metal flat fish which I saw as a fortune telling object.

CUR. Al, 5 - Fondness (desire) for luxury (waste) and grandeur.(distinction, fame)
Al, 6 - He would like to go travel in a great style.(luxury)

KALI-BR. Al, 3 - Decidedly insane; had delusions that lewd women had got into his mother's house; that he was pursued by the police; that his wife was threatened by members of the family; that he had thousands of dollars in gold sewed up in his clothing; (rich, wealth)

NUX-V. He, 37-...betraying (play false, feigning) great moral and physical languor (indifference),..launches into high-flying, fantastic plans, fancies himself rich (rank, position) and wants to make presents of thousands (squanders, waste), and makes large useless purchases; does not consider himself ill; ...,and takes in bad part if not allowed to read indictment (accusation) for said lawsuit, a confused irrational piece of work...
He, 37-...brooding all night long over a lawsuit by which he may gain or lose a million (megalomania) ; ..replies reluctantly and slowly to physician's questions, and takes it in bad part (offenses) if not allowed to read indictment (accusation) for said lawsuit, a confused irrational piece of work, on which he has been working all night.

OP. Al, 19-...; all the actors are happy, and each retires home in a total state of irrationality, but likewise in the entire and full enjoyment of happiness not to be procured by reason. Disregarding the ridicule of those they meet, who divert themselves by making them talk absurdly, each imagines looks and feels himself possessed of whatever he wishes...

PHOS. He, 31-...; indifference even towards dearest friends;... ; monomania de grandeur et de la richesse;...

PLB. Al, 61 - He had, some time back, illusions of vision; saw castles, palaces, but these have ceased since he entered the hospital.

PYROG. Al,N-8 - Hallucination that he is very wealthy (rich); remaining after fever.

STAPH. He, 15-...; firmly believed he would lose his fortune, constantly told his wife to be careful that they did not starve; thinks his wife will run away from him (deserted) (lost: position, rank), ... amuses himself by throwing into the fire any article near at hand, regardless of value; at times more violent, strikes at any one coming near him, ...tells his wife he will try not kill any one;...

SULPH. Al, 2 - Delirium; she destroys her things, throws them away, thinking that she has a superfluity (excess) of everything, wherewith she wastes(thin) to a skeleton.(wealth?)
Ha, 63 - Insanity; she spoils (ruin) her things and throws them away, imagining she has an abundance of everything; at the same time she becomes emaciated, like a skeleton.-(wealthy, rich X miserable, poor, destitute)
He, 38 - Destroys clothing; imagines she has everything in abundance. (wealth)

WICKED

Ambition; much, means, employed every possible: lyc.[30] plat.[30] ***verat.***[30]
Anxiety; murdered someone, as if he had, all night: phos.[36]
Anxiety; murdered someone, as if he had, mania, in: ***ars.***[54]
Charlatan: calc.[30] plat.[30] sulph.[30]
Cheerfulness; alternating with, vandalism: spong.[184]
Cheerfulness; morbidly: aur-s.[58]
Contrary; spiteful, just to be: tub.[162]
Cruelty, animals to: **ARS.**[162] ***bell.*** calc.[193] med.[162]
Cruelty, brutality, inhumanity: abrot. absin. alco.[36] <u>**ANAC.**</u>[122] androc.[222] ***ars.***[30] ***aur.*** bell.[102] bry.[102] canth.[102] carc.[207] chin.[5] choc.[222] croc. cur. **HEP.**[30] ***hyos.***[30] ***kali-i.***[58] kali-p.[5] ***lach.***[122] lap-mar-c.[194] med.[137] nicc.[30] ***nit-ac.***[102] nux-v. op. ***plat.*** sabad.[10] sel.[30] squil.[10] staph.[102] ***stram.***[102] tarent.[102] verat.[102]
Cruelty; family, to her: kali-p.[58]
Cruelty; religiousness, with: ***plat.***[54]
Cursing; laughing, with, immoderate: stram.[155]
Cut, mutilate, slit others, desire to: lyss. verat.[58]
Deceitful, sly: agar.[5] anac.[5] androc.[222] arg.[111] arg-n. ***ars.***[30] aur-s.[10] bell.[5] bufo calc.[30] chin.[30] chlol. coca ***cupr.***[5] dig.[1] dros. fl-ac.[122] ***hyos.***[5] ***lach.***[5] lap-mar-c.[194] lyc.[30] ***med.***[198] morph.[162] mosch.[58] ***nat-m.***[30] nux-v.[5] ***op.***[5] plat.[30] plb.[58] puls.[30] sep.[30] sil.[30] sulph.[30] ***tarent.***[122] thuj.[58] verat.[5]
Deceitful; corrupt, venal: ars.[30] chin.[30] lyc.[30] puls.[30] sulph.[30]
Deceitful; fraudulent: bell.[30] calc.[30] merc.[30]
Deceitful; perjured: hep.[30] nat-m.[30] nit-ac.[30]
Delirium tremens; oversensitiveness, with, nervous excitability and malicious vehemence: **NUX-V.**[54]
Delirium tremens; voices, heard continually on right side of occiput a loud voice, scolding, vituperating and accusing him of ungodliness, and also personifies voices: **STRAM.**[54]
Delusions; called before court, on account of wicked actions during climacteric period: ***zinc.***[54]
- criminal, that he is a: alum.[10] am-c.[10] ars.[10] carb-v.[10] caust.[10] chel.[5] cina[10] cob. coff.[10] cycl. dig. ferr.[10] graph.[10] hyos. ***ign.*** m-arct.[10] ***merc.*** nat-c.[10] nit-ac.[10] nux-v.[10] op. phos. puls.[10] ruta[10] sabad.[139] sarr. sil.[10] stront-c.[10] sulph.[10] thuj. verat.[10]
- criminals, about: alum. am-c. ***ars.*** bell. carb-v. caust. ***chel.*** cina ***cocc.*** coff. dig. ***ferr.*** graph. ***hyos.*** merc. nat-c. nit-ac. nux-v. puls. ruta sil. stront-c. sulph. verat.
- demoniacal, he is: ***anac.***[54] **HYOS.**[30]
- devils, connected to, he is, arrogant towards those who strive to purity, light and love: ozone[227]
- devils, he is a devil: anac. camph. cann-i. ***hyos.*** kali-br. stram.
- faces, scheming: anh.[119]
- foul, everything appears: cur.
- God, he is, then he is devil: **STRAM.**[54]
- honest, he is not: ***stram.***[8]
- injury, inflict, will, on someone: lap-c-b.[194]
- juggler, he is a: bell.
- lie, all she said is a: lac-c.
- murder, struck friends who came to help him: ***stram.***[54]
- obscene, actions of which she had not been guilty, accuses herself of.: ***phos.***
- spectres, sees, night, evil ones: ***hell.***[54]
- voices, hears, abusive and filthy language, voices from within him speaking in: ***zinc.***[54]
- voices, hears, steal and kill, that she must: lach.[58]
- wicked deed, she has committed a: cocc.[139]
- women, evil, are, and will injure his soul: puls.

Destructiveness: agar. anan. androc.[222] apis bac.[62] ***bell.*** bufo calc. ***camph.*** cand-a.[239] canth. carbn-s. carc.[207] chlol.[25] ***cimx.***[54] ***con.***[54] ***cupr.*** cur. fl-ac.[111] gall-ac.[162] hep.[58] hura ***hyos.*** iod.[54] kali-p.[193] lach. laur.

lil-t.[102] med.[40] merc-i-f. mosch. nux-v.[5] oena.[54] op. phos. plat. plb. prot.[136] sec.[102] sol-t-ae. staph. **STRAM.**[122] stront-c. sulph. ***tarent. tub. verat.*** verat-v.[102]

Destructiveness; cunning: ***tarent.***

Dreams; cruelty: ***ign.***[10] lil-t.[36] nat-m. nux-v. sel. sil. stann.

➤ cruelty, anger, without: lil-t.[36]

➤ cutting, trying to cut off finger of acquaintance: nicc.[36]

➤ killing: stram.[54]

➤ killing, children: thea.[144]

➤ murdering, young boys and girls in cold blood: thea.[36]

➤ rape, that he has committed: ***cench.*** kreos.[10] petr. sep.[10]

➤ remorse, want of: androc.[222]

➤ shameful: acon.[36] alum. am-c.[5] arn.[10] ***asar.***[5] con. erech.[36] hydrog.[222] led.[1] mag-m.[1] mosch.[5] mur-ac.[1] ozone[227] staph.[5] tub.[111]

➤ terrorists, of: ozone[227]

➤ wedding, women, with two: nat-c.[10]

Evil to others, wishes: nat-c.[1]

Fear; alone, of being, crime and cruelty would be committed, lest: kali-br.[172]

✦ animals, dogs, black, malicious: ***stram.***[54]

✦ killing, child, her: ars.[172] coff.[172] manc.[30] ***merc.***[185] ***nux-v.***[185] rhus-t.[172] sep.[185] sil.[172] ***sulph.***[185] **THEA.**[162]

✦ killing, of, delivery, parturition, during: acon.[172] ars.[172] coff.[172] plat.[172]

✦ killing, of, mother, her: der.[162]

✦ mischief, he might do (night on waking): canth.[172] ***phys.***

✦ moral obliquity alternating with sexual, excitement: lil-t.

Honor; sensation of honor, no: anac.[30] ars.[30] hyos.[30] lach.[30] psor.[168] verat.[30]

Impulse, morbid: alum.[5] anac.[5] arg-n.[111] ars.[5] bac.[62] caust.[5] hep.[5] iod.[5] lach.[5] lyc.[5] merc.[5]

Impulse; run, to, violence, and to: iod.[102]

Impulse; violence, to do: merc.[58]

Impulse; wrong, to do: hep.[85]

Inconsolable; actions, over all her, which she thinks are evil: sulph.[1]

Indifference; fine feeling, to: op.[10]

Insanity; malicious, malignant: agar.[10] cann-s.[10] ***cupr.*** lyc.[10]

Jesting; licentious: alco.[36]

Jesting; malicious: ars. choc.[222] lap-mar-c.[194]

Jesting; roguish: puls.[10]

Kill, desire to: agar. alco.[36] alum.[116] anac. androc.[222] ***ars. ars-i.*** bell. calc. camph. chin. cupr. cur. **HEP.**[122] **HYOS.** ***iod.*** kali-ar.[58] lach. ***lyc.***[30] lyss. ***med.***[184] merc. ***nux-v.*** op. ***petr. phos. plat.*** prot.[136] sec. sil.[122] ***staph.***[54] ***stram.*** syph.[122] thea. thyr.[85] x-ray[115]

Liar; lie, believes all she says is a: ***lac-c.***

Liar; never speaks the truth, does not know what she is saying: alco.[122] arg-n.[122] ***morph.***[122] **OP.**[122] ***syph.***[122] ***verat.***[122]

Loquacity; alternating with, maliciousness: ars-s-f.[58]

Love; anal coition with a woman: caust.[30] plat.[30]

Love; perversity: hura[36] ind.[85] kali-n.[36] nux-v.[85] plat.[85]

Love; perversity, animals, with, sodomy: ***plat.***[162]

Love; sadistic: thiop.[149]

Malicious, spiteful, vindictive: abrot. ***acon.*** agar. alco.[36] aloe am-c. am-m. ambr. **ANAC.**[122] androc.[222] arn. **ARS.**[122] ars-s-f.[58] ***aur.*** aur-ar.[58] bar-c. ***bell.*** berb. ***bor.*** bry.[85] bufo ***calc.*** calc-s. cand-a.[239] cann-s. canth. caps. carb-an. caust. cham.[111] chin. choc.[222] cic. clem. coca[30] cocc. coloc. com. con. croc. ***cupr.*** cycl.[10] cyna.[149] fl-ac.[30] gall-ac.[162] glon. guai. haem.[36] ***hep.*** hydr. ***hyos.*** ign. ilx-a.[120] ip.[10] kali-c.[10] kali-i. ***lac-c.*** lac-h.[229] ***lach.*** lap-c-b.[194] lap-mar-c.[194] ***led.*** levo.[149] ***lyc.*** mang. med.[189] merc. mosch. ***nat-c.***[122] **NAT-M.**[122] nicc. ***nit-ac.*** **NUX-V.** op. opun-a.[36] ozone[227] par. ped.[36] petr. ***ph-ac.***[30] phos. pitu-a.[164] plat. puls.[30] ran-b.[10] ***sac-alb.***[210] sarr.[36] sec. sep.[58] sol-m.[10] spong.[10] squil. stann. ***staph.***[30] **STRAM.** stront-c. sulph. syph.[122] tarent.[111] thuj.[5] **TUB.**[122] tus-f.[36] verat. zinc. zinc-p.[58]

Malicious; anger, during: anac.[10] bar-c.[10] calc.[54] canth.[10] ***caps.***[10] carb-an.[10] ***chin.***[10] hep.[10] ***lyc.***[10] ***nat-m.***[10] nicc.[10] petr.[30] zinc.[10]

Malicious; convulsions, after: ***cupr.***[54]

Malicious; convulsions, during: cham.[54]

Malicious; dogs, to: tub.[162]

Malicious; injure someone, desire to: androc.[222] levo.[149] osm.[36]

Malicious; insulting: hyos.[10] merc.[10]

Malicious; insults, long after: nit-ac.[60]

Malicious; laughing: cupr.[10] lap-mar-c.[194]

Malicious; loved ones, to: germ.[222] sep.[58]

Malicious; murder someone, as if she could: ***hep.***[54]

Malicious; sadness, in: **KALI-I.**[54]

Malicious; savage: cupr.[54]

Malicious; sweets, after: sac-alb.[210]

Mania; abuses, violent outburst, abuses her child, parturition, after, puerperal: ***camph.***[54]

Mania; destructive efforts, sudden foxlike, requiring utmost vigilance, followed by laughter and apologies: ***tarent.***[54]

Mischievous: ***agar.*** aloe **ANAC.** arn. ***ars.*** bar-c. bufo ***calc.*** calc-ar.[58] **CANN-I.** cann-s.[137] **CHAM.**[85] ***cupr.*** dam.[85] hep.[109] ***hyos.*** ign.[189] ***lach. merc.*** **NUX-V.** puls.[85] spong.[10] **STANN.**[30] ***stram. tarent.*** tub.[189] ***verat.***

Mischievous; play tricks with their elders: phos.[189]

Moral affections; criminal, disposition to become a; without remorse: ars.[30] bell.[30] hep.[30] lach.[30] merc.[30]

Moral affections; want of moral feeling: abrot.[102] acetan.[102] achy.[149] alco.[36] am-c.[36] ***anac.*** androc.[222] ars.[36] aster.[36] aur.[60] **BELL.**[137] bism. ***bufo***[5] cass.[36] cere-s.[102] cham.[137] chin.[5] choc.[222] clem.[36] ***coca***[98] ***cocain.***[102] cocc. coloc. con. convo-d.[36] croc. cur. germ.[222] hep.[30] hura[36] hyos. ***kali-br.*** kali-c.[60] kali-n.[36] lac-c. ***laur.*** lyc.[30] ***morph.***[102] nat-m.[5] nit-ac.[5] nit-s-d.[60] nux-v.[137] op. ozone[227] ped.[36] ph-ac.[137] pic-ac.[102] ***plat.***[5] psil.[149] raph.[36] sabad. ***sep.***[5] squil.[10] ***stram.***[5] stry-p.[102] ***tarent.***[5] thuj.[60] ***verat.***[5]

Moral affections; want of moral feeling, sadness, with: ***kali-br.***[54]

Necromania: **AGAR.**[185]

Play; dirty trick on others or their teachers, schoolboys p. a: lach.[30] zinc.[30]

Pleasure; waking from a dream of murder, on: thea.

Rage; malicious: ***bell.***[10] cann-s.[10] choc.[222] cocc.[10] cupr.[10] lyc.[10] mosch.[10] petr.[10] sec.[10]

Rage; mischievous: agar. bell.[10] cann-s.[10] cocc.[10] cupr.[10] lyc.[10] mosch.[10] petr.[10] sec.[10]

Religious affections; taciturnity, haughtiness, voluptuousness, cruelty, r. a with: ***plat.***[54]

Slander; disposition to sneak: ars.[30] lach.[30] nat-c.[30]

Slander; disposition to, hypocritical, and: phos.[30] sep.[30]

Temperament; choleric, ardent, disposed to anger, spite or deception, always irritable and impatient: **NUX-V.**[54]

Thoughts; persistent, injury to others, of doing: osm.[54]

Ugly behavior: bry.[137] bufo[107] ***cham.***[111] ***cina***[107] ***nux-v.***[111]

Undignified: alco.[36]

Unfeeling, hard-hearted: alco.[116] **ANAC.** androc.[222] arg.[102] ars.[30] bism.[10] cench.[58] choc.[222] con.[10] croc.[10] hep.[30] hyos.[10] lac-h.[229] ***lach.***[54] lap-mar-c.[194] ***laur.***[10] med.[137] op.[10] ozone[227] squil.[10] ***sulph.***[10] sumb.[36]

Unsympathetic, unscrupulous: am-c.[1] ***anac.***[5] androc.[222] ars.[30] calc.[1] carb-an.[1] carb-v.[1] ***cham.*** chin.[5] con.[1] **DIG.**[91] lac-h.[229] lap-gr-m.[194] lap-mar-c.[194] mag-m.[5] nat-m.[5] nit-ac.[5] op.[5] ozone[227] 0pall.[185] ***plat.*** puls.[30] ***sep.*** staph.[1] sumb.[36]

Voyeurism: bufo[171] hyos.[185] staph.[185]

Weeping; anger, with, violent quarreling, even to extreme malice and rage: ***mosch.***[54]

Wicked disposition: anac.[54] cocc. cub.[36] cur. nux-v.[1] sarr.[36]

Wicked, disposition, mental derangement before amenorrhea, in: ***cocc.***[54]

Witty; indecent, but: ***stram.***[54]

Writing; mean and contemptible things to her friends, all sorts of: ***lac-c.***[54]

ABROT. He, 12 - Exceedingly peevish, feels as if she would like to do something cruel (sadistic, torture); no humanity.

ADAM. Sh, 214 - I am fidgety and angry and very jealous of people. I feel cold and empty and very angry, almost cruel. 20, 1M, 02:XX:XX

AGAR. Al, 3 - Fearless, menacing, mischievous (rude) frenzy; also, frenzy which causes the patient to assail and injure himself, with great exertion of power.

Ha, 23 - Fearless, threatening, destructive frenzy, also such as turns against itself and injures itself, combined with great exertion of strength.

ALUM. Ha, 16 - Anxiety with external heat and restlessness, as if she had done something wicked. (immoral, evil)

ANAC. He, 40 - Uses profane language, swears, thinks himself a demon.

He, 32 - Disposed to malice, seems bent on wickedness.

ANDROC. Sh, 37 - Pushed kids out of bed with no compassion, would usually have felt very guilty doing this. (7)

Sh, 41 - Feels much more self centred — have given up all the permanent favours I do for people — I don't want to do any more. Feel I need more time for me. I must feel guilt but I don't think I do. I feel the nasty side of my character is emerging much more aggressive and domineering. I don't want peoples' good opinion of me as someone who is nice —very unusual. (7)

Sh, 97 - Very strong liking and disliking to people —very intense —ranging from immense sexual attraction to extreme hatred. Spoke with hatred and maliciousness about colleagues. (4)

Sh, 102 - Assertive, impatient, aggressive. Felt resentful and abused. Had no control over her temper. Bellowed and lashed out at everyone. In the evening, furious for no apparent reason. Wanted to kill her husband and children, banged doors and threw things. By bed-time, she felt fine but the intensity of her evil thoughts was very frightening. (7)

Sh, 103 - Had a very caustic conversation with someone she hardly knew. Enjoyed her rudeness and was surprised by it. (7)

Sh, 108 - Incredibly sensitive to noise, can't bear it, hundreds of thoughts pop in and out of my brain, thoughts of 'why are we here?', deep philosophical issues. Everyday things disappear from my mind. Am free from pressing, nagging responsibilities —just a black thunder sits within me, and I feel afraid of what I might do next. my eyes are staring and full of hate —just looking at the children sends them frantic. I have no control over my emotions. Then after 8:00 p.m., deadness resumes and I feel .k., but the end of myself as I usually am. (7)

Sh, 109 - Black, horrible moods which don't last long, but are frightening in their violence. (7)

Sh, 124 - In the street, he felt aggressive and very strong, that his umbrella was a knife, and desired to smash people up. (29)

Sh, 129 - It seemed as though he was a different person, very similar to the way he had been in adolescence, but in a much more powerful manner. These emotions were so intense he wanted to rip his chest apart to let them out. He lost all control over his emotions, which seemed to come from a deep and distant part of himself, a darker side. He desired to continue the proving for the rest of his life. (29)

ARS. Ha, 35 - He sees nothing but rogues in his room, and therefore always creeps under the bed.

He, 104 - Obstinacy, avarice, inclined to malice and satire.

BELL. Al, 34 - He took a piece of bread for a stone, and threw it far away, laughing violently and running about the room.

Ha, 1364 - Unrestrainedly and exuberantly merry, inclined to scold (criticize) without cause, and to insult (affront, offend) in a laughing humor.

He, 18 - When closing eyes, though not asleep, patient sees fierce (wild), wicked looking large animals with horns and bushy (scabrous) heads; room seemed to be full of strange men passing in and out, who would snatch (take hold) at her as they passed, which frightened her very much, she thought the men wanted to take her away from home ; she then saw children sitting on low benches (seat) in rows (line) as in a school-room. (purity)

BUFO. Al, 25 - Defiance (disobedience, challenger), duplicity (hypocrisy), spitefulness.(cruelty)

CALC. He, 70 - Excessive mischievousness, with obstinacy.

CAMPH. Al, 46-... There was no other feeling in my soul than that of my hopeless endless damnation (condemnation). I sank back upon the bed, believing that I was the spirit of evil in a world forsaken of God.

Al, 46-.... As I lay stretched on my couch, as the evil demon, and suffered all the anguish of a condemned and God-forsaken soul, ...I was forever deprived of the Divine protection, and of every consolation and every hope. Nothing remained to me but the conviction of my everlasting damnation...

CHOC. Sh, 328 - Humourless, intolerant -almost cruel. Scalded a child's hand out of anger, and nothing would make him apologise.[35], 30C, XX:XX:XX:

Sh, 329 - Felt anger at life, I wasn't getting anywhere. The world appeared a cruel place to me, and I felt I had no place in the scheme of things.[35], 30C, XX:XX:XX:

COB. Al, 5 - Condemned, mean feeling, as though guilty of some deed (action) of which others knew; as if he could not look one in the face. (shame, dishonored)

COCC. Al, 27 - Very much affected and offended by slight obliquities (immorality) and untruths (falsehood) of others.

He, 25 - Melancholy and sadness, with weeping and constant profound absorption in sorrowful thoughts; great apprehensive anxiety of conscience, and feeling at heart as after committing a wicked deed (act), with desire to escape.

CROC. Al, 11 - Sardonic (sarcastic, satirical) laughter, and attacks of morbid jollity.

CUPR-A. Al, 2 - Attacks of mania; he fancies that he is a military officer; a fancy that he is selling green vegetables; a fancy that he is repairing old chairs...he spits in the faces of the attendants, and laughs heartily at it.

CUPR. Ha, 27 - Fits of insanity, he spits into people's faces, and laughs heartily (soberly) over it.

He, 6 - Craziness (insanity); attacks with savage malice (evil), with proud (arrogant) bearing (posture),...

He, 10 - Mania with biting, beating, and tearing things to pieces; insane foolish gestures of imitation and mimicry; full of insane spiteful (cruelty, brutality) tricks (deceitful, false), ..unhappy, despairing...miserable look...

CUR. Al, 4 - Everything he sees appears foul and nasty. (dirty, dishonest, offensive, injurious, indecent)

Al, 17 - Irascibility, wicked disposition; desires to lie in wait in order to assault others, and even to kill and rob them.

DROS. Ha, 272 - Extremely uneasy, sad disposition, all day he imagined he was being deceived (deluded, defrauded) by spiteful (hateful), envious people.

Ha, 275 - He is sad and dejected about the ills (evil) of life, which people cause one another and himself, respecting which he is anxious and concerned;...(ethical)

Ha, 276 - He is dejected (unhappy) about the malice (rancor, hostility) of others on all hands, and at the same time disheartened (discouraged) and concerned about the future.(disgusted, revolted)

FERR. Ha, 272 - Anxiety at night, as she have done something bad; she could not sleep, tossed about the bed.

GERM. Sh, 6 - Difficult to accept my own feelings, accusing myself for letting them out, especially anger. Felt a rage, had to use all my power to control it. Lost my patience because of something my son did. I got angry with him, but at the same time despised myself for not having patience with him. I did not want to report this, because I feel unveiled - now everybody can see what awful person I am. I go completely mad of all my thoughts; can't bear it anymore. Inside me everything is chaos. Feel no power. 18, 30C, 18:XX:XX

Sh, 5 - Everything was heavy and felt impossible without meaning. Terrible anger. Bad conscience and crying afterwards. Could not do what I had planned to do, because I felt so terrible and everything was chaos. Was crying, but couldn't get it out - no release in it. 18, 30C, 176:XX:XX

Sh, 111 - If I were me, nobody would like me -so I try to be what I think others expect me to be. I don't think I can be loved with all the parts of me which are ugly and bad. Lonely feelings. Longing for love and understanding. Feel I am so unfriendly to myself. 18, 30C, 04:00:00

Sh, 137 - Entertain myself with mischievous reflections and realize that these are more thoughts of an outsider. 08, 12C, 02:14:10

HALI-L. Sh, 570 - Don't want to do anything but stay underground—"kick a can" around town. Feel angry about people who may be maligning me. 16, 10C, 14:XX:XX

Sh, 588 - I was in a gallows humor, cruel but funny. My friends had never seen that side of me before. Like I was on speed. I had no control. They asked me not to cut up vegetables, not to use a knife. I was waving the knife around. I threw the knife at a potato. 02, 30C, XX:XX:XX

Sh.589 - I wanted to really hurt somebody or something, no respect for the person, anyway that I could. There was another part of me that couldn't believe I was doing that. It was like a horror movie. I got to that place of no boundaries or responsibility to life. It didn't matter what I did. Indifferent. Like ice, no feeling. Just like if I killed someone there would be no regrets. Just the thought: This is what I have to do now. Desire to kill. It did not matter. Just do it. You've got to. I had no fear. I could do anything, whatever I was asked to do, I could do it then. I was a strong person. The me was the only thing that kept me from doing it. That's where I got scared. The last five days of the proving were in a black hole. I refused to write anything down. A god-like place or a devil-like place. Why do I have these things? Human things. 02, 30C, XX:XX:XX

Sh, 592 - Had a peculiar experience during the day. While playing with one of my dogs, I started to wonder what it would be like to crush her. Suddenly I thought how sensual it would be to crush its little head and rip its flesh. There was something very sensual about the idea of crushing flesh and bones of a soft creature that would not be able to fight me off. It was not a strong, powerful impulse, but there was something compelling about the idea. 04, 30C, 02:XX:XX

Sh, 594 - Yesterday and today, when I was playing with my puppy I felt like hurting her. Today while playing, the feeling was how much stronger I was than her and I could really hurt her. It's a strange feeling. I really love my puppy. This reminds me of when I was 20 years old and there was a child sitting on the steps. I felt I could crush her. I realized how strong I am. I'm not usually a psychopath. It's a feeling of violence. 04, 30C, 04:XX:XX

Sh, 607 - An urge to destroy my relationship, scream at people. It felt very destructive. 13, 30C, 04:06:30

Sh, 644 - The "fry an egg and eat it," repetitive, meaningless motion, reminds me of an extermination camp, of a killing machine; was about not caring; it's from the split or chasm. Not caring about anything, is part of what happens with the split. That's what evil is, that's really what it's about. 06, 6C, 01:00:XX

Sh, 648 - Down side, dark side, feels like the gates between the unconscious and conscious are open. Hurricane-like feeling of unconscious energy. Like the gates of hell are open. No barrier. Extreme amount of power. Darkness. Internal pressure. Dogs guard the gates of Hades. A lot of internal pressure-type feeling all day. 13, 30C, 10:XX:XX

Sh, 936 - I had a down morning, but had a good day out with a friend and her two sons, and many birds caged and uncaged at the Botanical Gardens. A very high and low day before they arrived. Tried not to see them, but was pleased when they came. Before they came, was feeling I must be a very bad person—different. 20, 30C, 15:XX:XX

HEP. Ha, 289 - The slightest thing put him into a violent passion, he could have murdered any one without hesitation.

He, 9 - Malicious (vindictive, malevolent) mood; feels as if he could murder someone whith pleasure.

He, 22 - Temper obstinate and cross, a ferocious spleen (irascible) which would lead to cold blooded murder even among those habitually gay and benevolent.

HURA. Al, 8 - He reproaches himself for all his bad actions, even the merest trifles.

HYDR. Al, 16 - Spiteful (cruel), angry disposition, with desire to snub (scorn) any one who differed in anything with me; lasting all day.

HYDROG. Sh, 220 - Laughter wicked and voice seemed low. 24, 30C, 02:XX:XX

Sh, 250 - I think I'm dangerous to people and they can't cope with me. 16, 30C, XX:XX:XX

HYOS. He, 46 - Sings amorous and obscene songs.

He, 69 - Lascivious mania, uncovers body, especially sexual parts; sings amorous songs.

HYPER. Al,S-3 - For a week past, impure ideas have very seldom presented themselves by day; the mind has been reposing on higher thoughts.

IOD. He, 15 - At night, especially when thinking of real or imaginary wrongs ...dares (try) to go home for fear of doing some dreadful (bad, wicked) deed (action); on one occasion was seized with an almost irresistible impulse to murder a woman who was acting as a guide (direct, conduct) for him, he having lost his way (direction);...must be constantly in action, in some laborious occupation. (lost; direction, correction, control)

KALI-BR. He, 15 - Frightful imaginings at night (in pregnant women during latter months), they are under impression that they have committed, or about to commit, some great crime and cruelty (brutality), such murdering their children or husbands.

He, 31-...religious delusions and feeling of moral deficiency; ...profound indifference and almost disgust for life.

He, 33 - Great despondency, with insanity, a feeling of moral deficiency, or a religious delusion, from anemia.

KALI-N. Al, 19 - Perverse hypochondriac mood; discontented with himself and the world, peevish irritable, ...

LAC-C. Al,N -8 - Is impressed with the idea that all she says is a lie; it seems to be very difficult to speak the truth (liar, dissimulator), but continually distrusts things (suspicious); when reading anything she rapidly changes the meaning, omitting or adding things. (mischievous)

Al,N-43 - Intense ugliness (repulsiveness, offensiveness) and hatefulness (odiousness, repellently); writes to her best friends all sorts of mean(vulgar) and contemptible things.

He, 11 - Imagines to be dirty. (obscene, vulgar, dishonorable)

He, 37 - Intense ugliness (repulsiveness, hideousness) and hatefulness (offensiveness); writes to her best friends all sorts of mean and contemptible things. (disdainful)

LACH. He, 52 - Malice; thinks only of mischief. (evil, harm, hurt)

LIL-T. Al, 10 - Profound mental depression; to the prover "the heavens seemed brass and the earth iron;" an apprehension of moral obliquity weighed grievously upon her, for about ten days after the sexual excitement,...

Al, 25 - While attending a lecture (speech), desire to hit the lecturer, and in the evening desirous of swearing and damning the fire and things generally, and to think and speak obscene things; disposed to strike and hit persons; as these feelings came, the uterine pains passed away.

LYC. He, 38 - Parsimonious (economical), greedy (avaricious), malicious (malevolent) and pusillanimous.(cowardice)

LYSS. Al, 15 - He cannot prevent ideas of something awful (terrible) about to happen, or as if he would do something awful (bad).

Al, 32 - Thought came into his mind to attack others in a mean way; to cut others with a knife he holds; to throw water he has in a tumbler into another's face.

NAT-M. Ha, 28 - Anxiety, as if she had done something wicked (immoral), with heat and night-sweat.

NEON. Sh, 176 - Got up late in a horrible mood and reproached my partner again. I hurt him but I didn't care. I felt indifferent, malicious and vindictive, full of hate. 02, 6C, 05:22:10

NUX-V. He, 8 - Suits very particular, careful,(prudent, meticulous) zealous (conscientious) persons, inclined to get angry or excited, or a spiteful (cruel), malicious disposition.

OSM. Al, 5 - Thoughts of accidents having happened to others, by a blow, a fall, or being dashed (crushed, hit, knock) to pieces; gradually these thoughts grow upon him, as if he were to do the same injuries to others.

PHOS. Al, 12-...; wherever he turned his eyes he saw faces; they swarmed (crowded, surrounded) by him in long panoramic succession; they leered (look lecherous) at him over the footboard of the bed; they squinted (look) at him though the windows, or came trooping (crowd) in when the doors were left ajar (open) (invade);..he fancied he was some one else, ...

He, 29 - Crazy deliria in a young woman who was strictly moral and unhappy in her love; accused herself of the most obscene (immoral, wicked) actions, of which she never was guilty; ....

PLAT. He, 16 - Very peevish and easily excited; he could have beaten any one without provocation.

He, 40 - Disturbed state of mind; religious, with taciturnity, haughtiness, voluptuousness (sensual) and cruelty.

PULS. He, 47-...; pangs (pain, anxiety) of conscience about religion and female sex; violent palpitation in the presence of women; abhors (detests, aversion) and hates the sex; must go out of their way for fear of injuring them; looks upon them as evil beings and is afraid (fear; temptation, seduction); considers their presence injurious (insulted, offended) to his soul; ... (sexual loathing)

RAPH. Al, 1 - Feeling of aversion towards all women; she is provoked by seeing women going and coming about her; their approach threw her into a fury; the mere contact with a woman's dress caused intolerable distress;...She is attracted to all men without distinction (nymphomania) ; when she gives her hand to a man, she feels great agitation,...When left alone for a hour in the evening, she gave herself a very deep wound in the lips with a penknife, in hopes to put an end to this condition (hurt, punishes). Moral feeling was completely extinct, the physical nature alone ruled and threw her into a frightful state (wild). From morning to noon she would not have been able to resist the advances even of a man for whom she had not the least friendly feeling; from noon to 6 p.m. she could not have held out against any man whatsoever; from 8 to 11 the demands of sense were so importunate as to silence the voice of shame and reason; ... and would have thrown herself into the arms of the first man she met...she was still unable to control her impulses;...

SAPIN. Al, 5 - Quite ill-natured and inclined to view matters in a disagreeable light; did not seem able to feel settled (decided) enough to know what to do; the crossness became so intense, that I felt myself getting very unreasonable, especially as to food, which seemed all wrong in some way;...

STICT. Al, 1 - She got very lively (active), told her father she felt as if she would like to strike out, only for fun; she would like it just for fun of it. After awhile she lay down on the lounge, and began, to use a common expression, to kick up her heels; her mother reproaching, said, " Bella, do behave, that is not ladylike"; when child responded: " Ma, I cannot help it; I feel exactly as if I want to fly away"...

STRAM. He, 107-...heard continually, on r. side of occiput, a loud voice, scolding, vituperating and accusing him of ungodliness (impious, sinful, irreligious, godless, profane); ....prayed expecting, with great anxiety, the flash of lightning which was to kill him;...(redemption, regeneration, salvation)

He, 178 - Pangs of conscience; thinks he is not honest. (dishonest)

He, 94-...fear of malicious animals, black dogs; ...

He, 119 - His thoughts ran upon obscene things, frequently put his hands to erect penis; sought to bite or to catch flies.

TARENT. He, 15 - Suddenly sprang (escape) away from her attendants and swept (clean) ornaments from mantelpiece (an ornamental facing around fireplace); said she was sorry, but could not help it; very mischievous and destructive, ...

VERAT. He, 47 - Anxiety as after committing an evil (immoral) deed (act)...

He, 5 - Never speaks the truth; does not know herself what she is saying.

He, 22 - Nymphomania, with violence and destructiveness; had been disappointed in love; melancholia; ...great desire for sexual intercourse; void (empty) of shame; obscenity; ....

ZINC. He, 46-...; believed herself to be called before court (judged) on account of her wicked (immoral) actions; ....;believe the devil is after her;...(persecution)

WIFE

Abusive; husband insults wife, children, and: lyss.[36]

Aversion; wife, to his: ars.[137] ***fl-ac.***[122] nat-s.[137] plat.[137] staph.[137]

Delusions; jealousy, lovers concealed behind stove wife has: ***stram.***[54]

Dreams; cutting, woman, of cutting a woman up for salting: calc-f.

➤ dead, people, of, wife: aran-ix.[119]

➤ old gentleman ran away from wife, suspected of having married another: sep.[36]

Estranged; wife, from his: ars. nat-c.[58] plat. staph.

Forsaken; feeling, beloved by his parents, wife, friends, feels of not being: ***ars.***[30] calc.[30] lyc.[30] ***mag-c.***[122] sep.[30] sil.[30] sulph.[30]

Jealousy; accuses wife of being faithless: ***stram.***[54]

Jealousy; strikes his wife: lach.[30] nux-v.[30]

Kill; threatens to k, wife and children: ***hep.***[54]

HEP. He, 8-...threatened to murder wife and children, attempted to set house on fire, and was with difficulty controlled; ... (pyromaniac) 0Scabies.

KALI-BR. Al, 3 - Decidedly insane; had

delusions that lewd women had got into his mother's house; that he was pursued by the police; that his wife was threatened by members of the family; that he had thousands of dollars in gold sewed up in his clothing; (rich, wealth)

LYSS. Al, 28 - Very cross, so much that my children expressed great surprise; took offense at the merest trifles; scolded (censorious) my wife and children; ....

Al,N-88 - Very cross, so much... he took offense at veriest trifles, scolding his wife and children, felt wretched, ...

He, 88 - Very cross, so much so that his children expressed great surprise; he took offense at veriest trifles, scolded his wife and children, felt wretched, ...

MED. He, 24 - Tendency to suicide, gets up in night and takes his pistol (gun), but his wife prevents him.

PLAT. Ha, 40 - Indifference, he felt unconcerned (careless, insensible) as to whether his absent wife would die or not.

STRAM. He, 145 - Wife complains of husband neglecting her; man accuses his wife of being faithless.

WILD

Animal consciousness: choc.[222] germ.[222]

Anxiety; control over senses is lost, with feeling that: acon.[210] gels.[210] manc.[210] ***merc.***[54] tarent.[210]

Anxiety; wild: sec.[54]

Cheerfulness; wildly: alum-p.[58] ant-t.[54]

Concentration difficult; crazy feeling in the top of head, wild feeling in head with confusion of ideas: lil-t.

Dancing; desire for; wild: androc.[222] ***bell.*** camph. tarent.

Delirium; wild: atro.[116] **BELL.** ***bry.***[116] ***calen.***[54] camph. canth. chlol. colch. cupr. gall-ac.[36] ***gels.***[54] hydr-ac. ***hyos. kali-br.***[54] lach. nat-sal.[36] oena.[144] ***op.***[122] **PLB. STRAM.** ***valer.***[54] vario.[54] ***verat.***

Delirium; wild, stab and bite, attempts to: **STRAM.**[54]

Delusions; alone, wilderness, being a. in a: stram.

- animals, fierce, with horns and bushy heads: ***bell.***[54]
- wild, he will go: lob.[139]
- wilderness, being in a: stram.[10]

Dreams; animals, boars, wild: merc.[36]

➤ animals, cats, wild: ozone[227]

➤ animals, horses, fearing to be bitten by a ferocious black: phos.[36]

➤ animals, horses, wild: lap-mar-c.[194]

➤ animals, pursued by, wild: allox.[119] alum. cench.[58] eupi. hipp.[36] ind. led.[36] nux-v. sil. ***sulph.*** tet.[36] verat.

➤ animals, wild: hyos.[10] lyc.[36] nux-v. sil. sulph. tarent.[36]

➤ desert, of: sil.[10]

➤ eating, live animals: hydrog.[222]

➤ lion, that he was a: phys.

➤ wild: aloe apis cann-i. dor. glon. kalm. op. ozone[227] pip-m.[36] tab.

Fancies; wild: cimic.[8] con.[36] phos.[58] rhus-v.[85] stram.[8]

Fear; animals, wild, in mania: ***stram.***[54]

✦ death, excitement, with wild, begs to know if he is to die and before answer drops into heavy sleep: vario.[172]

Foolish; behavior, hilarity, with riotous, and subsequent angry savageness, or tearful sorrow: op.[54]

Growling like a dog: alum. ***bell.*** hell. hyos.[162] lyss. mag-m. phos.[122]

Irrational: arg-n.[58] bell.[36] lil-t.[58] ***nux-v.***[8] op.[36] plb.[36] stram.[1]

Irrational; alternating with rationality: cann-i.[58]

Lasciviousness; animal, as if she were completely, mental power dormant: lach.[54]

Laughing; wildly: atro.[36] calc. cann-i.[25]

Malicious; savage: cupr.[54]

Mania; wild: kali-br.[54] ph-ac.[10]

Self-control; loss, of: anac.[137] androc.[222] anh.[119] apis[60] arg.[137] arg-n.[137] caust.[58] germ.[222] lac-h.[229] ***lach.***[54] lap-mar-c.[194] lyc.[109] med.[189] nat-m.[60] olnd.[137] ozone[227] sanic.[127] sil.[54] staph.[137] sulph.[8] tarent.[111]

Shrieking; wild, with disposition to bite and tear: ***verat.***[54]

Talk; wild: ars.[54] atro.[36] bell.[1] camph.[36] canth.[58] lyc.[36] plb.[36] spig-m.[36] stram.[8] ***verat-v.***[54]

Thoughts; wild: phos.[58] stram.[54]

Wild feeling in head: ambr.[111] bapt. ***cimic.***[111] lil-t. ***med.***

Wildness: acon. acon-l.[36] ant-t. apoc.[102] arag.[102] aur.[58] bapt. bell. calc-p. camph. canth. chin-ar.[58] chlf.[36] chlol.[36] croc. cupr. fagu.[36] hyos. lil-t.[5] ***lob.***[54] lyss.[54] m-aust.[10] med. mosch. nat-s.[58] op. petr. ph-ac. phos. ***stram.*** tab.[5] tarent.[36] vario.[54] ***verat.***

Wildness; bad news, from: calc-p.
Wildness; bright light, strong odors or touch, from: ***colch.***
Wildness; misdeeds of others, from: ***colch.***[36]
Wildness; sounds, on hearing any, as striking of clock, etc., dances about, must be held: verat.[54]
Wildness; vexation, from: ph-ac.

ADAM. Sh, 79 - Hurriedwild. Husband says I look wild, like a jungle child moving rapidly, jerky movements in different directions. Very excitable as if about to lose control. 10, 6C, 19:XX:XX

Sh, 158 - I feel detached and not sexual. I could bite my partner as a signal I loved her, not in a loving or hungry way. My partner said, "He is looking at me like a piece of steak, he wants to eat me. He looks like a cave man. He wants to nibble me." 7, 6C, 03:22:30

ANT-T. He, 41 - Gaiety, wild mirthfulness, with subsequent ill humor and anxiety for future.

ARS. Al-S, 2879 - Became very nervous, agitated, and delirious, suspecting people were about the house plotting (conspiracy, betrayed) against his life, jumps out of the bed suddenly and reaches after imaginary objects, and stares wildly and suspiciously around him,...

ATRO. Al, 3-...the mind would become filled with strange and fanciful ideas ...fits of wild, uncontrollable laughter...I fancied myself afflicted with epilepsy, and was constantly fearful lest others should discover my unfortunate condition; ...

BAPT. He, 4 - Cannot confine (control) his mind; a sort of wild, wandering feeling.

BELL. He, 18 - When closing eyes, though not asleep, patient sees fierce (wild), wicked looking large animals with horns and bushy (scabrous) heads; room seemed to be full of strange men passing in and out, who would snatch (take hold) at her as they passed, which frightened her very much, she thought the men wanted to take her away from home ; she then saw children sitting on low benches (seat) in rows (line) as in a school-room. (purity)

He, 70 - Instead of eating, bit wooden spoon in two, gnawed plate, and growled and barked like a dog.

He, 62 - Loud laughter, wild abandon, singing, whistling, lascivious conversation.

CAMPH. Al, 19 - Stripped naked, he danced wildly about, and attempted to jump out of the window.

CHOC. Sh, 228 - Thoughts about the 'veneer of civilisation' that inhibits how we really feel and keeps us from displaying what we're like beneath the surface. It seems a legitimate layer, but so is the layer beneath it, and I feel amused and happy to meet it. This feeling continued for a few days, a very graphic picture of a veneer - a layer of learned social behaviour lifting and detaching from a basis that is thick, dark, solid, instinctual animal.15, 30C, 00:00:30

Sh, 301 - Desire to bite my husband in a playful way. I bit him —I wanted to really sink my teeth in, but willed myself not to. It was an animal need in me.[15], 30C, 00:05:30

Sh, 302 - Tonight my husband committed a large annoyance. I felt rage rise up in me —he jumped back and cowered! I wanted to beat some sensibility into him, stopping short of actually wanting to kill him, I felt: 'its not fair', 'how inconsiderate and thoughtless to an extreme degree'. However, my will intervened before I made a scene. Its as if I'm more aware of my 'shadow side' and really feeling it, but precisely because I'm more aware of it, I can step in with my will and curb my behaviour if it looks as if I'm likely to hurt someone else.[15], 30C, 03:XX:XX

CROT-C. Al, 3-... hears a strange voice to her left, and behind her; she follows it, throws herself against closed doors, and scratches them with her nails...She cries out: " He is in the den, but the lions will not eat him"

CUPR. He, 6 - Craziness (insanity); attacks with savage malice (evil), with proud (arrogant) bearing (posture),...

He, 8 - Mania characterized by a wild look and fear; tries to escape.

GERM. Sh, 4 - Desperately angry. So intense that I could barely control it. I made noises like an animal, pushed my arms up and down - instead of hitting my children, which helped. Want to just leave the house and the kids. Felt completely mad, afraid of what the neighbors heard and thought. Very bad conscience afterwards, but no relief - didn't get the anger out. There are a lot of feelings inside that don't come out. 18, 30C, 02:09:00

Sh, 101 - I'm desperate. I want to die. Feel the power to kill. Feel like a wild animal locked in. It's strong, so intense. I hate so strong-feel a terrible disgust and I'm afraid of what I'm able to do. It's completely impossible to be in it and impossible to get out of it. 18, 30C, 190:XX:XX

HALI-L. Sh, 202 - There is a holding back of impulses. Usually impulsive, now unsure whether impulses will serve me. Feeling as if I am a wild horse, ready to gallop full force, and being held back. 02, 30C, 11:XX:XX

Sh, 428 - Realizing we haven't had any fun as a family in forever. Haven't had any fun myself either. Like a caged animal, snarling. I'm in a pressure cooker. Can't even imagine what would get me out of this mood, what actually would be fun. Don't want to do anything, or talk to anyone. Like a porcupine or sea urchin. "Don't tread on me." 09, 6C, 30:XX:XX

Sh, 597 - Reading about the Ring Cycle and how Siegfried tasted the blood of the slain dragon.[16], 10C, 22:XX:XX

Sh, 663 - In a total frenzy, like steaming horses that had escaped, running down the road. Very hard to keep any control, to be patient in traffic, or the grocery store. Couldn't handle it any longer. Put lip balm with camphor on, every ten minutes, and would feel calm momentarily. Finally got some tiger balm at a friend's house and used it two times. I was instantly calmer. Came back to being me. 02, 30C, 11:XX:XX

LACH. He, 33-...want of self control; lascivious; felt as if she was clear (pure) animal right through, whilst of all mental power was dormant; sensation as if hands of stronger power, as if charmed (enchanted), and as if could not break the spell (charm). (possessed, wildness)

LIL-T. Al, 16 - Worse on going to bed; can't go to sleep; wild (tumultuous, uncontrollable) feeling in the head as though I should go crazy (insane) and no one would take care of me (forsaken, helpless); thoughts of suicide; how much opium would put me to sleep forever, and who would find my body, and who would care; ... (friendless, abandoned, deserted)

He, 6 - Crazy feeling on top of head; wild feeling in head, with confusion of ideas.

MED. Al-N, 38-...;desire for rest and dread (fear) of change;...wild crazy feeling in brain...

Al,N-44 - The impatience, excitement, wild feelings; the unreal, dazed condition; the gloom (sadness) and fear in the dark;... are marked evidence of functional derangement of the nervous system.

Al,N-23 - Wild desperate feeling, as of incipient insanity.

He, 22 - Wild and desperate feeling, as of incipient insanity.

RAPH. Al, 1 - Feeling of aversion towards all women; she is provoked by seeing women going and coming about her; their approach threw her into a fury; the mere contact with a woman's dress caused intolerable distress;...She is attracted to all men without distinction (nymphomania) ; when she gives her hand to a man, she feels great agitation,...When left alone for a hour in the evening, she gave herself a very deep wound in the lips with a penknife, in hopes to put an end to this condition (hurt, punishes). Moral feeling was completely extinct, the physical nature alone ruled and threw her into a frightful state (wild). From morning to noon she would not have been able to resist the advances even of a man for whom she had not the least friendly feeling; from noon to 6 p.m. she could not have held out against any man whatsoever; from 8 to 11 the demands of sense were so importunate as to silence the voice of shame and reason; ... and would have thrown herself into the arms of the first man she met...she was still unable to control her impulses;...

STRAM. He, 66 - Woke suddenly in night and said there were snakes under and about her; looked wild, screamed and pointed to them.

He, 14-...thoughts of dying;...fear of wild animals and black dogs.

SULPH. Al, 3780 - At night, very vivid anxious dreams, as if was pursued by wild beasts.

TARENT. He, 12 - Sudden foxlike destruc-

tive efforts, requiring utmost vigilance to prevent damage;...
VAC. He, 5 - Fear of death; wild excitement and begging (implore) to know if he was to die,...

WILL

Casting off of people against her will: **PLAT.**[36]
Confusion of mind; will, strong effort of, amel.: glon.
Contemptuous; paroxysms against her will, in: ***plat.***
Delusions; die, about to, will, thinks there is but little time to make his: ***petr.***[54]
- will power, loss of: carb-v.[139] chin-s.[10] nit-ac.[139] pop.[139]
- wills, possessed of two: anac.[1] lach.[102]

Indifference; desires, has no, no action of the will: hell. ***verat.***[54]
Initiative, lack of: anh.[119] aur.[127] calc.[127] calc-f.[149] hydro-c.[149] ign.[127] iod.[30] lach.[30] lyc.[30] onop.[149] rhus-t.[30] saroth.[119] sil.[155] sulph.[30] thala.[149]
Suppression; will, by, in order to proper: sil.[162]
Thoughts; persistent, separated, will, thoughts separated from: anh.[119]
Undertakes; lacks will power to undertake anything: androc.[222] phos. ***pic-ac.***
Will; astonished of finding themselves not masters of their own acts: cann-i.[36]
Will; loss of: am-c.[30] am-m.[30] ***anh.***[119] bar-c.[30] ***bar-s.***[58] ***calc.***[10] calc-acet.[36] calc-sil.[58] camph.[36] chin-s.[10] clem.[36] coca[54] ***con.***[54] cortico.[149] croc.[10] des-ac.[149] foll.[1201] grat.[58] ***hell.***[54] hypoth.[149] lyc.[30] ***merc.***[36] naja[141] nat-br.[36] nat-c.[10] ***nat-m.***[54] nid.[149] op.[10] petr.[10] phos.[54] ***pic-ac.***[54] ***ptel.***[54] sil.[30] sulph.[30] thuj-l.[149]
Will; loss of, sadness, from: ***arg-n.***[54]
Will; muscles refuse to obey the w. when attention is turned away: ***hell.*** lil-t.[122]
Will; none of his own, has: bar-c.[162]
Will; weakness of: abrot.[102] acetan.[102] act-sp.[111] alum.[5] alum-sil.[58] am-c.[30] am-m.[30] ambr.[116] ***anac.***[5] ***anh.***[119] ant-c.[5] ***ars.***[5] asaf.[5] ***bar-acet.***[116] **BAR-C.**[5] bism.[116] bry.[5] buth-aust.[144] calc.[5] calc-acet.[116] cand-a.[239] cann-s.[116] caust.[30] cere-s.[102] chin.[5] cimic.[58] ***coca***[98] ***cocain.***[102] coff.[5] coloc.[5] ***con.***[30] ***cori-r.***[5] ***croc.***[5] dulc.[5] gels.[188] graph.[30] grat.[58] ***haem.***[116] ign.[5] ip.[5] irid.[5] kali-br.[102] kali-c.[5] kali-sil.[58] ***lach.***[10] laur.[5] lyc.[5] merc.[30] mez.[5] ***morph.***[102] nat-c.[5] nat-m.[5] nux-v.[116] op.[5] ***petr.***[5] pic-ac.[5] ***puls.***[5] rheum[5] sil.[30] staph.[116] stry-p.[102] sulph.[5] ***tarent.***[102]

ALOE. Al, 23 - Immediately, strong exhibition of will (disposition); he quarrels with every one who contradicts him; it seems as if he would permit himself to be torn (ruined) in pieces, sooner than give up his will. (lack; will, integration, union)
ALUM. Al, 4 - The boy weeps constantly against his will, for half a hour.
ANAC. He, 67 - Contradiction between reason and will.
APIS. Al, 23 - It seems to her as if she did not know what to do, as if she had no volition (desire) of her own, her head feels stupid.
ARG-N. He, 56 - Was utterly (complete) bereft(deprived) of all power of will.
CALC. He, NERVES, Sensation of power with lack (loss, want) of will (command, resolution, intention), force.
CON. He, 33 - Timid, cannot be persuaded to work ; want of proper will. (lack of: resolution) (vagabond)
DROS. Ha, 284 - Obstinate prosecution of resolutions he had formed.
LYSS. Al, 39 - A strange oppression and indifference, as if he was unable to do anything if he forces himself; there is no power of mind.
Al,N-7 - Thoughts of something terrible going to happen come into his mind against his will; feels impelled to do reckless (impulsive) things, such as throwing child, which he carries in his arms, through the window, and the like.
Al,N-64 - Disinclination to change position of head; two distinct trains of thought existing at one time in her mind, the idea that she was unable to move her head (when lying down) with the positive conviction that she has only to make up her mind that she will do it to achieve it.
He, 64 - Disinclination to change position of head; two distinct trains of thought existing at one time in her mind, the idea that she is unable to move her head (when lying down) with the positive conviction that she has only to make up her mind that she will do it to achieve it.

MERC. He, 3 - Loss of will (command, intentions, resolutions,) power.(vigor)
NAT-C. Al, 53 - Sensation of loss of will power, in the morning on waking.
NIT-AC. He, 7 - Feels as though he had partly lost his will-power.
NUX-V. Ha, 1254 - She cannot get over the smallest evil.
PETR. He, 11 - Melancholy mood, imagines but little time is left him to make his will.
PHOS. Ha, 78 - She has to laugh against her will, while she is sad.
PIC-AC. Al, 6 - Great indifference; lack of will power to undertake anything.
RHUS-T. Ha, 974 - He can restrain the rush of ideas at his will, follow out uninterruptedly any train of thought he chooses, without being troubled with other thoughts.

WORK

Activity; business, in: bor.[36] brom.[36] manc.[36]
Activity; creative: choc.[222] coff.[36] germ.[222]
Activity; work, at: benz-ac.[36]
Ailments from; business, cares: ambr.[137] calc.[58] caust.[137] kali-br.[85] nux-v.[36] ph-ac.[58] puls.[8] rhus-t.[1] sep.[8] sulph.[36]
Ailments from; business, failure: ***ambr.***[30] aur.[187] calc.[58] ***cimic.***[8] coloc.[30] ***hyos.***[8] ign.[8] kali-br.[56] nat-m.[30] nux-v.[30] ph-ac.[30] puls.[30] rhus-t.[30] sep.[30] sulph.[30] verat.[30]
Ailments from; busy, after being: acon.[30] arn.[30] bry.[30] rhus-t.[30] sulph.[30]
Ailments from; position, job, loss of: ***ign.***[30] ***nux-v.***[8] pers.[149] ***plat.***[30] staph.[30]
Ailments from; work, mental: agar.[58] ***alum-p.***[122] alum-sil.[58] ambr.[116] ***anac.***[54] ***arg-n.***[102] arn.[122] ars.[116] ***ars-i.***[85] ars-met.[85] aven.[116] bar-acet.[116] bell.[30] calc.[85] ***calc-p.***[85] calc-sil.[58] caps.[85] chin.[116] coca[83] cocc.[85] con.[116] **CUPR.**[54] cupr-acet.[85] cypr.[25] ***epig.***[116] epip.[85] fl-ac.[58] ***gels.***[102] graph.[1] ign.[58] iod.[58] iris[112] kali-br.[116] ***kali-c.***[116] **KALI-I.** **KALI-P.**[122] ***lach.***[116] lyc. mag-p.[85] med.[116] **NAT-C.**[122] nat-m. nat-p.[58] nux-m.[116] **NUX-V.**[122] ***ph-ac.***[122] phos. ***pic-ac.***[122] pip-m.[116] psor.[85] pyrog.[5] rhus-t.[116] sabad.[85] scut.[85] sel.[116] sep.[30] ***sil.***[5] **STAPH.**[30] **TUB.**[122] vinc.[85]
Ailments from; work, mental, manual, fine work: graph. iod.
Ailments from; work, mental, prolonged: agar.[58]
Ailments from; work, mental, writing: asaf.[54] laur.[5] med.[54] nux-m.[5] rhus-t.[5] sil.[1] stann.[149]
Ailments from; work, mental, writing, reading, and: sil.[1]
Anger; business, about: ip.[36]
Anger; work: nat-m.[36]
Anger; work, aversion: bov.[10] m-aust.[10]
Anger; work, cannot: calc-p.[54]
Anxiety; business, about: acet-ac.[102] anac. arn.[10] bac.[62] bar-c.[5] bry.[5] calc.[5] caust.[10] chel.[10] cimic.[172] dros.[10] ***graph.***[54] kali-m.[192] kali-p.[137] lac-h.[229] ***lil-t.***[54] mang.[10] nat-c.[10] nat-m.[10] **NUX-V.**[5] op.[10] ph-ac.[10] podo.[137] ***psor.***[122] puls. rhus-t.[10] sep.[10] spig.[10] stann.[10] sulph.[5] thuj.[10]
Anxiety; business, lawsuit, as if engaged in a: ***nit-ac.***[60]
Anxiety; nursing, after: ***cham.***[54] cocc.[58]
Anxiety; work, inclination to work, with: calc.[54]
Anxiety; work, manual, during: aloe anac. ***graph.*** iod.
Anxiety; work, preventing work: aloe[60] mosch.[36]
Business; averse to: acon-l.[122] agar. aloe[130] am-c. anac. androc.[222] arg-n.[137] arn.[5] ars. ars-h. asar.[54] aur-m. bapt.[137] ***brom.*** calc.[58] carb-v.[137] chel.[137] ***chin.***[137] chin-s. cimic. ***con.*** cop. cycl.[137] fl-ac. graph. ham.[137] hipp. kali-ar. kali-bi. kali-br. kali-c. kali-i. kali-s. lac-ac. ***lach.*** laur. lil-t. lyc.[1] mag-s. nat-ar.[58] nat-c.[30] **NAT-M.**[137] nux-v.[36] opun-a.[36] ***ph-ac.***[122] ***phos.***[137] ***phyt.*** psor.[137] ***puls.*** rhod.[58] rhus-t.[30] **SEP.** stann.[58] ***stram.***[5] ***sulph.***[58] syph.[58] ther.[54]
Business; desire for: ars.[36] ***carb-v.***[54] cere-b.[36] con.[36] fel.[36] lach.[36] tarent.[36]
Business; incapacity for: agn. am-c.[30] ars.[30] caust.[58] chin-s.[36] ferr.[30] kali-bi. lyc.[30] mag-c.[30] mit.[36] nux-v.[30] sel.[58] sil.[30] sul-i. tab.[36]
Business; neglects his: opun-a.[36] ptel.[144] ***sulph.***[36]
Business; talk of: ars. bell. **BRY.** canth. cimic. dor. ***hyos. med.***[184] mygal. op. phos. plb. stram. sulph.
Business; talk of, delirium, during: **BRY.**[54] canth.[116] dor.[36] **HYOS.**[54] op.[36] phos.[116] ***rhus-t.***[116]
Business; talk of, exploits, their: agar.[36]
Busy; fruitlessly: absin.[102] adax.[96] ***apis***[5] ***arg-n.***[102] ars.[102] bor.[5] calc.[5] canth.[102] ***kali-bi.***[54] kali-br.[137] lil-t.[122] stann. sulph.[102] tarent.[102] ther.[111] verat.[162]

Cares; full of, domestic affairs, about: bar-c. ***puls. sep.***
Cheerfulness; alternating with, aversion to work: spong.
Cheerfulness; work, during manual: ang.[54]
Deeds; he could do great, as if: cocain.[162] hell.
Delirium; fatigue, study, over-exertion, from: ***lach.***[54]
Delirium; loquacious, business of: ars.[36] bell.[111] **BRY.**[54] ***canth.***[111] dor.[54] **HYOS.**[54] op.[36] ***phos.***[111] **RHUS-T.**[111] stram.[36]
Delirium; mild, roaring over fields or hard at work, he thinks he is: ***rhus-t.***[54]
Delirium; night, business of the day, of: bry.[54]
Delirium; study, from excessive: hyos.[10] ***lach.***[54] nux-v.[10]
Delirium; work, of his: bell.[5] **BRY.**[5] ***canth.***[5] ***phos.***[5] **RHUS-T.**[5]
Delusions; business, accomplished, can not be: med.[139]
- business, doing, is: bell. ***bry.*** canth. cupr. op.[102] ***phos.*** rhus-t. verat.
- business, ordinary, they are pursuing: ars. atro. bell. plb. stram.
- business, unfit for, that he is: ***croc.***
- chairs, he is repairing old: cupr. cupr-acet.[36]
- machine, he is working a: plb.
- sick, he is, work, and for this reason will not: calc.[30] caust.[30] nux-v.[30] sep.[30]
- unfit for, work: cupr.[193] meph.[54]
- wheelwright, he is a, and starts to bore holes: stram.[54]
- wood, carries home, to manufacture brandy: stram.[54]
- work, accomplish the, he cannot: bry.[36]
- work, advance fast enough, does not: gamb.[36]
- work, harm, will do him: ***arg-n.***
- work, hindered, is: ***chin.***
- work, works too much, all work comes to him: ozone[227]

Dementia; business, worry from: lil-t.[137]
Desires; work, routine: bar-c.[162] kali-c.[162]
Despair; work, over his: anac.[58]
Discouraged; business, aversion to: puls.[10]
Dreams; business, absorbing: nux-v.[36]
➤ business, accomplish, cannot: mag-m. ***phos.*** sabad.
➤ business, difficulties, in: am-m.[137] ars.[137] ***bry.***[137] nux-v.[137] puls.[137] ***rhus-t.***[137]
➤ business, forgot during day, he: sel.[102]
➤ business, neglected: hyper. myris. sil. stann.
➤ business, of: aether[36] anac. apis arg.[163] arist-m.[36] ars.[163] asaf. bell. ***bry.*** bufo calc. calc-acet.[36] calc-f.[163] calc-sil.[58] camph. canth. carb-v. carc.[193] carl. ***chel.*** cic. cina[10] croc. ***cur.*** elaps fl-ac.[163] gels. graph.[163] hep. hura hyper.[36] kali-c. kali-chl.[163] ***lach. lyc.*** mag-c.[163] merc. **NUX-V.** phos. psor. ***puls.*** pyrog. **RHUS-T.** sang. sars. sel.[85] ***sil.*** stann.[163] staph. sulph.[163] tarent.
➤ business, operations on a large scale: hura[36]
➤ business, pressure of: hyper.[36]
➤ business, projects: camph.[36]
➤ business, vexatious: apis[36]
➤ excelling in mental work: acon. anac. arn. ***bry.*** camph. carb-an. graph. ***ign.*** lach. ***nux-v.*** puls. rhus-t. sabad. ***sabin. thuj.***
➤ farming: mag-s. merc-i-r.
➤ frightful, laborious: lil-t.[54]
➤ fruit, gathering in garden: mag-c.[36]
➤ snow, working in snow: bapt.
➤ wedding, preparing: ozone[227]
➤ work: ambr.[10] carc.[119] dicha.[144] gels.[36] ign.[1] lil-t.[36] ozone[227] ***phos.***[54] rhus-t.[116] sel.[149] spong.[1]

Dullness; alternating with, work, desire for: cycl.[10]
Dullness; cares for his business, from: ph-ac.[58]
Euphoria; working, when: dicha.[149]
Excitement; mental work, from: ambr.[85] ind. kali-p. med. nat-p.[1] tub.
Excitement; unemployed, when: sulph.[10]
Excitement; working, when: ang.[10] mur-ac. olnd.
Extravagance; work, with hard: paull.[36]
Fear; business, of: ***graph. lil-t.***[54]
✦ exertion, of: calad. calc-sil.[58] guai. mez. ph-ac. phos. phyt. sul-i. tab. thea.
✦ failure, business or work, in: acon.[172] arg-n.[58] arn.[162] ***aur.***[184] bry.[172] calc.[172] carb-an.[162] cimic.[172] gels.[162] iod.[162] ***kali-c.***[184] kali-p.[172] lac-c.[162] lyc.[58] nat-m.[162] nux-v.[172] phos.[162] ***psor.*** sil.[162] sulph.[162]
✦ mental exertion, after: calc-sil.[58]
✦ occupation, of: lyc.[172] sel. sil.[172]
✦ work, become unfit for, to: cean.[54]
✦ work, dread of: ***arg-n.*** aur-i.[58] cadm-s. calc. calc-sil.[58] cham. chin.[58] coloc.[1] ***con.***[54] graph.[1] hyos. ind. iod.[5] ***kali-c.*** kali-p.

kali-s. kali-sil.[58] lyc.[172] nat-m. nat-p.[58] ***nux-v.***[30] ozone[227] petr. phos.[1] plb.[30] ***puls.*** ran-b. sanic. sel. ***sil. sulph.*** tab. tarax. tong. zinc.[1]

✦ work, dread of, daily, of: calc-f.[119] nux-v.[58]

✦ work, dread of, literary, of: aloe[162] lyc.[172] ***nux-v.***[122] ***sil.*** sulph.

✦ work, dread of, mental, of: calc-p.[58] con.[116] graph.[58] nat-p.[58] ph-ac.[162] pic-ac.[162]

✦ work, dread of, mental, of: calc-p.[58] con.[116] graph.[58] nat-p.[58] ph-ac.[162] pic-ac.[162]

✦ work, dread of, persuaded to, cannot be: ***con.***[54]

✦ work, dread of, prolonged, of: con.[172] nat-m.[172]

Forgetfulness; business, of: fl-ac.[54] sel.[10]

Grief; business, when thinking of his, in morning: ***puls.***[54]

Heedless; business, about: myris.[36]

House-keeping, women inapt to: cit-l.[54] lyc.[30] nux-v.[30] pitu-a.[164] sil.[30] sulph.[30]

Hurry; mental work, in: ambr. aur. ign. ***kali-c.*** laur. op. ***sul-ac. thuj.***

Impatience; work, for: ***ip.***[54]

Impatience; work, in: ***nux-v.***[116] sep.[30]

Indifference; business affairs, to: aesc.[162] agar. ***arg-n. arn.***[10] bamb-a.[1184] ***fl-ac.*** ham.[122] ***kali-bi.*** kali-p.[58] myris. nat-ar. ***ph-ac.*** phys. phyt.[58] psil.[164] ***ptel. puls.*** rhus-t.[162] ***sep. stram. sulph.***

Indifference; money-making, to: chin.[30] kali-c.[30] merc.[30] nat-c.[30] sep.[30]

Indifference; work aversion to: agar.[10] allox.[119] androc.[222] camph.[54] ign.[10] kali-m.[192] lach.[10] rhod.[54] squil.[10] staph.[10]

Indolence; business, when transacting: nux-v.[36] opun-a.[36]

Indolence; housework, aversion to her usual: bamb-a.[1184] cench.[58] ***cit-ac.*** cit-l.[54] sep.[137] sul-i.[58]

Indolence; mania for work, changing to: aur-s.[58]

Industrious, mania for work: acon.[5] aeth.[102] agar. allox.[119] ***aloe***[5] amn-l.[119] ang.[5] ***apis***[5] arist-cl.[119] arn. ars. **AUR.** aur-ar.[58] ***bar-c.*** bell. ***brom.***[5] bry. bufo[170] calc. calc-acet.[36] calc-ar.[36] calc-f.[149] calc-p. ***cann-s.***[5] caps. carc.[154] caust.[30] cere-b. chin. choc.[222] cic.[5] cimic.[5] cit-v.[36] clem. cob-n.[149] coca ***co-cain.***[102] cocc. **COFF.**[5] cupr.[210] ***cycl.***[5] cypr.[25] dicha.[36] dig. ***eucal.***[102] euph.[36] euphr.[5] fl-ac.[5] gamb.[36] ***helon.***[5] hura hydrog.[222] ***hyos.*** hyper.[36] ***ign.*** indg. **IOD.**[5] ip. iris ***kali-br.***[5] kali-c.[122] kreos. ***lacer.***[102] ***lach.*** lap-mar-c.[194] laur.[5] led. lil-t.[5] **LYC.**[5] lycps.[25] m-arct. mag-c. mag-m.[5] manc.[36] mand.[119] med.[184] menth.[36] merc.[184] mez. mosch. mur-ac. murx.[36] nat-c. nat-m.[36] nat-s. nux-v.[5] ***op.*** ped.[36] phos. pic-ac.[5] pip-m. pisc.[102] plan.[36] plb. puls.[5] rhus-t. sars.[10] seneg.[10] ***sep. spig.***[30] stann. staph.[5] stram.[5] sul-ac. sulph.[5] **TARENT.** ther.[10] **TUB.**[122] ***valer.***[5] verat. verb.[36] viol-o.[5] zinc.[5]

Industrious; coition, after: calc-p.

Insanity; business, from failure in: ***cimic.***[54] ***lil-t.***[54]

Irritability; business, about: bor.[10] ip. nat-m.

Irritability; business, important, in a: ***bor.***

Irritability; business; proceed fast, when does not: ip.[36]

Irritability; working, when: plan.[36] tong.[36]

Laughing; overwork, after: ***cupr.***[54]

Loathing; general, business, his: ars-h.

Loathing; work, at: anac.[102] arg-n. arn. bar-c.[54] calc. carb-ac.[54] chin.[30] cob.[54] con.[30] croc.[30] hyos. ***kali-bi.***[54] kali-c. lach.[30] ***lil-t.***[54] merc.[30] nat-m. nit-ac.[1] petr. ***puls.*** ran-b. ***sil.*** stann.[58] sulph. tab. tarax. ther.[36] tub.[102]

Mania; business, discouragement, from: ***lil-t.***[54]

Mania; business, failure, from: ***cimic.***[54]

Mania; study, from too much: ***lach.***[60]

Memory; weakness, business, for: agn. androc.[222] chel. fl-ac. hyos. kali-c. kreos. mag-c.[10] phos. sabin. sel. sulph. tell. tep

Mistakes; makes, work, in: acet-ac. all-c. androc.[222] bell. chin-s. germ.[222] meli. nat-c. phos. sep.

Morose; business does not proceed fast, when: ip.[36]

Morose; work, with inclination: sars.[54]

Muttering; business matters, about: dor.[25] mygal.[25]

Postponing everything to next day, business seems so long lasting, or as if it never could be accomplished: med.[54]

Prostration; business, from: podo.[85]

Sadness; business, when thinking of: mez.[58] ***puls.*** syph.[122]

Sadness; overwork and excesses, by: ***coca***[11] ign.[109]

Sadness; work, aversion to, with: berb.[10] bov.[10] croto-t.[10] dros.[10] laur.[10] mez.[10] prun.[10] zinc.[10]

Singing; alternating with, hatred of work: spong.

Somnambulism; work of the day, to do: bry.[30] nat-m.[30] sil.[116] sulph.[30]
Talk; domestic affairs, of: hyos.[54]
Talk; sleep, in, business, of: com. rhus-t. sulph.
Thoughts; business at evening in bed of: bell.[10] cocc.[10] sulph.[10]
Thoughts; intrude and crowd around each other, work, while at: mur-ac. ***sulph.***
Thoughts; rush, business accomplished, evening of: sulph.[36]
Thoughts; vanishing, work, while at: ***asar.***[116] hep.[36]
Timidity; business, in transacting: op.[36]
Tranquillity; thoughts of business, from: coloc.[36]
Weeping; disturbed at work, when: ***puls.***
Work; aversion to mental, anger after: **NUX-V.**[54]
Work; aversion to mental, hypochondriasis, in: ***ip.***[54]
Work; aversion to mental, masturbation, after: ***dig.***[54]
Work; aversion to mental, sadness, in: ***arg-n.***[54]
Work; aversion to mental, thinks it will do him harm, he: ***arg-n.***[54]
Work; aversion to mental, wants to leave everything as soon as it is commenced: ***lac-c.***[54]
Work; crazy, seems to drive him, in mental occupation, owing to the impotency of his mind: ind. ***kali-p.*** med.
Work; desire for mental: aloe anth. arn. aur. bad. ***brom.*** carb-ac. carc.[187] chin. cic.[5] clem. cob. cob-n.[119] coca cypr.[25] dig.[10] eug.[36] gels. ham.[36] lach.[116] laur. lycps.[25] m-arct.[10] menth.[85] naja nat-m.[30] nat-p.[36] op.[5] opun-a.[36] ozone[227] ped.[36] pip-m.[116] plb.[5] rhus-t. seneg. sulph. sumb.[36] **TARENT.** ther. verat.[10] verb.[54]
Work; desire for mental, insane passion for: ***hyos.***[54]
Work; impossible, anger, after: calc-p.[54]
Work; impossible, sexual excesses, after: ph-ac.[116] pic-ac.[116] ***sel.***[116]

ACT-SP. He, 6 - Great desire to work, though incapacity of it.
AGAR. Ha, 17 - Disgust for all work which occupies the mind, ...
AGN. Al, 1-,...he feels as if nothing existed around him; he is dissatisfied with himself all the time; he is incapable of attending to any business; the things around him are entirely indifferent to him;...
ALOE. Al, 20 - Little inclination to labor; discouraged, apprehensive about his success.
ALUM. Ha, 23 - Excited, over-worked (industrious), and yet discontented, because not enough had been done. (duty)
ANAC. Ha, 20 - Indisposition to work; he is afraid to undertake anything, he has no pleasure in anything.
ARG-N. He, 40 - Melancholy since an undeserved slight (scorn); fixed idea that he was neglected and despised by his family; his callings (job, work) became indifferent to him.
He, 8 - To fix thoughts in anything, or to give his business any consideration, was impossible for him; on attempting it, it immediately got dark before his eyes and headache increased.
He, 31 - Does not work, thinking it will do him harm or that he is not able to stand it.
ARN. Al, 39-...;one feels as if one were prevented (suspend) from doing something which is extremely necessary, accompanied by a total want of disposition for any kind of work.
Al, 31 - Excessive inclination to perform many and long literary labors, without possessing the strength which is required to terminate them without injuring health.
Ha, 620 - Restlessness of body and mind, as if he was prevented (obstructed) doing something necessary, whith complete indisposition for occupation.
Ha, 623 - Over-busy, inclination and disposition for great and continuous literary work with no power to do it without injury to the health.
He, 23 - Excessive inclination to hard and long literary labors.(industrious)
He, 47 - All occupation had to be relinquished (quit) for the time, so intense were the sufferings. (impediment)
He, 49 - Inability to perform continued active work.
ARS. Ha, 53 - Dissatisfied all day and extremely vexed at himself; he thought he had not worked enough and reproached himself most bitterly.

ART-V. He, 7 - Gets up every night and does her daily work as a house servant, with closed eyes, lies down again and cannot remember anything next morning.

ASTER. Al, 5 - Melancholy, alternating with almost intolerable cerebral excitement; she is inclined to give herself up to mental or bodily work, to walk, or engage in a violent exercise;...

AUR-M. He, 3 - Inclined to suicide; frequent weeping; aversion to occupation.

AUR. Ha, 346 - Remorse about his idleness (indolence), and yet he cannot work at anything; it drives him out of the house, he must always moving.

Ha, 11 - Restlessness and hurried impulse to bodily and mental activity; he can not work fast enough; he could not act so as to satisfy himself.

BELL. Al, 54 - The delirium was of a busy (engaged, working), restless, vivid character, but generally rather pleasing than otherwise. The patient appeared to think they were pursuing (persevere) their ordinary occupations; one boy appeared eager (animated) in flying a kite (toy), another pulled tables and chairs about, thinking he was working in a coal-pit, and a woman appeared to be remarkably busy with her household duties...

Al, 109 - A tailor was poisoned with a belladona injection, and for fifteen hours, though speechless and insensible to external objects, went through all the customary operations of his trade with great vivacity and moved his lips as if in conversation.(busy)

A-S, 2554-..The patients appeared to think that they were pursuing their ordinary occupations;... the woman appeared remarkably busy with her ordinary household duties.

Ha, 1366 - Ridiculous grimaces; ...acts as if she were washing, at another as if counting money, ...

BOR. Ha, 20 - Disinclination to work, he only does what he has to do, as if compulsorily.

Ha, 21 - He fritters away the afternoon, without getting to any real work, goes from one work to another, from one room to another, without remaining in one thing.

BROM. Al, 1 - He becomes averse to his business; it seems as though he must relinquish (quit) it.

He, 6 - Aversion to any kind of work, even reading; takes no interest in household duties.

BRY. Ha, 777 - Cross; imagined she could not finish her work (obstruction) ; she always took hold (continued) of the wrong thing and constantly wished to take something else ; then a pressing aching headache in the forehead.

Al, 37 - Over-busy (industrious); she undertakes and works far too much.

Ha, 766 - Raving (insanity) about business for an hour.

Ha, 780 - Too busy; she wishes to undertake and to work at too many things.

He, 16 - Irrational talk or prattle of his business.

He, 10 - Nightly delirium; delirious talk, especially about business.< after 3 a.m.

He, 12 - Talking of business of day in his delirium at night.

CALC-A. Al, 10-...;he performed all his work with aversion and as if compelled (drive) to do so. (compulsive, obsessive)

Ha, 261 - Not without inclination to work, but indifferent to all external things; sunk in thought about the present and future.

Ha, 263 - Anxious disposition as if something evil had happened or he had to fear reproaches (censures); at the same time, however, persistent inclination to work. (industrious)

CALC. Ha, 13 - Anxious at heart, as if he had done wrong,(immoral) or had to apprehend reproaches (deserves), with constant inclination to work.

CANTH. Al, 14 - He talked deliriously when lying, sitting and walking, disconnectedly of his business and of people who had long since been dead.

CARB-V. Al, 25 - Exceedingly irritable; she seems to be overhurried (quick, fast) in her business.

Ha, 16 - Excessive excitation, as if she was too much hurried (fast), or over-worked (industrious) in business.

CAUST. Ha, 7 - Anxious, restlessness mood, as if something disagreeable (difficult) was impending (imminent), which keeps him from working.

CERE-B. Al, 1 - Desire to engage at work.
Al, 2 - Desire to have the time all employed. (work)
Al, 16 - Difficult to keep employed.
CHEL. He, 18 - Anxiety: allowing no rest at any employment (business) ; as if she had committed a crime; fear of getting crazy (insanity), with restlessness and heat.
CHIN. Ha, 1134 - Liking for work, reading, writing, and thinking; particularly well disposed and industrious.
CHOC. Sh, 205 - Though Previously lazy, became intensely obsessed with work for a long period of time. Put all my energy into work. 35, 30C, XX:XX:XX:
CIMIC. He, 34 - Mind disturbed by disappointed love, business failures.
COCC. Ha, 532 - She dawdles (indolent); in business she cannot accomplish anything nor finish anything, with contracted pupils.
CON. He, 33 - Timid, cannot be persuaded to work ; want of proper will. (lack of: resolution) (vagabond)
CROC. He, 3 - Greatly concerned about his life, believes that he will die, is no longer fit for business.
CUPR-A. Al, 2 - Attacks of mania; he fancies that he is a military officer; a fancy that he is selling green vegetables; a fancy that he is repairing old chairs...he spits in the faces of the attendants, and laughs heartily at it.
CUPR. Ha, 24 - Fits of insanity, he imagines (delirium) he has green herbs for sale.
Ha, 25 - Fits of insanity, he imagines he is repairing old chairs. (humility) (reparation, restitution)
Ha, 10 - Indisposition to work, and yet idleness is a burden to him.
CYCL. Al, 16 - Fretful and sad; has no desire to work ; she feels a great anxiety, as if some great misfortune were impending.
ELAPS. Al, 7 - She seeks a retired room to work in.
GERM. Sh, 182 - Engaged in my work and my music with fierce intensity. 08, 12C, 14:12:00
GRAT. Al, 16 - Irresolute; no persistence in work.
HALI-L. Sh, 157 - Called into work a half an hour early, for an emergency. Went into automatic overwhelm. Felt a lot of responsibilities. I didn't have the time to do all the things I wanted to do. 01, 30C, 01:23:XX
Sh, 183 - I feel good, charged. Had a surge of energy. Feel very industrious. Organizing things, cleaning out my room. Organizing stuff to give away to charity. 01, 30C, 00:01:00
Sh, 336 - Changed work shift. Didn't want to go to work. Don't like being at work at all. Frustrated at lack of ability to communicate with patient I was assisting. 02, 30C, 10:XX:XX
HYDROG. Sh, 155 - In the afternoon (during the full moon) I felt low and depressed, insecure and vulnerable. Could not cope with work load and didn't want to be alone. 12, 6C, 39:XX:XX
HYOS. He, 31 - Delirium; talks of business of imaginary wrongs.
He, 49 - Insane passion for work.
IGN. He, 41 - Altered appearance; made an unsuccessful attempt to end his most unendurable (intolerable) sufferings, by eating the phosphorus from matches; after business embarrassment.
IOD. Al, 22 - Apprehensiveness (fearful) after some manual labor, ...
Al, 31 - Mind feels tired, and does not care to work.
Ha, 10 - Apprehensiveness after some manual work; it goes off while sitting.
He, 15 - At night, especially when thinking of real or imaginary wrongs ...dares (try) to go home for fear of doing some dreadful (bad, wicked) deed (action); on one occasion was seized with an almost irresistible impulse to murder a woman who was acting as a guide (direct, conduct) for him, he having lost his way (direction);...must be constantly in action, in some laborious occupation. (lost; direction, correction, control)
IP. Al, 11 - Ill-humored and vexed that his business does not proceed fast enough.
LAC-AC. He, 2 - Averse to business or what formerly was pleasant to do; lazy (indolent); dislikes to read or think; finds fault, is sarcastic, exacting. (exigent, severe)
LACH. Al, 43 - He is impelled to productive work in the evening, although he had been much fatigued during the day ... writes with the greatest freedom and increased vigor about everything he knows;...

Al, 54 - Dilatory (slow); he cannot accomplish his business as usual.
He, 31 - Disinclined to his own proper work; complains of trifles.
LED. Ha, 338 - Calm and happy disposition with love for work and self-contented.
LIL-T. He, 7 - Dementia produced by business discouragements and sexual excesses.
LIM. Al, 3 - The great disinclination to work, and inability to accomplish much, which he had experienced since the sea-bath, disappeared completely during the day, and gave place to mental quiet and steadiness, with constancy and perseverance in performing very irksome duties.
LYC. He, 40 - Nervous action weakened; threatened softening of brain from overwork, or metastasis of ulcers suddenly healed.
MAG-M. Al, 709 - She becomes anxious in a dream about the work that she could not accomplish.
MED. He, 2 - Dullness of memory and desire to procrastinate (delay), because business seemed so long lasting (permanent), or as if it never could be accomplished. (postponing)
He, 20 - Is sure that she is worse, knows she is not going to live, cannot see any improvement, even when it is pointed out (antagonism); has no fear of death, speaks calmly about it, and gives directions as to the disposition of her affairs.
MEZ. Al, 8 - Very sad; every trifle affects him disagreeably; indifferent to the whole world; has no desire for anything; disinclined to work.
MUR-AC. Al, 21 - Deep reflection, and quiet absorption in himself, as if something disagreeable were impending, though with desire to work.
Ha, 8-...no work succeeds in his hands,...
NAT-AR. Al, 5 - Feel well; can study easily ; disposed to be reconciled to circumstances, favorable and unfavorable; feel like working hard; no undertaking too large for me.
NAT-C. Al, 56 - He has no desire to do anything, and can keep at nothing long.
NAT-M. Al, 132 - Irresolute at work; he could not see his way clearly.
Ha, 90 - Irresolution in doing mental work; he cannot easily find his way.
NUX-V. Al, 73 - Dread of that kind of literary work at which one must think and employ the ideas, ...
PETR. Al, 28 - No desire to work; no pleasure in objects of which he was usually fond (loving), hence intolerable ennui.
PH-AC. Ha, 668 - Inward restlessness hinders (delay) him in his work.
PHOS. Al, 38 - Told those about him repeatedly that he could not possibly recover, and gave some disjointed directions about his business affairs.
He, 22-...uneasy about one's health; paroxysms of anguish, when alone or in a stormy weather, with timorous disposition; told those about him repeatedly that he could not possibly recover, and gave some disjointed (incoherent) directions about his business affairs.
PSOR. Al, 19 - Despairing mood; he fears to fail in business.
Al,N-24 - Despairing mood; fears he will fail in business.
He, 24 - Despairing mood; fears he will fail in business.
He, 34-...;thinks he will not recover; has lost all hope; cannot apply his mind to business;...
PTEL. Al, 43 - Goes about his professional duties in a perfunctory (indifference) manner, very unlike (contradictory) his fiery (passionate) zeal with which he usually combats disease and his allopathic step-brethren (brotherhood).
PULS. Al, 5 - He wishes now for this, now for that employment, but when given to him he will have nothing to do with it.
Al, 44 - Shuns business, is irresolute, with sighing respiration and a feeling as if he were beside himself.
Ha, 1122 - Neglect of his business, hesitancy (indecision), sobbing (cry) respiration and loss of composure.(calm, serenity)
Ha, 1123 - Sometimes he wants to do one thing, sometimes another, and when he is given something to do, he will not do it.
He, 9 - Shuns business; irresolute; sighing respiration; feels as if he were beside himself.
RHUS-T. Al, 40 - Impatient desire to accomplish several kinds of business, chiefly intellectual,...

He, 5 - Low, mild delirium, thinks he is roaming (wander, travel) over fields, or hard at work.

SANT. Al, 6-...irresolution and want of confidence in my own powers as to render me quite unfit for work of any kind;

SEL. Al, 4 - Dread of people and of his occupation, but overcoming this he is able to continue his work.

SEP. Al, 92 - One dose of the medicine takes away my ambition; I simply do not want to do anything, either work or play; it is even an exertion to think.

He, 19 - Aversion to one's occupation (work) and family.

SPONG. Ha, 384 - She is not satisfied with her work; she cannot do her work properly, she is not successful with it.

He, 12 - Feels awkward (unskillful) about her work, which she cannot accomplish (succeed, prosper) satisfactorily.

STANN. Al, 20 - Fruitlessly busy, as if a rush of ideas prevented him from completing his work at a certain time; all sorts of things occur to him to be done.

Ha, 8 - Restless and distracted, no perseverance in her work (at once).

STRAM. Al, 123-...seemed to herself to be engaged in her usual avocation,...imitate in every respect the routine procedure of one thus engaged.

He, 40 - Aberration of mind; one carries home all sorts of wood in order to manufacture brandy (cognac) (busy, manufacturing) ; another placed two axes across each other in order to split wood in this way; a third burrowed in ground like a pig with his mouth (animal); a fourth alleged he was a wheelwright and began to bore holes; a fifth ran into forge to catch fish, which he saw swimming there; a lacemaker threw about her bobbins incessantly, and threw everything into confusion; another girl ran about the room and cried out that all evil spirits were pursuing her.(restoration, restitution)

SUL-AC. Al, 35 - Fretful, peevish, impatient, if his work is not done to suit.(unsatisfying)

Ha, 16 - Vexed, peevish, impatient, at once when he does not succeed in his work.

He, 6-... unfit for work, would sit and weep whole day long;...

SULPH. Al, 8 - Numerous morbid ideas, extremely disagreeable, causing rancor, though with also joyous thoughts (and melodies) mostly from the past, take possession of her they throng one upon another so that she cannot free herself from them during the day, with neglect of business,...

Al, 42-...discontented with himself and all about him, which made him unfit for any serious occupations...whole evening he was absorbed in himself and unable to command his thoughts to read...

Al, 100 - Thoughts of the business that had been accomplished thronged (crowd) upon her...

He, 8 - Numerous morbid ideas, extremely disagreeable, causing rancor; neglect of business;...

TAB. Al, 45 - He was incapacitated for business of any kind, weak irresolute, and despondent.

TARAX. Al, 6 - Irresolution and dread of work, though it progresses well as soon as he undertakes it.

He, 3 - Undecided, shunning (avoid) labor, but after beginning, works well.

WRONG

Anger; mistakes, about his: ars.[54] bell.[54] bry. carc.[193] ***nit-ac.*** nux-v.[30] ***staph. sulph.***

Anxiety; conscience, unpardonable sin, feels she has done the, and will be eternally lost: ***chel.***[54].

Delirium; wrongs, of fancied: hyos.

Delusions; disgraced, family or his absent friends, he disgraced his: sarr.[36]

- disgraced, family, she disgraced her: ***plat.***[8]
- names, calls things by wrong, his boots logs of wood, his bedroom the stable: stram.[54]
- read, it seems wrong to: lach.[36]
- right, does nothing: anac. arg-n. ***aur.*** nat-c.
- succeed, he cannot; does everything wrong: anac. ***arg-n.*** arn.[114] ***aur.***[122] bamb-a.[1184] bapt.[58] bar-c.[162] gels.[114] naja[130] nat-c. nat-m.[114] ozone[227] phos.[114] sulph.[137]
- writing is untidy, her: hydrog.[222]
- wrong, everything is: androc.[222] bac.[62] bamb-a.[1184] calc.[5] coloc. eug. hep.[5] kali-br.[139] ***naja*** nux-v.
- wrong, giving wrong things to people, causing their death: sulph.[102]

- wrong, he has done: alum.[36] ***ars. aur.*** aur-ar.[58] cand-a.[239] cina[130] cob.[139] cocc.[85] cycl. dig. digin.[36] germ.[222] ***hell.*** hyos.[122] ***ign. lach. lil-t.***[168] lyc. merc. myric.[144] naja[58] nat-ar. ***nux-m.***[137] puls. ruta[130] sarr.[36] sil.[116] sulph.[1] thuj. verat.[139]
- wrong, he has done, people are therefore against her: lil-t.[168]

Discontented; wrong, everything another does is: ***cham.***[54]

Distance; inaccurate judge of: agar.[5] anac.[5] ***arg-n.***[5] atro.[25] ***cann-i.*** cann-s.[5] carb-an.[85] coca[25] dat-m.[85] glon.[5] hyos.[1] lac-h.[229] magn-gr.[139] ***nux-m.***[122] onos.[137] op.[5] ozone[227] stann.[5] ***stram.***

Dreams; errors, mistakes: am-m.[5] ozone[227]

- ➤ friends, apartment, in wrong: ozone[227]
- ➤ incestuous: lap-mar-c.[194]
- ➤ mother, taking the wrong road: ozone[227]
- ➤ remorse, God was punishing her for her sins, that: aether[36]
- ➤ remorse, past mistakes, for: nat-m.[36]
- ➤ vexatious, wrong doings of others, over: dros.[54]
- ➤ wrong, doing: cocc.[5] ozone[227]
- ➤ wrong, everything goes: fago.[36]

Fear; say something wrong, lest he should: bamb-a.[1184] germ.[222] ***lil-t.*** med.[85]

- ✦ wrong, commit something, and kill herself: ***merc.***[54]

Impulse; wrong, to do: hep.[85]

Liar; makes wrong statements to herself, because she does not know what to say next, begins all right but does not know how to finish: ***med.***[54]

Reading; wrong, seems: lach.[36]

Remorse; indiscretion, over past: spira.[36]

Sadness; brooding over imaginary wrongs and misfortunes, by: naja[130]

Sadness; conscience, of, as if he had committed a bad action, or not done his duty: cycl.[54]

Sadness; fault, as if in: tarent.[36]

Sadness; wrong way, as if having done everything in, during headache: ***naja***[36]

Thoughts; thoughtful, errors of others, about the: cic.[36]

Wrong; doing things: ant-t.[36] hell.[137]

ACON. Ha, 516 - Inconsolable anxiety and piteous howling, with complaints and reproaches about (often triflings) evils.

ADAM. Sh, 246 - Cried with despair. Nothing I do is right. Rocking from side to side, sobbing. Desire to stab with a knife or scissors. Felt very different from other humans. Long, late phone call ameliorates. 16, 12C, 43:XX:XX

ALUM. He, 6 - Makes mistakes in speaking, using words not intended.

AM-C. Al, 33 - She found fault with everything.

ANT-T. Al, 13 - Bad humor, everything goes wrong.

APIS. Al, 17-... would have liked to kill a dog that barked at him, etc. ; everything went wrong; nothing could be done to please him.

Al, 19-...nothing appeared to satisfy him; everything out of place.

He, 48 - Constantly busily engaged doing this or that, but do nothing right; young girls.

ARS. Al, 95 - Very fretful (irritable) and contented with nothing; she finds fault (imperfection, error) with everything; ...

Ha, 20 - Continual anguish, like remorse of conscience, as if he had acted in violation (transgression, crime) of his duty, without knowing in what particular.

Ha, 1042 - Irritable state of the disposition, he vexes himself about trifles, and cannot leave off talking about the faults of others.

Ha, 1049 - Discontented with everything, finds fault with everything; everything is too strong and too irritating, all conversation, all noise, and all light.

He, 92 - Disposed to discuss the faults of others.

ATRO. Al, 42 - Morose, quarrelsome the whole day, everything went wrong; trifles usually passed unheeded irritated him to anger.

AUR. Ha, 19 - Dispirited and despondent; he thinks that everything goes awkwardly (incapacity, unfit) with him, and nothing will succeed with him.

He, 10 - Imagines he cannot succeed (perform, prosper) in anything, (failure) and he does everything wrong; he is in disunion whith himself.

BAR-A. Al, 9 - Dread (fear). When walking in the street, she imagines that people were criticizing her, and judging her wrongfully which makes her anxious, so that she will not look up, will look (aversion) at no one, and sweats all over.

BAR-C. Ha, 4 - She suspected, that when walking in the street, men found fault (defect) with her, and judged her amiss (wrong), which made her anxious, so that she dared not look up, she looked at nobody, and perspired all over.

BELL. Al, 178 - Fretfulness; nothing seemed right to him; he was vexed with himself.

Ha, 1401 - Peevishness, nothing was right for him; he was angry with himself.

He, 119 - Fretfulness; nothing seemed right to him; was vexed with himself.

BRY. Ha, 777 - Cross; imagined she could not finish her work (obstruction) ; she always took hold (continued) of the wrong thing and constantly wished to take something else ; then a pressing aching headache in the forehead.

Al, 25 - Fretful; she imagines that she cannot accomplish (realize) her work; constantly takes up the wrong piece, and always inclined to change and take another; ...

CACT. Al, 16 - Feeling of semi remorse at having done something wrong.

CALC-P. Al, 14 - Violent, irritable, and snappish; it affects him most to hear that someone has done wrong; indignation rises in him...

CALC. Ha, 13 - Anxious at heart, as if he had done wrong,(immoral) or had to apprehend reproaches (deserves), with constant inclination to work.

He, 86 - Easily offended; takes everything amiss.

CAMPH. Ha, 343 - Quarrelsomeness, insists he is right.

CAPS. Al, 1 - He makes reproaches and becomes angry at the faults of others; he becomes offended at trifles and finds fault.

Ha, 334 - He makes reproaches, and is indignant (angry) at the faults (errors) of others; he takes trifles ill and finds fault with them.

CAUST. Al, 12 - Anxiety the whole day, as if he had done something bad, or apprehended it, or as if he had been unfortunate (unsuccessful, umprosperous).

Ha, 6 - Anxiety the whole day, as if he had done something wrong, or to fear it, or as if a misfortune had happened.

CHAM. Al, 64 - He stammers (hesitate) uses wrong expressions, and corrects himself.

Ha, 465 - Very anxious; nothing she does seems to her to be right; she is irresolute; ...(indecisive)

He, 44 - Morose fretfulness; everything that another does is wrong; no one does anything to please him.

CIC. Al, 27 - Want of confidence in mankind; with misanthropy; he forsook society, remained alone and reflected upon their errors and about himself.

Ha, 238 - Want of trust (mistrust, skepticism) in people and anthrophoby,(misanthropy) he fled (escape) from them remained solitary, and thought seriously about their errors and about himself.

CIMIC. He, 27 - Irritable; the least thing that goes wrong makes her angry.

COCC. Al, 27 - Very much affected and offended by slight obliquities (immorality) and untruths (falsehood) of others.

Ha, 554 - He is very indignant and annoyed at slight faults and fibs (lie, falsify) of others.

COLOC. He, 10 - Extremely irritable and impatient; nothing seems right; gets angry on being questioned.

CUR. Al, 4 - Everything he sees appears foul and nasty. (dirty, dishonest, offensive, injurious, indecent)

DIG. Al, 21 - Anxiety, as though he had done wrong.

Ha, 425 - An anxious feeling as if he had done something bad.

Ha, 8 - Anxiety as if he had done wrong.

FERR. Ha, 272 - Anxiety at night, as she have done something bad; she could not sleep, tossed about the bed.

GERM. Sh, 134 - Felt uncomfortable if any one stood close to me. Felt uneasy and paranoid in class. Feel as if done something wrong. 10, 9C, 06:06:00

Sh, 115 - Very much in doubt whether I should take any more tablets. Whatever I do, I feel that somebody will criticize me, that I do something wrong. Difficult to make a decision. Afraid that other people will laugh at me or say, haven't you understood anything?" Crying. Don't want to get up. Don't want to bother the supervisor so early in the morning. I am a failure. 18, 30C, 01:06:30

Sh, 122 - It is difficult to describe the

symptoms-want to correct myself all the time. I am thinking too much. I get mad at all my thoughts. 18, 30C, 05:XX:XX

Sh, 81 - Wrote red instead of right. Said one word and understood another, husband said physician twice and twice I understood physicist. Talked about a patient who had a need for light and I thought photophobia. Wrote dylexist instead of dyslexic. Said amelioration occupates instead of occupation ameliorates. Quicked instead of quite. V Said nerve underneath sciatica instead of underneath thigh. 05, 6C, 02:XX:XX

Sh, 84 - I repeat adverbs very close together. "Lovely music by this lovely musician. I think its lovely" Lots of editing -I notice it when I'm reading it back. 13, 30C, XX:XX:XX

HALI-L. Sh, 928 - I'm only half aware. When I was doing things wrong, I was half aware I was doing them. 20, 30C, 14:XX:XX

HELON. Al, 4-.... could not endure the least contradiction or receive any suggestions in regard to any subject (fixed ideas) ;... what I most desired was to be left alone, reserved to myself the privilege of finding fault (imperfection) with everything around me;....

HEP. Al, 4 - Everything of which she only thought was disagreeable and not right.

Al, 16 - Irritable mood; everything that she undertook was wrong; she desired to be alone.

HYDROG. Sh, 15 - I felt in the presence of a totally pure energy, like meeting God and feeling totally unworthy or like meeting a lover and feeling unworthy — realizing all the mistakes of a lifetime. This pure energy was around for some time protecting me. I feel this unification cleared out lifetimes of symptomatology for me. The joining with this energy was as if a male energy joined with me sexually, but with no desire, pleasure or pain involved. This unification with the male energy lasted quite a few days — I'm not used to seeing myself as a man. The morning after this unifying with the higher presence, I collapsed in emotional overflow. All my grief and pain came out. I was doubled upon the floor and went into a deep state of catharsis. It is not possible to describe where I went as there are no concepts applicable. I felt overflowing love for humanity and wanted to give everything away. My mind turned to the Buddha. It was like seeing the complete picture instead of fragmented bits. (These primary effects lasted about 28 days, then changing to a paranoia state). 16, 30C, 07.XX.XX

Sh, 30 - The whole environment I am in feels wrong now as if my life doesn't fit anymore. 16, 30C, 08:XX:XX

Sh, 131 - Marked tendency to panic at little things that go wrong or small decisions to be made. 08, 30C, 00:XX:XX

HYOS. He, 31 - Delirium; talks of business of imaginary wrongs.

IGN. Al, 30 - Extremely morose, finds fault, and makes reproaches.

Al, 32 - He is discontented, morose, and obstinate towards evening; no one can do anything right or please him.

Ha, 749 - Anxiety as if he had done something bad.

Ha, 754-,... he cannot express himself in talking, write, or do anything as quickly as he wishes; ...he makes mistakes in speaking and writing, and does everything awkwardly...

Ha, 768 - Towards evening he is discontented, sulky, stubborn (obstinate), no one can do anything right, anything to please him.

Ha, 769 - Is extremely sulky; finds fault and makes reproaches.

He, 39 - Anxiety and disquiet as if she had done something wrong, or as if some great misfortune were about to happen, this so overpowers her that she can with difficulty refrain from weeping;...

IOD. Al, 28 - Peevish, fretful; nothing is done right.

He, 15 - At night, especially when thinking of real or imaginary wrongs ...dares (try) to go home for fear of doing some dreadful (bad, wicked) deed (action); on one occasion was seized with an almost irresistible impulse to murder a woman who was acting as a guide (direct, conduct) for him, he having lost his way (direction);...must be constantly in action, in some laborious occupation. (lost; direction, correction, control)

JAMB. He, 2 - Nothing seemed right, when sitting, he wanted to lie; when lying, he wanted to rise again.
KALI-CY. Al, 4 - For two days, desire to find fault; crossness almost uncontrollable on entering the room; while the cold air produces good spirits.
KALI-I. Al, 16 - Very peevish and excited; everything goes wrong, and she is ready to quarrel with every one.
LACH. Al, 23 - It frequently seems to him wrong to read long at a time, although the subject interests him.
He, 54 - A girl, after excessive study, uses exalted language; exceedingly particular about language she uses, often correcting after using a word, and substituting another of very similar meaning, talking about being under influence of a superior power. (possessed) 0 Mania.
LIL-T. Al, 49 - She dreads saying anything to anybody, lest she should say something wrong, and yet she wants to walk.
LYC. He, 36 - Distrustful, suspicious and fault (mistake) finding. (judgment)
LYSS. Al, 18-...caught myself saying to nephew, in severe tone, " If you do that again" etc., when he was not really in fault.
MAG-S. Al, 4 - Anxious as if conscious of some evil...
MANG. Ha, 325 - Cross and discontented with himself, and concerned about future..., considers himself very weak (stupid) in mind, and makes mistakes whenever he speaks.
MED. He, 13 - Seems to herself to make wrong statements (declaration), because she does not know what to say next, begins all right but does not know how to finish...
He, 31 - Dread of saying the wrong thing when she has headache.
He, 7 - Reads a letter and thinks the words look queer (inadequate) and are spelled wrong.
MERC. Al, 22 - A feeling as though he had done wrong, with loss of ideas.
Al, 36 - Quarrels with everything; would above all have everything right; quarrelsome.
Ha, 1237 - With absence of thought, (discernment, knowledge),he feels as if he had done something bad.
He, 22 - Great desire to murder (homicidal) or committed suicide ...is fearful that she may commit some wrong and kill herself (punishment); something urges her to kill her husband, of whom she is very fond (loving), and she implores him to hide his razor (knife).
MYRIC. Al, 9-...a constant desire to find fault (censorious); everything went wrong; looked upon (contemptuous) this world as a place not fit to live in any longer; considered himself better than the rest (great person, megalomania), in the morning; ...; condemned himself for various imaginary faults; ...
Al, 11 - Irritable, worried by little things; everything seemed to go wrong, in the morning.
NAJA. Al, 13-...I felt that everything that was done was done in a wrong way, and could not be rectified (corrected, revised); if I felt that I had some duty to perform (execute), I had at the same time a strong impulse not to do it, and I am extremely restless in consequence; I seemed to have an increased perception of what I ought to do, but, at the same time, an unaccountable inclination not to do it, to which I was irresistibly compelled to yield "I couldn't help it, didn't know why, but couldn't do it."
Al, 14 - Felt melancholy; began to form images of possible wrongs (mistaken) and misfortunes, over which the mind broods; very wretched at times;... a slight cause sets him in a perfect agony of mental suffering on another's behalf (welfare);...makes himself imaginary troubles and wrongs, and frets (bother) over them for two hours...
Al, 9 - Considerable depression of spirits, and a feeling of inability to exertion of any kind, and a conviction that all is going wrong;...
Al, 10 - Great depression of spirits this morning; everything for two or three hours appeared to go wrong with me, and to be without remedy;...
He, 3 - Melancholy; began to form images of possible wrongs (evils) and misfortunes over which the mind broods; very wretched (miserable) at times.
NAT-C. Al, 17 - Anxiety and restlessness; he

thought he could do nothing properly.(rightly, correctly)

Al, 22 - His fancy is mostly busy with apprehensions of the future; he often makes plans for half an hour at a time as if it would go wrong with him, wherewith he seeks to be alone for several days together.

Al, 41-..;the room seems too small for him, and even in open air he walks without anything seeming right to him;... (confined, limited, restricted)

Ha, 13 - Anxious and restless, he thinks he cannot do anything right.

NAT-M. Al, 59 - Anxiety, as if she had done something wrong, with heat and night sweat.

Al, 119 - The patient's mind was much weakened by disease and poison; her moral perceptions, her once keen (sharp) sense of honor, and of right and wrong, seemed blunted (dull); she was in turns vehement (angry) and passionate, and moody and silent.

He, 2 - Absent minded or distracted while talking; does not know what he ought (have to) say; awkward in talking; easily makes mistakes.

NEON. Sh, 173 - Anxious about everything and depressed about the anxiety and feel it's all wrong. 10, 6C, 18:XX:XX

NIT-AC. Al, 27 - Vexed at the least trifle, even at himself if he makes a mistake.

Ha, 44 - Vexed at the least trifle, also at himself, when he does something amiss.(wrong)

NUX-M. Al, 30 - While writing he omitted letters, wrote in different alphabets against his will and changed from one subject to another.

He, 14 - While writing he omitted letters, wrote in different alphabets against his will, and changed from one subject to another.

NUX-V. Al, 88 - Clear consciousness of his existence; fine, strong, correct feeling of right and wrong.

Ha, 1301 - Clear consciousness of his existence; delicate, strong proper (accurate, correct, exact) feeling of right and wrong. (sapience) (justice)

Ha, 1266 - Very much given to reproach others severely for their faults.

Ha, 1291 - Everything goes wrong with him. (everything goes contrary)

He, 5 - Very easily bewildered(confused); everything goes wrong.

He, 35 - From disappointed ambition, bewildered, (confused) talks incoherently; does everything he attempts (try) to do wrong;..

He, 39 - Mania puerperalis...constantly complaining, criticizing or explaining, ... as soon she recognized physician she spoke of imperfection of medical knowledge and declared it an error that one could not live without a heart, inasmuch as she felt very well without one, it having come away with the afterbirth to which it had grown fast, the nurse having separated the two before her eyes; complains of her husband, says he wishes to convince her she is sick, ... nymphomania,... frequently sips at a bowl of warm sugar-water, declaring it will form her a new heart; .(health, healing)...(expert)

OP. Al, 37 - Conscious of being possessed (seized) of two persons (double) of another self besides his real self, the Opium man does things which the real self considers wrong, and it is not always sure which will conquer the other.

PHOS. Al, 136 - Felt exceedingly petulant (irritable, contemptuous) all day; nothing went right; felt as dissatisfied with myself as with others; seemed as if everybody said or did something to provoke me.

PHYS. Al, 17 - Nothing was right; too many things in the room; continually counting them.

PSOR. Al, 19 - Despairing mood; he fears to fail in business.

PULS. Ha, 1140 - In the evening (about sunset), extraordinarily sulky, will not answer, and takes everything amiss.(wrong)

RUTA. Al, 3 - Very anxious all day, as though he had done something wrong; if any one opened the door he feared that some one had come to arrest (imprisonment, jailing) him.

Ha, 280 - All day long very anxious as if he had done something bad; when the door was opened, he feared that someone was coming to take him to prison. (incarcerated, punished)

SAPIN. Al, 4 - Very irritable; nothing goes right; fault-finding, dissatisfied with everything previously done, no matter how well it was done before; ...
Al, 5 - Quite ill-natured and inclined to view matters in a disagreeable light; did not seem able to feel settled (decided) enough to know what to do; the crossness became so intense, that I felt myself getting very unreasonable, especially as to food, which seemed all wrong in some way;...

SEP. Al, 96 - He thinks of things which he does not think of, uses expressions which he knows are incorrect, undertakes those things which are opposed to his intentions, and finds such contradictions with himself that it puts him in a very uncomfortable and uneasy mood.
Ha, 68 - He thinks, what he does not wish to think, uses expressions which he himself knows are incorrect; he resolves to do what is against his intention, and is thus in conflict with himself and, therefore in a disagreeable, restless mood. (lost: knowledge, correction)
Ha, 44 - She finds fault with everything, does not wish what others desire; with weeping ...

SIL. Al, 27 - Most excessive scruples of conscience about trifles frequently, as though he had done a great wrong.
Ha, 8 - He feels the greatest conscientious scruples about trifles; as if he had done a very great wrong.
He, 5 - Becomes confused, makes mistakes; she is unable to control himself.

SPIG. Ha, 666 - He is very cross and sensitive to everything that he thinks not good, for many hours.

STAPH. He, 9 - Very sensitive to least impression; least word that seems wrong (offenses) hurts her very much.

SULPH. Al, 69 - Extremely peevish and ill-humored; nothing seems right to her.
Ha, 24 - She imagines that she might give people something wrong, which might kill them.

THUJ. Al, 1 - She herself desires, with anxiety and despair, to be taken to an insane asylum, (imprisonment, confining) and there to be treated very harshly and strictly, (penalized), so that her fixed ideas may be subdued and banished (purified); she knows very well that she does wrong (conscience) and thinks all sorts of bad thoughts (immoral), but she will not take the trouble to banish such thoughts; therewith she indistinctly gives to understand that she is constantly obliged to think of taking her own life, but feels the sinfulness (wicked) of it, in order to avoid it, desires the strict restraint of the asylum;...
Al, 2 - She fancies that she has intentionally represented herself as insane (feigning) in the presence of others in order to palliate a wrong supposed to have been done (penitence, remorse), and that now she is punished, therefore, by real insanity.

VERAT. Al, 62 - He seeks out faults in others and contemplates (examine, inspect) them. (critical)
Ha, 690 - Anxiety as from a bad conscience, as if he had done something bad.
Ha, 706 - He searches for faults in others and taunts (ridicule, mockery) them with them.

YIELDING

Absent-mindedness; standing in one place, never accomplishes what he undertakes: med.[162] ***nux-m.***[54]
Delusions; enslaved, is: lap-c-b.[194]
- vegetable existence, he is leading a: cann-i.
- wait, he had to: anh.[119]
- waiting, he is: lap-c-b.[194]

Dependent; desires to be, at another's cost: lap-mar-c.[194]
Discontented; life, cut off from: bamb-a.[1184]
Discouraged; ambition, from loss of: nux-v.[137]
Discouraged; resignation: agar.[5] agn.[5] anh.[119] bry.[30] chin-b.[54] lyc.[54] nat-m.[30] nit-ac.[30] ***ph-ac.***[5] pic-ac.[5] sulph.[5] ***tab.***[5]
Dreams; people, influential persons, to whom he occupies position of servant or subordinate: lyss.[54]
➤ people, standing before window: merc.[36]
➤ subordination like a servant: lyss.[36]

Execution lost as the result of overpowering visual sensations: anh.[119]
Far away; as if, with apathy and indifference to the future: med.[137] syph.[54]
Grief; silent, submissiveness, with: **PULS.**[54]

Hypochondriasis; inert, takes no interest in his surroundings: euphr.[54]
Hysteria; mild, gentle, yielding, although whimsical and introverted: ***ign.***[54]
Independent; cannot be: calc.[30] kiss.[36] nat-m.[36]
Indifference; act for herself, no longer wishes to, in nervous weakness: ***cur.***[54]
Indifference; desires, has no, no action of the will: hell. ***verat.***[54]
Indifference; window, looks hours at: androc.[222] mez.[30]
Initiative, lack of: anh.[119] aur.[127] calc.[127] calc-f.[149] hydro-c.[149] ign.[127] iod.[30] lach.[30] lyc.[30] onop.[149] rhus-t.[30] saroth.[119] sil.[155] sulph.[30] thala.[149]
Mildness; complaining, bears suffering, even outrage without: ***ign.***[54]
No, cannot say: ***ambr.***[162] murx.[185] ozone[227] staph.[185]
Quiet disposition: abies-c. aesc.[25] aloe ***alum.*** am-c.[10] anh.[119] ars.[36] asar. aur.[10] ***bamb-a.***[1184] ***bell.*** bism.[10] brom.[10] bruc.[10] bufo[58] calc.[189] cand-a.[239] cann-i.[36] caps. ***caust.***[10] cham.[10] chel.[25] choc.[222] ***cic.*** clem. coca[36] cocc. cupr-s.[36] dios.[36] dros.[36] eryth.[36] euph. euphr.[10] fic.[102] ***gels.*** germ.[222] ***hell.***[10] hydrog.[222] ***hyos. ign.*** ip.[10] kali-m.[192] lac-h.[229] ***lach.*** lyc. mang. meny.[36] mur-ac. naja[36] nat-m.[1] nux-v. op.[10] petr. **PH-AC.** plat. ***plb.*** psil.[164] puls. rheum[10] sabad.[10] sars. scut.[25] sep. sil. stann. thuj.[54] tub.[85] valer.[54] viol-o. viol-t. zinc.
Quiet disposition; inactive, and, after losing his accustomed brightness: lyc.[8]
Sadness; quiet: ars.[30] ***hell.***[54] ign. nux-v. ph-ac.[30] puls.[30] ziz.[54]
Servile, obsequious, submissive: cham.[1] lyc.[85] m-arct.[85] **PULS.**[122] sil.[30] strept.[149] sulph.[30]
Spineless: am-c.[30] bar-c.[30] calc.[30] sil.[155]
Staring; thoughtless: androc.[222] brom.[54] carbn-s.[54] carc.[227] cench.[58] choc.[222] cic.[5] **HELL.**[54] ***hydr-ac.***[54] hyos.[58] ign.[8] lap-mar-c.[194] ***merc-c.***[54] ***puls.***[54] ran-b.[54] stram.[58]
Weeping; persuaded, when: bell.[10] calc.[10] ign.[10] plat.[10]
Yielding disposition: bamb-a.[1184] calc-sil.[58] cann-s.[122] carc.[193] cic.[58] ***cocc.***[5] ***cori-r.***[10] ***croc.***[10] cupr.[5] ign.[58] kiss.[36] **LYC.**[5] ***m-arct.***[5] murx.[102] nat-m.[189] ***nux-v.***[30] ph-ac.[102] phos.[5] **PULS.**[58] sep.[102] sil.[5] staph.[30]
Yielding disposition; children, in: bar-c.[162] fl-ac.[127] puls.[127]
Yielding; alternating with obstinacy: cupr.[137]

ADAM. Sh, 126 - I feel like I want to hibernate, not to be seen and keep warm. I want to curl up somewhere warm and forget the world. I could easily have stayed in bed. 7, 6C, 06:08:00
Sh, 184 - I didn't have any competitive feeling. All my senses went out and I didn't feel the need to get involved, so spent the evening observing and feeling. 7, 6C, 12:22:00
Sh, 188 - Lack of confidence. I feel worthless. I haven't got a life. All that I have revolves around boyfriend. If something happened to him I'd be at a loss. No direction. 22, 200C, 01:XX:XX
Sh, 262 - Resentful, feeling aware of being used by husband and family; having to fit into their demands rather than have a life of my own. 8, 6C, 17:XX:XX
Sh, 293 - Before taking the remedy I had said "Yes" to my husband about something I didn't want to do. After taking the remedy I felt angry about this, realized I didn't have to do it and changed my mind. 1, 12C, 00:00:45
ANAN. Al, 5 - Restless, suspicious, and very irritable character, or apathetic and as if besotted.(intoxicated)
ANDROC. Sh, 31 - Felt remote and ineffectual, a dreamy state. Felt more like a spectator than a participant. (25)
Sh, 34 - Much more untidy, the house was a mess and it didn't bother her. Made ineffectual efforts to tidy up and then lost interest. Desire to sit undisturbed and just look. (25)
Sh, 179 - Extreme anguish and restlessness, but at the same time felt like an observer of my condition, watching it all transpire without being able to change anything. Mind fixed on the physical anguish. It dominates my senses. (21)
BRASS. Sh, 14 - Very irritable with no cause, snapping at the children for no reason; apathy, can't be bothered to do anything; restless, twitchy, can't settle to anything 3I, 00:04:00
CHAM. Ha, 491 - Serious reservedness; calm submission to his profoundly felt fate (destiny).

CROT-H. He, 13 - Marked indifference, seems only half alive; utter apathy.

GELS. He, 33 - Effects (ailments from) of grief; cannot cry; when thinking of his symptoms (disease), also when spoken to of his loss ; >from diverting talk; oppression and palpitation of heart; feels a sense of peril (danger, harm, risk) ; face flushed; sleeplessness; subdued (subjugate, yielding) manner; ...

GERM. Sh, 120 - Easily led of others opinion, and provoked. Sensitive to others attempts at restricting me. Feel like a teenager, but I don't dare to protest. I just feel it inside. 18, 30C, 04:00:00

Sh, 151-.... I feel I have no real contact with people, I have no emotion at all except for a feeling of isolation and a concern that people may not like me. I wish someone would cuddle me. By 10 o'clock I have a definite aversion to people, especially certain people- the stubborn or authoritarian kind. I become deeply involved in my own thoughts and can be very irritable and even angry when the thoughts are interrupted by people, but I don't show any signs of anger or irritation. The fate of other people leaves me cold, but I know this is not right. My mind is blank and I feel I could just sit and stare. I have no feelings, no emotions! I think a lot about my state of mind and try to understand it; it puzzles me. What is missing? Eating removes this thoughtful mood. By afternoon and evening I become gradually more involved with what I am doing but still feel isolated even when in the company of other people. I don't mind listening to people, but I contribute little to conversation. This state lasted for three days. 16, 30C, 04:XX:XX

Sh, 37 - Difficult to concentrate, staring out of the window. Must find something to eat. Inefficient. I am feeling very far away. 18, 30C, 04:00:00

HALI-L. Sh, 143 - Organized. I feel if I could get things neat and organized the world would be perfect, but I can never get to that point, because there will be a flow. Trying to get things organized at home, which is like trying to get my eyes focused . Other times I just stared out the window, unfocussed. I either feel totally in flow with the universe, or floating aimlessly down a river. When I'm unfocussed, it's like a place where you can get lost, as if you're going to lose it. When I'm focused, I bring it all in, in the present, There. like meditating, or seeing God. When I'm unfocussed it's like I'll go into the abyss, and won't come back, go crazy. 08, 30C, 31:XX:XX

Sh, 375 - Just wants to crawl away, hide in a hole, do something else. Hard to get motivated. This feeling about one job she has to do spills over into everything else and she doesn't want to do anything. 09, 6C, 03:XX:XX

HYDROG. Sh, 171 - Feel more patient and accepting during my period. When water poured through the ceiling from an over-full bath, I just sat there and let it flood the floor because I didn't want to disturb the cat sitting on my knee. 12, 6C, 27:XX:XX

Sh, 184 - Feel despondent, indifferent, apathetic, separated from things and don't care. Deep sighing with sense of resignation. Can't be bothered to do things. 16, 30C, 02:XX:XX

IGN. He, 14 - Inclined to be very secretive (taciturn) and passive.(yielding)

He, 36 - Anxiety as though something terrible had happened cannot speak because of it; hurry, fearfulness, terror, alternating with irresolution and inertness.

He, 49 - Mild disposition; bears suffering, even outrage (offenses), without complaining.

IRID. Sh, 332 - On waking this morning was reminded of childhood illness. Same sense of not wanting to move, of not wanting to do anything, of not wanting to talk to anyone, just wanting to sleep and sleep the rest of my life away. In a way that feeling has always been with me and it is only by driving myself on that I have managed to achieve anything. It summarizes my feelings of everything being an effort, of spontaneous enthusiasm missing, of being too serious and lacking joy. A27

LYC. He, 29 - Want of self confidence; indecision; timidity; resignation.

MAG-M. Ha, 16 - Joyless and passive, whatever she looks at is repugnant (disgusting, offensive) to her, she answers very unwillingly,..

PULS. Ha, 18 - Mild, bashful, gentle, yielding disposition.
He, 19 - Silent mood; inclined to silent grief with submissiveness.
SIL. He, 16 - Yielding, faint-hearted, anxious mood.

YOUNG

Adolescent, felt he was again: androc.[222]
Childish behavior: acon. aeth.[137] ***agar.***[5] alco.[36] aloe[130] alum. ambr.[137] anac. ***apis*** ***arg-n.*** arn.[193] ars.[5] **BAR-C.**[122] ***bar-m.*** bell.[5] bov.[162] bufo calad. calc.[189] carb-an. carb-v. ***carbn-s.*** chlol. **CIC.** con.[137] ***croc.*** crot-c. germ.[222] ***hell.***[137] hyos.[5] ***ign.*** kali-br. kres.[144] lach.[137] lyc.[137] ***nat-c.***[137] ***nux-m.*** nux-v.[5] ***op.*** par. ***ph-ac.***[137] phos.[189] pic-ac.[137] plb.[137] puls. rhus-t. seneg. sep.[137] sil.[137] ***stram.*** sulfa.[114] sulph.[137] thyr.[137] tub.[193] verat.[137] viol-o.
Childish behavior, sadness, in: ***kali-br.***[54]
Childish behavior; body grows, but: bufo[130]
Dancing; desire for, fetus, of, to music: carc.[147]
Delirium; romping, with, children: agar.
Delusions; adolescent, he was again: androc.[222]
• born into the world and was overwhelmed with wonder at the novelty of his surroundings, feels as if newly: cori-r.[58]
• cat, kitten, an newly born: lap-mar-c.[194]
• child, he is again a, acts like a, and: ***cic.***
• child, sitting on low benches in rows as in a schoolroom: bell.[8]
• childish fantasies, has: lyc.
• companions, companions of his youth, is with the: aether.
• room, people in, sees, babies, full of white and colored: morph.[85]
Dreams; animals, dogs, many young dogs, fastening themselves tightly, in constant succession on various parts of his body: lyc.[36]
➤ childhood, about: ozone[227]
➤ childhood, about, past events mixed with present events: ozone[227]
➤ children, about, babies: choc.[222]
➤ children, about, younger, were ten years: ozone[227]
➤ children, became a three year old, and rejoiced much: mag-c.[36]
➤ excrements, youths defecating enormous amounts of: hydrog.[222]
➤ girl, that he is a: apis.
➤ houses, like the house of her youth: ozone[227]
➤ youth, time of: **SIL.**[36]
Helplessness; feeling of, infant, feels like a: hell.[54]
Irritability; old, childish people, in: sulph.[137]
Lewdness; man searching for little girls: caust.[30] phos.[30] plat.[30] verat.[30]
Religious affections; puberty, in: ***ars.***[122] ***calc.***[122] ***lach.***[122] ***sulph.***[122]
Sentimental; young persons, in: ant-c.[85] ign.[85]
Talk; childish: acon. ***arg-n.*** bar-c.[58] lyc.[122]

ADAM. Sh, 79 - Hurriedwild. Husband says I look wild, like a jungle child moving rapidly, jerky movements in different directions. Very excitable as if about to lose control. 10, 6C, 19:XX:XX
ANDROC. Sh, 129 - It seemed as though he was a different person, very similar to the way he had been in adolescence, but in a much more powerful manner. These emotions were so intense he wanted to rip his chest apart to let them out. He lost all control over his emotions, which seemed to come from a deep and distant part of himself, a darker side. He desired to continue the proving for the rest of his life. (29)
Sh, 155 - At night —brain revving away like crazy, thoughts racing through his head. Very interesting and exciting thoughts. Stayed awake til early morning, enjoying himself tremendously, and felt young again. (4)
HALI-L. Sh, 211 - I allowed my mother to mother me for the first time. It was a wonderful visit. For the first time ever I was allowing myself to be vulnerable and allowed her to love me. I had never felt I was the child with her before. These thoughts were foreign to me. 01, 30C, 21:XX:XX
Sh, 327 - I want to sleep. Want to be left alone, like a kid just before he goes to sleep. I don't want to bother with people anymore. 08, 30C, 34:XX:XX
Sh, 402 - I felt pathetic, defeated and vulnerable. I was reaching on a high shelf for pots for plants. All the pots and soil came tumbling down. Was knocked on the

head, on the vertex. Dirt all over me, and I thought, "This is perfect. This is exactly how I feel." I felt like I had to just give up —give up the bravado. I'm exhausted, I'm just going to rest. I just wanted to go into a little ball and lick my wounds. Felt very much like childhood symptoms. I felt very young. 01, 30C, 18:XX:XX

Sh, 727 - Overwhelming images of very wrinkled skin on bony naked legs and buttocks of premature babies covered in meconium. Wiping meconium off, and then it changed to naked featherless young birds — necks and upper bits of the birds. They were sitting in meconium. 20, 30C, 01:00:40

Sh, 867 - Memories of being fed as a child and having no choice of what to eat. 20, 30C, 08:23:50

Sh, 883 - Lying in bed this morning, inner vision of lifting up old clothes from a pile, ready to be given away, one by one. Underneath them, all an image of the inside of an egg without a shell and I could see fine, red veins on the membrane and one eye on an unhatched fledgling. The feathers were wet, and the membrane around it was complete. 20, 30C, 10:00:30

HYDROG. Sh, 34 - I felt myself really getting into my yoga and exploring new positions. At one point, I ended up playing with my toes like a baby. 08, 30C, 00:XX:XX

IRID. Sh, 102 - Just before sleep, image came into head from nowhere. Sitting on an air current as if it was a soft comfy settee foam cushion. Started to move over a landscape, took me high up, trees, towns, like the flying sequence from The Snowman. The air was so supportive, like floating on water. It had real substance but unlike water it was bouncy. There was no way I was going to fall. I was sitting back, not floating, tummy down. Felt like a child bouncing on the air. Fun —at the same time sense of awe, experiencing something for the first time. No sense of danger — trust. Floatiness experienced before with cannabis but then I was anxious, "Would I get back into body?" With this I was still in my body —no separation. G44

Sh, 103 - Felt light and young, found things fun and amusing. Walking effortlessly, easy, as if not touching the ground. Q1

NEON. Sh, 63 - I notice a foolish and irresistible desire to spy on my partner through the keyhole in the door to his study. I now remember doing this a couple of times yesterday (on the first day of the proving) as well. I am finding it ridiculous, laughing to myself. I feel like a mischievous child, doing something it shouldn't do, giggling away to myself. It makes me feel excited in a childish sense. I have never felt compelled to spy on anyone ever -be it through a keyhole or otherwise. Very strange. 02, 6C, 01:06:40

Sh, 69 - Recognized a change in awareness -a vaguely stoned,unreal feeling. Giggly, childish, grinning. Felt light. 05, 12C, 05:05:XX

Sh, 159 - Images of newborn babies crying. 20, 6C, 00:10:15

J.A. Mirilli, MD

In the very beginning of my homeopathic studies, I understood that because of the great amount of information that is part of the Repertory and the Materia Medica, I should dedicate myself also to organize better the homeopathic knowledge. Everybody recognizes that the homeopaths are not able to dispose in their mind all the homeopathic knowledge, needing, for this reason, instruments to help him in the search of symptoms. At this time, the Clinical Materia Medica and the Kent's Repertory were the main sources of studies for the most part of the homeopaths, and the homeopathic knowledge was transmitted in a dogmatic form. I wondered about the origin of Repertory and CMM's symptoms. Only when I got in touch with the Pure Materia Medica I saw the experimental nature of the homeopathic symptom, my studies were dedicated toward the foundation and organization of the symptoms from the PMM.

When I came close to the Thematic methodology study of the homeopathic symptoms, I saw a great possibility of this method to be applied to reorganize the PMM and the Repertories.

The classes I attended, formerly at the Kentian Course, after with Dr. Masi Elizaldi, himself, and later at the Training Course of the GEHSH, directed by Dr. Aldo Farias Dias, inspired and gave me the will to an integral dedication to the compilation of a Thematic Repertory able to express the thematic Philosophy of the study of homeopathic symptoms. It was a hard task to start the study of the PMMs from the beginning, searching to organize the symptoms by themes.

The result was amazing: totally revolutionary aspects were discovered. The Repertory symptoms were enriched with new medicines coming directly from PMMs, and new rubrics were suggested. The organization methodology itself was in check because of the thematic richness of PMM symptoms that was not supported by the entries of the repertories, and - the most surprising ! - the thematic classification gave us the possibility to observe the psychodynamics' of each medicine, relating the successive and consequent concatenation of themes that are part of the complete homeopathic symptoms from the PMMs. In the Repertory, the same did not happen because the symptoms were divided in parts and presented in alphabetical order. In the Barthel's Repertory, for example, we can observe that symptoms of *Pulsatilla* are related to the **forsaken** theme: - *Delusions; alone, she is always,, - Delusions; alone world, she is a. in the, - Delusions; deserted, forsaken, is - Delusions; neglected, of being, - Forsaken; isolation, sensation of.* In the Hahnemann's PMM, we have the complete symptom (Ha, 1143) : *"Her head is so quiet and all about her is so empty as if she were alone in the house and in the world; she does not wish to talk to any one, just as if all around her were no concern of her and she belonged to nobody."* In this case, we can see the symptoms apart from the Repertory, and psycodynamically presented.

The study of the **theme-words**, i.e. the most important words from the PMMs symptoms, gave us a broader richness of vocabulary in relation to that of the Repertory. For example, we can create new repertory entries based in theme-words from the PMMs, **Far away, sensation of**: Cann-s: *He, 5; Al, 44 (distance); Med: He, 9 (far); Syph: He, 11 (far-away); Thuj: AI, 5 (distance).* In this case the words **distance, far, far-away,** all refer to the sensation of far away that the patient relates.

The problem was how to transmit those conclusions to the Homeopaths, and, more than that, how to strengthen the possibilities of the right choice of medicines, based upon a greater evaluation of patient's homeophatical symptoms . It was logical that new tools should be created, making it possible to the Homeopaths to expand their horizons. Those new tools, necessarily, should be capable of showing the richness of the PMM symptoms and, at the same time, should be available for fast consultation, giving the Homeopaths the possibility of using them at their homeopathic clinics. This was an ambitious enterprise, because everybody recognizes the difficulties of studying the PMMs, where the symptoms are dispersed in dozens of volumes randomly presented, not to speak about the difficulties for the foreigners of reading texts in the English language. Since the beginning, I was aware that the work was not only to add more medicines to the rubrics, nor to create new entries, but to create a new concept of organization of homeopathic symptoms.

I started to organize by themes the symptoms from the main PMMs, dispersed among 25 volumes (4 Hahnemann, 10 T.Allen, 10 Hering, and 1 in the Nosodes de H. Allen). More than 4,000 symptoms from 17,000 that compound the PMMs' mental symptoms were selected. The result was amazing once more, since the Thematic Repertory (formed by 300 mental themes) was organized from almost 15.000 PMM citations (a single symptom can be pointed in different themes).

In a careful examination of PMM symptoms, we can observe that certain words give **significance** to symptoms, and these are the **theme words**. We can make a group of theme words and create thematic groups. Those theme groups are the same PMM symptoms linked by their most significant words. It was necessary to deeply scrutinize the meaning of most important words present in symptoms in the English language, and to search for their analogues, and look for resemblances. A Dictionary (a word index) with more than 4,000 words in the English language was created, with the main words of PMM mental symptoms, and their synonyms and similar words. Words, instead of being defined as Dictionary entries, are exemplified, in this case, by the symptoms in which they occur. Throughout the reading of many symptoms described by the same word, we can capture its meaning in the context of the homeopathic symptom (and not simply like a Dictionary definition). The word hypochondria, for example, in the PMM classical texts, can be, in some symptoms, similar to melancholia or other symptoms - fear of illness, or illusion of illness- like in the contemporary meaning of that word. These studies resulted in the compilation of the **Word Index**.

Now, I present an opportune combination of the Thematic Repertory and the Word Index in the same volume. Symptoms in the Word Index are listed by words, observing the alphabetical criteria of their main **theme-words**.

We can observe by thematic technique that symptoms, as a whole, have one or many **purposes,** that are **themes;** they are the subject that symptoms are about, in an explicit or implicit form; and we can see a **specificity** or **modality** that is the **theme-word**, i.e., the most important word that gives significance to a symptom, where we can find the **peculiarity** of each **theme**, in each medicine. We consider the Word Index as a Repertory of theme words, followed by the main theme words that compound the PMM symptoms.

I have used the Word Index in my clinic as a side repertory, extending the entry menu of

traditional Repertories. I can always remember the case of a child presenting a pattern of chronic allergy, in which the main local symptom was a night cough access, that condemned him (and his family) to insomnia. At the evaluation of mental symptoms, the most characteristic, after his mother, was that in games, he always wanted to win, and when frustrated, he suffered in excess, and because of this, he had a peculiar behavior. In the Repertory, there is not the **Winning, desire of,** and for that reason I looked for the word **win** in Word Index, and as I did not find it, so I looked for its opposite: **to lose,** and then, I found the symptom (Hering, 37, *Nux Vomica*) in which the patient spent all night suffering on a process in which he could **gain** or **lose** very much money. Afterwards, I verified that many symptoms of *Nux Vomica* are related to **money** and **ambition** themes. At additional consultations of this patient, I could evaluate general and local symptoms. I made a specific evaluation of coughing with particular local symptoms (more than 20), to arise other possible medicines related to that mental pattern. To my surprise, the most indicated medicine was *Nux Vomica* again. In high and spared doses it showed to be very efficient, reverting the principal mental symptoms and promoting a surprising psicophysical healing. As in this case, there were many others, where consulting the Thematic Repertory, and the Word Index,_opened to me new horizons.

It is very important to underline that results are very restricted in computer word - scanning of PMM and Repertory. In the Thematic Repertory and in the Word Index we can evaluate not only the words, but the **intentions** (themes) of symptoms. In the research of the word **abandon** in the PMMs, for example, only the symptoms that have the word abandon (or forsaken) are shown. In the Thematic Repertory, at the Forsaken theme, we have a lot of symptoms with the sense of forsaken but they do not present the word abandon (or forsaken). In the Word Index , theme-words are linked by a similar significance; otherwise, in computerized word research - in traditional homeopathic programs - many times symptoms are presented with the same words, but with different meanings and, The word **wrong** generally means **mistake**, but we can find the same word with the **injustice** meaning " Delusions; wrong, suffered, has"; "Dreams; accusations, crime, wrongful of" or wrong sas **misfortune** "Fear; wrong, of something, indescribable". For that reason, the pure research of words in PMMs and Repertory are restrict.

I hope this set of books can be helpful to the Homeopathic Community, and that they serve as a guide of symptoms, with the objective to alleviate human suffering, by the right choice of the most similar medicine prescriptions.

ABROT.

He,12- Exceedingly peevish, feels as if she would like to do something cruel (sadistic, torture); no humanity. Themes: sadism, wicked

He,2- No capacity for thinking, as if all bodily and mental power were gone. Themes: knowledge, energy

He,3- Thinks her brain is softening. (dissolving) Themes: disease, ruined, disintegration

He,4- Excited, loquacious, feels like shouting. Themes: talk, pleasure

ABSIN.

Al,4- Very tranquil as if brain were rounded (spherical) and symmetrical.(balanced, regular, organized) Themes: organization, perfection

Al,S-5- Terrifying hallucination of persons pursuing him. Themes: persecution

Al,S-6- Terrifying hallucinations, he sees all kinds of animals, cats and rats of all colors, grotesque animals, fancies that he is pursued by soldiers. Themes: animal, officer, horrible, ugly, persecution

Al,S-7- Hallucination of vision and of hearing, that is pursued by imaginary enemies; hallucinations of various kinds, of naked women, etc. Themes: enemy, persecution, sexual

Al,S-9- Fear of assassination. Themes: murdered

ACET-AC.

He,3- Fancies he has an ulcer in his stomach. Themes: disease

He,6- Anxiety; grieves about his sickness and his children. Themes: disease, grief, cares, others, child

ACON-F.

Al,3- In the intervals of relief from distressing symptoms, he laughed and joked about his very comical condition;...(proper disease) Themes: sarcasm, disease, pleasure

ACON.

Al,14- Excessive disagreeable restlessness; without occasion for hurrying, he is in the greatest haste, every obstacle that delays his rapid pace is excessively annoying; he knocks against some people who do not get out of his way fast enough, and runs in breathless haste up the steps;... Themes: restless, hurry, obstructed, impatience, time

Al,15- He raves, though awake; jumps out of bed and imagines he is driving sheep.(guide) Themes: conduct

Al,21- Unsteadiness (inconstant) of ideas; on attempting to think of one thing, another forces it out of the mind and this is supplanted by another, and so on, until he becomes quite confused. Themes: dispersion

Al,22- Restlessness, uninterrupted, unpleasant; he must now sit, now stand, now walk, he does not know what is the matter. Themes: movement, restless

Al,23- Excessive restlessness, all movements and actions are performed with great haste and hurry. Themes: restless, movement, hurry

Al,27- Alternate attacks of opposite moral symptoms. Themes: antagonism

Al,28- Variable humour, at one time gay, at another dejected. Themes: antagonism, sadness

Al,30- Now he doubts his recovery, now he is full of hope. (despair x hopeful) Themes: disease, doubtful

Al,46- Anxiety only transiently relieved by drinking cold water. Themes: water

Al,47- Anxiety as though a great misfortune would happen to him. Themes: misfortune

Al,49- Anxiety which does not allow him to remain in one place, he must constantly walk about. (restlessness) Themes: restless, movement

Al,53- Dolorous anxious complaints, with pusillanimous (cowardly) fears, despair, loud wailing (laments) and weeping, and bitter reproaches. Themes: conscience, despair, cowardice

Al,55- Flickering (spark, flash) before vision makes him anxious on street, he thinks he constantly jostles (press)the passers by. Themes: obstructed, touch

Al,56- Anxiety he believes he will soon die. Themes: death
Al,59- Feeling as if his last hour had come. Themes: death, time
Al,63- Dread of some accident happening. Themes: accidents, misfortune
Al,65- Fear that he might stagger and fall. Themes: fall
Al,66- Great timidity after a severe fright (fear), afraid to go out unattended (abandoned, helplessness) after dark, is unable to control his feelings of apprehensive fear. Themes: cowardice, go out, helplessness, dark, fearful
Al,67- Fear of ghosts. Themes: ghosts
Al,71- Dejected, as if she had no life in her. (lifeless) Themes: lifeless, sadness
Al,92-...feels that all the mental operations transpire (develop) in the region of the stomach; after two hours,...the thinking power returns again to the head. Themes: identity
Al,S-2- Some few hallucinations, such as imagining his head was three times its original size. Themes: great, grow
Ha,502- He does everything in a hurry (quick), and runs about the house. Themes: hurry,
Ha,505- Morose, as though she had no life in her. (animation) Themes: energy, lifeless
Ha,510- Sometimes he despairs of his recovery, sometimes he is full of hope. Themes: disease, hopeless, despair
Ha,511- After vomiting, immediate revival of hope. Themes: energy
Ha,514- Palpitation of the heart with great anxiety, oppression of the breathing and great weariness (lassitude) in all limbs... Themes: oppression, energy, heart
Ha,516- Inconsolable anxiety and piteous howling, with complaints and reproaches about (often triflings) evils. Themes: conscience, wrong, disease
Ha,517- Piteous (miserable), anxious complaints, with cowardly fears, despair, loud whining weeping, bitter complaints and reproaches. Themes: censorious, cowardice, conscience, despair
Ha,518- Fear lest he should fall. Themes: fall
Ha,521- Lucid vision: he says, now my beloved (70 miles away) must have sung the difficult passage (of Beethoven) that I was just singing. Themes: love, clairvoyance, music
Ha,523- The slightest noise is intolerable to him. Themes: noise
Ha,526- He takes every joke in bad part. Themes: offenses
Ha,535- Lively power of imagination. Themes: energy
Ha,538- Dread of impending death. Themes: death
Ha,539- Mortal anxiety recurring from time to time. Themes: death
Ha,540- Lamentable fears of impending death. Themes: fearful, death
Ha,541- Fear of some misfortune happening to him. Themes: misfortune
He,2- Clairvoyance; conscious that his beloved, miles away, was singing a certain piece. Themes: clairvoyance, love, union, music
He,21- Delirium, with talk about death. Themes: death, talk
He,23- Pains are so intolerable, they drive him crazy; he becomes very restless. Themes: insanity, disease, restless
He,28- Moaning, anxious lamentations; reproaches from trifling causes. Themes: conscience, conscientious
He,31- Restlessness, agony, internal anxiety; does everything in great haste (rapidity); must move about or change position often. Themes: restless, hurry, movement
He,35- Sadness with solicitude; concerned about future; about her recovery or fears loss of reason. (insanity) Themes: future, disease, insanity, sadness
He,36- Extreme timidity, especially after a fright; afraid (fear) in dark. Themes: fearful, timidity, cowardice, dark
He,37- Fears to go where is any excitement (tumult) or many people (crowd); thinks she is jostling (pressing) against everyone she meets (oppressed); countenance (expression) expressive of timidity; constant dread (fear) lest she stagger (vacillated) and fall. Themes: crowd, oppression, suffocation, cowardice, fall
He,38- fear of ghosts. Themes: ghosts
He,39- Fear of death; during pregnancy or confinement; with prolapsus uteri; with great loquacity or anxiety in region of

heart. Themes: death, heart, disease, talk
He,40 -Thrice he became blind and affirmed that death was at hand. Themes: disease, death, obstructed
He,41- Predicts day of death; bids (offer) her friends good-bye.(farewell) Themes: death, clairvoyance, friend
He,47- Vexed at trifles; takes every joke in bad part. Themes: bothered, offenses
He,51- Ailments from fright: afraid (fear) in dark; vertigo; faintness; trembling; cardiac weakness; threatened miscarriage (abortion); impending cessation of menstrual flow;.. Themes: fearful, fit, heart, dark, disease
He,53- Ailments from vexation (worry, care), with fear or vehemence: congestion; palpitation; fever; anxiety, beside himself; threatened miscarriage ; apoplectic congestion. Themes: bothered, heart, disease,
He,7- Memory lively, or weak; what has just been done seems like a remote dream; cannot remember dates. Themes: unreal
He,8- Ideas haunt (obsess) him, cannot get rid of them. Themes: dwells, seized, mortification

ACT-SP.

He,12- Hopeless; constant apprehension; anxious solicitude when quiet. Themes: hopeless
He,13- Anxiety with urging in heart. Themes: heart
He,14- Fear of death, especially at night in bed. Themes: death, dark
He,16- Desperation of success of every, even most trifling undertaking. Themes: succeed, failure, despair
He,17- Irresolution, inconstancy and caprice. Themes: doubtful, irresolution, dispersion, capricious
He,3- Judgment perplexed; bewildering fits, almost to insanity. Themes: justice, insanity
He,4- Self-deception; self-satisfaction. Themes: vanity, himself, haughty
He,6- Great desire to work, though incapacity of it. Themes: work, unfit
He,7- Inclined to debauchery.(seduction, lewdness) Themes: lascivious, sexual

ADAM.

Sh,1- I felt as if a heavy, gray cloud with red specks descended down to my chest entering into me. 7, 6C, 02:00:XX Themes: heavy, seized
Sh,100- Sensitive to music that I know and like — very nostalgic. 20, 1M, 11:XX:XX Themes: music, nostalgia, homesickness
Sh,105- I went shopping for a red sweater but couldn't find one bright enough. I never wear red. 7, 6C, 12:10:00 Themes: bright
Sh,106- Things are very black and white for me. 7, 6C, 04:19:00 Themes: antagonism
Sh,107- Wearing light things instead of dark. Want light next to my skin. Desire for yellow silk underwear. 16, 12C, 26:XX:XX Themes: light
Sh,108- I feel like burying myself in grass and earth. I love touching and covering my hands with earth. I want to be enclosed and hidden in the earth. 20, 1M, 08:XX:XX Themes: touch, fire
Sh,110- Intense feeling of wanting to break through. Felt it around the solar plexus. Just felt like I wanted to burst out. 6, 30C,10:XX:XX Themes: disintegration
Sh,111- Sense of waiting for things to explode, more in others than in me. 7, 6C, 59:00:XX Themes: disintegration
Sh,112- Thoughts, on waking, were that I was like a sponge that absorbs in the day and gets squeezed out at night via my dreams. 11, 30C, 06.XX.XX Themes: constriction
Sh,113- Waking, my hands were together, but I did not know which one was holding which; which fingers were next to each other. I did not know where everything was. I lay for several seconds wondering where my hands were, or what they were doing. Could hardly get together. 5, 30C, 00:12:50 Themes: disintegration
Sh,115- Averse company. I wanted to spend time alone, which lasted throughout the entire proving. 1, 12C, 00:00:50 Themes: company
Sh,119- Feel drawn in on myself; don't find it easy to extend outwards. 8, 6C, 04:XX:XX Themes: isolation
Sh,121- Wanting to be alone with own thoughts. Guilt over past event: daughter's back injury that occurred 22 years

ago as result of my taking her to a horse riding lesson. 5, 30C, 20:XX:XX Themes: company, conscience, past

Sh,122- I do not want to go out at all, just need to be on my own. Unusual for me and I feel drained. 12, 30C, 22:XX:XX. Themes: go out, energy

Sh,124- I want to be alone with things being done for me. For example, I didn't want to drive so I got a mini-cab. 7, 6C, 06:10:00 Themes: company

Sh,126- I feel like I want to hibernate, not to be seen and keep warm. I want to curl up somewhere warm and forget the world. I could easily have stayed in bed. 7, 6C, 06:08:00 Themes: company, yielding

Sh,127- I don't want to go out of the flat 7, 6C, 08:00:XX Themes: go out

Sh,128- I really need to escape, booked trip to France. 7, 6C 14:00:xx Themes: escape, travel

Sh,129- Irritability about intrusion of space by my house guest. I felt hemmed in. 11, 30C, 07.XX.XX Themes: invaded, bothered

Sh,130- I was angry at my house guest and wanted to be left alone, at breakfast.11, 30C, 12.XX.XX Themes: anger, company

Sh,132- Being told that I'm grumpy really irritates me. Why can't I be let alone and they can just go away. 7, 6C, 05:17:00 Themes: bothered, company

Sh,134- I am behaving differently with strangers, containing myself, letting them make the first move. 7, 6C, 07:21:30 Themes: reserved

Sh,135- I am less grumpy during the day. People are saying I am holding back, different, not so open. 7, 6C, 07:21:30 Themes: reserved

Sh,140- Does not like to talk. As if nothing needs to be said: it's all obvious so why talk about it. 2, 12C, 111:XX:XX Themes: talk

Sh,144- I don't want to be touched or talked to. 7, 6C, 04:08:00 Themes: touch, talk

Sh,150- Felt separate from friends today, which was unusual. I felt outside them. I was quiet. Definitely unusual. 5, 30C, 00:06:50 Themes: isolation, friend

Sh,151- The "cloud" feeling has left me with a sense of detachedness and separateness. 7, 6C, 04:08:00 Themes: isolation

Sh,152- I feel the separateness of me from the world, not my spirit from my body, the whole of me, I can't touch the world. 7, 6C, 04:08:00 Themes: isolation

Sh,153- I feel very irritated, I need to maintain separateness to keep the grumpiness to myself. 7, 6C, 04:08:00 Themes: isolation

154- Very selfish to other peoples needs and cares — unseeing in that way. I do not want to listen to my mother's problems, or my friends'. 20, 1M, 11:XX:XX Themes: egotism

Sh,155- I am feeling disconnected from what is going on in my relationship. It's hard to understand why she couldn't take my overall viewpoint. She seems stuck. I cut off and disconnected from her. 7, 6C, 14:00:XX Themes: isolation

Sh,156- The weekend started with me locking myself and the boys and one dog out of the house, and the keys and one dog still inside. I got very upset then and the weekend just got worse and worse. I had blazing rows with everybody. Thought I was getting the flu. Thought I was surrounded by dirt. Wanted to just go to bed and take my boys and the dogs with me. Couldn't or wouldn't go to work on Monday. 18, 30C, 31:XX:XX Themes: fight, dirty

Sh,157- I am allowing myself to be detached and not fighting it. 7, 6C, 04:19:00 Themes: isolation

Sh,158- I feel detached and not sexual. I could bite my partner as a signal I loved her, not in a loving or hungry way. My partner said, "He is looking at me like a piece of steak, he wants to eat me. He looks like a cave man. He wants to nibble me." 7, 6C, 03:22:30 Themes: isolation, sexual, bite, wild

Sh,159- I felt detached during coition. 7, 6C, 13:23:00 Themes: sexual, isolation

Sh,160- Disliked being touched and uninterested in any sexual relationship. Began to be repulsed by boyfriend. 20, 1M, XX:XX:XX Themes: touch, sexual, loathing

Sh,163- A distant feeling, as if I'm not totally here, with need to blink left eye as if to clear it. 8, 6C, 20:00:00 Themes: isolation, unreal

Sh,165- I feel like I'm looking at the world through half-closed eyes, like slits. 7, 6C, 09:00:XX Themes: disintegration, isolation,

Sh,166- I felt confused and not myself. 7, 6C, 02:00:XX Themes: identity

Sh,169- I realize that the remedy was, for me, about structure. With the cloud lifted I have got back a sense of structure which I had lost. This morning I know who I am and what I am doing. 7, 6C, 11:08:00 Themes: organization

Sh,170- Husband's description: "You are like Alice in Wonderland in an unreal world." 10, 6C, XX:XX:XX Themes: unreal, isolation

Sh,178- I see myself as being too intrusive with people. 7, 6C, 14:00:XX Themes: offensive

Sh,180- Generally fairly severe mood, very straightforward and will say what is needed to be said. Quite strict and harsh, yet not tactless or mean. 20, 1M, XX:XX:XX Themes: offensive

Sh,181- I realized I am observing a lot and have a feeling of being observed. The observer bit is female aspect, and the male bit is a critical voice. 7, 6C, 06:06:00 Themes: observed, censured

Sh,182- Feel disconnected and distanced from everything. It's like keeping something in reserve, more observing. 7, 6C, 06:22:30 Themes: isolation, reserved

Sh, 183- I couldn't get involved in the conversation at family supper. I didn't feel the need to. I spent most of the evening being there, but observing. It was a strange experience but I felt very calm and present. 7, 6C, 12:22:00 Themes: family, isolation

Sh,184- I didn't have any competitive feeling. All my senses went out and I didn't feel the need to get involved, so spent the evening observing and feeling. 7, 6C, 12:22:00 Themes: isolation, yielding

Sh,185- Feeling detached from things, observing again, not touching the world. 7, 6C, 44:00:XX Themes: isolation

Sh,188- Lack of confidence. I feel worthless. I haven't got a life. All that I have revolves around boyfriend. If something happened to him I'd be at a loss. No direction. 22, 200C, 01:XX:XX Themes: confidence, unfit, yielding

Sh,189- Low self esteem. Felt I am not worthy or not pretty or not interesting enough for people. 20, 1M, XX:XX:XX Themes: confidence, failure, unfit

Sh,190- Very unhappy with my body, I want to escape from it, to run away from myself. I want to go from me. 20, 1M, 08:XX:XX Themes: himself, loathing, escape, unfortunate

Sh,191- I feel like vomiting out all my insides. I want to get rid of everything inside me I physically feel like vomiting all my stomach and even all my breath. I want everything to get out of me. 20, 1M, 07:XX:XX Themes: loathing, himself

Sh,192- Feel fat!!! 25SA, 5MMb, 09:XX:XX Themes: heavy

Sh,193- Felt had spoiled the proving by spraining ankle. Blamed myself. 8, 6C, 02:XX:XX Themes: conscience, hurt

Sh,194- Felt ugly, miserable and generally fed up with myself during menses, more intensely than I usually would at this time. 8, 6C, 17:XX:XX Themes: ugly, miserable, loathing, himself

Sh,195- Bad paranoia, that people hate me, anyone just walking down the street hates me. I think they will hit me. 20, 1M, 07:XX:XX Themes: persecution, hurt, anger

196- Very nervous and little self-confidence. I think people are laughing at me and hate me. 20, 1M, 07:XX:XX Themes: confidence, despised, anger

197- Suspicious confusion that people are making a fool of me, laughing at me. 2, 12C, XX:XX:XX Themes: despised, suspicious

Sh,198- I wanted thanks and acknowledgment for a particular act and I didn't get it. I didn't get resentful but I got hesitant and don't want to repeat the act. 7, 6C, 12:00:XX Themes: confidence

Sh,199- The downside was that I also experienced hurt more keenly and felt mortally wounded more often than is good for me, in situations that I would normally have shrugged off. And when I felt bad, I felt rotten. 18, 30C, XX:XX:XX Themes: rotten, offended

Sh,200- I felt like I had been treated badly, a mixture of insult and humiliation. 15, 12C, 01:09:45 Themes: offended, despised

Sh,201- Sensation of being wronged, of being betrayed, which affects my social relationships. 15, 12C, 08:XX:XX Themes: betrayed, prejudiced

Sh,202- Preoccupied with the past on waking, concerning betrayal of trust in relationships. 15, 12C, 07:XX:XX Themes: betrayed, suspicious

Sh,203- Insulted. The worst insult is being told I've become like my father. 7, 6C, 05:17:00 Themes: offended, father

Sh,204- I feel overwhelmingly hard done by (mistreated) and need to feel heard and understood. 7, 6C, 13:00:XX Themes: offended, sensitive

Sh,205- Get angry when criticized, yet easily critical of others.20, 1M, 06:XX:XX Themes: offended, censured, censorious

Sh,207- I am feeling very critical, casting a critical eye. 7, 6C, 03:00:XX Themes: censorious

Sh,208- I wanted to sack the receptionist 15 times in the last hour for stupidity. 7, 6C, 03:00:XX Themes: anger

Sh,210- I complained to another therapist who got upset. I thought "I am going nuts." I was upset that he was upset. It was just a little thing. I couldn't see why he couldn't see my point of view. 7, 6C, 03:00:XX Themes: contradiction

Sh,211- I felt very impatient with my patients. I was making a lot of judgments. 7, 6C, 03:00:XX Themes: impatience, censorious

Sh,212- Sharp and brusque with people. 8, 6C, 04:XX:XX Themes: offensive

Sh,213- Furious cold anger when money stolen from me. 2, 12C, 73:XX:XX Themes: anger, money, robbed

Sh,214- I am fidgety and angry and very jealous of people. I feel cold and empty and very angry, almost cruel. 20, 1M, 02:XX:XX Themes: anger, jealousy, wicked

Sh,215- I feel very angry and extremely intolerant, cold and hard and I hate myself for feeling these harsh unkind feelings. 20, 1M, 02:XX:XX Themes: anger, offensive, conscience

Sh,216- Feel harder, more rebellious. I will do what I want. Inconsiderate and unsympathetic. Unfeeling in relationship and sexually. 22, 200C, 01:XX:XX Themes: offensive, revolutionary, sexual

Sh,217- Impatient and intolerant with others. 20, 1M, 00:XX:XX Themes: impatience

Sh,218- Red anger with irregularly pounding heart. 2, 12C 73:XX:XX Themes: anger, heart

Sh,219- I recognized a familiar uncomfortable feeling as being one of anger. 1, 12C, 00:00:45 Themes: anger

Sh,221- I felt angry on waking, noise of people upstairs sounds like elephants. I want to kill them. I wanted to complain to them. 7, 6C, 03:06:00 Themes: anger, homicidal, noise

Sh,223- Anger with aggressive attitude, short tempered and intolerant. I lashed out verbally when my partner invaded my space. I knew it was out of proportion at the time. 7, 6C, 30:00:XX Themes: invaded, anger

Sh,226- Angry at my daughter for ignoring that I want my time to do my things. 10, 6C, 17:XX:XX Themes: anger, time

Sh,227- Get very easily angry. Needed to assert myself and pick on someone who I neither know nor respect. My anger was very violent. 20, 1M, 10:XX:XX Themes: anger, violence

Sh,228- Resentful towards others. 20, 1M, 10:XX:XX Themes: resentment, anger

Sh,229- Feeling very angry towards others and hate people. I want to be alone and away from people who upset me. I hate feeling angry and resentful, a lot of it is directed to myself. 20, 1M, XX:XX:XX Themes: anger, himself, resentment, solitude

Sh,234- Swearing and cursing. A lot to do, finding it hard to set priorities in my work and the needs of my family. 10, 6C, 19:XX:XX Themes: offensive, family

Sh,237- Quite a lot of anger — a strange kind of energy. I feel like things are changing all around me, like life is speeding along. 20, 1M, 09:XX:XX Themes: anger

Sh,238- Quickly felt remorse after anger. 8, 6C, 04:XX:XX Themes: remorse, conscience, anger

Sh,239- Would like some support. Cannot tolerate the emotional demands made on me. I ask for help or remedy. 2, 12C, 72:XX:XX Themes: helplessness

Sh,240- Anger from lack of physical or emotional support. 2, 12C, 73:XX:XX Themes: helplessness, anger

Sh,241- I feel angry and want to be comforted. 7, 6C, 03:07:30 Themes: anger, helplessness

Sh,242- Feeling very pathetic and scared of

people getting angry with me. 20, 1M, 10:XX:XX Themes: fearful, anger

Sh,243- Anger at people putting lights on instead of opening curtains. 16, 12C, 18:XX:XX Themes: light, anger

Sh,244- Anger with my attraction to P. He's a walker and I wanted to walk with him. I didn't want to be attracted but was, as if enchanted. 16, 12C, 18:XX:XX Themes: seized, sexual, anger, antagonism

Sh,246- Cried with despair. Nothing I do is right. Rocking from side to side, sobbing. Desire to stab with a knife or scissors. Felt very different from other humans. Long, late phone call ameliorates. 16, 12C, 43:XX:XX Themes: wrong, suicidal, despair, strange

Sh,262- Resentful, feeling aware of being used by husband and family; having to fit into their demands rather than have a life of my own. 8, 6C, 17:XX:XX Themes: resentment, yielding

Sh,269- The beginning of many "help me" phone calls from people in difficult relationships which they need to leave and can't. 2, 12C, 00:00:10 Themes: helpful

Sh,277- Exceptionally strong desire to leave my marriage and children, to live a clear unmuddled life alone. 2, 12C, 74:XX:XX-160:XX:XX Themes: forsakes, loathing, dirty, union, child

Sh,278- Felt I would create irreparable damage if I said how I feel. Thought I would say the most awful things that the kids would never recover from. Supreme effort to keep silent. Didn't want to be here. The kids were a hassle. I felt old and tired. Desire to get away from the fighting. 16, 12C, 17:XX:XX Themes: prejudiced, conscience, offensive, suppressed

Sh,283- My husband has commented that I am talking more and cuddling less, and I realize I do not feel so dependent on him, I feel more of an individual. 12, 30C, 07.:XX:XX. Themes: liberty

Sh,29- "Perfect" and "ideal" — someone commented I was using these words a lot. 8, 6C, 20:XX:XX Themes: perfection

Sh,292- It's crystal clear! Clarifying female roles. Clarification of issues. Realization — anger and depression in the past, had to do with conditioning, not saying what I wanted, not having my needs met. 10, 6C, 47:XX:XX Themes: knowledge, liberty, suppressed

Sh,293- Before taking the remedy I had said "Yes" to my husband about something I didn't want to do. After taking the remedy I felt angry about this, realized I didn't have to do it and changed my mind. 1, 12C, 00:00:45 Themes: yielding

Sh,295- On sniffing the remedy, I had an immediate vision and feeling of the place where I feel most at ease and comfortable (a cottage in the woods). A feeling of being at home. 1, 12C, 00:00:01 Themes: nostalgia

Sh,296- Thinking a lot about a cottage in Hampshire that I'd wanted to buy and feeling sad that I hadn't. Feeling that it would have been so blissful to be alone there, and be creative in the garden. No sound except birds, just to relax and be alone. 1, 12C, 01:XX:XX Themes: nostalgia, home, peace

Sh,297- I didn't want to go away to teach. Wanted to be at home. Feel happy at home with children. 2, 12C, 05:XX:XX Themes: go out, home, nostalgia

Sh,299- Want desperately to be at home. 8, 6C, 01:10:00 Themes: homesickness

Sh,3- Feeling like a cloud is lifting, world becoming clearer again and not feeling so irritable and grumpy. 7, 6C, 48:00:XX Themes: floating

Sh,303- I feel connected with my children, that a barrier I've erected due to the fear of losing them has gone. 8, 6C, 20:XX:XX Themes: integration

Sh,306- Determined to help children recognize and free themselves from family patterns and to be themselves. 10, 6C, 34:XX:XX Themes: liberty

Sh,307- Still an enormous desire to nurture and feed people. In the last month I have fed sixty people weekly during a political campaign. Made many friends. 2, 12C, 57:XX:XX Themes: helpful, friendly

Sh, 308- A conversation about death with my children. A feeling that they need some insurance; and I thought I would make a will, to make provisions for them, to clarify the situation. 2, 12C, 05:XX:XX Themes: helpful, death

Sh,309- Vision: during meditation, image of deceased mother. Sobbed at the loss of her friendship and love. Later felt good — something had lifted. 5, 30C, 15:06:20 Themes: nostalgia

Sh,31- The proving experience was very clear. There was a sharpness in both how I felt and what I saw. Mostly this was pleasant: brilliant sunshine through the drops of water in a shower, candlelight bouncing off wine glasses, tiny detail on the chrome-work of cars. 18, 30C, XX:XX:XX Themes: bright, conscientious

Sh,310- Feel orphaned after an angry phone call from my parents. Feel unparented. Oh well, what the hell. 2, 12C, 26:XX:XX Themes: helplessness

Sh,313, I feel very tall and large. I am a giant, 12:30 a.m. - powerful feeling. 20, 1M, 09:XX:XX Themes: great, energy, greatness

Sh,314- Feeling of absolute power, invincible. 16, 12C, 14:14:00 Themes: greatness, inexpugnable

Sh,317- Enjoy the powerful night force. I can fly in the dark. 16, 12C, 35:XX:XX Themes: fly, energy

Sh,33- Went out to dinner in a restaurant. Was very struck by how everything sparkled. Really dazzling. Asked my friend if it was particularly striking, but she just said it was all of the liquids on the table (water and wine in bottles and glasses.) 18, 30C, 29:XX:XX Themes: bright

Sh,34- After taking the remedy again, I was very struck again by sparkling—this time the sun in the shower. Before I took it, I seemed to be surrounded by dark and dirt. 18, 30C, XX:XX:XX Themes: dirty, bright

Sh,345- Lack of irritability in a crowded store and able to focus and be positive, I usually would have left within minutes. Placid and patient although tired and in pain. 12, 30C, 00:07:30 Themes: crowd

Sh,35- Delusion of being an Indian prince, with a turban and jewel on his Third Eye. 16, 12C, 31:XX:XX Themes: greatness

Sh,357- I have a great desire to feed huge nourishing meals to my family; to spend money in the achievement of their dreams. 2, 12C, 26:XX:XX Themes: money, helpful

Sh,359- Feeling a sense of wealth of prosperity of a beneficent universe. 32SA, 200C, XX:XX:XX Themes: wealth, helpful

Sh,36- White frost this morning. At last some purity in this world. Every ice crystal sparkled like jewels. 16, 12C, 27:XX:XX Themes: dirty, pure, bright

Sh,365- I am obsessed about the future and what's going to happen to me. A feeling, nothing specific, of vulnerability. 7, 6C, 05:07:00 Themes: future, fragile

Sh,37- Great joy at the beauty of the snow, especially at night, reflecting light. Sparkled like jewels, purity. After the snow, joy at seeing greens again, appeared brighter and clearer than before the snow. 16, 12C, 67:XX:XX Themes: pure, bright

Sh,374- Joyless, desired death. Looked at a pair of scissors and thought of suicide. 16, 12C, 17:XX:XX Themes: suicidal, death, pointed

Sh,376- Cried with despair. Nothing I do is right. Rocking from side to side sobbing. Desire to stab with a knife or scissors. Felt very different from other humans. Long, late phone call ameliorates. 16, 12C, 43:XX:XX Themes: despair, suicidal, pointed, strange

Sh,378- I have lost my enthusiasm, not so much sadness, but a heavy depression. Prefer to be on my own. Everything is an effort, feel I am carrying a heavy weight. 12, 30C, 04:XX:XX. Themes: heavy, company

Sh,379- Tearful and vulnerable. A situation I would normally cope with seemed threatening. 8, 6C, 01:20:00 Themes: fragile, menaced

Sh,387- Got terribly distressed. Sharp and keen sense of grief (over past issues) with a lot of words. 18, 30C, 05:XX:XX Themes: grief

Sh,39- Drove (without a map) 120 miles to see a jewelry exhibition. Bought a wonderful book on minerals. Spent ages looking at the gems, but they all seemed too cloudy, except the Leopard stone. 2, 12C, 100:XX:XX Themes: obstructed

Sh,390- Sensitive to other people's problems and I feel very sad when people I care about tell me that something bad happened to them. Also people I don't know, I still feel very sorry for their sadness. 20, 1M, XX:XX:XX Themes: compassionate

Sh,393- Remember old days, dwelling on past, especially about when my friend who died was still alive. I can't seem to let him go, I don't ever want to accept that he has gone, though I know I should because it will free his spirit, yet I love him too much to accept his death and allow his soul to go. 20, 1M, 06:XX:XX Themes: nostalgia

Sh,4- The cloud is lifting from neck and shoulders but it is still over eyes and forehead. I feel as if I'm waking up. 7, 6C, 10:11:00 Themes: obstructed

Sh,40- Overwhelmed by beauty of Sumatran tiger on TV, especially his eyes. 16, 12C, 01:XX:XX Themes: perfection, animal

Sh,41- Desire to see pyrites. 2, 12C, 100:XX:XX Themes: bright

Sh,418- Anxiety regarding acting irresponsibly about my health. "This might affect the rest of my life." 8, 6C, 01:XX:XX Themes: conscience, health

Sh,419- Fear of breast cancer because of aching in the breast and arm. Feel a certainty of breast cancer. 2, 12C, 08:XX:XX Themes: disease

Sh,42- Using a lot of words that one might connect with crystals, e.g., clear, cold, shining, crystalline, sparkly, gem, jewel, cut, facet, incisive, penetrating, sharp. 2, 12C, 80:XX:XX Themes: bright

Sh,420- Informed that my father has cancer of cardiac sphincter. Feel sure I have cancer of the lymph nodes of interior axilla. Don't feel any emotion for my father, but weep with anger. 2, 12C, 26:XX:XX Themes: disease

Sh,422- I am concerned about my health. Think I have TB or pneumonia. I am sure I will die. 7, 6C, 28:00:XX Themes: disease

Sh,423- Extreme weakness, painful cough, weak chest. Feels like TB or wasting disease. 22, 200C, 01:XX:XX Themes: ruined, energy, disease

Sh,424- Mind alive but body feels wrecked. 7, 6C, 23:10:00 Themes: ruined

Sh,425- Despair about my health. 7, 6C, 31:22:00 Themes: health

Sh,426- Feeling proving is major setback to my long term health. 7, 6C, 43:00:XX Themes: prejudiced, health

Sh,428- Despair about health as I feel I am taking a long time to recover and I'm still coughing. 7, 6C, 75:00:XX Themes: health

Sh,429- Fear something could happen if I had a bath. Want to keep dry. 7, 6C, 20:09:00 Themes: water, disease, prejudiced

Sh,43- Feeling alone and tall and capable, like a beacon beaming out rays of light to all and sundry. 2, 12C, XX:XX:XX Themes: solitude, greatness, bright, light

Sh,431- I feel old and creaky. 7, 6C, 08:00:XX Themes: ruined, old

Sh,432- This remedy is prematurely aging me. I feel the youthful bounce has gone. 7, 6C, 21:00:XX Themes: old

Sh,434- Before a journey, fear of not being able to get home. 8, 6C, 01:09:00 Themes: travel, accidents

Sh,436- Very scared of driving in a car, obsessed with crashing and accidents and death. 20, 1M, XX:XX:XX Themes: accidents, death

Sh,438- Nearly backed into another car, which was double-parked, although checking very carefully. Felt as if I was going to have an accident. Didn't feel safe. 6,30C, 01:16:XX Themes: accidents, danger

Sh,44- Attracted to dark night skies. Stars seem more visible. 16, 12C, 23:XX:XX Themes: dark, bright

Sh,45- Sensation as if I am bubbling under the surface 7, 6C, 59:00:XX Themes: floating

Sh,46- Feel need to be outdoors, in air surrounded by trees even when raining, need air and space and beauty all around. 20, 1M, 04:XX:XX Themes: go out

Sh,47- Need air—fresh, cold, clean. I feel stuffy inside. This feeling is related to the feeling of food being dirty. 20, 1M, 06:XX:XX Themes: dirty, pure

Sh,49- Great desire to get my affairs in order, making phone calls without putting it off. Tidier mind. Better with homework, etc. I made a list of about 10 phone calls I had been putting off and then made each one. Paid all my outstanding bills, balanced my books, returned two questionnaires, prioritized work outstanding for school—in short, cleared my desk, and all in one day. 18, 30C, 09:XX:XX Themes: organization

Sh,51- Wanted to clean windows and wash clothes, enjoyed the cleaning. Most unusual. 12, 30C, 01.XX:XX Themes: organization, dirty

Sh,519- mages of nuclear mushroom clouds.

16, 12C, 00:04:25 Themes: disintegration
Sh,520- Thoughts of creativity and destruction. One does not exist without the other. 16, 12C, 30:XX:XX Themes: ruined, antagonism
Sh,521- After waking, pattern on walls became fluid in movement, in air. The wall lost solidity; could easily move through it. 16, 12C, 26:XX:XX Themes: disintegration
Sh,522- Wondered if I dematerialized, would I be able to regain the same form? 16, 12C, 26:XX:XX Themes: disintegration
Sh,523- Delusion animals are changing form, i.e. see a cat and when closer it's actually a dog. 16, 12C, 28:XX:XX Themes: transmutation, animal
Sh,525- Delusion I saw a man with a green face. I looked to see if his ears were pointed, but they were normal. Thought he might be a Vulcan. 16, 12C, 51:XX:XX Themes: stranger
Sh,527- Walking lopsided, sensation as if right side is elongated. 16, 12C, 00:13:20 Themes: grow
Sh,528- Feeling as if right side bigger than the left. 16, 12C, 05:03:55 Themes: grow
Sh,533- Feels like cycle of life has speeded up with no way of stopping. 16, 12C, 51:XX:XX Themes: hurry
Sh,536- With my eyes closed after meditating, to my right appeared a huge Tibetan deity. He appeared to know who I was. Felt it would be rude to ask his name. He said, "Do you want to know how powerful I am?" He was not friendly but powerful.... 16, 12C, 00:07:30 Themes: greatness, inexpugnable
54- Holding together, connecting, bonding. Interconnection in body, had body bonding points. Feel full, connected again.16, 12C, 03:07:45 Themes: disintegration
Sh,541- Feeling of absolute power, invincible.16, 12C, 14:14:00 Themes: inexpugnable
Sh,554- Image of reptilian dinosaur skins. Reached up and took his head off. Inside, a human was underneath dinosaur skin. The head was hanging down in shame. 16, 12C, 00:07:30 Themes: shame, transmutation, animal
Sh,555- Feel feminine and beautiful. 16, 12C, 26:XX:XX Themes: sexual
Sh,556- Feel bright, free and beautiful, more feminine, more fertile and voluptuous. 16, 12C, 24:XX:XX Themes: sexual, liberty, bright
Sh,557- Males finding me attractive. I'm finding others more attractive. 16, 12C, 31:XX:XX Themes: sexual
Sh,56- Everything seems to complement everything else; balance and harmony, and order and form in the universe. 16, 12C, 26:XX:XX Themes: perfection
Sh,58- Watching the infinite variety created from simple building blocks. Only subtly energy creating difference. 16, 12C, 28:XX:XX Themes: organization
Sh,6- Felt really strong love for children. Looking at daughter had a feeling of a barrier being lifted or a cloud lifted from me. Felt I could really see her, that she was mine; of me but separate. 8, 6C, 02:XX:XX Themes: obstructed, isolation, indifference
Sh,60- After waking, pattern on walls became fluid in movement, in air. The wall lost solidity, could easily move through it. 16, 12C, 26:XX:XX Themes: disintegration
Sh,61- Material objects appear to lack substance. I see molecules.16, 12C, 34:XX:XX Themes: disintegration, unreal
Sh,62- Wondered, if I dematerialized would I be able to regain the same form? 16, 12C, 26:XX:XX Themes: disintegration
Sh,63- Thought of female twins producing male twins. 16, 12C, 00:00:20 Themes: double
Sh,64- In Tai Chi asked to get into a pair, but formed a foursome which felt comfortable. We laughed. We all wanted to be together. I couldn't pair, needed to be four — very unusual. 16, 12C, 07:14:00 Themes: double
Sh,66- Delusion that I can see four sides, as if four faces. 16, 12C, 38:03:14 Themes: double
Sh,67- Delusion of galaxies spiraling. One, then two, then four. 16, 12C, 39:XX:XX Themes: double
Sh, 68- Delusion; I have two pairs of hands. 16, 12C, 45:XX:XX Themes: double
Sh,71- Extremely irritable and it seems as if I have a lot of work to do — the work of two.16, 12C, 35:XX:XX Themes: double
Sh,73- Feels like doing two things at once all the time.16, 12C, 67:XX:XX Themes: double
Sh,74- Unbelievable poles, further than I've stretched to before.16, 12C, 26:XX:XX Themes: antagonism

Sh,75- Feel like a square without corners.16, 12C, 67:XX:XX Themes: antagonism

Sh,76- Felt rushed; so much to do. Overwhelmed. 8, 6C, 04:XX:XX Themes: hurry, duty

Sh,78- Hurried. Family tells me to stop rushing. On a high, but I don't feel hurried inside.10, 6C, 05:XX:XX Themes: hurry

Sh,79- Hurried wild. Husband says I look wild, like a jungle child moving rapidly, jerky movements in different directions. Very excitable as if about to lose control. 10, 6C, 19:XX:XX Themes: wild, hurry, young

Sh,8- Watched past emotions float away in reverse order. 16, 12C, 00:00:20 Themes: inversion, past

Sh,81- I'm feeling impatient with patients. I'm using intuition more as I have a sense of not wanting to waste time. 7, 6C, 17:18:00 Themes: hurry

Sh,82- Finding it difficult to treat, finding I'm there for my patients too much. Sensation as if there's no time to wait to let them finish their story. 7, 6C, 18:00:XX Themes: hurry, time

Sh,83- Impatience for plans to come to fruition, but can't hurry the process. 2, 12C, 60:XX:XX Themes: impatience, hurry

Sh,86- Feels like cycle of life has speeded up, with no way of stopping. 16, 12C, 51:XX:XX Themes: hurry

Sh,89- Feeling of time passing slowly. I kept thinking it was earlier than it was. 8, 6C, 07:XX:XX Themes: time, slow

Sh,93- Notice slowness between thought and action. It has been happening for weeks. Have started to hesitate. 16, 12C, 61:XX:XX Themes: slow, confidence

Sh,95- Great difference between the thought of how long it will take and actuality. Thought much longer than actuality. 16, 12C, 22:XX:XX Themes: slow, time

Sh,97- At times, my awareness is not at the same speed as my head, it's faster.16, 12C, 29:XX:XX Themes: hurry

AESC.

Al,1- Great repugnance to the drug.(medicine) Themes: loathing, suspicious, poisoned

Al,6- Gloomy (dark) forebodings. Themes: pessimism

Al,8- Feels miserably cross. Themes: miserable, bothered

Al,9-...he had a feeling as if death was impending (imminent); but this was followed by an exalted condition of brain and nervous system... Themes: menaced, anticipation, death

AETH.

Al,15- The disposition becomes retiring (reserved) and tearful, as in nostalgia. Themes: reserved, homesickness

Al,28- A fixed idea, which she cannot throw off, of a garment (clothes) made the day previous; she also dreamed of it. Themes: clothes, dwells

Al,30- Loss of comprehension (understanding); a kind of stupefaction, as if there was a barrier (obstruction) between his organs of sense and external objects. (disconnection, interruption) Themes: knowledge, obstructed

Al,7- Imagined she saw rats run across the room. Themes: animal

Al,8- Delirium; he imagines he sees dogs and cats. Themes: animal

Al,9- Delirium; he jumps out of window. Themes: suicidal, height

Al,S-1- Imagined she saw rats run across the room. Themes: animal

Al,S-11- Disposition becomes retiring (reserved) and tearful, as in nostalgia. Themes: misanthropy, reserved, nostalgia

Al,S-2- A fixed idea, from which she could not free herself, of a garment (clothes) made the previous day, of which she also dreamed. Themes: dwells, clothes

He,14- Great sadness when alone. Themes: sadness, solitude

He,15- Anxiousness sensation as if a heavy load was lying on chest. Themes: heavy, heart, oppression

He,22- After social talking, all symptoms disappear. Themes: disease, talk, company

AGAR.

Al,13- She ran about the yard, romped (playing) with the children, threw them down, even hit them. Themes: child, violence, hurt

Al,14- He imagines himself at a gate of the hell and that the mushroom commands him to fall on his knees and confess his sins, which he does. (forgiveness, absolution) Themes: seized, penitence, conscience, salvation, religious, hell, dictatorial

Al,15- The father had fantasies; seemed to see his dead sister in heaven. Themes: lack, sister

Al,16-.... reciting (enumerate) before the beauties of the tribe their exploits (adventures) in war or the chase.(hunting) Their physical strength is increased...(boasting) Themes: vanity, energy, fight, hunter

Al,19- During the intoxication they lift and carry the heaviest loads, take long steps and jump over small objects, as if trunks of trees lay in their way. Themes: energy, heavy

Al,2- He becomes so furious that he can hardly be restrained from ripping up his bowels, as he fancies the mushroom had ordered him to do. Themes: seized, suicidal, anger, dictatorial, tear

Al,22- Some run and walk involuntarily in the most dangerous places.(defiant) Themes: fearless, defiant, danger

Al,29- Taken in moderation it excites the intellect and inspires cheerfulness and courage. Themes: knowledge, energy

Al,3- Fearless, menacing, mischievous (rude) frenzy; also, frenzy which causes the patient to assail and injure himself, with great exertion of power. Themes: fearless, menacing, wicked, hurt, energy,

Al,37- An impulse to laugh overcame him in bed, owing to an indescribably mixed sensation of happiness and misery.(duality) Themes: antagonism, unfortunate, pleasure, miserable

Al,4- He is intoxicated with fearless frenzy; forming bold (courageous, brave) and revengeful projects. Themes: revengeful, fearless, planning

Al,45- Anxiety, as though something unpleasant were going to happen to her. Themes: misfortune

Al,46- His mind is uneasy and anxious; he was constantly concerned only about himself, his present and future condition. Themes: himself, future, position

Al,56-...grew angry at the servant and felt inclined to fight. Themes: anger, fight

Al,57- She is vexed with herself and pities (compassion) herself. Themes: bothered, compassionate, himself

Al,8-...called for his hatchet; had to be confined alternated with religious excitement. Themes: anger, penitence, seized, conscience, imprisoned, religious

Al,9- Delirium; he imagines himself a military (martial) officer, commanding (dominant) at a drill (training) and directing the various maneuvers. Themes: officer, dictatorial, planning, greatness, organization

Ha,17- Disgust for all work which occupies the mind, ... Themes: loathing, work

Ha,20- Drunken fearless frenzy with bold (courageous), vengeful determinations. Themes: fearless, revengeful, violence

Ha,23- Fearless, threatening, destructive frenzy, also such as turns against itself and injures itself , combined with great exertion of strength. Themes: fearless, menacing, wicked, suicidal, energy, hurt, violence

Ha,27- Extravagant fancy, rapture (ecstasy), prophesying, making verses. Themes: clairvoyance, poetry, pleasure

Ha,28- Quiet, equable (tranquil), sociable, active, and glad of having done his duty. Themes: duty, pleasure, company, busy

Ha,3- Anxious forebodings (anticipation), as if she were about to experience something disagreeable. Themes: misfortune, anticipation

Ha,5- The mind is restless and troubled; he was always solely occupied with his present and his future condition. Themes: future, tormented, restless, mortification

He,23- Great selfishness. 0 Nymphomania. Themes: egotism, sexual

He,25- Protracted (postponed) mental application or exciting debates brought on vertigo. Themes: discussion, fit

AGN.

Al,1-,...he feels as if nothing existed around him; he is dissatisfied with himself all the time; he is incapable of attending to any business; the things around him are entirely indifferent to him;... Themes: unfit, work, unreal, indifference, himself, discontented

Al,2- He sometimes feels as if he were nobody (unimportant, insignificant, worthless), and would rather be dead than have that feeling; when possessed by that feeling he has no courage to undertake anything; and when free from it he feels exalted, would like to read like an orator, etc. Themes: confidence, contemptuous, death, greatness, cowardice, talk

Al,3- She is very sad, and keeps repeating that she will soon die. Themes: sadness, death

He,3- Low spirited, fears of approaching death. Themes: sadness, anticipation, death

He,4- Despairing sadness; keeps repeating that she will die, that there is no use doing anything. Themes: sadness, despair, doomed, death

AIL.

Al,4- Recklessness (careless) in regard (respect) to present and future. Themes: future, negligence

Al,5- Stoical indifference to whatever happens. Themes: indifference

He,1- Past events are forgotten, remembered as belonging to someone else, or as matters read. Themes: identity, past, separated, strange

ALL-S.

Al,4- Dread (fear) of being poisoned. Themes: poisoned

Al,5- Fears he will never get well. Themes: disease

Al,6- Fears of being unable to bear any medicine. Themes: unfit

He,3- Sadness when alone; moral uneasiness; afraid of never getting well; fear of not being able to bear any kind of medicine; fear of being poisoned... Themes: sadness, solitude, conscience, disease, poisoned, suspicious,

ALOE.

Al,1- Amorous (sexual) thoughts present themselves which are very annoying. Themes: tormented, sexual

Al,11- In the afternoon, he is disposed to become reconciled (pacify) where he would not otherwise have been so. Themes: peace, fight

Al,17- Great anxiety, timorousness, restlessness, dread (fear) of death, and great anguish, so that she cannot stay anywhere.(restlessness) Themes: fearful, restless, death, cowardice, movement

Al,2- Before taking it, the disposition is apprehensive, speculative, amorous, after taking it, quiet ...reflective, more self sufficient,... Themes: theorizing, sexual, meditation, confidence

Al,20- Little inclination to labor; discouraged, apprehensive about his success. Themes: work, succeed, failure

Al,21- Irritable, he cannot endure the visit of many people, they are repugnant to him. Themes: loathing, company

Al,25- Ill-humor; peevish (angry) about himself, so that he insults and blasphemes; worse afternoons. Themes: anger, himself, offensive

Al,23- Immediately, strong exhibition of will (disposition); he quarrels with every one who contradicts him; it seems as if he would permit himself to be torn (ruined) in pieces, sooner than give up his will. (lack; will, integration, union) Themes: will, fight, contradiction, contrary

Al,38- ...continually mocking the remarks (saying) of others;... Themes: contemptuous

Al,40-...wrap up in himself (introspection), as after a sickness or a fit of anger, which still gnaws (bite) internally, which one cannot express. Themes: disease, reserved, anger, ruined, suppressed

Al,5- Merry, self-contented; fraternized with the whole world. Themes: pleasure, union

Al,9- Contented with his station (position, rank) in life; it involuntarily occurs to him, that he is really much better off than many other people. Themes: position, greatness, haughty

He,11- Dissatisfied and angry about himself, more so when he is constipated or suffers from pain. Themes: anger, himself

He,12- An easily excited, angry, revengeful state of mind, could not brook opposition (contradiction), wanted to destroy object of wrath, relief from tea or milk stimulants;... Themes: anger, violence, revengeful, contradiction

He,2- She knew she would die in a week. (predicts, death) Themes: anticipation, death

He,3- life is a burden. (load) Themes: heavy, loathing
He,9- Restlessness and fear; fear of men. Themes: misanthropy

ALUM.

Al,10- He feels low-spirited on account of his disease. Themes: unfortunate, disease
Al,11- She is constantly possessed by bad thoughts which oblige her to weep; at the same time she feels apprehensive and uneasy, as if something evil were to happen to her; everything she only looks at, fills her with sadness. Themes: misfortune, pessimism, sadness
Al,16- Oppressive anxiety, attended with emptiness and confusion of the head... Themes: oppression
Al,17- Anxiety with external heat and uneasiness as if she had done something bad. Themes: restless, conscience
Al,19- Anxiety and fearfulness, as if he had committed a crime. Themes: fearful, conscience, criminal
Al,24- He is apprehensive of losing his thoughts, and his understanding. Themes: knowledge
Al,3- He takes everything in the worse sense, and weeps and howls for hours. Themes: offenses
Al,31- Is opposed to the wishes of other people. Themes: antagonism
Al,32- She is excessively peevish, and everything is offensive to her; she desires nothing but to quarrel and make a fuss,... Themes: offenses, fight
Al,33- He sneers (mock) at everybody contemptuously. Themes: contemptuous
Al,4- The boy weeps constantly against his will, for half a hour. Themes: antagonism, will
Al,41- Incapacity for connected thought. Themes: disintegration
Al,44- Great absence of mind and irresolution.(undecided) Themes: doubtful, irresolution
Al,6- Depressed and friendless; he wishes only to be left alone, in the forenoon. Themes: sadness, friendless, helplessness, solitude
Al,7- The person imagines only disagreeable, sad images. Themes: pessimism, sadness
Al,9- He believes he will not be able to recover his health. Themes: unfit, disease
Ha,1- Dejected and joyless; he only desires to be left alone, forenoon. Themes: solitude
Ha,10- She looks at everything in the worst light, and weeps and cries for hours. Themes: pessimism
Ha,16- Anxiety with external heat and restlessness, as if she had done something wicked. (immoral, evil) Themes: conscience, wicked
Ha,17- Anxiety and fearfulness, as if he had committed a crime. Themes: conscience, criminal, fearful
Ha,18- Restlessness in the evening, as if evil was imminent. Themes: misfortune, danger, menaced
Ha,20- In the morning, anxiety as if he were to have an attack of epilepsy in a few hours.(convulsion) Themes: disease, fit
Ha,21- Apprehension of losing his thoughts, his reason. Themes: insanity
Ha,22- She cannot see blood nor a knife without horrible thoughts pressing in upon her, as if she should, e. g. commit suicide; though she has the greatest horror of it. Themes: suicidal, antagonism, pointed, blood, horrible,
Ha,23- Excited, over-worked (industrious), and yet discontented, because not enough had been done. (duty) Themes: busy, duty, work, conscience
Ha,25 - Varying moods through the day, now confidence, then again faint-heartedness.(timid) Themes: confidence, fearful
Ha,32- She does not wish to do what others wish. Themes: contrary
Ha,33- She is extremely peevish, and everything is offensive to her; she only wishes to scold (criticize) and to raise a fuss (trouble) in the afternoon. Themes: offenses, censorious, fight
Ha,35- He laughs contemptuously at everything. Themes: sarcasm, pleasure, contemptuous
Ha,39- Great absent-mindedness and irresolution. Themes: irresolution, meditation
Ha,4- Dejected (depressed, unhappy) as to his disease._ Themes: sadness, disease
Ha,5- He thinks that he cannot get well again. Themes: disease, despair
Ha,52- Everything is easy to him, the powers

of his understanding and of his body seem excited. Themes: knowledge, energy

Ha,54- Numb (paralyzed) feeling in the head, with a fear that he would become unconscious. Themes: obstructed, fit

Ha,55- A numb (insensibility) feeling in the head as if his consciousness was outside of his body; when he says anything , he feels as if another person had said it; and when he sees anything , as if another person had seen it, or as if he could transfer himself into another, and only then could see. (transmigration) Themes: double, divided, identity, obstructed,

Ha,6- Fancy paints to itself nothing but disagreeable, sad pictures. Themes: sadness, mortification

Ha,7-...anxiety as if something bad would happen (misfortune) to her; whatever she looks at, fills her with sadness. Themes: misfortune, pessimism, sadness

He,10- Seeing blood on a knife, she has horrid ideas of killing herself, though she abhors the idea. Themes: suicidal, blood, pointed, antagonism

He,11- Crying, against his will. Themes: antagonism

He,16- Low-spirited, trifling things appeared insurmountable. (impossible) Themes: sadness, obstructed

He,18- Apprehensive of losing his reason. Themes: insanity

He,19- Uneasy evenings as from impending evil. Themes: menaced, misfortune

He,2- Consciousness (knowledge) of his personal identity (personality) confused. Themes: identity

He,20- Fears he is not to recover. Themes: disease

He,21- Dread (fear) of death, with thoughts of suicide. Themes: death, suicidal

He,23- Anguish, oppressive and vague fearfulness, or uneasiness as if he had committed a crime. Themes: fearful, oppression, conscience, criminal

He,25- Variable mood, at one time confident, at another timid. Themes: confidence, timidity

He,4- Inability to recollect things or follow up a train of thought. Themes: unfit, past, disintegration, dispersion

He,6- Makes mistakes in speaking, using words not intended. Themes: talk, wrong

He,7- Time passes too slowly; intolerable ennui; an hour seems half a day. Themes: impatience, time, tedium,

He,9- Mania to kill himself with a sharp weapon. Themes: suicidal, pointed

ALUMN.

Al,13- When thinking about his disease, he feels the heart beating. Themes: disease, heart

Al,2-...felt very much oppressed, anxious, and heavy, like a stone on the chest, with inclination to take a long breath. Themes: oppression, heavy,

Al,3- Great anxiety, and disbelief (doubt, suspicious) in the power of medicine to relieve him. Themes: hopeless, disease

Al,4- Feared to leave her sit in church, after feeling faint. Themes: fearful, fit

Al,9- Excitability of feeling, as when one is agitated by unpleasant news. Themes: restless, news

He,3- Feels like after unpleasant news. Themes: news

He,5- Thinking about her disease causes palpitation. Themes: disease, heart

He,6- Unpleasant (bad) news excites and causes nervous tremors. Themes: news

AM-C.

Al,11- Sad, low-spirited, apprehensive of evil... Themes: sadness, misfortune

Al,13- Kind of sadness not usual with me; no inclination to go out. Themes: sadness, go out

Al,16- The recollection of past disagreeable occurrences torments him. Themes: tormented, past

Al,19- She is anxious on account of her illness. Themes: disease

Al,20-...she knows not how to comfort (console) herself, what to do with her-self;... Themes: doubtful, confidence

Al,22- At night, attack of great anxiety, as if she had to die ,... she was unable to move her eyes or to speak,... Themes: death, doomed, paralysis

Al,23- Every afternoon, between five and six o'clock, she is seized with anguish, as if she had committed the greatest crime; towards evening the anguish passes off. Themes: conscience, criminal

Al,33- She found fault with everything.

Themes: wrong, censorious
Al,7- Very weeping mood, with thoughts of death. Themes: death
Ha,10- Severe compression of the heart, he knows not how to help himself. Themes: oppression, heart, helplessness
Ha,11- The mind is restless and feels uncanny. (mysterious, strange) Themes: restless, strange
Ha,12- She finds no rest (restlessness) , and prosper (realize, achieve) in nothing. Themes: restless, succeed,
Ha,16- Cloudy weather makes her very sad. Themes: sadness, storm
Ha,23- Can bear no contradiction. Themes: contradiction
Ha,3- Very lugubrious (sad), with thoughts of death. Themes: sadness, death
Ha,37- She cannot well arrange her ideas. Themes: organization
Ha,5- Thoughts of previous annoyances torment him. Themes: bothered, tormented, past
Ha,6- Anxious and distressed about her diseased condition. Themes: disease
Ha,7- Sad, dejected, feeling as if a misfortune was imminent,.. Themes: anticipation, misfortune
Ha,8- Every afternoon between 5 and 6 o'clock she is seized with anguish, as if she had committed the greatest crime; ... Themes: criminal, conscience
Ha,9- Many afternoons she is seized with weakness and timidity, so that she cannot control herself and knew not what to do;... Themes: timidity, energy, cowardice, confidence, irresolution
He,5- Gloomy, depressed, with feeling of impending trouble,... Themes: reserved, anticipation, danger
He,6- Anxious concern about one's sickness. Themes: disease
He,8- Anguish as if a crime had been committed. Themes: conscience, criminal

AM-M.

Ha,2- Anxious and melancholy, as if internal grief or sorrow were gnawing in her heart. Themes: sadness, grief, heart

AMBR

He,15- Hurries too much while engaged in mental labor. Themes: hurry

AMBR.

Al,2- Lewd fancies, even when dreaming; the mind and the sexual organs, however, do not feel excited by them. Themes: lascivious, sexual
Al,21- He is always as if he were in a dream. Themes: unreal
Al,3- She is excited, loquacious; talking fatigues her; she was enable to sleep at night; got a headache, as if she carried a large load upon her head... Themes: heavy
Al,4- Uncommonly long excitement. Themes: sexual
Al,N-11- Fears of becoming insane. Themes: insanity
Al,N-6- Distorted images, grimaces; diabolical faces crowd upon his fancy. Themes: devil, horrible
Al,N-8- Great sadness; despondent, does not want to live. Themes: sadness, hopeless, death
Al,N-9- Forced to dwell upon most disagreeable things; ... Themes: dwells
Ha,477- The imagination is occupied with many lascivious ideas, even in dreams, and yet the disposition and the sexual organs are but little excited by them. Themes: lascivious, sexual
Ha,478- Distorted fancies, grimaces, satanic faces take possession of the mind, and he cannot get rid of them. Themes: seized, devil, dwells
Ha,483- Sad thoughts take possession of him, with sinking feeling about the heart; he is for a long time depressed in spirits. Themes: energy, heart, sadness
He,10- Fear to become crazy. Themes: insanity
He,16- Embarrassed (inhibit) manner in company. Themes: timidity, company
He,18- The presence of other people aggravates the symptoms. Themes: company

AML-N.

Al,1- Anxiety, as if something might happen; must have fresh air. Themes: anticipation, misfortune

He,1- Mental confusion and dreamlike state. Themes: unreal

He,11- Cannot sit still for fear of something dreadful happening. Themes: restless, misfortune

He,13- Haunted (obsessed) many times a day with an indescribable dread and sensation as of an oncoming fit, although it came on only once or twice a week. Themes: seized, fearful, fit, disease

He,2- A trance like state, everything seeming unreal to her. Themes: unreal, seized

ANAC.

Al,1- Illusions of fancy; he imagines he has his name called by the voice of his far-distant mother and sister, accompanied by an apprehension of misfortune and anxiety. Themes: others, cares, mother, sister, nostalgia, misfortune, homesickness,

Al,11- When walking he felt anxious, as if some one were pursuing him; he suspected everything around him. Themes: persecution, suspicious

Al,15- The future appears dangerous to him, as if nothing but misfortune and danger were reserved for him; want of confidence in his strength (vigor, force) and despondency. Themes: future, danger, misfortune, doomed, confidence, energy,

Al,16- Anxiety in all his actions; everything appears to him more terrible; he imagine himself surrounded with enemies; then he feels warm and the blood seems to boil within him. Themes: pessimism, enemy, surrounded, blood

Al,26- Increased fancy; he constantly thinks of some new object to which the mind forcibly clings.(adhere) Themes: seized

Al,28- Extreme excitement of the fancy, with a number of projects, in the evening... Themes: planning

Al,8- Melancholic illusion; he imagines a bier in the side room, upon which either his friend or himself is lying. Themes: death, corpse, funeral, friend

Ha,10- In the forenoon, extremely hypochondriac, discouraged and despondent, with awkward (unskillful), helpless manner; ... Themes: sadness, unfit, helplessness

Ha,15- Very peevish and out of humor, with great sensitiveness to all offenses. Themes: sensitive, offenses

Ha,16- He takes everything ill and becomes violent. Themes: violence, offenses

Ha,17- Passionate and contrary. Themes: antagonism, passionate, contrary

Ha,18- Extremely passionate at a slight offense, breaking out into violence. Themes: passionate, offenses, violence

Ha,2- Anguish and apprehension as of imminent misfortune. Themes: misfortune

Ha,20- Indisposition to work; he is afraid to undertake anything, he has no pleasure in anything. Themes: succeed, confidence, work, unfit, failure

Ha,24- He laughs, when he ought to be serious. Themes: pleasure, antagonism

Ha,25- He is compelled to laugh, while engaged in very serious matters, ...;in laughable matters he can keep serious. (contrary) Themes: antagonism, pleasure, contrary

Ha,26- His thoughts leaves him.(empty) Themes: lack

Ha,29-...he has a lack of ideas, and loses subject quickly and without perceiving it. Themes: lack

Ha,3- Anxiety and apprehension in the evening, after cheerfulness during the day. Themes: anticipation, pleasure

Ha,33-Increased, greater keenness (acutely) of memory; even the least circumstances of times long past come back to him, without cause; he would also be now able to easily learn by heart... Themes: past, knowledge

Ha,36- His mind is very much oppressed, as if a cold in the head were coming on. Themes: oppression

Ha,37- He can only think when a subject is suggested to him; he does not of himself think of anything; he cannot independently determine anything. Themes: knowledge, lifeless, irresolution

Ha,38- Everything intellectual is hard for him, as in a dearth (lack) of ideas. Themes: lack

Ha,4- Internal anguish, which did not allow him to rest, he troubled himself about every trifle, as if it would cause great injure, with solicitude about the future. Themes: restless, conscientious, misfortune, future, conscience, damage

Ha,45- Delusions of fancy, he thought his name was called by the voice of his (far distant) mother and sister; at the same time an apprehension and anguish foreboding misfortune. Themes: misfortune, mother, sister, helplessness

Ha,46- Melancholy dejection and imagination, as if there was standing in the adjacent room a bier, on which a friend or he himself was lying. Themes: funeral, death, corpse, friend

Ha,47- He mixes up the present with the future. Themes: time, future

Ha,5- In walking and in standing, uneasiness, as if someone were coming behind him (persecuted); everything around him seemed to him suspicious. Themes: persecution, suspicious

Ha,6- Timorous in all his actions; he views everything more anxiously and timidly, always thinks of being surrounded by enemies, then he becomes hot, his blood seems to boil in his chest. Themes: fearful, surrounded, persecution, blood, enemy, cowardice, timidity,

Ha,7- Anxious apprehension and deep thoughts, on meditating over his present and his future fate. (destiny) Themes: future, meditation, mortification

Ha,8- The future seems to him very dangerous, as if nothing were imminent but misfortune and danger; distrust in his own power, and despondency. Themes: future, danger, misfortune, confidence, despair

Ha,9- He is at odds (quarreling) with the whole world, and has so little confidence in himself that he despairs of being able to accomplish (succeed) what is demanded of him. Themes: fight, confidence, unfit, succeed, failure, despair

He,1- Everything appears as in a dream. Themes: unreal

He,13- After having caressed her husband or child she pushes them away from her, as if they were not what she supposed. Themes: husband, child, forsakes,

He,2- Feeling as if spirit was separated from the body. Themes: divided, double

He,24- Imagines he hears voice of mother or sister, who are far away. Themes: mother, sister, homesickness

He,25- Has a devil in his ear whispering blasphemous words. Themes: offenses, seized, devil,

He,26- Idea as if everything perceived had no reality, all things appear as in a dream. Themes: unreal, strange

He,27- Thinks he is double. Themes: double

He,28- Fixed ideas: that mind and body are separated ; about redemption (salvation) of soul and about the devil; that a stranger is constantly by his side (pursued); that strange forms accompany him, one to his right and one to his left. Themes: divided, double, religious, stranger, persecution, salvation, devil, strange

He,29- Has the fixed idea that her husband is not her husband, her child not her child; now she fondles (caress) them and again pushes them away. (reject, repudiate) Themes: forsakes, identity, obstinate, husband, child,

He,30- Hallucination; delirium a demon sits on his neck and tells him most offensive things. Themes: seized, offenses, devil

He,32- Disposed to malice, seems bent on wickedness. Themes: wicked

He,39- Every five minutes he screams loudly, as if he would call someone. Themes: helplessness

He,40- Uses profane language, swears, thinks himself a demon. Themes: seized, identity, offensive, devil, wicked

He,46- Estrangement (separation) from individuals and society, with fear of future. Themes: separated, future

He,49- Sadness; looks on dark side of everything. Themes: sadness, pessimism

He,56- When walking he left anxious, as if some one were pursuing him; he suspected everything around him. Themes: persecution, suspicious,

He,57- Apprehensive (fear) of death being close at hand. Themes: death, anticipation

He,59- Fear of paralysis. Themes: paralysis

He,61- Anxiety and feeling of impending misfortune. Themes: misfortune

He,62- Internal anxiety, which did not leave him any peace; he felt solicitous (careful) on account of every trifle, as if it would lead to some great trouble (misfortune); with apprehension (fear) of future. Themes: peace, tormented, conscientious, misfortune, future

He,63- Despondency (desperation) and fear of approaching death. Themes: death, despair

He,64- Anxiousness; despairs of getting well.

Themes: despair, disease

He,66- He is separated (divided, disconnect, estranged) from the whole world and has so little confidence in himself that he despairs of being able to do that which is required of him. Themes: separated, confidence, unfit, despair

He,67- Contradiction between reason and will. Themes: will, antagonism, contradiction

He,68- Feels as though he had two wills (intentions), one commanding to do what the other forbids. Themes: antagonism, double, divided

He,69- In one ear a devil, in the other an angel, prompts (incite) him to do murder or acts of benevolence. (homicidal, x helpfulness, kindness) Themes: antagonism, seized, homicidal, devil, helpful, compassionate

ANAN.

Al,14- Ardent desire to travel. Themes: travel

Al,17- Persistent fear of death during all his sufferings. Themes: death

Al,2- Sadness and restlessness, with fear of death and of the future. Themes: fearful, death, future

Al,4- Hypochondria, with dread (fear) of society (people); he seeks solitude and obscurity; does not want to see or hear anything. Themes: solitude, dark, misanthropy

Al,5- Restless, suspicious, and very irritable character, or apathetic and as if besotted.(intoxicated) Themes: suspicious, yielding

Al,6- Disposition to anger, with desire to strike and destroy. Themes: anger, violence

Al,7- Quarrelsome and contrary humor, but after being angry he often regrets (remorse) what he has done. Themes: fight, bothered, anger, conscience, contrary

Al,8- Ungovernable jealousy; everything causes jealousy. Themes: jealousy

He,3- Hypochondriasis and dread of society. Themes: misanthropy

He,8- Monomania for doing same thing and frequenting same places. Themes: mania, obstinate

ANDROC.

Sh,101- Can't avoid shouting at people she was intolerant of, could not hide her feelings. More impatient with others and herself. (7) Themes: intolerance, impatience

Sh,102- Assertive, impatient, aggressive. Felt resentful and abused. Had no control over her temper. Bellowed and lashed out at everyone. In the evening, furious for no apparent reason. Wanted to kill her husband and children, banged doors and threw things. By bed-time, she felt fine but the intensity of her evil thoughts was very frightening. (7) Themes: resentment, impatience, offensive, homicidal, anger, husband, child, wicked

Sh,103- Had a very caustic conversation with someone she hardly knew. Enjoyed her rudeness and was surprised by it. (7) Themes: sadism, offensive, wicked

Sh,104- By evening, needing to avoid people, anger coming out, no restraint — I look for reasons but there aren't any. (7) Themes: anger

Sh,106- Desire to break things. (7) Themes: violence

Sh,108- Incredibly sensitive to noise, can't bear it, hundreds of thoughts pop in and out of my brain, thoughts of 'why are we here?', deep philosophical issues. Everyday things disappear from my mind. Am free from pressing, nagging responsibilities — just a black thunder sits within me, and I feel afraid of what I might do next. my eyes are staring and full of hate — just looking at the children sends them frantic. I have no control over my emotions. Then after 8:00 p.m., deadness resumes and I feel .k., but the end of myself as I usually am. (7) Themes: noise, philosophy, anger, wicked

Sh,109- Black, horrible moods which don't last long, but are frightening in their violence. (7) Themes: violence, wicked

Sh,111- Short tempered in afternoon, easily excited to anger, worse from being interrupted. (12) Themes: anger, obstructed

Sh,112- Became excited to anger and confrontation. She was not aware of hurting others' feelings and did not seem to care. Could not appreciate anyone else's feeling. Later she reflected on her actions and felt ashamed. (12) Themes: anger, fight, defiant, conscience, egotism

Sh,113- Argumentative. Pursued conflict almost with relish. (12) Themes: fight, discussion, pleasure

Sh,114- Intolerant of interruption and questions. (12) Themes: obstructed

Sh,115- When reflecting on her anger and arguments, was filled with remorse, although at the time she believed she was being perfectly reasonable. (12) Themes: anger, conscience, remorse

Sh,116- Impatient, snappy, shouting, felt trapped and despairing. Growled at her children. (12) Themes: impatience, caught, offensive, despair

Sh,117- Angry with her children and family. (7, 12, 17, 28) Themes: anger, family

Sh,118- Irritability, worse for noise and bright lights. (17) Themes: bright, light, noise

Sh,119- Critical and irritable. (21) Themes: censorious

Sh,121- When talking to friends felt 'paranoid', suspicious and guilty, when asked questions, he became hot and sweaty. He felt it was a game of who was cleverer, and tried to lie to and outwit his friend, though this gave no satisfaction. His friends reported that he seemed unusually distant and cool. (29) Themes: persecution, conscience, suspicious, liar, discussion, deceitful, isolation

Sh,122- When his friends were talking, he became very suspicious and fearful, but had no fear of strangers or the police. (29) Themes: suspicious, fearful

Sh,123- In the evening he became manic, stalked the streets and visited many friends for a short time only, but could not relax or relate to them. Was pleased when he found his friends were not at home. Spoke nonsense and tried to squeeze a laugh out of anything. (29) Themes: persecution, insanity, suspicious, friend

Sh,124- In the street, he felt aggressive and very strong, that his umbrella was a knife, and desired to smash people up. (29) Themes: energy, wicked, violence, pointed, homicidal

Sh,125- Desire to pick an argument or fight. (29) Themes: fight, discussion

Sh,126- Great hostility to those around him, which manifested in brooding and stinging observations and comments directed at his friends. (29) Themes: anger, dwells, offensive, friend

Sh,128- Desired alcohol and drugs, a feeling of wanting to escape. (29) Themes: escape

Sh,129- It seemed as though he was a different person, very similar to the way he had been in adolescence, but in a much more powerful manner. These emotions were so intense he wanted to rip his chest apart to let them out. He lost all control over his emotions, which seemed to come from a deep and distant part of himself, a darker side. He desired to continue the proving for the rest of his life. (29) Themes: identity, young, strange, energy, divided, wicked, passionate, dark

Sh,140- Very sensitive to music. During a black mood, almost any sort of music will shake me out of it. (7) Themes: music

Sh,141- Danced all night in a frenzy, could not keep still, and was frustrated when the music finished. (29) Themes: music, restless

Sh,144- Sadness and confusion, unable to see a solution to her problems. Worse 6:00 p.m. onwards. (28) Themes: sadness

Sh,145- She found that she was thinking or saying something at the same time or just before someone else was thinking or saying the same thing. (13) Themes: clairvoyance

Sh,147- Sensitive to others' emotions. I feel I know how people are feeling. (25) Themes: sensitive, compassionate

Sh,148- Sympathetic, took on other people's problems. (29) Themes: compassionate

Sh,150- Speech slurred, answered with difficulty, was indisposed to talk and averse to company. (16) Themes: talk, company, misanthropy

Sh,153- Words and thoughts tripped over themselves, but he laughed and enjoyed himself. (29) Themes: pleasure

Sh,154- Sighing — sighed deeply all day, as if trying to remove a sadness from his diaphragm. (29) Themes: sadness

Sh,155- At night — brain revving away like crazy, thoughts racing through his head. Very interesting and exciting thoughts. Stayed awake til early morning, enjoying himself tremendously, and felt young again. (4) Themes: insanity, young, pleasure

Sh,167- Pretended to feel well, although sick. (17) Themes: feigning, disease, antagonism

Sh,176- Fear of driving, especially fear of hurting someone else in an accident. (Clinical) Themes: accidents, others, hurt

Sh,179- Extreme anguish and restlessness, but at the same time felt like an observer of my condition, watching it all transpire without being able to change anything. Mind fixed on the physical anguish. It dominates my senses. (21) Themes: restless, divided, yielding

Sh,180- Desire to be out in the country, intense desire to be on the rocks. Desire to feel the rocks, to stick hand beneath the rocks, to crawl into or behind rocks. (Clinical) Themes: abroad, travel, nature

Sh,19- Feeling of separateness, usual sense of urgency gone. (15) Themes: isolation, danger

Sh,20- Felt detached from her stomach cramps. (6) Themes: divided

Sh,24- I feel entirely alone, that I am viewing the world through one hole, for it all seems just a picture, and the rest of the world share a different view finder together. I don't want to join theirs though. (7) Themes: solitude, isolation, misanthropy

Sh,25- Felt disconnected from the human race, as if everyone were another species. Directionless. (7) Themes: misanthropy, isolation

Sh,26- Totally detached — not from self but from surroundings. (10) Themes: isolation

Sh,29- Could not care what others thought of her. (17) Themes: indifference

Sh,30- Distant and staring. (20) Themes: isolation, indifference

Sh,31- Felt remote and ineffectual, a dreamy state. Felt more like a spectator than a participant. (25) Themes: unreal, yielding, isolation

Sh,34- Much more untidy, the house was a mess and it didn't bother her. Made ineffectual efforts to tidy up and then lost interest. Desire to sit undisturbed and just look. (25) Themes: organization, indifference, yielding

Sh,35- Felt 'stoned', tried to express himself to a friend but could not. Behaved in a dreamy absent minded way. His friends thought that he had taken drugs. (29) Themes: indifference, isolation

Sh,37- Pushed kids out of bed with no compassion, would usually have felt very guilty doing this. (7) Themes: wicked

Sh,38- Things she would normally feel guilt about don't bother her, (cured symptom?). (7) Themes: indifference

Sh,39- Cancelled an appointment without any remorse. Thought "maybe I shall feel guilt later". (7) Themes: conscience

Sh,40- She dreamt that she had murdered her grandfather by poking a knitting needle through his eyes while he slept. Though she felt no remorse, she wanted to be punished but no-one would accept her guilt. Was told by her friends that she had responsibilities and could not go to jail and the police refused to prosecute. Was frightened by the dream. (7) Themes: homicidal, punished, pointed, conscience, imprisoned

Sh,41- Feels much more self centred — have given up all the permanent favours I do for people — I don't want to do any more. Feel I need more time for me. I must feel guilt but I don't think I do. I feel the nasty side of my character is emerging much more aggressive and domineering. I don't want peoples' good opinion of me as someone who is nice — very unusual. (7) Themes: dictatorial, egotism, wicked

Sh,43- Felt she should forgive her parents for any blame of real or imagined slights, at the same time she felt as if knots were untying within her.(25) Themes: compassionate

Sh,45- Incredible upsurge of energy — laughing, felt very high, then low, then high again. (4, 29) Themes: energy, pleasure

Sh,48- Extremely accident prone, had to avoid driving the car. (10) Themes: accidents

Sh,49- Accident prone (10, 25) cut fingers frequently. (10) Themes: accidents, hurt

Sh,50- Did the shopping in a very disorganised way, started one thing, forgot it, then started something else. (25) Themes: organization, dispersion

Sh,52- Behaved as if drunk, swayed and

slurred her words with increased sexual desire. (25) Themes: sexual

Sh,57- In the evening felt very lonely and desolate, although not alone. She felt separated, detached, disconnected and unreal. (7) Themes: solitude, isolation, unreal

Sh,58-. Felt more love for her mother, friends and husband. (7) Themes: friendly, mother, friend, husband

Sh,59- Felt disappointed with people. (7) Themes: disappointment

Sh,60- Felt tense and absolutely alone, but sure that the rest of the world was mad, not her. She felt defiant with others and would not be manipulated. (7) Themes: solitude, contemptuous, isolation, suspicious, defiant, antagonism

Sh,61- Felt constrained and had a gloomy approach to everything, averse company, desire to be alone. I feel people will not want to talk or be with me. (28) Themes: solitude, forsaken, reserved, suppressed

Sh,62- A friend commented that she "looked strange and not at all like herself". (7) Themes: strange, identity

Sh,63- Desired company but could not be bothered to see anyone, felt lonely as if he didn't belong. (21) Themes: company, bothered, solitude, forsaken, isolation

Sh,65- Desired comfort and sympathy. (29) Themes: lack, friendly

Sh,72- My mind is concentrated on one objective and I push aside all distracting influences. A mental 'tunnel vision'. (12) Themes: obstinate

Sh,76- Mind blank when concentrating. Unable to think of more than one thing at a time. The current thought excludes all others, I often forget what I am doing and am easily side tracked. (25) Themes: disintegration

Sh,77- While cooking dinner, she remembered a ring she had lost and began searching for it in a very disorganised fashion, completely forgetting what she had previously been doing. (25) Themes: lost

Sh,79- Fear — as if something terrible would happen. (10) Themes: misfortune

Sh,80- On occasions experienced fear, especially of being attacked in the street. (1) Themes: attacked

Sh,81- Felt out of control, his emotions took over. Felt terror, panic, fear and that he could not cope. (2) Themes: unfit, fearful

Sh,82- Absolutely terrified of dog on street, for no apparent reason, with numbness and tingling through every part of his body, followed by a sick feeling in the stomach. He felt shaken for hours later. (2) Themes: fearful, animal

Sh,83- Woke at night to urinate. On going upstairs, all colours seemed incredibly bright and the walls were pulsating — in towards him and out again. This felt similar to an L.S.D. experience years ago. Did not know what to do, was stricken with panic. Terrified, he raced back to bed where he felt hot, so uncovered, then cold so covered, then hot, he uncovered and sat up and immediately felt better — no panic. As soon as he lay down he began to panic. Became afraid in the light and felt better in the dark with the lights off. He wanted to call someone for help, and felt angry about the proving. He then got up and walked around for a few minutes, got back to bed, and fell asleep. (2) Themes: bright, fearful, helplessness, light,

Sh,84- Overwhelmed by terror, panic and fear, like a psychic attack. Then specifically became fear of being psychically tested as if confronted by something absolutely horrible, as in a "cult initiation ordeal". He felt so scared he had to shut the door, with a feeling that something would appear from behind it if he left it open. (4) Themes: fearful, horrible, ordeal, persecution

Sh,86- Full of fear when driving, avoided it at all costs. (7) Themes: accidents

Sh,87- Panic stricken with her customers. (7) Themes: fearful

Sh,88- Intense but very rapid fear, immensely powerful and very upsetting. Avery deep fear and panic felt in abdomen. (10) Themes: fearful

Sh,90- Impatient, expected to be able to do everything immediately. (1) Themes: impatience, hurry

Sh,91- Impatient watching others, wanted to speed them up. (7) Themes: impatience, hurry

Sh,92- Time seemed to go slowly. (2, 25) Themes: time

Sh,93- Felt that she was driving very slowly. Could not judge the speeds of cars coming towards her. While playing the flute, she had the sensation that she was playing very slowly. Felt disconnected from the music but able to play. (25) Themes: time

Sh,96- Increased irritability, a "how dare you!" feeling. Felt like tearing offenders to pieces with his bare hands. He felt an enormous surge of violent emotions at trifles, and had to exercise great control to stop outbursts of violence and impulses to hurt someone. Felt that "everyone were creeps", could not be bothered with anyone. (2) Themes: offended, bothered, violence, anger, passionate

Sh,97- Very strong liking and disliking to people — very intense — ranging from immense sexual attraction to extreme hatred. Spoke with hatred and maliciousness about colleagues. (4) Themes: passionate, sexual, anger, wicked

Sh,98- A colleague thought he was being very sarcastic. (4) Themes: sarcasm

Sh,99- Felt angry, did not want to speak to anyone, in the evening with friends he felt very lively, self-confident and forceful, rather biting at times. (4) Themes: energy, reserved, anger

ANG.

Al,10- Discouragement; dissatisfaction with his situation; he does not bear a joke; slight offenses fill him with bitterness. Themes: offenses

Al,14-...internal uneasiness, such as is experienced by those who anticipate some great pleasure, or also owing to all sorts of plans crowding upon his mind. Themes: anticipation, planning, pleasure

Al,15-,...prevented by the intrusion upon his mind of a rather agreeable project which he almost believes to be real and feasible, and which exclusively absorbs all his attention; it is a sort of waking dream. Themes: dwells, planning, pleasure, obstructed

Al,16- Lively mood; he is confident he can achieve everything with vigor. Themes: confidence, energy

Ha,292- No confidence in himself to undertake and carry through voluntary movements. Themes: confidence, movement

Ha,298- Cheerfulness and self-confidence that he can undertake anything with power. Themes: energy, confidence, succeed

He,2- No confidence in use of voluntary muscles; could not finish what he attempted. Themes: unfit

He,3- Ill-humored, oversensitive to jokes, slight offenses fill him with bitterness. Themes: sensitive, offenses

He,4- The slightest offense, a mere trifle, irritates. Themes: offenses

He,8- Thinks about one project and nothing else, with great activity of mind. Themes: dwells, obstinate, planning

ANT-C.

Al,10-...the sound of the bells as well as the sight of that which surrounds him, moves him to tears;... Themes: sensitive, time,

Ha,18- Continuous state of enthusiastic love and ecstatic longing for an ideal woman, which quite filled his fantasy;... (perfection, utopian) Themes: union, perfection, love, pleasure,

Ha,23- Ecstasy and exalted love, with great anxiety about his fate (destiny, doom), and inclination to shoot himself;... Themes: pleasure, future, suicidal, love

Ha,28- Consequences of (ailments from) disappointed love. Themes: disappointment, love

Ha,7- Anxious meditation, during the day, about himself, his present and future fate. (doom, destine). Themes: meditation, future, himself

Ha,8- Decided impulse to shoot himself, at night, but no inclination to any other kind of suicide; ... Themes: suicidal,

He,18- Anxiety in relation to his present and future condition. Themes: future

He,20- Is driven to despair, resolved to drown himself. Themes: despair, suicidal, water

He,22- Sentimental mood in the moonlight, particularly ecstatic love. Themes: pleasure, love, light

He,24- Sentimental or distrustful mood. Themes: passionate, suspicious

He,26- Irresistible desire to talk in rhymes or verses. (poetry) Themes: talk, poetry

He,6- Inclined to suicide by shooting; at night he is obliged to get out of bed, because he cannot free himself of the idea. Themes: dwells, suicidal

He,8- Contradiction between mind and will. Themes: antagonism, contradiction

ANT-T.

Al,12- Dreaded (fear) to be left alone even for a few moments, lest he " should be dreadfully nervous and not know what to do with himself." Themes: fearful, solitude, confidence, helplessness
Al,13- Bad humor, everything goes wrong. Themes: wrong
Al,17- He rubs his eyes with his hands as if in a stupid sleep, and wakes in a very ill-humor e.g., if one looked at him he began to howl. Themes: observed
Al,19-...anxious thoughts about the future; she thinks she will remain in her present condition. Themes: future, disease
Al,2- Suicidal mood; he raves (talk incoherently) and does not know what he is doing. Themes: suicidal,
Al,5- Despondent and apprehensive about his recovery. (despair) Themes: despair, disease
He,16- Child clings (adhere) to those around, calls for help in a hoarse voice, with cough. Themes: child, helplessness
He,18- Fear and dread of being alone. Themes: solitude
He,22- Despondent and apprehensive (fear) that he would not recover. Themes: despair, disease
He,23- Hopelessness. despondency. Themes: hopeless
He,25- Hopeless and despairing when awake. Themes: despair
He,29- Despair of his recovery. Themes: disease, despair
He,30- Depression of mind and fear that he will never get well. Themes: sadness, disease, fearful
He,32- Great concern (care) about future with beating in stomach. Themes: future
He,38- Despair and hopelessness, with lethargy, with cold sweat. Themes: hopeless, despair
He,41- Gaiety , wild mirthfulness, with subsequent ill humor and anxiety for future. Themes: future, pleasure, wild
He,6- Apathy and indifference to everything, even death would have been welcome. Themes: indifference, death

ANTH.

Al,1- Very low spirits; feeling as if something were about to happen; as if would like to get alone, and unburden (relieve) himself by crying ... Themes: sadness, misfortune, solitude,
Al,4- Feeling as if something was about to happen to him. Themes: anticipation, misfortune
Al,5- Dislike to go out of doors. Themes: loathing, go out
Al,6- On going out of doors, in evening, felt nervous, and exceedingly afraid of being run over. Themes: fearful, go out, run over

ANTHR.

Al,N-6- Thinks she feels death approaching. Themes: death
He,5- Thinks she feels death approaching. Themes: anticipation, death

APIS.

Al,12- Dread (fear) of death, or sensation as if he should not be able to breathe again. Themes: death, suffocation
Al,13- Premonition of death arose after a few minutes; "he believes he is going". Themes: death, clairvoyance
Al,15- She thought she must die, she felt so strangely.(strange) Themes: death, anticipation, strange
Al,16- He says, after a few minutes, "I am a dead man". Themes: death, doomed
Al,17-... would have liked to kill a dog that barked at him, etc. ; everything went wrong; nothing could be done to please him. Themes: homicidal, failure, wrong, discontented
Al,19-...nothing appeared to satisfy him; everything out of place. Themes: discontented, wrong
Al,2- Laughs at every misfortune. Themes: misfortune, sarcasm, pleasure,
Al,23- It seems to her as if she did not know what to do, as if she had no volition (desire) of her own, her head feels stupid. Themes: irresolution, confidence, will, knowledge

Al,3-... He laughed at the greatest misfortune, as he would at a great comedy. (mockery) Themes: misfortune, sarcasm, pleasure
Al,5- Sad thoughts, with longing for death, forenoon. Themes: death
He,11- Lets everything fall out of her hand, or breaks things and laughs over it. Themes: fall, sarcasm, pleasure
He,18- Thinks he will die. 0 Organic disease of heart. Themes: death, disease, heart
He,19- A strange boy lying in bed with him prevents (restrict) sleep. Themes: strange, child, invaded
He,20- Anticipation (intuition) of death. Themes: anticipation, death
He,28- Manias (insanity) especially proceeding from a sexual cause in women. Themes: mania, sexual
He,29- Insanity, particularly nymphomania... Themes: insanity, sexual, lascivious
He,48- Constantly busily engaged doing this or that, but do nothing right; young girls. Themes: wrong, unfit
He,49- Cannot bear (endure) to be left alone. Themes: solitude
He,53- Eccentric cheerfulness, despondency, or hopelessness. Themes: stranger, pleasure, hopeless, despair
He,59- Dread of death or sensation as if he should not be able to breath again. Themes: death, suffocation
He,60- Dread (fear) of apoplexy. Themes: disease
He,61- Will not take spirits of camphor , fears she will be poisoned. Themes: poisoned
He,66- When asked if sick, he says: "Nothing is the matter". Themes: indifference, disease
He,76- Jealousy.(in women) Themes: jealousy
He,77- All her ideas turn around jealousy, very talkative (loquacity), sometimes disgusting salacious. (lascivious) Themes: jealousy, talk, sexual, betrayed, lascivious, loathing
He,81- Ailments from fright, rage, vexation, jealousy, or hearing bad news. Themes: fearful, jealousy, anger, news,

ARG-M.

Al,449- Anxious dreams; on waking up, he still felt so anxious that he imagined he had suffered the accident he had dreamed about. Themes: accidents
He,13- Great serenity, a heavenly sensation of peace. Themes: peace, perfection
He,16- Anxious about her health; full of care. Themes: disease, cares
He,19- Fear of concussion (hurt, injure) as if he might run against something, with pain in testicles. Themes: hurt, sexual, accidents
He,2-...as if he might have an apoplectic stroke, and could not finish this proving; with spasmodic contraction of heart. Themes: fit, disease, heart
He,4- Imagines things about the military which he never liked; long forgotten old songs come into his mind. Themes: officer, music, past, knowledge

ARG-N.

Al,1-... visions and distorted (deform) faces hover before his imagination... Themes: horrible, ugly
Al,6- He fells very much affected bodily and mentally; he does not undertake anything lest he should not succeed. Themes: succeed, failure
Ha,16- Anxiety that compels him to walk quickly. Themes: movement, hurry
He,10- ...; does not work because he thinks it will do him harm (hurt), or that he is not able to stand it. Themes: unfit, hurt, damage
He,12- The sight of high houses always made him dizzy (confused) and caused him stagger (hesitation) ; it seemed as if houses on both sides would approach and crush him. Themes: height, fit, crushed,
He,13- Frequently settle (decide, fix) upon time he should die. (death) Themes: time, death, clairvoyance
He,14- Thinks he has softening of brain, or some other incurable affection (disease), which almost drives him to despair. Themes: disease, ruined, despair
He,15- When walking gets nervous (anxiety), thinks he will have a fit (convulsion?) or die suddenly, which makes him walk faster,(rapid) but soon has to stop, because he gets tired. Themes: fit, death, hurry,

He,16- Possessed of distressing idea that all his undertakings will and must fail. Themes: succeed, failure, doomed
He,17- Refused food, saying one who does not work should not eat (punishment); but driven by hunger he tried to secretly procure it. Themes: starving, conscience, punished
He,18- Feels as if everything at home had changed and that his mind is weak. Themes: strange, energy
He,19- He wept and assured every one that he has lost beyond hope for this world; that no one could delude him in that respect, and no one could reason him out of it. Themes: despair, lost, hopeless
He,20- Thoughts about suicide. Themes: suicidal
He,21- Thinks about killing himself. Themes: suicidal
He,22- On crossing a bridge, almost irresistible desire to jump into river; meeting some one prevented it. Themes: suicidal, height, water
He,23- Often awakes his wife or child to have some one to talk to. Themes: company, talk
He,24- Constantly talking about his sufferings. 0Hypochondriasis Themes: disease
He,25- Impulsive, must walk very fast; frequent turns of anxiety. Themes: hurry, movement
He,27- If a time is set, becomes uneasy the day before; is worried and ready long before the time.(anticipation) Themes: restless, time, anticipation
He,29- Frequently remains in bed on slightest pretext of being "indisposed". 0 Hypochondriasis. Themes: disease, feigning
He,31- Does not work, thinking it will do him harm or that he is not able to stand it. Themes: work, disease, unfit, succeed, damage
He,35- Sad; fear of apoplexy. Themes: sadness, disease
He,40 - Melancholy since an undeserved slight (scorn); fixed idea that he was neglected and despised by his family; his callings (job, work) became indifferent to him. Themes: injustice, despised, forsaken, family, work, indifference
He,41- Despaired of help from himself or others. Themes: helplessness, despair
He,42- Fits of despondency and all kinds of fanciful (unreal) notions for example, that whilst walking along street he could not pass a given point without falling; frequently settled on the time he was to die. Themes: despair, fall, time, death
He,43- Alarmed by vertigo and weakness of left side. Themes: fit, energy
He,44- Apprehension of some serious disease. Themes: disease
He,45- Apprehension when ready to go to church or to opera; diarrhea sets in. Themes: go out
He,46- Easily frightened; fears disease may result seriously; weeping mood. Themes: disease, fearful
He,47- Fear or thinking brings on diarrhea.(ailments from) Themes: fearful
He,48- Great nervousness and prostration (lassitude); fears to be alone because he thinks he will die ; is apprehensive of some serious disease, which almost drives him to despair. Themes: solitude, death, disease, despair
He,49- Fears if passing a certain corner or building that he will drop down and create a sensation; is relieved by going in another direction. Themes: fall, crushed
He,5- In conversation, forgetting what he wanted to say, he looked around as if expecting some one to help (aid) him out. Themes: helplessness, confidence, knowledge
He,52- Frequent attacks of anxiety with weakness in legs, ... (walking?) Themes: energy
He,53- When walking, becomes faint (weak, fall?) with anxiety, which makes him walk faster. Themes: fit, hurry
He,56- Was utterly (complete) bereft(deprived) of all power of will. Themes: energy, will
He,59- Against whatever was proposed he had the queerest objections. 0 Melancholia. Themes: strange, antagonism
He,8- To fix thoughts in anything, or to give his business any consideration, was impossible for him; on attempting it, it immediately got dark before his eyes and headache increased. Themes: work, dispersion,

ARN.

Al,13- Anxiety about the present and the future. Themes: future
Al,16- Apprehension of future evils. Themes: misfortune, future
Al,17- Horror of instant death. Themes: death
Al,23- He is contradictory; nothing can be done to suit him. Themes: antagonism
Al,27- Sullen (morose) insolence and imperiousness. (dictatorial) Themes: misanthropy, dictatorial, offensive
Al,28- Obstinate and headstrong resistance to other people's opinions. Themes: obstinate, antagonism
Al,31- Excessive inclination to perform many and long literary labors, without possessing the strength which is required to terminate them without injuring health. Themes: knowledge, energy, unfit, work, disease, damage
Al,39- ...;one feels as if one were prevented (suspend) from doing something which is extremely necessary, accompanied by a total want of disposition for any kind of work. Themes: obstructed, duty, work
Ha,609- Anxious concern (care) about the present and the future. Themes: future
Ha,611 -Fright and starting at unexpected (accidental) trifles. Themes: fearful
Ha,619- Uncommonly peevish, everything is repugnant to her; everything annoys her. Themes: loathing, bothered
Ha,620 - Restlessness of body and mind, as if he was prevented (obstructed) doing something necessary, whith complete indisposition for occupation. Themes: restless, obstructed, duty, work, unfit
Ha,623- Over-busy, inclination and disposition for great and continuous literary work with no power to do it without injury to the health. Themes: busy, succeed, hurt, work, damage
Ha,625- Over- excitability; she could easily laugh when there was no occasion for it, and when one said something annoying to her, she got angry ... Themes: sensitive, anger, bothered
Ha,627- Surly, wants to have many things and then refuses them. Themes: ambition, capricious
Ha,630- He contradicts; is opinionative; no one can please him. Themes: contrary, censorious, discontented
Ha,633- Stiff-necked obstinacy. Themes: obstinate
Ha,634- Surly insolence and imperiousness. (domineering) Themes: offensive, dictatorial
Ha,637- Fears; anxious dread of coming evil. Themes: misfortune
He,11- Mind clear like that of a clairvoyant; quiet countenance (expression), pale as chalk, thinks her death unavoidable.(inevitable) Themes: clairvoyance, death, doomed
He,18- Says there is nothing the matter with him. Themes: disease, antagonism
He,23- Excessive inclination to hard and long literary labors.(industrious) Themes: busy, work
He,27- Prays quietly for her soul. (salvation) Themes: religious, salvation
He,32- Despondency and conviction of approaching death. Themes: hopeless, death, anticipation
He,34- Fears being struck (hit, hurt) by those coming towards him; fears even the possibility of being touched. Themes: hurt, attacked, touch, approached
He,36- Horror of instant death. With cardiac distress in night. Themes: death, heart
He,46- Sensation of being good for nothing. (incompetent, unable, incapable) Themes: unfit
He,47- All occupation had to be relinquished (quit) for the time, so intense were the sufferings. (impediment) Themes: disease, work
He,49- Inability to perform continued active work. Themes: unfit, work

ARS-H.

Al,1- Anxiety he believes his death is near, and despairs of being better... Themes: death, disease, despair
He,12- Full of care and fear about his complaint (disease) when he gets awake at night. Themes: disease
He,13- Afraid (fear) of being alone he thinks he will die. Themes: solitude, death
He,14- The fear of dying is gone on 3d day, notwithstanding all around him have doubts of his recovery. Themes: death, disease, fearless
He,15- Anxiety, he believes his death is near,

and despairs of being better... Themes: death, disease, hopeless

He,23- Thinking of water irritates him, as if he would have to vomit; it nauseates him. Themes: water, disease

ARS-MET.

He,11- Afraid (fear) she will be poisoned. Themes: poisoned

He,4- Fearful visions of spectres (ghosts) in bright daylight; she sees threatening people after her,... Themes: fearful, ghosts, menaced, persecution

He,5- Feels as if she had to run away (escape), far away , and as if she would hardly touch ground. Themes: escape, floating, touch

He,5- Feels as if she had to run away, far away, and as if she would hardly touch ground. Themes: escape, touch

He,6- She would very much like to die, or fall asleep (sleep), never to awaken. Themes: death, conscience, pleasure

ARS.

Al,108- Dissatisfied the whole day, and very fretful at himself for not having done enough. Themes: conscience, duty

Al,109- Indignation, alternating with mildness; in her indignation she looks at nobody, and does not want to hear anything; she also cries. Themes: indignation, mildness, noise

Al,34- Piteous (miserable) complainings (lamenting)... and excessive mental anguish took away his breath ... Themes: unfortunate, suffocation

Al,50- He despairs of his life.(recovery?) Themes: disease, despair

Al,51- He despairs and weeps and imagines no one can help him, that he must die;...(unprotected) Themes: helplessness, doomed, friendless, despair, death

Al,56- Anguish and despair driving from one place to another for relief. Themes: despair, movement

Al,57- Anguish from the heart, interrupted by attacks of weakness. Themes: heart, energy

Al,6- After midnight, a frequent desire to kill himself, by stabbing his heart through and through. Themes: suicidal, heart, pointed

Al,70- The anxiety and restlessness are indescribable; "Kill me", he cried, "or relieve my pains!".(help) Themes: restless, executed, death, disease, helplessness

Al,74- Continued anxiety, a mental anguish, as if he had not done his duty, without, however, knowing wherein. Themes: conscience, duty

Al,78- Anxiety and fear; he sees a absent acquaintance (friend) lying dead upon the sofa, and has great dread of him. Themes: fearful, corpse, friend, death, past

Al,83- Dread of death coming on suddenly when alone, or on going to bed. Themes: death, solitude

Al,84- The greatest fear and anguish; sees ghosts day and night. Themes: fearful, ghosts

Al,85- He is anxious and trembling, and is afraid he shall not be able to prevent himself from killing a person with a knife. Themes: homicidal, pointed

Al,86- He runs through the whole house at night in search of thieves. Themes: home, robber, suspicious

Al,87- He imagines that the whole house, and the space under the bed, are full of thieves, which causes, from fright, anxious cold sweat to break out over his body. Themes: robber, surrounded, fearful, home,

Al,88- He has so much fear that he jumps out of his bed and hides himself in the wardrobe, which he can hardly be induced to leave. Themes: hide, escape

Al,89- He sees thieves in his room, and therefore hides himself under the bed. Themes: robber, hide, escape

Al,90- He sees vermin and bugs crawl about his bed, from which he wants to escape, and constantly throws away whole handfuls of them. Themes: animal, crawling, persecution, escape,

Al,91-...she was afraid (fear) of solitude and death; the slightest cause was sufficient to put her into anger and rage, which especially occurred when one spoke of her complete recovery which she considered wholly impossible. Themes: solitude, death, disease, antagonism, anger

Al,94- Very fretful, indignant, capricious; every word offends her, and makes her very angry, when she should answer.

Themes: indignation, offenses, capricious, anger

Al,95- Very fretful (irritable) and contented with nothing; she finds fault (imperfection, error) with everything; ... Themes: censorious, wrong

Al,98- Indignation in the morning when in bed; pushes the pillows about indignantly uncovers himself, sees no one, and does not want to be spoken to. Themes: indignation

Al-S,2879- Became very nervous, agitated, and delirious, suspecting people were about the house plotting (conspiracy, betrayed) against his life, jumps out of the bed suddenly and reaches after imaginary objects, and stares wildly and suspiciously around him,... Themes: suspicious, betrayed, murdered, wild

Al-S,2893- The whole head sick, the heart faint, she awoke in the morning wretched, her life a burden (load) weariness the day's portion , and each succeeding day like its predecessor, unless (except) physic (laxative) helped her with its little aid. Themes: loathing, heart, miserable, energy

Ha,1008- He can find no rest in any place, continually changes his position in bed, will get out of one bed and into another, and lie now here, now there. Themes: restless, movement

Ha,1013- Anxiety so that he frequently fainted, besides a violent pain in the place, and black pocks on the spot . Themes: fit

Ha,1015- Talks little, only complains of anxiety. Themes: talk

Ha,1017-Precordial anxiety, interrupted by the occurrence of faintings. Themes: heart, fit

Ha,1019- Anxiety, trembling and quaking, with cold sweat in the face. Themes: movement

Ha,1020 -Anxiety and restlessness in the whole body. Themes: restless

Ha,1021- On account of increasing pains he appeared to lie at the last gasp (breath), with unspeakable anxiety. Themes: suffocation, death

Ha,1026- Piteous lamentations, that the most intolerable anxiety, with extremely disagreeable sensation in the whole abdomen, took away his breath and compelled him to curl (bend) himself together now here now there, then again to rise up and walk about.(dyspnea) Themes: suffocation

Ha,1027- Trembling, anxious, he is afraid (fear) that he cannot refrain (restrain) from killing some one with a sharp knife. Themes: homicidal, pointed

Ha,1031- He became furious, must be bound, and seeks to run away. Themes: escape, anger

Ha,1032- Mania; first headache, horrible anxiety, noise before the ears, as from a number of large bells, and when he opened the eyes, he always saw a man who had (formerly) hung himself (suicidal, justified) on the ground-floor of the house, who incessantly beckoned (call) him to cut him down (help); he ran thither (there) with a knife, but, as he could not cut him down, (rescue) he became overwhelmed (beaten) with despair (remorse?) and wished (as his friends assured him) to hang himself (punish); but being prevented (stop) from doing so, he became so restless that he could hardly be kept in bed,... and he knelt down and raised his hands in a supplicating manner. Themes: time, suicidal, helplessness, religious, conscience, unfit, doomed, salvation, noise, pointed, others

Ha,1034- Hypochondriac anxiety, ...as if it came from the upper part of the chest; without palpitation of the heart. Themes: heart, disease

Ha,1035- He is cold, shivers and weeps, and thinks, in his despair, (hopelessness, despairing) that nothing can help him, (helplessness) and he must die; followed by general exhaustion. Themes: helplessness, death, conscience, doomed, despair, energy

Ha,1036- In the evening, in bed, anxious sad fancies, e.g. that something bad (misfortune) must have happened to his relatives. Themes: misfortune, others, relatives

Ha,1038- When he is alone he is beset by thoughts about disease and other thoughts of an indifferent character, of which he cannot get rid. Themes: disease, solitude, mortification, tormented, dwells, liberty

Ha,1039- Persistent anxiety, like a qualm (doubt) of conscience, just as if he had failed (neglected) to do his duty, but without knowing wherein. Themes: conscience, duty, failure

Ha,1042- Irritable state of the disposition, he vexes himself about trifles, and cannot leave off talking about the faults of others. Themes: bothered, wrong, censorious
Ha,1044- Recurring fits of irresolution; he wishes something and when one attempts (try) to gratify his wish the merest trifle will alter his resolution, and he wishes it no longer. Themes: doubtful, irresolution
Ha,1045- Her desire is greater then her need ; she eats and drinks more than is good for her; she walks further than she need do or can bear. (avidity) Themes: ambition, voracity
Ha,1049- Discontented with everything, finds fault with everything; everything is too strong and too irritating, all conversation, all noise, and all light. Themes: discontented, wrong, censorious, noise, light
Ha,1056- Life appears to him naught (emptiness); he attaches no value (worth) to it. (insignificant, worthlessness) Themes: indifference, lifeless
Ha,1057- Uncommonly tranquil disposition; quite unconcerned about their approaching death, they neither hoped nor wished to recover. Themes: peace, indifference, death, disease,
Ha,1064- All day long discontented with himself and very cross with himself; he imagines he has not done enough, and reproaches himself bitterly. Themes: conscience, duty, himself, failure
Ha,1065- ...extreme anxiety, restlessness; he had a great dread (fear) of the effects of the poison and desired to life. Themes: poisoned, restless, death
Ha,20- Continual anguish, like remorse of conscience, as if he had acted in violation (transgression, crime) of his duty, without knowing in what particular. Themes: conscience, wrong, duty,
Ha,3- Sad, sorrowful ideas ,in the evenings in bed, as if some misfortune (disaster, accident) might have happened to one's relatives. Themes: grief, relatives, others
Ha,33- Anguish and fear; he sees an acquaintance who is not present lie dead on sofa, and is much afraid of him. Themes: death, corpse, fearful, friend
Ha,34- He sees nothing but worms and bugs crawling about on his bed, from which he desires to run away (escape) and of which he throws out whole hands full. Themes: crawling, escape, animal, invaded
Ha,35- He sees nothing but rogues in his room, and therefore always creeps under the bed. Themes: hide, invaded, wicked
Ha,36- His whole house, also under his bed, is full of rogues, which causes a cold sweat to break out, which runs down cold over his body. Themes: home, invaded, suspicious
Ha,37- In the night he runs all about the house, looking for thieves. Themes: home, invaded, robber, suspicious
Ha,38- The greatest fear and anguish; night and day he sees ghosts. Themes: ghosts
Ha,39- He jumps out of bed for fear, and hides away in a wardrobe.(closed) Themes: hide
Ha,40- Lack determination (indetermination); he desires something, and when the endeavor (try) is made to fulfill his desire; the merest trifle will change his determination and he is not willing to have it so. Themes: doubtful, irresolution
Ha,42- When he is alone he falls into thoughts about disease and other things, from which he can not easily tear himself away. Themes: disease, solitude
Ha,44- Desponding and weeping, he thinks that nothing can help him, and he would have to die anyhow; (in any way)... Themes: despair, helplessness, death
Ha,45- Super-sensitiveness and over-tenderness of mind; dejected, sad and lugubrious (unhappy), she is troubled and solicitous about the merest trifles. Themes: fragile, conscientious, sadness, sensitive
Ha,53- Dissatisfied all day and extremely vexed at himself; he thought he had not worked enough and reproached himself most bitterly. Themes: discontented, bothered, himself, conscience, duty, work, negligence
Ha,58- Very peevish and sensitive; the least thing insults him and angers him. Themes: sensitive, anger, offenses
Ha,60- Inclined to sarcastic mocking. Themes: contemptuous, sarcasm
Ha,71- During the first minutes great tranquillity of soul and serenity; but after half a hour excessive restlessness and

anxiety; he imagines that the effects of the poison would be dreadful and desires to remain alive.(in a despondent suicide). Themes: peace, restless, suicidal

He,10 -Fixed idea that he and his family will die of starvation. (hunger, privation, want) Themes: others, starving, poverty, family

He,101- The least thing offends him, and moves him to anger. Themes: offenses, anger

He,103- She became furious when something to eat was offered her while complaining of loss of appetite. Themes: anger, antagonism

He,1033- He despairs of his life. Themes: despair

He,104- Obstinacy, avarice, inclined to malice and satire. Themes: obstinate, avarice, wicked, contemptuous, sarcasm

He,15- Thinks he must die. Themes: death

He,16- Tormenting hallucination, as if there was one by his side who did that he was doing, eating ,washing etc. Themes: tormented, imitated, double

He,17- He sees all kinds of vermin (insects) on his bed, throws handfuls of them away, and tries to escape from them. Themes: animal, persecution, escape, attacked

He,18- He imagines that he sees burglars (robbers) in the room, and listens under the bed; he is bathed in cold sweat. Themes: robber, suspicious

He,22- In her delirium she thinks she is well; girl, aet.7. Themes: disease, antagonism

He,24- Delirium during heat, unconsciousness, mania, wants to be held; with a tearing headache. Themes: helplessness

He,25- Mania...sees a man who has hanged himself beckoning (call) him to cut him loose (rescue, deliverance, free, saving) on failing to accomplish this he attempts to hang himself (punish, penalize);...finally kneels down and lifts his hands in supplication.(forgiveness, absolution) Themes: suicidal, religious, failure, doomed, helplessness, salvation, conscience, penitence, liberty

He,26- Her desires are greater than her need; she eats and drinks more than is good for her, and walks farther (great distance) than she ought to do. Themes: ambition, voracity

He,27- Suicidal mania. Themes: suicidal

He,28- A barber felt inclination to cut his customer's throats. Themes: homicidal

He,42- Fear drives him out of bed; he hides in a closet. Themes: fearful, escape, hide

He,43- Runs about house at night looking for thieves. (search) Themes: suspicious, robber

He,48- Averse to meeting acquaintances, (friends) because he imagines he has formerly offended them, though knows not how. Themes: loathing, conscience, offensive, shame, friend

He,58- Melancholy; after financial losses; cannot be consoled; thinks he will have to die (sentenced), with his family, from starvation (hunger); sleepless nights; walks about wringing his hands, with moaning and groaning. Themes: failure, position, doomed, starving, poverty, family, mortification, money

He,59- Very peevish and passionate, capricious, she takes every word ill and is cross when she has to answer. Themes: anger, passionate, capricious, offenses, talk

He,61- Religious melancholy; hopelessness, despair. Themes: religious, hopeless, despair, sadness

He,62- Fear of being left alone. Themes: solitude

He,63- Dread (fear) of death when alone, or on going to bed. Themes: fearful, death, solitude,

He,7- When alone, he falls to thinking about disease and other things, which he can scarcely keep out of his mind. Themes: disease, mortification, solitude, dwells

He,75- Precordial anxiety, feels constricted. Themes: constriction

He,76- Anxiety like that of one who has committed murder; driven from place to place; avoids meeting persons, thinking that he has offended them. Themes: conscience, homicidal, restless, criminal, shame, offensive

He,77- Terrible anxiety ,flushing up; restless glance (look), no rest by day or night; inclination to commit suicide. Themes: restless, suicidal

He,8- Gloomy (dark) forebodings (premonition) while lying in bed, in evening, fears something may have happened to his relatives. Themes: others, misfortune, relatives, anticipation

He,89- Irritable, despondent (despairing) and anxious ; cardiac anxiety, with insupportable pain. Themes: heart

He,9- Thoughts of death and the incurability of his complaint. 0Cancerous inoculation Themes: death, disease, despair

He,92- Disposed to discuss the faults of others. Themes: discussion, wrong, censorious

He,95- Dissatisfied and angry with himself all day; thinks he has not accomplished enough, and reproaches himself bitterly. Themes: himself, conscience, duty, failure, anger, succeed

ART-V.

He,11- Picking (gathering) of bedcovers, making a fold (wrap) of skin on back of her mother's hand, saying that it will not come off (disconnected), wants a knife to cut it off. (stab, wound) Themes: clothes, pointed, union

He,18- Fright (fear) and other emotions are followed by epilepsy. Themes: fit, disease

He,7- Gets up every night and does her daily work as a house servant, with closed eyes, lies down again and cannot remember anything next morning. Themes: duty, busy, work

He,8- Inclination to steal.(rob, kleptomania) Themes: robber, criminal

ASAF.

He,10- Dislike for solitude. Themes: solitude, company

He,17- If he thinks of having taken drug, it brings on faintness. (medicine) Themes: fit, poisoned

He,4- Unsteady (inconstant) and fickle (changeable), cannot persevere in anything; wants now one thing, then another; walks hither and thither. Themes: capricious, dispersion

He,5- Anxious sadness and apprehensions (fear) of dying. Themes: sadness, death

He,8- With heart symptoms, fear of death. Themes: death, heart

He,9- Fear paralysis or softening of brain. Themes: disease, paralysis

ASAR.

Al,1- He imagines he is hovering (floating) in the air, when walking, like a spirit. Themes: floating

ASTER.

Al,5- Melancholy, alternating with almost intolerable cerebral excitement; she is inclined to give herself up to mental or bodily work, to walk, or engage in a violent exercise;... Themes: restless, movement, work, energy

Al,6- Feeling of excessive anguish...it seems as if some misfortune was impending, as if he was going to hear bad news ... Themes: misfortune, news

Al,7-...it seems as if some misfortune was about to happen to him, and that, should it actually (really) come upon him, he would weep, rather than brace (encourage) himself to meet it, or become angry. Themes: misfortune, cowardice

He,12- Paroxysms easily excited by any emotion, especially by contradiction. Themes: contradiction

He,15- Fear of fainting, with sensation of fullness in chest.(fit) Themes: fit,

He,17- Nervous agitation, with erotic thoughts and sexual desire. Themes: sexual, lascivious

He,2- ...hallucinations as if away from home in midst (middle) of strangers; hears voices to which he replies. Themes: stranger, home, abroad

He,7- Fear of apoplexy, followed by fever. Themes: disease

He,9- It seems as if some misfortune was impending, as if bad news was about to arrive... Themes: menaced, news, misfortune,

ATRO.

Al,15- The patient is busied with subjects which at other times occupy his mind, politics and struggles consequent on his relations in life. Themes: fight, discussion

Al,21- Keep his eyes closed, ..."Oh, I shall lose my train." Themes: lost, time

Al,22- Expostulates with those who try to lead him to bed; says he will lose the train, that all things are packed up, and that he must start immediately. Themes: discussion, lost, travel, time

Al,24- I imagined I had to go off by a railway train, which started at ten in the morning, and that the hour was approaching, whilst I had nothing ready for the journey; and I believed that I wished to dress and to pack my things, but was thwarted (stopped) and prevented by the people about me. At length I was persuaded, that it was too late to catch the train, and agreed to wait till evening. Themes: time, travel, obstructed

Al,3-...the mind would become filled with strange and fanciful ideas ...fits of wild, uncontrollable laughter...I fancied myself afflicted with epilepsy, and was constantly fearful lest others should discover my unfortunate condition; ... Themes: strange, wild, pleasure, disease, shame, unfortunate

Al,33- Mentally either very sad, depressed in constant anxiety and restlessness, fearful of misfortune, or angry and inclined to be alone, seldom lively. Themes: sadness, restless, misfortune, anger, solitude

Al,25- Insisted repeatedly that her blood did not circulate, and that her feet must put into warm or she should die. Themes: blood, stagnation, death

Al,42- Morose, quarrelsome the whole day, everything went wrong; trifles usually passed unheeded irritated him to anger. Themes: fight, wrong, anger

Ha,17- Sad and morose, preferring solitude and a dark room to society of friends. Themes: sadness, solitude, dark, friend, company

AUR-M.

Al,4- Sad mood as though a great misfortune impending. Themes: menaced, misfortune

Al,5- Disgust for life; inclination to suicide. Themes: loathing, suicidal

Al,6- Unreasonable contrariety. Themes: contradiction

He,1-...he imagines he has all possible diseases. Themes: disease

He,11- Loss of energy; diminished virility; unrefreshing sleep. Themes: energy, sexual

He,13- Insurmountable mental or bodily restlessness; he has to spend hours in street and in open air. 0 Angina pectoris. Themes: restless, movement, heart

He,15- Thinking about his disease brings on palpitation. Themes: disease

He,17- Ailments from violent chagrin. Themes: grief

He,2- If left alone he thinks about nothing but his ailments,... ; desires company. Themes: solitude, disease, company

He,3- Inclined to suicide; frequent weeping; aversion to occupation. Themes: suicidal, work

He,6- Everything is disagreeable, dreary (lugubrious, desolate, deserted), even nature around. Themes: solitude, nature, forsaken

He,7- Sadness as when homesick; sad as though a great misfortune impended. Themes: homesickness, menaced, misfortune, menaced

AUR.

Ha,10- Great anguish, mounting even to suicide with spasmodic contraction in the abdomen. Themes: suicidal

Ha,11- Restlessness and hurried impulse to bodily and mental activity; he can not work fast enough; he could not act so as to satisfy himself. Themes: hurry, movement, restless, work, conscience, discontented

Ha,12- He is driven to constant activity, and is sorry for his inaction, although he cannot do anything. Themes: restless, movement, busy, conscience, unfit, succeed

Ha,13- Restless and undecided, without perceptible ebullition of the blood; he always thinks he is neglecting something for which he will be reproached; he seems to carry with him this internal restlessness, and it took from him all perseverance and energy. Themes: doubtful, restless, negligence, duty, censured, conscience, energy

Ha,14- Anxiousness; even a noise before the door makes him anxious; he is afraid some one might come in; as if afraid of men. Themes: noise, invaded, attacked

Ha,18- Dispirited ill-humor; he thinks he cannot succeed in anything. Themes: despair, unfit, succeed, failure

Ha,19- Dispirited and despondent; he thinks that everything goes awkwardly (incapacity, unfit) with him, and nothing will succeed with him. Themes: wrong, despair, failure, pessimism, succeed

Ha,20 -Discouraged (despair) and at odds (quarreling) with himself.(antagonism) Themes: antagonism, himself

Ha,21- Crying and wailing (lamenting); she thinks that she is irretrievably lost. Themes: lost, doomed

Ha,28- Excessively disposed to take offense; even the least thing seeming offensive to him, affected him deeply and caused resentment. Themes: offenses, mortification, resentment

Ha,3- He believes that he has lost the love of others, and this mortifies him even to tears. Themes: forsaken, despised, mortification, love

Ha,33- He tries his best to quarrel with somebody and to revile (scold) him. Themes: fight, censured

Ha,330- All day long good humor; he was talkative and contented with himself. Themes: talk, conscience, himself

Ha,331 -Cheerful humor; he was always disposed to converse with others and was quite contented with his position.(rank) Themes: talk, position

Ha,334- Trembling agitation of the nerves as if under the influence of some joyous hope.(faith, optimism) Themes: pleasure

Ha,337- Very much given to feel offended; the slightest thing which he thought offensive affected him deeply, and caused him to resent it. Themes: offenses, resentment

Ha,338- Irascibility; he is very excitable, and the slightest contradiction excites the utmost anger. Themes: contradiction, anger

Ha,340 -He sits apart (separated), all by himself in a corner, wrapt up in himself, as if in the deepest melancholy, when left undisturbed; but the slightest contradiction excites the greatest heat and anger,... Themes: separated, contradiction, anger, sadness, solitude

Ha,342- Peevish (irritable) dejection; (sadness) he thinks nothing will succeed (prosper) with him. Themes: failure, succeed, pessimism,

Ha,344- Discontented with all circumstances; he imagines that he finds everywhere some obstacle (impediment ,restriction) in the way; at one time he thinks that this is owing to an unlucky (unfortunate) fate (destiny), at another that he himself is to blame (censured) for it ; when the latter was the case he was particularly mortified and dejected. Themes: discontented, obstructed, unfortunate, mortification, conscience, doomed, sadness

Ha,345- An urging to activity, bodily as well as mental; when he did anything, he thought he did not do it quick enough, and that he had a great deal (much) more to do; he could not live to his liking. (desire, aspiration) Themes: restless, hurry, time, succeed, duty, movement

Ha,346- Remorse about his idleness (indolence), and yet he cannot work at anything; it drives him out of the house, he must always moving. Themes: conscience, unfit, movement, negligence, work

Ha,347- Always very restless and undecided (doubtful) - thought he was neglecting something for which he must incur (obtain) reproach - ...he seemed to carry about this restlessness with him in his inmost (deepest) parts ; this condition deprived him of all perseverance , all energy. Themes: restless, doubtful, duty, censured, conscience, doomed, negligence, energy

Ha,348- A noise before the door made him anxious; he feared lest some one would come in; like anthropophobia. Themes: invaded, noise, misanthropy

Ha,350- Great anxiety that has its origin in the praecordial region; ... Themes: heart

Ha,351- Great weakness and anxiety, so that he is thought (delusion) to be near death. Themes: energy, death

Ha,352- Amid (in the middle) howling and crying she imagines herself to be irretrievably lost. Themes: doomed

Ha,353- He imagines he has forfeited (penalty, lost,) the affections of others, and this grieves him to tears. Themes: forsaken, despised, doomed, grief

Ha,355- He is discontented with himself and depressed in spirits. Themes: discontented, himself, sadness

Ha,356- Melancholy; he imagines he is unfitted (incompetent, unqualified) for the world ; he is filled (full) with intense delight when he thinks of death, so that he longs to die. (punishment) Themes: unfit, death, confidence, pleasure

Ha,4- Discontented with all conditions; he thinks that he everywhere finds an impediment, caused now by an opposing fate,(destiny) then again by himself, which latter mortifies him and renders him dejected.(sad) Themes: discontented, obstructed, doomed, sadness, mortification

Ha,5- Melancholy; he imagines that he is not fitted for the world, he therefore longs for death, of which he thinks with the most intense delight. Themes: unfit, death, pleasure

Ha,6- Great anxiety springing from the region of the heart, and which drives him from one place to another, so that he cannot long remain in a place. (restlessness) Themes: heart, movement, restless

Ha,7- Great anxiety and weakness, so that he is thought to be near death. Themes: death, energy

He,10- Imagines he cannot succeed (perform, prosper) in anything, (failure) and he does everything wrong; he is in disunion with himself. Themes: succeed, antagonism, failure, wrong,

He,12- Thinking of death, gives him intense joy. Themes: death, pleasure

He,17- Suicidal mania or melancholia, tedium vitae, with genital symptoms.(sexual) Themes: suicidal, tedium, sexual

He,18- Religious mania; prays all the time. Themes: religious, mania

He,22- Disposition to commit suicide. Themes: suicidal

He,29- He gets excited in his thoughts about some absent persons. Themes: nostalgia

He,40- Melancholic mood, disposed to shun people; if meeting some one it gives him a nervous trembling and has to weep. Themes: misanthropy

He,41- All the time a dark, hopeless mood, frequently anxiety and despair; life is a burden (load) to him. Themes: dark, hopeless, despair

He,43- Is very unhappy; continued thought of suicide. 0Puerperal mania. Themes: unfortunate, suicidal

He,49- Fearfulness, a longing for death. 0Hyperemia of brain. Themes: fearful, death

He,53- Great anguish increasing unto self-destruction, with spasmodic contraction of abdomen. Themes: suicidal

He,55- Great anguish coming from precordial region, and driving him from place to place, so that he can remain nowhere. Themes: heart, restless, movement

He,57- Despair of self and others. Themes: despair, himself

He,59- Disappointed love, with weeping and inclination to commit suicide. Themes: disappointment, suicidal, love

He,61- Has no confidence in herself, thinks others have none; this makes her unhappy. (merit, value) Themes: unfortunate, confidence

He,69- Becomes angry at absent persons while thinking of them. Themes: anger

He,72- Contradiction excites wrath; distrust. Themes: contradiction, anger, suspicious

He,79- Ailments from grief, disappointed love. Themes: grief, sadness, love, disappointment

He,8- Looks on dark side, weeps, prays, thinks she is not fit for this world, longs for death, strong inclination to commit suicide; desperate, desires to jump from a height. Themes: pessimism, religious, unfit, death, suicidal, despair, height

He,80- Ailments from fright, anger, contradiction, mortification, or vexation with dread, fear, reserved displeasure, or vehemence. Themes: fearful, contradiction, mortification, anger, suppressed, passionate reserved

BAPT.

He,16- Aversion... to hear conversation about sickness or injuries; feeble mind. (impressionable) 0Spasmodic stricture of esophagus. Themes: loathing, sensitive, disease, energy

He,17- A sensation as if some person touched him gently while dozing.(sleep) Themes: mildness, touch

He,19- Hopeless (despair) of recovery, and certain (inevitable) of death. Themes: hopeless, disease, death

He,4- Cannot confine (control) his mind; a sort of wild, wandering feeling. Themes: insanity, wild

He,5- Cannot go to sleep, because he cannot get himself together. 0Orchitis 0Typhoid Themes:

He,6- Sensation as if there was a second self

outside of patient. 0Typhus. Themes: double

He,7- Feels scattered about, and tosses about to get the pieces together. (dispersed, separated, reparation.) Themes: disintegration, divided

He,8- He thinks his legs are holding a conversation with each other. 0Gout. Themes: double, talk, identity

He,9- He thinks his gouty toe is holding a confab (conversation, talk) with his gouty thumb. Themes: double, talk, identity

BAR-A.

Al,10- An evil, fearful suspicion suddenly takes possession of her, as if, for example, a loved friend had been taken suddenly deathly ill. Themes: anticipation, fearful, cares, disease, friend, others, death

Al,13- He wavers for a long time between opposite resolutions.(irresolute, indecision) Themes: antagonism, doubtful, irresolution

Al,14- During the day she resolves to undertake a certain matter in the evening, but scarcely is the time come when she repents it, and is undecided whether she shall do it or not. Themes: succeed, doubtful, irresolution

Al,15- Extreme irresolution ; he proposes a short journey, but as soon as he makes preparation he changes his mind, and is inclined to remain at home. Themes: irresolution, travel, doubtful, home

Al,3- All of self confidence has disappeared. Themes: confidence

Al,5- Grief at every trifle. Themes: grief

Al,6- Great solicitude and anxious care. Themes: restless

Al,7- She is very anxious and careful about very insignificant things, which formerly were perfectly indifferent to her. Themes: conscientious

Al,8- Solicitous (careful) and fearful. The slightest noise in the street seems to him like a fire alarm, and he is frightened thereat, so that he starts in every limb. Themes: fearful, fire, noise, danger

Al,9- Dread (fear). When walking in the street, she imagines that people were criticizing her, and judging her wrongfully which makes her anxious, so that she will not look up, will look (aversion) at no one , and sweats all over. Themes: censured, injustice, shame, wrong

BAR-C.

Al,12- Great fear and cowardice. Themes: fearful, cowardice

Al,16- Great irresolution about small things; he wants to drink the cup of coffee, then again not, does not know what he shall do. Themes: doubtful, antagonism, confidence, irresolution

Al,2- Imagine he walks on his knees. Themes: confidence, fall

Al,5- Sad and fearful; he has all kinds of sad thoughts about his future state, and thinks that he is lost entirely; in the evening. Themes: sadness, pessimism, future, lost,

Al,9- Extremely despondent and depressed; she believes that she must die; cries. Themes: sadness, death, conscience

Ha,10- She is very anxious and solicitous about things quite trifling, which are indifferent to her. Themes: conscientious

Ha,11- Anxious and fearful; a little noise on the street seems to him at once like fire alarm, and he is frightened by it, so that it darts (move quickly) through all his limbs. Themes: noise, fire, danger, movement, fearful, restless

Ha,12- The greatest irresolution; he proposes to himself a brief journey, and as soon as he is to make his preparation, he is sorry for it and prefers to stay at home. Themes: doubtful, planning, confidence, travel, irresolution, go out

Ha,13- Long wavering between opposing resolutions. Themes: antagonism, doubtful, irresolution

Ha,14- During the day she determines to attend (take care) to some particular matter; but scarcely (just) has the time come, when she is sorry (give up) for it, and she knows not for irresolution what to do to leave undone. Themes: doubtful, succeed, antagonism, irresolution,

Ha,15- All self-confidence has vanished. Themes: confidence

Ha,16- Great timidity and cowardice. Themes: timidity, cowardice

Ha,17- Extremely discouraged and pusillanimous ;(cowardice) she thinks she will die, and weeps. Themes: despair, cowardice, death

Ha,4- She suspected, that when walking in the street, men found fault (defect) with her, and judged her amiss (wrong), which made her anxious, so that she dared not look up ,she looked at nobody, and perspired all over. Themes: suspicious, censured, injustice, shame, wrong, doomed, confidence, cowardice

Ha,6- Sad and anxious; all manner of gloomy (sad) ideas as to his future fate (destiny) rise in his mind, and believes himself totally forsaken (deserted); in the evening. Themes: future, forsaken, sadness

Ha,7- An evil fearful foreboding comes suddenly upon his soul, as if, e.g. a beloved friend might suddenly have fallen fatally ill. Themes: others, disease, anticipation, friend, death

He,11- Imagines he walks on his knees. Themes: confidence, fall

He,12- Walking in street she imagines men are laughing at her, criticizing to disadvantage; this makes her so timid that she dare (venture) not look up or at anybody, and she perspires over whole body. Themes: observed, despised, censured, shame

He,15- Mania; talks much and confusedly; wants to go out of house. 0during pregnancy. Themes: talk, go out

He,16- Inclined to make fruitless exertions of memory; tries to recollect past events. Themes: past

He,24- Extremely contrary, irritable humor, passionate about trifles . Themes: contrary, antagonism, passionate, conscientious

He,26- Anxious about most trivial affairs.(duty) Themes: duty, confidence

He,27- She is suddenly overwhelmed with an evil apprehension; she imagines, for instance, that a beloved friend has suddenly fallen sick and is dying. Themes: misfortune, friend, others, disease, death

He,28- Solicitude, about his future; about domestic affairs. Themes: future, duty, home

He,29- A peculiar dread of men. Themes: cowardice

He,34- Loss of self confidence; desponding: pusillanimous.(cowardice) Themes: cowardice, confidence, despair

He,36- Sudden ebullitions of anger, but coupled with cowardice. Themes: anger, cowardice

He,39- Thinking of one's complaints makes them worse. Themes: disease

He,5- Forgets what was just said, just done, or what he was going to do or get. Themes: talk

BAR-M.

He,1- The locality around him seems transformed.(strange, unfamiliar) Themes: unreal, strange

He,11- During an attack of fear, she says in a weak, husky voice, she must die. Themes: fearful, death

He,4- In every form of mania, as soon as the sexual desire is increased. (lascivious) Themes: mania, sexual, lascivious

He,6- Dejection and dread of men. Themes: suspicious, misanthropy

He,7- Sense of oppressive anxiety, accompanied by the illusory notion that he is walking on his knees, without legs. (inferiority, dwarf?) Themes: oppression, fall, confidence

BELL.

Ha,1432- Fearful mistrust. Themes: fearful, suspicious

Al,109- A tailor was poisoned with a belladona injection, and for fifteen hours, though speechless and insensible to external objects, went through all the customary operations of his trade with great vivacity and moved his lips as if in conversation.(busy) Themes: work, busy, duty, energy, talk

Al,121- Inclination to violent exercise and rapid travelling. Themes: travel, movement

Al,124- Dread (fear) of solitude, of ghosts and thieves. Themes: solitude, ghosts, robber

Al,127- Aversion to all fluids (liquid, water) so that she demeaned (conduct) herself frightfully (fear) at the sight of them. Themes: water, fearful

Al,134- Great mirthfulness (happy) after supper; the vital powers were increased to an extraordinary degree for a quarter of an hour, after which came drowsiness. Themes: pleasure, energy

Al,153- She is so anxious and confused that she fears she is about to die. Themes: death

Al,156- By day great anxiety; she has no peace anywhere; it seems to her as if she must flee away.(escape) Themes: peace, escape

Al,160- In her momentary lucid intervals she complains of intolerable anguish, so that she wishes to die. Themes: death

Al,161- In walking in the open air, she is overwhelmed with tearful anguish; she is weary of life, and inclines to drown herself. Themes: oppression, suicidal, loathing, water

Al,162- She begs the bystanders to kill her. Themes: executed, murdered, death

Al,165- Cowardice, distrust, suspicion, inclination to run away. Themes: cowardice, fearful, suspicious, escape

Al,166- He starts in affright very readily, especially when any one approaches him. Themes: fearful, approached

Al,167- Events which had been previously anticipated with pleasure appeared to him in an anxious light; he thought them fearful and dreadful. Themes: anticipation, pleasure, fearful

Al,170- He feared that death was near. Themes: death

Al,171- She is so anxious and confused that she fears she is about to die. Themes: death

Al,172- She tries to strangle herself, and begs the bystanders to kill her, because she believes that she will certainly die. Themes: suicidal, suffocation, death, executed, doomed

Al,174- He escaped, under some pretext, into the open field.(run away) Themes: liberty, escape, nature

Al,178- Fretfulness; nothing seemed right to him; he was vexed with himself. Themes: wrong, himself, conscience

Al,203- ..;he imagined himself rich, owner of a large house, etc. (great person) Themes: greatness, position, wealth, home

Al,34- He took a piece of bread for a stone, and threw it far away, laughing violently and running about the room. Themes: pleasure, wicked, heavy, hard

Al,35-...she acts as if she were washing or counting money, or as if she were drinking. Themes: dirty, busy, money,

Al,48- Very delirious; she would persist that there were very horrid monsters all over the room, staring at her. Themes: horrible, ugly, observed

Al,54- The delirium was of a busy (engaged, working), restless, vivid character, but generally rather pleasing than otherwise. The patient appeared to think they were pursuing (persevere) their ordinary occupations; one boy appeared eager (animated) in flying a kite (toy), another pulled tables and chairs about, thinking he was working in a coal-pit, and a woman appeared to be remarkably busy with her household duties... Themes: work, busy, duty, feigning, home

Al,55- The delirium was attended (followed) with phantasms (ghosts), and in this respect resembled that caused by alcohol, but the mind did not run on cats, rats, and mice, ...Sometimes the phantasms appeared to be in the air, and various attempts were made to catch them or chase them with the hands; at other times they were supposed to be on the bed.. One patient (a woman) fancied the sheets (cloths) were covered with cucumbers. Themes: ghosts, clothes

Al,57- ...ludicrous and fantastic spectacles were always uppermost in my mind...my mind was in a state of delightful exhilaration. Themes: pleasure

Al,58-... Passed a restless night, her sleep, she says, being disturbed by "miserable phantoms"... Themes: miserable, ghosts

Al,81- He imagines he sees birds flying off through the chimney, and wishes to follow them by the same route. (desire: fly, liberty, freedom) Themes: liberty, animal, fly, escape

Al,82- Delirious talk of dogs, as if they swarmed (crowd) about him. Themes: talk, surrounded, animal,

Al,85- Visions of wolves, dogs, giants, and fire. Themes: great, fire, animal

Al,86-...pointing with trembling fingers to swarms (crowd) of unclean (dirty) beasts which she fancied were scrambling (mix) all over the walls, beds, table, etc. of the wards. Themes: crawling, surrounded, dirty, animal,

Al,87- Fancied he saw ghosts and animals in

the fire. Themes: fire, ghosts, animal

Al,89- He imagines he is riding on an ox, or some such thing. Themes: conduct, animal

Al,90- It seems to her that her nose is transparent, and a spot on the left side of the head transparent and colored brown. Themes: fragile, dirty

Al,91- He raves as in a dream, and cries he must go home, because everything is burning up there. (rescue, saving) Themes: fire, home

Al,92- Lying in bed in the evening, it appears to him as if he were floating away with his couch; ten evenings in succession, he imagined, immediately after lying down, that he was floating in his bed. Themes: floating

Al,96- In his delirium he threw himself down from a height. Themes: suicidal, height

Al,S-2552-...the yellow corpse of a tall man, shrouded (dressed, clothes) in white, tried to share the patient's bed with him, and the unwelcome visitor was promptly ejected. A crimson serpent came from the foot of the bed, with the design of fastening upon the patient's neck... Themes: corpse, great, clothes, invaded, animal, attacked, suffocation

A-S,2554- ..The patients appeared to think that they were pursuing their ordinary occupations;... the woman appeared remarkably busy with her ordinary household duties. Themes: duty, work, busy, home

Al,S-2559- Seems to see birds flying past and wishes to follow them. Themes: fly, animal, liberty

Ha,1312- By day great anxiety; she cannot rest (restlessness) anywhere; she feels as if she should run away. Themes: restless, escape

Ha,1324- Events which hitherto he had hoped for with pleasure, now appear to him in an anxious light; they appear to him frightful and horrible. (attractive x horrible, terrible) Themes: pleasure, horrible

Ha,1325- In the momentary intervals, when free from fury, complaints of intolerable anxiety, so that she wished to die. Themes: anger, death

Ha,1329- Great restlessness, she cannot remain long seated in one place; she is driven all about. Themes: restless, movement

Ha,1337- He makes preparation to go home. Themes: homesickness, home

Ha,1338- He is delirious, and cries out in his dreams that he must go home, because everything is on fire there. Themes: fire, home

Ha,1339- Raves (delirious) about wolves being in the room; at the same time full pulse. Themes: invaded, animal

Ha,1340 -Delirious talk about dogs surrounding him. Themes: surrounded, animal

Ha,1351- Chattering (talk) lascivious. Themes: talk, sexual, lascivious

Ha,1357- Involuntary, almost loud laughter, without having any laughable thoughts. Themes: pleasure, antagonism

Ha,1361- She bursts out in loud laughter, sings, and touches things near her. Themes: touch, pleasure, music

Ha,1364- Unrestrainedly and exuberantly merry, inclined to scold (criticize) without cause, and to insult (affront, offend) in a laughing humor. Themes: censorious, offensive, pleasure, wicked

Ha,1365- Excessive gaiety (happiness) after supper, the vital powers extraordinarily increased for a quarter of a hour, followed by drowsiness. Themes: energy, pleasure

Ha,1366- Ridiculous grimaces; ...acts as if she were washing, at another as if counting money, ... Themes: ridiculous, work, feigning, busy, money, dirty

Ha,1372- He walks lifting his feet high, as if he must step over things in his path, like a drunken person. Themes: obstructed

Ha,1381- ...she is weary of life, and wishes to go into the water to drown herself. Themes: suicidal, water

Ha,1390- Excessive indifference, for hours; one might take her life, she would not stir. (move) (immobility) Themes: indifference, suicidal

Ha,1395- He wishes for solitude and quiet; all noise and visits from others are repugnant to him. Themes: company, solitude, loathing, noise, misanthropy, peace, company

Ha,1400- Great irritability and acuteness of the senses; everything tastes and smells

stronger; the sense of touch, the sight, and the rearing are more acute,... Themes: sensitive, touch, noise
Ha,1401- Peevishness, nothing was right for him; he was angry with himself. Themes: anger, himself, censorious, wrong
Ha,1419- Fury; he injures himself and others and strikes about him. (beat, hit) Themes: anger, himself, hurt, violence
Ha,1420- He tries to bite those about him at night. Themes: bite
Ha,1422- Along with burning heat of the body, with open, staring, and fixed eyes, such fury she must constantly be held fast in order to prevent her attacking others,... Themes: energy, anger, violence, hell
Ha,1426- Inclination to tear everything about her to pieces. Themes: tear
Ha,1430- So anxious and distracted (worried) that she apprehends the approach of death. Themes: death
Ha,1431- He fears death in night. Themes: death
Ha,1433- Fearful madness; he is afraid (fear) of an imaginary black dog, of the gallows. (hanging) Themes: insanity, fearful, executed, dark, animal
Ha,1434- Madness; he thinks that his living body is putrefying. (decay, degeneracy) Themes: insanity, rotten, disease
Ha,1436- He makes an excuse (pretext) and runs out into the open fields. Themes: liberty, escape, nature, go out
Ha,1437 -She tries to strangle herself, and begs those about her to kill her, for this time she must die. (redemption, regeneration, salvation) Themes: suicidal, executed, conscience, death, doomed
Ha,1439- Throws herself down from a height.(in delirium) Themes: suicidal, height
Ha,1440- Throws herself into water. (drowning) Themes: suicidal, water
He,102- Became fearful when persons approached him in street, and when they had passed, he insisted on it that he had stabbed them. Themes: fearful, approached, suspicious, homicidal, pointed
He,104- Fear of imaginary things, wants to run away from them. Themes: fearful, escape
He,105- Anxiety and fear of imaginary objects and hallucinations, ghosts, soldiers which come to take them away, black animals, rats, dogs, wolves, etc. Themes: ghosts, officer, imprisoned, dark, animal
He,106- Anxiety and fear of imaginary objects and hallucinations, ghosts, soldiers which come to take them away (arrest), black animals, rats dogs ,wolves, etc. Themes: ghosts, officer, imprisoned, animal, dark
He,108- By day great anxiety; has no peace anywhere; it seemed to her as if she must fly away. Themes: peace
He,109 - Anxious and confused, fears she is about to die. Themes: death
He,115- Intolerable anguish during time she is free from rage, with desire to die. Themes: anger, death
He,119- Fretfulness; nothing seemed right to him; was vexed with himself. Themes: wrong, conscience, bothered, himself
He,13- Timorous anxiety; he is afraid of a an imaginary black dog; of the gallows, etc. Themes: fearful, animal, executed, dark
He,18- When closing eyes, though not asleep, patient sees fierce (wild), wicked looking large animals with horns and bushy (scabrous) heads; room seemed to be full of strange men passing in and out, who would snatch (take hold) at her as they passed, which frightened her very much, she thought the men wanted to take her away from home ; she then saw children sitting on low benches (seat) in rows (line) as in a school-room. (purity) Themes: great, animal, wicked, horrible, caught, suspicious, attacked, stranger, invaded, home, child, wild, pure
He,20- Imagines he sees ghosts, hideous (horrible) faces and various insects. Themes: ghosts, horrible, ugly, animal
He,22- Frightful visions; she wishes (desires) to hide herself.(veil, cover) Themes: fearful, hide
He,24- Fixed ideas, thinks he is riding on an ox, uses a stick for a gun, growling and barking like a dog. Themes: travel, conduct, animal, identity
He,30- Delirium: with frightful figures and images before eyes; is afraid (fear) of imaginary things; sees monsters; talks of dogs as if they swarmed (crowded) about him; furious. Themes: fearful, animal, surrounded

He,33- In evening he was seized with such violent delirium, that required three men to confine him;... Themes: violence, seized

He,4- Memory lively; remembers things long gone by. Themes: past, knowledge

He,49- She rather (first) desires death than fears it. Themes: death

He,53- Weary of life, with desire to drown herself. Themes: suicidal, water

He,62- Loud laughter, wild abandon, singing, whistling, lascivious conversation. Themes: pleasure, wild, music, lascivious, sexual

He,67- ...suffered greatest anxiety and despaired of recovery. Themes: despair, disease

He,7- Likes to brood in silence, supreme indifference, nothing makes an impression. Themes: meditation, indifference

He,70- Instead of eating, bit wooden spoon in two, gnawed plate, and growled and barked like a dog. Themes: bite, animal, wild

He,74- Picking at bedclothes as if looking for something lost, with confused muttering. Themes: lost

He,80- The boy ran around room laughing immoderately, desired neither food nor drink; a piece of bread, which he took to be a stone, he threw far from him;... Themes: pleasure, hard

He,85- ...patient must do everything violently; she wishes those around her to kill her. (salvation, redemption) Themes: violence, executed, conscience

He,86- Sensation of floating or gliding along, as if in a boat; as if the body, or part of it was greatly enlarged. Themes: floating, grow, great

BENZ-AC.

Al,2- ...If he saw any one who was deformed (disfigured) it made him shudder. (tremor) Themes: ugly, horrible

BERB.

Al,3- Anxious mood, with great fear and fright...; in the twilight some dogs and children appeared as large again as natural. Themes: fearful, animal, grow, great, child

BISM.

Al,1- Solitude is unendurable. Themes: solitude

Al,3- He is morose and discontented with his condition (health, position) and complains about it. Themes: disease, discontented, position

Al,5- He commences one thing and then another, but keeps to one thing only a short time. Themes: succeed, dispersion

Ha,108- Solitude (isolation) is intolerable to him. Themes: solitude, company

He,10- Unstable-minded; begin now this, again that, holds but short time to any one thing. Themes: succeed, dispersion

He,11- Ill humor; he is morose and discontented with his condition (position), and complains about it. Themes: disease, himself, position, discontented

He,6- Desire for company; child holds on to its mother's hand. Themes: company, child, helplessness

He,7- Solitude is unbearable. Themes: solitude

BOR.

Al,14- Dread and fear of contagion. Themes: disease, infection

Al,18- ..contented with himself and the world, and looking cheerfully into the future. Themes: conscience, future, himself

Ha,14- ...reproaches people for slight matters, for several days. Themes: censorious

Ha,15- Passionate, cross, takes offense easily. Themes: passionate, bothered, offenses

Ha,20 - Disinclination to work, he only does what he has to do, as if compulsorily. Themes: loathing, duty, work

Ha,21- He fritters away the afternoon, without getting to any real work, goes from one work to another, from one room to another, without remaining in one thing. Themes: dispersion, succeed, work, movement

Ha,4- Very timid, in driving down a mountain (elevation); quite at variance with his customary bearing; he felt as if it would take his breath away. Themes: fearful, fall, suffocation

Ha,5- The child is timid while being dandled; when it is rocked up and down in the arms it makes a very frightened face...(fear, touch, caresses) Themes: fearful, child, movement

Ha,6- Apprehension and fear of infection. Themes: disease, infection

Ha,8- Timid, an anxious scream causes terror to fall on all his limbs. Themes: fearful, fall

He,3- The child becomes anxious when dancing; if one rocks it in arms it has an anxious expression of face during downward motion. Themes: movement

BOV.

Al,10- Great sensitiveness; became easily offended at everything. Themes: sensitive, offenses

Al,2- Very open-hearted; she spoke of her own failings, contrary to her custom. Themes: failure

Al,5- Very courageous and vigorous; he would like to fight with everybody. Themes: fearless, energy, fight, compassionate

Al,9- Anguish; she felt as if enveloped in a black vapor. (cloud, fog) Themes: surrounded, dark, obstructed

He,6- Sad, depressed and desponding when alone. Themes: sadness, solitude

BRASS.

Sh,1- General feeling of aloofness 08, 6C, 04:12:30 Themes: indifference, reserved, isolation

Sh,10- A very pleasant lack of thoughts; finding it harder to apply myself to the work I'm doing. Very difficult to describe the sensation, unable to find the right words, hard to explain things 08, 6C, 02:03:00 Themes: pleasure, lack

Sh,11- I began to feel a little depressed; I'm definitely not in a party mood, desire to be still and quiet, maybe listen to classical music, Bach, Chopin, something well composed and not Beethoven 08, 6C, 05:08:30 Themes: sadness, solitude, music

Sh,12- Called on a friend who was busy with funeral arrangements. Felt rejected when she had not time to talk to me; my head was saying "don't be silly" but my eyes filled with tears, and my wee heart felt very unloved 3I, 00:06:30 Themes: forsaken, despised

Sh,13- My wife was very emotional saying she would be happier if I left, yet my reaction was how inconvenient. I did not become emotionally involved. Also a friend at work asked me if I was alright as he thought I'd not been quite with it recently. The proving experience was generally pleasant for me, and I felt low coming back to my old self, rather like going away on holiday and coming back to a messy house and all the things you have to do. Prover's wife said he'd been unbearable all that week, Rremote and not with us at allS. It was his tendency anyway, but it had been exaggerated. 08, 6C, 10:00:00 Themes: isolation, reserved

Sh,14- Very irritable with no cause, snapping at the children for no reason; apathy, can't be bothered to do anything; restless, twitchy, can't settle to anything 3I, 00:04:00 Themes: indifference, yielding, restless

Sh,15- Feeling of "leave me alone" if John or the children came near. 3I, 00:06:30 Themes: forsakes

Sh,16- Prefer to be silent, not talk. There is much I could say but who really wants to listen 08, 6C, 05:00:00 Themes: reserved

Sh,2-Feeling of aloofness still present, feeling of separation from others not so noticeable when with the children 08, 6C, 05:00:00 Themes: reserved, isolation

Sh,3- Am feeling light-headed (frivolous); do not feel in such contact with the ground; I have stumbled a few times 08, 6C, 01:23:30 Themes: isolation, indifference

Sh,4- Still feeling spaced out but centered, notice it most when sitting still. 08, 6C, 03:03:00 Themes: isolation

Sh,7- Twice this week I have had my view obstructed by someone sitting in front of me, each time I have had to move twice. 06, 30C, 04:00:00 Themes: obstructed

Sh,8- Feeling of impending disaster, still cannot settle to anything 3I,00:08:00 Themes: misfortune, accidents

BROM.

Al,1- He becomes averse to his business; it seems as though he must relinquish (quit) it. Themes: work, loathing

He,2- In the evening when alone, felt as if he would see something if he should turn

around; as if some one was back of him. Themes: persecution
He,3- Expects to see something jump around floor. Themes: attacked, persecution
He,6- Aversion to any kind of work, even reading; takes no interest in household duties. Themes: loathing, work, home, duty

BRY.

Ha,777- Cross; imagined she could not finish her work (obstruction) ; she always took hold (continued) of the wrong thing and constantly wished to take something else ; then a pressing aching headache in the forehead. Themes: obstructed, succeed, work, wrong, unfit, dispersion
Al,13- Anxiety in the whole body, which compelled him to do something constantly, and wherever he went he found no rest. Themes: restless, movement, busy
Al,25- Fretful; she imagines that she cannot accomplish (realize) her work; constantly takes up the wrong piece, and always inclined to change and take another; ... Themes: succeed, doubtful, unfit, confidence, wrong, dispersion
Al,37- Over-busy (industrious); she undertakes and works far too much. Themes: work, succeed, busy,
Al,39- Imagination very sluggish (slow); it is impossible to make any plan for the future, even for the next day; the judgment (discernment), however, is unimpaired . Themes: future, obstructed, unfit, planning
Al,5-...a delirious frightful fantasy, as of soldiers cutting him down, that he was on the point of escaping;.. Themes: attacked, hurt, officer, escape
Ha,766- Raving (insanity) about business for an hour. Themes: insanity, work
Ha,770- Anxiety; he is apprehensive about the future. Themes: future
Ha,779- Morose; looking at everything with ill-will. Themes: sadness
Ha,780- Too busy; she wishes to undertake and to work at too many things. Themes: ambition, succeed, busy, work, dispersion
He,10- Nightly delirium; delirious talk, especially about business.< after 3 a.m. Themes: talk, work
He,12- Talking of business of day in his delirium at night. Themes: talk, work
He,13- The patient desires to go home. Themes: homesickness, home
He,14- Desire to get out of bed and go home. Themes: homesickness, lack
He,15- Desire for things that cannot be had, which are refused, or not wanted when offered. Themes: ambition, capricious
He,16- Irrational talk or prattle of his business. Themes: work, talk
He,20- Great sense of insecurity, with mental depression. Themes: confidence, sadness
He,22- Apprehensive, uneasiness and dread of future. Themes: confidence, fearful, future
He,25- Anxiety in whole body compelled him to do something constantly, wherever he went he found no rest. Themes: restless, movement
He,26- Anxiety about future, particularly in childbed (puerperal) or after. Themes: future
He,27- She fears not to have wherewithal (money, funds) to live. Themes: poverty, position, money
He,29- Fear of death, which he thinks is near. Themes: death, anticipation
He,30- Fear of death. Themes: death
He,33- Despair of recovery. Themes: disease, despair
He,4- So weak in mind that his ideas vanish (empty) as if he would faint, ... Themes: energy, fit
He,42- Contradiction easily provoked anger during whole proving. Themes: contradiction, anger
He,46- Restlessness: wants change; with fear of future; fear of death, which he thinks is near; with nocturnal heat. Themes: restless, future, death
He,47- Bad effects from mortification, violence and anger. Themes: mortification, violence, anger

BUFO-S.

Al,1- Aversion to work, with unfitness for it, ... Themes: loathing, work, unfit
Al,7- He is unable to act with decision (doubtful) ; he forms projects and does not accomplish (succeed) them. Themes: confidence, irresolution, unfit, planning, succeed,

BUFO.

Al,12- He is anxious about the state of his health; is afraid he will die or that some other misfortune will happen to him. Themes: disease, death, misfortune

Al,14- Very easily frightened; a bird or insect flying by causes a start. Themes: noise, animal, fly

Al,15- Fear of animals. Themes: fearful, animal

Al,16- Fear of catching diseases. Themes: fearful, disease

Al,22- He is irritable, anxious about his state of health, with great dread of death. Themes: fearful, disease, death

Al,25- Defiance (disobedience, challenger), duplicity (hypocrisy) , spitefulness.(cruelty) Themes: defiant, liar, wicked

Al,26- Anger with desire to strike and destroy. Themes: violence, anger

Al,7- Desires solitude, and yet is afraid of being left alone and dying forsaken. Themes: solitude, forsaken, death

He,1- Desire for solitude, to practice masturbation. Themes: sexual, solitude

He,12- Fear of disease, of animals, of death. Themes: disease, animal, death

CACT.

Al,16- Feeling of semi remorse at having done something wrong. Themes: conscience, wrong

Al,17- Feeling of doing violence (injury) to myself. Themes: hurt, suicidal, himself

Al,18- Fear of death extreme and continuous; he believes his disease to be incurable. Themes: fearful, death, disease

Al,19- Disposition to do deliberately (resolutely, carefully) whatever was undertaken. Themes: conscientious, duty, succeed

Al,3- Loves solitude; he avoids those around him who wish to comfort him. Themes: solitude, misanthropy

Al,4- Felt decided impulses to swallow large and unwholesome portions of medicine. Themes: suicidal

Al,6- Decided repugnance to take any more medicine. Themes: disease, suspicious, poisoned, loathing

Al,7- Was affected with impulses to do something facetious (comical), which were repelled. (rejected) Themes: pleasure, suppressed

Al,8- Impulses to do something bordering, on the grotesque.(bizarre, strange) Themes: strange

He,14- Fear of death; he believes his disease, incurable. Themes: death, disease

He,15- Indescribable fear that something terrible is going to happen to him. Themes: misfortune

He,16- During and after attack, great anxiety, fearing some organic lesion of heart which will cause sudden death. Themes: fit, death, disease, heart

He,3- Thinks she will not recover; weeps much; despondent. Themes: disease, despair

He,4- Feels she is dying and thinks she will not live till morning, but has no fear of death. (fearless) Themes: fearless, death

CAJ.

Al,S-60- Want to walk in a low and a very dignified (nobility, honored, proud, refined) manner, and prefer to walk alone. Themes: haughty, solitude

CALAD.

Al,14- Fear of cutting himself while shaving. Themes: hurt, confidence

Al,3- He is very apprehensive about his health, and about everything... Themes: fearful, disease

Al,5- Fear of cutting himself while shaving. Themes: hurt

He,12- Very careful about his health; apprehensive. Themes: disease, conscientious

He,13- Fear of catching scarlet fever when attending a case; a fear he never had before. Themes: disease, infection

He,15- Lascivious ideas. 0Gleet 0Impotence. Themes: sexual, lascivious

He,3- Opens her eyes and asks, “Where am I? what do you all want around me?” A few moments after Calad. 0typhus. Themes: lost, surrounded

He,4- Very forgetful; he cannot remember if what he ought to have done and written during the day is really accomplished until he convinces himself of it. Themes: duty, succeed

He,8- So averse to the medicine, that it required a desperate effort to overcome it. Themes: suspicious, poisoned

CALC-A.

Al,10-...;he performed all his work with aversion and as if compelled (drive) to do so. (compulsive, obsessive) Themes: loathing, work, duty, antagonism,

Al,253- Dreams vivid, full of strife (quarrel, fight) and anger. Themes: fight, anger

Al,255- Dreams of sick people, and dead people, with violent weeping in the sleep. Themes: death, disease, ghosts

Al,3- Sadness, almost to weeping, with solicitous cares for the present and future. Themes: future

Al,5- Anxious thoughts, which came and went, before going to sleep in the evening; with which the objects seemed like different (strange) objects; he dreaded (fear) the dark, and made an effort to look at the light; all of which was relieved after the passage of flatus. Themes: strange, dark

Al,7- Apprehensive, sad mood, as though he were awaiting some depressing news. Themes: sadness, news, misfortune

Ha,261- Not without inclination to work, but indifferent to all external things; sunk in thought about the present and future. Themes: work, indifference, future, dwells

Ha,262- Very grave (serious) and full of care (worry); busied with the present and the future; he becomes sad almost to tears. Themes: cares, future

Ha,263- Anxious disposition as if something evil had happened or he had to fear reproaches (censures); at the same time, however, persistent inclination to work. (industrious) Themes: misfortune, censured, conscience, busy, work

Ha,264- Very sad humor, as if he had to expect (anticipation) bad news. Themes: sadness, anticipation, news

Ha,265- ...very indifferent to the most important things; he did everything unwillingly (reluctant, averse) as if forced to do them. Themes: indifference, antagonism, duty, conscience

CALC-F.

Al,S-1-...tendency to look on the dark side of things, with much depression of spirits. Feeling of anxiety about money matters, or thought would come to want (lack), or would soon be "running astern" (reversed, failure) financially...disposition to set a higher value on money than natural to him (avarice?, poverty?). Themes: pessimism, sadness, poverty, failure, money, ambition, avarice

He,1- All day an unusual tendency to look on the dark side of things; with much depression of spirits. Themes: sadness, pessimism

He,2- Depression of spirits and disposition to set a higher value on money than natural to him. (avarice?) Themes: ambition, money

He,3- Feeling of anxiety about money matters; thought he would come to want (poverty) or would soon be "running astern" financially (entirely without occasion) Themes: money, poverty, failure

CALC-P.

Al,13- Grows very violent, if his opinion is differed from, or if contradicted, so that he is vexed not to have been able to control himself. Themes: violence, contradiction, anger, unfit

Al,14- Violent, irritable, and snappish; it affects him most to hear that someone has done wrong; indignation rises in him... Themes: violence, wrong, indignation

Al,15- A communication in which some one is justly reproached concerning his conduct, affects him very disagreeably; he grows violent, and holds up his faults to himself. Themes: censured, offenses, conscience, criminal, sensitive, compassionate, justice, violence, indignation

Al,16- Unpleasant news makes him beside himself; sweat breaks out; inclined to indignation and anger. Themes: news, indignation, anger

Al,19- He has a clearer oversight (observation), and more distinct views of many things. Themes: knowledge

He,11- Does not want to do what he has to do. Themes: antagonism, negligence, duty

He,12- Feels as if he had been

frightened.(terrorized) Themes: fearful
He,17- Feel complaints more when thinking about them. Themes: disease
He,18- Unpleasant news brings him beside himself; sweat breaks out. Themes: news
He,19- Ailments from grief, disappointed love. Themes: grief, disappointment, union, love

CALC-S.

Al,7- Excessive, bitter melancholy, with distressing apprehensions of evil to loved ones. Themes: sadness, misfortune, love, others

CALC.

Al,1-Illusion of fancy when going to sleep, as if she heard noises and clattering (noise) about her bed, which caused shuddering (tremor). Themes: noise
Al,15- Melancholy, not exactly a sad feeling, about the heart, without cause, with a kind of voluptuous trembling of the body. Themes: heart, sexual
Al,1557-Anxious dream that he would be bitten by a dog, which awoke him, after... Themes: bite, animal
Al,16- Sorrowful and peevish; she looked upon everything from the worst side, and imagined everything evil. Themes: grief, misfortune, pessimism
Al,17- She is very hypochondriac; she thinks that she is deadly sick, nevertheless can complain of nothing. Themes: disease, death
Al,18- Despairing mood, with dread of disease and suffering, with foreboding of sad events. Themes: despair, disease, pessimism, anticipation
Al,19- She despaired of her life, and believed that she must die, with a most sad mood, and weeping, and frequent sudden attacks of general heat, as if hot water had been dashed over her. Themes: despair, death, water
Al,21- Anxious at night as she would become insane, followed by shuddering chilliness for a few minutes, and a sensation as if the body were dashed (hit) to pieces. Themes: insanity, disintegration, divided
Al,22- Anxious, restless, and busy mood; she is undertaking much things but accomplish nothing... Themes: restless, busy, succeed, dispersion
Al,25- Frightened apprehensive mood, as if some misfortune were about to happen to him, or some one else, which he could in no way overcome. Themes: fearful, misfortune, doomed, obstructed
Al,30- Dread and anxiety of the future, with fear of consumption. Themes: disease, future, infection
Al,4- Repugnance, aversion, disgust for most persons. Themes: loathing, misanthropy
Al,54- Loss of consciousness, with illusion as regards place; it seems as if the room were a bower. Themes: nature
Al,7- Loneliness is very oppressive, with coldness of the face, hands, and feet. Themes: solitude, oppression
Al,9- Cries and complains about the long-past offenses. Themes: offenses, past
Ha,12- Anxious about the present and the future, with deep reflection, at the same time indifferent to things outside... Themes: future, meditation, indifference
Ha,13- Anxious at heart, as if he had done wrong,(immoral) or had to apprehend reproaches (deserves) ,with constant inclination to work. Themes: conscience, work, wrong, heart, censured
Ha,2- Melancholy, not really mournful (unhappy) feeling, about the heart, without cause, with a sort of voluptuous tremor all over the body. Themes: heart, sadness, unfortunate
Ha,21- Solitude is a burden (load) to him, with coldness of the face, of the hands and feet. Themes: solitude
Ha,22- Timid and restless, as if evil (harmful, misfortune) was impending (imminent) over her. Themes: restless, misfortune, cowardice, timidity
Ha,23- Fearful, anxious forebodings, as if evil would befall (happen) him or some one else, and as if he could in no way evade it. Themes: fearful, anticipation, misfortune, doomed
Ha,24- Anxious, sad mood, as if he had to expect sad news. Themes: news
Ha,25- His heart is agitated with fear and anxiety for the future, with fear of consumption.(tuberculosis, ruin) Themes:

future, disease, ruined, heart, infection, fearful
Ha,26- She is afraid of losing her reason. (sanity) Themes: insanity
Ha,27- She is afraid people may notice (observed) the confusion (disorder) in her head. Themes: shame, insanity, observed
Ha,28- Hypochondriac, she conceives herself fatally diseased, and yet cannot complain of anything. Themes: disease, death
Ha,29 -Despairing (hopeless) mood with fear of sickness (disease) and misery, with forebodings of sad events. (misfortune) Themes: disease, poverty, misfortune, despair, anticipation
Ha,3- Mournful (grief), almost to tears, with solicitous occupation with the present and the future. Themes: future, grief, cares
Ha,30- She despairs of her life and believes she has to die (punishment?) ; her heart is sad with weeping, and frequent attacks of sudden, general heat, as if she had hot water poured (flow) over her. Themes: doomed, conscience, water, despair, heart, sadness, death
Ha,40- As soon he is idle (unoccupied) and sits still, he becomes peevish and drowsy (tired), and everything goes against him. Themes: tedium, antagonism, contradiction
Ha,41- Peevish, morose, very cross and most indifferent to the most important things; he also did everything repugnantly and as if by compulsion. Themes: bothered, indifference, loathing
Ha,45- Everything is repugnant (offensive) to her, with much crossness. Themes: loathing
Ha,46- Troubled and cross, she looked at the worst side of things, and sought (pursued) out all the evil. Themes: bothered, pessimism, mortification
Ha,55- Thoughts of former vexations irritate him to anger. Themes: bothered, past, anger
Ha,56- Aversion, dislike and repugnance to most men. Themes: grief, sexual, loathing
Ha,62- He is cheerful, and would like to be among men, to walk with them. Themes: talk, company
Ha,65- Great weakness of the imaginative (creative) faculty; with a very slight exertion in speaking, he felt as if his brain was paralyzed, ...;he could not think , nor recollect what was spoken of, with muddled (confused) feeling in the head.(lost: imagination, thoughts) Themes: paralysis, obstructed, knowledge, energy, talk
Ha,69- Unconsciousness and delusion about her abode (home) as if her room were a hall (passage) in a garden. Themes: home, escape
Ha,70- In the evening, two fits of loss of consciousness in walking; she would have fallen down ,if she had not been held up. Themes: fit
Ha,9- Grief and complains over insults long past. Themes: grief, offenses, sadness, past
He, NERVES, Sensation of power with lack (loss, want) of will (command, resolution, intention), force. Themes: doubtful, will
He,15- Imagines someone is walking beside her (persecution); that something hanging over back of chair is a person sitting there, etc. Themes: persecution, observed
He,16- Feels as if she would lose her senses.0Megrim Themes: fit
He,18- Mental aberration with horrid visions before eyes and cardiac anxiety; he despairs of his salvation (pardon, rescue) and wants to stab himself. Themes: horrible, salvation, persecution, doomed, suicidal, heart, despair, pointed
He,21- Mania-a-potu, with delirious talk about fire, rats, mice and murder. Themes: talk, animal, fire, murdered
He,22- Mania; sees many curs (dogs) crowding (compress) around him, fights them off. (surrounded) Themes: surrounded, attacked, animal, fight
He,23- Desire to go home. Themes: homesickness, home
He,28- She thinks and talks of nothing but murder, fire, rats, etc. Themes: murdered, fire, animal
He,34- Does not care to get well, or to do anything to assist (aid) recovery. Themes: indifference, negligence, disease
He,38- Low-spirited and melancholy, with weeping and despair of life. Themes: sadness, death, despair
He,43- Hopelessness; despair. Themes: hopeless, despair
He,48- Anxious about getting well, during the intervals. (Epilepsy) Themes: disease
He,5- Buried in deep thought; anxiety about present and future.(destine) Themes: meditation, dwells, future

He,50- Apprehensive (fearful , worried) mood ; as if some misfortune was about to happen; about his health (vigour) ; that he might have an organic disease of the heart. Themes: misfortune, disease, heart
He,51 -Fear, that something sad or terrible will happen. Themes: sadness, misfortune
He,52- Fears she will lose her reason (insanity), or that people will observe her confusion of mind. Themes: insanity, shame, observed
He,53- Fear: of death; of consumption (decay, waste, tuberculosis); of misfortune (disaster) ; of being alone. (lonely) Themes: death, disease, misfortune, solitude, infection
He,55 -Concern (anxiety, care) about spiritual welfare.(salvation) Themes: salvation, religious
He,56- Feels awe-stricken (terror- injure) at night. 0 Diarrhea Themes: attacked, hurt, fearful
He,57- Anxiety, shuddering and dread (fear) as soon as evening comes on, with fear of death ; torments those around him day and night. Themes: death, bother
He,61- Anguish, with palpitation of heart. Themes: heart
He,62- Fear excited by reports (news) of cruelties.(brutality, barbarity). Themes: horrible,
He,65- Despairing; hopeless (unhappy, pessimistic) of ever getting well (health); with fear of death, tormenting all around day and night. Themes: hopeless, disease, death, bother
He,70- Excessive mischievousness, with obstinacy. Themes: obstinate, wicked
He,71- Voluptuous (sensual), lascivious fancies. Themes: sexual, lascivious
He,8- Mind full of concern about imaginary things that might happen to her. 0 Chlorosis. Themes: danger, misfortune, cares
He,86- Easily offended; takes everything amiss. Themes: offenses, wrong
He,96 -The slight effort of talking gave him sensation as if brain would be paralyzed (disable) ,mostly in occiput. Themes: paralysis, knowledge

CAMPH.

Al,17- He beats himself on the chest, and falls into a faint. Themes: fit, himself, hurt
Al,19- Stripped naked, he danced wildly about, and attempted to jump out of the window. Themes: wild, music, suicidal, height
Al,27- The child creeps (crawl) into a corner, howls and cries; everything that is said to him is taken as if one were ordering him, and he were considered naughty (disobedient) and should be punished. Themes: child, punished, doomed
Al,32- Indescribable wretchedness. (unhappiness) Themes: unfortunate, miserable
Al,37- Excessively fearful, especially in the dark. Themes: fearful, dark
Al,38- Dread of being alone in the dark. Themes: fearful, solitude, dark
Al,39- Indescribable dread of being drawn upwards. Themes: fearful, fall, height
Al,40- Afraid of the mirrors in the room, lest he should see himself in them; so excessive was this fear at times in the night that he would have got up and broken the mirrors, only that he was still more afraid to get up alone in the dark;... Themes: loathing, himself, bright, dark
Al,46- ..." I am death! No, I am not death! but indeed I must be dead!" And thus I flew round about myself like a top, with no other feeling than for the strong smell of the Camphor. The external world existed for me no longer.... Themes: death, unreal, strange,
Al,46-...The external world existed for me no longer. (solitude) My thoughts were gone; one single fearful one remained; I imagined myself transferred to another world (estranged, alienated); for me all else was extinguished... Themes: strange, unreal, stranger, solitude, separated, abroad
Al,46-...I sat up in bed, but all about me had indeed disappeared. I was alone in the great universe, the last of all things. My ideas of the world, God and religion, now seemed to me to have existed only in my imagination; the earth upon which yesterday I lived and moved, had run its appointed course, and I was the final and solitary fragment of the whole creation...(meaningless, unimportant, neglected, forsaken, loneliness, deserted) (godless) Themes: unreal, strange, solitude, forsaken, despised, religious, godless, helplessness

Al,46-... There was no other feeling in my soul than that of my hopeless endless damnation (condemnation). I sank back upon the bed, believing that I was the spirit of evil in a world forsaken of God. Themes: doomed, identity, forsaken, wicked, hopeless,

Al,46-... Faith and hope were gone. There was here no longer any God, or rather the Infinite himself, like all his works, had ceased to be... (hopeless, faithless, godless, privation, want, destitution) Themes: godless, hopeless, religious, unreal,

Al,46-... My misery was boundless; time itself was no more; in short, I suffered such fearful anguish as no fancy can comprehend. What soul could paint to itself my everlasting (eternal) dwelling as the Evil One (devil), alone in a vast universe, without faith or hope, and my heart forever broken by unimaginable tortures? (miserable, timeless, endless, solitude, forsaken, faithless, hopeless) Themes: unfortunate, time, solitude, godless, tortured, lack, forsaken, fearful, devil, hopeless, heart

Al,46-...For a moment I resolved to throw myself from the window and sweep through the domain of my infernal kingdom, but a weak glimmer of reason held me back... Themes: suicidal, height, hell, devil

Al,46-.... As I lay stretched on my couch, as the evil demon, and suffered all the anguish of a condemned and God-forsaken soul, ...I was forever deprived of the Divine protection, and of every consolation and every hope. Nothing remained to me but the conviction of my everlasting damnation... Themes: doomed, forsaken, helplessness, hopeless, seized, devil, conscience, wicked, godless, lack,

Al,46-...I feel a tendency to self contemplation; outer things vanish, and I behold myself in spirit freed from matter. Themes: meditation, divided, liberty, unreal

Al,46-... The sight increased my despair poor nature extinguished; the sky transparent and lifeless; the earth was still in the dim, dead light. I could not bear it. The sense of touch was gone, and my eyes protruded from their sockets. Themes: despair, ruined, nature, lifeless, dark, touch

Al,46- ...A fearful terror seized me, and I knew not whither to fly. I cried out aloud, "And so I am indeed dead; that hell I used to think about is no fiction, but a reality which I am doomed to experience forever... Themes: fearful, hell, seized, doomed, death, escape,

Al,46- ...And yet I confessed this every morning, and no heavy sin rests upon my conscience. And then came doubts about my doctrinal views, for I had never been of strong faith... Themes: penitence, conscience, religious

Al,46...I started up, ran out, and fell prostrate, with a loud shriek for help, not far from the door of a neighbor.... Themes: helplessness, danger

Al,46- ...I am alone. I feel a tendency to self contemplation; outer things vanished, and I behold myself in spirit freed from matter... Themes: solitude, meditation, unreal, liberty

Al,46-...I shriek and call for help, because it seems that a murderer stands at my bed side... Themes: danger, helplessness, murdered

Al,6- Often felt as if he ought (must) to kill people, when in the street, never felt the disposition to kill any of his own family, but thought he ought to kill somebody. Themes: homicidal

Ha,341- All external things are repugnant to him, and excite in him a repellent (repulsive) crossness. Themes: loathing, anger

Ha,342- The boy crawls into a corner and howls and weeps; he takes offense at everything one says to him, as if he thought he was being ordered (instructed) about, and he thinks he is insulted and affronted. Themes: offenses, indignation

Ha,343- Quarrelsomeness, insists he is right. Themes: fight, antagonism, wrong, dictatorial

He,11- Though he could remember the name of everything, when he looked at it, yet it was not without investigating its nature that he could discover its use. (dissociation; memory x vision x knowledge) Themes: knowledge

He,16- Monomania, with horrible visions and torturing ideas about religion, which he cannot shake off, although he is conscious that they are morbid.; is< at night. Themes: religious, tortured, dwells, mania, mortification

He,18- ...one evening he went to the piano with closed eyes and played with great precision what at other times he could not have done without his notes; several times he wrote letters in an acquired (learned) language more correctly than in a waking state;...(clairvoyance) Themes: music, perfection, knowledge

He,19- It was to him as if he moved in his own little world, in which all things were clear (pure, perfect) and defined; outside of which uncertain (doubtful) and undefined. (obscure) (purity x impurity) Themes: pure, perfection, confidence

He,21- Very nervous; imagined various things; that he would get yellow fever. Themes: disease, infection

He,35- Often felt as if he ought (must) to kill people, when in the street; never felt a disposition to kill any of his own family, but thought he ought to kill somebody. Themes: homicidal,

He,36- Impulse to jump out the window. Themes: suicidal, height

He,42- Was found much excited, screaming loudly, " I shall not faint! I can't faint, for if I do, I will have fits and never come out of them. Themes: fit

He,45- Cries for help, takes hold of others, will not be left alone. Themes: danger, helplessness, company

He,51- Strips (undress) himself (naked) , and tries to jump out of window. Themes: suicidal, height

He,52- He beats himself on chest, and falls into a faint. Themes: fit

He,53- ...everything that is said is taken as if one was ordering him, and he was considered naughty (disobedient) and would be punished. Themes: conscience, punished

He,60- Indescribable wretchedness. Themes: miserable

He,61- Felt a vague sense of impending danger to life,... Themes: menaced, death, danger

He,62- Dread of being alone in dark. Themes: solitude, dark

He,63- Afraid of mirrors in room, lest he should see himself in them (reflection) ; so excessive was his fear at times in night that he would have got up and broken mirrors, only that he was still (but) more afraid to get up alone in the dark. Themes: bright, himself, dark

He,69- An indifference whether the world (mankind) uses one well (suitable) or ill (depravity, wrong), everything is repulsive.(offensive) Themes: misanthropy, indifference, loathing

He,72- Palpitation; vexed by want of sympathy (compassion, aid), afraid to be alone a moment, fears death. Themes: bothered, helplessness, solitude, death, company

He,73- Dogmatical, easily offended. Themes: offenses, dictatorial

He,81- Thinks he is going to die; < when he thinks about it. Themes: death

CANN-I.

Al,23- He seemed to have the one idea that he should die and soon be dissected. Themes: mania, disintegration, death

Al,24-He seemed possessed with the idea that he did not know whether he himself existed, or whether men generally existed, or for what purpose (intention, mission, aim) he existed.(existence x nonexistence) Themes: unreal, knowledge

Al,25- He became possessed with the idea that he was about to die, from which he cried out, "I am dying; I shall be carried to my death-chamber." Themes: death, funeral

Al,25-...Now demoniac shapes clutched (grasp) at him from the darkness, cloaked (covered) from head to foot in inky (black) palls (mantle), glaring (staring, looking) at him with fiery eyes from beneath their cowls(mantle).... Themes: devil, caught, dark, seized, observed, fire

Al,25-...He seemed to be walking in a vast arena, encircled by tremendous walls... (confined, limited) Themes: imprisoned, surrounded

Al,25... The stars seemed to look upon him with pitying (compassion) human aspect, and to bewail (lament) his condition. Themes: compassionate, unfortunate, despised

Al,26- The idea that he must die returned several times, and seemed to be particularly connected with the sinking and disappearance of the pulse. (blood, circulation) Themes: death, sinking, blood, stagnation

Al,29- Looks under beds and tables, unlocks and relocks doors, for the fancies he hears strange noises, and that thieves are in the house. Themes: suspicious, strange, robber, noise, home

Al,30- When his friends went out of the room, he thought (delusion) they had left him to his fate (destiny, doom), and wrote "cowards" in his notes. Themes: helplessness, forsaken, friend, censorious

Al,31- Imagines men are bribed (suborn) to kill him. Themes: betrayed, murdered

Al,32- He thinks he can fly through the air like the birds. Themes: liberty, fly

Al,33- Said "he had been transported to heaven (paradise)"... Themes: pleasure, liberty, perfection

Al,34- All around and within seems to be a great mystery, and is terrifying. Themes: fearful, knowledge

Al,35- Despair, and fear of being eternally lost. Themes: doomed, despair, lost

Al,36- The sun seemed reeling (moving) from his place, and the clouds danced around him like a chorus. Themes: surrounded, music

Al,40- Had a feeling of duality. One of his minds would be thinking of something, while the other would laugh at it... Themes: double, antagonism, pleasure

Al,41- Felt as if he was a third person looking at himself and his friend. Themes: observed, double, friend

Al,42- The soul seemed to be separated from the body, and to look down upon it, and view all the motions of the vital processes, and to be able to pass and repass though the solid walls of the room, and to view the landscape (view) beyond. Themes: double, energy, liberty

Al,44- Extreme exaggerations of the duration of time and extent of space- a few seconds seem ages- the utterance (declaration) of a word seems as long as a whole drama, and a few rods are a distance which can never be passed it is so great.(distances) Themes: time, great

Al,48- Attention principally occupied by an hallucination that time was indefinitely prolonged. (infinite) Themes: time

Al,57- Strange feeling of isolation (solitude) from all around him, with great sense of loneliness (isolation), though surrounded by his friends. Themes: solitude, forsaken, friend, separated

Al,58- He imagines that he is possessed of infinite knowledge and power of vision, and then that he is Christ come to restore the world to perfect peace. (redemption, savior, rescuer) Themes: seized, knowledge, clairvoyance, greatness, salvation, peace, perfection

Al,59- He believes there is creative power in his own word, and that he has only to speak, and it will be done. Themes: greatness , talk

Al,61- Then he possesses the wealth of the world, and with a benevolence equal to his wealth, showers riches on all the needy around him. Themes: greatness, wealth, compassionate,

Al,62- It seemed as though I was transparent; the fire in the grate seemed to shine through me, and to warm the marrow of the bones. Themes: fire, bright, energy

Al,63- His body seemed to him become transparent, and he imagined he saw within his breast the hashish he had eaten in the form of an emerald, from which issued millions of little sparks. Themes: bright, wealth, energy

Al,64- Imagines he is gradually swelling, his body becoming larger and larger. Themes: grow, great

Al,65- Hallucinations which lead the patient to imagine that he is on horseback, is hunting, that he sees blue water, that he is swimming, or that he is captain of a vessel, that he is traveling, that he has no weight.(lightness) Themes: hunter, conduct, travel, water, dirty, light, officer

Al,66- Illusion that he was a pump-log, through which a stream of hot water was playing, and threatening his friend with a wetting. Themes: menacing, identity, friend, water

Al,67- Illusion that he was an inkstand, and that, as he lay on the bed, the ink might spill over the white counterpane. Themes: identity, dirty

Al,69- He seems to himself to be transformed into a vegetable existence, as a huge fern, and to be surrounded by clouds of music and perfume. Themes: identity, pleasure, lifeless, surrounded, pleasure, music

He,22- Uncontrollable laughter, till the face becomes purple, and back and loins ache. Themes: pleasure

He,14-... visions of a great sublimity (splendor) usually follow visions of a quiet, relaxing and recreating nature. Themes: peace, pleasure

He,15- ...he is gradually swelling, his body becomes larger and larger; that someone calls him; that he hears numberless bells ringing most sweetly; imagines he hears music; shuts his eyes, and is lost for some time in the most delicious thoughts and dreams. Themes: great, music, noise, grow, pleasure

He,16- Exaggeration of duration of time and extend of space; a few seconds seem ages; a few rods an immense distance. Themes: time

He,18- A sense of having two existences; double consciousness. Themes: double

He,25- Great apprehension of approaching (imminent) death. Themes: anticipation, death,

He,26- He was in constant fear he would become insane. Themes: insanity

CANN-S.

Ha,289- He fears he will fall to the ground... Themes: fall

Ha,303- Dreams of misfortunes happening to others. Themes: misfortune, cares, others

Ha,304- Dreams of disagreeable and frightful character, in which he is unsuccessful (unproductive, frustrated) in everything, which causes him great anxiety. Themes: failure

He,1- Seems to be in a dream, as if things were not real; feels as if she did not know where she was; objects seem strange; feels at times as if she was somebody else;... Themes: unreal, lost, strange, identity

He,5- Voices including her own, seem to come from a distance; her own voice seems strange, as if it was somebody else speaking. Themes: strange, identity, separated,

CANTH.

Al,14- He talked deliriously when lying, sitting and walking, disconnectedly of his business and of people who had long since been dead. Themes: talk, work, past, death

Al,16- Visions at night, when half awake; she heard soft steps in the room, then knocking under the bed, and the bed was raised up. Themes: noise, invaded, floating

Al,17- Visions...something took hold of her hand, and bent it several times up and down, then it seemed as if someone took her by the throat with ice-cold hands. Themes: touch, caught

Al,22-...; she feels as if newly (recently) born;... (innocent, naive, pure) Themes: pure, child, identity

Al,25- Extreme despondency and faintheartedness; she says she must die. Themes: fearful, death

Al,26- Distrust of himself, like a hypochondriac. Themes: suspicious, confidence, disease

Al,29- Anxiety in the morning, as if he expected something very important. Themes: anticipation

Al,36- He is anxious as if he had committed a murder (homicide); it seems to arise from the stomach. Themes: homicidal, conscience, criminal,

He,14- Constantly attempting (try) to do something, but accomplishing nothing. Themes: succeed, dispersion

He,15- Despondent and low-spirited, says she must die. Themes: despair, death

He,17- Great amativeness, amorous frenzy. Themes: lascivious, sexual

He,18- Unbounded frantic sexual desire. 0 Mania. Themes: lascivious, sexual

He,6- Strange ideas crowd on him against his will. Themes: antagonism, strange

CAPS.

Al,1- He makes reproaches and becomes angry at the faults of others; he becomes offended at trifles and finds fault. Themes: wrong, censorious, offenses, anger

Al,12- An excessively busy (occupied) uneasy mood. Themes: busy

Al,18- He is in a contented mood, is jocose, and sings, and still he becomes angry from

the slightest causes. Themes: anger, music, pleasure
Al,2- Even in the midst of joking he becomes offended at the slightest trifles. Themes: offenses
Al,6- Anxiety and apprehensiveness; he imagines that he will die. Themes: death
Ha,177- Vivid dreams about scientific subjects; straining of the thinking faculty when dreaming; he composed literary essays in thought and spoke aloud. Themes: knowledge
Ha,334- He makes reproaches, and is indignant (angry) at the faults (errors) of others; he takes trifles ill and finds fault with them. Themes: censorious, indignation, wrong, offenses
Ha,335- In the midst (center) of joking he takes the slightest trifle in bad part. Themes: offenses
He,10- Fear of censure. Themes: censured
He,12- Awakens with fright, screams, and remains full of fear. Themes: fearful
He,13- Anxiety and fear, as though he was going to die. Themes: death
He,14- Peevish, irritable angry; easily offended, takes everything in bad part. Themes: anger, offenses
He,4- Haunted (obsessed) by a disposition to suicide. Themes: suicidal
He,7- He is in a content mood, is jocose, and sings, and still he becomes angry from the slightest cause. Themes: anger, music, pleasure
He,8- Homesickness; with red cheeks and sleeplessness; ... Themes: homesickness

CARB-AC.

He,12- Entire disinclination to study; what he had accomplished seemed very trifling. (unimportant) Themes: loathing, succeed, failure, knowledge, contemptuous
He,17- Fear of impending sickness... Themes: disease

CARB-AN.

Al,1- Desire to be alone ; she is sad and reflective (thoughtful); avoids all conversation. Themes: solitude, talk, sadness, meditation
Al,10- Discouraged and sad (unhappy); everything seems so sad and lonely that she desires to weep. Themes: despair, solitude, sadness
Al,11- In the morning, he felt abandoned and homesick. Themes: forsaken, homesickness
Al,28- Sullen (unsociable, silent) mood and ill-humor about present and past events; this cannot be overcome ; it even amounts to weeping. Themes: anger, past, solitude
Ha,1- Extremely melancholy (depression, grief) mood, with a sensation of being deserted. Themes: forsaken, sadness
Ha,15- Timid and fearful (coward), all day. Themes: cowardice, fearful
Ha,16- He feels horror in the evening, even to shivering and weeping. Themes: fearful
Ha,17- Thoughts of death. Themes: death
Ha,177- Vivid dreams about scientific (precise, accurate) subjects; straining (efforts) of the thinking faculty when dreaming; he composed literary essays in thought and spoke aloud. Themes: knowledge, talk
Ha,2- He feels in the morning, as if he was deserted, and full of homesickness.(nostalgia, loneliness, isolation) Themes: forsaken, homesickness
Ha,25- Self-willed; no one can do anything to please him. Themes: contrary
Ha,3- Homesickness. Themes: homesickness
Ha,32- The objects on the street seem to him changed, e.g. , farther apart and brighter (vivid, brilliant) than usual, as an empty, abandoned city. Themes: strange, separated, bright, solitude, forsaken
Ha,5- Pusillanimous (cowardice) and sad; everything seems to her so lonely (alone, deserted) and sad, that she would like to weep. Themes: cowardice, solitude, forsaken, sadness,
Ha,6- Inclination to solitude (isolation), sad and introverted (egotistic), she always only wishes to be alone, and she shuns every conversation. Themes: solitude, reserved, misanthropy, talk
Ha,7- Morose thoughts and ill-humor, not to be driven away, concerning things present and past, even to weeping. Themes: sadness, mortification, past
He,1- Unclouded consciousness and great anguish with sinking of vital forces. Themes: energy
He,13- Homesick. Themes: nostalgia, homesickness

He,9- Fearful in the dark. Themes: fearful, dark

CARB-V.

Al,12- Anxiety in the evening after lying down, as from oppression of the chest, ...,a sensation as if the heart would be pressed downward; objects about her seem to become constantly narrower and smaller,... Themes: oppression, heart, small

Al,2- Immoderately jovial (sociable, friendly), though easily put out of humor.(irritable) Themes: pleasure

Al,25- Exceedingly irritable; she seems to be overhurried (quick, fast) in her business. Themes: hurry, work

Al,7- She desired death, she felt so unhappy. Themes: death, unfortunate

Ha,10- Great disposition to weep, he wishes to shoot himself. Themes: suicidal

Ha,11- She wishes to die, she feels so unhappy. Themes: death, unfortunate

Ha,16- Excessive excitation, as if she was too much hurried (fast), or over-worked (industrious) in business. Themes: hurry, busy, work

Ha,21- Peevish, impatient, desperate, so that he would like to shoot himself. Themes: despair, suicidal

Ha,3- Inexpressibly weighed down with anguish, every afternoon from four to six o'clock. Themes: oppression

Ha,37- Freedom of spirit, lightness and general good health (curative...) Themes: liberty, light

Ha,677- At night he wakes up several times on account of pulsation in the head and anxiety as if about to have a fit of apoplexy; ...and he felt that if he put off awaking longer he would have fainted. Themes: fit, disease,

Ha,678- ... feeling over the body as if some one stroked him with the hand, and as if ants were running over the skin, at every moment in bed... Themes: crawling, hurt, attacked, animal

Ha,679- In the evening, during sleep, deception of the hearing; he thought he heard some one approach his bed, this woke him up with anxiety. Themes: approached,

Ha,706- Anxious as if oppressed, for several days. Themes: oppression

Ha,711- Excessive irritation, as if she were too much hurried, or had too much to do. Themes: duty, hurry

Ha,714- Peevish, impatient and desperate, so much so that he would like to shoot himself. Themes: despair, suicidal

Ha,8- For restlessness and anguish every afternoon, he trembled all over the body; he felt as if he had committed a great crime, this dissolved itself into copious weeping, even before strangers on the street. Themes: conscience, criminal,

Ha,9- He felt like weeping, everything seemed to him dreadful (fearful), and he felt in despair. Themes: grief, fearful, misfortune, despair

He,13- Feels unhappy with every little pain. Themes: unfortunate

He,14- Nightly fear of ghosts. Themes: ghosts

He,18- Anxiety and uneasiness causing him to tremble all over, as if he had committed a crime, ending in weeping, even before strangers;... Themes: conscience, criminal

CARBN-O.

Al,11- After supper, felt buoyant (happy) and in good humor, an effect never produced by tea; this mental sensation soon passed over into an irritable and sarcastic one, so that I sharply criticized an article in a medical journal, which a few hours ago I hardly thought worth that trouble, and threw away in disgust a book of reference as flat and superficial, which I highly sluggish.(inactive) Themes: pleasure, sarcasm, censorious, grief, contemptuous

Al,7- Frightful anxiety, and instinctive impulse to seek change of air, while he felt powerless to overcome the paralysis of his muscles and move from where he sat. Themes: fearful, restless, paralysis, unfit

CARBN-S.

Al-S,754- Hallucinations (delirium) of vision and hearing, he seemed to see splendid spectacles of carriages, with magnificent objects, talked of the emperor, of money, and of grandeur, often incoherently. Themes: greatness, wealth, money

Al-S,753- At one time during the night he

seemed to be surrounded by enemies; persons were coming to harm him;... Themes: hurt, surrounded, enemy, attacked

CARL.

Al,10- Discouraged and anxious in the discharge (execution) of his domestic duties. Themes: despair, duty, home

Al,16- Very much disposed to take everything in bad part and to be critical.(especially after three weeks and later) Themes: offenses, censorious

Al,4- His nerves are so much affected that the sorrows of others cause him to weep easily. Themes: compassionate, others

Al,5- Mood very much depressed, like an excessive homesickness; at last violent weeping.(second day) (after four glasses) Themes: sadness, homesickness, nostalgia

CAST.

Al,2- Very melancholy and depressed, as if something evil would befall her, in the afternoon. Themes: sadness, anticipation

CAUST.

Al,11- Excessively sympathetic; she is beside herself, with weeping and sobbing and cannot be contented when listening to accounts of the hardships (misfortune, difficulty) of others. Themes: compassionate, others

Al,12- Anxiety the whole day, as if he had done something bad, or apprehended it, or as if he had been unfortunate (unsuccessful, umprosperous). Themes: wrong, conscience, anticipation, unfortunate

Al,18- Anxiety with the physical troubles. Themes: disease

Al,24- Anxious apprehension lest something evil should happen, with urging to stool. Themes: misfortune, danger,

Al,26- He was busy with thoughts of death, with uneasiness and great solicitude. Themes: death, anticipation

Al,27- Loss of courage. Themes: cowardice

Al,28- Fear and anxiety, so that she does not wish to live. (death) Themes: death, loathing

Al,36- Extreme irritability of mind; the slightest vexation affects her whole body, so that her knees sink under her. Themes: bothered, sinking, fall

Al,9- Sad, weeping mood, full of care, as if beside oneself. Themes: sadness

Ha,13- Anxiously careful (cautious, prudent) as to all occurrences. Themes: conscientious

Ha,14- Great apprehensions (forebodings) as to whatever happens. Themes: misfortune, anticipation

Ha,16- Lack of courage. Themes: cowardice

Ha,19- When she closes her eyes, she always sees frightful visages and distorted human faces before her. Themes: horrible, ugly

Ha,20 -Extreme anxious timidity; she is so much afraid (fear) of a dog near her, which did not harm (hurt, injure) her at all,...every noise in the street made her afraid, and when she saw boys climbing she was very uneasy lest they might get hurt. (care, others) Themes: timidity, fearful, cowardice, bite, hurt, compassionate, animal, fearful, noise, others,

Ha,21- Her fear and anxiety cause her to wish that she might not live.(death) Themes: fearful, death

Ha,22- He occupies himself with thoughts of death, with restlessness and great solicitude.(cares) Themes: death,

Ha,23- Extreme excitability of spirit; the least vexation (difficulty) darts through her body, so that her knees give way. Themes: contradiction, fall

Ha,24- Discontented with himself, of gloomy (melancholic) countenance. Themes: discontented, sadness

Ha,30- Peevish (angry) all day, at odds (quarrel) with himself, dissatisfied, anxious and yet not indisposed to mental work. Themes: fight, discontented, anger

Ha,39- Unbounded inclination to take things ill.(insulted) Themes: offenses

Ha,4- Excessively compassionate (sympathetic); at the relations of others and of the cruelties inflicted upon them, she is beside herself for weeping and sobbing, and cannot content herself. Themes: compassionate, others

Ha,6- Anxiety the whole day, as if he had done something wrong, or to fear it, or as if a misfortune had happened. Themes: conscience, misfortune, wrong

Ha,61- A sort of absent-mindedness; while doing one thing, he always felt as if he had to do something else, more importance, (duty) and yet he knew not what ; he reflected about it, and yet thought nothing. (lost: signification, value, purpose) Themes: separated, duty, knowledge
Ha,7- Anxious, restlessness mood, as if something disagreeable (difficult) was impending (imminent) , which keeps him from working. Themes: restless, menaced, obstructed, anticipation, work
Ha,9 - Anxiety about bodily ailments.(disease) Themes: disease
He,17- Great restlessness, which prompts him to run away. Themes: restless, escape
He,24- Chilly, with sad mood and apprehension of the future < in evening. Themes: separated, future
He,25- Sorrowful thoughts during night, during day weeping, anxiety and misgiving (doubt) about the future. Themes: sadness, future
He,27- Melancholy mood; sadness; hopelessness. Themes: sadness, hopeless
He,30- Melancholy; she looks upon the dark side of everything. O Amenorrhoea. 0 Menorrhagia. Themes: pessimism
He,32- Hopeless weeping mood, expecting death. Themes: despair, death
He,33- Anxious uneasy mood, as if something unpleasant impended (threaten, frighten); this unfits (incompetent) him for every kind of work.(lost: competence) Themes: restless, menaced, unfit, confidence
He,34- Becomes anxious, as though he would die. Themes: death
He,36- Fearfulness and distressed (anguish) feeling about heart. Themes: fearful, heart
He,37- Full of timorous fancies, evenings; child fears to go to bed alone. Themes: solitude, fearful
He,39- Ill effects of sudden emotions, fright, fear, etc. (ailments from) Themes: fearful, disease
He,40- Fear of death. 0 Paralysis. Themes: death
He,42- Great apprehension whenever anything happens; despondent, depressed, most excessive exhaustion and prostration. Themes: anticipation, fearful, energy
He,43- Apprehension of impending danger, with urging to stool. Themes: danger
He,52- Anxiety before falling asleep, as though attack of fainting would return and he would die. Themes: fit, death
He,54- Excessive sympathy for others. Themes: compassionate, others,
He,58- Irritable temper, disposition to take everything in bad part. Themes: offenses
He,61- Very suspicious and distrustful. Themes: suspicious, conscientious
He,62- Thinking of complains aggravates them. Themes: disease
He,69- Injurious (ailments from) effects of fear and vexation. (worry) Themes: fearful, bothered, contradiction

CEDR.

Al,5- Dread of friends.(in females, particularly) Themes: fearful, misanthropy, friend

CERE-B.

Al,1- Desire to engage at work. Themes: work, busy
Al,11- Arose feeling miserable. Themes: unfortunate, miserable
Al,16- Difficult to keep employed. Themes: dispersion, work
Al,2- Desire to have the time all employed. (work) Themes: time, busy, work
Al,3- Felt all day an astonishing (unusual) inclination to be engaged (work, busy) in something useful. (helpful) Themes: busy, helpful, compassionate
Al,4- Felt a desire to give something quite necessary to myself to another. (altruism, helpful, sympathetic) Themes: helpful, compassionate, cares, others
Al,5- Desire to be dissolved, (evaporate, disintegrate) especially the trunk. Themes: disintegration
Al,6- Reluctance (doubt) to take medicine. Themes: suspicious, poisoned
Al,8- A grateful feeling of dependence (need, faith, relation) on a divine spirit was experienced. (reverence, veneration, praise) Themes: pleasure, religious,

CHAM.

Al,13- Piteous moaning of a child because he cannot have what he wants. (contrariety)

Themes: capricious, child, lack
Al,15- Very depressed mood, with anxiety and oppression, as of impending evil. Themes: sadness, oppression, misfortune, anticipation,
Al,20- Great dread of wind. Themes: storm
Al,3- At night, it seems as though he hears the voices of absent persons. Themes: helplessness
Al,31- She makes conscientious scruples about everything. Themes: conscientious, conscience
Al,40- Ill-humor; he suspects that he has been imposed upon. Themes: suspicious, betrayed
Al,53- Disposed to anger scorn quarrelsomeness. (after two hours) Themes: anger, contemptuous, fight
Al,54- Morose inclined to scorn. Themes: contemptuous
Al,58- He cannot stop talking about old vexatious (unpleasant) circumstances. Themes: past, mortification
Al,6- Earnest (serious) and taciturn mood; reconciled to his fate (destiny), about which he is deeply affected (later action). Themes: reserved, doomed
Al,64- He stammers (hesitate) uses wrong expressions, and corrects himself. Themes: talk, wrong
Ha,458- He feels a sinking in the precordium; he is beside himself with anxiety,... Themes: sinking, heart
Ha,460-... The child makes itself stiff and bends backwards, stamps with its feet on the nurse's arm, cries in an uncontrollable way, and throws everything away. Themes: fit, capricious
Ha,461- Lachrymose restlessness; the child wants this thing and the other, and when given anything he refuses it or knocks it away from him. Themes: capricious, antagonism
Ha,465- Very anxious; nothing she does seems to her to be right; she is irresolute; ...(indecisive) Themes: wrong, doubtful, irresolution, confidence
Ha,469- Howling (scream) on account of a slight, even an imaginary insult, which indeed , occurred long ago. (past) Themes: offenses, past
Ha,470 -Cannot cease talking about old vexatious things. Themes: bothered, mortification, past, talk
Ha,471- Suspicion that he may have been insulted. Themes: offenses, suspicious
Ha,475- Sulky moroseness; everything others do is displeasing to him; no one does anything to please him. Themes: bothered
Ha,476- He vexes himself inwardly about every trifle. Themes: bothered
Ha,485- Quarrelsome crossness; she seeks for everything vexatious.(provoking) Themes: bothered, fight
Ha,488- She sits stiffly (rigid, petrified) on a chair like a statue, and seems to take no notice of anything about her. Themes: paralysis,
Ha,490- She has scruples of conscience about everything. Themes: conscientious, doubtful, confidence
Ha,491- Serious reservedness; calm submission to his profoundly felt fate (destiny). Themes: reserved, yielding, doomed
He,14-..., vows there is some dreadful beast under his bed or in the room, and will not be appeased (calm) until the gas is lit and the room is searched. Themes: invaded, horrible, animal
He,15- Piteous moaning of a child because he cannot have what he wants. Themes: child, capricious
He,16- Moaning on account of a very trifling offense, which had happened a long time ago. Themes: offenses, past, resentment
He,17- Whining (lamenting) restlessness; the child wants this and that, which, when offered, is refused or pushed away. Themes: capricious
He,25- Cannot endure being spoken to, or interrupted while speaking, ... Themes: talk
He,32- Very anxious; everything she undertakes is very unsatisfactory (disappointed) ; she is irresolute,...(indecision) Themes: failure, succeed, doubtful,
He,36- Thoughts of dying. Themes: death
He,41- Peevishness (cross, angry); she seeks a cause for being peevish at everything; can't return a civil (polite) answer.(impolite ,rude) Themes: bother
He,44- Morose fretfulness; everything that another does is wrong; no one does anything to please him. Themes: wrong, antagonism
He,49- Great impatience, everything seems to go too slowly. Themes: hurry, impatience, time

He,55- In all her sufferings there is a vein of ill humor; she can hardly speak pleasantly; feels like scolding (censorious, offensive) about everything; she often gives vent to her ill humor in spite of all restraint. Themes: censorious, suppressed
He,58- Insulting, cross and uncivil temper. Themes: offensive, bothered
He,59- Great tendency to quarrel, to speak in an obstreperous (rude, vulgar) manner. Themes: fight, talk, defiant
He,68- All bad effects following anger. (ailments, from) 0Convultions, 0chill, 0fever, 0bilious complaints Themes: anger
He,70- Bad effects of having feelings wounded. (ailments from) Themes: offenses

CHEL.

Al,24- Sad mood; she fears that she has ruined her health by the proving. Themes: disease, ruined,
Al,25- Sadness, even to weeping, and despondency (desperation) about the present and future. Themes: future, sadness, despair
Al,27- Extremely depressed; full of sad thoughts about the present and future, even to weeping; he had no rest of any kind. Themes: future, pessimism, sadness,
Al,43- Anxiety and fear of death, with desire to eructate, which he cannot do, at night. Themes: death
Al,51- Anxious about death and being a soldier (warrior, disputant), at night. Themes: death, officer
Al,53- Becomes frightened at the slightest noise, as if he had not a good conscience. Themes: fearful, conscience, noise
Al,54- Fear that pneumonia is coming on. Themes: disease, infection
Al,55 - Mood very irritable, daily outbreaks of anger without cause (causeless); feels as though she could beat the children, and trembles from rage because she has no reason for doing it. Themes: anger, conscience, violence, child,
Al,65- Fretful depressed, anxious, as if I had committed some evil (crime), which gave me no rest. (remorse) Themes: conscience, criminal
Al,74- It seems as though she could not think, and would lose her reason. (after three hours) Themes: obstructed, unfit, insanity
Ha,154- Extraordinarily depressed, full of gloomy (dark) thoughts about the present and future, causing him to weep;... Themes: future, pessimism, sadness,
Ha,155- Sad to weeping and depressed about the present and future. Themes: sadness, future
He,17- Restlessness and uneasiness of conscience; feels that she has committed the unpardonable sin (crime, transgression), and that she will be eternally lost. Themes: conscience, criminal, doomed, lost
He,18- Anxiety: allowing no rest at any employment (business) ; as if she had committed a crime; fear of getting crazy (insanity), with restlessness and heat. Themes: work, conscience, criminal, insanity
He,25- Is vexed (anger, irritated) about every trifle and has violent attacks of passionate outbursts of temper. Themes: bothered, passionate, anger
He,6- Imagines she cannot think and will lose her reason.(impediment) Themes: insanity, unfit
He,7- Thinks she must die. Themes: death, conscience

CHIN-B.

He,5- Feels abandoned and deserted. Themes: forsaken, despised

CHIN-S.

Al,16- Great anxiety, amounting to an apprehension, as if some evil would happen. Themes: anticipation, misfortune
Al,20-...; felt a gloom (darkness) come over me, as if some evil were impending; relieved by a specific trust in the Almighty;...(divine) (faithful, confiding, devoted) Themes: menaced, dark, misfortune, religious,
He,9- Recurrence of feeling of impending evil. Themes: menaced, misfortune

CHIN.

Al, DREAM .1105- ...;he imagines he is descending a precipice, on which account he awakes, but the dangerous place remains vividly before his fancy...Al,1109- At night frightful dreams of falling from a height, with waking full of uneasiness... Themes: height, fall, danger

Al, DREAM-1110- Dreamed that some one had stabbed his brother, and then called for his mother; that his mother was dead, and then he cried; that his mother's arms was hurt;... Themes: pointed, murdered, death, mother, brother, others, hurt

Al,35- Ill-humor, amounting to the most violent wrath (fury), so that he could have stabbed any one. Themes: anger, violence, homicidal, pointed

Al,39- Fretful and irresolute; she is unable to accomplish her aim, and consequently is indignant. (angry) Themes: anger, confidence, succeed, unfit, indignation

Al,47- Discontent; he considers himself unhappy and thinks he is hindered (obstructed) and tormented by everyone. (after five hours) Themes: discontented, obstructed, tormented, unfortunate, suppressed

Al,49- He despises everything. Themes: contemptuous

Al,56- A large number of projects. Themes: planning

Ha,1093-...;he jumps out of the bed and wants to make away with himself (suicide) , and yet he fears to go near and open window or to approach a knife. Themes: suicidal, height, pointed

Ha,1095- Too anxious caution. Themes: conscientious

Ha,1096- An over-anxious concern (care) about trifles. Themes: conscientious

Ha,1103- She falls time to time into a lachrymose humour, without external cause, from some self-made, trivial whim (caprice), e.q. from some imaginary want (lack, need), such as that she cannot eat enough... Themes: capricious, lack, poverty, starving

Ha,1105- What formerly appeared to him in a bright genial light, seems now to be lusterless (lifeless), unworthy (inutile), and shallow (superficial, stupid) Themes: bright, disappointment, knowledge, light

Ha,1110- Extremely disposed to be vexed, and to take every occasion to get cross; afterwards quarrelsome and disposed to vex others, and to make reproaches and give annoyance(irritation) to others. Themes: bothered, fight, censorious, offensive, bother

Ha,1113- Discontented; he thinks himself unfortunate (unsuccessful) ,and fancies he is opposed (confronted, hostilised), and tormented (molested) by everybody. Themes: unfortunate, bothered, tormented

Ha,1119- Humour gloomy, no wish to live. Themes: sadness, death

Ha,1134- Liking for work, reading, writing, and thinking; particularly well disposed and industrious. Themes: work, succeed, busy, pleasure

Ha,1135- He makes a number of grand (great) plans for the future. Themes: planning, greatness, future

Ha,1136- He makes many plans, and thinks over their accomplishment (execution, success), many ideas force themselves upon him at once. Themes: planning, succeed

Ha,1137- He has many ideas, undertakes (begin, try) to carry out (achieve, perform, execute) all sorts of things, builds castles in air.(fanciful) Themes: succeed, planning, greatness

Ha,1138- He has a number of plans in his head which he greatly desires to carry into execution (progress), in the evening. Themes: succeed, planning,

He,10- Fixed idea that he is unhappy, persecuted by enemies. Themes: persecution, unfortunate, enemy

He,11- She thinks she is very unfortunate and constantly harassed (molested, tormented) by enemies. Themes: unfortunate, persecution, bothered, enemy, tormented

He,16-...;wants to destroy himself, but lacks courage. Themes: suicidal, cowardice, lack

He,27- Inconsolable anxiety, even to suicide. Themes: suicidal

He,28- Dread of dogs and other animals at night. Themes: animal, dark

He,31- Inclined to reproach and vex (annoy, provoke) others. Themes: censorious, bother

He,55- He has many ideas, a variety of things occupy his mind; he builds castles in the air (after a few hours). Themes: planning

CHLOL.

Al,17-...a feeling as if he were now in one country and now in another, and with an anxious desire to go home.(abroad) Themes: homesickness, stranger, travel, home, nostalgia, abroad

Al,24-...knew that she was very ill, and herself insisted upon my being sent for...(ordered, dictatorial) Themes: disease

Al,3- A horrible state of mind, fears he will go crazy, fears he cannot make a living.(subsistence) Themes: insanity, poverty, starving

Al,5- Became delirious, and hurled (throw) a hot-water bottle at an imaginary figure which stood menacing her at the foot of the bed. Themes: menaced

He,10- Gorgeous (superb, beautiful) visions of arches, tapestry (decoration) and colors pass before the eyes when shut, or open in the dark. Themes: pleasure, wealth

He,3- Fixed despair of recovery; believes he will give his imaginary disease (syphilis) to others. Themes: despair, disease, infection, conscience, others

He,7-...inclined to wander and hide herself, avoiding shrewdly (astute) the vigilance of her friends... Themes: hide, persecution, escape, observed, friend

CHLOR.

Al,4-...he is afraid of becoming insane; thinks it is impossible to get through it. (obstruction , impediment) Themes: insanity

He,3- A horrible state of mind, fears he will go crazy, fears he cannot make a living.(subsistence) Themes: insanity, poverty, failure,

CHOC.

Sh,103- On looking at a bird in a cage, felt it should be out. Themes: liberty, imprisoned, compassionate

Sh,104- Rather than hearing the usual music I listen to, I wanted to hear a blackbird sing. The outdoors seems very familiar and my hands get excited at the thought of it. Themes: music, animal, nature

Sh,106- I feel excited —a purpose in me — as if geared up and something is about to happen. Is nice. There is no choice involved. It just is. A feeling that you know that every part of you is right and must be right to go forward. All the senses must be there, not like my old blithering-around in distraction. Just one objective — find food! Themes: eating

Sh,107- A strange feeling of being an animal, yet having this thinking. Themes: transmutation, identity, animal

Sh,109- In the night, heart stops beating. All very still inside. Themes: stagnation, heart

Sh,110- I really like my nose. It feels more useful in the dark. Themes: dark, sensitive

Sh,114- When I feel like a hedgehog, my heart is much faster, but when I feel the stillness, I don't feel my heart at all. Themes: animal, identity, transmutation, heart

Sh,116- 12:30pm - I feel less and less animal at the moment and I desire company. When it comes, its so intense, I almost lose what I am. I've never been there before. I feel very privileged, as if I can be on both sides at the same time. Themes: company, animal, identity, double

Sh,117- I thought how would an animal be if it had my body. What would they do with thought. I think I'm better off. Themes: identity, animal, transmutation

Sh,120- Felt as if I was hibernating — mouth sealed up perfectly and my tongue seems to fill all the space. I usually sleep with my mouth open as I cannot breathe through my nose, but now my mouth is perfectly sealed and nose free-flowing. Themes: animal, transmutation

Sh,121- I met a dog this morning and felt that I understood it now and it wasn't a threat, whereas earlier I had been uncertain and wary. Themes: animal, menaced

Sh,122- While looking out of the window, I realised I had the capacity to see from above and below at the same time — not a dividing in two from bottom to top, but a knowledge of both sides at once. Themes: sensitive, knowledge

Sh,124- I see things differently than before —

everything more clear and three-dimensional — more real. Textures and shapes seem different- like a new way of seeing. I seem to have a fascination with certain objects and textures, like wood on doors or colours of hair. Sense of smell very acute. I can smell what people drink from the other side of the room and where to locate it. Themes: sensitive

Sh,127- Before this, I never felt very comfortable with men. Now I feel much more comfortable. I feel I've lost that extreme feeling of totally female identity. I feel like a female animal, but its not really in my awareness, it just is. Desire to curl up over a man's back. It felt right and comfortable. Themes: sexual, animal, identity

Sh,128- The separation that I have always felt seems to be gone and I feel much more part of what's around. Themes: integration

Sh,130- I feel slightly less like a hedgehog today, but the picture is still in my mind. Human things seem so trivial — so much energy wasted when you are human. Nature is so efficient. It never wastes a seed and we just spend energy everywhere. Themes: animal, identity, nature, perfection

Sh,134- I felt small enough to get into a drawer in a desk full of rubbish and rout around under things, a kind of curiosity. Themes: small, identity

Sh,135- The earth has taken on a new meaning. Before it was just there, now it has everything. A desire to be in contact with the earth. Themes: integration, nature

Sh,139- Meditation is much smoother —an effortless zooming in. I feel much more comfortable in the world. Before I always wanted to get out. During meditation, felt a floating feeling, felt an opening and upwards movement in my back, as if wings were forming and I was just light. Themes: meditation, floating, fly, liberty, transmutation

Sh,14- Angry about being in city. When I look, I want to see far distances and sky, not houses. Went to estate agents to look at country houses. Themes: anger, distances, nature, travel

Sh,145- My fears around the kids — that they would die, etc. and that they were my total responsibility, like parasites — have gone and I know feel total trust that they will be o.k. Themes: duty, child, death, others

Sh,146- I find dark exciting and comfortable, whereas before I was fearful in the dark. Themes: dark

Sh,149- Hearing and smell still acute — nature seems wonderful. Saw nine magpies and they seemed much bigger than before. Themes: sensitive, perfection, animal, great

Sh,15- I see plants in the house differently, very aware of them and want to give them more light. Themes: compassionate, light, nature

Sh,150- People keep stopping me and saying they don't recognise me. I still have a silly grin on my face. Laugh more — so much joy inside and a sense of freedom very different to before the proving. Dogs seem to like me more and babies seem to like me more, and this was noticed by others too. Themes: friendly, liberty, pleasure

Sh,151- Still get images of creatures — thought a tomato was a grasshopper. Themes: identity, animal,

Sh,152- Wanted to eat slugs and grasshoppers. I could feel how they would be in my mouth while they were still alive and wriggling. (Has been vegetarian for twenty years). Themes: alive, eating

Sh,153- Since the proving, I know how it feels to be a animal or a plant. I know the feeling of daffodil, of flower, of hedgehog, of dog. Themes: animal, transmutation, identity

Sh,172- Dreams of fire. Themes: fire

Sh,179- Apprehensive about the shift in consciousness and nervous someone would notice. It is reminiscent of L.S.D., the 'shifting edges', before the full blown trip arrives — an uneasiness and unsureness about which way things will go. A desire to hide in case things go to pieces. 15, 30C, 00:00:50 Themes: shame, hide, disintegration, insanity

Sh,180- I felt that I was making exceptionally profound statements about life. 35, 30C, 03:XX:XX Themes: philosophy, theorizing

Sh,181- Attitude good, feel calm and philosophical about things45, 30C, 02:XX:XX Themes: philosophy

Sh,182- This remedy is making me look more

deeply into things. Found myself looking into a flower, plugging into its inner substance. 35, 30C, 05:XX:XX Themes: integration, nature

Sh,183- Thoughts of what's in all this for me? What am I getting out of this? Wondering about his life and why I continue with it. 45, 30C, 23:XX:XX Themes: philosophy

Sh,185- Religious like feeling. 45, 30C, 00:00:10 Themes: religious

Sh,186- It seems like ages ago I started the proving and I can hardly believe its only the fourth day. It seems like I'm going through a whole lifetime of emotions in a short time. 4 , 6C, 05:XX:XX Themes: time

Sh,188- While walking outside, became anxious in a self-conscious way, anxious and vulnerable as if being watched or observed by something or someone - the attention was on me - anxiety that something would happen. Immediately afterwards I was attacked by four dogs and bitten on the calf. 27, 100C, 01:XX:XX Themes: fragile, observed, clairvoyance, accidents

Sh,189- While outside became very weary of cars and people. Felt open and vulnerable. Fear of accidents, cars, or of someone leaping into the road and punching me. This anxiety was worse out of doors. 27, 100C, 01:XX:XX Themes: run over, accidents, attacked, fragile, go out, attacked, hurt

Sh,19- I feel very vulnerable in the base of the spine. Themes: fragile

Sh,190- While walking past a block of flats, I worried that it might blow over in the wind and fall on me. 27, 100C, 01:XX:XX Themes: accidents, hurt

Sh,191- I Since the being bitten by the dogs have developed a strong fear of dogs, and have been chased by one dog and growled at by another. This is coupled with a general fear of something happening. These fears are new to me and were better again after the proving. 27, 100C, 05:XX:XX Themes: attacked, hurt, menaced, animal, misfortune

Sh,192- I woke up and could not feel the usual sensation of my heart bulging or beating through my ribs while lying on my left side. I felt shock and thought 'perhaps I'm dead'. Groped for pulse and was reassured to be able to feel it. 15, 30C, 02:02:XX Themes: stagnation, heart, death

Sh,193- Husband wants to go out for a walk. I don't want to go. I feel paranoid that someone will see me and think 'on drugs' and arrest me or cart me off to an institution. 15, 30C, 00:02:00 Themes: persecution, imprisoned, conscience

Sh,195- No need to worry about money as usually do. 41, 6C, 00:XX:XX Themes: money

Sh,2- Feel very excited, very alive, bright and efficient. Had an image of a hedgehog's face. Themes: energy, alive, animal, bright

Sh,205- Though Previously lazy, became intensely obsessed with work for a long period of time. Put all my energy into work. 35, 30C, XX:XX:XX: Themes: obstinate, work

Sh,208- Felt rejected and oversensitive. Hid away from the world, felt my life would fall apart. 35, 30C, XX:XX:XX: Themes: forsaken, sensitive, isolation, hide, misanthropy

Sh,209- A desire to hide in case things go to pieces. 15, 30C, 00:00:50 Themes: hide, escape, disintegration

Sh,210- Felt totally isolated and averse to company. Estranged himself from his family and friends and stopped all communication with them for a long period. Did not reply to letters and left no address. He seemed to hide away and literally disappear. The state of Isolation resulted from feeling that "I didn't exist as a human being". This behaviour was in strong contrast to his normal sociable disposition. 35, 30C, XX:XX:XX: Themes: isolation, company, forsakes, misanthropy, family, friend, identity, reserved, hide

Sh,211- Feeling like I don't belong in a crowd. Conscious of all social and economic pressures on people nowadays and was glad to get home.41, 6C, 01:XX:XX Themes: isolation, stranger

Sh,212- Felt more desire to be alone and more able to live alone. 07, 100C, 19:XX:XX Themes: solitude

Sh,213- Unsociable — averse company and conversation.15, 30C, 04:XX:XX Themes: company, solitude, talk, loathing

Sh,218- Had a deep conversation with a friend and felt more mature, as if being detached, is helping me to understand her more.35, 30C, 04:XX:XX Themes: knowledge, friendly

Sh,227- The phone rings and I think 'How typical, how thoughtless, to ring at this moment'. It feels like an intrusion. I stay polite, but am thinking 'Oh tell the truth or shut up'. 1, 30C, 00:XX:XX Themes: misanthropy

Sh,228- Thoughts about the 'veneer of civilisation' that inhibits how we really feel and keeps us from displaying what we're like beneath the surface. It seems a legitimate layer, but so is the layer beneath it, and I feel amused and happy to meet it. This feeling continued for a few days, a very graphic picture of a veneer - a layer of learned social behaviour lifting and detaching from a basis that is thick, dark, solid, instinctual animal.15 ,30C, 00:00:30 Themes: feigning, suppressed, animal, wild, divided

Sh,23- A sensation of my back being larger and wider than what I know it to be. The sensation developed so that it seemed that my back moved higher up and outwards towards the scapula — as if opening out. Themes: grow

Sh,301- Desire to bite my husband in a playful way. I bit him — I wanted to really sink my teeth in, but willed myself not to. It was an animal need in me.15, 30C, 00:05:30 Themes: bite, animal, wild

Sh,302- Tonight my husband committed a large annoyance. I felt rage rise up in me — he jumped back and cowered! I wanted to beat some sensibility into him, stopping short of actually wanting to kill him, I felt: 'its not fair', 'how inconsiderate and thoughtless to an extreme degree'. However, my will intervened before I made a scene. Its as if I'm more aware of my 'shadow side' and really feeling it, but precisely because I'm more aware of it, I can step in with my will and curb my behaviour if it looks as if I'm likely to hurt someone else.15, 30C, 03:XX:XX Themes: anger, homicidal, violence, wild

Sh,303- I'm ready to speak my mind — I don't care if people cease to like me.15, 30C, 20:XX:XX Themes: offensive

Sh,304- Feels she has changed her attitude towards herself, less judgmental and pedantic, kinder to herself now. Eating more meat and feeling OK about it, previously had been vegetarian for health and moral reasons.13, 12C, XX:XX:XX Themes: censorious, himself

Sh,306- Her usual sensation of left right body split has been much more defined. Later on during the proving this "split" became more balanced than usual and felt much more integrated, (curative).13, 12C, 02:XX:XX Themes: divided, half, integration

Sh,307- Talking to a friend, noticed her mouth felt strange, almost as if she had two mouths, one on top of the other. No other part appeared double.27, 100C, 00:22:15 Themes: strange, double

Sh,308- I feel both more present and more distant. 29, 200C, 02:XX:XX Themes: isolation

Sh,309- A feeling of intoxication with double sensations. Colours are stronger and hearing is sharpened but at the same time feel absent and removed.29, 200C, 00:XX:XX Themes: double, bright, sensitive, isolation

Sh,310- On bending my head back, a sensation, or imagination, that the back of my head is horribly elongated. I can't get it out of my mind.15, 30C, 03:13:30 Themes: grow, great

Sh,311- On stepping out of the shower, a fleeting, momentary imagination of both arms crawling with insects. No physical sensation, purely an imagination.15, 30C, 00:02:XX Themes: crawling, animal

Sh,312- While reading small print in materia medica, I had a delusion that tiny insects were crawling down the page. 15, 30C, 03:XX:XX Themes: animal, crawling

Sh,313- Desire to see far — to a distant horizon. Desire to be outside more.01A, 30C, 00:XX:XX Themes: distances, go out

Sh,314- Talking about flying. I would like to be a bird or a bat or in a plane.01A, 30C, 00:12:XX Themes: fly, animal, liberty

Sh,315- Been on the move all day — painted a room blue. While lying in the bath looking out the window, the sky is the most glorious, vibrant blue — it seems like the most beautiful colour I've ever seen.

Almost wept for the beauty of it. Suddenly, while I'm lying in the bath, the colour blue seems very important — seems very potent. It has the same quality and intensity that I remember colours having on L.S.D. I am very moved by this blue. I wanted to dissolve into it.15, 30C, 03:05:XX Themes: bright, perfection, integration, pleasure

Sh,319- Felt emotionally numb and separated from things.35, 30C, XX:XX:XX: Themes: indifference, isolation

Sh,32- When I look in the mirror, I don't recognise myself. I look different, especially around and over the eyes — my face doesn't seem familiar. The area around my forehead feels more congested and bigger. Themes: strange, identity

Sh,322- Have lost interest in my husband, feel totally indifferent. I have hardly spoken to him all weekend, with a desire to avoid him. Don't want to discuss or share anything with him.15, 30C, 06:XX:XX Themes: indifference, sexual, loathing, solitude

Sh,324- Still snapping and resentful generally.15, 30C, 36:XX:XX Themes: anger, offensive, resentment

Sh,327- My humour has taken a sarcastic turn, mocking people, a bit aggressive in a joking way.35, 30C, 00:03:XX Themes: contemptuous, sarcasm, offensive

Sh,328- Humourless, intolerant - almost cruel. Scalded a child's hand out of anger, and nothing would make him apologise.35, 30C, XX:XX:XX: Themes: cruel, intolerant, wicked, sadism, anger

Sh,329- Felt anger at life, I wasn't getting anywhere. The world appeared a cruel place to me, and I felt I had no place in the scheme of things.35, 30C, XX:XX:XX: Themes: anger, cruel, isolation

Sh,331- I became selfish, impatient and intolerant. Behaved in a strange way - hard and quarrelsome - snapping at people. Could not stand people wasting time or being inefficient, I wanted things done immediately.35, 30C, XX:XX:XX: Themes: egotism, impatience, intolerant, offensive, fight, anger, hurry, conscientious

Sh,38- Sense of smell very acute. Hearing more acute, especially for deeper tones which have more resonance. Themes: sensitive

Sh,39- Felt a need to be covered up. Themes: hide

Sh,40- Became aware of a man's hair and had an intense desire to touch it, to make contact with it. Themes: sexual, touch

Sh,41- When hearing talk of babies, breasts aching with a sensation as if filling up with milk — an aching fullness. An image came to me where I found myself suckling young hairy babies, sometimes animals, especially hedgehogs. Themes: sexual, animal, eating

Sh,412- Much more sensitive to music — especially happy music. It gives me incredible pleasure.01A, 30C, XX:XX:XX Themes: music, pleasure

Sh,418- Feel affectionate and quiet in evening, less restless than usual.11, 6C, 00:XX:XX Themes: friendly, peace

Sh,42- Attracted to a man's beard. I could just feel his hair around the mouth. Themes: sexual

Sh,420- Urgency and strong desire to travel decreased since proving, (curative).11, 6C, XX:XX:XX Themes: hurry, travel

Sh,44- Dream — coming out of the station a huge black bird the size of a dog with black long soft feathers like those of an ostrich, and a very big beak. It took my left hand in his beak. There were two gypsies there and they stood in front of me and opened their hands and I saw that they held a gold metal flat fish which I saw as a fortune telling object. Themes: animal, dark, great, liberty, stranger, wealth

Sh,45- When I woke from the dream, I had a little panic, an unusual childhood memory came back in which I remembered having read as a child about being covered in clay, baked and eaten. The thought came to me of the spines on my back covered in clay and baked and eaten like a hedgehog. Themes: past, identity, animal, transmutation

Sh,50- Panic feeling of being trapped and enclosed — worse when curtains are closed and the light blocked out. Strong desire to be outside and moving, to be in the bright and warm sunlight. Kept having to move my feet, which I felt I wanted to move. Themes: caught, imprisoned, dark, liberty, light, movement

Sh,51- While out walking, saw a dog and became very scared. I felt very uncomfortable and unsympathetic to the dog. All very unusual. Themes: fearful, animal

Sh,52- My right hand feels bigger and wider and I feel more powerful. But my wrists feel weaker and flatter. Sensation of opening of hands and tightness in the forearm. Themes: energy, great, small

Sh,57- Keep getting a picture of the prickles of the start of the hairline of the hedgehog and am aware of this point in me —not discomfort, but keep pushing hair back and pulling my fingers backwards through my hair, thinking its nice that its not in my face. Keep getting pictures of faces of hedgehogs, (rather than the spiny bits) especially the nose, which seems so black and wet. Themes: animal, identity, transmutation

Sh,58- My nose has been running in the cold, dripping. It feels smaller. Themes: small

Sh,62- The blackness of the trees is bothering me. They seem dark and leafless. Themes: dark. bothered, lifeless

Sh,7- In the evening, felt angry with bristling down my back. Irritable with the kids, shouted a lot, slammed doors. Feeling very uncomfortable with my daughter near me. I made a huge issue over something small which I would normally leave. I wanted to leave and walk out of the door on them. Felt very unsympathetic to the children. "You either go, or go to bed". Couldn't cuddle the children and took longer to say "Its all right". I thought that their father should look after them instead of me (very unusual). The feeling I can't be where I want to be because of them. I want to be roaming outside without my possessions. Left kids alone in the house for the first time. I was surprised at how easily I let them go. My daughter liked it very much. Themes: anger, offensive, censorious, forsakes, escape

Sh,73- Feel I have to be alert, as if my total survival depended on me being alert — exhausting. Themes: danger, conscientious

Sh,74- I saw a rat. We stood looking at each other. I felt we both recognised each other. It was very exciting. Themes: integration, animal, identity

Sh,8- I felt like being outside, roaming around without any possessions, to have the freedom to go where I want to go when the feeling took me. I felt very restricted. Themes: liberty, suppressed

Sh,82- Dream that my daughter was there drying her hair. She was late for school and I was very distressed with her slowness. I felt she should be brushing her hair and not drying it. I went to switch off the drier, but the wall socket was open and exposed, with electrical bits everywhere, so I couldn't switch it off. Themes: hurry

Sh,86- On seeing a bristly carpet, started laughing excitedly — had a familiar feeling, like meeting a friend. The texture of the carpet was very spiky like a Hedgehog. Told friend that they should come and see it. It's such a wonderful carpet! Themes: animal, friend, identity, perfection

Sh,9- Had a vivid dream of worms —they were dark and fat, but I wished they were red and thin. I felt very excited by the worms. Themes: animal, dark, heavy

Sh,90- Concentration very sharp, as if my survival depended on it. I felt very focused. (During a lecture) My understanding was sharper. Normally I have many things going on in my head —too scattered — but in the last few days, narrower attention. Themes: danger, conscientious, knowledge

Sh,96- Everything seems right and in order now. I feel much better. Only survival matters, simpler. All the trivial affairs and worries of humans are irrelevant. The only things that matter are food and warmth. I need just enough to eat — red berries. On a walk I saw red berries and thought everything is there, no problem. I have no worries like humans have — no decision making — there isn't any choice. Themes: eating, transmutation

Sh,97- I feel my kids are ready to go, but I have to get back to the younger ones to feed. Felt I could walk home (300 miles), a feeling that I should never go further than I could walk. Themes: eating, child, walk

CIC.

Al,25- He believes he would die. Themes: death

Al,26- Contempt and scorn for mankind; he avoided them, abhorred their follies (stupidity) excessively, and his disposition seemed to tend towards misanthropy; he withdrew (retire) himself into solitude. Themes: loathing, contemptuous, indignation, solitude, misanthropy, haughty

Al,27- Want of confidence in mankind; with misanthropy; he forsook society, remained alone and reflected upon their errors and about himself. Themes: misanthropy, suspicious, forsakes, solitude, censorious, wrong, justice

Al,29- He was indifferent to everything, and began to doubt whether he was really in the condition which he found himself. Themes: indifference, unreal, strange

Al,9- He did not believe that he was living under ordinary relations; everything seemed strange and almost fearful to him; it seemed as though he has awakened from an acute fever... Themes: unreal, strange, horrible

Ha,226- He became indifferent to everything, and began to doubt whether this was really the condition in which he was. Themes: indifference, doubtful, unreal

Ha,227- He confounded the present with the past. Themes: time

Ha,228- He thought with anxiety of the future and was always sad. Themes: future, sadness

Ha,229- Anxiety; he was violently affected by sad stories. Themes: sadness

Ha,231- Excitement, with concern for the future, he represented to himself as dangerous everything that would happen to him. Themes: future, danger

Ha,232- When others were gay he was sad. Themes: antagonism, envy, others

Ha,235- ...; everything appeared to him strange and almost frightful; it was as if he woke up out of an acute fever and saw all sorts of figures, and yet he did not feel corporeally ill. Themes: strange, disease

Ha,237- Depreciation and contempt of mankind; he fled (desert) his fellow-creatures, was in the highest degree disgusted with their follies (stupidity), and his disposition seemed to change into misanthropy; he withdrew into solitude. Themes: contemptuous, forsakes, grief, solitude, loathing, misanthropy,

Ha,238- Want of trust (mistrust, skepticism) in people and anthrophoby,(misanthropy) he fled (escape) from them remained solitary, and thought seriously about their errors and about himself. Themes: suspicious, misanthropy, forsakes, himself, escape, solitude, wrong,

Ha,240- He felt like a child of seven or eight years old, objects were very dear and attractive to him, as toys are to a child. (purity) Themes: child, identity, pure, pleasure

Ha,241- Tranquillity of mind; he was extremely satisfied with his position, and with himself, and very cheerful. Themes: position, himself, pleasure

He,10- Feels as if he was in a strange place, which causes fear. Themes: strange

He,16- Thinks of the future with anxiety, and is constantly sad. Themes: future

He,18- Fondness (desire) for solitude; great disregard and dislike for society of others. Themes: solitude, contemptuous, misanthropy, company

He,30- Anxiety, excessively affected by sad stories. Themes: sensitive, sadness

He,33- Old man fear a long spell (time) of sickness before dying. Themes: disease, death

He,34- Is afraid (fear) of society, and wants to be alone. Themes: misanthropy, solitude, company

He,35- Excited, with apprehension concerning the future; everything that could befall him seemed to be dangerous. Themes: future, danger

He,36- Mistrust and shunning (avoid) of men; despises others. Themes: suspicious, misanthropy, contemptuous, loathing, others

He,7- He thinks himself a young child. (purity, juvenile, infant) Themes: pure, identity, child

He,8- He imagined he was not living in his usual condition and circumstances; everything appears to him strange and almost terrible. Themes: unreal, strange

He,9- She thinks she sees coming towards her a huge drunken man, who lies down alongside of her, she begs him to retire... Themes: invaded

CIMIC.

Al,3- Miserable, dejected (sad) feeling. Themes: miserable, sadness

He,1- Sensation as if a heavy black cloud (smoke) had settled (descent) all over her, and enveloped (surrounded, wrap) her head, so that all was darkness and confusion, while, at the same time, it weighed (heavy) like lead (metal) on her head. Themes: obstructed, surrounded, dark, heavy

He,10- Fear of death; fears those in house will kill him (murdered, by parents); saw wires encasing (lock, imprisoned) him; visions of rats and of strange objects. Themes: death, betrayed, murdered, suspicious, imprisoned, strange, animal, family

He,13- Desire for solitude, or to wander from place to place. Themes: solitude, travel

He,15- Declares she has been poisoned. Themes: poisoned, suspicious

He,20- Miserable dejected feeling; anxious weeping. Themes: miserable, sadness

He,21- Mental depression, with suicidal mood; also after checked neuralgia. Themes: suicidal, disease

He,24- Fears she will become crazy, with headache on vertex. Themes: insanity

He,25- Fear of death. Themes: death

He,26- Indifferent, taciturn, takes no interest in household matters. Themes: indifference, reserved, duty, home

He,27- Irritable; the least thing that goes wrong makes her angry. Themes: wrong, anger

He,29- Suspicious of everything, would not take medicine if she knew it. Themes: suspicious, poisoned, betrayed

He,34- Mind disturbed by disappointed love, business failures. Themes: love, disappointment, failure, work

He,5- Thinks she is going crazy. Themes: insanity

He,6- Often startled by illusion of a mouse running from under her chair. Themes: animal

He,7- Imagines strange objects about bed, as rats, sheep, etc. Themes: animal, strange

CIMX.

He,4- Sensation as if he would creep (slide) into himself, and on that account could not sufficiently crouch (bend, incline) together. Themes: reserved

CINA.

He,8- Great earnestness (serious) and sensitiveness; he is offended at slightest joke. Themes: offenses, sensitive

CINNB.

Al,1- Illusion of mind; he considers himself well. Themes: antagonism, disease

CIST.

He,3- Bad effects of vexation; feels as if paralyzed. Themes: contradiction, paralysis

CLEM.

Al,11- Very sad humor with thoughts of suicide. Themes: suicidal

Al,13- Buried in sad thought and in dread (fear) of impending misfortune. Themes: mortification, misfortune

Al,14- He seemed oppressed by some grief or sorrow, or the shadow of impending misfortune. Themes: oppression, grief, misfortune

Al,17- Anxious uneasiness, as though some evil would befall him. Themes: misfortune

Al,19- ...dreading to be alone, tired of living, full of thoughts of death, with fear that it would be speedy, longing however, for the repose of death; this mood was soon followed by apprehension, weeping, and homesickness, ... Themes: solitude, tedium, death, homesickness, peace

He,5- Fear of being alone, but disinclined to meet even agreeable company. Themes: solitude, company

He,6- Irritable, taciturn, does not want to go out. Themes: go out

He,8- Ailments from homesickness, or contrition (penitence, remorse) of spirit. Themes: homesickness, conscience, salvation

COB.

Al,4- Low-spirited; thinks too little of himself. Themes: sadness, himself, separated

Al,5- Condemned, mean feeling, as though guilty of some deed (action) of which others knew; as if he could not look one in the face. (shame, dishonored) Themes: conscience, wicked, shame, doomed,

COCA.

Al,17- When lifting anything, fear lest I should let it fall, in the morning (dropping) Themes: fall

COCC.

Al,10- She is absorbed in the saddest thoughts, and affronts (indignity) sink deep into her heart. Themes: dwells, sadness, offenses, heart

Al,11- Thoughts directed to an unpleasant object; she is absorbed in herself, and notices nothing about her. Themes: dwells, mortification

Al,15- Anxiety concerning the curability of a slight complaint, in the morning. Themes: disease

Al,16- Anxiety as if she had committed a great crime. Themes: conscience, criminal

Al,17- Great anxiety, as though he had done some evil. Themes: conscience, criminal

Al,26- She is offended at the slightest circumstance, often to weeping, with contraction of the pupils : after weeping loss of appetite. Themes: offenses

Al,27- Very much affected and offended by slight obliquities (immorality) and untruths (falsehood) of others. Themes: offenses, wrong, wicked, liar

Al,30- Great dissatisfaction with himself. Themes: discontented, conscience, himself

Al,9- Constant sad thoughts, as though he had suffered an insult. Themes: sadness, offenses

Ha,520- The thoughts are fixed on a single disagreeable subject; she is absorbed in thought and notices nothing about her. Themes: dwells

Ha,521- He is sunk in saddest thoughts, and insults he has received he takes deeply to heart. Themes: offenses, sinking, sadness

Ha,524- Continual sad thoughts, just as if he had received insults. Themes: offenses, sadness

Ha,523- Time passes too rapidly with him, several hours appears to him as short as one hour. Themes: time

Ha,529- Great discontent with himself. Themes: discontented, himself

Ha,531- Serious, and though caring little about his own health, he is very anxious about the illnesses of others. Themes: disease, others

Ha,532- She dawdles (indolent); in business she cannot accomplish anything nor finish anything, with contracted pupils. Themes: unfit, work, time, succeed

Ha,535- In the morning, anxiety respecting the incurability of a trifling malady. Themes: despair, disease, death

Ha,536- Anxiety as if she had committed a great crime. Themes: conscience, criminal

Ha,537- Great anxiety as if he had done something bad. Themes: conscience, criminal

Ha,547- Great sensitiveness of disposition; everything offends him. Themes: offenses

Ha,548- He cannot bear any interruption in conversation, nor any noise. Themes: noise, bothered

Ha,550- Everything angers and vexes him; after a few hours he becomes lively and disposed to make jokes. Themes: bothered, anger, pleasure

Ha,551- Easily annoyed; he takes everything in bad part. Themes: bothered, offenses

Ha,554- He is very indignant and annoyed at slight faults and fibs (lie, falsify) of others. Themes: indignation, offenses, wrong, liar, bothered

He,18- Intolerance of noise or any disturbing influence. Themes: noise

He,22- Great sorrowfulness, with constant inclination to sit in a corner buried in thought. Themes: misanthropy, grief, sadness, solitude

He,24- Melancholy and sad; indulges in sad reveries (daydream); is sensitive to insults, slights (despises) and disappointment. Themes: sensitive, offenses, disappointment, sadness, despised

He,25- Melancholy and sadness, with weeping and constant profound absorption in sorrowful thoughts; great apprehensive anxiety of conscience, and feeling

at heart as after committing a wicked deed (act), with desire to escape. Themes: sadness, grief, conscience, criminal, escape, wicked, heart
He,27- Apprehensive mood; fears death and unknown dangers. Themes: death, danger
He,28- Great fear of death. Themes: death
He,33- Tearful chagrin about least trifle. Themes: grief
He,39- Angry and indignant form of delirium. Themes: indignation, anger, insanity
He,42- Ill effects of anger and grief. (ailments from) Themes: anger, grief
He,545- He dreads any sudden surprise. Themes: news
He,9-...cannot bear least noise or contradiction. Themes: noise, contradiction

COFF-T.

Al,12- The power of judgment is increased. Themes: knowledge, justice
Al,15- It gives rise to a need of creative activity, a vivacity of thought, a versatility and ardor of desire, more favorable to the exaggerated expression of ideas previously formed, than to the quiet examination of new conceptions. Themes: greatness, planning, energy
Al,5- Desire to perform good deeds intensified. Themes: helpful, compassionate
Al,6- Veneration for Supreme Being. Themes: religious
Al,9- Timidity, and fear of sudden death;... Themes: cowardice, death
He,2- She is greatly excited and sure (inevitable) she will die. Themes: death
He,3- Full of apprehension of terrible things happening. Themes: misfortune
He,5- Begs that someone might end her life. (salvation, redemption) (murdered) Themes: executed, death, murdered

COFF.

Al,1- Lively fancies; full of plans for the future; contrary to his custom is very much charmed by the beauties of nature,... Themes: planning, seized, nature, pleasure
Al,4- He is able to hear many annoying things spoken of, without being affected or becoming offended thereby (curative action). Themes: offenses,
Al,7- Great anxiety, so that she does not know what she shall do with herself; she trembles, and cannot hold the pen still. Themes: confidence
He,1- Memory active, easy comprehension; increased power to think. Themes: knowledge
He,12- Weeping and complaining ,with fear of death; thinks that she will die. Themes: death
He,20- ...anxiety of mind and conscience filled with many fears. Themes: fearful
He,21- Fear of death. Themes: death
He,23- Fright from sudden pleasant surprises. Themes: news, pleasure
He,24-...fear of fresh air and of least noise... Themes: noise, nature
He,33- Ailments from excessive joy, excessive laughing and playing; from disappointed love; from anger, from vexations with vehemence or fright... Themes: pleasure, disappointment, love, anger, bothered
He,35- Affections after sudden emotions, particularly pleasant surprises.(ailments from) Themes: pleasure, news
He,5- Lively fancies; full of plans for the future. Themes: future, planning
He,7- Delirium tremens: unsteady running about; imagines he is not at home,... Themes: lack, home
He,8- Great loquacity, brain feels clear and is active, he feels strong enough to do anything, feels impelled to push things; veneration for the Supreme Being and love for family; benevolence excited. Themes: talk, love, helpful, greatness, energy, religious, compassionate

COLCH.

He,15- Ailments from grief of misbehavior of others. Themes: grief, offenses
He,5- Says nothing unless questioned, his condition does not seem to him dangerous. 0Typhus. Themes: talk, disease, danger

COLOC.

He,10- Extremely irritable and impatient; nothing seems right; gets angry on being questioned. Themes: impatience, wrong, anger

He,11- Morose mood; becomes offended at everything. Themes: offenses, sadness
He,12- Anger with indignation and extreme irritability; throws things out of his hands. Themes: anger, indignation
He,13- Indignation, with silent internal grief. Themes: indignation, suppressed, grief
He,14- Affections from anger, with indignation, particularly vomiting and diarrhoea ...(ailments from) Themes: anger, indignation

CON.

Al,10 - The husband, who had been somewhat addicted to liquor, saw all sorts of animals dancing upon the bed, and "picked straws" a little. Themes: animal, music
Al,11- Visions of her brother and child, who had died; at the same time, she saw distinctly persons in the room;... Themes: ghosts, brother, child, death,
Al,1276- Dreams of physical mutilation. Themes: mutilated
Al,1277- Dreams of wretched (miserable) diseases. Themes: disease, misfortune
Al,1278- Many dreams of dead people, and of the death of those living. Themes: ghosts, death
Al,15- Tendency to laugh, with loss of vital energy. Themes: energy, pleasure
Al,27- Frequent thoughts of death. Themes: death
Al,36- Very apprehensive thoughts, almost amounting (whole) to deathly anxiety, after midnight, while half awake. Themes: death
Al,38- Sunk in deep thought; he apprehensively considered the present and the future, and sought (wanted) to be alone. Themes: meditation, dwells, future, solitude
Al,39- Dread (fear) of men of their approach, yet with dread of being alone. Themes: fearful, approached, solitude
Al,40- Fear of thieves. Themes: robber
Al,43- ...a great guilt weighed upon him, with paralyzed feeling in all the limbs, indifference,.. Themes: conscience, paralysis, indifference
Al,45- Extremely fretful and anxious thoughts about dying, in the morning, with confusion of the head. Themes: death,
Al,46- Fretful mood; he does not knows how he shall busy himself; the times passes too slowly. (tedium) Themes: time, doubtful, tedium
Al,6- Delirious and stupid; they threw themselves into the water, thinking they were geese; for three years they remained partly paralytic, suffering from much pain. Themes: liberty, identity, paralysis, water, animal,
Ha,10- The propinquity (proximity) and the talk of people passing by is very offensive to him, and he feels impelled to assault and maltreat them. Themes: approached, offenses, offensive, violence
Ha,13- Fear of thieves. Themes: robber
Ha,14- He imagines that somebody has come in at the door by night. Themes: suspicious, invaded
Ha,16- Frequents thoughts of death. Themes: death.
Ha,18- Very morose; ...as if a great guilt weighed him down; at the same time a sensation of paralysis in all the limbs; ... Themes: sadness, conscience, paralysis
Ha,20- Peevish mood, he does not know what to do with himself, the time passes too slow for him. Themes: anger, irresolution, confidence, time
Ha,365- Sunk in deep thought, he cogitated timorously about the present and the future and sought (wants) solitude. Themes: meditation, future, solitude, fearful
Ha,366- Cross temper; everything about him made a disagreeable impression on him. Themes: bothered
Ha,367- Peevish disposition; he knows not what to occupy himself with, the times appears to pass too slowly. Themes: time, irresolution
Ha,8- Lost in deep meditation, he anxiously thought over the present and the future, and sought solitude. Themes: future, solitude, meditation
Ha,9- Shyness (timidity) at the approach of people, and yet also dread of being alone. Themes: timidity, approached, solitude
He,10 - Buried in thought; apprehensive (anxiety) respecting the present or future. Themes: meditation, future

He,14- Likes to wear his best clothes, (vanity) makes useless purchases, (squander) cares very little for things (indifferent), wastes or ruins them; does not want to work, prefers to play. (wanderer) Themes: vanity, squanders, indifference, ruined, negligence, pleasure, clothes

He,17- Dislike to society and yet a dread to be alone. (solitude) Themes: misanthropy, solitude, company

He,18- He is averse to being near people, and to the talk of those passing him (misanthropy); is inclined to seize hold of and abuse them. (insult, offend, curse) Themes: offensive, company, misanthropy, loathing, talk,

He,26- Great unhappiness of mind, recurring every fourteen days. Themes: unfortunate

He,28- Solicitude (anxiety) concerning the future; great concern (cares) about any little thing that may happen. Themes: future, misfortune

He,29- Hypochondriasis and hysteria from suppression of, or too free indulgence in, sexual instinct,...(ailments from) Themes: sexual, suppressed, disease

He,31- Great anxiety; precordial anguish; superstitious (careful, credulous, naive) and full of fear (coward) , with frequent thoughts of death... Themes: heart, conscientious, death, fearful, danger

He,32- Discouraged, despondent, and dissatisfied (discontented) with herself and her surrounds. Themes: hopeless, conscience, himself

He,33- Timid, cannot be persuaded to work ; want of proper will. (lack of: resolution) (vagabond) Themes: cowardice, work, negligence, will

He,35- ...a great grief weighed upon him, with paralyzed feeling in all the limbs, indifference and taking no interest in anything. Themes: paralysis, grief, indifference, heavy

He,36- Morose mood; everything about him impresses him unpleasantly. Themes: himself

He,38- Very much excited, passionate, domineering (dictatorial), quarrelsome, scolds (censorious) and will not bear contradiction. Themes: passionate, dictatorial, fight, censorious, contradiction, offensive

COP.

Al,2- Disgust (loathing) with life ,and at the same time fear of death. Themes: loathing, death, fearful, grief

Al,7- Anxiety about his health. Themes: disease

Al,9- Absurd recriminations about trifling and long -past occurrences. Themes: conscience, past, tortured, mortification

COT.

Al,1- ...a feeling as if there was no foot. The head felt exceeding light, as if there were no solid head, and she could not articulate for some time, although she endeavored to do so.... Themes: disintegration, mutilated, talk, paralysis, light

Al,11- Feels silly (ridiculous) and lost. Themes: lost, contemptuous, himself, ridiculous

Al,14- After taking the medicine, she feels lost; cannot collect herself; forgets what she is doing and saying; difficulty in expressing herself. Themes: lost, disintegration

Al,2- Awoke, early in the morning, in a state in which she felt as if she were going out of her mind. (insanity) Themes: insanity

CROC.

Al,10- Immoderate laughter, as if he would die. Themes: death, pleasure

Al,11- Sardonic (sarcastic, satirical) laughter, and attacks of morbid jollity. Themes: sarcasm, pleasure, wicked

Al,14- Very lively (happy) mood, witty, jocose, excessively talkative.(loquacious) Themes: sarcasm, pleasure, talk

Al,18- Irresistible inclination to joke and laugh, with great prostration, and great dilatation of the pupils. Themes: pleasure, energy

Al,2- Suddenly there arises before her fancy a concern (care) which she attended a long time since, as vividly as if were she listening to it;... Themes: past, mortification

Al,24- A slight cause which would usually have made her laugh, now causes a most violent ill-humor, almost rage, so that she frequently loses her consciousness; afterwards she is astonished at this out break. Themes: anger, fit

Al,28- Vacillating (hesitate) , peevish mood; the slightest cause excites his anger, for which, next moment, he is sorry (remorse), which however ,soon returns, because his calmness frets (disturbs) him and prevents (stop) his exposing his feelings (oppressed); usually he changes a hard word which he has on his tongue to a mild one, but the latter seems too mild, and now chooses a more severe word, ...(sorry, guilty, by anger, mildness, x harsh, rude) Themes: anger, conscience, offensive, mildness,

Al,29- He takes everything in anger and suddenly repents (apologize) of having injured (offend) others. Themes: anger, conscience, offensive, others

Al,3- An unpleasant sensation, as if he were longing (desire) for something without knowing what, with a kind of apprehension, ... Themes: capricious

Al,30-...the behavior of relatives and friends excites her to anger,...she is vexed with herself, and her anger becomes greater than ever;.. Themes: anger, friend, relatives, himself

Al,5- If any one happens to sing a single musical note, she begins involuntarily to sing, and then is obliged to laugh at herself; she however, soon sings in spite of her determination to stop. (sympathy) Themes: antagonism, music, imitated, sarcasm, ridiculous

He,12- Vexation, contradicted by bursts of laughter. Themes: pleasure, antagonism

He,13- He takes everything in anger and suddenly repents (sorry) of having injured (offensive) others. Themes: anger, conscience, offensive,

He,3- Greatly concerned about his life, believes that he will die, is no longer fit for business. Themes: death, unfit, work

CROT-C.

Al,1- Magnetic state; she hears nothing, and again sees the spectre of death, as a gigantic black skeleton. Themes: death, corpse, great, dark

Al,18- Her thoughts dwell on death; with great sadness. Themes: dwells, death, sadness

Al,19- Thoughts of death haunt (torment) her everywhere , especially when alone. Themes: death, solitude, seized

Al,3-... hears a strange voice to her left, and behind her; she follows it, throws herself against closed doors, and scratches them with her nails...She cries out: " He is in the den, but the lions will not eat him" Themes: seized, strange, persecution, wild, animal, bite

Al,4- Another attack of mental alienation; she hears voices, which she follows (obey); with copious tears. Themes: separated, seized

Al,5- She stands for ten minutes on the window-sill, and is arrested when on the point of throwing herself off. Themes: suicidal, height

Al,6- She fancies her eyes are falling out (tenth day). Themes: disease, fall

Al,7- He fancies he hears groans. (laments) Themes: helplessness

Al,8- He fancies he hears some one walking behind him. Themes: persecution

Al,9- While in a clairvoyant state, he speaks to some one who does not answer. Themes: clairvoyance, talk

CROT-H.

Al,7- For several days, a certain dread of selecting (choice) remedies, which is usually an agreeable occupation. Themes: confidence

He,10- Mania in zymotic (infectious) disease and when connected with puerperal or ovary-uterine disease. Themes: disease, infection

He,13- Marked indifference, seems only half alive; utter apathy. Themes: lifeless, indifference, half, yielding, alive

He,14- Sadness, her thoughts dwell on death continually. Themes: death, dwells

He,15- Oppression as if brain had been intoxicated by carbonic acid, or by degraded or non-oxygenated blood. Themes: oppression, poisoned, disease, blood, ruined

He,22- Suspicion and snappishness (irritable), or quiet indifference. Themes: suspicious, indifference

He,5-...imagines himself surrounded by enemies or hideous animals;... Themes: surrounded, enemy, animal, horrible

CROT-T.

He,2- Feeling of anxiety, as thought some personal misfortune would befall him. Themes: misfortune

He,5- Feeling as though one cannot think outside of himself, "feels all pent up" (restricted, limited, confined, circumscribed) inside, and no chance for thoughts to flow out; as if hidebound.(obstinate) Themes: reserved, suppressed, obstructed, imprisoned, surrounded

CUPR-A.

Al,2- Attacks of mania; he fancies that he is a military officer; a fancy that he is selling green vegetables; a fancy that he is repairing old chairs...he spits in the faces of the attendants, and laughs heartily at it. Themes: officer, greatness, contemptuous, work, money, wicked, pleasure

He,10- Awoke suddenly from sleep...and wished to escape...thinks she is about to die and desires to see the pastor;... Themes: escape, death, conscience, salvation, religious

He,15- Afraid of falling; holds on to his nurse's hair, hugs up to her, afraid of being injured,... Themes: fall, hurt, helplessness

He,16- Afraid of everyone who approaches him, shrinking away from them. Themes: approached

He,17- Feared bedclothes or house would catch fire. Themes: fire, home, clothes

He,4- Fixed idea that he sees persons connected with the law who are about to seize him (imprisoned),...at times sees thieves in the room, spirits, and various other immaterial objects;... Themes: officer, imprisoned, conscience, criminal, robber, ghosts

CUPR.

Al,13- Irresolute; satisfied with nothing; this only lasts as long as he is fretful. Themes: irresolution, discontented

Al,5- Melancholy; she shuns the sight of people (observed), seeks and loves to be alone, and becomes anxious about her death, which she supposes imminent and inevitable. Themes: shame, solitude, death, doomed

Al,8- Fearful; want of courage. Themes: fearful, cowardice

Ha,1- Melancholy; she shuns the sight of men, seeks and loves (desire) solitude, and troubles herself about her imminent death (impending) , which she supposes to be unavoidable. Themes: shame, solitude, death, doomed, misanthropy

Ha,10- Indisposition to work, and yet idleness is a burden to him. Themes: work, negligence

Ha,23- Fits of insanity, imagines he is a military commander. Themes: insanity, dictatorial, officer, greatness

Ha,24- Fits of insanity, he imagines (delirium) he has green herbs for sale. Themes: insanity, work, money

Ha,25- Fits of insanity, he imagines he is repairing old chairs. (humility) (reparation, restitution) Themes: insanity, work

Ha,27- Fits of insanity, he spits into people's faces, and laughs heartily (soberly) over it. Themes: insanity, contemptuous, pleasure, sadism, wicked

Ha,5- A kind of timidity; he felt as if he had to step softly, in order not to hurt himself, nor to disturb his room-mates. (friend) (cautious, prudent, gentle, delicate) Themes: hurt, cares, conscientious, friend, others

Ha,7- Irresolute (indecisive) and dissatisfied with everything, but only so long as he is peevish. (cross) Themes: bothered, doubtful, discontented

Ha,8- Peevishness, he himself does not know what he wants, he wishes to be alone;... Themes: solitude, company

He,10- Mania with biting, beating, and tearing things to pieces; insane foolish gestures of imitation and mimicry; full of insane spiteful (cruelty, brutality) tricks (deceitful, false) ,..unhappy, despairing...miserable look... Themes: bite, violence, wicked, insanity, deceitful, unfortunate, imitated, miserable

He,18- Unconquerable sadness, constant restlessness, as if some misfortune were approaching; fears he will lose his reason. Themes: sadness, misfortune, insanity, restless,

He,21- Afraid of and shrinking away from

everyone who approaches him; afraid of falling; clinging tightly to nurse;... Themes: fearful, approached, escape, fall

He,26- Loss of spirits (courage); anxiety; fits of anguish and fear of death. Themes: cowardice, fit, death

He,5- Delirium: afraid of every one who approached him, shrinking (retire) away from them; tries to escape; in evening and in the dark. Themes: approached, escape, dark

He,6- Craziness (insanity); attacks with savage malice (evil), with proud (arrogant) bearing (posture),... Themes: insanity, haughty, violence, wicked, wild

He,8- Mania characterized by a wild look and fear; tries to escape. Themes: fearful, escape, wild,

CUR.

Al,1- Paroxysm of insanity impelling him to attack himself; he strikes, scratches, and tears himself with a sort of relish, (enjoy) and without feeling any pain. Themes: insanity, hurt, tear, pleasure, himself

Al,10- Brooding sadness, frequent weeping, with desire for solitude. Themes: sadness, mortification, solitude

Al,11- Great despondency (grief) ; becomes reckless (careless) about himself. Themes: indifference, negligence

Al,12- Regrets (remorse) from the past. Themes: conscience, past

Al,13- Disposition to suicide. Themes: suicidal

Al,16- Excessive fear of death. Themes: death

Al,17- Irascibility, wicked disposition; desires to lie in wait in order to assault others, and even to kill and rob them. Themes: wicked, homicidal, robber

Al,3- Fits of ecstasy at night, as if caused by hearing music. Themes: pleasure, music

Al,4- Everything he sees appears foul and nasty. (dirty, dishonest, offensive, injurious, indecent) Themes: offenses, dirty, wrong, wicked

Al,5- Fondness (desire) for luxury (waste) and grandeur.(distinction, fame) Themes: greatness, ambition, wealth

Al,6- He would like to go travel in a great style.(luxury) Themes: travel, greatness, wealth

Al,9- Melancholy, egotistical, envious, obstinate... Themes: egotism, envy, obstinate

He,1- Indecision, no longer (more) wishes to think and act for herself. Themes: irresolution, doubtful, confidence

He,2- Very much depressed about herself, desire only to shut herself up away from people. Themes: sadness, himself, solitude, company

CYCL.

Al,10- Internal grief and anxiety of conscience, as though he had not done his duty, or had committed a crime. Themes: grief, conscience, duty, negligence, criminal

Al,13- Ill-humored, morose mood; he could easily take offense at every trifle and get very much exercised about it. Themes: offenses

Al,16- Fretful and sad; has no desire to work ; she feels a great anxiety, as if some great misfortune were impending. Themes: work, misfortune

Al,17- Very fretful (irritable) the whole day; disinclined to speak and insensible (indifferent), having very little feeling (emotion) in his body. Themes: talk, indifference, lifeless

Al,19- Sometimes he is very ill-humored and fretful, but suddenly he feels again a strange joyous sensation,... Themes: strange, pleasure

Al,28-...he constantly feels as though he had just suffered from an overwhelming (remarkable) affliction; only when he becomes excited is his mind somewhat clearer, and then he acts like one who has just awakened from slumber (sleep), and only half understands what is going on about him. Themes: knowledge, obstructed, unreal, half

Ha,188- He is always in a reverie (meditation, air castles) , and not inclined to speak. (talk, aversion) Themes: dispersion, talk

Ha,193- Peevish, morose disposition; he easily takes every trifle in bad part, and gets angry over it. Themes: offenses, anger

Ha,194- Sunk in deep thought (meditation), he sought (desire) solitude and thought about his future fate (destine, doom).

Themes: meditation, future, solitude

Ha,195- Deep thought about the present and future, so that he almost wept. Themes: meditation, future

Ha,196- Inward grief and anxiety of conscience, as if he had not done his duty or had committed a crime. Themes: grief, conscience, negligence, duty, criminal

Ha,197- Excessive sadness, as if he had done something bad and had neglected his duty. Themes: sadness, conscience, duty, negligence

Ha,201- All day long he is peevish not disposed to talk, and insensible, so that he feels little (inadequate, incompetent) in his body. Themes: indifference, talk, unfit

Ha,202- Towards evening there suddenly occurs a strange happy feeling and lively fancy, which conjures (remember) up agreeable pictures. Themes: strange, pleasure, past

He,12- Great sadness, as if he had committed a bad action or not done his duty. Themes: sadness, conscience, duty, negligence

He,17-...fear of death, or an illusion of being deserted or persecuted by every one. Themes: death, forsaken, persecution

He,20- Ill humored, morose mood; could easily take offense at every trifle. Themes: sadness, offenses

He,23- Ailments from inward grief and terrors of conscience. Themes: grief, conscience

He,4- Absorbed in deep thought, seeks solitude, thinks about his future. Themes: meditation, solitude, future

He,6- ...love of (desire) solitude;....;sensation as if room was too small, with reluctance to go into open air;... Themes: solitude, small, go out

CYPR.

He,2- Profound indifference to everything, even to his studies, duties and common courtesies (kindness, compassion) of life. Themes: indifference, knowledge, duty

DER.

Al,1- He fancies he is seasick. (nauseated) Themes: disease, travel

Al,2- He desires death and will attempt (try) suicide. Themes: death, suicidal

Al,3- He is discouraged and despairs of a cure (recovery), declaring himself a hypochondriac. Themes: disease, despair

Al,4- He dreads pain, and is averse to solitude with great anxiety. Themes: disease, solitude, company

Al,5- He is afraid of killing some one with a knife. Themes: homicidal, pointed

Al,6- He is disposed to strike, and inveighs against his dearest friends. Themes: violence, offensive, friend

DIG.

Al,19- Weeping sadness about many things which have disappointed him. Themes: sadness, disappointment

Al,21- Anxiety, as though he had done wrong. Themes: conscience, wrong

Al,22- Anxiety with great dread of the future, worse about 6 p.m. with sadness and weeping, which bring relief. Themes: future

Al,24- Internal anxiety, like pangs of conscience, as though he had committed a crime, or expected to be reproved, continuing nearly three months. Themes: conscience, criminal, censured

Al,31- Great irritability; everything especially sad things affected him very much, and the merest trifle can make him hopelessly despondent; lasting more than three months. Themes: sadness, hopeless

Al,43- Intellectual faculties seemed to be affected, as if I had taken more wine than usual. Themes: obstructed

Al,9- Great desire to be alone. Themes: solitude

Ha,11- Anxious apprehension (fear) of a sad kind, with great dejection, extremely aggravated by music. Themes: hopeless, music

Ha,14- ..he is much affected by everything, but especially by sad things, and the least trifle can throw him into disconsolate despair.(sensitive) Themes: sensitive, despair, sadness

Ha,421- He is sad and has a feeling of being very ill; all objects appear to him as in fever, just as if he had a perversion of the visual faculty as in fever. Themes: disease,

Ha,4- Tearful sorrow (grief) over many things which have failed (disappointment, frustration) with him. Themes: grief, failure

Ha,420- Lachrymose sadness about many things in which he has been unsuccessful. Themes: unfortunate, failure

Ha,424- Fear of death. Themes: death

Ha,425- An anxious feeling as if he had done something bad. Themes: conscience, wrong

Ha,7- Anxiousness, with great apprehension of the future... Themes: future

Ha,8- Anxiety as if he had done wrong. Themes: conscience, wrong

Ha,9- Internal anguish, like anguish (anxiety) of conscience, as if he had committed a crime, or had to expect reproaches... Themes: conscience, criminal, censured

He,10- Profound melancholy,...great fear of future; insane obstinacy and disobedience, with desire to escape. Themes: sadness, future, escape, obstinate

He,11- Melancholic, despondent, and constantly tortured by fear of death or loss of reason. Themes: despair, death, insanity, tortured

He,12- Desponding (sad) and irresolute.(indecisive) Themes: hopeless, irresolution

He,13- Great anxiety, like from troubled conscience. Themes: conscience

He,14- Gloomy, peevish and distrustful.(suspicious) Themes: sadness, suspicious

He,7- Lascivious fancies day and night. Themes: sexual, lascivious

DIOS.

Al,1- Desire to be alone; do not enjoy society (misanthropy); am usually quite fond of the society of ladies, but they now seem repulsive,... Themes: solitude, sexual, misanthropy, loathing, company

DIRC.

Al,1- Uneasy and sensation as if something unpleasant were to happen. Themes: misfortune

Al,2- In day time was constantly expecting some bad news; everything seemed worry and annoy. Themes: news, misfortune

Al,3- Sense of apprehension, throughout the proving, as of some trouble, which may have depended upon the morbid state of the mind at the same time of the proving. Themes: anticipation, disease

DROS.

Al,1- Joyful, good courage: he had no fear of evil, because he was conscious of having done right. (moral, virtuous, honest, fearless) Themes: conscientious, fearless, justice

Al,11- Anxiety as if his enemies allowed him no rest, but persecuted and pursued him. Themes: persecution, enemy,

Al,12- Restless mood and anxiety the whole day; full of distrust, as if he were dealing with none but false men. Themes: suspicious, betrayed

Al,13- Extremely uneasy, sad mood the whole day; he imagines that he would be deceived by tricky, designing (tricky) men. Themes: suspicious, betrayed

Al,14- Taciturn, quiet, and anxious; he was constantly in dread (fear) of hearing something unpleasant. Themes: misanthropy, reserved, offenses

Al,15- He is very much affected by offenses, with some vexation. Themes: offenses, contradiction

Al,266- Vivid frightful dreams about being maltreated (insulted, injured). Themes: offenses, hurt

Al,4- He is depressed by the persecutions of others on all sides, and also discouraged and solicitous about the future. Themes: sadness, persecution, cowardice, future

Ha,269- Anxiety with feeling of heat quickly running all over the body, but especially all over the face, as though he were about to receive bad news ...rigor all over the body, without heat and without thirst. Themes: energy, news

Ha,271- All day long, uneasiness of disposition and anxiety, full of mistrust (suspicious) as if he had to do with none but false (faithless) people. Themes: suspicious, betrayed

Ha,272- Extremely uneasy, sad disposition, all day he imagined he was being deceived (deluded, defrauded) by spiteful (hateful), envious people. Themes: betrayed, envy, suspicious, wicked

Ha,273- Silent and reserved, with anxiety he always feared he was about to learn (discover) something disagreeable. Themes: reserved, misfortune

Ha,274- Anxiety, as if his enemies would not leave him quiet, envied (competition, rivalry, opposition, spite) and persecuted him. Themes: enemy, persecution, envy, bother

Ha,275- He is sad and dejected about the ills (evil) of life, which people cause one another and himself, respecting which he is anxious and concerned;...(ethical) Themes: misfortune, sadness, despair, others, wicked

Ha,276- He is dejected (unhappy) about the malice (rancor, hostility) of others on all hands, and at the same time disheartened (discouraged) and concerned about the future.(disgusted, revolted) Themes: unfortunate, future, wicked,

Ha,277- Anxiety; ...,as if he were impelled to jump into the water in order to take his own life by drowning he was not impelled to any other mode of death. Themes: suicidal, water, death

Ha,278- Anxiety in solitude (alone) he wished to have someone always near him, could not bear to be without companions (friends, company), and was quieter when he had someone to speak to; but when they again left him in solitude, he was all the more anxious, until he fell asleep; on awaking the anxiety returned. Themes: solitude, lack, talk, company

Ha,281- He takes insults very resentfully, not without vexation. Themes: offenses, mortification, resentment, bothered

Ha,284- Obstinate prosecution of resolutions he had formed. Themes: obstinate, will

Ha,287- Happy steadfast (confiding) disposition; he dreaded no evil, because he was conscious of having acted honorably. Themes: pleasure, confidence, duty, justice

He,2- Depressed by persecutions of others on all sides, and also discouraged and solicitous about future. Themes: persecution, future

He,3- Anxiety: with flushes of heat; when alone (solitude), ...as if it would impel him to commit suicide by drowning. (water will purify?) Themes: solitude, suicidal, water

He,4- Dread (fear) of ghosts and of being alone. Themes: ghosts, solitude

He,5- Great mistrust. Themes: suspicious

He,7- Self-willed (inflexible); obstinate; insists upon carrying out his plans.(determination) Themes: obstinate, planning

DULC.

Al,3- She wakes early, as if called and sees the form of a ghost, which keeps enlarging until it disappears. Themes: grow, ghosts

Al,8- Anxiety and fear of the future after midnight. Themes: future

ELAPS.

Al,11- Depression of spirits; desires to be in a deep cavern, where he can see no one. Themes: solitude, misanthropy

Al,13- Fearfulness, dread (fear) of being alone, as though something would happen, or as though rowdies (revolution, rebellious) would break in. Themes: fearful, solitude, misfortune, fight, revolutionary

Al,14- Excessive horror of rain. Themes: fearful, storm, water

Al,16- Inclination to strike and pick a quarrel. Themes: violence, hurt, fight

Al,17- Peevish in the afternoon, did not want to be spoken to, even fretful (irritable) about herself. Themes: talk, anger

Al,2- Reveries in the daytime; he imagines he is being beaten. Themes: bite, hurt, attacked,

Al,4- She fancies she is falling forward, thought really quite still. Themes: fall

Al,5- Desire to go into to the country , and play about in the grass. (nature) Themes: nature, pleasure

Al,6- Desire to be alone; she takes refuge for days together in a corner of the antechamber. Themes: solitude, hide

Al,7- She seeks a retired room to work in. Themes: solitude, work

Al,9- She wishes to leave the house just when she is going to bed. Themes: go out, escape

He,2- Imagines he hears some one talking. Themes: talk

He,3- Depression of spirits, and desire for solitude. Themes: sadness, solitude

He,4- Fearful and apprehensive of some fatal disease. Themes: fearful, disease

He,5- Fear of being left alone, as if something horrible might happen; horror of rain. Themes: fearful, horrible, solitude, misfortune, storm, water
He,6- Angry about one's self, does not wish to be spoken to. Themes: anger, himself, talk

ELAT.

He,2- Irresistible propensity to wander from home, even in the night, and range (distance) in woods.(forest) Themes: movement, travel, nature
He,3- Fear of some approaching disaster. Themes: accidents, misfortune

ERY-A.

Al,1- Felt very queer (eccentric, inadequate) before completely dressed. Themes: strange, clothes

EUCAL.

He,2- Irresistible desire to move about, with a feeling of buoyancy (happiness) and increased strength. Themes: movement, energy, pleasure

EUP-PER.

He,1- Feels at night as if he was going out of his mind.(insanity) Themes: insanity

EUP-PUR.

He,7-... feeling like homesickness, though occupying her own home and surrounded by her own family,... Themes: nostalgia, homesickness, family,
He,9- Has a great fear of sickness. Themes: fearful, disease

EUPH.

Al,4- Anxiety as if he had taken poison.(venom) Themes: poisoned
Ha,2- Anxiety as if he had swallowed poison. Themes: poisoned
He,3- Temporary attacks of craziness, insists upon saying his prayers at the tail of his horse; knows his freaks (abnormality) and wants to be by himself and in silence. Themes: insanity, religious, solitude, salvation
He,4- Imagines he sees the same man walking after him that he sees walking before him. Themes: persecution, double

EUPHR.

Ha,127- Lazy, hypochondriacal; external objects had no charm (beauty), no life (animation) for him. (indifference) Themes: lifeless, indifference

FERR-MA.

Al-S,1- Walking along with a self-sufficient impression of importance. Themes: greatness, haughty
Al-S,4- Irresolute; he considers for a long time before commencing anything . Themes: irresolution, doubtful

FERR.

Al,12- She never complained or wept and was always plunged (fall) in deep melancholy when no one was about her. Themes: solitude, sadness, suppressed
Al,14- Anxiety as if something evil had happened to her. Themes: misfortune
Al,20 - Excited by the slightest opposition; ... even her children's caresses increased her bad temper; she was often rude to those about her, because she hated to see or talk to them, and wanted them to leave her in solitude, which alone was pleasing to her. Themes: contradiction, solitude, forsakes, loathing, talk, misanthropy, anger, pleasure
Al,21- Violence, quarrelsomeness; insists that he is right. Themes: violence, fight, obstinate
Al,3- My surroundings (material welfare) seem very large (big) and capacious (vast), and I am inclined to attribute great importance to trifles... Themes: great, conscientious
Al,4- Constant desire for solitude; horror of conversation, noise, visits, and even the society of her cherished friends. Themes: solitude, talk, noise, company, misanthropy, friend
Al,6- Temper more equable (regular) all through the proving. Themes: peace

Al,764- Did not sleep well, as sleep was much disturbed by dreams of old friends. Themes: friend, past

Al,766- Dreams he is in battle, that he has fallen into the water, etc. Themes: fight, fall, water

Al,769- Rested well, but dreamed a great deal of meeting with old schoolmates, of student life, etc. Themes: nostalgia, past, friend

Ha,270 - Dreams that he is in battle , that he has fallen into the water... Themes: fight, fall, water

Ha,272- Anxiety at night, as she have done something bad; she could not sleep, tossed about the bed. Themes: wrong, wicked, conscience,

Ha,290 -Low spirits (sad) as if from bowels being too relaxed. Themes: sadness

Ha,291- Violence, quarrelsomeness (litigious, combative), positiveness (obstinate, emphatic, resolute) Themes: violence, fight, obstinate

Ha,295- Anxiety as if she had done something bad. Themes: conscience

He,10- Anxiety as after committing a crime. Themes: conscience, criminal

He,12- Nervous, hysterical feeling; fear of apoplexy. Themes: disease

He,14- Pettish(irritable), quarrelsome, disputative (litigious), easily excited, least contradiction angers. Themes: fight, contradiction, anger

He,15- Excited by slightest opposition; everything irritates or depresses her. Themes: sadness, contradiction

He,16- Vehement; quarrelsome; anxious. Themes: dictatorial, fight

He,17- Haughtiness; proud, self-contented look. Themes: haughty,

He,18- Ailments from anger. Themes: anger

He,8- Mental depression, gloomy (dark) foreboding thoughts. Themes: anticipation, sadness, pessimism

He,9- Mind in highest degree oppressed; despondent (sad); great solicitude (cares) about those belonging to him (relatives, family), with constant thoughts of death. Themes: despair, oppression, death, others, relatives, family,

FL-AC.

Al,1- Great disposition, when alone, to repulsive fantastic imaginations, particularly in regard to persons with whom he stands in near relations, or with whom he is connected (united, joined); it seems , for example, as though he must get rid (discard, repudiate, reject) of all the servants, children must go out of house, a betrothal must be broken off, a marriage should be dissolved. (broke; vows) Themes: loathing, family, child, home, union, suspicious, forsakes, liberty

Al,12- During the tottering (tremble) sensation he has a decided though not anxious expectation, as if there was to happen something awful (horrible), but he feels no anxiety. Themes: misfortune, fearless

Al,13- Sensation as if dangers did menace (threaten) him, but without being afraid;... Themes: danger, menaced, fearless

Al,15- During the fourth week very irritable towards people, even to the greatest hatred, which he does not hesitate to give vent to in words, but as soon as he sees them everything is forgotten, and he has an entirely different opinion of them. Themes: anger, offensive, antagonism, solitude

Al,16- Whilst (while) considering what might happen he gets into a most ungovernable anger, but only in his thoughts;..(lost relation; anger x action) Themes: anger, suppressed

Al,18- In the evening he is very discontented; he looks at everything in the worst light; ... Themes: discontented, pessimism

Al,5- Feeling of perfect happiness within (inside) and without.(outside) Themes: pleasure, perfection

Al,9- Satisfaction, he desires no better state of things; all is right. Themes: perfection, justice

Al,8- All nature seems to smile in the morning. Themes: pleasure, nature

He,12- Sensation as if danger menaced (threatened) him, but without fear. (fearless) Themes: danger, menaced, fearless

He,13- Felt certain (inevitable) that something dreadful would happen,... Themes: misfortune, doomed

He,14- Fear of apoplexy. Themes: disease, fit

He,6- Feeling of indifference towards those he loves best; has no objection to their presence but does not care to converse with them, yet if strangers or mere acquaintances come in will enter into animated conversation.... Themes: forsakes, others, union, love, indifference,

He,7- Aversion to his own family, bordering on insanity. Themes: family, insanity, loathing

FORM.

Al,4- During the day remarkably happy and able to study; everything seemed easy to be accomplished. Themes: knowledge, succeed, pleasure

Al,5-...sudden but momentary spells of unhappiness; everything looks dark.(obscure) Themes: dark, unfortunate

Al,7- Sudden and unexpected return of sense of mortification and grief, with vivid recollection of circumstances long since passed, which had caused great mortification and pain, and which had rendered several years of his life unhappy; this was caused by the transactions (doing) of a near relative; this grief continues... Themes: mortification, past, grief, unfortunate, money, relatives

GELS.

Al,2- General vivacity after rising. Themes: energy

Al,20 -The sensorial modification consisted of a mistiness (fog, cloudiness) within the brain, not much affecting the lucidity (precision) of thought, but somewhat confusing the perceptions, so that I experienced some difficulty in attending to the physical details connected with my practice.(lost, connections) Themes: obstructed, knowledge,

Al,22-...I could not pursue one train of thought for any time, the ideas would vanish (disappear) and leave a vacancy (empty) of mind...(lost, ideas, thoughts) Themes: disintegration

He,10- Unconnected (disconnection, separation) ideas, cannot follow any idea for any length of time; if he attempts to think consecutively (step by step), he is attacked by a painful, vacant feeling of the mind. Themes: disintegration, organization,

He,13- Confusion; when attempting to move, the muscles refuse to obey the will; head giddy. Themes: movement, antagonism

He,18- Desires to be quiet, does not wish to speak, nor have any one near her for company, even if the person be silent. Themes: loathing, talk, solitude, company

He,22- Solicitude (anxiety) about the present and the future. Themes: future

He,23- Fear of death; has no courage. (cowardice) Themes: death, cowardice

He,27 -Mental exertions cause a sense of helplessness (disability) from brain-weakness; inability to attend to anything requiring thought. Themes: helplessness, unfit, energy, knowledge

He,28- Great lack of courage. Themes: cowardice, lack

He,29- Every exciting news causes diarrhea ; bad effects from fright and fear. (ailments from) Themes: news, cowardice, fearful

He,30- Bad effects (ailments) from suddenly hearing bad news; from fright(fear); diarrhea, abortion etc. Themes: news, fearful

He,31- Nervous dread (fear) of appearing in public; singers and speakers.(talking?, acting?) Themes: confidence, talk,

He,32- Complaints: (ailments) from exciting or bad news; sudden emotions; the anticipation of any unusual ordeal (difficulty) ; general depression from heat of sun or summer. Themes: news, confidence, anticipation, sadness

He,33- Effects (ailments from) of grief; cannot cry; when thinking of his symptoms (disease), also when spoken to of his loss ; >from diverting talk; oppression and palpitation of heart; feels a sense of peril (danger, harm, risk) ; face flushed; sleeplessness; subdued (subjugate, yielding) manner; ... Themes: grief, sadness, disease, lack, oppression, heart, danger, yielding,

He,42- When attempting (effort) to move, the muscles refuse to obey the will; giddy, confused, lack of muscular co-ordination. Themes: conduct, disintegration

He,43- Child dizzy, when carried seizes hold of nurse, fearing that it will fall. Themes: fall, child

He,6- After losing son, inclined to brood

over her loss; at times becomes unconscious, or , rather, "rapt"; in imagination thinks herself at the grave; smothered pressure on chest after the spell. Themes: lack, dwells, seized, funeral, death, child, suffocation

GERM.

Sh,10- Reacted very strongly to a very close friend. Something quite small sparked it off and I hung up the phone. Just felt I'd had enough. It's an issue feeling that's been built up for months, but tonight I flipped inside. Only our third argument in years. I still feel indignant and angry 1 hour later, even after going and working in the garden. Won't answer her calls. 13, 30c, 06:08:30 Themes: indignation, anger

Sh,100- Cannot feel pleasure or sorrow. Everything is Chaos. Cannot restore my energy. Totally meaningless. Feels like an empty battery. Cannot take care of the kids as I should. 18, 30C, 183:XX:XX Themes: indifference, energy

Sh,101- I'm desperate. I want to die. Feel the power to kill. Feel like a wild animal locked in. It's strong, so intense. I hate so strong-feel a terrible disgust and I'm afraid of what I'm able to do. It's completely impossible to be in it and impossible to get out of it. 18, 30C, 190:XX:XX Themes: despair, death, homicidal, wild, animal, imprisoned, identity, anger, violence

Sh,102- Everything is my fault - I asked for 'drubbing' (beating) and I have got it. The kids are afraid of me, and I feel insecure about what I'm able to do. I called my sister - the only person I could talk to - but she was not at home. With an enormous effort, with heart palpitations, pain in the stomach, trembling and aggravation of headache I rang another prover. But I didn't get through - it was occupied. 18, 30C, XX:XX:XX Themes: conscience, punished, confidence

Sh,103- Felt closed in. My every movement and thought controlled. Didn't know where to go for help. Felt like a coward . Felt afraid of violence. I don't know who I am. 04, 6C, XX:XX:XX Themes: isolation, helplessness, cowardice, fearful, violence

Sh,108- Hopeless, helpless, gloom and doom. Weeping and self pity. 14, 30C, 23:00:00. Themes: hopeless, helplessness, sadness, doomed, miserable

Sh,109- Feeling a total failure, I would prefer to die. Very unmotivated. 05, 6C, 360:XX:XX Themes: failure, death

Sh,11- Feeling detached when involved in a row with husband. No guilt that I'm not pleasing him . 04, 6C, 09:XX:XX Themes: isolation, discussion

Sh,110- I don't like to be me. Want to be different. Have a distant feeling to myself yet long for physical contact, a boyfriend. Not able to do something about it. 18, 30c, 02:10:00 Themes: sexual, identity, isolation

Sh,111- If I were me, nobody would like me - so I try to be what I think others expect me to be. I don't think I can be loved with all the parts of me which are ugly and bad. Lonely feelings. Longing for love and understanding. Feel I am so unfriendly to myself. 18, 30C, 04:00:00 Themes: forsaken, despised, contemptuous, himself, confidence, ugly, wicked, helplessness, love, lack, solitude

Sh,112- Don't see why I am here. I can't bear it. I go mad. I hate myself. I want to beat myself and I do it. Tear my hair. Stop when it hurts too much. It is like hell !!! 18, 30C, 20:XX:XX Themes: loathing, himself, anger, hell, hurt, tear, conscience, punished

Sh,113- Sometimes I don't want to show my strength. I keep it back. I am afraid that others will feel inferior and I don't want them to, because I feel it so much myself. 18, 30C, 26:XX:XX Themes: greatness, contemptuous, energy

Sh,114- Difficult to feel joy, pleasure. It is more safe to be sad, unhappy, to suffer. Because joy doesn't last. 18, 30C, 85:XX:XX Themes: sadness, unfortunate

Sh,115- Very much in doubt whether I should take any more tablets. Whatever I do, I feel that somebody will criticize me, that I do something wrong. Difficult to make a decision. Afraid that other people will laugh at me or say, haven't you understood anything?" Crying. Don't want to get up. Don't want to bother the supervisor so early in the morning. I am a failure. 18, 30C, 01:06:30 Themes: censured, wrong, doubtful, despised, shame, bother

Sh,116- Blaming myself for having taken too many doses. Was afraid that I would not get the symptoms out strongly enough. Maybe I spoiled the whole proving. Still accusing myself. I felt it does not matter how much I suffer - it's what other think of me that is important. I think that I ought to suffer a good deal. 18, 30C, 01:08:15 Themes: remorse, conscience, unfit, confidence, punished

Sh,117- I am probably incurable and that's my own fault. The thoughts are repeating themselves again and again in my head. 18, 30C, 46:XX:XX Themes: conscience, disease

Sh,118- Just want to cry. Feeling embarrassed. I do not believe in my own feelings and decisions. So afraid of what others think of me. 18, 30C, 01:09:15 Themes: confidence, censured

Sh,120- Easily led of others opinion, and provoked. Sensitive to others attempts at restricting me. Feel like a teenager, but I don't dare to protest. I just feel it inside. 18, 30C, 04:00:00 Themes: yielding, offended, sensitive, fragile, confidence, unfit

Sh,121- Very strong longing for excitement and some love adventure. I planned to go out, but though I probably would be disappointed, so I stayed at home and was depressed instead. Feel like drinking - to get away from myself and everything. 18, 30C, 04:00:00 Themes: love, disappointment, sadness, isolated

Sh,122- It is difficult to describe the symptoms- want to correct myself all the time. I am thinking too much. I get mad at all my thoughts. 18, 30C, 05:XX:XX Themes: wrong

Sh,123- Don't understand anything, the meaning of life. Feel also strength somewhere inside. I wish a change could happen, I ought to bring myself together and change. It is silly of me to go on like this. I despise myself. I am hard to myself, but I don't deserve anything else. I think other people are silly too. 18, 30C, 06:XX:XX Themes: punished, contemptuous, conscience, himself

Sh,124-. I was supposed to talk seriously, but started to laugh instead. I couldn't stop it, the laughter bubbled inside and had to come out. Laughing when supposed to talk seriously, nervous laughter, quite near weeping. Felt I held back something, tried to avoid an ugly noise - something which touched me deeply inside, something unveiling. 18, 30C, 07:XX:XX Themes: ugly, suppressed

Sh,126- I have a guilty feeling if I get too much attention. I am afraid of bothering others. 18, 30C, 13:XX:XX Themes: conscience, timidity, shame, bother

Sh,127- Feel like a prisoner. 18, 30C, 15:XX:XX Themes: imprisoned

Sh,128- Afraid of the police of being caught and unveiled. 18, 30C, 02:10:00 Themes: officer, criminal, imprisoned, conscience

Sh,129- Felt not enough space in bed. It's a big bed. I felt spacy, out of focus, odd, slightly, not there. Maybe in a dream. 05 ,6C, 06.00.00 Themes: grow, unreal

Sh,129- I felt spacy, out of focus, odd, slightly, not there. Maybe in a dream. 05 ,6C, Themes: unreal

Sh,130- While standing felt my spirit step backwards. The kitchen seems smaller and lower down. 04, 6C, 00.10.00. Themes: divided, double, small

Sh,131- Suddenly aware of my feet standing on the ground and feeling very connected to the ground through my feet. Rooted to the spot. Wanted to stay that way. Good feelings. Feet feeling at one with the ground. 04, 6C, 00.13.30. Themes: integration, pleasure

Sh,132- Feeling of being pushed backwards, floating backwards in space, as if weightless. 10, 9C, 00:00:10 Themes: floating, light

Sh,134- Felt uncomfortable if any one stood close to me. Felt uneasy and paranoid in class. Feel as if done something wrong. 10, 9C, 06:06:00 Themes: approached, persecution, wrong, conscience

Sh,135- I see a stranger who looks so familiar . 08, 12C, 11:04:20 Themes: stranger, friendly

Sh,136- Feeling lonely like an alien freak. 08, 12C, 22:00:00 Themes: solitude, stranger, isolation, ugly

Sh,137- Entertain myself with mischievous reflections and realize that these are more thoughts of an outsider. 08, 12C, 02:14:10 Themes: stranger, wicked, seized

Sh,138- Feeling of revulsion for many people

especially young parents with children, while wandering through town. Feel people are stuck in their lives. What a waste. 10, 9C, 00:05:00 Themes: loathing, child, family, forsaken

Sh,139- Feel angry hostile and tearful easily. Someone says that I have behaved as if I am from another planet. 08, 12C, 30:00:00 Themes: anger, stranger, offensive

Sh,140- Feel I am in an impossible situation. Nobody to talk to who understands me. I can't say things as they are because I have to take others feelings into consideration. I need comfort and encouragement, but no one can give me. Weeping. 18, 30C, 36:XX:XX Themes: helplessness, forsaken, solitude

Sh,141- Painfully aware of the feelings of being an outcast. 08, 12C, 02:00:10 Themes: forsaken, solitude, despised

Sh,142- Observe the world as being shabby. I feel separated from people and places. I feel an intense yearning for the feminine. 08, 12C, 08:04:50 Themes: contemptuous, isolation, sexual

Sh,143- I Don't belong. I don't feel at home any place. Strong desire for finding a place to stay, to make a home for me and my kids. 18, 30C, 30:XX:XX Themes: homesickness, nostalgia, isolation

Sh,144- I have an intense feeling of estrangement and isolation, with a desire to start my life again. 08, 12C, 11:06:50 Themes: strange, isolation

Sh,145- I am easily offended by being told that I look strange. 08, 12C, 18:06:10 Themes: strange, offended

Sh,146- Slightest criticism and I am broken hearted. Almost started to cry among all the people, very doubtful about relationships. It kills my confidence. Deep sigh. 21, 12C, 41:XX:XX Themes: offended, censured, sensitive, confidence

Sh,148- The last days I have had moments when I have felt I have been united to the world and people - to humanity. Have felt more love and reconciliation towards myself and other people. Started to be more conscious about the environment and what I can do to our mutual benefit. Something is happening within me. I wish to get more contact with my feelings. 18, 30C, 64:XX:XX Themes: integration, union, friendly, nature

Sh, 149- Feel lonely. I nearly always feel special - always on the side outside of others. Either better or smaller than others. 18, 30C, 46:XX:XX Themes: solitude, greatness, stranger, isolation

Sh,15- Wake feeling anxious, increasingly. Legs tremble and shake. I have to get out of bed. I am scared that a heart attack is imminent and cannot be prevented. It's to late to do anything. I walk from room to room, thirsty, chilly and in turmoil. Accompanied by a desire for stool and flatulence. 08, 12C, 80:00:00 Themes: fearful, heart, disease, fit, restless

Sh,150- I only want to cry. Don't know what to do. Feel terrible and lonely. Cannot describe how I feel. Want attention, but don't dare to ask for it. Soon there is no more energy left. 18, 30C, 182:XX:XX Themes: solitude, lack, friendless

Sh,151-.... I feel I have no real contact with people, I have no emotion at all except for a feeling of isolation and a concern that people may not like me. I wish someone would cuddle me. By 10 o'clock I have a definite aversion to people, especially certain people- the stubborn or authoritarian kind. I become deeply involved in my own thoughts and can be very irritable and even angry when the thoughts are interrupted by people, but I don't show any signs of anger or irritation. The fate of other people leaves me cold, but I know this is not right. My mind is blank and I feel I could just sit and stare. I have no feelings, no emotions! I think a lot about my state of mind and try to understand it; it puzzles me. What is missing? Eating removes this thoughtful mood. By afternoon and evening I become gradually more involved with what I am doing but still feel isolated even when in the company of other people. I don't mind listening to people, but I contribute little to

conversation. This state lasted for three days. 16, 30C, 04:XX:XX Themes: isolation, indifference, solitude, despised, lack, misanthropy, loathing, anger, obstructed, yielding,

Sh,152- Aversion to people. Abrupt when obliged to speak. Had a consultation at 10 o'clock and really messed it up. I wish everybody would just go away and leave me alone. No contact. 16, 30C, 07:04:00 Themes: loathing, misanthropy, offensive, solitude

Sh,153- Thought nobody understood me and cared for what I felt. Felt it was unfair. I was presented with complaints about something others had done. Felt I was standing between two fighting parts. Felt awkward about it, embarrassed. Difficult to argue about such strong outburst. Thoughts about the day's arguing milling in my head all evening and night. 21, 12C, 32:XX.XX. Themes: solitude, despised, forsaken, injustice, accused, fight, helplessness, antagonism

Sh,154- When outside and looking at people thought to myself I know them. People were friendlier to me. Thought I could start a conversation with strangers . 07, 30C, 00.06.00. Themes: integration, friendly

Sh,156- At night on closing the eyes I have a vision of a pair of eyes looking at me, then suddenly I saw the face very clearly. The face had an asking expression. 16, 30C, 07:04:00 Themes: observed

Sh,158- Some persistent feelings coming up. Feel envious of a colleague who I feel manages so well. When I compare with myself I feel worthless and nothing. I feel like talking badly about her to my friends and I do this, even though she is not present. It takes a lot of my attention and energy. 21, 12C, 67:XX:XX. Themes: envy, contemptuous, himself, deceitful, liar

Sh,159- People seem friendlier in the streets in London. Felt like I'd made some sort of contact - people smile at me and were chatty. 13, 30C, 02:XX:XX Themes: friendly, integration

Sh,163- Felt lack of romance in my life. Desired romantic love, to be loved. 05, 6C, 41:XX:XX Themes: friendly, love, lack

Sh,168- Indignation. Think all falls on me. 21, 12C, 36:XX:XX. Themes: indignation, offended, injustice

Sh,169- Depressed, wonder how I would manage economically. 21, 12C, 39:XX:XX Themes: sadness

Sh,171- Heavy sighing in the morning. Critical and irritable with son. Feel I can't handle him. 21, 12C, 40:XX:XX. Themes: censorious

Sh,172- Sad, indifferent and hopeless feeling. Want to cry but it won't come. 18, 30C, 00:14:00 Themes: sadness, indifference, hopeless

Sh,173- Sadness from the pains. Not irritable, just gently sad. 05, 6C, 25:00:00 Themes: sadness

Sh,174- Hopeless. There no hope for me. My fate is not to get well. 18, 30C, 36:XX:XX Themes: hopeless, doomed, disease

Sh,176- Woke up and could not relax. Thought about how to solve problems, found a plan at last. 21, 12C, 34:XX:XX. Themes: planning

Sh,177- Twice while driving I had an illusion - part of a stationery car on the right moved through my field of vision. 02, 6C, 01:XX:XX Themes: movement, disintegration

Sh,178- Generally a sense of unreality. A kind of fuzzy sensation around the periphery of where I imagined my brain to be in my head i.e. just below the surface. 02, 6C, 01:XX:XX Themes: unreal, disintegration

Sh,179- Sensation of being very slightly aware of having a brain. A kind of fuzzy sensation around the periphery of where I imagined my brain to be in my head i.e. just below the surface. 02, 6C, 01:XX:XX Themes: disintegration

Sh,180- Woke up early 3.30 am. had strong feeling, like a visualization. I picture myself lying on floor in fetal position and being shot in the head like a horse or a dog. Almost welcomed it. Then thought my children still need me. A very strong feeling of failure accompanied this. I felt I did not deserve to live. Better crying next day when talking to husband. This feeling of depression carried on for several nights. As soon as I wake up in the early morning, my mind is active and a feeling of inadequacy comes on strongly. 05 ,6C, 28:XX:XX Themes: hurt, duty, failure, conscience, punished, doomed

Sh,181- Ten minutes seemed like an hour. Time seemed to pass slowly. 06, 6C, 06.09.00 Themes: time

Sh,182- Engaged in my work and my music

with fierce intensity. 08, 12C, 14:12:00 Themes: work, music

Sh,186- While walking felt round-shoulder like a bodybuilder, worse after rising. 15, 30C, Themes: greatness, grow, great

Sh,187- Head jumped inside when there was a sudden noise. 07, 30C, 00.09.30 Themes: noise, fall, sinking

Sh,191- Feeling in a rather poetical mood. I feel I can almost capture the essence of the feeling I have been going through: it's an eructation! As if a marble lands somewhere, chest, stomach, brain and sucks to it all the matter around it in a radius of 3-4 cm and packs it tighter and tighter. It gets hard and brittle, then suddenly it grows with a zoomy feeling, steadily becoming less dense and suddenly it bursts and spreads a cloud of relief. I think the remedy is Champagne. 16, 30C, 03:14:00 Themes: poetry, oppressed, heavy

Sh,200- Constant need for cuddles without sexual desire. 16, 30C, 07:04:00 Themes: touch, lack

Sh,21- Contemplative, like nice things, sees beauty in stones and nature. Good at instinctive understanding, compassionate. 16, 30C, 01:XX:XX Themes: nature, compassionate, knowledge, pleasure, perfection

Sh,26- Feel more aware and connected looking at the sun trees and sky colors. 04, 6C, 01.00.00. Themes: integration, nature

Sh,27- Felt very quiet and calm. Almost detached. More patient and less irritable. 11, 12C, 00:04:05 Themes: peace, isolation

Sh,3- Reacted angrily to husband's demands. 14, 30C, 26:00:00. Themes: anger, bothered

Sh,37- Difficult to concentrate, staring out of the window. Must find something to eat. Inefficient. I am feeling very far away. 18, 30C, 04:00:00 Themes: yielding, isolation

Sh,39- Concentration difficult. I lost my pen. I am careful, afraid of doing or saying something silly. 16, 30C, 00:06:00 Themes: lost, conscientious

Sh,4- Desperately angry. So intense that I could barely control it. I made noises like an animal, pushed my arms up and down - instead of hitting my children, which helped. Want to just leave the house and the kids. Felt completely mad, afraid of what the neighbors heard and thought. Very bad conscience afterwards, but no relief - didn't get the anger out. There are a lot of feelings inside that don't come out. 18, 30C, 02:09:00 Themes: anger, wild, forsakes, conscience, insanity, censured, shame

Sh,42- Can't decide what to buy. Don't know where to put things. Head in the clouds. 09, 9C, 01:09:00. Themes: doubtful

Sh,45- Loss of concentration. Lost my thoughts while driving, nearly causing two accidents. 05, 6C, 08:XX:XX Themes: accidents

Sh,46- Accident prone at work because of not thinking about what I am doing. Close miss accident driving a fork lift. 16, 30C, 00:04:00 Themes: accidents

Sh,5- Everything was heavy and felt impossible without meaning. Terrible anger. Bad conscience and crying afterwards. Could not do what I had planned to do, because I felt so terrible and everything was chaos. Was crying, but couldn't get it out - no release in it. 18, 30C, 176:XX:XX Themes: anger, conscience, wicked

Sh,6- Difficult to accept my own feelings, accusing myself for letting them out, especially anger. Felt a rage, had to use all my power to control it. Lost my patience because of something my son did. I got angry with him, but at the same time despised myself for not having patience with him. I did not want to report this, because I feel unveiled - now everybody can see what awful person I am. I go completely mad of all my thoughts; can't bear it anymore. Inside me everything is chaos. Feel no power. 18, 30C, 18:XX:XX Themes: conscience, anger, remorse, contemptuous, wicked

Sh,69- Want to sit alone in front of fire listening to music by myself. Fed up with people everywhere I go irritating me. Want to be looked after. 09, 9C, 01:11:00. Themes: solitude, music, bothered, helplessness

Sh,7- Recurrent rows triggered by my detachment. Felt despair and utter confusion about what was related to the proving and what was reality. 04, 6C, 14.00.00. Themes: disintegration, despair

Sh,8- Weeping. Feeling very offended

towards father who had objected because I had bought something expensive for myself. Felt anger because of my reaction, but also curiosity to find out why I reacted. Feel anxiety about all my responsibilities. Everything feels like too much. 21, 12C, 26:XX:XX. Themes: offended, conscience, duty, passionate

Sh,81- Wrote red instead of right. Said one word and understood another, husband said physician twice and twice I understood physicist. Talked about a patient who had a need for light and I thought photophobia. Wrote dylexist instead of dyslexic. Said amelioration occupates instead of occupation ameliorates. Quicked instead of quite. V Said nerve underneath sciatica instead of underneath thigh. 05, 6C, 02:XX:XX Themes: wrong, antagonism

Sh,84- I repeat adverbs very close together. "Lovely music by this lovely musician. I think its lovely" Lots of editing - I notice it when I'm reading it back. 13, 30C, XX:XX:XX Themes: wrong

Sh,9- Carried out a threat to fold son's homework which creased it, but I didn't feel guilty. 04, 6C, 01.06.00 Themes: menacing

Sh,94- Did not know which way to go on a well known route. 05, 6C, 08:XX:XX Themes: lost

Sh,99- Came in contact with very much hate and disgust within, and it made a deep impression on me. I have to be reconciled with those parts of me. I think that power can be used in a different way - not so destructive. I am no person. Feel I have no power when I meet people. Sometimes I feel I disappear. I am not in my body. My hands feel gone. My feet are cold; I don't like them. Yet I feel I have great power inside, especially I feel it when I get angry or when I sing. 18, 30C, 46:XX:XX Themes: anger, loathing, himself, disintegration, unfit, energy, music

GINS.

Al,3- Mind generally calm; still there are impatient impulses and fear of accidents, with, at times, disposition to weep, or to be anxious about the future. Themes: impatience, accidents, future

GLON.

Al,12- Though naturally cheerful she became apprehensive of her approaching death. Themes: fearful, death

Al,13-...fear she had been poisoned, and that no one would catch her taking any more. Themes: poisoned, betrayed, suspicious

Al,14- Recalls old grievances...; he was constantly thinking of persons who had offended him, with determination to justify (excuse, defend) his own conduct. Themes: offenses, conscience, justice, past, mortification

Al,15- My intellect returned almost immediately, and I remember saying, " This has nothing to do with homeopathy ,but with a very powerful poison." Themes: knowledge, poisoned

Al,18- Immediate effect, confusion of ideas, and loss of strength; with diminished power of tongue. Themes: energy

Al,19- Confusion of ideas so great that he could not tell where he was. Themes: lost

Al,20 -When the effect (in head and arms), which she exactly described, ceased after five minutes, it seemed to her as if she awoke from a dream; ... Themes: unreal

Al,21- As he returned home through the streets, after the headache, everything seemed strange to him, not as familiar as usual; he was obliged to look about him every few moments to convince himself of being in the right street; it seemed to him as if the houses were not in their right places, on the same route that he had passed over at least four times a day for years. Themes: strange, unreal, lost

Al,8- Feeling of impending misfortune, with a sensation in the chest. Themes: misfortune

He,10-...looked as if he were contemplating some afflicting (torment) sight,... Themes: horrible

He,12- Great mental agitation; attempts to run away; attempted to spring from window. Themes: restless, escape

He,15- Fear; throat feels swollen; chest as if screwed together; apprehensive of approaching death; fears she has been poisoned. Themes: crushed, death, poisoned

He,16- Bad effects of mental excitement, fright, fear, mechanical contusions and their consequences.(ailments from) Themes: fearful, hurt, accidents

He,2- Recognized no one; repulsed her husband and children; raved, screamed, and wished to rush from house; jumped out of bed, but fell because her knees gave way. Themes: loathing, forsakes, fall, husband, child, escape, home,

He,3- She could not remember which side of the street her house was on. Themes: lost, home

He,4- Well-known street seem strange; way home too long. Themes: strange, lost

He,5- Loses his way in the known streets. Themes: lost

He,6- The chin (jaw) feels too long. Themes: grow, great

He,7- Loss of location (locating); commencement about ten years ago; loses himself, even when walking in streets that he has traveled in for years;... Themes: lost

He,8- Long forgotten old offenses come back to him. Themes: offenses, past

He,9- Frantic; attempted to jump from the window. Themes: suicidal, height

GRAN.

Al,10- Inclined to get angry at offenses. Themes: offenses, anger

Al,11- Inclined to criticize and blame. Themes: censorious, offensive

GRAPH.

Al,12- Grief about the slightest occurrences (trifle), even to despair. Themes: grief, despair

Al,17- Anxiety and hastiness (hurry) drive him about like an evil- doer.(criminal) Themes: criminal, hurry

Al,22- At night, after lying down, thoughts full of care, from which she could not free herself, ... Themes: mortification

Al,27- Extreme apprehensiveness, so that she did not know how to overcome (succeed) it, disappearing after weeping. Themes: fearful, obstructed,

Al,3- Sadness, with thoughts of nothing but death. Themes: sadness, death

Al,23- He awoke at 2 a. m. with restless mood; everything that could injure him happened, and made him anxious, so that frequently he did not know where he should turn,... Themes: restless, offenses

Al,43- Extreme hesitation (doubtful); she is unable to make up her mind about anything. Themes: confidence, irresolution, unfit

Al,45- She was usually very quick to resolve, but soon after taking was very slow of thought and resolution. Themes: irresolution

Ha,14- Extraordinary apprehensiveness, so that she cannot compose (calm) herself; it goes off on weeping. Themes: fearful

Ha,17- Great anguish, so that she trembles all over, for several minutes. Themes: oppression

Ha,19- Great anguish in the evening, as if a misfortune had happened,... Themes: misfortune

Ha,20- He often feels as if his end was near (death), or as if the greatest misfortune impended over him. Themes: anticipation, death, misfortune

Ha,22- Anguish and hurry (quick) chase (pursue, follow) him about, like a criminal. Themes: hurry, criminal, conscience

Ha,25- Though usually quick to decide, she, soon after taking the medicine, becomes slow of recollection (memory) and resolution.(determination) Themes: time, irresolution

Ha,26- Extreme scrupulousness (careful, prudent); she cannot take anything lightly.(casually) Themes: conscientious,

Ha,35- Very peevish; everything vexes him and makes him indignant.(anger) Themes: bothered, indignation

Ha,36- He would like to be alone, every disturbance vexes him. Themes: solitude, bothered

Ha,46- Only obscure remembrance, even of what has just passed. Themes: past

Ha,6- Grief even to despair, about the most trifling matters. Themes: grief, despair

Ha,7- Very much disposed to grieve and to weep, in the evening; while in the morning, contrary to her wont, she laughs (smile) at every trifle. Themes: grief, antagonism, pleasure

Ha,8- Mournfulness (sorrowful), with nothing but thoughts of death. Themes: death, grief

He,12- Extreme apprehensiveness, so that she did not know how to overcome it. Themes: obstructed

He,13- It frequently seemed to him as though his end was near, or the greatest misfortunes were impending. Themes: misfortune, death, menaced
He,15- Solicitude (anxiety) concerning spiritual welfare. Themes: religious, salvation
He,19- Extreme hesitation; she is unable to make up her mind about anything; timidity. Themes: confidence, doubtful, unfit, timidity
He,22- Extremely fretful; everything angers and offends him. Themes: offenses, anger
He,27- Ailments from grief. Themes: grief
He,6- Sadness, with thoughts of nothing but death. Themes: sadness, death
He,9- Feels miserable, unhappy. Themes: unfortunate, miserable

GRAT.

Al,16- Irresolute; no persistence in work. Themes: irresolution, work, succeed
Al,8- Fretful, irritated by every contradiction, angry outbreaks, misanthropic, with solicitude about his own health. Themes: disease, contradiction, anger, misanthropy
He,1- Irresolute (wavering); want of perseverance. (determination) Themes: doubtful, irresolution, dispersion
He,6- Ill humor, tired (weary) of life, apprehensive of the future. Themes: future
He,9- Mental troubles from overweening (presumptuous, arrogant, haughty) pride. (ailments) Themes: haughty

GUAI.

Al,5- Loss of ideas; he stands in one place, and looks in front of him without thought,... Themes: lost
Ha,125- Dreams as if she would be stabbed with knives. Themes: murdered, pointed
Ha,126- Dreams of fighting. Themes: fight
Ha,129- In the evening in bed (when slumbering?) he felt as if some one threw a towel at his face, so that he started up in affright at it. Themes: fearful, attacked
Ha,130- Frequent waking from sleep, as from a fright; he felt as if he were falling. Themes: fall\plain
Ha,131- Whilst he lay asleep on his back, he dreamt that some one was lying on him; from anxiety he could not fetch his breath nor cry out; ... Themes: double, suffocation

HALI-L.

Sh,1-Vision on waking of orange-red colored circles on my abdomen like the skin on an orange when it gets old and dry. 08, 30C, 00:07:00 Themes: old
Sh,10- Sensation as if floor suddenly dropped down another few inches, after left foot landed on the floor. 09, 6C, 16:XX:XX Themes: fall
Sh,11- Sensation that my right leg was lengthening. 16, 10C, 00:XX:XX Themes: grow
Sh,110- In the evening I felt very different in relating in bed with my husband. It hasn't been nice for a long time because of my long-standing resentment towards him. It was as if there was no history between us, relating more in the moment. It was nice to be cuddling without feeling pressured by him or myself. We were communicating. 09, 6C, 01:05:25 Themes: resentment
Sh,12- Returning home after dropping kids off at school, I feel light, my legs feel springy, the weight on my feet more forward, feel like I am floating around the house. Still calm. 09, 6C, 03:XX:XX Themes: light, floating
Sh,13- Increased sense of sensuality to the skin, pulling on jeans is a luxury, I feel like a kitten, soft, cuddly and warm. 09, 6C, 03:XX:XX Themes: sexual, touch
Sh,139- During a massage on her abdomen, felt as if she were going into shock. Had this feeling before at age 19 when she had a bad fall with broken ribs, and punctures to the liver, with internal bleeding, which resulted in surgery and the unnecessary removal of her spleen. Never had this kind of experience during massage before... 09, 6C, 04:XX:XX Themes: hurt
Sh,14- Delusion—Small white animal, sweet and cuddly, has been living in a chair in my living room. 16, 10C, 04:XX:XX Themes: animal, love
Sh,140- Went to co-counseling feeling happy and suddenly started crying. I was focused while I was crying. A part of me was above myself crying, watching me crying. 08, 30C, 21:XX:XX Themes: double

Sh,141- The drama was clear; the good guy and bad guys. During the proving, I realized it all leads to the same thing. Withdraw. Acting watching. A Chosen separation. Zen state of watching and witnessing, but I could see how it could become sociopathic. My kids were fighting and I grabbed them and spanked them. Normally, I would be wracked with guilt. It was lovely to be a parent without guilt for awhile. 09, 9C, XX:XX:XX Themes: antagonism, indifference

Sh,142- Good guys and bad guys. Drama of evil is set up by the bad guys. They always win, always a struggle to just keep going. That is where I came from. During the proving, I saw that even engaging in that struggle gives it power and meaning. If you stop and watch the game, eventually there won't be anyone playing anymore. Good and bad were still positions, but it was all the same game. 09, 9C, XX:XX:XX Themes: antagonism, indifference

Sh,143- Organized. I feel if I could get things neat and organized the world would be perfect, but I can never get to that point, because there will be a flow. Trying to get things organized at home, which is like trying to get my eyes focused . Other times I just stared out the window, unfocussed. I either feel totally in flow with the universe, or floating aimlessly down a river. When I'm unfocussed, it's like a place where you can get lost, as if you're going to lose it. When I'm focused, I bring it all in, in the present, There. like meditating, or seeing God. When I'm unfocussed it's like I'll go into the abyss, and won't come back, go crazy. 08, 30C, 31:XX:XX Themes: organization, yielding

Sh,144- Woke feeling fearful, anxious and out of sorts. I thought of what motivates me to be good, and then the ugly feeling. I felt as if the good things were like a mirror to the other side. 08, 30C, 21:XX:XX Themes: antagonism

Sh,15- My pillow smelled like mouse excrement. 16, 10C, XX:XX:XX Themes: dirty

Sh,150- Is this true calm or the calm of the dead? I'm not feeling so much, which is a relief because I was feeling so negative before. 09, 6C, 04:XX:XX Themes: death, indifference

Sh,152- I used to always be ready to tangle. Loved to argue even if it was a topic I didn't care about. Since the proving that is gone. I now actually enjoy listening to people express opinions I don't necessarily agree with. I continue to feel calm, able to listen, and not get caught up in the fray. 03, 12C, 62:XX:XX Themes: discussion

Sh,153- In retrospect, over the last few days, it seems as if the past and the future have collapsed into the present. The past was unimportant, and I don't concern myself over the future. 09, 6C, 08:XX:XX Themes: time, indifference

Sh,155- Thoughts in the morning of our house when we lived in Japan. I can remember certain details so vividly. The carpet, kitchen, bath; the back door we never used, and the back yard I only went into three times. A feeling of longing for the past. 09, 6C, 08:14:XX Themes: nostalgia\plain

Sh,156- A person is late to meet me. This is unusual, as I am almost always late. I think, "This is why I am always late, so I don't have to wait. This is what it feels like for other people when I keep them waiting." I have sympathy for people whom I have kept waiting. 09, 6C, 10:06:40 Themes: time

Sh,157- Called into work a half an hour early, for an emergency. Went into automatic overwhelm. Felt a lot of responsibilities. I didn't have the time to do all the things I wanted to do. 01, 30C, 01:23:XX Themes: duty, work, time

Sh,16- Had a superstitious thing happen. A white moth flew up by me in class and I had a strong sense someone close to me had died. 13, 30C, 01:04:XX Themes: death, clairvoyance

Sh,161- I feel like I should write down, "Pandora's box," in my journal. I feel like something started and I don't know where the end is. It's an endless feeling. 06, 6C, 00:12:30 Themes: time

Sh,163- Sitting down watching things pass you by. Time is a factor. You only have a certain amount of time to get there. After a certain time you've blocked yourself from the opportunity to have made a move. 18, 30C, 17:XX:XX Themes: time

Sh,165- Tremulous heart center sensation. Feeling for people, puppies and just feel my heart. Emotional pressure over sternum and heart. I was more empathic, feeling other people's pain, almost to the point of weepiness. 13, 30C, 06:XX:XX Themes: compassionate

Sh,166- Very sensitive to people. If I looked at them I would see their emotions written on them. I worked on one patient and felt his deep seated grief. Intense hypersensitivity to people. 13, 30C, 06:XX:XX Themes: sensitive

Sh,167- Clairvoyance about people and what was going on with them. 13, 30C, 12:XX:XX Themes: clairvoyance

Sh,168- We are adopting a toddler from China. I want to do it for the girls in China. Three hundred a day are abandoned. 01,30C, XX:XX:XX Themes: compassionate

Sh,170- More self confident and self accepting than in the past. Questioning the times I'm not confident, and what to do about it. Instead of viewing it in a paranoid way, I'm treating it in a more matter of fact way. My feelings changed about certain people at work who have bothered me. Bouncing back quicker. Before, hours and hours would pass thinking about it. 18, 30C, 01:13:30 Themes: resentment, confidence

Sh,171- Made a decision to play cards with my friend at work even though a guard who has been hassling me was nearby. She makes me uncomfortable. Decided not to let that person's presence get in the way of my life. Did it very confidently. Very confident! Confidence to accept and to go about my business without making detours. 18, 30C, 03:02:00 Themes: conscience, negligence

Sh,172- I have an inner sense of confidence. I feel good about the things I do. I am able to let my friend go and not torment myself about things which haven't working out. 08, 30C, 19:XX:XX Themes: conscience, tormented

Sh,175- Date with the local Catholic priest who has a thing for me. I haven't had a date in years and now this—a priest! 16, 10C, 41:XX:XX Themes: conscience

Sh,18- Woke up and thought I smelled burnt wood. 08, 30C, 16:XX:XX Themes: fire

Sh,182- Not doing enough. Feel somewhat critical of myself. Not getting anything done. Want to be in a structured, organized place and can't get there. I'd like to be really busy. I have more ideas in my head than I can do. I need to get active again, structure things, and set goals. 08, 30C, 03:XX:XX Themes: unfit, busy, duty, organization, planning

Sh,183- I feel good, charged. Had a surge of energy. Feel very industrious. Organizing things, cleaning out my room. Organizing stuff to give away to charity. 01, 30C, 00:01:00 Themes: organization, work

Sh,184- Totally in gear. Cleaned and organized my whole house. Wanted everything in order. If everything is in order then life will be great. It will go well. 08, 30C, 08:XX:XX Themes: organization, house

Sh,185- I have a higher energy and things happen. I think of something and immediately someone hands it to me. The power is greater so I have to make sure the goals are right. Have to be in perfect order because goals will happen. 08, 30C, 12:XX:XX Themes: justice, energy

Sh,186- I've never been this clean for this long. I want to use up everything, all the leftovers. Everything has to be done and clean. Very methodically using up old things, like old jars of beans. I want everything to be in order and neat. 08, 30C, 22:XX:XX Themes: organization, dirty

Sh,187- I want more from school. Ethics and education are very important. I want things done to a very high standard. To be methodical and well thought out. Want higher quality. 08, 30C, 25:XX:XX Themes: justice, perfection, conscientious

Sh,189- Mad at a friend. Was at his house organizing stuff for him. I had the system organized and then he brought a whole other set of things and dumped them in. I was so furious, I left and got a headache from being angry. 08, 30C, 41:XX:XX Themes: organization, anger

Sh,190- Something is changing like the feeling of a door opening. Wanting to get on with what I am doing in general. Cleaning up loose ends, and clutter and getting on top of daily details. More matter of fact. 11, 30C, 15:XX:XX Themes: organization

Sh,191- Frustration. Slight feeling of being hurried. 11, 30C, 15:XX:XX Themes: hurry

Sh,192- Ran up an down a beach yelling and screaming to get it out of me. 02, 30C, XX:XX:XX Themes: escape

Sh,194- Uptight, jittery, as from a lot of coffee. Inner agitation, tension. Anxious agitation welling up. 06, 6C, 05:13:00 Themes: restless

Sh,197- I was flowing in the car. Driving to a destination and not being driven. More a sense like floating without the tension of driving. 09, 9C, XX:XX:XX Themes: floating

Sh,2- Looking in the mirror is weird. Feel ugly. Very pale. I feel I look ugly, pale, big body and butt. Throughout the whole day I kept catching myself in the mirror and felt this all day. 01, 30C, 01:XX:XX Themes: ugly, ridiculous

Sh,20- See the beginnings of rainbows in the sky. On second glance nothing is there. A sense of a rainbow starting to form, squinting I see faint pink & blue. Also see wavy motion in the sky, like a ripple of wind, like five lines of horizontal smoke but nothing is there. Periodically I see colors and motion. It is movement without an object. It occurs in the daytime, looking out from inside or when outside looking into the sky. pleasant sensation. 03, 12C, 02:XX:XX Themes: light

Sh,201- Very speedy feeling, anxious inside regarding relationship. Trying to get car fixed so I can go see her. 02, 30C, 07:XX:XX Themes: hurry

Sh,202- There is a holding back of impulses. Usually impulsive, now unsure whether impulses will serve me. Feeling as if I am a wild horse, ready to gallop full force, and being held back. 02, 30C, 11:XX:XX Themes: impulsive, wild

203- Feel like a rushing train. Like diving from a high dive and there is no water in the pool. 02, 30C, 16:XX:XX Themes: hurry

Sh,205- Aggravated driving to work. Why don't these people get out of my way? Frustrated with the world, angry with the world. I don't want any red lights. Want everything to be smooth. I used to feel this way years ago when I used to drink. 02, 30C, 10:XX:XX Themes: impatience, hurry, anger

Sh,206- Feeling on an emotional roller coaster. 02, 30C, 05:XX:XX Themes: hurry

Sh,208- Daughter home sick. I'm enjoying just hanging around with her being. "Mom." Realize I still don't feel like her mom. I'm not Mom; I'm just me. But to them, I'm Mom. Does my mom feel the same? 09, 6C, 23:XX:XX Themes: identity

Sh,208- Daughter home sick. I'm enjoying just hanging around with her being. "Mom." Realize I still don't feel like her mom. I'm not Mom; I'm just me. But to them, I'm Mom. Does my mom feel the same? 09, 6C, 23:XX:XX Themes: love, compassionate

Sh,21- Preoccupied with right eye awareness. Staring at the rainbow colors on the beveling of a stained glass window. Excited to discover what might occur with my right eye. 03, 12C, 03:XX:XX Themes: bright, light

Sh,211- I allowed my mother to mother me for the first time. It was a wonderful visit. For the first time ever I was allowing myself to be vulnerable and allowed her to love me. I had never felt I was the child with her before. These thoughts were foreign to me. 01, 30C, 21:XX:XX Themes: live, young

Sh,212- Out of the blue, a friend called to see if I want to adopt another child and I said, "Yes I do." It shocked me. 01, 30C, 21:XX:XX Themes: compassionate

Sh, 213- I wanted to do more mothering while I was being mothered and at the same time not mothering the son I do have. Feeling envy of all families who had more children. Constant state of desire for something other than what I had. If busy, I wanted to be not busy. If no one calls, I felt nobody cares about me. Could find no comfort anywhere and felt isolated alone. 01, 30C, , 21:XX:XX Themes: envy, family, forsaken, solitude

Sh,215- Made up a meditation before going to bed. Felt both parents at the bedside. I am being totally held and loved by my father, wrapped up in blankets like I'm a baby. He is adoring me, cooing over me with my mother looking on. This calms my nerves and the sad feeling moves outward. This feels the same as swimming to me. The water on my skin calms my nerves. 08, 30C, 23:XX:XX Themes: love, family, water

Sh,216- Had an extreme emotional shift about my Dad and what he did to me in the past. Cried and cried and cried. Went into a deep place of far past stuff that I've rarely talked about. Surprised, because I didn't think I had anything to say. Went to co-counseling feeling happy and suddenly started crying. I was focused while I was crying. I had to tell everything and not stop until I was done, even though it went overtime. A part of me was above myself crying, watching me crying. 08, 30C, 21:XX:XX Themes: grief, past, double

Sh,217- Skin feels softer, a hardness is gone from it. Feels squishier, more pliable. It reminds me of my mother's skin, which gives me the creeps. Not wanting to be like my mother. 09, 6C, 02:XX:XX Themes: touch, hard

Sh,22- Sense of a rainbow at the edge of my right eye when looking outside, but there's nothing there. Noticed phenomenon of seeing color in the sky and having a second look and no color there. Now eager and expectant to see or sense it again. 03, 12C, 03:XX:XX Themes: light

Sh,221- I feel heavy and earthbound — why don't I fit? 20, 30C, XX:XX:XX Themes: heavy

Sh,222- Increased sensitivity to the shopping mall environment. It seems destructive, unpleasant. I feel over stimulated, easily distracted, not knowing what I wanted. Feeling ungrounded and out of body; walking but not seeing, aimless, without a mind of my own. 09, 6C, 04:XX:XX Themes: lost

Sh,223- Don't feel I have any direction. Usually I have a direction though I might not know where it is going to lead. Now I feel lost, like I have no ground under me. I have no idea. 08, 30C, 28:XX:XX Themes: lost

Sh,227- Pictures of the mountains make me homesick. Deeper than homesick. Feeling low, remembering the freedom of going to them. Missing mountains and the outdoors. 02, 30C, 07:01:XX Themes: homesickness, nature, sadness

Sh,228- Homesick for home before I go away to NY—I don't want to go. 16, 10C, 27:XX:XX Themes: homesickness

Sh,229- Walk at night in the moonlight; hard to come back into the house. I have no fear, it's so beautiful. 16, 10C, 30:XX:XX Themes: go out

Sh,25- While listening to a patient grieve, had a return of increased awareness of right eye, especially the socket. I had a strong image of how my mother's right eye was knocked out when she was hit by a truck and killed 30 years ago. Feel a very strong sense of connection with her. Telling this to my proving supervisor later, I realized I had never said this to anyone. This was an aspect of her death I had suppressed. It had always been so horrifying to me I couldn't deal with it. I cried gently with lots of tears. Feeling very sad and some remorse that I couldn't have been with my mother when she died. Felt very calm with all of this. 03, 12C, 18:XX:XX Themes: death, lack, mother, compassionate, horrible

Sh,26- My eyes feel wide open when they are not. Unusual that I'm feeling the width and depth of the wide openness. I feel as if my eyes are taking in a lot of light. Repositories of light. 18, 30C, 00:11:30 Themes: light

Sh,27- Eyes feel like receptors to light the way a satellite dish is a receptor for stellar signals or microwaves, as if they are meant to capture light or receive it. Odd feeling. Sensitive to light but at the same time wide open to it, as if it is meant to be. 18, 30C, 03:XX:XX Themes: light

Sh,29- I kept seeing deep purple light — amazingly deep. Watched the sun rise over the house — I had a desire for symmetry in the sky. I felt there should be two suns. Strange because it's been so hot. An image of light radiating towards me — white lightfull spectrum. 20, 30C, XX:XX:XX Themes: light

Sh,3- Feel like abdomen is much bigger, but husband says it's not. 09, 6C, 00:XX:XX Themes: big

Sh,30- After I looked at the sun, I saw four suns in a ring connected to each other, and another one above with strings of light. One had two lesser ones. 20, 30C, XX:XX:XX Themes: light, bright

Sh,300- Like being outside at night. 16, 10C, 33:XX:XX Themes: go out

Sh,301- Want to move to mountains, but I

can't do it in one day. 08, 30C, 30:XX:XX Themes: greatness

Sh,305- I could hear something on a railroad traveling from east to west across the States. I was above looking down. 20, 30C, XX:XX:XX Themes: travel

Sh,306- When I'm focused I bring it all in, in the present, There. like meditating, or seeing God. When I'm unfocussed it's like I'll go into the abyss, and won't come back, go crazy. 08, 30C, 31:XX:XX Themes: religious, god, fall, insanity

Sh,312- Eyes feel nearsighted. Don't want to look far away. Don't want to go far out of my house either, not even to the market. Don't want to go far outside my territory. 08, 30C, 15:XX:XX Themes: go out

Sh,316- I start something and get bored with it. I need three things going on at the same time and rotate from one to the other. Can't stick to anything. 08, 30C, 34:XX:XX Themes: dispersion

Sh,317- Feel overwhelmed when deciding what art supplies to order. Hard to make limited choices among many good things. Usually very decisive. 03, 12C, 08:XX:XX Themes: doubtful

Sh,318- Procrastinated doing grocery shopping. Debated which day to go, and which store. Decided much later to go to neither place, and just pick up what I absolutely needed. 03, 12C, 15:XX:XX Themes: postponing

Sh,319- Very difficult to decide what to eat. 03, 12C, 15:XX:XX Themes: doubtful

Sh,324- Don't feel I have any direction. Usually I have a direction though I might not know where it is going to lead. Now I feel lost, like I have no ground under me. I have no idea. 08, 30C, 28:XX:XX Themes: lost

Sh,326- Unconsciously, I have taken on the characteristics of the speech of a guy I work with; an actual copying of a certain vernacular. When he talks, he stretches a word. I don't do it consciously, but when it happens, I'm aware I've adopted a small part of that personality. The way he gestures, the way he uses his teeth—enunciates—the gestures of his language. I feel I'm malleable. I don't like it. It feels like I don't have my own personality, no true identity. In fact I might even believe that. I'm more outward with actual copying. It's something I like in him, so when I do it, it makes me feel good about myself. I realize it then try to combat it. I don't want to be like a piece of clay that can be pressed this way and that way. 18, 30C, 17:XX:XX Themes: identity

Sh,327- I want to sleep. Want to be left alone, like a kid just before he goes to sleep. I don't want to bother with people anymore. 08, 30C, 34:XX:XX Themes: company, young

Sh,330- Bored and superior feeling with an old friend. 16, 10C, 22:XX:XX Themes: friend, contemptuous, greatness

Sh,331- Don't like people and they don't like me. Feel over exposed. 16, 10C, 33:XX:XX Themes: loathing

Sh,333- Aversion to going out of the house. 16, 10C, 07:XX:XX Themes: go out, loathing

Sh,334- Sad. Can't break from therapist. Don't want to go out because I feel like I would be over exposed. 16, 10C, 10:XX:XX Themes: fragile

Sh,336- Changed work shift. Didn't want to go to work. Don't like being at work at all. Frustrated at lack of ability to communicate with patient I was assisting. 02, 30C, 10:XX:XX Themes: talk, work

Sh,337- Talked to a friend who didn't understand me and didn't understand my goals. I felt degraded and wanted to really yell at him. In the end, he understood me, and I expressed my frustration with him. Frustrated that I couldn't make him get what I was saying. So furious. They didn't give me any respect. I deserve more. Frustrated. I do so much more than he thought, and he didn't understand. 08, 30C, 37:XX:XX Themes: despised

Sh,338- Getting curt with people. Abrupt in conversation, cutting things off sooner. 09, 6C, 14:17:XX Themes: offensive

Sh,341- Can't be bothered to write symptoms down because they seem so minor. Feel this is too private. 02, 30C, 04:XX:XX Themes: reserved

Sh,347- In response to a question from the supervisor started yelling, " I'm getting irritated with these conversations . Why can't we just get on with it ?! Why can't you understand what I am saying?!" 02,

30C, 09:XX:XX Themes: bothered

Sh,349- I said I was moody. It wasn't as qualitative as she wanted, and she was asking for more details and I yelled, " A stupid five year old would understand what I was saying." I became sarcastic and very belligerent. I thought I was being simplistic and clear. I gave what I had to give. I was in a depressed state, lost my good feeling and was angry at being asked to explain the depression. She asked me what do you mean and I said, "XXXX off. If you don't understand that, too bad. Do you understand that?! Do you know the English language?" 18, 30C, 04:14:00 Themes: sarcasm, fight, offensive, anger, contemptuous

Sh,350- ... "Considered committing suicide. Feeling that life has passed me by. Thinking about my mortality. Terrified of dying. My time has run out." ...18, 30C, 05:XX:XX-16:XX:XX Themes: time, suicidal, death, fearful

Sh,375- Just wants to crawl away, hide in a hole, do something else. Hard to get motivated. This feeling about one job she has to do spills over into everything else and she doesn't want to do anything. 09, 6C, 03:XX:XX Themes: hide, yielding

Sh,376- Lethargic, spaced out. It feel like I don't have the impetus to move. Inertia. I just want to sleep, but there's this tension inside. 06, 6C, 00:11:00 Themes: movement

Sh,384- There is some kind of barrier or buffer. Everything's kind of distant, like being wrapped in cotton wool. There's a distance between me and everything outside. Things weren't up close. Something between me and everything else. 07, 30C, 04:00:30 Themes: isolation, obstructed

Sh,386- I feel removed and everything is in slow motion and I couldn't really contact reality. I felt like I was compensating for the lack of motion. (On this page of her journal she has doodled a picture of a slanted cube with vertical bars on it. It looks like an animal cage leaning to the right.) 01, 30C, 15:XX:XX Themes: isolation, imprisoned

Sh,389- Hadn't studied for exams; normally would be extremely anxious. This time totally centered, hunkered down into hips, knew I didn't know the material. It was a nice exam. Enjoyed it. Feel no anxiety regarding exams. 02, 30C, 05:XX:XX Themes: negligence

Sh,390- While making the schedule, instead of working hard to fill every spot, I left some blanks to be filled in at the staff meeting. It felt good to let go of the responsibility. 02, 30C, 01:04:XX Themes: duty

Sh,391- Staff meeting was awful. Everyone feeling frustrated due to extra work, but I did not feel any blame. Normally I would have felt responsible, but this time I felt it was not my fault. 02, 30C, 01:10:XX - 01:12:XX Themes: duty

Sh,391- Staff meeting was awful. Everyone feeling frustrated due to extra work, but I did not feel any blame. Normally I would have felt responsible, but this time I felt it was not my fault. 02, 30C, 01:10:XX - 01:12:XX Themes: indifference

Sh,4- Feel fat. 16, 10C, 18:XX:XX Themes: heavy

Sh,401- Worried feeling. Tearful but can't cry. Want to be with someone. Can't let it go that a friend yelled at me two days ago. I'm more sad than I should be. I don't want to be by myself. Want to cry but can't. Feel better with people and worse being alone. This is happening during my period; usually happens before menses. 08, 30C, 17:XX:XX Themes: company, solitude

Sh,402- I felt pathetic, defeated and vulnerable. I was reaching on a high shelf for pots for plants. All the pots and soil came tumbling down. Was knocked on the head, on the vertex. Dirt all over me, and I thought, "This is perfect. This is exactly how I feel." I felt like I had to just give up — give up the bravado. I'm exhausted, I'm just going to rest. I just wanted to go into a little ball and lick my wounds. Felt very much like childhood symptoms. I felt very young. 01, 30C, 18:XX:XX Themes: fragile, dirty, young, failure

Sh,403- For three weeks I was in a depression, unlike anything I have felt for a long time. Deep sense of low self-worth. Feeling invisible, uncared for and envious. I was lethargic, couldn't do anything. My practice dropped, patients just didn't show up. I felt I sunk as low as I needed to go, unmotivated. Felt unappreciative of all I have. Unappreciative of my life which I usually adore. Anger, dissatisfaction with life, isolating. I wasn't seeing anyone not even my husband, exhaustive. Had no dreams during the depression — unusual. I am emerging from it now. 01, 30C, 30:XX:XX-50:XX:XX Themes: sadness, envy, contemptuous, helplessness, isolation

Sh,410- Feel as low now as I was high. An opposite. More serious. It's a little overbearing. It shouldn't be so serious. I have a place to go. Old issues looked upon detrimentally—maybe. Hard to dispel or find my place with them. Maybe I should lighten up a little. Issues are pressing, weighty. 18, 30C, 03:11:XX Themes: serious

Sh,411- The way I'm feeling today is aggravated and slightly depressed; mostly aggravated about financial things. Reflecting on a bigger picture now, need to do something about it. More on my mind than before. It has to do with my position and place in life; where I am at this particular point in life. Am I pleased? Am I happy? Am I disgruntled? Of course I'm disgruntled. A switch happened. I wasn't looking so detrimentally on my feelings about position and place. The remedy lightened everything, seasoned it, not as bland as I thought. Now things are bland—not spiced up or happy. 18, 30C, 03:11:XX Themes: position, money

Sh,412- Somewhat apathetic with an undercurrent of depression. Neither here nor there. I was water. Moody as a rainy day, down, blue, depressed, easily aggravated. 18, 30C, 04:13:30 Themes: sadness

Sh,414- Every thing back to yucky normal. 09, 6C, 00:15:XX Themes: dirty

Sh,416- Feel really dull with the rain. I think I'm in a mild depression. I'm not visiting friends, just hanging around. No goals, not doing things. 08, 30C, 03:XX:XX Themes: water, sadness

Sh,417- Frustrated and depressed. Feeling lonely, friendless and unaccomplished. 18, 30C, 15:XX:XX Themes: failure, sadness, friendless, helplessness

Sh,427- Luckily, this legal dispute is not happening to me personally. But I feel it is. I imagine them laughing at us and doing their worst to squash us. Never felt so helpless in my life. 09, 6C, 26:XX:XX Themes: helplessness, despised

Sh,428- Realizing we haven't had any fun as a family in forever. Haven't had any fun myself either. Like a caged animal, snarling. I'm in a pressure cooker. Can't even imagine what would get me out of this mood, what actually would be fun. Don't want to do anything, or talk to anyone. Like a porcupine or sea urchin. "Don't tread on me." 09, 6C, 30:XX:XX Themes: imprisoned, isolation, wild

Sh,430- Get a call from a friend that the utility district is at it again. Don't know what, but expect the worst in negotiations with them. Can't win. So tired of fighting the losing battle. Can't raise the energy to do anything. Rage inside. Hopeless. Daydreams of blowing up the utility district, of shooting them. Only option left to desperate people and I feel desperate. we're a rag-tag group without luck, or leadership, fighting a losing battle. Feels like we're the American Indians. "Here's 24 dollars worth of beads for your island, idiot." In the pit of despair. 09, 6C, 25:XX:XX Themes: failure, fight, anger, hopeless, despair

Sh,431- The first thing that happened was I became very depressed and fearful. I was weak and couldn't resolve my issues. I became a laughable matter. The next thing I knew, I became embittered at all those I thought were laughing at me. During the last week of the proving, the vindictive side of reacting to that depression came out. 18, 30C, 7:XX:XX Themes: revengeful, despised, sadness

Sh,432- I am deeply in touch with a self—destructive sense inside. The part of me that wants to disintegrate and die. Disintegrate; the opposite of integral oneness, the opposite direction. I'll have another egg to ground me. 06, 6C, 10:XX:XX Themes: disintegration, death

Sh,433- Feel self-destructive, like eating greasy fatty junk food, not exercising, slowly kill myself that way. Why care? 06, 6C, 10:XX:XX Themes: suicidal, dirty

Sh,434- Usually I enjoy my exercise; today it's going against what my will wants to do. The exercise practice equals life and health. I feel like going the opposite way.

06, 6C, 10:XX:XX Themes: antagonism

Sh,435- I was feeling very self-destructive. I wanted to do crappy things to myself. The border's breaking loose. I know I have a part of me that does this. It's just rising up. Screw it all, the futility of it all; the futility of working toward the positive, of caring for my health, of doing good things. What for? My big fear is that I'm really crazy, that I'm making all this up, that I'm just crazy (i.e., that the remedy is a placebo). 06, 6C, 11:XX:XX Themes: ruined, insanity, antagonism

Sh,436- About suicide; I would never have entertained a thought to do something like this. The thought of suicide was destined to make me look beyond it. It wasn't a game. It was just part of a phase that was passing—the last rung of it. 18, 30C, 35:XX:XX Themes: suicidal

Sh,437- Remedy brought up tendency to look at my lack of self-benefaction, and I became depressed looking at that picture. "What you need to do is do it. Get on with your life. Concentrate on the moves for your future." 18, 30C, 35:XX:XX Themes: helplessness

Sh, 5- Feel like I'm gaining weight, but am actually losing weight. 08, 30C, 05:XX:XX Themes: heavy

Sh,507- Having some trouble speaking. Using the wrong words, or lacking words at times. Just keep it simple. Husband told the kids. We all laughed. I guess that's what you can say for adversity. If it happens enough you learn to get used to it. If it's not too hard. Began thinking about one of my kids dying—that would be too hard. I don't want to do that to find out. 09, 6C, 16:XX:XX Themes: death, misfortune, family

Sh,510- Still having difficulty thinking. Nothing there. In shock about missing court filing deadline. Paralyzed about what to do. Mixes up words when talking. Drifting off. Unable to hold a train of thought. But not getting critical or depressed the way I would have been in the past. It's like fighting an enemy you can't see that keeps hitting you from behind. It's nasty. Observing. Just being, brain completely diffused. Can't keep thoughts on track. 09, 6C, 18:XX:XX Themes: betrayed

Sh,512- Feeling slightly hysterical, on and off through the day, as if disconnected and fragile. Not an overpowering sensation, but distinct. It was a sensation as if some danger was near. 04, 30C, 01:XX:XX Themes: danger, fragile

Sh,513- On my way home, while it was dark, I saw a glow in the sky and immediately I thought my house was burning. I was very scared and I should have realized that the glow came from the town behind the ridge, but it took me a while to get that. 04, 30C, 03:XX:XX Themes: fire, house

Sh,517- Dread of upcoming legal battle. 09, 6C, 15:XX:XX Themes: justice, discussion

Sh,518- Feeling obsessed with the question of whether it will rain. I'm planning my son's birthday party outside for tomorrow with 17 children, and am afraid it will rain. 01, 30C, 11:12:30 Themes: accidents

Sh,519- I was anxious about so much rain. There was severe flooding in our valley, washing the bridge out that connected us to the rest of the world. I felt isolated; lives were decimated. I felt frantic because I couldn't be helpful. 01, 30C, 30:XX:XX—53:XX:XX Themes: helpful

Sh,520- When the rain came down hard, there was a roaring from the creek outside. Awful sleep. I'd wake up with each roar, envisioning the water rising up, fearing the creek was backed up and would overflow its banks. I'd listen till the sound died down, then I could go back to sleep. 08, 30C, 06:XX:XX Themes: accidents, water

Sh,521- Fear of death. 16, 10C, 05:XX:XX Themes: death

Sh,522- Fear for the life of my cat. 16, 10C, 08:XX:XX Themes: death

Sh,523- Sense of fear. Vision: The shadow of death creeping in, like it did in the movie, Ten Commandments". 16, 10C, 09:XX:XX Themes: death

Sh,525- Big fear on icy road. Scared driving on "Separate Road". Went to see a friend, had a quick hello and good-bye. All wanted to do was go home. 16, 10C, 36:XX:XX Themes: accidents

Sh,526- Fear of death came up more than usual during the proving. It wasn't the fear of aging. It was fear of the finality, that one day you won't see the light, or breathe the air, or live to contemplate overcoming your problems. 18, 30C, 35:XX:XX Themes: death

Sh,536- I have been really pissed off again since the proving ended. Every two months, I get this thing on the 13th to the 16th. Something lightly ruffling happens. It's an unusual amount of anger. An Everest of emotions. 02, 30C, XX:XX:XX Themes: anger

Sh,527- I was paying attention to the obituaries at this time. Noticed people dying in the newspaper. I would get very angry and frustrated. For a short time, was looking at death notices on a daily basis, during the last week or so of the proving. My anger towards death. How unfair. I don't want it. I shouldn't have to have it. There should never be a day where the morning is taken from me. 18, 30C, 35:XX:XX Themes: justice, death, anger

Sh,528- Noticed in the paper all cancer related deaths, particularly prostate, mostly men between 40-60. Seemed to be men who were very loved. Seemed most unfair. Fear that if I drank too much coffee I would get a headache, and the thought was cancer related. 18, 30C, 35:XX:XX Themes: death, justice, disease

Sh,529- There was definitely someone else inside of me. The essence of that person was trying to get out, escaping, trying to get away. It felt like I was in prison or the thing in me was in prison. I was saying, "go," and it wouldn't get out of there. My supervisor got worried about me. On purpose, I made sure I was unavailable. If anyone asked me details, I would get angry. I won't explain it to you. I'm feeling that now a little, talking about it. 02, 30C, XX:XX:XX Themes: escape, imprisoned

Sh,530- Trying to do the work schedule; it won't click in like normal. Get stuck, then go away from it, get stuck again. Want to run away. Left the schedule until the next morning. 02, 30C, 00:04:XX Themes: escape

Sh,532- I started to speed up emotionally, got really pissed off at supervisor for getting in touch with me, beeping me. Wanted to escape and fly away. Phoned the airlines, trying to fly away. Hiding. Difficult to be with patients, with their stupid emotions. 02, 30C, XX:XX:XX Themes: hide, escape, hurry

Sh,533- Boxed in feeling with no way to express anger. Start taking it out on the kids, as if they are trying to break me, to get me. Better getting out, going away from home and family. 09, 6C, 20:XX:XX Themes: suppressed, anger, prejudiced

Sh,534- The thing about the proving, I see now, was the intense trapped feeling. I felt trapped by people and situations. People who are being weird. Before, I would just let things slide, or roll off of me, like water off a duck's back. During the proving, I needed to break out, a screeching feeling. I had to speak out to change the situation. I had to stop letting things slide. 13, 30C, 7 months Themes: imprisoned, liberty

Sh,537- While asleep in bed, my husband touched my leg and I started from sleep. Oversensitive to touch and sound. Aversion to being touched. I just wanted to be left alone. Too irritable. 06, 6C, 00:05:00 Themes: touch, company

Sh,55- I usually relate to people who make a lot less money than me. I had an argument with a friend who is in a high class about money. Am thinking about taking a job that would put me in a high class, but don't know if I would want to work with those kind of people—downtown people into their careers who make hundreds of thousands. They make me nervous. Afraid they will snub me. So much to do with worth. What am I worth? 08, 30C, 42:XX:XX Themes: position, despised

Sh,557- I feel like everybody's judging me or in my face. 07, 30C, 04:22:30 Themes: censured

Sh,56- Lately thinking over my worth and friendships. Who are my friends and where am I wasting my time. What is my position in society in relationship to career, how friends view me and relationships with men? I find myself going back to having older friends and finding them to be true to me. 08, 30C, 42:XX:XX Themes: friends, position

Sh,560- I don't feel cranky, but I have no idea how I'd feel if someone criticized me or tried to lecture me. 07, 30C, 07:06:00 Themes: censured

Sh,561- Felt insulted and taunted by a bitchy patient all day. 16, 10C, 02:XX:XX Themes: offended

Sh,563- Patient called and I felt I had no patience for her. Wanted to be more present for her, but felt she was too weepy and needy. Couldn't be bothered. Couldn't be bothered with all the patients the rest of the day. Felt overwhelmed. Trying to be nice at work, hard to do. 02, 30C, 00:06:XX Themes: bothered

Sh,565- Really angry at the swimming club commissioner for planning our morning swim against the tide and not telling me. So angry, I couldn't even look at his face. It was such a hard swim, I knew I couldn't make it and had to be pulled in by a boat. Really furious. 08, 30C, 18:XX:XX Themes: anger

Sh,567- Had to leave my house to study elsewhere, due to an unpleasant visitor at home. Someone I can't stand being around came to visit my partner and see our puppies. He wouldn't ask her to leave. I didn't want to engage with her, because there is no way you can win. If I had said, "It's time to go, now," then I am the ogre. There are no boundaries. 13, 30C, 00:06:00 Themes: go out, bothered, invaded

Sh,569- About 5:00 p.m. felt an irascibility again about people not paying me, but now it feels like an easily moving type of rage, not suppressed. 13, 30C, 01:11:XX Themes: money, anger

Sh,570- Don't want to do anything but stay underground— "kick a can" around town. Feel angry about people who may be maligning me. 16, 10C, 14:XX:XX Themes: prejudiced, hide, wicked

Sh,571- At sacred ceremony, but want to be alone. See a friend there who is rude, disrespectful, and obnoxious at this sacred ceremony, and I feel annoyed. 16, 10C, 15:XX:XX Themes: company, bothered

Sh,572- Dwell on past disagreeable occurrences. Hold a grudge. 16, 10C, 33:XX:XX Themes: resentment, past, offended

Sh,573- Back into usual blaming and being critical of children and family. Also being very self critical and dissatisfied. 09, 6C, 27—34:XX:XX Themes: censorious

Sh,575- Very angry with the children, who have done no chores. Irritated and yelled at them. I get so angry my nervous system refuses to calm down. I take their behavior personally, plus I'm angry at myself for my own response to them. 09, 6C, 05:04:XX Themes: duty, anger

Sh,577- Children are an obstacle to enlightenment. 09, 6C, 05:XX:XX Themes: knowledge, obstructed, children

Sh,580- Spent most of today thinking about how I am surrounded by idiots, (my family), who are showing no attempts to think for themselves, letting me run the show. They don't care to figure things out. I'm in hyper-drive. I know a lot and I'm right. I've been extremely productive or at least active, balancing several major projects all at the same time, and they can't seem to tidy a table properly. This includes my husband, who continually interrupts me (or so it seems) for some trivial question. I'm coming across with too much force. I find myself shouting at everyone much more than usual. Like a crazy person. Impatient over others' slowness. Almost an arrogance. I want them to THINK! (Obviously, the way I do). or get off the ship and drown yourself. A hard anger, more intense that usual. Feel like leaving them all—they just take and give back little. More trouble than support. This isn't complaining or victimizing talking. This is how it is. I'm healing myself and leaving my family in the dust. I've passed on to them my bad habits, bad parenting. They are content to be idiots. 09, 6C, 13:XX:XX Themes: greatness, contemptuous, hurry, haughty, forsakes

Sh,581- At a meeting for parents and children, I am very critical of my daughter and myself, comparing her to other kids, myself to other moms. Cringe when she sits with her mouth open, pulling on her hair and twisting it into braids. Want to warn her, don't do that! She looks to me like she's bossing someone. Compare myself to other woman who has perfectly put together hair, clothes, nails, boots, bracelets. Very angry and jealous. Make excuses for myself and tear her down inside. 09, 6C, 14:00:XX Themes: contemptuous, censorious, greatness, jealous

Sh,582- Enforcing deadlines and rules with kids. Son wants to sing me a song but his work's not done so I "don't have time" to listen. Feel I am neglecting my family. 09,

6C, 15:00:XX Themes: dictatorial, forsakes
Sh,588- I was in a gallows humor, cruel but funny. My friends had never seen that side of me before. Like I was on speed. I had no control. They asked me not to cut up vegetables, not to use a knife. I was waving the knife around. I threw the knife at a potato. 02, 30C, XX:XX:XX Themes: pointed, wicked
Sh.589- I wanted to really hurt somebody or something , no respect for the person, anyway that I could. There was another part of me that couldn't believe I was doing that. It was like a horror movie. I got to that place of no boundaries or responsibility to life. It didn't matter what I did. Indifferent. Like ice, no feeling. Just like if I killed someone there would be no regrets. Just the thought: This is what I have to do now. Desire to kill. It did not matter. Just do it. You've got to. I had no fear. I could do anything, whatever I was asked to do, I could do it then. I was a strong person. The me was the only thing that kept me from doing it. That's where I got scared. The last five days of the proving were in a black hole. I refused to write anything down. A god-like place or a devil-like place. Why do I have these things? Human things. 02, 30C, XX:XX:XX Themes: violence, wicked, homicidal, devil
Sh,590- While I was in the shower, I just wanted to kill. 02, 30C, 11:XX:XX Themes: homicidal
Sh,591- I have to kill the children. They are not obeying me. 09, 6C, 06:XX:XX Themes: homicidal
Sh,592- Had a peculiar experience during the day. While playing with one of my dogs, I started to wonder what it would be like to crush her. Suddenly I thought how sensual it would be to crush its little head and rip its flesh. There was something very sensual about the idea of crushing flesh and bones of a soft creature that would not be able to fight me off. It was not a strong, powerful impulse, but there was something compelling about the idea. 04, 30C, 02:XX:XX Themes: wicked, crushed, violence, animal
Sh,594- Yesterday and today, when I was playing with my puppy I felt like hurting her. Today while playing, the feeling was how much stronger I was than her and I could really hurt her. It's a strange feeling. I really love my puppy. This reminds me of when I was 20 years old and there was a child sitting on the steps. I felt I could crush her. I realized how strong I am. I'm not usually a psychopath. It's a feeling of violence. 04, 30C, 04:XX:XX Themes: violence, wicked
Sh,595- I look at rabbits and birds in a different light. Wondering how a rabbit would taste raw. What would the fur taste like? 20, 30C, XX:XX:XX Themes: animal, eating
Sh,596- Drive through New Mexico. Long scary dirt road. Stop to look at a dead lamb by the side of the road and the stink of the carrion smelt good. I am intoxicated by the smell; I can't get enough of it. 16, 10C, 16:XX:XX Themes: rotten
Sh,597- Reading about the Ring Cycle and how Siegfried tasted the blood of the slain dragon.16, 10C, 22:XX:XX Themes: blood, animal, wild
Sh,598- Calmness continued, with the exception of seeing ants in my house. They had invaded my house, and I was irritated that I had to kill them and clean them up. I don't like to kill anything. My heart was racing and my face was sweaty while doing this. 03, 12C, 00:XX:XX Themes: invaded, conscience
Sh,599- Recall a detail I'd forgotten before—like the mist parting. Looked through my desk again and found the missing package. Recalled losing something earlier this week, probably thrown out. No one else saw it except me. The strangest feeling to remember having seen something, remembered the color of the paper, and the picture, and the wording, and yet not be able to confirm its existence with anyone. Beginning to doubt if it was really real, and yet I know it was. 09, 6C, 11:04:40 Themes: unreal, lost
Sh,6- Feeling old, really old. 02, 30C, 07:01:XX Themes: old
Sh,601- Back feels split as if two planes are pulled apart, like after an earthquake; the planes are off with a sharp delineation between the two. 09, 6C, 03:XX:XX Themes: disintegration

Sh,602- Have had experience of split personas before, but during the proving all the bits and pieces that seemingly had unique personalities of their own were simply more broken up. I call it a movement. It happened only when I was alone. 18, 30C, 35:XX:XX Themes: disintegration

Sh,603- The remedy brought up episodes from the past. After each episode I'd create and act out. I'd step to the side and say, "This is not you. You can't do this. You know you can't do this." And as it went on, I pulled things together and got integrated. 18, 30C, 35:XX:XX Themes: disintegration

Sh,604- Since the remedy, I took over and the physical manifestation of personas splitting off would only come out when I was alone. Did these drawings. The figure in the box was my death — captured, buried and can't get out. The first drawing is a depressed boy, the second is the buried man, the third is an x-ray figure. After that the depression abated. I did another drawing of a negative being laughing at me. It has no arms, no movement. 18, 30C, 35:XX:XX Themes: disintegration, death, imprisoned, despised

Sh,605- The remedy accelerated the personas out of me, and along with them, all these other problems. It forced me to look at all of it. Then my "I" came out! Has happened before but this was much more magnified. With the remedy, none of the fragmented personalities were willing to get behind the wheel and drive. It was like being driven, without going anywhere. Then, I slowly started seeing that these personas were just rationalizations that just didn't suffice. It helped me to come out to face them. With the remedy, I quickly pulled them together. 18, 30C, 35:XX:XX Themes: disintegration, integration

Sh,606- No more sense of sensuality, no more connection with my husband. I'm back in my head when it comes to relating to others. Damn it, it's gone. It slipped through my fingers. 09, 6C, 06:XX:XX Themes: sexual

Sh,607- An urge to destroy my relationship, scream at people. It felt very destructive. 13, 30C, 04:06:30 Themes: offensive, wicked

Sh,608- Sad that there is a crack, a possibility my relationship might end. 02, 30C, 00:14:XX Themes: union

Sh,610- Want to stay in integrity with myself and not run after my lover. We talked about commitment and she got scared. I got angry. This is it. I told her I'm not going all over the place with you. Want you XX per cent here. Feel angry at her indecision and confusion. Feel I want to hit and shake her. Ran on the beach instead. 02, 30C, 02:09:XX Themes: haughty, dictatorial, violence

Sh,612- Anxious all day. Feel my relationship is on the rocks as if partner is emotionally abusing me. 02, 30C, 05:XX:XX Themes: prejudiced, union

Sh,614- Full of energy in the morning. Run and walk in the sea, amazed at my high energy. Feel like I have to let out lack of sex. Want partner badly but mad at her and at myself for being so open. Feel speedy. 02, 30C, 08:03:XX Themes: sexual, energy, hurry

Sh,615- Don't have the guts to tell partner to stick it out a little longer, that it might work out. Feel totally devastated, but have a lot of energy to deal with it, to stick up for my rights. Felt quite centered, as if I can take care of it. Feels like being on a roller coaster, up and down, in and out. Partner wants to be friends, but not sexual. Feeling emotionally abused. 02, 30C, 09:XX:XX Themes: justice, prejudiced

Sh,618- I was trying to connect with husband. He starts sharing with me about his seminar. Daughter was calling me, "Mom, Mom.... Dinner on the table." There was this glass wall between us that neither one of us could traverse. 01, 30C, 03:09:30 Themes: obstructed

Sh,619- Explosive fight. Communication not good. I felt trapped. We didn't have a common language and we usually do. It was like two needy babies. I had my plan and he wasn't playing his part, and he had his plan and I wasn't playing my part. 01, 30C, 03:XX:XX Themes: dictatorial

Sh,623- I don't meet people like my girlfriends do. I walk around the world not seeing people look my way. Being unrecognized. It's like I'm not there. No one misses me when I'm gone. It's really uncomfortable. I never cared before. Now I want to be recognized, but I'm not. 08, 30C, 03:XX:XX Themes: isolation

Sh,625- I find that I don't have a real friend. I have acquaintances, but not a friend. That has been bothering me. A new realization. The friends I have cultivated are caught up in their own lives, and they don't have time for me. This is different— now I have time to think about it. I'm seeing for myself. At times I'm extremely lonely. I like my own place but sometimes it's nice to have a friend. 18, 30C, 17:XX:XX Themes: friendless, solitude

Sh,629- Broke things off with a friend. Felt sad then angry. Felt he degraded me. It was unhealthy to have that energy around me anymore. Very angry. No respect from him. 08, 30C, 36:XX:XX Themes: despised, anger

Sh,632- In the body a lot of splits. Lower lumbar, felt a definite line. Same split with my vision, a break. We were having a lot of earthquakes, the huge earthquake in Kobe the day the proving started. I am very connected to Japan, having lived there. Felt a shift, along a fault line, along the spine. Split was at the waist lower back. Vision was split on horizon. 09, 9C, XX:XX:XX Themes: divided, disintegration

Sh,624- Companionship. The idea that you had your chance and it didn't work out, and you're just going to be alone, and there's nothing you can do about it. 18, 30C, 17:XX:XX Themes: failure

Sh,634- Like being in the edge of an abyss, a crevice that's cracking deeper all the time. A crack that gets deeper and longer. 06, 6C, 00:12:30 Themes: fall, disintegration

Sh,637- If I had known this was going to happen, I wonder if I would have taken the remedy. I thought I must be crazy (after taking remedy last night). I would like to fling that vial of remedy to the ends of the universe. 06, 6C, 00:12:30 Themes: fly, distances

Sh,640- A lot of agitation and irritability on the surface. Underneath there was a crevice, a crack... in my soul or the universe. Dread or anticipation of what else could happen if this process went on. If the process went on, it could lead to complete insanity, completely being out of touch with reality. 06, 6C, 01:00:XX Themes: insanity, disintegration

Sh,642- I read prayers for safety before bed because I was afraid of what might happen when I went to sleep. When I came to the phrase "God is One" I realized that was the crux of it— the universe was cracked or split instead of one. Saying that prayer feels healing. Oneness is about caring; the split is about not caring. It's evil in a way. 06, 6C, 01:00:XX Themes: disintegration, integration, antagonism

Sh,644- The "fry an egg and eat it," repetitive, meaningless motion, reminds me of an extermination camp, of a killing machine; was about not caring; it's from the split or chasm. Not caring about anything, is part of what happens with the split. That's what evil is, that's really what it's about. 06, 6C, 01:00:XX Themes: wicked, indifference

Sh,645- Caring equals oneness. A scary point about that acute phase yesterday— there was no caring. It didn't matter. Nothing mattered. I was alone and wanted to be that way. To have caring, there must be an attunement with the oneness of the universe. Is that where Hitler came from? The crack in the universe? 06, 6C, 01:09:00 Themes: indifference, integration, god, disintegration

Sh,647- Life seems like hell. The beauty and order are gone. I feel awful, tense, overwhelmed, anxious with nausea. My sense of well being is gone.06, 6C, 16:XX:XX Themes: hell

Sh,648- Down side, dark side, feels like the gates between the unconscious and conscious are open. Hurricane-like feeling of unconscious energy. Like the gates of hell are open. No barrier. Extreme amount of power. Darkness. Internal pressure. Dogs guard the gates of Hades. A lot of internal pressure-type feeling all day. 13, 30C, 10:XX:XX Themes: hell, energy, dark, wicked

Sh,649- Aware of being pulled in two different directions, as if being pulled by two elephants, two strong forces. 02, 30C, 06:XX:XX Themes: antagonism

Sh,650- It was like a horror movie. That's where I got scared. The last five days of the proving were in a black hole. A god-like place or a devil-like place. Why do I have these things? Human things. 02, 30C, XX:XX:XX Themes: horrible, devil, god

Sh,651- When I'm focused, I bring it all in, in the present. There, like meditating, or seeing God. When I'm unfocussed, it's like I'll go into the abyss, and won't come back; go crazy. 08, 30C, 31:XX:XX Themes: god, height, fall, insanity

Sh,659- Less maniacal type feeling but still high amount of energy. Excessive energy but not uncontrollable. Strong sense of well being. Meditation very strong. 13, 30C, 08:XX:XX Themes: energy

Sh,662- I can't stand it any longer. Spiraled and spiraled and spiraled. Feel like I'm going mad, like there's no escaping out of this. Pull, pull, like a hypoglycemic who hasn't eaten, and just wants to scream and yell. While I was in the shower I just wanted to kill. Feel like I'm going to lose it. Going stir crazy;...02, 30C, 11:XX:XX Themes: insanity, homicidal

Sh,663- In a total frenzy, like steaming horses that had escaped, running down the road. Very hard to keep any control, to be patient in traffic, or the grocery store. Couldn't handle it any longer. Put lip balm with camphor on, every ten minutes, and would feel calm momentarily. Finally got some tiger balm at a friend's house and used it two times. I was instantly calmer. Came back to being me. 02, 30C, 11:XX:XX Themes: wild, insanity, escape

Sh,664- Feel deflated, calmer and flatter. The feeling of going mad goes back to when I was drinking 15 years ago. That feeling of not being able to decide what to do. Today feeling flat, exhausted; a wonderful day outside, unable to enjoy it. Feeling unenergized, although glad the craziness is gone. I felt I was on speed with emotions. I'm glad I antidoted that thing; feel like an empty balloon. It could have gotten down to a dangerous place. Reminded me of going mad; like the energy it gave me. Felt hooked on the remedy. 02, 30C, 12:XX:XX Themes: insanity, energy, danger

Sh,670- When I was alone in my apartment with the lights on, I manifested many fragmented personalities, probably around five or six. Never did before like this. What was different was nobody was in the room to make a chain reaction. I was alone. Needed no provocation to make a change, or experience a change. I talk outloud, and talk to the person in a number of different ways. Fearful Joe, Vindictive Joe, One That's Just Like Someone Else Joe — each will act out in a number of different ways. 18, 30C, 35:XX:XX Themes: fearful, revengeful, disintegration, double

Sh,676- The remedy worked very directly on my will. Fragmentation is the denial of will. Integration is the use of will. All separate states under a unified country. 18, 30C, 35:XX:XX Themes: disintegration, integration

Sh,676- The remedy worked very directly on my will. Fragmentation is the denial of will. Integration is the use of will. All separate states under a unified country. 18, 30C, 35:XX:XX Themes: light, heart

Sh,679- Sun rose over house, felt there should be two suns. Desire for symmetry in the sky. 20, 30C, 00:00:20 Themes: double, perfection

Sh,683- I am parallel to myself, with myself; dual, but not divided. 20, 30C, 00:00:50 Themes: double

Sh,690- Seeing faces—I do sometimes anyway. These were human faces, broadened in the middle and the eyes went round the sides. They changed from human to birds to fish . Image of human face becoming alien looking as eyes became less central and changed to bird to fish then, as bird. 20, 30C, 00:01:14 Themes: transmutation

Sh,691- Do fish, as well as birds, pair for life? I don't think so— a free for all. 20, 30C, 00:01:14 Themes: liberty, money

Sh,7- My left arm feels like a broken wing. 01, 30C, 21:XX:XX Themes: animal, identity, hurt

Sh,719- Not sure whether asleep or not — inner vision. I'm high up and there is water below me and I have an image of a few of my breast feathers floating on the water. Between the breast feathers, the reflection of a very pink dawn. Noticed all birds in pairs. 20, 30C, 00:23:30 Themes: animal, identity

Sh,720- Thoughts of flying — Icarus! 20, 30C, 00:23:30 Themes: fly

Sh,721- Inner vision; I was sunning my

wings in the dawn sun. I'm not flapping-soaring — not dusk, at dawn — not for dark, of Light. 20, 30C, 00:23:50 Themes: fly, animal, identity

Sh,722- Looking out the window, on waking, and a huge bird outside the window. Birds look bigger than they really are. 20, 30C, 00:23:50 Themes: grow

Sh,726- Then I heard a milkman clinking bottles. I felt the sound in my upper arm bones. My upper arm bones felt hollow, and the sound resonated in them. Bone felt and sounded hollow. 20, 30C, 01:00:34 Themes: empty

Sh,727- Overwhelming images of very wrinkled skin on bony naked legs and buttocks of premature babies covered in meconium. Wiping meconium off, and then it changed to naked featherless young birds — necks and upper bits of the birds. They were sitting in meconium. 20, 30C, 01:00:40 Themes: young, transmutation

Sh,728- Felt a tremendous power. Me in bed with my arms stretched out in the shape of a cross. The horizontal line across was powerful. 20, 30C, 01:00:58 Themes: energy

Sh,729- Delusions — sees eagles. They were rooks and crows really. They looked bigger. 20, 30C, 01:00:58 Themes: animal, great

Sh,733- Upper body feels strong, chest and shoulders. Lower back feels weak and tired. 20, 30C, 01:02:00 Themes: divided

Sh,741- A five year old boy, friend of daughter, said I looked strange, different. He said I was staring at him. I said, "It's all right. I have the eye of an eagle." 20, 30C, 01:12:00 Themes: identity, animal

Sh,783- On waking, my arms felt like wings. I was spread-eagled across the bed, front and back. Normally I would sleep on my side, but I can't get the right position on my arms. 20, 30C, 03:23:00 Themes: transmutation, identity

Sh,791- Desire to find a mate. I'm feeling sexual and just want a mate. 03:23:00 Themes: sexual

Sh,792- Parallel universes—all happening somewhere else. Everything in home, food, etc.: carry in. I felt maybe I was in a parallel universe and it's all happening the same somewhere else. Not lonely. Just what happens. 20, 30C, 03:23:00 Themes: supernatural

Sh,794- A very pleasurable sensation, walking around with the top half of body naked, and feeling the skin under my arms. Great pleasure with naked of softness of underarm against side of body. 20, 30C, 04:01:36 Themes: pleasure, touch

Sh,796- Head felt disproportionately small compared with side of shoulders and arms when washing hair. When I touched my head this morning, when washing my hair, it felt very small in relation to my arms and shoulders. It was a shock. 20, 30C, 04:02:30 Themes: small

Sh,8- Delusions legs feel shorter by a foot while laying in bed. 09, 6C, 00:05:00 Themes: small

Sh,802- A guy told me I was hugging him like a nun. I didn't want my genitals to touch his. 20, 30C, 04:XX:XX Themes: sexual, touch

Sh,803- I feel like a sexual nun. 20, 30C, 04:XX:XX Themes: sexual, religious

Sh,812- My bones feel lighter than the outside of me. I don't like this fat anymore. 20, 30C, 04:XX:XX Themes: light, heavy

Sh,817- I feel regal and generous. 20, 30C, 05:01:XX Themes: greatness, helpful

Sh,819- Why am I mostly on my own? I'm not lonely with so much beauty but desire a mate - a parallel. Together, but still space in between. 05:01:XX Themes: sexual

Sh,84- Sensitive to energy. A lot of synchronicity going on. At a seminar, the teacher talked about the same topic I wrote a paper on. I met people from the same town I grew up in. When I wanted to get on to another subject, someone else would bring it up. I'd just answer the teacher's questions and it would be right. 08, 30C, 12:XX:XX Themes: energy, integration

Sh,847- The next image (in my head) was of a huge sphere = the sun. Two enormous birds of prey were holding a bright sphere of sun aloft by great talons on either side — beautiful. Then the sphere became a hoop of flames, and they were still holding on. It was very windy outside, and the sky was baby pink. 20, 30C, 06:20:00 Themes: bright

Sh,852- Feel twice as wide as high (line drawing of long outspread arms, tiny head, shorter spine, no legs, just feet). 20, 30C, 07:XX:XX Themes: transmutation

Sh,86- Even now, two years later I have an occasional return of the eagle state. Clarity to my vision. Usually my eyes have a soft focus, but since the proving, every so often they clear up and the focus is sharp. Normally I walk around in a fog, thinking, in my head. In the proving state, there is an outward focus. I'm aware of people, and how they're moving, and what they're doing. Conscious of them and how they might effect me and I might effect them. Normally, I don't care. I like to be in this altered state. The ability to be in that state intensified since taking eagle. An animal awareness, very conscious of other people as animals. 09, 6C, XX:XX:XX Themes: conscientious

Sh,862- Clear and bright, an eagle soared, an amazing bird high up in the sky, when I was lying naked on my back. It wasn't flapping, it just soared. coming from the east towards me then flew into the sun. As I lay there, unbelieving, he soared out again, circled again and then disappeared into the radiance of the sun. I felt like the proving was finished. It felt like a good-bye. My vision had changed. I feel more like me. 20, 30C, 08:08:XX Themes: bright, animal, fly

Sh,867- Memories of being fed as a child and having no choice of what to eat. 20, 30C, 08:23:50 Themes: eating, young

Sh,869- Realized that the wind is more nourishing than food. 20, 30C, 09:XX:XX Themes: eating

Sh,877- Inner vision—more images of courting copulating birds soaring together, playing with talons locked, plummeting, sounds of beaks, whooshing wind, magnificently exhilarating. 20, 30C, 09:XX:XX Themes: sexual

Sh,883- Lying in bed this morning, inner vision of lifting up old clothes from a pile, ready to be given away, one by one. Underneath them, all an image of the inside of an egg without a shell and I could see fine, red veins on the membrane and one eye on an unhatched fledgling. The feathers were wet, and the membrane around it was complete. 20, 30C, 10:00:30 Themes: young

Sh,887- I called Daughter a parasite last night, because of money. 20, 30C, 10:XX:XX Themes: money, avarice

Sh,889- I'm ripping all my clothes. I'm so much fatter that I'm not aware of my width, and I'm catching on things. 20, 30C, 10:XX:XX Themes: grow, heavy

Sh,900- It was or is ? As if I'm not really used to domestic duties. I can't really do anything for any other, just hopefully glimpses of illumination. All on own—with everything. Just to give—Does it really help? Doesn't it make others expect, or more needy? They lose freedom—independence. 20, 30C, 10:XX:XX Themes: unfit, liberty, avarice

Sh,901- Sensation of such harmonious balance when on the wing, Such power in these almost weightless wings. Sensation of deep warmth echoing the sun. 20, 30C, 10:XX:XX Themes: perfection, pleasure, fly, transmutation

Sh,913- 6:30 a.m. Sitting up in bed to meditate. The dawn came and I felt majestic. 20, 30C, 12:00:30 Themes: greatness

Sh,917- Air very hot today. All day, desire to create a storm, but one is not forecast for two days. That night we had a storm. I wanted thunder and lightning. 20, 30C, 12:XX:XX Themes: storm

Sh,923- Any sudden noise was like painful shocks through my body, like my body being blasted. 20, 30C, 13:XX:XX Themes: noise

Sh,927- I've felt lonely over the last three to four days. This morning I realized how great the girls were and burst into tears — emotional, but separate. 20, 30C, 14:XX:XX Themes: isolation, solitude

Sh,928- I'm only half aware. When I was doing things wrong, I was half aware I was doing them. 20, 30C, 14:XX:XX Themes: half, wrong

Sh,933- I don't recognize myself as human. I don't know who I am. 20, 30C, 15:XX:XX Themes: identity

Sh,934- As I woke, I decided I should be a nun. Strange. I feel like I've got my wings clipped when I think about men. 20, 30C, 15:XX:XX Themes: religious, sexual, obstructed

Sh,936- I had a down morning, but had a good day out with a friend and her two sons ,and many birds caged and uncaged at the Botanical Gardens. A very high and low day before they arrived. Tried not to see them, but was pleased when they came. Before they came, was feeling I must be a very bad person— different. 20, 30C, 15:XX:XX Themes: wicked

Sh,937- I don't know what or who to be. I'm not human. I feel that I'm trapped in a body that's not mine. I related to the birds at the Botanical Gardens more than the people, but felt sad because they are caged. 20, 30C, 15:XX:XX Themes: identity, compassionate

Sh,938- I feel so heavy and earthbound, stuck with human desires that are not my own. Why don't I fit? Where is the truth and justice they talk about? Why do humans lie and deceive? I feel a big thing about truth and justice. "Why don't these people just tell me the truth?" It feels like a game, not telling me what they really want and need. 20, 30C, 15:XX:XX Themes: heavy, justice, unfit,

Sh,942-Don't feel part of the human race. Overwhelming gratitude that I could walk and not be in a wheelchair. 20, 30C, 15:XX:XX Themes: identity

Sh,943- Excited by the sounds of beaks clicking together, even empty pistachio nut cases clicking together in the palm of my hand excited me. 20, 30C, 15:XX:XX Themes: noise

Sh,944- Big doubts about doing Homeopathy. If you can make people healthy, then the balance must be that someone else gets sicker. 20, 30C, 15:XX:XX Themes: antagonism, health

Sh,946- Inner vision: I was a male Indian. I thought, "I'm not a brave. I don't deserve this feather". 20, 30C, 15:XX:XX Themes: conscience, contemptuous, justice

Sh,948- I can't identify other bird calls here, as if I'm in the wrong country. All unfamiliar. 20, 30C, 16:XX:XX Themes: abroad

Sh,950- This morning a friend brought me three condor feathers. I was standing wrapped in a towel, wet from the bath and the friend said I looked like a wet fledgling. 20, 30C, 17:XX:XX Themes: identity

Sh,951- Phoned a friend to hear what I already knew. As I heard the words, I felt a sensation as if hit by a thunderbolt through the vertex, down to hit my heart then spread up and across my shoulders out to my hands. (Drawing shows hands like wing tips). 20, 30C, 17:XX:XX Themes: storm, heart

Sh,952- Today felt ordinary. It felt like my head cleared. Like it's open again. It felt like it was blasted open from the sky coming downwards, like a thunderbolt — hot, sharp, and sudden — through the vertex while I was talking to someone. I just understood what's been happening the last couple of weeks, even the breast dreams. There was just clarity and I could see how I'd been in the wrong shape all these years. 20, 30C, 17:XX:XX Themes: storm, knowledge

Sh,953- Memories triggered off by the sensation in my head back and feet. Twenty three years ago in the States, I fell off a wall and smashed lots of vertebrae together. I was told I would never walk again. At the time, I got an internal explosion in my head opposite to what happened yesterday with the lightning in my vertex. 20, 30C, 18:XX:XX Themes: healing, storm

Sh,954- My feet hurt — sharp — down the inside, all along the big toe joint when I started walking again 23 years ago. I had the same pain again last night. 20, 30C, 18:XX:XX Themes: hurt

Sh,958- This morning, my bones in my arms felt different — lighter and less dense. 20, 30C, 18:XX:XX Themes: transmutation

Sh,958- This morning, my bones in my arms felt different — lighter and less dense. 20, 30C, 18:XX:XX Themes: transmutation

Sh,96- Feeling spacey and disoriented, stoned, far away from reality; am I making this up? I'm aware of my body, my breasts going up and down with my breath. I'm relaxed and sleepy. Time is very slowed down. I'm in the moment. Am I hot or cold? I don't know, I think it's kind of warm heat I'm feeling. Who is writing this anyway? 06, 6C, 00:00:05 Themes: isolation, time

Sh,966- I'm so slow and heavy on earth and so light and swift in the air. 20, 30C, 19:XX:XX Themes: heavy, light

Sh,97- I get energy rushes like from a good meditation or a martial arts workout. I felt in the moment. Every moment is an eternity. Being very still, in the moment, every thing was really slow. Time had slowed down. 06, 6C, 00:01:00 Themes: time

Sh,973- I was told I was an opportunist shopper. I went in at the end of the day and got all the food they were throwing out. 20, 30C, 20:XX:XX Themes: avarice

Sh,975- As I woke up, the sun had just come up and I felt I had purpose and direction. I really need the sun. 20, 30C, 20:XX:XX Themes: direction, bright

Sh,977- Tears come easily, just on looking at an exhibition of wildlife — sobbing. It was beautiful and lit from the back. It was so beautiful I couldn't contain it. There were pictures of a bald eagle and of a hedgehog right next to each other. 20, 30C, 20:XX:XX Themes: nature, animal

Sh,992- I know things so clearly before they happen. 20, 30C, 31:XX:XX Themes: clairvoyance

Sh,993- I was traveling around inside my head last night — Israel, the States, New Zealand and Scotland. All places I've never been, but all the same sort of terrain, like barren, down South, New Zealand. I was looking for a new home. 20, 30C, 31:XX:XX Themes: house, travel

HAM.

Al,1- Feeling that she ought (have) to be reverenced (honored, venerated) by all around her and have great respect (regard) paid to her opinions; lasting about an hour. Themes: flattery, greatness, haughty

Al,14- I became impatient, and resolved not to take anymore of the medicine; felt as if I did not care whether I attended (guard) to my practice or not; did not want any one to call at the office for medicine. Themes: impatience, negligence, duty

Al,15- Was afraid to risk (danger) another dose (medicine); his mind was in a fearful condition. Themes: fearful, danger, poisoned

Al,18- Quick perception of anything out of shape or disproportioned. Themes: organization, perfection

Al,9- Regretful (sorry) in mind for having had emissions at night. Themes: sexual, conscience

He,5- Felt as if he was going out of his mind. Themes: insanity

HELL.

Al,10- He becomes melancholy on beholding (observe) a cheerful person, and then, for the first time, feels very unhappy. Themes: sadness, unfortunate, envy, pleasure

Al,12- Such anxiety , nausea , and distress that he thinks he will die. Themes: death

Al,15- Dread of death (in a sufferer from religious melancholy). Themes: death, religious, sadness,

Al,16- He is doubtful (uncertain) about his own life. Themes: confidence, disease, death

Al,17- Extremely inclined to be irritable, the most trifling things which goes contrary to his wishes excites anger. Themes: contradiction, bothered, anger

Al,19- Dread of death.(in a sufferer from religious melancholy) Themes: fearful, death, religious

Al,5- Homesickness. Themes: homesickness

Al,7- Sad mood, on account of his present condition (restriction, limitation) ,everything seems shallow (stupid, superficial) and has no incentive for him. (lost :motive ,purpose, force, mission,) -(lost: depth, profundity, perception.) Themes: sadness, indifference, tedium

Al,S-1 Happy carelessness about everything; feel indifferent to family. Themes: indifference, family, negligence

Ha,277- He could neither sit, stand nor lie, and always pointed to his heart. Themes: heart

Ha,276- Such anxiety, nausea and suffering, that he thinks he is going to die. Themes: death

Ha,278- Restless and anxious, as if anticipating misfortune. Themes: restless, misfortune, anticipation

Ha,281- He despairs of his life. Themes: despair

Ha,284- On seeing a happy person he becomes melancholy and then only he feels very unhappy. Themes: envy, unfortunate, sadness

Ha,286- Sad disposition respecting his present position, everything seems to him so insipid (tedious, boring,) and nothing interests him. Themes: sadness, position, indifference, tedium

Ha,287- Wrapped (envelop) up in his own

thoughts, silent humour, all the afternoon. Themes: meditation, reserved

He,11- Psychical conditions occupying a place between melancholia and mania, and in conditions where true depression and weakness is present, in which the patient is governed by a fixed idea. Themes: obstinate, sadness, insanity, mania, energy

He,12- An old woman having been accused of theft by the women around, took it so much to heart that she hanged herself. This suicide produced a profound effect upon the women of the village. One after another accused herself of having caused the death of the old woman by their insinuations; they wept and howled, ran about day and night wringing their hands and despairing of salvation on account of their sin (error); they became quite irrepressible and deranged (disordered) In this way twenty - four or twenty five women were affected, every fresh case being followed by another. Hysterical mania. Themes: salvation, doomed, conscience, suicidal, censorious, religious, insanity, despair

He,19- Tries to escape, to throw herself into the river. Themes: water, suicidal, escape

He,20- After typhoid, ...sits quietly in bed and seems lost in brooding;...constantly seeks (try) to escape, ...;without a word quietly climbs out of the window, and if she succeeds in escaping goes in direction of river; finally threw herself into privy (toilet), from which she was rescued. Themes: meditation, dwells, escape, suicidal, water

He,24- Dread of dying ; feels unhappy in presence of cheerful faces. (spite) Themes: death, unfortunate, envy,

He,9- Mania demoniac; sees evil (harmful) spirits at night. Themes: ghosts, devil, mania

HELON.

Al,2- Reaction (from feeling of general wellness) began, and for a fortnight I was in a mental hell; it was the most profound mental depression I have ever known; I was plunged into the most abject despair. Themes: sadness, miserable, despair, hell

Al,4- .... could not endure the least contradiction or receive any suggestions in regard to any subject (fixed ideas) ;... what I most desired was to be left alone, reserved to myself the privilege of finding fault (imperfection) with everything around me;.... Themes: contradiction, solitude, reserved, censorious, wrong, misanthropy

He,5- Irritable; cannot endure the least contradiction or receive suggestions in relation to any subject. Themes: contradiction, obstinate

HEP.

Al,1- Ghostly image of one who was dead, in the morning, in bed, after waking and while conscious, which frightened him; it also seemed as though he saw his neighbor's house burning, which also frightened him. Themes: ghosts, fire, death, home, others, fearful

Al,10- Fearful concerning sickness in the family, especially when walking alone in the open air. Themes: fearful, family, others, disease, solitude

Al,15- Extremely discontented and fretful about his pains, and discouraged (unhappy). Themes: disease, despair

Al,16- Irritable mood; everything that she undertook was wrong; she desired to be alone. Themes: conscience, solitude, wrong, failure

Al,19- Contrary mood, he does not wish to see the members of his own family. Themes: antagonism, company, family, contrary

Al,4- Everything of which she only thought was disagreeable and not right. Themes: conscience, wrong

Al,5- She remembers everything that has been unpleasant during her life. Themes: mortification

Ha,11- Dissatisfied with oneself. Themes: discontented, himself

Ha,12- She thinks about everything disagreeable that happened to her in her lifetime. Themes: mortification, past

Ha,13- Whatever she thought about was unsatisfactory (disappointed) and did not suit (satisfy) her. Themes: discontented

Ha,289- The slightest thing put him into a violent passion, he could have murdered any one without hesitation. Themes: passionate, homicidal, violence, wicked

Ha,296- In the evening a frightful anxiety for two hours; he thought he must be ruined (lost, failed), and was sad to that degree that he could have killed himself. Themes: ruined, sadness, suicidal

Ha,298- In the morning in bed after waking, when conscious, he had the visionary appearance of a deceased (dead, defunct) person, which frightened him, and he also imagined he saw a neighboring house in flames, which terrified him. Themes: fearful, ghosts, fire, home

Ha,4- Fearful anguish, in the evening, for two hours; he thought he had to perish (die), and was sad even so that he could have committed suicide. (redemption, salvation) Themes: death, conscience, suicidal, doomed, sadness

Ha,5- Fear about the illness of his family, especially while walking in the open air. Themes: cares, disease, family, others

Ha,7- Contrary mood; he does not like to look at his folks. (relatives) Themes: bothered, family, loathing, contrary

Ha,9- Irritable mood; whatever she started to do, was not satisfactory, she wished to be alone. Themes: discontented, solitude

He,10- Repulsive (offensive) mood, with desire to be left alone. Themes: loathing, solitude, misanthropy

He,14- Low spirited, even to thoughts of suicide. Themes: sadness, suicidal

He,17- Impelled by unaccountable attacks of internal anguish, which sometimes come on quite suddenly, to attempt suicide. Themes: suicidal

He,20- Violent, passionate fretfulness; she spoke with such volubility that one could not always get a chance to reason with her, and she would not listen to the most just remarks. Themes: passionate, talk, violence, obstinate

He,22- Temper obstinate and cross, a ferocious spleen (irascible) which would lead to cold blooded murder even among those habitually gay and benevolent. Themes: anger, obstinate, homicidal, violence, wicked, blood

He,23- Wrathful irritability, even to the most extreme violence, threatening to end in murder and arson.(firing pyromania) Themes: anger, fire, violence, menacing, homicidal

He,5- Frightful visions of fire and of dead persons. Themes: fearful, fire, ghosts

He,8-...threatened to murder wife and children, attempted to set house on fire, and was with difficulty controlled; ... (pyromaniac) 0Scabies. Themes: menacing, homicidal, fire, wife, child, home,

He,9- Malicious (vindictive, malevolent) mood; feels as if he could murder someone with pleasure. Themes: wicked, homicidal, sadism, pleasure

HIPP.

Al,1- Lascivious fancies in the forenoon. Themes: sexual, lascivious

Al,15- He feels as though he would fight with any one. Themes: fight

Al,2- Homesickness in the evening. Themes: homesickness

Al,3- Apprehensiveness, anxiety about the future, in the evening. Themes: future

Al,6- Fretful, discontented with himself almost lachrymose, in the morning. Themes: anger, himself, conscience

Al,8- Ill-humored, weary of life, even to suicide, in both provings. Themes: loathing, suicidal

He,1- Melancholy; a young man sits in the corner and does not want to have anything to do with the world. (alienated) Themes: solitude, separated, misanthropy

HURA.

Al,1- Much excited and oppressed as if by some great misfortune. Themes: suppressed, misfortune, oppression

Al,10- Sadness, melancholy; she thinks despondingly of the future. Themes: future, despair, sadness

Al,12- Flow of sad thoughts; she fancies she is about to lose a dear friend. Themes: death, sadness, friend,

Al,15- Hypochondria, sadness, despair; he fancies he is repudiated and deserted by his relations. (rejected, refused) Themes: despised, forsaken, sadness, relatives

Al,16 - She fancies she is left alone (lonely, solitary, forsaken) in the world and is lost. Themes: solitude, forsaken

Al,17- Feeling much affected, and she sighs a good deal. (very much) Themes:

Al,19- Inclination to weep, chest constrict, as

from emotion...the least thing disturbs her and makes her sad;... Themes: constriction, unfortunate

Al,20- Unusual inclination to weep, even when singing, followed by a suffocative feeling... Themes: suffocation, music

Al,23- Anxiety about his salvation, during the nervous attack. Themes: salvation, religious, conscience

Al,25- Irritated by the least opposition. Themes: contradiction

Al,26- Since taking the drug, the least thing irritates her, and then she feels oppressed, with desire to weep;... Themes: constriction

Al,28- Impatience, anger; she bites her hands, and gets into passion because her ideas come too slowly. Themes: impatience, hurt, anger, bite, obstructed, knowledge

Al,3- Every paroxysm of pain excites a nervous laugh, with moanings like those of a sick child. Themes: pure, disease, child

Al,4- She weeps every little while, and especially for two days past, fancies she sees the dead person before her eyes. (ghost) Themes: ghosts, death

Al,7- During and after the fainting spell (trance) , disposed to love everybody, especially those about him; he often thinks of death, but does not fear it; he feels as though he could die without regret.(fearless) Themes: seized, death, fearless, love, conscience

Al,700- Dream about children and the release (liberty) of prisoners. Themes: imprisoned, liberty, child, criminal

Al,709- Restless night; dream about crimes, dead bodies (corpse), and children lying with their heads half cut off, while others were being decapitated. Themes: criminal, corpse, mutilated, executed, child

Al,8- He reproaches himself for all his bad actions, even the merest trifles. Themes: conscience, conscientious, wicked

HYDR-AC.

He,3- Could not remain in middle of road when he saw a vehicle approaching him even at a considerable distance,... (run over) Themes: approached, run over, accidents

HYDR.

Al,16- Spiteful (cruel), angry disposition, with desire to snub (scorn) any one who differed in anything with me; lasting all day. Themes: wicked, contemptuous, anger

Al,26-...forget, for a few seconds, what was wanted, which makes me very angry and feel like damning (swearing) and cursing (blaspheme) everything and anybody who bothered me the least. Themes: anger, offensive, bother, obstructed

Al,4- In high spirits; everything looked bright; felt happy, and wanted to sing. Themes: pleasure, music, bright

He,5- Depression of spirits, sure of death and desires it. Themes: sadness, death

HYDROG.

Sh,1- It dawned on me that it was as if there was a shift in the universe. 12, 6C, 07:XX:XX Themes: identity

Sh,10- I feel a bit unreal — like taking drugs — a weird spaced-outness. The top of my head feels very clear — seeing and hearing clear and remote, but from the sinus down, I feel muzzy and warm. 08, 30C, 00:01:XX Themes: unreal, strange, clairvoyance

Sh,100- I was having problems assimilating the notion of time, outside time seemed beyond description. I Couldn't differentiate between backwards and forwards in time. Felt I had got stuck in time. 16, 30C, 10:XX:XX Themes: time, integration

Sh,103- Feel like a crippled old man. 38, 200C, 18:XX:XX Themes: disease, old, paralysis

Sh,104- Don't want to move at all — want to be still and warm and lie around in a heap all day. like what it must feel to be old. I do feel old. 16, 30C, 02:XX:XX Themes: time, old

Sh,105- I felt better when driving the car fast with company and loud music. 24, 30C, 03:XX:XX Themes: music, hurry

Sh,107- Charged around like a bull in a china shop. 22, 12C, 04:XX:XX Themes: anger

Sh,108- Doing everything faster — driving

faster than usual. 24, 30C, 100:XX:XX Themes: hurry

Sh,11- I felt I had gone mad, possessed, hysterical laughter, singing and a feeling of non-reality, as if in a dream, out of the body — like my mind went out of the window. High one minute and then low. People asked if I was on speed. After seven hours, in the evening (7:30p.m.), the feeling changed to an angry mood and very irritable with a dry furry mouth,...l. 24, 30C, 00:00:45 Themes: insanity, seized, music, unreal, double, disintegration

Sh,114- I feel quite resentful about having to hurry. 08, 30C, 09:XX:XX Themes: hurry, resentment, conscience

Sh,12- Driving home I felt odd, as if I was hardly in my body. Feel like my body's working on automatic but I'm not really there. Driving along I kept forgetting where I was. Now I feel I'm really more "absent" than normal and feel quite afraid of losing my mind or having an accident. I feel my connection with the physical world is very loose, as though my soul was separated from my body. I have thoughts that this is a bit like dying — not unpleasant. 10, 200C, 13:02:XX Themes: lost, unreal, double, insanity, accidents, separated, disintegration

Sh,13- Falling in love on a very deep level. 16, 30C, XX:XX:XX Themes: love, passionate

Sh,130- Anxiety about money and fear of poverty. 24, 30C, 100:XX:XX Themes: money, poverty

Sh,131- Marked tendency to panic at little things that go wrong or small decisions to be made. 08, 30C, 00:XX:XX Themes: wrong, irresolution, confidence

Sh,14- I felt so much love I didn't know how to focus it. Its like being in another state of consciousness. No one can come near and its frightening me. 16, 30C, 25:XX:XX Themes: love, passionate

Sh,144- Feeling I want to isolate myself — want to be alone. 12, 6C, 27:XX:XX Themes: isolation, solitude

Sh,145- Feel that I could get on with everything alright if those around me would either leave me alone or help constructively. 04, 12C, 19:XX:XX Themes: solitude, bothered, obstructed

Sh,147- Aversion to being touched. 24, 30C, 01:XX:XX Themes: loathing, touch

Sh,15- I felt in the presence of a totally pure energy, like meeting God and feeling totally unworthy or like meeting a lover and feeling unworthy — realizing all the mistakes of a lifetime. This pure energy was around for some time protecting me. I feel this unification cleared out lifetimes of symptomatology for me. The joining with this energy was as if a male energy joined with me sexually, but with no desire, pleasure or pain involved. This unification with the male energy lasted quite a few days — I'm not used to seeing myself as a man. The morning after this unifying with the higher presence, I collapsed in emotional overflow. All my grief and pain came out. I was doubled upon the floor and went into a deep state of catharsis. It is not possible to describe where I went as there are no concepts applicable. I felt overflowing love for humanity and wanted to give everything away. My mind turned to the Buddha. It was like seeing the complete picture instead of

fragmented bits. (These primary effects lasted about 28 days, then changing to a paranoia state). 16, 30C, 07.XX.XX Themes: energy, god, unfit, miserable, wrong, conscience, sexual, compassionate, religious, union, integration, grief, love,

Sh,150- Feeling weepy and vulnerable — want someone to "manage" things for me. Feel so fed up of having to do it all myself. 18, 200C, 26:XX:XX Themes: fragile, helplessness, solitude, vexation

Sh,152- Feel helpless, as if I may need to be looked after because I don't feel I can do anything. 16, 30C, 00:00:30 Themes: helplessness, unfit

Sh,153- Insecurity and self doubt. 16, 30C, XX:XX:XX Themes: confidence, doubtful

Sh,155- In the afternoon (during the full moon) I felt low and depressed, insecure and vulnerable. Could not cope with work load and didn't want to be alone. 12, 6C, 39:XX:XX Themes: sadness, confidence, fragile, work, unfit, solitude

Sh,156- Felt extremely ill at ease and embarrassed when spoken to by male hairdresser. 12, 6C, 23:XX:XX Themes: sexual

Sh,158- Thoughts of death and suicide. 16, 30C, 25:XX:XX Themes: death, suicidal

Sh,159- Thoughts of dead bodies made me feel slightly sick. 10, 200C, 00:XX:XX Themes: corpse, death

Sh,16- I felt I could see more deeply into people — beyond the roles they were playing. 16, 30C, XX:XX:XX Themes: union, clairvoyance

Sh,160- Wrote a letter to my son, 'to be opened after my death', not morbid, nor do I feel a premonition of death. Its something I've always meant to do — a sort of resolving. Wept with emotion as I wrote it. 12, 6C, 25:XX:XX Themes: death, organization

Sh,161- I am aware of some ridiculous thoughts coming into my mind, odd unconnected sentences such as about killing a 13 year old girl. 12, 6C, 22:XX:XX Themes: homicidal, sexual

Sh,162- The remedy "made me think of formaldehyde and dead things". 10, 200C, 00:XX:XX Themes: death, corpse

Sh,163- Thoughts of death — thoughts went back to doing dissection as a medical student.10, 200C, 00:XX:XX Themes: death, corpse

Sh,164- Delusion — saw black masses. 24, 30C, 100:XX:XX Themes: crowd, dark

Sh,165- I thought I could see energy moving around in the air. Colours looked bright and everything looked beautiful. 16, 30C, 25:XX:XX Themes: energy, bright, perfection

Sh,166- Sensation of being larger. 10, 200C, 11:XX:XX Themes: grow, great

Sh,167- Thought or vision that I was taller or stronger than I was. 28, 200C, 02:01:XX Themes: great, energy, greatness

Sh,168- Sensation of being smaller than normal, while making porridge. 10, 200C, 13:20:XX Themes: small

Sh,169- Thought there was a large insect, a locust, on the back of my head and put up my hand to check. 16, 30C, 01:XX:XX Themes: great, animal

Sh,17- Feeling of great release — catharsis — my whole time scale has changed since taking the remedy. Even my work on Homeopathy has opened up — boundaries have disappeared. Lost a lot of boundaries on time. All sorts of things have clicked into place since yesterday. Feel wonderful. Now I don't actually feel slowed down. Didn't hurry, just did things in my own time. Normally would have pulled out all the stops and rushed around. It doesn't matter if I'm late. 08, 30C, 06:XX:XX Themes: hurry

Sh,170- Sensation as if something is crawling on my head. Checked for lice, but can't find any. 32, 9C, 09:XX:XX Themes: animal, crawling

Sh,171- Feel more patient and accepting during my period. When water poured through the ceiling from an over-full bath, I just sat there and let it flood the floor because I didn't want to disturb the cat sitting on my knee. 12, 6C, 27:XX:XX Themes: yielding, impatience, conscientious

Sh,172- Felt distant and detached. 32, 9C, 04:XX:XX Themes: isolation

Sh,174- Emotionally cold and non-communicable with anger felt in stomach. 12, 6C, 17:XX:XX Themes: anger, reserved, indifference, isolation

Sh,175- At the family celebration, I could not feel that I belonged. 12, 6C, 34:XX:XX Themes: isolation, family

Sh,176- Feel distant and separated from things and they feel unreal. 16, 30C, 01:XX:XX Themes: isolation, unreal

Sh,177- Upset husband by telling him what I thought of the way he'd been behaving. I felt curiously uninvolved. Indifference to husband. Felt a little 'dead', uninvolved, wasn't really responding in any way — not in a good way or a bad way. Didn't feel cross, affectionate or anything. Very peculiar, like I was watching and its nothing to do with me. Like looking at somebody else, almost as if I wasn't there. Felt emotionally numb and unable to respond — as if I wasn't there. Like a living dead being alive and not being able to make the appropriate responses. Real total detachment. 08, 30C, 10:XX:XX Themes: isolation, indifference, husband

Sh,18- Sometimes I think there isn't much of me left anymore — as if I left myself behind ages ago. 16, 30C, XX:XX:XX Themes: lost, past

Sh,180- Indifference, despair and hopelessness— no way out. 32, 9C, 03:XX:XX

Themes: indifference, despair, hopeless

Sh,182- A feeling of boredom and depression at 10:00p.m., whilst in company — very distressful. I didn't talk at all, friends thought something had greatly upset me. 24, 30C, 01:10:XX Themes: tedium, sadness, company, bothered

Sh,184- Feel despondent, indifferent, apathetic, separated from things and don't care. Deep sighing with sense of resignation. Can't be bothered to do things. 16, 30C, 02:XX:XX Themes: indifference, isolation, yielding

Sh,188- On getting up in the morning, I feel very angry and bad about myself. I feel I can't cope. What's the use of trying? I feel like giving up. I think for a moment I'd like to die. 10, 200C, 09:XX:XX Themes: anger, himself, failure, death

Sh,189- As if in a dream, not there, difficult to stay with it all while driving home — very conscious of the blackbirds flying across the motorway. Better taking a nap and fresh air from opening the window. Concomitant to finger abscess. 02, 6C, 54:XX:XX Themes: unreal, isolation, animal, fly, solitude

Sh,19- The general impression is that the prover entered a larger totality dimension in terms of space and time, whereupon all previous or smaller totalities became trivial and alien. A conflict of understanding and behaviour arose. 16, 30C, XX:XX:XX Themes: time, knowledge

Sh,192- During palpitations, extreme fear — thought I was having a heart attack. Frightened the living daylights out of me. 24, 30C, 100:XX:XX Themes: fearful, heart, disease

Sh,194- Fear I may lose my mind, or even die. Fear about the proving. Feel I could bash the car so I have to make a real effort. 10, 200C, 12:XX:XX Themes: death, insanity, accidents, damage

Sh,195- Apprehensive, panicky, with cold sweat on palms. Feel extremely vulnerable emotionally — like an egg that has just broken. Frightened, anything can happen. 16, 30C, 05:XX:XX Themes: fearful, fragile, misfortune

Sh,198- Growing irritability. Anger below the surface if something is on the floor in my way or if something goes wrong. 12, 6C, 05:00:30 Themes: misfortune, anger, obstructed

Sh,2- I can honestly say I'll never be the same again — a bit like having a baby. Amazing how my whole perception seems to have altered one degree, which makes everything different. 08, 30C, 100:XX:XX Themes: identity

Sh,20- Distortion of reality — that other places seemed a million times more real than the real world. Everything seemed a long way away. 16, 30C, 04:XX:XX Themes: distances, unreal, isolation

Sh,202- The instant I woke I felt angry, felt like throwing the clock at the wall. Didn't feel like talking to anyone and felt a desire to kick the furniture — seemed the only way to let my anger out. 10, 200C, 16:XX:XX Themes: anger, violence

Sh,207- Stormy and acrimonious (hash) row (fight) with girlfriend. Quarrelling continued throughout the day. Cried a lot — generally feeling rough with loss of appetite — heart pounding and sunk feeling in abdomen though I can't eat. 04, 12C, 01:00:30 Themes: offensive, fight

Sh,21- I feel I have moved into a different state of consciousness and there aren't any guiding posts or means of navigation — a bit like being lost in space. 16, 30C, 06:XX:XX Themes: lost, unreal

Sh,210- I was shouting down the phone, but dead quiet with friends. I thought "Why are they talking? They haven't anything to say". I was very sarcastic. 24, 30C, 01:XX:XX Themes: offensive, contemptuous, sarcasm, reserved

Sh,219- Things seem ridiculous and amusing, ordinary things like birds. Laughing at them. Everything seemed so absurd or futile. 16, 30C, 02:XX:XX Themes: ridiculous, animal, unreal, contemptuous

Sh,220- Laughter wicked and voice seemed low. 24, 30C, 02:XX:XX Themes: wicked, pleasure

Sh,222- Feel that the things we do are on different levels. Some of them are on higher and more meaningful levels — the real me — and others are just a trivial game. Laughing at the absurdity of notions — everything seems ridiculous. 16, 30C, 09:XX:XX Themes: ridiculous, feigning

Sh,223- Tried to talk to someone who is afraid of dying and I wanted to laugh. Thought I shouldn't talk to anybody in case I laugh. 16, 30C, 04:XX:XX Themes: sarcasm

Sh,23- Feel as if I've been somewhere else and coming back into my body is a shock. 16, 30C, 10:XX:XX Themes: divided, disintegration

Sh,231- Silent, morose and introverted, with headache. 12, 6C, 05:06:45 Themes: reserved

Sh,233- Feel a blanket of depression over me. 08, 30C, 09:XX:XX Themes: sadness

Sh,234- Developed a self pitying, very tearful depression through the morning. I was unable to communicate any of these feelings and this led to a fierce row with girlfriend. 04, 12C, 30:XX:XX Themes: miserable, sadness, fight, reserved

Sh,235- Feel a bit depressed and frustrated by present circumstances. Feel like the unappreciated victim. 04, 12C, 14:XX:XX Themes: sadness, miserable, despised

Sh,236- Dwells on past disagreeable occurrences. 16, 30C, XX:XX:XX Themes: past, dwells

Sh,240- I feel life is a serious thing. When putting children to bed, I felt serious and uncompromising. I wanted them to do exactly as I said and, if not, threatened to hit them. 32, 9C, 03:XX:XX Themes: obstinate, menacing, dictatorial

Sh,241- I'm afraid to go out because I think I frighten people. 16, 30C, XX:XX:XX Themes: go out, offensive, ugly

Sh,242- Felt vulnerable to criticism — felt people were getting at me. Felt people were not taking notice of poor little me — over-reacting — upset and hurt. 02, 6C, XX:XX:XX Themes: fragile, censured, helplessness, miserable

Sh,243- Fear that someone was trying to find out if I was home so that they could come and rape and murder me. 16, 30C, XX:XX:XX Themes: invaded, attacked, hurt, sexual, murdered

Sh,244- Paranoid feeling with cold perspiration. 16, 30C, XX:XX:XX Themes: persecution

Sh,245- Feel I can't trust anyone — 'paranoia'. 24, 30C, 100:XX:XX Themes: persecution, suspicious

Sh,246- I felt mistrust, suspicion and paranoia. 16, 30C, Letter Themes: suspicious, persecution

Sh,247- I feel people are playing games with me. Everything is out of balance. (prejudiced)16, 30C, XX:XX:XX Themes: suspicious, damage

Sh,248- While sitting in a restaurant, felt progressively more cut off from friends at the table. I began to feel detached and paranoid. I felt disliked by people. They seemed to look at me menacingly. I became concerned that my lecture this afternoon had created conflict, mayhem and destruction, that my friends in the audience did not like me any more. I became aware of a dull ache in my sacrum making me want to shift backwards and forwards. At the same time, the people round the table seemed further away and smaller, as if I had moved four feet back from the table. I felt very uncomfortable and wanted to get out. I put my head down and rushed out without saying goodbye, feeling a sense of relief at getting away (all very unusual for me). Outside, I felt relief and my mind cleared and I walked home alone. 22, 12C, 04:XX:XX Themes: isolation, persecution, misanthropy, suspicious, menaced, offensive, conscience, forsaken, damage

Sh,249- I think that no one likes me. I felt betrayed and everything went haywire. 16, 30C, Themes: forsaken, betrayed

Sh,25- A hovering numbness hit with a sensation that my mind was being pulled from the top of the head downwards, like internal pressure being pulled down inside of me — as after a fright. Incredible sensation. 24, 30C, 00:XX:45 Themes: floating, divided, disintegration

Sh,250- I think I'm dangerous to people and they can't cope with me. 16, 30C, XX:XX:XX Themes: conscience, wicked, danger, offensive

Sh,251- A spark of a paranoid thought — "maybe I'm being poisoned". 10, 200C, 00:00:00 Themes: suspicious, poisoned

Sh,253- I was defensive and angry. I thought my friend didn't understand me. I had to apologize. I felt vulnerable and deeply hurt by her. 16, 30C, 05:XX:XX Themes: anger, offended, damage, fragile

Sh,254- When shopping, felt people did not accept me as belonging to the community. Felt isolated in the shop. Feeling unacceptable, 'as if I was a marked person' — but later felt better on my own. 12, 6C, 19:XX:XX Themes: forsaken, despised, isolation, solitude

Sh,255- Very worried that people don't like me and can't cope with me — that they will think I am insane. I think maybe I am insane. This is frightening me. 16, 30C, 25:XX:XX Themes: forsaken, insanity, despised, fearful

Sh,256- Thought someone was telling someone else that I was mad and asking what should be done about it. 16, 30C, 25:XX:XX Themes: suspicious, censured, insanity

Sh,257- Feeling suspicious all day. Anxious and conscious of vulnerability. (Asked husband to move out if he was thinking of being unfaithful). 12, 6C, 06:XX:XX Themes: suspicious, fragile, betrayed

Sh,258- Felt cut off from people and suspicious. 22, 12C, 06:XX:XX Themes: isolation, forsaken, suspicious

Sh,259- Fear and desperation about being pregnant — period 16 days late — felt terrible all day. So despairing. 08, 30C, 50:XX:XX Themes: despair, double, divided

Sh,26- Felt inspired that the potential within is so great and we have a possibility of becoming whole and suddenly it comes crashing down into a sort of mundane realization — that the physical world would never reach the potential possible — like losing a dream. This is really bringing me down. 16, 30C, 08:XX:XX Themes: integration, union

Sh,261- Almost the impression that I am pregnant — many old sensations and emotions from previous pregnancies recurred. Like having another person inside of me. All physical symptoms of pregnancy. Went for a test. 08, 30C, 01:XX:XX Themes: dwells, past, double, divided

Sh,263- Turned to Christianity in which he had never had interest before. 24, 30C, 100:XX:XX Themes: religious

Sh,264- Talking to God about the state of my heart and asking for it to be healed. 16, 30C, XX:XX:XX Themes: God, heart, disease, healing

Sh,265- Greatly increased tendency to theorize and philosophize, especially concerning esoteric matters. 16, 30C, 05:XX:XX Themes: theorizing, philosophy

Sh,266- While talking, restless, impatient and ill at ease, as if wanting to leave. 22, 12C, 06:XX:XX Themes: restless, impatience

Sh,27- There is a very fine line at this time between enlightenment and insanity — a split consciousness. The dark side is horrendous, but the positive side of the proving has been well worth it. The positive aspects are beautiful. Its a shame we need to come down. I guess the price of going into the heavens is a trip to hell. 16, 30C, XX:XX:XX Themes: religious, insanity, disintegration, divided, hell, dark, perfection

Sh,272- Sudden thoughts of making love while cuddling child and listening to old song — very vivid. 08, 30C, 00:00:XX Themes: sexual, touch, music

Sh,273- Sexual desire for men (in a man). 24, 30C, 100:XX:XX (homosexuality) Themes: sexual

Sh,274- Developed an aversion to the idea of sex — confused about sexual issues and identity. Became aware of being bi-sexual or homosexual (in a man). "I want to find out who I am. I should know at 23. I used to know. What am I sexually?" Very confused. This led to suicidal depression. 24, 30C, 100:XX:XX Themes: loathing, sexual, identity, suicidal, sadness

Sh,275- Sexually totally closed when my girlfriend kissed me. I felt as if it was a sin. 24, 30C, 00:08:XX Themes: sexual, suppressed, doomed

Sh,276- Feelings of vulnerability and anxiety about being masculine, both in looks and in behaviour roles. Hope it doesn't get more. To counteract this, I have been stressing the feminine. I spent lots of money on silk clothing and spent a lot of time making myself up, curling hair, etc. People comment that I look softer, but I feel harder inside. I feel confused about my sexual identity. This is in contrast to my previous proving of the remedy, when people commented that my moustache disappeared and breasts grew. 12, 6C, 30:XX:XX (homosexuality) Themes: fragile, sexual, identity, vanity

Sh,277- I've been looking at other men in a sexual light. 08, 30C, 10:XX:XX Themes: sexual

Sh,278- Taking very big deep sighs over the last ten to fourteen days. It feels as if the sigh has to go deep down into my lungs so that sometimes it almost hurts. 02, 6C, 109:XX:XX Themes: damage

Sh,28- I felt an incredible clarity before and now I feel it may all have been a illusion. I am uncertain, don't know how I am anymore. I don't recognize what is happening. It's as if I have made a step into the unknown. I feel I'm in an unknown area without protection. Fear is the biggest limitation. 16, 30C, 05:XX:XX Themes: unreal, knowledge. identity

Sh,281- Felt benevolent — wanted to do something for someone else. Went out and spent a lot of money on food which I then gave to old people. 16, 30C, 03:XX:XX Themes: compassionate, helpful

Sh,282- During the proving, developed a true sympathy for the weakness of others. 08, 30C, 100:XX:XX Themes: compassionate

Sh,283- I feel more in touch with people, more sympathetic to the rest of the world. Feel more understanding. 08, 30C, 14:XX:XX Themes: compassionate, friendly

Sh,284- While talking to friends, felt less weighed down by their problems. I feel less absorbed into people, more able to let go of things that bother me. (cured symptom). 28, 200C, 00:04:XX Themes: compassionate

Sh,285- More charitable and sympathetic than usual. 08, 30C, 04:XX:XX Themes: helpful, compassionate

Sh,286- Generous in my feelings towards my husband. 02, 6C, 04:XX:XX Themes: compassionate, friendly

Sh,287- Feel relaxed, like a jellyfish — no bones in my body. 16, 30C, 00:XX:XX Themes: fragile

Sh,29- I've experienced a lot more egotism in the last few weeks. I feel frustrated by the limitations of the ego. 16, 30C, XX:XX:XX Themes: egotism

Sh,294- Spirits uplifted by wonderful weather. Felt strong, positive and adventurous. 04, 12C, 32:XX:XX Themes: fearless, nature, pleasure, energy

Sh,30- The whole environment I am in feels wrong now as if my life doesn't fit anymore. 16, 30C, 08:XX:XX Themes: wrong, unfit

Sh,32- Depressed — like seeing a window open and unable to go through it. 16, 30C, 08:XX:XX Themes: sadness, unfit

Sh,33- About two months after beginning the proving, developed an extreme range of mental symptoms that he had never had before. These included severe depression with strong alternations of moods, & high then low &, with suicidal tendency, desire to jump from a high building or cut wrist, confusion of identity (especially concerning sex and homosexuality) and became more religious. He moved away from his parents home (which he had never before been able t o do) and shut himself away in a small flat. This condition lasted for another six or seven months and was finally antidoted by Phosphorus 200. Before that, he had tried to anti-dote it with acupuncture, to no avail. 24, 30C, 60:XX:XX Themes: sadness, suicidal, height, identity, sexual, religious

Sh,34- I felt myself really getting into my yoga and exploring new positions. At one point, I ended up playing with my toes like a baby. 08, 30C, 00:XX:XX Themes: young, child

Sh,37- Have given up my normal planning and making lists. I used to organize all the time (curative). 08, 30C, 09:XX:XX Themes: organization

Sh,38- Decided to clean the kitchen floor and to move my things into the new study for the first time — both unusual. 02, 6C, 00:03:XX Themes: organization

Sh,4- Feeling spacey, lightheaded. 28, 200C, 00:03:45 Themes:

Sh,45- Feel grubby even after a shower. 16, 30C, 02:XX:XX Themes: dirty

Sh,6- Feeling of being out of reality. 24, 30C, 02:XX:XX Themes: unreal

Sh,63- "Oh God, what shall I do? Where do things go from here? What way shall I go? Feel I'm cracking up". Emotional confusion. Try to find a path to be happy, but unsure of what I'm doing. 24, 30C,

100:XX:XX Themes: lost, doubtful, disintegration

Sh,64- Irresolution about what she is going to do with her life. 14, 15C, 04:XX:XX Themes: irresolution

Sh,75- Tendency to lose things and blamed myself. Became frantic searching for them. Tore open a friend's bag to find paper and wouldn't have cared if the bag had ripped. 22, 12C, 04:XX:XX Themes: lost, conscience

Sh,8- I felt slightly high, removed from reality, yet very alert, clear and calm. Very aware of the colour of the sky, the light, birds singing, flowers — like a pastoral ideal. Feeling of expansiveness, mentally cool, airy and light. 28, 200C, 00:04:XX Themes: unreal, nature, light, religious

Sh,93- I can't believe its only a week ago I took the remedy. It seems like an aeon. 16, 30C, 08:XX:XX Themes: time

Sh,94- Time sense seems warped. 12, 6C, 09:XX:XX Themes: time

Sh,95- I looked at the clock. I think it was about an hour clock time. Time is different on this level, its moving very quickly. 16, 30C, Letter Themes: time

Sh,96- Looking at my life from a distance and thinking probably only thirty or forty summers left to be around, and it looked like a short time and very unimportant. A lifetime is a very short space of time. 16, 30C, 02:XX:XX Themes: time

Sh,97- My whole time scale has changed since taking the remedy, I've lost a lot of boundaries on time. Don't hurry, just do things in my own time. 08, 30C, 06:XX:XX Themes: time, hurry

Sh,98- It seems as if all the days became one. 16, 30C, XX:XX:XX Themes: time, integration

HYOS.

Al,139- He remembers persons and occurrences which he does not try to recollect. Themes: antagonism, past

Al,14- Thought he was in his own home, and desire to go out and make visits. Themes: home, go out, company

Al,28- The people in the room seemed to assume grotesque appearances; ... Themes: horrible, ugly

Al,42- In his delirium he acts as though he were frightening away peacocks with his hands. Themes: animal

Al,48- Laughed and said he was exceedingly well. Themes: antagonism, pleasure, disease

Al,5-...suspicious of those about him; he became delirious, saw policeman coming into the house; heard them speaking about the hall;... Themes: suspicious, invaded, officer,

Al,53- They laughed aloud because all persons seemed ridiculous;...the old woman talked of future,... Themes: ridiculous, contemptuous, future

Al,58- He sings amorous and obscene songs. Themes: sexual, music

Al,60-... Then he wandered into the country and suddenly pulling up a leg, exclaimed, " Take care; give me your hand; that is a very deep step"... Themes: helpful, conscientious

Al,67- He prattles and makes preparations for his wedding. Themes: talk, union

Al,73- In speaking, used very fine language, so that the usually quiet and indolent peasant (farmer) was scarcely recognized. Themes: greatness, talk

Al,77- He reproaches himself, and has conscious scruples. Themes: conscience, conscientious

Al,78- He considers himself a criminal. Themes: conscience, criminal

Al,80- Anxiety, soon after dinner, as though a sad occurrence impended. Themes: menaced, misfortune

Al,82- In despair, he wishes to drown himself. Themes: despair, suicidal, water

Al,85- Excessive fear of death, becoming a monomania,... Themes: fearful, mania, death

Al,86- He complained that he had been poisoned. Themes: poisoned

Al,87- Remarkable fear that he had been devoured by animals. Themes: fearful, animal, bite, death

Al,89- Dread of water. Themes: water

Al,9- Madness as if possessed by a devil. Themes: insanity, seized, devil

Al,90- ...called on various absent persons by name, with whom imagined himself to be in debate. Themes: discussion

Al,94- He reproaches others, and complains of a supposed injury done him. Themes: offenses, censorious

Ha,485- He is in danger of becoming senseless. Themes: danger, fit
Ha,489- Bereft (deprived) of all his senses, he sits in bed immovable, like a statue. Themes: paralysis
Ha,517- Over-busy: he thought he was more active and stronger (powerful, Herculean) than he actually was. Themes: busy, energy, greatness
Ha,519- In the confusion of his fancy he thinks men are swine.(pigs) Themes: contemptuous, animal, identity
Ha,525- Chattering he prepares for a journey. Themes: travel, talk
Ha,526- Chattering he makes preparation for a wedding. Themes: talk, union
Ha,529- Comical confusion of mind: they perform all sorts of ridiculous antics (jokes), like monkeys. Themes: feigning, ridiculous, animal
Ha,533- He gesticulates like a harlequin. (buffoon) (foot-note: "like an actor" - Hughes). (feigning) Themes: feigning, ridiculous
Ha,535- In his mania, he acts as if he must drive away peacocks with his hands.(conduct) Themes: insanity, animal
Ha,539- They cried out that near objects were going to fall, and seized hold of them. Themes: fall
Ha,541- Mania, as if possessed by the devil. Themes: seized, devil
Ha,544- Naked and enveloped in a fur cloak, he senselessly wanders about to a great distance in the summer heat. Themes: camouflage, clothes, travel
Ha,545- Ridiculously solemn acts in improper clothing, mixed with fury. (In a priest's cassock, put on over nothing but a shirt, and in fur boots, he wishes to go to church, in order to preach and perform clerical offices there, and furiously attacks those who try to prevent him.) Themes: ridiculous, anger, clothes, feigning, religious, violence, greatness, insanity
Ha,550- He displays uncontrollable strength in his fury. Themes: energy, anger
Ha,559- Fury; he tries to inflict injury on and hurt others. Themes: anger, hurt, violence
Ha,562 -Extreme fury: he rushes at people with knives. Themes: anger, homicidal, pointed, violence
Ha,563- He strikes and tries to murder those he meets. Themes: hurt, homicidal, violence
Ha,573- He complains that he has been poisoned. Themes: poisoned
Ha,574- He considers himself a criminal. Themes: conscience, criminal
Ha,575- Peculiar fear of being bitten (hurt) by beasts. Themes: fearful, attacked, hurt, bite, animal
Ha,577- He reproaches himself and has scruples of conscience. Themes: conscience, conscientious
Ha,578- He reproaches others, and complains of injustice that he imagines has been done him. Themes: censorious, injustice, justice
Ha,579- In despair he wishes to take his life, and throw himself into the water.(suicidal) Themes: despair, suicidal, water
Ha,582- Impatient: he thought he should die when he had to wait for something of quite trivial nature. Themes: death, impatience, time
Ha,67- Amativeness; nymphomania; erotomania.(sexual) Themes: sexual, lascivious
He,11- Thinks he is in the wrong place. Themes: lost
He,13- Does not know whether or not to take what is offered. Themes: suspicious, irresolution
He,14- Dread of drinks; of water. Themes: water, poisoned
He,16- Fears: being left alone (solitude, deserted); poison, or being bitten (hurt); being poisoned or sold; being betrayed, or injured; wishes to run away. (escape) Themes: solitude, poisoned, hurt, betrayed, offenses, bite, escape, forsaken
He,17- Complains of having been poisoned. Themes: poisoned, suspicious
He,19- Very suspicious. Themes: suspicious
He,31- Delirium; talks of business of imaginary wrongs. Themes: work, conscience, wrong
He,34- Scolds (censorious); raves; abuses those about him. Themes: censorious, offensive
He,41- Comical alienation of mind; ludicrous actions like monkeys; makes ridiculous gestures like a dancing clown;... Themes: feigning, music, animal, ridiculous
He,46- Sings amorous and obscene songs.

Themes: love, sexual, lascivious, music, wicked

He,49- Insane passion for work. Themes: work

He,50- Tendency to action: wants to kill somebody or himself. Themes: movement, homicidal, suicidal

He,52- Bite, scratch (hurt) and nip (pinch) everyone interfering with them. Themes: bite, contradiction

He,54- Tries to injure those around him; convulsions after trying to swallow. Themes: hurt, violence, fit

He,57- Delirium tremens:...averse to light and company; visions as if persecuted preceded by an epileptic attack;... seeks to escape from men by whom he imagines himself surrounded and who are trying to capture him; does not recognize his wife who is standing by his side, but imagines he sees her under a distant bed. Themes: persecution, light, company, fit, escape, surrounded, imprisoned, separated

He,59- ...constantly pointing to serpents (snakes) which she saw creeping up towards her... Themes: animal, persecution, crawling, attacked

He,60-... wants to run away for fear of being persecuted by police;... Themes: persecution, escape, criminal, officer

He,62- Jealousy: with rage and delirium; with attempt (try) to murder. Themes: jealousy, anger, homicidal

He,63- Erotic mania accompanied by jealousy. Themes: mania, sexual, jealousy

He,64- Serious illness (ailments) from jealousy and grief about faithless lover;... Themes: disease, jealousy, grief, betrayed, love

He,65- Violent and threatening...; mind nearly deranged; disturbed by unfounded jealousy. Themes: violence, jealousy, menacing, suspicious, betrayed,

He,66- A gentle, lovable woman became extremely jealous of her husband, and although fully realizing that she did him injustice, she was so filled with grief that she found no rest day or night... (remorse) Themes: jealousy, conscience, injustice, betrayed, husband, grief

He,68- Onanism since childhood; has always been greatly attracted by opposite sex and prematurely busied himself with thoughts of marriage;... secretly wrote his love affairs; mania,...one idea rapidly follow another, all in some away concerning love, masturbates at every opportunity...(satyriasis) Themes: sexual, child, union, love, lascivious

He,69- Lascivious mania, uncovers body, especially sexual parts; sings amorous songs. Themes: lascivious, sexual, music, love, wicked

He,72- He lies in bed nude and chatters; walks about insane, naked, wrapped in a skin during summer heat. Themes: talk, camouflage, insanity

He,74- Disappointed love followed by: epilepsy, melancholy, rage, or inclination to laugh at everything; despair and propensity to drown himself. (ailments from) Themes: love, disappointment, anger, sarcasm, suicidal, water, despair, sadness, fit

He,76- After a fit of passion, melancholia,... appetite gone;... Themes: passionate, sadness

He,77- After a fit of passion and sudden fear, became so melancholy and timorous as to hide himself in every corner,... Themes: passionate, sadness

He,78- Groundless suspicion of being watched (observed, spied) by members of family with whom he had some slight misunderstanding (dispute); to avoid being recognized by them, clothed himself differently every day,...watching his relations suspiciously and imagining he might be poisoned;... (disguise, camouflage) Themes: suspicious, observed, family, discussion, camouflage, feigning, poisoned, betrayed, hide, clothes

He,78-...fixing himself to correspond with the points of the compass and looking through his fingers; tracing the pattern of carpet with his feet and twisting his legs till he nearly fell down;...(direction) Themes: organization

He,79 - After being harshly (severe) accused of theft (crime), continual delirium; fancies surrounded by objects of a terrifying nature; not a moment quiet, continual calling out that she saw the devil; denies herself guilty of theft (innocent, injustice), or that she has any concern with witches; ... Themes: accused, criminal, surrounded, restless, devil, injustice, indignation, conscience, offenses

He,81- ...attempts to escape from room; frightful hallucinations of figures coming to seize him, hens (chicken) bound (imprisoned) with chains,... Themes: escape, seized, imprisoned, animal, caught

He,83-...imagining that her deceased sister was sitting by her bedside, and talking with this imaginary person... Themes: ghosts, sister, talk

He,84- ...constant talking, particularly on religious subjects; believes himself poisoned, or that there is a stinking odor from his mouth;... Themes: talk, religious, poisoned, dirty, rotten

He,85-...repelled with rage and seeming disgust his mother, of whom, in natural state, he was dotingly (loving) fond, did not know her, said she was not his mama;...0Maniacal fury. Themes: loathing, forsakes, love

He,87-...; refused medicine, and cunningly (skill) evaded all stratagems to give it; escaped from room, ... Themes: suspicious, poisoned, escape, feigning

He,90- Looks at men as hogs.(pigs) Themes: contemptuous, animal

HYPER.

Al,S-3- For a week past, impure ideas have very seldom presented themselves by day; the mind has been reposing on higher thoughts. Themes: dirty, conscience, wicked

He,3- Erotic ideas; brain excited, as after tea. Themes: sexual

IBER.

Al,1- Frightened mood; fears she has taken too much of the drug; in the evening.(medicine) Themes: fearful, poisoned

Al,2- Feels frightened; ...as if she had taken a dangerous dose.(medicine) Themes: fearful, poisoned, danger

IGN.

Al,15- Anxiety as if he had committed a crime. Themes: conscience, criminal

Al,2- He fancies that he is unable (incapable, powerless) to proceed (progress, advance), that he cannot walk. Themes: unfit, paralysis

Al,20 -Fearfulness timidity; she has no confidence in herself, gives up (desist) everything. Themes: confidence, succeed, fearful, cowardice, timidity

Al,21- Fear of thieves, on waking after midnight. Themes: robber

Al,22- She fears that she will have an ulcer in the stomach. Themes: disease

Al,27- Slight blame or contradiction excites him to anger, and this makes him angry with himself. Themes: contradiction, conscience, himself, anger, censured,

Al,28- Contrary to his will, thinks of vexatious and peevish things, and dwells upon them. Themes: antagonism, bothered, dwells

Al,3- A fixed idea, which he pursues in his thoughts, or expatiates (talk) upon with great earnestness and exhaustiveness in conversation (after two hours). Themes: talk, obstinate

Al,30- Extremely morose, finds fault, and makes reproaches. Themes: censorious, wrong

Al,32- He is discontented, morose, and obstinate towards evening; no one can do anything right or please him. Themes: obstinate, discontented, wrong

Al,5- Desires improper (inappropriate) things, and cries aloud when they are refused. Themes: capricious, contradiction

Ha,749- Anxiety as if he had done something bad. Themes: wrong, conscience

Ha,753- Extreme anxiety, which prevents (restrain) speaking. Themes: talk, obstructed

Ha,754-,... he cannot express himself in talking, write, or do anything as quickly as he wishes; ...he makes mistakes in speaking and writing, and does everything awkwardly... Themes: talk, hurry, failure, wrong, time

Ha,755- Excessively busy: he restlessly sets about doing first one thing then another. Themes: busy, restless, succeed, dispersion

Ha,757- He imagines he cannot get on (succeed), cannot walk. Themes: obstructed, paralysis, confidence

Ha,758 - She fears she will get an ulceration of the stomach. Themes: disease

Ha,759- Fearfulness, cowardice cannot trust himself to do anything, considers all is lost . Themes: fearful, confidence, failure, cowardice, succeed
Ha,760- On waking, after midnight, has fears of thieves. Themes: robber
Ha,762- Fears every trifle, is specially afraid of objects coming near him. Themes: fearful, approached
Ha,764 -Slight blame (censuring) or contradiction excites him to quarrel, and he is vexed at himself for doing so. Themes: contradiction, fight, conscience, shame, censured, bothered
Ha,765- From the slight contradiction he is irritated and angry. Themes: contradiction, anger
Ha,768- Towards evening he is discontented, sulky, stubborn (obstinate), no one can do anything right, anything to please him. Themes: discontented, obstinate, wrong
Ha,769- Is extremely sulky; finds fault and makes reproaches. Themes: wrong, censorious
Ha,770- Fickle, impatient, irresolute, quarrelsome. Themes: dispersion, impatience, irresolution, fight, doubtful
Ha,774- Desires improper things, and weeps aloud when they are denied him. Themes: capricious
Ha,775- When one hesitates in the least to do what she wishes, or remonstrates (censures) much with her, though in a mild friendly manner, or endeavor to persuade her, or wishes differently from what she wishes, she weeps aloud. Themes: capricious, contradiction, censured
Ha,791- Thinks against his will of annoying, vexatious things, and dwells on them. Themes: bothered, antagonism, dwells, mortification
Ha,792- Delicate disposition (character), with very clear consciousness (justice, judgment, equity) Themes: mildness, conscientious, justice
Ha,793- Sensitive disposition, delicate conscientiousness (careful ,scrupulous) Themes: sensitive, mildness, conscientious
He,10- Spasms and insanity after fright; imagines her soul cannot be saved (rescued), and cries very much; ...(lost, sentenced) Themes: doomed, religious, salvation
He,11- ...believes herself married (connected) and pregnant; is tormented by remorse of imagined crimes; seeks constantly to escape to drown (suicide) herself; ...;is only quiet when lying undisturbed and brooding over her troubles, which she rehearses (tell) in a doleful (unhappy) tone ;..." I am neglecting my duty, breaking my vow" (promise, engagement)...;conscientious scruples after eating. Themes: union, tormented, conscience, criminal, suicidal, water, unfortunate, duty, conscientious, mortification, escape, negligence,
He,14- Inclined to be very secretive (taciturn) and passive.(yielding) Themes: reserved, suppressed, yielding
He,2- ...;sees everything as if through a fog (obscurity) ; sits quietly, with a vacant gaze (expression), always thinking of the mortification endured,... prefers to be alone; thinking of the past mortification...0Melancholy after mortification. Themes: dark, obstructed, mortification, sadness, solitude
He,22- Melancholia from suppressed mental sufferings, with much sighing; desire to be alone (solitude) so as to give way to her real or imaginary grief; weeps bitterly. Themes: grief, suppressed, mortification, sadness, solitude
He,24- Melancholy after disappointed love, always combined with spinal symptoms. Themes: disappointment, love
He,26- Great grief after losing persons or objects very dear. Themes: lack, death, sadness,
He,27- Unhappy love with silent grief. Themes: disappointment, unfortunate, love, grief
He,28- Senseless (illogical) staring at one object, with sighing and moaning; remorse about imaginary crimes, intolerance to noise; great inclination to have fixed ideas. Themes: conscience, criminal, obstinate, noise,
He,30- Became bilious, nervous, depressed, and would scarce move from the fire, for days together. Morbid grief Themes: anger, sadness, fire, grief
He,31- A peculiar trembling of hands disturbs her very much in writing, most when she has to write in any one's presence

(public), gets worse as soon as she fancies any one might notice it. (observed) Themes: confidence, observed, shame,

He,33- Dread of every trifle, especially of things coming near him. Themes: fearful, approached

He,34- Fear of thieves, on waking after midnight. Themes: robber

He,35- Fearfulness; does not like to talk; prefers to be alone. Themes: talk, solitude, fearful, company

He,36- Anxiety as though something terrible had happened cannot speak because of it; hurry, fearfulness, terror, alternating with irresolution and inertness. Themes: misfortune, talk, irresolution, confidence, hurry, fearful, yielding

He,37- Tears wept inwardly, the pain and penalty (forfeit) of unrequited (unrecompensed) love; desires solitude so that one may nourish inward grief;... Themes: conscience, disappointment, solitude, mortification, love, sadness, grief

He,38- Anxiety as if he had committed some crime. Themes: conscience, criminal

He,39- Anxiety and disquiet as if she had done something wrong, or as if some great misfortune were about to happen, this so overpowers her that she can with difficulty refrain from weeping;... Themes: restless, wrong, conscience, misfortune, anticipation

He,40- Anxiety, sleeplessness, despair; severe palpitation; loss of appetite; constipation. Themes: despair

He,41- Altered appearance; made an unsuccessful attempt to end his most unendurable (intolerable) sufferings, by eating the phosphorus from matches; after business embarrassment. Themes: suicidal, work

He,42- A state of anguish in which she shrieks (scream) for help, with suffocating constriction of throat... Themes: helplessness, suffocation, constriction

He,44-...;indifference to things she loved best ; sits alone and weeps, imagines things, a especially that she might go crazy; .. Themes: love, forsakes, insanity, indifference, solitude

He,49- Mild disposition; bears suffering, even outrage (offenses), without complaining. Themes: mildness, yielding, offenses, suppressed

He,50- Jealousy, disappointed love. Themes: jealousy, disappointment, love

He,52- The slightest contradiction irritates. Themes: contradiction

He,53- Slight blame (censure) or contradiction excites him to anger, and this makes him angry with himself. Themes: censured, contradiction, anger, himself

He,55- Anger, followed by quiet grief or sorrow. Themes: anger, grief, sadness

He,6- Brooding over imaginary or real troubles; is wrapped in thought. Themes: meditation, dwells

He,61- Melancholia after great grief and domestic trouble; complete sleeplessness; suicidal thoughts and desire to escape. Themes: grief, duty, cares, suicidal, sadness, home, escape

He,62- Ill effects (ailments) from hearing bad news; from vexation with reserved displeasure ; from grief , or suppressed mental sufferings; of shame and disappointed love. Themes: news, suppressed, grief, shame, disappointment, mortification, sadness, love, reserved

IND.

Al,4- Felt almost crazed when attempting to study... Themes: insanity, knowledge

INDG.

Al,1- Illusion of sensation; it constantly seems to her as though she had a large goiter, which was very prominent; she was constantly obliged to look down and feel whether it was so. Themes: disease

IOD.

Al,16- Anxiety and prostration; the patients busy themselves for the most part about the future. Themes: future

Al,21- He fears that from every trifle some misfortune would arise. Themes: misfortune,

Al,22- Apprehensiveness (fearful) after some manual labor, ... Themes: work

Al,27- Is cross and irascible; feels stupid.(obtuse) Themes: bothered, anger, contemptuous, himself

Al,28- Peevish, fretful; nothing is done right. Themes: anger, wrong

Al,31- Mind feels tired, and does not care to work. Themes: work, indifference, duty

Al,39- Feels unfitted for everything. Themes: unfit

Al,6- Remarkably lively and talkative, no one else is able to get in a word. Themes: talk, energy

Al,8- Disposition mild, scrupulous (careful) and timid (irresolute), with blunted (dull) sensibilities. Themes: mildness, conscientious, obstructed, timidity, cowardice

Ha,10- Apprehensiveness after some manual work; it goes off while sitting. Themes: work

Ha,15- Oppression, and tightness of the chest. Themes: oppression

Ha,16- Anxiety and dejection; the patients generally busy themselves with the present. Themes: busy

Ha,17- Restless moving about; she runs about incessantly and does not get to sit down, nor does she sleep at night, so that she has to be considered as crazy. Themes: restless, movement, insanity

Ha,18- Restlessness, which keeps the body in constant activity. Themes: restless, movement

Ha,21- He is afraid at every trifle, that one or another mishap (accident) may rise from it. Themes: misfortune

Ha,25- He feels unable to do anything. Themes: unfit

Ha,26- Her phlegmatic disposition has disappeared; she has become blooming (growing), stronger and more lively. Themes: energy

Ha,27- Peevish, cross, she is not suited by anything... Themes: bothered

Ha,6-...oppressive sensation in the throat and chest, as when one is about to weep. Themes: oppression

He,1- Feeling as of having forgotten something and does not know what. Themes: lost

He,13- Excessive kind of impatience, she is running about all the time and never sits down or sleeps at night. Themes: impatience, restless

He,14- Consequences of amorousness.(passionate, libidinous)(ailments from) Themes: sexual

He,15- At night, especially when thinking of real or imaginary wrongs ...dares (try) to go home for fear of doing some dreadful (bad, wicked) deed (action); on one occasion was seized with an almost irresistible impulse to murder a woman who was acting as a guide (direct, conduct) for him, he having lost his way (direction);...must be constantly in action, in some laborious occupation. (lost; direction, correction, control) Themes: wrong, home, wicked, seized, conscience, homicidal, indignation, busy, movement, lost, work

He,3- Must keep in motion day and night (restlessness), brain felt as if it was stirred (agitation) up, felt as if going crazy. Themes: restless, movement, insanity

He,4- Restless, inclined to move about not permitting to sit or sleep; thought she could tear everything to pieces. Themes: movement, tear

He,7- Apprehends an accident from every trifle. Themes: accidents

He,8- Fear of evil with over carefulness. Themes: misfortune, conscientious

He,9- Fear and anxiety shuns (avoid) even the doctor. Themes: suspicious, loathing

IP.

Al,11- Ill-humored and vexed that his business does not proceed fast enough. Themes: work, succeed, hurry, time

Al,12- Ill-humored, quiet, retired in himself, scorning everything. Themes: solitude, contemptuous

Al,7- His courage sinks, and he is extremely inclined to be peevish and ill-humored. Themes: cowardice

Al,8- He is thoughtful, fearful, and thinks trifles are very important. Themes: fearful, conscientious

Al,9- Ill- humored; he thinks that he is very unhappy. Themes: unfortunate

Ha,215- He has no pleasure in nothing, nothing is agreeable to him. Themes: discontented

Ha,216- Everything is repugnant to him. Themes: loathing

Ha,218- Repugnance to literary work; thoughts fail him. Themes: loathing, unfit, knowledge, knowledge

Ha,219 -Sullen unsociable moroseness, that makes him disdain (reject) everything.

Themes: solitude, forsakes, misanthropy, loathing, contemptuous

Ha,221- Sulky humor, that despises (scorn, intolerant, antipathy) everything, and he desires that others also should not esteem or care for anything. Themes: contemptuous, envy, others

Ha,222- Moroseness: he considers himself unfortunate.(unlucky, unsuccessful) Themes: misanthropy, unfortunate

Ha,223- He is scrupulous (careful, conscientious), apprehensive, and thinks trifles of importance. Themes: conscientious

Ha,224- He is morose and vexed that his business is not performed quick enough. (time) Themes: hurry, succeed, duty, time,

Ha,227- He lets (permit) his courage sink (fail), and is greatly given to be vexed and to get angry. Themes: cowardice, anger, bothered

Ha,228- His disposition is full of wishes and longing he knows not for what. Themes: capricious

Ha,229- He very often gets angry about the merest trifle, and can just as easily and quickly become calm. Themes: anger

He,12- Morose mood that scorns everything, and desires also that others shall not appreciate or value anything. Themes: contemptuous, envy

He,13- Ailments from vexation (worry) and reserved displeasure. Themes: contradiction, suppressed, grief, reserved

He,3- Full of inexpressible desires. Themes: capricious

He,8- Peevish; irritable; impatient; morose, scornful mood. Themes: impatience, contemptuous

He,9- Ill humor, despises everything. Themes: contemptuous

IRID.

Sh,101- Went into pet shop. There was a budgie chirping in a cage. I was so upset. "Oh God, I want to let this bird out." I felt it was crying to be let out. Took me all my control not to let it out or shout at the man to do it. Then thought, "This is silly. It would get hurt, he'll think I'm mad." I slunk out of the shop thinking I'd really let that bird down. Distracted and nearly in tears. Walked round town in a daze, should I go back and ask him to at least open the door, knew that wasn't on. It might get out of the shop and die. Felt a real coward. Set up a train of thought —condor in bird garden —a notice justifying its captivity —it only flies for food —it's quite happy to be there because food comes to it. Weeping as I write this. Birds in cages can't lean on the air currents and be blown away. G6 Themes: liberty, compassionate, helpful, conscience, cowardice

Sh,102- Just before sleep, image came into head from nowhere. Sitting on an air current as if it was a soft comfy settee foam cushion. Started to move over a landscape, took me high up, trees, towns, like the flying sequence from The Snowman. The air was so supportive, like floating on water. It had real substance but unlike water it was bouncy. There was no way I was going to fall. I was sitting back, not floating, tummy down. Felt like a child bouncing on the air. Fun —at the same time sense of awe, experiencing something for the first time. No sense of danger — trust. Floatiness experienced before with cannabis but then I was anxious, "Would I get back into body?" With this I was still in my body — no separation. G44 Themes: floating, flying, liberty, young

Sh,103- Felt light and young, found things fun and amusing. Walking effortlessly, easy, as if not touching the ground. Q1 Themes: young, light, pleasure, floating

Sh,106- Mental image: I am inside an egg —a bird, wet feathers, at the point it is smashing through its shell, bursting out; a chick, wet crumpled and hot, shell flying all over. The relief —getting to the air, refreshing, cool. Inside it was humid, stifling. Stretching vast wings, enjoying feeling the air dry them out. G5 Themes: pleasure, imprisoned, liberty, flying, animal, identity

Sh,107- On waking, hands joined by first fingers; hands fused to become wings; thumbs crossed in the form of a heart. Q2 Themes: transmutation

Sh,108- Realized I had called my ex-partner a chicken for pulling out of an arrangement to go together to a school fundraising event. G5 Themes: contemptuous, animal

Sh,109- Sensation as if wings 3 —4 p.m. Q5 Themes: transmutation, flying, liberty

Sh,110- Meditating, vision of an angel, face and wings. Q6 Themes: meditation, religious, liberty

Sh,112- Sensation as if winged ankles, while wind blowing through house. Thought, "back to earth." Q17 Themes: flying, liberty, transmutation

Sh,113- Feel as if growing wings in back. SENSATION AS IF body wanting to change form, mainly in chest, face, back. Q4 Themes: transmutation, liberty

Sh,114- Felt I had been given the role of messenger, wasn't always in English. Q3 Themes: travel, abroad

Sh,115- Inner vision, rows upon rows of letters. Thought, "This looks Greek to me." Q8 Themes: abroad, strange

Sh,116- On going to sleep, asked the question, "Who am I." Message on waking, that my name was Iris. QXX Themes: identity

Sh,117- Attention wanders to messages that I hear in my head to pass onto people. QXX Themes: talk

Sh,118- Thoughts: Wind is breath of the spirit; love is the greatest of all messages between heaven and earth. Yes, go to heaven, but return to the world transformed by the light of experience, transcend and return; Metals —immortality; need knowledge of their names; Iridescence, oil mother of pearl metal, rainbow, seven plus seven, cosmic joke, messages in other languages —language of angels?; Seven heavens, seven earths. I adore these territories, not so much new as forgotten. Q20 Themes: love, knowledge, bright, supernatural

Sh,122-Sensation as if seven stars in a ring around my head. QXX Themes: bright

Sh,125- Attracted to men with pale skins, appear even more beautiful, luminosity, light shining forth. Q5 Themes: sexual, bright, light

Sh,126- Euphoric, others look gray, I am many-colored. Q1 Themes: bright

Sh,127- Bright cold day. My attention was taken by the light reflected off the wet road. The brightness meant I wasn't seeing the tree or road at all. It added to the feeling of detachment. B3 Themes: isolation, bright

Sh,128- People said "You look radiant today." People came and chatted to me. Felt incredibly clear and colourful. Such a big grin on my face, my face hurts. Q1 Themes: bright

Sh,13- Would like to sit down and go to sleep. Want to go and hibernate, go to bed. Feel happy to sit and stare at a blank wall and reduce input. A3 Themes: isolation

Sh,138- Crossing road, thought wouldn't it be nice to see a rainbow. Saw van belonging to "F. Rainbow and Son" —a removal company. Company I've never seen before. Q17 Themes: bright

Sh,140- Felt flat, not much energy. Will be glad when it's daylight. When daylight comes you feel lifted. D6 Themes: energy, bright

Sh,145- Time goes too fast. I'm late for tutorial by half an hour, not like me. E1 Themes: slow

Sh,146- Am realizing that time is passing very quickly. Thursday now, and Monday seems only yesterday. G18 Themes: time

Sh,15- Don't feel like reading paper or working on the train. Very unusual; just want to look out of window at the snow. E2 Themes: isolation, distance

Sh,150- Feeling of moving in slow motion. Mum left jobs for me to do, could usually do them in the time but I didn't today. The more I tried to do the slower I became. B7 Themes: slow

Sh,151- I feel slow and down and far away. E.1 Themes: isolation, slow

Sh,153- Time seems to have gone extremely slowly; it feels like weeks have passed since proving started. Time either goes fast or slow, it feels a bit warped. E5 Themes: time, slow

Sh,154- Felt quick and was frustrated at the slowness of others. Q4 Themes: hurry

Sh,155- Very restless night, not insomnia, just kept rising into consciousness, thinking it had to be morning now. Knew I had to be up at 6.30 a.m., and the night seemed so long, I kept checking to see if the alarm was working. Even at 1.30 a.m., thought it was morning; shocked it was so early. Night seemed elastic. The night stretched and stretched and seemed so long. E7 Themes: time

Sh,169- Did teaching by myself. Bit anxious

but nothing like usual. The video didn't work. I would have panicked. I thought, "Let's be systematic about this." Found the problem and it was fine. Much more confident risking it. Very relaxed about how the time was going, not in such a rush. A student called me chicken for taking only one tablet. G4 Themes: cowardice

Sh,18- Sitting still and staring into space, feeling very defined and contained in my body again, as if in an invisible capsule. Warm in my own air and lack of thoughts inside. This state tends to happen when I'm in a warmish place, don't think it could happen outside. People's chatter washes over me, I don't notice them or their talk. Body feels exactly like when you've just woken up and don't want to move. E7 Themes: integration

Sh,19- Still didn't feel much like talking. Feel very contained and self contained and my mind feels still. Unintellectual, unthinking, heavy. I wanted to be pre-verbal like the cat. Words too much effort. E1 Themes: transmutation, animal, talk

Sh,195- Panicked about servicing car before a long journey. Felt anxiety that car might break down as it hadn't been running smoothly. However found that car didn't need a service for another two thousand miles. Over-conscientious about getting jobs done on car. A3 Themes: accidents, disintegration

Sh,197- There's a slight element of confusion and a faint glimmer of not being able to cope. The feeling of not coping came on this afternoon. I've got lots to do and I've done nothing. I don't feel like doing anything but the concern is will I ever be able to focus my mind long enough to get anything done! M4 Themes: failure, unfit

Sh,198- The class I was teaching did not go well and left me feeling upset. I did not perform well and I felt low after it. I identified myself as the problem. I began to doubt the work I'm doing was being valued. Wasn't myself. It was the thirteenth time I'd done similar material and it was as if I had never done it before. I tripped over words, couldn't concentrate on what I was doing. (Added at a later date: "This was like I was pregnant.") No one in class had noticed anything was wrong. It was more my own perception. B2 Themes: confidence, unfit

199- Feelings of self-doubt crept in during the morning. Helped out at school and found myself checking with others over little things. Unable to make small decisions, spellings, etc., things I wouldn't be concerned about normally, usually feel sure of my own judgment. B4 Themes: doubtful

Sh-2- Felt similar to being in water or asleep, as if almost asleep or in a trance, aware, but floating in inner self, uncommunicative; like a near death experience, inner self is primary and separate. E1 Themes: death, isolation, water

Sh,20- Skin to skin, started stroking arms, arms to face, hands to arms to face, then down body acutely aware of boundaries of body. Q1 Themes: integration

Sh,200- Waking frequently, every hour, feeling very alert and wide awake, worried that I had forgotten something, not put the guard on the fire, closed down the stove, locked the doors, etc. Feels like I would take ages to get off to sleep. In reality got to sleep quickly. A19 Themes: fire, accidents, conscientious

Sh,201- Visited friends and although I was happy, calm, relaxed in their company, I was reticent to put forward my views. Was worried that what I had to say was not relevant or good enough. These women are good friends. I usually feel on a par with them. We chatted easily, up to the point when I felt inadequate in the conversation. (She later added, "I was acting as if this familiar situation was a new one.") B8 Themes: confidence

Sh,203- Being driven home, I felt the feeling of imminent danger on waking. I kept waking with a start six or seven times during the journey. Nervous because too near the car in front. B7 Themes: accidents

Sh,204- All day, woke with sense of foreboding as if something bad was going to happen. Feeling quite shaky, butterflies in tummy, a bit nauseous. I14 Themes: misfortune, fearful

Sh,21- The edges of my body felt very defined as if surrounded by warm skin or air. Very pleasant. The edges very clear, especially the back and top of arms, my neck and my back as if I've just woken in my own little capsule of warmth. E11 Themes: integration

Sh,214- Very strong protective feeling towards daughters. Hen and chicks image. Feel more tender towards them then usual. It feels like they are on the brink of adolescence and very vulnerable. Very strong protective feeling, not felt their vulnerability since they were born and very little. G42 Themes: fragile, compassionate

Sh,22- I feel whole and connected to everything, yet at the same time I feel I unreal, my boundaries don't feel the same. I1 Themes: integration, unreal

Sh,25- Feeling of being on the outside. F9 Themes: unreal, identity, transmigration

Sh,26- Felt detached in company, reticent to speak my mind. Sat and listened but didn't speak at the moments I usually would. Felt "sidelined," watching what's going on, rather than being a part of it. Felt detachment and self-doubt. I didn't speak because didn't feel I would be able to answer them (subject matter was my area of expertise). B9 Themes: isolation, talk

Sh, 29- Feel like not talking at all. A far-away-from-others-deep-in-me feeling. E1 Themes: isolation

Sh,3- The heavy feeling is more earthed than spaced. I don't feel spacey, more interior, like in a dream or under water. E1 Themes: heavy

Sh,30- Feel as if I am the only person. E3 Themes: greatness, isolation

Sh,300- I feel snappy, as though I could bite someone's head off. Feel really ratty. I2 At 5.00 a.m., I felt very resentful at having to get up. This mood lasted for at least two hours. At 9.15 a.m., went back to bed, slept for two hours, had frustrating, agitated dreams about the car. Things kept going wrong. Seem to be attracting aggravation. L8 Themes: anger, bite

Sh,309- I have found that voices are sounding really loud. I have turned the television down again, as I wish I could turn the children down and off. I feel really irritated around them. I feel better on my own. J4 Themes: noise

Sh,318- Still feeling down, irritable, restless, frustrated and bored. I Feel heavy, everything is an effort. Feel totally unloved, dejected, unwanted, "nobody likes me" feeling. I34 Themes: forsaken

Sh,320- Full of anger, like fire burning away inside me. Less tolerant with people. Normally I would say it's okay, but I haven't, and I feel very strong like I could chop any one down who got in the way. Feel very emotional. I would burst into tears if someone said the wrong thing. Similar to the feeling I used to have at school when I was being bullied, a defiant, "I'll show you one day!" type of feeling. I5 Themes: anger, passionate

Sh,322- Had row with partner over work, money, and time off. I was storming about. I said, "You can't say that to me." I went storming after partner went into another room. I was overwhelmed with fury. I cried with fury. D13 Themes: anger, fight

Sh,325- Stroppy —felt more frustrated, did not want to communicate at all, shouting and abusive. N7 Themes: offensive

Sh,327- Had a massive argument with friend. For first time in my life really stood my ground. Went hot. Said, "This is my point and I am sticking to it." Burst into floods of tears. It was as though a volcano had erupted. Anger and grief were coming out. My friend had done this on purpose. I got on high horse. We parted friends and sorted it all out. I4 Themes: fight, obstinate, passionate

Sh,332- On waking this morning was reminded of childhood illness. Same sense of not wanting to move, of not wanting to do anything, of not wanting to talk to anyone, just wanting to sleep and sleep the rest of my life away. In a way that feeling has always been with me and it is only by driving myself on that I have managed to achieve anything. It summarizes my feelings of everything being an effort, of spontaneous enthusiasm missing, of being too serious and lacking joy. A27 Themes: yielding

Sh,344- Feels like I have lost something, feels like I am grieving. It is a bit of a swine really. I11 Themes: grief, lack

Sh,36- Went to a 40th birthday celebration. One very good friend said I didn't seem to be there. They seemed like strangers to me. I was looking at the situation, which needed jollying up, but was unable to do anything about it because I felt distanced from them. It felt strange as if I'd gone out with people I didn't want to be with. H3 Themes: strange, isolation, friends

Sh,37- I kept distancing myself from people, more than I normally do. For example, if I was in a group of people then I would be stood apart from the rest of the group or sat on my own at a distance. The remedy heightened my separation and isolation from people. I24 Themes: isolation

Sh,39- I am less reserved than normal, more confident; but my boundaries have altered. I get less drawn into other people's emotional problems, less sympathetic. I26 Themes: reserved, compassionate

Sh-4- This remedy makes me feel settled in one place, planted. No desire to move. E1 Themes: movement

Sh,40- Hairdresser cut my hair. I felt quite close to her though I don't really know her. Had these feelings of being closer to people. D11 Themes: integration

Sh,41- Bumped into people I hadn't seen for ages, some for maybe six years. D24 Themes: integration

Sh,42- I wanted to sit with the rest of my family. This is unusual for me; usually sit on my own. I1 Themes: family, company, homesickness

Sh,43- Overall felt better for animated conversation. O13 Themes: talk, company

Sh,44- Better for company. It felt better to be with the family. D2 Themes: company, family

Sh,45- "I want you to hold my hand." B3 Themes: helplessness

Sh,46- Went to bed and clung to husband, needed him to hold me (due to depression). We made love out of need rather than passion. B9 Themes: helplessness

sh,48- Desire to touch backs of hands on face. Enjoy touch on skin. Old memories of gentleness, delightfully feminine. Wearing bright pink (unusual!) and stroking my legs. Enjoying my skin, touching bottom, stroking it. Dancing erotically at 8.00 a.m. (one hour after remedy). Particularly joyous. Q1 Themes: past, sexual, touch, music

Sh,49- Skin felt very alive, tactile, fingertips felt "awake." Feathers felt amazing. Skin to skin; very aware of contact of surfaces. More erotic dancing, morning. Q2 Themes: sexual, touch, music

Sh,5- I want to be a home-bird this week. I don't want to go out at all. D9 Themes: go out, isolation

Sh,50- When a friend visited, she touched me a lot, and I noticed it. I've not touched people as much as I normally do. B4 Themes: touch

Sh,52- Woke in white softness, like rabbit's fur. Q3 Themes: touch

Sh,54- Getting dressed, didn't want to put clothes on, wanted the freedom of nakedness, chose clothes for their lack of restriction. G 6 Themes: liberty, clothes

Sh,55- Memories and associations of giving birth, and of being born. Warm nakedness. Marriage? Old memories of marriage and wedding day. Gently erotic and sensual. Q1 Themes: sexual, union, past, pleasure

Sh,56- Delight at seeing my own female form in mirror, desire to shave legs so they would be smooth. Highly sexual, more refined, dressed in best clothes today. Desire to dance naked in moonlight. Q6 Themes: sexual, fine, vanity, touch

Sh,57- On the bus a woman turned to me and said, "Your eyes are the same as my daughter's." Baby like me. I knew we had met before, knew that I knew her. She knew me as well. A wonderful moment. Q7 Themes: integration, pleasure, identity

Sh,58- Felt child-like, innocent, happy as though seeing things from a child's perspective. Sat watching a milk tanker, it looks just like a child's toy. Felt like I could pick it up and brrrm brrrm it up the lane. I9 Themes: pure, child, identity, pleasure

Sh,59- Woke from a dream about wedding, feeling of unease, remembered my own wedding day, got a letter of proposal from former lover. Went ahead despite. What did I do? Q7 Themes: union, love, past

Sh,60- Patient said she was going to get married, I thought "big mistake." Q17 Themes: envy

Sh,61- I feel buzzy and vibrating, feels as if my hair is stood on end. I keep talking about being a dog. H1 Themes: animal, identity, transmutation

Sh,65- Motivation difficult, Sensation as if trapped in magnetic fields. Curled up stroking body, especially legs, feet together, Feeling as if they were magnetic. Desire for a young man. Thought that the feminine form is rounded and curved due to magnetism; arcs due to magnetic forces. Q2 Themes: imprisoned, sexual

Sh,67- Sensation of movement in face as if head, face and skin full of magnetism. Sense of alignment. Q2 Themes: integration, perfection

Sh,68- Woke up thinking my alarm clock was a hedgehog. I wondered what the spiky sound was. I10 Themes: animal, noise, transmutation

Sh-7- Abnormal mental awareness, very conscious of nature, everything seemed very vivid, very lovely. Profound feeling. F22 Themes: integration, love

Sh,70- Felt cold water running through my arms and legs and out; though it didn't make me feel cold. D34 Themes: water

Sh,71- Feel more sexually stimulated. More aware of it. Sensitive to others' sexuality since proving. A9 Themes: sexual

Sh,72- Very sexual thoughts on waking (male prover). More sexual than I have been for several weeks. K5 Themes: sexual

Sh,73- I imagined being naked, not having sex, with female houseguest. (Male prover) K5 Themes: sexual

Sh,74- No desire to touch, make love to husband all week in spite of easy, relaxed week. I feel detached from him, as if this is a problem within me. B20 Themes: sexual, isolation, loathing

Sh,75- While watching TV felt feelings of attraction to older men. I would not normally be attracted to older men. I6 Themes: sexual, old

Sh,76- Twice now I have overtaken cars going up the hill out of town which were going only marginally slower than me. Had to get past them, urgency to get to the top out of the valley. G7 Themes: nature, hurry

Sh,77- A sudden, very deep desire for wilderness, space and air and height. E15 Themes: nature, height

Sh,78- Today I noticed how narrow my life feels, and what I feel like doing is making my life even narrower. E2 Themes: imprisoned

Sh,79- Had this longing to find real wilderness. Britain is too full, nothing is really alive anymore except people. The world really feels too oppressed with people and roofs. I kept saying to partner, "Why do we live in this dreary, ugly place, where people know nothing about freedom, and certainly nothing about discovery or mystery, just tarmac and roofs." It struck me that the world was too small for me, and thought "That's got to be something about the remedy, something around pressure." E5 Themes: nature, imprisoned. liberty, small

Sh,80- I felt all closed in like I couldn't move, I couldn't breathe. I felt oppressed by being in this room, there's no space. It's funny but I felt like that tonight when I was sitting outside. There were lots of clouds in the sky and it felt like they were coming down on me. Like the sky had been really close and the clouds in the sky were nearer to me; I noticed it because I was watching the moon waxing. It was like I hadn't really noticed the clouds at night before. J5 Themes: imprisoned, suffocation,

Sh,81- Feel hemmed in by ex-partner's needs, feel I'm being fitted into the little spaces in his life. Can no longer shrug and say, "Well this is how it is." G5 Themes: liberty, imprisoned

Sh,82- Last three Fridays, since proving began, have gone to bed very early. Really exhausted. Realized that part of the going to bed is to be by myself —needed space in bed, alone and quiet. Rare for me to go to bed and leave daughters up watching TV. Could hear it and felt it invading my space. G26 Themes: invaded, liberty

Sh,83- It feels like my personality has been invaded, taken over. I7 Themes: seized, invaded, identity

Sh,84- Morning getting dressed, didn't really want to put clothes on, felt I was taking the first gulp of air that the first breathing animal took as it came out of the water, bursting through the surface, lungs expanding. As with the egg image (day 5), the movement is forceful, BURSTING with great relief. G6 Themes: transmutation, animal

Sh,85- Have noticed a difference in my spatial awareness. Am misjudging distances when driving not to a dangerous degree. Keep bumping into things and people in the house and street. B ? Themes: distances

Sh,87- Somerset countryside not big enough. E14 Themes: nature

Sh,88- Forgot to race downhill again. Voice sounded deeper. My immediate reaction, "Oh God, I'm turning into a man." Felt I was overwhelming colleague so didn't ask if I really was. I seemed to take up a lot of space in the room so I drew back and left. G5 Themes: grow, great, transmutation

Sh,89- Sensation as if tall. Q3 Themes: great, grow

Sh-9- Partner said, "I've never seen you so still. You look like a stone Buddha. Your speech is irritating, you can barely get to the end of your sentences." E1 Themes: isolation, talk

Sh,90- Feeling extremely tall. Feeling as if kitchen table too low. Q6 Themes: grow, great

Sh,91- Felt very low again, like being covered by a heavy blanket. I felt weighed down by it. B3 Themes: small, heavy

Sh,93- Felt the blanket descending on me again (happened exactly one week ago), and I suddenly felt exhausted. Lay down and slept for half an hour. Woke and felt heavy feelings in arms and legs. Felt panicky as I recognized same feelings of despair that characterized events of last week. B9 Themes: heavy

Sh,97- Had a big clearout in the cellar (note: on the same day I was constipated!) .Enjoyed this spring cleaning and throwing loads of stuff away. I was making space for ex-partner to store stuff he still has in house which is suffocating me. I need the space to breathe. Feeling that if he doesn't put his things into the space in the cellar I shall explode. Generally not as lax about things, giving people the "hard word." G11 suffocation, organization Themes: suffocation, organization

Sh,98- Feeling as if my right and left were equal, previously feeling as if my right side bigger. Q1 Themes: grow

Sh,99- Sat at the bus stop. Felt like a really small, frightened rabbit, with a large shadow of this great bird hovering over ready to pounce. G8 Themes: attacked, animal, transmutation, fearful, identity

IRIS.

Al,3- Despondency; thinks he is going to be very sick, then a disposition to laugh at his fears, which, however, soon return. Themes: fearful, disease, pleasure

Al,5- Vexed, irritable mood, disposed to find fault. Themes: bothered, censorious

He,2- Fears approaching illness. Themes: disease

JAMB.

He,1- Constantly desirous of sitting alone and reflecting. Themes: solitude, meditation

He,2- Nothing seemed right, when sitting, he wanted to lie; when lying, he wanted to rise again. Themes: wrong, movement, restless

He,4- Sudden great change in him after micturition, everything seems more beautiful and bright, sky and trees more joyous and clear; but after quarter of an hour everything became gloomy again. Themes: perfection, bright, pleasure

JATR.

Al,3- An ecstasy, as if an ideal had appeared to a poetic painter, or like that which sometimes comes to a dying person, ...a feeling of lovely warmth and ethereal lightness... Themes: perfection, pleasure, poetry

KALI-AR.

He,1- Scolding (censorious) morose, retired, quarrelsome and discontented, jealous, indifferent to everything,... Themes: reserved, censorious, jealousy, fight, discontented, indifference

He,2- Thought her head felt larger. Themes: great, grow

KALI-BI.

He,2- Misanthropy and ill humor, even to disgust of life. Themes: misanthropy, loathing

KALI-BR.

Al,11- ...gloomy ideas relative to his present and future condition, if an opinion could be formed from the signs of distress, such as weeping, moaning, and wringing his hands,... Themes: future, pessimism

Al,14- Great mental depression, a feeling (sensation) of approaching death. Themes: sadness, death

Al,16- A consciousness that the currents or sources of psychical force are hampered...(obstructed) sometimes makes an intellectual patient who is moderately bromized, reason himself into depression.... Themes: energy, obstructed, sadness

Al,19- Painful sadness, profound indifference, and almost disgust for life. Themes: sadness, indifference, grief

Al,2- General delirium, with hallucinations; delusions about persecution and violence. Themes: persecution, violence

Al,24- The patient, who has been violently excited, glorying (adoration) in his imaginary power of body and mind, becomes desponding sullen, melancholic, and frequently lachrymose, often even despairing. Themes: greatness, sadness, despair, vanity

Al,25- At times he cried most bitterly, yet twelve hours previously he was singing and dancing, saying he was "the happiest man alive". Themes: pleasure, perfection, music, unfortunate

Al,3- Decidedly insane; had delusions that lewd women had got into his mother's house; that he was pursued by the police; that his wife was threatened by members of the family; that he had thousands of dollars in gold sewed up in his clothing; (rich, wealth) Themes: lascivious, sexual, invaded, mother, home, officer, persecution, menaced, position, greatness, wife, family, money, wealth, clothes

Al,3- ...his character also had undergone a radical change, from having been very frank and brave, he had become excessively timid, and suspicious of every trifling circumstance; ...several times he attempted to throw himself from a window and battered down a door with an axe, in order to escape from some imaginary danger;... Themes: cowardice, suspicious, suicidal, height, escape, danger

Al,4- He imagined that he had been specially singled out (select) for divine vengeance... deploring his sad fate (destiny),...he informed me that he had been accused of robbing a friend, and that the officers were in search of him.... Themes: doomed, anger, accused, criminal, officer, persecution, friend, robber

Al,44- Felt as if everything that I feel, see or think, had been experienced before, as in a dream; this delusion is so strong that I could swear I dreamt it all. Themes: clairvoyance, unreal

Al,5- She had the erroneous idea that she was deserted by all her friends, and as a consequence she passed all her waking moments, which are not many in tears;...delusion that her child was dead, had taken fixed possession of her mind;...she declared that she saw it dead (corpse) before her, and when it was brought to her, she refused to acknowledge that it was hers, or had any resemblance to the one she imagined was dead. Themes: forsaken, friend, child, death, mortification, corpse, dwells

Al,6-...she fancied that the boarders in the hotel insulted her, and imagined that the weekly bills of the landlord (owner) were evidences of a conspiracy which had been got up against her father; ... while standing on the guards of the boat ...declared she had seen her brother fall overboard;... Themes: offenses, betrayed, fall, accidents, brother

He,10- Imagines he is singled out as an object of divine wrath (fury, rage); extreme drowsiness. Themes: anger, doomed, religious

He,11- Imagines she is a devil; cannot sleep; fears to be alone. Themes: devil, seized, identity, solitude

He,15- Frightful imaginings at night (in pregnant women during latter months), they are under impression that they have committed, or about to commit, some great crime and cruelty (brutality), such murdering their children or husbands. Themes: conscience, criminal, homicidal, wicked, child, husband

He,17- Delirium with delusions; thinks he is

pursued (hunt); will be poisoned; is selected (designated) for divine vengeance (revenge); that her child is dead, etc. Themes: persecution, poisoned, doomed, religious, child, death

He,22- Feels as if he would go out of his mind. Themes: insanity

He,23- ...constantly brooding over loss of a daughter; almost crazy; ... (child) Themes: mortification, lack, death, child, insanity, dwells

He,24- Hands constantly busy; all sorts of fearful delusions; walks the room groaning, bemoaning his fate (destine, doom); full of fear; unsteady.(inconstant) Themes: busy, fearful, doomed, confidence

He,29-... dread of impending destruction of all near her. Themes: misfortune

He,30- Great despondency; "feel as if they should go out of their minds." Themes: despair, insanity

He,31- ...religious delusions and feeling of moral deficiency; ...profound indifference and almost disgust for life. Themes: conscience, wicked, religious, indifference, grief

He,33- Great despondency, with insanity, a feeling of moral deficiency, or a religious delusion, from anemia. Themes: wicked, religious, insanity

He,37- Timid, suspicious, full of fear. Themes: timidity, fearful, suspicious

He,38- Much concerned (anxiety) about health; complains without cause;...uncontrollable sensation of fear and anxiety, thinks she is becoming deranged (insanity) ; change of life. Themes: disease, insanity, fearful

He,39-...fear and apprehension that she is losing her mind (insanity);...makes her utterly (completely) miserable to be looked at or spoken to; fear to see people; always depressed and low spirited;... Themes: fearful, insanity, approached, miserable, misanthropy, disappointment, unfortunate, approached, sadness

He,4-...constant worry, fears to see people or to be spoken to;...failure of mental and bodily strength;...constantly busy, tying his shoes, fumbling in his pockets, picking threads, etc. Themes: misanthropy, talk, busy, energy

KALI-C.

Al,13- He has anxious presentiments, in the evening. Themes: anticipation

Al,14- Sad presentiments of the future. Themes: misfortune, future

Al,15- At night after lying down, sad forebodings overtake him, on account of which he is unable to sleep. Themes: anticipation, sadness

Al,17- Fearful and anxious about her disease. Themes: fearful, disease

Al,19 - Fears that she cannot recover. Themes: disease

Al,2- Dread of being alone. Themes: solitude

Al,20- Apprehensiveness and aversion to society. Themes: misanthropy, solitude

Al,21- Apprehensiveness and great sadness. Themes: sadness

Al,22- Faint-hearted and despondent to an excessive degree. Themes: timidity, despair

Al,25- She is frightened with a loud cry, by an imaginary apparition (as for example, of a bird flying to the window). Themes: fearful, liberty, animal, fly, noise

Al,4- Very much depressed; she was obliged to weep much, because it was constantly in her thoughts that she must die. Themes: sadness, death, conscience

Al,44- Disagreeable mood; he is obstinate and frequently does not himself know what he wishes. Themes: obstinate, capricious

Al,45- Disagreeable mood; she longs for things with impetuosity; is contented with nothing, is beside herself, and gets into rage if everything does not go according to her wishes, and frequently does not herself know what she really wishes to have. Themes: impatience, discontented, anger, contradiction, capricious

Al,7- Sad, lonely (solitary) ; she seeks society in order to enliven (animate) herself. Themes: sadness, solitude, company, lack

Ha,11- Anxiety and dislike company. Themes: company, loathing

Ha,14- He is afraid that he might not get well. Themes: disease

Ha,15- Apprehensive and anxious about her disease. Themes: disease

Ha,17- Troubled ideas about the future. Themes: future

Ha,20- Irresolution. Themes: irresolution

Ha,23- Fearful about being alone. Themes: solitude
Ha,25- Readily frightened, especially by a slight touch of the body. Themes: fearful, touch
Ha,26- She is frightened by an imaginary appearance (e.g. as if a bird was flying toward the window) and she utters a loud scream. Themes: fearful, animal, liberty, fly
Ha,30- Peevish mood, as if she could not do anything to suit (satisfy) herself. Themes: anger, discontented, himself
Ha,31- She is always in antagonism with herself; she knows not what she wants, and feels exceedingly unhappy. Themes: himself, antagonism, doubtful, unfortunate
Ha,32- Contrary disposition; he is self-willed (obstinate) and often does not know himself what he wishes. (indecision) Themes: antagonism, obstinate, doubtful, confidence, contrary
Ha,33- Contrary mood; she demands (order, command) impetuously; is not satisfied with anything (dissatisfied) ; she is beside herself, and furiously angry; if everything does not go according to her wishes, and often does not herself know what she really wants. Themes: antagonism, dictatorial, anger, contradiction, doubtful, contrary
Ha,41- Very peevish, she has no pleasure in anything. Themes: anger
Ha,44- Cross and angry thoughts, in the morning, on awaking, so that he gnashes with his teeth. Themes: anger, bothered
Ha,49- Changeful mood, now good and quiet, then passionate and angry about trifles; often hopeful, often despondent. Themes: passionate, hopeless, anger,
Ha,5- Sad, she feels lonesome (solitary, lonely); she seeks for company to cheer her up. Themes: solitude, company, pleasure
Ha,51- Lack of presence of mind; he cannot proceed right along in his business. Themes: dispersion, unfit, succeed
Ha,8- Very ill-humored; she has to weep much, because it was constantly on her mind that she had to die. (doomed, sentenced) Themes: death, doomed
He,10- Timid and apprehensive of future and about her disease. Themes: cowardice, disease, future
He,11- Fear of being alone; fears she will die. Themes: solitude, death
He,16- Very easily frightened; shrieks about imaginary appearances; starts when touched. Themes: ghosts, touch, fearful
He,17- Is frightened and cries out whenever he is touched lightly on his feet. Themes: fearful, touch
He,5- Imagines seeing birds flying in room; he tries to catch them. (seize) Themes: animal, liberty, fly
He,6- Great aversion to being alone. Themes: company
He,9- ...constantly in antagonism which herself; frequently hopeful, frequently despondent; frets (worry) about everything; peevish impatient, contented with nothing. Themes: antagonism, himself, despair, bothered, discontented, impatience

KALI-CY.

Al,3- Had occasion to get angry, but could not; felt more like laughing instead. Themes: anger, pleasure, antagonism
Al,4- For two days, desire to find fault; crossness almost uncontrollable on entering the room; while the cold air produces good spirits. Themes: wrong, bothered, censorious
Al,5- At 7 p.m., while walking out of doors, feelings of crossness; carries on a kind of conversation within himself, as if quarreling with someone with whom he had previously disagreed; thinks what he will reply in case certain things are said to him. Themes: bothered, antagonism, offenses, discussion, fight, himself

KALI-FCY.

Al,1- Feeling of sadness and some disposition to tears, caused by an impression that he was soon to die and leave his friends; disposition to take a sad view of the beauties of autumn; the apprehension of approaching sickness and death can be overcome by reason, but soon returns. Themes: sadness, friend, nature, death, lack, disease, helplessness

KALI-I.

Al,11- Very apprehensive and lachrymose, as if some evil were impending, ... Themes: misfortune, anticipation, menaced

Al,12- He dreads to return of dawn (morning), and the most trivial details of daily life seem insupportable to him. Themes: loathing

Al,16- Very peevish and excited; everything goes wrong, and she is ready to quarrel with every one. Themes: anger, wrong, fight

Al,17- Feelings easily disturbed, as if something was always happening to trouble her. Themes: bothered

Ha,8- Whining; apprehensive as from threatened accident. Themes: menaced, accidents

He,6- Very great irritability and unwonted harshness of demeanor (behavior); his children, to whom he is devoted and attached, become burdensome to him; very passionate and spiteful temper;...constant apprehension of impending evil. Themes: offenses, child, forsakes, bothered, misfortune, passionate, revengeful

KALI-N.

Al,19- Perverse hypochondriac mood; discontented with himself and the world, peevish irritable, ... Themes: wicked, himself, discontented

Al,4- Depressed; she thinks she must die. Themes: death

KALI-P.

He,15- Profound hypochondria and melancholia, weariness of life and fear of death, suspiciousness... Themes: sadness, death, suspicious

He,17- Homesickness, morbid activity of memory, haunted (obsessed) by visions of past, and longing after them. Themes: homesickness, past, nostalgia, seized

He,3- Delirium tremens; horrors of drunkards; fear, sleeplessness, ... and suspicion; rambling (incoherent) talk... Themes: suspicious

He,4- Says she is eternally and irretrievably damned;...food and medicine must be forcibly administered. 0 Melancholia religious. Themes: conscience, doomed, suspicious

He,5- Anxiety, nervous dread without special cause, gloomy moods, fancies, taking dark views of things, dark forebodings. Themes: pessimism, anticipation

KALM.

Al,1- A feeling of anxiety; feel as though something dreadful (calamitous) was going to happen to me. Themes: misfortune

Al,3- Feels like scolding (censure) everybody... Themes: censorious

KEROSE.

Al,1- As you breathe the vapor you seem to float into a wavy maze (labyrinth, puzzle), with a sense of complete loneliness; there appears to be but one object in the universe, and that object is yourself; on recovery the first thing seen is deemed (judge, conclude) the next only existence in the universe; ... Themes: floating, solitude

KREOS.

Al,10- When she undertakes to accomplish anything and has gone ten or twelve steps, she remains standing, and does not know what she had intended (planned) to do. Themes: lost

Al,4- She was depressed; the longing (desire) for death constantly became greater. Themes: death

Al,5- Towards evening her spirits were much depressed, and she was doubtful whether she would ever be well again. Themes: sadness, doubtful, disease

He,11- Seeks for unpleasant things and broods over them. Themes: mortification, dwells

He,4- Thinks herself well. 0 Metritis Themes: disease, antagonism

He,5- Sorrowful mood, inclined to weep or longing (desire) for death;... Themes: death

LAC-AC.

He,2- Averse to business or what formerly was pleasant to do; lazy (indolent); dislikes to read or think; finds fault, is sarcastic, exacting. (exigent, severe) Themes: loathing, work, censorious, sarcasm

LAC-C.

Al,N-18- After menses, imagines all sorts of things about snakes. Themes: animal

Al,N-19- Wakes at night with a sensation that she was lying on a large snake. Themes: great, animal

Al,N -8- Is impressed with the idea that all she says is a lie; it seems to be very difficult to speak the truth (liar, dissimulator), but continually distrusts things (suspicious); when reading anything she rapidly changes the meaning, omitting or adding things. (mischievous) Themes: liar, wicked, suspicious, deceitful, feigning,

Al,N-11- Thinks that she is looked down upon (despised) by every one, that she is of no importance in life, and feels insulted thereat. (unimportant, worthless) Themes: despised, contemptuous, himself, offenses

Al,N-15- Feels very short in morning; while walking; same in evening. Themes: small, confidence

Al,N-28- Fear of disease; of consumption; of heart disease. (tuberculosis) Themes: disease, heart, infection

Al,N-33- Depression of spirits, doubts her ability and success, thinks she will have heart disease and die of it. Themes: sadness, confidence, unfit, succeed, disease, heart, death

Al,N-36- Fears she will become unable to perform her duties. Themes: duty, unfit

Al,N-37- Fear of death, with anxious expression of countenance. Themes: death

Al,N-39- Wakes distressed, and obliged to rise and occupy herself in some manner; fears she will be crazy. Themes: duty, busy, insanity

Al,N-40- Has a great fear of falling down stairs at times. Themes: fall

Al,N-43- Intense ugliness (repulsiveness, offensiveness) and hatefulness (odiousness, repellently); writes to her best friends all sorts of mean(vulgar) and contemptible things. Themes: contemptuous, loathing, friend, wicked

He,10- Imagine he wears some one's nose. Themes: double, identity

He,11- Imagines to be dirty. (obscene, vulgar, dishonorable) Themes: dirty, wicked

He,12- Imagines to see spiders. Themes: animal

He,13- Woke at daylight feeling that she is a loathsome (repulsive), horrible mass of disease (while the breasts were affected); could not bear to look at any portion of her body (loathing, himself), not even hands, as it intensified feeling of disgust and horror; could not bear to have any part of her body touch another , had to keep even fingers apart; felt that if she could not in some way get out of her body, she should soon become crazy . Themes: horrible, disease, touch, insanity, ugly, loathing,

He,14-..;sometimes imagines heart or breathing are going to stop, or otherwise frightens himself, and this makes heart beat violently; occasionally very depressed, and fancies he is going out of his mind. (insanity) Themes: stagnation, death, heart, insanity

He,15- Sensation or delusion as if surrounded by myriads of snakes, some running like lightning up and down inside the skin ; some that are inside feel long and thin; fears to put her feet on floor, lest she should tread (walk) on them and make them squirm (shake) and wind (round) around her legs; is afraid to look behind her, for fear that she will see snakes there, does not dream of them and is seldom troubled with them after dark; on going to bed she was afraid to shut her eyes for fear that a large snake, the size of her arm, would hit her in the face. Themes: surrounded, crawling, persecution, touch, animal, attacked, dark, bite

He,16- Worries (care) herself lest (fear) pimples (boil) which appear during menses will prove to be little snakes, and twine and twist around each other. Themes: disease, animal,

He,17- On lying down either by day or night begins to think how horrible it would be if a very sharp pain, like a knife, should go through her, and thought of it causes great mental distress. Themes: hurt, attacked, horrible, pointed

He,19- Cannot bear to be left alone for an instant. Themes: solitude, company

He,20- No desire to live. Themes: loathing

He,21- Sits and looks under chairs, table, sofa and everything in room, expecting yet dreading (fear) to see some terrible monster creep forth and feeling all the time , that if it does, it will drive her raving mad; she is not afraid in dark, it is only in light where she can imagine that she can see them. Themes: fearful, horrible, crawling, insanity, light

He,24- When paroxysms of intense nervousness (anxiety) come on, feels like tearing off her clothes; takes off her rings; cannot bear anything to touch her, ... Themes: touch, loathing, tear, clothes

He,25- Had to keep her fingers apart from each other. Themes: touch

He,26- Depression of spirits, doubts her ability (competence, aptitude) and success (prospering, progressing, achieving) , thinks she will have heart disease and die of it. Themes: sadness, unfit, confidence, succeed, disease, heart, death

He,27- Chronic "blue" condition; everything seems so dark that it can grow no darker. Themes: sadness

He,29- Fears she will become unable to perform (achieve, accomplish) her duties.(responsibility) Themes: unfit, succeed, duty

He,30- Fear of death, with anxious expression of countenance.(face) Themes: death

He,31- Very nervous; constant dread; a feeling as if she was going to become unconscious (faint, fit) Themes: fit

He,32- Wakes distressed, and obliged to rise and occupy herself in some manner; fears she will be crazy. Themes: busy, insanity

He,33- Has a great fear of falling down stairs at times. Themes: fall, height

He,36- Feels insulted because she thinks she is looked down (scorn, despised) upon by everyone. Themes: offenses, despised

He,37- Intense ugliness (repulsiveness, hideousness) and hatefulness (offensiveness); writes to her best friends all sorts of mean and contemptible things. (disdainful) Themes: offensive, contemptuous, wicked, friend

He,40- Feels weak, and nerves so thoroughly out of order, that she cannot bear one finger touch another. Themes: energy, touch, loathing

He,5- Very restlessness; cannot concentrate her thoughts or mind to read; wants to leave everything as soon as it is commenced. Themes: unfit

He,6- Is impressed with idea that all she says is a lie. (false) Themes: liar

He,7- Every time a symptom appears she feels very confident that it is not attributable to medicine, but that it is some settled disease. Themes: disease

He,8- Sensation as if she was going deranged, when sitting still and thinking; sometimes she has most horrible sights presented to her mental vision (not always snakes), feels horribly afraid that they will take objective form and show themselves to her natural eye. Themes: insanity, horrible, fearful

He,9- Thinks she is looked down (contempted, scorned, despised) upon by everyone, that she is of no importance in life. (self-contemptuous) Themes: despised, contemptuous, himself

LAC-D.

Al,N-1- Depression of spirits; don't care to live (indifferent) ; question as to quietest and most certain way of hastening (accelerate) one's death. Themes: sadness, indifference, suicidal

Al,N-10- Has no fear of death but is sure is going to die. Themes: death, fearless

Al,N-4- Imagines that all her friends will die and that she must go to a convent. (purification, solitude) Themes: friend, penitence, solitude, death, religious, lack

Al,N-9- Great despondency on account of the disease, is sure he is going to die in 24 hours. Themes: hopeless, disease, death

He,10- Has no fear (fearless) of death but is sure he is going to die. Themes: death, fearless

He,2- Depression of spirits; don't care to live, question as to quietest and most certain way of hastening one's death. Themes: indifference, death, suicidal

He,5- Imagines that all her friends will die and that she must go to a convent. (purification, salvation) Themes: penitence, solitude, death, religious, friend, others, forsaken

He,9- Great despondency on account of the disease, is sure he is going to die in twenty-four hours. Themes: death, disease, doomed

LAC-F.

Al,N-3- Fear falling down stairs, but without vertigo. Themes: fall

Al,N-4- Morbid conscientiousness; every little fault appeared a crime. Themes: criminal, conscientious, conscience

Al,N-5- Mental illusion that the corners of furniture, or any pointed object near her, were about to run into eyes;... Themes: hurt, pointed

LACH.

Al,11- An unusual inclination to be communicative. (affectionate) Themes: talk

Al,15- The more cause for fretfulness, the greater inclination for humour, jest, satire, and humorous fancies. Themes: sarcasm, pleasure

Al,19- So great apprehensiveness while riding in the open air that it seemed to him some great evil (hurtful, injurious) was impending (imminent), like an evil foreboding; it torments him for more than an hour. Themes: menaced, tormented, anticipation,

Al,22- Sudden doubts (indecision) arise about truths (veracity) of which he had hitherto (before) been convinced (converted), in the afternoon. Themes: doubtful, knowledge, confidence

Al,23- It frequently seems to him wrong to read long at a time, although the subject interests him. Themes: conscience, wrong, knowledge

Al,25- Towards evening very unusual almost crazy jealousy, as foolish as it is irresistible. Themes: jealousy, insanity, ridiculous

Al,28- At times, can only think for a long time of some fancied worry. Themes: mortification

Al,30- Impatient; desires positive answers when this is not practicable. Themes: impatience, obstinate

Al,32- Becomes easily peevish and mistrustful; believes himself intentionally injured (hurt, prejudice) by all his environments, and attaches the most hateful significance to the most innocent occurrences. Themes: suspicious, offenses, persecution, damage

Al,33- Unusually contentious (hostile) and obstinate, so that he quarrels with everything about him. Themes: fight, obstinate, discussion

Al,34- So quarrelsome that he disputes with a mother about the age of her daughter, and affirms the younger to be the elder. Themes: fight, antagonism, discussion

Al,41- Need of being very busy, without the slightest perseverance. Themes: busy, dispersion

Al,43- He is impelled to productive work in the evening, although he had been much fatigued during the day ... writes with the greatest freedom and increased vigor about everything he knows;... Themes: liberty, energy, knowledge, work,

Al,44- Increased power of originality in all mental work, increased activity of fancy; scenes and occurrences throng to him in an unusual amount. Themes: knowledge

Al,45- No sooner does one idea occur to him then a number of others follow in succession while he is writing down, so that he is unable to finish the record. Themes: dispersion, unfit, knowledge

Al,5- A kind of ecstasy, as after sublime impressions, or excessive joy, throughout the day; he constantly wishes to talk and do much, and even more seems to be at his command.(control, domination) Themes: pleasure, greatness, busy, talk, seized, planning

Al,54- Dilatory (slow); he cannot accomplish his business as usual. Themes: work, succeed

Al,66- It became extremely difficult for him to listen to others, though his hearing was not impaired; The words just spoken seemed obliterated. Themes: obstructed

Al,7- It seems to him during the day that he has dreamed everything that has happened, only somewhat different.(d,j... vu) Themes: clairvoyance

He,12- Delirium; fears she will be damned. Themes: conscience, doomed

He,14- Delirium from overwatching, overfatigue; loss of fluids; excessive study. Themes: duty, energy

He,16- Most extraordinary loquacity, making speeches in very select (finest, excellent) phrases (pretentious), but jumping off to most heterogeneous subjects; at the same time proud (haughty), full of mistrust. 0Mania. Themes: talk, haughty, suspicious, greatness

He,17- Religious monomania, fear of being damned (condemned to eternal punishment). Themes: religious, doomed, mania

He,19- Insane jealousy. Themes: jealousy

He,21-...imagines he is followed by enemies who are trying to harm him; attempts to leave room as if frightened by visions behind him. Themes: enemy, persecution, hurt, attacked, escape

He,22- She is tempted to commit suicide. Themes: suicidal

He,24- Inclination to be communicative; vivid imagination; extremely impatient at tedious and dry (arid) things. Themes: talk, bother, impatience

He,25- Is morbidly talkative and gives a rambling (discursive) account of her ailments. Themes: disease, talk

He,26- Jealousy, with frightful images, great tendency to mock, to satire and ridiculous ideas. Themes: jealousy, contemptuous, ridiculous, sarcasm

He,30- Undertakes many things, perseveres in nothing. Themes: succeed, dispersion

He,31- Disinclined to his own proper work; complains of trifles. Themes: loathing, work

He,32- Aversion of women to marry. Themes: loathing, sexual, union

He,33- ...want of self control; lascivious; felt as if she was clear (pure) animal right through, whilst of all mental power was dormant; sensation as if hands of stronger power, as if charmed (enchanted), and as if could not break the spell (charm). (possessed, wildness) Themes: lascivious, sexual, energy, seized, animal, greatness, wild, identity

He,34-...repugnance to society and dislike to talk; solicitude about future, with disgust of life; inclination to doubt everything; mistrusts (suspicious) and misconstrues (misjudge) ...0 Melancholia. Themes: talk, grief, future, doubtful, suspicious, misanthropy, loathing

He,35- Feels extremely sad, unhappy and distressed in mind on waking in morning. Themes: sadness, unfortunate

He,39- Weak and unhappy ,particularly in morning, when she feels, on awaking, friendless and forsaken; ...(deserted) has had domestic troubles. 0 Melancholia Themes: forsaken, unfortunate, friendless, home, sadness

He,40- He wishes to do a great deal; begins many things. (undertakes) Themes: succeed, busy

He,41- Dread (fear) of death, fears to go to bed ; fears of being poisoned. Themes: fearful, death, suspicious, poisoned

He,43- Weary of life, looks at everything from dark side;... Themes: tedium, loathing, pessimism

He,44- Satiety (loathing?) of life with longing (desiring) for death. Themes: tedium, death, loathing

He,45- She is tormented by the idea that her better principles (ideals) might be overcome (beaten) by irresistible desire to suicide. (lost: moral) 0 Mania. Themes: tormented, seized, suicidal

He,47- Amorousness; amativeness. Themes: sexual, lascivious

He,5- Quick comprehension; mental activity, with almost prophetical (oracular, predictive) perception; ecstasy; a kind of trance. Themes: clairvoyance, seized, knowledge

He,51- Proud; jealous, suspicious; developing into mania. Themes: jealousy, suspicious, haughty, mania

He,52- Malice; thinks only of mischief. (evil, harm, hurt) Themes: wicked

He,54- A girl, after excessive study, uses exalted language; exceedingly particular about language she uses, often correcting after using a word, and substituting another of very similar meaning, talking about being under influence of a superior power. (possessed) 0 Mania. Themes: seized, knowledge, perfection, greatness, wrong

He,55- Nightly attacks of anxiety; afraid of chorea, gets cramps in calves from fear; nausea, heavy feeling in abdomen... Themes: disease, infection

He,59- Ailments from fright (fear), disappointed love or jealousy. Themes: fearful, disappointment, jealousy, love

He,60- After a jealous quarrel, she put both hands to her chest and cried out "Oh! my heart!" then fell down and was in an asphyxiated state for nearly twenty- four hours;... Themes: jealousy, fight, disease, feigning, heart, suffocation

He,8- Thinks: she is somebody else in the hands (seized) of a stronger power; (supremacy, superiority).or that she is dead, and preparations are made for funeral (cortege) or that she is nearly dead and wishes some one would help her off; herself pursued by enemies, or fears medicine is poison; there are robbers in house and wants to jump out the window; herself under super-human control; visions real, he will die. (helplessness, desire; aid, comfort, salvation) Themes: death, funeral, helplessness, seized, persecution, poisoned, suicidal, identity, greatness, enemy, robber, home,

He,9- Imagines he is followed (pursued) by enemies who are trying to harm (hurt, injure) him; attempts to leave room as if frightened by visions behind him. Themes: persecution, hurt, escape, enemy, attacked

LACHN.

Al,5- Became much excited over a trifle; he had suppressed his anger, in the evening. Themes: anger, suppressed

LAM.

Al,1- Weeping mood; she wept as if she had been abandoned. (forsaken) Themes: forsaken

Al,2- Extraordinary sadness; he thought he had been blamed for reverses (failure) for which he was blameless, and in consequence was obliged to suffer;... Themes: sadness, conscience, mortification, injustice

Al,5-...,(fixed ideas) so that at last she becomes sad about it, and thinks she shall lose her reason. Themes: mania, insanity

LAUR.

Al,8-Very lachrymose and despondent (sad) mood; he would rather die than live. Themes: hopeless, death

He,6- Fear and anxiety about imaginary evils; despondency.(desperation) Themes: misfortune, sadness

LED.

Al,10- Fretful; he went by himself, and almost weeping wished to die. Themes: helplessness, death

Al,11- Morose mood, with much uneasiness and irresolution; he is unable to reflect constantly upon anything, or work with a quiet mind. Themes: restless, irresolution, unfit, meditation

Al,12- Discontented all day with his companions, which at last amounts to misanthropy. Themes: misanthropy, friend, discontented

Ha,329- All day long; discontented with his fellow-creatures (friend, relations), which at last amounted to misanthropy. Themes: discontented, solitude, misanthropy

Ha,333- Cross: he retired into solitude, and almost weeping he longed for death. Themes: bothered, solitude, death

Ha,335- Passionate: he easily gives way to angry expressions. Themes: passionate, anger

Ha,336- All day long great seriousness(gravity); he regarded everything that happened to him in a serious and thoughtful (meditative) manner. Themes: meditation

Ha,338- Calm and happy disposition with love for work and self-contented. Themes: peace, pleasure, work

He,2- After nightmare, fears to go to sleep lest she die. Themes: fearful, death

He,4- Discontented; morose; hates his fellow beings. Themes: discontented, anger, misanthropy

LEPI.

Al,1- She fancies herself alone in a graveyard, pursued by a ghost, and screams so that her voice is lost next day; yet nobody hears her. (helpless) Themes: solitude, funeral, persecution, ghosts, helplessness

Al,6- Deep melancholy; with thoughts of sickness. Themes: sadness, disease

LIL-T.

Al,10 -Profound mental depression; to the prover "the heavens seemed brass and the earth iron;" an apprehension of moral obliquity weighed grievously upon her, for about ten days after the sexual excitement,... Themes: conscience, wicked, sexual

Al,15- Apprehensive as from impending disease or calamity (misfortune); fears insanity; fears heart disease; fears she is incurable; often with moderate or sub acute uterine or ovarian inflammation. Themes: disease, misfortune, menaced, insanity, heart,

Al,16- Worse on going to bed; can't go to sleep; wild (tumultuous, uncontrollable) feeling in the head as though I should go crazy (insane) and no one would take care of me (forsaken, helpless); thoughts of suicide; how much opium would put me to sleep forever, and who would find my body, and who would care; ... (friendless, abandoned, deserted) Themes: insanity, helplessness, suicidal, friendless, wild, forsaken

Al,17-... and expressed to her sister great fear of insanity.(through the proving) Themes: sister, insanity

Al,19- Apprehension of some calamity or serious disease very much increased. Themes: disease, misfortune

Al,2- Excitement, weeping, feeling as if she were two persons, at night. Themes: double, identity

Al,24- ..a feeling of irritation and of something wrong in abdomen and pelvic organs (disease); feels hurried (fast) and yet incapable (incompetent), as if she had a great deal (busy) to do and cannot do it. Themes: disease, hurry, unfit, succeed, duty

Al,25- While attending a lecture (speech), desire to hit the lecturer, and in the evening desirous of swearing and damning the fire and things generally, and to think and speak obscene things; disposed to strike and hit persons; as these feelings came, the uterine pains passed away. Themes: violence, offensive, hurt, fire, sexual, wicked

Al,27- Symptoms came down on her like a sudden cloud, ...she lost vigor and snap (vitality), ...with all this depression comes a desire for fine (quality) things of all kinds; she is dissatisfied with what she has and is envious of others. (sophistication) Themes: energy, envy, ambition

Al,3- A sense as if she were going to be crazy, if she did not hang on to herself, and hold tight. Themes: insanity, helplessness

Al,30- Constant hurried (precipitation) feeling as of imperative duties and utter inability to perform them; during the sexual excitement. Themes: hurry, duty, unfit, sexual,

Al,32- Perceptive and reflexive faculties seem benumbed (confused), whereas at first she was overactive and seemed to be two individuals. Themes: obstructed, double

Al,351- The sexual desire, dormant hitherto, was so strongly aroused that the prover said, "I am afraid of myself, I seem possessed of a demon." Themes: sexual, lascivious, seized, devil

Al,40-...I can see around me any number of things I must do, but cannot force myself to do anything. Themes: duty, unfit

Al,45- She can't think; acts without thought; keeps walking fast as though by instinct; feels hurried, but doesn't know why; is forgetful, can't decide for herself; must depend on others. Themes: obstructed, hurry, irresolution, unfit, knowledge

Al,47- Everything seems unreal to me. Themes: unreal

Al,49- She dreads saying anything to anybody, lest she should say something wrong, and yet she wants to walk. Themes: talk, wrong, confidence

Al,9- Depression of spirits; constant inclination to weep, with fearfulness, and apprehension of suffering from some terrible internal disease, already seated. Themes: sadness, disease, fearful,

He,10- Aversion to being alone, and yet no dread felt. Themes: company, solitude

He,12- Listless, inert, yet does not want to sit still (quiet); restless, yet does not want to walk; hurried manner, desire to do something, yet feels no ambition; feeling as of imperative duties and utter (complete) inability (incapacity, incompetence) to perform them; sexual excitement. Themes: paralysis, restless, hurry, duty, sexual, succeed, unfit

He,13-...indifference about everything being done for her.(help) Themes: indifference

He,14- Anxiety; fearful that the symptoms

indicate an internal organic disease; very marked in both male and female. Themes: disease

He,16- Doubts her salvation; thinks she is doomed to expiate her sins and those of her family; ... (redemption, salvation) (sacrifice) Themes: religious, doomed, salvation, family, penitence

He,4- Believes her disease to be incurable; that she has some organic disease that nobody understands. (misunderstanding, misjudged) Themes: disease, knowledge

He,5- Tormented about her salvation. Themes: tormented, salvation, religious,

He,6- Crazy feeling on top of head; wild feeling in head, with confusion of ideas. Themes: insanity, wild

He,7- Dementia produced by business discouragements and sexual excesses. Themes: work, insanity, hopeless, sexual, failure

He,8- Disposition to weep, with pain in back; has to keep very busy to repress (control) sexual desire. Themes: sexual, suppressed

He,9- Disposed to curse, to strike, to think of obscene things; as these mental states came, uterine irritation abated.(reduced) Themes: offensive, hurt, lascivious, violence, sexual

LIM.

Al,3- The great disinclination to work, and inability to accomplish much, which he had experienced since the sea-bath, disappeared completely during the day, and gave place to mental quiet and steadiness, with constancy and perseverance in performing very irksome duties. Themes: loathing, unfit, duty, succeed, work

LIPP.

Al,2- Feeling of great apprehension, while riding in a carriage; a kind of anxiety in the heart, as of impending misfortune, together with a kind of homesickness. Themes: heart, menaced, accidents, misfortune, homesickness

LITH.

He,2- Disposed to weep about lonesome condition. Themes: solitude

LOB-S.

He,1- Much depressed, tearful, unhappy. Themes: sadness, unfortunate

He,2- Bad effects from grief.(ailments from) Themes: grief, disease

He,4- Great depression of spirits; unhappy state of mind,... Themes: sadness, unfortunate

LYC.

Al,10- He cries and howls, at first about past and then about future troubles. Themes: future, past

Al,113- Excited, busy mood in the evening, without perseverance, changing from one subject to another, with difficulty of fixing the thoughts, and greater difficulty in accomplishing anything; while reading fell asleep... Themes: restless, dispersion, succeed

Al,12- If one looks at her to say anything serious she is obliged to laugh. Themes: antagonism, pleasure

Al,127- Indecision and loss of confidence. Themes: confidence, doubtful, irresolution

Al,128- He is unable to do anything, cannot think; passes his time with trifles, without being able to make up his mind what to do. Themes: confidence, doubtful, unfit

Al,2- Delirious, raging, envious, reproachful, presumptuous, and imperious. Themes: anger, envy, censorious, haughty, greatness, dictatorial

Al,32- She became very miserable... Themes: miserable, unfortunate

Al,36- Hypochondriac, complaining mood; he feels unhappy. Themes: unfortunate

Al,4- A kind of living (presence) outside of herself, as in the commencement of fever. Themes: double

Al,40 -If people come near her, she is immediately attacked with anxiety at the pit of the stomach. Themes: approached, suspicious

Al,43- Anxious thoughts, as if she were about to die, for which she even prepared by thinking of her farewell messages, in the morning... Themes: death, organization
Al,44- Loss of confidence in his own vigor. Themes: confidence, energy
Al,45- While walking in open air, apprehensiveness and attacks of vertigo. Themes: fit
Al,49- Fear of going to bed in the evening. (sleep?) Themes: fearful
Al,50- In the evening on entering a room he is attacked with fear, as though he saw some one; even during the day he believes that he hears some one in the room. Themes: noise, fearful, invaded, suspicious
Al,51- In the evening, in the dark, he is seized with fear when a door that he wishes to open moves with difficulty. Themes: dark, seized, imprisoned
Al,52- Great fear of frightful images which her fancy conjures(charm) up, in the evening, and lachrymose during the day. Themes: fearful, horrible, seized
Al,55- She flees from her own children. Themes: forsakes, child
Al,6- Desires to be alone. Themes: solitude
Al,89- She cannot endure the slightest opposition, and is speedily beside herself from peevishness (cross). Themes: contradiction, anger
Al,91- She is overpowered (defeat) by many unpleasant recollections (memory), about which she becomes vexed; even at night on waking. Themes: seized, past, mortification, bothered
Al,92- Easily roused to anger and scorn. Themes: contemptuous, anger
Al,94- Indolent, obstinate (inflexible), rebellious (revolutionary, dissident), passionate, wrathful. (angry) Themes: antagonism, anger, obstinate, passionate,
Al,96- Quarrelsome rage, partly at herself partly at others. Themes: himself, anger, fight, others
Al,97- As if out of her mind, she seeks quarrels, makes unfounded reproaches, is most exceedingly violent, and strikes those whom she thus insults. Themes: fight, offensive, violence, hurt
Ha,1- Hypochondriac, tormenting mood; he feels unhappy. Themes: tormented, unfortunate
Ha,18- He weeps and cries, at first, about the past, then about the coming evils. Themes: misfortune, past
Ha,19- Great oppression in the scrobiculus cordis from vexation. Themes: oppression, bothered
Ha,25- Great fear of phantoms, (ghosts) which crowd upon her fancy in the evening; during the day she is disposed to weep. Themes: ghosts, surrounded
Ha,26- In the evening in the dark, he is frightened because a door he wants to open, opens with difficulty. (confined, restricted) Themes: fearful, imprisoned, dark
Ha,27- He is afraid (fear) in the evening, on entering a room, as if he saw somebody; by day also he sometimes imagines he hears somebody in the room. Themes: fearful, suspicious, invaded
Ha,28- She is afraid of being alone. Themes: solitude
Ha,32- Lack of confidence in his strength.(power, vigor) Themes: confidence, energy
Ha,34- Distrustful, suspicious, inclined to take things ill. Themes: suspicious
Ha,35- Extremely distrustful and suspicious. Themes: suspicious
Ha,47- She thinks of a number of disagreeable occurrences in former(past) times, which vex her, even at night, when she wakes up. Themes: past, mortification
Ha,48- He has trouble to conceal (mask, hide) his internal obstinacy and vexation. (dissimulated) Themes: obstinate, suppressed
Ha,50- He smiles without being merry, capricious. Themes: feigning, capricious, antagonism
Ha,55- She cannot bear the least contradiction, and at once gets beside herself for vexation. Themes: contradiction, bothered
Ha,56- Angry fury, partly against himself, and partly against others. Themes: himself, anger, others
Ha,58- He quarrels in mind with absent persons. Themes: fight
Ha,59- Insanity and fury, breaking out in envy, pretensions (inflated) and ordering (dictatorial) others about. Themes: greatness, envy, dictatorial, anger, haughty
Ha,60- As if insane she seeks for quarrels, makes ungrounded reproaches abuses

(insulting) most violently and beats the person whom she abuses. Themes: censorious, offensive, fight, violence, anger

Ha,68- After being anxious, there is a great inclination to laugh about trifles, for several hours, and then weeping for half an hour without cause. Themes: pleasure, sadness

Ha,78- He cannot do nor think anything; he spends his time in trifling, and is not able to resolve to do what he has to do. Themes: dispersion, unfit, duty

Ha,8- When other persons come too near her she feels anguish in the scrobiculus cordis. Themes: approached

Ha,9- She flees (desert) from her own children. Themes: forsakes, child

He,14- Dread (fear) of men ; of solitude, irritability and melancholy. Themes: fearful, misanthropy, solitude, sadness

He,17- ...imperiousness(domineering, despotic) ; speaks with an air of command (ordering, domination) ; manner stiff (severe ,obstinate) and pretentious;... Themes: greatness, dictatorial, obstinate, talk

He,20- Melancholy: has doubts about her salvation; before catamenia; in mild (pacific) characters. Themes: religious, salvation, mildness

He,24- Easily frightened (afraid) and starts up; feels frightened at everything, even ringing of door bell. Themes: fearful, noise

He,25- Anthropophobia (in children); fear of phantoms in evening, with anguish. Themes: misanthropy, child, ghosts

He,26- Anxious thoughts, as if about to die, for which she prepares farewell (departure, adieu) messages. Themes: death, organization

He,28- Amativeness or amorousness. Themes: sexual, love

He,29- Want of self confidence; indecision; timidity; resignation. Themes: confidence, doubtful, yielding, timidity, doubtful

He,30- Loss (want) of confidence; in his own vigor (vitality, strength); in physician and remedies. Themes: confidence, energy, disease

He,31- Sensitive, irritable disposition; peevish and cross on getting awake; easily excited to anger; cannot endure slightest opposition, and is speedily beside herself. Themes: sensitive, anger, bothered, contradiction

He,32- Obstinate, defiant (contrary), arbitrary (capricious?); seeks disputes. Themes: defiant, obstinate, fight, dictatorial, contrary

He,35- Misanthropic; flies even from his own children. Themes: misanthropy, forsakes, child

He,36- Distrustful, suspicious and fault (mistake) finding. (judgment) Themes: fearful, suspicious, wrong

He,37- Haughty, reproachful and overbearing.(despotic) Themes: haughty, censorious, dictatorial

He,38- Parsimonious (economical), greedy (avaricious), malicious (malevolent) and pusillanimous.(cowardice) Themes: egotism, avarice, cowardice, wicked

He,39- Ailments from fright, anger, mortification, or vexation, with reserved displeasure. Themes: fearful, mortification, anger, suppressed, grief, bothered, reserved

He,40- Nervous action weakened; threatened softening of brain from overwork, or metastasis of ulcers suddenly healed. Themes: work, disease

He,9- Absent minded; supposes to be in two places at a time. Themes: separated, double

LYSS.

Al,12- Feeling as if I had heard, or was about to hear something bad... Themes: news, misfortune

Al,13- Mind much depressed; felt as if something disagreeable was about to happen. Themes: misfortune

Al,14- Feeling as if something annoying was about to happen; goes off when thinking of it. Themes: bother

Al,15- He cannot prevent ideas of something awful (terrible) about to happen, or as if he would do something awful (bad). Themes: misfortune, conscience, wicked

Al,16- An indescribable idea, which I could not shake off, (fixed idea) of something dreadful (calamitous) about to happen to me; all day feeling as if some great misfortune were about to occur. Themes: misfortune

Al,18- ...caught myself saying to nephew, in severe tone, " If you do that again" etc., when he was not really in fault. Themes: menacing, wrong

Al,2- Exaltation; thinks he has something of importance. Themes: greatness, haughty

Al,28- Very cross, so much that my children expressed great surprise; took offense at the merest trifles; scolded (censorious) my wife and children; .... Themes: offenses, bothered, censorious, wife, child

Al,30- Offended at everything; gives offensive answers. Themes: offenses, offensive

Al,32- Thought came into his mind to attack others in a mean way; to cut others with a knife he holds; to throw water he has in a tumbler into another's face. Themes: wicked, homicidal, violence, pointed

Al,34- There seems to be two distinct trains of thought operating at one and the same time. Themes: double, identity

Al,36- Undecided about little things. Themes: irresolution, doubtful

Al,39- A strange oppression and indifference, as if he was unable to do anything if he forces himself; there is no power of mind. Themes: strange, oppression, indifference, unfit, will

Al,6- Exhilarated, felt as if he had received joyful intelligence, all day. Themes: knowledge, pleasure

Al,N-10- They appreciate the formidable character of the disease and speak frequently with a remarkable quick and sharp articulation of the impending fatal results. Themes: disease, sadism

Al,N-11-...presentiment of impending death begged them to pray for him and not to leave him alone. (absolution, redemption) Themes: death, company, religious, salvation, penitence

Al,N-116- Attacks of nervous headache become awful and insupportable if he hears water run out of a hydrant. Themes: noise, water

Al,N-118- When he hears water poured out, or if he hears it run, or if he sees it, he becomes very irritable, nervous;... Themes: noise, water,

Al,N-12- The majority of patients have no adequate conception of real origin of their malady, and affirm in decided terms that the scar is of no significance whatever and causes them no pain. Themes: disease, antagonism

Al,N-121- Mortifying news affects him very much. Themes: sensitive, misfortune, news, mortification

Al,N-124- Every offense she feels very much. Themes: offenses

Al,N-127- Thinking of fluids of any kind, even of blood, brings on convulsions. Themes: disease, water, fit, blood

Al,N-129- Hyperesthesia, current of air, bright light, sight of any shining object, slightest touch, even conversation in vicinity of patient, may throw him into a most violent agitation and bring on severe convulsions. Themes: restless, bright, touch, disease, noise, fit, light, talk

Al,N-14- Is astonished (surprised) in his dream at the readiness with which he can express himself in elegant Latin. Themes: knowledge, stranger

Al,N-15- It seems to her as if two entirely different trains of thought influenced her at the same time. Themes: double

Al,N-22- Believe that they are reduced to their present wretched (miserable) condition by the instrumentality (aid) of those about them. Themes: miserable, betrayed

Al,N-23- Imagine that they are being abused (injured, offended), and energetically defend themselves against attacks and insults, ... Themes: offenses, injustice,

Al,N-24- Fancies he is being blown (hit, hurt) at by several persons, some of whom are not present. Themes: attacked, hurt

Al,N-26- Thinks he is a dog or a bird, and runs up and down chirping and twittering...(liberty?) Themes: identity, animal, liberty

Al,N-28- Complains bitterly that a fire has been lighted and that the stove is smoking, although there is no fire; another continually directed a window to be closed, which was not opened. (fear suffocation?) Themes: fire, invaded, suspicious

Al,N-31- ...Fancies doctors were two young girls who had come in to see her. Themes: disease

Al,N-33- ...Thinks he is a man of great authority.(power, command, expert) Themes: greatness, haughty, dictatorial

Al,N-34- ....to stab his flesh with the knife he is holding, and the like. Themes: hurt, suicidal, pointed

Al-N,37-Inclined to use insulting language, scold his friends, beat and abuse those near him. Themes: offensive, friend, hurt

Al,N-40- A strong and uncontrollable impulse to do certain acts; to spring at and bite any moving object that came within reach; dog. Themes: bite, animal

Al,N-42- Deny, with great obstinacy, that they have ever been bitten. Themes: obstinate, bite, disease

Al,N-45- Wrote to doctor: I am waiting with impatience that you give me and my young ones something to eat. Themes: impatience, helplessness, starving, child, lack

Al,N-46- After fainting (weak) spell he wrote on paper: I am forsaken by all; even the birds of heaven, they do not look at me (despised), do not fed me if hungry (helplessness) ; I hunger with the young ones and am thirsty with their she ones (starving); my nest (house) is made out of dirt (soiled), not gotten by my own exertions (efforts), but by driving them out of their nests (home) and sitting there with the females and the young. Themes: energy, forsaken, despised, helplessness, starving, dirty, animal, child, poverty, home

Al,N-50- Declares amid violent sobs that she is suffering the torments of hell. Themes: hell, doomed, tormented

Al,N-58- Ordered her husband to go away(forsakes) , as she wanted to bite him, and joining (associated) act to threat(menace), she bit herself in arm. Themes: husband, bite, forsakes, menacing, hurt,

Al,N-62- He cautioned people around him not to inhale his exhaled air, it was spoiled (dirty), stinking (smelling) like rotten (putrefying) eggs, worse than cholera, and could injure. (contaminates, infects) Themes: others, infection, dirty, disease, rotten

Al,N-64- Disinclination to change position of head; two distinct trains of thought existing at one time in her mind, the idea that she was unable to move her head (when lying down) with the positive conviction that she has only to make up her mind that she will do it to achieve it. Themes: double, antagonism, paralysis, will

Al,N-7- Thoughts of something terrible going to happen come into his mind against his will; feels impelled to do reckless (impulsive) things, such as throwing child, which he carries in his arms, through the window, and the like. Themes: misfortune, homicidal, child, height, will

Al,N-72- An attack of mental depression and indifference quite (very) strange to him; feels as if he could do nothing; if he forces himself he lacks mental power. Themes: sadness, indifference, unfit, energy

Al,N-75- He feels as if he had heard unpleasant news, or would soon hear it; until 4 p.m. Themes: news

Al,N-76- Felt as if she was going to get a fit. Themes: fit

Al,N-77- Lyssophobia; fear of becoming mad. (hydrophobia) Themes: insanity, water

Al,N-78- Feels as if he cannot physically endure his fears much longer, and shall be compelled to go into an insane asylum. Themes: fearful, insanity

Al,N-79- ...terror ...by endeavoring to take a drink of water, ...attacks...induced by running of water,... Themes: noise, water

Al,N-8- Could not get rid of the indescribable tormenting feeling that something terrible was going to happen to him. Themes: tormented, misfortune

Al,N-80- Felt as if she was going to die, as if she was going to sink away.(decline) Themes: death, sinking, ruined

Al,N-88- Very cross, so much... he took offense at veriest trifles ,scolding his wife and children, felt wretched, ... Themes: bothered, offenses, offensive, miserable, wife, child

Al,N-89- After attacks of fury, evinces (manifest) great regret at his behavior, making earnest (ardent) apologies, warning those about him not to allow him to bite them. Themes: anger, conscience, bite

Al,N-92- Exalted state of smell, taste and touch, with a feeling of anxiety and a fear of being alone. Themes: sensitive, touch, solitude

He,10- They appreciate the formidable (terrible) character of the disease and speak frequently with a remarkable (unusual) quick and sharp articulation of the impending fatal results. Themes: disease, pleasure, sadism, death

He,15- It seems to her as if two entirely different trains of thought influenced her at the same time. Themes: seized, double

He,22- Believe that they are reduced to their present wretched condition by the instrumentality (aid) of those about them. Themes: miserable, damage, unfortunate

He,23- Imagine that they are being abused (hurt, injured), and energetically defend themselves against attacks and insults, which in reality are products of their own fancy. Themes: hurt, offenses, attacked, injustice

He,24- Fancies he is being blown (strike) at by several persons, some of whom are not present. Themes: hurt, attacked

He,26- Thinks he is a dog or a bird, and runs up and down, chirping and twittering, until he falls down fainting. Themes: liberty, animal, identity, fit

He,28- Complains bitterly that a fire has been lighted and that the stove is smoking, although there is no fire; another continually directed a window to be closed, which was not opened. Themes: fire

He,33- Makes speeches in delirium; thinks he is a man of great authority. Themes: talk, dictatorial, greatness, haughty

He,40- A strong and uncontrollable impulse to do certain acts; to spring at and to bite any moving object that came within reach; ... Themes: bite, movement, approached

He,50- Declares amid violent sobs that she is suffering the torments of hell. Themes: tormented, hell

He,62- He cautioned people around him not to inhale his exhaled air, it was spoiled, stinking like rotten eggs, worse than cholera, and could injure. Themes: infection, rotten, disease, damage

He,64- Disinclination to change position of head; two distinct trains of thought existing at one time in her mind, the idea that she is unable to move her head (when lying down) with the positive conviction that she has only to make up her mind that she will do it to achieve it. Themes: double, antagonism, paralysis, will, movement, unfit

He,7- Thoughts of something terrible going to happen come into his mind against his will; feels impelled to do reckless (impulsive, precipitated) things, such as throwing child, which he carries in his arms, through the window, and the like. Themes: misfortune, antagonism, homicidal, height, child,

He,72- An attack of mental depression and indifference quite strange to him; feels as if he could do nothing; if he forces himself he lacks mental power. Themes: sadness, indifference, unfit, energy

He,76- Felt as if she was going to get a fit; at 11 p.m. Themes: fit

He,78- Feels he cannot physically endure his fears much longer, and shall be compelled to go into an insane asylum. Themes: fearful, insanity

He,80- Felt as if she was going to die; as if she was going to sink away. Themes: death, sinking, ruined

He,84- Indecision even in small matters. Themes: irresolution

He,88- Very cross, so much so that his children expressed great surprise; he took offense at veriest trifles, scolded his wife and children, felt wretched, ... Themes: bothered, offenses, offensive, miserable, censorious, wife, child

MACRO.

Al,2- She feels miserable; words cannot express how badly she feels. Themes: miserable

Al,4- Fear of impending danger. Themes: danger, menaced

Al,5- More or less fear; apprehensive; thinks she has some incurable disease. Themes: disease

Al,6- Suspicious of everybody; thinks she has not told the truth (veracity) in regard to himself. (secretive, pretend) Themes: suspicious, conscience, liar

MAG-C.

Al,13- Tremulous anxiety and fright, as if she apprehended some misfortune, disappearing in the evening in bed. Themes: anticipation, misfortune

Al,22- So fretful (irritable) that she does not know what she shall undertake...(begin) Themes: succeed

Al,8- She was very anxious several nights in

succession, and the bed felt as hard as though she were lying upon stones,... Themes: hard

Al,816- Dream that some one came to murder her; that she jumped from a window,... Themes: murdered, escape

Al,923- Dream that she had become a child three years old, which rejoiced her very much. (youngish) Themes: child, pure, pleasure

Al,926- Dream of gathering fruit in a garden. Themes: nature

Al,927- A pleasant dream of receiving money. Themes: money

Al,928- Dream that she invested money in a lottery. Themes: money

Al,929- Dream of very small horses, that she exerted herself to reflect upon, after midnight. Themes: small, animal, meditation

Al,930- Dreams of masks (false) in fools'(idiot) clothes, which they soiled.(dirty) Themes: dirty, clothes, deceitful

Al,931- Dream that she was at a ball (dance) where they did not dance enough; also at first she could not get ready (fitted) with her dress. Themes: unfit, music, clothes

Al,932- Dream of flowers, clothes, and other things; she had to make up the clothes, but had no inclination to do it, and besides did not understand how; she also saw many foreign plants, but during this she became soaked (wet) with rain. Themes: nature, clothes, duty, unfit, stranger, water, abroad

Al,933- Dream that she has to marry one she did not like, which she violently resisted;... Themes: union, antagonism, love

Al,935- Dream of her hair falling out, which made her very sad. Themes: ruined, fall

Al,936- Dream of the dangerous carrying of glasses. Themes: danger

Al,937- Dream she had something contraband, and wanted to snatch (seize) it away from those looking at it, and lock it up. Themes: shame, conscience, criminal

Al,940- Dream of a fire, at which she was present. Themes: fire

Al,941- Anxious dream of a fire, being arrested etc. Themes: fire, imprisoned

Al,943- Dream of danger by water. Themes: danger, water

Al,944- Dream of a flood, which flowed across the market-place, from which she woke in fright. Themes: storm, water

Al,945- Anxious dream, that a child was bathing in boiling water. (purification?) Themes: child, water, fire, dirty

Al,946- Dream that she made a long journey, and at last could go no farther (distance), at which she became very anxious. (limited, restricted) Themes: travel, obstructed

Al,947- Anxious dream as if he was unable to find his way in his own house. Themes: lost, unfit, home

Al,948- Anxious dreams of the misfortune of relatives. Themes: misfortune, relatives, others

Al,950- Dream that she burnt her back by some one throwing hot roast (meat) pigeons (bird) at her. Themes: fire, attacked, animal

Al,951- Frightful dream, that she burnt her cheek by the light. Themes: fearful, light, fire, bright

Al,952- Dream that he had an epileptic fit. Themes: disease, fit

Al,953- Dream that she was sadly disturbed in company, where especially her grandmother was taken with spasms, and at last had apoplexy. Themes: company, disease, fit, others

Al,955- Dream that she was weeping about the death of a near relative. Themes: death, relatives, others

Al,956- Dream that her mother had died, at which she woke, and believed that she was still weeping. Themes: death, mother,

Al,957- Dream that she saw her dead grandmother. Themes: death

Al,958- Anxious dream of a fight with robbers. Themes: fight, robber

Al,959- Dream of thieves who broke into the house and tried to kill her. Themes: robber, invaded, murdered

Al,964- Dream of funeral; she was obliged to dress the hair of the company; also of balls and marriages. Themes: funeral, union, company, music, vanity

Al,965- Dream of a grave in a cemetery, into which, after voluntary preparation, she was to be thrown. Themes: funeral, death

Al,969- Dream...he quarreled with a beggar. Themes: fight, poverty

Al,942- Anxious dream of a bright fire, at which she shrieked out violently and cried "fire". Themes: bright, fire

Ha,1- Trembling anguish and fear, as if evil was threatening (menacing, endangering); it passes off in the evening in bed. Themes: menaced, misfortune

Ha,16- Lack of tone (character, personality) in spirit, mind and body. Themes: disintegration

He,4- Trembling, anguish and fear, as if some accident would happen;... Themes: accidents

MAG-M.

Al,709- She becomes anxious in a dream about the work that she could not accomplish. Themes: unfit, work, duty

Al,710- Dream that she became confused in a forest, and for a long time could not find her way. Themes: nature, lost

Al,711- An anxious dream; she was lying in a strange house, where rubbish (garbage) was constantly falling upon her; she tried to cry out and could not, because there was too great heaviness on the chest. Themes: strange, dirty, oppression, obstructed, home, heavy

Al,714- Frightful dreams; that she was pursued by robbers; that she burned her hand by washing ... Themes: fearful, persecution, robber, fire, water, dirty

Al,715- Dream that someone cut away one side of her face; that a skin was being taken from a dead body and the like. Themes: mutilated, corpse, death

Ha,16- Joyless and passive, whatever she looks at is repugnant (disgusting, offensive) to her, she answers very unwillingly,.. Themes: yielding, loathing

Ha,18- He hated to talk; he desired to follow his thought in solitude. Themes: anger, talk, solitude

Ha,20- Fanciful (fantastic) delusions: As if while she was reading in a book, another person was reading after her, and compelled her to read more quickly, with humming and buzzing (murmur) around her...(faster) Themes: imitated, hurry, noise

Ha,20-....when she raised her head up she seemed to see great clouds and rocks above her, ... Themes: menaced, crushed

Ha,3- Apprehensive and melancholic, lonely (isolated, abandoned) ; she is homesick and weeps. Themes: sadness, solitude, homesickness, home

He,2- Tearful, inclined to weep; sad and homesick. Themes: sadness, homesickness

He,6- While reading, felt as if some one was reading after her and she must read faster and faster. (imitated) Themes: imitated, double, hurry

MAG-S.

Al,11-..while knitting she constantly saw strange persons about (surround) her, though she knew it was an illusion. Themes: strange, surrounded,

Al,4- Anxious as if conscious of some evil... Themes: misfortune, wrong

Al,5- Apprehensive (fear), fearful, very gloomy; she thought some misfortune would happen to her;... Themes: misfortune

MANC.

Al,4- Disposed to take everything in good part (first day). Themes: pleasure

Al,5- feeling of tenderness (friendship) and deep compassion.(sympathy) Themes: compassionate

He,3- Fear of getting crazy; of evil spirits; of being taken (possessed) by the devil. Themes: insanity, ghosts, seized, devil

He,5- ...about midnight attacks of fear and trembling; afraid of evil spirits, of being taken (possessed) hold of by the devil;... Themes: ghosts, seized, devil

MANG.

Al,3- Constant uneasiness (restlessness), as if he apprehended something sad. Themes: sadness

Ha,14- Embittered humor; irreconcilable and long-continued resentment against those who injure him. Themes: resentment, offenses

Ha,2- Constant restlessness, as if he apprehended some sad news. Themes: restless, anticipation, news

Ha,3- Great restlessness of body and mind, as if something was tormenting him. Themes: restless, tormented

Ha,324- Cross reflective, silently reserved, wrapped up in himself, with discomfort in the whole body, ... Themes: bothered, meditation, reserved, dwells

Ha,325- Cross and discontented with himself, and concerned about future..., considers himself very weak (stupid) in mind, and makes mistakes whenever he speaks. Themes: bothered, conscience, future, energy, wrong

Ha,326- Persistent restlessness of disposition, just as if he were going to hear some bad news. Themes: restless, news

Ha,327- Ill-humored, so that the most joyful music does not cheer (joy) him, but he feels as if refreshed by the most melancholy music. Themes: pleasure, music, sadness

Ha,329- Embittered humor; he could not forget injustice done to him; he fostered (support) resentment for a long time. Themes: injustice, mortification, resentment

Ha,330- Great restlessness of body and disposition, as if something bothered him. Themes: restless, bothered

Ha,7- Everything she thinks of is annoying (irritating)to her. Themes: bothered

He,6- Everything she even thinks of makes her fretful. Themes: himself

MED.

Al,N-20- Fears he is going to die. Themes: death

Al,N-22- Sensation as if all life was unreal, like a dream. Themes: unreal

Al,N-23- Wild desperate feeling, as of incipient insanity. Themes: despair, insanity, wild

Al,N-25- Tendency to suicide, gets up in night and takes his pistol, but his wife prevents him. Themes: suicidal

Al-N,38- ...;desire for rest and dread (fear) of change;...wild crazy feeling in brain... Themes: insanity, wild

Al,N-40- Always wakens tired in the morning; hates to do anything that must be done (duty), even nice things; gets nervous and excited about riding and driving as soon the time is fixed. Themes: negligence, duty, succeed, time,

Al,N-41- Constant state of anguish. Always a feeling of impending danger, but knows not what. There is no cause for such feelings, as she is not obliged to do anything when disinclined; is so situated that nothing need cause her trouble. Themes: menaced, danger, succeed

Al,N-43- Forgetful, cannot remember the least thing any length of time; writes everything down of any importance; cannot trust herself to remember it; great irritability and disgust with life. Themes: confidence, grief

Al,N-44- The impatience, excitement, wild feelings; the unreal, dazed condition; the gloom (sadness) and fear in the dark;... are marked evidence of functional derangement of the nervous system. Themes: impatience, wild, insanity, unreal, dark, organization

Al,N-47- It feels the evil coming to it, and the bad news before it arrives (clairvoyance), of course it is selfish, and it is easily hurt by a harsh (rude) word. Themes: misfortune, news, clairvoyance, offenses

Al,N-48- It is also introspective, self-accusative, remorseful. Time moves slowly to it, therefore it is hurried. Themes: reserved, conscience, time, hurry

Al,N-50- It is always anticipating, fearing evil will happen, loss of reason or suicide. Themes: misfortune, suicidal, anticipation, insanity

Al,N-52- Feeling of desperation; did not care if he went to heaven or hell. Themes: despair, religious, hell

Al,N-59- Time moves so slowly that things done an hour ago appear to have occurred a year since; asked the time of day, and in five minutes insisted that half an hour had elapsed and could not believe it had till she had seen the watch. Themes: time, past,

He,13- Seems to herself to make wrong statements (declaration), because she does not know what to say next, begins all right but does not know how to finish... Themes: doubtful, confidence, wrong

He,17- Thinks some one is behind her, (pursued) hear whispering; sees faces that peer (observe) at her from behind bed and furniture.(spied) Themes: persecution, observed

He,18- Persons come in, look at her (observed), whisper, and say "come". (spied, called) Themes: observed, seized

He,19- One night saw large (big) people in

room; large rats running; felt a delicate hand smoothing her head from front to back. (caressed) Themes: great, invaded, animal, touch

He,2- Dullness of memory and desire to procrastinate (delay), because business seemed so long lasting (permanent), or as if it never could be accomplished. (postponing) Themes: postponing, duty, succeed, work, time, unfit

He,20- Is sure that she is worse, knows she is not going to live, cannot see any improvement, even when it is pointed out (antagonism); has no fear of death, speaks calmly about it, and gives directions as to the disposition of her affairs. Themes: death, disease, antagonism, organization, pessimism, work

He,21- Sensation as if life was unreal, like a dream. Themes: unreal

He,22- Wild and desperate feeling, as of incipient insanity. Themes: insanity, wild, despair

He,24- Tendency to suicide, gets up in night and takes his pistol (gun), but his wife prevents him. Themes: suicidal, wife

He,25- Is in a great hurry; when doing anything is in such a hurry that she gets fatigued. Themes: hurry, time

He,28- Spirits in the depths, weighed down with heavy, solid gloom (sadness),> by torrents of tears. Themes: sadness, heavy

He,29- Is always anticipating; feels most matters sensitively before they occur and generally correctly. (predicts) Themes: anticipation, clairvoyance

He,30- Anticipates death. (predicts) Themes: anticipation, death, clairvoyance

He,31- Dread of saying the wrong thing when she has headache. Themes: talk, wrong, confidence

He,32- Everything startles her, news coming to her seems to touch her heart before she hears it. Themes: news, sensitive

He,33- Woke at an early hour with a frightened sensation, as if something dreadful had happened;... as if she must do something to rid her mind of this torture. Themes: fearful, misfortune, tortured

He,34- Fear of the dark. Themes: dark

He,35- Feeling as if he had committed the unpardonable sin and was going to hell. Themes: conscience, doomed, hell

He,36- A word or look of seeming harshness (reproach) put her in despondency for hours. (sensitive) Themes: despair, censured,

He,37- Feeling of desperation, did not care if he went to heaven or hell. Themes: despair, religious, salvation, hell

He,7- Reads a letter and thinks the words look queer (inadequate) and are spelled wrong. Themes: wrong, strange

He,8- Time moves too slowly. Themes: time

He,9- Dazed (confused) feeling; a far (distant) sensation, as though things done today occurred a week ago.(time) Themes: time

MELI.

He,8- Religious melancholy of four months' standing; ... Themes: sadness, religious

MENY.

Al,2- Quiet mood; contented with his circumstances. (chances) Themes: position

Al,3- Quiet, reserved, contented with himself all day. Themes: reserved

Al,8- Apprehensive sensation about the heart, as of impending evil, and as if he had to endure some hardship. (adversity, privation, suffering) Themes: heart, misfortune, menaced

Ha,285- Anxious feeling about the heart, as if something bad were about to happen, and he had to undergo (experience) a calamity. (cataclysm, disaster) Themes: heart, misfortune,

Ha,286- Cross, ill-humored and discontented with himself and his position (rank); anxiety drives him from one place to another.(restlessness) Themes: discontented, himself, position, conscience, restless

Ha,290- Melancholy humor; his thoughts are disposed to dwell on past sad disagreeable things. Themes: dwells, past, mortification

Ha,295- Tranquil disposition; he was contented with his position. Themes: position

He,2- Anxiety about heart, as if some evil was going to happen. Themes: heart, misfortune

MERC-I-F.

Al,1- While in bed, he imagined that a man was in his room who intended to perforate his throat with a gimlet;... Themes: invaded, murdered, pointed

MERC.

Al,1......she puts small stones into her mouth without swallowing them, and complains that they cut her intestines; ... Themes: poisoned, hurt

Al,10- Great seriousness, with much indifference all day; he was much offended if others laughed over a trifle, and yet was extremely indifferent to everything that took place about him. Themes: offenses, antagonism, indifference

Al,22- A feeling as though he had done wrong, with loss of ideas. Themes: wrong, conscience

Al,30- Fretful and peevish all day; he imagined that all his efforts would at last miscarry. (fail) Themes: failure

Al,31- Fretful all day; very much out of sorts and discontented with himself; he had no desire to talk or joke. Themes: discontented, himself, talk

Al,36- Quarrels with everything; would above all have everything right; quarrelsome. Themes: fight, justice, wrong

Al,37- While taking a walk, he has a strong inclination to pinch the noses of the strangers he meets. Themes: hurt

Ha,1125- Anxious dreams; of being bitten by dog, of getting up a revolution (revolutionary , revolting, radical) after midnight. Themes: bite, revolutionary, animal

Ha,1127- She dreams that people are before the window , and on being woke up thereby be cannot persuaded that they were not there. (observed) Themes: observed, suspicious, persecution

Ha,1130- Frightful dreams, in which he started up; he imagined he was not in his own house, sat up in bed and spoke about a distant village. Themes: home, travel, stranger

Ha,1222- Restlessness, he cannot remain quiet in any place; he can neither stand nor lie, and is as if mad, or as if he had committed a great crime. Themes: restless, conscience, insanity, criminal, movement

Ha,1224. Indescribable sensation of an internal, intolerable ill, during which he remains silent and will not get up from bed. Themes: disease

Ha,1225- Imagines he is enduring the tortures (torment) of hell, without being able to account for it (explain). -(lost understanding , judgment) Themes: tortured, doomed, hell, conscience

Ha,1227- Much anxiety and ebullition in the blood at night, and shooting in the blood vessels. Themes: blood, movement

Ha,1229- Anxiety as if he had committed a crime. Themes: conscience, criminal

Ha,1231- He has no rest, and must go hither and thither, and cannot remain long in one place. Themes: restless, movement

Ha,1234- Anxiety and apprehension in the blood, he knew not how to compose (control) himself; he felt as if he had committed a crime, without heat, also at the same time as if he was not quite master,(commander). of his senses all day. (lost: mastering, commander) Themes: restless, blood, organization, criminal

Ha,1235- Anxiety that could drive him far away, as if he had committed a crime or some misfortune were about to happen to him.- (transgression) Themes: movement, restless, criminal, misfortune, conscience

Ha,1236- He thinks he is losing his reason,(intelligence, capacity) that he is going to die ; with illusions of imagination, e.g. he sees water flowing where there is none (in the morning). (water- 1 origin, genesis) Themes: insanity, death, water

Ha,1237- With absence of thought ,(discernment, knowledge),he feels as if he had done something bad. Themes: knowledge, criminal, conscience, wrong

Ha,1241- He wished to die, was indifferent to everything, even to what he took most delight in. Themes: death, indifference

Ha,1242- All day long great seriousness with much indifference; he got angry when others laughed at a trifle, and at the same time was extremely indifferent to all about him. Themes: indifference, anger, offenses

Ha,1243- He is indifferent to everything in the world, has no desire to eat, and yet when he does eat he relishes (like) his food and can partake (eat) of what is required.(necessary) Themes: indifference

Ha,1248- Without cause he is very discontented with himself and his position. Themes: discontented, himself, position

Ha,1249- All day long depression of spirits combined with anxiety; he always thought he was going to hear of something disagreeable. Themes: misfortune, sadness

Ha,1251- All day long cross and peevish; he believed that all his efforts (endeavor) would finally fail. Themes: failure

Ha,1253- Very cross and intolerant, easily irritated, very suspicious. Themes: bothered, suspicious

Ha,1254- Quarreling with everyone, opinionative, (doctrinal) quarrelsome. Themes: fight, dictatorial

Ha,1256- All day long sulky and distrustful (suspicious); he almost insulted those about him, and regarded them all as his greatest enemies.(opponent, rival) Themes: suspicious, offensive, enemy

Ha,1257- During the whole day cross, as if at variance and dissatisfied with himself, and had no inclination for speaking and joking. Themes: bothered, discontented, himself, talk

Ha,1259- An almost irresistible desire to travel (explore, wandering) away to a distance. Themes: travel

Ha,1261- He talked nonsense: look! you strike a fly on your hand, and you had previously forbidden me to do so (which was not the case). Themes: censured

Ha,1262- He is silly , acts like a buffoon , ...he lit (burning) his fire, laid swords across one another, and put candles in one corner of the room, in the other boots (shoe),all this quite gravely...(serious) Themes: ridiculous, fire, organization, feigning

Ha,1263- Mania; she throws off the clothes at night, tears the straw about, and scolds; by day she leaps (jump) up high like a petulant extravagant person...she talks and scolds much to herself,...spits frequently and spreads the saliva out with her feet, and licks some of it up again; she often licks cow dung (excrements) and the mud of ponds (lake); she often takes little stones in her mouth, without swallowing them, and at the same time complains that they are cutting her bowels; much clotted blood passes with her motion; ... Themes: clothes, tear, offensive, defiant, dirty, hurt, disease, blood

Ha,1264- When taking a walk he felt a strong inclination to catch (capture) by the nose strangers whom he met. Themes: conduct

He,14- Believes he is losing his reason, thinks he is dying, with illusions of fantasy; sees water running where there is none. Themes: insanity, death, water

He,16- Great restlessness as if he had committed a great crime; ...considers everybody his enemy;...great inclination when walking to take people by the nose;...(desire: conduct, direct, guide) Themes: restless, conscience, criminal, suspicious, conduct, enemy,

He,19- Homesickness (nostalgia, isolation), or desire to travel; wants to go abroad (absent, nomad); nightly anxiety and perspiration.(wander) Themes: homesickness, travel, abroad

He,20- After suppression of foot sweat, whenever he sees an open window or cutting instruments breaks into a sweat, with great heat of head, and is seized with an almost uncontrollable desire to commit suicide. Themes: suicidal, pointed, height, seized

He,21- Desire to kill the person contradicting her. Themes: contradiction, homicidal

He,22- Great desire to murder (homicidal) or committed suicide ...is fearful that she may commit some wrong and kill herself (punishment); something urges her to kill her husband, of whom she is very fond (loving), and she implores him to hide his razor (knife). Themes: homicidal, suicidal, conscience, wrong, husband, seized

He,27- Fear of being alone. Themes: solitude

He,28- Anxiety and restless change of place; ebullitions, sweat; apprehensive, imaginary fears; fears he will lose his mind;...(sanity). Themes: restless, fearful, insanity

He,29- Anxiety and apprehension; did not know what to do ; it seemed as though he had committed a crime ; without heat; also with a feeling that he had not control over his senses. Themes: confidence, criminal, conscience, irresolution

He,3- Loss of will (command, intentions, resolutions,) power.(vigor) Themes: energy, will

He,30- Anxiety driving her to suicide ; thoughts of suicide; ...desire for death; great indifference even to those she formerly loved;... Themes: suicidal, death, indifference, forsakes, love

He,32- Much wretchedness (miserable, unhappy) and dejection (sadness) of spirits, with diarrhea. Themes: unfortunate, sadness

He,33- Hysterical melancholia, with inclination to murder. Themes: sadness, homicidal

He,34- Inexpressive pain of soul and body, anxious restlessness, as if some evil impended ...; disgusted (revolt) with himself, has not courage (cowardice) to live; constant suspicion (distrust), considering everybody his enemy. Themes: danger, misfortune, suspicious, himself, cowardice, enemy

He,35- Grief, with fear at night: disposition to quarrel; complaining of relations and surroundings. (living conditions) Themes: grief, discussion, discontented, family, position

He,35- Grief, with fear at night; disposition to quarrel; complaining of relations and surroundings. Themes: grief, fight, censorious, discontented

He,37- Morose and mistrustful; treated his associates almost insultingly, looked upon every one as his worst enemy. Themes: suspicious, offensive, enemy

He,38- Great restlessness, must constantly change her place; fear, with desire to escape, as if she had committed some crime. Themes: restless, escape, criminal, conscience

He,44- Ailments from mortification; from insults; from egotism. Themes: mortification, offenses, egotism

He,49- Ailments from mortification; from insults; from egotism. Themes: offenses, mortification, egotism

MEZ.

Al,10- Great discontent with himself and his surroundings (living, conditions, position) for several weeks... Themes: discontented, himself, position

Al,14- Indifferent to everything; he could scarcely compel himself to note the symptoms beyond brief annotations (as a sea-sickness) Themes: dispersion, indifference

Al,2- No rest when alone; he desires company. Themes: solitude, company

Al,20- Apprehensiveness in the pit of the stomach, as though expecting something disagreeable. Themes: anticipation

Al,23- Very irritable mood; very averse to everything; desire to run away. Themes: loathing, escape

Al,32- Is inclined to get angry with others about trifling and perfectly harmless things; everything vexes him, and he wants to say all kinds of annoying and vexatious things. Themes: offenses, bothered, anger, offensive

Al,33- Violent outbreak of anger about trifles, which he soon regrets.(remorse) Themes: conscience, anger

Al,34- Inclined to reproach others. Themes: censorious

Al,36- Quiet and contemplative; weary of life, and longing for death. Themes: meditation, loathing, death

Al,38- It becomes difficult for him to make a resolution. Themes: irresolution, confidence

Al,47- He looked out of the window for hours without thought, and without knowing what he was looking at. Themes: lack, knowledge, time

Al,8- Very sad; every trifle affects him disagreeably; indifferent to the whole world; has no desire for anything; disinclined to work. Themes: indifference, loathing, work

Ha,14- Disposed to reproach others. Themes: censorious

Ha,16- Violent boiling over with passion about trifles, for which he is soon sorry. Themes: passionate, conscience

Ha,17- He finds it difficult to come to a determination. Themes: irresolution

Ha,2- ...everything seemed to him as if dead, and nothing made a vivid impression on him. Themes: death, indifference, lifeless

Ha,23- He would vacantly (empty) look through the windows for hours, without becoming conscious of what he saw, and without then thinking about anything. Themes: time

Ha,4- Apprehensiveness in the scrobiculus cordis, as if he expected something disagreeable. Themes: misfortune

Ha,7- Restless when alone, he wishes to be in company. Themes: restless, solitude, company

Ha,8- Introverted, tired of life and longing for death. Themes: loathing, reserved, death

He,10-...; everything seems to him dead (lifeless, inert) and nothing makes a vivid impression upon his mind. Themes: lifeless, death

He,11- Inclined to get angry with others about trifles; everything vexes him, he wants to say annoying and vexatious things; is soon sorry for it. Themes: anger, bothered, offensive, conscience

He,4- Irresolute (undecided); mind easily confused, unable to recollect; thinking is difficult. Themes: irresolution, obstructed, past

He,5- No rest when alone; wants to be in company ...unable to repeat what has been learned by heart; looks through window for hours, without being conscious of objects around; knows not what she is about; forgets what she is about to utter (talk); looks ill humored, pale, wretched, fallen away; ......expecting some very unpleasant news. Themes: restless, solitude, news, knowledge, unfortunate, company, talk, unreal, miserable, misfortune

He,8- Despairs of eternal salvation. Themes: religious, despair, salvation

MORPH.

Al,13- Complete melancholy, so that he desired to commit suicide. Themes: sadness, suicidal

MOSCH.

Al,11- He was extremely anxious about the death;...."this is my death" became deathly pale, and in ten minutes fell down in a faint. Themes: death, fit

Al,12- She spoke of nothing but that she must die. (from triturating ten minutes) Themes: death

Al,19- She sits in thought, strikes her hands together, makes various gestures, so that others fear she will lose her reason,... Themes: meditation, insanity

Al,7- Anxiety, as if something were about to happen. Themes: misfortune

He,1- Great anxiety with palpitation of heart; feeling of anxious expectancy.(anticipation) Themes: anticipation, heart

He,11- Great tendency to be frightened, trembling, palpitation of heart, and dread of death. Themes: fearful, heart, death

He,3- Scolding; keeps it up till her lips turn blue, eyes stare, and she falls down fainting. Themes: fit, offensive

He,4- Great dread (fear) of death, with paleness of face, fainting; talks only of approaching (nearing) death. Themes: fearful, death, fit, talk

He,5- Hypochondriacal complaints having their origin in sexual system. Themes: disease, sexual

MUR-AC.

Al,10- Anxious thoughtfulness; he cannot free himself from the slightest trouble. Themes: meditation, tormented, mortification

Al,15- The brightness (lively, vivid) of his disposition constantly diminished , until in the evening he became very fretful (irritable). Themes: bright, energy, lifeless

Al,2- Joyous trustful (hopeful) mood. Themes: pleasure

Al,21- Deep reflection, and quiet absorption in himself, as if something disagreeable were impending, though with desire to work. Themes: meditation, menaced, misfortune, work

Al,4- Sad, quiet, and discontented with his lot.(destiny) Themes: sadness

Al,5- Sad absorbed in herself, as if there were no life (inert, lifeless) in her during menses. Themes: reserved, lifeless

Al,6- During the menses she is sad, taciturn, as if she had no life. Themes: sadness, lifeless

Al,637- Dream that she had lice, which made her very much ashamed.(shame) Themes: shame, disease, infection

Ha,1 -Sad taciturn and discontented with his fate. (destiny, doom) Themes: discontented, doomed

Ha,2- Sad and introverted, as if she had no

life in her, during the menses. Themes: sadness, lifeless, reserved

Ha,266- Silent reserve, with anxious concern about the present and future. Themes: reserved, future

Ha,267-...anxiety and restlessness in the upper extremities (as if in the blood vessels)... Themes: restless, blood,

Ha,269- Sunk in profound thought, as if something disagreeable were about to happen,... Themes: anticipation, meditation, misfortune

Ha,270- Anxious scrupulosity (careful) (immediately) all day; he cannot get over the slightest misfortune or become contented; after 72 hours more cheerful, less scrupulous (caution), and more courageous than at ordinary times. Themes: conscientious

Ha,279- Very tranquil, calm and free from care. Themes: peace

Ha,4- Deep reflection, and quiet introversion, as if something unpleasant was impending,... Themes: meditation, menaced, reserved, misfortune

Ha,5- Anxious apprehension; he cannot get over the slightest misfortune. Themes: misfortune, obstructed

Ha,8- ...no work succeeds in his hands,... Themes: work, succeed

He,2- Taciturn, introverted and quiet; anxious care about future. Themes: misanthropy, reserved, future

MURX.

Al,2- Great depression of spirits; it seemed to her that she was hopelessly ill. Themes: sadness, disease, hopeless

Al,4- It made me miserable; I was so low-spirited that I gave up everything; I had no strength left. Themes: miserable, sadness, energy

He,2- Deep sadness at approach of menses, all her symptoms gave her great concern (care); seemed to her she was hopelessly ill; she gave up everything. Themes: sadness, sexual, disease, hopeless

MYRIC.

Al,11- Irritable, worried by little things; everything seemed to go wrong, in the morning. Themes: wrong

Al,12- Exceedingly irritable; the slightest thing fretted (bother) and irritated him; ungovernable petulance.(rudeness) Themes: bother

Al,6- Miserable dejected (unhappy) feeling all day. Themes: unfortunate, miserable

Al,8-...;did not care about anything or for any friends; was perfectly wretched, beyond description. Themes: miserable, indifference, friend

Al,9-...a constant desire to find fault (censorious); everything went wrong; looked upon (contemptuous) this world as a place not fit to live in any longer; considered himself better than the rest (great person, megalomania), in the morning; ...; condemned himself for various imaginary faults; ... Themes: censorious, contemptuous, greatness, conscience, wrong

NAJA.

Al,10- Great depression of spirits this morning; everything for two or three hours appeared to go wrong with me, and to be without remedy;... Themes: sadness, wrong, failure

Al,11- Great depression of mind, with the distress, about the generative organs. (sexual) Themes: sadness, sexual

Al,12- Sadness or serious disposition; sadness and irresolution. Themes: sadness, irresolution

Al,13- ...I felt that everything that was done was done in a wrong way, and could not be rectified (corrected, revised); if I felt that I had some duty to perform (execute), I had at the same time a strong impulse not to do it, and I am extremely restless in consequence; I seemed to have an increased perception of what I ought to do, but, at the same time , an unaccountable inclination not to do it, to which I was irresistibly compelled to yield "I couldn't help it, didn't know why, but couldn't do it." Themes: wrong, duty, antagonism, restless, conscience, helplessness, negligence,

Al,14- Felt melancholy; began to form images of possible wrongs (mistaken) and misfortunes, over which the mind broods; very wretched at times;... a slight cause sets him in a perfect agony of mental suffering on another's behalf (welfare);...makes himself imaginary troubles and wrongs, and frets (bother) over them for two hours... Themes: wrong, dwells, miserable, conscience, compassionate, misfortune, unfortunate, mortification, others

Al,3-...having an axe in his hand,...he suddenly split his head in two; he had become insane. Themes: suicidal, insanity

Al,9- Considerable depression of spirits, and a feeling of inability to exertion of any kind, and a conviction that all is going wrong;... Themes: sadness, unfit, wrong, failure

He,3- Melancholy; began to form images of possible wrongs (evils) and misfortunes over which the mind broods; very wretched (miserable) at times. Themes: wrong, conscience, dwells, miserable, misfortune

He,5-...imagines she is in a terrible rainstorm, complains of being so cold (coldness), and that the carriage has turned over and hurt her head. (accident) Themes: storm, hurt, accidents

NAT-AR.

Al,15- Requires an effort to attend to accustomed duties; feels dull; tries to write, but it requires an effort to form each word. Themes: duty, succeed, obstructed

Al,22-...mind not fit for study ... Themes: unfit, knowledge

Al,3- Feeling as something was impending, which caused him to move about. Themes: menaced, movement

Al,5- Feel well; can study easily ; disposed to be reconciled to circumstances, favorable and unfavorable; feel like working hard; no undertaking too large for me. Themes: work, succeed

NAT-C.

Al,11- Intolerable melancholy and apprehension; she was wholly occupied with sad thoughts. Themes: sadness, mortification

Al, DREAM ,1102-..;of marrying two women, of parties, walks, entertainments, and excursions on horseback, afterwards they were frequently anxious, of going astray (lost),of murders, having his ears cut off; also vexatious dreams; he would take a journey and could not get away from the place,(immobilization) and when has reached the first station was obliged to turn back, on account of something he had forgotten. Themes: love, travel, mutilated, murdered, paralysis, lack, stranger, union, pleasure, lost, obstructed

Al,DREAM,1111- Dream of a flood (current, inundate), and threatening danger. Themes: storm, danger, water, menaced

Al,DREAM,1113- Anxious, vivid, frightful dreams of thieves, from which he started up with loud cry, and when awake could scarcely realize that his fears were groundless. Themes: fearful, robber,

Al,1114- Dream of a quarrel, in which he stabbed his antagonist (enemy) in the chest with a large knife. Themes: fight, homicidal, enemy, pointed

Al,1116- Dream that she saw a corpse, at which she woke in fright, when it seemed as though a dead acquaintance stood before her, which made her scream aloud, afterwards she fell asleep again . Themes: ghosts, corpse, friend

Al, DREAM, 1117- Illusions of fantasy, in the evening, while half asleep; she sees figures, visions of soldiers marching in the air;.. Themes: officer, organization

Al,14- Anxious, solicitous about himself.(cares) Themes: himself

Al,17- Anxiety and restlessness; he thought he could do nothing properly.(rightly, correctly) Themes: restless, confidence, wrong

Al,18- Anxiety and hasty (fast) restlessness all day; he could not keep the limbs still, especially the arms; obliged to stretch them; it seemed as though they would be torn (cut) asunder. (in two divided). Themes: restless, hurry, movement, mutilated, divided, disintegration

Al,22- His fancy is mostly busy with apprehensions of the future; he often makes plans for half an hour at a time as if it would go wrong with him, wherewith he seeks to be alone for several days together. Themes: separated, future, planning, unfortunate, failure, solitude, time, wrong, misanthropy

Al,24- She does not know what to do, on account of apprehensiveness and ennui and thinks that she is quite lonely (alone,

solitary, insulated) and forsaken, all day. Themes: doubtful, confidence, solitude, forsaken, tedium
Al,28- He is very timid, and starts at the slightest noise. Themes: timidity, fearful, noise
Al,29- Anthropophobia and fearfulness. Themes: misanthropy, solitude, fearful
Al,3- Every event makes a strong impression upon her; a wavy trembling in the nerves, with a sensation of faintness. Themes: sensitive, fit
Al,30- He shuns (avoid) mankind. Themes: misanthropy, solitude
Al,41-..;the room seems too small for him, and even in open air he walks without anything seeming right to him;... (confined, limited, restricted) Themes: small, wrong
Al,42- Very fretful and discontented with whole world; he constantly felt as though he could beat (punish ?) himself, his whole life angered him , and he preferred to have no existence at all; he was solicitous about the future, and inclined to despair, all day. Themes: discontented, conscience, future, hurt, himself, anger, despair
Al,48- He is angry, and inclined to fight and strike, and cannot tolerate contradiction,... Themes: anger, fight, violence, contradiction
Al,53- Sensation of loss of will power, in the morning on waking. Themes: lack, energy, will
Al,56- He has no desire to do anything, and can keep at nothing long. Themes: work, succeed, negligence, dispersion
Ha,10- His fancy is mostly anxiously occupied with the future; he paints to himself what misfortunes might happen to him; and he seeks solitude for several days. Themes: future, misfortune, solitude, misanthropy
Ha,11- Less anxious than usual during a thunderstorm. Themes: storm
Ha,13- Anxious and restless, he thinks he cannot do anything right. Themes: succeed, confidence, wrong
Ha,14- Anxiously solicitous about himself. Themes: himself,
Ha,23- Restlessness and unsteadiness (inconstant); he knew not what he wanted, nor what he should do or leave undone. Themes: restless, doubtful, succeed, duty, irresolution, confidence
Ha,24- Sensation of irresolution, in the morning. Themes: irresolution
Ha,3- Dread of men and timidity. Themes: misanthropy, cowardice, timidity
Ha,48- Peevish and cross, dissatisfied with all the world; he could have kicked (self censure) himself; he would rather not live at all ; at the same time solicitous about the future, so that he is ready to despair. Themes: bothered, death, future, himself, conscience
Ha,5- Great melancholy and apprehensiveness; only occupied with sad thoughts. Themes: sadness, mortification
Ha,52- Passionate; disposed to quarrel and fight, and cannot bear any contradiction. Themes: passionate, fight, contradiction
Ha,8- Apprehensive and ennui (tedium, monotony), so that she cannot contain herself; she deems (believe), herself altogether (entirely) lonely (solitary) and forsaken. Themes: solitude, forsaken, tedium, anticipation
He,13- Constant fear and forebodings. Themes: anticipation, fearful
He,4- Aversion to mankind and society; estrangement (separation, alienation) from individuals and society; even from her husband and family. Themes: misanthropy, stranger, solitude, forsakes, separated, husband, family
He,6- Intolerable melancholy and apprehension; she is wholly occupied with sad thoughts. Themes: pessimism, misfortune
He,9- Restlessness, with attacks of anxiety, especially during a thunderstorm; < from music. Themes: restless, storm, music

NAT-M.

Al,103- Hatred of people who had insulted him. Themes: offenses, anger
Al,109- Offended by a joke. Themes: offenses, despised
Al,11- Constant laughing; everything in the room looked so ridiculous. Themes: ridiculous, contemptuous, sarcasm
Al,119- The patient's mind was much weakened by disease and poison; her moral perceptions, her once keen (sharp) sense of honor, and of right and wrong, seemed blunted (dull); she was in turns

vehement (angry) and passionate, and moody and silent. Themes: disease, poisoned, knowledge, justice, wrong, obstructed, passionate

Al,12- She laughed so immoderately at something not ludicrous, that she could not be quieted, and tears come into her eyes, so that she looked as though she had been weeping. Themes: pleasure, antagonism,

Al,132- Irresolute at work; he could not see his way clearly. Themes: irresolution, work, confidence, knowledge

Al,18- If one only looked at him, he was obliged to weep. Themes: miserable, unfortunate, observed

Al,2761- In a dream he reproached himself for past mistakes, full of restlessness and anxiety. Themes: conscience, past, himself, restless

Al,35- Sad as if sick (suffering), in the afternoon. Themes: sadness, disease

Al,39- Melancholy mood; she has preferred to be alone for several days past. Themes: sadness, solitude

Al,42- Melancholic depression, and sad apprehension, and disheartened (depress, discourage) all day, without definite cause, with constant palpitation, without physical infirmity. Themes: sadness

Al,44- The more he was consoled, the more he was affected. (aggravate) Themes: unfortunate

Al,45- If she only thinks of a want (need, lack) long since past, tears come into her eyes. Themes: lack, nostalgia, past

Al,47- Full of grief; he tormented himself; he seemed to prefer disagreeable thoughts, which prostrated him very much. Themes: grief, tormented, mortification

Al,5- Great excitement, followed by falling asleep and deadness of the limbs. Themes: paralysis

Al,51- Attacks of complete hopelessness and internal despair, that deprived him of all power. Themes: hopeless, despair, energy

Al,59- Anxiety, as if she had done something wrong, with heat and night sweat. Themes: conscience, wrong

Al,6- She talked more than usual, but did not like so much to be talked to; when she had nothing to say, she became depressed and melancholy. Themes: talk, sadness

Al,61- Very anxious, as if he would fall, while walking. Themes: fall

Al,62- Woke at 2A.M. in perspiration, and with a distressing anxiety, as though he were shut up (lock) in a dark cellar; this sensation only disappeared on perceiving light through the window.(confined, restricted, incarcerated) Themes: imprisoned, dark, separated, light

Al,63- When alone, she becomes uneasy (discontent) about herself, and must weep. Themes: himself, solitude

Al,64- She often looks into the mirror, and imagines that she looks wretched. (miserable, unhappy) Themes: miserable

Al,65- Extremely solicitous about the future. Themes: future

Al,66- Lost for hours in thought as to what would become of him. Themes: future, meditation

Al,70 -In the evening it seemed as though he became paralyzed from a fright (terrify) ; afterwards he seemed horrified, and apprehended some misfortune. Themes: paralysis, fearful, misfortune

Al,71- Fear of insanity. Themes: fearful, insanity

Al,72- Anxious fear of dying. Themes: death

Al,79- Easily vexed, pettish; he will not bear opposition for several evenings. Themes: contradiction

Al,93- Ill- humored does not want to go into society for fear of vexing others; feels that he could easily give offense. Themes: company, offensive, conscience, solitude, bother

Al,97- She takes everything in bad part, and weeps and cries much. Themes: offenses

Ha,10- In his thought he constantly recalls former disagreeable occurrences, so as to worry himself by thinking about them. Themes: past, mortification

Ha,11- She takes everything in bad part, and weeps and cries. Themes: offenses

Ha,12- When alone, she calls up disagreeable thoughts and has to weep. Themes: mortification, solitude

Ha,13- If she merely thinks of troubles past, tears come into her eyes. Themes: mortification, past

Ha,14- From the looks of everyone, he concludes that people pity (compassion, sympathy) him for his misfortune, and he

weeps.(miserable) Themes: misfortune, unfortunate, miserable
Ha,15- He had to weep as soon as anyone merely looked at him. (pitied) Themes: unfortunate, miserable
Ha,21- Attacks of entire hopelessness (despairing) and internal despondency (despair) which take away all her strength. Themes: energy, hopeless, despair
Ha,22- Hypochondriac, even to being tired of life. Themes: tedium, loathing
Ha,23- Anxiously solicitous about the future. Themes: future
Ha,24- Anxious about becoming insane. Themes: insanity
Ha,25- He is afraid he will have to die. Themes: death
Ha,26- She often looks into the looking-glass, (mirror) and thinks she looks wretched (miserable, contemptible). Themes: unfortunate, miserable
Ha,28- Anxiety, as if she had done something wicked (immoral), with heat and night-sweat. Themes: conscience, wicked
Ha,4- Melancholy mood; he cannot remove from his thoughts injuries (insults) he has inflicted on others , or which have been inflicted on him, which depressed him so much that he had no pleasure in anything. (remorse) Themes: offensive, offenses, conscience, mortification, others
Ha,5- Melancholy dejection and sorrowful anxious despondency all day, without any known cause, with unceasing palpitation,... Themes: sadness, grief, despair
Ha,54- In the evening, he was, as it were, paralyzed by a fright, then he became horrified and apprehensive. Themes: paralysis, fearful
Ha,57- Offended by a joke. Themes: offenses, despised
Ha,58- Apt to be peevish and abrupt; he does not endure opposition. Themes: offensive, contradiction
Ha,59- He feels peevish and avoids company , because he foresees that he might easily annoy (bother, molest) others. (intrude) Themes: bother, company, conscience, solitude
Ha,64- Injuries which he had inflicted on others, or which others had done to him, always dwelled in his thoughts; he could not get rid of them, and this annoyed him, so that he had no pleasure in anything. Themes: offensive, offenses, dwells, conscience, mortification, tormented, damage
Ha,68- Hatred (rancor, resentment) against persons, who had formerly offended him. Themes: offenses, anger, resentment
Ha,8- He sorrowfully torments (torture) himself, by continually looking for disagreeable ideas, which weakens him. Themes: grief, tormented, mortification, energy, conscience
Ha,9- For hours, immersed in thoughts, as to what would become of him. Themes: meditation, dwells, future
Ha,90- Irresolution in doing mental work; he cannot easily find his way. Themes: irresolution, work, lost
Ha,93- Loss of memory; he could not recall anything about yesterday and was afraid he had lost his mind. Themes: insanity
Ha,97- Lack of memory, so that he thought his mother (present continually) had died, because he did not remember to have seen her. Themes: death, mother, lack
He,11-, ...uttered the most atrocious blasphemes, swore (blaspheme, curse) against God (divine) and the elements (environment), and after raging for awhile became exhausted,... Themes: offensive, godless, anger, nature
He,13-Taciturnity; offended at every word (easily); avoids company; hates persons because they have offended him; spleen. Themes: offenses, solitude, company, anger, misanthropy
He,15- Whenever alone she wished to cry, she did not know why. Themes: solitude
He,2- Absent minded or distracted while talking; does not know what he ought (have to) say; awkward in talking; easily makes mistakes. Themes: talk, doubtful, irresolution, wrong, knowledge
He,21- Gloomy thoughts, recalls (remember),insults long since suffered; likes to dwell upon past unpleasant occurrences. Themes: offenses, mortification, past, dwells
He,32- Apprehension, feels as if something was going to happen. Themes: anticipation
He,33- Brain fag (weakness), with sleeplessness, gloomy (dark) forebodings, exhaustion after talking, embarrassment (confusion) of brain. Themes: misfortune,

anticipation, pessimism

He,34- A pregnant woman saw a man who had a disfiguring nasal cancer; this haunted (obsessed) her, and she was sure her child would be marked; she was melancholy, avoided society, wept continually. Themes: horrible, seized, doomed, solitude, child, misanthropy, sadness

He,35- Fear of loss of reason.(sanity) Themes: insanity

He,36- Despairing, hopeless feeling about the future. Themes: despair, hopeless, future

He,42- Quarrelsome fretfulness, gets into passion about trifles; passionate vehemence. Themes: fight, anger, passionate

He,43- Hateful and vindictive nature. Themes: resentment, anger, revengeful

He,48- Consequences (ailments) of fright, anger, vexation, mortification, or reserved displeasure. Themes: fearful, anger, bothered, mortification, suppressed, grief, reserved

He,5- Haunted with thoughts that something unpleasant will happen. Themes: anticipation, seized

He,51- After violent fits of passion, paralysis. Themes: passionate, paralysis, fit

He,6- Tries to recollect past disagreeable occurrences for the purpose of thinking on them and indulging (suffer) the grief which it causes. Themes: past, mortification, grief

NAT-P.

Al,1- Awakes at night, and imagines pieces of furniture are persons. Themes: alive

Al,10- Awakens; fears his child, who has a trifling ailment (disease), is dead; he goes to her room to relieve the otherwise ineffaceable (perpetual) impression. Themes: child, disease, death, others, dwells

Al,6- Very despondent; imagined he was going to be sick, to have typhoid fever. Themes: sadness, disease, infection

Al,7- Felt anxious about home (homesickness?); had misgivings (worry) ; feared bad news. Themes: news, home,

Al,8- Worries (cares) about the health, about the future. Themes: disease, future

Al,9- Apprehensive (fear) of some approaching evil. Themes: misfortune

NAT-S.

Al,12- Nothing that she undertakes succeeds well, and she does not know why. Themes: succeed, failure

Al,4- Lachrymose; thinks only of sad things. Themes: sadness, pessimism

Al,5- Very much disheartened; tired (weary) of life; despairs of getting well. (recovery) Themes: despair, disease

Al,6- Great fear, with dread of a misfortune. Themes: misfortune

He,4- Satiety (weary) of life; must use all self-control to prevent shooting himself. Themes: loathing, suicidal

NEON.

Sh,50- I have superbly fluid and graceful motions, as if I were moving in water instead of air. I have much pleasure in the right shoulder being free. 20, 6C, 05:XX:XX Themes: water, floating

Sh, 1- I was overwhelmingly agitated, amazed, confused, and upset about a neon tube discarded across the road. I couldn't believe that people could use these things. Where would the dustmen throw it? I thought, "It's the worst kind of light possible." I could not believe people would want it. 20, 6C, 00:03:05 Themes: light, dirty

Sh,10- Walking up a long gradual incline, I felt every stride was covering great distances. I felt I was doing the usual 20 minute walk in seconds. I felt like a titan in 7-league boots, but then I couldn't decide which league boots they were and I wanted an even number. My thoughts went titan-titanium-uranium-Uranus-clouds-clouds-where is the sky? 20, 6C, 01:12:20 Themes: greatness, great, grow

Sh,100- On a cloudy day, I really wanted blue. I looked for the blue sky and remembered the blue flash on the wings of a duck I had seen. I was very excited about anything blue that I could see, especially vibrant blues. I felt I had never seen blues in that way before. Also excited by yellow, limey green fluorescent colors. 20, 6C, 01:03:28 Themes: bright

Sh,102- My daughter commented that I looked brown and that my eyes looked clear, blue and bright. 20, 6C, 01:09:55 Themes: bright

Sh,108- I went to the market to buy food and instead I bought lots of material, two pairs of boots and no food. One pair of boots were Canadian arctic boots for 40 degrees below zero. They had a thick felt lining the color of the bright night sky. From a distance I saw the second pair hanging up. It was love at first sight. There they hung under the neon lights. They glowed a fluorescent greenyyellow. They fit perfectly and felt amazing. I thought, "These are my wingless boots." When I unpacked them at home, they were yellow. 20, 6C, 06:04:XX Themes: bright

Sh,109- Caught sight of a (black and white) cardboard box in the kitchen and momentarily thought it was a black and white dog (day time). 05, 12C, 08:XX:XX Themes: animal

Sh,11- Doing research on Uranus, I found that the planet has a tilt. For 42 years one side is in the dark and then comes into the light for 42 years. Interesting that I am now 43. Uranus feels very near, like a friend. The quasars are much further out and it was a real stretch for me to go so far. 20, 6C, XX:XX:XX Themes: integration, half, knowledge

Sh,12- I had many thoughts of the second day of creation. 20, 6C, 03:XX:XX Themes: greatness

Sh,123- Immediately after taking the remedy, everything stopped. I become very subdued and depressed. It felt like a void. No joy in birds singing. "How can I lift it?" 20, 6C, 00:00:00 Themes: sadness, music

Sh,13- Thoughts of twos and water. Saw images of Noah's ark. 20, 6C, 08:01:30 Themes: past, water, double

Sh,14- After a shower, I felt enormous, massive, yet in proportion. I was amazed at how huge I was. 20, 6C, 03:00:00 Themes: great, grow

Sh,15- I've been feeling huge the last few days, due to eating biscuits. Feel like my legs have gone all fleshy. 02, 6C, 07:XX:XX Themes: grow, great

Sh,159- Images of newborn babies crying. 20, 6C, 00:10:15 Themes: young

Sh,16- When I first put the remedy in my mouth I felt as if I had shrunk, particularly the legs. 02, 6C, 00:00:00 Themes: small

Sh,163- My head above the eyes cleared. It felt like a very wide opening from the top of my head outward. I felt a total synchronicity. I didn't have to get to a thought, bring it up, act. I was observing the mechanics of thought instead of needing them. It was effortless. While I felt I wasn't having thoughts, I was still doing everything I usually do. Everything was more beautiful. There was total order in space, more stable. This was a contrast for me. I usually feel chaotic. 20, 6C, XX:XX:XX Themes: integration

Sh,164- One of our visitors had gone out to buy a newspaper. When he came back I could not recognize him, although I've known him for 12 years. It took 30 seconds or more, not just a flash, thinking he was a total stranger. 02, 6C, 15:XX:XX Themes: stranger

Sh,165- I felt alone and as if everyone perceived me as odd. I felt strange, like an outsider and could not connect on any level. 02, 6C, 22:XX:XX Themes: solitude, abroad, strange

Sh,166- I paid the cobbler with a œ5 note. I could not recognize the money. My whole thought process seemed to be in slow motion. I felt the cobbler thought I was weird. 02, 6C, 23:XX:XX Themes: slow

Sh,169- Averse to doing practical jobs and put them off. I have not panicked as usual because I haven't done them. 10, 6C, 01:XX:XX Themes: negligence

Sh,17- Legs felt shorter.20, 6C, 00:02:40 Themes: small

Sh,173- Anxious about everything and depressed about the anxiety and feel it's all wrong. 10, 6C, 18:XX:XX Themes: wrong

Sh,175- I've been in a rotten mood all day, dwelling on past offenses. I just can't let go, it's making me angry. I feel like I hate that bastard; it's not an emotion I've had before. Now I feel vindictive, really awful; I feel that if I ever found out that he had been lying to me again I would say to him, "I'll kill you," "I'll slit your throat." These violent feelings were much eased when alone. 02, 6C, 04:22:40 Themes: offended, resentment, anger, homicidal, violence, revengeful, pointed

Sh,176- Got up late in a horrible mood and reproached my partner again. I hurt him but I didn't care. I felt indifferent, malicious and vindictive, full of hate. 02, 6C, 05:22:10 Themes: censorious, wicked, anger, indifference, revengeful

Sh,177- I feel like writing a letter to Jeremy and reproaching him about the proving. I just realized that I want to reproach people. I reproach my partner as well. 02, 6C, 05:XX:XX Themes: offensive, censorious

Sh,182- Had an explosion for not being the perfect person. I was really pissed off at the situation. I felt out of control, helpless, and lashed out with vehemence and anger at the situation and myself. I'm in the "Valley of Discontent" and want to get out of Sacramento. 31, 12C, 16:XX:XX Themes: perfection, anger, helplessness

Sh,191- I suddenly thought about my grandfather and cried over his unfortunate life. Suddenly I was cheerful and joking again. 02, 6C, 16:XX:XX Themes: compassionate

Sh,193- Feel sad and depressed while walking outside in the cold, clear, open air. I don't want to be outside, and walk with head down. On returning inside, I feel in suspended animation. Listless, low energy. Want to close my eyes, which are dry, with heavy, slightly numb lids. I don't feel like working and would just like to go to sleep or read a good book in bed under covers. I still feel chilly from 5 minute walk outside though I've been inside and dressed warmly for 5 minutes. 06, 12C, 00:01:00 Themes: sadness, go out, shame, energy

Sh,196- I got nominated for a scholarship and I couldn't generate any excitement about it. I thought "I probably won't get it." 35, 6C, 02:XX:XX Themes: indifference

Sh,197- This morning I felt indifference about the dirty house. I left the dishes, and dirty hair in the bath. 02, 6C, 05:XX:XX Themes: dirty

Sh,198- Received a long letter from a patient today; haven't even read it, can't be bothered. Very unusual. In terms of indifference, I have felt disgusted with myself; one of these violent and malicious feelings. God, I feel so wretched. 02, 6C, 05:XX:XX Themes: indifference, conscience, wretched, violence, loathing

Sh, 2- I took a deep breath of relief as I saw the dustmen come for the neon strip light. 20, 6C, 00:04:30 Themes: dirty, light

Sh,20- I had thoughts of albatrosses circumnavigating the earth without having to touch the ground. 20, 6C, 03:02:14 Themes: animal, distances, fly

Sh,200- I feel that nobody is there for me when I need them; I'm there for everyone when they need me but no one is ever there for me. 13, 30C, 07:00:00 Themes: helplessness, forsaken

Sh,201- Mental symptoms accompanying cystitis: I was very withdrawn, grouchy, wanted to be alone. Stayed in bed a lot and did a lot of mental work withdrawn from emotions. This is how I always was during my many past bouts of cystitis. 06, 12C, XX:XX:X Themes: solitude

Sh,203- Had thoughts of sex over 2 days; mentally planned scenarios of a clandestine meeting with an old boyfriend (more in the evening). 08, 30C, 00:00:20 Themes: sexual, lascivious

Sh,204- While dancing with a slightly known acquaintance felt sexually aroused; unusual for me. 08, 30C, 00:12:30 Themes: sexual

Sh,205- Sexy thoughts with increased desire; made love, felt nicely physical. 08, 30C, 00:00:40 Themes: sexual

Sh,21- Walking was effortless, light and free, with a sensation of walking uniformly. I feel so different in my body. I am all in the now, especially in lower legs and feet. At last, I touch the earth. 20, 6C, 03:01:00 Themes: integration, light, liberty

Sh,24- I feel invincible when upright. No wavering- like a laser. 20, 6C, 04:02:XX Themes: inexpugnable

Sh,29- While drifting in and out of sleep between 6:30 and 7:30 am, I had a fleeting sensation that part of me was parchment-like, i.e., thin, somewhat stiff, somewhat brittle in appearance but actually not brittle. Appearing weak but not weak. 06, 12C, 01:22:XX Themes: fragile

Sh,30- I had a fleeting image of being split down the middle (left and right sides split). 06, 12C, 01:22:XX Themes: divided, double

Sh,31- On closing eyes to relieve a bad headache, sensation that top of head and headache seemed to rise as I and the rest of my body sank, like a horizontal separation. Felt sick and exhausted 7:30 PM. 06, 12C, 18:XX:XX Themes: disintegration

Sh,33- I had intense pleasure at hearing the wind and I thought, "It will clear the skies." 20, 6C, 05:00:XX Themes: dirty

Sh,34- I feel more stable now that my feet touch the earth while still having my head touching the heavens. 20, 6C, 04:XX:XX Themes: integration

Sh,35- Feel like I have been kissed by heaven. 10, 6C, 07:01:XX Themes: pleasure, love

Sh,36- Now I felt no resistance, a harmony between heaven and earth. 20, 6C, XX:XX:XX Themes: peace

Sh,37- On walking in the fresh air I suddenly felt as if I was cruising along on an energy which was not of my own muscular power. It seemed as if it was coming from somewhere else. It seemed effortless and unreal. I felt as if I was passing everyone else. 02, 6C, 13:XX:XX Themes: energy, unreal, seized

Sh,38- I have always felt comfortable with the division between the dark and the light. What I now need is the division of heavens and oceans. Thoughts about my love for the Pacific Ocean. 20, 6C, 06:XX:XX Themes: love, nature

Sh,39- During the night, in a semi-sleep state, I had many thoughts of the second day of creation. I was aware that my form and weight were appropriate. 20, 6C, 03:XX:XX Themes: greatness, perfection

Sh,4- I have been living without a partner for 10 years, which I really enjoyed. Now I have an uncomfortable feeling of needing a partner. Usually I only want a partner because I have so much that I want to share it. This is a feeling of only being half and needing another. 20, 6C, 01:03:40 Themes: union, half

Sh,40- Twice thought I heard someone at the door but when I checked there was no one there. Thought there might have been a noise which suggested somebody was there. This happened twice during the proving. 05, 12C, 01:06:20 Themes: persecution

Sh,41- Twice at 5.45 am I was awakened by hearing a doorbell - leapt out of bed to open the door but no one was there.09, 12C, 17:XX:XX Themes: persecution

Sh,44- Dreamed that I was knocking on many different doors. Nobody opened them. 20, 6C, 19:XX:XX Themes: despised

Sh,46- Had the strong thought, "my connection with the past is dissolving" at 2.15 pm. 05, 12C, 05:05:35 Themes: past, disintegration

Sh,47- Lay in bed and body felt insubstantial starting with hands and forearms - as if I was dematerializing "beaming down." 05, 12C, 00:14:20 Themes: disintegration

Sh,48- A phrase from a Lewis Carroll poem repeated itself over and over in my mind: "Come tell me aged man he cried, come tell me how you live. And his answer trickled through my brain like water through a sieve." I felt this was about dissolving, which related to my feeling in the proving. 05, 12C, 05:05:XX Themes: water, disintegration

Sh,49- I have lost the delusion, which I have always had, that I could walk on water. 20, 6C, 04:XX:XX Themes: floating, water, greatness

5- I've always really liked odd numbers. I suddenly felt the capacity to be even. Even numbers were much more attractive. It felt like I'd never known even numbers and now I did. Half was missing. Now, it was like a new toy of evenness. Before I had gaps and I was jumping; now I could move smoothly. It's like there was too big a gap at the synapses. Now there was no gap between the source and the action. 20, 6C, 01:01:17 Themes: integration

Sh,51- I have many thoughts of freezing. "Why would people want to deep freeze themselves? Why not freeze dry them?" 20, 6C, 05:XX:XX Themes: water

Sh,52- Thoughts of rivers and oceans and being very happy by them. 20, 6C, 08:XX:XX Themes: pleasure, water

Sh,53- While lying awake in bed last night I heard a dinging sound, like glass or the sound of icicles tapping against each other. I looked but couldn't locate it. I tried to ignore it but the sound increased. I got up, went to the bedroom window and looked over the back garden. It was a fantastic cold, clear night. With a thrill of excitement I watched all the stars in the sky above and I just knew that the noise I'd heard was the stars trying to communicate with me. The noise seemed to last for ages. The thrill lasted for as long as I stood by the window. When I went back to bed I felt wonderful. The noise stopped. 02, 6C, 06:XX:XX Themes: integration

Sh,54- I just long for some clear nights, so I can see my stars. If I could reconnect, then everything would be all right. 02, 6C, 11:XX:XX Themes: nature, integration

Sh,55- Looking out of the window at the night sky, it suddenly cracked open and a great darkness revealed itself. Infinity was blackness. It was deeply disturbing. 02, 6C, 67:XX:XX Themes: disintegration

Sh,57- Felt wonderful. Kept going outside during the night, between midnight and 3 am. At last the sky was clear, moon brilliant, stars familiar, air cold. I felt so much a part of everything again. 20, 6C, 06:19:XX Themes: integration

Sh,58- Image of being inside my iris and looking through. That is, I see a large iris and I was looking through it. From the center of it light was radiating out. 20, 6C, 07:XX:XX Themes: bright, light

Sh,6- Occasional thoughts about numbers: I had always felt comfortable with odd numbers. Now, being both gave a whole other dimension. To have had half missing for so long! What is different? From 3 to 1, slight tension. From 2 to 1, effortless natural progression. I had many thoughts on potency. It was important to chose the potency precisely, not to be so random in choosing a 9, 12, 15 etc. 20, 6C, 02:01:02 Themes: half, integration

Sh,60- During the proving the prover separated from her partner of 13 years. She had attempted this several times previously, unsuccessfully. I asked her what had changed: "Somehow I had a very profound realization that this is my own life time. My usual feelings of guilt shifted and I was able to take responsibility for my own life. There was a sudden clarity. During the proving I wore my glasses more and had dreams of windows. As though there had been a shift of focus to my own needs." 02, 6C, XX:XX:XX Themes: liberty, union

Sh,63- I notice a foolish and irresistible desire to spy on my partner through the keyhole in the door to his study. I now remember doing this a couple of times yesterday (on the first day of the proving) as well. I am finding it ridiculous, laughing to myself. I feel like a mischievous child, doing something it shouldn't do, giggling away to myself. It makes me feel excited in a childish sense. I have never felt compelled to spy on anyone ever - be it through a keyhole or otherwise. Very strange. 02, 6C, 01:06:40 Themes: young, child

Sh,65- While looking at a star map, it looked unfamiliar, as if I had always been seeing the stars from the other side. 20, 6C, 08:09:XX Themes: strange

Sh,69- Recognized a change in awareness - a vaguely stoned, unreal feeling. Giggly, childish, grinning. Felt light. 05, 12C, 05:05:XX Themes: young, child, unreal, light

Sh,7- I saw two points of white light merging together, becoming one. 20, 6C, 03:03:22 Themes:

Sh,77- I don't quite seem to know where my body is in space, tripping and falling. 06, 12C, 00:05:00 Themes: lost

Sh,79- Heard the sound of my foot move but was not aware of it moving. I did not know where I was. 20, 6C, 00:06:30 Themes: lost

Sh,8- I had thoughts of odd and even numbers. I felt I had always jumped up from 3 to 1. That made me too high. I now feel that I need to work my way down, 1-2-3. In the past, it was easier for me to go up than come down. Now I feel that I can go down or either way. 20, 6C, 06:03:XX Themes: integration

Sh,84- Repeated prophetic notions of daily events before hearing of them, causing anxiety and discomfort; thoughts of a person not seen for months and found he had phoned a few days before, depression and sadness unexplained until heard of sad family news that had already happened. 10, 6C, 01:XX:XX Themes: clairvoyance, sadness, compassionate

Sh,85- Feel out of control, as if time is moving relentlessly and remorselessly forward and I'm stuck behind, unable to keep up. Panic, guilt, constant anxiety that I won't get it all done, including keeping up this journal. 10, 6C, 12:XX:XX Themes: time, duty, conscience, unfit

Sh,86- A friend observed that my eyes were wider open, not so soft. She said they looked very forward and excited. She also observed that I seemed excited in company. I felt very speedy, and could not get words out fast enough, tripping over my words. I was speaking faster than I could articulate the words. 20, 6C, 01:08:45 Themes: hurry

Sh,88- I remembered the incidences in dreams in the reverse order in which they happened—very unusual for me. 20, 6C, 01:01:55 Themes: inversion

Sh,89- Husband comments that I seem "far away and long ago." He hasn't seen me this "gone" in a long time. 06, 12C, 00:04:55 Themes: isolation

Sh,91- I'm finding it hard to judge how long ago recent events were. Can't seem to judge time in the past. Can't think back through the days. It's as if I've lost the thread with the past that connects all past days together. It has dissolved. I seem to be more in the moment and less hurried. I usually look at my watch often, but today I forgot I had put it on, and kept asking a friend the time. Was surprised when I discovered I'd been wearing it all day. Very unusual. 05, 12C, 05:XX:XX Themes: past, disintegration, time

Sh,92- I had a sense of timelessness and wanted to find the clock but could not. I had no reference points and thought that if I could find the time, it would be a reference point in the void. 20, 6C, 00:00:30 Themes: time

Sh,93- I was confused about my watch. I couldn't tell which way was up on the clock face. 20, 6C, 00:01:50 Themes: inversion

Sh,97- Then I had the image like the inside of a body. I was in the dark but it was bright, like an amazing landscape. There were gently undulating folds of membrane. It was shiny and beautiful with bright points (nuclei of each cell) sparkling like tiny jewels. The tiny points of light were like the points of light that sun makes on snow. 'Epithelium' came to mind. 20, 6C, 00:01:30 Themes: bright

Sh,99- Image of folds of membrane inside a body like a landscape, and it sparkled like tiny jewels, like sun shining in snow. I thought 'epithelium,' and these are the nuclei. 20, 6C, 07:01:30 Themes: bright

NICC.

Al,1- Very angry and quarrelsome mood; she was inclined to quarrel with and contradict everyone, in the evening. Themes: anger, fight, contradiction, antagonism

Al,2- Quarrelsome and impatient; she could tolerate no contradiction;... Themes: impatience, contradiction, fight

Al,6 - Apprehensive and despondent, as if some misfortune were impending. Themes: despair, misfortune, menaced

Al,9- Tremulous, fearful, with inclination to be alone all day. Themes: fearful, solitude

He,1- Low-spirited, tearful; fears something evil will happen. Themes: sadness, misfortune

He,2- Vexed and very angry from least contradiction. Themes: anger, contradiction

NIT-AC.

Al,17- At once she is taken which peculiar anguish, runs to her physician, but he is not at home, hires a carriage to drive to the house where she expects to find him; during her ride all the anguish is gone; arrived at home she feels as bad as ever, and feels herself thus forced to drive about the whole day, till all the effects of the Nitric acid have passed off. Themes: disease, helplessness, home, travel, go out

Al,18- Satiety of life with fear of death. Themes: tedium, death

Al,2- Attacks of rage and despair, with curses and imprecations.(blasphemy) Themes: anger, despair, offensive

Al,20- Anxiety, like palpitation, with nausea, without efforts to vomit, as if she had committed a crime, at night in bed; ...(conscience) Themes: conscience, criminal

Al,24- More anxious than usual during a storm. Themes: storm

Al,27- Vexed at the least trifle, even at himself if he makes a mistake. Themes: bothered, conscience, wrong, himself, conscientious

Al,30- Anxious oppression, like nightmare,

as if some one were lying under him and holding him fast with the arms about his abdomen, so that he could not free himself, immediately after falling asleep. (constriction, immobilization) Themes: oppression, imprisoned, caught

Al,33- Depressed, as if despondent and as if in deep thought. Themes: sadness, despair, mortification

Al,43- She wishes for death and yet dreads it. Themes: death, antagonism

Al,5- Long-continued rancor, insensible to apologies and excuses. Themes: resentment, anger

Al,60- Could scarcely free himself from sad thoughts. Themes: mortification

Al,62- Discontented, despising (scorn) life. Themes: discontented, loathing

Ha,12- She falls to thinking over an anxious occurrence long past, and cannot rid herself of it, almost like as if in a waking dream; from time to time she, as it were, awakes from it startled, but is always absorbed in these ideas, without being able, in spite of strenuous efforts of thinking of anything else. Themes: mortification, past, dwells

Ha,15- Apprehensiveness, with stitches above the heart, and a fancy as if he was talking deliriously, with coldness of the body and a tendency to fall down. Themes: heart, talk, insanity, fall

Ha,16- Anxiety, as if he was engaged in a disquieting lawsuit or contest. (conflict, debate, competition) Themes: discussion, justice, fight

Ha,18- In the evening, he feels apprehensive; he cannot sit still, but has to walk about. Themes: restless, movement

Ha,19- More apprehensive during a thunderstorm than usually. Themes: storm

Ha,2- Dejected, as if desponding and as if lost in thoughts. Themes: sadness, despair, lost

Ha,25- She imagines she will die soon, but has no bodily indisposition. Themes: death, disease

Ha,27- She wishes to die, and nevertheless she is afraid of death. Themes: death, antagonism

Ha,28- Discontented despising life. Themes: discontented, loathing, discontented

Ha,33-Discontented with oneself, dissolving in tears, which gives relief. Themes: discontented, himself

Ha,38- Very ill- humored and vexed at himself. Themes: bothered, himself

Ha,4- He cannot get rid of his sad thoughts. Themes: mortification, tortured

Ha,42- Peevishness with sadness and a crabbed (irritable) humor with restlessness, so that she knows not where to turn (drive) Themes: restless, movement

Ha,44- Vexed at the least trifle, also at himself, when he does something amiss.(wrong) Themes: conscience, conscientious, wrong, himself

Ha,46- When disputing (debate), there is trembling in all the limbs. Themes: discussion

Ha,47- He is inclined to be passionate and contentious.(quarrelsome) Themes: passionate, fight, discussion

Ha,48- Passionateness, venting itself in abuse. (insult) Themes: passionate, offensive

Ha,49- He gets violently excited about trifles, all the day, and has then to laugh at himself. Themes: passionate, himself, pleasure

Ha,5- homesickness. Themes: homesickness

Ha,51- Long-continued rancor; insensible to apology and excuses. Themes: anger, resentment

Ha,6- Inclined to be violent and to quarrel. Themes: fight, violence, discussion

Ha,9- At the least admonition (censure), the child begins to weep piteously. Themes: censured

He,10- Sadness, great fear of death, sensation of extreme weakness, even to trembling. Themes: death, energy

He,13- Hopeless despair. Themes: hopeless, despair

He,14- Often anxious about his illness; constantly thinks about his past troubles; mind weak and wandering. Themes: disease, mortification, energy, past, dispersion

He,15- Anxiety as if he was engaged in a lawsuit or dispute, causing uneasiness. Themes: justice, discussion,

He,16- Anxiety about his disease, with fear of death; morbid fear of cholera. Themes: disease, death, infection

He,17- After continued loss of sleep, long-lasting anxiety, over-exertions of mind and body from nursing the sick, great anguish of mind from loss of his dearest friend. Themes: lack, death, friend,

He,19- ...headstrong (obstinate); trembling while quarreling; fits of rage with curses and maledictions; inveterate ill-will, unmoved by apologies. Themes: anger, offensive, resentment, obstinate, fight

He,22- Discontent with himself induces violent weeping. Themes: himself, discontented

He,5- Fancies she will die soon, yet is not physically ill. Themes: death, disease, anticipation

He,6- Raving, as if delirious, with coldness of body and inclination to fall. Themes: anger, fall

He,7- Feels as though he had partly lost his will-power. Themes: will, energy

He,8- Taciturn, disinclined to communicate anything; moody in morning. Themes: misanthropy, solitude, company

NUX-M.

Al,16- Great fear of death. Themes: death

Al,24- Variable mood; at one time he wishes to do something, but when he is about to accomplish it changes his mind. Themes: succeed, irresolution,

Al,27- As soon as she lay down felt a sinking sensation, as though she were going to die, with no fear, however, being perfectly at ease (peace) in mind,... Themes: sinking, death, fearless, peace

Al,30- While writing he omitted letters, wrote in different alphabets against his will and changed from one subject to another. Themes: stranger, wrong, antagonism

Al,31- The words he employed to express his sensations remarkable for the merit of being the opposite (contrary) to what he should have used;... Themes: talk, antagonism

Al,32- Many ridiculous or extravagant acts or expressions, like idiocy, while she seemed perfectly conscious, and at the next moment would appear chagrined at her conduct, and said she could not control her actions... Themes: ridiculous, conscience, grief, shame

Al,48- He never accomplishes what she undertakes, but remains standing in one place, absent minded; he appears quite changed to his companions. Themes: reserved, succeed, dispersion,

Al,49- It became difficult to recall to mind things learned shortly before; for many such things the mind seemed paralyzed for many days together. Themes: knowledge, paralysis

Al,56-...he went to the theater, which was at some distance; the way seemed to have no end (endless, interminable); ... Although he was, at times, quite unconscious, his limbs did not fail to their service; he went straight on, without recognizing the streets that crossed his way; he was concerned about the time, he feared to come too late..., fancy and reality battle (fight) with each other. Themes: time, lost, antagonism, unreal

Al,60- State of mind similar to that of the opium-eater, entertaining no apprehension of the result, although aware of the presence of some danger. Themes: fearless, danger, indifference

He,14- While writing he omitted letters, wrote in different alphabets against his will, and changed from one subject to another. Themes: antagonism, wrong

He,15- Surroundings seemed changed; fanciful, dreamy images; does not recognize the known street. Themes: lost, unreal, strange

He,17- The outer world had no existence for her; automatically she attended to her household duties, and on awaking from this condition she had not the slightest recollection of what she had done; ... Themes: indifference, duty, unreal, home

He,24- Fitful mood, changing from deepest sorrow to most frolicsome (happy) behavior; now grave (serious), now gay. Themes: grief, pleasure, antagonism

He,25- Fickle (capricious); irresolute and wavering in his undertakings. Themes: irresolution, doubtful, confidence, succeed

He,26- Aware of danger, but no apprehension. Themes: danger, fearless

He,6- Never accomplishes what he undertakes, but remains standing in one place, absent-minded... Themes: dispersion, suppressed, separated

NUX-V.

Al,1- Anxious delirious fantasies, in the evening in bed, in the ninth hour, as if some one would get into his bed,(base, foundation) and there was no room (space) in it; or as if some one had sold his bed etc. Themes: invaded, robber

Al,21- Great aversion to fluids, which were swallowed with great difficulty and often not at all. Themes: water, loathing

Al,3- Rushed into the room, exclaiming that her mother had been murdered. Themes: death, murdered, mother

Al,39- Great anxiety; he had to rise from any place and wished rather (first) to die. Themes: restless, death

Al,4- He is hasty; looked angrily at anyone who asked him a question without answering, as though he was obliged to restrain himself to avoid being insulting; he was in such an irritable and unrestrained mood that it seemed as though he would like to strike any one in the face who spoke a word to him. Themes: hurry, anger, bother, offensive, suppressed, violence, indignation

Al,41- Anxiety; an anxious solicitude, as though something serious (dangerous) were dreaded, in the morning and afternoon.. Themes: fearful, danger

Al,45- Anxiety, caused by a suspicious and apprehensive condition of mind, especially during the afternoon hours. Themes: suspicious

Al,5- (Suicide; she throws herself down from a height) Themes: suicidal, height

Al,53- She believes that she is near death. Themes: death

Al,54- She was in great alarm, kept fast hold on her husband and refused to let him go. Themes: fearful, helplessness, danger

Al,6- The usual pain seems intolerable; she would rather take her life. Themes: disease, suicidal

Al,60- Everything miscarriages (failure) with him; it seems to go contrary. Themes: failure

Al,68- Irresolution; constant fickleness in his plans. Themes: irresolution, confidence

Al,69- Dawdles (delay) and is irresolute. Themes: postponing, doubtful, irresolution

Al,71- She wishes to accomplish much, but thinks it will not succeed. Themes: ambition, failure, succeed

Al,73- Dread of that kind of literary work at which one must think and employ the ideas, ... Themes: work, knowledge, confidence

Al,88- Clear consciousness of his existence; fine, strong, correct feeling of right and wrong. Themes: justice, wrong

Ha,1235- ...anxiety and anxious solicitude (care), as if something important were to be feared (afraid). Themes: fearful, misfortune, danger

Ha,1236- Anxiety and anguish as if he had committed some crime. Themes: conscience, criminal

Ha,1237- Great anxiety; he cannot rest in any place, (restlessness) and would rather die. Themes: death, restless

Ha,1238- After midnight very violent palpitation of the heart with extreme anxiety, which urges (impulse) him to commit suicide. Themes: suicidal, heart

Ha,1239 -She deems (believe) the pain she suffers intolerable and will rather take her own life. Themes: suicidal, disease

Ha,1240- Anxiety with impulse to commit suicide. Themes: suicidal

Ha,1241- (Suicide; she throws herself from a height.) Themes: suicidal, height

Ha,1246- He fears death. Themes: fearful, death

Ha,1247- She thinks herself near death. Themes: death

Ha,1248- Wrapped up in sorrow and care. Themes: mortification, grief

Ha,1253- Pains are not borne without loud whining and lamenting, mixed with reproaches and scolding. Themes: censorious, offensive.

Ha,1254- She cannot get over the smallest evil. Themes: will, obstructed, unfit

Ha,1255- Anxious solicitude and inconsolableness, which breaks out in loud weeping complaints and reproaches... Themes: censorious

Ha,1256- Anxious solicitude (care) and irresolution. Themes: irresolution

Ha,1257- Anxiety from suspicious and timorous (timidity) solicitude, especially in the hours after midnight. Themes: suspicious, fearful

Ha,1262- She cannot bear the least contradiction, nor suffer the most reasonable representations (narration) to induce her to alter her conduct; they put her beside herself. Themes: contradiction, censured

Ha,1263- He is peevish solicitous, takes everything amiss (erroneous), and readily breaks out into scolding and abuse. Themes: offenses, offensive

Ha,1266- Very much given to reproach others severely for their faults. Themes: censorious, wrong

Ha,1267- Scolding, reproaches, abuse, jealous invectives (accusation), mixed with indelicate expressions - then soon howling and loud weeping. Themes: jealousy, censorious, offensive

Ha,1269- He obstinately opposes what others wish. Themes: obstinate, antagonism

Ha,1270- He is hasty (careless, rapid), looks malignantly (deadly) at any one who asks (asked) him anything, without answering, just as if he must control himself in order to avoid becoming coarse (rude) , it seems as if he would like to strike any one in the face who speaks a word to him, so irritable and uncontrollable in his disposition. Themes: indignation, violence, anger, suppressed, hurry, bothered

Ha,1272- Over-sensitiveness to impressions of the senses; he cannot bear strong odors and bright light. Themes: sensitive, bright, light

Ha,1273- He cannot bear any noise or speaking; music and singing affect him strongly. Themes: music, talk, noise, sensitive

Ha,1283- Ennui; time seems to him intolerably long. Themes: time, tedium

Ha,1288- Irresolution, constant hesitation in his intentions. Themes: irresolution, doubtful, confidence

Ha,1289- She wishes to do much, but thinks she will not succeed. Themes: succeed, failure

Ha,1289- She wishes to do much, but thinks she will not succeed. Themes: succeed, confidence, failure

Ha,1290- He thinks that everything will go wrong.(failure) Themes: failure

Ha,1291- Everything goes wrong with him. (everything goes contrary) Themes: wrong, failure

Ha,1294- Something, he knows not what, hinders (opposed ,obstructed) him, specially in scientific occupations. Themes: obstructed, knowledge

Ha,1296- In the morning, dread of those literary occupations in which he must think for himself and unfold ideas from his own mind in order either to commit them to writing or to express them orally; but reading and learning by heart are not distasteful to him. Themes: confidence, knowledge

Ha,1301- Clear consciousness of his existence; delicate, strong proper (accurate, correct, exact) feeling of right and wrong. (sapience) (justice) Themes: knowledge, justice, perfection, wrong

He,10-...every harmless word offends, every little noise frightens, anxious and beside themselves, cannot bear even the least suitable medicine. (contrary) Themes: offenses, suspicious, noise, contrary

He,11- Cannot bear reading or conversation; irritable and wishes to be alone. Themes: talk, solitude, sensitive

He,12- Inclined to find fault and scold (reprove); morose; stubborn; (obstinate) an insane desire when alone with her husband, whom she adores, to kill him. Themes: censorious, offensive, obstinate, homicidal, husband

He,13- Irritable, angry disposition, anxious concern about little things. (trifles) Themes: anger, conscientious

He,16- Ill-humored, resists obstinately the wishes of others. Themes: obstinate, antagonism

He,17- He quarrels, reproaches, scolds, insults, from jealousy, mingled with unchaste (obscene) expressions; ... Themes: fight, censorious, jealousy, offensive

He,19- ...; imagines himself surrounded by persons who carry on all sorts of pranks (joke, jest), or ply (covering) him with questions which he thinks he is compelled (forced) to answer (proved, questioned, interrogated);..; answers questions rationally and is conscious of his condition; ...appears to be haunted (obsessed) by a great fear. Themes: surrounded, despised, offenses, bother, knowledge, fearful

He,20- Desire to talk about one's condition, with anxious reflections about it. Themes:

talk, disease, himself, meditation

He,21- Anxiety with irritability and inclination to commit suicide, but is afraid to die. Themes: suicidal, death, antagonism

He,23- Great anxiety of mind without particular cause; thinks she will not be able to get along (prosper) in life; caducity; (senility)... Themes: unfit, succeed, failure

He,26- Melancholic in consequence of losing his position (rank),...the least contradiction puts him out entirely...(ailments from) Themes: sadness, position, failure, contradiction

He,30- Ailments after continued mental exertion; indisposition to it, particularly to that form which involves elaboration and connection of subjective ideas independently of external objects. Themes: knowledge, disintegration, unfit

He,33- Mental disturbance, patient tortured with fixed idea. Themes: tortured, mortification

He,35- From disappointed ambition, bewildered, (confused) talks incoherently; does everything he attempts (try) to do wrong;.. Themes: ambition, failure, wrong

He,37- ...betraying (play false, feigning) great moral and physical languor (indifference),..launches into high-flying, fantastic plans, fancies himself rich (rank, position) and wants to make presents of thousands (squanders, waste), and makes large useless purchases; does not consider himself ill; ...,and takes in bad part if not allowed to read indictment (accusation) for said lawsuit, a confused irrational piece of work... Themes: helpful, greatness, feigning, planning, position, squanders, wealth, helpful, offenses, censorious, justice

He,37-...brooding all night long over a lawsuit by which he may gain or lose a million (megalomania) ; ..replies reluctantly and slowly to physician's questions, and takes it in bad part (offenses) if not allowed to read indictment (accusation) for said lawsuit, a confused irrational piece of work, on which he has been working all night. Themes: dwells, justice, wealth, offenses, discussion, ambition

He,38- Three months ago mental shock, since then fears to be alone,...fears as if she would choke (suffocation)...fears to be alone, fear of knives and the like, (similar) lest she should kill herself or others... Themes: solitude, suicidal, homicidal, suffocation, pointed

He,39- Mania puerperalis...constantly complaining, criticizing or explaining, ... as soon she recognized physician she spoke of imperfection of medical knowledge and declared it an error that one could not live without a heart, inasmuch as she felt very well without one, it having come away with the afterbirth to which it had grown fast, the nurse having separated the two before her eyes; complains of her husband, says he wishes to convince her she is sick, ... nymphomania,... frequently sips at a bowl of warm sugar-water, declaring it will form her a new heart; .(health, healing)...(expert) Themes: censorious, perfection, wrong, grow, knowledge, disease, heart, husband, sexual,

He,4- Cannot read or calculate, for she loses the connection of ideas; thinks she will lose her reason. Themes: disintegration, insanity, knowledge

He,5- Very easily bewildered(confused); everything goes wrong. Themes: wrong

He,6- Ennui; the time seems intolerably long, passes slowly. Themes: tedium, time

He,8- Suits very particular, careful,(prudent, meticulous) zealous (conscientious) persons, inclined to get angry or excited, or a spiteful (cruel), malicious disposition. Themes: conscientious, anger, wicked,

OENA.

Al,14- It seemed to her as if she were flying. Themes: fly

Al,21- She thought that she was transported to a very great elevation.(elevated) Themes: height

OLND.

Al,15- While studying he had constantly other thoughts; he found himself dreaming of the future, and busying himself with beautiful images concerning it. Themes: future, pleasure, perfection

Al,5- Loss (want) of confidence in himself, and on that account a sad mood. Themes: confidence,

Al,6- He immediately became overheated; he became passionate, though he immediately repented (sorry) of it. Themes: passionate, conscience

Al,7- He cannot tolerate contradiction. Themes: contradiction

Ha,348- Want of self confidence, and hence serious sad disposition. Themes: confidence,

Ha,350- He cannot bear contradiction. Themes: contradiction

Ha,352- The heat rapidly overcomes him; he breaks out in anger, but repents (sorry) immediately afterwards. Themes: anger, conscience

He,6- Despondency and lack of self-confidence. Themes: hopeless, confidence

OP.

Al,137- Appeared jealous and afraid (fear) of people around. Themes: jealousy, suspicious

ml,148-...his mind to be not only clear and active, but filled with gigantic schemes and theories, the realization of which seems to him quite natural and easy; his faculties are remarkably keen (sharp)... Themes: planning, greatness, theorizing

Al,16- ...started up in a fright on account of fancied swordsmen (rival, competitor) who threatened to stab him; became angry if any one argued him or thought him delirious; however, he blamed (reproaches) himself while in delirium for his folly. Themes: menaced, pointed, murdered, conscience, hurt, anger, attacked

Al,187- The memory and mental powers generally became greatly impaired, attended by a miserable depression of spirits. Themes: energy, miserable, sadness

Al,19-...each possessing some imaginary bliss (happiness) which " the dull (dark) reality of life" could never give....they are wrapped in an elysium, (heaven) from which they are only to be awakened by the miserable reaction which must, sooner or later recall them to existence. Themes: seized, pleasure, religious, perfection

Al,19- ...; all the actors are happy, and each retires home in a total state of irrationality, but likewise in the entire and full enjoyment of happiness not to be procured by reason. Disregarding the ridicule of those they meet, who divert themselves by making them talk absurdly, each imagines looks and feels himself possessed of whatever he wishes... Themes: greatness, pleasure, wealth, perfection, ridiculous

Al,29- A half intoxicated and excited condition , so that I came near being run over by a carriage, and at another time of running into a horse, though I had seen it coming from some distance. Themes: run over

Al,36- Mind in a state of great confusion; at one moment she was sensible (conscious) to her crime, called for assistance (comfort, aid, help) ; at another she resisted the means used to save her. Themes: conscience, criminal, helplessness, antagonism

Al,37- Conscious of being possessed (seized) of two persons (double) of another self besides his real self, the Opium man does things which the real self considers wrong, and it is not always sure which will conquer the other. Themes: seized, double, conscience, antagonism, wrong,

Al,39- ...threatened alternately self-destruction and injury to others. Themes: suicidal, hurt, violence, menacing

Al,43- In walking I was hardly sensible that my feet touched the ground; it seemed as if I slid (floating) along the ground impelled by some invisible agent, and that my blood was composed of some ethereal fluid which rendered my body lighter than air. Themes: floating, blood, unreal, light

Al,44- He seems to be flying or floating in the air, and to whirl (rotate) with everything about him. Themes: fly, floating

Al,45- Sensation as if he had been taken to heaven; vivid, lovely fantasies float before his vision like a waking dream, which the slumber (sleep) drives away. Themes: pleasure, unreal, perfection,

Al,68- Criminals (in India) lose their fear of death and go courageously to their execution.(fearless) Themes: criminal, fearless, executed, death

Al,69- Great strength, courage, contentment with himself. Themes: energy, himself, conscience

Al,70- Sensation of courage with activity, as if he could forcibly accomplish whatever was required without dread or fear, with a peculiar sensation of lustiness. (strong) Themes: sexual, energy, succeed, fearless, duty

Al,78- Fear of impending death. Themes: death

Ha,601- Tranquil indifference to earthly things; she cared for nothing in comparison with ecstasies of the fantasy. Themes: indifference, duty, pleasure

Ha,621- Feeling of courage and merriment (joy), so that he is as if he would carry out what was required with energy, without repugnance or fear, with a peculiar feeling of voluptuousness...(sensuality) Themes: pleasure, energy, sexual,

Ha,637- She was troubled when awake with the supposed sight of ghosts, devils and spectres, which she believed to be surrounding her bed... Themes: surrounded, ghosts, devil

Ha,638 - He chattered all sorts of unconnected stuff and pointed with his fingers to imaginary masked people approaching him; ...he started at imaginary swordsmen, who might kill him ; ... Themes: approached, attacked, pointed, murdered, death

He,11- Thinks he is not in his own house; imagines himself living in a locality three hours distant from his house; detains all passers-by and wishes to take them into his house; ...he does not recognize friends;... (estranged, alien) Themes: home, homesickness, helplessness, stranger, friend

He,12- Said many disconnected things and pointed to masked people who seemed to approach him. Themes: approached, suspicious

He,13- Sees frightful ghosts; easily frightened. Themes: ghosts, fearful

He,16- Imagines parts of body very large. Themes: great

He,17- Thinks she is not at home. Themes: home

He,20- ...declares he is not alone in bed; ..desire to escape; says a regiment of horsemen are upon his bed and that he fears to be trodden upon (run over, crushed); when told that horses are very careful, answered that he feared he would be crushed by the wagons that followed them. Themes: invaded, officer, run over, crushed, danger, accidents, attacked

He,21-...in old, emaciated persons; sees animals coming towards him; people want to hurt him, execute him ; creeping under covers or jumping out of bed; in "old sinners" (criminals) whose long lives of excess have thoroughly destroyed their constitutions; ...; believe themselves to be murderers or criminals to be executed; want to run away (escape) ;... Themes: attacked, animal, hurt, murdered, hide, conscience, criminal, executed, escape, hide

He,22-... feeling of great strength; contempt of death;...indifference to joy and suffering. Themes: greatness, energy, inexpugnable, death, pleasure, contemptuous, indifference

He,27- Anxiety; apprehension; fear of impending death. Themes: death

He,30- Grief over insults is followed by convulsions. Themes: grief, offenses, fit

He,7- Drunkenness, with stupor; as if from smoke in brain;.. Themes: obstructed

OPUN-V.

Al,2- The mind appears to be much affected, and does not appreciate any of its morbid condition; much tempted to do things one should not do. Themes: duty, conscience, conscience

Al,4- In a few minutes, desire to be at prayer; go there, and in a minute or two desire to go out and "tidy" up; soon went out on an errand downstairs, then come up and go again to prayer. Themes: go out, religious, vanity

Al,5- Fit of swearing (cursing) at evening after coming home; praying in the morning, swearing (cursing) on disappointment in plans; fit of rage, on thwarting (frustrating) of plans. Themes: offensive, religious, menacing, disappointment, planning, anger, failure

Al,6- In the afternoon, fit of petulance, angry at near relatives, swearing mood, not at all pleased, cannot get over the thought of injuries done by friends. Themes: offenses, anger, relatives, offensive, friend

Al,8- Very vindictive at night. Themes: revengeful

OSM.

Al,5- Thoughts of accidents having happened to others, by a blow, a fall, or being dashed (crushed, hit, knock) to pieces; gradually these thoughts grow upon him, as if he were to do the same injuries to others. Themes: accidents, others, fall, hurt, wicked, crushed

OX-AC.

Al,19- Philoprogenitiveness, greater love of his children, in one in whom this feeling was always predominating; a decidedly expressed and clearly distinguishable symptom, it being not traceable to any other cause. (love creation of child) Themes: love, child, sexual

Al,28- Great distress and fear of death. Themes: death

Al,32- Greater presence of mind; the relations of the world seem to be clearer to him. Themes: organization. knowledge

PAEON.

He,1- Anxious, afraid (fear) to talk with any one; much affected by bad news, after pinching in belly. Themes: sensitive, talk, news

PALL.

He,2- Time seems longer to him, as if contained more; when he looks at the clock far less has been spent than he expected. Themes: time

He,1- Extremely fatigued in evening; feels mentally gone; is averse to speaking a foreign language which at other times he speaks fluently; it is too much of an exertion, he is tired of it. (lack of communication) Themes: lost, energy, talk, stranger,

He,12- Greatly inclined to use strong and violent expressions. Themes: offensive, violence

He,14- She tries to appear as amiable as possible, but is obstinate. Themes: mildness, feigning, obstinate

He,15- Depressing news makes all her symptoms worse. Themes: sadness, news

He,18- Feels best in company and wants to be flattered. Themes: flattery, company

He,3- When walking in street in evening, it seems to him as if he had grown taller. (enlarged, grow) Themes: great, grow

He,5- They set great store (deposit) on other people's opinion, and attach great importance to what others think, hence they are very excitable in company and their complaints are worse next day. (sensitive, judgment) Themes: company,

He,6- Apprehension (fear) as if something horrible would happen. Themes: horrible, misfortune

He,8- Imagines herself neglected (scorned, despised); wounded pride. Themes: despised, offenses, forsaken

PETR.

Al,10 - Anxiety at a noise of a crowd of many people. Themes: crowd, noise

Al,12- Fear of death. Themes: death

Al,28- No desire to work; no pleasure in objects of which he was usually fond (loving), hence intolerable ennui. Themes: work, indifference, tedium

Al,8- Violent irritable, offended at trifles. Themes: violence, offenses

Ha,1- Sad and dispirited, with a sick (suffering) feeling owing (due) to weakness of the heart. Themes: heart, disease, sadness, energy

Ha,10- He does not know how to stop talking about a thing. Themes: talk, doubtful

Ha,14- Ill-humor; strong tendency to be hypochondriac with a feverish condition for fourteen days. Themes: disease

Ha,27- The whole day, he is only half conscious, as if only half alive. Themes: divided, double, alive, half

Ha,4- Anxiety in the bustle (confusion) of many men. crowd Themes: company, crowd

He,5- Since confinement two weeks ago when in bed, in dark room, at night, delusion that there is another baby (small, tiny) in bed which requires attention also that she has a third leg which would not remain quiet. Themes: double, helplessness, dark, child, restless

Ha,8- The greatest irresolution. Themes: irresolution

Ha,9- Lack of determination.(resolution) Themes: irresolution, confidence

He,11- Melancholy mood, imagines but little time is left him to make his will. Themes: time, sadness, will

He,12- Sensation as if there were a cold stone in heart.(indifferent, careless) Themes: hard, oppression, heart,
He,13- Towards evening anxiety and apprehension about his family which he left behind while going on a short journey; the anxiety increases until he becomes inconsolable. Themes: family, others, travel
He,3- Did not know where she was in the street. Themes: lost
He,4- Delirium; thinks another person lies alongside (close) of him, or that one limb is double. Themes: double, organization
He,6- Excitable, irritable with inclination to be angry and to scold; anxious and irresolute. Themes: irresolution, doubtful, anger, offensive
He,7- Violent irritable, offended at trifles. Themes: violence, offenses

PH-AC.

Al,10- Sadness and feeling of solitude, as if she would be sick. Themes: sadness, solitude, disease
Al,12- Sad , earnest, discouraged only when walking in the open air, the farther (great distance) he walks the more it increases; in the house it gradually disappears. Themes: sadness
Al,17- He was constantly complaining about his illness. Themes: disease
Al,8- Lachrymose, as from homesickness. Themes: homesickness
Al,9- Sad and solicitous concerning the future. Themes: sadness, future
Ha,13- Hurried in talking; he cannot get anything fast enough. Themes: talk, hurry, time
Ha,20- Discontented with himself, reproaches himself. Themes: discontented, conscience
Ha,22- He looks very ill-humored and peevish, so that everyone asks him what is the matter with him; but he was not sick. (appearance) Themes: disease
Ha,25- At a slight offense, he is, as it were, beside himself and passionate. Themes: offenses, passionate
Ha,3- Sad and full of solicitude (anxiety), afraid she might fall ill. Themes: sadness, disease
Ha,34- He cannot get his ideas into their proper connection. Themes: organization, disintegration
Ha,35- He cannot get rid of one thought, and the other thoughts to be connected therewith do not come in. Themes: dwells
Ha,4- Restless and full of anxiety, that she might get ill. Themes: disease
Ha,40- While reading, a thousand other thoughts crowd into his mind (dispersion) ; he could not comprehend anything , what he read was dark to him, and he forgot everything at once, with difficulty in recollecting what he had known a long time already. (lost: memory, concentration, comprehension, knowledge) Themes: dispersion, knowledge, dark, past
Ha,41- Illusion of the senses, as if he heard the clock strike or as if lofty (tall, elevated) things lying out of his horizon were moving near him. Themes: noise, time, approached, height
Ha,42- In the evening, while sitting down, nothing but numbers appeared before his eyes, he felt stupid and ill in the head, and at last very hot. Themes: insanity
Ha,47- Muddled (confused) feeling of the head, as from excessive coitus, for three days. Themes: sexual
Ha,5- Continually brooding over his disease. Themes: dwells, mortification, disease
Ha,6- Sad and solicitous about the future. Themes: future
Ha,654- Internal heat and anxiety; he feels as if the chest were too narrow. Themes: constriction
Ha,662- A trifling vexation makes him very angry and hot. Themes: contradiction, anger
Ha,668- Inward restlessness hinders (delay) him in his work. Themes: restless, work
Ha,670- Sad humor, on account of concern for the future. Themes: future
Ha,673- Disposition lachrymose, as from homesickness. Themes: homesickness
Ha,674- Discontented with himself, self-reproaches. Themes: discontented, himself, conscience, censorious
Ha,7- Tendency to weep, as from homesickness. Themes: homesickness
Ha,8- Sad serious, disheartened (depressed), only while walking in the open air, increasing the longer he walks; at home it gradually passed of and he became more serene. Themes: sadness, movement, home

He,11- Ailments from care, grief, sorrow, chagrin, homesickness; or disappointed love;... Themes: sadness, cares, homesickness, disappointment, love, grief

He,12- Anxiety and doubt concerning his recovery... Themes: doubtful, disease

He,18- Dread (fear) of the future; brooding over one's condition. Themes: future, disease, dwells

He,8- Homesickness, with inclination to weep. Themes: homesickness

PHEL.

Al,9- Sad mood and fear the whole day, as from impending misfortune; she wept, and was prone to think upon sad subjects. Themes: menaced, sadness, misfortune

PHOS.

Al,1- ..this delirium, which preceded death, was erotic, with indications of great, excitement of the sexual system... Themes: death, sexual, lascivious

Al,100- She is made anxious by a disagreeable event, mingled with fear and vexation, and inclined to weep. Themes: bothered, news

Al,101- Anxiety all night without heat, as if he had murdered some one, with constant tossing about. Themes: homicidal, conscience, criminal, restless

Al,104- Anxiety, as from impending misfortune. Themes: menaced, misfortune

Al,107- Anxiety and internal restlessness, without grounds (reason) therefor. Themes: restless

Al,108- Anxiously solicitous concerning the unfortunate termination of her illness. Themes: unfortunate, disease, despair, doomed

Al,109- Discouraged about his health. Themes: despair, disease

Al,111- Horrible fearfulness, late in the evening, as if a horrible face were looking out from every corner. Themes: horrible, persecution, observed, ugly, fearful

Al,115- Frightened feeling, as if I was about to be run over by a locomotive. (crushed, smash) Themes: run over, accidents, crushed

Al,116- The world was frightful (fearful, offensive) to him, only weeping could relieve him;... Themes: fearful

Al,118- Felt nervous, as if I were going to die. Themes: death

Al,12-...; wherever he turned his eyes he saw faces; they swarmed (crowded, surrounded) by him in long panoramic succession; they leered (look lecherous) at him over the footboard of the bed; they squinted (look) at him though the windows, or came trooping (crowd) in when the doors were left ajar (open) (invade);..he fancied he was some one else, ... Themes: persecution, surrounded, wicked, organization, observed, invaded, identity, suspicious

Al,136- Felt exceedingly petulant (irritable, contemptuous) all day; nothing went right; felt as dissatisfied with myself as with others; seemed as if everybody said or did something to provoke me. Themes: discontented, offenses, wrong, contemptuous

Al,150- My wants were numerous and variable. Themes: capricious

Al,38- Told those about him repeatedly that he could not possibly recover, and gave some disjointed directions about his business affairs. Themes: despair, disease, organization, duty, work

Al,4- Delirium with fear of death,... Themes: death

Al,40- As the darkness of night began to enclose (surround) the earth, my peace was disturbed by the most frightful visions and thoughts; constant fear of death, with an almost uncontrollable desire to commit suicide. Themes: death, suicidal, dark, surrounded

Al,46- Imagines he has hydrothorax. Themes: disease

Al,69- Sadness and melancholic, as if some misfortune had happened. Themes: misfortune, sadness

Al,71- Filled with gloomy forebodings. Themes: anticipation, pessimism

Al,80- Mental depression, and a most uncommon fearfulness or timidity, with a great sense of fatigue. Themes: cowardice, sadness, fearful, energy, timidity

Al,86-...; a feeling of dread (fear), as if awaiting something terrible, yet unable to resist or move (terrifying, scaring), overcame me; sometimes it seemed as if I was beginning to bloat (inhalant, inflate, vanity?), and then I could hear a multitude of voices saying in high glee, "Fill him up a little more and he will burst," (blow up) followed by demoniacal laughter, which made the cold chills run over me... I imagined myself an aurora borealis, and could distinctly hear voices shouting, "Beautiful! Oh , was not that splendid?"... Themes: misfortune, paralysis, great, disintegration, greatness, grow, devil, bright, identity

Al,90- Apprehensive, as if were grieving about something, frequently recurring. Themes: grief

Al,94- Anxiety; oppressed, as if I had heard unpleasant (bad) news. Themes: news, oppression

Al,96- Great anxiety and irritability when alone. Themes: solitude

Ha,12- The world seemed dreadful to him; only weeping could relieve him, soon afterward apathy and indifference. Themes: fearful, indifference

Ha,17- Apprehension, as if she was grieved about something, frequently recurring. Themes: grief, offenses

Ha,20- Anguish at times in the evening, as if about to die. Themes: death

Ha,21- Apprehensiveness, like the foreboding (anticipation) of misfortune. Themes: misfortune, anticipation

Ha,23- Anxiously solicitous, about the unfortunate (unlucky) issue (subject) of her disease. Themes: unfortunate, disease

Ha,27- ....Talks in a vehement, (impetuous) commanding (dictatorial) tone; spits at nurse, lifts up her clothes (naked) and kisses hotly all who come near her;... Themes: talk, dictatorial, sexual, lascivious, clothes

Ha,31- Dreadful fearfulness, late in the evening, as if a horrid face was looking out of every corner. Themes: persecution, observed, fearful, ugly, horrible

Ha,43- Depressed on account of his health. Themes: sadness, disease

Ha,5- Sad and melancholy, as if some accident had happened to his beloved ones. Themes: accidents, misfortune, sadness, others

Ha,59- When he thinks of anything disagreeable, he is seized with a sort of apprehension, felt most in the scrobiculus cordis. Themes: anticipation

Ha,62- Very irritable mood, she takes every word ill and becomes pusillanimous (coward) from it. Themes: fearful, cowardice, pessimism

Ha,71- Exaltation of the sense of common brotherhood.(fraternity) Themes: compassionate

Ha,76- Freedom (liberty) of spirit,... everything seems brighter (luminous, vivid) to him. Themes: liberty, bright

Ha,78- She has to laugh against her will, while she is sad. Themes: antagonism, pleasure, sadness, will

Ha,79- In the evening, usually of so vivid an imagination that the mere representation of disagreeable things causes horror with her. Themes: sensitive, horrible, fearful

Ha,82- Indifferent to her child, whom at other times she dearly loved. Themes: indifference, forsakes, child, love

Ha,89- Delirious fantasies, while slumbering (sleep) and when awake, as if she was on a distant island (isolation, segregation), as if she had a large business, was a distinguished (important, rank) lady, etc. Themes: solitude, greatness, position, separated, forsaken

He,1- Excited imagination; zoomagnetic (animal magnetism) condition; ecstasy; clairvoyance. Themes: clairvoyance, pleasure, energy

He,14- Apathy; indifferent even to his own children;... Themes: forsakes, indifference, child

He,18- Does not like to be alone. Themes: company, solitude

He,19- Weary of life; full of gloomy (dark) forebodings. Themes: loathing, anticipation, misfortune, pessimism

He,21- Dejection (sadness); thought he would die. Themes: sadness, death

He,22- ...uneasy about one's health; paroxysms of anguish, when alone or in a stormy weather, with timorous disposition; told those about him repeatedly that he could not possibly recover, and gave some disjointed (incoherent) directions about his business affairs. Themes: disease, solitude, storm, organization, despair, fearful, work

He,25- Amativeness; erotic mania. Themes: mania, sexual

He,28- ...;erotic with indications of great excitement of sexual system; ... fancied he was in several pieces and could not get the fragments properly adjusted.(disconnection, fragmentation, split, disconnected, divided) Themes: lascivious, disintegration, sexual, divided,

He,29- Crazy deliria in a young woman who was strictly moral and unhappy in her love; accused herself of the most obscene (immoral, wicked) actions, of which she never was guilty; .... Themes: lascivious, unfortunate, sexual, wicked, conscience, disappointment, love,

He,31-...; indifference even towards dearest friends;... ; monomania de grandeur et de la richesse;... Themes: mania, greatness, friend, indifference, wealth

He,34- ...full of fear, especially at piano; constantly on lookout (look carefully) for something to happen; ...sexual dreams and violent sexual excitement. Themes: fearful, music, menaced, sexual

He,7- Anxious: filled with gloomy (dark) forebodings; as if about to die; about termination (conclude) of her illness (disease); and restless ; at twilight; when alone; about future; during a thunder-storm; .. Themes: death, disease, future, storm, misfortune, pessimism, restless

He,8- Fear and dread: in evening; of death; as if something were creeping out of every corner; late in evening as if a horrible face were looking out of every corner. Themes: death, crawling, persecution, observed, horrible, ugly,

He,9- Mental depression and a most uncommon fearfulness or timidity with great sense of fatigue. Themes: timidity, fearful, energy

PHYS.

Al,17- Nothing was right; too many things in the room; continually counting them. Themes: wrong

Al,3- Felt great anxiety about friends at home; could not get them out of mind. Themes: friend, others

He,3- ...feels as if she must lose her mind and become insane or despondent;...;thinks she is a castaway (repudiated, discarded, rejected, forsaken);....fears she is crazy or will certainly lose her mind;... Themes: insanity, despair, forsaken, despised, insanity

PHYT.

He,4- Great fear; is sure she will die. Themes: death

PIC-AC.

Al,1- While enjoying the society of gentlemen, the idea of marriage (wedding) seemed unendurable. Themes: union, love, loathing

Al,6- Great indifference; lack of will power to undertake anything. Themes: indifference, will

PIP-N.

Al,S-3- Amorous (passionate, ardent) thoughts and desires, with hypochondria. Themes: sexual

Al,S-4- Hypochondriac, with fear of being poisoned. Themes: poisoned

PLAN.

Al,19- Feeling great desire to be at home when abroad. Themes: homesickness, travel, abroad

PLAT.

Al,11- Contemptuous, pitiful looking down upon people usually venerated, with a kind of casting (reject, discard) them off in paroxysms, against her will. Themes: contemptuous, forsakes, antagonism, compassionate, loathing

Al,23- Feeling as if he would die soon, with shuddering (tremor) at the thought. Themes: death

Ha,11- Great restlessness of mind, so that she knows not where to stay (indecision), with gloominess (melancholy) which spoils even what should be most enjoyable; she imagines she is not fit (unfit, incapable) for this world, is tired (weary) of life, but has a great horror of the death she believes to be approaching. Themes: restless, unfit, death, confidence, anticipation

Ha,15- At odds (quarreling) with all the world, everything is too close (near, intimate) for her, with inclination to weep. (persecution) Themes: fight, separated, invaded

Ha,17- Sad and sullen, she sits solitary, without speaking and she cannot ward off sleep; then inconsolable weeping, especially when she is addressed. Themes: solitude, unfortunate

Ha,18- Taciturnity and involuntary weeping, even after the most friendly address (communication), so that she gets vexed (anger) about it herself. Themes: approached, sadness, himself, bothered

Ha,19- Tendency to weep and weeping, after a mild reproach. Themes: censured

Ha,2- She imagines herself deserted (abandoned) and standing alone in the world. Themes: solitude, forsaken

Ha,21- She thinks all persons are demons. Themes: suspicious, contemptuous, devil

Ha,25-...felt like embracing everybody and could have laughed over the most sad things. Themes: love, union, pleasure

Ha,33- Very cross and irritated at harmless matters and words; so that she at times would have liked to have beaten herself and friends. Themes: offenses, bothered, anger, violence, hurt, himself, friend

Ha,35- Illusion of the imagination; on entering the room after walking for an hour, everything around her seemed very small and all persons physically and bodily inferior to her, but she herself great and lofty (distinguish, elevated) in body;... Themes: small, great, greatness, contemptuous, haughty

Ha,36- Contemptuous, pitying looking down on people at other times respected, with a certain disdain (scorn, arrogance), in paroxysms, against her will. (antagonism) Themes: compassionate, contemptuous, haughty, antagonism

Ha,37- During the caprice of contempt, suddenly a voracious hunger... Themes: capricious, offensive, contemptuous, starving

Ha,38- Haughty, proud feelings. Themes: haughty, greatness

Ha,39- Indifference, cold (reserved), abstracted (separated) in company of friends,.. Themes: forsakes, separated, indifference, friend, company

Ha,40 -Indifference, he felt unconcerned (careless, insensible) as to whether his absent wife would die or not. Themes: indifference, death, wife

Ha,41- She feels as if she did not at all belong to her family (stranger); after a short absence everything appears to be quite changed. (unfamiliar) Themes: separated, stranger, strange, family

Ha,7- Anguish as if about to die, as if unconsciousness (insensible) would ensue (result),... Themes: death, fit

Ha,9- Sensation as if she would have to die soon (immediately), with horror at the thought. Themes: death, doomed, anticipation

He,10- Cold, haughty, too well satisfied with one's self, and not at all anxious about the future. (presumptuous ,egotistic, inexpugnable, safe) Themes: indifference, haughty, himself, future, inexpugnable

He,11- Contemptuous, pitiful, looking down upon people usually venerated, with a kind of casting (forsakes) them off, in paroxysms against her will. Themes: contemptuous, compassionate, forsakes, antagonism

He,12- Dislikes her children; calls them too little. Themes: loathing, child, forsakes

He,15- Deadly anxiety, as if her senses would vanish, ...(disappear) Themes: fit

He,16- Very peevish and easily excited; he could have beaten any one without provocation. Themes: hurt, violence, wicked

He,17- After anger alternate laughing and weeping, with great anguish and fear of death. Themes: anger, pleasure, death

He,2- Inclination to embrace everybody. (contact) Themes: touch, love

He,20- Everything seems strange and horrible to her. Themes: strange, horrible, ugly

He,23- Satiety of life, with taciturnity and fear of death. Themes: death, loathing, reserved

He,24- Much anguish; she feels as if she would lose her senses and die soon. Themes: fit, death

He,25- Out of sorts (irritated) with the whole world; everything seems too narrow (restricted, confined, near) ; weeping mood. Themes: separated, stranger

He,28- Thinks she is left entirely to herself

and stands alone in the world. (loneliness) Themes: solitude, forsaken, helplessness
He,29-...thought she had no place in the world; life was wearisome (boring), but had great dread of death, which she believed near at hand. Themes: forsaken, separated, tedium, death
He,3- Attacks of cheerfulness; increased feeling of strength. Themes: pleasure, energy
He,35- Precordial anguish with palpitation and fear of death and imaginary forms, ghosts. Themes: death, ghosts, heart
He,36- While suffering from a slight erysipelas faciei, took leave (quit, abandon) of her children, exhorted her husband to join (unite, combine) church, wanted people to join her in prayer (beg), felt happy to join her Redeemer. Themes: union, forsakes, disease, religious, salvation, child, penitence
He,37- ...depressed condition of physical powers; ...fear of approaching death; ... aversion to coition and yet dreams of intense lasciviousness,... Themes: energy, death, sexual, lascivious
He,39- It seems to her as if she does not belong to her own family; ... Themes: separated, stranger, family
He,40- Disturbed state of mind; religious, with taciturnity, haughtiness, voluptuousness (sensual) and cruelty. Themes: religious, haughty, wicked, sexual, lascivious
He,41- Delirium, with fear of men (people); often changing, with overestimation (haughty) of oneself. Themes: greatness, haughty, misanthropy, sexual
He,42- Mania; with great pride; fault-finding; unchaste (sensual) talk; ...(chaste = moral, pure) Themes: mania, greatness, haughty, censorious, sexual, talk, lascivious
He,44- Talks almost continually about fanciful things or such as have really occurred; of faithless love; of her teacher and old school days; ... Themes: love, betrayed, nostalgia, past, disappointment
He,45-...melancholy with great fear of death, imagines himself superior to his wife;... Themes: greatness, contemptuous, death
He,46- ...;suffers unspeakable pangs (anxiety) of conscience in consequence of a faux (fault, mistake, embarrassing mistake?) pass when thirty-two years old; says she has brought disgrace upon her family ,and that she has incurred the penalty of damnation; (doomed) in order to do penance (penitence) gave away whatever she could lay her hands upon, (redemption) so that she had to be constantly watched; after her confessor asserted that she could not hope for pardon or heaven (condemnable), she seemed in absolute despair ; bemoaned her misery throughout the night, wringing her hands and beseeching (implore) that she might be delivered (free) from the hell of her conscience; twice attempted self-destruction (suicide);...wished to live and do penance (penitence, purgation, purification) in order to mitigate her eternal punishment. Themes: conscience, doomed, ruined, miserable, hell, penitence, religious, unfortunate,
suicidal, salvation, liberty
He,48- Mental depression from onanism. (masturbation) Themes: sadness, sexual
He,49- Affections from pride. (ailments from) Themes: haughty
He,50- Puerperal mania...assumed or seemed to feel herself a person of great superiority;... Themes: vanity, haughty, greatness
He,8- Arrogant, reserved, absent-minded. Themes: haughty, reserved, greatness, separated
He,9- Pride (haughty) and overestimation of one's self, looking down with haughtiness on others. Themes: haughty, greatness, contemptuous

PLB.

Al,112- He is very sad, has no desire to live, and has threatened to destroy himself, and is very fault-finding (severe, critical) with his friends. Themes: sadness, death, suicidal, censorious, friend
Al,114-...he imagined his disease incurable, and gave way to the gloomy thoughts which the fear of death excited, and to repinings (sadness) caused by the dread of his journey to Valencia. Themes: disease, death, sadness, travel,
Al,118- Much depressed, fearing to die if left alone. Themes: death, solitude
Al,127- Longing (deprived, wanting) for a

distant friend, in the evening... Themes: lack, homesickness, friend

Al,20- He was at time delirious, very restless, and manifested great concern (care) for his affairs. Themes: insanity, duty

Al,23-...His delirium turned chiefly upon the idea that his life was in danger from assassination or poisoning, and that every one about him was a murderer... Themes: death, danger, murdered, poisoned, suspicious

Al,38- Begged and prayed to be released from the strait-waistcoat, "for", he said, "I am not mad; but the idea of being forcibly restrained is enough to drive me crazy". Themes: liberty, imprisoned, insanity

Al,53-...; he fancied one of the patients called to him, ran headlong (hurry) to help him, ... Themes: helplessness, hurry, others, helpful

Al,59- ...;he fancied that a cavalry regiment was about to fall upon him (attacked); or that he was in the presence of his employer, who was finding fault with him. Themes: officer, attacked, censured

Al,60-...; he hears everywhere threatening voices, officers come to arrest him, to seize his furniture (movables), (confiscated, expropriated) and to expel (eject) him from his lodgings (home) (expulsion, exiled) ; the voices come from the pillow, the mattress (bed); they enter by the window, where he sees people, and they consult about him with closed doors (secretive) ; ... Themes: menaced, officer, imprisoned, robber, home

Al,61- He had, some time back, illusions of vision; saw castles, palaces, but these have ceased since he entered the hospital. Themes: greatness, wealth

Al,63- The patient imagined that he was constantly followed (persecuted), and that he heard voices coming from the chimney... ; this man after a few days wished to leave the hospital and go home, because he was convinced that there were fiends in the building that pursued him and sought (want) his life. Themes: persecution, suspicious, menaced, murdered, ghosts, devil

Al,65- Often getting out of bed and wishing to go home; sometimes not recognizing his family; thought they were conspiring to kill him. Themes: betrayed, murdered, family,

Al,66- Hallucinations of mind, she seemed to see her dead husband and child in a tree out of the window. Themes: death, husband, child, nostalgia

Al,69- On first recovering consciousness the people in the ward (hospital) seemed to him as small as dolls (toy, little) , and the opposite of the room seemed to be sunk (under, below) forty feet below his own level. Themes: contemptuous, small

Al,75-..imagined he was going to be poisoned; that his bed was full of ants. Themes: poisoned, animal

He,13- Thought his life was in danger from assassination or poison and every one about him was a murderer. Themes: death, danger, murdered, poisoned, suspicious

He,15-...; despair of her salvation...; fixed idea that could only obtain peace and safety though absolution by a priest of the papal church, although she had been a zealous Protestant; ....brooded over any forbidden thing; would steal (leave) from house in servant's cloak (coat, camouflage) and bonnet (hat) to obtain stimulants (drugs), but from the moment their prohibition was withdrawn (retired) ceased to have any desire for them; after being permitted to visit a priest and converse with him ceased to talk and think of the church. (desire; redemption, absolution) Themes: despair, salvation, obstinate, dwells, religious, conscience, feigning, doomed, salvation, criminal, camouflage, penitence, clothes, clothes

He,16- Mental disturbance of eight or ten years' duration in a man addicted to masturbation; has several times attempted suicide; has been in seclusion (solitude); greatest dejection and despair;...; believes himself lost (condemned) ; has the sounds of hell constantly in his ears; hears voices and sees shadows of demons, great disposition to make away (suicide) with himself or do himself some bodily injury; Themes: solitude, doomed, despair, noise, lost, hurt, sexual, suicidal, devil, hell

PODO.

He,3- Depression: imagines he is going to die or be very ill;... Themes: sadness, death, disease

POLYG-H.

He,2- Gloomy (dark) views of life, dislike of change (evolution, transformation) and excessive dread (fear) of death. Themes: pessimism, dark, death,

PSOR.

Al,13- She is so downhearted (unhappy) that she could commit suicide, then is full of phantasms. Themes: sadness, suicidal, ghosts

Al,14- Very melancholy and despairing; he wishes to die in spite of his good luck. Themes: despair, sadness, death, antagonism

Al,19- Despairing mood; he fears to fail in business. Themes: despair, work, failure, wrong

Al,22- She is very irritable, easily angered; thinking always of dying. Themes: anger, death

Al,24- ...only disagreeable things affect him, agreeable impressions he passes without noticing them. Themes: mortification, pleasure, indifference

Al,32- Great disinclination to ride in a carriage; then at once she wants to ride all the time , even in bad weather. Themes: travel, accidents

Al,5- He pictures the future in the brightest colors. Themes: bright, future, pleasure

Al,8- Full of forebodings very restless, with trembling of the hands. Themes: anticipation,

Al,9- Unusual anxiety when riding in a carriage. Themes: travel, accidents

Al,N-10- Intolerable self-willed (obstinate), annoys those about him; a boy suffering from an eruption. Themes: bother, obstinate

Al,N-11- She is very irritable, easily angered; always thinks of dying. Themes: anger, death

Al,N-14- Anxious, full of fear, melancholic; evil forebodings. Themes: fearful, sadness, anticipation, pessimism

Al,N-15- Great fear of death; anxiety about heart ... Themes: death, heart

Al,N-16- Believe the stitches in heart will kill him if they do not cease. Themes: heart, disease, death

Al,N-21- Very depressed, sad, suicidal thoughts. Themes: sadness, suicidal

Al,N-22- Depressed in spirits and hopeless. Themes: sadness, hopeless

Al,N-24-Despairing mood; fears he will fail in business. Themes: despair, work, failure, confidence

Al,N-25- Much depression on account of an eruption on dorsum of hand which appears over night. Themes: disease, sadness

Al,N-26- Greatest despondency (grief), making his own life and that of those about him intolerable;... Themes: grief, bother

Al,N-27- Is so downhearted she could commit suicide, then is so full of phantasms. Themes: sadness, suicidal

Al,N-28- Great depression of mind during climaxes, with chronic abdominal disorders. Themes: sadness, disease

Al,N-31- Despairs of recovery; thinks he will die; hopeless,... Themes: disease, death, hopeless

Al,N-32- Melancholy after suppressed itch;...seeks solitude, despairs of recovery; ... Themes: sadness, disease, solitude, despair

Al,N-34-....thinks he will not recover; has lost all hope;...formication and crawling, with pricking and smarting on scalp, and some on extremities; tongue white. Themes: disease, hopeless

Al,N-35- Driving to despair with excessive itching. Themes: despair

Al,N-44- Mania of self-destruction. Themes: mania, hurt, himself, suicidal

Al,N-46- Attacks of fear; fear of fire, of being alone, of apoplexy, of becoming insane. Themes: fearful, fire, solitude, disease, insanity

Al,N-48- Fright caused by the merest trifles; this often causes perspiration and trembling. Themes: fearful, cowardice

He,11- She is very irritable, easily angered; always thinks of dying. Themes: anger, death

He,13- Anxious, full of fear, melancholic; evil forebodings. Themes: fearful, anticipation, pessimism

He,15- Great fear of death; anxiety about heart and dyspnea,... Themes: death, heart, suffocation
He,16- Believes the stitches in heart will kill him if they do not cease. Themes: heart, death, disease
He,21- Very depressed, sad, suicidal thoughts. Themes: sadness, suicidal
He,22- Depressed in spirits and hopeless. Themes: sadness, hopeless
He,24- Despairing mood; fears he will fail in business. Themes: despair, failure, confidence, work
He,26- Greatest despondency (desperation), making his own life and those about him intolerable;... Themes: despair, bother
He,27- Is so downhearted she could committed suicide, then is full of phantasms. Themes: suicidal, surrounded, ghosts
He,31- Despairs recovery; thinks he will die; hopeless; especially after typhus... Themes: disease, death, infection, hopeless
He,32- Melancholy after suppressed itch;...seeks solitude, despair of recovery;... Themes: disease, solitude, despair
He,34-...;thinks he will not recover; has lost all hope; cannot apply his mind to business;... Themes: disease, hopeless, work

PTEL.

Al,2- Depression of spirits, and a feeling of anxiety about some unknown thing, with the severe headache, in the afternoon. Themes: sadness, anticipation
Al,20- In writing a letter, felt a curious and unusual disposition to hurry (run, hasten, speed) through with it as quickly as possible, hardly taking time to write the words. Themes: hurry, time
Al,21- Able to examine the papers, but inclined to hurry with it, and in selecting the remedy, inclined to follow Fred Humphrey's rule, "First impressions are the best". (hastily, rapidly, quickly) (heedless) Themes: hurry, negligence
Al,43- Goes about his professional duties in a perfunctory (indifference) manner, very unlike (contradictory) his fiery (passionate) zeal with which he usually combats disease and his allopathic step-brethren (brotherhood). Themes: duty, work, indifference, disease, passionate,

PULS-N.

Al,3- Great depression of spirits, in the afternoon; a kind of homesickness, with despondency.(grief) Themes: sadness, homesickness, grief

PULS.

Al,10- Everything disgusts him; he seems averse to everything. Themes: loathing, antagonism
Al,12- Nightly anxiety on waking as if he had committed a crime. Themes: conscience, criminal
Al,16- Anxiety thinks to die. Themes: death
Al,18- Anxiety as if would have apoplexy, in the evening, after lying down, ... Themes: fit, disease
Al,19- Tremulous anxiety, as if death were imminent.(destined) Themes: death, doomed
Al,21- Anxiety as if he were in a hot atmosphere. Themes:
Al,22- Anxious solicitude about his health. Themes: disease
Al,25- It seems so quiet (silent) in her head and everything feels so empty that she seems alone in the house and in the world; she will speak to no one, just as if her surroundings did not exist (estrange), and she paid attention to no one. (left, solitary) Themes: lifeless, solitude, strange, separated, home
Al,28- He sinks into a condition of sadness and despondency from disagreeable news. Themes: sadness, despair, news
Al,32- Extremely morose, will not answer, takes everything in bad part, in the evening towards sundown. Themes: sadness, offenses
Al,44- Shuns business, is irresolute, with sighing respiration and a feeling as if he were beside himself. Themes: work, irresolution, confidence
Al,47- He cannot at all get rid of a thought that he once grasped. Themes: dwells, liberty
Al,5- He wishes now for this, now for that employment, but when given to him he will have nothing to do with it. Themes: work, dispersion, capricious, indifference
Al,8- Extremely capricious and peevish at

everything, even at himself. Themes: capricious, himself, anger
Al,9- Envious, avaricious, unsatisfied, greedy, he would gladly have everything, to himself. Themes: envy, avarice, ambition
Ha,1101- Anxious heat as if hot water were thrown over him, with cold forehead. Themes: water
Ha,1110- When it becomes evening ... he began to be afraid of ghosts; ... Themes: ghosts
Ha,1113- Anxiety, thinks he will be ruined.(decay, perdition) Themes: future, ruined, doomed
Ha,1114- Anxiety in the region of the heart, with suicidal impulse, and feeling or inclination to vomit in the scrobiculus cordis. Themes: suicidal, heart
Ha,1115- Anxiety, as if threatened with apoplexy, in the evening after lying down, ... Themes: fit, disease, menaced
Ha,1116- Trembling anxiety, as if about to die. Themes: death
Ha,1116- Trembling anxiety, as if about to die. Themes: death
Ha,1117- Anxious solicitude about his health. Themes: disease
Ha,1118- Solicitude about his domestic concerns, in the morning. Themes: duty, home
Ha,1119- Cannot think without fretting (anguish) about his affairs (duty, responsibility), in the morning. Themes: duty, conscience
Ha,1120 - Restless state of the disposition, as if did not do his duty properly. Themes: duty, conscience, negligence
Ha,1122- Neglect of his business, hesitancy (indecision), sobbing (cry) respiration and loss of composure.(calm, serenity) Themes: confidence, duty, doubtful, negligence, work
Ha,1123- Sometimes he wants to do one thing, sometimes another, and when he is given something to do, he will not do it. Themes: dispersion, work, negligence
Ha,1125- Envious, avaricious, dissatisfied, greedy, wants to have everything for himself. Themes: envy, ambition, avarice
Ha,1131- On hearing some disagreeable news he became affected with sadness and despondency. Themes: news, sadness, despair
Ha,1133- Cross, takes in bad part what others say. Themes: bothered, offenses
Ha,1140- In the evening (about sunset), extraordinarily sulky, will not answer, and takes everything amiss.(wrong) Themes: wrong
Ha,1142- Everything disgusts him; everything is repugnant to him. Themes: discontented, loathing
Ha,1143- Her head is so quiet and all about her is so empty as if she were alone (solitude, loneliness) in the house and in the world; she does not wish to talk to any one, just as if all around her were no concern (relation) of hers and she belonged to nobody. (lonely, missed) Themes: solitude, forsaken, separated, home
Ha,1147- Inattention, acts with precipitancy (hurry), does something different to what he wished to do. Themes: hurry, antagonism
Ha,18- Mild, bashful, gentle, yielding disposition. Themes: mildness, timidity, yielding
He,13- Extremely capricious and peevish about everything, himself included. Themes: capricious, himself
He,16- ...easily moved to tears or laughter; well one hour, miserable (unhappy) the next. Themes: miserable
He,19- Silent mood; inclined to silent grief with submissiveness. Themes: grief, suppressed, yielding
He,21- Continuous crying with great melancholy and fear of losing her reason, or that she might commit suicide. Themes: suicidal, insanity, sadness
He,23- Disposition mild and gentle, never cross. Themes: mildness
He,25- Weary of life; thinks with pleasure of drowning. (suicide, water) Themes: suicidal, loathing, water, pleasure
He,26- Anxiety: thinks to die; does not know what to do; as if in a hot atmosphere; in region of heart; even to suicide;... Themes: death, doubtful, suicidal, heart
He,27- Anguish in region of heart, sometimes increasing to a desire for suicide. Themes: suicidal, heart
He,28- Tremulous anguish: as if death were near;... Themes: death
He,29- When evening comes begins to dread

ghosts. Themes: fearful, ghosts
He,36- Mistrust; envy; covetousness (avidity); dislike to people. Themes: suspicious, avarice, envy, misanthropy, loathing
He,39- Children are extremely affectionate, which they manifest by kissing and caressing. Themes: child, love
He,40- Religious mania; sees the devil coming to take her; the world on fire during night; fear, rage in spells, or weeping... (captured, possessed) Themes: religious, seized, fire, mania, devil, anger
He,42- ...full of anxiety, forebodings of impending (imminent, destined) disaster; ... Themes: misfortune, anticipation, accidents
He,43- Sleepless nights on account of great fear and anxious restlessness; despairs of her salvation and seeks aid in constant prayer;... Themes: restless, fearful, religious, salvation, helplessness
He,46- Dark suspicious and reserved manner; disturbed look on face; sleepless; looks for her bed in the yard (lost?); hides in a corner to escape from a little gray man who wanted to pull out her leg;... Themes: reserved, suspicious, lost, home, hide, persecution, attacked, mutilated, escape
He,47- ...; pangs (pain , anxiety) of conscience about religion and female sex; violent palpitation in the presence of women; abhors (detests, aversion) and hates the sex; must go out of their way for fear of injuring them; looks upon them as evil beings and is afraid (fear; temptation, seduction); considers their presence injurious (insulted, offended) to his soul; ... (sexual loathing) Themes: conscience, religious, suspicious, contemptuous, offenses, sexual, loathing, violence, devil, wicked
He,48- ...despaired of her soul's salvation; did not believe she would be restored to health ; ... Themes: salvation, religious, disease, hopeless, despair, doomed
He,5- Fancies a naked man is wrapped in her bedclothes; dreams of men. Themes: sexual
He,50 -After slight emotions, difficult breathing; bad effects from fright, mortification or excessive joy.(ailments from) Themes: mortification, fearful, pleasure
He,51- Sinks into a condition of sadness and despondency (grief) from disagreeable news.(ailments from) Themes: sadness, grief, news
He,52- After mortification, sad gloomy (melancholy) and weary (disgusted) of life;...thinks of drowning with great pleasure;... Themes: sadness, loathing, suicidal, mortification, pleasure, water
He,53- ...afraid of everybody; considers every one her enemy, despairs of everything; ...;trusts no one;.. (suspicious) Themes: fearful, suspicious, enemy, despair
He,9- Shuns business; irresolute; sighing respiration; feels as if he were beside himself. Themes: negligence, work, irresolution,

PYROG.

Al,N-5- Sensation as if she covered the whole bed; knew her head was on pillow, but did not know where the rest of her body was. Themes: divided, disintegration
Al,N-6- Feels when lying on one side that she is one person, and another person when turning on the other side. Themes: double, identity,
Al,N-7- Sensation as though crowded with arms and legs. Themes: double, identity
Al,N-8- Hallucination that he is very wealthy (rich); remaining after fever. Themes: wealth, greatness
Al,N-9- Increased buoyancy (happy) of spirits, although he felt ill. Themes: pleasure, disease

RAN-B.

Al,1- Fearfulness in the evening, she does not want to remain alone, she is afraid she may be haunted (seized) by ghosts. Themes: solitude, seized, ghosts
Al,2- Vexed and inclined to be angry; quarrels and scolds when the slightest cause is offered (after two hours). Themes: bothered, offensive, fight, anger, censorious
Al,3- Ill humored, and disposed to quarrel and scold the first forenoon; in the evening is desponding, apprehensive, sensitive, discontented; on the second day he again inclines to be provoked by innocent jests

of his friends, etc.;... Themes: offensive, fight, offenses, sadness, sensitive, discontented, friend

Al,7- The objects of his feelings, for instance, chagrin, occupy his mind long after the occurrence took place; one sees that he is thinking of those things; he talks to himself, gesticulates in his anger... Themes: grief, dwells, mortification, anger

He,4- Afraid of ghosts; does not like to remain alone. Themes: ghosts, solitude

RAPH.

Al,1- Feeling of aversion towards all women; she is provoked by seeing women going and coming about her; their approach threw her into a fury; the mere contact with a woman's dress caused intolerable distress;...She is attracted to all men without distinction (nymphomania) ; when she gives her hand to a man, she feels great agitation,...When left alone for a hour in the evening, she gave herself a very deep wound in the lips with a penknife, in hopes to put an end to this condition (hurt, punishes). Moral feeling was completely extinct, the physical nature alone ruled and threw her into a frightful state (wild). From morning to noon she would not have been able to resist the advances even of a man for whom she had not the least friendly feeling; from noon to 6 p.m. she could not have held out against any man whatsoever; from 8 to 11 the demands of sense were so importunate as to silence the voice of shame and reason; ... and would have thrown herself

into the arms of the first man she met...she was still unable to control her impulses;... Themes: loathing, sexual, approached, anger, touch, hurt, conscience, shame, wicked, seized, wild, lascivious,

Al,16- Her condition troubles her , and for a moment cannot believe it to be owing to the medicine; she forgets it entirely, and believes she has a disease which is not recognized. (unknown, undiscovered) Themes: disease, strange, knowledge

Al,17- Extreme anxiety, she thought she would die. Themes: death

Al,18- Apprehension and fear of death. Themes: death

Al,2- ...she fears she will become a burden (load) to everyone. (flat, tiresome) Themes: bother, heavy

Al,7- ...dangerous fancies assail (attacks) her, but she restrains (suppress) herself from putting them into execution. Themes: danger, suppressed

He,1- Anguish with dread (fear) of death, which supposed to be near. Themes: death

RHOD.

He,4- Nervous persons who dread a storm and are particularly afraid of thunder. Themes: storm

RHUS-T.

Al,1382 DREAM- ...it seemed to her that the head was hanging out of the bed and the blood was streaming (flow) into it, so that she could hear it flow; together with the appearance of a horrible image which she was obliged to accompany. Themes: blood, movement, horrible, ghosts

Al,1385 -Fearful dreams, for example, that the world was on fire, with palpitation on waking. Themes: fearful, fire

Al,26- Anxiety at night; he would flee (leave) from bed and seek help (aid), on account of an indescribable distressing sensation. Themes: helplessness

Al,27- Anxiety, with loss of strength (power, energy, force) , as if he would die, more after midnight than before. Themes: energy, death

Al,31- Fear and despair on account of sad thoughts, which she could not get rid of. Themes: despair, mortification

Al,32- He thought an enemy want to poison him. Themes: enemy, suspicious, poisoned

Al,33- He is frightened (afraid, fear) by a trifle (insignificance) (on falling asleep) as if he had dreaded (worry) the greatest misfortune. Themes: fearful, misfortune

Al,4- Full of sad thoughts, anxious and fearful, wherewith she gradually lost strength, and was obliged to lie down for hours in order to regain vigor. Themes: sadness, fearful, energy

Al,40- Impatient desire to accomplish several kinds of business, chiefly intellectual,... Themes: hurry, impatience, succeed, work, duty

Al,41- Confusion of mind, he thought he would die. Themes: death

Al,5- Melancholy, ill-humor, and anxiety, as if a misfortune (disgrace) would happen, or as if she were alone (solitary), and all about her were dead (lifeless, inert) and still (silent, quiet), or as if she had been forsaken by a near friend; worse in the house, relieved by walking in the open air. Themes: misfortune, solitude, forsaken, lifeless, friend

Al,9- Satiety (surfeit) of life, with desire to die without sadness. Themes: death, loathing

Ha,946- He is frightened (afraid, fearful) (on going to sleep) at a trifle, as if he had to fear the greatest calamity (disaster, misfortune) from it. Themes: misfortune, misfortune

Ha,950- He could not be pleased, was indifferent to society. Themes: indifference, misanthropy

Ha,952- Sadness, making him prefer quiet solitude. Themes: sadness, solitude

Ha,953- Melancholy, sad, and anxious, as if about to hear of a calamity,(misfortune, disaster) or as if she were solitary (lonely, alone) and all around her were dead (lifeless, extinct) and silent (quiet) ; or as if she had bid farewell (separation) to an intimate friend ; worst in the room, diminished by walking in a open air. Themes: misfortune, solitude, lifeless, forsaken, lack, movement, sadness, death, friend

Ha,956- Along with sinking (descend, submerge) of the strength, (vigor, energy ,force) anxiety as if he must die, worse after than before midnight. Themes: energy, death

Ha,957- Without sadness, as if tired of life, with desire to die. Themes: loathing, death

Ha,959- ...;true cardiac anxiety; she could not to sleep half the night on account of great anguish, and was always so anxious that she perspired. Themes: heart,

Ha,960- On account of inward (inside) uneasiness (agitation) she could not sit still, but must rock (shake) herself to and fro on her chair, and move all the limbs a little. Themes: movement, restless

Ha,961- Very restless disposition, and anxiety and anguish, so that she had always a clutching (grasp) at the heart, with dyspnea. Themes: restless, heart, constriction

Ha,962- She did not sleep half the night, was timorous (timid, fearful) full of anguish and cardiac anxiety. Themes: fearful, heart

Ha,963- Ill-humored, dejected, and as if in despair. Themes: sadness, despair

Ha,964- Full of sad thoughts, anxious and timorous (timid) , during which she always lost her strength, (power) and must lie down for hours; in order to recover her strength. (inert, motionless) Themes: sadness, fearful, energy

Ha,965- He imagines an enemy seeks to poison him. Themes: poisoned, suspicious, enemy

Ha,967- She was inexpressibly anxious; she had pressure at the heart and tearing (cut) in the sacrum. Themes: constriction, heart

Ha,970- In the dusk, towards evening, anxiety and anguish, as if he would kill himself, for an hour. Themes: suicidal

Ha,971- Confusion of the reason; he thinks he is dying. Themes: death

Ha,972- From sad thoughts, which she could not get rid of, she became timorous and fainthearted.(coward, fearful) Themes: fearful, cowardice, sadness

Ha,973- When she had disagreeable thoughts in her head she could not get rid of them. Themes: mortification, tortured, liberty

Ha,974- He can restrain the rush of ideas at his will, follow out uninterruptedly any train of thought he chooses, without being troubled with other thoughts. Themes: will, knowledge, organization

Ha,(curative) 975 -He can master (leading, chief) his thoughts and think calmly (tranquillity) of any subject he will and as long as he likes, and at his pleasure take up some other topic, with tranquil, slow inspiration. Themes: peace, restless

He,11- Anxiety: while sitting was obliged to take hold (grasp, keep) of something because she did not think she could keep up (support) on account of the beating and drawing pains in limbs; and apprehension as if he wished to take his own life; with loss of strength (vigor, vitality) as if he would die. Themes: helplessness, suicidal, energy, death

He,12- Fear and despair on account of sad thoughts, which she could not get rid of. (fixed ideas) Themes: mortification, despair, sadness

He,13- Fear: that he will die; with anxiousness and sighing; of being poisoned. Themes: death, poisoned,

He,14- Fretful; general unhappiness of temper. Themes: anger, unfortunate

He,18- Disgust of life: thoughts of suicide; wants to drown (immerse) himself; with fear of death: with desire to die, without sadness. Themes: grief, suicidal, water, death, antagonism

He,22- ... great restlessness and anguish as if she had committed a crime or as if she thought some terrible calamity impended; these feelings drove her from one place to another; could not rest quietly at night in bed; was robbed of sleep and all desire to live;... Themes: restless, conscience, criminal, misfortune, movement, death, menaced

He,23- Restlessness and anxiety about heart as if she had committed a crime or as if some great misfortune was in store (reserved) for her, is driven from one place to another; deprived of sleep and all desire to live; ... Themes: restless, conscience, criminal, misfortune, movement, death

He,24- ...a week later she told her mother to not look at her (observed) ; seemed to be distrustful (suspicious) and did not wish to see any one; she came running in from the street and said people were looking at her; ....; cries without cause, imagines people are finding fault (misconduct, criticized, censured) with her because she is earning (succeed, prosper, reach) nothing, acts in a childish manner;... Themes: observed, suspicious, censured, succeed, despised,

He,5- Low, mild delirium, thinks he is roaming (wander, travel) over fields, or hard at work. Themes: travel, nature, work

RHUS-V.

Al,1- Great sadness, no desire to live, everything seems gloomy. Themes: sadness, loathing, death

ROB.

Al,10- Love and excited passions, leading him to the grossest (obscene, rude) excesses, even to homicide. Themes: love, violence, homicidal, passionate

Al,11- Strong disposition to be obscene, to gormandize (gluttony, voracity), and for all kinds of orgies. Themes: sexual, pleasure, lascivious, voracity

Al,12- Anxiety to seek honors (distinction) ; excessive pride (haughtiness, arrogance) ; he considers himself better than an emperor. Themes: flattery, greatness, haughty,

Al,13- Hypochondriac grief; he seeks pleasures and tries to divert his mind, without succeeding. Themes: grief, pleasure, sadness

Al,3- Moral agitation, great restlessness; he is always under the impression that he will be disgraced. Themes: conscience, restless, miserable

Al,6- Fear and confusion (anxiety ?) of conscience, as if he had committed a crime,... Themes: conscience, criminal

Al,7- Dread of everything that is somber and black. Themes: dark

Al,9- Bacchanalian (love to be drunken), erotic, or religious madness. Themes: religious, sexual

RUMX.

Al,4- Depression, as if some evil was impending. Themes: sadness, menaced

He,1- Low-spirited: with serious expression of face; with suicidal mood. Themes: suicidal

RUTA.

Al,11- Much dissatisfied (discontented) by everything that happened to him, and especially with whatever he did himself, and great inclination to weep. Themes: himself, conscience

Al,3- Very anxious all day, as though he had done something wrong; if any one opened the door he feared that some one had come to arrest (imprisonment, jailing) him. Themes: wrong, conscience, imprisoned

Al,8- Peevish and mistrustful (suspicious) all day; he no longer trusted his best friends, he thought that he was constantly deceived.(deluded) Themes: suspicious, betrayed, friend

Ha,270-...anxiety as if he must die,... Themes: death

Ha,275- Very frequent anxiety with desponding (sad) thoughts and fears. Themes: fearful

Ha,276- Very discontented and very much disposed to weep over everything that happens about him and especially over what he himself has done. Themes: discontented, conscience

Ha,280- All day long very anxious as if he had done something bad; when the door was opened, he feared that someone was coming to take him to prison. (incarcerated, punished) Themes: wrong, conscience, criminal, imprisoned

Ha,286- All day long cross and suspicious; he would no longer trust (mistrust) his best friend, and imagined he was always being deceived. Themes: suspicious, betrayed, friend,

He,1- Inclination to contradict and quarrel. Themes: contradiction, fight

He,2- Dissatisfied with himself and others. Themes: discontented, himself, others

SABAD.

Al,2- He imagines all sorts of strange things about his own body, for instance, that it had shrunk (dry, wrinkled) like that of dead persons (corpse), that his stomach was corroded (degeneracy, decomposition), that the scrotum was swollen (enlarged), etc.;... Themes: strange, ruined, corpse, death, disease, grow

Al,6- Gloomy mood, as if he were the greatest criminal,... Themes: conscience, criminal

He,2- Erroneous impressions as to the state of his body. Themes: identity, disease

Al,3- Imagines: himself sick; parts shrunken (small wrinkled) ; that she is pregnant (important?), when she is merely swollen from flatus; that she has some horrible throat disease which will end fatally. (incurable) Themes: disease, ruined, death

SABIN.

Al,1- Great anxiety, as if he apprehended some evil. Themes: misfortune

Al,5-...music was intolerable, it penetrated marrow and bone,...feeling of weakness, debility. Themes: music, loathing, energy

Al,7- Ill-humor, with sensation as if he had taken cold. Themes: disease

He,4- Great tiredness and laziness, with a feeling of deep-seated inward trouble, which makes him melancholy and sad. Themes: disease, sadness

SAMB-C.

Al,1- ...an indefinable fear as if the horse (a very gentle animal) might run away, or the wagon break at any moment; a dread of some undefined danger. Themes: animal, danger, accidents, misfortune

SANG.

He,11- It seems to her ...she is in a railroad car and begs others to hold her. Themes: travel, helplessness, lost

He,8- Sensation as if paralyzed and unable to move while lying on her back, ... Themes: paralysis

He,9-..."what will become of my condition, shall I have typhoid fever, inflammation of the brain, or shall I remain paralyzed?". Themes: disease, infection, paralysis

SANT.

Al,6-...irresolution and want of confidence in my own powers as to render me quite unfit for work of any kind; Themes: irresolution, confidence, energy, unfit, work

SAPIN.

Al,4- Very irritable; nothing goes right; fault-finding, dissatisfied with everything previously done, no matter how well it was done before; ... Themes: wrong, censorious, discontented

Al,5- Quite ill-natured and inclined to view matters in a disagreeable light; did not seem able to feel settled (decided) enough to know what to do; the crossness became so intense, that I felt myself getting very unreasonable, especially as to food, which seemed all wrong in some way;... Themes: wicked, pessimism, doubtful, bothered, confidence, wrong

SARS.

Al,18- Extremely ill-humored even vexed " by the fly on the wall". Themes: bothered, animal

Al,19- Every word may offend him. Themes: offenses

Al,7- The soul is affected inordinately by the pains; the mind is depressed the mood dull; he feels wretchedly, and moans involuntarily. Themes: miserable, unfortunate

Ha,14- Extremely peevish, the fly on the wall vexes him. (insects) Themes: animal, bothered

Ha,16- Readily insulted by a word. Themes: offenses

Ha,3- The soul is extraordinarily affected by the pains, the spirit is oppressed, the mind troubled; he feels unhappy and groans involuntarily. Themes: oppression, unfortunate

He,6- Thinking about the food he has been eating makes him sick. (indigestion) Themes: poisoned, disease

He,8- She thinks she cannot bear (support, endure) the headache. Themes: disease

SCROPH-N.

Al,1- Desponding (sad), much troubled (worried) about the past, and very apprehensive of the future, which passed off after a few days, and left the intellect clear. Themes: despair, past, future

Al,2- A miserable and sluggish (inactive, lethargic) feeling of the mind when moving about. Themes: miserable, movement

SEC.

Al,1- Delirium; she abandons (reject, forsakes) her relatives and does absurd things. Themes: forsakes, relatives

Al,10- Raving (talk wildly), with an attempt to jump into the water. Themes: anger, suicidal, water

Al,19-...There were two sick persons in the bed, one of whom recovered and the other did not. Themes: double, disease

Al,20- She was conscious, but the room (space) presented to her the impression of water excessively agitated on its surface. She could compare it only to the "foaming of a troubled sea" (storm, tempest) Themes: water, storm, restless

Al,27- Strong desire to recover. Themes: disease

Al,28- Constant moaning and fear of death, with strong desire to live. Themes: death

Al,36- The greatest depression of mind and loss of strength, a very sick feeling. Themes: sadness, energy, disease

Al,4- Muttering delirium, very restless, agitated ,and fearful of death. Themes: death

Al,45- Anxiety and fear of death. Themes: death

Al,46- Hypochondria; patient says she must have something to relieve her or she must die. Themes: disease, death

Al,47- Hypochondria; patient says she must have something to relieve her or she must die. Themes: death, disease

Al,57- The only expression that he gave utterance (say) to was a stupid kind of "I am hungry". Themes: starving

Al,N-13- Paralytic mental diseases; treats his relations contemptuously and sarcastically. Themes: paralysis, contemptuous, sarcasm

Al,N-18- Anticipated misfortunes, as though about to lose something of great value.(estimate) Themes: anticipation, misfortune

Al,N-6- Fear of death. Themes: death

He,10- Constant moaning and fear of death. Themes: death

He,12- Paralytic mental diseases; treats his relations contemptuously and sarcastically;... Themes: paralysis, contemptuous, sarcasm

He,4- Mania; with inclination to bite; with inclination to drown. Themes: suicidal, bite, water

SEL.

Al,4- Dread of people and of his occupation, but overcoming this he is able to continue his work. Themes: fearful, work, suspicious

He,8- Lascivious thoughts with impotence. Themes: sexual, lascivious
He,9- Dread of society. Themes: misanthropy

SENEG.

Al,13- Phlegmatic; inclines to quarrel and give offense. Themes: indifference, offensive, fight
Al,14- He recollects (remember) suddenly, without any cause, unimportant regions (places) which he had long seen ago, and which had never made a deep impression upon him. Themes: past

SEP.

Al,1- So excited from anger that she fears an apoplectic fit; everything becomes black (evil) before the eyes. Themes: disease, fit, anger, dark
Al,100-...seems as if my mind were hedged (enclose) in, as if it were circumscribed,...(encircle, confined) Themes: obstructed, knowledge, imprisoned
Al,101- Dullness of comprehension; inability to collect or express his thoughts; constantly building air-castles or running on future events. Themes: knowledge, planning, future
Al,112- Memory so poor I cannot remember the least thing, and it makes me feel very miserable. Themes: miserable,
Al,20- Internal loathing of life. Themes: loathing
Al,2162 - Anxious dreams as if the body were disfigured.(distort, deface) Themes: ugly
Al,22- Sadness about her health. Themes: sadness, disease
Al,24- Feel very low-spirited, and don't care what becomes of me. Themes: sadness, indifference
Al,28- Gloominess (melancholy); she felt unfortunate, without cause. Themes: unfortunate
Al,29- Dark forebodings about his disease in regard to the future. Themes: anticipation, pessimism, disease, future
Al,3- Attacks of anger over past times come on involuntarily, through which he becomes so excited that he does not know what to do, accompanied by anxiety, palpitation of the heart, and sweat of the whole body. Themes: past, restless, anger, heart
Al,30- All her troubles appear to her mind in a very gloomy light, so that she is fearful. Themes: pessimism, fearful
Al,31-...I cannot recall things which I know very well; the thoughts will not come... Themes: knowledge
Al,33- Received news of the slight illness of a friend, which caused great mental depression (at another time it would not have made slightest impression); this condition grew on me until I became so nervous that I felt that unless I held on something, I should scream. Themes: news, friend, sensitive, others, sadness, disease, indifference, helplessness
Al,34- Feel very much depressed, at 7 A.M.; feel like quarreling with everybody; became very much excited about a mere trifle, and said some very sharp things. (feeling ashamed of it at the same time) Themes: sadness, fight, offensive, conscience, shame
Al,36- The greatest loathing of life; it seemed to him as if he could not endure so miserable an existence any longer, and as if he would pine away (longing, wanting) if he did not kill himself. (pine = intense longing or grief) Themes: loathing, miserable, grief, suicidal
Al,38- He feels oppressed in sultry weather, but becomes more cheerful when it thunders and lightens. Themes: oppression, storm, pleasure
Al,39- She wishes to be alone and lie with closed eyes. Themes: solitude
Al,48- Great anguish, as if in the blood. Themes: blood
Al,52- She is filled with concern about her health; thinks she will have consumption and soon die. Themes: disease, death, infection
Al,53- Concerned about her health, anxious, irritated, and very weak. Themes: disease, energy
Al,58- Fearfulness when riding in a carriage. Themes: fearful, conduct, accidents
Al,66- She finds fault and desires nothing which others want, accompanied by

weeping and heat of face. Themes: censorious, contradiction, capricious,
Al,76- Peevish mood, as after suppressed anger. Themes: suppressed, anger
Al,82- Great indifference toward everything; no proper sense of life. Themes: indifference, lifeless, separated
Al,92- One dose of the medicine takes away my ambition; I simply do not want to do anything, either work or play; it is even an exertion to think. Themes: ambition, indifference, pleasure, work
Al,94- Inclination of the mind to wonder over future events. Themes: future
Al,95- The recollection of past unpleasant circumstances puts him in an extreme ill-humor. Themes: past, mortification
Al,96- He thinks of things which he does not think of, uses expressions which he knows are incorrect, undertakes those things which are opposed to his intentions, and finds such contradictions with himself that it puts him in a very uncomfortable and uneasy mood. Themes: antagonism, wrong, conscience, contradiction
Ha,10- All her troubles present themselves in a very sad light to her mind, so that she is despondent.(sad, depressed) Themes: pessimism, despair, sadness,
Ha,11- If he only thinks of his past troubles, his pulse is quickened and his breath fails him. Themes: mortification, past
Ha,16- Melancholy, she feels unhappy without cause. Themes: unfortunate
Ha,17- Dread of men. Themes: misanthropy, sexual
Ha,18- She wishes to be by herself and to lie with closed eyes. Themes: solitude
Ha,19- He must not be alone for a moment. Themes: solitude, company
Ha,27- Great internal restlessness, for many days, with hastiness (hurried); he wants to be done with his work even as he begins it. Themes: restless, hurry, impatience
Ha,28- Restless and lacking serenity, for many days; occupied with sad memories, and anxious, she has not the patience to stay long in place. Themes: restless, past, impatience
Ha,31- Extreme loathing of life (existence he felt as if he could not any longer bear this miserable (wretched, unhappy) existence, and as if he would pine away (ruined) unless he made away with himself.-(suicidal) Themes: unfortunate, ruined, suicidal, loathing, miserable,
Ha,34- Very readily offended. Themes: offenses
Ha,37- Sorrowful mood, as after secret vexation. Themes: suppressed, grief
Ha,42- The remembrance of past trouble puts him into extreme ill humor. Themes: past, mortification
Ha,43- Vexatious occurrences from past times keep recurring of themselves, which makes him so irritated ... Themes: past, mortification
Ha,44- She finds fault with everything, does not wish what others desire; with weeping ... Themes: wrong, censorious, antagonism
Ha,45- She finds fault in everything, approves of nothing. Themes: censorious
Ha,5- Sad (despair) about her health.(vitality) Themes: disease, sadness
Ha,51- (Ailments) From vexation, she is so excited that she fears an apoplectic fit, and everything turns black before her eyes. Themes: bothered, disease, dark, fit
Ha,55- A trifle produces a violent ebullition of anger, with trembling. Themes: anger
Ha,59- Great indifference to everything, no real vital feeling. Themes: indifference, energy, lifeless
Ha,6- Troubled (worries) thoughts about his disease and about the future.(destine) Themes: disease, future
Ha,68- He thinks, what he does not wish to think, uses expressions which he himself knows are incorrect; he resolves to do what is against his intention, and is thus in conflict with himself and, therefore in a disagreeable, restless mood. (lost: knowledge, correction) Themes: wrong, antagonism, himself,
Ha,8- Troubled (worried) about her health (vigor) anxious, irritated and very weak. Themes: disease, energy
Ha,9- She has none but troubled thoughts about her health, thinks she is getting the consumption (tuberculosis, degenerate, decomposition) and will die soon. Themes: disease, death, infection, ruined
He,11- Sad about her health and domestic affairs, discontented with everything. Themes: disease, duty, discontented, sadness, home

He,12- Gloominess; she feels unfortunate (unhappy) without cause. Themes: unfortunate,

He,13- Dark forebodings about his disease in regard to the future. Themes: disease, future, pessimism

He,14- Felt that unless he held on to something he should scream. Themes: helplessness, touch

He,19- Aversion to one's occupation (work) and family. Themes: work, family, loathing

He,20- Dread of being alone. Themes: solitude

He,21- Anxiety; with fear, flushes of heat over face; about real or imaginary evils... Themes: misfortune

He,22- Great indifference to one's family, to those they love best. Themes: indifference, forsakes, family, love

He,23- Is easily offended and inclined to be vehement.(intense) Themes: offenses, dictatorial

He,28- Propensity to suicide from despair about his miserable (wretched, unfortunate) existence. Themes: suicidal, miserable, despair

He,29- Fear to starve,(hunger) is peevish, and feels mortified (disgraced), easily frightened and full of evil forebodings. Themes: starving, pessimism, mortification

He,3- Felt all day as if he did not care what happened; ... Themes: indifference

He,31- Contradictory, quarrelsome, complaining about others. Themes: antagonism, fight, censorious

He,34- Greatest irritability from slightest causes; very easily offended. Themes: offenses

He,38- ...everything seems strange (unusual, unfamiliar) to her;...; it seems as if she could not understand (realize) anything and would have to learn anew everything she wished to do;...(lost: knowledge); greatest indifference to everything, the death of a near relative, or some happy occurrence, leaves her equally unaffected; no trace of her former love for friends or even for her child; aversion for social intercourse amounting to contempt;... Themes: strange, knowledge, indifference, forsakes, death, relatives, love, friend, child, misanthropy, contemptuous, others

He,6- Great indifference to everything; no proper sense of life. Themes: indifference, lifeless

SIL.

Al,11- Gloominess; she felt as if she would die, and for the time lost her memory. Themes: sadness, death

Al,17- Self-willed. Themes: obstinate

Al,21- He woke with great anxiety about midnight, could not move in spite of every effort, and imagined that thieves were breaking in; on rising he became quiet, after lying down the anxiety returned. Themes: invaded, robber, paralysis

Al,27- Most excessive scruples of conscience about trifles frequently, as though he had done a great wrong. Themes: conscience, conscientious, wrong

Al,37- Whimsical (capricious) and fault - finding. Themes: censorious, capricious

Al,40- She could and would do nothing on account of ill-humor. Themes: succeed, unfit

Al,58- Distraction of mind; he is almost always trying to think of two things at the same time. Themes: double.

Ha,11- Sensitive to noise, which makes him apprehensive. Themes: noise, sensitive

Ha,12- Loud talking is oppressive to him. Themes: noise, sensitive, oppression

Ha,14- She could not and would not attend to anything. Themes: succeed

Ha,16- Internal surfeit (satiety) of life. Themes: loathing, grief

Ha,18- Capricious and disposed to take things ill. Themes: capricious, offenses

Ha,26- The child becomes self-willed, obstinate and headstrong. Themes: obstinate

Ha,3- Longing for home. Themes: homesickness, home

Ha,34- Distracted, he is almost always, as to his mind, in two places at time. Themes: double

Ha,36- Even from little conversation, his head at once becomes muddled (confusion) and there is general exhaustion,... Themes: talk, energy

Ha,5- The least remark makes her weep. Themes: censured

Ha,6- He is frequently seized by anguish, so

that he cannot sit still.(silent) Themes: seized

Ha,8- He feels the greatest conscientious scruples about trifles; as if he had done a very great wrong. Themes: conscientious, conscience, wrong

He,13- Desponding, melancholy, tired of life. Themes: hopeless, sadness, tedium

He,14- Gloomy, feels as if she would die. Themes: pessimism, death

He,15- Wishes to drown herself. Themes: suicidal, water

He,16- Yielding, faint-hearted, anxious mood. Themes: yielding, fearful, timidity

He,19- When crossed has to restrain himself to keep from doing violence. Themes: bother, violence

He,23- ...believes she has swallowed pins, and asks those about her whether she has not done so; seeks for hours for lost pins; ...and careful examined her food for fear of pins; very indifferent to friends and former amusements;... Themes: conscientious, pointed, suspicious, friend, pleasure, indifference

He,4- Reading and writing fatigue, cannot bear to think. Themes: talk, energy, unfit

He,5- Becomes confused, makes mistakes; she is unable to control himself. Themes: unfit, wrong

He,6- Affections from egotism. (ailments from) Themes: egotism

He,7- Compunction (remorse) of conscience about trifles. Themes: conscience, conscientious

He,8- Overanxious about himself; low-spirited... Themes: sadness, himself

He,9- Longing for his relations and home. Themes: homesickness, nostalgia, lack, relatives, home

SIN-N.

He,3- From fright during coition, impotence. Themes: sexual

SOL-T-AE.

Al,1- She rises in the night, imagining that thieves are hidden behind the curtains; but she not dare (risk) to look for them, and begs some one else to do so. Themes: robber, cowardice, helplessness, hide,

Al,5- She is much concerned (care, anxiety) about her future, destiny, which she fancies will be wretched.(miserable) Themes: future, miserable, unfortunate

SPIG.

Al,10- Deep thought about his future. Themes: future

Al,15- Earnestness; he is vexed if one jokes in the least with him. Themes: offenses

Al,17- Extreme ill humor in the evening; he could kill himself, with chilliness of the body. Themes: suicidal

Al,3- Lively contented, and trustful mood, alternating with palpitation and anxious oppression of the chest. Themes: energy, oppression

Al,8- Anxious forebodings, therewith inclination to a peevish indolent mood. Themes: anticipation, negligence

Al,9- Anxiety and apprehensive solicitude for the future. Themes: future

Ha,657- Anxiety and anxious concern about the future. Themes: future

Ha,658- Profound reflection about his future fate. (destiny) Themes: meditation, future

Ha,659- Anxious forebodings (premonition) about the future,... Themes: anticipation, future

Ha,664- Great dejection, in the evening; he could have killed himself... Themes: suicidal

Ha,665- Serious humor, he gets cross if the slightest joke is attempted on him. Themes: bothered, despised, offenses

Ha,666- He is very cross and sensitive to everything that he thinks not good, for many hours. Themes: sensitive, wrong, bothered

He,3- Restless and anxious; solicitude about the future. Themes: restless, future

He,4- Gloomy suicidal mood. Themes: suicidal

He,5- Afraid (fear) of pointed things, pins, etc. Themes: hurt, pointed

He,6- Easily irritated or offended. Themes: offenses

SPIRAE.

Al,1- At 1 A.M. he was attacked with remorse over a long-past slight indiscretion (mistake, wrong), with most fearful qualms (anxiety) of conscience and loathing of himself; .... Themes: conscience, past, loathing, himself

SPONG.

Al,11- She is dissatisfied with what she accomplishes; she cannot rightly help herself at work (helpless) (incompetent) ; she does not succeed. Themes: succeed, helplessness, failure, unfit,

Al,5- Anxiety as if a misfortune would befall him, which he seemed to foresee. (predict, prophesy) Themes: misfortune, clairvoyance

Al,6- She is very fearful, and tormented by a frightful image of a past sad event. Themes: fearful, horrible, tormented, past

Al,7- She was very easily frightened, and started at every trifle; it always seemed to shoot (discharge) into her feet, and afterwards they seemed to remain heavy. Themes: heavy

Ha,377- Every day, several fits of heat, with anxiety, pain in the cardiac region, weeping and inconsolable; she would like to die there and then. Themes: fit, heart, death

Ha,381- She is timorous (fearful) and particularly pursued and incessantly plagued (disturbed, bothered) by a frightful picture out of a melancholic past. Themes: fearful, tormented, past, mortification, seized

Ha,382- Anxious as if misfortune (disaster) threatened (endangered) him and he had a foreboding of it. Themes: anticipation, misfortune, danger, menaced

Ha,384- She is not satisfied with her work; she cannot do her work properly, she is not successful with it. Themes: work, unfit, succeed, failure

He,11- Crazy feeling, head feels blown up. Themes: insanity, disintegration

He,12- Feels awkward (unskillful) about her work, which she cannot accomplish (succeed, prosper) satisfactorily. Themes: work, unfit, succeed

He,15- Inconsolability, would rather die on the spot (immediate); with the heat. Themes: death

He,19- She is very fretful and anxious about her condition, fears she will die of suffocation. Themes: disease, suffocation, death

He,21- She is very timid, and is especially pursued and incessantly tormented by a frightful scene of some mournful (unhappy) event of the past. Themes: timidity, fearful, persecution, tormented, past, misfortune

He,22- She is very timorous (fearful), and starts at every trifle, which affects her feet, so as to make them feel heavy. Themes: fearful, heavy

He,24- Terror and fear: of approaching death; that she will die of suffocation; with heart disease;... Themes: death, suffocation, heart, disease

He,25- He is anxious as if some misfortune would occur of which he has a presentiment. Themes: anticipation, misfortune

He,26- Apprehension of a fatal termination of his disease. Themes: disease, death

He,29- Nervous; despondent about loss of sexual power. Themes: despair, sexual

He,6- Fear of future, tired of life.(ennui) Themes: future, tedium

SQUIL.

He,1- Great anxiety of mind, with fear of death. Themes: death

STANN.

Al,1- Excited and inclined to storms of anger. Themes: anger

Al,20- Fruitlessly busy, as if a rush of ideas prevented him from completing his work at a certain time; all sorts of things occur to him to be done. Themes: busy, work, obstructed, duty, succeed, time, dispersion

Al,21- Indolent and irritable, with heat in the face; would do everything , but really does nothing. Themes: postponing, duty, negligence

Al,7- Quite absorbed in himself, solicitous for the future. Themes: meditation, future

Ha,10 -He is ineffectually (inefficiently) busied, as if he was prevented (obstructed) by super abundance of ideas from finishing his work at a certain time; he thinks of a number of things which he ought yet to attend to. Themes: obstructed, busy, succeed, dispersion

Ha,16- The mind is quiet, introverted, solicitous (anxiety) about the future. Themes: reserved, future

Ha,3- Aversion and distaste for human society. Themes: loathing, misanthropy

Ha,638- Dawdling and irritable, with heat of face; she wished to do all sorts of things and could accomplish nothing. Themes: succeed, unfit

Ha,639- Busy uselessness (inefficiency) : he exerts (use) himself to get a necessary task (duty) done at the appointed hour, and cannot accomplish it, as though prevented (interrupted) by an over-crowding of thoughts, during which one thing and another occur to him which he wishes to do... Themes: busy, duty, failure, succeed, obstructed, dispersion

Ha,640- Peevish: nothing was done according to his wish. Themes: anger, capricious, contradiction

Ha,648- Silent reserved disposition; he thought about the present and the future and was much concerned (care) about the latter. Themes: future, reserved,

Ha,649- Aversion from and dread (fear) of people. Themes: misanthropy, loathing

Ha,655- In the first three days he is rather calm and his vexation quickly passes off, does not fly into a passion, is rather quickly sensitive; the fourth day he is disposed to stormy anger and to fly into a passion... Themes: bothered, anger, passionate

Ha,659- Calm, collected disposition: he was reconciled to his fate (destiny) and was perfectly contented with his lot. (destiny, doom) Themes: doomed, misfortune

Ha,7- Dawdling (indolent) and irritated, with heat in the face; she wanted to do a number of things, but accomplished (complete) nothing. Themes: succeed, dispersion

Ha,8- Restless and distracted, no perseverance in her work (at once). Themes: restless, work, succeed, dispersion

He,1- Sadness, with aversion to men and disinclination to talk. Themes: sexual, talk,

He,3- Uneasy, does not know what to do with himself pains > by walking, yet so weak he soon must die. Themes: confidence, doubtful, energy, death

He,6- A woman, age 39, pregnant in fourth month;...inability to do anything as she cannot muster sufficient courage,...great palpitation of heart and anxiety, especially if she has to give directions in her domestic affairs; thinking makes her feel wretched, ...(unable, incapable) Themes: cowardice, heart, home, miserable, duty, unfit

STAPH.

Al,1- He was joyous, enjoyed society, and was good-humored. Themes: company, pleasure

Al,15- Anxious thoughts and events in the past came to him as if the past were present before him, which caused anxiety...then it became black before his eyes; he did not know whether the images were real or illusory, then everything seemed different, and he lost all desire to live. Themes: past, mortification, unreal, strange, loathing, obstructed

Al,21- Quiet fretfulness (irritable) ; he is vexed at everything which even does not concern him. Themes: bothered

Al,6- Sad; he fears the worst results from slight causes, and cannot quiet himself. Themes: pessimism

Ha,691- Serious, silent, occupied with himself, he speaks but little. Themes: reserved, talk

Ha,692- The most attractive things made no impression on him. Themes: indifference

Ha,693- Phlegmatic (indifferent), prostrate mind and sad disposition, unsympathetic, indifferent to all externals, yet not cross or exhausted. Themes: reserved, energy, indifference

Ha,695- As if dead (decease, lifeless, inert) in mind and sad, but not to weeping. Themes: lifeless, death, sadness

Ha,696- He does not know if what is hovering before his imagination like something in his memory has actually taken place or whether he only dreamt it. Themes: unreal

Ha,697- When he walks quickly he feels as if some one were following him; this caused anxiety and fear, and he must always look about him. Themes: hurry, persecution, suspicious

Ha,700- All day long peevish and cross; he did not know what to do for ill-humor, and was extremely pensive. Themes: bothered, meditation

Ha,701- Silent peevishness; he gets cross about everything, even what does not concern him. Themes: bothered

Ha,703- Anxious thoughts and things long

past come before him as if they were actually present and stood before him, which causes anxiety and the sweat of anguish - Then blackness comes before his eyes; he knows not if what he sees is true (real) or deception (false, unreal) , then he regards (suppose) everything as something different to what it is (strange), and he loses all wish to live. (lost; discernment, perception) Themes: mortification, death, obstructed, past, dark, unreal

Ha,704- Great inward anxiety, so that he cannot remain in one place, but he says nothing about it.(restlessness) Themes: restless, movement

Ha,706- Great anxiety; he dreads the future. Themes: future

Ha,707- Hypochondriacal humor; everything is indifferent to him; he would like to die. Themes: death, indifference

Ha,708- Sad, he apprehends (perceive) the worst consequences from slight (trivial) things and cannot calm himself. Themes: misfortune, pessimism, conscience

Ha,716- She was all day long full of grief; she was afflicted (torment) to weeping about her circumstances (position), and she cared for nothing in the world. Themes: tortured, indifference

He,11- Great indignation about things done by others or by himself; grieves about consequences. (remorse) Themes: injustice, indignation, offenses, conscience

He,12- Ailments from indignation and vexation, or reserved displeasure ;sleeplessness. Themes: indignation, suppressed, grief, reserved

He,13- Continual concern about the future. Themes: future

He,14- ...; was insulted (slandered, defamed, calumniated) being too dignified (reserved, lordly,) to fight (contest), subdued (control) his wrath(anger) and went home sick,.. (ailments, from offenses) Themes: offenses, haughty, indignation, anger, suppressed, disease, fight, reserved

He,15- ...; firmly believed he would lose his fortune, constantly told his wife to be careful that they did not starve; thinks his wife will run away from him (deserted) (lost: position, rank), ... amuses himself by throwing into the fire any article near at hand, regardless of value; at times more violent, strikes at any one coming near him, ...tells his wife he will try not kill any one;... Themes: failure, position, starving, forsaken, fire, violence, homicidal, wealth,

He,2- Indifference, low-spirited, dullness of mind; after onanism.(masturbation) Themes: indifference, sadness, sexual

He,4- Sad distressing thoughts about one's illness. Themes: disease, sadness, cares

He,6- Hypochondriasis (depression);...;caused by unmerited insults (offenses, affronts, abuses) sexual excesses, or by persistently dwelling on sexual subjects. Themes: offenses, injustice, sexual, dwells, lascivious

He,7- Suffering from pride, envy (spite) or chagrin (shame, dishonor) . Themes: haughty, envy, grief

He,9- Very sensitive to least impression; least word that seems wrong (offenses) hurts her very much. Themes: sensitive, offenses, wrong, injustice

STICT.

Al,1- She got very lively (active), told her father she felt as if she would like to strike out, only for fun; she would like it just for fun of it. After awhile she lay down on the lounge, and began, to use a common expression, to kick up her heels; her mother reproaching, said, " Bella, do behave, that is not ladylike"; when child responded: " Ma, I cannot help it; I feel exactly as if I want to fly away"... Themes: pleasure, wicked, sadism, fly, liberty

He,2- Great desire to talk about anything and everything, does not care whether any one listens or not, she must talk; feels as if she cannot keep her tongue still. Themes: talk

STRAM.

Al,120...all his ideas seemed to consist of mere reproductions (duplication); there was nothing original (creative) and there were no new combinations. Themes: imitated

Al,122- For some days the patient was affected with hallucinations and thought that one side of him was alive, while the other side was buried. Themes: lifeless, double, death, half, alive

Al,123- ...seemed to herself to be engaged in her usual avocation,...imitate in every respect the routine procedure of one thus engaged. Themes: work, busy, feigning, imitated

Al,126- The boy repeatedly said there were" big sores" on him. Themes: disease

Al,130- The apartment seemed all on fire. Themes: fire

Al,136-Delirium...seeming to dread the approach of some imaginary monster, and giving utterance in the most piteous appeals for help, protection. Themes: approached, attacked, helplessness

Al,206- Fear of being in the dark and a less extent of being alone, in the evening after sunset. Themes: dark, solitude

Al,207- His whole conduct and countenance was like that of a child severely frightened and apprehending some terrible calamity. Themes: anticipation, fearful, child, misfortune

Al,23- Violent delirium; with was alternately mirthful, furious or dolorous (sad), directed to some imaginary source of pleasure or repugnance, and accompanied which corresponding gesticulations. Themes: anger, loathing, pleasure, insanity

Al,24- Much excited and rather delirious, under the impression of some immediate danger, clinging to the person who had him in her lap. Themes: danger, helplessness

Al,45- ...seemed to forget herself...seemed to sit like a perfect idiot (fool),... Themes: perfection

Al,48- She is all the time inconsolable; much affected by trifles; makes much fuss about trifles; disposed to weep, and sometimes also very easily vexed; now and then neglects her duties; now and then thinks she is not fitted for her position ; after the fall equinox...; she wants light and company. Themes: duty, unfit, position, conscience, negligence, confidence, light, company

Al,53-...throw the hands about the head as if attempting to ward off some threatening evil;...escape from the imaginary object ... Themes: danger, menaced, persecution, escape

Al,63-...I was assailed (attacked) by imaginary spectres, in the most hideous forms and menacing attitudes; and what was still to my torment my bed was suspended and tantalized (charmed) like a feather (plumage) between two floors. Themes: attacked, ghosts, horrible, ugly, menaced, tormented, floating

Al-S,1684-...Constant fear of sudden death. At times believed herself dying... Themes: death

Ha,360- Sensation in the arms and legs as if the limbs were completely severed (separated, detached, cut of) from the body. Themes: disintegration, mutilated

Ha,361- Sensation as if every portion of the limbs were completely severed in the joints from the other parts and could not be joined together again. Themes: disintegration, mutilated

Ha,363- He feels his hands and feet as if separated in the joints, and he is inconsolable on account of this sensation. Themes: disintegration, mutilated, despair

Ha,499- In this slumber he hears two persons talking but knows not who they are. Themes: talk, double

Ha,503- After waking all objects seem to him new (strange, unusual) even his friends as though he had never in his life seen them before. Themes: strange, friend

Ha,504- He appears to himself large and tall, but surrounding objects appear small to him. Themes: great, contemptuous, greatness, small

Ha,507 -He fears he is losing his senses. (sanity) Themes: insanity

Ha,519- He speaks to absent persons as though they were present, and addresses(talk) lifeless objects (e.g. chessmen) by the names of those persons, but does not notice any of those around him. Themes: talk, lifeless

Ha,520 - Loquacious madness; he complains of a dog biting and tearing the flesh off his chest. Themes: tear, bite, attacked, animal

Ha,524- He dances at night in the churchyard. Themes: music, funeral

Ha,542- Exertion of strength: a strong man could scarcely hold him down in bed. Themes: energy

Ha,544- Great desire to bite and tear everything with his teeth that comes near his mouth, even his own limbs. Themes: bite, tear, himself, hurt

Ha,546- Furious endeavors to kill people. Themes: anger, homicidal

Ha,547- Furious endeavor to kill himself. Themes: anger, suicidal

Ha,548- Nonsensical idea, as though he were killed, roasted, and being devoured. Themes: murdered, attacked

Ha,549- He thinks he is dying, and that he will not live over the evening , he rejoices that he is dying, and gives directions about his funeral, otherwise he is rational and does not feel particularly ill. Themes: death, organization, funeral, pleasure

Ha,550- At night he jumps out of the bed and cries out that the disease is breaking out of his head. Themes: disease, disintegration

Ha,551- She sometimes cries out about cats, dogs and rabbits, which were approaching (pursuing) her from above, from the side and from the middle of the room. Themes: attacked, animal, surrounded, approached

Ha,553- Frightful pictures of the imagination; he fancies he sees ghosts. Themes: fearful, ghosts

Ha,556- In the evening after lying in bed very sad, with thoughts of death and violent weeping. Themes: death

Ha,559- She fancies she sees a number of people who are not present, and she grasps at them. Themes: caught, helplessness, lack

Ha,561- In the moments of consciousness he begged to be held as he was falling. Themes: helplessness, fall

Ha,562- His surroundings appear to him quite strange; (unfamiliar) although in the first minutes he knows that he is surrounded by his friends, he forgets this in the second minute, and imagines he is quite alone (solitary, deserted) in a desert (wildness), and is afraid (fearful) ; figures of beasts suddenly spring out of the ground at his side, so that he moves to the other side, where, however, other similar figures pursue him, and he runs forward. Themes: strange, solitude, forsaken, attacked, persecution, surrounded, friend, animal

Ha,563- As a rule he has more imaginary figures at his side than in front of him, they all inspire him with horror. Themes: fearful, surrounded, ghosts

Ha,564- He always imagines he is alone (solitary, lonely) and is afraid. Themes: solitude, forsaken, fearful

Ha,565- Nowhere has he rest, is startled by dream-pictures, even when his eyes are open, which in the form of big dogs, cats and other horrible beasts, grow (expand) out of the ground at his side, and from which he jumps away to the side with signs of terror (fear), and knows not how to save (rescue, free) himself. (cornered, corralled) Themes: attacked, horrible, animal, grow, escape, salvation, fearful

He,100- ...threatens to knock everybody down, to break furniture, to throw himself out of window. Themes: menacing, hurt, violence, suicidal, height

He,101- Mania for light and company, cannot bear to be alone. Themes: mania, solitude, company, light

He,102- Mania with insomnia ; very talkative; thinks he has every imaginable disease; that he has power (powerful) over all disease; masturbates, fills his pockets with anything he can find (lack?), thinks he has snakes in him. Themes: disease, ruined, inexpugnable, sexual, animal

He,103- Had many strange fancies, such as imagining his wife had lovers concealed (hidden) behind stove; ...afterward had a fit that looked so much like apoplexy that he was bled.(blood) Themes: suspicious, betrayed, fit, blood, disease, jealousy

He,107-...heard continually ,on r. side of occiput, a loud voice, scolding, vituperating and accusing him of ungodliness (impious, sinful, irreligious, godless, profane); ....prayed expecting, with great anxiety, the flash of lightning which was to kill him;...(redemption, regeneration, salvation) Themes: accused, godless, executed, conscience, wicked, salvation, death, light, censured, offenses, penitence

He,108-...spoke of lizards and worms being on his clothes,... Themes: animal, clothes

He,11- Stupor: weakened intellect; torpor and fits; extreme excitement of sexual parts,... Themes: energy, fit, sexual

He,110-...frightful dreams about fighting and killing; takes offensive in imaginary quarrels, and attacks aggressor; runs against supposed object to attack it;... Themes: fight, homicidal, violence, hurt, homicidal

He,111- Nymphomania; with diaphragmitis; violent attacks, even to rage; exalted sexual passion. Themes: lascivious, sexual, anger, passionate

He,112- Religious mania; pious (divine) looks, praying; restless nights; inspired talking, singing; despairs of her salvation. Themes: religious, feigning, seized, music, despair, salvation

He,113- Hydrophobia; water, a mirror, or anything bright, excites convulsion...,afraid to be alone;... Themes: water, bright, fit, solitude

He,114- ...seeing rats and cats in room,...wanted a razor;... Themes: animal, pointed

He,117- Ceaseless talking mostly devout; very earnestly beseeching. (supplicating) Themes: talk, salvation, religious

He,119- His thoughts ran upon obscene things, frequently put his hands to erect penis; sought to bite or to catch flies. Themes: lascivious, sexual, bite, hunter, animal, wicked

He,122- Excessive loquacity each time during menses; tears and prayers and earnest (ardent) supplications. Themes: talk, religious, salvation

He,130- Talks in a foreign tongue. Themes: talk, stranger, abroad

He,14-...thoughts of dying;...fear of wild animals and black dogs. Themes: wild, death, animal, dark

He,145- Wife complains of husband neglecting her; man accuses his wife of being faithless. Themes: husband, despised, forsaken, betrayed, wife

He,151- Making all kinds of faces and imitating motions, gestures and voices of different animals. Themes: imitated, feigning, animal

He,155- Disposition to suicide; wanted a razor (blade, knife) to cut his throat. Themes: suicidal

He,156- Endeavors to escape, imagines he is alone all the time, and is afraid. (loneliness, isolation) Themes: solitude, escape, fearful

He,161- While sitting on a sofa, fancied she was falling off, kept holding on to everything; while in bed said that bed was being drawn from under her. Themes: fall, helplessness

He,162- In his conscious moments, he asked to be held because he was falling. Themes: helplessness, fall

He,163- Cries out fearfully, hides face in pillow, is terrified by presence or approach of physician; after attack of typhoid. Themes: fearful, suspicious, attacked, hide, attacked, approached

He,171- Crying mood, with inclination to give offense and to feel offended. Themes: offensive, offenses

He,172- Downcast and full of anguish, believes herself unworthy of eternal bliss, because she is unable to perform her duties. Themes: sadness, unfit, duty, religious, conscience

He,175- Sad; apprehends evil consequences from trifling things. Themes: conscientious, pessimism

He,176- Melancholia,...complains her husband has neglecting her. Themes: husband, despised, forsaken

He,177-...sometimes vexed; neglects her duties, thinks she is not fitted for her position;... Themes: bothered, negligence, duty, unfit, position, conscience

He,178- Pangs of conscience; thinks he is not honest. (dishonest) Themes: conscience, wicked

He,29- Talking in Jewish jargon.(cliche,) Themes: talk, stranger, feigning

He,32- After getting out of bed, vertigo and loss of thought; everything hovers dimly and distantly before his memory, there seems to be a veil before his eyes. Themes: obstructed, separated

He,40- Aberration of mind; one carries home all sorts of wood in order to manufacture brandy (cognac) (busy, manufacturing) ; another placed two axes across each other in order to split wood in this way; a third burrowed in ground like a pig with his mouth (animal); a fourth alleged he was a wheelwright and began to bore holes; a fifth ran into forge to catch fish, which he saw swimming there; a lacemaker threw about her bobbins incessantly, and threw everything into confusion; another girl ran about the room and cried out that all evil spirits were pursuing her.(restoration, restitution) Themes: busy, feigning, persecution, organization, work, animal, hunter, devil,

He,47- He is like one enchanted and beside himself. Themes: seized

He,49- After spasms she fell into a trance, says she is under influence(seized) of spirits ,and has had conversation with spirits, communications from God; delivers emphatic sermons, prophecies. (missionary) Themes: seized, religious, greatness, clairvoyance

He,51- ...converses with spirits who approach his bed, lays hold of a stick and strikes about him,...great sexual excitement. Themes: talk, approached, ghosts, violence, sexual

He,53- Hallucinations which terrify patient; sees ghosts, hears voices back his ear; sees strangers. Themes: ghosts, seized, stranger

He,55- He thinks that he is dying and that he will not live over night, rejoices (celebrate) and gives directions about his funeral. Themes: death, funeral, organization

He,56- Believes to be in his grave; shrives,(confess) prays, asks to be killed (justified); accuses his wife of infidelity; scolds (cursing), strikes at everybody who wishes to restrain him; thinks they are dogs and barks at them to make himself understood. Themes: funeral, death, executed, suspicious, betrayed, censorious, contemptuous, conscience, religious, animal, jealousy, violence, offensive

He,57- Strange absurd ideas; thinks herself tall, double or lying crosswise; one half of body cut off (divided); bed is full of creases (wrinkle) (disorganization); that he was killed roasted and being eaten. Themes: strange, great, double, divided, murdered, disintegration, half, mutilated, organization

He,58- Imagines he is alone, and is frightened. Themes: solitude, fearful

He,59- ...clings to her mother with as much desperation as if she were going to be thrown from a precipice. Themes: despair, fall, helplessness, mother, caught, height

He,61- Thinks she is not fitted for her position. Themes: unfit, position, confidence

He,63- An old lady had a vision every night since six weeks, in which many persons, all strangers, came into her room and to her bedside, causing her such fear that she had to leave bed. Themes: stranger, invaded, persecution, escape

He,65-"There", he replied, "A long train of bedbugs, and after them a procession of beetles and here come crawling over me a host (crowd) of cockroaches"; sank back in alarm, then suddenly said:" I believe I know they are not really bugs, but, except once in a while, they seem real to me. (organization, association, union) Themes: organization, union, crawling, animal, fearful

He,66- Woke suddenly in night and said there were snakes under and about her; looked wild, screamed and pointed to them. Themes: surrounded, animal, attacked, wild

He,68- Hears dancing, music, sees men and hears them talk in foreign tongues. Themes: music, talk, stranger

He,69- Hallucinations as if near r. mastoid process a voice were scolding (censured, reproved), her < at night, sometimes voice seemed to be under bed. Themes: censured, seized,

He,71- Fears; he will lose his senses (insanity); his lips will grow together; to suffocate; of falling; everything is falling on her. Themes: insanity, suffocation, fall, crushed

He,77- Patient had a constant vision of an executioner(hangman, lynches) standing before him in spite of which he was lively, talkative, laughed and joked about his hallucination, yet it seemed to him a reality. Themes: executed, contemptuous, murdered, pleasure, menaced,

He,79- Boy seemed to see black objects, spoke of black people and black clouds, and grasped at air. Themes: dark, helplessness, caught

He,81-...attempts to stab and bite;...with sexual excitement; fear as if a dog were attacking him;... Themes: homicidal, animal, bite, sexual, attacked, pointed, violence

He,85-...seemed to dread approach of some imaginary monster, and giving utterance to most piteous appeals for help. Themes: approached, helplessness, danger, attacked

He,87- After a dreadful shock, occasioned by death of his brother, who fell dead in his arms,...struck all at around him...spoke at one time in Hungarian, and then in Wallachian language; sang Latin paternosters, declared he was God, and then that he was the devil;... Themes: death, brother, hurt, stranger, greatness, seized, religious, devil

He,92- Mania:... complains that a dog is biting and tearing flesh off his chest; merry exaltation; with pride (haughty) and affectation; runs about, complains of violent headache; ...;steals from his roommates...; disposition to scold persons whom he otherwise loved. Themes: animal, bite, tear, haughty, criminal, offensive, attacked, censorious, pleasure, greatness,

He,93- Mania; thinks he is lying on his sepulchre (tomb); confessing, praying, wants to be killed (redemption, salvation, regeneration); laughs as if tickled (excited); wants to be kissed; accuses his wife of being faithless (betrayed); scolding (censure) beating in a rage, will not be taken hold of by attendants (suspicious?) ; takes them for dogs (contemptuous), and barks at them; talking in Jewish jargon; (rank?, stranger?) supposes his house to be surrounded by carts (vehicle), Jews (Judaism) and geese, offending him, ... - (strange, foreign, alien) Themes: funeral, death, executed, betrayed, suspicious, censorious, contemptuous, stranger, offenses, conscience, religious, salvation, surrounded,

He,94-...fear of malicious animals, black dogs; ... Themes: fearful, animal, dark, wicked

He,98 - Mania; affects (pretend) being a distinguished (label) person, of high rank (position, nobility) ; is full of fear. Themes: feigning, greatness, position,

He,99- Acute mania; tears his clothing;... threatens to use knife on those about him. Themes: tear, clothes, menacing, pointed, homicidal

STRONT-C.

Al,2- Apprehensive and anxious, as from a bad conscience. Themes: conscience

He,1- Apprehensive and anxious as from a bad conscience. Themes: conscience

STRY.

Al,3- Shouted out, "They are coming for me". Themes: persecution

Al,30- He had a feeling of dread, and begged he might not be left alone. Themes: solitude, helplessness

Al,31- A fear of something about to occur. Themes: misfortune

Al,5- A peculiar nervous erethism, almost resembling what I had seen in a case of hydrophobia ...wandering when left to himself, and begged most piteously (miserable) that I would not hurt him...fear of being injured... Themes: disease, solitude, hurt

SUL-AC.

Al,28- Very fearful; extremely mistrustful. Themes: fearful, suspicious

Al,35- Fretful, peevish, impatient, if his work is not done to suit.(unsatisfying) Themes: impatience, work, failure, duty, conscience

Al,5- He was roused (waken) with difficulty , and when roused, resisted fiercely, saying in a hoarse muffled (deaden) voice, "Let me alone, let me die". Themes: death, solitude

Al,9- Hasty (hurried, fast) mood; nothing that she does can be finished quickly enough, though she makes unusual effort. Themes: time, hurry, succeed, duty

Ha,10- So irritable and affected that she gets frightened at everything. Themes: fearful

Ha,12- Hastiness (fast) ; everything she does, she cannot accomplish fast enough; but it fatigues her exceedingly. Themes: hurry, time, succeed

Ha,16- Vexed, peevish, impatient, at once when he does not succeed in his work. Themes: bothered, succeed, work, failure

Ha,7- Fearing many things, exceedingly suspicious. Themes: suspicious

He,2- Must do everything in a great hurry; nothing can be finished quickly enough. Themes: hurry, duty, succeed, time

He,6-... unfit for work, would sit and weep whole day long;... Themes: unfit, work

SULPH.

Al,10- Vexatious and morbid ideas of the past arise from the most indifferent thoughts, and from every occurrence in life, which continue to be united with new vexations, so that she cannot free herself from them, together with a courageous mood which is ready for great resolution. Themes: mortification, dwells, liberty

Al,100- Thoughts of the business that had been accomplished thronged (crowd) upon her... Themes: work, conscience, duty

Al,11- She fancies that she is becoming emaciated.(skeletal) Themes: fragile, disease

Al,12- She fancies that she has beautiful (refined) clothes; old rags look like fine things, a coat like a beautiful jacket, a cap like a beautiful hat. Themes: greatness, vanity, clothes,

Al,2- Delirium; she destroys her things, throws them away, thinking that she has a superfluity (excess) of everything, wherewith she wastes(thin) to a skeleton.(wealth?) Themes: greatness, fragile, wealth, starving,

Al,28- Depressed about his illness and out of humor. Themes: disease

Al,29- She does not know what to do with herself on account of internal discouragement. Themes: confidence

Al,3772-...it was disturbed by dreams of fire and death. Themes: fire, death

Al,3780- At night, very vivid anxious dreams, as if was pursued by wild beasts. Themes: persecution, animal, wild

Al,3784- At night, vivid dreams of a comic character, with loud laughter, ... Themes: pleasure

Al,3799- An anxious dream, that fire came down from heaven. Themes: fire

Al,3800-....(DREAM) she walked about like a somnambulist, thought there was a fire, dressed herself, talked out of the window, and was frightened as she heard that it was nothing; for three days afterwards she was very weak, and felt bruised(hurt). Themes: fire, hurt, clothes, fearful, energy

Al,3802- Frightful, anxious dreams of danger of death, and of dead people. Themes: danger, death, ghosts

Al,3813- At night uncomfortable dreams of murders. Themes: murdered

Al,3815- At night, horrible dreams, with great palpitation or heart, and on awaking, sometimes rigor, sometimes heat and fear of robbers. Themes: robber, heart, horrible,

Al,3816- Frightful dream that he had been bitten by a dog. Themes: fearful, attacked, bite, animal

Al,3824- The first three nights he rose from bed in a somnambulistic way, as if unconscious; cried, "My head, my head! I am crazy!" grasped his forehead; ... Themes: insanity\plain

Al,41- Frequently during the day she has attacks of melancholy, lasting a few minutes, when she feels extremely unhappy, without cause; she wishes to die. Themes: sadness, unfortunate, death

Al,42-...discontented with himself and all about him, which made him unfit for any serious occupations...whole evening he was absorbed in himself and unable to command his thoughts to read... Themes: discontented, himself, unfit, work,

Al,44- Anxiety as if he would cease to live. Themes: death

Al,45- Anxious disposition I could not free myself from the anticipation of some great misfortune, though I had no ground for such fear,... Themes: anticipation, misfortune

Al,56- She is apprehensive for others, and anxious. Themes: others

Al,57- During the proving I was much concerned (anxiety) about my state of health, and feared lest I might really get ill. Themes: disease

Al,58- The condition seems very distressing, and she is apprehensive of the future. Themes: future

Al,59- Awoke in a hour in great fright and distress; horror of instant death. Themes: fearful, death

Al,60- Fear that he would take cold in the open air; he did not know whether it was illusive or physical. Themes: disease, infection

Al,69- Extremely peevish and ill-humored; nothing seems right to her. Themes: anger, wrong

Al,8- Numerous morbid ideas, extremely disagreeable, causing rancor, though with also joyous thoughts (and melodies) mostly from the past, take possession of her they throng one upon another so that she cannot free herself from them during the day, with neglect of business,...

Themes: mortification, pessimism, anger, tormented, past, duty, resentment, music, work, negligence, liberty

Al,84- He is vexed at everything, gets angry and out of humor at every word, thinks he must be defended (protect) and becomes exasperated. Themes: bothered, anger, offenses

Al,85- He could tear himself to pieces from vexation. Themes: anger, clothes, bothered, tear

Al,87- Embittered mood as if he had been injured. Themes: offenses, injustice

Al,9- She imagines that people injure her, and she will die in consequence. Themes: death, hurt

Al,94- He sits for hours immovable and indolent, without definite thought, though he has much to accomplish. Themes: duty, succeed, negligence

Ha,11- She finds her state very agonizing and she is apprehensive about the future. Themes: future

Ha,15- Apprehension, as if he had to lose his life at once. Themes: death

Ha,24- She imagines that she might give people something wrong, which might kill them. Themes: homicidal, conscience, wrong, confidence

Ha,25- She is apprehensive for others, with anxiety. Themes: others

Ha,26- Anxiety with heat in the head and cold feet, so that he does not know what to do; he forgets every moment what he desired to do. Themes: dispersion

Ha,30- He greatly feels the need of tranquillity of spirit, as his spirit is ever active. Themes: restless, peace

Ha,35- He imagines he is getting thin (weak). Themes: disease, fragile

Ha,38- He gets vexed about everything, takes every word ill and gets insulted (dishonored, degraded), he imagines he ought (must) to defend himself and gets angry. Themes: bothered, offenses, indignation, anger

Ha,39- He allows himself to be carried away by vexation. Themes: contradiction

Ha,4- Often during the day, attacks lasting for several minutes, when she feels herself utterly (completely) miserable, without any cause, like melancholy; she desires to die. Themes: death, miserable, sadness

Ha,43- Ill-humored; she becomes vexed at herself. Themes: antagonism, himself

Ha,44- Ill-humored and in a criticizing mood. Themes: censorious

Ha,5- Sad pusillanimous, full of weariness (fatigue) of life. Themes: sadness, loathing, cowardice

Ha,51- For hours he sits motionless and indolent, without any definite thoughts, though he has many things to attend to. Themes: indifference, duty, negligence

Ha,53- He is so peevish and obstinate, that he will not give an answer to anybody, he cannot bear to have anyone around him, and cannot get quickly enough what he wants. Themes: anger, obstinate, approached, hurry, capricious

Ha,55-...cannot do anything to please herself, is obstinate and unyielding (rigorous), without herself knowing why. Themes: discontented, obstinate

Ha,56- The mind is embittered, as if he had been insulted. Themes: offenses

Ha,57- His mood is quarrelsome and contentious (hostile) about everything. Themes: fight, offensive

Ha,58- ..She thinks of nothing but anxious, annoying and dejecting thoughts, which she cannot get rid of; this makes her apprehensive and peevish unto tears. Themes: sadness, mortification, liberty

Ha,59- A number of ideas from her past life, mostly disagreeable, causing indignation and mortification...come into her mind;...so that she cannot get rid of them, while she has nothing to do;... Themes: indignation, mortification, injustice, past, tortured

Ha,60- Indifferent things and such things as naturally occur in life are attended in her mind with annoying, mortifying ideas from her past, which continually connect themselves with recent annoyances of which she cannot rid herself. This attended (accompanied) with a resoluteness of mind, which is ready for great resolves.(determination) Themes: bothered, mortification, confidence, past, tortured,

Ha,61- Great inclination to philosophic and religious ravings.(insanity) Themes: religious, meditation, philosophy, insanity

Ha,62- She imagines that she has beautiful

clothes, she takes old rags for beautiful clothes , she takes a coat for a jacket, a cap for a hat. Themes: vanity, greatness, feigning, clothes

Ha,63- Insanity; she spoils (ruin) her things and throws them away, imagining she has an abundance of everything; at the same time she becomes emaciated, like a skeleton.-(wealthy, rich X miserable, poor, destitute) Themes: squanders, greatness, ruined, wealth, starving

He,11- Foolish happiness and pride(haughtiness),thinks himself in possession of beautiful (attractive) things; even rags seem beautiful. (rank, position, distinction) Themes: haughty, greatness, clothes, vanity

He,13- A little girl with religious insanity, takes passages of Scripture literally and acts upon them. (fanatical) (virtuous, noble, elevated) Themes: insanity, religious, obstinate, mania

He,21- Satiety of life, longing for death. Themes: tedium, loathing, death

He,29- ...is filled with anxious, despondent (sad) thoughts, from which she cannot free herself, they make her suspicious, peevish and lachrymose. Themes: despair, mortification, tortured, suspicious,

He,3-...feels as if crazy; does not know whether she has done what she intended (planned) or whether objects seen are really there, or whether she only imagines them to be, until she has touched them;... Themes: insanity, duty, unreal, touch

He,31- Depressed about her illness, and out of humor. Themes: disease, sadness

He,32- Melancholy mood; dwelling on religious or philosophic speculations; anxiety about soul's salvation; indifference about lot (destiny) of others. Themes: sadness, religious, conscience, dwells, theorizing, philosophy, salvation, indifference, others

He,33- Sleepless, disgusted with life, fears the future, where she sees nothing but misery (wretchedness, poverty) and suffering (misfortune). 0 Melancholia. Themes: grief, fearful, future, poverty, unfortunate, pessimism, mortification

He,34-...; profound melancholy; considers herself disgraced (dishonor, degradation) ; speaks of dying , finds life insupportable;... Themes: unfortunate, death, loathing, sadness, unfortunate,

He,35-...,strong impulsive tendency to suicide, by drowning or by precipitating herself from window;...(high, water) Themes: suicidal, height, water

He,36-..., feels extremely unhappy without cause, she wishes to die. Themes: unfortunate, death

He,37- Great dejection,(grief), with thoughts of suicide; feels inferior (mediocre, lower) to everybody; can decide nothing;... Themes: grief, suicidal, despised, unfortunate, doubtful, confidence

He,38- Destroys clothing; imagines she has everything in abundance. (wealth) Themes: greatness, clothes, wealth

He,39- Too lazy (indolent) to rouse (animate) himself up, and too unhappy to live. Themes: unfortunate

He,43- Vexations and morbid ideas of past arise from most indifferent thoughts, and from every occurrence in life, which continue to be united with new vexations, so that she cannot free herself from them. Themes: tormented, past, mortification, bothered

He,46- Great anxiety, fear lest she should come to ruin (destruction); ..tried to run away... Themes: ruined, escape

He,47- Anxiety;...as if some great misfortune were impending (threatening);... Themes: misfortune, menaced

He,50- Irritable mood; easily excited and always absorbed in himself. Themes: meditation, himself

He,51- Dread of being washed. Themes: water, dirty

He,53- Ill-humored and fault-finding. Themes: censorious

He,55- Ill-humored; vexed with herself; everything makes her impatient. Themes: bothered, himself, impatience

He,56- He could tear himself to pieces with vexation. Themes: tear, himself

He,59- Egotism. Themes: egotism

He,8- Numerous morbid ideas, extremely disagreeable, causing rancor; neglect of business;... Themes: mortification, anger, work, resentment, negligence, work

He,9- Rack (torture) their brains about metaphysical subtleties (nuances). Themes: theorizing, tormented, philosophy

SUMB.

Al,2- More cheerful in humor and more disposed for intellectual occupation; he felt in the happy enthusiastic state of mind that accompanies the consciousness of having performed a noble (generous, virtuous) deed; this sort of medicinal intoxication went away in a few hours. Themes: duty, pleasure, helpful

Al,8- ...fond (love) of the society of women; ...sympathy with suffering seems robbed of its pain...nervous excitement and heat, especially in head from listening (hearing) to a disputation, ...humor depressed with despair of future...melancholy despondency, as if ill-treated by everyone purposely... mildness, amiability Themes: sexual, compassionate, discussion, despair, future, despised, mildness, damage

He,2- Happy disposition with continued smiling; expression idiotic; fear of becoming insane. Themes: pleasure, insanity

SYPH.

Al,N-12- Terrible dread (fear) of night, ...death is preferable ; she fears to prepare for night and is positively in abject fear of suffering,... Themes: fearful, death, disease, dark

Al,N-5-... violent on being opposed, has tremors, seems on the verge of convulsions,...always washing her hands. Themes: dirty, contradiction, violence, fit

Al,N-7- Very despondent, does not think he will ever get better. Themes: hopeless, disease

Al,N-8- Feeling as if going insane, or about to be paralyzed. Themes: paralysis, insanity

He,10- Feeling as if going insane, or about be paralyzed. Themes: paralysis, insanity

He,11- A far-away feeling, with apathy and indifference to future. Themes: separated, indifference, future

He,8- Very despondent, does not think will ever get better. (hopeless) Themes: hopeless, disease

He,9- Terrible dread of night, ...it is intolerable, death is preferable. She fears to prepare for night and is positively in abject fear of suffering... Themes: fearful, death, disease

TAB.

Al,19- Low spirits, want of resolution and general hypochondriasis. Themes: irresolution, sadness,

Al,2- He went to sleep in the cabin, which was full of large packages of tobacco, ...His inability to move was not accompanied by any pain or uneasiness but he felt as if the principle of life had entirely departed from his frame.(body) Themes: paralysis, divided, lifeless

Al,20- Gloom, hypochondria, apprehensions of sudden death. Themes: sadness, death

Al,28- Anxiety of being alone at night. Themes: solitude

Al,30- Uneasiness and anxiety in the afternoon, as if some misfortune would occur. Themes: misfortune

Al,34- Apprehensive, faint-hearted, and despondent, with nausea; she thought she would die, ... Themes: cowardice, death

Al,35- Great apprehension with oppression of the chest, and a very despondent, sad mood, as if apprehended some misfortune,... Themes: oppression, misfortune, despair

Al,36- Apprehension, anxiety, and despondency, as if she dreaded death at 4 p.m. two days in succession. Themes: hopeless, death

Al,38- Terrible apprehensions (fear) of immediate death. Themes: fearful, death

Al,41- From having been one of the most healthy and fearless of men, he had become sick all over, and was timid as a girl; he could not even present a petition in Congress, much less say a word concerning it; ...by any ordinary noise, he was startled or thrown into tremulousness, and afraid to be alone at night. Themes: fearful, timidity, noise, talk, confidence

Al,42- Evenness and mildness of temper, notwithstanding he felt very uneasy about his health. Themes: mildness, disease

Al,45- He was incapacitated for business of any kind, weak irresolute, and despondent. Themes: work, irresolution, doubtful, unfit, energy

Al,51- Exalted action of the brain; copious flow of ideas; ...leaving me in the morning worn-out and sick, I would conceive and elaborate about twenty undertakings, of which probably not one would ever come to light. Themes: planning, succeed, greatness, disease, energy, dispersion

TARAX.

Al,4- Without occupation he is quite gloomy; does not know what to do, and cannot make up his mind to do anything. Themes: irresolution, doubtful, confidence, energy

Al,6- Irresolution and dread of work, though it progresses well as soon as he undertakes it. Themes: irresolution, work, doubtful, succeed

He,3- Undecided, shunning (avoid) labor, but after beginning, works well. Themes: irresolution, work, succeed

TARENT.

Al,1- ...threatening words of destruction and death; she believes she is insulted; ... Themes: menacing, violence, homicidal, death, offenses

Al,11- Visions of monsters or animals, that frightened him. Themes: fearful, animal, horrible

Al,12-...Hallucinations (delirium) sees strangers (aliens) in the room. Themes: stranger, invaded

Al,14- Feigned (simulate) paroxysms; a girl simulating fainting and insensibility, looks sideways to watch the effect produced on those around her. (manipulation) Themes: feigning, fit, disease

Al,16- Great taciturnity and irritability; desire to strike himself and others. Themes: hurt, violence

Al,18- Fourteen days after taking the medicine, the happy mood reached the borders of mania; the disposition to joke and laugh was extreme. Themes: pleasure, insanity

Al,2- Insanity on account of an unfortunate love. Themes: insanity, disappointment, union, love, unfortunate

Al,34- Lamentation, with oppressive pain in the heart, as if a misfortune had befallen her. Themes: oppression, misfortune, heart,

Al,35- Weeping, with oppression and pain in the heart, as from misfortune;... Themes: heart, oppression, misfortune

Al,40- Excessive grief, accompanied in the afternoon by thoughts of death. Themes: grief, death

Al,46- Sadness, lamentation, as if a misfortune had befallen him;... Themes: sadness, misfortune

Al,52- Worried (troubled) and greatly vexed (disturbing), with much weeping, as if one could not realize (accomplish, complete) something earnestly (ardently) desired. Themes: succeed, failure

Al,55- Fear, which could not be stopped, in a young lady; questioned about it, she tried to find a cause, and leaves others to think there is one; but really there was none. Themes: fearful, feigning, liar

Al,56- Fear and shaking; the patient cannot find a suitable place where to hide himself; thinks he is going to be assaulted. Themes: escape, robber, hide

Al,57- Fear of getting "typhus fever". Themes: disease, infection

Al,60- Irritable and cross at the least contradiction. Themes: bothered, contradiction

Al,65-...great haste in whatever I undertook, from a constant fear that something would happen to prevent my finishing it;...fear that something would fall on me (doom, disgrace);...fear of striking it against some imaginary object which appeared to be suspended....(hurt) Themes: hurry, misfortune, crushed, obstructed, failure, restless, misfortune, hurt

Al,65-... Great fear of an imaginary impending calamity (cataclysm, catastrophe) great desire of be alone, fear of being alone... Themes: misfortune, solitude, antagonism

Al,76-...changeable mind, tears , singing, and irresoluteness.(In a woman, twenty-six years old, who complained of violent sexual appetite.) Themes: sexual, irresolution, lascivious

He,12- Sudden foxlike destructive efforts, requiring utmost vigilance to prevent damage;... Themes: violence, wild

He,14- Paroxysms of insanity; restlessness of legs; threatening words of destruction and death. Themes: restless, menacing, violence, homicidal

He,15- Suddenly sprang (escape) away from her attendants and swept (clean) ornaments from mantelpiece (an ornamental facing around fireplace); said she was sorry, but could not help it; very mischievous and destructive, ... Themes: escape, conscience, organization, wicked, violence

He,16- Attacks of hystero-mania... hits and abuses everyone, destroys whatever she can lay hold of,...mocks aged people with their old age, ... Themes: offensive, violence, contemptuous

He,2- Great taciturnity and irritability; desire to strike himself and others. Themes: reserved, violence, himself, hurt

He,5- Mental chorea; hyperaemia and hyperesthesia of female sexual organs. Themes: sexual

TAX.

Al,10 -State of profound stupor and helplessness. Themes: helplessness

Al,5- Impatient disposition, which scarcely allows of the least intellectual contest.(discussion) Themes: impatience, discussion

TELL.

Al,2- Her disposition is particularly quiet, being otherwise very lively, anxious and full of care. Themes: restless

Al,3- He forgets and neglects (ignores, indifference) much; also the writing down, and even the observing of symptoms ...when thinking of the one, or of any business, he forgets everything else, and on account of this he neglects much that is necessary. Themes: negligence, duty

He,2- Fear of being touched in sensitive places. Themes: touch

TER.

He,12- Suicide by hanging, in two cases followed washing of laces in oil of turpentine and alcohol. Themes: suicidal

He,14- Fears apoplexy; fullness and pressure in head. Themes: disease

THEA.

Al,10- A most uncomfortable state of nervousness and want of confidence, relieved by beer... Themes: confidence

Al,11- The sound of the "night bell" made me terribly nervous. Themes: time, noise

Al,19- Appeared to be actuated by the greatest terror, and said: "I have called upon you to request you would let me in and allow me to die in your house". Themes: fearful, death, home, helplessness

Al,20- Nocturnal fright; sinister thoughts; invincible propensity to analyze his life, to look at it on the dark side, and to resolve it into its most hopeless realities. Themes: mortification, pessimism, meditation, hopeless

Al,3- Delirium with great ecstasy; the patient laughed incessantly talked constantly in rhyme, showed us that he felt extraordinarily well. Themes: pleasure, talk, poetry

Al,4- Sensation as if impelled by some uncontrollable power to commit suicide, to jump out of window, to put her baby in the boiler with the clothes, to cut its throat while cutting bread, to throw it downstairs (in a woman who kept a pot of tea boiling on the stove and drank several bowlfuls every day; cured with tea cm, Finckle) Themes: seized, suicidal, height, homicidal, pointed, child, fire

THER.

Al,3- Time appears to him to pass more rapidly, although he does very little. Themes: time, succeed

Al,7- Despair; want of confidence; he gives himself up. Themes: despair, confidence, himself

THUJ.

Al,1- She herself desires, with anxiety and despair, to be taken to an insane asylum, (imprisonment, confining) and there to be treated very harshly and strictly, (penalized), so that her fixed ideas may be subdued and banished (purified); she knows very well that she does wrong (conscience) and thinks all sorts of bad thoughts (immoral), but she will not take the trouble to banish such thoughts; therewith she indistinctly gives to understand that she is constantly obliged to think of taking her own life, but feels the sinfulness (wicked) of it, in order to avoid it, desires the strict restraint of the asylum;... Themes: insanity, despair, obstinate, imprisoned, conscience, doomed, religious, suicidal, seized, helplessness, salvation, wrong

Al,10-,...; his whole existence consists of only

extremes, wherewith he is always irresistibly inclined to agreeable (pleasing) exciting, heating drinks, but without intoxication; these happy and exalted reveries constantly increase from day to day, overstepping (exceed) all bounds and becoming a joyful, dizzy intoxication, with entire extinction of reason.(torpid)(ludicrous) Themes: pleasure

Al,11- He often dreamed in a clear day, with open eyes...; in this he especially reveled in a overpowering selfishness, himself the central point about which everything must turn, with an intoxicated feeling of the most joyous self-satisfaction, ... (egotism) Themes: egotism, pleasure

Al,16- The child is excessively obstinate; on the slightest contradiction it throws itself in the ground in rage and loses its breath. Themes: obstinate, contradiction, capricious, anger

Al,2- She fancies that she has intentionally represented herself as insane (feigning) in the presence of others in order to palliate a wrong supposed to have been done (penitence, remorse), and that now she is punished, therefore, by real insanity. Themes: feigning, insanity, conscience, doomed, wrong, penitence

Al,20- Uneasiness of mind for many days, everything seems burdensome and distressing. Themes: bothered

Al,3- She feels and says that she is deranged (insane, disordered) and unfit (unsuitable) to life, as a punishment for a fault (penitence) which she cannot name, ... Themes: unfit, doomed, conscience

Al,34- While talking, she is unable to go on in spite of every effort; she begins to weep bitterly, and says she can no longer think or live. Themes: talk, obstructed, unfit, death

Al,4- She fancies that she has committed a sin.(wrong) Themes: conscience, religious,

Al,49- Sudden rising of dark thoughts (pessimism) causing uneasiness, apprehension (foreboding) of misfortune, with fancied scruples of conscience, ... Themes: dark, misfortune, conscience, pessimism, anticipation

Al,5- She has a decided sensation that her soul is separated from her body (split), and in such a condition hears and feels everything as from distance. Themes: divided, double, separated

Al,51- Remarkable indifference to the opposite sex. (sexual) Themes: indifference, sexual

Al,57- Apprehension of becoming sick. Themes: disease

Al,58- Continual thoughts of dying (death), with increasing weakness. Themes: death, energy

Al,59- Presentiment of death. Themes: anticipation, death

Al,6- She often fancies that someone is sitting near her, with whom she talks aloud while she is lying quite wide awake with open eyes, and wonders when she is asked with whom she is talking, then she does not know what to think of it. (double) Themes: double

Al,62- Averse to everything; anxious and solicitous about the future. Themes: loathing, future

Al,64- Frightful anxiety, like death agony; a nameless internal ache, as if the soul were escaping from the body (split), with most terrible uneasiness, frightful orgasm of blood, at night, even to suffocation. Themes: death, divided, suffocation, blood, double, disintegration

Al,67- Sudden unaccountable (strange) anxiety in the head, which against her will, compels her to call some one. Themes: helplessness, antagonism

Al,7- She constantly longs for the offices of the church in order to banish her sinful thoughts of suicide. (redemption, salvation) Themes: religious, suicidal, penitence, salvation

Al,72- Constant anxiety, as if he had committed a great crime, with forgetfulness and general trembling, even to disturbing sleep. Themes: conscience, criminal,

Al,74- Constant great despair changes at last to complete indifference. Themes: indifference, despair

Al,76- Dread that she would be attacked with apoplexy, ... Themes: fit, disease

Al,8- At night, while lying awake with closed eyes, she seems to see ghosts, and also now and then all kinds of animals brilliantly illuminated, coming from her... Themes: ghosts, bright, animal,

Al,9- While half awake...cannot move a limb (paralyzed), with a sensation as though the whole body were as heavy as lead (heaviness), then she tries to call for help; can utter no sound, and lies with open eyes ... Themes: paralysis, heavy, helplessness,

Al,90- Excited mood; he is irritable, especially if any one says anything of which he does not exactly approve. Themes: contradiction, antagonism

Al,91- Morose, quarrels about a harmless joke. Themes: fight, offenses, discussion

Ha,628- Prolonged thoughtfulness about the merest trifle. Themes: meditation, conscientious

Ha,629- Everything is distasteful (unpleasant) to him; he is anxious and concerned about the future. Themes: future

Ha,630- Walking is performed with extreme ease; she feels as though her body were borne up by wings; she ran many miles in an uncommonly short time, and with unusual high spirits. Themes: floating, travel, fly, energy

He,10- Fixed ideas: as if a strange person were at his side; as if soul and body were separated (split) ; that body, particularly limbs, are made of glass (frail) and will readily break (weakness); as if a living animal were in abdomen ;talks about being under the influence of a superior power. (possessed) Themes: strange, divided, fragile, double, alive, seized, disintegration, greatness, animal

He,12- Insane women will not be touched or approached. Themes: touch, approached

He,13- Nervousness to such a degree that approach of a stranger gave her sudden twitches... Themes: approached, stranger

He,23- Mental depression, after childbirth (puerperal), in consequence of being told that there had been a slight rupture (division, hurt) of perineum; grows quiet; thinks she must die;...wants to jumps the window; does not care for children or her relatives (careless) ;..(sensitive to disrupt, partition) Themes: disintegration, divided, death, suicidal, forsakes, sadness, height, child, relatives, disease

He,27- Extremely scrupulous (conscientious, careful) about small things. Themes: conscientious

He,29- Feels as if she cannot exist any longer; quiet, shunning everybody. Themes: death, doomed, misanthropy

He,9- Sensation as if whole body were thin and delicate, (weak, fragile, frail) and could not resist least attack (illness); as if continuity of body would be dissolved. Themes: fragile, disease, disintegration, ruined

THYR.

Al,N-1-...at times dangerous and homicidal, would put her arms round the necks of other patients so tightly as almost to strangle them (in this case the insanity was primary and the myxedema secondary; both conditions were removed). Evinced increased vivacity by quarreling with another patient about a trifling difference of opinion. Themes: homicidal, violence, fight, contradiction, discussion, energy

Al,N-4-"All progressed cases of myxedema ... delusions ...suspicion, and persecution". Themes: suspicious, persecution

Al,N-5- Delirium of persecution (three cases observed, one fatal, the result of taking Thyro in tablets to reduce obesity). Themes: persecution

TIL.

Al,19- Irritable, critical mood, inclined to quarrel and get angry, even from the slightest difference of opinion. Themes: censorious, fight, anger, contradiction

Al,2- Lovesick (passion, fervor); all his thoughts centered upon an ideal woman; in this revelry he was possessed by a sweet melancholy... Themes: love, perfection, union,

TUB.

Al,N-10- Does not like to be disturbed by people; trembling of hands. Themes: bothered

Al,N-11- Felt positively ugly (repulsive, spiteful); personal aversions became almost a mania. Themes: loathing, ugly, insanity, himself

Al,N-13- Very irritable, want to fight; no hesitancy in throwing anything at anyone, even without cause. Themes: fight, hurt

Al,N-16- Great anxiety for future, otherwise

marked indifference. Themes: future, indifference

Al,N-25- Everything in the room seems strange, as though in a strange place. Themes: strange

Al,N-27- With every little ailment whines and complains; easily frightened, particularly by dogs; screams in terror when approached by a dog. Themes: fearful, approached, animal

Al,N-36- Somnolence; loss of vital power; great physical weakness. (vigor) Themes: energy,

Al,N-38- Soporous, dazed condition; unable to find the right way (lost); is confused; surroundings appear strange. Themes: unfit, lost, strange

Al,N-45- Insanity; acute or chronic, with a family history of tubercular affections. Themes: insanity, infection, disease

Al,N-46- When the best selected remedy fails to relieve or permanently cure in a marked tubercular diathesis, with a tubercular family history. Themes: infection, disease

Al,N-47- Despondent, discouraged, feel as if I would rather die than live. Themes: despair, death

He,2- Fretful (irritable), ailing (sick), whines (moan) and complains; mind given to be frightened (fearful), particularly by dogs. Themes: fearful, animal

UPA.

Al,4- Melancholic; has to force the tears back; cold towards his friends, repelling everyone. Themes: suppressed, indifference, forsakes, friend

UST.

He,2- Very sad, cries frequently; excessively prostrated from sexual abuse and loss of semen; sleep restless. Themes: sadness, sexual, energy

VAC.

He,5- Fear of death; wild excitement and begging (implore) to know if he was to die,... Themes: death, wild

VALER.

Al,1- Extremely delirious, attempting to get out of the window, ... imagined himself away from home, and beset (surrounded) with all sorts of danger, from which he was attempting to escape, although unable to walk without staggering from side to side. Themes: home, suicidal, surrounded, danger, escape

Al,11- Anxious, hypochondriac feeling, as if the objects around him had been estranged from him; the room appears to him desolate (isolated), he does not feel at home in the room, he is impelled to leave it. Themes: strange, solitude, home, unreal, go out, separated, forsaken

Al,12- Fearfulness in the evening when sitting in the dark (imagining that some one might hurt him). Themes: fearful, dark, hurt, attacked

He,11- Feels light as if flying in air. Themes: fly, light, floating

He,4- Erroneous ideas; thinks she is some one else,...; imagines animals lying near her which she fears she may hurt. Themes: animal, hurt, identity, conscientious

He,7- Fear, especially evening in dark,... Themes: dark

VERAT-V.

Al,6- Great fear of death. Themes: death

He,3- From sudden cerebral congestion: quarrelsome delirium; great mental depression and fear of death;... Themes: sadness, death, fight

He,4- Puerperal mania: silent, suspicious; will not see physician, he seems to terrify her; fears being poisoned;... Themes: reserved, suspicious, poisoned

He,6-Loquacity, with exaltation of ideas, or an exalted opinion of her own ideas and powers; everything seems clear to her; now clearly understands former mysterious things; wants no medicine, as that will restore her to former condition;... Themes: greatness, knowledge, suspicious, energy

VERAT.

Al,12- He thinks that he is dumb and blind, and has a cancer. Themes: disease, obstructed

Al,2- Slight delirium; ...he prattles about religious subjects and about vows to be performed, prays, believes that he is not in his own house. Themes: talk, religious, duty, home

Al,23- He groans, is beside himself; does not know what to do with himself. Themes: doubtful

Al,4- He imagines that he is a prince (noble) and behaves in a very haughty manner. (proud, arrogant) Themes: position, greatness, haughty

Al,44- Anxiety as from a bad conscience, as if he had committed a crime. Themes: conscience, criminal

Al,45- Anxiety as if he dread a misfortune, as if some evil were impending. Themes: misfortune, doomed

Al,49- Anxiety with fear of apoplexy during an evacuation of the bowels. Themes: disease

Al,62- He seeks out faults in others and contemplates (examine, inspect) them. (critical) Themes: censorious, wrong, others

Ha,664- Cursing and making a noise all night, and complains of being stupid, with headache and flow of saliva. Themes: offensive, noise, contemptuous, himself

Ha,671- Mania: he alleges that he is a hunter.(pursue) Themes: hunter, identity

Ha,672- He pretends (simulate, feigning) he is a prince, and gives himself airs (affectation, pretentious) accordingly. Themes: greatness, position, feigning, identity, haughty

Ha,673- He asserts (declare) that he is deaf and blind (obstructed) and that he has got cancer. Themes: disease, obstructed, feigning

Ha,674- She asserts that she has labour pains (pregnant).(important?) Themes: feigning, sexual

Ha,675- She boasts (exult, triumph) that she is pregnant. Themes: vanity, greatness, feigning

Ha,676- She announces her imminent confinement. Themes: sexual, feigning

Ha,688- She is inconsolable (unhappy) about an imaginary misfortune, ... Themes: misfortune

Ha,690- Anxiety as from a bad conscience, as if he had done something bad. Themes: conscience, criminal, wrong,

Ha,691- Anxiety as though he anticipated (expected) misfortune, as if threatened with some calamity.(disaster) Themes: menaced, misfortune, anticipation

Ha,692- A feeling in his whole being , as if he must gradually come to an end, but with calmness. (death) Themes: death

Ha,706- He searches for faults in others and taunts (ridicule, mockery) them with them. Themes: wrong, contemptuous, others

Ha,709- He is too lively (energetic), eccentric, extravagant.(wasteful) Themes: energy, strange

Ha,713- Busy restlessness; he undertakes many things, but becomes always tired of them, nothing succeeds with him. Themes: restless, succeed, dispersion

He,1- Is conscious only as in a dream. Themes: unreal

He,10 - Suicidal tendency from religious despair. Themes: religious, suicidal, despair

He,11- Thinks himself distinguished (classify) ; squanders (futile) his money; proud (haughty) of his position. Themes: greatness, squanders, haughty, position, money, vanity

He,13- After severe illness, aversion to husband and children; desire to leave house: hallucinations, room appeared full of people, crowding in, there was no longer room... Themes: loathing, forsakes, invaded, husband, child, go out, home

He,16-... prattles about religious subjects and about vows (promise) to be performed, prays, believes that he is not in his own house. Themes: religious, duty, homesickness, home,

He,19- A woman, ...hopeless despair, ...brought on by sexual excitement. Themes: despair, hopeless, sexual

He,21- Mania; with desire to cut and tear everything, especially clothes; with lewdness and lascivious talk; religious or amorous; de grandeur. Themes: tear, clothes, lascivious, talk, sexual, religious, greatness

He,22- Nymphomania, with violence and destructiveness; had been disappointed in love; melancholia; ...great desire for sexual intercourse; void (empty) of shame; obscenity; .... Themes: sexual, violence, love, union, disappointment, lascivious, wicked, sadness,

He,24- Disposed to silence, or to talk about faults of others; if irritated scolding and calling names. Themes: reserved, talk, censorious, offensive

He,26- Chases (pursue, hunt) his family out of house ; declares the sun travels around the earth (geocentric); fear of death, restlessness, despair... Themes: persecution, egotism, death, home, despair

He,28- Talks much on religious subjects; praying; is overconscientious. Themes: talk, religious, conscientious

He,29-...prays says it is a secret (secretive, mysterious) and a misfortune; ...saying she must strengthen (encourage) herself, ...imagines herself in heaven (elevated, sublime, noble) talking with God. Themes: religious, misfortune, greatness, energy

He,3- Fancies herself pregnant, or that she will be delivered (liberation) soon; that she is in throes (spasms) of childbirth.(labor) Themes: sexual, feigning,

He,4- Erroneous and haughty notions. Themes: haughty, greatness

He,44- Cold sweat on forehead, with anguish and fear of death. Themes: death

He,45-... he is tormented by fearful anxiety, wherewith forehead becomes covered with cold sweat and he becomes sick to vomiting. Themes: tormented, fearful

He,46- Anxiety as from a bad conscience, as if he had committed a crime. Themes: conscience, criminal

He,47- Anxiety as after committing an evil (immoral) deed (act)... Themes: conscience, wicked

VIOL-T.

He,2- Low spirited about domestic affairs. Themes: duty, home

He,5- Very sensitive and inclined to scold. Themes: offensive

VIP.

Al,12- Premonition of death. Themes: clairvoyance, death

YUC.

Al,6- 4 p.m. irresolute, changing mind once in fifteen minutes; don't know what to do; can't keep easy. Themes: irresolution, confidence

ZINC.

Al,24- Anxious mood, as from a misfortune. Themes: misfortune

Al,26- Very uneasy mood, as though he had committed a crime. Themes: conscience, criminal

Ha,11- Fear of thieves or of horrible phantoms, seen while waking as if in a feverish fancy. Themes: robber, ghosts, horrible

Ha,13- Apprehension and ennui; she seeks company. Themes: tedium, company

Ha,15- Tranquil thoughts of dying, in the afternoon, when weary. Themes: fearless, death

Ha,26- He would like to have some one, on whom he might wreak (vent) his (causeless) anger. Themes: anger

Ha,47- Illusion of fancy, when holding down her head, as if she had a large goitre, which prevented her looking beyond it. Themes: disease, obstructed

He,10- Anxiety on account of thieves or horrible apparitions, while awake, like a feverish fancy. Themes: robber, horrible

He,13- Anxious mood as from a misfortune. Themes: misfortune

He,14- Very uneasy mood as if he had committed a crime. Themes: criminal, conscience

He,29-...;sad, weeps frequently; despairs of her recovery;... Themes: disease, sadness, despair

He,43- Great fear, as if persecuted by men or the devil, on account of crimes he has never done (injustice); is afraid of becoming imprisoned, or poisoned, or shot, or buried (inter) alive...0 Delirium tremens. Themes: devil, persecution, criminal, injustice, imprisoned, poisoned, murdered, suffocation, funeral, alive

He,46- ...; believed herself to be called before court (judged) on account of her wicked (immoral) actions; ....;believe the devil is after her;...(persecution) Themes: criminal, persecution, conscience, wicked, justice, devil

He,7- Stares (look) as if frightened on waking, head rolls (turn) from side to side. Themes: fearful

Abelmoschus	abel.
Abies canadensis	abies-c.
Abies nigra	abies-n.
Abroma augusta	abrom-aug.
Abrotanum	abrot.
Abrus precatorius	abr.
Absinthium	absin.
Abuta	abut.
Acalypha indica	acal.
Acanthus mollis	aca-m.
Acetanilidum	acetan.
Aceticum acidum	acet-ac.
Acetonum	aceton
Achyranthes aspera	achy-a.
Achyranthes calea	achy.
Aconitinum	aconin.
Aconitum anthora	acon-a.
Aconitum cammarum	acon-c.
Aconitum ferox	acon-f.
Aconitum lycoctonum	acon-l.
Aconitum napellus	acon.
Aconitum septentrionale	acon-s.
Acorus calamus	acor-c.
Actea spicata	act-sp.
Adamas	adam.
Adansonia digitata	adan.
Adaxukah	adax.
Adelheid aqua	adel.
Adeps suillus	adeps-s
Adlumia fungosa	adlu.
Adonidinum	adonin.
Adonis aestivalis	adon-ae.
Adonis vernalis	adon.
Adoxa moschatellina	adox.
Adrenalinum	adren.
Aegle folia	aegle-f.
Aegle marmelos	aegle.
Aegopodium podagraria	aego-p.
Aesculus carnea	aesc-c.
Aesculus glabra	aesc-g.
Aesculus hippocastanum	aesc.
Aether	aether
Aethiops antimonialis	aethi-a.
Aethiops mineralis	aethi-m.
Aethusa cynapium	aeth.
Aethylum bromidum	aethyl-br.
Aethylum nitricum	aethyl-n.
Aethylum sulphuricum dichloratum	aethyl-s.
Agapanthus orientalis	aga.
Agerati	ager.
Agaricinum	agarin.
Agaricus campanulatus	agar-cpn.
Agaricus campestris	agar-cps.
Agaricus citrinus	agar-cit.
Agaricus emeticus	agar-em.
Agaricus muscarius	agar.
Agaricus pantherinus	agar-pa.
Agaricus phalloides	agar-ph.
Agaricus procerus	agar-pr.
Agaricus semiglobatus	agar-se.
Agaricus stercoranius	agar-st.
Agaricus vernus	agar-v.
Agave americana	agav-a.
Agave tequilana	agav-t.
Agnus castus	agn.
Agraphis nutans	agra.
Agrimonia eupatoria	agr-B.
Agrimonia eupatoria	agri.
Agrostemma githago	agro.
Agrostis alba	agros.
Ailanthus glandulosa	ail.
Alchemilla vulgaris	alch-v.
Alcoholus	alco.
Alcoholus sulphuris	alco-s.
Aldehyde	ald.
Aletris farinosa	alet.
Alfalfa	alf.
Allium cepa	all-c.
Allium sativum	all-s.
Allium ursinum	all-u.
Alloxanum	allox.
Alnus rubra	aln.
Aloe socotrina	aloe
Alpha-dinitrophenol	a-dnphen.
Alpinia officinarum	alpi.
Alstonia constricta	alst-c.
Alstonia scholaris	alst-s.
Althaea officinalis	alth.
Alumen	alumn.
Aluminium aceticum	alum-acet.
Aluminium bromatum	alum-br.
Aluminium metallicum	alum-met.
Aluminium muriaticum	alum-m.
Aluminium oxydata	alum.

Aluminium phosphorica	alum-p.
Aluminium silicata	alum-sil.
Aluminium sulphuricum	alum-s.
Ambra grisea	ambr.
Ambrosia artemisiefolia	ambro.
Ammi visnaga	ammi-v.
Ammoniacum gummi	ammc.
Ammonium aceticum	am-acet.
Ammonium benzoicum	am-be.
Ammonium bromatum	am-br.
Ammonium carbonicum	am-c.
Ammonium causticum	am-caust.
Ammonium fluoratum	am-f.
Ammonium formaldehyde	am-form.
Ammonium iodatum	am-i
Ammonium muriaticum	am-m.
Ammonium nitricum	am-n.
Ammonium phosphoricum	am-p.
Ammonium picricum	am-pic.
Ammonium sulphuricum	am-s.
Ammonium tartaricum	am-t.
Ammonium valerianicum	am-val.
Ammonium vanadinicum	am-van.
Amnii liquor	amn-l.
Amorphophallus rivieri	amor-r.
Ampelopsis quinquefolia	ampe-qu
Ampelopsis trifoliata	ampe-tr.
Amphisbaena vermicularis	amph.
Amygdalae amarae aqua	amyg-am.
Amygdalus persica	amyg-p.
Amylaminum hydrochloricum	amylam.
Amylenum nitrosum	aml-n.
Anacardium occidentale	anac-oc.
Anacardium orientale	anac.
Anagallis arvensis	anag.
Anagyris foetida	anagy.
Anantherum muricatum	anan.
Andersonia rohitika	ander.
Androctonos amurreuxi hebraeus	androc.
Andrographis peniculata	androg-p.
Androsace lactea	andr.
Anemone nemorosa	ane-n.
Anemone ranunculoides	ane-r.
Anemopsis californica	anemps.
Anethum graveolens	anet-g.
Angelica atropurpurea	ange.
Angelica brasiliensis	ange-b.
Angelica sinensis radix	ange-s.
Angophora lanceolata	ango.
Angustura vera	ang.
Anhalonium lewinii	anh.
Anilinum	anil.
Anilinum sulphuricum	anil-s.
Anisum stellatum	anis.
Anthemis cotula	anth-c.
Anthemis nobilis	anth.
Anthoxanthum odoratum	antho.
Anthracinum	anthr.
Anthrokokali	anthro.
Antimonium arsenicosum	ant-ar.
Antimonium crudum	ant-c.
Antimonium fluoratum	ant-f.
Antimonium iodatum	ant-i.
Antimonium metallicum	ant.
Antimonium muriaticum	ant-m.
Antimonium natrum lacticum	ant-n-l.
Antimonium nitricum	ant-n.
Antimonium oxydatum	ant-o.
Antimonium sulphuratum aureum	ant-s.
Antimonium sulphuratum rubrum	ant-s-r.
Antimonium tartaricum	ant-t.
Antipyrinum	antipyrin.
Aorta	aorta
Aphis chenopodii glauci	aphis.
Aphtosinum	aphto.
Apiolum	apiol.
Apis mellifica	apis
Apisinum	apisin.
Apium graveolens	ap-g.
Apocynum androsemifolium	apoc-a.
Apocynum cannabinum	apoc.
Apomorphini hydrochloridum	apom.
Aqua marina	aq-mar.
Aqua petra	aq-pet.
Aqua pura	aq-pu.
Aqua silicata	aq-sil.
Aquila chrysaetos	aqui-c.
Aquilegia vulgaris	aquil.
Aragallus lamberti	arag.
Aralia hispida	aral-h.
Aralia racemosa	aral.
Aranea diadema	aran.
Aranea ixobola	aran-ix.

Aranea scinencia	aran-s.
Arbutinum	arbin.
Arbutus andrachne	arbu.
Areca catechu	arec.
Arenaria rubra	aren-r.
Argemone mexicana	arge.
Argentum bromatum	arg-br.
Argentum carbonicum	arg-c.
Argentum cyanatum	arg-cy.
Argentum fluoratum	arg-f.
Argentum iodatum	arg-i.
Argentum metallicum	arg.
Argentum muriaticum	arg-m.
Argentum nitricum	arg-n.
Argentum oxydatum	arg-o.
Argentum phosphoricum	arg-p.
Argentum sulphuricum	arg-s.
Argomon aulaga	argom.
Argon	argo.
Aristolochia clematitis	arist-cl.
Aristolochia milhomens	arist-m.
Arnica montana	arn.
Arsenal	arsenal
Arsenicum album	ars.
Arsenicum bromatum	ars-br.
Arsenicum hydrogenisatum	ars-h.
Arsenicum iodatum	ars-i.
Arsenicum metallicum	ars-met.
Arsenicum nitricum	ars-n.
Arsenicum sulphuratum flavum	ars-s-f.
Arsenicum sulphuratum rubrum	ars-s-r.
Arsenicum tersulphuratum	ars-t-s.
Artemisia tridentata	art-tri.
Artemisia vulgaris	art-v.
Arteria	arte.
Arum arisarum	arum-a.
Arum dracontium	arum-d.
Arum dracunculus	arum-dru.
Arum italicum	arum-i.
Arum maculatum	arum-m.
Arum triphyllum	arum-t.
Arundo mauritanica	arund.
Asafoetida	asaf.
Asai	asai
Asarum canadense	asar-c.
Asarum europaeum	asar.
Asclepias cornuti	glyc-g.
Asclepias incarnata	asc-i.
Asclepias tuberosa	asc-t.
Asimina triloba	asim.
Askalabotes laevigatus	ask.
Asparagus officinalis	aspar.
Aspen	asp-B.
Aspergilus fumigatus	asperg-f.
Aspergilus niger	asperg-n.
Asperula odorata	asper.
Aspidosperminum	aspin.
Astacus fluviatilis	astac.
Astatinum	asta.
Asterias rubens	aster.
Astragalus exscapus	astra-e.
Astragalus menziesii	astra-me.
Astragalus mollisimus	astra-mo.
Astur cachinnaus	astur
Athamanta cretensis	atha.
Atista indica	atista
Atrax robustus	atra-r.
Atriplex hortensis	atri
Atropinum purum, sulphuricum	atro.
Augopora	aug.
Aurum arsenicicum	aur-ar.
Aurum bromatum	aur-br.
Aurum fluoratum	aur-f.
Aurum fulminans	aur-fu.
Aurum iodatum	aur-i.
Aurum metallicum	aur.
Aurum muriaticum	aur-m.
Aurum muriaticum kalinatum	aur-m-k.
Aurum muriaticum natronatum	aur-m-n.
Aurum nitricum	aur-n.
Aurum phosphoricum	aur-p.
Aurum sulphuratum	aur-s.
Autonosodes	auto.
Avena sativa	aven.
Azadirachta indica	aza.
B.C.G	bcg
Baccharis crista	bacch.
Bacillinum Burnett	bac.
Bacillinum testium	bac-ts.
Bacillus dysenteriae	dys-co.
Bacillus seven	ba-sv.
Bacillus sycoccus by Paterson	syc-co.
Bacillus ten	ba-tn.
Bad Ems	ems
Badiaga	bad.
Baja	baj.

Balnea maritima	baln.
Balsamodendron mukul	balsa.
Balsamum peruvianum	bals-p.
Balsamum toluiferum	bals-t.
Bambusa arundinacea	bamb-a.
Banisteria caapi	bani-c.
Baptisia confusa acetica	bapt-c.
Baptisia tinctoria	bapt.
Barbae cyprini ova	barb.
Barosma crenata	baros.
Bartfelder aqua	bart.
Baryta metallica	bar.
Baryta acetica	bar-acet.
Baryta arsenicosa	bar-ar.
Baryta bromata	bar-br.
Baryta carbonica	bar-c.
Baryta fluorica	bar-f.
Baryta iodata	bar-i.
Baryta muriatica	bar-m.
Baryta nitrica	bar-n.
Baryta oxydatum	bar-o.
Baryta phosphorica	bar-p.
Baryta sulphurica	bar-s.
Baryta silicata	bar-sil.
Beech	beech-B.
Belladonna	bell.
Bellis perennis	bell-p.
Benzinum	benzin.
Benzoicum acidum	benz-ac.
Benzoinum oderiferum	benzo.
Benzolum Benzolum	benz.
Benzolum dinitricum	benz-d.
Benzolum nitricum	benz-n.
Berberinum	berbin.
Berberis aquifolium	berb-a.
Berberis vulgaris	berb.
Beryllium metallicum	beryl.
Beryllium muriaticum	beryl-m.
Beryllium sulphuricum	beryl-s.
Beta vulgaris	beta.
Betainum muriaticum	betin.
Betula alba	betul.
Bismuthum metallicum	bism-met.
Bismuthum subnitricum	bism.
Bitis arietans	biti-a.
Bixa orellana	bix.
Blatta americana	blatta-a.
Blatta orientalis	blatta
Blumia odorata	blum-o.
Boerhavia diffusa	boerh.
Boldo fragrans	bold.
Boletus laricis	bol.
Boletus luridus	bol-lu.
Boletus satanas	bol-s.
Bombyx chrysorrhea	bomb-chr.
Bombyx processionea	bomb-pr.
Bondonneau aqua	bond.
Borago officinalis	borag.
Borax veneta	bor.
Boricum acidum	bor-ac.
Boron metallicum	bor-met.
Boswelia serrata	bos-s.
Bothriocephalus latus	bothr-l.
Bothrops atrox	both-a.
Bothrops lanceolatus	both-l.
Botulinum	botul.
Bovista lycoperdon	bov.
Bowdichea major	bowd.
Brachyglottis repens	brach.
Brahmi	brahmi
Branca ursina	bran.
Brassica napus	brass.
Brassica oleracea	brass-o.
Bromium	brom.
Bromium acidum	brom-ac.
Bromus ramosus	bromu.
Brucea antidysenterica	bruc.
Brucella melitensis	brucel.
Brucinum nitricum	brucin.
Bryonia alba	bry.
Bufo rana	bufo
Bufo sahytiensis Mure	bufo-s.
Bulbinum	bulb.
Bulbocapnin	bulbin.
Bungarus caeruleus	bung-c.
Bungaris fasciatus	bung-f.
Bunias orientalis	buni-o.
Buthus australis	buth-aust.
Butyricum acidum	but-ac.
Buxus sempervirens	bux.
Carbon dioxide	c-di-o.
Cacao	cac.
Cactina	cactin.
Cactus grandiflorus	cact.
Cadmium arsenicosum	cadm-ar.
Cadmium bromatum	cadm-br.

Cadmium fluoricum	cadm-f.
Cadmium iodatum	cadm-i.
Cadmium metallicum	cadm.
Cadmium muriaticum	cadm-m.
Cadmium nitricum	cadm-n.
Cadmium oxidatum	cadm-o.
Cadmium phosphoricum	cadm-p.
Cadmium sulphuratum	cadm-s.
Caela zacatechichi	cael.
Caeruleum iritis solis	caer-i-s.
Caesalpinia bonducella	caesal.
Caesium metallicum aut sulphuricum	caes.
Cahinca racemosa	cahin.
Cajuputum	caj.
Caladium seguinum	calad.
Calaguala	calag.
Calcarea acetica	calc-acet.
Calcarea arsenicosa	calc-ar.
Calcarea bromata	calc-br.
Calcarea calcinata	calc-cal.
Calcarea carbonica Hahnemanni	calc.
Calcarea caustica Segini	calc-caust.
Calcarea chlorinata	calc-chln.
Calcarea fluorata	calc-f.
Calcarea hypophosphorosa	calc-hp.
Calcarea iodata	calc-i.
Calcarea lactica	calc-l.
Calcarea lactica natronata	calc-l-n.
Calcarea lactica phosphorica	calc-l-p.
Calcarea muriatica	calc-m.
Calcarea metallica	calc-met.
Calcarea nitrica	calc-n.
Calcarea ovi testae	calc-o-t.
Calcarea oxalica	calc-ox.
Calcarea phosphorica	calc-p.
Calcarea picrica	calc-pic.
Calcarea silicata	calc-sil.
Calcarea stibiato-sulphurata	calc-st-sula.
Calcarea sulphurica	calc-s.
Calculus bilialis	calcul-b.
Calculus renalis	calcul-r.
Calendula officinalis	calen.
Calliandra houstoni	calli.
Calluna vulgaris	callun.
Calotropis gigantea	calo.
Calotropis lactum	calo-l.
Caltha palustris	calth.
Camphora	camph.
Camphora bromata	camph-br.
Camphoricum acidum	camph-ac.
Canchalagua	canch.
Candida parapsilosis	cand-p.
Canna angustifolia	canna
Cannabis indica	cann-i.
Cannabis sativa	cann-s.
Cantharidinum	canthin.
Cantharis vesicatoria	canth.
Capparis coriacea	capp.
Capsicum annuum	caps.
Carbo animalis	carb-an.
Carbo vegetabilis	carb-v.
Carbolicum acidum	carb-ac.
Carbondioxide	carb-ac.
Carboneum	carbn.
Carboneum chloratum	carbn-chl.
Carboneum hydrogenisatum	carbn-h.
Carboneum oxygenisatum	carbn-o.
Carboneum sulphuratum	carbn-s.
Carcinosinum Burnett	carc.
Cardamine pratense	carda.
Cardiazol	cardz.
Cardiospermum halicacabum	cardi-h.
Carduus benedictus	card-b.
Carduus marianus	card-m.
Carex arenaria	care-a.
Carissa schimperi	cari.
Carlsbad aqua	carl.
Carpinus betulus	carp.
Cartilago suis	cartil-s.
Cartilago	cartil.
Carum carvi	caru.
Carya alba	cary.
Cascarilla	casc.
Cassada	cass.
Cassia alata	cassi-a.
Cassia medica	cassi-m.
Cassia sophera	cassi-s.
Castanea vesca	cast-v.
Castor equi	cast-eq.
Castoreum canadense	cast.
Catalpa bignonioides	catal.
Cataria nepeta	catar.
Catuaba	cat.
Caulophyllum thalictroides	caul.
Causticum Hahnemanni	caust.

Ceanothus americanus	cean.
Ceanothus trysiflorus	cean-tr.
Cecropia mexicana	cecr.
Cecropia palmata	cecr-p.
Cecropia petata	cecr-pe.
Cedron	cedr.
Celtis occidentalis	celt.
Cement	cem.
Cenchris contortrix	cench.
Centaurea tagana	cent.
Centaurium umbellatum	cent-u.
Cephalandra indica	cephd.
Cephalanthus occidentalis	ceph.
Cerato	cer-B.
Cerebellum cortex	cereb-cort.
Cerebellum	cereb.
Cerefolius	ceref.
Cereus bonplandii	cere-b.
Cereus serpentinus	cere-s.
Cerium metallicum	cer.
Cerium oxalicum	cer-ox.
Cervus brasilicus	cerv.
Cetonia	ceto.
Cetraria islandica	cetr.
Chamaedrys	chamae.
Chamomilla vulgaris	cham.
Chaparro amargoso	chap.
Chasmanthera palmata	chasm.
Chaulmoograe	chaul.
Cheiranthus cheiri	cheir.
Chelidoninum	chelin.
Chelidonium glaucum	chel-g.
Chelidonium majus	chel.
Chelone glabra	chelo.
Chenopodium anthelminthicum	chen-a.
Chenopodium vulvaria	chen-v.
Cherry plum	cher-p-B.
Chestnut buds	ch-bd-B.
Chicory	chic-B.
Chimaphila maculata	chim-m.
Chimaphila rotundifolia	chim-rot.
Chimaphila umbellata	chim.
China boliviana	chin-b.
China officinalis	chin.
Chinaria canadensis	chinar.
Chinidinum hydrochloricum	chinid.
Chininum arsenicosum	chin-ar.
Chininum hydrocyanicum	chin-hydr.
Chininum muriaticum	chin-m.
Chininum salicylicum	chin-sal.
Chininum sulphuricum	chin-s.
Chininum valerianicum	chin-val.
Chionanthus virginica	chion.
Chloralum hydratum	chlol.
Chloramphenicolum	chloram.
Chloroformum	chlf.
Chlorophyllum	chlph.
Chlorpromazinum	chlorpr.
Chlorum	chlor.
Chocolate	choc.
Cholesterinum	chol.
Cholinum	cholin.
Cholos terrapina	cho.
Chopheenee	choph.
Chromicum acidum	chr-ac.
Chromium metallicum	chr.
Chromium muriaticum	chr-m.
Chromium oxidatum	chr-o.
Chromium phosphoricum	chr-p.
Chromium sulphuricum	chr-s.
Chrysanthemum leucanthemum	chrysan.
Chrysarobinum	chrysar.
Chrysis	chrysi.
Chrysophanicum acidum	chrys-ac.
Cicer arietinum	cice.
Cichorium intybus	cich.
Cicuta maculata	cic-m.
Cicuta virosa	cic.
Ciguatera	cigua.
Cimex lectularius	cimx.
Cimicifuga racemosa	cimic.
Cina maritima	cina
Cinchoninum sulphuricum	cinch.
Cineraria maritima	cine.
Cinnabaris	cinnb.
Cinnamomum ceylanicum	cinnam.
Cistus canadensis	cist.
Citricum acidum	cit-ac.
Citrus decumana	cit-d.
Citrus limonum	cit-l.
Citrus vulgaris	cit-v.
Cladonia pyxidata	clad-p.
Clematis	clem-B.
Clematis recta	clem.
Clematis virginiana	clem-vir.
Clematis vitalba	clem-vit.

Clerodendron infortunatum	cler-i.
Cobaltum chloridum	cob-chl.
Cobaltum fluoratum	cob-f.
Cobaltum iodatum	cob-i.
Cobaltum metallicum	cob.
Cobaltum muriaticum	cob-m.
Cobaltum nitricum	cob-n.
Cobaltum oxydatum	cob-o.
Cobaltum phosphoricum	cob-p.
Cobaltum silicatum	cob-sil.
Cobaltum sulphuratum	cob-s.
Coca	coca
Cocainum hydrochloricum	cocain.
Coccal co Paterson	coccal
Coccinella septempunctata	cocci-s.
Cocculus indicus	cocc.
Coccus cacti	coc-c.
Cochlearia armoracia	coch.
Cochlearia officinalis	coch-o.
Codeinum purum, phosphoricum, sulphuricum	cod.
Coenzym A	coenz-a.
Coffea cruda	coff.
Coffea tosta	coff-t.
Coffeinum	coffin.
Colchicinum	colchin.
Colchicum autumnale	colch.
Coleus aromaticus	col-a.
Coli by Paterson	mut.
Colibacillinum, anti-colibacillair serum	coli.
Collinsonia canadensis	coll.
Colocynthinum	colocin.
Colocynthis	coloc.
Colon	colon
Colostrum	colos.
Comocladia dentata	com.
Conchiolinum	conch.
Coniinum bromatum	conin-br.
Coniinum pura	conin.
Conium maculatum	con.
Conjunctiva	conj.
Convallaria majalis	conv.
Convolvulus arvensis	convo-a.
Convolvulus duartinus	convo-d.
Convolvulus stans	convo-s.
Copaiva	cop.
Corallium rubrum	cor-r.
Corallorhiza odontorhiza	corh.
Cordia coffeoide	cord.
Coriaria myrtifolia	cori-m.
Coriaria ruscifolia	cori-r.
Cornus alternifolia	corn-a.
Cornus circinata	corn.
Cornus florida	corn-f.
Cornus sericea	corn-s.
Corpus luteum	corp-l.
Corticotropinum	cortico.
Cortisonum	cortiso.
Corydalis cava	cory-c.
Corydalis formosa	cory.
Cosmoline	cosm.
Costus pisonis	cost-p.
Coto bark	coto
Cotyledon umbilicus	cot.
Crab Apple	crb-a-B.
Crassula obliqua	cras-o.
Crataegus oxyacantha	crat.
Cristalinum	cristal.
Crocus sativus	croc.
Crotalus cascavella	crot-c.
Crotalus horridus	crot-h.
Croton campestris	croto-ca.
Croton chloralum	croto-chlol.
Croton tiglium	croto-t.
Cryptopinum	cryp.
Cubeba officinalis	cub.
Cucurbita citrullus	cuc-c.
Cucurbita pepo	cuc-p.
Culex musca	culx.
Cumarinum	cumin.
Cundurango	cund.
Cuphea viscosissima	cuph.
Cupressus australis	cupre-aust.
Cupressus lawsoniana	cupre-l.
Cuprum metallicum	cupr.
Cuprum aceticum	cupr-acet.
Cuprum ammoniae sulphuricum	cupr-am-s.
Cuprum arsenicosum	cupr-ar.
Cuprum carbonicum	cupr-c.
Cuprum cyanatum	cupr-cy.
Cuprum fluoratum	cupr-f.
Cuprum muriaticum	cupr-m.
Cuprum nitricum	cupr-n.
Cuprum oxydatum nigrum	cupr-o.
Cuprum phosphoricum	cupr-p.

Cuprum silicatum	cupr-sil.
Cuprum sulphuricum	cupr-s.
Curare woorari	cur.
Curcuma javanensis	curc.
Cyclamen europaeum	cycl.
Cyclosporine	cyclos.
Cydonia vulgaris	cyd.
Cymarinum	cymin.
Cynara scolymos	cyna.
Cynodon dactylon	cyn-d.
Cynoglossum officinale	cyno.
Cypripedium pubescens	cypr.
Cyrtus	cyrt-p.
Cystinum	cystin.
Cytisinum	cytin.
Cytisus laburnum	cyt-l.
Damiana aphrodisiaca	dam.
Daoboia russelli	dao-r.
Daphne indica	daph.
Datisca cannabina	datis.
Datura arborea	dat-a.
Datura ferox	dat-f.
Datura metel	dat-m.
Datura sanguinea	dat-s.
Daturinum	datin.
Daucus carotis	dauc.
Delphinus amazonicus	del.
Dematium petraeum	dema.
Dendroaspis polytepis	dendro-p.
Dens humane	dens
Derma	derma
Derris pinnata	der.
Desmodium gangeticum	desm-g.
Desmoncus rudentum	des-r.
Desoxyribonucleinicum acidum	des-ac.
Dialium ferrum	dial.
Diaphragma	diaphr.
Dichapetalum Thunbergh	dicha.
Dictamnus albus	dict.
Digitalinum	digin.
Digitalis purpurea	dig.
Digitoxinum	digox.
Dioscorea petrea	dios-p.
Dioscorea villosa	dios.
Dioscorin	diosin.
Diosma lincaris	diosm.
Diphtheria Pertussis Tetanus vaccine	dpt
Diphtherinum	diph.
Diphtherotoxinum	diphtox.
Dipodium punctatum	dip.
Dipsacus silvester	dips-s.
Dirca palustris	dirc.
Discus intervertebrales	disc-i.
Ditainum	ditin.
Dolichos pruriens	dol.
Doryphora decemlineata	dor.
Drosera rotundifolia	dros.
Drymis winteri	drym.
DTTAB	dttab.
Duboisinum	dubin.
Duboisinum sulphuricum	dubin-s.
Dulcamara	dulc.
Duodenum	duod.
Eaux bonnes aqua	eaux
Eberthinum	eberth.
Echinacea angustifolia	echi.
Echinacea purpurea	echi-p.
Echis carinatus	echi-c.
Echites suberecta	echit.
Egg-vaccine	egg-vac.
Eichornia crassipes	eich-c.
Elaeis guineensis	elae.
Elaps corallinus	elaps
Elaterium officinarum	elat.
Electricitas	electr.
Elemuy gauteria	elem.
Elm	elm-B.
Elmen Soolbad	elmen
Embelia ribes	emb.
Embelica officinalis	emb-off.
Embryo suis	embry.
Emetine	emetin.
Enterococcinum	enteroc.
Eosinum	eos.
Ephedra vulgaris	ephe.
Ephedrin	ephin.
Epigea repens	epig.
Epihysterinum	epih.
Epilobium angustifolium	epil-a.
Epilobium palustre	epil.
Epiphegus virginiana	epip.
Equisetum arvense	equis-a.
Equisetum hyemale	equis.
Eranthis hymnalis	eran.
Erechthites hieracifolia	erech.

Ergotinum	ergot.
Erigeron canadensis	erig.
Erinacea species	erin.
Eriodictyon glutinosum	erio.
Erodium cicutarium	erod.
Ervum ervilla	erv.
Eryngium aquaticum	ery-a.
Eryngium maritimum	ery-m.
Erythrinus	eryth.
Erythrophlaeum judiciale	eryt-j.
Eschscholtzia californica	esch.
Eserinum	esin.
Eserinum salicylicum	esin-sal.
Espeletia grandiflora	esp-g.
Ethylicum	ethyl-a.
Eucalyptolum	eucol.
Eucalyptus globulus	eucal.
Eucalyptus tereticortis	eucal-t.
Eugenia jambosa	eug.
Euonyminum	euonin.
Euonymus atropurpurea	euon-a.
Euonymus europea	euon.
Eupatorium aromaticum	eup-a.
Eupatorium cannabinum	eup-c.
Eupatorium dendroides	eup-d.
Eupatorium perfoliatum	eup-per.
Eupatorium purpureum	eup-pur.
Euphorbia amygdaloides	euph-a.
Euphorbia corollata	euph-c.
Euphorbia cyparissias	euph-cy.
Euphorbia herophylla	euph-her.
Euphorbia heterodoxa	euph-he.
Euphorbia hypericifolia	euph-hy.
Euphorbia ipecacuanha	euph-ip.
Euphorbia lathyris	euph-l.
Euphorbia linearis	euph-li.
Euphorbia marginata	euph-m.
Euphorbia peplus	euph-pe.
Euphorbia pilulifera	euph-pi.
Euphorbia polycarpa	euph-po.
Euphorbia prostata	euph-pr.
Euphorbia resinifera	euph.
Euphrasia officinalis	euphr.
Eupionum	eupi.
Eysenhardtia polystachia	eys.
Fabiana imbricata	fab.
Faecalis alcaligenes	faec.
Fagopyrum esculentum	fago.
Fagus silvatica	fagu.
Fatpoison	fat.
Fel tauri	fel.
Feldspar	feld.
Ferrum aceticum	ferr-acet.
Ferrum arsenicosum	ferr-ar.
Ferrum bromatum	ferr-br.
Ferrum carbonicum	ferr-c.
Ferrum citricum	ferr-cit.
Ferrum cyanatum	ferr-cy.
Ferrum fluoratum	ferr-f.
Ferrum iodatum	ferr-i.
Ferrum lacticum	ferr-l.
Ferrum magneticum	ferr-ma.
Ferrum metallicum	ferr.
Ferrum muriaticum	ferr-m.
Ferrum nitricum	ferr-n.
Ferrum oxidatum rubrum	ferr-o-r.
Ferrum phosphoricum	ferr-p.
Ferrum phosphoricum hydricum	ferr-p-h.
Ferrum picricum	ferr-pic.
Ferrum protoxalatum	ferr-prox.
Ferrum pyrophosphoricum	ferr-py.
Ferrum silicatum	ferr-sil.
Ferrum sulphuricum	ferr-s.
Ferrum tartaricum	ferr-t.
Ferrum valerianicum	ferr-val.
Ferula glauca	ferul.
Fibrinum	fibrin.
Ficus carica	fic-c.
Ficus indica	fic-i.
Ficus religiosa	fic.
Ficus venosa	fic-v.
Filix-mas	fil.
Fluor	fl.
Flavus	flav.
Flor de piedra	flor-p.
Fluoformum	fluoform.
Fluoricum acidum	fl-ac.
Foeniculum sativum	foen.
Folliculinum	foll.
Formalinum	formal.
Formica rufa	form.
Formicicum acidum	form-ac.
Fragaria vesca	frag.
Framboesinum	fram.
Franciscaea uniflora	franc.
Franzensbad	franz.

Fraxinus americana	frax.
Fraxinus excelsior	frax-e.
Friedrichhaller aqua	fried.
Fuchsinum	fuch.
Fucus vesiculosus	fuc.
Fuligo ligni	fuli.
Fumaria officinalis	fum.
Funiculus umbilicalis suis	funi-umb.
Furfur iritici	furf-i.
Gadus morrhua	gad.
Gaertner by Bach	gaert.
Galanthus nivalis	gala.
Galega officinalis	galeg.
Galeopsis segetum	galeo.
Galinsoga parviflora	galin.
Galium aparine	gali.
Gallicum acidum	gall-ac.
Gallium fluoratum	gall-f.
Gallium metallicum	gall.
Gallium muriaticum	gall-m.
Gallium oxydatum	gall-o.
Gallium phosphoricum	gall-p.
Gallium sulphuricum	gall-s.
Galphimia glauca	galph.
Galvanismus	galv.
Gambogia	gamb.
Gastein aqua	gast.
Gaultheria procumbens	gaul.
Gelatinum	gelin.
Gelsemium sempervirens	gels.
Gemiasma verdans	gemi.
Genatosan	genat.
Genista tinctoria	genist.
Gentian	gent-B.
Gentiana cruciata	gent-c.
Gentiana lutea	gent-l.
Gentiana quinqueflora	gent-q.
Geoffroya vermifuga	geo.
Geranium maculatum	ger.
Geranium robertianum	ger-r.
Germanium metallicum	germ.
Gettysburg aqua	get.
Geum rivale	geum
Ginkgo biloba	gink.
Ginseng	gins.
Glandula pinealis	pineal.
Glechoma hederacea	glech.
Glonoinum	glon.
Glycerinum	glyc.
Glycyrrhiza glabra	glyc-g.
Gnaphalium polycephalum	gnaph.
Gomprhena officinalis	gomph.
Gonotoxinum	gonotox.
Gorse	gors-B.
Gossypium herbaceum	goss.
Granatum	gran.
Graphites naturalis	graph.
Gratiola officinalis	grat.
Grindelia robusta	grin.
Guaco	gua.
Guaiacolum	guajol.
Guaiacum officinale	guai.
Guaninum	guan.
Guano australis	guano
Guarea trichiloides	guare.
Guatteria gaumeri	guat.
Guipsine	guipsin.
Gunpowder	gunp.
Gymnema sylvestre	gymne.
Gymnocladus canadensis	gymn.
Haematoxylon campechianum	haem.
Haffkine	haff.
Hafnium metallicum	hafn.
Haliaceetus leucocephalus	hali-l.
Hall aqua	hall
Haloperidol	halo.
Hamamelis macrophylla	ham.
Haplopappus baylahuen	hapl-b.
Harpagophytum procumbens	harp.
Heather	heath-B.
Hecla lava	hecla.
Hedeoma pulegioides	hedeo
Hedera helix	hed.
Hedysarum ildefonsianum	hedy.
Heleninum	helin.
Helianthemum species	helia-m.
Helianthus annuus	helia.
Heliotropium peruvianum	helio.
Helium	heli.
Helix tosta	helx.
Helleborus foetidus	hell-f.
Helleborus niger	hell.
Helleborus orientalis	hell-o.
Helleborus viridis	hell-v.
Helmintochortos	helm.
Heloderma horridus	helo.

Helonias dioica	helon.
Hemidesmus indica	hemid.
Hemoglobinum	hemog.
Heuchera americana	heuch.
Hepar sulphuris calcareum	hep.
Hepatica triloba	hepat.
Hepatinum	hepar
Herniaria glabra	hern-g.
Heroinum	herin.
Hieracium pilosella	hier-p.
Hiloropium peruvianum	hilo.
Hippomanes	hipp.
Hippozaeninum	hippoz.
Hippuricum acidum	hip-ac.
Hirudo medicinalis	hir.
Histaminum muriaticum	hist.
Histidinum	histid.
Hoang-Nan	ho.
Hoitzia coccinea	hoit.
Holly	holly-B.
Homarus gammarus	hom.
Homeria collina	home.
Honeysuckle	honey-B.
Hornbeam	horn-B.
Hottonia palustris	hott.
Humea elegans	hume.
Hura brasiliensis	hura
Hura crepitans	hura-c.
Hydrangea arborescens	hydrang.
Hydrastininum muriaticum	hydrin-m.
Hydrastininum sulphuricum	hydrin-s.
Hydrastinum muriaticum	hydr-m.
Hydrastis canadensis	hydr.
Hydrobromicum acidum	hydrobr-ac.
Hydrocotyle asiatica	hydrc.
Hydrocyanicum acidum	hydr-ac.
Hydrogenum	hydrog.
Hydroiodicum acidum	iod-ac.
Hydrophis cyanocinctus	hydro-c.
Hydrophyllum virginianum	hydro-v.
Hymosa	hymosa
Hymenea coubaril	hym-c.
Hyoscinum bromhydricum	hyosin.
Hyoscyamus niger	hyos.
Hypericum perforatum	hyper.
Hypothalamus of the ox	hypoth.
Hyssopus officinalis	hyssop.
Iaspis	ias.
Iberis amara	iber.
Ichthyolum	ichth.
Ictodes foetida	ictod.
Ignatia amara	ign.
Ilex aquifolium	ilx-a.
Ilex casseine	ilx-c.
Ilex vomitoria	ilx-v.
Illecebrum	illec.
Immunoglobulin A	ig-a.
Impatiens	imp-B.
Imperatoria ostruthium	imp.
Incajea	inca.
Indigo tinctoria	indg.
Indium metallicum	ind.
Indolum	indol.
Influenzinum	influ.
Ingluvinum	ingluv.
Insulinum	insulin
Interleukin	il-two
Inula helenium	inul.
Iodoformum	iodof.
Iodothyrinum, thryroiodinum	iodot.
Iodium acidum	iod-ac.
Iodium purum	iod.
Ipecacuanha	ip.
Ipomoea purpurea	ipom.
Ira terror	ira
Iridium metallicum	irid.
Iridium muriaticum	irid-m.
Iris factissima	iris-fa.
Iris florentina	iris-fl.
Iris foetidissima	iris-foe.
Iris germanica	iris-g.
Iris pseudacorus	iris-ps.
Iris tenax	iris-t.
Iris versicolor	iris
Irisinum	irisin.
Isoleucinum	i-leuc.
Itu	itu
Jaborandi	jab.
Jacaranda caroba	jac-c.
Jacaranda gualandai	jac.
Jalapa	jal.
Jasminum officinale	jasm.
Jatropha curcas	jatr.
Jatropha urens	jatr-u.
Jatzfeld	jatz.
Jequiritolum	jeqol.

Joanesia asoca	joan.
Juglandinum	juglin.
Juglans cinerea	jug-c.
Juglans regia	jug-r.
Juncus effusus	junc.
Juncus pilosus	junc-p.
Juniperus brasiliensis	juni-b.
Juniperus communis	juni-c.
Juniperus virginianus	juni.
Justicia adhatoda	just.
Justicia rubrum	just-r.
Kalamegh	kalam.
Kali aceticum	kali-acet.
Kali arsenicosum	kali-ar.
Kali bichromicum	kali-bi.
Kali bitartaricum	kali-bit.
Kali bromatum	kali-br.
Kali carbonicum	kali-c.
Kali chloricum	kali-chl.
Kali chlorosum	kali-chls.
Kali chromicum	kali-chr.
Kali citricum	kali-cit.
Kali cyanatum	kali-cy.
Kali ferrocyanatum	kali-fcy.
Kali fluoricum	kali-f.
Kali hypophosphoricum	kali-hp.
Kali iodatum	kali-i.
Kali lacticum	kali-l.
Kali manganicum	kali-ma.
Kali metallicum	kali.
Kali muriaticum	kali-m.
Kali nitricum	kali-n.
Kali oxalicum	kali-ox.
Kali oxydatum	kali-o.
Kali phosphoricum	kali-p.
Kali picricum	kali-pic.
Kali picronitricum	kali-picn.
Kali salicylicum	kali-sal.
Kali silicicum	kali-sil.
Kali sulphuratum	kali-sula.
Kali sulphuricum	kali-s.
Kali sulphuricum chromicum	kali-s-chr.
Kali tartaricum	kali-t.
Kali telluricum	kali-tel.
Kali xanthogenicum	kali-x.
Kalmia latifolia	kalm.
Kamala	kam.
Kaolinum	kaol.
Karaka	kara.
Karwinskia humboldtiana	karw-h.
Kerosenum	kerose.
Kerosolenum	keroso.
Ketoglutaricum acidum	keto-ac.
Kissingen aqua	kiss.
Knautia arvensis	knau.
Kola	kola.
Kosen Soolbad	kosen
Kousso	kou.
Kreosotum	kreos.
Kresolum	kres.
Kronthal aqua	kron.
Krypton	kryp.
Kurchi	kurch.
Labyrinthum	labyr.
Lac caninum	lac-c.
Lac delphinum	lac-del.
Lac equis	lac-eq.
Lac felinum	lac-f.
Lac humanum	lac-h.
Lac leonis	lac-leo.
Lac ursinum	lac-urs.
Lac vaccini flos	lac-v-f.
Lac vaccinum	lac-v.
Lac vaccinum butyricum	lac-v-b.
Lac vaccinum coagulatum	lac-v-c.
Lac vaccinum defloratum	lac-d.
Lacerta agilis	lacer.
Lachesis muta	lach.
Lachnanthes tinctoria	lachn.
Lacticum acidum	lac-ac.
Lactuca elongata	lact-e.
Lactuca sativa	lact-s.
Lactuca virosa	lact.
Laetril	laetr.
Lager beer	lager
Laminaria digitata	lamin.
Lamium album	lam.
Landeck aqua	land.
Langebrunnen aqua	lang.
Lanolinum	lanol.
Lanthanum metallicum	lant.
Lanthanum nitricum	lant-n.
Lanthanum oxydatum	lant-o.
Lanthanum sulphuricum	lant-s.
Lapathum acutum	lapa.
Lapis albus	lap-a.

Lappa arctium	lappa
Lapsana communis	laps.
Larch	lar-b.
Lathyrus sativus	lath.
Latrodectus hasellti	lat-h.
Latrodectus katipo	lat-k.
Latrodectus mactans	lat-m.
Laurocerasus officinalis	laur.
Lavandula vera	lav-v.
Lecithinum	lec.
Ledum palustre	led.
Lemna minor	lem-m.
Lens culinaris	len-c.
Leonurus cardiaca	leon.
Lepidium bonariense	lepi.
Leprominium	lepro.
Leptandra virginica	lept.
Leptolobium elegans	leptol.
Leptospira	leptos.
Lespedeza capitata	lesp-c.
Lespedeza sieboldii	lesp-s.
Leucas aspera	leuc-a.
Leucinum	l-leuc.
Levico aqua	lev.
Levisticum officinale	levi-o.
Levomepromazine	levo.
Liatris spicata	liatr.
Ligustrum vulgaris	lig-v.
Lilium superbum	lil-s.
Lilium tigrinum	lil-t.
Limulus cyclops	lim.
Linaria vulgaris	lina.
Linum catharticum	linu-c.
Linum usitatissimum	linu-u
Lippia mexicana	lip.
Lippspringe aqua	lipp.
Lithium benzoicum	lith-be.
Lithium bromatum	lith-br.
Lithium carbonicum	lith-c.
Lithium chloricum	lith-chl.
Lithium iodatum	lith-i.
Lithium lacticum	lith-l.
Lithium metallicum	lith.
Lithium muriaticum	lith-m.
Lithium phosphoricum	lith-p.
Lithium salicylicum	lith-sal.
Lithium sulphuricum	lith-s.
Loasa tricolor	loa.
Lobelia cardinalis	lob-c.
Lobelia dortmanna	lob-d.
Lobelia erinus	lob-e.
Lobelia inflata	lob.
Lobelia purpurescens	lob-p.
Lobelia syphilitica	lob-s.
Lobelinum	lobin.
Lolium temulentum	lol.
Lonicera caprifolium	lon-c.
Lonicera periclymenum	lon-p.
Lonicera xylosteum	lon-x.
Luffa actangula	luf-act.
Luffa amara	luf-a.
Luffa bindal	luf-b.
Luffa operculata	luf-op.
Luna	luna
Lupulinum	lupin.
Lupulus humulus	lup.
Luteinum	lutein.
Lycopersicum esculentum	lycpr.
Lycopodium clavatum	lyc.
Lycopus virginicus	lycps.
Lymphatica	lymph.
Lysidinum	lysid.
Lysimachia nummularia	lysim.
Lyssinum	lyss.
Lythrum salicaria	lythr-s.
Macrotinum	macrin.
Macrozamia spiralis	macroz.
Magnesia acetica	mag-acet.
Magnesia borocitrica	mag-bcit.
Magnesia bromata	mag-br.
Magnesia carbonica	mag-c.
Magnesia fluorata	mag-f.
Magnesia iodata	mag-i.
Magnesia lactica	mag-l.
Magnesia metallica	mag.
Magnesia muriatica	mag-m.
Magnesia nitricum	mag-n.
Magnesia oxydatum	mag-o.
Magnesia phosphorica	mag-p.
Magnesia silicata	mag-sil.
Magnesia sulphurica	mag-s.
Magnesia usta	mag-u.
Magnetis artificialis	m-art.
Magnetis poli ambo	m-p-a.
Magnetis polus arcticus	m-arct.
Magnetis polus australis	m-aust.

Magnolia glauca	magn-gl.
Magnolia grandiflora	magn-gr.
Makaradhwaja	maka.
Malaiatoxinum	malatox.
Malandrinum	maland.
Malaria officinalis	malar.
Malt	malt
Malus pumila	mal-p.
Malva sylvestris	malv.
Malvine	malvin.
Mamma glandula	mamm.
Mancinella venenata	manc.
Mandragora officinarum	mand.
Manganum colloidale	mang-coll
Manganum iodatum	mang-i.
Manganum lacticum	mang-l.
Manganum metallicum	mang-met.
Manganum muriaticum	mang-m.
Manganum oxydatum nativum	mang-o.
Manganum phosphoricum	mang-p.
Manganum sulphuricum	mang-s.
Mangifera indica	mangi.
Mannitol	mannit.
Mantis religiosa	mant-r.
Manzanita	manz.
Marienbader Kruzbunner	marien.
Marrubium album	marr.
Mate	mate
Matico	mati.
Matricaria discoidea	matr-d.
Matthiola graeca	matth.
Meconinum	mec.
Medorrhinum	med.
Medulla ossea	medul-o.
Medulla spinalis	medul-s.
Medusa	medus.
Meinberg Pyrmont aqua	mein.
Mel cum sale	mel-c-s.
Mel	mel
Melaleuca hypericifolia	melal.
Melastoma ackermani	mela.
Melilotus alba	meli-a.
Melilotus officinalis	meli.
Melissa officinalis	melis.
Melitagrinum	melit.
Meloe majalis	meloe
Meningococcinum	meningoc.
Menispermum canadense	menis.

Mentha piperita	menth.
Mentha pulegium	menth-pu.
Mentha viridis	menth-v.
Mentholum	menthol
Menyanthes trifoliata	meny.
Mephitis putorius	meph.
Mercurialis perennis	merl.
Mercurius aceticus	merc-acet.
Mercurius auratus	merc-aur.
Mercurius biniodatus cum kali iodatum	merc-k-i.
Mercurius bromatus	merc-br.
Mercurius corrosivus	merc-c.
Mercurius cyanatus	merc-cy.
Mercurius dulcis	merc-d.
Mercurius fluoratus	merc-f.
Mercurius iodatus flavus	merc-i-f.
Mercurius iodatus ruber	merc-i-r.
Mercurius methylenus	merc-meth.
Mercurius nitrosus	merc-n.
Mercurius phosphoricus	merc-p.
Mercurius praecipitatus albus	merc-pr-a.
Mercurius praecipitatus flavus	merc-pr-f.
Mercurius praecipitatus ruber	merc-pr-r.
Mercurius rhodanatus	merc-r.
Mercurius solubilis Hahnemanni	merc.
Mercurius sulphocyanatus	merc-s-cy.
Mercurius sulphuricus	merc-s.
Mercurius tannicus	merc-tn.
Mesembrianthemum cristallinum	mese-c.
Methioninum	methion.
Methylenum bichloratum	methyl-chl.
Methylenum coeruleum	methyl.
Methylenum salicylicum	methyl-sal.
Methylium aethyloaethereum	meth-ae-ae.
Methysergidum	methys.
Mezereum	mez.
Mica	mica
Micromeria douglasii	micr.
Mikania setigera	mika.
Millefolium	mill.
Mimosa humilis	mim-h.
Mimosa pudica	mim-p.
Mimulus	mimul-b.
Mimulus	mimul.
Mimulus luteus	mimul-l.

Mississquoi aqua	miss.	Naphtha	napht.
Mitchella repens	mit.	Naphthalinum	naphtin.
Molybdaenum metallicum	moly.	Narceinum	narcin.
Molybdaenum muriaticum	moly-m.	Narcissus poeticus	narc-po.
Momordica balsamica	mom-b.	Narcissus pseudonarcissus	narc-ps.
Momordica charantia	mom-ch.	Narcotinum aceticum	narcot-acet.
Momordica purgans	mom-p.	Narcotinum muriaticum	narcot-m.
Monilia albicans	moni.	Narcotinum pura	narcot.
Monotropa uniflora	mono.	Narzan aqua	narz.
Monsonia ovata	mons.	Nasturtium aquaticum	nast.
Monstera pertusa	monst.	Natrum aceticum	nat-acet.
Morbillinum	morbill.	Natrum aethylosulphuricum	nat-ae-s.
Morgan Gaertner	morg-g.	Natrum arsenicum	nat-ar.
Morgan pure by Paterson	morg.	Natrum arsenicum gaertner	nat-a-g.
Morphinum aceticum	morph.	Natrum bicarbonicum	nat-bic.
Morphinum muriaticum	morph-m.	Natrum bromatum	nat-br.
Morphinum sulphuricum	morph-s.	Natrum cacodylicum	nat-cac.
Morus nigra	mor-n.	Natrum carbonicum	nat-c.
Moschus moschiferus	mosch.	Natrum causticum	nat-caust.
Mucob.	Mucobacter	Natrum choleinicum	nat-ch.
Mucobacter	Mucob.	Natrum fluoratum	nat-f.
Mucor mucedo	mucor	Natrum hypochlorosum	nat-h.
Mucosa nasalis	muc-nas.	Natrum hyposulphuricum	nat-hchls.
Mucotoxinum	mucot.	Natrum hyposulphurosum	nat-hsulo.
Mucuna urens	muc-u.	Natrum iodatum	nat-i.
Murex purpurea	murx.	Natrum lacticum	nat-l.
Muriaticum acidum	mur-ac.	Natrum metallicum	nat.
Murure leite	muru.	Natrum muriaticum	nat-m.
Musa sapientum	musa	Natrum marinum	nat-mar.
Musanna	musan.	Natrum nitricum	nat-n.
Muscarinum	muscin.	Natrum nitrosum	nat-ns.
Mustard	must-B.	Natrum oxydatum	nat-o.
Mutabile	mut.	Natrum oxalaceticum	nat-ox.
Mygale lasiodora	mygal.	Natrum phosphoricum	nat-p.
Myocardium	myocard.	Natrum salicylicum	nat-sal.
Myosotis arvensis	myos-a.	Natrum selenicum	nat-sel.
Myosotis symphytifolia	myos.	Natrum silicicum	nat-sil.
Myrica cerifera	myric.	Natrum silicofluoricum	nat-sil-f.
Myricin	myrin.	Natrum succinicum	nat-suc.
Myristica sebifera	myris.	Natrum sulphocarbolicum	nat-s-c.
Myrrha	myrrh.	Natrum sulphuratum	nat-sula.
Myrtus cheken	myrt-ch.	Natrum sulphuricum	nat-s.
Myrtus communis	myrt-c.	Natrum sulphurosum	nat-sulo.
Myrtus pimenta	myrt-p.	Natrum taurocholicum	nat-taur.
Norleucinum	n-leuc.	Natrum telluricum	nat-tel.
Nabalus serpentaria	nabal.	Natrum uricum	nat-uric.
Naja tripudians	naja	Naxolone	nax.
Napellin	napin.	Nectandra amare	nect.

Nectrianinum	nectrin.
Negundium americanum	neg.
Nelubrium luteum	nelu.
Neon	neon
Nepenthes distillatoria	nep.
Nepeta cataria	nepet.
Nerium odorum	neri-o.
Nervus auditorius	nerv-au.
Neurinum	neur.
Niccolum bromatum	nicc-br.
Niccolum carbonicum	nicc.
Niccolum fluoratum	nicc-f.
Niccolum oxydatum	nicc-o.
Niccolum silicatum	nicc-sil.
Niccolum sulphuricum	nicc-s.
Nicotinamide adenine dinucleotide	nad
Nicotinum	nicot.
Nidus edulis	nid.
Nigella damascena	nig-d.
Nigella sativa	nig-s.
Niobium metallicum	niob.
Niobium muriaticum	niob-m.
Nitri spiritus dulcis	nit-s-d.
Nitricum acidum	nit-ac.
Nitro benzenum	nitro-benz.
Nitrogenum oxygenatum	nitro-o.
Nitrogenum purum	nitro.
Nitromuriaticum acidum	nit-m-ac.
Notechis scutatus	note-s.
Nuphar luteum	nuph.
Nux absurda	nux-a.
Nux moschata	nux-m.
Nux vomica	nux-v.
Nyctanthes arbor-tristis	nyct.
Nycterinia capensis	nycte.
Nymphaea alba	nym-a.
Nymphaea odorata	nym.
Oak	oak-B.
Ocimum basilicum	oci-b.
Ocimum canum	oci.
Ocimum caryophyllatum	oci-c.
Ocimum gratissimum	oci-g.
Ocimum sanctum	oci-s.
Oenanthe crocata	oena.
Oenothera biennis	oeno.
Oestrus cameli	oest.
Okoubaka aubrevillei	okou.
Oldenlandia herbacia	old-h.
Olea europea	olea
Oleander	olnd.
Oleum animale aethereum Dippeli	ol-an.
Oleum caryophyllatum	ol-car.
Oleum jecoris aselli	ol-j.
Oleum jofar	ol-jo.
Oleum myristicae	ol-myr.
Oleum patchouli	ol-p.
Oleum santali	ol-sant.
Oleum succinum	ol-suc.
Olive	oliv-B.
Oniscus asellus	onis.
Ononis spinosa	onon.
Onopordon acanthium	onop.
Onosmodium virginianum	onos.
Operculina turpethum	oper.
Opium	op.
Oplia farinosa	opl.
Opuntia alba spina	opun-a.
Opuntia vulgaris	opun-v.
Orchitinum	orch.
Oreodaphne californica	oreo.
Origanum majorana	orig.
Origanum vulgare	orig-v.
Ornithogalum umbellatum	orni.
Oroticum acidum	oro-ac.
Orthosiphon stamineus	orthos.
Os	oste.
Oscillococcinum	oscilloc.
Osmium metallicum	osm.
Osteo Arthritic Nosode	o-a-n.
Ostrya virginiana	ost.
Ouabainum	ouabin.
Ovarium	ovar.
Ovi gallinae pellicula	ovi-g-p.
Ovininum	ov.
Oxalicum acidum	ox-ac.
Oxalis acetosella	oxal.
Oxydendron arboreum	oxyd.
Oxygenium	oxyg.
Oxytropis lamberti	oxyt.
Oxyuranus microlepidotus	oxyu-m.
Oxyuranus scuttellatus	oxyu-s.
Ozonum	ozone
Paeonia officinalis	paeon.
Palladium fluoratum	pall-f.

Palladium metallicum	pall.
Palladium muriaticum	pall-m.
Palladium oxydatum	pall-o.
Paloondo	palo.
Panacea arvensis	pana.
Pancreatinum	pancreat.
Papaver rhoeas	pap-r.
Papaverinum	papin.
Papaya vulgaris	pap-v.
Paraffinum	paraf.
Paraphenylene diamine	paraph.
Parathion	paron.
Parathyreoid glands	parath.
Parathyreoidinum	parathyr.
Paratyphoidinum B	parat.
Pareira brava	pareir.
Parietaria officinalis	pariet.
Paris quadrifolia	par.
Paronichia illecebrum	paro-i.
Parotidinum	parot.
Parthenium hysterophorus	parth.
Passiflora incarnata	passi.
Pastinaca sativa	past.
Paullinia pinnata	paull-p.
Paullinia sorbilis	paull.
Pecten jacobaeus	pect.
Pedicularis canadensis	pedi-can.
Pediculus capitis	ped.
Peganum harmala	peg-h.
Pelargonium reniforme	pelarg.
Pellitierinum	pellin.
Penicillinum	penic.
Penthorum sedoides	pen.
Pepsinum	pep.
Perhexiline	perh.
Periploca graeca	peri.
Pernus canaliculus	pern-c.
Persea americana	pers.
Pertussinum	per.
Pestinum	pest.
Petiveria tetrandra	peti.
Petroleum	petr.
Petroselinum sativum	petros.
Phallus impudicus	phal.
Phaseolus nanus	phase.
Phellandrium aquaticum	phel.
Phenacetinum	phenac.
Phenobarbitalum	phenob.

Phenylalaninum D-phenylalaninum	d-phenyl.
Phenylalaninum L-phenylalaninum	l-phenyl.
Phleum pratense	phle.
Phlorizinum	phlor.
Phosphoricum acidum	ph-ac.
Phosphorus hydrogenatus	phos-h.
Phosphorus muriaticus	phos-pchl.
Phosphorus Phosphorus	phos.
Phosphorus triiodatus	phos-i.
Physalia physalis	physala-p.
Physalis alkekengi	physal.
Physostigma venenosum	phys.
Phytolacca berry	phyt-b.
Phytolacca decandra	phyt.
Picea excelsa	pice-e.
Picricum acidum	pic-ac.
Picrotoxicum acidum	pictx-ac.
Picrotoxinum	picro.
Pilocarpinum hydrochloricum	piloc.
Pimenta officinalis	pime.
Pimpinella anisum	pimp-a.
Pimpinella saxifraga	pimp.
Pine	pine-B.
Pineal gland	pineal.
Pinus cupressus	pin-c.
Pinus lambertiana	pin-l.
Pinus sylvestris	pin-s.
Piper methysticum	pip-m.
Piper nigrum	pip-n.
Piperazinum	pipe.
Piscidia erythrina	pisc.
Pituitaria glandula	pitu-gl.
Pituitaria glandula anterior	pitu-a.
Pituitaria glandula posterior	pitu-p.
Pix liquida	pix.
Placenta suis	plac-s.
Placenta humana	plac.
Plantago major	plan.
Plantago minor	plan-m.
Platanus occidentalis	platan.
Platinum fluoratum	plat-f.
Platinum metallicum	plat.
Platinum muriaticum	plat-m.
Platinum muriaticum natronatum	plat-m-n.
Plectranthus fruticosus	plect.

Plumbago europaeus	plumbg-eu.
Plumbago littoralis	plumbg.
Plumbum metallicum	plb.
Plumbum aceticum	plb-acet.
Plumbum tetraethylicum	plb-ae.
Plumbum arsenicosum	plb-ar.
Plumbum chromicum	plb-chr.
Plumbum fluoratum	plb-f.
Plumbum iodatum	plb-i.
Plumbum muriaticum	plb-m.
Plumbum nitricum	plb-n.
Plumbum oxidatum	plb-o.
Plumbum phosphoricum	plb-p.
Plumbum sulphuricum	plb-s.
Plumeria celinus	plume.
Plutonium nitricum	plut-n.
Pneumococcus	pneu.
Podophyllin	podin.
Podophyllum peltatum	podo.
Pollantinum	poll.
Polonium metallicum	polo.
Polyandra poligama	polya.
Polygala amara	poly-a.
Polygonatum officinale	polygo-o.
Polygonum aviculare	polyg-a.
Polygonum hydropiperoides	polyg.
Polygonum persicaria	polyg-pe.
Polygonum sagittatum	polyg-s.
Polymnia uvedalia	polym.
Polypodium vulgare	pol-v.
Polyporus nigricans	polyp-n.
Polyporus pinicola	polyp-p
Polytrichum juniperinum	polytr.
Populus candicans	pop-c.
Populus tremuloides	pop.
Potentilla anserina	pot-a.
Potentilla aurea	pot-au.
Potentilla reptans	pot-r.
Potentilla tormentilla	pot-t.
Prenanthes serpens	pren.
Primula farinosa	prim-f.
Primula obconica	prim-o.
Primula veris	prim-v.
Primula vulgaris	prim-vul.
Prinos verticillatus	prin.
Prolina	prol.
Propanolol	propol.
Propolis	propo.
Propylaminum	prop.
Prostatinum	prost.
Proteus	prot.
Prunella vulgaris	prune.
Prunus cerasus	prun-c.
Prunus domestica	prun-d.
Prunus mahaleb	prun-m.
Prunus padus e cortice	prun-p.
Prunus spinosa	prun.
Prunus virginiana	prun-v.
Psilocybe caerulescens	psil.
Psoralea bituminosa	psoral.
Psoralea corylifolia	psoral-c.
Psorinum	psor.
Ptelea trifoliata	ptel.
Ptychopetalum olacoides	ptych-o.
Pulex irritans	pulx.
Pullus gallinaceus	pull-g.
Pulmo anaphylacticus	pulm-a.
Pulmo pura	pulm.
Pulmo vulpis	pulm-v.
Pulmonaria officinalis	pul-o.
Pulsatilla nigricans	puls.
Pulsatilla nuttalliana	puls-n
Pyrarara	pyrar.
Pyrethrum officinarum	pyre-o.
Pyrethrum parthenium	pyre-p.
Pyrethrum roseum e floribus	pyre-r.
Pyrola rotundifolia	pyro-r.
Pyrogenium	pyrog.
Pyrola rotundifolia	pyrol.
Pyrolignosum acidum	pyro-ac.
Pyrus americanus	pyrus
Pyrus malus	pyrus-m.
Quassia amara	quas.
Quebracho	queb.
Quercus e glandibus	querc.
Quillaya saponaria	quill.
Radium bromatum	rad-br.
Radon	rado.
Rajania subsamarata	raja-s.
Ranunculus acris	ran-a.
Ranunculus bulbosus	ran-b.
Ranunculus ficaria	ran-fi.
Ranunculus flammula	ran-fl.
Ranunculus glacialis	ran-g.
Ranunculus repens	ran-r.
Ranunculus sceleratus	ran-s.

Raphanistrum arvense	raphani.	Ruthenium metallicum	ruth.
Raphanus sativus	raph.	Ruthenium muriaticum	ruth-m.
Ratanhia peruviana	rat.	Sabadilla officinalis	sabad.
Rauwolfia serpentina	rauw.	Sabal serrulata	sabal.
Red Chestnut	rd-ch-B.	Sabatia angularis	saba.
Reinerz aqua	rein.	Sabina officinalis	sabin.
Ren	ren	Sacharinum	sacchin.
Rescue remedy	resc-B.	Sacharum lactis	sac-l.
Reserpine	reser.	Sacharum officinale	sac-alb.
Resorcinum	res.	Sal marinum	sal-mar.
Retina	ret.	Salamandra lacerta	salam-l.
Rhamnus californica	rham-cal.	Salamandra maculosa	salam.
Rhamnus cathartica	rham-cath.	Salicinum	salin.
Rhamnus frangula	rham-f.	Salicylicum acidum	sal-ac.
Rhamnus purshiana	rham-p.	Salix alba	salx-a.
Rhenium metallicum	rhen.	Salix mollissima	salx-m.
Rheum palmatum	rheum	Salix nigra	salx-n.
Rhodium metallicum	rhodi.	Salix purpurea	salx-p.
Rhodium oxydatum nitricum	rhodi-o-n.	Salix vitellina	salx-v.
Rhododendron chrysanthum	rhod.	Salol	salol.
Rhus aromatica	rhus-a.	Salvia officinalis	salv.
Rhus cotinus	rhus-c.	Salvia sclarea	salv-sc.
Rhus diversiloba	rhus-d.	Samarsite	samars.
Rhus glabra	rhus-g.	Sambucus canadensis	samb-c.
Rhus laurina	rhus-l.	Sambucus ebulus	samb-e.
Rhus toxicodendron	rhus-t.	Sambucus nigra	samb.
Rhus venenata	rhus-v.	Sanguinaria canadensis	sang.
Ribes nigrum	ribs-n.	Sanguinarinum nitricum	sanguin-n.
Ribonucleinicum acidum	rib-ac.	Sanguinarinum pura	sanguin.
Ricinus communis	ric.	Sanguinarinum tartaricum	sanguin-t.
Rizophora mangle	rizo.	Sanguisorba officinalis	sanguis.
Robinia pseudacacia	rob.	Sanicula aqua	sanic.
Rock rose	rck-r-B.	Sanicula europaea	sani-eu.
Rock water	rck-w-B.	Santalum album	santa.
Rosa canina	ros-ca.	Santoninum	sant.
Rosa centifolia	ros-ce.	Sap soda	sap-sod.
Rosa damascena	ros-d.	Saponaria officinalis	sapo.
Rosmarinus officinalis	rosm.	Saponinum	sapin.
Rubia tinctorum	rub-t.	Sarcolacticum acidum	sarcol-ac.
Rubidium metallicum	rubi.	Sarothamnus scoparius	saroth.
Rubidium muriaticum	rubi-m.	Sarracenia purpurea	sarr.
Rubus chamaemorus	rubu-ch.	Sarsaparilla officinalis	sars.
Rubus fructicosus	rubu-f.	Sassafras officinalis	sass.
Rubus villosus	rubu.	Satureja hortensis	sat-h.
Rumex acetosa	rumx-a.	Saururus cernuus	saur.
Rumex crispus	rumx.	Saxifraga granulata	saxi-g.
Russula foetens	russ.	Saxonite	saxon.
Ruta graveolens	ruta	Scabiosa succisa	scab-s.

Scammonium	scam.
Scandium metallicum	scan.
Scarlatininum	scarl.
Schinus molle	schin.
Scirrhinum	scirr.
Scleranthus	scler-B.
Scleranthus annuus	scler-a.
Scolopendra morsitans	scol.
Scolopendrium vulgare	scolo-v.
Scopolia carniolica	scopo.
Scorpio italicus	scorp.
Scrophularia nodosa	scroph-n.
Scutellaria laterifolia	scut.
Secale cornutum	sec.
Secretinum	secret.
Sedinha	sedi.
Sedum acre	sed-ac.
Sedum repens	sed-r.
Sedum telephium	sed-t.
Selaginella species	sela.
Selenium	sel.
Semen tiglii	sem-t.
Sempervivum tectorum	semp.
Senecinum	senecin.
Senecio aureus	senec.
Senecio jacoboea	senec-j.
Senega officinalis	seneg.
Senna	senn.
Sepia succus	sep.
Sepin	sepin
Septicaeminum	septi.
Sequoia sempervirens	seq-s.
Serotoninum	serot.
Serpentaria aristolochia	serp.
Serum anguillae	ser-ang.
Serum anti-colibacillum	ser-a-c.
Serum equi	ser-eq.
Shucks	shucks
Siegesbeckia orientalis	sieg.
Silica marina	sil-mar.
Silica terra	sil.
Silicium metallicum	sil-met.
Silphion cyrenaicum	silpho.
Silphium laciniatum	silphu.
Simaruba amara	sima.
Simaruba versicolor	sima-v.
Sinapis alba	sin-a.
Sinapis arvensis	sin-ar.
Sinapis nigra	sin-n.
Sinusitisinum	sinusin.
Sisyrinchium glaxoides	sisy.
Sium latifolium	sium
Skatolum	skat.
Skookum chuck aqua	skook.
Slag	slag
Smilacinum	smilin.
Sol	sol
Solaninum aceticum	solin.
Solanum arrebenta	sol-a.
Solanum carolinense	sol-c.
Solanum integri	sol-i.
Solanum mammosum	sol-m.
Solanum nigrum	sol-n.
Solanum oleraceum	sol-o.
Solanum pseudocapsicum	sol-ps.
Solanum tuberosum	sol-t.
Solanum tuberosum aegrotans	sol-t-ae.
Solanum xanthocarpus	sol-x.
Solidago virga aurea	solid.
Sorbus aucuparia	sorb-au.
Sphingurus martini	sphing.
Spigelia anthelmia	spig.
Spigelia marilandica	spig-m.
Spiraea ulmaria	spirae.
Spiranthes autumnalis	spira.
Splenum	splen.
Spongia tosta	spong.
Squilla maritima	squil.
Stachys betonica	stach.
Stannum iodatum	stann-i.
Stannum metallicum	stann.
Stannum muriaticum	stann-m.
Stannum sulphuricum	stann-s.
Staphylococcinum	staphycoc.
Staphylotoxicum	staphytox.
Staphysagria	staph.
Star of Bethlehem	star-b-B.
Stellaria media	stel.
Sticta pulmonaria	stict.
Stigmata maydis	stigm.
Stillingia sylvatica	still.
Stomachus	stom.
Stovaine	stovain
Stramonium	stram.
Strepto-enterococcus	strept-ent.
Streptococcinum	strept.

Streptomycinum sulphuricum	strep-s.
Strontium bromatum	stront-br.
Strontium carbonicum	stront-c.
Strontium iodatum	stront-i.
Strontium metallicum	stront.
Strontium muriaticum	stront-m.
Strontium nitricum	stront-n.
Strontium oxydatum	stront-o.
Strophanthus hispidus	stroph.
Strophanthus sarmentosus	stroph-s.
Strychninum	
Strychninum arsenicosum	stry-ar.
Strychninum et ferri citras	stry-f-c.
Strychninum nitricum	stry-n.
Strychninum phosphoricum	stry-p.
Strychninum purum	stry.
Strychninum sulphuricum	stry-s.
Strychninum valerianicum	stry-val.
Succinum acidum	succ-ac.
Succinum purum	succ.
Succus fruti	succ-fr.
Sulfanilamide	sulfa.
Sulfonalum	sulfon.
Sulfonamide	sulfonam.
Sulphur	sulph.
Sulphur lotum	sulph.
Sulphur hydrogenisatum	sul-h.
Sulphur iodatum	sul-i.
Sulphur terebinthinatum	sul-ter.
Sulphuricum acidum	sul-ac.
Sulphuricum acidum aromaticum	sul-ac-ar.
Sulphurosum acidum	sulo-ac.
Sumbulus moschatus	sumb.
Suprarenalis glandula	supren.
Suprarenalis cortex	supren-cort.
Sweet chestnut	sw-ch-B.
Swertia chirata	swer-ch.
Symphoricarpus racemosus	sym-r.
Symphytum officinale	symph.
Syphilinum	syph.
Syringa vulgaris	syr.
Syzygium jambolanum	syzyg.
Tabacum	tab.
Tamarindus indica	tama.
Tamus communis	tam.
Tanacetum vulgare	tanac.
Tanghinia venenifera	tang.

Tannicum acidum	tann-ac.
Tantalum fluoratum	tant-f.
Tantalum metallicum	tant.
Taraxacum officinale	tarax.
Tarentula cubensis	tarent-c.
Tarentula hispanica	tarent.
Tartaricum acidum	tart-ac.
Taurine	taurin.
Taxus baccata	tax.
Technetium metallicum	tech.
Teinach aqua	tein.
Tela araneae	tela
Telluricum acidum	tell-ac.
Tellurium	tell.
Teplitz aqua	tep.
Terebenum	terebe.
Terebinthina chios	tere-ch.
Terebinthiniae oleum	ter.
Terminalia arjuna	term-a.
Terminalia chebula	term-c.
Terpini hydras	terp-h.
Testis	testis
Tetanotoxinum	tetox.
Tetradymitum	tet.
Teucrium marum verum	teucr.
Teucrium scorodonia	teucr-s.
Thalamus	thala.
Thallium fluoratum	thal-f.
Thallium metallicum	thal.
Thallium muriaticum	thal-m.
Thallium nitricum	thal-n.
Thallium oxydatum	thal-o.
Thallium sulphuricum	thal-s.
Thapsia garganica	thap-g.
Thea sinensis	thea.
Thebainum	thebin.
Theridion curassavicum	ther.
Thevetia nerifolia	thev.
Thiocticum acidum	thio-ac.
Thioproperazine	thiop.
Thiosinaminum	thiosin.
Thiotepa	thiot.
Thlaspi bursa pastoris	thlaspi
Threonine	threnin.
Thuja lobii	thuj-l.
Thuja occidentalis	thuj.
Thymi glandulae extractum	thym-gl.
Thymol	thymol.

Thymus serpyllum	thymu.
Thyreotropinum	thyreotr.
Thyroidinum	thyr.
Tilia europea	til.
Tinospora cordifolia	tinos.
Tipida aqua	tip.
Titanium metallicum	titan.
Titanium oxydatum	titan-o.
Titanium sulphuricum	titan-s.
Tongo	tong.
Torula cerevisiae	torul.
Toxicophloea thunbergi	tox-th.
Toxoplasms gondi	toxo.
Trachinus draco	trach.
Tradescantia diuretica	trad.
Triatema infestans	triat.
Tribulus terrestris	trib.
Trichosanthes dioica	trich-d.
Trifolium arvense	trif-a.
Trifolium pratense	trif-p.
Trifolium repens	trif-r.
Trigonella foenum graecum	trig-f-g.
Trigonocephalus piscivorus	trig-p.
Trillium cernuum	tril-c.
Trillium pendulum	tril.
Trimeresurus wagleri	trim.
Trinitrotoluene	trinit.
Trional	trion.
Triosteum perfoliatum	trio.
Triticum repens	tritic.
Trito	trito
Triumfetta semitriloba	triu-s.
Trombidium muscae domesticae	trom.
Tropaeolum majus	trop.
Tuba fallopii	tuba
Tuberculinum avis	tub-a.
Tuberculinum bovinum Kent	tub.
Tuberculinum denys	tub-d.
Tuberculinum koch	tub-k.
Tuberculinum laricus	tub-lar.
Tuberculinum marmoreck	tub-m.
Tuberculinum residuum Koch	tub-r.
Tuberculinum spengler	tub-sp.
Tungsten metallicum	tung.
Tungsten muriaticum	tung-m.
Tussilago farfara	tus-fa.
Tussilago fragrans	tus-f.
Tussilago petasites	tus-p.
Tylophora indica	tylo-i.
Typha latifolia	typh.
Tyraminum	tyr.
Tyrosinum	tyrin.
Ulmus fulva	ulm.
Ulmus procera	ulm-p.
Upas antiaris	upa-a.
Upas tieuté	upa.
Uranium arsenicicum	uran-ar.
Uranium metallicum	uran.
Uranium muriaticum	uran-m.
Uranium nitricum	uran-n.
Urea nitrica	urea-n.
Urea pura	urea
Uricum acidum	ur-ac.
Urinum	urine
Urotropinum	urotrop.
Urtica crenulata	urt-c.
Urtica gigas	urt-g.
Urtica urens	urt-u.
Usnea barbata	usn.
Ustilago maydis	ust.
Uterus	uter.
Uva-ursi	uva.
Uvaria triloba	uvar.
Uzara	uza.
Vaccin attenu bili	v-a-b.
Vaccinium myrtillus	vacc-m.
Vaccinotoxinum	vac.
Valeriana officinalis	valer.
Valinum	vali.
Vanadium metallicum	vanad.
Vanadium fluoricum	vanad-f.
Vanadium oxydatum	vanad-o.
Vanadium sulphuricum	vanad-s.
Vanilla aromatica	vanil.
Variolinum	vario.
Vena	vena
Venus mercenaria	ven-m.
Veratrinum	verin.
Veratrum album	verat.
Veratrum nigrum	verat-n.
Veratrum viride	verat-v.
Verbascum nigrum	verb-n.
Verbascum thapsus Hahnemanni, thapsiforme	verb.
Verbena hastata	verbe-h.
Verbena urticaefolia	verbe-u.

Vernonia anthelminthica	vern-a.
Veronal	veronal
Veronica arvensis	vero-a.
Veronica beccabunga	vero-b.
Veronica officinalis	vero-o.
Verrucinum	verr.
Vervain	verv-B.
Vesica urinaria	ves-u.
Vesicaria communis	vesi.
Vespa crabro	vesp.
Vibhuti	vibh.
Viburnum oderatissinum	vib-od.
Viburnum opulus	vib.
Viburnum prunifolium	vib-p.
Viburnum tinus	vib-t.
Vichy aqua grande grille	vichy-g.
Vichy aqua hospital	vichy-h.
Vinca minor	vinc.
Vincetoxicum officinale	vince.
Vinum	vine-B.
Viola odorata	viol-o.
Viola tricolor	viol-t.
Vipera aspis	vip-a.
Vipera berus	vip.
Vipera redi	vip-r.
Viscum album	visc.
Viscum quercinum	visc-q.
Vitamine A	vita-a.
Vitamine D	vita-d.
Vitamine E	vita-e.
Vitex trifolia	vit.
Vitis vinifera	vitis
Vitrum antimonii	vitr.
Voeslau aqua	voes.
Walnut	waln-B.
Water violet	wat-v-B.
Weilbach aqua	weil.
White chestnut	wh-ch-B.
Wiesbaden aqua	wies.
Wild oat	wld-o-B.
Wild rose	wld-r-B.
Wildbad aqua	wild.
Willow	will-B.
Wisteria species	wist.
Withania somnifera	with-s.
Wyethia helenoides	wye.
X-rays	x-ray
Xanthium spinosum	xanth.
Xanthorrhiza apifolia	xanrhi.
Xanthorrhoea arborea	xanrhoe.
Xanthoxylum fraxineum	xan.
Xenon	xeno.
Xerophyllum	xero
Yersin	yersin
Yohimbinum	yohim
Yttrium metallicum	yttr.
Yttrium oxydatum	yttr-o.
Yucca filamentosa	yuc.
Zea italica	zea-i.
Zincum aceticum	zinc-acet.
Zincum arsenicosum	zinc-ar.
Zincum bromatum	zinc-br.
Zincum carbonicum	zinc-c.
Zincum chromatum	zinc-chr.
Zincum cyanatum	zinc-cy.
Zincum ferrocyanatum	zinc-fcy.
Zincum fluoratum	zinc-f.
Zincum iodatum	zinc-i.
Zincum metallicum	zinc.
Zincum muriaticum	zinc-m.
Zincum nitricum	zinc-n.
Zincum oxydatum	zinc-o.
Zincum phosphoricum	zinc-p.
Zincum picricum	zinc-pic.
Zincum sulphuricum	zinc-s.
Zincum silicatum	zinc-sil.
Zincum valerianicum	zinc-val.
Zingiber officinale	zing.
Zirconium metallicum	zirc.
Zizia aurea	ziz.
Zizia italica	ziz-i.

abel.	Abelmoschus
abies-c.	Abies canadensis
abies-n.	Abies nigra
abrom-aug.	Abroma augusta
abrot.	Abrotanum
abr.	Abrus precatorius
absin.	Absinthium
abut.	Abuta
acal.	Acalypha indica
aca-m.	Acanthus mollis
acetan.	Acetanilidum
acet-ac.	Aceticum acidum
aceton	Acetonum
achy-a.	Achyranthes aspera
achy.	Achyranthes calea
aconin.	Aconitinum
acon-a.	Aconitum anthora
acon-c.	Aconitum cammarum
acon-f.	Aconitum ferox
acon-l.	Aconitum lycoctonum
acon.	Aconitum napellus
acon-s.	Aconitum septentrionale
acor-c.	Acorus calamus
act-sp.	Actea spicata
adam.	Adamas
adan.	Adansonia digitata
adax.	Adaxukah
adel.	Adelheid aqua
adeps-s	Adeps suillus
adlu.	Adlumia fungosa
adonin.	Adonidinum
adon-ae.	Adonis aestivalis
adon.	Adonis vernalis
adox.	Adoxa moschatellina
adren.	Adrenalinum
aegle-f.	Aegle folia
aegle.	Aegle marmelos
aego-p.	Aegopodium podagraria
aesc-c.	Aesculus carnea
aesc-g.	Aesculus glabra
aesc.	Aesculus hippocastanum
aether	Aether
aethi-a.	Aethiops antimonialis
aethi-m.	Aethiops mineralis
aeth.	Aethusa cynapium
aethyl-br.	Aethylum bromidum
aethyl-n.	Aethylum nitricum
aethyl-s.	Aethylum sulphuricum dichloratum
aga.	Agapanthus orientalis
ager.	Agerati
agarin.	Agaricinum
agar-cpn.	Agaricus campanulatus
agar-cps.	Agaricus campestris
agar-cit.	Agaricus citrinus
agar-em.	Agaricus emeticus
agar.	Agaricus muscarius
agar-pa.	Agaricus pantherinus
agar-ph.	Agaricus phalloides
agar-pr.	Agaricus procerus
agar-se.	Agaricus semiglobatus
agar-st.	Agaricus stercoranius
agar-v.	Agaricus vernus
agav-a.	Agave americana
agav-t.	Agave tequilana
agn.	Agnus castus
agra.	Agraphis nutans
agr-B.	Agrimonia eupatoria
agri.	Agrimonia eupatoria
agro.	Agrostemma githago
agros.	Agrostis alba
ail.	Ailanthus glandulosa
alch-v.	Alchemilla vulgaris
alco.	Alcoholus
alco-s.	Alcoholus sulphuris
ald.	Aldehyde
alet.	Aletris farinosa
alf.	Alfalfa
all-c.	Allium cepa
all-s.	Allium sativum
all-u.	Allium ursinum
allox.	Alloxanum
aln.	Alnus rubra
aloe	Aloe socotrina
a-dnphen.	Alpha-dinitrophenol
alpi.	Alpinia officinarum
alst-c.	Alstonia constricta
alst-s.	Alstonia scholaris
alth.	Althaea officinalis
alumn.	Alumen
alum-acet.	Aluminium aceticum
alum-br.	Aluminium bromatum
alum-met.	Aluminium metallicum
alum-m.	Aluminium muriaticum
alum.	Aluminium oxydata

alum-p.	Aluminium phosphorica
alum-sil.	Aluminium silicata
alum-s.	Aluminium sulphuricum
ambr.	Ambra grisea
ambro.	Ambrosia artemisiefolia
ammi-v.	Ammi visnaga
ammc.	Ammoniacum gummi
am-acet.	Ammonium aceticum
am-be.	Ammonium benzoicum
am-br.	Ammonium bromatum
am-c.	Ammonium carbonicum
am-caust.	Ammonium causticum
am-f.	Ammonium fluoratum
am-form.	Ammonium formaldehyde
am-i	Ammonium iodatum
am-m.	Ammonium muriaticum
am-n.	Ammonium nitricum
am-p.	Ammonium phosphoricum
am-pic.	Ammonium picricum
am-s.	Ammonium sulphuricum
am-t.	Ammonium tartaricum
am-val.	Ammonium valerianicum
am-van.	Ammonium vanadinicum
amn-l.	Amnii liquor
amor-r.	Amorphophallus rivieri
ampe-qu	Ampelopsis quinquefolia
ampe-tr.	Ampelopsis trifoliata
amph.	Amphisbaena vermicularis
amyg-am.	Amygdalae amarae aqua
amyg-p.	Amygdalus persica
amylam.	Amylaminum hydrochloricum
aml-n.	Amylenum nitrosum
anac-oc.	Anacardium occidentale
anac.	Anacardium orientale
anag.	Anagallis arvensis
anagy.	Anagyris foetida
anan.	Anantherum muricatum
ander.	Andersonia rohitika
androc.	Androctonos amurreuxi hebraeus
androg-p.	Andrographis peniculata
andr.	Androsace lactea
ane-n.	Anemone nemorosa
ane-r.	Anemone ranunculoides
anemps.	Anemopsis californica
anet-g.	Anethum graveolens
ange.	Angelica atropurpurea
ange-b.	Angelica brasiliensis
ange-s.	Angelica sinensis radix
ango.	Angophora lanceolata
ang.	Angustura vera
anh.	Anhalonium lewinii
anil.	Anilinum
anil-s.	Anilinum sulphuricum
anis.	Anisum stellatum
anth-c.	Anthemis cotula
anth.	Anthemis nobilis
antho.	Anthoxanthum odoratum
anthr.	Anthracinum
anthro.	Anthrokokali
ant-ar.	Antimonium arsenicosum
ant-c.	Antimonium crudum
ant-f.	Antimonium fluoratum
ant-i.	Antimonium iodatum
ant.	Antimonium metallicum
ant-m.	Antimonium muriaticum
ant-n-l.	Antimonium natrum lacticum
ant-n.	Antimonium nitricum
ant-o.	Antimonium oxydatum
ant-s.	Antimonium sulphuratum aureum
ant-s-r.	Antimonium sulphuratum rubrum
ant-t.	Antimonium tartaricum
antipyrin.	Antipyrinum
aorta	Aorta
aphis.	Aphis chenopodii glauci
aphto.	Aphtosinum
apiol.	Apiolum
apis	Apis mellifica
apisin.	Apisinum
ap-g.	Apium graveolens
apoc-a.	Apocynum androsemifolium
apoc.	Apocynum cannabinum
apom.	Apomorphini hydrochloridum
aq-mar.	Aqua marina
aq-pet.	Aqua petra
aq-pu.	Aqua pura
aq-sil.	Aqua silicata
aqui-c.	Aquila chrysaetos
aquil.	Aquilegia vulgaris
arag.	Aragallus lamberti
aral-h.	Aralia hispida
aral.	Aralia racemosa
aran.	Aranea diadema
aran-ix.	Aranea ixobola

aran-s.	Aranea scinencia
arbin.	Arbutinum
arbu.	Arbutus andrachne
arec.	Areca catechu
aren-r.	Arenaria rubra
arge.	Argemone mexicana
arg-br.	Argentum bromatum
arg-c.	Argentum carbonicum
arg-cy.	Argentum cyanatum
arg-f.	Argentum fluoratum
arg-i.	Argentum iodatum
arg.	Argentum metallicum
arg-m.	Argentum muriaticum
arg-n.	Argentum nitricum
arg-o.	Argentum oxydatum
arg-p.	Argentum phosphoricum
arg-s.	Argentum sulphuricum
argom.	Argomon aulaga
argo.	Argon
arist-cl.	Aristolochia clematitis
arist-m.	Aristolochia milhomens
arn.	Arnica montana
arsenal	Arsenal
ars.	Arsenicum album
ars-br.	Arsenicum bromatum
ars-h.	Arsenicum hydrogenisatum
ars-i.	Arsenicum iodatum
ars-met.	Arsenicum metallicum
ars-n.	Arsenicum nitricum
ars-s-f.	Arsenicum sulphuratum flavum
ars-s-r.	Arsenicum sulphuratum rubrum
ars-t-s.	Arsenicum tersulphuratum
art-tri.	Artemisia tridentata
art-v.	Artemisia vulgaris
arte.	Arteria
arum-a.	Arum arisarum
arum-d.	Arum dracontium
arum-dru.	Arum dracunculus
arum-i.	Arum italicum
arum-m.	Arum maculatum
arum-t.	Arum triphyllum
arund.	Arundo mauritanica
asaf.	Asafoetida
asai	Asai
asar-c.	Asarum canadense
asar.	Asarum europaeum
glyc-g.	Asclepias cornuti
asc-i.	Asclepias incarnata
asc-t.	Asclepias tuberosa
asim.	Asimina triloba
ask.	Askalabotes laevigatus
aspar.	Asparagus officinalis
asp-B.	Aspen
asperg-f.	Aspergilus fumigatus
asperg-n.	Aspergilus niger
asper.	Asperula odorata
aspin.	Aspidosperminum
astac.	Astacus fluviatilis
asta.	Astatinum
aster.	Asterias rubens
astra-e.	Astragalus exscapus
astra-me.	Astragalus menziesii
astra-mo.	Astragalus mollisimus
astur	Astur cachinnaus
atha.	Athamanta cretensis
atista	Atista indica
atra-r.	Atrax robustus
atri	Atriplex hortensis
atro.	Atropinum purum, sulphuricum
aug.	Augopora
aur-ar.	Aurum arsenicicum
aur-br.	Aurum bromatum
aur-f.	Aurum fluoratum
aur-fu.	Aurum fulminans
aur-i.	Aurum iodatum
aur.	Aurum metallicum
aur-m.	Aurum muriaticum
aur-m-k.	Aurum muriaticum kalinatum
aur-m-n.	Aurum muriaticum natronatum
aur-n.	Aurum nitricum
aur-p.	Aurum phosphoricum
aur-s.	Aurum sulphuratum
auto.	Autonosodes
aven.	Avena sativa
aza.	Azadirachta indica
bcg	B.C.G
bacch.	Baccharis crista
bac.	Bacillinum Burnett
bac-ts.	Bacillinum testium
dys-co.	Bacillus dysenteriae
ba-sv.	Bacillus seven
syc-co.	Bacillus sycoccus by Paterson
ba-tn.	Bacillus ten
ems	Bad Ems
bad.	Badiaga
baj.	Baja

baln.	Balnea maritima
balsa.	Balsamodendron mukul
bals-p.	Balsamum peruvianum
bals-t.	Balsamum toluiferum
bamb-a.	Bambusa arundinacea
bani-c.	Banisteria caapi
bapt-c.	Baptisia confusa acetica
bapt.	Baptisia tinctoria
barb.	Barbae cyprini ova
baros.	Barosma crenata
bart.	Bartfelder aqua
bar.	Baryta metallica
bar-acet.	Baryta acetica
bar-ar.	Baryta arsenicosa
bar-br.	Baryta bromata
bar-c.	Baryta carbonica
bar-f.	Baryta fluorica
bar-i.	Baryta iodata
bar-m.	Baryta muriatica
bar-n.	Baryta nitrica
bar-o.	Baryta oxydatum
bar-p.	Baryta phosphorica
bar-s.	Baryta sulphurica
bar-sil.	Baryta silicata
beech-B.	Beech
bell.	Belladonna
bell-p.	Bellis perennis
benzin.	Benzinum
benz-ac.	Benzoicum acidum
benzo.	Benzoinum oderiferum
benz.	Benzolum Benzolum
benz-d.	Benzolum dinitricum
benz-n.	Benzolum nitricum
berbin.	Berberinum
berb-a.	Berberis aquifolium
berb.	Berberis vulgaris
beryl.	Beryllium metallicum
beryl-m.	Beryllium muriaticum
beryl-s.	Beryllium sulphuricum
beta.	Beta vulgaris
betin.	Betainum muriaticum
betul.	Betula alba
bism-met.	Bismuthum metallicum
bism.	Bismuthum subnitricum
biti-a.	Bitis arietans
bix.	Bixa orellana
blatta-a.	Blatta americana
blatta	Blatta orientalis
blum-o.	Blumia odorata
boerh.	Boerhavia diffusa
bold.	Boldo fragrans
bol.	Boletus laricis
bol-lu.	Boletus luridus
bol-s.	Boletus satanas
bomb-chr.	Bombyx chrysorrhea
bomb-pr.	Bombyx processionea
bond.	Bondonneau aqua
borag.	Borago officinalis
bor.	Borax veneta
bor-ac.	Boricum acidum
bor-met.	Boron metallicum
bos-s.	Boswelia serrata
bothr-l.	Bothriocephalus latus
both-a.	Bothrops atrox
both-l.	Bothrops lanceolatus
botul.	Botulinum
bov.	Bovista lycoperdon
bowd.	Bowdichea major
brach.	Brachyglottis repens
brahmi	Brahmi
bran.	Branca ursina
brass.	Brassica napus
brass-o.	Brassica oleracea
brom.	Bromium
brom-ac.	Bromium acidum
bromu.	Bromus ramosus
bruc.	Brucea antidysenterica
brucel.	Brucella melitensis
brucin.	Brucinum nitricum
bry.	Bryonia alba
bufo	Bufo rana
bufo-s.	Bufo sahytiensis Mure
bulb.	Bulbinum
bulbin.	Bulbocapnin
bung-c.	Bungarus caeruleus
bung-f.	Bungaris fasciatus
buni-o.	Bunias orientalis
buth-aust.	Buthus australis
but-ac.	Butyricum acidum
bux.	Buxus sempervirens
c-di-o.	Carbon dioxide
cac.	Cacao
cactin.	Cactina
cact.	Cactus grandiflorus
cadm-ar.	Cadmium arsenicosum
cadm-br.	Cadmium bromatum

cadm-f.	Cadmium fluoricum
cadm-i.	Cadmium iodatum
cadm.	Cadmium metallicum
cadm-m.	Cadmium muriaticum
cadm-n.	Cadmium nitricum
cadm-o.	Cadmium oxidatum
cadm-p.	Cadmium phosphoricum
cadm-s.	Cadmium sulphuratum
cael.	Caela zacatechichi
caer-i-s.	Caeruleum iritis solis
caesal.	Caesalpinia bonducella
caes.	Caesium metallicum aut sulphuricum
cahin.	Cahinca racemosa
caj.	Cajuputum
calad.	Caladium seguinum
calag.	Calaguala
calc-acet.	Calcarea acetica
calc-ar.	Calcarea arsenicosa
calc-br.	Calcarea bromata
calc-cal.	Calcarea calcinata
calc.	Calcarea carbonica Hahnemanni
calc-caust.	Calcarea caustica Segini
calc-chln.	Calcarea chlorinata
calc-f.	Calcarea fluorata
calc-hp.	Calcarea hypophosphorosa
calc-i.	Calcarea iodata
calc-l.	Calcarea lactica
calc-l-n.	Calcarea lactica natronata
calc-l-p.	Calcarea lactica phosphorica
calc-m.	Calcarea muriatica
calc-met.	Calcarea metallica
calc-n.	Calcarea nitrica
calc-o-t.	Calcarea ovi testae
calc-ox.	Calcarea oxalica
calc-p.	Calcarea phosphorica
calc-pic.	Calcarea picrica
calc-sil.	Calcarea silicata
calc-st-sula.	Calcarea stibiato-sulphurata
calc-s.	Calcarea sulphurica
calcul-b.	Calculus bilialis
calcul-r.	Calculus renalis
calen.	Calendula officinalis
calli.	Calliandra houstoni
callun.	Calluna vulgaris
calo.	Calotropis gigantea
calo-l.	Calotropis lactum
calth.	Caltha palustris
camph.	Camphora
camph-br.	Camphora bromata
camph-ac.	Camphoricum acidum
canch.	Canchalagua
cand-p.	Candida parapsilosis
canna	Canna angustifolia
cann-i.	Cannabis indica
cann-s.	Cannabis sativa
canthin.	Cantharidinum
canth.	Cantharis vesicatoria
capp.	Capparis coriacea
caps.	Capsicum annuum
carb-an.	Carbo animalis
carb-v.	Carbo vegetabilis
carb-ac.	Carbolicum acidum
carbn.	Carboneum Carboneum
carbn-chl.	Carboneum chloratum
carbn-h.	Carboneum hydrogenisatum
carbn-o.	Carboneum oxygenisatum
carbn-s.	Carboneum sulphuratum
carc.	Carcinosinum Burnett
carda.	Cardamine pratense
cardz.	Cardiazol
cardi-h.	Cardiospermum halicacabum
card-b.	Carduus benedictus
card-m.	Carduus marianus
care-a.	Carex arenaria
cari.	Carissa schimperi
carl.	Carlsbad aqua
carp.	Carpinus betulus
cartil-s.	Cartilago suis
cartil.	Cartilago
caru.	Carum carvi
cary.	Carya alba
casc.	Cascarilla
cass.	Cassada
cassi-a.	Cassia alata
cassi-m.	Cassia medica
cassi-s.	Cassia sophera
cast-v.	Castanea vesca
cast-eq.	Castor equi
cast.	Castoreum canadense
catal.	Catalpa bignonioides
catar.	Cataria nepeta
cat.	Catuaba
caul.	Caulophyllum thalictroides
caust.	Causticum Hahnemanni
cean.	Ceanothus americanus

cean-tr.	Ceanothus trysiflorus
cecr.	Cecropia mexicana
cecr-p.	Cecropia palmata
cecr-pe.	Cecropia petata
cedr.	Cedron
celt.	Celtis occidentalis
cem.	Cement
cench.	Cenchris contortrix
cent.	Centaurea tagana
cent-u.	Centaurium umbellatum
cephd.	Cephalandra indica
ceph.	Cephalanthus occidentalis
cer-B.	Cerato
cereb-cort.	Cerebellum cortex
cereb.	Cerebellum
ceref.	Cerefolius
cere-b.	Cereus bonplandii
cere-s.	Cereus serpentinus
cer.	Cerium metallicum
cer-ox.	Cerium oxalicum
cerv.	Cervus brasilicus
ceto.	Cetonia
cetr.	Cetraria islandica
chamae.	Chamaedrys
cham.	Chamomilla vulgaris
chap.	Chaparro amargoso
chasm.	Chasmanthera palmata
chaul.	Chaulmoograe
cheir.	Cheiranthus cheiri
chelin.	Chelidoninum
chel-g.	Chelidonium glaucum
chel.	Chelidonium majus
chelo.	Chelone glabra
chen-a.	Chenopodium anthelminthicum
chen-v.	Chenopodium vulvaria
cher-p-B.	Cherry plum
ch-bd-B.	Chestnut buds
chic-B.	Chicory
chim-m.	Chimaphila maculata
chim-rot.	Chimaphila rotundifolia
chim.	Chimaphila umbellata
chin-b.	China boliviana
chin.	China officinalis
chinar.	Chinaria canadensis
chinid.	Chinidinum hydrochloricum
chin-ar.	Chininum arsenicosum
chin-hydr.	Chininum hydrocyanicum
chin-m.	Chininum muriaticum
chin-sal.	Chininum salicylicum
chin-s.	Chininum sulphuricum
chin-val.	Chininum valerianicum
chion.	Chionanthus virginica
chlol.	Chloralum hydratum
chloram.	Chloramphenicolum
chlf.	Chloroformum
chlph.	Chlorophyllum
chlorpr.	Chlorpromazinum
chlor.	Chlorum
choc.	Chocolate
chol.	Cholesterinum
cholin.	Cholinum
cho.	Cholos terrapina
choph.	Chopheenee
chr-ac.	Chromicum acidum
chr.	Chromium metallicum
chr-m.	Chromium muriaticum
chr-o.	Chromium oxidatum
chr-p.	Chromium phosphoricum
chr-s.	Chromium sulphuricum
chrysan.	Chrysanthemum leucanthemum
chrysar.	Chrysarobinum
chrysi.	Chrysis
chrys-ac.	Chrysophanicum acidum
cice.	Cicer arietinum
cich.	Cichorium intybus
cic-m.	Cicuta maculata
cic.	Cicuta virosa
cigua.	Ciguatera
cimx.	Cimex lectularius
cimic.	Cimicifuga racemosa
cina	Cina maritima
cinch.	Cinchoninum sulphuricum
cine.	Cineraria maritima
cinnb.	Cinnabaris
cinnam.	Cinnamomum ceylanicum
cist.	Cistus canadensis
cit-ac.	Citricum acidum
cit-d.	Citrus decumana
cit-l.	Citrus limonum
cit-v.	Citrus vulgaris
clad-p.	Cladonia pyxidata
clem-B.	Clematis
clem.	Clematis recta
clem-vir.	Clematis virginiana
clem-vit.	Clematis vitalba
cler-i.	Clerodendron infortunatum

cob-chl.	Cobaltum chloridum
cob-f.	Cobaltum fluoratum
cob-i.	Cobaltum iodatum
cob.	Cobaltum metallicum
cob-m.	Cobaltum muriaticum
cob-n.	Cobaltum nitricum
cob-o.	Cobaltum oxydatum
cob-p.	Cobaltum phosphoricum
cob-sil.	Cobaltum silicatum
cob-s.	Cobaltum sulphuratum
coca	Coca
cocain.	Cocainum hydrochloricum
coccal	Coccal co Paterson
cocci-s.	Coccinella septempunctata
cocc.	Cocculus indicus
coc-c.	Coccus cacti
coch.	Cochlearia armoracia
coch-o.	Cochlearia officinalis
cod.	Codeinum purum, phosphoricum, sulphuricum
coenz-a.	Coenzym A
coff.	Coffea cruda
coff-t.	Coffea tosta
coffin.	Coffeinum
colchin.	Colchicinum
colch.	Colchicum autumnale
col-a.	Coleus aromaticus
mut.	Coli by Paterson
coli.	Colibacillinum, anti-colibacillair serum
coll.	Collinsonia canadensis
colocin.	Colocynthinum
coloc.	Colocynthis
colon	Colon
colos.	Colostrum
com.	Comocladia dentata
conch.	Conchiolinum
conin-br.	Coniinum bromatum
conin.	Coniinum pura
con.	Conium maculatum
conj.	Conjunctiva
conv.	Convallaria majalis
convo-a.	Convolvulus arvensis
convo-d.	Convolvulus duartinus
convo-s.	Convolvulus stans
cop.	Copaiva
cor-r.	Corallium rubrum
corh.	Corallorhiza odontorhiza
cord.	Cordia coffeoide
cori-m.	Coriaria myrtifolia
cori-r.	Coriaria ruscifolia
corn-a.	Cornus alternifolia
corn.	Cornus circinata
corn-f.	Cornus florida
corn-s.	Cornus sericea
corp-l.	Corpus luteum
cortico.	Corticotropinum
cortiso.	Cortisonum
cory-c.	Corydalis cava
cory.	Corydalis formosa
cosm.	Cosmoline
cost-p.	Costus pisonis
coto	Coto bark
cot.	Cotyledon umbilicus
crb-a-B.	Crab Apple
cras-o.	Crassula obliqua
crat.	Crataegus oxyacantha
cristal.	Cristalinum
croc.	Crocus sativus
crot-c.	Crotalus cascavella
crot-h.	Crotalus horridus
croto-ca.	Croton campestris
croto-chlol.	Croton chloralum
croto-t.	Croton tiglium
cryp.	Cryptopinum
cub.	Cubeba officinalis
cuc-c.	Cucurbita citrullus
cuc-p.	Cucurbita pepo
culx.	Culex musca
cumin.	Cumarinum
cund.	Cundurango
cuph.	Cuphea viscosissima
cupre-aust.	Cupressus australis
cupre-l.	Cupressus lawsoniana
cupr.	Cuprum metallicum
cupr-acet.	Cuprum aceticum
cupr-am-s.	Cuprum ammoniae sulphuricum
cupr-ar.	Cuprum arsenicosum
cupr-c.	Cuprum carbonicum
cupr-cy.	Cuprum cyanatum
cupr-f.	Cuprum fluoratum
cupr-m.	Cuprum muriaticum
cupr-n.	Cuprum nitricum
cupr-o.	Cuprum oxydatum nigrum
cupr-p.	Cuprum phosphoricum

cupr-sil.	Cuprum silicatum
cupr-s.	Cuprum sulphuricum
cur.	Curare woorari
curc.	Curcuma javanensis
cycl.	Cyclamen europaeum
cyclos.	Cyclosporine
cyd.	Cydonia vulgaris
cymin.	Cymarinum
cyna.	Cynara scolymos
cyn-d.	Cynodon dactylon
cyno.	Cynoglossum officinale
cypr.	Cypripedium pubescens
cyrt-p.	Cyrtus
cystin.	Cystinum
cytin.	Cytisinum
cyt-l.	Cytisus laburnum
dam.	Damiana aphrodisiaca
dao-r.	Daoboia russelli
daph.	Daphne indica
datis.	Datisca cannabina
dat-a.	Datura arborea
dat-f.	Datura ferox
dat-m.	Datura metel
dat-s.	Datura sanguinea
datin.	Daturinum
dauc.	Daucus carotis
del.	Delphinus amazonicus
dema.	Dematium petraeum
dendro-p.	Dendroaspis polytepis
dens	Dens humane
derma	Derma
der.	Derris pinnata
desm-g.	Desmodium gangeticum
des-r.	Desmoncus rudentum
des-ac.	Desoxyribonucleinicum acidum
dial.	Dialium ferrum
diaphr.	Diaphragma
dicha.	Dichapetalum Thunbergh
dict.	Dictamnus albus
digin.	Digitalinum
dig.	Digitalis purpurea
digox.	Digitoxinum
dios-p.	Dioscorea petrea
dios.	Dioscorea villosa
diosin.	Dioscorin
diosm.	Diosma lincaris
dpt	Diphtheria Pertussis Tetanus vaccine
diph.	Diphtherinum
diphtox.	Diphtherotoxinum
dip.	Dipodium punctatum
dips-s.	Dipsacus silvester
dirc.	Dirca palustris
disc-i.	Discus intervertebrales
ditin.	Ditainum
dol.	Dolichos pruriens
dor.	Doryphora decemlineata
dros.	Drosera rotundifolia
drym.	Drymis winteri
dttab.	DTTAB
dubin.	Duboisinum
dubin-s.	Duboisinum sulphuricum
dulc.	Dulcamara
duod.	Duodenum
eaux	Eaux bonnes aqua
eberth.	Eberthinum
echi.	Echinacea angustifolia
echi-p.	Echinacea purpurea
echi-c.	Echis carinatus
echit.	Echites suberecta
egg-vac.	Egg-vaccine
eich-c.	Eichornia crassipes
elae.	Elaeis guineensis
elaps	Elaps corallinus
elat.	Elaterium officinarum
electr.	Electricitas
elem.	Elemuy gauteria
elm-B.	Elm
elmen	Elmen Soolbad
emb.	Embelia ribes
emb-off.	Embelica officinalis
embry.	Embryo suis
emetin.	Emetine
enteroc.	Enterococcinum
eos.	Eosinum
ephe.	Ephedra vulgaris
ephin.	Ephedrin
epig.	Epigea repens
epih.	Epihysterinum
epil-a.	Epilobium angustifolium
epil.	Epilobium palustre
epip.	Epiphegus virginiana
equis-a.	Equisetum arvense
equis.	Equisetum hyemale
eran.	Eranthis hymnalis
erech.	Erechthites hieracifolia

ergot.	Ergotinum
erig.	Erigeron canadensis
erin.	Erinacea species
erio.	Eriodictyon glutinosum
erod.	Erodium cicutarium
erv.	Ervum ervilla
ery-a.	Eryngium aquaticum
ery-m.	Eryngium maritimum
eryth.	Erythrinus
eryt-j.	Erythrophlaeum judiciale
esch.	Eschscholtzia californica
esin.	Eserinum
esin-sal.	Eserinum salicylicum
esp-g.	Espeletia grandiflora
ethyl-a.	Ethylicum
eucol.	Eucalyptolum
eucal.	Eucalyptus globulus
eucal-t.	Eucalyptus tereticortis
eug.	Eugenia jambosa
euonin.	Euonyminum
euon-a.	Euonymus atropurpurea
euon.	Euonymus europea
eup-a.	Eupatorium aromaticum
eup-c.	Eupatorium cannabinum
eup-d.	Eupatorium dendroides
eup-per.	Eupatorium perfoliatum
eup-pur.	Eupatorium purpureum
euph-a.	Euphorbia amygdaloides
euph-c.	Euphorbia corollata
euph-cy.	Euphorbia cyparissias
euph-her.	Euphorbia herophylla
euph-he.	Euphorbia heterodoxa
euph-hy.	Euphorbia hypericifolia
euph-ip.	Euphorbia ipecacuanha
euph-l.	Euphorbia lathyris
euph-li.	Euphorbia linearis
euph-m.	Euphorbia marginata
euph-pe.	Euphorbia peplus
euph-pi.	Euphorbia pilulifera
euph-po.	Euphorbia polycarpa
euph-pr.	Euphorbia prostata
euph.	Euphorbia resinifera
euphr.	Euphrasia officinalis
eupi.	Eupionum
eys.	Eysenhardtia polystachia
fab.	Fabiana imbricata
faec.	Faecalis alcaligenes
fago.	Fagopyrum esculentum
fagu.	Fagus silvatica
fat.	Fatpoison
fel.	Fel tauri
feld.	Feldspar
ferr-acet.	Ferrum aceticum
ferr-ar.	Ferrum arsenicosum
ferr-br.	Ferrum bromatum
ferr-c.	Ferrum carbonicum
ferr-cit.	Ferrum citricum
ferr-cy.	Ferrum cyanatum
ferr-f.	Ferrum fluoratum
ferr-i.	Ferrum iodatum
ferr-l.	Ferrum lacticum
ferr-ma.	Ferrum magneticum
ferr.	Ferrum metallicum
ferr-m.	Ferrum muriaticum
ferr-n.	Ferrum nitricum
ferr-o-r.	Ferrum oxidatum rubrum
ferr-p.	Ferrum phosphoricum
ferr-p-h.	Ferrum phosphoricum hydricum
ferr-pic.	Ferrum picricum
ferr-prox.	Ferrum protoxalatum
ferr-py.	Ferrum pyrophosphoricum
ferr-sil.	Ferrum silicatum
ferr-s.	Ferrum sulphuricum
ferr-t.	Ferrum tartaricum
ferr-val.	Ferrum valerianicum
ferul.	Ferula glauca
fibrin.	Fibrinum
fic-c.	Ficus carica
fic-i.	Ficus indica
fic.	Ficus religiosa
fic-v.	Ficus venosa
fil.	Filix-mas
fl.	Fluor
flav.	Flavus
flor-p.	Flor de piedra
fluoform.	Fluoformum
fl-ac.	Fluoricum acidum
foen.	Foeniculum sativum
foll.	Folliculinum
formal.	Formalinum
form.	Formica rufa
form-ac.	Formicicum acidum
frag.	Fragaria vesca
fram.	Framboesinum
franc.	Franciscaea uniflora
franz.	Franzensbad

frax. Fraxinus americana
frax-e. Fraxinus excelsior
fried. Friedrichhaller aqua
fuch. Fuchsinum
fuc. Fucus vesiculosus
fuli. Fuligo ligni
fum. Fumaria officinalis
funi-umb. Funiculus umbilicalis suis
furf-i. Furfur iritici
gad. Gadus morrhua
gaert. Gaertner by Bach
gala. Galanthus nivalis
galeg. Galega officinalis
galeo. Galeopsis segetum
galin. Galinsoga parviflora
gali. Galium aparine
gall-ac. Gallicum acidum
gall-f. Gallium fluoratum
gall. Gallium metallicum
gall-m. Gallium muriaticum
gall-o. Gallium oxydatum
gall-p. Gallium phosphoricum
gall-s. Gallium sulphuricum
galph. Galphimia glauca
galv. Galvanismus
gamb. Gambogia
gast. Gastein aqua
gaul. Gaultheria procumbens
gelin. Gelatinum
gels. Gelsemium sempervirens
genat. Genatosan
genist. Genista tinctoria
gent-B. Gentian
gent-c. Gentiana cruciata
gent-l. Gentiana lutea
gent-q. Gentiana quinqueflora
geo. Geoffroya vermifuga
ger. Geranium maculatum
ger-r. Geranium robertianum
germ. Germanium metallicum
get. Gettysburg aqua
geum Geum rivale
gink. Ginkgo biloba
gins. Ginseng
pineal. Glandula pinealis
glech. Glechoma hederacea
glon. Glonoinum
glyc. Glycerinum
glyc-g. Glycyrrhiza glabra
gnaph. Gnaphalium polycephalum
gomph. Gomprhena officinalis
gonotox. Gonotoxinum
gors-B. Gorse
goss. Gossypium herbaceum
gran. Granatum
graph. Graphites naturalis
grat. Gratiola officinalis
grin. Grindelia robusta
gua. Guaco
guajol. Guaiacolum
guai. Guaiacum officinale
guan. Guaninum
guano Guano australis
guare. Guarea trichiloides
guat. Guatteria gaumeri
guipsin. Guipsine
gunp. Gunpowder
gymne. Gymnema sylvestre
gymn. Gymnocladus canadensis
haem. Haematoxylon campechianum
haff. Haffkine
hafn. Hafnium metallicum
hali-l. Haliceetus leucocephalus
hall Hall aqua
halo. Haloperidol
ham. Hamamelis macrophylla
hapl-b. Haplopappus baylahuen
harp. Harpagophytum procumbens
heath-B. Heather
hecla. Hecla lava
hedeo Hedeoma pulegioides
hed. Hedera helix
hedy. Hedysarum ildefonsianum
helin. Heleninum
helia-m. Helianthemum species
helia. Helianthus annuus
helio. Heliotropium peruvianum
heli. Helium
helx. Helix tosta
hell-f. Helleborus foetidus
hell. Helleborus niger
hell-o. Helleborus orientalis
hell-v. Helleborus viridis
helm. Helmintochortos
helo. Heloderma horridus
helon. Helonias dioica

hemid.	Hemidesmus indica
hemog.	Hemoglobinum
heuch.	Heuchera americana
hep.	Hepar sulphuris calcareum
hepat.	Hepatica triloba
hepar	Hepatinum
hern-g.	Herniaria glabra
herin.	Heroinum
hier-p.	Hieracium pilosella
hilo.	Hiloropium peruvianum
hipp.	Hippomanes
hippoz.	Hippozaeninum
hip-ac.	Hippuricum acidum
hir.	Hirudo medicinalis
hist.	Histaminum muriaticum
histid.	Histidinum
ho.	Hoang-Nan
hoit.	Hoitzia coccinea
holly-B.	Holly
hom.	Homarus gammarus
home.	Homeria collina
honey-B.	Honeysuckle
horn-B.	Hornbeam
hott.	Hottonia palustris
hume.	Humea elegans
hura	Hura brasiliensis
hura-c.	Hura crepitans
hydrang.	Hydrangea arborescens
hydrin-m.	Hydrastininum muriaticum
hydrin-s.	Hydrastininum sulphuricum
hydr-m.	Hydrastinum muriaticum
hydr.	Hydrastis canadensis
hydrobr-ac.	Hydrobromicum acidum
hydrc.	Hydrocotyle asiatica
hydr-ac.	Hydrocyanicum acidum
hydrog.	Hydrogenum
iod-ac.	Hydroiodicum acidum
hydro-c.	Hydrophis cyanocinctus
hydro-v.	Hydrophyllum virginianum
hymosa	Hymosa
hym-c.	Hymenea coubaril
hyosin.	Hyoscinum bromhydricum
hyos.	Hyoscyamus niger
hyper.	Hypericum perforatum
hypoth.	Hypothalamus of the ox
hyssop.	Hyssopus officinalis
ias.	Iaspis
iber.	Iberis amara

ichth.	Ichthyolum
ictod.	Ictodes foetida
ign.	Ignatia amara
ilx-a.	Ilex aquifolium
ilx-c.	Ilex casseine
ilx-v.	Ilex vomitoria
illec.	Illecebrum
ig-a.	Immunoglobulin A
imp-B.	Impatiens
imp.	Imperatoria ostruthium
inca.	Incajea
indg.	Indigo tinctoria
ind.	Indium metallicum
indol.	Indolum
influ.	Influenzinum
ingluv.	Ingluvinum
insulin	Insulinum
il-two	Interleukin
inul.	Inula helenium
iodof.	Iodoformum
iodot.	Iodothyrinum, thryroiodinum
iod-ac.	Iodium acidum
iod.	Iodium purum
ip.	Ipecacuanha
ipom.	Ipomoea purpurea
ira	Ira terror
irid.	Iridium metallicum
irid-m.	Iridium muriaticum
iris-fa.	Iris factissima
iris-fl.	Iris florentina
iris-foe.	Iris foetidissima
iris-g.	Iris germanica
iris-ps.	Iris pseudacorus
iris-t.	Iris tenax
iris	Iris versicolor
irisin.	Irisinum
i-leuc.	Isoleucinum
itu	Itu
jab.	Jaborandi
jac-c.	Jacaranda caroba
jac.	Jacaranda gualandai
jal.	Jalapa
jasm.	Jasminum officinale
jatr.	Jatropha curcas
jatr-u.	Jatropha urens
jatz.	Jatzfeld
jeqol.	Jequiritolum
joan.	Joanesia asoca

juglin.	Juglandinum
jug-c.	Juglans cinerea
jug-r.	Juglans regia
junc.	Juncus effusus
junc-p.	Juncus pilosus
juni-b.	Juniperus brasiliensis
juni-c.	Juniperus communis
juni.	Juniperus virginianus
just.	Justicia adhatoda
just-r.	Justicia rubrum
kalam.	Kalamegh
kali-acet.	Kali aceticum
kali-ar.	Kali arsenicosum
kali-bi.	Kali bichromicum
kali-bit.	Kali bitartaricum
kali-br.	Kali bromatum
kali-c.	Kali carbonicum
kali-chl.	Kali chloricum
kali-chls.	Kali chlorosum
kali-chr.	Kali chromicum
kali-cit.	Kali citricum
kali-cy.	Kali cyanatum
kali-fcy.	Kali ferrocyanatum
kali-f.	Kali fluoricum
kali-hp.	Kali hypophosphoricum
kali-i.	Kali iodatum
kali-l.	Kali lacticum
kali-ma.	Kali manganicum
kali.	Kali metallicum
kali-m.	Kali muriaticum
kali-n.	Kali nitricum
kali-ox.	Kali oxalicum
kali-o.	Kali oxydatum
kali-p.	Kali phosphoricum
kali-pic.	Kali picricum
kali-picn.	Kali picronitricum
kali-sal.	Kali salicylicum
kali-sil.	Kali silicicum
kali-sula.	Kali sulphuratum
kali-s.	Kali sulphuricum
kali-s-chr.	Kali sulphuricum chromicum
kali-t.	Kali tartaricum
kali-tel.	Kali telluricum
kali-x.	Kali xanthogenicum
kalm.	Kalmia latifolia
kam.	Kamala
kaol.	Kaolinum
kara.	Karaka
karw-h.	Karwinskia humboldtiana
kerose.	Kerosenum
keroso.	Kerosolenum
keto-ac.	Ketoglutaricum acidum
kiss.	Kissingen aqua
knau.	Knautia arvensis
kola.	Kola
kosen	Kosen Soolbad
kou.	Kousso
kreos.	Kreosotum
kres.	Kresolum
kron.	Kronthal aqua
kryp.	Krypton
kurch.	Kurchi
labyr.	Labyrinthum
lac-c.	Lac caninum
lac-del.	Lac delphinum
lac-eq.	Lac equis
lac-f.	Lac felinum
lac-h.	Lac humanum
lac-leo.	Lac leonis
lac-urs.	Lac ursinum
lac-v-f.	Lac vaccini flos
lac-v.	Lac vaccinum
lac-v-b.	Lac vaccinum butyricum
lac-v-c.	Lac vaccinum coagulatum
lac-d.	Lac vaccinum defloratum
lacer.	Lacerta agilis
lach.	Lachesis muta
lachn.	Lachnanthes tinctoria
lac-ac.	Lacticum acidum
lact-e.	Lactuca elongata
lact-s.	Lactuca sativa
lact.	Lactuca virosa
laetr.	Laetril
lager	Lager beer
lamin.	Laminaria digitata
lam.	Lamium album
land.	Landeck aqua
lang.	Langebrunnen aqua
lanol.	Lanolinum
lant.	Lanthanum metallicum
lant-n.	Lanthanum nitricum
lant-o.	Lanthanum oxydatum
lant-s.	Lanthanum sulphuricum
lapa.	Lapathum acutum
lap-a.	Lapis albus
lappa	Lappa arctium

laps.	Lapsana communis
lar-B.	Larch
lath.	Lathyrus sativus
lat-h.	Latrodectus hasellti
lat-k.	Latrodectus katipo
lat-m.	Latrodectus mactans
laur.	Laurocerasus officinalis
lav-v.	Lavandula vera
lec.	Lecithinum
led.	Ledum palustre
lem-m.	Lemna minor
len-c.	Lens culinaris
leon.	Leonurus cardiaca
lepi.	Lepidium bonariense
lepro.	Leprominium
lept.	Leptandra virginica
leptol.	Leptolobium elegans
leptos.	Leptospira
lesp-c.	Lespedeza capitata
lesp-s.	Lespedeza sieboldii
leuc-a.	Leucas aspera
l-leuc.	Leucinum
lev.	Levico aqua
levi-o.	Levisticum officinale
levo.	Levomepromazine
liatr.	Liatris spicata
lig-v.	Ligustrum vulgaris
lil-s.	Lilium superbum
lil-t.	Lilium tigrinum
lim.	Limulus cyclops
lina.	Linaria vulgaris
linu-c.	Linum catharticum
linu-u	Linum usitatissimum
lip.	Lippia mexicana
lipp.	Lippspringe aqua
lith-be.	Lithium benzoicum
lith-br.	Lithium bromatum
lith-c.	Lithium carbonicum
lith-chl.	Lithium chloricum
lith-i.	Lithium iodatum
lith-l.	Lithium lacticum
lith.	Lithium metallicum
lith-m.	Lithium muriaticum
lith-p.	Lithium phosphoricum
lith-sal.	Lithium salicylicum
lith-s.	Lithium sulphuricum
loa.	Loasa tricolor
lob-c.	Lobelia cardinalis
lob-d.	Lobelia dortmanna
lob-e.	Lobelia erinus
lob.	Lobelia inflata
lob-p.	Lobelia purpurescens
lob-s.	Lobelia syphilitica
lobin.	Lobelinum
lol.	Lolium temulentum
lon-c.	Lonicera caprifolium
lon-p.	Lonicera periclymenum
lon-x.	Lonicera xylosteum
luf-act.	Luffa actangula
luf-a.	Luffa amara
luf-b.	Luffa bindal
luf-op.	Luffa operculata
luna	Luna
lupin.	Lupulinum
lup.	Lupulus humulus
lutein.	Luteinum
lycpr.	Lycopersicum esculentum
lyc.	Lycopodium clavatum
lycps.	Lycopus virginicus
lymph.	Lymphatica
lysid.	Lysidinum
lysim.	Lysimachia nummularia
lyss.	Lyssinum
lythr-s.	Lythrum salicaria
macrin.	Macrotinum
macroz.	Macrozamia spiralis
mag-acet.	Magnesia acetica
mag-bcit.	Magnesia borocitrica
mag-br.	Magnesia bromata
mag-c.	Magnesia carbonica
mag-f.	Magnesia fluorata
mag-i.	Magnesia iodata
mag-l.	Magnesia lactica
mag.	Magnesia metallica
mag-m.	Magnesia muriatica
mag-n.	Magnesia nitricum
mag-o.	Magnesia oxydatum
mag-p.	Magnesia phosphorica
mag-sil.	Magnesia silicata
mag-s.	Magnesia sulphurica
mag-u.	Magnesia usta
m-art.	Magnetis artificialis
m-p-a.	Magnetis poli ambo
m-arct.	Magnetis polus arcticus
m-aust.	Magnetis polus australis
magn-gl.	Magnolia glauca

magn-gr.	Magnolia grandiflora
maka.	Makaradhwaja
malatox.	Malaiatoxinum
maland.	Malandrinum
malar.	Malaria officinalis
malt	Malt
mal-p.	Malus pumila
malv.	Malva sylvestris
malvin.	Malvine
mamm.	Mamma glandula
manc.	Mancinella venenata
mand.	Mandragora officinarum
mang-coll	Manganum colloidale
mang-i.	Manganum iodatum
mang-l.	Manganum lacticum
mang-met.	Manganum metallicum
mang-m.	Manganum muriaticum
mang-o.	Manganum oxydatum nativum
mang-p.	Manganum phosphoricum
mang-s.	Manganum sulphuricum
mangi.	Mangifera indica
mannit.	Mannitol
mant-r.	Mantis religiosa
manz.	Manzanita
marien.	Marienbader Kruzbunner
marr.	Marrubium album
mate	Mate
mati.	Matico
matr-d.	Matricaria discoidea
matth.	Matthiola graeca
mec.	Meconinum
med.	Medorrhinum
medul-o.	Medulla ossea
medul-s.	Medulla spinalis
medus.	Medusa
mein.	Meinberg Pyrmont aqua
mel-c-s.	Mel cum sale
mel	Mel
melal.	Melaleuca hypericifolia
mela.	Melastoma ackermani
meli-a.	Melilotus alba
meli.	Melilotus officinalis
melis.	Melissa officinalis
melit.	Melitagrinum
meloe	Meloe majalis
meningoc.	Meningococcinum
menis.	Menispermum canadense
menth.	Mentha piperita
menth-pu.	Mentha pulegium
menth-v.	Mentha viridis
menthol	Mentholum
meny.	Menyanthes trifoliata
meph.	Mephitis putorius
merl.	Mercurialis perennis
merc-acet.	Mercurius aceticus
merc-aur.	Mercurius auratus
merc-k-i.	Mercurius biniodatus cum kali iodatum
merc-br.	Mercurius bromatus
merc-c.	Mercurius corrosivus
merc-cy.	Mercurius cyanatus
merc-d.	Mercurius dulcis
merc-f.	Mercurius fluoratus
merc-i-f.	Mercurius iodatus flavus
merc-i-r.	Mercurius iodatus ruber
merc-meth.	Mercurius methylenus
merc-n.	Mercurius nitrosus
merc-p.	Mercurius phosphoricus
merc-pr-a.	Mercurius praecipitatus albus
merc-pr-f.	Mercurius praecipitatus flavus
merc-pr-r.	Mercurius praecipitatus ruber
merc-r.	Mercurius rhodanatus
merc.	Mercurius solubilis Hahnemanni
merc-s-cy.	Mercurius sulphocyanatus
merc-s.	Mercurius sulphuricus
merc-tn.	Mercurius tannicus
mese-c.	Mesembrianthemum cristallinum
methion.	Methioninum
methyl-chl.	Methylenum bichloratum
methyl.	Methylenum coeruleum
methyl-sal.	Methylenum salicylicum
meth-ae-ae.	Methylium aethyloaethereum
methys.	Methysergidum
mez.	Mezereum
mica	Mica
micr.	Micromeria douglasii
mika.	Mikania setigera
mill.	Millefolium
mim-h.	Mimosa humilis
mim-p.	Mimosa pudica
mimul-b.	Mimulus
mimul.	Mimulus
mimul-l.	Mimulus luteus
miss.	Mississquoi aqua
mit.	Mitchella repens

moly.	Molybdaenum metallicum
moly-m.	Molybdaenum muriaticum
mom-b.	Momordica balsamica
mom-ch.	Momordica charantia
mom-p.	Momordica purgans
moni.	Monilia albicans
mono.	Monotropa uniflora
mons.	Monsonia ovata
monst.	Monstera pertusa
morbill.	Morbillinum
morg-g.	Morgan Gaertner
morg.	Morgan pure by Paterson
morph.	Morphinum aceticum
morph-m.	Morphinum muriaticum
morph-s.	Morphinum sulphuricum
mor-n.	Morus nigra
mosch.	Moschus moschiferus
mucor	Mucor mucedo
muc-nas.	Mucosa nasalis
mucot.	Mucotoxinum
muc-u.	Mucuna urens
murx.	Murex purpurea
mur-ac.	Muriaticum acidum
muru.	Murure leite
musa	Musa sapientum
musan.	Musanna
muscin.	Muscarinum
must-B.	Mustard
mut.	Mutabile
mygal.	Mygale lasiodora
myocard.	Myocardium
myos-a.	Myosotis arvensis
myos.	Myosotis symphytifolia
myric.	Myrica cerifera
myrin.	Myricin
myris.	Myristica sebifera
myrrh.	Myrrha
myrt-ch.	Myrtus cheken
myrt-c.	Myrtus communis
myrt-p.	Myrtus pimenta
n-leuc.	Norleucinum
nabal.	Nabalus serpentaria
naja	Naja tripudians
napin.	Napellin
napht.	Naphtha
naphtin.	Naphthalinum
narcin.	Narceinum
narc-po.	Narcissus poeticus
narc-ps.	Narcissus pseudonarcissus
narcot-acet.	Narcotinum aceticum
narcot-m.	Narcotinum muriaticum
narcot.	Narcotinum pura
narz.	Narzan aqua
nast.	Nasturtium aquaticum
nat-acet.	Natrum aceticum
nat-ae-s.	Natrum aethylosulphuricum
nat-ar.	Natrum arsenicum
nat-a-g.	Natrum arsenicum gaertner
nat-bic.	Natrum bicarbonicum
nat-br.	Natrum bromatum
nat-cac.	Natrum cacodylicum
nat-c.	Natrum carbonicum
nat-caust.	Natrum causticum
nat-ch.	Natrum choleinicum
nat-f.	Natrum fluoratum
nat-h.	Natrum hypochlorosum
nat-hchls.	Natrum hyposulphuricum
nat-hsulo.	Natrum hyposulphurosum
nat-i.	Natrum iodatum
nat-l.	Natrum lacticum
nat.	Natrum metallicum
nat-m.	Natrum muriaticum
nat-mar.	Natrum marinum
nat-n.	Natrum nitricum
nat-ns.	Natrum nitrosum
nat-o.	Natrum oxydatum
nat-ox.	Natrum oxalaceticum
nat-p.	Natrum phosphoricum
nat-sal.	Natrum salicylicum
nat-sel.	Natrum selenicum
nat-sil.	Natrum silicicum
nat-sil-f.	Natrum silicofluoricum
nat-suc.	Natrum succinicum
nat-s-c.	Natrum sulphocarbolicum
nat-sula.	Natrum sulphuratum
nat-s.	Natrum sulphuricum
nat-sulo.	Natrum sulphurosum
nat-taur.	Natrum taurocholicum
nat-tel.	Natrum telluricum
nat-uric.	Natrum uricum
nax.	Naxolone
nect.	Nectandra amare
nectrin.	Nectrianinum
neg.	Negundium americanum
nelu.	Nelubrium luteum
neon	Neon

nep.	Nepenthes distillatoria
nepet.	Nepeta cataria
neri-o.	Nerium odorum
nerv-au.	Nervus auditorius
neur.	Neurinum
nicc-br.	Niccolum bromatum
nicc.	Niccolum carbonicum
nicc-f.	Niccolum fluoratum
nicc-o.	Niccolum oxydatum
nicc-sil.	Niccolum silicatum
nicc-s.	Niccolum sulphuricum
nad	Nicotinamide adenine dinucleotide
nicot.	Nicotinum
nid.	Nidus edulis
nig-d.	Nigella damascena
nig-s.	Nigella sativa
niob.	Niobium metallicum
niob-m.	Niobium muriaticum
nit-s-d.	Nitri spiritus dulcis
nit-ac.	Nitricum acidum
nitro-benz.	Nitro benzenum
nitro-o.	Nitrogenum oxygenatum
nitro.	Nitrogenum purum
nit-m-ac.	Nitromuriaticum acidum
note-s.	Notechis scutatus
nuph.	Nuphar luteum
nux-a.	Nux absurda
nux-m.	Nux moschata
nux-v.	Nux vomica
nyct.	Nyctanthes arbor-tristis
nycte.	Nycterinia capensis
nym-a.	Nymphaea alba
nym.	Nymphaea odorata
oak-B.	Oak
oci-b.	Ocimum basilicum
oci.	Ocimum canum
oci-c.	Ocimum caryophyllatum
oci-g.	Ocimum gratissimum
oci-s.	Ocimum sanctum
oena.	Oenanthe crocata
oeno.	Oenothera biennis
oest.	Oestrus cameli
okou.	Okoubaka aubrevillei
old-h.	Oldenlandia herbacia
olea	Olea europea
olnd.	Oleander
ol-an.	Oleum animale aethereum Dippeli
ol-car.	Oleum caryophyllatum
ol-j.	Oleum jecoris aselli
ol-jo.	Oleum jofar
ol-myr.	Oleum myristicae
ol-p.	Oleum patchouli
ol-sant.	Oleum santali
ol-suc.	Oleum succinum
oliv-B.	Olive
onis.	Oniscus asellus
onon.	Ononis spinosa
onop.	Onopordon acanthium
onos.	Onosmodium virginianum
oper.	Operculina turpethum
op.	Opium
opl.	Oplia farinosa
opun-a.	Opuntia alba spina
opun-v.	Opuntia vulgaris
orch.	Orchitinum
oreo.	Oreodaphne californica
orig.	Origanum majorana
orig-v.	Origanum vulgare
orni.	Ornithogalum umbellatum
oro-ac.	Oroticum acidum
orthos.	Orthosiphon stamineus
oste.	Os
oscilloc.	Oscillococcinum
osm.	Osmium metallicum
o-a-n.	Osteo Arthritic Nosode
ost.	Ostrya virginiana
ouabin.	Ouabainum
ovar.	Ovarium
ovi-g-p.	Ovi gallinae pellicula
ov.	Ovininum
ox-ac.	Oxalicum acidum
oxal.	Oxalis acetosella
oxyd.	Oxydendron arboreum
oxyg.	Oxygenium
oxyt.	Oxytropis lamberti
oxyu-m.	Oxyuranus microlepidotus
oxyu-s.	Oxyuranus scuttellatus
ozone	Ozonum
paeon.	Paeonia officinalis
pall-f.	Palladium fluoratum
pall.	Palladium metallicum
pall-m.	Palladium muriaticum
pall-o.	Palladium oxydatum
palo.	Paloondo

pana.	Panacea arvensis
pancreat.	Pancreatinum
pap-r.	Papaver rhoeas
papin.	Papaverinum
pap-v.	Papaya vulgaris
paraf.	Paraffinum
paraph.	Paraphenylene diamine
paron.	Parathion
parath.	Parathyreoid glands
parathyr.	Parathyreoidinum
parat.	Paratyphoidinum B
pareir.	Pareira brava
pariet.	Parietaria officinalis
par.	Paris quadrifolia
paro-i.	Paronichia illecebrum
parot.	Parotidinum
parth.	Parthenium hysterophorus
passi.	Passiflora incarnata
past.	Pastinaca sativa
paull-p.	Paullinia pinnata
paull.	Paullinia sorbilis
pect.	Pecten jacobaeus
pedi-can.	Pedicularis canadensis
ped.	Pediculus capitis
peg-h.	Peganum harmala
pelarg.	Pelargonium reniforme
pellin.	Pellitierinum
penic.	Penicillinum
pen.	Penthorum sedoides
pep.	Pepsinum
perh.	Perhexiline
peri.	Periploca graeca
pern-c.	Pernus canaliculus
pers.	Persea americana
per.	Pertussinum
pest.	Pestinum
peti.	Petiveria tetrandra
petr.	Petroleum
petros.	Petroselinum sativum
phal.	Phallus impudicus
phase.	Phaseolus nanus
phel.	Phellandrium aquaticum
phenac.	Phenacetinum
phenob.	Phenobarbitalum
d-phenyl.	Phenylalaninum D-phenylalaninum
l-phenyl.	Phenylalaninum L-phenylalaninum
phle.	Phleum pratense
phlor.	Phlorizinum
ph-ac.	Phosphoricum acidum
phos-h.	Phosphorus hydrogenatus
phos-pchl.	Phosphorus muriaticus
phos.	Phosphorus Phosphorus
phos-i.	Phosphorus triiodatus
physala-p.	Physalia physalis
physal.	Physalis alkekengi
phys.	Physostigma venenosum
phyt-b.	Phytolacca berry
phyt.	Phytolacca decandra
pice-e.	Picea excelsa
pic-ac.	Picricum acidum
pictx-ac.	Picrotoxicum acidum
picro.	Picrotoxinum
piloc.	Pilocarpinum hydrochloricum
pime.	Pimenta officinalis
pimp-a.	Pimpinella anisum
pimp.	Pimpinella saxifraga
pine-B.	Pine
pineal.	Pineal gland
pin-c.	Pinus cupressus
pin-l.	Pinus lambertiana
pin-s.	Pinus sylvestris
pip-m.	Piper methysticum
pip-n.	Piper nigrum
pipe.	Piperazinum
pisc.	Piscidia erythrina
pitu-gl.	Pituitaria glandula
pitu-a.	Pituitaria glandula anterior
pitu-p.	Pituitaria glandula posterior
pix.	Pix liquida
plac-s.	Placenta suis
plac.	Placenta humana
plan.	Plantago major
plan-m.	Plantago minor
platan.	Platanus occidentalis
plat-f.	Platinum fluoratum
plat.	Platinum metallicum
plat-m.	Platinum muriaticum
plat-m-n.	Platinum muriaticum natronatum
plect.	Plectranthus fruticosus
plumbg-eu.	Plumbago europaeus
plumbg.	Plumbago littoralis
plb.	Plumbum metallicum
plb-acet.	Plumbum aceticum

plb-ae.	Plumbum tetraethylicum
plb-ar.	Plumbum arsenicosum
plb-chr.	Plumbum chromicum
plb-f.	Plumbum fluoratum
plb-i.	Plumbum iodatum
plb-m.	Plumbum muriaticum
plb-n.	Plumbum nitricum
plb-o.	Plumbum oxidatum
plb-p.	Plumbum phosphoricum
plb-s.	Plumbum sulphuricum
plume.	Plumeria celinus
plut-n.	Plutonium nitricum
pneu.	Pneumococcus
podin.	Podophyllin
podo.	Podophyllum peltatum
poll.	Pollantinum
polo.	Polonium metallicum
polya.	Polyandra poligama
poly-a.	Polygala amara
polygo-o.	Polygonatum officinale
polyg-a.	Polygonum aviculare
polyg.	Polygonum hydropiperoides
polyg-pe.	Polygonum persicaria
polyg-s.	Polygonum sagittatum
polym.	Polymnia uvedalia
pol-v.	Polypodium vulgare
polyp-n.	Polyporus nigricans
polyp-p	Polyporus pinicola
polytr.	Polytrichum juniperinum
pop-c.	Populus candicans
pop.	Populus tremuloides
pot-a.	Potentilla anserina
pot-au.	Potentilla aurea
pot-r.	Potentilla reptans
pot-t.	Potentilla tormentilla
pren.	Prenanthes serpens
prim-f.	Primula farinosa
prim-o.	Primula obconica
prim-v.	Primula veris
prim-vul.	Primula vulgaris
prin.	Prinos verticillatus
prol.	Prolina
propol.	Propanolol
propo.	Propolis
prop.	Propylaminum
prost.	Prostatinum
prot.	Proteus
prune.	Prunella vulgaris
prun-c.	Prunus cerasus
prun-d.	Prunus domestica
prun-m.	Prunus mahaleb
prun-p.	Prunus padus e cortice
prun.	Prunus spinosa
prun-v.	Prunus virginiana
psil.	Psilocybe caerulescens
psoral.	Psoralea bituminosa
psoral-c.	Psoralea corylifolia
psor.	Psorinum
ptel.	Ptelea trifoliata
ptych-o.	Ptychopetalum olacoides
pulx.	Pulex irritans
pull-g.	Pullus gallinaceus
pulm-a.	Pulmo anaphylacticus
pulm.	Pulmo pura
pulm-v.	Pulmo vulpis
pul-o.	Pulmonaria officinalis
puls.	Pulsatilla nigricans
puls-n	Pulsatilla nuttalliana
pyrar.	Pyrarara
pyre-o.	Pyrethrum officinarum
pyre-p.	Pyrethrum parthenium
pyre-r.	Pyrethrum roseum e floribus
pyro-r.	Pyrola rotundifolia
pyrog.	Pyrogenium
pyrol.	Pyrola rotundifolia
pyro-ac.	Pyrolignosum acidum
pyrus	Pyrus americanus
pyrus-m.	Pyrus malus
quas.	Quassia amara
queb.	Quebracho
querc.	Quercus e glandibus
quill.	Quillaya saponaria
rad-br.	Radium bromatum
rado.	Radon
raja-s.	Rajania subsamarata
ran-a.	Ranunculus acris
ran-b.	Ranunculus bulbosus
ran-fi.	Ranunculus ficaria
ran-fl.	Ranunculus flammula
ran-g.	Ranunculus glacialis
ran-r.	Ranunculus repens
ran-s.	Ranunculus sceleratus
raphani.	Raphanistrum arvense
raph.	Raphanus sativus
rat.	Ratanhia peruviana
rauw.	Rauwolfia serpentina

rd-ch-B.	Red Chestnut
rein.	Reinerz aqua
ren	Ren
resc-B.	Rescue remedy
reser.	Reserpine
res.	Resorcinum
ret.	Retina
rham-cal.	Rhamnus californica
rham-cath.	Rhamnus cathartica
rham-f.	Rhamnus frangula
rham-p.	Rhamnus purshiana
rhen.	Rhenium metallicum
rheum	Rheum palmatum
rhodi.	Rhodium metallicum
rhodi-o-n.	Rhodium oxydatum nitricum
rhod.	Rhododendron chrysanthum
rhus-a.	Rhus aromatica
rhus-c.	Rhus cotinus
rhus-d.	Rhus diversiloba
rhus-g.	Rhus glabra
rhus-l.	Rhus laurina
rhus-t.	Rhus toxicodendron
rhus-v.	Rhus venenata
ribs-n.	Ribes nigrum
rib-ac.	Ribonucleinicum acidum
ric.	Ricinus communis
rizo.	Rizophora mangle
rob.	Robinia pseudacacia
rck-r-B.	Rock rose
rck-w-B.	Rock water
ros-ca.	Rosa canina
ros-ce.	Rosa centifolia
ros-d.	Rosa damascena
rosm.	Rosmarinus officinalis
rub-t.	Rubia tinctorum
rubi.	Rubidium metallicum
rubi-m.	Rubidium muriaticum
rubu-ch.	Rubus chamaemorus
rubu-f.	Rubus fructicosus
rubu.	Rubus villosus
rumx-a.	Rumex acetosa
rumx.	Rumex crispus
russ.	Russula foetens
ruta	Ruta graveolens
ruth.	Ruthenium metallicum
ruth-m.	Ruthenium muriaticum
sabad.	Sabadilla officinalis
sabal.	Sabal serrulata

saba.	Sabatia angularis
sabin.	Sabina officinalis
sacchin.	Sacharinum
sac-l.	Sacharum lactis
sac-alb.	Sacharum officinale
sal-mar.	Sal marinum
salam-l.	Salamandra lacerta
salam.	Salamandra maculosa
salin.	Salicinum
sal-ac.	Salicylicum acidum
salx-a.	Salix alba
salx-m.	Salix mollissima
salx-n.	Salix nigra
salx-p.	Salix purpurea
salx-v.	Salix vitellina
salol.	Salol
salv.	Salvia officinalis
salv-sc.	Salvia sclarea
samars.	Samarsite
samb-c.	Sambucus canadensis
samb-e.	Sambucus ebulus
samb.	Sambucus nigra
sang.	Sanguinaria canadensis
sanguin-n.	Sanguinarinum nitricum
sanguin.	Sanguinarinum pura
sanguin-t.	Sanguinarinum tartaricum
sanguis.	Sanguisorba officinalis
sanic.	Sanicula aqua
sani-eu.	Sanicula europaea
santa.	Santalum album
sant.	Santoninum
sap-sod.	Sap soda
sapo.	Saponaria officinalis
sapin.	Saponinum
sarcol-ac.	Sarcolacticum acidum
saroth.	Sarothamnus scoparius
sarr.	Sarracenia purpurea
sars.	Sarsaparilla officinalis
sass.	Sassafras officinalis
sat-h.	Satureja hortensis
saur.	Saururus cernuus
saxi-g.	Saxifraga granulata
saxon.	Saxonite
scab-s.	Scabiosa succisa
scam.	Scammonium
scan.	Scandium metallicum
scarl.	Scarlatininum
schin.	Schinus molle

scirr.	Scirrhinum
scler-B.	Scleranthus
scler-a.	Scleranthus annuus
scol.	Scolopendra morsitans
scolo-v.	Scolopendrium vulgare
scopo.	Scopolia carniolica
scorp.	Scorpio italicus
scroph-n.	Scrophularia nodosa
scut.	Scutellaria laterifolia
sec.	Secale cornutum
secret.	Secretinum
sedi.	Sedinha
sed-ac.	Sedum acre
sed-r.	Sedum repens
sed-t.	Sedum telephium
sela.	Selaginella species
sel.	Selenium
sem-t.	Semen tiglii
semp.	Sempervivum tectorum
senecin.	Senecinum
senec.	Senecio aureus
senec-j.	Senecio jacoboea
seneg.	Senega officinalis
senn.	Senna
sep.	Sepia succus
sepin	Sepin
septi.	Septicaeminum
seq-s.	Sequoia sempervirens
serot.	Serotoninum
serp.	Serpentaria aristolochia
ser-ang.	Serum anguillae
ser-a-c.	Serum anti-colibacillum
ser-eq.	Serum equi
shucks	Shucks
sieg.	Siegesbeckia orientalis
sil-mar.	Silica marina
sil.	Silica terra
sil-met.	Silicium metallicum
silpho.	Silphion cyrenaicum
silphu.	Silphium laciniatum
sima.	Simaruba amara
sima-v.	Simaruba versicolor
sin-a.	Sinapis alba
sin-ar.	Sinapis arvensis
sin-n.	Sinapis nigra
sinusin.	Sinusitisinum
sisy.	Sisyrinchium glaxoides
sium	Sium latifolium
skat.	Skatolum
skook.	Skookum chuck aqua
slag	Slag
smilin.	Smilacinum
sol	Sol
solin.	Solaninum aceticum
sol-a.	Solanum arrebenta
sol-c.	Solanum carolinense
sol-i.	Solanum integri
sol-m.	Solanum mammosum
sol-n.	Solanum nigrum
sol-o.	Solanum oleraceum
sol-ps.	Solanum pseudocapsicum
sol-t.	Solanum tuberosum
sol-t-ae.	Solanum tuberosum aegrotans
sol-x.	Solanum xanthocarpus
solid.	Solidago virga aurea
sorb-au.	Sorbus aucuparia
sphing.	Sphingurus martini
spig.	Spigelia anthelmia
spig-m.	Spigelia marilandica
spirae.	Spiraea ulmaria
spira.	Spiranthes autumnalis
splen.	Splenum
spong.	Spongia tosta
squil.	Squilla maritima
stach.	Stachys betonica
stann-i.	Stannum iodatum
stann.	Stannum metallicum
stann-m.	Stannum muriaticum
stann-s.	Stannum sulphuricum
staphycoc.	Staphylococcinum
staphytox.	Staphylotoxicum
staph.	Staphysagria
star-b-B.	Star of Bethlehem
stel.	Stellaria media
stict.	Sticta pulmonaria
stigm.	Stigmata maydis
still.	Stillingia sylvatica
stom.	Stomachus
stovain	Stovaine
stram.	Stramonium
strept-ent.	Strepto-enterococcus
strept.	Streptococcinum
strep-s.	Streptomycinum sulphuricum
stront-br.	Strontium bromatum
stront-c.	Strontium carbonicum
stront-i.	Strontium iodatum

stront.	Strontium metallicum
stront-m.	Strontium muriaticum
stront-n.	Strontium nitricum
stront-o.	Strontium oxydatum
stroph.	Strophanthus hispidus
stroph-s.	Strophanthus sarmentosus
stry-ar.	Strychninum arsenicosum
stry-f-c.	Strychninum et ferri citras
stry-n.	Strychninum nitricum
stry-p.	Strychninum phosphoricum
stry.	Strychninum purum
stry-s.	Strychninum sulphuricum
stry-val.	Strychninum valerianicum
succ-ac.	Succinum acidum
succ.	Succinum purum
succ-fr.	Succus fruti
sulfa.	Sulfanilamide
sulfon.	Sulfonalum
sulfonam.	Sulfonamide
sulph.	Sulphur
sulph.	Sulphur lotum
sul-h.	Sulphur hydrogenisatum
sul-i.	Sulphur iodatum
sul-ter.	Sulphur terebinthinatum
sul-ac.	Sulphuricum acidum
sul-ac-ar.	Sulphuricum acidum aromaticum
sulo-ac.	Sulphurosum acidum
sumb.	Sumbulus moschatus
supren.	Suprarenalis glandula
supren-cort.	Suprarenalis cortex
sw-ch-B.	Sweet chestnut
swer-ch.	Swertia chirata
sym-r.	Symphoricarpus racemosus
symph.	Symphytum officinale
syph.	Syphilinum
syr.	Syringa vulgaris
syzyg.	Syzygium jambolanum
tab.	Tabacum
tama.	Tamarindus indica
tam.	Tamus communis
tanac.	Tanacetum vulgare
tang.	Tanghinia venenifera
tann-ac.	Tannicum acidum
tant-f.	Tantalum fluoratum
tant.	Tantalum metallicum
tarax.	Taraxacum officinale
tarent-c.	Tarentula cubensis
tarent.	Tarentula hispanica
tart-ac.	Tartaricum acidum
taurin.	Taurine
tax.	Taxus baccata
tech.	Technetium metallicum
tein.	Teinach aqua
tela	Tela araneae
tell-ac.	Telluricum acidum
tell.	Tellurium
tep.	Teplitz aqua
terebe.	Terebenum
tere-ch.	Terebinthina chios
ter.	Terebinthiniae oleum
term-a.	Terminalia arjuna
term-c.	Terminalia chebula
terp-h.	Terpini hydras
testis	Testis
tetox.	Tetanotoxinum
tet.	Tetradymitum
teucr.	Teucrium marum verum
teucr-s.	Teucrium scorodonia
thala.	Thalamus
thal-f.	Thallium fluoratum
thal.	Thallium metallicum
thal-m.	Thallium muriaticum
thal-n.	Thallium nitricum
thal-o.	Thallium oxydatum
thal-s.	Thallium sulphuricum
thap-g.	Thapsia garganica
thea.	Thea sinensis
thebin.	Thebainum
ther.	Theridion curassavicum
thev.	Thevetia nerifolia
thio-ac.	Thiocticum acidum
thiop.	Thioproperazine
thiosin.	Thiosinaminum
thiot.	Thiotepa
thlaspi	Thlaspi bursa pastoris
threnin.	Threonine
thuj-l.	Thuja lobii
thuj.	Thuja occidentalis
thym-gl.	Thymi glandulae extractum
thymol.	Thymol
thymu.	Thymus serpyllum
thyreotr.	Thyreotropinum
thyr.	Thyroidinum
til.	Tilia europea
tinos.	Tinospora cordifolia

tip. Tipida aqua
titan. Titanium metallicum
titan-o. Titanium oxydatum
titan-s. Titanium sulphuricum
tong. Tongo
torul. Torula cerevisiae
tox-th. Toxicophloea thunbergi
toxo. Toxoplasms gondi
trach. Trachinus draco
trad. Tradescantia diuretica
triat. Triatema infestans
trib. Tribulus terrestris
trich-d. Trichosanthes dioica
trif-a. Trifolium arvense
trif-p. Trifolium pratense
trif-r. Trifolium repens
trig-f-g. Trigonella foenum graecum
trig-p. Trigonocephalus piscivorus
tril-c. Trillium cernuum
tril. Trillium pendulum
trim. Trimeresurus wagleri
trinit. Trinitrotoluene
trion. Trional
trio. Triosteum perfoliatum
tritic. Triticum repens
trito Trito
triu-s. Triumfetta semitriloba
trom. Trombidium muscae domesticae
trop. Tropaeolum majus
tuba Tuba fallopii
tub-a. Tuberculinum avis
tub. Tuberculinum bovinum Kent
tub-d. Tuberculinum denys
tub-k. Tuberculinum koch
tub-lar. Tuberculinum laricus
tub-m. Tuberculinum marmoreck
tub-r. Tuberculinum residuum Koch
tub-sp. Tuberculinum spengler
tung. Tungsten metallicum
tung-m. Tungsten muriaticum
tus-fa. Tussilago farfara
tus-f. Tussilago fragrans
tus-p. Tussilago petasites
tylo-i. Tylophora indica
typh. Typha latifolia
tyr. Tyraminum
tyrin. Tyrosinum
ulm. Ulmus fulva
ulm-p. Ulmus procera
upa-a. Upas antiaris
upa. Upas tieuté
uran-ar. Uranium arsenicicum
uran. Uranium metallicum
uran-m. Uranium muriaticum
uran-n. Uranium nitricum
urea-n. Urea nitrica
urea Urea pura
ur-ac. Uricum acidum
urine Urinum
urotrop. Urotropinum
urt-c. Urtica crenulata
urt-g. Urtica gigas
urt-u. Urtica urens
usn. Usnea barbata
ust. Ustilago maydis
uter. Uterus
uva. Uva-ursi
uvar. Uvaria triloba
uza. Uzara
v-a-b. Vaccin attenu bili
vacc-m. Vaccinium myrtillus
vac. Vaccinotoxinum
valer. Valeriana officinalis
vali. Valinum
vanad. Vanadium metallicum
vanad-f. Vanadium fluoricum
vanad-o. Vanadium oxydatum
vanad-s. Vanadium sulphuricum
vanil. Vanilla aromatica
vario. Variolinum
vena Vena
ven-m. Venus mercenaria
verin. Veratrinum
verat. Veratrum album
verat-n. Veratrum nigrum
verat-v. Veratrum viride
verb-n. Verbascum nigrum
verb. Verbascum thapsus
Hahnemanni, thapsiforme
verbe-h. Verbena hastata
verbe-u. Verbena urticaefolia
vern-a. Vernonia anthelminthica
veronal Veronal
vero-a. Veronica arvensis
vero-b. Veronica beccabunga
vero-o. Veronica officinalis

verr.	Verrucinum
verv-B.	Vervain
ves-u.	Vesica urinaria
vesi.	Vesicaria communis
vesp.	Vespa crabro
vibh.	Vibhuti
vib-od.	Viburnum oderatissinum
vib.	Viburnum opulus
vib-p.	Viburnum prunifolium
vib-t.	Viburnum tinus
vichy-g.	Vichy aqua grande grille
vichy-h.	Vichy aqua hospital
vinc.	Vinca minor
vince.	Vincetoxicum officinale
vine-B.	Vinum
viol-o.	Viola odorata
viol-t.	Viola tricolor
vip-a.	Vipera aspis
vip.	Vipera berus
vip-r.	Vipera redi
visc.	Viscum album
visc-q.	Viscum quercinum
vita-a.	Vitamine A
vita-d.	Vitamine D
vita-e.	Vitamine E
vit.	Vitex trifolia
vitis	Vitis vinifera
vitr.	Vitrum antimonii
voes.	Voeslau aqua
waln-B.	Walnut
wat-v-B.	Water violet
weil.	Weilbach aqua
wh-ch-B.	White chestnut
wies.	Wiesbaden aqua
wld-o-B.	Wild oat
wld-r-B.	Wild rose
wild.	Wildbad aqua
will-B.	Willow
wist.	Wisteria species
with-s.	Withania somnifera
wye.	Wyethia helenoides
x-ray	X-rays
xanth.	Xanthium spinosum
xanrhi.	Xanthorrhiza apifolia
xanrhoe.	Xanthorrhoea arborea
xan.	Xanthoxylum fraxineum
xeno.	Xenon
xero	Xerophyllum

yersin	Yersin
yohim	Yohimbinum
yttr.	Yttrium metallicum
yttr-o.	Yttrium oxydatum
yuc.	Yucca filamentosa
zea-i.	Zea italica
zinc-acet.	Zincum aceticum
zinc-ar.	Zincum arsenicosum
zinc-br.	Zincum bromatum
zinc-c.	Zincum carbonicum
zinc-chr.	Zincum chromatum
zinc-cy.	Zincum cyanatum
zinc-fcy.	Zincum ferrocyanatum
zinc-f.	Zincum fluoratum
zinc-i.	Zincum iodatum
zinc.	Zincum metallicum
zinc-m.	Zincum muriaticum
zinc-n.	Zincum nitricum
zinc-o.	Zincum oxydatum
zinc-p.	Zincum phosphoricum
zinc-pic.	Zincum picricum
zinc-s.	Zincum sulphuricum
zinc-sil.	Zincum silicatum
zinc-val.	Zincum valerianicum
zing.	Zingiber officinale
zirc.	Zirconium metallicum
ziz.	Zizia aurea
ziz-i.	Zizia italica

*	Kent from subrubrics	56349
1	Hahnemann S.	49379
2	Stapf E.	70
3	Caspari	3
4	Noack A.	8
5	Bönninghausen C. von	134598
8	Hering C.	5825
10	Jahr. G.	14434
11	Lilienthal S.	32
13	Seidel E.	2
15	Hempel Ch.	47
16	Popham	4
20	Teste A.	101
22	Lippe A.	38
23	Vulpian	4
25	Hale E.	640
26	Minton H.	2043
28	Dunham C.	99
29	Fincke B.	36
30	Gallavardin J.P.	3544
31	Guernsey H.N.	1401
32	Ruddock E.H.	3
34	Gilchrist J.G.	1650
35	Gross H.	10
36	Allen T.F.	33642
37	Hoyne T.S.	429
38	Hughes R.	765
39	Bell J.B.	61
40	Berridge E.W.	17
41	Angell H.C.	4
42	James B.W.	66
44	Simmons B.	33
45	Macfarlan M.	43
46	Burt W.	327
47	Farrington E.A.	364
48	Gentry W.	43
49	Hale R.D.	7
51	Cowperthwaite A.C.	208
52	Skinner T.	3
53	Fellows H.B.	16
54	Knerr C.B.	30496
55	Swan S.	99
56	Allen H.C.	930
57	Guernsey Wm. J.	22
58	Kent J.T. Materia Medica	28955
59	King Jno.	141
60	Lippe C.	895
61	Schuessler W.H.	12
62	Burnett J.C.	677
63	Lee E.J.	30
64	Armstrong W.P.	59
65	Allen W.A.	178
66	Evans W.H.	3
70	Winterburn G.W.	47
71	Fisher C.E.	44
72	Boericke W.	2242
73	Case E.E.	23
75	Shultz	3
76	Snader E.R.	2
77	Anshutz E.P.	622
78	Dewey W.A.	26
79	Lutze F.H.	1
80	Morgan A.R.	3
81	Santee E.M.	4
82	Smith C.C.	4
83	Dudgeon R.E.	485
85	Clarke J.H.	14985
86	Holcombe A.W.	1
88	Yingling W.A.	69
89	Deschere	3
91	Pulford A.	89
92	Wood J.C.	5
93	Hansen O.	54
94	Allen J.H.	34
95	Mersch	27
96	Hayes R.E.S.	17
97	Ghose S.C.	107
98	Gladwin F.E.	77
99	Stearns G.B.	4
100	Blackwood A.L.	284
101	Dienst G.E.	17
102	Boericke O.	44457
103	Nash E.B.	124
104	Duprat H.	27
105	Rice P.	3
106	Burgess Webster M.	55
107	Moffat J.L.	28
108	Tyler M.L.	98
109	Vannier L., Poirier J.	98
110	Grimmer A.H.	31
111	Boger C.M.	6869
112	Weir J.	23
113	Griggs W.B.	19
114	Royal G.	67
115	Schulz H.	9
116	Stauffer K.	3344
117	Leeser O.	85
118	Neatby E.A., Neatby T.M.	1
119	Stephenson J.	5312
120	Bach E.	14
121	Olds S.C.L.	6
122	Schmidt P.	7543
123	Ward J.W.	102
125	McLaren K.A.	1
126	Wright-Hubbard E.	16

127	Borland D.M.	231
128	Schmidt R.A.	5
129	Waffensmidt J.W.	1
130	Del Mas R.	73
132	Divanji V.G.	2
133	Pfleiderer	1
134	Ross T.D.	6
135	Lathoud J.A.	65
136	Paterson J.	2470
137	Phatak S.R.	21697
138	Templeton W.L.	39
139	Roberts H.A.	578
140	Green J.	49
141	Bhanja K.C.	20
142	Voisin H.	583
143	Gutman W.	1
144	Mezger J.	3844
146	Foubister D.M.	120
147	Paschero P.	23
148	Künzli J.	253
149	Julian O.	4192
150	Rogers R.T.	1
151	Zissu R.	20
152	Lodispoto A.	241
153	Vijnovksy B.	12
154	Hui Bon Hoa J.	18
155	Gibson D.M.	47
156	Sankaran P.	77
157	Seror R.	2
159	Imhäuser H.	21
160	Mathur K.N.	34
161	Whitmont E.	35
162	Vithoulkas G.	2399
163	Flury R.	352
164	Flores Toledo D.	1777
166	Pladys A.	18
167	Schepens E.	1
168	Blackie M.G.	199
169	Imberechts J.	2
170	Ortega P.S.	12
171	Choudhuri N.M.	1260
172	Fayazuddin M.	826
173	Keller G. von	5
175	Eizayaga F.	124
176	Masi Elizalde A.	2
178	Boyd H.	2
179	Candegabe E.	38
181	Vrijlandt A.	113
182	Mundy D.	15
183	Gray B.	7
184	Geukens A.	358
185	Ghegas V.	358
186	Lamothe J.	7
187	Morrison R.	379
188	Vermeulen F.	27
189	Coulter C.R.	172
190	Degroote P.	7
192	CCRH	655
193	Dockx R., Kokelenberg G.	2692
194	Eising N.	1274
195	Bishambar Das	1
196	Shore J.	10
197	Prakash V.	2
198	Zaren A.	182
201	Collins D.	37
202	Guess G.	6
205	Klein L.	3
206	Logan R.	9
207	Micklem R.	330
209	Scholten J.	84
210	Smits T.	325
212	Herscu P.	120
214	Sankaran R.	45
215	Shah Y.	2
216	Banerjea S.K.	1
219	Digby B.	2
220	Moskowitz D.	16
222	Sherr J.	4209
223	Murphy R.	14
224	Coppé Y.	16
225	Heudens H.	3
226	Witzig F.	33
227	Schadde A.	2170
228	King L., Lawrence B.	33
229	Houghton J., Halahan E.	103
230	Birch K, Rockwell J.	32
231	Mangialavori M.	103
233	Müller K.	12
234	Aleem M.	14
237	Masci P.	42
239	Riefer M.	455
1020	Hamilton E.	8
1021	Demeures	1
1030	Wade J.L.	1
1033	Houat L.T.	1
1057	Breyfogle W.M.L.	1
1062	Carleton Smith C.	3
1065	Schlegel E.	2
1072	Sherbino G.W.	6
1073	Meyhoffer C.	3
1074	Guild-Legget S.L.	2
1076	Cooper R.T.	2
1083	Kunze H.	1
1085	Gilbert Ch.B.	1
1092	Roberts T.G.	1
1095	Krichbaum J.W.	2

1096	Campbell A.B.	2
1097	Fitz-Mathews J.	1
1101	Farrington H.	2
1102	Pierce W.I.	17
1105	Leonard W.H.	1
1111	Macfarlan D.	2
1114	Rabe R.F.	1
1117	Fields A.M.	4
1144	Roy M.	1
1158	Klunker W.	7
1179	Cooper D.J.	4
1184	Schuster B.	1886
1192	Agrawal M.L.	1
1201	Assilem M.	66
1212	Becker J.	9
2016	Mure J.B.	29
2021	Rhees	1
2103	Taylor E.A.	1
2111	Dugan J.	1
2147	Raeside J.R.	113
2189	Swoboda F.	1
3021	Toothaker C.G.	1
3070	Fornias S.	203
3087	Shannon S.F.	1

Al, *(The symptom's number) .Allen, T.F.*, Encyclopedia of Pure Materia Medica, *New York / Philadelphia , Boericke & Tafel, 1879.*

Al-S, for the supplementary symptoms of the tenth volume

Al-N, *Allen, H.C.* The Materia Medica of the Nosodes, *Philadelphia, Boericke & Tafel, 1910.*

Ha, *<200 - Hahnemann, S.* The Chronic Diseases, *Translated by Tafel ,Annotations by Hughes Jain Publishing, 1986.*

Ha, *>200 - Hahnemann, S.* Materia Medica Pura, *Translated by Dudgeon, Annotations by Hughes Jain Publishing,1986.*

He, *Hering, C.* Guiding Symptoms of Our Materia Medica, *Philadelphia 1879-1891.*

Sh, *Sherr,Jeremy* Dynamic Provings *Dynamis School 1997*

The symptom's codes at the end of the symptoms:

- The first number listed is the number of the prover, the next is the potency of the remedy that they received, and the next is the time the symptom occurred, in digital time. DD:HH:MM for days, hours and minutes. The proving of Iridium, by the Sheffield College, they have used a prover letter, followed by the date, i.e. G3 is prover G, on day three.